Volume 2

SECTION 8
Problems of Ingestion, Digestion, Absorption, and Elimination

SECTION 9
Problems of Urinary Function

SECTION 10
Problems Related to Regulatory and Reproductive Mechanisms

SECTION 11
Problems Related to Movement and Coordination

SECTION 12
Nursing Care in Critical Care Settings

APPENDIXES

NINTH EDITION

MEDICAL-SURGICAL NURSING

Assessment and Management of Clinical Problems

Volume 1

Sharon L. Lewis, RN, PhD, FAAN
Professor Emerita
University of New Mexico
Albuquerque, New Mexico;
Former Castella Distinguished Professor
School of Nursing
University of Texas Health Science Center at San Antonio
San Antonio, Texas;
Developer and Consultant
Stress-Busting Program for Family Caregivers

Shannon Ruff Dirksen, RN, PhD, FAAN
Associate Professor
College of Nursing and Health Innovation
Arizona State University
Phoenix, Arizona

Margaret McLean Heitkemper, RN, PhD, FAAN
Professor and Chairperson, Biobehavioral Nursing and Health Systems
Elizabeth Sterling Soule Endowed Chair in Nursing
School of Nursing;
Adjunct Professor, Division of Gastroenterology
School of Medicine
University of Washington
Seattle, Washington

Linda Bucher, RN, PhD, CEN, CNE
Emerita Professor
School of Nursing
University of Delaware
Newark, Delaware;
Consultant/Mentor
W. Cary Edwards School of Nursing
Thomas Edison State College
Trenton, New Jersey;
Per Diem Staff Nurse
Emergency Department
Virtua Memorial Hospital
Mt. Holly, New Jersey

Special Editor
Mariann M. Harding, RN, PhD, CNE
Associate Professor of Nursing
Kent State University at Tuscarawas
New Philadelphia, Ohio

ELSEVIER

ELSEVIER
MOSBY

3251 Riverport Lane
St. Louis, Missouri 63043

MEDICAL-SURGICAL NURSING: ASSESSMENT AND MANAGEMENT OF CLINICAL PROBLEMS ISBN: 978-0-323-10089-2

Part Number: 999-608-8820

Notices

Knowledge and best practice in this field are constantly changing. As new research and experience broaden our understanding, changes in research methods, professional practices, or medical treatment may become necessary.

Practitioners and researchers must always rely on their own experience and knowledge in evaluating and using any information, methods, compounds, or experiments described herein. In using such information or methods they should be mindful of their own safety and the safety of others, including parties for whom they have a professional responsibility.

With respect to any drug or pharmaceutical products identified, readers are advised to check the most current information provided (i) on procedures featured or (ii) by the manufacturer of each product to be administered, to verify the recommended dose or formula, the method and duration of administration, and contraindications. It is the responsibility of practitioners, relying on their own experience and knowledge of their patients, to make diagnoses, to determine dosages and the best treatment for each individual patient, and to take all appropriate safety precautions.

To the fullest extent of the law, neither the Publisher nor the authors, contributors, or editors, assume any liability for any injury and/or damage to persons or property as a matter of products liability, negligence or otherwise, or from any use or operation of any methods, products, instructions, or ideas contained in the material herein.

Library of Congress Cataloging-in-Publication Data

Lewis, Sharon Mantik, author.
Medical-surgical nursing : assessment and management of clinical problems / Sharon L. Lewis, Shannon Ruff Dirksen, Margaret McLean Heitkemper, Linda Bucher ; special editor, Mariann M. Harding. – Ninth edition.
p. ; cm.
Preceded by: Medical-surgical nursing : assessment and management of clinical problems / Sharon L. Lewis … [et al.]. 8th ed. c2011.
Includes bibliographical references and index.
ISBN 978-0-323-10089-2 (two volume set, pbk. : alk. paper)
I. Dirksen, Shannon Ruff, author. II. Heitkemper, Margaret M. (Margaret McLean), author. III. Bucher, Linda, author. IV. Harding, Mariann, editor. V. Title.
[DNLM: 1. Nursing Care. 2. Nursing Assessment. 3. Perioperative Nursing. WY 100]
RT41
617'.0231–dc23

2013036087

Executive Content Strategist: Kristin Geen
Content Manager: Jamie Randall
Associate Content Development Specialist: Melissa Rawe
Content Coordinator: Hannah Corrier
Publishing Services Manager: Jeff Patterson
Senior Project Manager: Mary G. Stueck
Designer: Maggie Reid

Printed in Canada

Last digit is the print number: 9 8 7 6 5 4 3 2

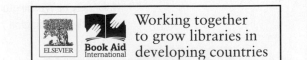

ABOUT THE AUTHORS

SHARON L. LEWIS, RN, PhD, FAAN

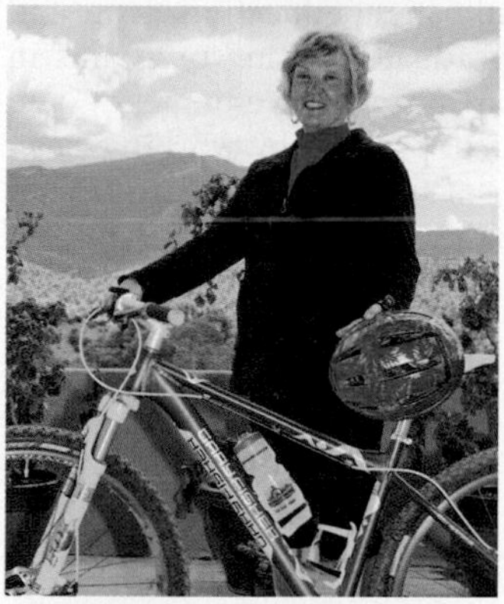

Sharon Lewis received her Bachelor of Science in nursing from the University of Wisconsin–Madison, Master of Science in nursing with a minor in biological sciences from the University of Colorado–Denver, and PhD in immunology from the Department of Pathology at the University of New Mexico School of Medicine. She had a 2-year postdoctoral fellowship from the National Kidney Foundation. Her more than 40 years of teaching experience include inservice education and teaching in associate degree, baccalaureate, master's degree, and doctoral programs in Maryland, Illinois, Wisconsin, New Mexico, and Texas. Favorite teaching areas are pathophysiology, immunology, and family caregiving. She has been actively involved in clinical research for the past 30 years, investigating altered immune responses in various disorders and developing a stress management program for family caregivers. Her primary professional responsibility is disseminating the Stress-Busting for Family Caregivers Program that she developed. Her free time is spent biking, landscaping, gardening, and being a grandmother.

SHANNON RUFF DIRKSEN, RN, PhD, FAAN

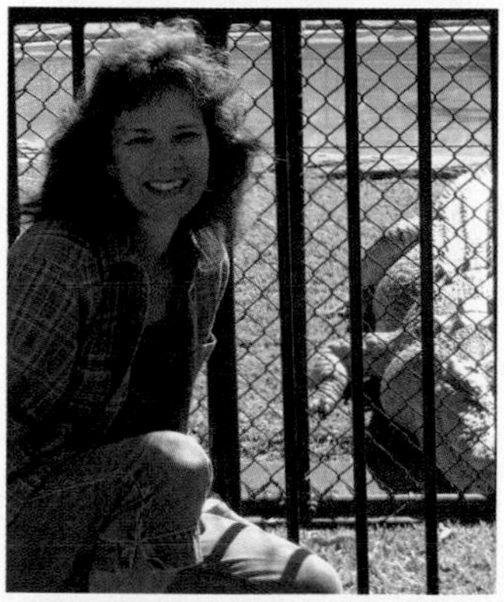

Shannon Dirksen is Associate Professor at the College of Nursing and Health Innovation, Arizona State University. She received her Bachelor of Science in nursing from Arizona State University, Master of Science in nursing from the University of Arizona, and doctorate in clinical nursing research with a minor in psychology from the University of Arizona. She has over 25 years of undergraduate and graduate teaching experience at the University of Arizona, Edith Cowan University (Western Australia), Intercollegiate College of Nursing–Washington State University, and University of New Mexico. She has been on the faculty at Arizona State University since 1996. She currently teaches nursing theory and research, including evidence-based practice. Her research for the past 25 years has focused on quality of life among individuals diagnosed with cancer. Her free time is spent traveling, gardening, bicycling, and reading.

MARGARET McLEAN HEITKEMPER, RN, PhD, FAAN

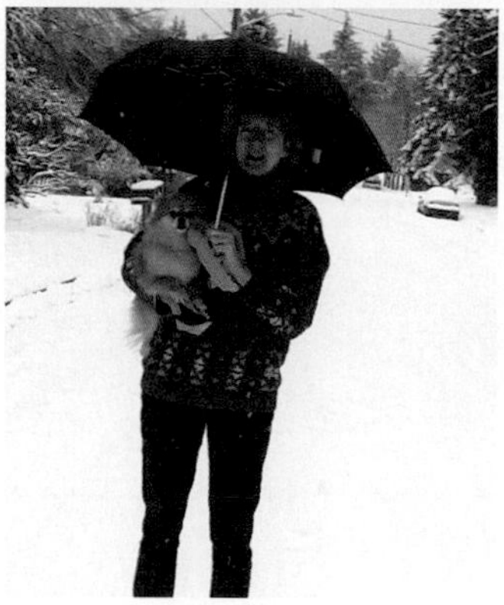

Margaret Heitkemper is Professor and Chairperson, Department of Biobehavioral Nursing and Health Systems at the School of Nursing, and Adjunct Professor, Division of Gastroenterology at the School of Medicine at the University of Washington. She is also Director of the National Institutes of Health-National Institute for Nursing Research–funded Center for Research on Management of Sleep Disturbances at the University of Washington. In the fall of 2006, Dr. Heitkemper was appointed the Elizabeth Sterling Soule Endowed Chair in Nursing. Dr. Heitkemper received her Bachelor of Science in nursing from Seattle University, a Master of Nursing in gerontologic nursing from the University of Washington, and a doctorate in Physiology and Biophysics from the University of Illinois–Chicago. She has been on faculty at the University of Washington since 1981 and has been the recipient of three School of Nursing Excellence in Teaching awards and the University of Washington Distinguished Teaching Award. In addition, in 2002 she received the Distinguished Nutrition Support Nurse Award from the American Society for Parenteral and Enteral Nutrition (ASPEN), in 2003 the American Gastroenterological Association and Janssen Award for Clinical Research in Gastroenterology, and in 2005 she was the first recipient of the Pfizer and Friends of the National Institutes for Nursing Research Award for Research in Women's Health.

LINDA BUCHER, RN, PhD, CEN, CNE

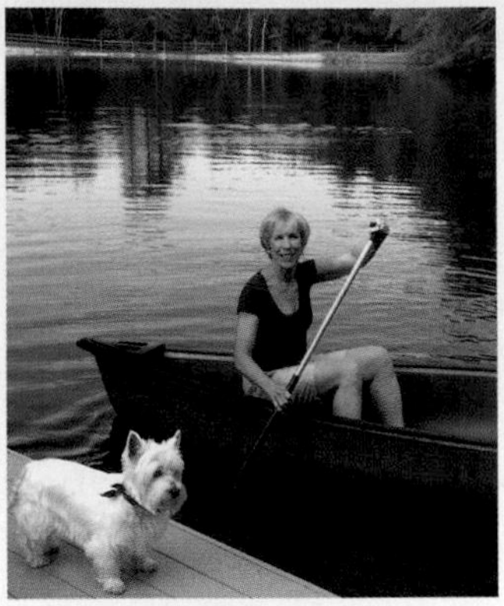

Linda Bucher is an Emerita Professor in the School of Nursing at the University of Delaware in Newark, Delaware. She also is a consultant/mentor in the W. Cary Edwards School of Nursing at Thomas Edison State College. She received her Bachelor of Science in nursing from Thomas Jefferson University in Philadelphia, her Master of Science in adult health and illness from the University of Pennsylvania in Philadelphia, and her doctorate in nursing from Widener University in Chester, Pennsylvania. Her 37 years of nursing experience has spanned staff and patient education, acute and critical care nursing, and teaching in associate, baccalaureate, and graduate nursing programs in New Jersey, Pennsylvania, and Delaware. Her preferred teaching areas include emergency and cardiac nursing and evidence-based practice. She maintains her clinical practice by working as an emergency nurse, is an active member of the American Association of Critical Care Nurses, and enjoys working as a volunteer nurse for Operation Smile. In her free time she enjoys traveling and skiing with her family.

CONTRIBUTORS

Richard Arbour, RN, MSN, CCRN, CNRN, CCNS, FAAN
Critical Care Clinical Nurse Specialist
Albert Einstein Healthcare Network
Philadelphia, Pennsylvania

Margaret Baker, RN, PhD, CNL
Associate Professor
University of Washington School of Nursing
Seattle, Washington

Elisabeth G. Bradley, RN, MS, ACNS-BC
Clinical Leader Cardiovascular Prevention Program
Christiana Care Health System
Newark, Delaware

Lucy Bradley-Springer, RN, PhD, ACRN, FAAN
Associate Professor
University of Colorado–Denver, Anschutz Medical Campus
Denver, Colorado

Jormain Cady, DNP, ARNP, AOCN
Nurse Practitioner
Virginia Mason Medical Center
Department of Radiation Oncology
Seattle, Washington

Paula Cox-North, RN, PhD, NP-C
Harborview Medical Center
Seattle, Washington

Anne Croghan, MN, ARNP
Nurse Practitioner
Seattle Gastroenterology Associates
Seattle, Washington

Betty Jean Reid Czarapata, MSN, ANP-BC, CUNP
Nurse Practitioner
Urology Wellness Center
Gaithersburg, Maryland

Judi Daniels, PhD, FNP, PNP
Advanced Practice Registered Nurse
Kentucky Polk-Dalton Clinic
Lexington, Kentucky;
Course Coordinator
Frontier Nursing University
Richmond, Kentucky

Rose DiMaria-Ghalili, RN, PhD, CNSC
Associate Professor of Nursing
College of Nursing and Health Professions
Drexel University
Philadelphia, Pennsylvania

Angela DiSabatino, RN, MS
Manager, Cardiovascular Clinical Trials
Christiana Care Health System
Newark, Delaware

Laura Dulski, MSN, RNC-HROB, CNE
Assistant Professor
Resurrection University
Chicago, Illinois

Susan J. Eisel, RN, MSEd
Associate Professor of Nursing
Mercy College of Ohio
Toledo, Ohio

Deborah Hamolsky, RN, MS, AOCNS
Clinical Nurse IV
Carol Franc Buck Breast Care Center
UCSF Helen Diller Family Comprehensive Cancer Center
San Francisco, California

Mariann M. Harding, RN, PhD, CNE
Associate Professor of Nursing
Kent State University at Tuscarawas
New Philadelphia, Ohio

Jerry Harvey, RN, MS, BC
Assistant Professor of Nursing
Liberty University
Lynchburg, Virginia

Carol Headley, RN, DNSc, ACNP-BC, CNN
Nephrology Nurse Practitioner
Veterans Affairs Medical Center
Memphis, Tennessee

Teresa E. Hills, RN, MSN, ACNP-BC, CNRN
Neurosurgery Critical Care Nurse Practitioner
Christiana Care Health System
Newark, Delaware

Christine Hoch, RN, MSN
Nursing Instructor
Delaware Technical Community College
Newark, Delaware

David M. Horner, CRNA, MS, APN
Nurse Anesthetist
Virtua Hospital
Marlton, New Jersey

Joyce Jackowski, MS, FNP-BC, AOCNP
Nurse Practitioner
Virginia Cancer Specialists
Arlington, Virginia

Kay Jarrell, RN, MS, CNE
Clinical Associate Professor
College of Nursing and Health Innovation
Arizona State University
Phoenix, Arizona

Sharmila Johnson, MSN, ACNS-BC, CCRN
Cardiovascular Clinical Nurse Specialist
Christiana Care Health System
Newark, Delaware

Jane Steinman Kaufman, RN, MS, ANP-BC, CRNP
Advanced Senior Lecturer
University of Pennsylvania School of Nursing
Philadelphia, Pennsylvania

Katherine A. Kelly, RN, DNP, FNP-C, CEN
Assistant Professor
School of Nursing
California State University
Sacramento, California

Lindsay L. Kindler, RN, PhD, CNS
Research Associate
Kaiser Permanente Center for Health Research
Portland, Oregon

Judy Knighton, RN, MScN
Clinical Nurse Specialist–Burns
Ross Tilley Burn Centre
Sunnybrook Health Sciences Centre
Toronto, Ontario, Canada

Mary Ann Kolis, RN, MSN, ANP-BC, APNP
Instructor
Gateway Technical College
Kenosha, Wisconsin

Catherine N. Kotecki, RN, PhD, APN
Associate Dean
W. Cary Edwards School of Nursing
Thomas Edison State College
Trenton, New Jersey

Nancy Kupper, RN, MSN
Associate Professor
Tarrant County College
Fort Worth, Texas

Jeffrey Kwong, DNP, MPH, ANP-BC
Assistant Professor of Nursing at CUMC
Program Director, Adult-Gerontology Nurse Practitioner Program
Columbia University
New York, New York

Carol A. Landis, RN, DNSc
Professor
Biobehavioral Nursing and Health Systems
University of Washington
School of Nursing
Seattle, Washington

Susan C. Landis, RN, MSN
Lecturer
Biobehavioral Nursing and Health Systems
University of Washington School of Nursing
Seattle, Washington

Janice Lazear, DNP, CRNP, CDE
Assistant Professor
School of Nursing
University of Maryland
Baltimore, Maryland

Catherine (Kate) Lein, MS, FNP-BC
Assistant Professor
Michigan State University College of Nursing
East Lansing, Michigan

Janet Lenart, RN, MN, MPH
Senior Lecturer
University of Washington School of Nursing
Seattle, Washington

Nancy MacMullen, PhD, APN/CNS, RNC, HR-OB, CNE
Associate Professor
Governors State University
Oak Forest, Illinois

Dorothy (Dottie) M. Mathers, RN, DNP, CNE
Professor
School of Health Sciences
Pennsylvania College of Technology
Williamsport, Pennsylvania

De Ann F. Mitchell, RN, PhD
Professor of Nursing
Tarrant County College
Trinity River East Campus
Fort Worth, Texas

Carolyn Moffa, MSN, FNP-C, CHFN
Clinical Leader
Heart Failure Program
Christiana Care Health System
Newark, Delaware

Janice Neil, RN, PhD
Associate Professor and Chair, Undergraduate Nursing Science Junior Division
College of Nursing
East Carolina University
Greenville, North Carolina

DaiWai Olson, RN, PhD, CCRN
Associate Professor of Neurology and Neurotherapeutics
University of Texas Southwestern
Dallas, Texas

Rosemary C. Polomano, RN, PhD, FAAN
Associate Professor of Pain Practice
Department of Biobehavioral Health Sciences
University of Pennsylvania School of Nursing;
Associate Professor of Anesthesiology and Critical Care
University of Pennsylvania Perelman School of Medicine
Philadelphia, Pennsylvania

Kathleen A. Rich, RN, PhD, CCNS, CCRN-CSC, CNN
Cardiovascular Clinical Specialist
Indiana University Health La Porte Hospital
La Porte, Indiana

Dottie Roberts, RN, MSN, MACI, CMSRN, OCNS-C, CNE
Instructor
University of South Carolina College of Nursing
Columbia, South Carolina

Sandra Irene Rome, RN, MN, AOCN, CNS
Clinical Nurse Specialist
Hematology/Oncology/BMT
Cedars-Sinai Medical Center
Los Angeles, California

Jennifer Saylor, RN, PhD, ACNS-BC
Clinical Instructor
University of Delaware
Wilmington, Delaware

Marilee Schmelzer, RN, PhD
Associate Professor
University of Texas at Arlington College of Nursing
Arlington, Texas

Maureen A. Seckel, RN, APN, MSN, ACNS-BC, CCNS, CCRN
Clinical Nurse Specialist Medical Pulmonary Critical Care
Christiana Care Health System
Newark, Delaware

Virginia (Jennie) Shaw, RN, MSN
Associate Professor
University of Texas Health Science Center School of Nursing
San Antonio, Texas

Anita Jo Shoup, RN, MSN, CNOR
Perioperative Clinical Nurse Specialist
Swedish Edmonds
Edmonds, Washington

Dierdre D. Wipke-Tevis, RN, PhD
Associate Professor
PhD Program Director, Coordinator of Clinical Nurse Specialist Area of Study
Sinclair School of Nursing
University of Missouri
Columbia, Missouri

Mary Wollan, RN, BAN, ONC
Orthopaedic Nurse Educator
Twin Cities Orthopaedic Education Association
Spring Park, Minnesota

Meg Zomorodi, RN, PhD, CNL
Clinical Associate Professor
University of North Carolina at Chapel Hill School of Nursing
Chapel Hill, North Carolina

Damien Zsiros, RN, MSN, CNE, CRNP
Nursing Instructor
The Pennsylvania State University School of Nursing
Fayette/The Eberly Campus
Uniontown, Pennsylvania

REVIEWERS

Lakshi M. Aldredge, RN, MSN, ANP-BC
Portland, Oregon

Katrina Allen, RN, MSN, CCRN
Fairhope and Bay Minette, Alabama

Carol C. Annesser, RN, MSN, BC, CNE
Toledo, Ohio

Debra Backus, RN, PhD, CNE, NEA-BC
Canton, New York

Jo Ann Baker, RN, MSN, FNP-C
Dover, Delaware

Kathleen M. Barta, RN, EdD
Fayetteville, Arkansas

Cecilia M. Bidigare, RN, MSN
Beavercreek, Ohio

Beth Perry Black, RN, PhD
Chapel Hill, North Carolina

Kathleen Blais, RN, EdD
Wilton Manors, Florida

Mary Blessing, RN, MSN
Albuquerque, New Mexico

Danese M. Boob, MSN/ED, RN-BC
Hershey, Pennsylvania

Barbara S. Broome, RN, PhD, FAAN
Mobile, Alabama

Anna M. Bruch, RN, MSN
Oglesby, Illinois

Carmen Bruni, RN, MSN
Laredo, Texas

Jean Burt, RN, MSN
Chicago, Illinois

Michelle M. Byrne, RN, PhD, CNE, CNOR
Dahlonega, Georgia

Carol Capitano, RN, PhD
Albuquerque, New Mexico

Ronald R. Castaldo, CRNA, MBA, MS, CCRN
New Castle, Delaware

Phyllis Christianson, MN, APRN-BC, GNP
Seattle, Washington

Katie Clark, RD, MPH, CDE
San Diego, California

Bernice Coleman, PhD, ACNP-BC, FAHA
Los Angeles, California

Deborah Marks Conley, RN, MSN, APRN-CNS, GCNS-BC, FNGNA
Omaha, Nebraska

Mary A. Cox, RN, MS
Dayton, Ohio

Paula Cox-North, RN, PhD, NP-C
Seattle, Washington

Betty Jean Reid Czarapata, MSN, ANP-BC, CUNP
Washington, D. C.

Julie Darby, RN, MSN
Memphis, Tennessee

Evelyn Dean, RN, MSN, ACNS-BC, CCRN
Kansas City, Missouri

Fernande E. Deno, RN, MSN, CNE
Coon Rapids, Minnesota

David J. Derrico, RN, MSN
Gainesville, Florida

Julie Dittmer, RN, MSN
Bettendorf, Iowa

Marci Ebberts, RN, BSN, CCRN
Kansas City, Missouri

Susan J. Eisel, RN, MSEd
Toledo, Ohio

Dana R. Epstein, RN, PhD
Phoenix, Arizona

Marianne Ferrin, MSN, ACNP-BC
Philadelphia, Pennsylvania

Shelley Fess, RN, MS, AOCN, CRNI
Rochester, New York

Eleanor Fitzpatrick, RN, MSN, CCRN
Philadelphia, Pennsylvania

Amanda J. Flagg, PhD, ACNS-BC, CNE
San Antonio, Texas

Jan Foecke, RN, MS, ONC
Kansas City, Missouri

Margie Francisco, RN, MSN, EdD
Oglesby, Illinois

Lori Godaire, RN-BC, MS, CCRN, CNL
Norwich, Connecticut

Debra B. Gordon, RN-BC, DNP, ACNS-BC, FAAN
Seattle, Washington

Claudia C. Grobbel, RN, DNP
Rochester, Michigan

Dianne Travers Gustafson, RN, PhD
Omaha, Nebraska

Elizabeth E. Hand, RN, MS
Tulsa, Oklahoma

Carla V. Hannon, MS, APRN, CCRN
New Haven, Connecticut

Mariann M. Harding, RN, PhD, CNE
New Philadelphia, Ohio

Shannon T. Harrington, RN, PhD
Norfolk, Virginia

Jerry Harvey, RN, MS, BC
Lynchburg, Virginia

Mimi Haskins, RN, MS, CMSRN
Buffalo, New York

Kay Helzer, RN, MSN
Phoenix, Arizona

Saundra J. Hendricks, RN, MS, FNP, BC-ADM
Houston, Texas

Margie Hesson, RN, MSN
Rapid City, South Dakota

Kathleen M. Hill, RN, MSN, CCNS
Cleveland, Ohio

Misty Hobart, RN, MSN, ARNP
Spokane, Washington

Patricia Hong, RN, MA
Seattle, Washington

Teressa Sanders Hunter, RN, PhD
Langston, Oklahoma

Janet E. Jackson, RN, MS
Peoria, Illinois

Suzanne L. Jed, MSN, FNP-BC
Los Angeles, California

Jane Faith Kapustin, PhD, CRNP, BC-ADM, FAANP
Baltimore, Maryland

Nancy Karnes, RN, MSN, CCRN, CDE
Bellevue, Washington

Christina D. Keller, RN, MSN
Radford, Virginia

Katherine A. Kelly, RN, DNP, FNP-C, CEN
Sacramento, California

Lisa Kiper, RN, MSN
Morehead, Kentucky

Teri Lynn Kiss, RN, MS, MSSW, CCRN
Fairbanks, Alaska

Tracy H. Knoll, RN, MSN
St. Louis, Missouri

Mary Ann Kolis, RN, MSN, ANP-BC, APNP
Kenosha, Wisconsin

Krista Krause, MSN, FNP-C
Syracuse, New York

Regina Kukulski, RN, MSN, ACNS, BC
Trenton, New Jersey

Vera Kunte, RN-BC, MSN
Trenton, New Jersey

Marci Lagenkamp, RN, MS
Piqua, Ohio

Catherine (Kate) Lein, MS, FNP-BC
East Lansing, Michigan

Linda R. Littlejohns, RN, MSN, CNRN, FAAN
San Juan Capistrano, California

Sarah Livesay, RN, DNP, ACNP, CNS-A
Houston, Texas

Erin M. Loughery, MSN, APRN
Norwich, Connecticut

Beth Lucasey, RN, MA
Kansas City, Missouri

Barbara Lukert, MD
Kansas City, Kansas

Jane A. Madden, RN, MSN
Colorado Springs, Colorado

Laura Mallett, RN, MSN
Laramie, Wyoming

Angela M. Martinelli, RN, PhD, CNOR
Fort Detrick, Maryland

Carole Martz, RN, MS, AOCN, CBCN
Highland Park, Illinois

Dorothy (Dottie) M. Mathers, RN, DNP, CNE
Williamsport, Pennsylvania

Phyllis A. Matthews, RN, MS, ANCP-BC, CUNP
Denver, Colorado

Molly L. McClelland, RN, PhD
Detroit, Michigan

Tara McMillan-Queen, RN, MSN, ANP, GNP
Charlotte, North Carolina

Molly M. McNett, RN, PhD
Cleveland, Ohio

Doreen Mingo, RN, MSN
Waterloo, Illinois

Heidi E. Monroe, RN, MSN, CPAN, CAPA
Green Bay, Wisconsin

Anna Moore, RN, MS
Richmond, Virginia

Amanda Jones Moose, RN, BSN
Taylorsville, North Carolina

Arlene H. Morris, RN, EdD, CNE
Montgomery, Alabama

Brenda C. Morris, RN, EdD, CNE
Phoenix, Arizona

Jason Mott, RN, MSN
Green Bay, Wisconsin

C. Denise Neill, RN, PhD, CNE
Victoria, Texas

Geri B. Neuberger, EdD, APRN-CNS
Kansas City, Kansas

Lorraine Nowakowski-Grier, MSN, APRN, BC, CDE
Newark, Delaware

Patricia O'Brien, RN, ACNS-BC, MA, MSN
Albuquerque, New Mexico

Margaret Ochab-Ohryn, RN, MS, MBA, CRNA
Farmington Hills, Michigan

Devorah Overbay, RN, MSN, CNS
Newberg, Oregon

Judith A. Paice, RN, PhD
Chicago, Illinois

Steven J. Palazzo, RN, PhD
Seattle, Washington

Trevah A. Panek, RN, MSN, CCRN
Loretto, Pennsylvania

Brenda Pavill, RN, PhD, FNP
Dallas, Pennsylvania

Rosalynde D. Peterson, RN, DNP
Tuscaloosa, Alabama

Barbara Pope, RN, MSN, PPCN, CCRN
Philadelphia, Pennsylvania

Tammy Ann Ramon, RN, MSN
University Center, Michigan

Patricia S. Regojo, RN, MSN
Philadelphia, Pennsylvania

Lynn F. Reinke, PhD, ARNP
Seattle, Washington

Tammy C. Roman, RN, EdD, CNE
Rochester, New York

Susan A. Sandstrom, RN, MSN, BC, CNE
Omaha, Nebraska

Marian Sawyier, RN, MSN
Albuquerque, New Mexico

Jennifer Saylor, RN, PhD, ACNS-BC
Wilmington, Delaware

Sally P. Scavone, RN, MS
Buffalo, New York

Mary Scheid, RN, MSN, OCN, CBCN
Greeley, Colorado

Cynthia Schoonover, RN, MS, CCRN
Kettering, Ohio

Teresa J. Seright, RN, PhD, CCRN
Bozeman, Montana

Shellie Simons, RN, PhD
Lowell, Massachusetts

Sarah Smith, RN, MA, CRNO, COT
Oxford, Iowa

Clemma K. Snider, RN, MSN
Richmond, Kentucky

Helen Stegall, RN, BSN, CORLN
Iowa City, Iowa

Elaine K. Strouss, RN, MSN
Monaca, Pennsylvania

Mindy B. Tinkle, RN, PhD, WHNP-BC
Albuquerque, New Mexico

Susan Turner, RN, MSN, FNP
Gilroy, California

Mark R. Van Horn, BS
High Point, North Carolina

Cheryl A. Waklatsi, RN, MSN
Cincinnati, Ohio

Danette Y. Wall, ACRN, MSN, MBA/HCM
Tampa, Florida

Daryle Wane, PhD, ARNP, FNP-BC
New Port Richey, Florida

Lisa A. Webb, RN, MSN, CEN
Charleston, South Carolina

Judith A. Widdoss, RN, MSN, CNE
Bethlehem, Pennsylvania

Sharon A. Willadsen, RN, PhD
Cleveland, Wisconsin

Julie Willenbrink, RN, MSN
Piqua, Ohio

Linda Wilson, RN, PhD, CPAN, CAPA, BC, CNE
Philadelphia, Pennsylvania

Mary Wollan, RN, BAN, ONC
Spring Park, Minnesota

Karen M. Wood, RN, DNSc, CCRN, CNL
Evergreen Park, Illinois

Patricia Worthington, RN, MSN, CNSC
Philadelphia, Pennsylvania

Susan Yeager, RN, MS, CCRN, ACNP
Columbus, Ohio

Amber Young, RN, MSN
Green Bay, Wisconsin

Damien Zsiros, RN, MSN, CNE, CRNP
Uniontown, Pennsylvania

To the Profession of Nursing and to the Important People in Our Lives

Sharon
My husband Peter and our grandchildren Malia, Halle, Aidan, Cian, and Layla

Shannon
My husband John, our children Marshall and Meaghan, my mother Marilyn, and my siblings Michael, Barbara, and Brian

Margaret
My husband David, our daughters Elizabeth and Ellen, and our grandson Jaxon James

Linda
My brother, Rich, who was always so proud of my accomplishments but not near as much as I was of him in his courageous fight against cancer

PREFACE

The ninth edition of *Medical-Surgical Nursing: Assessment and Management of Clinical Problems* has been thoroughly revised to incorporate the most current medical-surgical nursing information in an easy-to-use format. More than just a textbook, this is a comprehensive resource containing essential information that students need to prepare for lectures, classroom activities, examinations, clinical assignments, and the safe, comprehensive care of patients. In addition to the readable writing style and full-color illustrations, the text and accompanying resources include many special features to help students learn key medical-surgical nursing content, including patient and caregiver teaching, gerontology, collaborative care, cultural and ethnic considerations, patient safety, genetics, nutrition and drug therapy, evidence-based practice, and much more.

The comprehensive and timely content, special features, attractive layout, and student-friendly writing style combine to make this the number one medical-surgical nursing textbook used in more nursing schools than any other medical-surgical nursing textbook.

The strengths of the first eight editions have been retained, including the use of the nursing process as an organizational theme for nursing management. Numerous new features have been added to address some of the rapid changes in practice. Contributors have been selected for their expertise in specific content areas; one or more specialists in the subject area have thoroughly reviewed each chapter to increase accuracy. The editors have undertaken final rewriting and editing to achieve internal consistency. All efforts have been directed toward building on the strengths of the previous edition while preparing an even more effective new edition.

ORGANIZATION

Content is organized into two major divisions. The first division, Section 1 (Chapters 1 through 11), discusses general concepts related to adult patients. The second division, Sections 2 through 12 (Chapters 12 through 69), presents nursing assessment and nursing management of medical-surgical problems.

The various body systems are grouped to reflect their interrelated functions. Each section is organized around two central themes: assessment and management. Chapters dealing with assessment of a body system include a discussion of the following:

1. A brief review of anatomy and physiology, focusing on information that will promote understanding of nursing care
2. Health history and noninvasive physical assessment skills to expand the knowledge base on which treatment decisions are made
3. Common diagnostic studies, expected results, and related nursing responsibilities to provide easily accessible information

Management chapters focus on the pathophysiology, clinical manifestations, diagnostic studies, collaborative care, and nursing management of various diseases and disorders. The nursing management sections are organized into assessment, nursing diagnoses, planning, implementation, and evaluation. To emphasize the importance of patient care in various clinical settings, nursing implementation of all major health problems is organized by the following levels of care:

1. Health Promotion
2. Acute Intervention
3. Ambulatory and Home Care

CLASSIC FEATURES

- **Nursing management** is presented in a consistent and comprehensive format, with headings for Health Promotion, Acute Intervention, and Ambulatory and Home Care. Over 60 nursing care plans on the Evolve website and in the text incorporate Nursing Interventions Classification (NIC) and Nursing Outcomes Classification (NOC) in a way that clearly shows the linkages among NIC, NOC, and nursing diagnoses, and applies them to nursing practice.
- **Cultural and ethnic health disparities** content and boxes in the text highlight risk factors and important issues related to the nursing care of various ethnic groups. A special Culturally Competent Care heading denotes cultural and ethnic content related to diseases and disorders. Chapter 2: *Health Disparities and Culturally Competent Care* discusses health status differences among groups of people related to access to care, economic aspects of health care, gender and cultural issues, and disease risk.
- **Collaborative care** is highlighted in special Collaborative Care sections in all management chapters and Collaborative Care tables throughout the text.
- **Coverage on delegation and prioritization** includes the following:
  - Delegation Decisions boxes throughout the text highlight specific topics and skills related to delegation
  - Delegation and priority questions in case studies and Bridge to NCLEX® Examination Questions
  - Nursing interventions throughout the text are listed in order of priority
  - Nursing diagnoses in the nursing care plans are listed in order of priority
- **Focused Assessment boxes** in all assessment chapters provide brief checklists that help students do a more practical "assessment on the run" or bedside approach to assessment. They can be used to evaluate the status of previously identified health problems and monitor for signs of new problems.
- **Safety Alert boxes** highlight important patient safety issues and focus on the National Patient Safety Goals.
- **Pathophysiology Maps** outline complex concepts related to diseases in flowchart format, making them easier to understand.
- **Chapter 8: *Sleep and Sleep Disorders*** expands on this key topic that impacts multiple disorders and body systems as well as nearly every aspect of daily functioning.
- **Patient and caregiver teaching** is an ongoing theme throughout the text. Chapter 4: *Patient and Caregiver Teaching* emphasizes the increasing importance and prevalence of

patient management of chronic illnesses and conditions and the role of the caregiver in patient care.
- **Gerontology and chronic illness** are discussed in Chapter 5: *Chronic Illness and Older Adults,* and included throughout the text under Gerontologic Considerations headings and in Gerontologic Assessment Differences tables.
- **Nutrition** is highlighted throughout the book. Nutritional Therapy tables summarize nutritional interventions and promote healthy lifestyles in patients with various health problems.
- ***Healthy People* boxes** present health care goals as they relate to specific disorders such as diabetes and cancer.
- **Extensive drug therapy content** includes Drug Therapy tables and concise Drug Alerts highlighting important safety considerations for key drugs.
- **Genetics in Clinical Practice boxes** summarize the genetic basis, genetic testing, and clinical implications for genetic disorders that affect adults.
- **Gender Differences boxes** discuss how women and men are affected differently by conditions such as pain and hypertension.
- A separate chapter on **complementary and alternative therapies** (CAT) addresses current issues in today's health care settings related to these therapies. Complementary & Alternative Therapies boxes expand on this information and summarize what nurses need to know about therapies such as herbal remedies, acupuncture, and biofeedback.
- **Ethical/Legal Dilemmas boxes** promote critical thinking for timely and sensitive issues that nursing students may deal with in clinical practice—topics such as informed consent, advance directives, and confidentiality.
- **Home care/community-based care** is found in special Ambulatory and Home Care sections in the nursing management chapters.
- **Emergency Management tables** outline the emergency treatment of health problems most likely to require emergency intervention.
- **Assessment Abnormalities tables** in assessment chapters alert the nurse to frequently encountered abnormalities and their possible etiologies.
- **Nursing Assessment tables** summarize the key subjective and objective data related to common diseases. Subjective data are organized by functional health patterns.
- **Health History tables** in assessment chapters present key questions to ask patients related to a specific disease or disorder.
- Student-friendly pedagogy includes the following:
  - **Learning Outcomes** and **Key Terms** at the beginning of each chapter help students identify the key content for that chapter.
  - **Evolve website boxes** in chapter openers alert students to supplemental online content and exercises, making it easy for students to facilitate online learning.
  - **Bridge to NCLEX® Examination Questions** at the end of each chapter are matched to the learning outcomes and help students learn the important points in the chapter. Answers are provided just below the questions for immediate feedback, and rationales are provided on the Evolve website.
  - **Case Studies with photos** at the end of chapters bring patients to life. Multiple disorders are incorporated so students learn how to prioritize care and manage patients in the clinical setting. Discussion questions with a focus on prioritization, delegation, and evidence-based practice are included. Answer guidelines are provided on the Evolve website.
- **Resources** at the end of most chapters include websites for nursing and health care organizations that provide patient teaching and disease and disorder information.
- A **glossary** of key terms and definitions is provided at the back of the text. An expanded version of the glossary with audio pronunciations is included on the Evolve website.

NEW FEATURES

- Once again, each chapter has been carefully revised to ensure a **lower reading level** and more reader-friendly and understandable content than ever. Essential content has been streamlined to help students more effectively learn critical content.
- **Unfolding case studies** in every assessment chapter are an engaging tool that help students apply nursing concepts to real-life patient care.
- **Managing Multiple Patients Case Studies** at the end of each section help students learn to prioritize, delegate, and manage patient care.
- **Informatics boxes** discuss how technology is used by nurses and patients in health care settings.
- **Expanded evidence-based practice content** includes new Applying the Evidence boxes, updated Translating Research Into Practice boxes, and evidence-based practice-focused questions in the case studies.
- **Safety Alerts** have been expanded throughout the book to cover surveillance for high-risk situations.
- New content in Chapter 1 covers **teamwork and interdisciplinary teams,** as this is a key component of QSEN.
- An **increased focus on genetics** includes:
  - A new **genetics chapter** that focuses on practical application of nursing care as it relates to this important topic
  - **Genetic Risk Alerts** in the assessment chapters call attention to important genetic risks
  - **Genetic Link headings** in the management chapters highlight the specific genetic bases of many disorders
- **Expanded coverage of delegation** includes additional Delegation Decision boxes covering issues such as hypertension and postoperative patient care.
- Coverage of **legal considerations has been expanded** in the revised Ethical/Legal Dilemmas boxes.
- **New art** enhances the book's visual appeal and lends a more contemporary look throughout.

LEARNING SUPPLEMENTS FOR STUDENTS

- The handy ***Clinical Companion*** presents approximately 200 common medical-surgical conditions and procedures in a concise, alphabetical format for quick clinical reference. Designed for portability, this popular reference includes the essential, need-to-know information for treatments and procedures in which nurses play a major role. An attractive and functional two-color design highlights key information for quick, easy reference.

- An exceptionally thorough ***Study Guide*** contains over 500 pages of review material that reflect the content found in the book. It features a wide variety of clinically relevant exercises and activities, including NCLEX-format multiple choice and alternate format questions, case studies, anatomy review, critical thinking activities, and much more. It features an attractive two-color design and many alternate-item format questions to better prepare students for the NCLEX examination. An answer key is included to provide students with immediate feedback as they study.
- The **Evolve Student Resources** are available online at *http://evolve.elsevier.com/Lewis/medsurg* and include the following valuable learning aids organized by chapter:
  - Printable Key Points summaries for each chapter
  - 1000 NCLEX Examination Review Questions
  - Pre-Tests for every chapter
  - Answer Guidelines to the case studies in the textbook
  - Rationales for the Bridge to NCLEX® Examination Questions in the textbook
  - 55 Interactive Case Studies with state-of-the-art animations and a variety of learning activities, which provide students with immediate feedback. Ten of the case studies are enhanced with photos and narration of the clinical scenarios.
  - Customizable Nursing Care Plans
  - Concept Map Creator and concept maps for selected case studies in the textbook
  - Audio glossary of key terms, available as comprehensive alphabetical glossary and organized by chapter
  - Stress-Busting Kit
  - Animations, video clips, and audio clips
  - Fluids and Electrolytes Tutorial
  - Content Updates
  - Additional resources, including tables, figures, and clinical references
- **Virtual Clinical Excursions** (VCE) is an exciting learning tool that brings learning to life in a "virtual" hospital setting. VCE simulates a realistic, yet safe, nursing environment where the routine and rigors of the average clinical rotation abound. Students can conduct a complete assessment of a patient and set priorities for care, collect data, analyze and interpret data, prepare and administer medications, and reach conclusions about complex problems. Each lesson has a textbook reading assignment and online activities based on "visiting" patients in the hospital. Instructors receive an implementation manual with directions for using VCE as a teaching tool.
- More than just words on a screen, **Pageburst eBooks** come with a wealth of built-in study tools and interactive functionality to help students better connect with the course material and their instructors. Plus, with the ability to fit an entire library of books on one portable device, Pageburst gives students the ability to study when, where, and how they want.

TEACHING SUPPLEMENTS FOR INSTRUCTORS

- The **Evolve Instructor Resources** (available online at *http://evolve.elsevier.com/Lewis/medsurg*) remain the most comprehensive set of instructor's materials available, containing the following:
  - **TEACH for Nurses Lesson Plans** with electronic resources organized by chapter to help instructors develop and manage the course curriculum. This exciting resource includes:
    - Objectives
    - Teaching focus
    - Key terms
    - Nursing curriculum standards
    - Student and instructor chapter resource listings
    - Detailed chapter outlines
    - Teaching strategies with learning activities and links to resources in the image collection, PowerPoint presentations, animations, etc.
    - Case studies with answer guidelines
  - The **Test Bank** features over 2000 NCLEX Examination test questions with text page references and answers coded for NCLEX Client Needs category, nursing process, and cognitive level. The ninth edition test bank has been completely updated and reviewed, and it now includes hundreds of prioritization, delegation, and multiple patient questions. All alternate item format questions are included. The ExamView software allows instructors to create new tests; edit, add, and delete test questions; sort questions by NCLEX category, cognitive level, nursing process step, and question type; and administer and grade online tests.
  - The **Image Collection** contains more than 800 full-color images from the text for use in lectures.
  - An extensive collection of **PowerPoint Presentations** includes over 125 different presentations focused on the most common diseases and disorders. The presentations have been thoroughly revised to include helpful instructor notes/teaching tips, unfolding case studies, new illustrations and photos not found in the book, new animations, and updated audience response questions for use with iClicker and other audience response systems.
  - Course management system.
  - Access to all student resources listed above.
- The **Simulation Learning System (SLS)** is an online toolkit that helps instructors and facilitators effectively incorporate medium- to high-fidelity simulation into their nursing curriculum. Detailed patient scenarios promote and enhance the clinical decision-making skills of students at all levels. The SLS provides detailed instructions for preparation and implementation of the simulation experience, debriefing questions that encourage critical thinking, and learning resources to reinforce student comprehension. Each scenario in the SLS complements the textbook content and helps bridge the gap between lecture and clinical. The SLS provides the perfect environment for students to practice what they are learning in the text for a true-to-life, hands-on learning experience.

ACKNOWLEDGMENTS

The editors are especially grateful to many people at Elsevier who assisted with this major revision effort. In particular, we wish to thank the team of Kristin Geen, Jamie Randall, Mary Stueck, Jeff Patterson, and Maggie Reid. In addition, we want to thank the marketing team of Pat Crowe, Katie Schlesinger, and Becky McBride.

Special thanks and appreciation go to Peter Bonner who assisted with many details of manuscript preparation and review and photography for the book and interactive case studies.

We are particularly indebted to the faculty, nurses, and student nurses who have put their faith in our book to assist them on their path to excellence. The increasing use of this book throughout the United States, Canada, Australia, and other parts of the world has been gratifying. We appreciate the many users who have shared their comments and suggestions on the previous editions. All feedback is welcome.

We also wish to thank our contributors and reviewers for their assistance with the revision process. We sincerely hope that this book will assist both students and clinicians in practicing truly professional nursing.

Sharon L. Lewis
Shannon Ruff Dirksen
Margaret McLean Heitkemper
Linda Bucher

AUTHORS OF TEACHING AND LEARNING RESOURCES

TEST BANK

Barbara Bartz, MN, ARNP, CCRN
Nursing Instructor
Yakima Valley Community College
Yakima, Washington

Linda Bucher, RN, PhD, CEN, CNE
Emerita Professor
School of Nursing, University of Delaware
Newark, Delaware;
Consultant/Mentor
W. Cary Edwards School of Nursing
Thomas Edison State College
Trenton, New Jersey;
Per Diem Staff Nurse
Emergency Department,
Virtua Memorial Hospital
Mt. Holly, New Jersey

Debra Hagler, RN, PhD, ACNS-BC, CNE, CHSE, ANEF, FAAN
Clinical Professor
College of Nursing and Healthcare Innovation
Arizona State University
Phoenix, Arizona

Christina D. Keller, RN, MSN
Instructor
Radford University School of Nursing
Clinical Simulation Center
Radford, Virginia

Jo A. Voss, RN, PhD, CNS
Associate Professor
South Dakota State University
Rapid City, South Dakota

PRE-TESTS

Debra Hagler, RN, PhD, ACNS-BC, CNE, CHSE, ANEF, FAAN
Clinical Professor
College of Nursing and Healthcare Innovation
Arizona State University
Phoenix, Arizona

CASE STUDIES

Interactive, Managing Multiple Patients, and Assessment Case Studies

Dorothy (Dottie) M. Mathers, RN, DNP, CNE
Professor
School of Health Sciences
Pennsylvania College of Technology
Williamsport, Pennsylvania

TEACH for Nurses Case Studies

Elizabeth Day, RN, MSN, CHPN
Nursing Faculty
Fresno City College and Madera Center
Fresno, California

Heidi E. Monroe, RN-BC, MSN, CPAN, CAPA
Assistant Professor of Nursing
Bellin College
Green Bay, Wisconsin

POWERPOINT PRESENTATIONS

Dorothy (Dottie) M. Mathers, RN, DNP, CNE
Professor
School of Health Sciences
Pennsylvania College of Technology
Williamsport, Pennsylvania

Jane E. Oehme, RN, MS
Associate Professor of Nursing
Pennsylvania College of Technology
Williamsport, Pennsylvania

Michelle A. Latshaw, RN, MSN
Associate Professor of Nursing
Williamsport, Pennsylvania

PowerPoint Presentations and Glossaries

Cory Shaw Retherford, MOM, LAc.
Former Research Assistant
University of Texas Health Science Center at San Antonio
San Antonio, Texas

TEACH FOR NURSES

Mariann M. Harding, RN, PhD, CNE
Associate Professor of Nursing
Kent State University at Tuscarawas
New Philadelphia, Ohio

AUDIENCE RESPONSE QUESTIONS

Jo A. Voss, RN, PhD, CNS
Associate Professor
South Dakota State University
Rapid City, South Dakota

NCLEX® EXAMINATION REVIEW QUESTIONS

Susan A. Sandstrom, RN, MSN, BC, CNE
Associate Professor in Nursing, Retired
College of Saint Mary
Omaha, Nebraska

STUDY GUIDE

Susan A. Sandstrom, RN, MSN, BC, CNE
Associate Professor in Nursing, Retired
College of Saint Mary
Omaha, Nebraska

CLINICAL COMPANION

Shannon Ruff Dirksen, RN, PhD, FAAN
Associate Professor
College of Nursing and Health Innovation
Arizona State University
Phoenix, Arizona

Sharon L. Lewis, RN, PhD, FAAN
Professor Emerita
University of New Mexico
Albuquerque, New Mexico;
Former Castella Distinguished Professor
School of Nursing
University of Texas Health Science Center at San Antonio
San Antonio, Texas;
Developer and Consultant
Stress-Busting Program for Family Caregivers

ETHICAL/LEGAL DILEMMAS BOXES

Kathy Lucke, RN, PhD
Clinical Professor
University at Buffalo
School of Nursing
Buffalo, New York

Rosemary J. Mann, RN, CNM, MS, JD, PhD
Clinical Professor
School of Nursing
University at Buffalo
Buffalo, New York

DELEGATION DECISIONS BOXES

Barbara Bartz, MN, ARNP, CCRN
Nursing Instructor
Yakima Valley Community College
Yakima, Washington

EVIDENCE-BASED PRACTICE BOXES

Applying the Evidence Boxes

Linda Bucher, RN, PhD, CEN, CNE
Emerita Professor
School of Nursing
University of Delaware
Newark, Delaware;
Consultant/Mentor
W. Cary Edwards School of Nursing
Thomas Edison State College
Trenton, New Jersey;
Per Diem Staff Nurse
Emergency Department
Virtua Memorial Hospital
Mt. Holly, New Jersey

Translating Research Into Practice Boxes

Shannon Ruff Dirksen, RN, PhD, FAAN
Associate Professor
College of Nursing and Health Innovation
Arizona State University
Phoenix, Arizona

INFORMATICS BOXES

Mariann M. Harding, RN, PhD, CNE
Associate Professor of Nursing
Kent State University at Tuscarawas
New Philadelphia, Ohio

NURSING CARE PLANS

Patricia O'Brien, RN, ACNS-BC, MA, MSN
Albuquerque, New Mexico

SPECIAL PROJECTS

Peter Bonner, MS
DSI
Placitas, New Mexico

CONTENTS

VOLUME 1

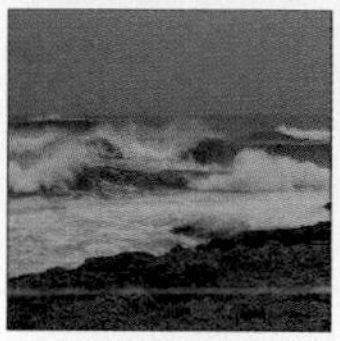

SECTION 1
Concepts in Nursing Practice

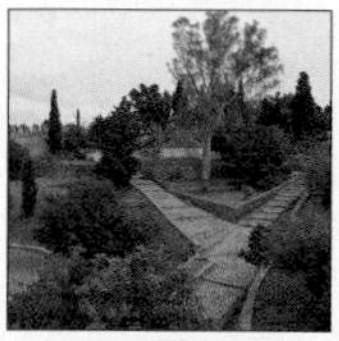

SECTION 2
Pathophysiologic Mechanisms of Disease

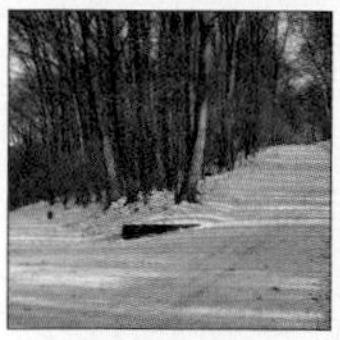

SECTION 3
Perioperative Care

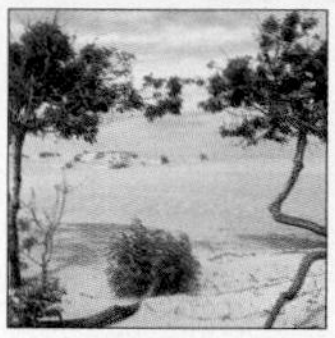

SECTION 4
Problems Related to Altered Sensory Input

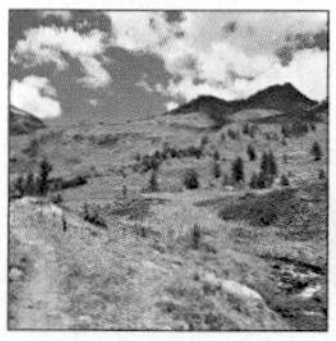

SECTION 5
Problems of Oxygenation: Ventilation

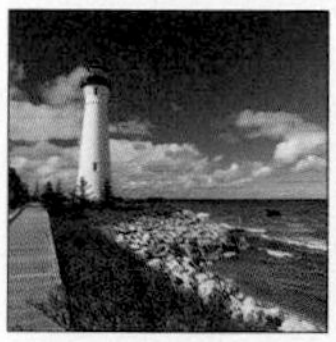

SECTION 6
Problems of Oxygenation: Transport

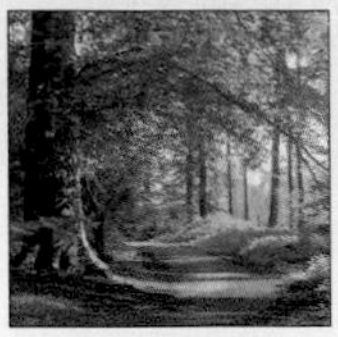

SECTION 7
Problems of Oxygenation: Perfusion

VOLUME 2

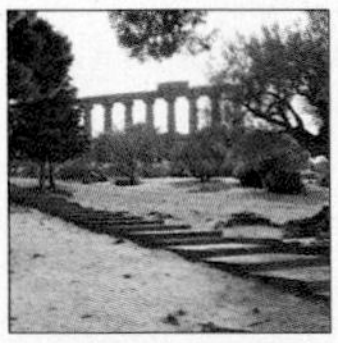

SECTION 8
Problems of Ingestion, Digestion, Absorption, and Elimination

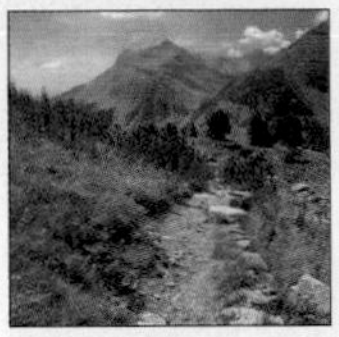

SECTION 9
Problems of Urinary Function

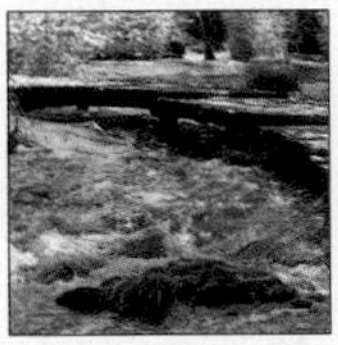

SECTION 10
Problems Related to Regulatory and Reproductive Mechanisms

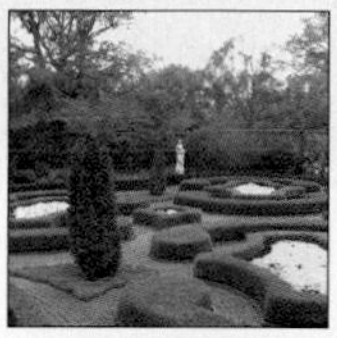

SECTION 11 Problems Related to Movement and Coordination

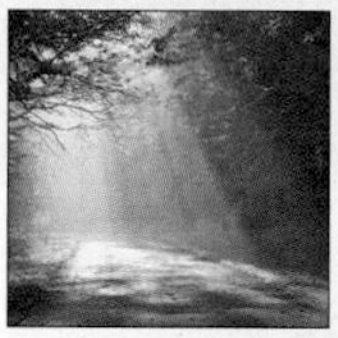

SECTION 12 Nursing Care in Critical Care Settings

APPENDIXES

SPECIAL FEATURES

ASSESSMENT ABNORMALITIES TABLES

CASE STUDIES

End-of-Chapter Case Studies

Managing Multiple Patients Case Studies

Assessment Case Studies

COLLABORATIVE CARE TABLES

COMPLEMENTARY & ALTERNATIVE THERAPIES BOXES

CULTURAL & ETHNIC HEALTH DISPARITIES BOXES

DELEGATION DECISIONS BOXES

DIAGNOSTIC STUDIES TABLES

DRUG THERAPY TABLES

EMERGENCY MANAGEMENT TABLES

ETHICAL/LEGAL DILEMMAS BOXES

EVIDENCE-BASED PRACTICE

Applying the Evidence Boxes

EVIDENCE-BASED PRACTICE

Translating Research Into Practice Boxes

FOCUSED ASSESSMENT BOXES

GENDER DIFFERENCES BOXES

GENETICS IN CLINICAL PRACTICE BOXES

GERONTOLOGIC ASSESSMENT DIFFERENCES TABLES

HEALTH HISTORY TABLES

HEALTHY PEOPLE BOXES

INFORMATICS IN PRACTICE BOXES

NURSING ASSESSMENT TABLES

NURSING CARE PLANS

NUTRITIONAL THERAPY TABLES

PATIENT & CAREGIVER TEACHING GUIDE TABLES

*Evolve On Evolve website.

SECTION 1

Concepts in Nursing Practice

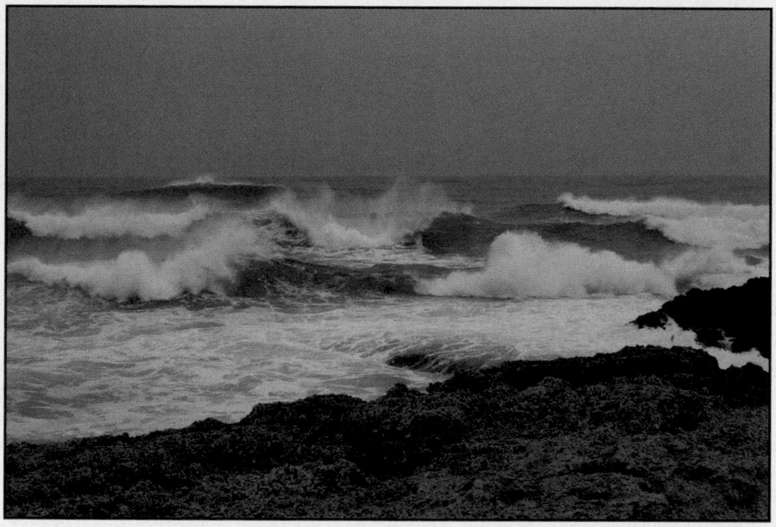

Peter Bonner

The journey is the reward.
Tao saying

CHAPTER

1

The road to knowledge begins with the turn of the page.
Anonymous

Professional Nursing Practice

Mariann M. Harding

evolve WEBSITE

http://evolve.elsevier.com/Lewis/medsurg

- NCLEX Review Questions
- Key Points
- Pre-Test
- Rationales for Bridge to NCLEX Examination Questions
- Concept Map Creator
- Glossary
- Content Updates

eFigures

- eFig. 1-1: Screen from a patient's electronic health record
- eFig. 1-2: Decision tree for delegation to unlicensed assistive personnel (UAP)

eTables

- eTable 1-1: Practice Settings for Transitional Care
- eTable 1-2: Practice Settings for Long-Term Care
- eTable 1-3: Overview of Delegation, Assignment, and Supervision

LEARNING OUTCOMES

1. Describe professional nursing practice in terms of domain, definitions, and recipients of care.
2. Compare the different scopes of practice available to professional nurses.
3. Analyze the effect of expanding technology and knowledge, changing populations, consumerism, and evolving health care systems on professional nursing practice.
4. Describe the role of critical thinking skills and use of the nursing process to provide patient-centered care.
5. Explain how standardized nursing terminologies for nursing diagnoses, patient outcomes, and nursing interventions can be used and linked.
6. Evaluate the role of informatics and technology in nursing practice.
7. Apply concepts of evidence-based practice to nursing practice.
8. Discuss the role of integrating safety and quality improvement processes into nursing practice.
9. Explore the role of the professional nurse in delegating care to licensed practical/vocational nurses and unlicensed assistive personnel.

KEY TERMS

advanced practice nurse (APN), p. 3
case management, p. 14
clinical (critical) pathway, p. 15
clinical reasoning, p. 6
collaborative problems, p. 8
concept map, p. 8
critical thinking, p. 6
delegation, p. 15
electronic health record (EHR), p. 10
evidence-based practice (EBP), p. 11
***Healthy People*, p. 5**
nursing, p. 3
nursing informatics, p. 10
nursing process, p. 6
telehealth, p. 11
unlicensed assistive personnel (UAP), p. 15

This chapter presents an overview of professional nursing practice, discussing the wide variety of roles and responsibilities nurses fulfill to meet the health care needs of society.

PROFESSIONAL NURSING PRACTICE

Domain of Nursing Practice

Nursing practice today consists of a wide variety of roles and responsibilities necessary to meet society's health care needs. As a nurse, you are the frontline professional of health care (Fig. 1-1). You practice in virtually all health care settings and communities across the country. You have never been more important to health care than you are today. As a nurse, you (1) offer skilled care to those recuperating from illness or injury, (2) advocate for patients' rights, (3) teach patients so that they can make informed decisions, (4) support patients and their caregivers at critical times, and (5) help them navigate the increasingly complex health care system. Although the majority of nurses are employed in acute care facilities, many nurses practice in long-term care, home care, primary and preventive care, ambulatory clinics, and community health. Wherever you practice, recipients of your care include individuals, groups, families, or communities.

The American Nurses Association (ANA) declares that the authority for the practice of nursing is based on a contract with society that acknowledges professional rights and respon-

Reviewed by Claudia C Grobbel, RN, DNP, Assistant Professor, Oakland University, Rochester, Michigan; Elizabeth E. Hand, RN, MS, Adjunct Faculty, Tulsa Community College, School of Nursing, Tulsa, Oklahoma; and Patricia O'Brien, RN, ACNS-BC, MA, MSN, Retired Instructor, University of New Mexico, College of Nursing and Central New Mexico Community College, Albuquerque, New Mexico.

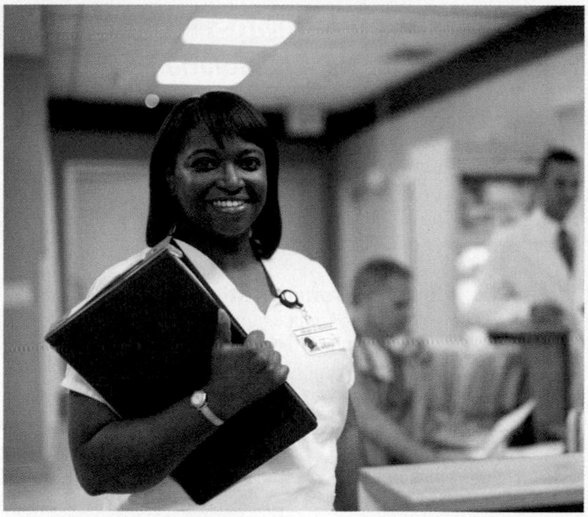

FIG. 1-1 Nurses are frontline professionals of health care. (Thomas Northcut/Digital Vision/Thinkstock)

sibilities, as well as mechanisms for public accountability.[1] The knowledge and skills that comprise nursing practice are derived from society's expectations and needs. Nursing practice continues to evolve according to society's health needs and as knowledge and technology expand. This chapter introduces concepts and factors that affect professional nursing practice.

Definitions of Nursing

Several well-known definitions of nursing indicate that the basic themes of health, illness, and caring have existed since Florence Nightingale described nursing. Following are two such examples:

- Nursing is putting the patient in the best condition for nature to act (Nightingale).[2]
- The nurse's unique function is to assist patients, sick or well, in the performance of those activities contributing to health or its recovery (or to peaceful death) that they would perform unaided if they had the necessary strength, will, or knowledge—and to do this in such a way as to help them gain independence as rapidly as possible (Henderson).[3]

In 1980 the ANA defined **nursing** as "the diagnosis and treatment of human responses to actual and potential health problems."[1] In this context, a nurse caring for a person with a fractured hip would focus on the patient's possible responses to immobility, pain, and loss of independence.

The widely accepted ANA definition of nursing was reaffirmed in the 2010 edition of the ANA's *Nursing: A Social Policy Statement* to reflect the continuing evolution of nursing practice:

> ***Nursing*** *is the protection, promotion, and optimization of health and abilities, prevention of illness and injury, alleviation of suffering through the diagnosis and treatment of human response, and advocacy in the care of individuals, families, communities, and populations.*[1]

This definition reflects nurses' increasing role in promoting health and wellness and advocating for the recipients of care.

Nursing's View of Humanity

Nursing theorists are in widespread agreement that an individual has physiologic (or biophysical), psychologic (or emotional), sociocultural (or interpersonal), spiritual, and environmental components or dimensions. In this text the human individual is considered "a biopsychosocial spiritual being in constant interaction with a changing environment."[4] The individual is composed of dimensions that are interrelated and not separate entities. Thus a problem in one dimension may affect one or more of the other dimensions. An individual's behavior is meaningful and oriented toward fulfilling needs, coping with stress, and developing one's self. However, at times an individual needs help to meet these needs, cope successfully, or develop his or her unique potential.

Scope of Nursing Practice

Like all health care professions, nursing's scope of practice has a flexible boundary that reflects the changing needs of society and advancement of knowledge. The essential core of nursing practice is to deliver holistic, patient-centered care. It includes assessment and evaluation, administration of a variety of interventions, patient and family teaching, and being a member of the interdisciplinary (also referred to as the interprofessional) health care team.

The extent that individual nurses engage in the scope of practice depends on their educational preparation, experience, and role, and is guided by individual state laws. To enter into practice, a nurse must complete an accredited program and pass an examination verifying the nurse has the skills necessary to provide competent care. Entry-level nurses with associate or baccalaureate degrees are prepared to function as generalists. At this level, nurses provide direct health care and focus on ensuring coordinated and comprehensive care to patients in a variety of settings. They work collaboratively with other health care providers to manage the needs of individuals and groups.[5,6]

With experience and continued study, nurses may specialize in an area of practice. Certification is a formal way for nurses to obtain professional recognition for their expertise in a specialty area. A variety of nursing organizations offer certification in a number of nursing specialties.[7] Certification usually requires a certain amount of clinical experience and successful completion of an examination. Recertification usually requires ongoing clinical experience and continuing education. Common nursing specialties include ambulatory care; cardiovascular care; critical care; women's health; diabetes education; nursing informatics; and geriatric, medical-surgical, perinatal, emergency, psychiatric/mental health, and community health nursing.

Additional formal education and experience can prepare nurses for advanced practice. An **advanced practice nurse (APN)** or *advanced practice registered nurse (APRN)* is a nurse with at least a master's degree in nursing; advanced education in pathophysiology, pharmacology, and health assessment; and expertise in a specialized area of practice. Examples of APNs/APRNs are clinical nurse specialists, clinical nurse leaders, nurse practitioners, nurse midwives, and nurse anesthetists. In addition to managing and delivering direct patient care, APNs/APRNs have roles in health promotion, case management, administration, research, and interdisciplinary health systems.[7] Nurses with a PhD typically serve as faculty in schools of nursing, policy analysts, and researchers. However, they are being increasingly employed in clinical settings as clinical experts and health care system executives.

In response to patient care needs and in anticipation of the needs of the current and future health care system, the doctorate of nursing practice (DNP) degree was endorsed in 2004 by the American Association of Colleges of Nursing (AACN). The DNP moves the educational preparation for advanced nursing practice from the master's degree to the doctoral level. It is designed for nurses seeking a practice-focused terminal degree in nursing. The DNP degree moves nursing in the direction of other health professions that offer practice doctorates (e.g., pharmacy [PharmD], psychology [PsyD], and physical therapy [DPT]).[8]

INFLUENCES ON PROFESSIONAL NURSING PRACTICE

Complex Health Care Environments

Expanding Knowledge and Technology. Rapidly changing technology and dramatically expanding knowledge are adding to the complexity of health care environments. Advanced communication technologies have created a more global environment that affects the delivery of health care worldwide. The number and complexity of patient care technologies are transforming how care is delivered. The human genome project and advances in genetics affect the prevention, diagnosis, and treatment of health problems. With advances in knowledge, ethical dilemmas and controversy arise regarding the use of new scientific knowledge and the disparities that exist in patients' access to more technologically advanced health care. Throughout this book, expanding knowledge and technology's impact on nursing practice are highlighted in genetics, informatics, and ethical/legal boxes.

Diverse Populations. Patient populations are more diverse than ever. Americans are living longer, in part due to advances in medical science, technology, and health care delivery. As the population ages, the number of patients with chronic conditions increases. Unlike those who receive acute, episodic care, patients with chronic conditions have a multitude of needs. They see a variety of health care providers in various settings over an extended period. Nurses are also caring for a more culturally and ethnically diverse population. Immigrants, particularly undocumented immigrants and refugees, often lack the resources necessary to access health care. Inability to pay for health care is associated with a tendency to delay seeking care, resulting in illnesses that are more serious. Boxes throughout this book emphasize the influence of such factors as gender, culture, and ethnicity on nursing practice.

Consumerism. Health care is a consumer-focused business. Patients today are active participants in their health care and expect high-quality, coordinated, and financially reasonable care. Health information is readily available. Many patients eagerly seek information about their health problems and health care from media and Internet sources. They gather information so that they can have a voice in making decisions about their health care. As a nurse, you must be able to help patients access and use appropriate health care information (Fig. 1-2).

Influences on Health Care Systems

Health Care Financing. Many changes in health care systems that influence nursing care delivery were initiated by the government, employers, insurance companies, and regulating agencies in an effort to provide more cost-effective health care. Historically, the most notable event related to changing reimbursement patterns was the institution of prospective payment systems in the Medicare program. With these changes, hospitals were no longer reimbursed for all costs. Instead, payment for hospital services for Medicare patients was based on flat fees determined by the diseases and problems treated during the admission. Private and other public health care systems followed suit by introducing managed care systems that use prospective payment as a means of offering cost-effective health care delivery. In health maintenance organizations (HMOs) and

ETHICAL/LEGAL DILEMMAS

Social Networking: HIPAA Violation

Situation

You log into a closed group on a social networking site and read a posting from a fellow nursing student. The posting describes in detail the complex care the student provided to an older patient in a local hospital the previous day. The student comments on how stressful the day was and asks for advice on how to deal with similar patients in the future.

Ethical/Legal Points for Consideration

- Protecting and maintaining patient privacy and confidentiality are basic obligations defined in the Nursing Code of Ethics, which nurses and nursing students should uphold.
- As outlined in the Health Insurance Portability and Accountability Act (HIPAA), a patient's private health information is any information that relates to the person's past, present, or future physical or mental health. This includes not only specific details such as a patient's name or picture, but also information that gives enough details that someone may be able to identify that person.
- You may unintentionally breach privacy or confidentiality by posting patient information (diagnosis, condition, or situation) on a social networking site. Using privacy settings or being in a closed group does not guarantee the secrecy of posted information. Others can copy and share any post without your knowledge.
- Potential consequences for improperly using social networking vary based on the situation. These may include dismissal from a nursing program or civil and criminal actions.
- A student nurse who experienced a stressful day and was looking for advice and support from peers (e.g., "Today my patient died. I wanted to cry.") could share the experience by clearly limiting the posts to the student's personal perspective and not sharing any identifying information.

Discussion Questions

1. How would you deal with the situation involving the fellow nursing student?
2. How would you handle a situation where you observed a staff member who violated HIPAA?

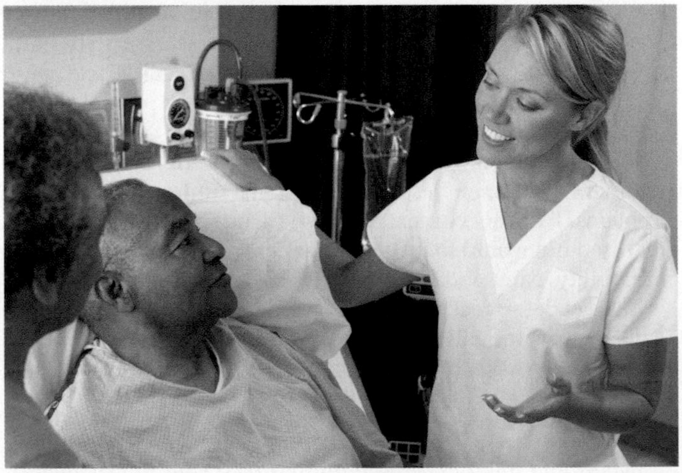

FIG. 1-2 The patient, family, and nurse collaborate as part of coordinating high-quality care. (Hemera/Thinkstock)

preferred provider organizations (PPOs), charges are negotiated in advance of the delivery of care using predetermined reimbursement rates or capitation fees for medical care, hospitalization, and other health care services.

These same third-party payers demand outcome-based quality care that is provided at a price affordable for both individuals and society. Payment for health care services or pay-for-performance programs reimburse hospitals for their performance on quality-of-care measures. These measures include clinical outcomes, patient safety, patient satisfaction, adherence to evidence-based practice, and adoption of information technology. Payment for care can be withheld if a patient develops certain health care conditions during a hospital stay (e.g., pressure ulcer) or if something happens to the patient that is considered preventable (e.g., acquiring a catheter-related urinary tract infection).[9]

***Healthy People* Initiative.** For the past 30 years the U.S. government has been active in establishing goals and objectives for promoting health and health care delivery for the nation through an initiative known as *Healthy People*.[10] The vision of *Healthy People* is a society in which all people live long, healthy lives. *Healthy People* is a broad-based program that involves government, private, public, and nonprofit organizations. Individuals, groups, and organizations are encouraged to integrate *Healthy People* goals and focus areas into current programs, special events, publications, and meetings. These activities can further the health of all members of a community. The overarching goals of the *Healthy People 2020* initiative are presented in Table 1-1. *Healthy People* boxes related to these goals are integrated throughout this book.

The *Healthy People* initiative is a significant challenge for nursing. Both nursing education programs and clinical nursing practice must respond to major trends in health care. Educational programs for entry-level nurses now place a greater emphasis on health promotion; maintenance; and cost-effective care that responds to the needs of older adults, culturally diverse groups, and underserved populations. Today's nurses must address the identified health problems, developments in health care delivery, research outcomes, and new technologies in order to meet *Healthy People* goals. As a reflection of nursing's contract with society, you are responsible for improving the health status of the public and reducing health disparities. (Health disparities are discussed in Chapter 2.)

Supporting Professional Practice

Professional Nursing Organizations. The American Nurses Association is the primary professional nursing organization. There are numerous professional specialty organizations, such as the American Association of Critical-Care Nurses (AACN), Association of periOperative Registered Nurses (AORN), and Oncology Nursing Society (ONS). Professional organizations have numerous roles in promoting quality patient care and professional nursing practice. These include developing standards of practice and codes of ethics, supporting research, and lobbying for legislation and regulations. Major nursing organizations also promote research into the causes of errors, develop strategies to prevent future errors, and address nursing issues that affect the nurse's ability to deliver patient care safely. Many nurses join a professional organization to keep current in their practice and network with others who are interested in a particular practice area.

QSEN. In 2003 the Institute of Medicine (IOM) commissioned an interdisciplinary task force to study the educational preparation of health care professionals to see whether new graduates were prepared for today's reality of practice.[11] What they found was that all health professions, including nursing, needed to review and revise their curricula and focus on developing specific competencies that serve as a basis for practice. In nursing this is done through a project known as *Quality and Safety Education for Nurses (QSEN) (www.qsen.org)*. QSEN consists of six core competencies: (1) patient-centered care, (2) informatics and technology, (3) evidence-based practice, (4) quality improvement, (5) safety, and (6) teamwork and collaboration. The remainder of this chapter discusses how professional nursing practice is focusing on acquiring the knowledge, skills, and attitudes within each competency.

TABLE 1-1 *HEALTHY PEOPLE 2020*

Overarching Goals

- Attain high quality, longer lives free of preventable disease, disability, injury, and premature death.
- Achieve health equity, eliminate disparities, and improve the health of all groups.
- Create social and physical environments that promote good health for all.
- Promote quality of life, healthy development, and healthy behaviors across all life stages.

Source: US Department of Health and Human Services: *Healthy People* 2020. Retrieved from *www.healthypeople.gov*.

PATIENT-CENTERED CARE

Nurses have long demonstrated that they truly deliver patient-centered care based on each patient's unique needs and understanding of the patient's preferences, values, and beliefs. Patient-centered care is interrelated with both quality and safety. In the patient-centered care model, patients and caregivers seek care from competent and knowledgeable health care professionals. Patients and caregivers are involved in making care decisions and managing the patient's care.

Delivery of Nursing Care

Nurses deliver patient-centered care in collaboration with the interdisciplinary health care team and within the framework of a care delivery model. Today a variety of care delivery models are being used in view of nursing shortages, state-mandated nurse-patient ratios, economic issues, and increased acuity of patient conditions.

A *team nursing* model uses a professional nurse as a team leader. As a team leader, you organize and manage the care for a group of patients with other ancillary workers such as licensed practical/vocational nurses (LPN/LVNs) and unlicensed assistive personnel (UAP). In this model, you have the authority and accountability for the quality of care delivered by team members during a work period.

In a *total patient care* model, you assume accountability for the complete care of a patient or group of patients during the assigned shift. In this model, you are responsible for planning and providing all care.

In a *primary nursing* model, you are responsible for a patient or caseload of patients over a period of time.[12] You provide care during assigned shifts, and coordinate and communicate all aspects of patient care with other disciplines and those who provide care when you are absent. Care delivered within a primary care model strengthens the nurse-patient relationship through a focus on continuity of care and interdisciplinary collaboration.

Continuum of Patient Care

Depending on their health status, patients often move among a multitude of different health care settings. Decisions regarding the most appropriate setting for obtaining health care frequently depend on the cost of care and constraints of a patient's health care insurance plan. Although the hospital remains the mainstay for acute care interventions within this continuum, community-based settings offer patients the opportunity to live or recover in settings that maximize their independence and preserve human dignity. For example, a person may be hospitalized in a trauma unit of an acute care hospital following a motor vehicle crash. After the person is stabilized, he or she may be transferred to a general medical-surgical unit and then to an acute rehabilitation facility. After a period of rehabilitation the person may be discharged to his or her home to continue with outpatient rehabilitation, with follow-up by home health care nurses and care in an outpatient clinic.

The continuum of care does not always include hospitalization. Some patients receive community-based care without experiencing an acute problem requiring hospitalization. Community-based settings where health care is provided include ambulatory care, transitional care, and long-term care. Transitional care settings provide care in between the acute care and the home or long-term care setting (see eTable 1-1 on the website for this chapter). Patients may receive transitional care at an acute rehabilitation facility after head trauma or a spinal cord injury. Long-term care refers to the care of patients for a period greater than 30 days (see eTable 1-2 on the website for this chapter). It may be required for individuals who are severely developmentally disabled, are mentally impaired, or have physical deficits requiring continuous medical or nursing management (e.g., patients who are ventilator dependent or have Alzheimer's disease). Long-term care facilities include skilled nursing facilities, intermediate care facilities, retirement communities, and residential care facilities.

Critical Thinking

Complex health care environments require that you use critical thinking and clinical reasoning skills to make decisions that lead to the best patient outcomes. Although no standard definitions of critical thinking or methods of teaching and evaluating critical thinking have been accepted, critical thinking is recognized as a broad term for a learned skill. **Critical thinking** has been described as knowing how to learn, reason, think creatively, generate ideas, make decisions, and solve problems.[13] Critical thinking is not memorizing a list of facts or the steps of a procedure; instead it is the ability to solve problems by making sense of information. Learning and using critical thinking is a continual process that occurs inside and outside of the clinical setting.

Clinical reasoning is a problem-solving activity in which critical thinking is used to examine patient care issues. It is a process that involves using knowledge from many fields to understand the medical and nursing implications of a patient situation when making decisions regarding patient care.[14] You use clinical reasoning when you identify a change in a patient's status, take into account the context and concerns of the patient and caregiver, and decide what to do about it.

Given the complexity of patient care today, nurses are required to learn and implement critical thinking and clinical reasoning skills long before they gain those skills through the experience of professional practice. Clinical experiences during nursing education provide opportunities for you to learn and make decisions about patient care. To promote practice in critical thinking and clinical reasoning, various education models and techniques have been developed, including exercises in simulation laboratories and interactive scenarios. Throughout this book, select boxes, case studies, and review questions promote your use of critical thinking and clinical reasoning skills.

Nursing Process

Nurses provide patient-centered care using an organizing framework called the nursing process. The **nursing process** is a problem-solving approach to the identification and treatment of patient problems that is the foundation of nursing practice. The nursing process framework provides a structure for the delivery of nursing care and the knowledge, judgments, and actions that nurses use to achieve best patient outcomes. Once started, the nursing process is not only continuous but also cyclic in nature.

The nursing process consists of five phases: assessment, diagnosis, planning, implementation, and evaluation (Fig. 1-3).

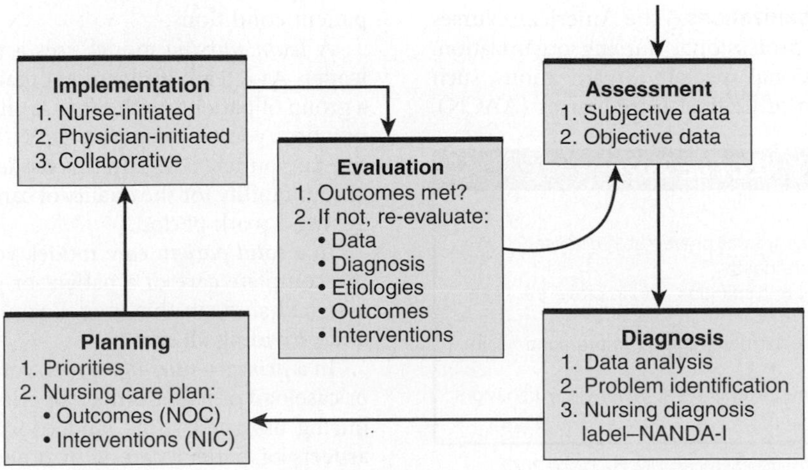

FIG. 1-3 Nursing process.

There is a basic order to the nursing process, beginning with assessment. *Assessment* is the collection of subjective and objective patient information on which to base the plan of care. *Nursing diagnosis* is the act of analyzing the assessment data and making a judgment about the nature of the data. It includes identifying and labeling human responses to actual or potential health problems or life processes. During *planning* the nursing diagnosis directs the development of patient outcomes or goals and identification of nursing interventions to accomplish the outcomes. *Implementation* is the activation of the plan with the use of nursing interventions. *Evaluation* is a continual activity in the nursing process. Evaluation determines whether the patient outcomes have been met as a result of nursing interventions. If the outcomes were not met, a review of the steps of the process is necessary to determine why not. Revision may be needed in assessment (data collection), the nursing diagnosis, planning (determining patient outcomes), or implementation (nursing interventions).

Standardized Nursing Terminologies

The demands of the current health care system challenge the nursing profession to define its practice and its impact on the health and health care of individuals, families, and communities. The nursing profession is asking questions such as the following: What do nurses do? How do they do it? Does it make a measurable difference in the health of those for whom they care? How can nurses best document their care? What happens as a result of their care?

In response to these questions, nursing has moved toward using standardizing nursing terminology (also called *nomenclatures, classification systems,* and *taxonomies*) to clearly define and evaluate nursing care. This can promote continuity of patient care and provide data to support the value of the profession. Instead of using a wide variety of words and methods to describe the same patient problems and nursing interventions, nurses use a readily understood common language to improve communication among themselves. In addition, standardized languages help identify the most effective nursing interventions.[15] For example, do the patient problems of pressure ulcer, decubitus ulcer, and skin breakdown all mean the same thing? What interventions can prevent these problems? Does turning the patient every 2 hours mean the same thing as repositioning the patient every 2 hours? If the patient is turned or repositioned every 2 hours, what happens as a result? How are the results described? Are the results different if a patient is placed on a pressure-relieving mattress or placed on a standard mattress and only turned? How are the results documented, and how do you know what works best?

Standardized terminologies offer ways to organize and describe nursing phenomena. A variety of languages have been developed that address different areas of nursing. Table 1-2 lists the classification systems recognized and approved by the ANA. The Omaha System and the Home Health Care Classification have been developed for community-based and home health care nursing, respectively. The Perioperative Nursing Dataset (discussed in Chapter 19) is used by perioperative nurses. The Nursing Management Minimum Data Set is available for use by nurse managers and administrators.

Three of the nursing terminologies recognized by the ANA are used to describe patient responses, patient outcomes, and nursing interventions: (1) NANDA International: Nursing Diagnoses, Definitions, and Classification; (2) the Nursing Outcomes Classification (NOC); and (3) the Nursing Interventions Classification (NIC). Each of these classification systems focuses on one component of the nursing process. Patients' responses or problems can be labeled using the nursing diagnoses classified and defined by NANDA-I.[16] Nursing interventions, or treatments, can be selected and implemented from NIC,[17] and nursing-sensitive patient outcomes can be identified and evaluated by selecting appropriate NOC outcomes.[18]

TABLE 1-2 ANA-RECOGNIZED NURSING TERMINOLOGIES

- NANDA International Nursing Diagnoses
- Nursing Interventions Classification (NIC)
- Nursing Outcomes Classification (NOC)
- Clinical Care Classification (CCC)
- Omaha System
- Nursing Management Minimum Data Set (NMMDS)
- PeriOperative Nursing Data Set (PNDS)
- SNOMED CT
- Nursing Minimum Data Set (NMDS)
- International Classification for Nursing Practice (ICNP)
- Logical Observation Identifiers Names and Codes (LOINC)

Source: American Nurses Association: *Recognized languages for nursing,* Washington, DC, 2010, The Association. Retrieved from *www.nursingworld.org/Terminologies.*

NANDA-I Nursing Diagnoses. NANDA International (NANDA-I) is a nursing organization that develops a standardized nursing terminology for identifying, defining, and classifying patients' actual or potential responses to health problems.[16] The two main purposes of NANDA-I are to develop a diagnostic classification system or taxonomy and to identify and accept nursing diagnoses. The use of the standardized terminology of nursing diagnoses documents the analysis and synthesis required in making a nursing diagnosis. It verifies nursing's contribution to cost-effective, efficient, quality health care.

The current NANDA-I nursing diagnoses are listed in Appendix B (NANDA-I nursing diagnoses are updated every 2 years). The nursing diagnoses used in this textbook are NANDA-I approved. The NANDA-I list is continually evolving as research results are interpreted and as nurses identify new human responses.

Nursing Outcomes Classification (NOC). Nursing Outcomes Classification (NOC) is a list of concepts, definitions, and measures that describe patient outcomes influenced by nursing interventions. A nursing-sensitive patient outcome is defined as an individual, family, or community state, behavior, or perception that is measured along a continuum in response to a nursing intervention(s).[18] The impact of your nursing practice on patient outcomes can be identified and measured when you choose a NOC outcome. Currently more than 385 coded outcomes have been organized into 7 domains and 34 classes. Each outcome has a label, a definition, a set of specific indicators to be used in rating the outcomes, and a five-point scale for rating the overall outcome and the specific indicators.

Nursing Interventions Classification (NIC). Nursing Interventions Classification (NIC) includes independent and collaborative interventions that you carry out, or direct others to carry out, on behalf of patients. It includes treatments that you perform in all settings and in all specialties. Because each intervention has a coded number, the use of NIC interventions facilitates electronic collection of standardized nursing data to evaluate the effectiveness of the interventions.

TABLE 1-3 **EXAMPLE OF NANDA-NOC-NIC LINKAGE**

NANDA-I Nursing Diagnosis: *Impaired skin integrity:* A state in which the individual has altered epidermis and/or dermis

NANDA-I–Related Factors	NOC Outcomes	NIC Interventions
Pressure	Tissue integrity: skin and mucous membranes	Pressure management Skin surveillance
Nutritional deficit	Nutritional status: food and fluid intake	Nutrition monitoring Nutrition therapy
Knowledge deficit	Knowledge: illness care	Teaching: disease process

Source: Nursing Diagnoses—Definitions and Classification 2012-2014. © 2012, 1994-2012 by NANDA International. Used by arrangement with Blackwell Publishing Limited, a company of John Wiley & Sons, Inc.
NANDA-I, NANDA International; *NIC*, Nursing Interventions Classification; *NOC*, Nursing Outcomes Classification.

NIC includes more than 500 interventions with a label name, a definition, and a set of activities for you to choose from to carry out the intervention. The interventions are grouped into 7 domains and 30 classes. Although more than 500 interventions may seem overwhelming, you will soon discover those interventions that are used most often in your particular specialty or with your patient population.[17] When planning care for a patient, choose specific interventions from the domain or class that is appropriate for the patient based on the nursing diagnosis and patient outcomes. Each intervention has a list of activities, and you select the appropriate activities from the list to implement the intervention. NIC does not prescribe interventions for specific situations. You are responsible for making the important decision of when and which interventions to use for a specific patient and situation based on your knowledge of the patient and the patient's condition.

NANDA-NOC-NIC Linkages. NANDA, NOC, and NIC (NNN) linkages show how the three distinct nursing terminologies can be connected and used together when planning care for patients. Linkages may assist in determination of a nursing diagnosis, projection of a desired outcome, and selection of interventions to achieve the desired outcome. Because each outcome or intervention has a coded number, the use of NNN facilitates electronic collection of standardized nursing data to evaluate the effectiveness of nursing care. An example of an NNN linkage is found in Table 1-3. The integration of NNN into the nursing process is illustrated in Fig. 1-4.

Nursing Care Plans

The nursing process is usually recorded and documented differently in nursing education when compared to clinical nursing practice. In nursing education the nursing process is frequently recorded in nursing care plans similar to those presented in this textbook. You practice and learn the nursing process by collecting assessment data, identifying nursing diagnoses, and selecting patient outcomes and nursing interventions—all of which are recorded on specific forms. Rationales for the selected interventions are also identified. These nursing care plans are used as teaching and learning tools.

In clinical practice, nursing care plans are often adapted for a specific setting. Electronic and written standardized care plans are used as guides for routine nursing care and are individualized to each patient's unique needs and problems.

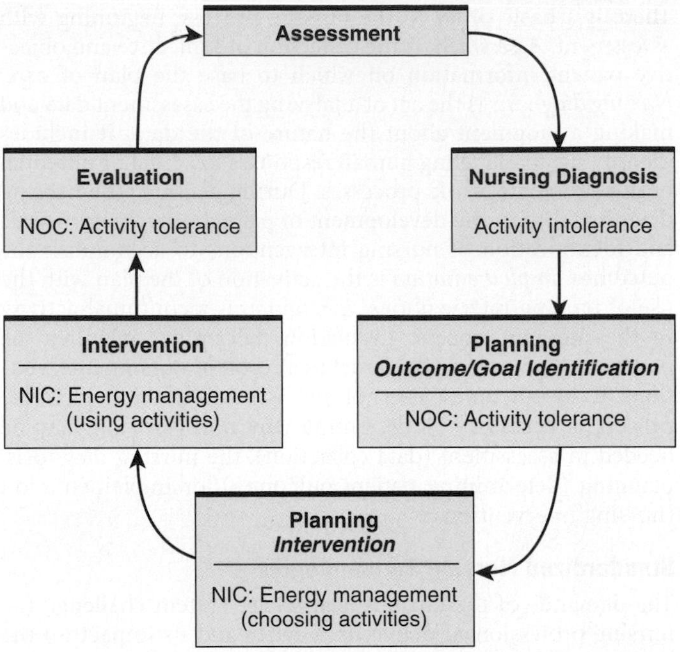

FIG. 1-4 Integration of NANDA, NIC, and NOC into the nursing process.

The nursing care plans presented throughout this book use the NANDA-I–approved nursing diagnoses, listed in order of priority, with NOC outcomes and NIC interventions (NCP 1-1). When any of these care plans are used, they should be individualized for a specific patient. You must use critical thinking to continually evaluate the situation and revise the diagnoses, outcomes, and interventions to fit each patient's unique care needs. All of the nursing care plans for this textbook are available in electronic format on the website at *http://evolve.elsevier.com/Lewis/medsurg*.

Collaborative problems are potential or actual complications of disease or treatment that nurses treat with other health care providers (e.g., physicians, APNs, speech therapists).[19] During the diagnosis phase of the nursing process, you identify these risks for physiologic complications in addition to nursing diagnoses. Identification of collaborative problems requires knowledge of pathophysiology and possible complications of medical treatment. Collaborative problem statements are usually written as "potential complication: ______" or "PC: ______" without a *"related to"* statement. An example is PC: pulmonary embolism. When potential complications are used in this textbook, *"related to"* statements have been added to increase understanding and relate the potential complication to possible causes.

A **concept map** is another method of recording a nursing care plan. In a concept map care plan the nursing process is recorded in a visual diagram of patient problems and interventions that illustrates the relationships among clinical data. Concept mapping is most useful in nursing education to teach nursing process and care planning.

Various formats are used for concept maps, and a variety of shapes, colors, and connecting arrows are used to identify concepts and relationships. In one example, assessment data are used to identify the patient's primary reason for seeking health care. That health state (often a medical diagnosis) is positioned centrally on the map. Positioned around the reason for seeking health care are nursing diagnoses that represent the patient's responses to the health state. Listed with each nursing diagnosis

NURSING CARE PLAN 1-1

*Patient with Heart Failure**

NURSING DIAGNOSIS **Activity intolerance** *related to* imbalance between oxygen supply and demand secondary to cardiac insufficiency and pulmonary congestion *as evidenced by* dyspnea, shortness of breath, weakness, increase in heart rate on exertion, and/or patient's statement, "I am too tired to get out of bed. I have no energy."

PATIENT GOAL Achieves a realistic program of activity that balances physical activity with energy-conserving activities

Outcomes (NOC)	Interventions (NIC) and *Rationales*
Activity Tolerance • Pulse rate with activity ____ • O_2 saturation with activity ____ • Respiratory rate with activity ____ • Systolic BP with activity ____ • Diastolic BP with activity ____ • Ease of breathing with activity ____ • Ease of performing ADLs ____ • Skin color ____ **Measurement Scale** 1 = Severely compromised 2 = Substantially compromised 3 = Moderately compromised 4 = Mildly compromised 5 = Not compromised	***Energy Management*** • Encourage alternate rest and activity periods *to reduce cardiac workload and conserve energy.* • Provide calming diversionary activities to promote relaxation *to reduce O_2 consumption and to relieve dyspnea and fatigue.* • Monitor patient's O_2 response (e.g., pulse rate, cardiac rhythm, and respiratory rate) to self-care or nursing activities *to determine level of activity that can be performed.* • Teach patient and caregiver techniques of self-care *that will minimize O_2 consumption* (e.g., self monitoring and pacing techniques for performance of ADLs). ***Activity Therapy*** • Collaborate with occupational and/or physical therapists *to plan and monitor activity and exercise program.* • Determine patient's commitment to increasing frequency and/or range of activities and exercise *to provide patient with obtainable goals.*

ADLs, Activities of daily living; *NIC,* Nursing Interventions Classification; *NOC,* Nursing Outcomes Classification.
*This example presents one nursing diagnosis for heart failure. The complete nursing care plan for heart failure is NCP 35-1 on pp. 780-781.

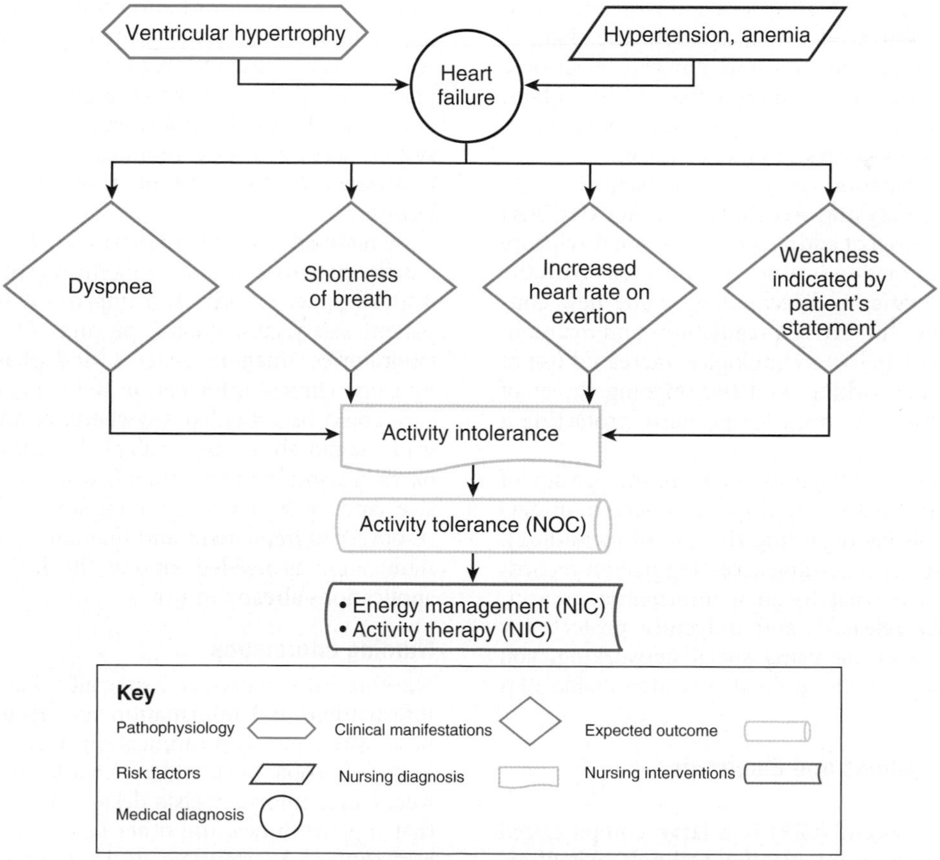

FIG. 1-5 Concept map.

are the assessment data that support the nursing diagnosis. Diagnostic testing data, treatments, medications, and nursing interventions may be listed with the nursing diagnoses or may be identified in separate areas and connected to the nursing diagnoses with arrows.[20] Fig. 1-5 illustrates a simplified version of a concept map for the patient with heart failure. For selected case studies at the end of the management chapters, related concept maps are available on the website at *http://evolve.elsevier.com/Lewis/medsurg.* In addition, a concept map builder is available online on the website.

INFORMATICS AND TECHNOLOGY

Information and Technology in Practice

Nursing is an information-intense profession. Advances in health information technology have changed the way nurses plan, deliver, document, and evaluate care. All nurses, regardless of their setting or role, use informatics and technology every day in practice. The incorporation of technologies into practice has changed how you obtain and review diagnostic information, make clinical decisions, communicate with patients and caregivers, and provide clinical interventions.[21]

Using information technology is becoming increasingly important in providing safe, quality patient care. For example, medication administration applications have been shown to improve patient safety by flagging potential errors, such as look-alike and sound-alike medications and adverse drug interactions, before they can occur. Computerized provider order entry (CPOE) systems can eliminate errors caused by misreading or misinterpreting handwritten instructions. Sensor technology is used to decrease the incidence of falls in high-risk patients.

Being able to use technology skills to communicate and access information is now an essential component of your professional nursing practice. You must be able to use word processing software, communicate by e-mail and text messaging, access the Internet to find information, and follow security and confidentiality rules.[22] You need to demonstrate the skills to safely use patient care technologies and navigate electronic health records and clinical information systems. Throughout this book suggestions on how to use informatics in your practice are highlighted in Informatics in Practice boxes.

Protected health information (PHI) is highly sensitive. The Health Insurance Portability and Accountability Act (HIPAA) is part of federal legislation that addresses the use and disclosure of PHI so that such information is properly protected. With the increased use of informatics and technology come new concerns for how to comply with HIPAA regulations and maintain a patient's privacy. New wireless technologies, increased use of e-mail and computer networking, and the ongoing threat of computer viruses increase the need for properly protecting a patient's privacy.

As a nurse, you have an obligation to ensure the privacy of your patient's health information. To do so, you need to understand your agency's policies regarding the use of technology. You need to know the rules regarding accessing patient records and releasing PHI, know what to do if information is accidently or intentionally released, and diligently protect any passwords you use. If you are using social networking, you must be careful not to place any individually identifiable PHI online.

Clinical Information Systems and Electronic Health Records

A clinical information system (CIS) is a large computerized system that integrates various information technology applications into a centralized repository of information related to patient care.[23] These systems support many types of activities related to patient care, including care documentation, order entry, and the retrieval of results, across various locations. Some examples of CISs including laboratory, nursing, pharmacy, long-term care, and emergency department systems and electronic health records.

An **electronic health record (EHR)** is a computerized record of PHI generated by one or more encounters in any care delivery setting.[24] Information that should be in an EHR includes patient demographics, progress notes, problems, medications, vital signs, past medical history, immunizations, laboratory data, and radiology reports (eFig. 1-1 available on the website for this chapter).

An *electronic medical record (EMR)* is a set of computerized data collected by a health care agency, such as an individual hospital or physician's office, which contributes to a record that is owned and used by that agency. In turn, an EHR is created when information from records created by a variety of agencies under different ownership is made available to other health care providers regardless of the location or affiliation of the health care provider. In practice, the terms *EHR* and *EMR* are often used interchangeably.[25]

The federal government was instrumental in the early adoption of EHRs because of its role in the delivery and payment of health care for millions of Americans through Medicare, the armed services, and the Department of Veterans Affairs (VA). The VA EHR system was one of the first implemented nationwide and today is a prototype for other providers. Patient records in the VA's electronic health system are fully electronic, portable, and readily accessible. The VA's EHR system provides a single place for health care providers to review and update a patient's health record and order medications, special procedures, nursing orders, diets, and diagnostic and laboratory tests. All aspects of a patient's record are integrated, including active problems, allergies, current medications, laboratory results, vital signs, hospitalizations, and outpatient clinic history. The system also provides reminders, cautions, and the ability to review data at sites remote from the original site of data collection.[26]

A national uniform EHR similar to the VA's health record has the potential to reduce medical errors associated with traditional paper records and improve clinical decision making, patient safety, and quality of care. As EHRs, entry systems, laboratories, imaging systems, and pharmacies are all linked into one clinical information network, many types of patient care could be provided anywhere, at anytime, since the "care grid" would always be available.[11] Unfortunately, a number of barriers stand in the way of a national system. EHRs are expensive and technologically complex, requiring a number of resources to implement and maintain. In addition, better communication is needed among the large number of software applications already in use.

Nursing Informatics

Nursing informatics is a specialty that integrates nursing, its information, and information management with information processing and communication technology to support the health of people worldwide.[27] An informatics nurse has a diverse role. Nurse informatacists design and build computer systems that support nurses and other health care providers in all roles and settings to improve decision making and enhance the quality of patient care. Other responsibilities of a nurse informatacist may include training health care providers and implementing, evaluating, and maintaining computer systems.

Computer Languages

When using applications such as an EHR, it is important to use a comprehensive, standardized medical vocabulary. One such standardized vocabulary is the Systematized Nomenclature of Medicine—Clinical Terms (SNOMED CT). In 2004 the federal government's licensure of SNOMED CT made the vocabulary available, free of charge, to all health care providers through the National Library of Medicine.[28] Uses for SNOMED CT include EHRs, intensive care monitoring, clinical decision support, medical research studies, clinical trials, CPOE, disease surveillance, and consumer health information services.

The use of SNOMED CT is of significant value to nursing in that the vocabulary includes the NANDA-I, NIC, and NOC (NNN) terminologies of nursing. With the use of SNOMED CT, nursing diagnoses, interventions, and outcomes can be recorded using the NNN terminologies. Following the links among diagnosis, interventions, and outcomes will greatly advance evidence-based practice (EBP). For example, when you choose the NANDA-I diagnosis of *fatigue* on a computer, the code 00093 is added to a database. Then you might select the NOC outcome of *endurance,* and the code 0001 would also be added to the database. You could select the NIC interventions of *energy management (0180)* and *exercise promotion (0200),* and these codes would also be incorporated. The coded data can be separated from the patient's name, thus providing for patient anonymity. Links that result from these data can be analyzed and serve not only to improve practice, but also to demonstrate the effectiveness of nursing interventions and formulate nursing research questions. This provides a continuing evaluation of nursing's efficacy.

Today many informatics nurses are concerned that, unless nursing care data are stored electronically, CISs or EHRs will contain no data about the decisions that nurses make. As a result, nursing data will not be used in health care planning and policies. Information about identified nursing problems, independent nursing interventions, and improved patient outcomes will not be apparent, and nursing's role in and contribution to health care will be invisible.[29]

Documenting the nursing process is a critical part of the patient's record. This is important because it provides evidence that nursing practice standards related to the nursing process have been maintained during the care of the patient.

All nurses must work to ensure that nursing data are stored electronically and become part of the EHR. Many different electronic documentation methods and formats are used. However, few agencies have implemented the use of standardized nursing terminologies for documenting nursing care. Using nursing terminologies for documenting nursing practice provides an efficient, consistent way to communicate nursing knowledge. It allows nurses to track, improve, and report on the outcomes of nursing care.[15] If nursing data are to be part of the data analyzed from EHRs, nurses need to decide what data should be included in the EHR and what terminology should be used to record the data so that the meaning is clear, consistent, and valuable.

Telehealth

Increasingly, technology is allowing nurses and other health care providers to deliver patient care services in a wider range of settings. **Telehealth** is the use of videoconferencing or other communication technologies to provide care when patients and health care providers are geographically separated. Telehealth care has many applications, not only in the assessment, diagnosis, and treatment of illness, but also in health promotion, follow-up, and coordination of care. Nurses engaged in telehealth nursing practice continue to assess, plan, intervene, and

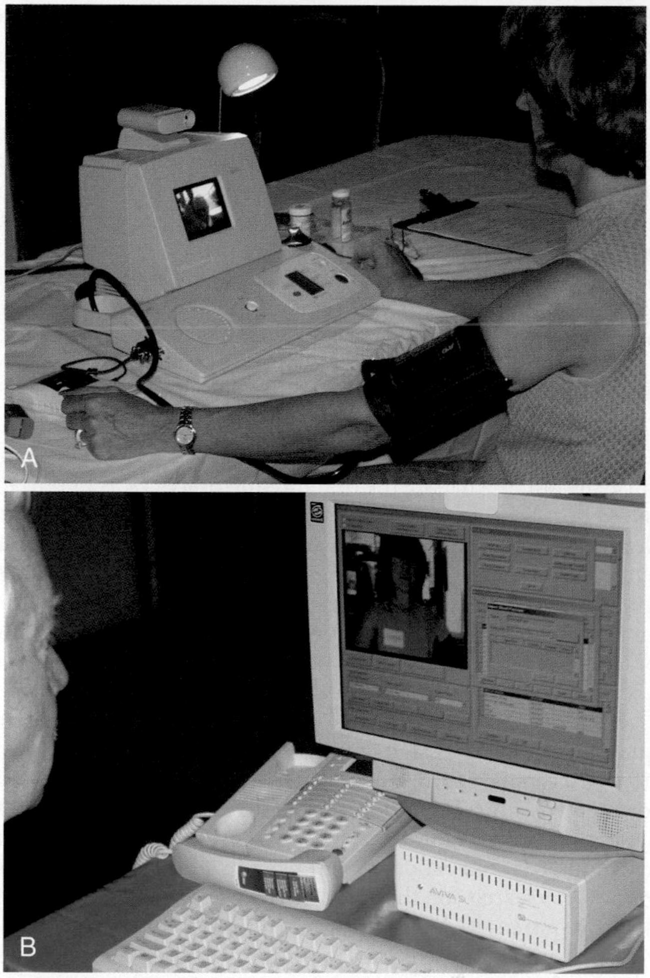

FIG. 1-6 Telemonitoring. **A,** Remote blood pressure monitoring. **B,** Videoconference with health care provider.

evaluate the outcomes of nursing care. However, they do so using technologies such as the Internet, computers, telephones, digital assessment tools, and telemonitoring equipment[30] (Fig. 1-6).

Home care is seeing significant changes as the result of rapidly expanding remote patient monitoring. A growing number of biomedical devices can collect, monitor, and report patient data in real time. These devices include blood glucose monitors, peak flow meters, scales, stethoscopes, and automated blood pressure cuffs. Video cameras with magnifying capabilities are used to assess wounds and monitor the status of healing. Nurses practicing telehealth can provide patient and caregiver teaching and emotional support through videoconferencing.

EVIDENCE-BASED PRACTICE

Evidence-based practice (EBP) is a problem-solving approach to clinical decision making. It involves the use of the best available evidence (e.g., research findings, data from quality improvement projects, professional organization standards) in combination with clinician expertise and patient preferences and values to achieve desired patient outcomes.[31] The most important reason to use EBP is the delivery of the highest quality of care for the best patient outcomes. Expectations for high-quality, cost-effective care and the increased accessibility of health information have contributed to a need for all health disciplines to provide care based on the best evidence. Regulatory and accrediting agencies, including The Joint Commission (TJC), require documentation of the effective use of evidence in clinical care decisions.

EBP does not mean that you need to conduct a research study. Instead, EBP is a process that involves finding, appraising, and applying research conducted by others in an effort to answer a specific clinical question. The use of technology supports EBP by providing you with access to data. You can easily search a number of online resources and collect large amounts of clinical information or evidence to identify the best patient care practices.

Steps of EBP Process

The EBP process has seven critical steps (Table 1-4).

Step 0 of EBP. Creating a spirit of inquiry, or an ongoing curiosity about what are the best nursing practices, is important to support the other stages of EBP. Positive patient outcomes depend on you taking an active role in using the best available evidence when delivering care. When you possess a spirit of inquiry, you routinely ask questions about your patient's care and recognize when more information is needed. When your practice is based on valid evidence, you are solving problems and supporting best patient outcomes.[32]

Step 1 of EBP. Step 1 of the EBP process is asking a clinical question in the PICOT format. Formulating the clinical question is the most important step in the EBP process.[33] A well-formulated clinical question that is searchable and answerable creates the context for integrating best available evidence, clinical judgment, and patient preferences. In addition, the question guides the search for the most current literature and the evidence required.

An example of a clinical question in PICOT format is, "In adult cardiac surgery patients (**P** = patients/population) is morphine (**I** = intervention) or fentanyl (**C** = comparison) more effective in reducing pain (**O** = outcome) on the first postoperative day (**T** = time period)?" A properly stated clinical question may not have all components of PICOT in the statement. Some may only include the first four components, PICO without the T, because the (T) timing for the (I) intervention to support the (O) outcome is not always pertinent. The (C) component of PICOT might include a comparison with a specific intervention, the usual standard of care, or no intervention at all.

Step 2 of EBP. Step 2 of the EBP process is a thorough search for and collection of evidence based on the clinical question. The content and type of question direct the clinician to the most appropriate databases. The search begins with the strongest external evidence to answer the question. Preappraised evidence such as systematic reviews and evidence-based clinical practice guidelines are time- and effort-saving resources in the EBP process (see Table 1-4).

Systematic reviews of randomized controlled trials (RCTs) are considered the strongest level of evidence to answer questions about interventions (i.e., cause and effect). Systematic reviews, which include the critical analysis and synthesis of methods and findings from multiple studies, are available for only a limited number of clinical topics and may not suit all types of clinical questions. If the clinical question involves how a patient experiences or copes with a health change, searching for a meta-synthesis of qualitative evidence may be the appropriate approach.

Clinical practice guidelines are helpful for translating research findings into specific interventions. However, these published guidelines vary in comprehensiveness and credibility. Guidelines are produced by a variety of authoring groups such as professional health care societies, patient advocacy organizations, and government agencies.

When insufficient research exists to guide practice, recommendations from expert committees, authority figures, and opinion authorities may be the best evidence available. When care decisions must depend on this type of evidence, ongoing and rigorous outcome data should be collected to provide stronger evidence.

Step 3 of EBP. Step 3 of the EBP process is critically appraising and synthesizing evidence found in the search. The purpose of critical appraisal is to determine the value of the research in actual practice. A successful critical appraisal process focuses on three essential questions: (1) What are the results? (2) Are the results reliable and valid? and (3) Will the results help me in caring for my patients? You must determine the strength of the evidence and synthesize the findings related to the clinical question to conclude what is the best practice.

Step 4 of EBP. Step 4 of the EBP process may differ depending on the strength and breadth of the evidence to answer the question. Recommendations from sufficient, strong evidence such as the meta-analysis of well-designed RCTs can be implemented into practice interventions in combination with clinicians' expertise and patient preferences. For example, although evidence supports the use of morphine as an effective analgesic, it may not be appropriate to use in a patient with renal failure. In another example, although their concerns are not supported by evidence, patients may be worried about perceived addictive effects of morphine and prefer an alternative to opioids for their pain management. These types of decisions must be made by combining knowledge of the best available evidence, clinician judgment, and application if the recommendations to the individual patient's circumstances and preferences.

Many areas in practice do not have an established evidence base or have inconsistent evidence. When evidence is insufficient to guide practice, the fourth step would be to generate data to answer the question. One way for data to be gathered is through the conduct of rigorous research. Health care providers can collaborate with researchers to conduct research and generate knowledge that identifies the best patient care practices.

Step 5 of EBP. Step 5 of the EBP process is evaluation of identified outcomes in the clinical setting. Outcomes to be measured must match the clinical project objective that has been

TABLE 1-4 STEPS OF EVIDENCE-BASED PRACTICE (EBP) PROCESS

0. Cultivate a spirit of inquiry.
1. Ask the burning clinical question using the **PICO** or **PICOT** format:
   Patients/population
   Intervention
   Comparison or comparison group
   Outcome(s)
   Time period (as applicable)
2. Collect the most relevant best evidence.
3. Critically appraise and synthesize the evidence.
4. Integrate all evidence with clinical expertise and patient preferences and values in making a practice decision or change.
5. Evaluate the practice decision or change.
6. Share the outcomes of the decision or change.

implemented. For example, evaluating only the cost of each medication for pain control does not provide data about clinical effectiveness. Outcomes must reflect all aspects of the implementation and capture the interdisciplinary contributions obtained by the EBP process. For example, an EBP initiative related to pain control might involve patients and caregivers, nurses, physicians, pharmacists, physical and respiratory therapists, and other team members. Some outcomes expectations may be shared, whereas other goals may be different for each team member.

Step 6 of EBP. The last step in EBP is to share the outcomes of the EBP change. If you do not share the outcomes of EBP, then other health care providers and patients cannot benefit from what you learned from your experience. Information is shared locally using unit- or hospital-based newsletters and posters and regionally and nationally through journal publications and presentations at conferences.

Implementing EBP

To implement EBP, you must develop the skills to continually seek and then incorporate into practice the scientific evidence that supports best patient outcomes. The incorporation of evidence, balanced with clinical expertise, should take into account the patient's unique circumstances and preferences. EBP closes the gap between research and practice, providing more reliable and predictable care than that based on tradition, opinion, and trial and error. It provides you with an effective process to manage the wealth of information and newly introduced technologies, while balancing concerns about health care costs and an increasing emphasis on quality and patient outcomes.

Throughout this book, two different types of EBP boxes are used to show how EBP is used in nursing practice. The Translating Research into Practice boxes provide initial answers to specific clinical questions. These boxes contain the clinical question, critical appraisal of the supportive evidence, implications for nursing practice, and the source of the evidence. Applying the Evidence boxes provide an opportunity for you to practice your critical thinking skills in applying EBP to patient scenarios.

To assist you in identifying the use of evidence incorporated throughout this book, an asterisk (*) is used in the reference list at the end of each chapter to indicate evidence-based information for clinical practice.

SAFETY AND QUALITY IMPROVEMENT

As the complexity of the environments in which health care is delivered increases, patient safety and communication among health care professionals are affected. In 1999 the IOM issued a report that indicated that at least 44,000 people, and perhaps as many as 98,000 people, die in hospitals each year as a result of preventable medical errors. The report described medical errors as an epidemic and concluded that it was not acceptable for patients to be harmed by a health care system that is supposed to offer healing and comfort.[34]

Since the IOM report, a series of organizations and commissions have provided safety goals for health care organizations and identified a number of safety competencies for health professionals. By implementing various procedures and systems to improve communication and health care delivery to meet safety goals, health care systems are creating a culture of safety that minimizes the risk of harm to the patient. Because you have the greatest amount of interaction with patients, you are a vital part of promoting this culture of safety by providing care in a manner that reduces errors and actively promotes patient safety.

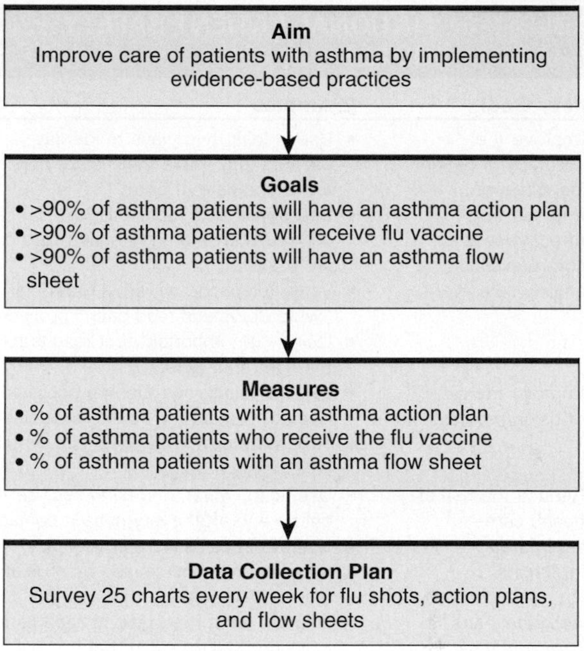

FIG. 1-7 Quality improvement system.

Patient-centered care is interrelated with both quality and safety—the higher the culture of safety, the better the quality of care. Health care systems focused on quality outcomes use practice standards and protocols based on best evidence while considering the patient's unique preferences and needs at the moment. Your role is to coordinate and integrate the complex aspects of patient care, including the care delivered by others, and identify issues that are associated with poor quality and unsafe care.

As part of professional nursing practice, you are responsible for collecting data, using data to monitor patient outcomes, and implementing interventions to improve quality of care. An example of a quality improvement system is shown in Fig. 1-7. You need to be able to assess current practices and compare them with relevant better practices elsewhere as a means of identifying areas for improving care and formulating clinical questions for EBP.

National Patient Safety Goals

The Joint Commission (TJC), the accrediting agency for health care organizations, issues National Patient Safety Goals (NPSGs) for each of its accreditation programs.[35] The NPSGs promote specific improvements in patient safety by providing health care organizations with evidence-based solutions to persistent safety problems. The 2013 goals are listed in Table 1-5. Safety alerts that highlight safety information related to patient care and the NPSGs are integrated throughout the textbook.

TEAMWORK AND COLLABORATION

Interdisciplinary Team Members

To deliver high-quality care, you need to establish effective working relationships with members of the health care team. A

TABLE 1-5 NATIONAL PATIENT SAFETY GOALS*

Safety Goal	Examples
1. Improve the accuracy of patient identification.	• Use at least two ways to identify patients (e.g., have them state full name and date of birth).
2. Improve the effectiveness of communication among caregivers.	• Use SBAR (see Table 1-7) for communication among health care professionals. • Verify telephone or verbal orders by "write down and read back" procedure. • Quickly get important test results to the right staff person.
3. Improve the safety of using medications.	• Label all medicines that are not already labeled. Discard any found unlabeled. • Take extra care with patients who take anticoagulant drugs.
4. Reduce the risk of health care–associated infections.	• Use soap, water, and hand sanitizer before and after every patient contact. • Use evidence-based practices to prevent infections caused by multidrug-resistant organisms.
5. Accurately and completely reconcile medications across the continuum of care.	• Find out what medications each patient is taking. Make certain that it is safe for the patient to take any new medicines with his or her current medicines. • Give a list of the patient's medicines to his or her next caregiver. Give the list to the patient's regular physician before the patient goes home. • Give a list of the patient's medicines to the patient and caregiver before they go home. Explain the list.
6. Reduce the risk of patient harm resulting from falls.	• Evaluate patients for fall risk. • Take action to reduce risk of injury.
7. Prevent health care–related pressure ulcers (decubitus ulcers).	• Assess patients at risk for pressure ulcers on admission and on a regular basis throughout their care.
8. The organization identifies safety risks inherent in its patient population.	• Assess patients at risk for suicide. • Assess any risks for patients who are getting home oxygen therapy, such as fires.
Universal Protocol (UP)	
• Preprocedure verification • Mark procedure site • Performance of time-out	• Conduct a time-out before the start of any invasive or surgical procedure, • Confirm correct patient, procedure, and site.

Adapted from The Joint Commission (TJC): 2013 National patient safety goals, Oakbrook Terrace, Ill. Retrieved from www.jointcommission.org/PatientSafety/NationalPatientSafetyGoals.
*The numbering system is correct and resulted from renumbering by TJC.

health care team may consist of physicians, nurses, pharmacists, occupational and physical therapists, social workers, and others (Table 1-6). As part of your interdisciplinary nursing practice, you will collaborate in many ways by exchanging knowledge, sharing responsibility for problem solving, and making patient care decisions. You may be responsible for coordinating care among the team members and initiating appropriate referrals when you anticipate that expertise in specialized areas is needed to help the patient. To do so, you need to be aware of the knowledge and skills of other team members and be able to communicate effectively among them.

TABLE 1-6 INTERDISCIPLINARY TEAM MEMBERS

Team Member	Description of Services Provided
Dietitian	Provides general nutrition services, including dietary consultation regarding health promotion or specialized diets
Home health aide	Assists patients with their personal care needs, such as bathing, dressing, and hair washing, or with some homemaking activities (e.g., meal preparation or light housekeeping)
Occupational therapist (OT)	May assist patient with fine motor coordination, performance of activities of daily living, cognitive-perceptual skills, sensory testing, and the construction or use of assistive or adaptive equipment
Pastoral care	Offers spiritual support and guidance to patients and caregivers
Pharmacist	Prepares medications and infusion products
Physical therapist (PT)	Works with patients on improving strength and endurance, gait training, transfer training, and developing a patient education program
Physician (medical doctor [MD])	Practices medicine and treats illness and injury by prescribing medication, performing diagnostic tests and evaluations, performing surgery, and providing other medical services and advice
Respiratory therapist	May assist with oxygen therapy in the home, provide specialized respiratory treatments, and instruct patient or caregiver regarding the proper use of respiratory equipment
Social worker	Assists patients with developing coping skills, meeting caregiver concerns, securing adequate financial resources or housing assistance, or making referrals to social service or volunteer agencies
Speech therapist	Focuses on treatment of speech defects and disorders, especially through the use of physical exercises to strengthen muscles used in speech, speech drills, and audiovisual aids that develop new speech habits

Coordinating Care Among Health Care Team Members

Communication. Communication is a key component of facilitating teamwork and care across the care continuum, which is essential for fostering a culture of safety. There is evidence that the majority of patient safety issues result from breakdown in communication.[35] Enhancing communication among the health care team requires a systematic approach. One model used for reporting and hand-off communications is the **SBAR (Situation-Background-Assessment-Recommendation)** technique (Table 1-7). This technique provides a mechanism for framing critical communication about a patient's condition between members of the health care team.[36] Other ways to enhance communication include "time-outs" before surgical procedures or during a busy day on a nursing unit to identify risks and develop a plan for delivering care.

Case Management. Case management is a collaborative process that involves assessing, planning, facilitating, and advocating for health services to meet an individual's and/or caregiver's needs through communication and use of available resources to promote cost-effective quality outcomes. Although health care agencies define case management in various ways, the concept of case management involves managing the patient's

TABLE 1-7 GUIDELINES FOR COMMUNICATING USING SBAR

Purpose: SBAR is a model for effective transfer of information by providing a standardized structure for concise factual communications from nurse-to-nurse, nurse-to-physician, or nurse-to–other health professionals.

Steps to Use: Before speaking with a physician or other health care professional about a patient problem, assess the patient yourself, read the most recent physician progress and nursing notes, and have the patient chart available.

S **Situation**	What is the situation you want to discuss? What is happening at the present time? • Identify self, unit. **State:** I am calling about: *patient, room number.* • Briefly state the problem: what it is, when it happened or started, and how severe it is. **State:** I have just assessed the patient and I am concerned about: *identify why you are concerned.*
B **Background**	What is the background or circumstances leading up to the situation? **State** pertinent background information related to the situation that may include • Admitting diagnosis and date of admission • List of current medications, allergies, IV fluids • Most recent vital signs • Date and time of any laboratory testing and results of previous tests for comparison • Synopsis of treatment to date • Code status
A **Assessment**	What do you think the problem is? What is your assessment of the situation? **State** what you think the problem is: • Changes from prior assessments • Patient condition unstable or worsening
R **Recommendation/ Request**	What should we do to correct the problem? What is your recommendation or request? **State** your request. • Specific treatments • Tests needed • Patient needs to be seen now

Source: Kaiser Permanente of Colorado: SBAR technique for communication: a situational briefing model, Institute for Health Care Improvement. Retrieved from *www.ihi.org/knowledge/Pages/Tools/SBARTechniqueforCommunicationASituationalBriefingModel.aspx.*

care across multiple care settings and levels of care.[37] The goals of case management are to provide quality care along a continuum, decrease fragmentation of care across many settings, enhance the patient's quality of life, and contain costs.

A professional nurse often serves as the case manager. The nurse assesses the needs of an individual or caregiver, coordinates services for them, makes referrals as appropriate, and evaluates progress to ensure that short- and long-term goals are met. For example, a patient with severe coronary artery disease may be assigned a nurse as a case manager in an outpatient clinic. When the patient is hospitalized for coronary artery bypass graft surgery, the same case manager coordinates care so that all health care providers understand the patient's unique needs. When the patient is discharged, the case manager determines whether home health care or other services are necessary for the patient.

Clinical Pathways. Care related to common health problems experienced by many patients is delineated and documented using clinical (critical) pathways. A **clinical (critical) pathway** directs the entire health care team in the daily care goals for select health care problems. It includes an interdisciplinary care plan, and goals and interventions specific for each day of hospitalization. The case types selected for clinical pathways are usually those that occur in high volume and are highly predictable, such as myocardial infarction and surgical procedures, including joint replacements, cholecystectomies, and appendectomies.

The clinical pathway describes the patient care required at specific times. An interdisciplinary approach moves the patient toward desired outcomes within an estimated length of stay. The exact content and format of clinical pathways vary among institutions. If clinical pathways are used by an institution, they are usually evidence based and specifically developed by that institution. Nurse- and physician-initiated interventions designed to achieve the patient outcomes are identified throughout the pathway. The interdisciplinary approach can be seen in the referral to and consultation with other health professionals. If a nursing-specific care plan is included in the clinical pathway, it is usually documented with the use of nursing diagnoses and evaluation of patient outcomes. Many pathways are computerized, making them a permanent part of the patient's record.

Delegation and Assignment. As a registered nurse (RN), you will delegate nursing care and supervise others who are qualified to deliver care. **Delegation** is transferring the authority or responsibility to perform a selected nursing task in a selected situation to a competent individual.[38] The delegation and assignment of nursing activities from the professional nurse (the RN) to nonprofessional and/or unlicensed health care personnel is a process that, when used appropriately, can result in safe, effective, and efficient nursing care. Delegating can allow you more time to focus on complex patient care needs.

Delegation typically involves tasks and procedures that **unlicensed assistive personnel (UAP)** and licensed practical/vocational nurses (LPN/LVNs) perform. Nursing interventions that require independent nursing knowledge, skill, or judgment such as assessment, patient teaching, and evaluation of care are your responsibility and cannot be delegated. UAP are unlicensed individuals who assist the RN, the professional nurse. UAP may include nursing aides, orderlies, nursing assistants, attendants, or technicians. Professional nurses are responsible for supervising the education, training, and use of UAP in providing direct patient care. As a nurse, you use professional judgment to determine appropriate activities to delegate based on the patient's needs, the UAP's education and training, and extent of supervision required.[38] In addition, some state boards of nursing identify specific activities that may be delegated to UAP such as obtaining routine vital signs on stable patients, feeding and assisting patients at mealtimes, ambulating stable patients, and helping patients with bathing and hygiene. eFig. 1-2 (available on the website for this chapter) shows a decision tree for delegation to UAP.

Delegation may also involve the LPN/LVN, whose scope and standards of practice are defined by the state nursing practice act and regulated by state agencies. However, you may also delegate specific tasks to the LPN/LVN. You must know the legal scope of practical/vocational nursing practice and delegate and assign nursing functions appropriately. In most states, LPN/LVNs may administer medications, perform sterile

TABLE 1-8 FIVE RIGHTS OF NURSING DELEGATION

1. The *right* task
2. Under the *right* circumstances
3. To the *right* person
4. With the *right* direction and communication
5. Under the *right* supervision and evaluation

Source: Joint Statement on Delegation: American Nurses Association (ANA) and the National Council of State Boards of Nursing (NCSBN), 2007. Retrieved from *https://www.ncsbn.org/Joint_statement.pdf*.

procedures, and provide a wide variety of interventions planned by the RN.

Assignment is different from delegation in that assignment is the distribution of work that each staff member is responsible for during a given work period. Therefore the term *assign* is used when you direct a person to do something that he or she is authorized to do. Assignments occur when an RN directs other RNs, LPN/LVNs, or UAP to perform care that is within their scope of practice. Whether you delegate or are working with staff to which you assign tasks, you are responsible for the patient's total care during your work period. You are responsible for the supervision of the UAP or LPN/LVN and remain accountable for ensuring that the delegated tasks are completed in a competent manner. This supervision includes guidance and direction, oversight, evaluation, and follow-up by the RN.[38]

Delegation is a skill that is learned and must be practiced for you to be proficient in managing patient care. You need to use critical thinking and professional judgment to ensure that the Five Rights of Nursing Delegation are implemented (Table 1-8). This book presents delegation decisions in boxes in appropriate chapters and provides delegation questions in case studies at the end of the management chapters.

DELEGATION DECISIONS

Delegation Decisions Boxes Throughout Book

BRIDGE TO NCLEX EXAMINATION

The number of the question corresponds to the same-numbered outcome at the beginning of the chapter.

1. An example of a nursing activity that reflects the American Nurses Association's definition of nursing is
   a. diagnosing a patient with a feeding tube as being at risk for aspiration.
   b. establishing protocols for treating patients in the emergency department.
   c. providing antianxiety drugs for a patient who has disturbed sleep patterns.
   d. identifying and treating dysrhythmias that occur in a patient in the coronary care unit.
2. A nurse working on the medical-surgical unit at an urban hospital would like to become certified in a medical-surgical specialty. The nurse knows that this process would most likely require
   a. a bachelor's degree in nursing.
   b. formal education in advanced nursing practice.
   c. experience for a specific period in medical-surgical nursing.
   d. membership in a medical-surgical nursing specialty organization.
3. A nurse is providing care to a patient after right hip surgery. Within a pay-for-performance system, a critical role of the nurse is to
   a. ensure that care is provided using a minimal amount of supplies.
   b. discharge the patient at completion of the number of approved days of care.
   c. implement measures to decrease the risk of the patient acquiring an infection.
   d. assess the patient's ability to pay for health care services at the time of admission.
4. The nurse is assigned to care for a newly admitted patient. Number in order the steps for using the nursing process to prioritize care. (Number 1 is the first step, and number 5 is the last step.)
   ___ Evaluate whether the plan was effective.
   ___ Identify any health problems.
   ___ Collect patient information.
   ___ Carry out the plan.
   ___ Determine a plan of action.

5. The linkages among NANDA-I nursing diagnoses, NOC patient outcomes, and NIC nursing interventions can be used to
   a. evaluate patient outcomes.
   b. provide guides for planning care.
   c. predict the results of nursing care.
   d. shorten written care plans for individual patients.
6. Advantages of the use of informatics in health care delivery are *(select all that apply)*
   a. reduced need for home care nurses in rural areas.
   b. increased patient anonymity and confidentiality.
   c. the ability to achieve and maintain high standards of care.
   d. improved communication of the patient's health status to the health care team.
   e. access to standardized plans of care that are available for most types of health problems.
7. When using evidence-based practice, the nurse
   a. must use clinical practice guidelines developed by national health agencies.
   b. should use findings from randomized controlled trials to plan care for all patient problems.
   c. uses clinical decision making and judgment to determine what evidence is appropriate for a specific clinical situation.
   d. statistically analyzes the relationship of nursing interventions to patient outcomes to establish evidence for the most appropriate patient interventions.
8. The nurse's role in addressing the National Patient Safety Goals established by The Joint Commission includes *(select all that apply)*
   a. using side rails and alarm systems as necessary to prevent patient falls.
   b. memorizing and implementing all the rules published by The Joint Commission.
   c. verifying telephone and verbal orders using the "write down and read back" procedure.
   d. encouraging patients to be actively involved in and question their own health care.
   e. obtaining a complete list of the patient's medications and monitoring their use throughout the continuum of care.
9. The nurse is caring for a diabetic patient in the ambulatory surgical unit who has just undergone debridement of an infected toe. Which task is most appropriate for the nurse to delegate to unlicensed assistive personnel (UAP)?
   a. Check the patient's vital signs.
   b. Evaluate the patient's awareness.
   c. Monitor the site of the patient's IV catheter.
   d. Evaluate the patient's tibial and pedal pulses.

1. a, 2. c, 3. c, 4. 5, 2, 1, 4, 3, 5. b, 6. c, d, e, 7. c, 8. a, c, e, 9. a.

evolve

For rationales to these answers and even more NCLEX review questions, visit *http://evolve.elsevier.com/Lewis/medsurg*.

REFERENCES

1. American Nurses Association: *Nursing: a social policy statement*, ed 3, Washington, DC, 2010, The Association. (Classic)
2. Nightingale F: *Notes on nursing: what it is and what it is not (facsimile edition)*, Philadelphia, 1946, Lippincott. (Classic)
3. Henderson V: *The nature of nursing*, New York, 1966, Macmillan. (Classic)
4. Roy S, Andrews H: *The Roy adaptation model*, ed 2, Stamford, Conn, 1999, Appleton & Lange. (Classic)
5. American Association of Colleges of Nursing: Essentials of baccalaureate education for professional nursing practice. Retrieved from *www.aacn.nche.edu*.
6. Sportsman S: Competency education and validation in the United States: what should nurses know? *Nurs Forum* 45:140, 2010.
7. American Nurses Credentialing Center: Certification. Retrieved from *www.nursecredentialing.org/certification.aspx*.
8. American Association of Colleges of Nursing: The essentials of doctoral education for advanced nursing practice. Retrieved from *www.aacn.nche.edu/DNP/index.htm*.
9. Cromwell J, Trisolini MG, Pope GC, et al: *Pay for performance in health care: methods and approaches*, Research Triangle Park, NC, 2011, RTI Press Publications.
10. US Department of Health and Human Services: Healthy People 2020. Retrieved from *www.healthypeople.gov*.
11. Committee on the Robert Wood Johnson Foundation Initiative on the Future of Nursing at the Institute of Medicine: *The future of nursing: leading change, advancing health*, Washington, DC, 2011, National Academies Press.
12. Jost SG, Bonnell M, Chacko SJ, et al: Integrated primary nursing: a care delivery model for the 21st-century knowledge worker, *NAQ* 34:208, 2010.
13. Alfaro-LeFevre R: *Critical thinking and clinical judgment*, ed 5, St Louis, 2012, Saunders.
14. Benner P, Sutphen M, Leonard D, et al: *Educating nurses: a call for radical transformation*, San Francisco, 2009, Jossey-Bass.
15. Jones D, Lunney M, Keenan G, et al: Standardized nursing languages: essential for the nursing workforce, *Annu Rev Nurs Res* 28:253, 2010.
16. NANDA International: *Nursing diagnoses: definitions and classification 2012-2014*, Kaukauna, Wisc, 2011, The Association.
17. Bulechek GM, Butcher HK, Dochterman JM: *Nursing interventions classification (NIC)*, ed 5, St Louis, 2008, Mosby.
18. Moorhead S, Johnson M, Maas M, et al: *Nursing outcomes classification (NOC)*, ed 4, St Louis, 2008, Mosby.
19. Carpenito-Moyet L: *Nursing diagnosis: application to clinical practice*, ed 13, Philadelphia, 2009, Lippincott Williams & Wilkins.
20. Kostovich CT, Poradzisz M, Wood K, et al: Learning style preference and student aptitude for concept maps, *J Nurs Educ* 46:225, 2007.
21. McGonigle D, Mastrian K: *Nursing informatics and the foundation of knowledge*, ed 2, Burlington, Mass, 2012, Jones & Bartlett Learning.
22. QSEN: Informatics. Retrieved from *www.qsen.org/ksas_prelicensure.php#informatics*.
23. Zerwekh J, Garneau A: *Nursing today: transitions and trends*, ed 7, St Louis, 2011, Saunders.
24. Thomes J: Avoiding the trap in the HITECH Act's incentive timeframe for implementing the EHR, *J Health Care Finance* 37:91, 2010.
25. Staggers N, Weir C, Phanaslkar S: Patient safety and health information technology: role of the electronic health record. In *Patient safety and quality: an evidence-based handbook for*

nurses, Rockville, Md, 2008, Agency for Healthcare Research and Quality. Retrieved from *www.ahrq.gov/qual/nurseshdbk*.
26. World VistA: About VistA. Retrieved from *http://worldvista.org*.
27. American Nurses Association: *Scope and standards for nursing informatics practice*, Washington, DC, 2008, The Association.
28. International Health Terminology Standards Development Organization: *Introducing SNOMED CT*, Copenhagen, 2010, The Organization.
29. Thede L: Informatics: the electronic health record: will nursing be on board when the ship leaves? *OJIN* 13:3, 2008. Retrieved from *www.nursingworld.org/MainMenuCategories/ANAMarketplace/ANAPeriodicals/OJIN/Columns/Informatics/ElectronicHealthRecord.aspx*.
30. Schlachta-Fairchild L, Elfrink V, Deickman A: Patient safety, telenursing, and telehealth. In *Patient safety and quality: an evidence-based handbook for nurses*, Rockville, Md, 2008, Agency for Healthcare Research and Quality. Retrieved from *www.ahrq.gov/qual/nurseshdbk*.
31. Melnyk B, Fineout-Overholt E: *Evidence-based practice in nursing and healthcare: a guide to best practice*, ed 2, Philadelphia, 2010, Lippincott Williams & Wilkins.
32. Malloch K, Porter-O'Grady T: *Introduction to evidence-based practice in nursing and health care*, Sudbury, Mass, 2010, Jones & Bartlett.
33. Stillwell S, Fineout-Overholt E, Melnyk B, et al: Asking the clinical question: a key step in evidence-based practice, *Am J Nurs* 110:58, 2010.
34. Institute of Medicine: *To err is human: building a safer health system*, Washington, DC, 2000, National Academy Press. (Classic)
35. The Joint Commission: National patient safety goals. Retrieved from *www.jointcommission.org/standards_information/npsgs.aspx*.
36. Kaiser Permanente of Colorado: SBAR technique for communication: a situational briefing model. Retrieved from *www.ihi.org/knowledge/Pages/Tools/SBARTechniqueforCommunicationASituationalBriefingModel.aspx*.
37. Case Management Society of America: Definition of case management. Retrieved from *www.cmsa.org*.
38. American Nurses Association: Joint statement on delegation: American Nurses Association (ANA) and the National Council of State Boards of Nursing (NCSBN). Retrieved from *www.ncsbn.org/Joint_statement.pdf*.

RESOURCES

American Nurses Association
www.nursingworld.org

American Nursing Informatics Association
www.ania.org

Canadian Nurses Association
www.cna-nurses.ca

Center for Nursing Classification and Clinical Effectiveness
www.nursing.uiowa.edu/center-for-nursing-classification-and-clinical-effectiveness

Healthy People
www.healthypeople.gov

NANDA International
www.nanda.org

National Association of Hispanic Nurses
www.thehispanicnurses.org

National Black Nurses Association, Inc.
www.nbna.org

National Student Nurses' Association
www.nsna.org

QSEN (Quality and Safety Education for Nurses)
www.qsen.org

CHAPTER

2

Health Disparities and Culturally Competent Care

Janet Lenart

Injustice anywhere is a threat to justice everywhere.
Dr. Martin Luther King, Jr.

evolve WEBSITE

http://evolve.elsevier.com/Lewis/medsurg

- NCLEX Review Questions
- Key Points
- Pre-Test
- Answer Guidelines for Case Study on p. 33
- Rationales for Bridge to NCLEX Examination Questions
- Concept Map Creator
- Glossary
- Content Updates

eTables

- eTable 2-1: Ethnic Differences in Response to Drugs
- eTable 2-2: Cultural Assessment Guide

LEARNING OUTCOMES

1. Identify the key determinants of health and equity.
2. Describe the primary factors that contribute to health disparities and health equity.
3. Define the terms *culture, values, acculturation, ethnicity, race, stereotyping, ethnocentrism, cultural imposition, transcultural nursing, cultural competency, folk healer,* and *culture-bound syndrome.*
4. Explain how culture and ethnicity may affect a person's physical and psychologic health.
5. Describe strategies for successfully communicating with a person who speaks a language that you do not understand.
6. Apply strategies for incorporating cultural information in the nursing process when providing care for patients from different cultural and ethnic groups.
7. Describe the role of nursing in reducing health disparities.
8. Examine ways that your own cultural background may influence nursing care when working with patients from different cultural and ethnic groups.

KEY TERMS

This chapter addresses health disparities and cultural issues. Nursing has a key role in recognizing and reducing health disparities and providing culturally competent care.

DETERMINANTS OF HEALTH

Why are there differences in the health status of people in America? How do these differences occur? The **determinants of health** are factors that (1) influence the health of individuals and groups (Fig. 2-1) and (2) help explain why some people experience poorer health than others.[1] Where people are born, grow up, live, work, and age helps determine their health status, behaviors, and care.

Health status describes the health of a person or a community. Many measures make up the concept of health status. For individuals, this means the sum of their current health problems plus their coping resources (e.g., family, financial resources). For a community, health status is the combination of health measures for all individuals living in the community. Community health measures include birth and death rates, life expectancy, access to care, and morbidity and mortality rates related to disease and injury.

Reviewed by Michelle M. Byrne, RN, PhD, CNE, CNOR, Professor of Nursing, North Georgia College & State University, Dahlonega, Georgia; Doreen Mingo, RN, MSN, Assistant Professor, Coordinator, Office of Diversity Services, Nursing Workforce Diversity Grant Project Director, Allen College, Waterloo, Illinois; and Kathleen M. Barta, RN, EdD, Associate Professor, University of Arkansas, Eleanor Mann School of Nursing, Fayetteville, Arkansas.

Factors in a person's social and physical environment, including personal relationships, workplace, housing, transportation, and neighborhood violence, all contribute to health status.[1] For example, the risk of youth homicide is much higher in neighborhoods with gang activity and high crime rates. The physical environment in which one lives, works, and plays may expose a person to such risks as environmental hazards (workplace injuries), toxic agents (chemical spills, industrial pollution), unsafe traffic patterns (lack of sidewalks), or absence of fresh and healthy food choices.

An individual's behavior is influenced by his or her environment, education, and economic status. Behaviors such as tobacco and illicit drug use are strongly linked to a number of health conditions (e.g., lung cancer, liver disease). An individual's biologic makeup such as genetics and family history of disease (e.g., heart disease) can increase the risk for specific diseases.

The amount and quality of health care available also contribute to an individual's health. For example, in some states, health care organizations have reduced the number of Medicaid patients they will cover. Although the use of emergency departments (EDs) for health care is increasing, they are not usually set up to provide primary or long-term follow-up care. In addition, the number of EDs, particularly in rural areas, is decreasing.[2] These determinants of health can either improve a person's health status or put an individual at risk for disease, injury, and mental illness.

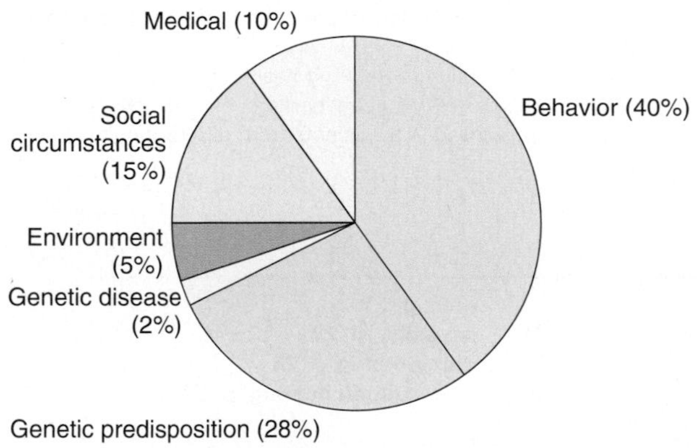

FIG. 2-1 Determinants of health.

HEALTHY PEOPLE

Access to Health Services

- Increase the proportion of people
  - With health insurance.
  - With a usual primary care provider.
  - Who receive appropriate evidence-based clinical preventive services.
- Increase the proportion of insured people with coverage for clinical preventive services.
- Ensure that all people have access to rapidly responding, prehospital emergency medical services.
- Reduce the proportion of individuals who are unable to obtain or delay in obtaining necessary medical care, dental care, or prescription medicines.
- Decrease the time people
  - Spend waiting in physicians' offices and emergency departments.
  - Wait between identifying a need for specific tests and treatments and actually receiving those services.

The vision of the government's *Healthy People 2020* is to create a society in which all people live long, healthy lives (see Table 1-1). This report (discussed in Chapter 1 on p. 5) includes measures that can be used to reflect the health status of the U.S. population.[3]

HEALTH DISPARITIES AND HEALTH EQUITY

Health disparities are differences in the incidence, prevalence, mortality rate, and burden of diseases that exist among specific population groups in the United States because of social, economic, or environmental disadvantages. Health disparities can affect population groups based on gender, age, ethnicity, socioeconomic status, geography, sexual orientation, disability, or special health care needs.[4,5] **Health equity** is achieved when every person has the opportunity to attain his or her health potential and no one is disadvantaged.

Factors and Conditions Leading to Health Disparities

Many factors and conditions can lead to the development of health disparities (Table 2-1). Awareness of these factors will assist you in providing optimal care for your patients.

ETHICAL/LEGAL DILEMMAS

Health Disparities

Situation

E.M., a 47-year-old Mexican American woman with type 2 diabetes mellitus, comes to the clinic to have her blood glucose measured. It has been 12 months since her last visit. At that time the nurse requested that she bring along her glucometer and strips to demonstrate how she checks her blood glucose because her glucose values were high at her previous visits.

When you check E.M.'s equipment and glucose strips, it is clear that the strips are for a different machine and they expired more than 2 years ago. When you inquire about the situation, E.M. explains that she cannot afford to come to the clinic or to buy new equipment and supplies to check her blood glucose level. During the day E.M. cares for her three grandchildren so her daughter can work. E.M. spends most of her income on food for her family, so little money is left over for her own health care.

Ethical/Legal Points for Consideration

- Ethnic minorities and other vulnerable or disadvantaged groups experience certain chronic illnesses at higher rates. Limited access to high-quality, accessible, and affordable health care services is clearly associated with an increased incidence of illness and complications, as well as a reduced life span.
- People with certain health problems such as diabetes may have difficulty obtaining health care insurance. These issues must be considered in the broader context of social justice.
- In many states the legal definition of the role of the professional nurse includes patient advocacy. Advocacy includes the obligation to provide adequate follow-up care for all patients, especially those who are experiencing health care disparities.
- When disparities are observed in an individual patient and family, as a nurse you must consider the possibilities of discrimination and abuse. Professional nurses are legally and ethically responsible for patient advocacy. When failure to fulfill this obligation results in harm to the patient, the nurse may incur legal liability.

Discussion Questions

1. How would you work with E.M. to help her obtain the necessary resources and knowledge to care for her diabetes?
2. What can you do to begin working on the problems of health disparities in your community?

TABLE 2-1 FACTORS AND CONDITIONS LEADING TO HEALTH DISPARITIES

• Ethnicity and race	• Age
• Place	• Sexual orientation
• Income status	• Disability status
• Education	• Health care provider attitudes
• Occupation or unemployment	• Lack of health care services access
• Health literacy	• Language barrier
• Gender	

Ethnicity and Race. The terms **ethnicity** and **race** are subjective and based on self-report. These terms are used interchangeably in conversation and cannot be defined by genetic markers. Social context and lived experiences influence people's decision about the ethnic and race category to which they belong. For example, ethnic and race categories may differ on a person's birth and death certificates.

People are asked to identify their own ethnicity and race for the purpose of health data collection (e.g., for birth and death certificates). Collection of health data based on self-reported ethnic and race categories is important for research, to inform policy, and to understand and eliminate disparities. For example, federal agencies are required to list a minimum of two ethnicities for people who self-identify as either *Hispanic or Latino* and *Not Hispanic or Latino.* A Hispanic or Latino is typically a person of Cuban, Mexican, Puerto Rican, South or Central American, or other Spanish descent, regardless of race.

In addition, federal agencies are required to list a minimum of five race categories: white, black or African American, American Indian or Alaska Native, Asian, and Native Hawaiian or other Pacific Islander.[6] People are asked to identify their race using one or more categories. In this book the terms *ethnicity* and *race* are used interchangeably or together.

Despite dramatic improvements in treatments to prolong life and improve quality of life for most individuals, racial and ethnic minorities have benefited far less from these advances. Disparities are generally determined by comparing population groups. Currently in the United States, based on the latest census, racial and ethnic minority groups include Hispanics/Latinos 16.3%, African Americans 12.6%, Asian Americans 4.8%, Native Hawaiians and other Pacific Islanders 0.2%, Native Americans and Native Alaskans 0.9%, and two or more races 2.9% of the U.S. population.[7] The percentages for most of these groups are expected to increase in the coming decades.

Obesity and chronic illness rates for diabetes, hypertension, chronic obstructive pulmonary diseases, cancer, and stroke are higher among minority people. Racial, ethnic, and cultural differences exist in health services, treatments provided, and access to health care providers. For example, African American men are less likely to be offered intervention procedures for cardiovascular disease and stroke.[8,9] African American and Hispanic women are less likely to have mammography for breast cancer screening.[6] Differences in access to screening and treatment exist even when minority groups are insured at the same level as whites. When patient groups are given the same care, the treatment outcomes are similar across racial and ethnic groups.[8,9]

Disease risk and outcomes are also influenced by race and ethnicity. For example, compared with U.S. white and African American populations, Native Americans have a higher incidence of stroke and are more likely to die as a consequence.[9]

CULTURAL & ETHNIC HEALTH DISPARITIES

Cultural & Ethnic Health Disparities Boxes Throughout Book

Breast and cervical cancer mortality rates are higher in Hispanic and African American women than in other American women.[10-12] African Americans are three times more likely to die from heart disease compared with whites. Fortunately, numerous strategies are underway to promote health equity and reduce disparities.

Place and Health. **Place** refers to the geographic and environmental location where a person is born, grows, lives, works, and ages. Place affects the use of health services, health status, and health behaviors.

Approximately 25% of Americans live in nonurban or rural areas.[7] Three percent of Americans live in designated frontier counties. Differences in access to health care services among frontier, rural, and urban settings can create geographic health disparities. For example, rural populations and Native Americans living on reservations may need to travel long distances to receive health care. This can result in inadequate or less frequent access to health care services. Some parts of the rural United States are considered "medically underserved" because of decreased numbers of health care providers per population.

People living in rural areas have higher rates of cancer, heart disease, diabetes, depression, and injury-related deaths than people living in urban areas. For example, in rural Appalachia the rates of lung, colon, cervical, and rectal cancer are higher than the national average.[13] Rural populations tend to be older than urban populations. Many rural areas have higher rates of obesity and chronic disease. Rural Americans are less likely to work for employers who provide health insurance.[12,13] As a group, rural populations have lower literacy rates and poorer health behaviors (e.g., increased smoking rates, increased substance abuse, higher rates of obesity, lower rates of physical activity). Generally, smaller and more isolated rural communities with low economic resources experience greater difficulties accessing high-quality health care.

Living in urban centers may also predispose a person to health disparities. Concerns about personal safety (e.g., clinics located in high-crime neighborhoods) can make patients reluctant to visit health care providers. At the same time, health care providers such as home health nurses working in high-risk areas may experience distress when they witness crime, drug use, or other illegal activities.[14] Among the most obvious health behaviors affected by place are physical activity and nutrition. Safe, walkable neighborhoods with playgrounds and sources of healthy foods promote physical activity and healthy eating. Social support and networks are related to health and coping with illness. Social networks are more likely to be found in communities where neighbors interact and rely on one another. Place may have more influence on the incidence of hypertension, diabetes, and obesity for women than race or ethnicity.[15]

Income, Education, and Occupation. People of lower income, education, or occupational status experience worse health. In addition, they die at a younger age than those who are more affluent. In fact, adults without a high school diploma or equivalent are three times more likely to die before age 65 than those with a college degree.[16] Health care costs are one of the important factors that contribute to health disparities. Individuals who have no insurance, are underinsured, or lack financial resources to pay for treatment of diseases may forgo health care visits and treatments (Fig. 2-2). Patients who lack the knowledge to apply for government assistance programs (e.g., Medicaid) are also at risk. The number of uninsured Americans has increased over the past decade.[17] Hazardous work environments and high-risk occupations of laborers also increase health risk and contribute to higher rates of illness, injury, and death.

Health literacy is defined as the degree to which individuals have the capacity to obtain, process, and understand basic health information and services needed to make appropriate health decisions. This includes the ability to read, comprehend, and analyze information; understand instructions; weigh risks and benefits; and ultimately make decisions and take action. Approximately 80 million Americans have limited healthy literacy.[16,18] Low health literacy is associated with more hospitalizations, greater use of emergency department care, decreased use of cancer screening and influenza vaccine, decreased ability to use medications correctly, and higher mortality rates among older adults. On a daily basis, patients need to self-manage conditions such as diabetes and asthma. For example, patients with diabetes may not be able to maintain adequate blood glucose levels if they cannot read or understand the numbers on the home glucose monitoring system. The inability to read and understand medication labels can result in taking medications at the wrong time or in the wrong dose. Health literacy is discussed further in Chapter 4.

Gender. Health disparities exist between men and women. Adult women use health care services more than men. At the same time, women are less likely than men to have medical insurance. Women may not receive the same quality of care (Fig. 2-3). For example, women are less likely than men to receive procedures (e.g., coronary angiography) for cardiovascular disease.[19] When gender is combined with racial and ethnic differences, the disparities are even greater. (Gender Differences boxes are presented throughout this book that highlight gender differences in disease risk, manifestations, and treatment.)

Age. Older adults are at risk for experiencing health disparities in the number of diagnostic tests performed and aggressiveness of treatments used. Biases toward older adults that affect their care, or *ageism,* are discussed in Chapter 5. Older women are less likely to be offered mammograms. Older people of low socioeconomic status experience greater disability, more limitations in activities of daily living, and more frequent and rapid cognitive decline.[20] Older adults who belong to minority groups are less likely than their white counterparts to receive screening for prostate and colorectal cancer.[21]

Sexual Orientation. Sexuality is defined as a person's romantic, emotional, or sexual attraction to another person. Gay, lesbian, and bisexual orientation places an individual at risk for health disparities due to their social, economic, or environmental disadvantages. With the repeal of the military's "don't ask, don't tell" legislation in 2010, the focus on the rights and specific health care needs of lesbian, gay, bisexual, and transgender (LGBT) individuals has increased.

Lesbian women are more likely to be obese when compared with their heterosexual counterparts. Lesbian and bisexual

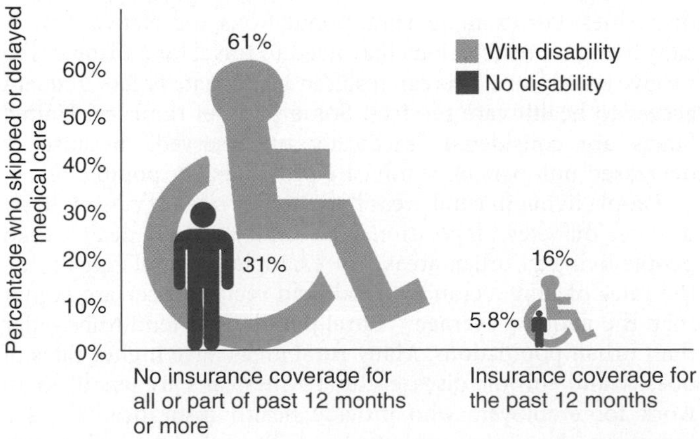

FIG. 2-2 Percentage of adults ages 18 to 64 years old who skipped or delayed medical care because of cost. The data are displayed by disability and insurance coverage status.

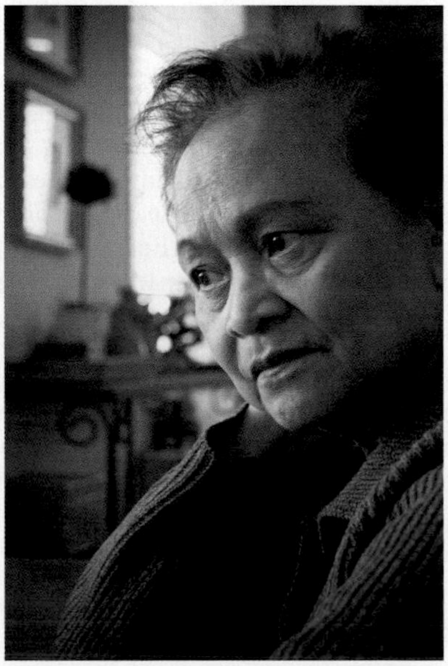

FIG. 2-3 Older Asian women are especially at risk for health disparities. (iStockphoto/Thinkstock)

women have increased risk factors for cardiovascular disease.[22] Gay men have higher rates of human immunodeficiency virus and hepatitis infections than other groups. Gay men and lesbian women have higher smoking rates than heterosexuals.

Understanding the cause of these disparities among LGBT individuals is essential to providing safe and high-quality care. One of the barriers to accessing high-quality health care by LGBT adults is the current lack of providers who are knowledgeable about their health needs. LGBT patients may also experience fear of discrimination in health care settings.[23] Within many, but not all, health care settings, LGBT health care issues are now more visible. The Joint Commission requires that patients be allowed the presence of the support individual of their choice. In addition, hospitals need to adopt policies that bar discrimination based on factors such as sexual orientation and gender identification and expression. *Healthy People 2020* has added an objective on LGBT health *(www.healthypeople.gov/2020/topicsobjectives2020/overview.aspx?topicid=25)*.

Health Care Provider Attitudes. Certain behaviors and biases of the health care provider can contribute to health disparities. Factors such as bias and prejudice can affect health care–seeking behavior in minority populations.[24] The health care system itself may also contribute to the problem of health disparities. For example, a clinic located in an area with a large Vietnamese immigrant population that does not provide translators or educational materials and financial forms in Vietnamese may limit these families' ability to understand how to access health care.

Discrimination and *bias* based on a patient's race, ethnicity, gender, age, sexual orientation, or ability to pay are likely to result in less aggressive or negative treatment practices. Sometimes discrimination is difficult to identify, especially when it occurs at the institutional level. Because a health care provider's overt discriminatory behavior may not be immediately evident to the patient or yourself, it may be difficult to confront. Even well-intentioned providers who try to eliminate bias in their care can demonstrate their prior beliefs or prejudices through nonverbal communication. Many policies are in place to eliminate discrimination, but it still exists.[25]

CULTURE

Culture is a way of life for a group of people. It includes the behaviors, beliefs, values, traditions, and symbols that the group accepts, generally without thinking about them. This way of life is passed along by communication and imitation from one generation to the next. You can also think of culture as cultivated behavior that is acquired through social learning. It is the totality of a person's learned, accumulated experience that is socially transmitted. The four classic characteristics of culture are described in Table 2-2.

Values are the sets of rules by which individuals, families, groups, and communities live. They are the principles and standards that serve as the basis for beliefs, attitudes, and behaviors. Although all cultures have values, the types and expressions of those values differ from one culture to another. These cultural values develop over time, guide decision making and actions, and may affect a person's self-esteem. Cultural values are often unconsciously developed early in life as a child learns about acceptable and unacceptable behaviors. The extent to which a person's cultural values are internalized influences that person's tendency toward judging other cultures, while usually using his or her own culture as the accepted standard. Table 2-3 provides some examples of cultural characteristics of different ethnic groups in the United States.

Although individuals within a cultural group have many similarities through their shared values, beliefs, and practices, there is also diversity within groups (Fig. 2-4). Each person is culturally unique. Such diversity may result from different perspectives and interpretations of situations. These differences may be based on age, gender, marital status, family structure, income, education level, religious views, and life experiences. Within any cultural group, there are smaller groups that may not hold all of the values of the dominant culture. These smaller cultural groups have experiences that differ from those of the dominant group. These differences may be related to ethnic background, residence, religion, occupation, health, age, gender,

TABLE 2-2 BASIC CHARACTERISTICS OF CULTURE

- *Dynamic* and ever-changing
- *Not always shared* by all members of a cultural group
- *Adapted* to specific conditions such as environmental factors
- *Learned* through oral and written histories, as well as socialization

TABLE 2-3 DISTINCT CULTURAL CHARACTERISTICS OF DIFFERENT ETHNIC GROUPS IN THE UNITED STATES

Native American
- Folk healing
- Living in harmony with people and nature
- Respect for all things living
- Returning what is taken from nature
- Doing the honorable thing
- Respect for tribal elders and children
- Spiritual guidance

Hispanic/Latino
- Cultural foods
- Folk healing
- Extended family valued
- Involvement of family in social activities
- Religion and spirituality highly valued
- Respect for elders and authority
- Interdependence and collectivism

African American
- Cultural foods
- Family networks
- Folk healing
- Importance of religion
- Interdependence within ethnic group
- Music and physical activities valued

European American
- Individualistic and competitive
- Equal rights of genders
- Independence and freedom
- Materialistic
- Self-reliance valued
- Technology dependent
- Youth and beauty valued

Asian American
- Cultural foods
- Folk healing
- Respect for one's parents and ancestors
- Family loyalty
- Respect for elders
- Harmonious relationships
- Harmony and balance within body vital for preservation of life energy

Pacific Islander American
- Kinship alliance among nuclear and extended family
- Natural order and balanced relationships
- Collective concern and involvement
- Knowledge is collective; belongs to group, not individual

Adapted from Andrews MM, Boyle JS: *Transcultural concepts in nursing care,* ed 5, Philadelphia, 2008, Wolters Kluwer-Lippincott Williams & Wilkins; and Giger JN, Davidhizar RE: *Transcultural nursing: assessment and intervention,* ed 6, St Louis, 2012, Mosby.

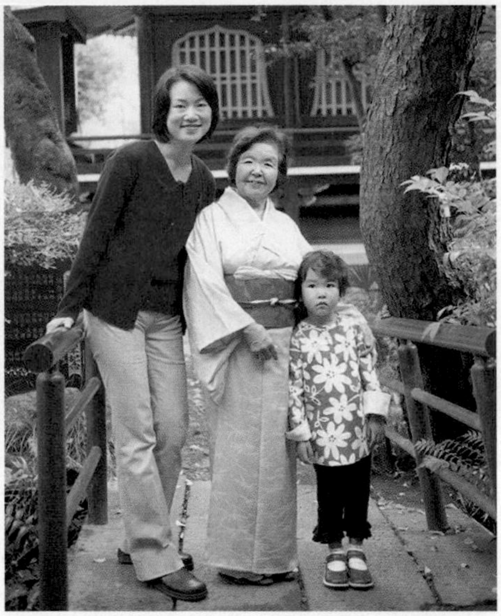

FIG. 2-4 Members of this family share a common heritage. (Jupiterimages/Photos.com/Thinkstock)

education, or other factors that unite the group. Members of a subculture share certain aspects of culture that are different from those of the overall cultural group. For example, among Hispanics, some seek professional health care immediately when symptoms appear, other Hispanics rely first on folk healers, and yet other Hispanics first seek the opinion of family and friends before seeking formal health care.

Cultural beliefs about symptom tolerance and health care–seeking behavior can contribute to health disparities. Some cultures consider pain something to be endured or ignored, and as a result, the patient does not seek help. Some cultures may view diseases or problems fatalistically; that is, people see no reason to seek treatment because they believe it is unlikely to have any benefit. Some cultures view the signs and symptoms of an illness as "God's will" or as a punishment for some prior behavior.[26]

Fatalism is higher in individuals with lower socioeconomic status. Fatalistic beliefs are associated with reduced cancer prevention activities such as exercising, not smoking, and following a healthy diet.[27] In some cultures it may not be acceptable to see a health care provider who is not of the same gender or ethnic group. Such beliefs can result in delays in seeking health care or inadequate treatment.

Acculturation is the life-long process of incorporating cultural aspects of the contexts in which a person grows, lives, works, and ages.[28,29] Acculturation is often bidirectional. In other words, the context also changes as it is influenced by a person's culture. Change may be in attitudes, behaviors, and values. For example, a sedentary person who loves to cook may change his or her attitude toward exercise when living with athletic roommates, who in turn also change as they begin to appreciate cooking. Behaviors change when an immigrant child learns the local language while also influencing the conduct of classmates. Lastly, a deeply held value such as self-sufficiency may change for a person exposed to a culture where reliance on others dominates.

Newcomers may adopt both the strengths and the limitations of the dominant culture. This is relevant when considering health behaviors of individuals and the quality of health care delivered by professionals. For example, an immigrant may be negatively influenced by a dominant cultural context in which unhealthy eating habits prevail. As a new nurse, you may be negatively or positively influenced by the culture of care that is most prevalent in the workplace.[30]

The result of acculturation for the individual may be new cultural variations in attitudes, behaviors, and values. All people participate in this process over their lives. People who move to a new cultural context are more aware of the acculturation experience than people who are not exposed to new experiences. Exposure to new cultural contexts increases the cultural competency of nurses.

Stereotyping refers to an over-generalized viewpoint that members of a specific culture, race, or ethnic group are alike and share the same values and beliefs. This oversimplified approach does not take into account the individual differences that exist within a culture. Being a member of a particular cultural, ethnic, or racial group does not make the person an expert on other members of that same group. Such stereotyping can lead to false assumptions and affect a patient's care. For example, it would be inappropriate for you to assume that just because a nurse is Mexican American, he would know how a Mexican American patient's beliefs might affect that patient's health care practices. A young nurse born and raised in a large city has experienced a different culture than the older patient who was born and raised in a rural area of Mexico.

Ethnocentrism refers to the belief that one's own culture and worldview are superior to those of others from different cultural, ethnic, or racial backgrounds.[31] Comparing others' ways to your own can lead to seeing others as different or inferior. Health care providers' ethnocentrism can result in poor communication, patient alienation, and potentially inadequate treatment. To avoid ethnocentrism, you need to remain open to a variety of perspectives and maintain a nonjudgmental view of the values, beliefs, and practices of others. Failure to do this can result in ethnic stereotyping or cultural imposition.

Cultural imposition occurs when one's own cultural beliefs and practices are imposed on another person or group of people. In health care it can result in disregarding or trivializing a patient's health care beliefs or practices. Cultural imposition may happen when a health care provider is unaware of the patient's cultural beliefs and plans and implements care without taking them into account.

Cultural safety describes care and advocacy that prevent cultural imposition. Culturally safe practice requires cultural competency and action to ensure that cultural histories, experiences, and traditions of patients, their families, and communities are valued and shape health care approaches and policies.[29,31]

The term **transcultural nursing** was coined by Madeleine Leininger in the 1950s. Transcultural nursing is a specialty that focuses on the comparative study and analysis of cultures and subcultures. The goal of transcultural nursing is the discovery of culturally relevant facts that can guide the nurse in providing culturally appropriate care.[31]

CULTURAL COMPETENCE

Cultural competence is the ability to understand, appreciate, and work with individuals from cultures other than your own. It involves an awareness and acceptance of cultural differences, self-awareness, knowledge of the patient's culture, and adaptation of skills to meet the patient's needs. The four components of cultural competence are (1) cultural awareness, (2) cultural knowledge, (3) cultural skill, and (4) cultural encounter[31] (Table 2-4).

Specific information is presented throughout this book to assist you in developing an awareness of cultural differences and learning assessment skills for different cultural groups. Table 2-7 (later in this chapter) presents a cultural assessment guide. Review cultural characteristics associated with a group when preparing to interview a patient. However, it is essential to seek information from patients about their culture because they may not exhibit the typical cultural characteristics.

Providing culturally competent care increases patient satisfaction, reduces health disparities, increases patient safety, and prevents misunderstandings between you and your patients. It also involves integrating cultural practices into Western medicine. For example, before some diagnostic procedures and interventions, it is typical to have patients remove personal objects that are worn on the body. Ask patients whether they wear personal objects and the significance of their removal, since they may have cultural or spiritual significance. You also need to know whether wearing these objects will compromise patient safety, test results, or outcomes of the intervention.

TABLE 2-4 HOW TO DEVELOP CULTURAL COMPETENCE

Description	Role of Nurse
Cultural Awareness	
• Ability to understand patients' unique cultural needs	• Identify your own cultural background, values, and beliefs, especially as related to health and health care. • Examine your own cultural biases toward people whose cultures differ from your own culture.
Cultural Knowledge	
• Process of learning key aspects of a group's culture, especially as it relates to health and health care practices • Patients as the best source of information about their culture	• Learn basic general information about predominant cultural groups in your geographic area. Cultural pocket guides can be a good resource. • Assess patients for presence or absence of cultural traits based on an understanding of generalizations about a cultural group. • Do not make assumptions based on cultural background because the degree of acculturation varies among individuals. • Read research studies that describe cultural differences. • Read ethnic newspaper articles and books. • View documentaries about cultural groups.
Cultural Skill	
• Ability to collect relevant cultural data • Performance of a cultural assessment	• Be alert for unexpected responses with patients, especially as related to cultural issues. • Become aware of cultural differences in predominant ethnic groups. • Develop assessment skills to do a competent cultural assessment for any patient.* • Learn assessment skills for different cultural groups, including cultural beliefs and practices.
Cultural Encounter	
• Direct cross-cultural interactions between people from culturally diverse backgrounds • Extended contact with a cultural group to enhance understanding of its values and beliefs	• Create opportunities to interact with predominant cultural groups. • Attend cultural events, such as religious ceremonies, significant life passage rituals, social events, and demonstrations of cultural practices. • Visit markets and restaurants in ethnic neighborhoods. • Explore ethnic neighborhoods, listen to different types of ethnic music, and learn games of various ethnic groups. • Visit or volunteer at health fairs in local ethnic neighborhoods. • Learn about prominent cultural beliefs and practices, and incorporate this knowledge into planning nursing care.

*See Table 2-7 later in the chapter.

CULTURAL DIVERSITY IN THE HEALTH CARE WORKPLACE

Poorer health outcomes for minorities are linked to the shortage of culturally and ethnically diverse health care providers, who have historically been underrepresented in the health professions.[32] A diversity gap exists between the ethnic composition of the health care workforce and the overall population in the United States (Fig. 2-5). The diversity of nurses in the United States is increasing but still lags behind that of the population. African Americans, Hispanic/Latino Americans, and Native Americans make up more than 27% of the population but only 17% of the nation's nurses.

Cultural differences exist in how well patients believe they can communicate with their health care provider. Communication issues include not understanding the health care provider, feeling that they are not listened to, and having questions but not asking them. In the United States approximately 25% to 33% of minority patients have difficulty communicating with their health care provider, compared with 16% of white patients. Similarly, minority patients are less likely than whites to have a regular health care provider. African Americans are more likely to receive outpatient care in the emergency department (ED) and have fewer physician visits.[33]

When health care providers from different cultures work together as members of the health care team, opportunities for miscommunication and conflict can occur. This is termed *cultural conflict.* The cultural origins of miscommunication and

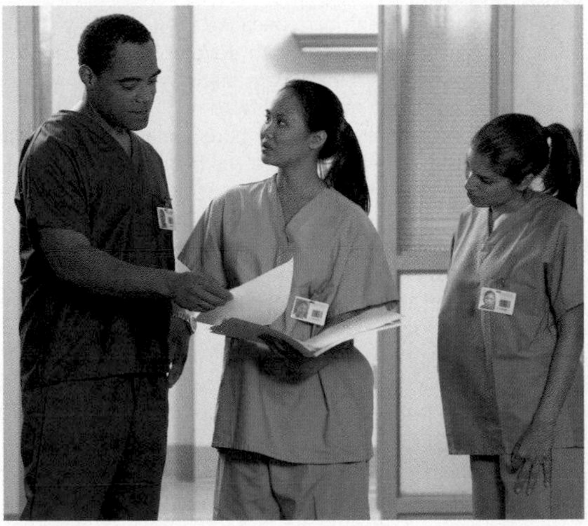

FIG. 2-5 Nurses working together in a multicultural health care environment. (Fuse/Thinkstock)

conflict in the workplace are often interconnected with cultural beliefs, values, and etiquette. Seeking clarification about misperceptions and misunderstandings is a communication strategy to foster effective teamwork among a multicultural health care team. To ensure the recruitment and retention of nurses from minority populations, all members of the health care team and leadership must create an environment that promotes effective cross-cultural communication and reduces bias and discrimination.

CULTURAL FACTORS AFFECTING HEALTH AND HEALTH CARE

Many cultural factors affect the patient's health and health care. Several potential factors are presented in Table 2-5.

Folk Healers

Many cultures have **folk healers,** who are also known as *traditional healers.* Most folk healers speak the person's native language and cost less than conventional health care providers. Among the many folk healers found worldwide, Hispanics may turn to a *curandero* (or *curandera*), African Americans may visit a *hougan,* Native Americans may seek help from a medicine man or *shaman,* and Asian Americans may use the services of a Chinese herbal therapist. In addition to folk healers, some cultures involve lay midwives (e.g., *parteras* for Hispanic women) in the care of pregnant women.

Folk medicine is a form of prevention and treatment that is culturally based and traditionally relies on oral transmission of healing techniques from one generation to the next. The patient may not use the term *folk medicine* but thinks of these as cultural home remedies or treatment practices. Folk medicine may be practiced in the home without the guidance of a folk healer. It is important to assess whether the patient is practicing traditional or folk healing.

Spirituality and Religion

Spirituality and religion are aspects of culture that may affect a person's beliefs about health, illness, and end-of-life care. They may also play a role in nutrition and decisions related to health, wellness, and how to respond to or treat an illness.

Spirituality refers to a person's effort to find purpose and meaning in life. It is influenced by a person's unique life experiences and reflects one's personal understanding of life's mysteries. Spirituality relates to the soul or spirit more than to the body, and it may provide hope and strength for an individual during an illness.

Religion is a more formal and organized system of beliefs, including belief in or worship of God or gods. Religious beliefs include the cause, nature, and purpose of the universe and involve prayer and rituals. Religion is based on beliefs about life, death, good, and evil. You can use several interventions to meet a patient's religious and spiritual needs, including prayer, scripture reading, listening, and referral to a chaplain, rabbi, or priest.[34]

Many patients find that rituals help them during times of illness. Rituals help a person make sense of life experiences and may take the form of prayer, meditation, or other rituals that the patient may create. With appropriate training, you may

TABLE 2-5 CULTURAL FACTORS AFFECTING HEALTH AND HEALTH CARE

Time Orientation
- For some cultures it is more important to attend to a social role than to arrive on time for an appointment with a health care provider.
- Some cultures are future oriented; others are past or present oriented.

Language and Communication
- Patients may not speak English and may not be able to communicate with the health care provider.
- Even with interpreters, communication may be difficult.

Economic Factors
- Patients may not get health care because they cannot pay for it or because of the costs associated with travel for health care.
- Refugee or undocumented immigrant status may deter some patients from using the health care system.
- Immigrant women who are heads of households or single mothers may not seek health care for themselves because of child care costs.
- Patients may lack health insurance.

Health Care System
- Patients may not make or keep appointments because of the time lag between the onset of an illness and an available appointment.
- Hours of operation of health care facilities may not accommodate patients' need to work or use public transportation.
- Requirements to access some types of care may discourage some patients from taking the steps to qualify for health care or health care payment assistance.
- Some patients have a general distrust of health care professionals and health care systems.
- Lack of ethnic-specific health care programs may deter some individuals from seeking health care.
- Transportation may be a problem for patients who have to travel long distances for health care.
- Adequate interpreter services may be unavailable.
- Patients may not have a primary health care provider and may use emergency departments or urgent care centers for health care.
- Shortages of health care providers from specific ethnic groups may deter some people from seeking health care.
- Patients may lack knowledge about the availability of existing health care resources.
- Facility policies may not be culturally competent (e.g., hospital policy may limit the number of visitors, which is problematic for cultures that value having many family members present).

Beliefs and Practices
- Care provided in established health care programs may not be perceived as culturally relevant.
- Religious reasons, beliefs, or practices may affect a person's decision to seek (or not seek) health care.
- Patients may delay seeking health care because of fear or dependence on folk medicine and herbal remedies.
- Patients may stop treatment or discontinue visits for health care because the symptoms are no longer present, and they believe that further care is not required.
- Some patients associate hospitals and extended care facilities with death.
- The patient may have had a previous negative experience with culturally incompetent health care providers or discriminatory practices.
- Some people mistrust the majority population and institutions dominated by them.
- Some patients may feel apprehensive about unfamiliar diagnostic procedures and treatment options.

include spiritual questions in the complete assessment of the patient and plan care based accordingly. (Table 10-5 has a spiritual assessment guide that may be used with patients.) Table 2-6 summarizes health-related beliefs and practices of selected religious groups.

Cross-Cultural Communication

Communication refers to an organized, patterned system of behavior that may be verbal or nonverbal (Fig. 2-6). *Verbal communication* includes not only one's language or dialect, but also voice tone, volume, timing, and ability to share thoughts and feelings. More than 45 million people in the United States speak a language other than English in their home, with Spanish being the most common. Hispanics who do not speak English at home are less likely to receive a variety of health care services regardless of whether they are comfortable speaking English.[35]

Nonverbal communication may take the form of writing, gestures, body movements, posture, and facial expressions. Nonverbal communication also includes eye contact, use of touch, body language, style of greeting, and spatial distancing. Eye

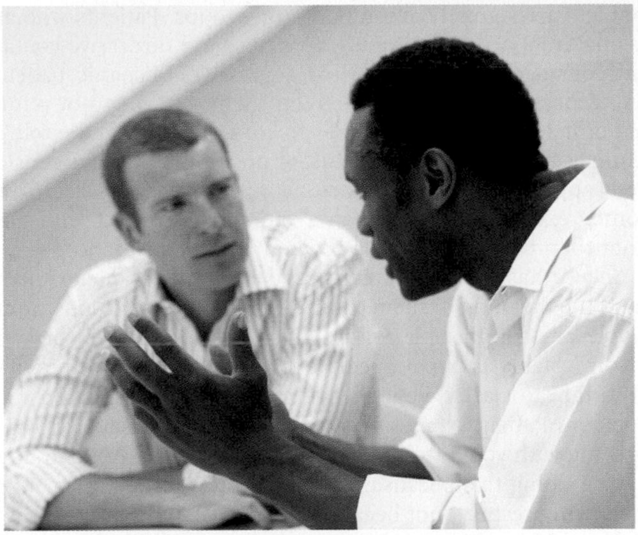

FIG. 2-6 Co-workers from different cultures communicate with verbal and nonverbal cues. (BananaStock/Thinkstock)

TABLE 2-6 HEALTH-RELATED BELIEFS AND PRACTICES OF SELECTED RELIGIOUS GROUPS

Amish
- Alcoholic beverages and drugs are prohibited unless prescribed by health care professional.
- Abortion, artificial insemination, and stem cell use are prohibited.
- Amish seldom purchase commercial health insurance.

Catholicism
- Many fast and abstain from meat and meat products on Ash Wednesday and the Fridays of Lent.
- Artificial contraception and direct abortion are prohibited. Indirect abortion (e.g., treatment of uterine cancer in a pregnant woman) may be morally justified.
- Sacrament of the Sick includes anointing of sick with oil, blessing by a priest, and communion (unleavened wafer made of flour and water).

Church of Jesus Christ of Latter-Day Saints (Mormons)
- Strict dietary code called Word of Wisdom prohibits all alcoholic beverages, hot drinks (nonherbal teas and coffee), tobacco, and illegal or recreational drugs.
- Fasting for 24-hour period occurs monthly on "Fast Sunday."
- During hospitalization or serious illness, an elder anoints the ill person with oil while a second elder seals the anointing with a prayer and blessing (laying on of hands).
- Abortion is prohibited except when the mother's life is in danger.

Hinduism
- Eating meat is prohibited because it involves harming a living creature.
- Cremation is most common form of body disposal, but fetuses or newborns are sometimes buried.

Islam
- Fasting during daytime hours occurs during a month-long period called Ramadan.
- Ritual cleansing with water before eating and before prayer is practiced.
- Eating pork or taking medicines with pork derivatives is prohibited.
- Drinking alcoholic beverages is prohibited.
- Artificial insemination is permissible only if from the husband to his own wife.

Jehovah's Witness
- Transfusions of blood in any form or agents in which blood is an ingredient are not acceptable. Blood volume expanders are acceptable if they are not derivatives of blood.
- Transplants that involve bodily mutilation are prohibited.
- Therapeutic and on-demand abortions are prohibited.
- Artificial insemination is prohibited for both donors and recipients.

Judaism
- Strictly observant Jews never eat pork, shellfish, or predatory fowl and never mix milk dishes and meat dishes in preparing foods. Fish with fins and scales are permissible.
- Certain foods and drink are designated as kosher, which means "proper." All animals must be ritually slaughtered.
- On the eighth day after birth, boys are circumcised in a ritual called Brit Milah, and girls are given a dedication ceremony involving prayers and blessings.
- Abortion is morally unacceptable except when the mother's life is in danger.
- Organized support system for the sick includes a visit from the rabbi. The rabbi may pray with the sick person alone or in a minyan, a group of 10 adults over age 13.
- If an autopsy is performed, all body parts must be returned for burial.

Seventh-Day Adventism
- Vegetarian diet encouraged.
- Nonvegetarian members refrain from eating foods derived from any animal having a cloven hoof that chews its cud (e.g., pigs, goats). Eating fish with fins and scales is acceptable, but consuming shellfish is prohibited.
- Consumption of alcoholic beverages is prohibited.
- Fasting is practiced and involves abstaining from food or liquids by healthy members of the church.

Buddhism*
- Consumption of alcoholic beverages and illicit drugs is prohibited.
- Moderation in diet and avoidance of extremes are practiced.
- Central tenets are maintaining right views, intentions, speech, actions, livelihood, effort, mindfulness, and concentration.

*Data from Andrews MM: Religion, culture, and nursing. In MM Andrews, JS Boyle, editors: *Transcultural concepts in nursing care,* ed 6, Philadelphia, 2012, Lippincott Williams & Wilkins.

contact varies greatly among cultural groups. Patients who are Asian, Arab, or Native American may avoid direct eye contact and consider it disrespectful or aggressive. Hispanic patients may expect you to look directly at them, but may not return that direct gaze. Other variables to consider include the role of gender, age, acculturation, status, or position on what is considered appropriate eye contact. For example, Muslim-Arab women exhibit modesty when avoiding eye contact with men other than their husbands and when in public situations.

Silence has many meanings, and it is important to understand the meaning of silence for different cultural groups. Some people are comfortable with silence, whereas others become uncomfortable and may speak to decrease the silent times. It is important to clarify what silence means in an interaction with a patient. Patients sometimes nod their head or say "yes" as if agreeing with you or to indicate they understand. Actually, they may be doing this because it is a culturally acceptable manner of showing respect, not because they understand or agree.

Many Native Americans are comfortable with silence and interpret silence as essential for thinking and carefully considering a response. In these interactions, silence shows respect for the other person and demonstrates the importance of the remarks. In traditional Japanese and Chinese cultures, the speaker may stop talking and leave a period of silence for the listener to think about what has been said before continuing. Silence may be intended to show respect for the speaker's privacy, whereas in some cultures (e.g., French, Spanish, Russian) the person may interpret silence as meaning agreement. Asian Americans may use silence to demonstrate respect for elders, whereas African Americans may use silence as a response to what is perceived to be an inappropriate question.

Family Roles and Relationships

Family roles differ from one culture to another (Fig. 2-7). It is important for you to determine who should be involved in communication and decision making related to health care. Some cultural groups emphasize interdependence rather than independence. In the United States many in the mainstream culture have strong beliefs related to autonomy. An individual is expected to sign consent forms when receiving health care. In other cultural groups a family member may be expected to make health care decisions. When you encounter a family that values interdependence over independence, the health care system may have difficulty adapting to how decisions are made. Treatment may need to be delayed while the patient waits for significant family members to arrive before giving consent for a procedure or treatment. In other instances the patient may make a decision that is best for the family despite adverse outcomes for the patient. Being aware of such values will better prepare you to advocate for the patient.

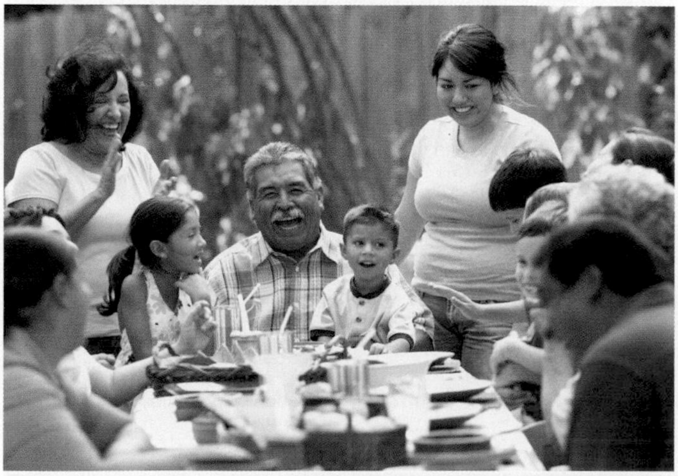

FIG. 2-7 Family roles and relationships differ from one culture to another. (Jack Hollingsworth/Photodisc/Thinkstock)

Some cultural differences relate to expectations of family members in providing care. In some cultures, family members expect to provide care for the patient even in the hospital. The patient may expect that the family, along with the health care providers, will provide all care. This view is the opposite of the predominant Western expectation that the patient will assume self-care as quickly as possible.

Ask about culturally relevant gender relationships. For example, in some cultures, such as many Arab groups, it is not appropriate for a man to be alone with a woman other than his wife. Nor is it appropriate for a woman other than a man's wife to provide physical care for him. The clinical implication of this cultural belief is that for many patients from Arab cultures, nurses cannot provide direct physical care for patients of the opposite gender. In some instances, procedures or treatments may be carried out for patients from the opposite gender but only if a third party is present.

Personal Space

Personal space zones refer to the preferred distances between two individuals. Personal space distances vary from culture to culture, as well as within a culture. For European Americans in the United States, the *intimate distance* ranges from 0 to 18 inches, and the *personal distance* ranges from 18 inches to 4 feet. The personal distance is the one experienced with friends. Social distance ranges from 4 to 12 feet, and public distance is 12 feet or more.[36] As a nurse, you often interact with patients in the intimate or personal zones, which might be uncomfortable for the patient.

Cultural groups have wide variations in their perception of appropriate distances. Whereas an American nurse of European descent may be comfortable with a certain distance, a person from a Hispanic or Middle Eastern background may believe that the distance is too far and will move closer, perhaps causing you to feel uncomfortable. If you then move away to a more comfortable distance, this may cause the other person to think that you are unfriendly, or the person may be offended. Personal space distance also varies within cultures.

Touch

Physical contact with patients conveys various meanings depending on the culture. To do a comprehensive assessment, touching a patient is necessary. Many people of Asian and Hispanic heritage believe that touching a person's head is a sign of disrespect, especially because the head is believed to be the source of one's strength and/or soul. Numerous people in the world believe in the evil eye, or *mal ojo.* In one culture-bound syndrome the illness, usually in a child or a woman, is believed to result from excessive admiration by another person. In some cultures the proper way to ward off the evil eye is to touch the area of admiration. For example, if the person admires the hair, the top of the head may be touched. It is important for you to ask permission before touching anyone, particularly if it is necessary to touch the person's head.

Nutrition

An important part of cultural practices is food, including both the foods that are eaten and rituals and practices associated with food. Muslims fast during the daytime during the Islamic month of Ramadan. Such practices may affect when and how medications are taken. Patients may be asked to make major changes in their diets because of health problems, or alternatively food may be used to cope with life changes such as homesickness. Specific foods may be considered essential to good health during pregnancy or other life stages. It is important that the health care provider take into account food-related cultural beliefs, practices, and habits when discussing nutrition with patients and planning their diets.

When individuals and families immigrate to an area that is very different from their country of origin, they may experience unfamiliar foods, food-storage systems, and food-buying habits. They also may come from countries that have limited food supplies because of poverty, wars, and poor sanitation. They may arrive with conditions such as general poor nutrition, hypertension, diarrhea, and dental caries. Other problems may develop after the person arrives in the new country. For example, second-generation Hispanic immigrants have a greater chance of becoming overweight than their first-generation counterparts. The increase in weight is related to the degree of acculturation experienced by the immigrant.[37]

Immigrants and Immigration

Migration is driven by a number of conditions, such as overcrowding, natural disasters, geopolitical conflict, persecution, and economic forces. Because of these migrations, a rich diversity of cultures exists in many communities and countries today (Fig. 2-8).

Recent immigrants may be at risk for physical and mental health problems for many reasons. Conditions in their countries of origin (e.g., malnutrition, poor sanitation, civil war) may have resulted in chronic health problems. In addition, recent immigrants are at increased risk for health problems after arriving in a new area. Relocation is associated with many losses and can cause economic hardship, physical stress, and mental distress.

As new immigrants go through the acculturation process, many experience cultural stress as they adjust to their new environment, especially if they have left relatives behind or are unable to return to their home country. Older immigrants are especially affected by changes in role and social position. This may result in depression. Posttraumatic stress disorder is seen in immigrants who have survived wars and violence. Immigrants may face barriers to social acceptance, such as prejudice or discrimination, and experience a lack of ethnic and cultural resources. For some, it may mean loss of the social status that they experienced in their countries of origin.

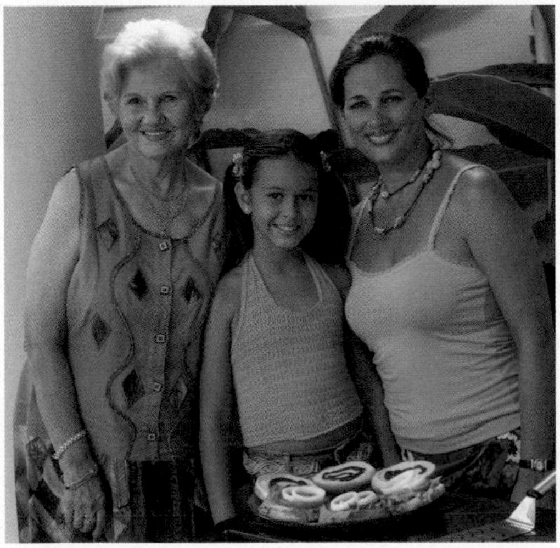

FIG. 2-8 Recently arrived immigrants join a neighbor for a barbecue, a common American tradition. (Jack Hollingsworth/Photodisc/Thinkstock)

Another potential problem is tuberculosis (TB). More than half of the TB cases in the United States occur in individuals born outside the country. Individuals who have recently immigrated from areas that have a high endemic rate of TB are more likely to have TB.[38] Foreign-born Hispanics and Asians combined account for 48% of the nation's TB cases. The top five countries of origin of foreign-born people with TB were Mexico, Philippines, Vietnam, India, and China. The *Refugee Health Guidelines* from the Centers for Disease Control and Prevention supports early identification and treatment.[39]

During the past 40 years, the migration pattern of North America has shifted. Whereas once most immigrants came from Europe, now most immigrants originate from Asia, Latin America, and Africa. Additionally, an increased number of first- and second-generation immigrants enter the United States after visiting friends and relatives. These individuals have a higher risk for malaria, typhoid fever, cholera, and hepatitis A than native-born Americans. Many immigrants lack health insurance and may primarily obtain their health care in emergency departments and urgent care clinics. Therefore nurses in all settings need to be aware of refugee health screening, treatment recommendations, and resources for access to health care.

Medications

Genetic differences among people from diverse ethnic or racial groups may explain differences in medication selection, dosage, or administration. For example, some medicines are more effective in certain ethnic groups than others. Side effects may vary among individuals from diverse backgrounds. eTable 2-1 on the website for this chapter highlights some ethnic differences in reaction to medications.

Genetic variations can affect how the body processes a drug and the overall effect of selected drugs on the body. Although race and ethnicity are imprecise indicators of genetic differences, they can be helpful in anticipating variations in the response to medications. (Genetics and drug metabolism are discussed in Chapter 13.)

Regardless of their cultural origins, many people use both cultural remedies and prescription drugs to treat their illnesses. Problems can result from interactions of these substances. For example, Chinese Americans who take ginseng as a stimulant and an antihypertensive drug may suffer adverse effects. Some Mexican Americans may treat gastrointestinal problems with preparations that contain lead. Individuals may self-treat their depression with St. John's wort, which can result in adverse effects if prescription antidepressants are also taken.

Patients may avoid standard Western medicine until herbal and other remedies become ineffective or the illness becomes acute. The challenge for you is to try to accommodate the patient's desire for traditional aspects of care while also using evidence-based approaches as appropriate and as acceptable to the patient. Evaluate the safety and appropriateness of the patient's traditional cultural healing therapies.

Develop a collaborative, trusting relationship with patients and encourage them to discuss their traditional approaches to healing. Seek out information on potential drug and herbal product interaction from the pharmacist. Honor the patient's choices, if safe and effective, since this will enhance collaboration and may have a positive impact on health outcomes.

Psychologic Factors

Symptoms are interpreted through a person's cultural norms and may vary from the recognized interpretations of Western medicine. All symptoms have meaning, and the meanings may vary from one culture to another. It is important to ask patients what their illness means to them, what they believe is the cause, and what they think is the best treatment (Table 2-7).

Culture-bound syndromes are illnesses or afflictions that are recognized only within a cultural group (Table 2-8). The symptoms, course of the illness, and people's reactions to the illness are limited to specific cultures. Culture-bound syndromes are expressed through psychologic or physical symptoms.

TABLE 2-7 CULTURAL ASSESSMENT*

A cultural assessment should include the following:

- Brief history of the cultural group with which person identifies
- Values orientation
- Cultural sanctions and restrictions
- Communication
- Health-related beliefs and practices
- Nutrition
- Socioeconomic considerations
- Organizations providing cultural support
- Educational background
- Religious affiliation
- Spiritual considerations

Adapted from Jarvis C: *Physical examination and health assessment*, ed 6, Philadelphia, 2012, Saunders.
*A comprehensive cultural assessment guide is available (eTable 2-2) on the website for this chapter.

NURSING MANAGEMENT
REDUCING HEALTH DISPARITIES AND INCREASING CULTURAL COMPETENCY

NURSE'S SELF-ASSESSMENT

The first step in reducing health disparities and providing culturally competent care is for you to assess your own cultural background, values, and beliefs, especially those that are related to health and health care. Many tools are available to assist you with this process *(http://nccc.georgetown.edu)*.

Table 2-4 suggests ways for you to improve your cultural competence. This information can help you better understand patients and provide culturally competent care. It is important to understand that cultures evolve and change over time. Culturally competent care requires continual learning and self-reflection.[40] Many other important aspects of culture related to

TABLE 2-8 CULTURE-BOUND SYNDROMES

Syndrome	Description
Hispanics/Latinos	
Bilis* or *colera	Caused by strong anger or rage. Many Hispanic/Latino groups believe that anger affects the body balance of hot and cold. Symptoms include acute nervous tension, headache, trembling, screaming, stomach disturbances, and, in severe cases, loss of consciousness.
Ataque de nervios	Brought on by a stressful family event (e.g., death, divorce). Symptoms may include uncontrollable shouting, crying and trembling, and verbal or physical aggression.
Empacho	Condition described as food forming into a ball that clings to the stomach or intestines, causing pain and cramping.
Susto	Sometimes referred to as "fright sickness" or "soul loss." A traumatic anxiety-depressive state that may result from a frightening experience, such as a loud sound or some threat. Can cause anxiety, insomnia, listlessness, loss of appetite, and social withdrawal. One treatment is to have the affected person lie on the floor. The healer then sweeps indigenous herbs over the person's body while praying to release the evil wind.
Native Americans	
Ghost sickness	Condition sometimes associated with witchcraft and a preoccupation with death. Symptoms include general weakness, loss of appetite, a feeling of suffocation, recurring nightmares, and a pervasive feeling of terror.
Chinese	
Shenjing shuairuo	Characterized by physical and mental fatigue, headaches and other pains, dizziness, sleep disturbances, and concentration difficulties.
European Americans (Appalachians)	
States of blood	Blood can exist in four states that are arranged into two sets of extremes: high and low blood, and thick and thin blood. The healthy person has blood that is balanced among these four states. A person with an imbalance lacks vitality; symptoms are fatigue, dizziness, pale complexion, and listlessness.
African Americans	
Brain fag	Term describing brain "fatigue" caused by the challenges of school. Symptoms include difficulties concentrating, remembering, and thinking.
Thin blood	Affects older adults, women, and children. Generally weakens an individual and increases susceptibility to illness.
Caribbean and Southern United States	
Falling out	Characterized by a sudden collapse, which may sometimes be preceded by dizziness or "swimming" in the head. The person can hear but is unable to move.
Cambodians	
Koucharang* or *Kit chroeun	Translates as "thinking too much," brought about by having witnessed or experienced a horrific trauma. Characterized by physical and emotional exhaustion, immobilization, and constant preoccupation with past suffering and loss.
Koreans	
Hwa-byung	Ailment characterized by resentment that is brought about by bitterness and discontent.

health care are included in the Culturally Competent Care sections throughout this book.

In today's increasingly multicultural environment, you will meet patients, families, significant others, and members of the health care team from many different cultures. You will find yourself in patient care situations that require an understanding of the patient's cultural beliefs and practices. Even when you provide care for patients from your own cultural background, you may be from a different subculture than the patient. For example, there are more than 550 federally recognized Native American tribes in the United States, so it would be inappropriate for you to assume that a Native American nurse can give culturally appropriate care to a Native American patient when both may be from different tribes. A white nurse from an urban upbringing may find cultural differences with a white patient from a rural community.

PATIENT ASSESSMENT

Health care providers play an important role in reducing health disparities. However, the causes of health disparities are not always easy to identify. Assess patients for their risk for reduced health care services because of limited access, inadequate resources, age, or low health literacy.

A cultural assessment should be included in the nursing process. Table 2-7 lists important components of the assessment. A comprehensive cultural assessment guide is available in eTable 2-2, which is available on the website for this chapter. Determine (1) the patient's health beliefs and health care practices; and (2) the patient's perspective of the meaning, cause, and preferred treatment of illness.[41] Ask questions that you are comfortable with based on your own culture.

How can you be aware of the differences among ethnic groups? Using guides to cultural assessment will facilitate the nursing process when working with patients, families, or other groups who are from different cultures. Although guides can assist in this process, you need to be careful not to stereotype or assume that common cultural characteristics pertain to each individual patient. Use guides to explore the degree to which patients share commonalities with the traits generally attributed to their cultural group. You need to be informed about traditional characteristics of cultural groups while recognizing that culture is constantly evolving and unique for each individual.

NURSING IMPLEMENTATION

Although the issues associated with health disparities can seem overwhelming, a number of strategies are available to reduce and ultimately eliminate health disparities. Table 2-9 presents nursing interventions to reduce health disparities.

ADVOCACY. The solutions to reduce health disparities often rest with the policy makers. Economic issues often determine health care delivery. Access and public policy decisions determine who is eligible for federal and state health insurance coverage. You, along with the social worker, can help by identifying key resources in the community, including transportation services, reduced-fee screening programs, and appropriate federal and state offices for Medicaid and Medicare.

You can be an advocate by finding and evaluating information on appropriate and individualized treatment and in navigating the health care system. One powerful strategy for reducing health disparities is to increase the number of underrepresented populations in the health care professions (Fig. 2-9).

TABLE 2-9 NURSING INTERVENTIONS TO REDUCE HEALTH DISPARITIES

- Treat all patients equally.
- Be aware of your own biases or prejudices and work toward eliminating them.
- Learn about services and programs that focus on specific cultural/ethnic groups.
- Inform patients about health care services available for their specific cultural/ethnic group.
- Make sure the same standards of care are followed for all patients regardless of culture or ethnicity.
- Identify health care practices and cultural practices that are important to cultural and ethnic identity.
- Participate in research focused on understanding and improving care to culturally and ethnically diverse populations.
- Identify stereotypic attitudes toward a culture/ethnic group that may interfere with getting appropriate health care.
- Support patients of specific cultural/ethnic groups who are fearful about traveling outside the accepted neighborhood for health care services.
- Advocate for patients of specific cultural/ethnic groups to receive health care services that pay special attention to English-language limitations and cultural health practices.
- Learn advocacy and interpersonal strategies from leaders of specific cultural/ethnic groups. For example, African Americans may respond to themes such as "do it for your loved ones." Asian Americans may respond to fear of dependency themes.
- Ensure availability of culturally appropriate patient educational resources.

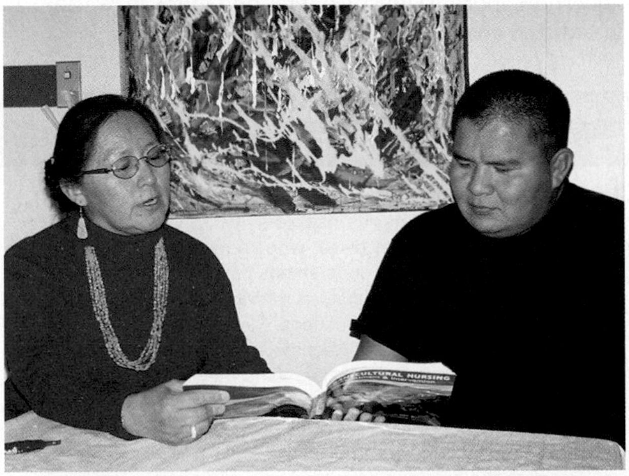

FIG. 2-9 A Navajo nurse instructs a Navajo patient.

STANDARDIZED GUIDELINES. The use of standardized evidence-based care guidelines can reduce disparities in diagnosis and treatments. For example, guidelines for the management of hypertension are based on the patient's blood pressure, symptoms, history, and laboratory values rather than other characteristics such as gender, age, or culture. Racial or cultural differences in outcomes are reduced when the guidelines are followed. In addition, recommendations related to cultural competency will guide you in your learning and practice.[41]

The National Standards for Culturally and Linguistically Appropriate Services in Health Care (CLAS standards) are guidelines that improve the quality of health care. The CLAS standards provide practical guidance for care of people with limited English proficiency and of diverse cultural backgrounds. These recommendations and resources for health care providers and organizations are available at the Think Cultural Health website listed in the Resources at the end of this chapter.

COMMUNICATION. Improving interpersonal skills is an important first step in reducing health disparities and providing culturally competent care. Effective communication between you and your patient is most likely to occur when both parties understand the meaning of that communication, whether it is through gestures, spoken words, or voice tones. To show respect for the patient, you should take into account the patient's usual communication style. For instance, a health history should start out in an unhurried manner and in a way that is appropriate for the culture. In some cultures it is best to start with general rather than direct questions. For some cultures it is most effective to engage in "small talk," with the discussion including answers that may seem to be unrelated to the questions. If you appear to be "too busy," communication may be impaired.

When meeting a patient or family member, introduce yourself and indicate how you would like them to address you—whether they should use first names; Mr., Ms., or Mrs.; or a title, such as nurse. Also ask the patient how he or she prefers to be addressed. This shows respect and will help you begin the relationship in a culturally appropriate manner.

If you need to gather personal information, it is important to understand the most effective approach to use. For instance, when talking with people from some cultural groups, it is imperative that you take time to establish trust and listen to the patient's responses to questions. There may be long silences as the person thinks about the question, showing respect by giving the question appropriate consideration before answering. Take time to listen and help establish trust.

TABLE 2-10 USING A MEDICAL INTERPRETER

Choosing an Interpreter

- Use an agency interpreter if possible.
- Use a trained medical interpreter who knows how to interpret, has a health care background, understands patients' rights, and can help with advice about the cultural relevance or appropriateness of the health care plan and instructions.
- Use a family member only if necessary. Be aware of limitations if the family member does not understand medical terms, is younger or a different gender than the patient, or is not aware of the health care procedures or medical ethics.
- Interpreter should be able to do the following:
  - Translate the patient's nonverbal as well as verbal communication.
  - Translate the message into understandable terms.
  - Act as a patient advocate to represent the patient's needs to the health care team.
  - Be culturally competent and understand how to provide teaching instructions.

Strategies for Working With an Interpreter

- If possible, have the interpreter meet with the patient ahead of time to establish rapport before the interpreting begins.
- Speak slowly.
- Maintain eye contact with the patient.
- Talk to the patient, not the interpreter.
- Use simple language with as few medical terms as possible.
- Speak one or two sentences at a time to allow for easier translation.
- Avoid raising your voice during the interaction.
- Obtain feedback to be certain the patient understands.
- Plan on taking twice as long to complete the interaction.

Some cultures, such as the Hmong, rely on oral communication. When working with patients who are from an oral culture, it is important to include oral instructions during the teaching-learning process.

Do not try to serve as an interpreter if your patient does not understand English because this could lead to misunderstandings. Get the assistance of a person who is qualified to do medical interpretation when you cannot speak the patient's primary language (Table 2-10). Interpreters are available by phone anywhere in the United States through a fee-based service and should be used rather than a family member. Table 2-11 provides guidelines for communicating when no interpreter is available. With the large number of immigrants and the many

TABLE 2-11 GUIDELINES FOR COMMUNICATING WHEN NO INTERPRETER IS AVAILABLE

1. Be polite and formal.
2. Pronounce name correctly. If unsure, ask about the correct pronunciation of the name. Use proper titles of respect, such as "Mr.," "Mrs.," "Ms.," "Dr." Greet the person using the last or complete name.
   Gesture to yourself and say your name.
   Offer a handshake or nod. Smile.
3. Proceed in an unhurried manner. Pay attention to any effort by the patient or family to communicate.
4. Speak in a low, moderate voice and avoid excessive hand gestures. Remember that there is a tendency to raise the volume and pitch of your voice when the listener appears not to understand. The listener may perceive that you are shouting or angry.
5. Use any words that you might know in the person's language. This indicates that you are aware of and respect his or her culture.
6. Use simple words, such as "pain" instead of "discomfort." Avoid medical jargon, idioms, and slang. Avoid using contractions (e.g., don't, can't, won't). Use nouns repeatedly instead of pronouns.
   Example:
   Do not say: "He has been taking his medicine, hasn't he?"
   Do say: "Does Juan take medicine?"
7. Pantomime words and simple actions while you verbalize them.
8. Give instructions in the proper sequence.
   Example:
   Do not say: "Before you rinse the bottle, sterilize it."
   Do say: "First, wash the bottle. Second, rinse the bottle."
9. Discuss one topic at a time. Avoid using conjunctions.
   Example:
   Do not say: "Are you cold and in pain?"
   Do say: "Are you cold [while pantomiming]? Are you in pain?"
10. Validate whether the person understands by having him or her repeat instructions, demonstrate the procedure, or act out the meaning.
11. Write out several short sentences in English and determine the person's ability to read them.
12. Try a third language. Many Indochinese people speak French. Europeans often know two or more languages. Try Latin words or phrases. Use English words that have Latin roots (e.g., use precipitation instead of rain).
13. Ask the person's family and friends who could serve as an interpreter.
14. Use websites that translate words from one language to another. Some of them also have audio to help you know how to say the word correctly.
15. Obtain phrase books from a library or bookstore, make or purchase flash cards, contact hospitals for a list of interpreters, and use both a formal and an informal network to locate a suitable interpreter.

Source: Jarvis C: *Physical examination and health assessment,* ed 6, Philadelphia, 2012, Saunders.

different cultural groups, it is highly likely that you will encounter patients who do not speak English.

A dictionary that translates from both your language and the patient's language (e.g., Spanish-English and English-Spanish dictionary) is helpful. You can look up questions and potential answers in several languages using these types of dictionaries. Many websites translate words and documents from one language into another (see Informatics in Practice box).

It is helpful to have resources for those cultural groups who frequently use the health care facility. This is especially beneficial when a qualified medical interpreter is not readily available and you need to learn important phrases in another language.

INFORMATICS IN PRACTICE

Use of Translation Applications

- Communication barriers can negatively affect the type of care received by non–English-speaking patients.
- Use a language translation app to help you translate one language into another language.
- Some apps allow you to speak critical phrases and have the translation immediately spoken back to you or the patient in a natural human voice with the proper accent.
- Check the policy of the health care institution on the use of medical interpreters or translators, including the use of apps for translation.

CASE STUDY

Health Disparities

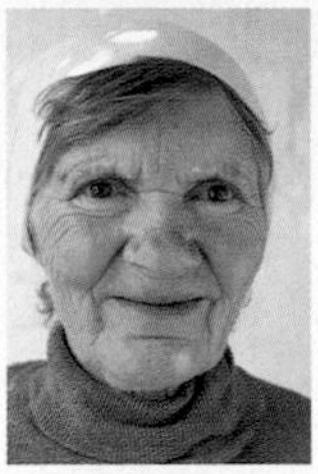

iStockphoto/ Thinkstock

Patient Profile

A.Z. is a 75-year-old woman who came to the United States from Russia 10 years ago with her daughter, her son-in-law, and their five children. She has a number of health problems, including coronary artery disease, osteoarthritis in her left hip, and diabetes. Her daughter is the primary caregiver and frequently brings her to the urban community health clinic for a variety of health-related complaints. Recently A.Z. has been experiencing memory problems.

The visits to the clinic tend to be chaotic and time consuming for the clinic staff. The entire family comes to the health clinic with A.Z. Because English is a second language for all of the adult family members, the staff relies on the oldest granddaughter to translate.

At this clinic visit A.Z. is complaining of shortness of breath. Through her granddaughter's translation, she tells the nurse that she is having trouble walking up the stairs in the apartment building and can no longer attend her Russian Orthodox church. The nurse does the history and assessment; checks her blood glucose, which is within normal limits; and advises that she get more exercise. Given A.Z.'s memory problems and limited English, the nurse does not complete a 24-hour dietary recall or counsel her or the family about diabetes management. A.Z. is scheduled for an appointment with the cardiologist for an evaluation of her cardiac disease. Two weeks later, when she is seen by the cardiologist, her shortness of breath is much worse and she is having chest pain. She is hospitalized immediately.

Meanwhile, the clinic supervisor is completing a chart audit for the clinic's quality review program. She is reviewing A.Z.'s chart and notices that, although she has been a patient in the clinic for 3 years, she has never received instructions on blood glucose monitoring or general diabetes management. The clinic has a nurse diabetes educator who teaches individual patients and groups of patients with diabetes. The clinic manager reviews these findings with the nurse and asks why she has not recommended that A.Z. see the diabetes educator. The nurse states that with all of the chaos in the family, A.Z.'s memory problems, and the language barrier, she just assumed that A.Z. would not benefit from the consultation.

Discussion Questions

1. What type of health disparity has A.Z. experienced?
2. What factors led to her not receiving the standard of care?
3. What additional assessment should have been done at the initial visit?
4. What strategies might have worked to enhance patient education?
5. How would you assess A.Z.'s religious and spiritual needs?
6. If you were the clinic manager, how would you recommend that the nurse improve her practice?

evolve Answers available at *http://evolve.elsevier.com/Lewis/medsurg.*

BRIDGE TO NCLEX EXAMINATION

The number of the question corresponds to the same-numbered outcome at the beginning of the chapter.

1. What is the leading determinant of a patient's health?
   a. Behavior
   b. Family history of disease
   c. Home and work environment
   d. Type and quality of medical care received
2. In identifying patients at the greatest risk for health disparities, the nurse would note that
   a. patients who live in urban areas have readily available access to health care services.
   b. cultural differences exist in patients' ability to communicate with their health care provider.
   c. a patient receiving care from a health care provider of a different culture would have decreased quality of care.
   d. men are more likely than women to have their cardiovascular disease symptoms ignored by their health care provider.
3. Forcing one's own cultural beliefs and practices on another person is an example of
   a. stereotyping.
   b. ethnocentrism.
   c. cultural relativity.
   d. cultural imposition.
4. Which statement most accurately describes cultural factors that may affect health?
   a. Diabetes and cancer rates differ by cultural/ethnic groups.
   b. Most patients find that religious rituals help them during times of illness.
   c. There are limited ethnic variations in physiologic responses to medications.
   d. Silence during a nurse-patient interaction usually means that the patient understands the instructions.

5. When communicating with a patient who speaks a language that the nurse does not understand, it is important to first attempt to
   a. have a family member translate.
   b. use a trained medical interpreter.
   c. use specific medical terminology so there will be no mistakes.
   d. focus on the translation rather than nonverbal communication.
6. As part of the nursing process, cultural assessment is best accomplished by
   a. judging the patient's cultural values based on observations.
   b. using a cultural assessment guide as part of the nursing process.
   c. seeking guidance from a nurse from the patient's cultural background.
   d. relying on the nurse's previous experience with patients from that cultural group.
7. Nurses play an important role in reducing health disparities. One important mechanism to do this is to
   a. discourage use of evidence-based practice guidelines.
   b. insist that patients adhere to the *Healthy People 2020* guidelines.
   c. teach patients to use the Internet to find resources related to their health.
   d. engage in active listening and establish relationships with patients and families.
8. What is the first step in developing cultural competence?
   a. Create opportunities to interact with a variety of cultural groups.
   b. Examine the nurse's own cultural background, values, and beliefs about health and health care.
   c. Learn about a multitude of folk medicines and herbal substances that different cultures use for self-care.
   d. Learn assessment skills for different cultural groups, including cultural beliefs and practices and physical assessments.

1. a, 2. b, 3. d, 4. a, 5. b, 6. b, 7. d, 8. b.

evolve

For rationales to these answers and even more NCLEX review questions, visit *http://evolve.elsevier.com/Lewis/medsurg*.

REFERENCES

1. World Health Organization: Health impact assessment. Retrieved from *www.who.int/hia/en*.
2. Hsia RY, Kellerman AL, Shen YC: Factors associated with closures of emergency departments in the United States, *JAMA* 305:1978, 2011.
3. US Department of Health and Human Services: Healthy People 2020. Retrieved from *www.healthypeople.gov*.
4. National Partnership for Action to End Health Disparities. Retrieved from *http://minorityhealth.hhs.gov/npa*.
5. Centers for Disease Control and Prevention: Chronic disease prevention and health promotion. Retrieved from *www.cdc.gov/chronicdisease/healthequity*.
6. Heurtin-Roberts S: Race and ethnicity in health and vital statistics, presented to National Committee on Health and Vital Statistics, Washington, DC. Retrieved from *www.ncvh.hhs.gov/040902p1*.
7. US Census Bureau: Population estimates. Retrieved from *www.census.gov/popest/estimates.php*.
8. Bhalla R, Yongue BG, Currie BP, et al: Improving primary percutaneous coronary intervention performance in an urban minority population using a quality improvement approach, *Am J Med Qual* 25:370, 2010.

*9. Cruz-Flores S, Rabinstein A, Biller J, et al: Racial-ethnic disparities in stroke care: the American experience: a statement for healthcare professionals from the American Heart Association/American Stroke Association, *Stroke* 42:2091, 2011.

*10. Byrne SK, Mary ES, DeShields T: Factors associated with why African-American women from one urban county use mammography services less, *J Natl Black Nurses Assoc* 22:8, 2011.

11. Health policy brief: achieving equity in health, *Health Affairs*. Retrieved from *www.healthaffairs.org/healthpolicybriefs/brief.php?brief_id=53*.

*12. National Cancer Institute, Center to Reduce Cancer Health Disparities: Examples of health disparities. Retrieved from *http://crchd.cancer.gov/disparities/examples.html#C4*.

13. Pfeifer G: Finding solutions to advance rural health, *Am J Nurs* 111:15, 2011.
14. Galinsky T, Feng HA, Streit J, et al: Risk factors associated with patient assaults of home healthcare workers, *Rehabil Nurs* 35:206, 2010.

*15. LaVeist T, Pollack K, Thorpe R, et al: Place, not race: disparities dissipate in southwest Baltimore when blacks and whites live under similar conditions, *Health Affairs* 30:1880, 2011.

16. Robert Woods Johnson Foundation: Health policy brief: achieving equity in health, *Health Affairs*. Retrieved from *http://rwjf.org/files/research/72893.disparities.pdf*.
17. Henry Kaiser Family Foundation: The uninsured: key facts about Americans without health insurance. Retrieved from *www.kff.org/uninsured/upload/7451-07.pdf*.
18. Centers for Disease Control and Prevention: Health disparities in cancer. Retrieved from *www.cdc.gov/cancer/healthdisparities/index.htm*.
19. Kones R: Recent advances in the management of chronic stable angina I: approach to the patient, diagnosis, pathophysiology, risk stratification, and gender disparities, *Vasc Health Risk Manag* 9:635, 2010.

*20. Choi NG, Ha JH: Relationship between spouse/partner support and depressive symptoms in older adults: gender differences, *Aging Ment Health* 15:307, 2011.

21. He J, Efron JE: Screening for colorectal cancer, *Adv Surg* 45:31, 2011.
22. Institute of Medicine of The National Academies: *The health of lesbian, gay, bisexual, and transgender people: building a foundation for better understanding*, Washington, DC, 2011, National Academies Press. Retrieved from *www.nap.edu*.
23. Narayan MC: Culture's effects on pain assessment and management, *Am J Nurs* 110:38, 2010.
24. Bralock AR, Farr NB, Kay J, et al: Issues in community-based care among homeless minorities, *J Natl Black Nurses Assoc* 22:57, 2011.

*Evidence-based information for clinical practice.

25. Centers for Disease Control and Prevention, Office of Minority Health & Health Disparities: American Indian and Alaska Native (AI/AN) populations. Retrieved from *www.cdc.gov/omhd/Populations/AIAN/AIAN.htm*.
26. Royse D, Dignan M: Fatalism and cancer screening in Appalachian Kentucky, *Fam Community Health* 34:126, 2011.
27. Li C, Balluz LS, Okoro CA, et al: Surveillance of certain health behaviors and conditions among states and selected local areas—Behavioral Risk Factor Surveillance System, United States, 2009, *MMWR Surveill Summ* 19:1, 2011.
28. Lopez-Class M, Castro FG, Ramirez AG: Conceptions of acculturation: a review and statement of critical issues, *Soc Sci Med* 72:1555, 2011.
29. Giger JN, Davidhizar RE: *Transcultural nursing: assessment and intervention*, ed 6, St Louis, 2012, Mosby.
30. Douglas MK, Pierce JU, Rosenkoetter M, et al: Standards of practice for culturally competent nursing care: 2011 update, *J Transcult Nurs* 22:317, 2011.
31. Andrews MM, Boyle JS: *Transcultural concepts in nursing care*, ed 5, Philadelphia, 2008, Lippincott Williams & Wilkins.
32. Gilliss CL, Powell DL, Carter B: Recruiting and retaining a diverse workforce in nursing: from evidence to best practice to policy, *Policy Polit Nurs Pract* 11:294, 2010.
*33. Karve SJ, Balkishnan R, Mohammad YM: Racial/ethnic disparities in emergency department waiting time for stroke patients in the United States, *J Stroke Cerebrovasc Dis* 20:30, 2011.
34. Sartori P: Exploring how to address patients' spiritual needs in practice, *Nurs Times* 106:23, 2010.
35. Maxwell J, Cortes DE, Schneider KL, et al: Massachusetts' health care reform increases access to care for Hispanics, but disparities remain, *Health Affairs* (Millwood) 30:1451, 2011.
36. Hall E: Proxemics: the study of man's spatial relationships. In Gladstone I, editor: *Man's image in medicine and anthropology*, New York, 1963, New York International University Press. (Classic)
*37. Singh GK, Siahpush M, Hiatt RA, et al: Dramatic increases in obesity and overweight prevalence and body mass index increase among ethnic-immigrant and social class groups in the United States, 1976-2008, *J Community Health* 36:94, 2011.
*38. Guh A, Sosa L, Hadler L, et al: Missed opportunities to prevent tuberculosis in foreign-born people, Connecticut, 2005-2008, *Int J Tuberc Lung Dis* 15:1044, 2011.
39. Centers for Disease Control and Prevention: Refugee health guidelines. Retrieved from *www.cdc.gov/immigrantrefugeehealth/guidelines/refugee-guidelines.html.*
40. Clark L, Calvillo E, dela Cruz F, et al: Cultural competencies for graduate nursing education, *J Profess Nurs* 127:133, 2011.
41. Higginbottom GM, Richter MS, Mogale RS, et al: Identification of nursing assessment models/tools validated in clinical practice for use with diverse ethno-cultural groups: an integrative review of the literature, *BMC Nurs* 10:16, 2011.

RESOURCES

American Association of Colleges of Nursing, Cultural Competency in Nursing Education
www.aacn.nche.edu/education-resources/cultural-competency

Center for Cross-Cultural Research
www.wwu.edu/culture

Cross Cultural Health Care Program
www.xculture.org

Health Literacy Universal Precautions Toolkit
www.nchealthliteracy.org/toolkit

National Center for Cultural Competence
http://nccc.georgetown.edu

National Partnership for Action to End Health Disparities
https://minorityhealth.hhs.gov/npa

Office of Minority Health
https://minorityhealth.hhs.gov

Think Cultural Health: Advancing Health Equity at Every Point of Contact
https://www.thinkculturalhealth.hhs.gov

Transcultural C.A.R.E. Associates
www.transculturalcare.net

Transcultural Nursing Society
www.tcns.org

CHAPTER

3

Strength does not come from physical capacity.
It comes from an indomitable will.
Mahatma Gandhi

Health History and Physical Examination

Jennifer Saylor and Linda Bucher

evolve WEBSITE

http://evolve.elsevier.com/Lewis/medsurg

- NCLEX Review Questions
- Key Points
- Pre-Test
- Rationales for Bridge to NCLEX Examination Questions
- Concept Map Creator
- Glossary
- Video
    - Physical Examination: General Inspection and Measurements
- Content Updates

eTables

- eTable 3-1: Recording Findings of a Normal Physical Examination of Healthy Adult
- eTable 3-2: Head-to-Toe (Total Body) Assessment Checklist
- eTable 3-3: Focused Assessments

LEARNING OUTCOMES

1. Explain the purpose, components, and techniques related to a patient's health history and physical examination.
2. Obtain a nursing history using a functional health pattern format.
3. Select appropriate techniques of inspection, palpation, percussion, and auscultation for physical examination of a patient.
4. Differentiate among comprehensive, focused, and emergency types of assessment in terms of indications, purposes, and components.

KEY TERMS

auscultation, p. 42
database, p. 36
functional health patterns, p. 38
inspection, p. 41
nursing history, p. 37
objective data, p. 37
palpation, p. 41
percussion, p. 41
subjective data, p. 37

You will obtain a patient's health history and perform a physical examination during the assessment phase of the nursing process. The findings of your assessment (1) contribute to a database that identifies the patient's current and past health status and (2) provide a baseline against which future changes can be evaluated. The purpose of the nursing assessment is to enable you to make clinical judgments or diagnoses about your patient's health status.[1] Assessment is identified as the first step of the nursing process, but it is performed continually throughout the nursing process to validate nursing diagnoses, evaluate nursing interventions, and determine whether patient outcomes and goals have been met.

The language of assessment is complex, with many overlapping and confusing terms. In this text, *assessment* describes a hands-on data collection process, whereas a *database* identifies a specific list of information (data) to be collected. For example, a *comprehensive database* would be completed for a patient who is being admitted to a hospital by doing a physical examination, a health history, and a psychosocial assessment.

DATA COLLECTION

In the broadest sense, the **database** is all the health information about a patient. This includes the nursing history and physical examination, the medical history and physical examination, results of laboratory and diagnostic tests, and information contributed by other health professionals. The nurse and physician both perform a patient history and a physical examination, but they use different formats and analyze the data based on their discipline's focus.

Medical Focus

A *medical history* is designed to collect data to be used primarily by the physician to determine risk for disease and diagnose medical conditions. The medical history is usually collected by a member of the health care team (e.g., physician, advanced practice nurse [APN], resident, physician's assistant, medical student). The health care provider's physical examination and laboratory and diagnostic tests assist in establishing medical

Reviewed by Misty Hobart, RN, MSN, ARNP, Department Chair, Nursing, Spokane Community College, Spokane, Washington; and Vera Kunte, RN-BC, MSN, Nurse Educator, Thomas Edison State College, Cary Edwards School of Nursing, Trenton, New Jersey.

diagnoses and evaluating treatments. The information collected and reported by the health care provider is also used by nurses and other members of the health care team (e.g., pharmacist, physical therapist, dietitian, social worker) within the focus of their care. For example, the abnormal results of a neurologic examination by an APN may assist in the diagnosis of a stroke. You may use the same results of the neurologic examination to identify a nursing diagnosis of risk for falls. A physical therapist may also use this information to plan therapy involving exercise and ambulatory aids.

Nursing Focus

The focus of nursing care is the diagnosis and treatment of human responses to actual or potential health problems or life processes. The information obtained from the **nursing history** and physical examination is used to determine the patient's strengths and responses to a health problem. For example, for the patient with a medical diagnosis of diabetes mellitus, the patient's responses may include anxiety or a lack of knowledge about self-management of the condition. This patient may also experience the physical response of fluid volume deficit because of the abnormal fluid loss caused by hyperglycemia. These human responses to the condition of diabetes are diagnosed and treated by nurses. During the nursing history interview and physical examination, you will obtain and record the necessary data to support the identification of nursing diagnoses (Fig. 3-1).

Types of Data

The database includes both subjective and objective data. **Subjective data,** also known as *symptoms,* are collected by interviewing the patient and/or caregiver during the nursing history. This type of data includes information that can be described or verified only by the patient or caregiver. It is what the person tells you either spontaneously or in response to direct questioning.

Objective data, also known as *signs,* are data that can be observed or measured. You obtain this type of data using inspection, palpation, percussion, and auscultation during the physical examination. Objective data are also acquired by diagnostic testing. Usually subjective data are obtained by interview, and objective data are obtained by physical examination.

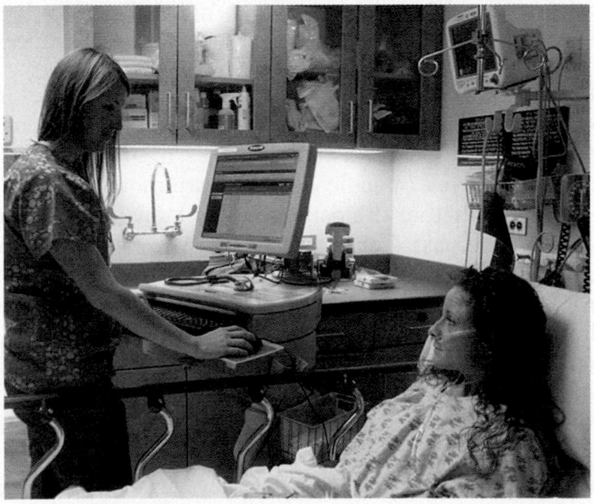

FIG. 3-1 Obtaining and recording data from a nursing history and physical examination using a computer.

However, patients often provide subjective data while you are performing the physical examination. You will also observe objective signs while interviewing the patient. All of the findings related to a specific problem, whether subjective or objective, are known as *clinical manifestations* of that problem.

Interview Considerations

The purpose of the patient interview is to obtain a health history (i.e., subjective data) about the patient's past and present health state. Effective communication is a key factor in the interview process. Creating a climate of trust and respect is critical to establishing a therapeutic relationship.[2] You need to communicate acceptance of the patient as an individual by using an open, responsive, nonjudgmental approach. You communicate not only through language but also in your manner of dress, gestures, and body language. Modes of communication are learned through one's culture, influencing not only the words, gestures, and postures one uses, but also the nature of information that is shared with others (see Chapter 2). In addition to understanding the principles of effective communication, you need to develop a personal style of relating to patients. Although no single style fits all people, your wording of questions can increase the probability of eliciting the needed information. The ease of asking questions, particularly those related to sensitive areas such as sexual functioning, comes with experience.

The amount of time you need to complete a nursing history varies with the format used and your experience. The nursing history may be completed in one or several sessions, depending on the setting and the patient. For example, you may need to plan several short sessions for an older adult patient with a low energy level to allow time for the patient to provide the needed information. You must also make a judgment about the amount of information collected on initial contact with the patient. In interviews with patients with chronic disease, patients in pain, and patients in emergency situations, ask only those questions that are pertinent to a specific problem. You can complete the health history interview at a more appropriate time.

Judge the reliability of the patient as a historian. An older adult may give a false impression about his or her mental status because of a prolonged response time or visual and hearing impairments. The complexity and long duration of health problems may make it difficult for an older adult or a chronically ill younger patient to be an accurate historian.

It is important for you to determine the patient's priority concerns and expectations, since your priorities may be different from the patient's. For example, your priority may be to complete the health history, whereas the patient is interested only in relief from symptoms. Until the patient's priority need is met, you will probably be unsuccessful in obtaining complete and accurate data.

Symptom Investigation

At any time during the assessment the patient may report a symptom such as pain, fatigue, or weakness. Symptoms experienced by the patient are not necessarily observed, so the symptom must be investigated. Table 3-1 shows a mnemonic (PQRST) to help you remember the areas to investigate if a symptom is reported. The information you receive may help determine the cause of the symptom. A common symptom that you will assess is pain (see Chapter 9). For example, if a patient states that he has "pain in his leg," you would assess and record the data using PQRST.

TABLE 3-1 INVESTIGATION OF PATIENT-REPORTED SYMPTOM

	Factor	Questions for Patient and Caregiver	Record
P	Precipitating and Palliative	Were there any events that came before the symptom? What makes it better? Worse? What have you done for the symptom? Did this help?	Influence of physical and emotional activities. Patient's attempts to alleviate (or treat) the symptom.
Q	Quality	Tell me what the symptom feels like (e.g., aching, dull, pressure, burning, stabbing).	Patient's own words (e.g., "Like a pinch or stabbing feeling").
R	Radiation	Where do you feel the symptom? Does it move to other areas?	Region of the body. Local or radiating, superficial or deep.
S	Severity	On a scale of 0-10, with 0 meaning no pain and 10 being the worst pain you could imagine, what number would you give your symptom?	Pain rating number (e.g., 5/0-10 scale).
T	Timing	When did the symptom start? Any particular time of day, week, month, or year? Has the symptom changed over time? Where are you and what are you doing when the symptom occurs?	Time of onset, duration, periodicity, and frequency. Course of symptoms. Where patient is and what patient is doing when the symptom occurs.

Has right midcalf pain that usually occurs at work when climbing stairs after lunch **(P)**. Pain is alleviated by stopping and resting for 2 to 3 minutes. Patient states he has been "eating a banana every day for extra potassium" but "it hasn't helped" **(P)**. Pain is described as "stabbing" and is non-radiating **(Q, R)**. Pain is so severe (rating 9 on 0-10 scale) that patient cannot continue activity **(S)**. Onset is abrupt, occurring once or twice daily. It last occurred yesterday while cutting the lawn **(T)**.

Data Organization

Assessment data must be systematically obtained and organized so you can readily analyze and make judgments about the patient's health status and any health problems. Some assessment forms are organized using body systems. Although helpful, these types of forms may be incomplete because they omit areas such as health promotion behaviors, sleep, coping, and values.

Functional health patterns, developed by Gordon,[3] provide the framework used throughout this textbook for obtaining a nursing history. This format includes an initial collection of important health information followed by assessment of 11 areas of health status or function (see Table 3-2). Data organized in this format promote the identification of areas of wellness (or positive function), as well as health problems.[2]

CULTURALLY COMPETENT CARE

ASSESSMENT

The process of obtaining a health history and performing a physical examination is an intimate experience for both you and the patient. As noted earlier in the chapter, one's culture influences patterns of communication and what information is shared with others. During the interview and physical examination, be sensitive to issues of eye contact, space, modesty, and touching, as discussed in Chapter 2. Adhering to cultural practices related to male-female relationships and gender identification is especially important during the physical examination. To avoid violating any culturally based practices, ask the patient about cultural values and whether the patient would like to have someone present during the history or physical examination.[1]

NURSING HISTORY: SUBJECTIVE DATA

Important Health Information

Important health information provides an overview of past and present medical conditions and treatments. Past health history, medications, allergies, and surgery or other treatments are included in this part of the history.

DELEGATION DECISIONS

Assessment and Data Collection

Ongoing data collection is expected of all members of the health care team. In acute care the initial (admission) nursing assessment must be completed by the registered nurse (RN).

Role of Registered Nurse (RN)
- On admission, do a comprehensive assessment (see Table 3-6).
- Obtain patient's health history by interviewing patient and/or caregiver.
- Perform physical examination using inspection, palpation, percussion, and auscultation as appropriate.
- Document findings from the health history and physical examination in the patient's record.
- Organize patient data into functional health patterns.
- Develop and prioritize nursing diagnoses and collaborative problems for the patient.
- Throughout hospitalization, perform focused assessments based on patient's history or clinical manifestations (see Table 3-6).

Role of Licensed Practical/Vocational Nurse (LPN/LVN)
- Collect and document specific patient data as delegated by the RN (after the RN has developed the plan of care based on the admission assessment).
- Perform focused assessment based on patient's history, clinical manifestations, or as instructed by the RN (see Table 3-6).

Role of Unlicensed Assistive Personnel (UAP)
- Take and document vital signs.
- Measure and document patient's height and weight.
- Report abnormal vital signs to RN.
- Report patient's subjective complaints to RN.

Past Health History. The past health history provides information about the patient's prior state of health. Ask the patient about major childhood and adult illnesses, injuries, hospitalizations, and surgeries. Specific questions are more effective than simply asking whether the patient has had any illness or health problems in the past. For example, "Do you have a history of diabetes?" will elicit better information than "Do you have any chronic illnesses?"

Medications. Ask the patient for specific details related to past and current medications, including prescription drugs, over-the-counter drugs, vitamins, herbal products, and dietary supplements. Patients frequently do not consider herbal products and dietary supplements as drugs. It is important to specifically ask about their use because they can interact adversely with existing or newly prescribed medications (Complementary & Alternative Therapies box).

COMPLEMENTARY & ALTERNATIVE THERAPIES

Assessment of Use of Herbs and Dietary Supplements

Why Assessment Is Important

- Herbal products and dietary supplements may have side effects or may interact adversely with prescription or OTC medications.
- Patients at high risk for drug-herb interactions include those taking anticoagulant, antihypertensive, antidepressant-psychotic, or immune-regulating therapy and patients undergoing anesthesia.
- Many patients do not tell health care providers that they are using herbal products and dietary supplements. They may fear health care professionals will disapprove of their use.
- Many herbal preparations contain a variety of ingredients. Ask the patient or caregiver to bring labeled containers to the health care site to determine the composition of the products.

Nurse's Role

- Patients typically share this information with you if they are specifically asked.
- Create an accepting and nonjudgmental attitude when assessing use of or interest in herbal products or dietary supplements.
- Use open-ended questions such as, "What types of herbs, vitamins, or supplements do you take?" and "What effects have you noticed from using them?"
- Respond to patients with comments that invite an open-minded discussion.
- Document the use of any herbal product(s) or dietary supplements in the patient record.

Question older adult and chronically ill patients about medication routines. Polypharmacy; changes in absorption, metabolism, reaction to drugs, and elimination of drugs; and surgery and concurrent disease can pose serious potential problems for these patients.[4]

Allergies. Fully explore the patient's history of allergies to medications, contrast media, food, and the environment (e.g., latex, pollen). Include a detailed description of any allergic reaction(s) reported by the patient.

Surgery or Other Treatments. Record all surgeries along with the date of the event, the reason for the surgery, and the outcome. The outcome includes whether the problem was completely resolved or has residual effects. Be sure to ask about and record any blood products the patient received.

Functional Health Patterns

Assess the patient's functional health patterns to identify positive, dysfunctional, and potential dysfunctional health patterns. Dysfunctional health patterns result in nursing diagnoses, and potential dysfunctional patterns identify risk conditions for problems. In addition, you may identify patients with effective health function who express a desire for a higher level of wellness. Examples of specific questions to ask the patient related to the functional health patterns are presented in Table 3-2.

Health Perception–Health Management Pattern. Assessment of the health perception–health management functional health pattern focuses on the patient's perceived level of health and well-being and on personal practices for maintaining health. Ask the patient to describe his or her personal health and any concerns about it. Explore the patient's feelings of effectiveness at staying healthy by asking what helps and what hinders his or her well-being. Ask the patient to rate his or her health as excellent, good, fair, or poor. Be sure to record this information in the patient's own words.

Next, while being culturally sensitive, ask about the type of health care provider the patient uses. For example, if the patient is Native American, a medicine man may be considered the primary health care provider. If the patient is of Hispanic origin, a *curandero* (Hispanic healer who uses folk medicine, herbal products, or magic to treat patients) may be the primary health care provider (see Chapter 2).

The questions for this pattern also seek to identify risk factors by obtaining a thorough family history (e.g., cardiac disease, cancer, genetic disorders), history of personal health habits (e.g., tobacco, alcohol, drug use), and history of exposure to environmental hazards (e.g., asbestos). If the patient is hospitalized, ask about the expectations for this experience. Have the patient describe his or her understanding of the current health problem, including its onset, course, and treatment. These questions obtain information about a patient's knowledge of the health problem and ability to use appropriate resources to manage the problem.

Nutritional-Metabolic Pattern. The processes of ingestion, digestion, absorption, and metabolism are assessed in this pattern. Obtain a 24-hour diet recall from the patient to evaluate the quantity and quality of foods and fluids consumed. If a problem is identified, ask the patient to keep a 3-day food diary for a more careful analysis of dietary intake. Assess the impact of psychologic factors such as depression, anxiety, stress, and self-concept on nutrition. Additionally, determine socioeconomic and cultural factors such as food budget, who prepares the meals, and food preferences. Determine whether the patient's present condition has interfered with eating and appetite by exploring any symptoms of nausea, intestinal gas, or pain. Food allergies should be differentiated from food intolerances, such as lactose or gluten intolerance.

Elimination Pattern. Assess bowel, bladder, and skin function in this pattern. Ask the patient about the frequency of bowel and bladder activity, including laxative and diuretic use. The skin is assessed in the elimination pattern in terms of its excretory function.

Activity-Exercise Pattern. Assess the patient's usual pattern of exercise, work activity, leisure, and recreation. Question the patient about his or her ability to perform activities of daily living and note any specific problems. Table 3-2 includes a scale for rating the functional levels of common activities.

Sleep-Rest Pattern. This pattern describes the patient's perception of his or her pattern of sleep, rest, and relaxation in a 24-hour period. This information can be elicited by asking, "Do you feel rested when you wake up?"

Cognitive-Perceptual Pattern. Assessment of this pattern involves a description of all of the senses and cognitive functions. In addition, assess pain as a sensory perception in this pattern. (See Chapter 9 for details on pain assessment.) Ask the patient about any sensory deficits that affect the ability to perform activities of daily living. Discuss and record ways in which the patient compensates for any sensory-perceptual problems. To plan for patient teaching, ask the patient how he or she communicates best and what he or she understands about the illness and treatment plan. (See Chapter 4 for details on patient teaching.)

Self-Perception–Self-Concept Pattern. This pattern describes the patient's self-concept, which is critical in determining the way the person interacts with others. Included are attitudes about self, perception of personal abilities, body image, and general sense of worth. Ask the patient for a self-description

TABLE 3-2 HEALTH HISTORY

Functional Health Pattern Format

Demographic Data
Name, address, age, occupation, gender
Race, ethnicity, culture

Important Health Information
Past health history
Medications, supplements
Allergies
Surgery or other treatments

Health Perception–Health Management Pattern
1. Reason for visit?
2. General state of health?
3. Number of colds in past year?
4. Most important things done to keep healthy? Testicular self-examination? Colorectal cancer, hypertension, and cardiac disease risk screening? Papanicolaou (Pap) test? Immunizations such as tetanus, pneumonia, hepatitis, and flu vaccines?
5. Who is your primary care physician or health care provider?
6. Health compliance problems?
7. Cause of illness? Action taken? Results?
8. Things important to you while here?
9. Family health history (e.g., cardiovascular disease, hypertension, cancer, diabetes mellitus, psychiatric illness, genetic disorders)?
10. Illness and injury risk factors (e.g., sexual abuse, intimate partner abuse, violence, use of cigarettes or alcohol, substance abuse)?

Nutritional-Metabolic Pattern
1. Typical daily food intake (describe)? Supplements?
2. Typical daily fluid intake (describe)?
3. Weight loss or gain (amount, time span)?
4. Desired weight?
5. Appetite?
6. Food or eating: Discomfort? Diet restrictions?
7. Change in appetite with anxiety?
8. Heal well or poorly?
9. Skin problems: Lesions? Dryness?
10. Dentition: Dental problems? Well-fitting dentures?
11. Food preferences?
12. Food allergies?

Elimination Pattern
1. Bowel elimination pattern (describe): Frequency? Character? Discomfort? Laxatives? Enemas?
2. Urinary elimination pattern (describe): Frequency? Problem in control? Diuretics?
3. Any external devices?
4. Excess perspiration? Odor problems? Itching?

Activity-Exercise Pattern
1. Sufficient energy for desired or required activities?
2. Exercise pattern? Type? Regularity?
3. Spare time (leisure) activities?
4. Dyspnea? Chest pain? Palpitations? Stiffness? Aching? Weakness?
5. Perceived ability for (rate Functional Level 0-III for each):
   Feeding __ Cooking __ Grooming __
   Bed mobility __ Bathing __ Dressing __
   Toileting __ Shopping __ General mobility __

   Functional Levels
   Level 0: Full self-care
   Level I: Requires use of equipment or device
   Level II: Requires assistance or supervision from another person
   Level III: Is dependent and does not participate

Sleep-Rest Pattern
1. Generally rested and ready for daily activities after sleep?
2. Sleep onset problems? Aids? Dreams (nightmares)? Early awakening?
3. Usual sleep rituals?
4. Usual sleep pattern?

Cognitive-Perceptual Pattern
1. Hearing difficulty? Hearing aids?
2. Vision? Wear glasses? Last checked?
3. Any change in taste? Any change in smell?
4. Any recent change in memory?
5. Easiest way to learn things?
6. Any discomfort? Pain (rating on scale of 0-10)? How managed?
7. Ability to communicate?
8. Understanding of illness?
9. Understanding of treatments?

Self-Perception–Self-Concept Pattern
1. Self-description? Self-perception?
2. Effect of illness on self-image?
3. Relieving factors?

Role-Relationship Pattern
1. Live alone? Family/caregiver? Family structure diagram?
2. Difficult family problems?
3. Family problem solving?
4. Family dependence on you for things? How managing?
5. Family's and others' feelings about illness or hospitalization?*
6. Problems with children? Difficulty handling?*
7. Belong to social groups? Have close friends? Feel lonely (frequency)?
8. Work (school) satisfaction? Income sufficient for needs?*
9. Feel part of or isolated from neighborhood where living?

Sexuality-Reproductive Pattern
1. Any changes or problems in sexual relations?*
2. Effect of illness?
3. Use of contraceptives? Problems?
4. When menstruation started? Last menstrual period? Menstrual problems? Gravida? Para?†
5. Effect of present condition or treatment on sexuality?
6. Sexually transmitted infections?

Coping–Stress Tolerance Pattern
1. Tense a lot of the time? What helps? Use any medications, drugs, alcohol?
2. Have someone to confide in? Available to you now?
3. Recent life changes?
4. Problem-solving techniques? Effective?

Value-Belief Pattern
1. Satisfied with life?
2. Religion important in your life?
3. Conflict between treatment and beliefs?

Other
1. Other important issues?
2. Questions?

Modified from Gordon M: *Manual of nursing diagnosis*, ed 12, Boston, 2010, Jones & Bartlett.
*If appropriate.
†For women.

and about how his or her health condition affects self-concept. Patients' expressions of hopelessness or loss of control frequently reflect an inability to care for oneself.

Role-Relationship Pattern. This pattern reveals the patient's roles and relationships, including major responsibilities. Ask the patient to describe family, social, and work roles and relationships and to rate his or her performance of the expected behaviors related to these. Determine whether patterns in these roles and relationships are satisfactory or whether strain is evident. Note the patient's feelings about how the present condition affects his or her roles and relationships.

Sexuality-Reproductive Pattern. This pattern describes satisfaction or dissatisfaction with personal sexuality and describes reproductive issues. Assessing this pattern is important because many illnesses, surgical procedures, and medications affect sexual function. A patient's sexual and reproductive concerns may be expressed, teaching needs and treatable problems may be identified, and normal growth and development may be monitored through information obtained in this pattern.

Obtaining information related to sexuality may be difficult for you. However, it is important to take a health history and screen for sexual function and dysfunction in order to provide information or refer the patient to a more experienced professional.

Coping–Stress Tolerance Pattern. This pattern describes the patient's general coping pattern and the effectiveness of the coping mechanisms. Assessment of this pattern involves analyzing the specific stressors or problems that confront the patient, the patient's perception of the stressors, and the patient's response to the stressors. Document any major losses or stressors experienced by the patient in the previous year. Note strategies used by the patient to deal with stressors and relieve tension, as well as individuals and groups that make up the patient's social support networks.

Value-Belief Pattern. This pattern describes the values, goals, and beliefs (including spiritual) that guide health-related choices. Document the patient's ethnic background and the effects of culture and beliefs on health practices. Note and honor the patient's wishes about continuation of religious or spiritual practices and the use of religious articles.

PHYSICAL EXAMINATION: OBJECTIVE DATA

General Survey

After the nursing history, make a *general survey statement.* This is your general impression of a patient, including behavioral observations. This initial survey is considered a scanning procedure that begins with your first encounter with the patient and continues during the health history interview.

Although you may include other data that seem pertinent, the major areas included in the general survey statement are (1) body features, (2) mental state, (3) speech, (4) body movements, (5) obvious physical signs, (6) nutritional status, and (7) behavior. Vital signs and body mass index (BMI) (calculated from height and weight [kg/m^2]) may be included. The following is a sample of a general survey statement:

> A.H. is a 34-year-old Hispanic woman, BP 130/84, P 88, R 18. No distinguishing body features. Alert but anxious. Speech rapid with trailing thoughts. Wringing hands and shuffling feet during interview. Skin flushed, hands clammy. Overweight relative to height (BMI = 28.3 kg/m^2). Sits with eyes downcast and shoulders slumped and avoids eye contact.

Physical Examination

The *physical examination* is the systematic assessment of a patient's physical status. Throughout the physical examination, explore any positive findings using the same criteria used during the investigation of a symptom in the nursing history (see Table 3-1). A *positive finding* indicates that the patient has or has had the particular problem or sign under discussion (e.g., if the patient with jaundice has an enlarged liver, it is a positive finding). Relevant information about this problem should then be gathered.

Negative findings may also be significant. A *pertinent negative* is the absence of a sign or symptom usually associated with a problem. For example, peripheral edema is common with advanced liver disease. If edema is not present in a patient with advanced liver disease, this should be specifically noted as "no peripheral edema."

Techniques. Four major techniques are used in performing the physical examination: inspection, palpation, percussion, and auscultation. The techniques are usually performed in this sequence, except for the abdominal examination (inspection, auscultation, percussion, and palpation). Performing percussion and palpation of the abdomen before auscultation can alter bowel sounds and produce false findings. Not every assessment area requires the use of all four assessment techniques (e.g., musculoskeletal system requires only inspection and palpation).

Inspection. **Inspection** is the visual examination of a part or region of the body to assess normal conditions or deviations. Inspection is more than just looking. This technique is deliberate, systematic, and focused. Compare what is seen with the known, generally visible characteristics of the body part that you are inspecting. For example, most 30-year-old men have hair on their legs. Absence of hair may indicate a vascular problem and the need for further investigation, or it may be normal for a patient of a particular ethnicity (e.g., Filipino men have little body hair). Always compare one side of the patient's body to the other to assess bilaterally for any abnormal findings.

Palpation. **Palpation** is the examination of the body using touch. Using light and deep palpation can yield information related to masses, pulsations, organ enlargement, tenderness or pain, swelling, muscular spasm or rigidity, elasticity, vibration of voice sounds, crepitus, moisture, and texture. Different parts of the hand are more sensitive for specific assessments. For example, use the palmar surface (base of fingers) to feel vibrations, the dorsa (backs) of your hands and fingers to assess temperature, and tips of your fingers to palpate the abdomen[1] (Fig. 3-2).

Percussion. **Percussion** is a technique that produces a sound and vibration to obtain information about the underlying area (Fig. 3-3). Evaluate the sounds and vibrations relative to the underlying structures. Deviation from an expected sound may indicate a problem. For example, the usual percussion sound in the right lower quadrant of the abdomen is tympany. Dullness in this area may indicate a problem that should be investigated. (Specific percussion sounds of various body parts and regions are discussed in the appropriate assessment chapters.)

Auscultation. **Auscultation** is listening to sounds produced by the body with a stethoscope to assess normal conditions and deviations from normal. This technique is particularly useful in evaluating sounds from the heart, lungs, abdomen, and vascular

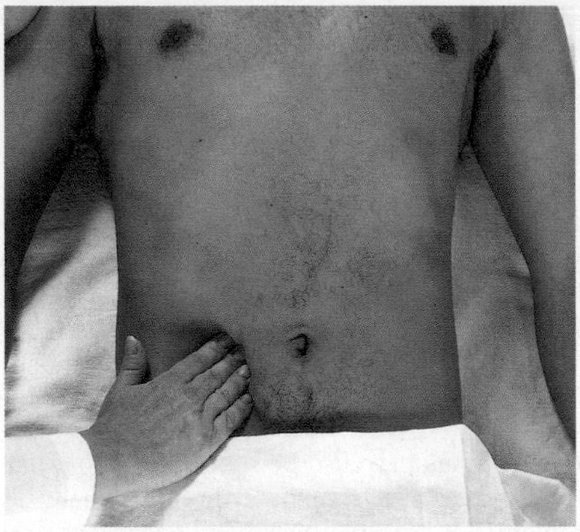

FIG. 3-2 Palpation is the examination of the body using touch. (From Jarvis C: *Physical examination and health assessment,* ed 6, St Louis, 2012, Saunders.)

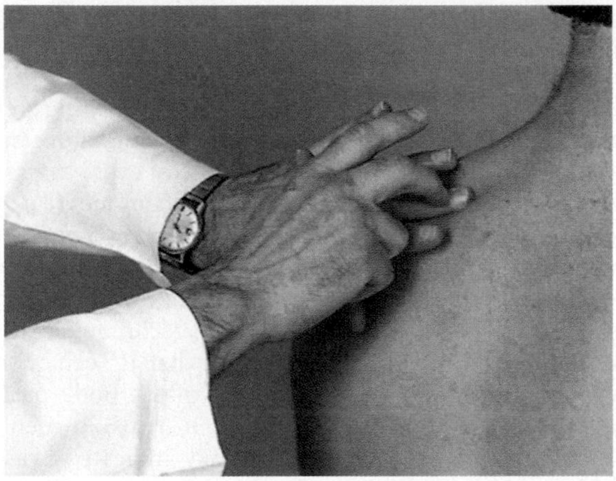

FIG. 3-3 Percussion technique. Tapping the interphalangeal joint. Only the middle finger of the nondominant hand should be in contact with the skin surface.

system. The bell of the stethoscope is more sensitive to low-pitched sounds (e.g., heart murmurs). The diaphragm of the stethoscope is more sensitive to high-pitched sounds (e.g., bowel sounds). Some stethoscopes have only a diaphragm, designed to transmit low- and high-pitched sounds. To listen for low-pitched sounds, hold the diaphragm lightly on the skin. For high-pitched sounds, press the diaphragm firmly on the skin[1] (Fig. 3-4). (Specific auscultatory sounds and techniques are discussed in the appropriate assessment chapters.)

Equipment. The equipment needed for the physical examination should be easily accessible (Table 3-3). Organizing equipment before the examination saves time and energy for you and the patient. (The uses of specific equipment are discussed in the appropriate assessment chapters.)

Organization of Examination. Perform the physical examination systematically and efficiently. Provide explanations to the patient as the examination proceeds, and consider the patient's comfort, safety, and privacy. You are less likely to forget a procedure, a step in the sequence, or a portion of the body if you follow the same sequence every time. Table 3-4 presents an outline for a physical examination that is organized and complete.

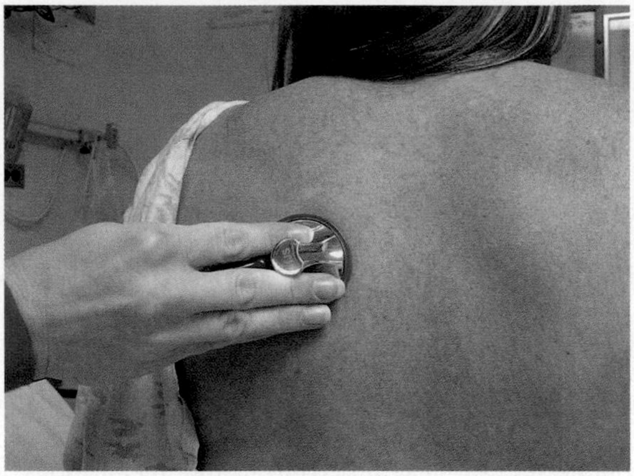

FIG. 3-4 Auscultation is listening to sounds produced by the body to assess normal conditions and deviations from normal.

TABLE 3-3 EQUIPMENT FOR PHYSICAL EXAMINATION*

• Stethoscope (with bell and diaphragm or a dual-purpose diaphragm; tubing 15-18 inches [38-46 cm])	• Pocket flashlight
• Watch (with second hand or digital)	• Tongue blades
• Blood pressure cuff	• Cotton balls
• Eye chart (wall chart or Snellen pocket eye card)	• Percussion hammer
	• Alcohol swabs
	• Patient gown
	• Paper cup with water
	• Examining table or bed

*These are examples of commonly used equipment; other equipment may be used depending on the situation.

Adaptations of the physical examination are often useful for the older adult patient, who may have age-related problems such as decreased mobility, limited energy, and perceptual changes.[5] An outline listing some of the useful adaptations is found in Table 3-5.

Recording Physical Examination. Only record abnormal findings during the actual examination. At the conclusion of the examination, combine the normal and abnormal findings in a carefully compiled record. An example of how to record findings of a physical examination of a healthy adult can be found in eTable 3-1 on the website for this chapter. See Table 5-6 to locate age-related assessment findings in the book.

TYPES OF ASSESSMENT

Various types of assessment are used to obtain information about a patient. These approaches can be divided into three types: comprehensive, focused, and emergency (Table 3-6 on p. 45). You need to decide what type of assessment to perform based on the clinical situation (e.g., admission history and physical examination, start of shift, throughout shift). Sometimes the health care agency provides guidelines, and other times it is a nursing judgment.

Comprehensive Assessment

A *comprehensive assessment* includes a detailed health history and physical examination of one body system or many body systems (see Table 3-6). This is typically done on admission to the hospital or onset of care in a primary care setting.

TABLE 3-4 OUTLINE FOR PHYSICAL EXAMINATION

1. General Survey

Observe general state of health (patient is seated).
- Body features
- Level of consciousness and orientation
- Speech
- Body movements and carriage
- Physical appearance
- Nutritional status
- Stature

2. Vital Signs

Record vital signs.
- Blood pressure—both arms for comparison
- Apical/radial pulse
- Respiration
- Temperature
- Record height and weight; calculate body mass index (BMI)

3. Integument

Inspect and palpate skin for the following:
- Color
- Breakdown, lacerations, lesions
- Scars, tattoos, piercings
- Bruises, rash
- Edema
- Moisture
- Texture
- Temperature
- Turgor
- Vascularity

Inspect and palpate nails for the following:
- Color
- Lesions
- Size
- Flexibility
- Shape
- Angle
- Capillary refill time

4. Head and Neck

Inspect and palpate head for the following:
- Shape and symmetry of skull
- Masses
- Tenderness
- Hair
- Scalp
- Skin
- Temporal arteries
- Temporomandibular joint
- Sensory (CN V, light touch, pain)
- Motor (CN VII, shows teeth, purses lips, raises eyebrows)
- Looks up, wrinkles forehead (CN VII)
- Raises shoulders against resistance (CN XI)

Inspect and palpate (occasionally auscultate) neck for the following:
- Skin (vascularity and visible pulsations)
- Symmetry
- Range of motion
- Pulses and bruits (carotid)
- Midline structure (trachea, thyroid gland, cartilage)
- Lymph nodes (preauricular, postauricular, occipital, mandibular, tonsillar, submental, anterior and posterior cervical, infraclavicular, supraclavicular)

Inspect and lightly palpate eyes for the following:
- Visual acuity
- Eyebrows
- Position and movement of eyelids (CN VII)
- Visual fields
- Extraocular movements (CN III, IV, VI)
- Cornea, sclera, conjunctiva
- Pupillary response (CN III)
- Red reflex

Inspect and palpate nose and sinuses for the following:
- External nose: shape, blockage
- Internal nose: patency of nasal passages, shape, turbinates or polyps, discharge
- Frontal and maxillary sinuses

Inspect and palpate ears for the following:
- Placement
- Pinna
- Auditory acuity (whispered voice, ticking watch) (CN VIII)
- Mastoid process
- Auditory canal
- Tympanic membrane

Inspect and palpate mouth for the following:
- Lips (symmetry, lesions, color)
- Buccal mucosa (Stensen's and Wharton's ducts)
- Teeth (absence, state of repair, color)
- Gums (color, receding from teeth)
- Tongue for strength (asymmetry, ability to stick out tongue, side to side, fasciculations) (CN XII)
- Palates
- Tonsils and pillars
- Uvular elevation (CN IX)
- Posterior pharynx
- Gag reflex (CN IX and X)
- Jaw strength (CN V)
- Moisture
- Color
- Floor of mouth

5. Extremities

Observe size and shape, symmetry and deformity, involuntary movements. Inspect and palpate arms, fingers, wrists, elbows, shoulders for the following:
- Strength
- Range of motion
- Joint pain
- Swelling
- Pulses (radial, brachial)
- Sensation (light touch, pain, temperature)
- Test reflexes: triceps, biceps, brachioradialis

Inspect and palpate legs for the following:
- Strength
- Range of motion
- Joint pain
- Swelling, edema
- Hair distribution
- Sensation (light touch, pain, temperature)
- Pulses (dorsalis pedis, posterior tibialis)
- Test reflexes: patellar, achilles, plantar

6. Posterior Thorax

Inspect for muscular development, scoliosis, respiratory movement, approximation of AP diameter.
- Palpate for symmetry of respiratory movement, tenderness of CVA, spinous processes, tumors or swelling, tactile fremitus
- Percuss for pulmonary resonance
- Auscultate for breath sounds
- Auscultate for egophony, bronchophony, and whispered pectoriloquy

7. Anterior Thorax
- Assess breasts for configuration, symmetry, dimpling of skin
- Assess nipples for rash, direction, inversion, retraction
- Inspect for apical impulse, other precordial pulsations
- Palpate the apical impulse and the precordium for thrills, lifts, heaves, tenderness
- Inspect neck for venous distention, pulsations, waves
- Palpate lymph nodes in the subclavian, axillary, and brachial areas
- Palpate breasts
- Auscultate for rate and rhythm; character of S_1 and S_2 in the aortic, pulmonic, Erb's point, tricuspid, mitral areas; bruits at carotid, epigastrium

AP, Anteroposterior; *CN*, cranial nerve; *CVA*, costovertebral angle.

Continued

TABLE 3-4 OUTLINE FOR PHYSICAL EXAMINATION—cont'd

8. Abdomen
- Inspect for scars, shape, symmetry, bulging, muscular position and condition of umbilicus, movements (respiratory, pulsations, presence of peristaltic waves)
- Auscultate for peristalsis (i.e., bowel sounds), bruits
- Percuss then palpate to confirm positive findings; check liver (size, tenderness), spleen, kidney (size, tenderness), urinary bladder (distention)
- Palpate femoral pulses, inguinofemoral nodes, and abdominal aorta

9. Neurologic

Observe motor status.
- Gait
- Toe walk
- Heel walk
- Drift

Observe coordination:
- Finger to nose
- Romberg sign
- Heel to opposite shin

Observe the following:
- Proprioception (position sense of great toe)

10. Genitalia*

Male External Genitalia
- Inspect penis, noting hair distribution, prepuce, glans, urethral meatus, scars, ulcers, eruptions, structural alterations, discharge
- Inspect epidermis of perineum, rectum
- Inspect skin of scrotum; palpate for descended testes, masses, pain

Female External Genitalia
- Inspect hair distribution; mons pubis, labia (minora and majora); urethral meatus; Bartholin's, urethral, Skene's glands (may also be palpated, if indicated); introitus; any discharge
- Assess for presence of cystocele, prolapse
- Inspect perineum, rectum

*If the nurse has the appropriate education, the speculum and bimanual examination of women and the prostate gland examination of men would be performed after this inspection.

TABLE 3-5 GERONTOLOGIC ASSESSMENT DIFFERENCES

Adaptations in Physical Assessment Techniques

General Approach
Keep patient warm and comfortable because loss of subcutaneous fat decreases ability to stay warm. Adapt positioning to physical limitations. Avoid unnecessary changes in position. Perform as many activities as possible in the position of comfort for the patient.

Skin
Handle with care because of fragility and loss of subcutaneous fat.

Head and Neck
Provide a quiet environment free from distraction because of possible sensory impairments (e.g., decreased vision, hearing).

Extremities
Use gentle movements and reinforcement techniques. Avoid having patient hop on one foot or perform deep knee bends because of patient's limited range of motion of the extremities, decreased reflexes, and diminished sense of balance.

Thorax
Adapt examination for changes related to decreased force of expiration, weakened cough reflex, and shortness of breath.

Abdomen
Use caution in palpating patient's liver because it is readily accessible because of a thinner, softer abdominal wall. The older adult patient may have diminished pain perception in the abdominal wall.

Focused Assessment

A *focused assessment* is a more abbreviated history and examination. It is used to evaluate the status of previously identified problems and monitor for signs of new problems. It can be done when a specific problem (e.g., pneumonia) is identified. The patient's clinical manifestations should alert you to the appropriate focused assessment. For example, abdominal pain indicates the need for a focused assessment of the abdomen. Some problems necessitate a focused assessment of more than one body system. A complaint of headache may indicate the need to do musculoskeletal, neurologic, and head and neck examinations. Examples of focused assessments for various body systems can be found in eTable 3-3 on the website for this chapter.

Emergency Assessment

In an emergency or critical situation an *emergency assessment* may be done. This involves the rapid examination and specific questioning of a patient while maintaining vital functions.

Using Assessment Approaches

Assessment in a hospital inpatient setting, particularly in acute care, is markedly different from assessment in other settings. Focused assessment of the hospitalized patient is frequent and performed by many different people. Such a team approach demands a high degree of consistency among different health care professionals.

As you provide ongoing care for a patient, you will be constantly refining your mental image of the patient. As you gain experience, you will form a mental image of a patient's status from a few basic details, such as "85-year-old woman admitted for COPD [chronic obstructive pulmonary disease] exacerbation." Your picture of her becomes clearer as you receive a more complete verbal report, such as length of stay, recent laboratory results, physical findings, and vital signs. Next, perform your own assessment using a focused approach. During your assessment, you will confirm or revise the findings that you read in the medical record and what you heard from other health care professionals.

Keep in mind that the process does not end once you have done your first assessment on a patient during your rounds. You will continue to gather information about all your patients throughout your shift. Everything that you learned previously about each patient is considered in the light of new information. For example, when you are doing a respiratory assessment on your patient with COPD, you hear crackles in her lungs. This finding should lead you to do a cardiovascular assessment because cardiac problems (e.g., heart failure) can also cause crackles. As you gain experience, the importance of new findings will be more obvious to you. Assessment case

TABLE 3-6 TYPES OF ASSESSMENT

The following describes types of assessment that you may use in various situations.

Description	When and Where Performed	Where to Find in Book
Comprehensive		
• Detailed assessment of one body system or many body systems, including those not directly involved in presenting problem or admission diagnosis • Used for head-to-toe assessment	• Onset of care in primary or ambulatory care setting • On admission to hospital or long-term care setting • On initial home care visit	• Assessment chapters for each body system • Outline for physical examination (see Table 3-4) • Head-to-toe (total body) assessment checklist (see eTable 3-2, available on the website for this chapter)
Focused		
• Abbreviated assessment that focuses on one or more body systems that are the focus of care • Includes an assessment related to a specific problem (e.g., pneumonia, specific abnormal laboratory findings) • Monitors for signs of new problems	• Throughout hospital admission—at beginning of a shift and as needed throughout shift • Revisited in ambulatory care setting or home care setting	• Focused assessment boxes in each assessment chapter (all boxes available in eTable 3-3 on website) • Tables on nursing assessment of specific diseases throughout book
Emergency		
• Limited to assessing life-threatening conditions (e.g., inhalation injuries, anaphylaxis, myocardial infarction, shock, stroke) • Conducted to ensure survival; focuses on airway, breathing, circulation, and disability • After lifesaving interventions are initiated, perform brief systematic assessment to identify any and all other injuries or problems	• Performed in any setting when signs or symptoms of a life-threatening condition appear (e.g., emergency department, critical care unit, surgical setting)	• Chapter 69, Table 69-3 and Table 69-5 • Emergency management tables throughout the book and listed in Table 69-1

studies are integrated into all of the assessment chapters for this book to help you develop your assessment skills and knowledge.

Table 3-7 shows how you can perform different types of assessments based on a patient's progress through a given hospitalization. When a patient arrives at the emergency department in acute distress, you will perform an emergency assessment based on the principles of airway, breathing, circulation, disability, and exposure/environmental control (see Chapter 69, Table 69-3). Once the patient is stabilized, you can begin a focused assessment of the respiratory and related body systems. Once the patient is admitted, a comprehensive assessment of all body systems, whether or not they are involved in the current clinical problem, is obtained.

PROBLEM IDENTIFICATION AND NURSING DIAGNOSES

After completing the history and physical examination, analyze the data to develop a list of nursing diagnoses and collaborative problems. See Chapter 1 for a description of the nursing process, including the identification of nursing diagnoses and collaborative problems.

TABLE 3-7 CLINICAL APPLICATION OF VARIOUS TYPES OF ASSESSMENT

The following is an example of how various types of assessment would be used for a patient progressing from the emergency department to a clinical unit of a hospital.

Timeline	Type of Assessment
Emergency Department (ED)	
Patient arrives in acute respiratory distress.	Perform emergency assessment (see Table 69-3).
Problem is identified and critical interventions are performed; patient stabilizes.	Conduct a focused assessment of the respiratory and related body systems (e.g., cardiovascular). May begin comprehensive assessment of all body systems.
Clinical Unit	
Patient is admitted to a monitored clinical unit.	Complete comprehensive assessment of all body systems within proper timeframe.
Reassess throughout shift. New nurse arrives at change of shift.	Perform focused assessment of respiratory system and other related body systems (to determine if new problems have arisen).

BRIDGE TO NCLEX EXAMINATION

The number of the question corresponds to the same-numbered outcome at the beginning of the chapter.

1. The patient health history and physical examination provide the nurse with information to primarily
   a. diagnose a medical problem.
   b. investigate a patient's signs and symptoms.
   c. classify subjective and objective patient data.
   d. identify nursing diagnoses and collaborative problems.
2. The nurse would place information about the patient's concern that his illness is threatening his job security in which functional health pattern?
   a. Role-relationship
   b. Cognitive-perceptual
   c. Coping–stress tolerance
   d. Health perception–health management
3. The nurse is preparing to examine a patient's abdomen. Identify the proper order of the steps in the assessment of the abdomen, using the numbers 1-4 with 1 = the first technique and 4 = the last technique:
   ___Inspection
   ___Palpation
   ___Percussion
   ___Auscultation
4. Which situation would require the nurse to obtain a focused assessment *(select all that apply)*?
   a. A patient denies a current health problem.
   b. A patient reports a new symptom during rounds.
   c. A previously identified problem needs reassessment.
   d. A baseline health maintenance examination is required.
   e. An emergency problem is identified during physical examination.

1. d, 2. a, 3. 1, 4, 3, 2, 4. b, c.

evolve

For rationales to these answers and even more NCLEX review questions, visit *http://evolve.elsevier.com/Lewis/medsurg.*

REFERENCES

1. Jarvis C: *Physical examination and health assessment*, ed 6, St Louis, 2012, Saunders.
2. Wilson S, Giddens J: *Health assessment for nursing practice*, ed 4, St Louis, 2009, Mosby.
3. Gordon M: *Manual of nursing diagnosis*, ed 12, Boston, 2010, Jones & Bartlett.
4. Lehne R: *Pharmacology for nursing care*, ed 7, St Louis, 2010, Mosby.
5. Eliopoulos C: *Gerontological nursing*, ed 7, Philadelphia, 2009, Lippincott Williams & Wilkins.

Tell me and I'll forget;
show me and I may remember;
involve me and I'll understand.
Chinese proverb

CHAPTER 4

Patient and Caregiver Teaching

Linda Bucher and Catherine N. Kotecki

evolve WEBSITE

http://evolve.elsevier.com/Lewis/medsurg

- NCLEX Review Questions
- Key Points
- Pre-Test
- Rationales for Bridge to NCLEX Examination Questions
- Concept Map Creator
- Glossary
- Content Updates

eFigures

- eFig. 4-1: Plan of care and education record
- eFig. 4-2: Supplemental plan of care—deficient knowledge

eTable

- eTable 4-1: Writing Learning Objectives/Goals

LEARNING OUTCOMES

1. Prioritize patient teaching goals for diverse patients and caregivers.
2. Analyze teaching implications related to the diverse needs of adult learners.
3. Apply strategies to manage challenges to nurse-teacher effectiveness.
4. Evaluate the role of the caregiver in patient teaching.
5. Apply the teaching-learning process to diverse patient populations.
6. Relate the physical, psychologic, and sociocultural characteristics of the patient and caregiver to the teaching-learning process.
7. Select appropriate teaching strategies for diverse patient populations.
8. Select appropriate methods to evaluate patient and caregiver teaching.

KEY TERMS

caregivers, p. 50
health literacy, p. 53
learning, p. 48
learning needs, p. 54
motivational interviewing, p. 48
positive reinforcement, p. 54
self-efficacy, p. 49
teaching, p. 48
teaching plan, p. 48
teaching process, p. 52

This chapter describes the process of patient and caregiver teaching. In addition, it discusses the strategies and methods that contribute to successful teaching and learning experiences.

ROLE OF PATIENT AND CAREGIVER TEACHING

Patient and caregiver (family member or significant other) teaching is an interactive and dynamic process that involves a change in a patient's knowledge, behavior, and/or attitude to maintain or improve health. You will find that teaching is one of your most challenging and rewarding roles. Teaching patients is a key nursing intervention that makes a difference in their lives.

General goals of patient teaching include health promotion, prevention of disease, management of illness, and appropriate selection and use of treatment options. In patients with acute and chronic health problems, teaching can prevent complications and promote recovery, self-care, and independence. Seventy percent of the deaths in the United States are due to chronic illnesses, illnesses with which patients often live for many years.[1] Whether patients adequately manage their health problems and maintain quality of life depends on what they learn about their conditions and what they choose to do with this knowledge. Patients who understand their discharge teaching, including how to take their medicines and when to follow-up with their health care providers, are 30% less likely to be readmitted or visit the emergency department than patients who did not receive this information.[2]

Teaching may occur wherever you work. Although institutions may employ advanced practice nurses and patient educators to establish and oversee patient teaching programs, you

Reviewed by Kathleen M. Barta, RN, EdD, Associate Professor, University of Arkansas, Eleanor Mann School of Nursing, Fayetteville, Arkansas; Regina Kukulski, RN, MSN, ACNS, BC, Nurse Educator Consultant, Thomas Edison State College, Capital Health Medical Center, Trenton, New Jersey; and C. Denise Neill, RN, PhD, CNE, Assistant Professor and RN-BSN and MSN Program Coordinator, University of Houston–Victoria, Victoria, Texas.

are always responsible for patient and caregiver teaching.[3-5] It is a responsibility that cannot be delegated to unlicensed assistive personnel.

Every interaction with a patient and a caregiver is a potential *teachable moment.* On any given day, more informal opportunities to teach will occur than formal opportunities. Take advantage of all of these moments. For example, when you teach a patient with asthma how to use a peak flow meter, you do not require a formal teaching plan. However, when your patient has a specific learning need about health promotion or management of a health problem, you should develop a teaching plan. A **teaching plan** includes (1) assessment of the patient's ability, need, and readiness to learn; and (2) identification of problems that can be resolved with teaching. Then develop goals with the patient, provide teaching interventions, and evaluate the effectiveness of the teaching.

TEACHING-LEARNING PROCESS

Teaching is not just imparting information. **Teaching** is a process of deliberately arranging conditions to promote learning that results in a change in behavior.[6] Teaching can be a planned or informal experience. It uses a combination of methods such as instruction, counseling, and behavior modification.

Learning is acquiring knowledge and/or skills. It can result in a permanent change in a person.[6] Observation of this change is an indication that learning has occurred. Learning may also result in a potential or capability to change behavior. This is seen in a patient who understands the instruction and is fully informed, but chooses not to change behavior. In this case, teaching gives the patient the capability to make a decision to change behavior, but the decision is the patient's.

Although learning may occur without teaching, teaching helps to organize information and skills to make learning more efficient. In patient teaching the teaching-learning process involves the patient, the patient's caregiver(s), and you.

Adult Learner

Adult Learning Principles. Understanding how and why adults learn is important for you to effectively teach patients and their caregivers. Many of the theories of adult learning have risen from the work of Malcolm Knowles, who identified six principles of *andragogy* (adult learning) that are important for you to consider when teaching adults[7] (Table 4-1).

Models to Promote Health. When a change in health behaviors is recommended, patients and their caregivers may progress through a series of steps before they are willing or able to accept the change. Prochaska and Velicer proposed six stages of change in their *Transtheoretical Model of Health Behavior Change*[8] (Table 4-2). This model is frequently used to help patients stop smoking, manage diabetes, and lose weight.

Motivational interviewing (see *www.motivationalinterview.org*) uses nonconfrontational interpersonal communication techniques to motivate patients to change behavior.[9] This strategy includes the use of any intervention that enhances the

TABLE 4-1 ADULT LEARNING PRINCIPLES APPLIED TO PATIENT AND CAREGIVER TEACHING

Principles	Teaching Implications for the Nurse	Examples
The learner's need to know	• Patients need to know why they should learn something, what they need to learn, and how it will benefit them. • Ask the patient questions such as, "What do you think you need to learn about this topic?"	Your patient and his caregiver have requested specific information on exercise guidelines after a heart attack.
The learner's readiness to learn	• Readiness and motivation to learn are high when facing new tasks. • Health crises provide opportunities for patients to learn and change behavior. • Stress and anxiety may interfere with learning, thus requiring frequent reinforcement of content.	While recovering from a transient ischemic attack, your patient tells you that she is ready to learn about the changes she needs to take to reduce her risk for stroke.
The learner's prior experiences	• Motivation is increased when patients already know something about the subject from past experiences. • Identification of past knowledge and experiences can help find familiar ground to increase patients' confidence.	Your patient needs to begin injections of enoxaparin (Lovenox). She tells you that she gives her father insulin injections and is ready to learn how to administer this medication.
The learner's motivation to learn	• Patients prefer to apply learning immediately. • Long-term goals may have less appeal than short-term goals. • Focus teaching on information that the patient views as being needed right now.	Your patient is scheduled to be discharged in the morning. Both she and her caregiver have received instruction on wound care and have watched the procedure. The caregiver tells you that he wants to perform the wound care this evening.
The learner's orientation to learning	• Patients seek out various resources for specific learning and prefer to have choices. • When the patient does not recognize the relevancy of the teaching, offer explanations of the value of the learning. • Teaching should target the specific problem or circumstance.	Your patient, who is newly diagnosed with diabetes mellitus, tells you that he is worried about the diet changes he will need to make. Share several options with him to learn about diet changes (e.g., cooking classes, Internet-based tutorials, individual sessions with the dietitian, brochures).
The learner's self-concept	• Patients need control and self-direction (sense of autonomy) to maintain their sense of self-worth. • Patients do not learn when they are treated like children and told what they must do.	Your patient has a temporary colostomy. She says she is not ready to look at the stoma. Work out a schedule with her for learning colostomy care that meets her need for control and prepares her for self-care.

TABLE 4-2 STAGES OF CHANGE IN TRANSTHEORETICAL MODEL

Stage	Patient Behavior	Nursing Implications
1. Precontemplation	Is not considering a change. Is not ready to learn.	Provide support, increase awareness of condition. Describe benefits of change and risks of not changing.
2. Contemplation	Thinks about a change. May verbalize recognition of need to change; says "I know I should," but identifies barriers.	Introduce what is involved in changing the behavior. Reinforce the stated need to change.
3. Preparation	Starts planning the change, gathers information, sets a date to initiate change, shares decision to change with others.	Reinforce the positive outcomes of change, provide information and encouragement, develop a plan, help set priorities, and identify sources of support.
4. Action	Begins to change behavior through practice. Tentative and may experience relapses.	Reinforce behavior with reward, encourage self-reward, discuss choices to help minimize relapses and regain focus. Help patient plan to deal with potential relapses.
5. Maintenance	Practices the behavior regularly. Able to sustain the change.	Continue to reinforce behavior. Provide additional teaching on the need to maintain change.
6. Termination	Change has become part of lifestyle. Behavior no longer considered a change.	Evaluate effectiveness of the new behavior. No further intervention needed.

Adapted from Prochaska J, Velicer W: The transtheoretical model of health behavior change, *Am J Health Promot* 12:38, 1997. (Classic)

patient's motivation for change (Table 4-3). The techniques used in motivational interviewing are linked to the stages of change as identified by Prochaska and Velicer.

During the process of change, relapse and recycling through the stages are expected. Sometimes patients do not change behaviors or return to previous behaviors after a period of change. This may indicate that the interventions used did not consider the patient's stage of change.[10] Identify the patient's current stage of readiness for change and the stage to which the patient is moving. Patients who are in the early stages of change need and use different kinds of motivational support than patients at later stages of change.

For example, a patient who smokes cigarettes who is hospitalized is often in the *precontemplation* or *contemplation* stage of change. In the precontemplation stage, patients are not concerned about their substance use and are not considering changing their behavior. During this stage, help the patient increase awareness of risks and problems related to smoking and create doubt about the use of cigarettes. Ask the patient what he or she thinks could happen if the behavior is continued, provide evidence of the problem (e.g., x-ray changes), and offer factual information about the risks of smoking. Although patients may not be ready to change behavior while experiencing an acute health problem, the seeds of doubt are sown. In other cases, such as when a patient experiences a life-threatening condition (e.g., heart attack), there may be an immediate awareness of the problem and motivation to change.

TABLE 4-3 KEY ASPECTS OF MOTIVATIONAL INTERVIEWING

- Listen rather than tell.
- Adjust to, rather than oppose, patient resistance.
- Express empathy through reflective listening.
- Focus on the positive. Do not criticize the patient.
- Gently persuade with the understanding that change is up to the patient.
- Focus on the patient's strengths to support the hope and optimism needed to make changes.
- Avoid argument and direct confrontation, which can cause defensiveness and a power struggle.
- Help the patient recognize the "gap" between where he or she is and where he or she hopes to be.

A patient in the *contemplation* stage of change often experiences ambivalence. The patient understands that the behavior is a problem and that change is necessary. However, he or she believes that change is too difficult or that the pleasures of the behavior are worth the risks. This is seen in the patient who says, "I know that I have to stop smoking. This heart attack really scared me. I know I need to lose weight and start exercising, but I can't change everything all at once. Smoking helps me control my eating—I can't stop until I lose some weight." During this stage of change, help the patient consider the positive and negative aspects of his or her behavior (e.g., substance use), gently trying to tip the balance in favor of positive behavior. Helping the patient discover internal motivators in addition to those external motivators (e.g., second heart attack, lung disease) that push the patient toward change can move the patient from contemplating change to preparation and action. Throughout this process, emphasize the patient's personal choices and responsibilities for change.

As the patient moves from contemplation to *preparation,* a commitment to change is strengthened by helping the patient develop **self-efficacy,** which is the belief that one can succeed in a given situation. In this case it is the patient's belief that substance-use behaviors can be changed. Support even the smallest effort to change. Movement through action and maintenance stages of change requires continued support to increase the patient's involvement and participation in treatment. A comprehensive discussion of motivational interviewing is presented in the Treatment Improvement Protocols available at *www.ncbi.nlm.nih.gov/books/NBK14856.*

The resolution of acute health problems or discharge from the hospital often occurs before the patient moves to the preparation and action stages of change. As the patient develops readiness to change in the contemplative stage of change, continue to support him or her with referral to appropriate community and outpatient resources.

Nurse as Teacher

Required Competencies

Knowledge of Subject Matter. Although it is impossible to be an expert in all subject areas, develop confidence as a teacher by becoming knowledgeable about the subject to be taught. Information can be obtained through reliable sources such as journals and books. For example, if you are teaching patients about the management of hypertension, you must be able to explain what hypertension is and why it is important to treat it. Also teach patients what they need to know about exercise, diet, and side effects of medications. Teach the patient and the caregiver how to use blood pressure (BP) equipment to monitor BP and to identify situations that need to be reported to health care providers. Finally, provide the patient with additional resources, such as written brochures, appropriate websites, and information about support organizations (e.g., American Heart Association).

Sometimes you will not be able to answer patients' or caregivers' questions. Clarifying their questions may help if you are unsure of what they are asking. When it is apparent that you do not have the knowledge to answer the question, admit this to the patient and caregiver and seek help from co-workers, patient educators, and other reliable sources.

Communication Skills. Patient teaching depends on effective communication between you and the patient or caregiver. *Medical jargon* is intimidating and frightening to most patients and their caregivers. Introduce medical words with definitions of their meaning. Consider carefully before using acronyms (e.g., CABG for coronary artery bypass graft) and abbreviations (e.g., IV) when talking with patients. Have the patient and caregiver clarify their understanding of the disease process. Have them explain what they know in their own words. For example, if a patient is told that he has leukopenia, explain this diagnosis in words that mean something to him. Use word roots, explaining that *leuko* refers to a leukocyte, a white blood cell that fights infections, and that *penia* means deficiency or shortage. To enhance learning, use a brief explanation such as, "You have a shortage of white blood cells, the cells that fight infection."

Nonverbal communication is critical when teaching. Nonverbal communication is often guided by cultural practices. For example, in Western culture, sitting in an open, relaxed position facing the patient with eyes at the same level delivers a positive, nonverbal message (Fig. 4-1). In a hospital setting this may require raising the patient's bed or sitting in a chair at the bedside. Open body gestures communicate interest and a willingness to share. With patients from Eastern cultures, you may need to avoid direct eye contact and provide health information to a family spokesperson rather than directly to the patient.

Also develop the art of *active listening* by paying attention to what is said, observing the patient's nonverbal cues, and not interrupting. Nod in response to the patient's statements and rephrase and reflect what the patient is saying to help clarify communication.

Empathy is the courage to enter into the world of another in a manner that does not judge or correct but where understanding is the goal. Empathy means putting aside your own self and stepping into the patient's shoes. When combined with the skill of empathy, active listening is a powerful way to communicate caring and prepare the patient to learn.

Challenges to Nurse-Teacher Effectiveness. Teaching patients and caregivers has many challenges, including (1) lack of time, (2) your own feelings as a teacher, (3) nurse-patient differences in learning goals, and (4) early discharge from the health care system.

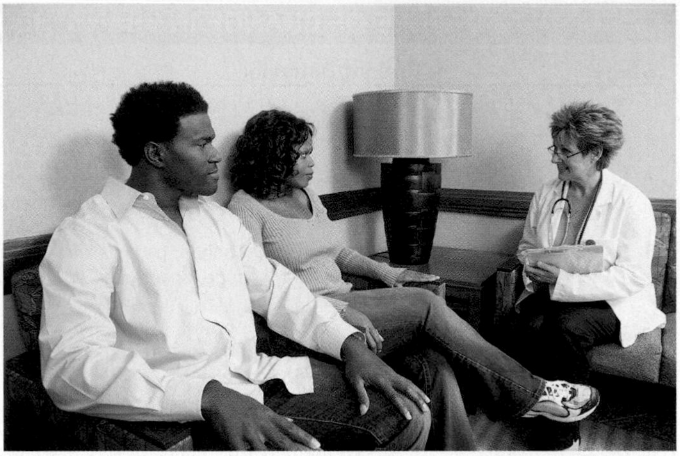

FIG. 4-1 Open, relaxed positioning of patient, spouse, and nurse at eye level promotes communication in teaching and learning. (Jupiterimages/Photos.com/Thinkstock.)

Lack of time can be a barrier to effective teaching. For example, the patient's physical needs may compete for time that could be used for teaching. To make the most of limited time, it is critical to set learning priorities with the patient. Tell the patient at the beginning of the interaction how much time you can devote to the session. Teaching can be delivered or reinforced during every contact with the patient or caregiver. For example, when giving medications, explain the purpose and side effects of each drug. Reinforcing small pieces of information over time is an effective teaching strategy, especially if information is new or complex.

Additional barriers are your *own feelings as a teacher* and insecurity about your own knowledge and competence. Teaching is a skill that takes time to master. Become familiar with the various resources for patient teaching that are available at your agency. Consult with nurse educators for further help with developing your teaching skills.

Also, disagreements can arise among the patient, the caregiver, and you regarding the expectations or outcomes of teaching. Having realistic discussions about discharge plans, identifying timelines, and exploring home care options can bring urgency to the teaching situation. For example, after a diagnosis of chronic heart failure as a result of aortic valve insufficiency and subsequent emergent valve surgery, the patient and the caregiver may reject teaching efforts until they accept and realize the seriousness of the patient's health problem.

Finally, another important challenge to patient teaching relates to patients having early and quick discharges from the health care system. Shortened lengths of hospital stays and hurried outpatient clinic visits have resulted in patients only having basic teaching plans implemented.

Caregiver Support in the Teaching-Learning Process

The teaching and learning process is applicable to the caregiver as well as the patient. **Caregivers** are people who care for those who cannot care for themselves. Most common, caregivers are family members or significant others who (1) give or assist with direct patient care; (2) provide emotional, social, spiritual, and possibly financial support for the patient; and (3) manage and coordinate health care services.

Approximately one in four American adults provides care to someone on a daily basis. Caregivers are often categorized by their relationship to the patient. The most common types of caregivers are spouses, adult children, parents, grandparents, and life partners. Although older adult women are the most common family caregivers, other examples include husbands who care for wives with Alzheimer's disease, adult children who care for a parent with a stroke, grandparents who care for a grandchild with a developmental disorder, parents who care for an adult child with a spinal cord injury, and life partners who care for loved ones with a variety of health problems.[11]

Identify the key caregiver(s) for the patient. Assess the caregiver's roles and relationships to the patient. The patient's health problem affects family roles and functions. Identify the needs of caregivers, whether it is in the acute care setting, during the transition to home, or in a home setting[12] (Table 4-4).

Consider cultural differences when assessing the caregiver. In some cultures a male family member may be the designated spokesperson. This person would receive and communicate information among family members and the patient. In planning for discharge to home, it is important to include caregivers who will actually provide the care for the patient, along with the family spokesperson.[12]

As much as possible, teach the caregiver along with the patient. Explain the goals of the teaching plan clearly to both of them. Caregivers may need assistance to learn the physical and technical requirements of care, find resources for home care, locate equipment and supplies, and rearrange the home environment to accommodate the patient. Sources of support for the transition from hospital to home include community-based agencies, Medicare and Medicaid offices, and case managers at the hospital and insurance companies.[13] Patients and caregivers may have different teaching needs. For example, the first priority of an older diabetic patient with a large leg ulcer may be to learn how to transfer from a bed to a chair in the least painful manner. On the other hand, the caregiver may be most concerned about learning the technique for dressing changes. Both the patient's and the caregiver's learning needs are important. The patient and the caregiver may also have differing or conflicting views of the illness and treatment options. Developing a successful teaching plan requires you to view the patient's needs within the context of the caregiver's needs. For instance, you may teach a patient with right sided *paresis* (weakness) self-feeding techniques with special implements, but at a home visit you find the patient being fed by the caregiver. On questioning, the caregiver reveals that it is too difficult to watch the patient struggle with feeding, it takes too long, and it is messy. As a result, the caregiver decides that it is easier to just feed the patient. This is an example of a situation in which both the patient and caregiver need additional teaching about the goals of self-care.

Finally, discuss the potential that support groups, networks of family and friends, and community resources have for providing ongoing support and continuing education. Support groups help by sharing experiences and information, offering understanding and acceptance, and suggesting solutions to common problems and concerns. Encourage the caregiver to seek help from the formal social support system on matters such as housing, health coverage, finances, and respite care. Respite care, which is planned temporary care for the patient, includes adult day care, in-home care, and assisted living services.

Caregiver Stress. Caregiver responsibilities are usually taken on gradually with the progression of the patient's illness. As the caregiving responsibilities become more demanding, caregivers often realize that their lives have changed because of this experience. Overwhelmingly, caregivers want to continue their usual activities (e.g., work) despite the hardships they face in caring for acute and chronically ill patients.[14,15]

Prolonged periods of caregiving coupled with a patient's life-limiting illness can contribute to stress and burnout. Some common caregiver stressors are listed in Table 4-5. As caregiving progresses, stressors may change. For example, a caregiver may initially need only to adjust work schedules to accommodate a patient's health care appointments. Later, as the patient's condition worsens, the caregiver may have to reduce work hours, incurring financial hardships.

Caregiving is an experience for which most people are not prepared. It is common for caregivers to become physically, emotionally, and economically overwhelmed by the responsibilities and demands of caring for a family member. The stress of caregiving may result in emotional problems such as depression, anger, and resentment. Signs of caregiver stress include irritability, inability to concentrate, fatigue, and sleeplessness. The caregiver often experiences decreased social interactions and may be at risk for social isolation. Multiple commitments, fatigue, and, at times, the patient's socially inappropriate behaviors contribute to the caregiver's social isolation. Stress can progress to burnout and result in negligence and abuse of the

TABLE 4-4 ASSESSMENT OF CAREGIVER NEEDS

Assess caregivers using the following questions:

1. How are you coping with your caregiver role?
2. Do you have any difficulties performing your caregiver responsibilities?
3. How much support do you get from outside sources (e.g., other family members, friends)?
4. Are you aware of and do you use community resources (e.g., disease-specific professional organizations [such as Alzheimer's Association, American Heart Association], adult day care centers, church, synagogue)?
5. Do you know about resources that are available for respite (someone caring for your loved one while you have time to yourself)?
6. What kind of help or services do you need now and in the near future?
7. How can I or other health care professionals help you in your caregiving role?

TABLE 4-5 CAREGIVER STRESSORS

- Change in roles and relationships within family unit
- Lack of respite or relief from caregiving responsibilities
- Need to juggle day-to-day activities, decisions, and caregiving
- Change in living conditions to accommodate family member
- Conflict in the family unit related to decisions about caregiving
- Other people's lack of understanding of the time and energy needed for caregiving
- Inability to meet personal self-care needs, such as socialization, sleep, eating, exercise, and rest
- Financial depletion of resources as a result of a caregiver's inability to work and the increased cost of health care
- Inadequate information or skills related to specific caregiving tasks, such as bathing, drug administration, wound care

patient by the caregiver. See Chapter 5 for information on elder mistreatment and abuse.

In the family system an illness experienced by one family member affects the entire family and alters family interactions. Often family members do not communicate with each other about the patient's needs, and this results in tension. Family conflicts regarding how patient care should be given can lead to disagreements and conflict within the family.

At the same time, many family members involved in direct caregiver activities also identify rewards associated with this role. Positive aspects of caregiving include (1) knowing that their loved one is receiving good care (often in a home environment), (2) learning and mastering new skills, and (3) finding opportunities for intimacy. The tasks involved in caregiving often provide opportunities for family members to gain greater insights into each other and strengthen their relationships.

Encourage caregivers to take care of themselves.[16] Suggest journaling or joining a support group (also available online) to help them share feelings that may be difficult to express. Remind caregivers that getting regular exercise and eating balanced meals at regular times will enhance their well-being. Encourage contact with others to provide emotional support. Finally, humor is important, and sometimes its use by caregivers can provide distraction and relieve stress-filled situations.

Regulatory Mandates for Patient Teaching

Several important agencies have provided specific mandates related to teaching hospitalized patients. The Joint Commission's (TJC's) accreditation standards, National Patient Safety Goals,[3] and the American Hospital Association's Patient Care Partnership[17] clearly state that patients have a fundamental right to receive written information about their care. This information includes their diagnosis, treatment, and prognosis in terms that they can reasonably be expected to understand. For example, this means that written materials must be appropriate for the patient's reading level. One program initiated by TJC, called Speak Up, was developed to encourage patients to become more involved and informed about their plan of care[18] (Table 4-6). Another program proposed by the National Patient Safety Foundation is called **Ask Me 3**.[19] A variety of resources that prompt patients to ask specific questions about their care are available as a part of these initiatives (*www.jointcommission.org/speakup.aspx, www.npsf.org/for-healthcare-professionals/programs/ask-me-3).*

TABLE 4-6 THE JOINT COMMISSION'S SPEAK UP™ INITIATIVE

Speak up if you have questions or concerns. If you still do not understand, ask again. It is your body and you have a right to know.
Pay attention to the care you get. Always make sure you are getting the right treatments and medicines by the right health care professionals. Do not assume anything.
Educate yourself about your illness. Learn about the medical tests you get and your treatment plan.
Ask a trusted family member or friend to be your advocate (advisor or supporter).
Know what medicines you take and why you take them. Medicine errors are the most common health care mistakes.
Use a hospital, clinic, surgery center, or other type of health care organization that has been carefully checked out.
Participate in all decisions about your treatment. You are the center of the health care team.

Source: The Joint Commission: To prevent health care errors, patients are urged to Speak Up (poster). Retrieved from *http://www.jointcommission.org/assets/1/18/SpeakUp_Poster.pdf.*

PROCESS OF PATIENT TEACHING

Many different models and approaches are used in the process of patient teaching. However, the approach used most frequently by nurses parallels the nursing process. The **teaching process** and the nursing process both involve the development of a plan that includes assessment, setting of patient goals or outcomes, intervention, and evaluation. The teaching process, like the nursing process, may not always flow in sequential order, but the steps serve as checkpoints.

Assessment

During the general nursing assessment, gather data to determine if the patient has learning needs. For example, what does the patient know about the health problem? How does he or she perceive the problem? If a learning need is identified, a more detailed assessment is needed, and that problem is addressed with the teaching plan. Assessment also includes the caregivers to determine their role and ability to care for the patient at home.[12] Key questions to use in the assessment are included in Table 4-7.

Physical Factors. The patient's age is an important factor to consider in the teaching plan. Age affects the patient's experiences, rate of learning, and ability to retain information.[20] The effects of increased age may be obvious, but the inexperience of younger individuals can also affect learning. For example, a man in his twenties who has never thought about his own mortality may be unable to accept the long-term health implications of diabetes mellitus.

Sensory impairments (e.g., hearing or vision loss) decrease sensory input and can alter learning. Magnifying glasses, bright lighting, and materials printed in a large font may help the patient with impaired vision read teaching materials. Hearing loss can be helped with hearing aids and teaching techniques that use more visual stimuli. Cognitive function may be affected by disorders of the nervous system, such as stroke and head trauma, and also by other diseases, such as liver impairment and heart failure. Patients with alterations in cognitive function may have difficulty learning and may require greater caregiver involvement in the teaching process. Manual dexterity is needed to perform procedures such as self-administration of injections or BP monitoring. Problems performing manual procedures might be resolved by using adaptive equipment.

Pain, fatigue, and certain medications also influence the patient's ability to learn. No one can learn effectively when in pain. When the patient is experiencing pain, provide only brief explanations and follow up with more detailed instruction when the pain has been managed. A fatigued and weakened patient cannot learn effectively because of the inability to concentrate. Sleep disruption is common during hospitalization, and patients are frequently exhausted at the time of discharge. Drugs that cause central nervous system depression, such as opioids and sedatives, cause a general decrease in mental alertness and can affect the patient's ability to learn new information. Adjust the teaching plan to accommodate these factors by setting high-priority goals based on need-to-know information and realistic expectations. The patient may need a referral for follow-up teaching so that learning is continued and reinforced after discharge.

TABLE 4-7 ASSESSMENT OF FACTORS AFFECTING PATIENT TEACHING

Factors and Key Questions

Physical
- What is the patient's age and gender?
- Is the patient acutely ill?
- Is the patient fatigued or in pain?
- What is the primary diagnosis?
- Are there additional medical problems?
- What is the patient's current mental status?
- What is the patient's hearing ability? Visual ability? Motor ability?
- What drugs does the patient take that may affect learning?

Psychologic
- Does the patient appear anxious, afraid, depressed, defensive?
- Is the patient in a state of denial?
- What is the patient's level of motivation? Self-efficacy?

Sociocultural
- What are the patient's beliefs regarding his or her illness or treatment?
- Is proposed teaching consistent with the patient's cultural values?
- What is the patient's educational experience, reading ability, primary language?
- What is the patient's present or past occupation?
- How does the patient describe his or her financial status?
- What is the patient's living arrangement?
- Does the patient have family or close friends?

Learner
- What does the patient already know?
- What does the patient think is most important to learn first?
- What prior learning experiences establish a frame of reference for current learning needs?
- What has the patient's health care provider told the patient about the health problem?
- Is the patient ready to change behavior or learn?
- Can the patient identify behaviors and habits that would make the problem better or worse?
- How does the patient learn best? Through reading, listening, doing things?
- In what kind of environment does the patient learn best? Formal classroom? Informal setting, such as home or office? Alone or among peers?
- In what way should the caregiver(s) be involved in patient teaching?

Psychologic Factors. Psychologic factors have a major influence in the patient's ability to learn. Anxiety and depression are common reactions to illness. Although mild anxiety increases the learner's perceptual and learning abilities, moderate or severe anxiety limits learning. Both anxiety and depression can negatively affect the patient's motivation and readiness to learn. For instance, the patient newly diagnosed with diabetes mellitus who is depressed about the diagnosis may not listen or respond to instructions about blood glucose testing. Discussions with the patient about these concerns or referrals to an appropriate support group may enable the patient to learn that management of diabetes is possible.

Patients also respond to the stress of illness with a variety of defense mechanisms such as denial, rationalization, or even humor. A patient who denies having cancer will not be receptive to information related to treatment options. Similarly, a caregiver may have difficulty accepting a terminal diagnosis. A patient using rationalization will imagine any number of reasons for avoiding change or for rejecting instruction. For example, a patient with heart disease who does not want to change dietary habits will relate stories of people who have eaten bacon and eggs every morning and lived to be 100. Some patients also use humor to filter reality or decrease anxiety. They may use laughter to escape from the experience of facing threatening situations. Humor in the teaching process is important and useful, but determine when humor is used excessively or inappropriately to avoid reality.

One important determinant of successful adoption of new behaviors is the patient's sense of self-efficacy. There is a strong relationship between self-efficacy and outcomes of illness management.[21,22] Self-efficacy increases when a person gains new skills in managing a threatening situation, but decreases when the individual experiences repeated failure, especially early in the course of events. Plan easily attainable goals early in the teaching sessions. Proceed from simple to more complex content to establish a feeling of success.

Sociocultural Factors

Health Literacy. *Literacy* is the ability to use printed and written information to function in society. The recent focus on the literacy rates of the U.S. population and their effects on health and health care have major implications for patient and caregiver teaching. The most recent national literacy survey reported that 43% of the general population and 66% of people older than 60 have basic to below basic literacy skills, and another 5% are nonliterate in English.[4] Assessment of literacy is challenging, since patients rarely admit they have difficulty reading because of feelings of inadequacy and low self-esteem.[23]

Health literacy is the degree to which individuals have the capacity to obtain and understand basic health information needed to make appropriate health decisions.[3] Patients with limited literacy have trouble understanding and acting on health information, leading to health illiteracy. Even patients with higher general literacy can have low health literacy when trying to understand complex health information. Health illiteracy results in poor patient outcomes, nonadherence with treatment plans, limited self-management skills, and increased health disparities.[24]

Easy-to-use assessment tools are available to determine a patient's health literacy. The Single-Item Literacy Screener (SILS) uses one question to identify adults who need help with reading.[25] The question is, "How often do you need to have someone help you when you read instructions, pamphlets, or other written material from your doctor or pharmacy?"

Patient teaching materials should be written at the fifth-grade or lower reading level.[23-25] TJC has established that patient teaching should be tailored to the patient's literacy needs. For example, patients should be taught in their primary language. This is accomplished using medical interpreters (translators)[26] (Fig. 4-2). (Medical interpreters are discussed in Chapter 2 on pp. 32 to 33.) Many patient teaching materials are currently available in languages other than English.

Cultural Considerations. Learning is influenced by the wider culture to which a patient belongs. Health practices, beliefs, and behavior are influenced by one's cultural traditions. These traditions, which can affect patient teaching, can be identified in a cultural assessment (see Table 2-7). TJC requires that patient teaching be tailored to the patient's cultural needs.[26] To prevent stereotyping patients, it is important to simply ask if there is a cultural group with which the patient identifies. Ask patients to describe their beliefs regarding health and illness.

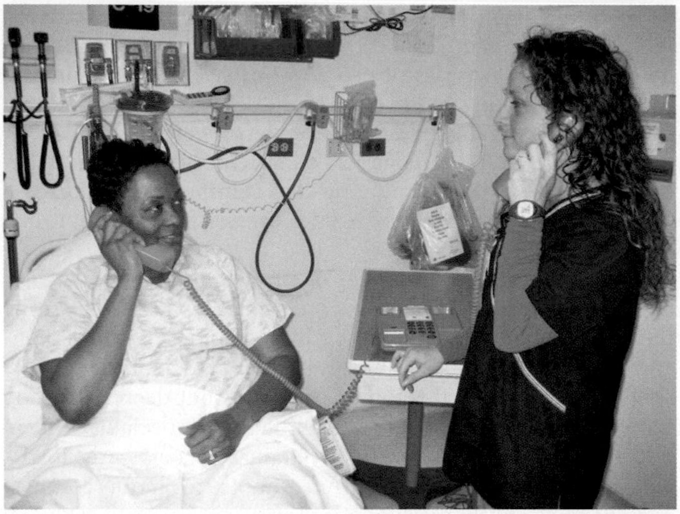

FIG. 4-2 Nurse communicating with a non-English-speaking patient using a translation phone service.

One cultural element that specifically affects the teaching-learning process is a conflict between the patient's cultural beliefs and values and the behaviors promoted by the health care team. For example, a patient who values a trim figure can be taught to use diet and exercise to retain that figure while at the same time improving BP control. However, in another patient's culture, being heavier may be valued as a sign of financial success and sexuality. This patient may have more difficulty accepting the need for diet and exercise unless the importance of BP control is understood.

Also assess the patient's use of cultural remedies and folk healers. For teaching to be effective, incorporate cultural health practices into the teaching plan. Also consider the cultural remedies that may interfere with or are contraindicated by the treatment plan.

In addition, it is important to know who has authority in the patient's culture. The patient may defer to the authority, such as an elder or a spiritual leader, for decisions. In this case, identify and work with the decision makers in the patient's cultural group. (See Chapter 2 for more information on cultural competence.)

Socioeconomic Considerations. A variety of socioeconomic factors are considered when preparing to teach patients. Knowing the patient's present or past occupation may assist you in determining the vocabulary to use during teaching. For example, an auto mechanic might understand the volume overload associated with heart failure as flooding an engine. An engineer may understand the principles of physics associated with gravity and pressures when discussing vascular problems.

Ask the patient about living arrangements. Whether the patient lives alone, with friends, or with family will influence who is included in the teaching process. You may need to modify the teaching plan if the patient does not have access to electricity or phones. If the patient has unmet learning needs by the time of discharge, arrange for continued teaching after discharge.

Learner Factors. Finally, assess learner factors, including the patient's learning needs, readiness to learn, and learning style.

Learning Needs. Learning needs are the new knowledge and skills that an individual must have to meet a goal. The assessment of learning needs should first determine what the patient already knows, whether the patient has misinformation, and any past experiences with health problems. Patients with long-standing health problems may have different learning needs from those patients with newly diagnosed health problems.

What a patient should learn about managing an illness or what behaviors need to be changed to promote health may seem obvious to you. However, what you think is important may be different from what patients want to know. Remember that adults learn best when the teaching provides information that they view as being needed immediately (see Table 4-1). Ask patients to prioritize what they see as the most critical information. For example, give the patient a list of the recommended topics to choose from. Also ask the patient to identify other topics not on the list. Having patients prioritize their own learning needs allows you to begin with the patient's most important needs. When information regarding life-threatening complications is needed, promote the priority of learning this content by explaining why the information is "need to know." Tailor your teaching to meet your patient's individual learning needs, especially when time is limited.

Readiness to Learn. Readiness to learn and motivation depend on multiple factors, such as perceived need, attitudes, and beliefs. When teaching adults, identify what information the person values. Readiness to learn is increased if the patient perceives a need for information, has a belief that a behavior change has value, or perceives the learning activities as new and stimulating.[27]

Before implementing the teaching plan, determine where the patient is in the stages of change process (see Table 4-2). If the patient is only in the precontemplation stage, just provide support and increase the patient's awareness of the problem until the patient is ready to consider a change in behavior. Nurses in outpatient settings and home health care can continue to evaluate the patient's readiness to learn and implement the teaching plan as the patient moves through the stages of change. Reinforcement is a strong motivational factor for achieving a desired behavior and needs to be incorporated throughout the change process. Positive reinforcement involves rewarding the target behavior with positive feedback or other rewards to maintain the behavior.[8]

Learning Style. Each person has a distinct style of learning that is as individual as his or her personality. The three general learning styles are (1) *visual* (reading, pictures), (2) *auditory* (listening), and (3) *physical* (doing things). People often use more than one learning style to acquire new information or skills. To assess a patient's learning style, ask how the patient prefers to learn and how the patient has learned in the past.[28] During assessment of the patient's learning style, identify the patient who does not read or who has limited health literacy. For example, the patient may tell you that he or she does not read much, but likes to learn from television programs. If possible, always use auditory and visual methods (e.g., CDs/DVDs) when patients specifically identify them as preferred methods of learning.

Planning

Prioritize the patient's learning needs and agree on learning goals. If the patient's physical or psychologic condition interferes with his or her participation, the patient's caregiver(s) can assist you in the planning phase.

Setting Goals. It is important to write clear, attainable, and measurable learning objectives or goals. Learning goals relate to the intended outcome of the learning process, guide the selection of teaching strategies, and help evaluate the patient's progress. Learning goals are parallel to patient outcomes in the nursing care plan (NCP). Many settings provide standardized NCPs that contain preset goals and interventions for specific learning needs. Modify these NCPs based on the patient's unique sociocultural and learner characteristics.

Standardized teaching plans are often included in care management guides and clinical practice guidelines. Standardized teaching plans frequently contain evidence-based information and skills that a patient and caregiver need to know concerning a specific health problem or procedure. However, as with NCPs, individualize these plans to meet the patient's specific needs. (See eFig. 4-1, eFig. 4-2, and eTable 4-1 on the website for this chapter for information on writing objectives or goals and examples of standardized teaching plans.)

EVIDENCE-BASED PRACTICE

Translating Research Into Practice

Are Decision Aids Helpful in Making Decisions About Health Care?

Clinical Question

For patients (P) with treatment and screening decisions, what is the effect of decision aids (I) versus usual teaching interventions (C) on outcomes associated with decisions about health care (O)?

Best Available Evidence

Systematic review of randomized controlled trials (RCTs).

Critical Appraisal and Synthesis of Evidence

- 86 RCTs ($n = 20{,}209$) of adults comparing use of decision aids versus usual care interventions on decision making attributes and behavioral outcomes.
- Decision aids provide information about treatment or screening options that may be valued differently by patients. Aids may be pamphlets, videos, or Internet-based tools.
- Knowledge, decisional conflict, patient-provider communication, and effect on behavior and health care system were measured.
- Decision aids significantly improved knowledge; reduced patient passivity and feelings of being uninformed; positively affected patient-provider communication; and reduced patient elective choices for invasive surgery, prostate specific antigen (PSA) screening, and menopausal hormone usage.

Conclusion

- Decision aids are valuable in helping patients decide among various treatments and screening options.

Implications for Nursing Practice

- Provide decision-making aids and collaboratively engage in communication with patients who face choices in treatment and screening.
- Involve patients in the decision-making process by sharing realistic perceptions of benefits and harms of options.
- Clarify with patients their personal values when exploring health care choices.

Reference for Evidence

Stacy D, Bennett C, Barry M, et al: Decision aids for people facing health treatment or screening decisions, *Cochrane Database Syst Rev* 10: CD00143, 2011.

P, Patient population of interest; *I*, intervention or area of interest; *C*, comparison of interest or comparison group; *O*, outcomes of interest; *T*, timing (see p. 12).

Selecting Teaching Strategies. Three factors that determine teaching strategies are (1) patient characteristics (e.g., age, educational background, culture, language skills), (2) subject matter, and (3) available resources. Table 4-8 provides a summary of the various learner characteristics and recommended teaching strategies based on the generation of the patient or caregiver.[29,30]

Various teaching strategies are used to enhance learning (Table 4-9). Frequently, several teaching strategies are used together (Fig. 4-3). Discussion is the most common type of interaction used in teaching patients and caregivers. Another type of group teaching involves *peer teaching*, as found in support groups. Patients dealing with common problems such as cancer, alcoholism, and eating disorders can benefit from peer teaching.

Learning Materials. Use learning materials that are provided in multiple formats (see Table 4-9). To use this strategy, know what materials are available within the facility, from support agencies, and from professional groups. The use of CDs/DVDs is extremely beneficial, particularly when teaching content that is largely visual, such as the steps of a procedure (e.g., suctioning a tracheostomy). The health care facility's television system may also deliver patient teaching programs (see Fig. 4-3). A

TABLE 4-8 LEARNER CHARACTERISTICS AND TEACHING STRATEGIES BY GENERATION

Birth Year	Learner Characteristics	Recommended Teaching Strategies
Millennials		
1981-2000	• Autonomous • Multitaskers • Prefer interactive and virtual environments • Technologically focused • Integrative thinking • Short attention span	• Provide access to Internet in patient's room. • Discuss reliable websites. • Download health information to cell phones, iPods, or similar devices. • Use video games and game systems to teach health behaviors (e.g., Wii Fit).
Generation X		
1965-1980	• Interaction with groups • Self-directed learning • Self-reliant	• Use group teaching sessions. • Recommend support groups. • Suggest role playing. • Provide Internet-based education materials.
Baby Boomers		
1946-1964	• Emphasis on self-knowledge • Acquisition of knowledge from authoritative sources	• Consider lecture or lecture-discussion (e.g., PowerPoint presentation). • Use patient education TV channels. • Provide printed materials.
Veterans		
Born before 1946	• Emphasis on rote learning • Memorization of knowledge	• Consider lecture or lecture-discussion. • Use pictures and printed materials such as books.

Compiled from Rose J: Designing training for Gen Y: learning style and values of Generation Y, 2007. Retrieved from *http://trainingpd.suite101.com/article.cfm/designing_training_for_gen_y;* and Educational strategies in generational designs, *Prog Transplant* 16(1):8, 2006.

TABLE 4-9 COMPARISON OF TEACHING STRATEGIES

Description	Advantages	Limitations
Discussion ("Teach Back")		
• Purpose is to exchange points of view about a topic or to arrive at a decision or conclusion. • Can be done with patient, with patient and caregiver, or with group. *Example:* Weight loss	• Allows for an active exchange of information and previous experiences among participants. • Good choice when patients have previous experience with subject and have information to share. • Nonthreatening format. • Can use peers (patients with common problems) to teach.	• May require additional time depending on topic and number of participants.
Lecture-Discussion		
• Commonly used when group of patients and caregivers can benefit from basic information. • Lecture portion is short (i.e., 15-20 minutes). • Discussion ("teach back") follows lecture. *Example:* Basic principles of cardiac rehabilitation (e.g., exercise, nutrition)	• Combines short lecture to present basic information with time for discussion. • Provision of printed material related to lecture content is useful and recommended.	• Need to limit number of lecture topics to 5-7. • May require additional time depending on topic and number of participants.
Demonstration/Return Demonstration ("Show Back")		
• Purpose is to teach patient and caregiver to perform a skill. • Through return demonstration ("show back") can evaluate patient's ability to perform skill (see Fig. 4-4). *Examples:* Dressing change, injection	• Provides for learning and practice of physical skills. • Dividing skill into series of smaller steps facilitates mastery and provides reinforcement.	• May require additional time for practice needed to master skill. • Patients with limited manual dexterity may have difficulty.
Role Play		

• Used when patients need to
  • Examine attitudes and behaviors
  • Understand viewpoints of others
  • Practice carrying out ideas or decisions
Example: Wife who rehearses how to talk with husband about need to quit smoking
	• Allows participants to rehearse variety of situations involving difficult decisions, attitudes, behaviors, etc.
	• Practicing ahead of time may increase self-efficacy.
		• May not be appropriate for all learners, since a certain level of maturity, confidence, and flexibility is required.
		• Requires adequate time for feedback and evaluation.

Learning Materials		

• Use of audiovisual materials to supplement teaching including
  • Printed materials (e.g., brochures)
  • CDs/DVDs
• Hospital-based TV
• Internet-based programs
	• Enhance the presentation through visual and/or auditory stimulation.
	• Best used in combination with other teaching strategies.
	• Use of the Internet for health information is the preferred choice for many.
	• Internet access in hospitals (including patient rooms) is increasing.
		• Materials must be previewed and evaluated (e.g., accuracy, completeness, reading level) before using.
		• Sites must be previewed and evaluated for validity of information.
		• Problems include limited access and inaccurate information.
		• May not be appropriate for all learners (e.g., lack of interest, decreased mental capacity).

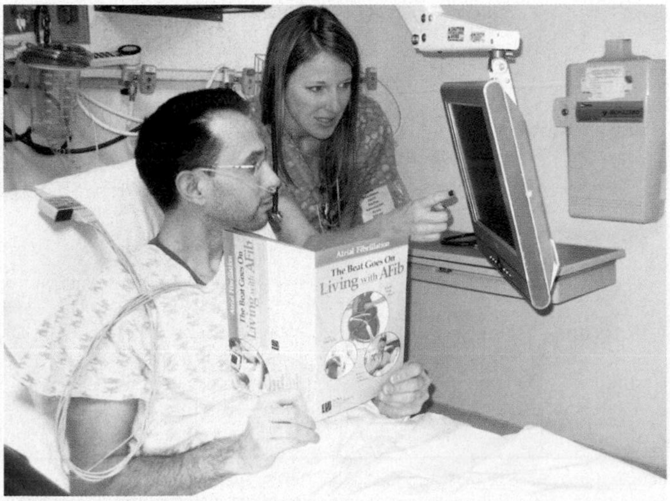

FIG. 4-3 Effective teaching using a variety of strategies (written materials, video-based patient education programs).

dedicated channel may be available and contain high-quality, professionally produced programs provided on demand or on a rotating schedule. Alternatively, education programs produced by the health care facility may be available on a hospital-based channel and provide content tailored to the patient experience.

Printed educational materials are widely used for teaching patients and caregivers. These materials are most often used in combination with previously discussed teaching strategies. For instance, after a discussion on the effects of smoking on heart disease, you might use a pamphlet from the American Cancer Society to reinforce the pathophysiologic effects of smoking. For a patient who has had surgery for breast cancer, you might provide a book or magazine article written by a woman who has had a mastectomy. Suggest that the patient read this material to prepare for other teaching sessions. Recommend written materials for patients whose preferred learning style is reading.

Before using written materials with patients, evaluate the readability level if it is not indicated on the materials. Several word processing programs (e.g., Microsoft Word) can assess the readability level of written materials. The use of Internet-based programs (e.g., *www.wordscount.info*) also can help you determine the readability and grade level of printed materials.

When writing teaching materials, use several techniques to keep the reading level at a fifth-grade level, including the following: (1) give key information first using bold or italics; (2) use short, common words of one or two syllables; (3) define medical words in simple language if they must be used; (4) keep sentences under 10 words if possible, and 15 at the most; (5) use pictures or drawings; and (6) use an active voice in the manner you would normally say something.[31] Pictographs (simple line drawings) combined with simplified text are an effective tool to improve discharge education for older adults with low literacy.[32]

Major resources for acquiring relevant printed material include the hospital or care facility library, pharmacies, public libraries, federal and state agencies, universities, voluntary organizations, research centers, and websites. Review written materials, including computer-based programs, before using them. In addition to reading level, review the material to determine whether it (1) is accurate, (2) is complete, (3) meets specific learning goals, (4) uses pictures and diagrams to stimulate interest, (5) uses one main idea or concept per pamphlet or program, (6) contains information the patient would like to know, and (7) is culture and gender sensitive and appropriate.[4]

Patients' use of the Internet to obtain health information continues to increase. Patients can quickly do an Internet search and have access to information about their disease, medications, treatments, and surgeries. Your job is to help the patient sift through the wide variety of information to find information that is valid, reliable, and usable. Understanding the principles of web searching for medical information and instructing the patient in finding valid information are critical. An estimated 80% of the people who use the Internet use it to gather health information. Factors that predict use of the Internet for this purpose include access to high-speed connections, younger age, some college education, and confidence in using technology.[33,34] Patients who are chronically ill are more likely to base health decisions on information that they find on the Internet.[33] Encourage patients to use Internet sites established by the government, universities, or reputable health-related associations (e.g., American Diabetes Association, American Heart Association, National Institutes of Health, U.S. Food and Drug Administration). Resources at the end of the chapter identify selected reliable websites for you to review and use for patient teaching.

Although older adults are using the Internet in greater numbers, many may not have the mental capacity, patience, or technical skills to successfully find information. Organizations dedicated to improving the quality of life for older adults are promoting the development of user-friendly websites (available at *www.nlm.nih.gov/pubs/checklist.pdf*) and publishing guides to help older adults evaluate web-based health information.

Obstacles to successful use of the Internet by many patients include limited access, lack of interest, and inaccurate information.[35] The presence of Internet connections in many hospital rooms provide an opportunity for you to teach patients about their illness and how to use the Internet to find health-related information.

The quantity and complexity of health care technology that patients and you have access to for patient teaching are increasing. Telehealth, interactive video, wireless technology, and podcasting are just some of the current technologies that patients may use to manage their health care. *Telehealth* is the delivery of health-related services and information via telecommunications technologies. Telehealth is used to monitor patients' cardiac rhythms, weights, and vital signs and to provide education (see Fig. 35-6). Wireless technology also may be used to monitor patients' blood glucose levels. Always educate yourself about these technologies before teaching patients.

Implementation

During the implementation phase, use the planned teaching strategies to present information and teach new skills (see Table 4-9). Incorporate verbal and nonverbal communication skills, active listening, and empathy into the process. Based on the assessment of the patient's physical, psychologic, sociocultural, and learner characteristics, determine how much the patient can participate. Whenever possible and appropriate, involve the patient's caregiver(s) in the teaching-learning process.

In implementing the teaching plan, remember the principles and characteristics of the adult learner. Reinforcement and reward are important, but be aware that phrases such as "Aren't you doing well?" in a tone one would use with a child can be condescending to adult learners.

Evaluation

Evaluation, the final step in the learning process, is a measure of the degree to which the patient has achieved the learning goals. Various evaluation techniques can be used (Table 4-10). Use techniques such as "teach back" and "show back" to determine the knowledge and skill levels of the patient and/or caregiver throughout the teaching and learning process[27,36] (Fig. 4-4). If certain goals are not reached, reassess the patient and revise the teaching plan accordingly.

For example, an older man with diabetes mellitus entered the hospital with a blood glucose level of 550 mg/dL (30.53 mmol/L). When the student nurse began to prepare his insulin injection, the nurse asked, "Are you going to have him give his own insulin and observe his technique?" "Oh, no," replied the student nurse, "He has been diabetic for 20 years!" The assumption was that a patient with diabetes would know how to perform this task

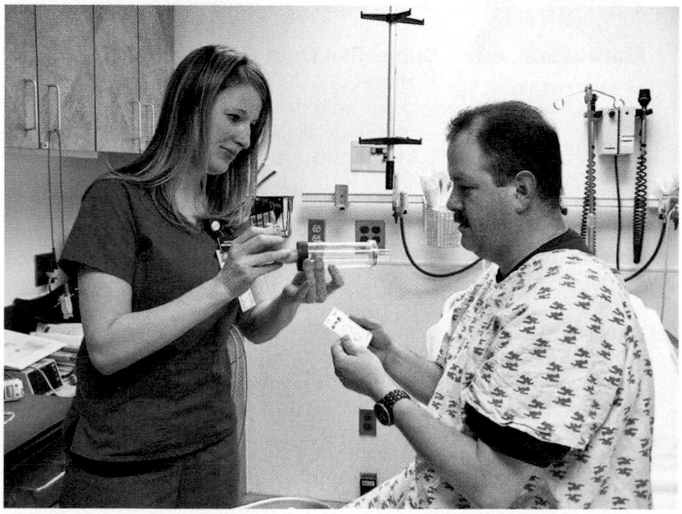

FIG. 4-4 Teaching using demonstration and return demonstration ("show back") increases successful learning by the patient.

TABLE 4-10 **TECHNIQUES TO EVALUATE PATIENT AND CAREGIVER LEARNING**

Technique	Strategy and Examples

Observe patient or caregiver directly.	• Ask person to show you how to change the dressing.
	• Return demonstration ("show back") determines whether
	  • Skill has been mastered.
	  • Further instruction is needed.
	  • Patient and caregiver are ready for new or additional content.

Observe verbal and nonverbal cues.	• Teaching may need to be delayed, further teaching is needed, or different strategy should be used if patient or caregiver
	  • Asks you to repeat instructions
	  • Loses eye contact
	  • Begins to doze in chair or bed
	  • Becomes restless or fidgety
	  • Does not speak English

Ask open-ended questions ("teach back").	• Open-ended questions provide more information about understanding than close-ended questions that require only a "yes" or "no."
	• Ask questions such as
	  • "How often do you need to change the dressing?"
	  • "What will you do if you develop chest pain after returning home?"

Talk with caregiver ("teach back").	• Involve caregiver in the evaluation process.
	• Ask questions such as
	  • "What medications is she taking?"
	  • "How often does he use his oxygen?"

Seek the patient's self-evaluation of progress.	• Ask patient's opinion about his or her progress.
	  • What evidence does the patient have that the goals are being met?
	  • Is the patient ready to go forward with learning new material?

correctly. The nurse and the student nurse returned to the patient's room and asked him to prepare an insulin injection ("show back"). The patient filled the syringe with 30 units of insulin and 10 units of air, instead of 40 units of insulin. After correcting the dose and questioning the patient more fully ("teach back"), the nurses concluded that the patient knew his correct dosage of insulin but could not accurately see the markings on the syringe. The patient most likely had been administering insufficient insulin to himself for some time. The patient's vision was not as good as it had been 20 years ago, and special equipment was now necessary for him to safely and accurately administer the insulin. The lesson here is that assumptions regarding a patient's knowledge and skills are dangerous. Evaluate all past and new learning as well as present abilities.

Long-term evaluation of learning goals often requires follow-up after discharge. Provide a written schedule of visits and other appropriate referrals for the patient before he or she leaves the hospital or clinic. The patient's caregiver(s) also must be familiar with the follow-up plan, so that everyone involved in the patient's long-term progress is on the same page.[18,37]

Documentation is an essential and required component throughout the entire teaching-learning process. Record everything from the assessment through plans for evaluation and follow-up. Because various members of the health care team use these records in different settings and for different reasons, the teaching goals, strategies, and evaluation results need to be clear, complete, and available to all members of the health care team.

CASE STUDY

Patient and Caregiver Teaching

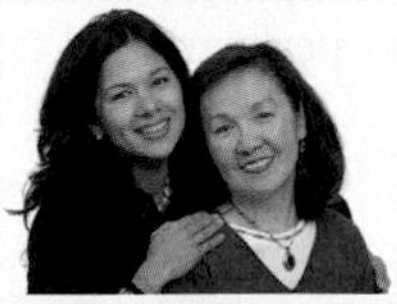

Thomas M Perkins/ Shutterstock.com

Patient Profile

M.L., a 60-year-old Asian woman, is admitted to the hospital with a diagnosis of exacerbation of chronic obstructive pulmonary disease (COPD).

Subjective Data

- History of COPD for 10 years; reports a chronic cough, and denies any recent change in color of sputum; states "I stopped smoking last year but my son-in-law smokes"
- Past medical history: gastroesophageal reflux disease; macular degeneration in right eye
- Social history: widowed 5 years ago and since then has lived with daughter and son-in-law who work full time; cares for two young grandchildren after school; English is M.L.'s second language

Objective Data

Physical Examination

- Alert, cognitively intact, anxious, thin woman with dyspnea on minimal exertion; speaking in short phases or sentences; states "I have no energy"
- Using oxygen via nasal cannula at 2 L/min
- Weight 100 lb, height 5 ft 2 in
- Wears glasses

Diagnostic Studies

- Chest x-ray negative for acute infection
- Arterial blood gases on room air: pH 7.35, $PaCO_2$ 47 mm Hg, PaO_2 75 mm Hg, HCO_3^- 30 mEq/L
- O_2 saturation (via pulse oximetry) during 6-minute walk test on room air = 83%
- Forced expiratory volume in 1 second of expiration (FEV_1) = 60% of predicted

Collaborative Care

- Medications: bronchodilator therapy (inpatient nebulizer therapy, inhalers on discharge), oral corticosteroids
- Long-term home O_2 therapy: O_2 at 2 L/min via nasal cannula
- Pulmonary rehabilitation: inpatient and outpatient

Discussion Questions

1. ***Priority Decision:*** Given M.L.'s history, what are the priority learning needs?
2. What factors (e.g., sociocultural, physical, psychologic) may influence M.L.'s response to teaching?
3. What potential challenges might you expect when planning to teach M.L.? How would you manage them?
4. ***Priority Decision:*** Identify two priority nursing diagnoses. Develop a teaching plan for M.L. based on these nursing diagnoses.

evolve Answers available at *http://evolve.elsevier.com/Lewis/medsurg.*

BRIDGE TO NCLEX EXAMINATION

The number of the question corresponds to the same-numbered outcome at the beginning of the chapter.

1. What would be the priority teaching goal for a middle-aged Hispanic woman regarding methods to relieve symptoms of menopause?
   a. Prevent the development of future disease.
   b. Maintain the patient's current state of health.
   c. Change the patient's cultural belief regarding the use of herbs.
   d. Provide information for selection and use of treatment options.
2. When planning teaching with consideration of the diverse learning needs of adults, the nurse's best approach would include
   a. presenting material in an efficient lecture format.
   b. recognizing that adults enjoy learning regardless of the relevance to their personal lives.
   c. providing opportunities for the patient to learn from other adults with similar experiences.
   d. postponing practice of new skills until the patient can independently practice the skill at home.
3. Which is the priority patient teaching strategy when limited time is available?
   a. Setting realistic goals that have high priority for the patient
   b. Referring the patient to a nurse educator in private practice for teaching
   c. Observing more experienced nurse-teachers to learn how to teach faster and more efficiently
   d. Providing reading materials for the patient instead of discussing information the patient needs to learn
4. The nurse needs to include caregivers in patient teaching primarily because *(select all that apply)*
   a. they provide most of the care for patients after discharge.
   b. they might feel rejected if they are not included in the teaching.
   c. patients have better outcomes when their caregivers are involved.
   d. the patient may be too ill or too stressed to fully understand the teaching.
   e. caregivers are responsible for the overall management of the patient's care.
5. Which technique is most appropriate when using motivational interviewing with a patient who tells you that he is ready to start a weight loss program?
   a. Confirm that the patient is serious about losing weight.
   b. Insist that the patient consider an organized group weight loss program.
   c. Focus on the patient's strengths to support his optimism that he can successfully lose weight.
   d. Ask a prescribed set of questions to increase the patient's awareness of his dietary behaviors.
6. Which patient characteristic enhances the teaching-learning process?
   a. Moderate anxiety
   b. High self-efficacy
   c. Being in the precontemplative stage of change
   d. Being able to laugh about the current health problem
7. A patient tells the nurse that she enjoys talking with others and sharing experiences, but easily falls asleep when reading. Which teaching strategy would be most effective with this patient?
   a. Role play
   b. Group teaching
   c. Lecture-discussion
   d. Discussion supplemented with computer programs
8. The nurse has taught a patient's caregiver how to administer insulin to her husband. Evaluation of the nurse's teaching effectiveness before discharge would include
   a. arranging for follow-up with a home care nurse.
   b. monitoring the patient's glucose readings before discharge.
   c. asking the caregiver to "show back" her ability to administer insulin.
   d. asking the caregiver what she found helpful about the teaching experience.

1. d, 2. c, 3. a, 4. c, d, 5. c, 6. b, 7. b, 8. c.

evolve

For rationales to these answers and even more NCLEX review questions, visit *http://evolve.elsevier.com/Lewis/medsurg.*

REFERENCES

1. National Center for Chronic Disease Prevention and Health Promotion: *Chronic disease overview*, Washington, DC, 2010, Centers for Disease Control and Prevention. Retrieved from *www.cdc.gov/nccdphp/overview.htm.*
2. Jack BW, Chetty VK, Anthony D, et al: A reengineered hospital discharge program to decrease rehospitalization: a randomized trial, *Ann Intern Med* 150:178, 2009.
3. The Joint Commission: 2011 Hospital national patient safety goals. Retrieved from *www.jointcommission.org/assets/1/6/HAP_NPSG_6-10-11.pdf.*
4. The Joint Commission: What did the doctor say? Improving health literacy to protect patient safety, 2007. Retrieved from *www.jointcommission.org/assets/1/18/improving_health_literacy.pdf.*
5. American Nurses Credentialing Center, Magnet Recognition Program Model: Exemplary professional practice: nurses as teachers, 2011. Retrieved from *http://nursecredentialing.org/Magnet/ProgramOverview/New-Magnet-Model.aspx#ExemplaryProfessionalPractice.*
6. Redman BK: *The practice of patient education*, ed 10, St Louis, 2007, Mosby.

7. Knowles MS, Holton EF, Swanson RA: *The adult learner: the definitive classic in adult education and human resource development*, ed 7, St Louis, 2011, Mosby.
8. Cancer Prevention Research Center: Detailed overview of the transtheoretical model. Retrieved from *www.uri.edu/research/cprc/TTM/detailedoverview.htm*.
9. Rollnick S, Miller WR, Yahne CE: *Motivational interviewing in health care: helping patients change behavior*, New York, 2008, Builford Press.
10. Miller WR: *Enhancing motivation for change in substance abuse treatment: Treatment Improvement Protocol (TIP) series 35, DHHS pub no (SMA) 99-3354*, Rockville, Md, 1999, US Department of Health and Human Services. Retrieved from *www.ncbi.nlm.nih.gov/books/NBK14856*. (Classic)
11. Feinberg L, Reinhard SC, Houser A, et al: Valuing the invaluable: 2011 update—the growing contributions and costs of family caregiving, AARP Public Policy Institute. Retrieved from *http://assets.aarp.org/rgcenter/ppi/ltc/i51-caregiving.pdf*.
12. Levine C: Supporting family caregivers: the hospital nurse's assessment of family caregiver needs, *Am J Nurs* 111:47, 2011.
13. Naylor MD, Aiken LH, Kurtzman ET, et al: The care span: the importance of transitional care in achieving health reform, *Health Affairs* 30:746, 2011.
*14. White K, D'Andrew N, Auret K, et al: Learn now: live well: an educational programme for caregivers, *Int J Palliative Nurs* 14(10):497, 2008.
15. Caregiver stress, 2011. Retrieved from *www.caregiversupport.org/caregiver_stress.cfm*.
16. Pagan CN: A caregiver's guide to staying well, *Arthritis Today* 25(6):80, 2011.
17. American Hospital Association: The patient care partnership: understanding expectations, rights and responsibilities, 2003. Retrieved from *www.aha.org/advocacy-issues/communicatingpts/pt-care-partnership.shtml*.
18. The Joint Commission: Speak up initiatives, 2011. Retrieved from *www.jointcommission.org/speakup.aspx*.
19. National Patient Safety Foundation: Ask me 3. Retrieved from *www.npsf.org/for-healthcare-professionals/programs/ask-me-3*.
*20. Kelley K, Abraham C: Health promotion for people aged over 65 years in hospitals: nurses' perceptions about their role, *J Clin Nurs* 16(3):569, 2007.
*21. Farrell K, Wicks MN, Martin JC: Chronic disease self-management improved with enhanced self-efficacy, *Clin Nurs Res* 13(4):289, 2004. (Classic)
*22. Resnick B: A longitudinal analysis of efficacy expectations and exercise in older adults, *Res Theory Nurs Pract* 18(4):331, 2004. (Classic)
23. Barclay L: Screening questions may help predict limited health literacy, *Ann Fam Med* 7:24, 2009.
*24. Villaire M, Mayer G: Low health literacy: the impact on chronic illness management, *Prof Case Manage* 12(4):213, 2007.
25. Morris NS, MacLean CD, Chew LD, et al: The single item literacy screener: evaluation of a brief instrument to identify limited reading ability, *BMC Fam Pract* 7:21, 2006. (Classic)
26. Wilson-Stronks A, Lee KK, Cordero CL, et al: One size does not fit all: meeting the health care needs of diverse populations, Oakland Terrace, Ill, 2008, The Joint Commission. Retrieved from *www.jointcommission.org/assets/1/6/HLCOneSizeFinal.pdf*.
27. Nigolian CJ, Miller KL: Teaching essential skills to family caregivers, *Am J Nurs* 111:52, 2011.
28. Inott T, Kennedy BB: Assessing learning styles: practical tips for patient education, *Nurs Clin North Am* 46:313, 2011.
29. Rose J: Designing training for Gen Y: learning style and values of Generation Y, 2007. Retrieved from *http://trainingpd.suite101.com/article.cfm/designing_training_for_gen_y*.
30. Educational strategies in generational designs, *Prog Transplant* 16(1):8, 2006.
31. Medline Plus: How to write easy-to-read health materials, 2011. Retrieved from *www.nlm.nih.gov/medlineplus/etr.html*.
32. Choi J: Literature review: using pictographs in discharge instructions for older adults with low-literacy skills, *J Clin Nurs* 20:2984, 2011.
33. Fox S: Pew Internet and American Life Project: the engaged e-patient population, 2008. Retrieved from *www.pewinternet.org/Reports/2008/The-Engaged-Epatient-Population.aspx*.
34. Watson A, Bell A, Kvedar J, et al:. Reevaluating the digital divide: current lack of Internet use is not a barrier to adoption of novel health information technology, *Diabetes Care* 31(3):433, 2008.
35. Anderson A, Klemm P: The Internet: friend or foe when providing patient education? *Clin J Oncol Nurs* 12(1):55, 2008.
36. National Center for Ethics in Health Care: "Teach back": a tool for improving provider-patient communication, *In Focus: Topics in Health Care Ethics*, 2006. Retrieved from *www.ethics.va.gov/docs/infocus/InFocus_20060401_teach_Back.pdf*.
37. Agency for Healthcare Research and Quality: Implementing re-engineered hospital discharges (Project RED): frequently asked questions, 2009. Retrieved from *www.ahrq.gov/news/kt/red/redfaq.htm*.

*Evidence-based information for clinical practice.

RESOURCES

Family Caregiver Alliance
www.caregiver.org

GetWellNetwork
www.getwellnetwork.com/index.asp

Implementing Re-engineered Hospital Discharges (Project Red)
www.ahrq.gov/news/kt/red/redfaq.htm

The Joint Commission—Speak Up Initiatives
www.jointcommission.org/speakup.aspx

Mayo Clinic Health Information
www.mayoclinic.com/health-information

National Family Caregivers Association
www.nfcacares.org

U.S. Department of Health and Human Resources—Healthfinder
www.healthfinder.gov

U.S. National Library of Medicine and National Institutes of Health—MedlinePlus
www.nlm.nih.gov/medlineplus

WebMD
www.webmd.com

CHAPTER 5

Aging is not "lost youth" but a new stage of opportunity and strength.
Betty Friedan

Chronic Illness and Older Adults

Margaret Baker and Margaret McLean Heitkemper

evolve WEBSITE

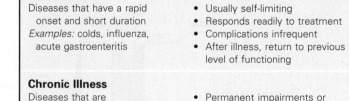

http://evolve.elsevier.com/Lewis/medsurg

- NCLEX Review Questions
- Key Points
- Pre-Test
- Answer Guidelines for Case Study on p. 76
- Rationales for Bridge to NCLEX Examination Questions
- Concept Map Creator
- Glossary
- Content Updates

eTable

- eTable 5-1: Geriatric Depression Scale (Short Form)

LEARNING OUTCOMES

1. Describe the prevention and major causes of chronic illness.
2. Explain the characteristics of a chronic illness.
3. Define *ageism*.
4. Explain the needs of special populations of older adults.
5. Describe nursing interventions to assist older adults with chronic conditions.
6. Describe common problems of older adults related to hospitalization and acute illness and the nurse's role in assisting them.
7. Differentiate among care alternatives to meet needs of older adults.
8. Describe the nurse's role in health promotion, disease prevention, and managing the special needs of older adults.

KEY TERMS

ageism, p. 65
chronic illness, Table 5-1, p. 61
elder mistreatment, p. 68
ethnogeriatric, p. 67
frail older adult, p. 64
gerontologic nursing, p. 71
Medicaid, p. 69
Medicare, p. 68
old-old adult, p. 64
young-old adult, p. 64

This chapter discusses issues related to chronic illness and aging. The population of older adults is growing quickly and they often have increased health care needs and problems that you need to consider.

CHRONIC ILLNESS

Illness can be categorized as either acute or chronic (Table 5-1). Today the U.S. health care system faces a growing burden of chronic illness as the population ages. Chronic diseases account for 70% of all deaths in the United States.[1] Chronic illness results in limitations in physical functioning, work productivity, and quality of life for nearly 1 out of 10 Americans, or about 31 million people. Older adults often live with more than one chronic illness. A significant portion of U.S. health care dollars go toward the treatment of chronic illnesses.[1] The management of a chronic illness can profoundly affect the lives and identities of the patient, family, and caregiver. Table 5-2 presents the impact of some chronic illnesses.

TABLE 5-1 CHARACTERISTICS OF ACUTE AND CHRONIC ILLNESS

Description	Characteristics
Acute Illness	
Diseases that have a rapid onset and short duration *Examples:* colds, influenza, acute gastroenteritis	• Usually self-limiting • Responds readily to treatment • Complications infrequent • After illness, return to previous level of functioning
Chronic Illness	
Diseases that are prolonged, do not resolve spontaneously, and are rarely cured completely *Examples:* see Table 5-2	• Permanent impairments or deviations from normal • Irreversible pathologic changes • Residual disability • Special rehabilitation required • Need for long-term medical and/or nursing management

Reviewed by Kathleen Blais, RN, EdD, Professor Emerita, Florida International University, College of Nursing and Health Sciences, Wilton Manors, Florida; Deborah Marks Conley, RN, MSN, APRN-CNS, GCNS-BC, FNGNA, Gerontological Clinical Nurse Specialist, Nebraska Methodist Hospital and Assistant Professor of Nursing, Nebraska Methodist College, Omaha, Nebraska; and Mary A. Cox, RN, MS, Professor, Nursing, Sinclair Community College, Dayton, Ohio.

TABLE 5-2 IMPACT OF CHRONIC ILLNESSES

Chronic Illness	Impact	Content in Book: Chapter	Content in Book: Page
Alzheimer's disease	• Affects 5.4 million people • 6th leading cause of death	60	1445
Arthritis	• Affects 1 in 5 people • One of most common chronic illnesses	65	1562
Cancer	• 2nd leading cause of death	16	247
Chronic obstructive pulmonary disease	• Affects many older adults • 3rd leading cause of death	29	579
Coronary artery disease	• Affects about 17 million adults • Leading cause of death	34	731
Diabetes	• Affects >25.8 million Americans • 7.0 million do not know they have the disease • 7th leading cause of death	49	1153
Heart failure	• Most common reason older adults are hospitalized	35	766
Obesity	• Affects >35% of adults • Major contributor to other health problems	41	906
Stroke	• Affects about 7 million adults, 15%-30% disabled • 4th leading cause of death	58	1388

Data from Centers for Disease Control and Prevention: Quick facts: economic and health burden of chronic disease. Retrieved from *www.cdc.gov/nccdphp/press/index.htm#3*; and Heart Disease and Stroke Statistics—2011 update.

TABLE 5-3 CHRONIC ILLNESS TRAJECTORY

Phases	Description
Onset	• Signs and symptoms are present. • Disease diagnosed.
Stable	• Illness course and symptoms controlled by treatment regimen. • Person maintains everyday activities.
Acute	• Active illness with severe and unrelieved symptoms or complications. • Hospitalization may be required for management.
Comeback	• Gradual return to an acceptable way of life.
Crisis	• Life-threatening situation occurs. • Emergency services are necessary.
Unstable	• Unable to keep symptoms or disease course under control. • Life becomes disrupted while patient works to regain stability. • Hospitalization not required.
Downward	• Gradual and progressive deterioration in physical or mental status. • Accompanied by increasing disability and symptoms. • Continuous alterations in everyday life activities.
Dying	• Patient has to relinquish everyday life interests and activities, let go, and die peacefully. • Immediate weeks, days, hours preceding death.

Source: Woog P: *The chronic illness trajectory framework: the Corbin and Strauss nursing model,* New York, 1992, Springer.

In addition to people living longer, other societal changes have contributed to the increase in chronic illnesses, including insufficient physical activity, lack of access to fresh fruits and vegetables, tobacco use, and alcohol consumption.[1]

Trajectory of Chronic Illness

Chronic illnesses may have acute exacerbations in which an individual moves from a level of optimum functioning, with the illness well controlled, to a period of instability during which the individual may need assistance. Corbin and Strauss proposed a view of chronic illness as a trajectory (Fig. 5-1) with overlapping phases[2] (Table 5-3). This trajectory characterizes the common course of most chronic illnesses. In addition,

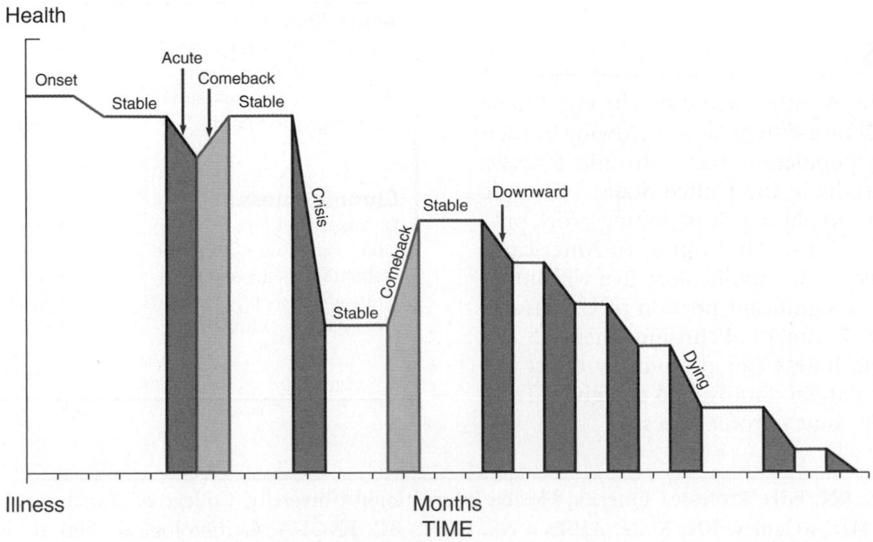

FIG. 5-1 The Chronic Illness Trajectory is a theoretical model of chronic illness. The trajectory model of chronic illness recognizes that chronic illness will have many phases (see Table 5-3).

TABLE 5-4 SEVEN TASKS OF PEOPLE WITH CHRONIC ILLNESS

1. Prevent and manage a crisis.
2. Carry out prescribed treatment regimen.
3. Control symptoms.
4. Reorder time.
5. Adjust to changes in course of disease.
6. Prevent social isolation.
7. Attempt to normalize interactions with others.

Source: Corbin JM, Strauss A: A nursing model for chronic illness management based upon the trajectory framework, *Sch Inq Nurs Pract* 5:155, 1991.

TABLE 5-5 CHARACTERISTICS OF TREATMENT REGIMENS

Characteristic	Example
Difficult	Managing a home hemodialysis unit
Time consuming	Dressing changes done four times daily
Painful or uncomfortable	Injecting heparin daily in the abdomen
Unsightly appearance	Tracheostomy
Slow rate of effectiveness	Lowering blood cholesterol level with medication or diet

Corbin and Strauss identified the seven tasks of those who are chronically ill[2] (Table 5-4). These tasks are discussed in the following sections.

Preventing and Managing a Crisis. Most chronic illnesses have the potential for an acute exacerbation of symptoms, which may result in further disability or death. Examples include the patient with heart disease who has another myocardial infarction or the patient with asthma who has a severe attack. A major task for both the patient and the caregiver is to learn to prevent or manage the crisis. First, the patient and caregiver need to understand the potential for the crisis to occur. Second, they need to know ways to prevent or modify the threat. This often involves adherence to a prescribed medical regimen. Patients also need to know the signs and symptoms of the onset of a crisis. Depending on the chronic illness, signs and symptoms may occur suddenly (e.g., seizure in a patient with seizure disorder) or slowly (e.g., heart failure in a patient with untreated hypertension). It is important for the patient and caregiver to develop a plan to manage a crisis that is likely to occur.

Carrying Out Prescribed Treatment Regimens. Treatment regimens vary in degree of difficulty and the impact that they have on the person's lifestyle. Characteristics of treatment regimens are included in Table 5-5.

Controlling Symptoms. An important task for those with chronic illnesses is to learn to control symptoms so that desired activities may be continued. Some individuals redesign their lifestyle by learning to plan ahead, such as the person with irritable bowel syndrome choosing to go only to events where there are restrooms near the seating area. Others may redesign their living space. Patients and their families or caregivers need to learn about the pattern of symptoms, such as typical onset, duration, and severity, so that lifestyle can be changed accordingly.

Reordering Time. Patients with chronic illness often report having too much or too little time. Treatment plans that require large amounts of time for the patient, as well as caregivers, may necessitate changing schedules or eliminating other activities.

Adjusting to Changes in Course of Disease. Some diseases, such as multiple sclerosis, have unpredictable courses that make planning activities difficult. Part of the patient's task is to develop a personal identity that includes the chronic illness and adjust to the lifestyle changes it necessitates.

Preventing Social Isolation. Social isolation may occur with chronic illness because the individual chooses to withdraw from previous activities or because others withdraw from the chronically ill person. An example is a man who has aphasia secondary to a stroke who may be unwilling to go out in public because he is embarrassed because of communication problems.

Attempting to Normalize Interactions With Others. Most individuals with chronic illness attempt to manage symptoms so that they can hide their disabilities or disfigurement. This may involve wearing a prosthesis or demonstrating that they can function the same as a person without a disability or chronic illness. An example of this is the man with chronic lung problems who stops walking to catch his breath, but appears to be inspecting a plant or looking in a store window.

Prevention of Chronic Illness

Chronic illnesses are often preventable. *Primary prevention* refers to measures such as proper diet, proper exercise, and immunizations that prevent the occurrence of a specific disease. *Secondary prevention* refers to actions aimed at early detection of disease that can lead to interventions to prevent disease progression. *Tertiary prevention* refers to activities that limit disease progression, such as rehabilitation.[3]

NURSING MANAGEMENT CHRONIC ILLNESS

Diagnosis and treatment of the acute phase or acute exacerbations of a chronic illness are sometimes done in a hospital. Other phases of a chronic illness are managed in an ambulatory care setting, at home, in an assisted living facility, or in a skilled nursing facility. The course of chronic illness is often unpredictable. The management of a chronic illness can profoundly affect the lives of the patient, caregiver, and family.

An assessment of health status includes an individual's level of daily functioning and his or her perception of relative health or illness. This health assessment includes activities of daily living (ADLs), such as bathing, dressing, eating, toileting, and transfer. It also includes instrumental ADLs (IADLs), such as using a phone, shopping, preparing food, housekeeping, doing laundry, arranging transportation, taking medications, and handling finances.

Because the majority of chronic illnesses are treated in an ambulatory care setting, it is increasingly important for patients and caregivers to understand and manage their own health. The term *self-management* refers to the individual's ability to manage his or her symptoms, treatment, physical and psychosocial consequences, and lifestyle changes in response to living with a long-term disorder.[4]

You play an important role in the management of individuals with chronic illness. This begins with planning care, teaching the patient and caregiver regarding the treatment plan, implementing strategies for symptom management, and assessing patient outcomes.

Family caregivers (e.g., spouses, adult children, partners) often have important roles in the life of the chronically ill person. The ideal situation is one in which family caregivers work together with the patient to manage the illness. This collaboration begins under the direction of the health care team at the time of diagnosis. When the caregiver is a spouse who is also older, he or she may have a chronic illness as well, which complicates the situation.[5] The stresses and needs of family caregivers are discussed in Chapter 4 and Table 4-5.

OLDER ADULTS

DEMOGRAPHICS OF AGING

In the past three decades the older adult population (those 65 years of age and older) has grown twice as fast as the rest of the population. Almost 40 million people, or 13% of the population, are age 65 or older.[6] Nearly one in five U.S. residents is expected to be 65 or older by 2030. The number of Americans age 85 or older is expected to more than triple, from 5.8 million to 19 million, between 2010 and 2050.[6] This dramatic increase is in part due to aging of the *Baby Boomers* (those born between 1946 and 1964) who began to turn 65 in 2011.

Upcoming cohorts of older adults will be better educated than previous cohorts and have greater access to technology and resources. In the United States 13% of people over age 65 are people of color, including 8% African Americans; 3% Asian/Pacific Islanders; and less than 1% American Indians, Eskimos, and Aleuts. People of Hispanic/Latino ethnicity (who may be of any race) represent 7% of the older population.[1] By 2030 the proportion of older adults who are people of color will increase 160% (Latinos 202%; African Americans 114%; American Indians, Eskimos, and Aleuts 145%; and Asian/Pacific Islanders 145%), while growth in the European-American population will increase by only 59%.[6]

Other factors add to the overall increase in the older population. Common diseases of the early to mid-twentieth century that killed many people before they reached older age, such as influenza and diarrhea, are now less common. Declining infant mortality, new drug therapies, mechanical devices, improved surgical interventions, health promotion, and earlier detection and treatment of diseases have contributed to the increase in life span.

The U.S. Census Bureau predicts life expectancy to continue to increase for both men and women. Men and women born in 1950 who reach age 65 can expect, on average, another 12.8 and 15.8 years of life, respectively.[1,7] Whether this gender difference is due to differences in health behaviors (e.g., smoking, alcohol use) or occupation is not known.[8]

The fastest-growing segment of older Americans is people ages 85 or older. Since the 1960s, this group has increased 250%. The terms **young-old adult** (65 to 74 years of age) and **old-old adult** (85 years of age and older) describe two groups of older adults with different characteristics and needs. The old-old adult is often a woman who is widowed, divorced, or single and dependent on family for support. Many have outlived children, spouses or partners, and siblings. Old-old adults are often characterized as hardy, elite survivors. Because old-old adults have lived so long, they may have become the family icon, the symbol of family tradition and legacy.

Nearly 6% of individuals age 65 to 74 and 25% of those 85 and older live in nursing homes.[8] The **frail older adult** is usually over age 75 and has physical, cognitive, or mental dysfunctions that may interfere with independently performing ADLs.[9] (Older frail adults are discussed later in this chapter.)

EVIDENCE-BASED PRACTICE

Translating Research Into Practice

What Is the Effectiveness of Chronic Illness Strategies for Asian/Pacific Islanders?

Clinical Question

What is the effectiveness (O) of self-management interventions (I) on chronic illness in Asian/Pacific Islanders (P)?

Best Available Evidence

Systematic review of randomized controlled trials (RCTs)

Critical Appraisal and Synthesis of Evidence

- 21 RCTs (*n* = 4446) related to chronic illness self-management and self-care in male and female Asian/Pacific Islanders, including Asians from Far East, Southeast Asia, or Indian subcontinent, and Pacific Islanders from Hawaii, Guam, and Samoa.
- Many chronic health conditions were examined, with diabetes mellitus being the most common.
- Alternative therapies (exercise and body-mind-spirit), cognitive-behavioral interventions (CBI), and health education programs lasting from 1 month to 2 years were included.
- All interventions, especially CBI, resulted in positive and significant health outcomes, including improvements in mood and quality of life.

Conclusion

- Self-management interventions assist Asian/Pacific Islanders in restoring and maintaining health while preventing disease.

Implications for Nursing Practice

- Tailor self-management interventions for ethnically diverse groups and monitor outcomes.
- Teach and assist patients in caring for themselves.
- Support patient self-management strategies that promote health.

Reference for Evidence

Inouye J, Braqinsky N, Kataoka-Yahiro M: Randomized clinical trials of self-management with Asian/Pacific Islanders, *Clin Nurs Res* 20:366, 2011.

P, Patient population of interest; *I*, intervention or area of interest; *O*, outcomes of interest (see p. 12).

ATTITUDES TOWARD AGING

Who is old? The answer to this question often depends on the respondent's age and attitude. It is important to understand that aging is normal and is not related to pathology or disease. Age is established by a date in time and is influenced by many factors, including emotional and physical health, developmental stage, socioeconomic status, culture, and ethnicity.[10]

As people age, they are exposed to new and different life experiences. The accumulation of these differences makes older adults more diverse than any other age-group. As you assess older adults, consider and value their diversity and life history. Also assess their own perceptions of what it means to be an older adult. Older adults with poor health report a higher perceived age and lower sense of well-being when compared with healthy older adults. The majority of older adults report having good-to-excellent health despite having a chronic illness. Age is important, but it may not be the most relevant factor in determining appropriate care of an individual older adult patient.

Myths and stereotypes about aging are often supported by media reports of older adults who are "problematic." These commonly held misconceptions may lead to errors in assessment and unnecessary limitations or interventions. For example, if you think that all older people are rigid in their thinking, you

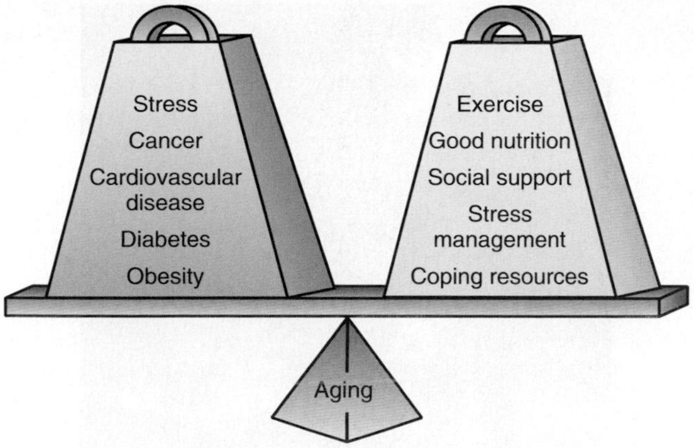

FIG. 5-2 The aging process can be viewed as a balance between negative and positive factors.

may not present new ideas to a patient.[11] **Ageism** is a negative attitude based on age. Ageism leads to discrimination and disparities in the care given to older adults. If you demonstrate negative attitudes, it may be because you fear your own aging process or you are not knowledgeable about aging and the health care needs of the older adult. Therefore it is important to gain knowledge about normal aging and have increased contact with older adults who are healthy and live independently. Also, it is your role as a nurse to dispel myths of aging.

BIOLOGIC AGING

From a biologic view, *aging* is defined as the progressive loss of function. The exact cause of biologic aging is unknown. Biologic aging is a multifactorial process involving genetics, diet, and environment.[12] In part, biologic aging can be viewed as a balance of positive and negative factors (Fig. 5-2).

Research is directed at increasing both the average life span and the quality of life of older adults. The hope is that new antiaging therapies will be developed to slow down or reverse age-related changes that result in chronic illness and disability. Based on numerous laboratory studies in rodents, caloric restriction (reducing dietary intake by 25% to 50%) has been consistently shown to significantly extend the life span.[13] It may be that caloric restriction results in changes in body composition, metabolism, and hormones that are conducive to long life. Caloric restriction in humans is associated with decreases in the incidence of obesity, diabetes, hypertension, and cancer, all of which are associated with aging.[13,14]

A number of nutrients have been tested for their potential benefits in reducing the impact of aging. Examples include β-carotene, selenium, vitamin C, and vitamin E. To date, research has failed to show that large doses of these supplements prevent chronic illness, such as heart disease or diabetes.[15] However, much more research is needed before it is determined whether any of these substances will delay aging or enhance the functional ability of older adults.

AGE-RELATED PHYSIOLOGIC CHANGES

Age-related changes affect every body system. These changes are normal and occur as people age. However, the age at which specific changes occur differs from person to person and within the same person. For instance, a person may have gray hair at age 45 but relatively unwrinkled skin at age 80. In your role as a nurse, assess for age-related changes. Table 5-6 presents a list of tables where specific age-related assessment findings can be found throughout the book.

TABLE 5-6 GERONTOLOGIC ASSESSMENT DIFFERENCES

Summary of Tables

Body System	Table Number	Page
Visual	21-1	371
Auditory	21-7	380
Integumentary	23-1	417
Respiratory	26-4	481
Hematologic	30-3	619
Cardiovascular	32-1	691
Gastrointestinal	39-5	871
Urinary	45-2	1051
Endocrine	48-3	1141
Reproductive	51-3	1225
Nervous	56-4	1344
Musculoskeletal	62-1	1494

SPECIAL OLDER ADULT POPULATIONS

Chronically Ill Older Adults

Daily living with chronic illness is a reality for many older adults. The incidence of chronic illness triples after age 45. Most people 65 years of age and older have at least one chronic condition, and many have multiple conditions.[1] The most common chronic conditions in older adults are hypertension, osteoarthritis, heart disease, cancer, and diabetes. Other common chronic conditions include Alzheimer's disease, vision and hearing deficits, osteoporosis, hip fractures, stroke, Parkinson's disease, and depression.

Older Adult Women

For the aging woman, the impact of an aging body and being a woman is considered double jeopardy. Many factors have a significant negative impact on the health of older women (see Gender Differences box). Many of these factors are directly

GENDER DIFFERENCES

Older Adults

Men
- More likely to be living with spouse
- More likely to have health insurance
- Higher income after retirement
- Less likely to be involved in caregiving activities
- Generally have fewer chronic health problems than women

Women
- More likely to live alone
- Loss of spouse more common
- Less likely to have health insurance
- More likely to live in poverty
- Poverty rates highest among minority women
- Lack of formal work experience leading to lower income
- More likely to rely on Social Security as major source of income
- More likely to be caregiver of ill spouse
- Have a higher incidence of chronic health problems such as arthritis, hypertension, stroke, and diabetes

TABLE 5-7 GERONTOLOGIC ASSESSMENT DIFFERENCES

Cognitive Function

Cognitive Function	Effect of Aging
Fluid intelligence	Declines during middle age
Crystallized intelligence	Improves
Vocabulary and verbal reasoning	Improves
Spatial perception	Constant visuospatial perception Declines in spatial navigation tasks
Synthesis of new information	Declines during middle age
Mental performance speed	Declines during middle age
Short-term recall memory	Declines during old age
Long-term recall memory	Constant

related to reduced financial resources and the greater longevity of women compared with men. Thus older women often experience disparities, including unequal access to quality health care. (Health disparities are discussed in Chapter 2.) As a nurse, you are in an excellent position to be an advocate for equity for older women in the health care system. Advocacy organizations, such as the Older Women's League (OWL) and the Society for Women's Health Research, can be helpful in this process.

Cognitively Impaired Older Adults

Most healthy older adults have no noticeable decline in cognitive abilities (Table 5-7). Older adults may experience memory lapses or benign forgetfulness, which is significantly different from cognitive impairment. This is also referred to as *age-associated memory impairment.* Encourage older adults with memory loss to be evaluated by their primary care provider, and to use memory aids, attempt recall in a calm and quiet environment, and actively engage in memory improvement techniques. Memory aids include clocks, calendars, notes, marked pillboxes, safety alarms on stoves, and identity necklaces or bracelets. Memory techniques include word association, mental imaging, and mnemonics.

Declining physical health is an important factor that influences cognitive impairment. Older adults who experience sensory loss, heart failure, or cerebrovascular disease may show a decline in cognitive functioning.[16] Cognitive impairment, delirium, and dementia are discussed in Chapter 60.

Rural Older Adults

People over age 65 are less likely to live in metropolitan areas than younger people. Five barriers to health care access for older adults are transportation, limited supply of health care workers and facilities, lack of quality health care, social isolation, and financial limitations.[17,18] Rural older adults are often stressed by declining self-care abilities. Particularly vulnerable are older adults of color living in rural areas, who have even less access to health care providers. In addition, older adults who live in rural areas may be less likely to engage in health-promoting activities.

When you work with older adults in rural areas, recognize lifestyle values and practices of rural life (Fig. 5-3). In planning care, be aware that transportation is the number one barrier to health care for rural older adults. Alternative service approaches such as computer-based Internet sources and chat rooms, DVDs, radio, community centers, and church social events can be used to promote healthful practices or to conduct health screening (Fig. 5-4). The development of telehealth devices for

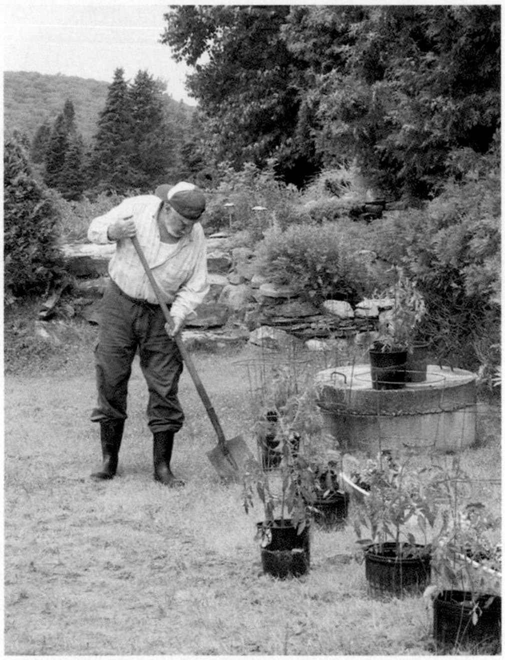

FIG. 5-3 Older adults living in rural areas often enjoy outside activities, such as gardening. (iStockphoto/Thinkstock)

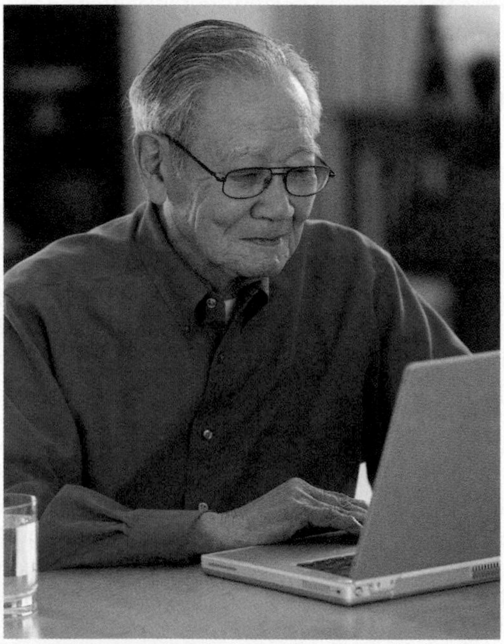

FIG. 5-4 Older adults are using computers more frequently and accessing health care information on the Internet. (Comstock Images/Thinkstock)

INFORMATICS IN PRACTICE

Older Adults and Internet Use

- Forty percent of older adults use the Internet to look for health information.
- Older adults are more likely to accept as true what they read on a Web page. This is related to a lack of Internet experience and confusion from the large amounts of available information.
- Teach patients who use the Internet as a source of information how to assess the credibility of a website.
- Suggest the use of websites that include senior-friendly design elements.

monitoring patients in their home environments has enhanced the ability to provide care to isolated individuals.[19] Innovative models of nursing practice must continue to be developed to assist the rural older adult.[20]

Homeless Older Adults

The number of older adults who are homeless is increasing. Key factors associated with homelessness include (1) having a low income, (2) having reduced cognitive capacity, (3) living alone, and (4) living in a community that lacks affordable housing. Homeless older adults may be chronically homeless or recently homeless because of a crisis in either health or economic status.[21]

Mortality rates for homeless older adults are three times higher than for older adults who have housing. Older adults who are homeless have more health problems and appear older. They are also at additional risk because many aging network services are not designed to reach out to people who are homeless. Older people who are homeless are less likely to use shelters or meal site services than younger homeless people.[22] Long-term care placement is often an alternative to homelessness, especially when the person is cognitively impaired and alone. Fear of institutionalization may explain why homeless older adults do not use shelter and meal site services. Care for homeless older adults requires an interdisciplinary approach (including nurses, physicians, social workers, clerical workers, and transporters) that links shelters with outreach, primary care clinics, Medicare and Medicaid offices, and pharmacies.

Frail Older Adults

Frailty is a geriatric syndrome in which three or more of the following are present: advanced age, unplanned weight loss (10 lb or more in the past year), weakness, poor endurance and energy, slowness, and low activity levels. Risk factors include disability, multiple chronic illnesses, and dementia. People are more likely to become frail if they smoke, have a history of depression or long-term medical health problems, or are underweight. The old-old population (85 years of age or older) is most at risk for frailty, although many in this age-group remain healthy and robust.

Older frail adults have difficulty coping with declining functional abilities and decreasing daily energy. When stressful life events (e.g., death of a pet) and daily strain (e.g., caring for an ill spouse) occur, frail older adults often cannot cope with the effects of stress and, as a result, may become ill. Common health problems of frail older adults include mobility limitations, sensory impairment, cognitive decline, falls, and increasing frailty.[23]

Frail older adults tire easily; have little physical reserve; and are at risk for disability, elder mistreatment, and institutionalization. Frail older adults are especially at risk for malnutrition and dehydration, which are related to factors such as living alone, depression, and low income. Other factors, such as declining cognitive status, inadequate dental care, sensory decreases, physical fatigue, and limited mobility, increase the risks of malnutrition and dehydration. Monitor frail older adults for adequate calorie, protein, iron, calcium, vitamin D, and fluid intake. Because medications may interfere with nutrition, perform a thorough medication review, including prescription drugs, over-the-counter drugs, vitamins, minerals, supplements, herbal remedies, and cultural remedies.

TABLE 5-8 SCALES: NUTRITIONAL ASSESSMENT OF OLDER ADULTS

The acronym SCALES can remind you to assess important nutritional indicators:

Sadness, or mood change
Cholesterol, high
Albumin, low
Loss or gain of weight
Eating problems (e.g., mechanical problems such as impaired swallowing, poor dentition)
Shopping and food preparation problems

A tool to assess the risk factors for poor nutritional status in older adults is presented in Table 5-8. Once an older adult's nutritional needs are identified, common interventions include home-delivered meals, dietary supplements, food stamps, dental referrals, and vitamin supplements.

CULTURALLY COMPETENT CARE

OLDER ADULTS

The term **ethnogeriatric** describes the specialty area of providing culturally competent care to older adults.[24] As American society changes, ethnic institutions and neighborhoods may also change. For the older adult with strong ethnic and cultural roots, there may be a loss of friends who speak the "mother tongue," a loss of the religious institution that supports social ethnic activities, and a loss of stores that carry desired ethnic foods. This sense of loss is increased when children and others deny or ignore ethnic and cultural practices. Support for older adults of color is most frequently found in the family, religious practices, and isolated geographic or community ethnic clusters. In the old-old population, members of an ethnically diverse group often live with extended family and continue to speak their native language.

Ethnic populations of older adults face unique problems. Because older adults often live in older neighborhoods, physical security and personal safety related to crime may be a concern. Individuals with ethnic identities often have disproportionately lower incomes and may not be able to afford Medicare deductibles or drugs needed to treat chronic illnesses.[25] Perceptions of health may also differ by ethnic group. Among older adults, fewer African Americans and Hispanic/Latinos rate their health as excellent or good as compared with white older adults.[26]

Assess each older adult's ethnic and cultural orientation. Do not assume that ethnicity and culture are or are not of value to the patient and the patient's family until you do an assessment. For you to be effective with the ethnic older adult, a sense of respect and clear communication are critical. Nursing interventions to assist in meeting the needs of ethnic populations are described in Table 2-9. (Culturally competent care is discussed in Chapter 2.)

SOCIAL SUPPORT FOR OLDER ADULTS

Social support for older adults occurs at three levels. First, family members are the primary and preferred providers of social support. Second, a semiformal level of support is found in clubs, religious (or faith-based) organizations, neighborhoods, and senior citizen centers. Third, older adults may be linked to formal systems of social welfare agencies, health facilities, and government support. Generally, you, as a nurse, are part of the formal support system.

Family Caregivers

Many older adults require caregiving by family members. Other older adults may take on the role of caregiver for someone in their family, usually their spouse or partner. Many family caregivers caring for older adults are themselves age 65 or over.[27] The challenges of caregiving are discussed in Chapter 4 on pp. 51 to 52.

Elder Mistreatment or Abuse

Elder mistreatment (EM) describes intentional acts of omission or commission by a caregiver or "trusted other" that cause harm or serious risk of harm to a vulnerable older adult. EM may occur in community (home or assisted living facility) or long-term care (institutional) settings.

Approximately 2% to 10% of community-dwelling older adults in the United States are abused, neglected, or exploited by trusted others.[28] The prevalence of EM in institutional settings is unknown, but it is thought to be widespread. Although EM rates are similar in women and men, the majority of victims are women because of the predominance of women in older age cohorts. Victims of EM have a mortality risk that is three times higher than that of nonmistreated peers. The higher mortality risk is not due to the abuse or neglect itself, but rather may be due to stress-related illnesses associated with prolonged mistreatment.[29]

EM is a hidden problem. For every reported case in the community setting, more than five cases go unreported. Underreporting may be higher based on immigration status, ethnic background, or sexual orientation. Victims are unlikely to report mistreatment by "trusted others" because of isolation; impaired cognitive or physical function; feelings of shame, guilt, or self-blame; fear of reprisal; pressure from family members; fear of nursing home placement; or cultural norms. Health care providers also underreport, possibly because of failure to suspect or recognize EM, perceived inability to successfully intervene, desire to avoid responsibility for further action, or ageism.

Much of domestic EM is family violence that involves power and control dynamics. Family members are responsible for up to 90% of domestic EM. Adult children who abuse, neglect, or exploit their parents are usually dependent on their parent(s) for housing and financial support, have a history of violence, are unemployed, and/or are disabled from substance abuse or mental illness. Abusive spouses or partners may either initiate intimate partner violence in older age or continue a lifelong pattern of abuse.[30]

Many factors put community-dwelling older adults at risk for domestic EM. These include (1) physical or cognitive dysfunction that leads to an inability to perform ADLs (and therefore produces dependence on others for care), (2) any psychiatric diagnoses (especially dementia and depression), (3) alcohol abuse, and (4) decreased social support.[31] In long-term care settings the same factors that lead to institutionalization are risk factors for mistreatment by staff, visitors, and others. These include dependence on others for care because of physical or cognitive dysfunction (especially conditions that produce aggressive behaviors). Residents of long-term care facilities are also at risk for harmful aggression by other residents.[32]

Types of EM, characteristics, and manifestations are shown in Table 5-9. EM types frequently co-occur, and up to 70% of cases involve neglect. In institutional settings EM includes the types described in Table 5-9, but also includes failure to follow the plan of care, unauthorized use of physical or chemical restraints, overuse or underuse of medication, or isolation as punishment.

Assess for and consider EM if you observe any of these characteristics or manifestations. Perform a thorough history and physical examination that includes screening for mistreatment. Follow your organization's protocols for EM screening and interventions. Tools that are helpful in assessment include the Elder Mistreatment Assessment and the American Medical Association's Diagnostic and Treatment Guidelines on Elder Abuse and Neglect (see Resources at the end of this chapter).

It is important that you interview patients alone because, if mistreatment is occurring, they may not disclose in the presence of the person who accompanied them, especially if that person is the abuser. Be especially attentive to explanations about injuries that are not consistent with what you observe, contradictory explanations between the patient and the caregiver, or behavioral clues that suggest the patient is being threatened or intimidated. Additional nursing interventions are listed in Table 5-10. In most states, health care workers and others are mandated to report suspected or actual EM to Adult Protective Services and/or law enforcement. Know your legal responsibilities by checking the laws in your state.

Self-Neglect

Despite the prevalence of mistreatment of older adults by trusted others, the majority of referrals made to Adult Protective Services are for self-neglect. Older adults who self-neglect are likely to live alone; refuse or are unable to meet their basic needs; have multiple, untreated medical or psychiatric conditions; and live in squalor. Like EM, older community-dwelling adults who self-neglect face a higher risk of mortality than peers who do not self-neglect. Nursing interventions include assessment for possible self-neglect, referrals for long-term multidisciplinary case management, and referral to Adult Protective Services.[33]

SOCIAL SERVICES FOR OLDER ADULTS

A network of services supports older adults both in the community and in health care facilities. In the United States most older adults are the beneficiaries of at least one social or governmental service. To understand the older adult's situation, learn about government structures that fund and regulate programs for older adults. The Administration on Aging (AoA), which is part of the Department of Health and Human Services, is the federal agency responsible for many older adult programs. Funding from the AoA is funneled to state and local Area Agencies on Aging.[34]

MEDICARE AND MEDICAID

Medicare is a federally funded health insurance program for people ages 65 years or older, as well as for people under age 65 with certain disabilities and people of any age with end-stage kidney disease requiring dialysis or a kidney transplant. Nursing documentation is critically important for adequate reimbursement of services.

TABLE 5-9 TYPES OF ELDER MISTREATMENT

Characteristics	Manifestations
Physical Abuse	
Slapping, striking; restraining; incorrect positioning; oversedation with medications	Bruises, bilateral injuries (ankles, wrists), repeated injuries in various stages of healing; oversedation; use of several emergency departments
Neglect	
Failure or refusal to provide basic life needs, including food, water, medications, clothing, hygiene; failure to provide physical aids such as dentures, eyeglasses, hearing aid; failure to ensure safety	Older adult's reports of being neglected; untreated or infected pressure ulcers on sacral area, heels; loss of body weight; laboratory values showing dehydration (e.g., ↑ Hct, ↑ serum sodium), malnutrition (↓ serum protein); poor personal hygiene; lack of adherence with medical treatment
Failure to provide social stimulation; leaving alone for long periods; failure to provide companionship	Depression, withdrawn behavior; agitation; ambivalent attitude toward caregiver or family member
Psychologic Abuse	
Berating verbally; harassment; intimidation; threats of punishment or deprivation; childlike treatment; isolation	Depression, withdrawn behavior; agitation; ambivalent attitude toward caregiver or family member
Sexual Abuse	
Nonconsensual sexual contact, including touching inappropriately; forced sexual contact	Older adult's report of sexual abuse; unexplained vaginal or anal bleeding; bruised breasts; unexplained STIs or genital infections
Financial Abuse	
Denying access to personal resources, stealing money or possessions; coercing to sign contracts or durable power of attorney; making changes in will or trust	Living situation below level of personal resources; sudden change in personal finances; sudden transfer of assets
Violation of Personal Rights	
Denying right to privacy or right to make decisions regarding health care or living environment; forcible eviction	Sudden inexplicable changes in living situation; confusion
Abandonment	
Desertion of an older person by an individual who has assumed responsibility for providing care or by a person with physical custody	Older adult's reports of being abandoned; desertion of an older adult at a hospital or nursing facility, shopping center, or other public place

Hct, Hematocrit; *STIs*, sexually transmitted infections.

TABLE 5-10 NURSING ASSESSMENT

Mistreatment

- Screen for possible elder mistreatment, including domestic violence.
- Conduct a thorough history and head-to-toe assessment. Document your findings, including any statements made by the older adult or accompanying adult.
- If the older adult appears to be in immediate danger, develop and implement a safety plan in collaboration with the interdisciplinary team involved in the person's care.
- Identify, collect, and preserve physical evidence (e.g., dirty or bloody clothing, dressings, or sheets).
- After obtaining consent, take photographs to document physical findings of suspected abuse or neglect. If possible and appropriate, do this before treating or bathing the alleged victim.
- If you suspect that mistreatment is occurring, report your findings to the appropriate state agency and/or law enforcement as mandated by the laws in your state.
- Initiate social work, forensic nursing, and other consultations as appropriate.

Medicare has four options for coverage: A, B, C, and D. Part A covers inpatient hospital care and partially covers skilled nursing facility care, hospice, and home health care. Part A coverage is "free" because workers support Medicare through payroll taxes.[35] Medicare Part B partially covers outpatient care, physicians' services, and home health care. It also covers some preventive services, such as mammograms. Medicare Part B is voluntary and has a monthly premium and an annual deductible before payment begins. Medicare Advantage Plans, sometimes called "Part C" or "MA Plans," are offered by private companies approved by Medicare to provide Part A and Part B benefits. Part D is available to Medicare enrollees and provides a prescription drug benefit. Members pay a yearly deductible, a monthly premium, and a copayment. People with lower incomes and limited assets may qualify for extra help to pay for prescriptions.

Medicare does not cover long-term care, custodial ADLs or IADLs care, dental care or dentures, hearing aids, or eyeglasses. (More information is available at *www.Medicare.gov.*) These costs, plus the Medicare deductible, account for the fact that some older adults pay for 50% of their health care costs yearly.

Medicaid is a state-administered, needs-based program to assist eligible low-income people, including Medicare beneficiaries, with certain medical expenses. Individuals who qualify for both Medicare and Medicaid are frequently referred to as "dual-eligibles." Eligibility and coverage vary by state. For Qualified Medicare Beneficiaries, Medicaid pays Medicare premiums, deductibles, and co-insurance, as well as long-term care and home health expenses. In the United States the majority of long-term care is paid for by Medicaid or private pay. (More information is available at *www.medicaid.gov.*)

CARE ALTERNATIVES FOR OLDER ADULTS

Older adults with special care needs include people who are homeless, in need of assistance with ADLs, cognitively impaired, homebound, or no longer able to live at home. Older adults may be served by adult day care, adult day health care, home health care, and long-term care.

Adult Day Care and Adult Day Health Care

Adult day care centers provide social, recreational, and health-related services to individuals in a safe, community-based environment (Fig. 5-5). This includes daily supervision, social activities, opportunities for social interaction, and ADLs assistance for two major groups of adults: those who are cognitively impaired, and those who have problems independently performing ADLs. Services offered in adult day care programs are individualized based on need. Programs designed for adults who are cognitively impaired offer therapeutic recreation, support for family, family counseling, and social involvement.

Adult day health care centers are similar to adult day care but are designed to meet the needs of older adults and people with disabilities who need a higher level of care. This might include health monitoring, therapeutic activities, one-on-one ADLs training, and personal services.

Adult day care centers and adult day health care centers may provide respite to allow continued employment for the caregiver and delay institutionalization of older adults. Centers are regulated, and standards are set by the state. Medicare does not cover costs. Adult day health care is tax deductible as dependent care. Appropriate placement in adult care programs that match participants' needs is important. Caregivers and adults with self-care deficits are often uninformed about adult day centers and their services as an alternative care option. You can assist by knowing the available centers in your area and assessing the needs of older adults and their families. You will then be in a position to assist older adults and their families in making good decisions about their care.

Home Health Care. Home health care (HHC) can be a cost-effective care alternative for older adults who are homebound, have health needs that are intermittent or acute, and have supportive caregiver involvement. HHC is not an alternative for adults in need of 24-hour ADLs assistance or continuous safety supervision. (Private duty care may be an alternative in these situations.) HHC services require physician orders and skilled nursing care for Medicare reimbursement. Unless these requirements are met, assistance by home health aides for ADLs management or assistance by a homemaker for IADLs management will not be paid by Medicare.

In addition to HHC, respite, personal care, and homemaker services are often sought by caregivers through organizations that provide nonmedical assistance. These services help older adults stay at home.

Long-Term Care Facilities

Practice settings for long-term care are presented in eTable 1-2. Three factors appear to precipitate placement in a long-term care facility: (1) rapid patient deterioration, (2) caregiver inability to continue care because of stress and burnout, and (3) an alteration in or loss of the family support system. Deteriorating cognition, incontinence, or a major health event (e.g., stroke) can accelerate placement.

The conflicts and fears faced by older adults and their families make placement a difficult transition. Common caregiver concerns include: (1) Will the older adult resist the admission process?; (2) Will the level of care given by staff be insufficient?; (3) Will the resident be lonely?; and (4) Will nursing care be affordable?

This time of disruption is exacerbated by the physical relocation of the older adult and may result in adverse health effects for them. *Relocation stress syndrome* is a nursing diagnosis that is associated with the disruption, confusion, and challenges that older adults face when moving from one environment to a new environment. Older adults may experience anxiety, depression, and disorientation. Appropriate interventions can reduce the effects of relocation. Whenever possible, involve older adults in the decision to move and fully inform them about the location. Caregivers can share information, pictures, or a video recording of the new location. Personnel at the institution can send a welcome message. On arrival, new residents can be greeted by staff members to provide orientation. To bridge the relocation, new residents can be "buddied" with seasoned residents (Fig. 5-6).

LEGAL AND ETHICAL ISSUES

Legal assistance is a concern for many older adults. Legal concerns include advance directives, estate planning, taxation issues, appeals for denied services (e.g., disability), financial decisions, or exploitation by strangers or "trusted others." Legal aid is available to older adults with low income by contacting a local senior center.

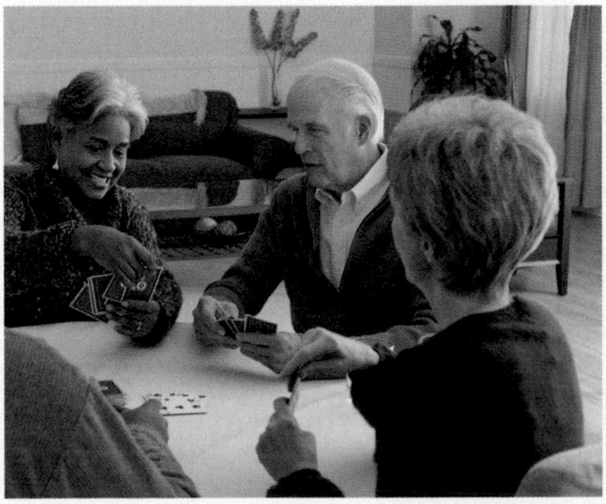

FIG. 5-5 Senior centers offer places for older adults who live independently to meet and gather with friends. (Jupiterimages/Comstock/Thinkstock)

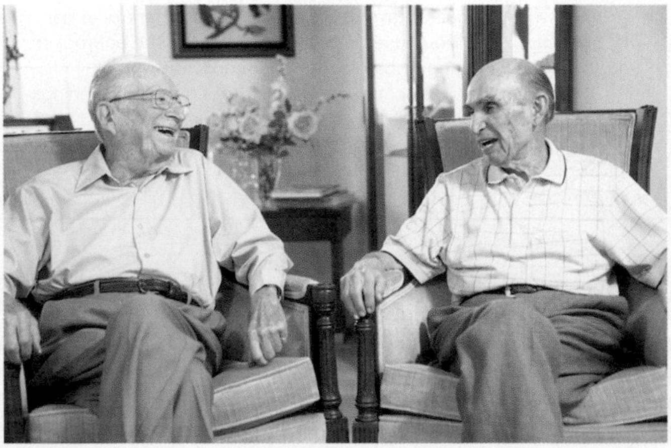

FIG. 5-6 Social interaction and acceptance are important for older adults. (Hemera/Thinkstock)

Advance directives are written statements of a person's wishes regarding medical care. These documents allow patients to more specifically direct their own care at end of life. Advance directives are discussed in detail in Chapter 10 and Table 10-6.

When working with older adults, you may find several ethical issues that influence practice, such as use of physical or chemical restraints or the assessment of older adults' ability to make decisions. Other ethical issues related to end-of-life care include decisions about resuscitation, treatment of infections, nutrition and hydration, and transfer to more intensive treatment units. These situations are often complex and emotionally charged. You can assist the patient, family, and other health care workers by (1) acknowledging when an ethical dilemma is present, (2) keeping current on the ethical issues, and (3) advocating for an institutional ethics committee to help in the decision-making process.

NURSING MANAGEMENT OLDER ADULTS

Gerontologic nursing is the care of older adults based on the specialty body of knowledge of gerontology and nursing. These specialty nurses approach older adults with a whole-person (physical, psychologic, developmental, socioeconomic, cultural) perspective. Care of older adults is complex and presents challenges that require skilled assessment and creative nursing interventions tailored to this population.

Diseases and conditions in older adults may be difficult to accurately assess and diagnose. Older adults may underreport symptoms and "treat" these symptoms by altering their functional status. For example, a man having loss of feeling in his feet because of neuropathy may start using a walker to get around. At the same time, he does not report the symptom to his health care provider. The older adult may attribute a new symptom to "aging" and ignore it. The older adult may eat less, sleep more, or "wait it out."

In older adults, disease symptoms are often atypical. Complaints of an "aching joint" may actually be a broken hip. Asymptomatic cardiac disease may be diagnosed when the patient is being treated for a urinary tract infection. Pathologic conditions with similar symptoms are often confused. For example, depression may be misdiagnosed and treated as dementia.

In older adults a *cascade disease pattern* may occur. For example, a patient who experiences insomnia treats the condition with a hypnotic medication, becomes lethargic and confused, falls, breaks a hip, and subsequently develops pneumonia. You play a vital role in preventing this downward trajectory.

Older adults may face health problems with fear and anxiety. They may view health care workers as helpful, but perceive institutions as negative and potentially harmful places. Communicate a sense of concern and care by use of direct and simple statements, appropriate eye contact, direct touch, and gentle humor. These actions help the older adult relax in this stressful situation.

NURSING ASSESSMENT

Before beginning the assessment process, first attend to primary needs. For example, make certain that the patient is comfortable and does not need to urinate. Place all assistive devices, such as glasses and hearing aids, within reach. Evaluate your patient's level of fatigue and stop the interview if necessary. Allow adequate time to offer information to the patient and time for the patient to respond to questions. Interview both the older adult and his or her family or caregivers. This can be done separately unless the patient is cognitively impaired or specifically requests the caregiver's presence. The medical history may be lengthy. Review medical records and determine what information is relevant.

The focus of a comprehensive geriatric assessment is to determine appropriate interventions to maintain and enhance the functional abilities of older adults. Comprehensive geriatric assessment is interdisciplinary and, at a minimum, includes the medical history, physical examination, functional assessment, medication review, cognitive and mood evaluation, and social resources. Comprehensive geriatric assessment is often conducted by an interdisciplinary geriatric assessment team. The interdisciplinary team may include many disciplines, but at least a nurse, a physician, and a social worker. After the assessment is complete, the interdisciplinary team meets with the patient and family to present the team's findings and recommendations.[32]

Elements in a comprehensive nursing assessment include a history using a functional health pattern format (see Chapter 3), physical assessment, mood assessment, assessment of ADLs and IADLs, mental status evaluation, and a social-environmental assessment. Evaluation of mental status is particularly important for older adults because these results often determine the potential for independent living. SPICES, an effective tool for obtaining assessment data in older adults, should be the basis of nursing assessment when working in any setting (Fig. 5-7).

Evaluation of the results of a comprehensive nursing assessment helps determine the service and placement needs of older adults. Collect data regarding community resources that are needed to assist older adults and their caregivers in maintaining maximal functioning. The goal is to plan and implement actions that help older adults remain as functionally independent as possible.

PLANNING

When setting goals with older adults, it is helpful to identify their strengths and abilities. Include caregivers in planning. Priority goals for older adults might include gaining a sense of control, feeling safe, and reducing stress.

NURSING IMPLEMENTATION

When carrying out a plan of action for older adults, modify your approach and actions based on their physical and mental status. Small body size, common in older adults who are frail,

Patient name:	Date:	
	EVIDENCE	
SPICES	Yes	No
Sleep disorders		
Problems with eating or feeding		
Incontinence		
Confusion		
Evidence of falls		
Skin breakdown		

FIG. 5-7 SPICES.

may necessitate the use of pediatric equipment (e.g., blood pressure cuff). As with all patient groups, safety is a primary concern when caring for an older adult. Bone and joint changes often require transfer assistance, altered positioning, and use of gait belts and lift devices. Older adults with declining energy reserves may require additional time to complete tasks. A slower approach and the use of other adaptive equipment may be necessary.

Cognitive impairment, if present, requires that you offer careful explanations and a calm approach to avoid producing anxiety and resistance in the older adult. Depression can result in apathy and poor cooperation with the treatment plan.

HEALTH PROMOTION. Health promotion and prevention of health problems for older adults focus on three areas: (1) reduction in diseases and problems, (2) increased participation in health promotion activities (Fig. 5-8), and (3) increased targeted services that reduce health hazards. Programs have been successfully developed for screening for chronic health conditions, tobacco cessation, geriatric foot care, vision and hearing screening, stress reduction, exercise programs, drug usage, crime prevention, elder mistreatment, and home hazards assessment. You can carry out and teach older adults about the need for specific preventive services.

Health promotion and prevention can be included in nursing interventions at any location or level where nurses and older adults interact. You can use health promotion activities to increase self-care, personal responsibility for health, and independent functioning that will enhance the well-being of older adults. Resources available to you are listed at the end of the chapter. Teaching is an important tool for you to use to enhance self-care practices by older adults. (Patient teaching is discussed in Chapter 4.)

ACUTE CARE. Frequently the hospital is the first point of contact for older adults and the formal health care system. Conditions that most commonly result in hospitalization include falls, dysrhythmias, heart failure, stroke, fluid and electrolyte imbalances (e.g., hyponatremia, dehydration), pneumonia, urosepsis, and hip fractures. Older adults are often hospitalized with multiple system problems.

When older adults are being cared for in the acute care setting, both patients and caregivers need assistance with a variety of functions (Table 5-11). The outcome of hospitalization for older adults varies. Of particular concern are problems of high surgical risk, acute confusional state, health care–associated infection, and premature discharge in an unstable condition. Geriatric nursing considerations sections throughout this book emphasize special needs and interventions for older adult patients.

Care Transitions. At the time of a care transition to another setting (e.g., acute care hospital to rehabilitation), many older adults are in an unstable condition. (Transitional care settings are presented in eTable 1-1.) Frail older adults and patients over 85 years of age are particularly vulnerable during care transitions. Most of these patients are transitioned under Medicare regulations that require a registered nurse or qualified person to develop a plan for discharge. Care transition plans are periodically reassessed, and caregivers and patients must be counseled to prepare the patient for posthospital care. Safe, effective, and efficient care transitions are most likely to occur when interdisciplinary team members work together to coordinate care.

Rehabilitation. The goal of rehabilitation is to help older adults adapt to or recover from disability. Rehabilitation may occur in acute inpatient rehabilitation or long-term care settings. With proper training, assistive equipment, and attendant personal care, people with disabilities often live independently. Older adults, primarily through Medicare reimbursement, can receive rehabilitative assistance through acute inpatient rehabilitation (limited days) and home health care programs (Fig. 5-9).

TABLE 5-11 CARE OF THE HOSPITALIZED OLDER ADULT

- Identify adults over age 85 with or without frailty and patients at risk for iatrogenic (due to medical/surgical treatment) problems.
- Consider discharge needs early in the hospital stay, especially assistance with ADLs, IADLs, and medications.
- Encourage the development and use of interdisciplinary teams, special care units, and individuals who focus on the special needs of older patients.
- Implement standard protocols to screen for at-risk conditions commonly present in the hospitalized older adult, such as urinary tract infection and delirium.
- Implement mobility programs to prevent functional decline. ("The bed is not your friend.")
- Advocate for referral of the patient to appropriate community-based services.

ADLs, Activities of daily living; *IADLs,* instrumental activities of daily living.

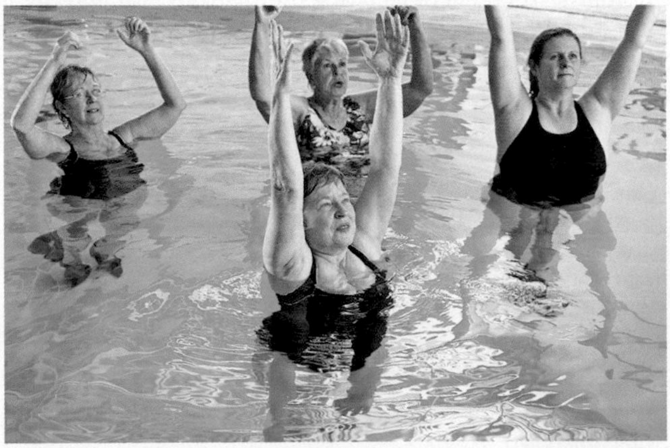

FIG. 5-8 Water aerobics is an example of a health promotion activity for older adults. (Jupiterimages/Photos.com/Thinkstock)

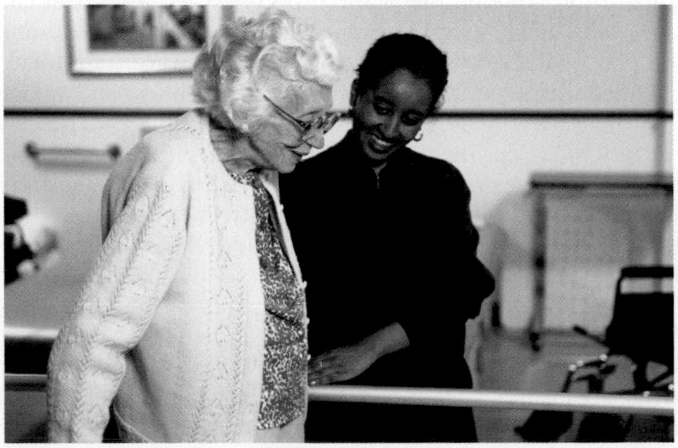

FIG. 5-9 The nurse assists a patient in a geriatric rehabilitation facility. (Keith Brofsky/Photodisc/Thinkstock)

Older adults with chronic conditions, such as stroke, arthritis, and heart disease, have increased risk of becoming functionally limited. These disabilities lead to increased self-care deficits, higher mortality rates, increased rates of institutionalization, and decreased life span. Reducing disability through geriatric rehabilitation is important to the quality of life of older adults.

Often older adults have specific fears and anxieties related to falling. Older adults are limited in the rehabilitation process by sensory-perceptual deficits, other health problems, impaired cognition, poor nutrition, and financial problems. Encouragement, support, and acceptance from all members of the health care team and their caregivers can assist older adults in remaining motivated for the hard work of rehabilitation.

Rehabilitation of older adults is influenced by several factors. First, preexisting problems associated with reaction time, visual acuity, fine motor ability, physical strength, cognitive function, and motivation affect the rehabilitation potential of older adults.

Second, older adults often lose function because of inactivity and immobility. This *deconditioning* can occur as a result of unstable acute medical conditions, environmental barriers that limit mobility, and a lack of motivation to stay in condition. The effect of inactivity clearly leads to "use it or lose it" consequences. Older adults can improve flexibility, strength, and aerobic capacity even into very old age. Passive and active range-of-motion exercises are used with all older adults to prevent deconditioning and subsequent functional decline.

Last, the goal of rehabilitation is to strive for maximal function and physical capabilities considering the individual's current health status. When an older adult demonstrates suboptimal health, screen and evaluate for risk behaviors. For example, on admission to any acute or long-term care facility and home health services, assess for fall risk, initiate appropriate fall prevention interventions, and evaluate for ongoing risk. Conduct accurate and comprehensive foot assessments for older adults with diabetes and arrange appropriate follow-up care.

Assistive Devices. Consider the use of assistive devices as interventions for older adults. Using appropriate assistive devices such as dentures, glasses, hearing aids, walkers, wheelchairs, adult briefs or protectors, adaptive utensils, elevated toilet seats, and skin protective devices can decrease disability. Include these tools and devices in the older adult's care plan when appropriate, and provide instruction in the proper use of the devices. For example, using a cane inappropriately may increase the risk for a fall.

Technology can assist with rehabilitation and living with functional impairments.[36] For example, electronic monitoring equipment can be used to monitor heart rhythms and blood pressure. Monitoring can also locate a person with dementia who has wandered away from home or a long-term care facility. Computerized assistive devices can be used to help patients with speech difficulties following stroke, and small electronic devices can serve as memory aids.

Safety. Safety is crucial in the health maintenance of older adults. When compared to younger adults, older adults are at higher risk for accidents because of normal sensory changes, slowed reaction time, decreased thermal and pain sensitivity, changes in gait and balance, and medication effects. Most accidents occur in or around the home. Falls, motor vehicle accidents, and fires are common causes of accidental death in older adults. Another environmental problem arises from the older person's impaired thermoregulation system that cannot adapt to extremes in environmental temperatures. The bodies of older adults can neither conserve nor dissipate heat as efficiently as younger adults. Therefore both hypothermia and hyperthermia occur more readily. This age-group accounts for the majority of deaths during severe cold spells and heat waves.

You can provide valuable counsel regarding environmental changes, which may improve safety for older adults. Measures such as colored step strips, tub and toilet grab bars, and stairway handrails can be effective in "safety-proofing" the living spaces of older adults. You can also advocate for home fire and security alarms. Uncluttered floor space, railings, and increased lighting and night-lights are some of the easiest and most practical adaptations.

Older adults who are new to inpatient or long-term care settings need a thorough orientation to the environment. Reassure the older adult that he or she is safe, and attempt to answer all questions. Foster orientation by displaying large-print clocks, avoiding complex or visually confusing wall designs, clearly designating doors and exits, and using simple bed and nurse-call controls. Provide diffuse lighting while avoiding glare. Environments that provide consistent caregivers and an established daily routine increase an older adult's sense of comfort and safety.

Medication Use. Medication use in older adults requires thorough and regular assessment, care planning, and evaluation. Nonadherence to medication regimens by older adults is common. Four of ten older adults are unable to read prescription drug labels, and two thirds are unable to understand the health information that is provided to them.[37]

Age-related changes alter the pharmacodynamics and pharmacokinetics of drugs. Drug-drug, drug-food, and drug-disease interactions all influence the absorption, distribution, metabolism, and excretion of drugs. The most dramatic changes with aging are related to drug metabolism (Fig. 5-10). Overall, by age 75 to 80, there is a 50% decline in the renal clearance of drugs. Hepatic blood flow decreases markedly with aging, and the enzymes largely responsible for drug metabolism are decreased as well. As a result, drug half-life is increased in older adults as compared with younger adults. This leads to drug toxicity and adverse drug events.

In addition to changes in the metabolism of drugs, older adults may have difficulty due to cognitive impairment, altered sensory perceptions, limited hand mobility, and the high cost of many prescriptions. Common reasons for drug errors made by older adults are listed in Table 5-12. *Polypharmacy* (the use of multiple medications by a person who has more than one health problem), overdose, and addiction to prescription drugs are recognized as major causes of illness in older adults.[37]

The effects of medications in older adults with multiple health problems are particularly challenging to assess and manage. As one disease is treated, another may be affected. For

TABLE 5-12 DRUG THERAPY

Common Causes of Medication Errors by Older Adults

- Decreased vision
- Forgetting to take drugs
- Use of nonprescription over-the-counter drugs
- Use of medications prescribed for someone else
- Lack of financial resources to obtain prescribed medication
- Failure to understand instructions or importance of drug treatment
- Refusal to take medication because of undesirable side effects

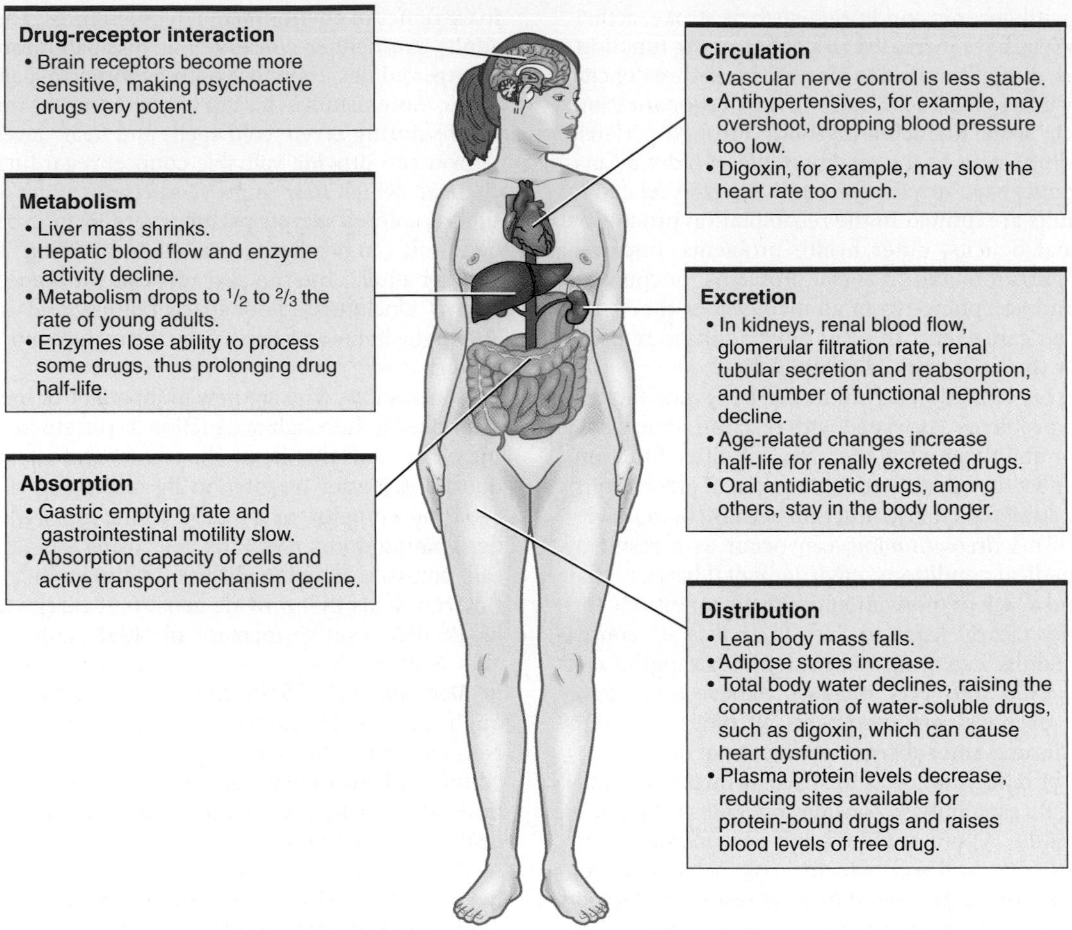
Drug-receptor interaction
• Brain receptors become more sensitive, making psychoactive drugs very potent.
Metabolism
• Liver mass shrinks.
• Hepatic blood flow and enzyme activity decline.
• Metabolism drops to 1/2 to 2/3 the rate of young adults.
• Enzymes lose ability to process some drugs, thus prolonging drug half-life.
Absorption
• Gastric emptying rate and gastrointestinal motility slow.
• Absorption capacity of cells and active transport mechanism decline.
Circulation
• Vascular nerve control is less stable.
• Antihypertensives, for example, may overshoot, dropping blood pressure too low.
• Digoxin, for example, may slow the heart rate too much.
Excretion
• In kidneys, renal blood flow, glomerular filtration rate, renal tubular secretion and reabsorption, and number of functional nephrons decline.
• Age-related changes increase half-life for renally excreted drugs.
• Oral antidiabetic drugs, among others, stay in the body longer.
Distribution
• Lean body mass falls.
• Adipose stores increase.
• Total body water declines, raising the concentration of water-soluble drugs, such as digoxin, which can cause heart dysfunction.
• Plasma protein levels decrease, reducing sites available for protein-bound drugs and raises blood levels of free drug.

FIG. 5-10 The effects of aging on drug metabolism.

example, the use of a drug such as oxybutynin (Ditropan), which is prescribed for overactive bladder, may cause confusion. To accurately assess medication use and knowledge, ask older adults to bring all medications (over-the-counter drugs, prescription drugs, vitamins and supplements, and herbal remedies) that they take regularly or occasionally to their health care appointment. You will then be able to accurately assess all medications the patient is taking, including drugs that the person may have omitted or thought unimportant. Additional nursing interventions to assist older adults in following a safe medication routine are listed in Table 5-13.

Depression. Depression is not a normal part of aging. However, it is often an underrecognized problem in older adults. Approximately 15% of older adults living in their homes have symptoms of depression. Rates of depressive symptoms in older adults in institutional settings are higher. Older adults commit 20% of the suicides in the United States, and older men who are white have the highest rate of suicide.[38]

Depression is associated with female gender, divorced or separated marital status, low socioeconomic status, poor social support, and a recent adverse and unexpected event. Depression in older adults tends to arise from a loss of self-esteem and may be related to life situations, such as retirement or loss of a spouse or partner. Problems such as physical complaints, insomnia, lethargy, agitation, weight loss, decreased memory, and inability to concentrate are common.

Late-life depression often co-occurs with medical conditions, such as heart disease, stroke, diabetes, and cancer. Depression can exacerbate medical conditions by affecting adherence

TABLE 5-13 DRUG THERAPY

Medication Use by Older Adults

- Evaluate cognitive function and ensure ability to self-administer medication.
- Attempt to reduce medication use that is not essential by consulting the health care provider and pharmacist.
- Assess medication use, including prescription drugs; over-the-counter drugs; antihistamines; cough syrups; vitamins, minerals, and supplements; and herbal remedies.
- Assess alcohol and illicit drug use.
- Encourage the use of written or electronic medication-reminder systems.
- Encourage the use of one pharmacy.
- Work with health care providers and pharmacists to establish routine drug profiles on all older adult patients.
- Advocate (with drug companies) for low-income prescription support services.

with diet, exercise, or drug regimens. It is important that your assessment include physical examination and interpretation of laboratory results for physical disorders that may have symptoms similar to those of depression (e.g., thyroid disorders, vitamin deficiencies). The Geriatric Depression Scale is easy to administer and is the gold standard assessment tool (see eTable 5-1 on the website for this chapter).

Encourage older adults who exhibit depressive symptoms to seek treatment. Because older adults with depression may feel unworthy, withdrawn, and isolated, the support of the family or others in encouraging older adults to seek treatment is important. Assist older adult caregivers who exhibit depressive symptoms to seek medical attention, and assist them in securing respite services and support for their caregiving role. (Family caregiving is discussed in Chapter 4 on pp. 50 to 52.)

Use of Restraints. *Physical restraints* are devices, materials, and equipment that physically prevent individuals from moving freely, such as walking, standing, lying, transferring, or sitting. *Chemical restraints* are medications that prevent a patient's voluntary movement.

Restraints may be used only to ensure the person's safety or the safety of others. Physical and chemical restraints are a last resort in the care of older adults. If physical or chemical restraints are used in the hospital or long-term care setting, use of the least restrictive restraint is required. Restraints require an order from a physician or an independently licensed advance practice nurse. In addition, frequent scheduled reviews of the ongoing necessity of the restraint are needed. There are additional regulatory requirements for restraint use, including time limit, observation and care, and alternatives to the use of restraints. Long-term care regulations and The Joint Commission set standards for restraint usage.

Carefully document restraint use and the behaviors that require this intervention. It is not appropriate to use restraints based on fall risk or irritating behaviors, such as calling out. The current standard is to provide safe care without using restraints of any form, whether physical or chemical.[39]

To achieve this standard, evaluate the patient's behavior. Behavioral symptoms, such as crying and shouting, may arise from co-morbidities, pain, medication toxicity, unmet needs, or environmental factors. When behavioral symptoms are evident, ask the following questions to better understand the patient's behavior: Is the person able to verbalize what she or he needs and wants? People with dementia may respond by speaking, gesturing, nodding, or making eye contact.[38] Questions that use "yes" or "no" answers are better than open-ended questions for gathering assessment information. Ask family, friends, or staff members from previous care settings about the patient's history; usual communication style and cues to indicate pain, fatigue, hunger, or a need to urinate or defecate; abilities in ADLs; and daily routines (e.g., "Is he often awake at night or an early riser?" "Does she prefer breakfast before dressing? Take an afternoon nap? Have a routine for dressing?").

Evaluate whether disruptive behaviors signal unmet physiologic or psychosocial needs. For example, a patient who tries to get out of bed without help may be trying to reach the toilet. A toileting schedule will help to curtail such attempts and prevent incontinence. In critical care settings, patients emerging from sedation may be alarmed by an inability to speak or the presence of inserted tubes. Consider how treatments feel to the patient and pay attention to gestures, actions, and words to ascertain their meaning.

Restraint alternatives require vigilant, creative, and sensitive nursing care. Restraint alternatives include low beds, body props, and electronic devices (such as bed alarm signaling). Such approaches support the development of a "restraint-free" environment.

Sleep. Adequacy of sleep is often a concern for older adults because of altered sleep patterns. Older people experience a marked decrease in deep sleep and are easily aroused. Many older adults report difficulty initiating sleep and maintaining prolonged sleep; they may state they feel "unrefreshed" after sleep. (Sleep problems of older adults are discussed in Chapter 8.)

EVALUATION

The evaluation phase of the nursing process is similar for all patients. The results of evaluation direct you to continue the plan of care or revise as indicated. When evaluating nursing care with older adults, focus on functional improvement. Useful questions to consider when evaluating the plan of care for older adults are included in Table 5-14.

TABLE 5-14 EVALUATING NURSING CARE FOR OLDER ADULTS

Use the following questions to evaluate the effectiveness of care for older adults.

- Is there an identifiable change in ADLs, IADLs, mental status, or disease signs and symptoms?
- Does the patient consider his or her health state to be improved?
- Does the patient think the treatment is helpful?
- Do the patient and caregiver think the care is worth the time and cost?
- Can you document positive changes that support the interventions?
- Does change adequately meet the required mandates for reimbursement?

ADLs, Activities of daily living; *IADLs*, instrumental activities of daily living.

CASE STUDY

Older Adults

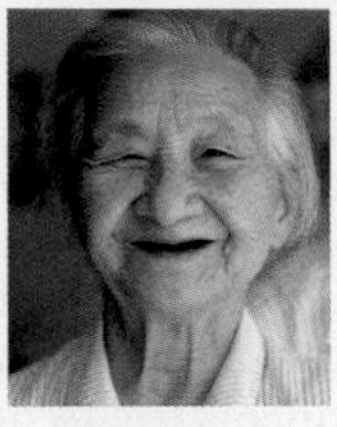

iStockphoto/Thinkstock

Patient Profile

L.X., a 79-year-old Chinese woman, was admitted through the emergency department with shortness of breath. She was diagnosed with community-acquired pneumonia. Her history also indicates she has chronic obstructive pulmonary disease (COPD), hypertension, diabetes, mild cognitive impairment, depression, macular degeneration, and significant hearing loss.

Subjective Data

- Had a stroke 5 years ago and has right-sided weakness
- Has a 100 pack-year history of tobacco use but quit smoking after her stroke
- Has not seen primary care physician in 1 year
- In past year has had an unplanned weight loss of 20 pounds
- Spends her days either in bed or in a recliner watching television

Psychosocial Data

- Came to the United States 15 years ago from China.
- Speaks Mandarin with limited English proficiency.
- Lives with her unemployed adult son who provides assistance with ADLs and IADLs.
- Has three daughters who live within a 2-hour drive.
- Has limited financial resources but has Medicare and Medicaid benefits.
- Her son has not visited her in the hospital, but her daughters raise concerns about their mother's care and safety at home, given their brother's history of anger issues and a gambling addiction.
- When daughters ask their brother about how he is caring for his mother, he says, "I'm doing the best I can. She refuses help. She refuses to go to the doctor. What do you want me to do? She's old. She's crazy. She's going to die anyway!"

Objective Data

- Matted hair, poor oral hygiene, overgrown toenails
- Two stage III sacral ulcers
- Unstageable right heel ulcer
- Multiple small bruises on her forearms and shins
- 5 × 10-cm bruise in the middle of her back

Discussion Questions

1. Compare L.X.'s experience as an older woman to known gender differences for older adults.
2. Identify the stage(s) of Corbin and Strauss chronic illness trajectory that describe L.X.'s current status. Which stage(s) is the goal of your nursing care?
3. Given the tasks of people with chronic illness as described by Corbin and Strauss, what is your assessment of L.X.'s ability to successfully complete these tasks? What will you include in your care planning to optimize her ability to complete these tasks?
4. Define *ageism,* and explain how it may be manifested in this case.
5. What risk factors does L.X. have for development of frailty? Which of these factors are modifiable?
6. ***Priority Decision:*** Based on your assessment of L.X., what are the priority nursing diagnoses?
7. ***Priority Decision:*** What are the priority nursing interventions for L.X.?
8. Explain ethnogeriatrics considerations that affect L.X. and how they will influence your nursing care.
9. Based on your knowledge of care alternatives for older adults, what setting(s) might be appropriate for L.X. on hospital discharge?
10. What risk factors does L.X. have for becoming a victim of elder mistreatment?

evolve Answers available at *http://evolve.elsevier.com/Lewis/medsurg.*

BRIDGE TO NCLEX EXAMINATION

The number of the question corresponds to the same-numbered outcome at the beginning of the chapter.

1. Examples of primary prevention strategies include
   a. colonoscopy at age 50.
   b. avoidance of tobacco products.
   c. intake of a diet low in saturated fat in a patient with high cholesterol.
   d. teaching the importance of exercise to a patient with hypertension.
2. A characteristic of a chronic illness is that it *(select all that apply)*
   a. has reversible pathologic changes.
   b. has a consistent, predictable clinical course.
   c. results in permanent deviation from normal.
   d. is associated with many stable and unstable phases.
   e. always starts with an acute illness and then progresses slowly.
3. Ageism is characterized by
   a. denial of negative stereotypes regarding aging.
   b. positive attitudes toward the elderly based on age.
   c. negative attitudes toward the elderly based on age.
   d. negative attitudes toward the elderly based on physical disability.
4. An ethnic older adult may feel a loss of self-worth when the nurse
   a. informs the patient about ethnic support services.
   b. allows a patient to rely on ethnic health beliefs and practices.
   c. has to use an interpreter to provide explanations and teaching.
   d. emphasizes that a therapeutic diet does not allow ethnic foods.
5. An important nursing action to help a chronically ill older adult is to
   a. avoid discussing future lifestyle changes.
   b. assure the patient that the condition is stable.
   c. treat the patient as a competent manager of the disease.
   d. encourage the patient to "fight" the disease as long as possible.
6. Older adults who become ill are more likely than younger adults to
   a. complain about the symptoms of their problems.
   b. refuse to carry out lifestyle changes to promote recovery.
   c. seek medical attention because of limitations on their lifestyle.
   d. alter their daily living activities to accommodate new symptoms.

7. An appropriate care choice for an older adult who lives with an employed daughter but requires help with activities of daily living is
   a. adult day care.
   b. long-term care.
   c. a retirement center.
   d. an assisted living facility.

8. Nursing interventions directed at health promotion in the older adult are primarily focused on
   a. disease management.
   b. controlling symptoms of illness.
   c. teaching positive health behaviors.
   d. teaching regarding nutrition to enhance longevity.

1. b, 2. c, 3. d, 4. c, 5. d, 6. c, 7. a, 8. c.

evolve

For rationales to these answers and even more NCLEX review questions, visit *http://evolve.elsevier.com/Lewis/medsurg.*

REFERENCES

1. Centers for Disease Control and Prevention: Chronic diseases and health promotion, Retrieved from *www.cdc.gov/chronicdisease/overview/index.htm.*
2. Corbin JM, Strauss A: A nursing model for chronic illness management based upon the Trajectory Framework, *Sch Inq Nurs Pract* 5:155, 1991. (Classic)
3. Centers for Disease Control and Prevention: Skin cancer module: practice exercises. Retrieved from *www.cdc.gov/excite/skincancer/mod13.htm.*
*4. Inouye J, Braqinsky N, Kataoka-Yahiro M: Randomized clinical trials of self-management with Asian/Pacific Islanders, *Clin Nurs Res* 20:366, 2011.
5. Stajduhar KI, Funk L, Wolse F, et al: Core aspects of "empowering" caregivers as articulated by leaders in home health care: palliative and chronic illness contexts, *Can J Nurse Res* 43:78, 2011.
6. Administration on Aging: A profile of older Americans. Retrieved from *www.aoa.gov/aoaroot/aging_statistics/Profile/2010/3.aspx.*
7. US Census Bureau: Facts for features and special editions. Retrieved from *www.census.gov/newsroom/releases/archives/facts_for_features_special_editions.*
8. Administration on Aging: Projected future growth of the older population. Retrieved from *www.aoa.gov/AoARoot/AgingStatistics.*
*9. Vermeulen J, Neyens JC, van Rossum E, et al: Predicting ADL disability in community-dwelling elderly people using physical frailty indicators: a systematic review, *BMC Geriatr* 11:33, 2011.
10. Luo Y, Waite LJ: Mistreatment and psychological well-being among older adults: exploring the role of psychosocial resources and deficits, *J Gerontol B Psychol Sci Soc Sci* 66:217, 2011.
11. Scott G: Ageism is rife in health care, *Nurs Stan* 25:1, 2011.
12. Kourtis N, Tavernarakis N: Cellular stress response pathways and ageing: intricate molecular relationships, *EMBO J* 30:2520, 2011.
13. Barnes SK, Ozanne SE: Pathways linking the early environment to long-term health and lifespan, *Prog Biophys Mol Biol* 106:323, 2011.
14. Weiss EP, Fontana L: Caloric restriction: powerful protection for the aging heart and vasculature, *Am J Physiol Heart Circ Physiol* 301:H1205, 2011.
*15. Dunn-Lewis C, Karemer WJ, Kupchak BR, et al: A multi-nutrient supplement reduced markers of inflammation and improved physical performance in active individuals of middle to older age: a randomized, double-blind, placebo-controlled study, *Nutr J* 10:90, 2011.
16. Nowrangi MA, Rao V, Lyketsos CG: Epidemiology, assessment, and treatment of dementia, *Psychiatr Clin North Am* 34:277, 2011.
*17. Thorpe JM, Thorpe CT, Kennelty KA, et al: Patterns of perceived barriers to medical care in older adults: a latent class analysis, *BMC Health Serv Res* 3:11, 2011.
18. Griffin SF, Williams JE, Hickman P, et al: A university, community coalition, and town partnership to promote walking, *J Public Health Manag Pract* 17:358, 2011.
19. McIlhenny CV, Guzic BL, Knee DR, et al: Using technology to deliver healthcare education to rural patients, *Rural Remote Health* 11:1798, 2011.
*20. Nkosi ZZ, Asah F, Pillay P: Post-basic nursing students' access to and attitudes toward the use of information technology in practice: a descriptive analysis, *J Nurs Manag* 19:876, 2011.
21. Fargo J, Metraux S, Byrne T, et al: Prevalence and risk of homelessness among US veterans: a multisite investigation: the selected works of Dennis P. Culhane. Retrieved from *www.works.bepress.com/dennis_culhane/107.*
22. Brown RT, Kiely DK, Bharel M, et al: Geriatric syndromes in older homeless adults, *J Gen Internal Med* 27:16, 2012.
23. Xue QL: The frailty syndrome: definition and natural history, *Clin Geriatr Med* 27:1, 2011.
24. McBride M: Ethnogeriatrics and cultural competence for nursing practice. Retrieved from *consultgerirn.org/topics/ethnogeriatrics_and_cultural_competence_for_nursing_practice/want_to_know_more.*
*25. Kim G, Worley CB, Allen RS, et al: Vulnerability of older Latino and Asian immigrants with limited English proficiency, *J Am Geriatr Soc* 59:1246, 2011.
26. August KJ, Sorkin DH: Racial and ethnic disparities in indicators of physical health status: do they still exist throughout late life? *J Am Geriatr Soc* 58:2009, 2010.
27. National Family Caregivers Association: Who are America's family caregivers? Retrieved from *www.nfcacares.org/who_are_family_caregiver.*
*28. Acierno R, Hernandez MA, Amstadter AB, et al: Prevalence and correlates of emotional, physical, sexual, and financial abuse and potential neglect in the United States: the National Elder Mistreatment Study, *Am J Public Health* 100:292, 2010.
*29. Lachs M, Bachman R, Williams CS, et al: Resident-to-resident elder mistreatment and police contact in nursing homes:

*Evidence-based information for clinical practice.

findings from a population-based cohort, *J Am Geriatr Soc* 55:840, 2007. (Classic)

30. US Department of Health and Human Services: The national elder abuse incidence study. Retrieved from *http://purl.access.gpo.gov/GPO/LPS104188.*
*31. Cisler JM, Amstadter AB, Begle AM, et al: Elder mistreatment and physical health among older adults: the South Carolina Elder Mistreatment Study, *J Trauma Stress* 23:461, 2010.
*32. Ellis G, Whitehead MA, O'Neill D, et al: Comprehensive geriatric assessment for older adults admitted to hospital, *Cochrane Database Syst Rev* 7:CD006211, 2011.
33. Mosqueda L, Dong X: Elder abuse and self-neglect: "I don't care anything about going to the doctor, to be honest…," *JAMA* 306:532, 2011.
34. HealthCare.gov: Improving care transitions. Retrieved from *www.healthcare.gov/compare/partnership-for-patients/safety/transitions.html#BackgroundonCareTransitions.*
35. Medicare.gov: Medicare basics. Retrieved from *www.medicare.gov/navigation/medicare-basics/medicare-basics-overview.aspx.*
36. Thompson HJ, Demiris G, Rue T, et al: A holistic approach to assess older adults' wellness using e-health technologies, *Telemed J E Health* 17(10):794, 2011.
37. Medication Use Safety Training for Seniors: Facts: older adults and medicine use. Retrieved from *www.mustforseniors.org/facts.jsp.*
38. National Institute of Mental Health: Older adults: depression and suicide facts. Retrieved from *www.nimh.nih.gov/health/publications/older-adults-depression-and-suicide-facts-fact-sheet/index.shtml.*
*39. Enmarker I, Olsen R, Hellzen O: Management of person with dementia with aggressive and violent behavior: a systematic literature review, *Int J Older People Nurs* 6:153, 2011.

RESOURCES

AARP
www.aarp.org
Administration on Aging
www.aoa.gov
American Geriatrics Society
www.americangeriatrics.org
American Society on Aging
www.asaging.org
Best Practices in Nursing Care to Older Adults
www.consultgerirn.org
Centers for Disease Control and Prevention—Healthy Aging
www.cdc.gov/aging
Centers for Medicare and Medicaid Services
www.cms.gov
Hartford Institute for Geriatric Nursing
www.hartfordign.org
National Caucus and Center on Black Aged
www.ncba-aged.org
National Center on Elder Abuse
www.ncea.aoa.gov/ncearoot/Main_Site/index.aspx
National Gerontological Nursing Association
www.NGNA.org
National Hispanic Council on Aging
www.nhcoa.org
National Indian Council on Aging
www.nicoa.org
National Institute on Aging
www.nia.nih.gov

CHAPTER 6

It's supposed to be a secret, but I'll tell you anyway.
We doctors do nothing. We only help and encourage the doctor within.
Albert Schweitzer, MD

Complementary and Alternative Therapies

Virginia (Jennie) Shaw

evolve WEBSITE

http://evolve.elsevier.com/Lewis/medsurg

- NCLEX Review Questions
- Key Points
- Pre-Test
- Rationales for Bridge to NCLEX Examination Questions
- Concept Map Creator
- Glossary
- Stress-Busting Kit for Nursing Students
- Content Updates

LEARNING OUTCOMES

1. Compare and contrast the conventional model and the integrative model for health care.
2. Describe four categories of complementary and alternative therapies.
3. Choose the key concepts to include when teaching patients about herbal supplements.
4. Name three commonly used herbal products and their indications for use.
5. Describe the nurse's role related to complementary and alternative therapies.
6. Explain how the nurse can assess a patient's use of complementary and alternative therapies.
7. Describe ways that the nurse can use complementary and alternative therapies to provide self-care.

KEY TERMS

acupuncture, p. 83
complementary and alternative therapies, p. 80
herbal therapy, p. 81
holistic nursing, p. 80
massage, p. 83

Historically wellness has been viewed as incorporating the physical, emotional, mental, and spiritual realms. Hippocrates, the father of medicine, advised a daily aromatic bath and fragrant massage for the maintenance of health. Florence Nightingale believed that nursing puts patients in the best condition for nature to act on them. The concepts of holism and balance guided the belief that the body heals itself and works to maintain homeostasis. The concepts of spirituality and harmony with nature were inseparable from the concepts of health and wellness.

This view of "wholeness" began to change with the works of René Descartes (1596–1650) and Sir Isaac Newton (1642–1727). They postulated that the body is a series of parts that can be broken down and studied. This mechanistic approach views the body as a machine; whatever part is broken is analyzed and then repaired, without regard for other aspects of the person involved. The *conventional model* of health care is based on this approach. Health care focuses on the physical body, often to the exclusion of the mind and the spirit. Emphasis is placed on what can be seen, measured, and quantified.

This conventional model has guided American health care for more than 100 years. About 40 years ago Americans began to explore health care therapies that were outside this model. This consumer-led movement fostered development of a new model of health care, a more "integrative" model. In this model, consumers combine the use of complementary and alternative therapies with conventional therapies. The conventional and integrative health care models are compared in Table 6-1.

The *integrative model* focuses on (1) personal responsibility for health; (2) joining of mind-body-spirit; and (3) use of natural, less invasive modalities. This model promotes health and wellness, not just treatment of diseases. Consumers desire more involvement in their health care decisions. They desire modalities that are more natural, less costly, and safer. The rise of chronic diseases and stress-related disorders has also led to consumers' interest in complementary and alternative therapies.

Reviewed by Jane A. Madden, RN, MSN, Professor of Nursing, Pikes Peak Community College, Colorado Springs, Colorado.

TABLE 6-1 COMPARISON OF CONVENTIONAL AND INTEGRATIVE HEALTH CARE MODELS

Conventional Health Care Model	Integrative Health Care Model
• Focus on physical body	• Focus on mind-body-spirit
• Focus on treatment of symptoms using medications and surgery	• Focus on self-healing of the body using herbs, exercise, nutrition, stress management
• Health care provider directs care	• Individual directs care; personal responsibility for health encouraged
• Focus on disease states	• Focus on health and wellness
• Technologic, invasive	• Noninvasive
• Increasing cost	• Lower cost
• Little focus on prevention	• Focus on prevention

COMPLEMENTARY AND ALTERNATIVE THERAPIES

Complementary and alternative therapies (CAT) are a group of diverse medical and health care systems, practices, and products that are not generally considered part of conventional medicine.[1] This definition highlights what might be considered "complementary and alternative" in one country or at one period of history might be considered "conventional" in another place or time. What is classified as complementary and alternative therapies is constantly changing. When these therapies are proven safe and effective, they are often adopted into conventional medicine.

Terms frequently used to describe health-related approaches that are outside the dominant system of health care include *alternative, complementary,* and *integrative. Alternative therapies* are therapies used in place of conventional medicine, whereas *complementary therapies* are used in conjunction with conventional medicine. *Integrative therapies* combine treatments from conventional medicine with complementary and alternative therapies that have evidence of safety and effectiveness.

Many complementary and alternative therapies are harmonious with the values of nursing. Nurses emphasize healing, recognize the provider-patient relationship as a partnership, and focus on health promotion and illness prevention. The American Holistic Nurses Association (AHNA) was established to focus nursing care on the whole person—recognizing the interconnectedness of body, mind, spirit, and environment. The AHNA highlights the practice of holistic nursing.

Holistic nursing is based on a body of knowledge; evidence-based research; sophisticated skill sets; defined standards of practice; and a philosophy of living and being that is grounded in caring, relationship, and interconnectedness.[2] AHNA *(www.ahna.org)* advances the profession of holistic nursing by providing continuing education in holistic nursing, helping to improve the health care workplace through the incorporation of the concepts of holistic nursing, educating professionals and the public about holistic nursing and integrative health care, and promoting research and scholarship in the field of holistic nursing.[3]

Health care professionals have raised important questions about the effectiveness and safety of complementary and alternative approaches in the face of their increased use. In response to this need, the National Center for Complementary and Alternative Medicine (NCCAM) was established *(http://nccam.nih.gov)*. A branch of the National Institutes of Health (NIH), NCCAM serves as the federal government's lead agency for scientific research on complementary and alternative therapies. The mission of NCCAM is to define, through rigorous scientific investigation, the usefulness and safety of complementary and alternative medicine interventions and their roles in improving health and health care.[4]

NCCAM has four areas of focus: (1) advancing scientific research, (2) training CAM researchers, (3) sharing news and information, and (4) supporting integration of proven CAM therapies. The website provides a wealth of information for consumers and professionals, including clinical practice guidelines and literature reviews for the health care professional.

A large study conducted by NCCAM and the National Center for Health Statistics (as a part of the National Health Interview Survey [NHIS]) showed that approximately 38% of adults used CAT within the past 12 months.[5] In another survey Americans were asked why they use CAT, and 55% responded they believed their health would be improved if conventional medical treatments were combined with CAT.[6] Because of this growing use of CAT, you need to have a basic understanding of this topic and know where to find reliable in-depth information. A list of helpful websites is provided at the end of the chapter.

NCCAM CATEGORIES

Because the field of CAT is broad and ever changing, it is helpful to place therapies into broad categories. NCCAM groups these therapies into four broad categories, recognizing that one therapy may fit into more than one category (Table 6-2).

TABLE 6-2 NCCAM CATEGORIES OF COMPLEMENTARY AND ALTERNATIVE THERAPIES

Category	Description	Examples
Natural products	Practices that use substances found in nature for their impact on health and wellness.	Herbal therapy, dietary supplements, vitamins, minerals, probiotics, aromatherapy
Mind-body medicine	Techniques that enhance mind's ability to affect the physical body. Science of psychoneuroimmunology demonstrates strength of mind-body connection.	Meditation, yoga, acupuncture, relaxation breathing, guided imagery, hypnotherapy, prayer, journaling, art therapy
Manipulative and body-based practices	Practices that are based on the manipulation and/or movement of one or more parts of the body.	Massage, chiropractic therapy, yoga
Other CAT practices	Wide variety of practices.	Movement therapies (e.g., Pilates), traditional healers, manipulation of energy fields (e.g., Healing Touch), whole medical systems (Table 6-3)

Source: *http://nccam.nih.gov.*
CAT, Complementary and alternative therapies; *NCCAM,* National Center for Complementary and Alternative Medicine.

Natural Products

The category of natural products includes herbal therapy, dietary supplements, vitamins, minerals, and other "natural products." The NHIS found that 17.7% of American adults had used a natural product in the previous year. These products were the most commonly used CAT.[5]

Herbal therapy is the use of individual herbs or combinations of herbs for therapeutic benefit. An *herb* is a plant or plant part (bark, roots, leaves, seeds, flowers, or fruit) that produces and contains chemical substances that act on the body. It is estimated that approximately 25,000 plant species are used medicinally throughout the world, and approximately 30% of modern prescription drugs are derived from plants. Botanical medicine is the oldest form of medicine; archaeologic evidence suggests that Neanderthals used plant-based remedies 60,000 years ago. Today about 80% of the world's population relies extensively on plant-derived remedies.

Medicinal plants work in much the same way as drugs; both are absorbed and trigger biologic effects that can be therapeutic. Many have more than one physiologic effect and thus have more than one condition for which they can be used. The range of action of herbs is extensive.

Overall the use of herbal therapy continues to increase. Although most herbal products can safely be used without professional assistance, side effects and interactions with prescription drugs have been described. There is concern that side effects from the use of herbal products are underreported, thus promoting the impression that herbal products are completely safe to use.

Because consumers tend not to share their use of herbal products with their primary health care provider, herb-drug interactions may also be underreported. Patients who are scheduled for surgery should be advised to stop taking herbal products 2 to 3 weeks before surgery. Patients who are being treated with conventional drug therapy should be advised to discontinue herbal products with similar pharmacologic effects because the combination may lead to an excessive reaction or to unknown interaction effects. Patient teaching guidelines related to herbal therapy are presented in Table 6-4.

TABLE 6-3 WHOLE MEDICAL SYSTEMS

Examples	Description
Traditional Chinese Medicine (TCM)	Based on restoring and maintaining balance of vital energy *(Qi)*. One of the world's oldest, most complete medical systems.
Ayurveda	Based on balance of mind, body, and spirit. Developed in India. Views disease as an imbalance between a person's life force *(prana)* and basic metabolic condition *(dosha)*.
Homeopathy	Based on "like cures like." Remedies are specially prepared from the same substance that causes the symptom or problem. Extremely small amounts of the substance are used for the remedy. Remedies are believed to work through an energy transfer.
Naturopathy	Based on promotion of health rather than symptom management. Focuses on enhancing the body's natural healing response using a variety of individualized interventions such as nutrition, herbology, homeopathy, physical therapies, and counseling. Naturopathic physicians are graduates of accredited naturopathic medical schools, and licensing varies by state.

TABLE 6-4 PATIENT & CAREGIVER TEACHING GUIDE

Herbal Therapies

- Ask the patient about use of herbal therapies. Take a complete history of herbal use, including amounts, brand names, and frequency of use. Ask the patient about allergies.
- Investigate whether herbs are used instead of or in addition to traditional medical treatments. Find out whether herbal therapies are used to prevent disease or to treat an existing problem.
- Instruct the patient to inform health care provider before taking any herbal treatments.
- Make the patient aware of the risks and benefits associated with herbal use, including drug reactions when taken in combination with other drugs.
- Advise the patient using herbal therapies to be aware of any side effects while taking herbal treatments and to immediately report them to health care provider.
- Make the patient aware that moisture, sunlight, and heat may alter the components of herbal treatments.
- Advise the patient to determine the reputation of the manufacturers of herbal products and the safety of the product before buying herbal treatments.
- Encourage the patient to read labels of herbal therapies carefully. Advise the patient not to take more of an herb than is recommended.
- Inform the patient that most herbal therapies should be discontinued at least 2 to 3 weeks before surgery.
- Inform the patient that the employees of health food stores are not trained health care professionals.

COMPLEMENTARY & ALTERNATIVE THERAPIES

Complementary & Alternative Therapies Boxes Throughout Book

Information related to various complementary and alternative therapies can be found in the following boxes throughout the book.

TABLE 6-5 COMMONLY USED HERBS*

Name	Uses Based on Scientific Evidence	Comments
Aloe	Constipation	• Short-term use only. • May cause electrolyte imbalances. • May lower blood glucose.
Cranberry	Prevention of urinary tract infection	• Drinking cranberry juice appears to be safe. • Excessive amounts can lead to gastrointestinal upset or diarrhea.
Echinacea	May reduce incidence and duration of upper respiratory tract infections	• Short-term use is recommended. • Use with caution in patients with conditions affecting immune system. • Use cautiously in patients with asthma because of increased risk of allergic reaction.
Evening primrose	Eczema, skin irritation	• Contraindicated in individuals with seizure disorders.
Feverfew	Migraine headache prevention	• May increase risk of bleeding. • Long-term users may experience withdrawal symptoms.
Garlic	May decrease cholesterol and low-density lipoproteins (studies have been inconsistent)	• May increase risk of bleeding. • May lower blood glucose.
Ginger	Nausea and vomiting of pregnancy	• May increase risk of bleeding. • May lower blood glucose. • Use in pregnancy should not exceed 1 g/day. • Supervision by health care provider is recommended for pregnant women considering use of ginger.
Ginkgo biloba	Symptoms of claudication	• Generally well tolerated in recommended dosages for up to 6 months. • May increase risk of stroke. • May increase risk of bleeding. • May affect blood glucose levels.
Ginseng (*Panax* species)	May improve mental performance May enhance immune system May lower blood glucose	• May increase or decrease blood pressure. • May increase risk of bleeding. • Avoid use in patients with hormone-sensitive conditions such as breast cancer.
Hawthorn	Mild to moderate heart failure	• May add to the effects of cardiac glycosides, antihypertensives, and cholesterol-lowering agents.
Kava	Anxiety	• FDA has issued warning of severe liver damage linked to use. • Avoid use in patients with liver problems and patients taking medications that affect liver. • May increase drowsiness. • Use cautiously with herbs or supplements that are metabolized by kidneys.
St. John's wort	Short-term treatment of depression (studies on benefits of use are contradictory)	• Well tolerated in recommended dosages for 1–3 months. • May lead to serious interactions with herbs, supplements, OTC drugs, or prescription drugs. • Interferes with metabolism of drugs that use cytochrome P450 enzyme system. • May lead to increased side effects when taken with other antidepressants. • Advise patients to consult health care professional before self-medicating with St. John's wort.
Zinc	Upper respiratory tract infections	• Relatively safe. • Should not be taken with dairy products or caffeine, which will reduce its absorption.

Source: Data from *www.naturalstandard.com*.
*Advise patients who are pregnant or lactating to consult a health care practitioner before using any herbs. There is limited scientific evidence for the use of most herbs during pregnancy or lactation.
FDA, Food and Drug Administration; *OTC*, over-the-counter.

Commonly used herbs are presented in Table 6-5. Although herbs are derived from plants, most individuals administer them in the form of a pill or capsule (Fig. 6-2). Commonly used dietary supplements are found in Table 6-6 on p. 84. Complementary and alternative therapy boxes related to specific herbs and dietary supplements are found throughout the book (see summary box on previous page).

Mind-Body Medicine

Mind-body medicine therapies focus on the interaction between the mind, the body, and behavior, with the intent to promote health. Examples of these therapies include meditation, yoga, relaxation breathing, guided imagery, and acupuncture. Because some of these therapies are used in stress management, they are discussed in Chapter 7.

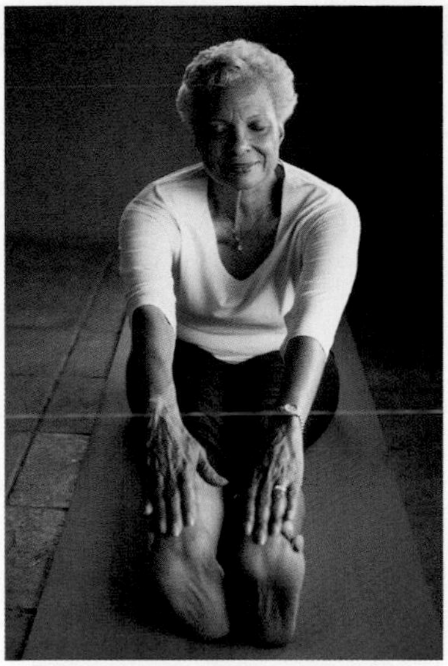

FIG. 6-1 Yoga is an example of both mind-body medicine and manipulative and body-based practices. (Jupiterimages/Comstock/Thinkstock)

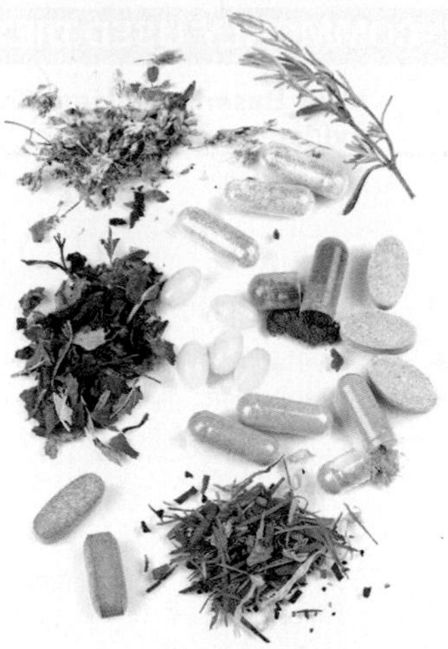

FIG. 6-2 Herbs are most commonly administered as a pill or capsule, but the source is a plant, such as echinacea. (iStockphoto/Thinkstock)

COMPLEMENTARY & ALTERNATIVE THERAPIES

Yoga

Yoga is an ancient system of relaxation, exercise, and healing with its origins in Indian philosophy. The goal of yoga is physical and mental well-being achieved through the use of stretching, postures, breathing practices, and meditation.

Scientific Evidence

There is evidence to support use of yoga to treat hypertension and to reduce stress and anxiety.*

Nursing Implications

- Regardless of the type of yoga, deep abdominal relaxation breathing is a main component and helps one to focus on the inner self and to promote the relaxation response (Fig. 6-1).
- Yoga is often used to promote relaxation, decrease stress, improve flexibility, and enhance overall health.
- Yoga is generally considered safe. Some postures should not be used by patients with certain medical conditions or illnesses.

*Based on a systematic review of scientific literature, available at *www.naturalstandard.com.*

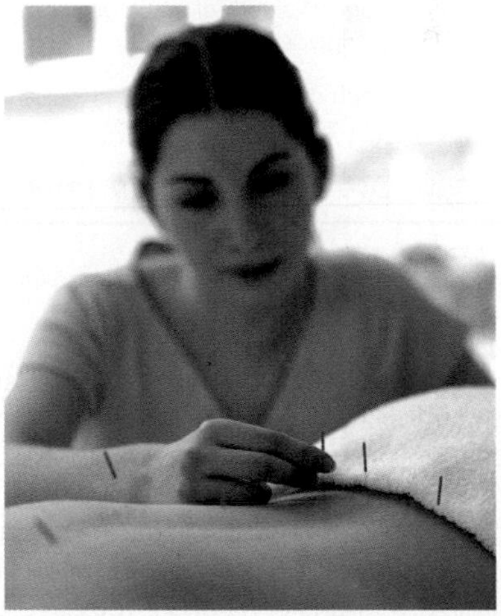

FIG. 6-3 Acupuncture showing the placement of acupuncture needles. (Creatas/Thinkstock)

Acupuncture. Acupuncture involves the insertion of fine needles into the circulation of Qi underneath the skin's surface (Fig. 6-3). Specific points are selected based on the diagnosis and nature of the complaint. With proper point selection and manipulation, acupuncture corrects disruptions in the flow of Qi.

Acupuncture has benefits for osteoarthritis, chronic pain, postoperative pain, headaches, fibromyalgia, postoperative nausea, and nausea and vomiting after chemotherapy.[7]

Acupuncture is considered a safe therapy when the practitioner has been appropriately trained and uses disposable needles. Patients should review their practitioner's credentials. The practitioner should have at least a master's degree in Oriental Medicine and be registered to practice acupuncture in that state. The practitioner should have passed the National Certification Commission for Acupuncture and Oriental Medicine examinations.

Manipulative and Body-Based Practices

Manipulative and body-based practices include interventions and approaches that are based on manipulation or movement of the body. Massage is one of the body-based methods commonly used by nurses.

Massage. Massage includes a range of techniques that manipulate the soft tissues and joints of the body. Involving touch and movement, massage is typically delivered with the hands, although elbows, forearms, feet, or various devices may be used. Massage techniques are used in bodywork, sports training, physical therapy, nursing, chiropractic therapy, osteopathy, and naturopathy.

Benefits of massage relate to its effects on the musculoskeletal, circulatory, lymphatic, and nervous systems. Massage also positively affects mental and emotional states. Massage therapy continues to grow in popularity, with most people using it as a means to reduce stress.

Until the 1970s, nurses were taught to perform "PM care," which consisted of a back rub and other measures to promote

TABLE 6-6 COMMONLY USED DIETARY SUPPLEMENTS*

Name	Uses Based on Scientific Evidence	Comments
Chondroitin sulfate	Osteoarthritis	• Well tolerated for up to 3 years. • Avoid in patients with prostate cancer or those at increased risk for prostate cancer. • Use with caution in patients with bleeding disorders or those taking anticoagulants.
Coenzyme Q_{10}	Hypertension	• May decrease blood glucose levels.
Fish oil/omega-3 fatty acids	Hypertriglyceridemia Hypertension	• May increase risk of bleeding. • May increase blood glucose levels.
Glucosamine	Osteoarthritis	• Use with caution in patients taking insulin or diabetes medications. • May increase risk of bleeding.
Melatonin	Jet lag Decrease sleep latency (time to fall asleep)	• May increase risk of bleeding. Use with caution in patients with bleeding disorders or those taking anticoagulant drugs. • May decrease blood pressure. • Use with caution in patients with diabetes. • Avoid in patients taking antiseizure medications or central nervous system depressants.
Probiotics (live bacteria or yeast)	Acute diarrhea related to antibiotic therapy Upper respiratory tract infections	• Use with caution in patients with compromised immune systems or gastrointestinal disorders.
Red yeast rice	High cholesterol and high triglycerides	• Some products contain monacolin K, which is the active ingredient in the cholesterol-lowering drug lovastatin.
Soy	High cholesterol	• Use with caution in patients with hormone-sensitive cancers. • May interact with medications taken for diabetes, diarrhea, hypertension, high cholesterol, obesity, or cardiovascular disorders. • Advise patients to consult a health care professional.

Data from *www.naturalstandard.com.*
*Advise patients who are pregnant or lactating to consult a health care professional before using any supplements. There is limited scientific evidence for use during pregnancy or lactation.

relaxation and sleep. After that time, PM care and back rubs became the exception rather than the rule. Yet today, with the increased focus on providing holistic care, nurses are again recognizing the benefits of massage. Massage is an important form of touch. It is also a form of caring, communication, and comfort. Your role related to massage differs from that of the registered massage therapist. Whereas massage therapists can provide more comprehensive therapies, nurses can use specific massage techniques as part of nursing care. For example, you can give a back massage to help promote sleep. For a bedridden patient, gentle massage can stimulate circulation and help prevent skin breakdown.

When you have determined that massage may be useful in meeting a patient goal, first assess the patient's preference regarding touch and massage. Consider cultural and social beliefs, and discuss potential benefits with the patient. Then you can implement the indicated plan of care (e.g., hand massage, back massage) with reassessment after the massage.

Massage Techniques. Nursing use of massage typically begins with *effleurage,* or gliding strokes, to promote relaxation. Stroking is done from distal to proximal, along the long axis of the muscle. After relaxing the muscles with effleurage, you may use *petrissage,* or a "kneading" stroke, to gently lift and knead the muscle. Gently scented lotions or diluted essential oils may be included in the massage.

A simple hand massage (Fig. 6-4) can have a calming and relaxing effect, especially for patients who are anxious or agitated. When a patient is frustrated or agitated, a hand massage can provide a distraction and calm the patient.

Family members can be taught to perform massage on their loved one, providing an excellent way for them to participate in patient care. This can be therapeutic for both the patient and the family, even when the loved one is cognitively impaired or unresponsive. Massage is beneficial throughout the life continuum. During end-of-life care, hospice nurses may incorporate massage into their nursing care, since the massaging touch can lessen pain and restlessness.

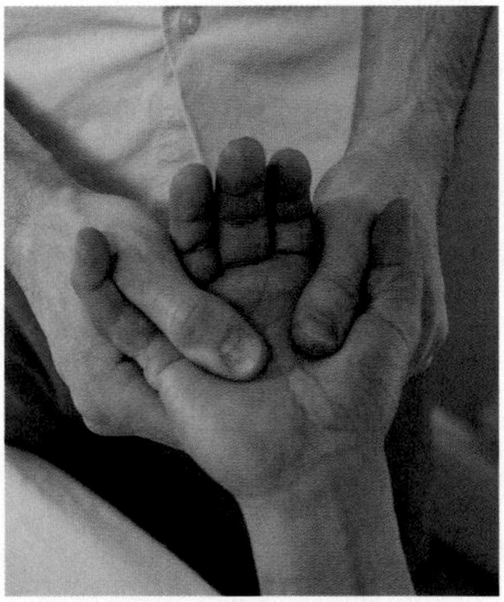

FIG. 6-4 Hand massage can be a helpful tool to calm down an agitated or nervous patient. (Jupiterimages/Photos.com/Thinkstock)

Massage is contraindicated in patients who have recent injuries or trauma, recent surgery, open wounds, deep vein thrombosis, inflammation or infections, bleeding, edema, or decreased sensation. Massage is also contraindicated when someone has used alcohol or recreational drugs.

Other CAT Practices

This broad category incorporates many practices, including movement therapies, practices of traditional healers, energy therapies, and whole body systems (see Table 6-3).

Energy Therapies. Energy therapies involve the manipulation of energy fields. They focus on energy fields originating within the body (biofields) or those from other sources (electromagnetic fields). Biofield therapies are based on the theory that energy systems in and around the body need to be balanced to enhance healing. Examples of energy therapies include Healing Touch, Therapeutic Touch, and Reiki.

Healing Touch (HT) is a nurse-based program founded in the 1980s by a nurse, Janet Mentgen. In HT, the nurse gently places his or her hands on or near the patient's clothed body. Based on established guidelines, the nurse assesses the patient's energy field, realigns energy flow, eliminates energy blockages, reactivates the mind-body-spirit connection, and then evaluates the process. It is an organized system designed to assist the patient to self-heal. The patient, not the nurse, determines effectiveness.

Information on classes, resources, and research findings is available at the Healing Touch International website *(www.healingtouchinternational.org)*.

GERONTOLOGIC CONSIDERATIONS

COMPLEMENTARY AND ALTERNATIVE THERAPIES

Older adults with non–life-threatening, chronic conditions are likely to use complementary and alternative therapies. For the older adult, safety concerns involve herb-drug interactions or toxicity related to polypharmacy and age-related changes in pharmacokinetics. Decreased renal or liver function may slow metabolism and excretion of herbs and dietary supplements. Since older adults are a more vulnerable population, it is critical that you discuss the risks and benefits of using herbal products, while encouraging patients to inform their health care provider of any herbal product or dietary supplement they are taking.

NURSING MANAGEMENT
COMPLEMENTARY AND ALTERNATIVE THERAPIES

The professional nurse can use complementary and alternative therapies in professional practice and also in self-care practice.

PROFESSIONAL PRACTICE

In professional practice, be knowledgeable of these therapies, assess their use in patients, and promote their safety. You can incorporate many of these therapies into your professional nursing practice.

KNOWLEDGE OF THERAPIES. The use of complementary and alternative therapies continues to grow, and your patients expect you to know about them. Nursing schools are incorporating content relating to complementary and alternative therapies into their curriculum. Questions related to this topic are on the National Council Licensure Examination (NCLEX).

It is important for you to understand the commonly used CAT. This includes their clinical uses and scientific-based evidence for their uses. In addition, you need to know about the personal, cultural, and spiritual dimensions related to these therapies. As a nurse, you have been educated as a critical thinker and problem solver. You need to seek ongoing education regarding complementary and alternative therapies and to continually evaluate the evidence for use of these therapies.

You need to provide information on both conventional therapies and complementary and alternative therapies. Advise patients that complementary and alternative therapies do not replace conventional therapies, but can often be used in combination with them. By providing this information, you help patients make informed decisions. You are well positioned to become the "link" between conventional therapy and complementary and alternative therapies.

ASSESSMENT OF COMPLEMENTARY AND ALTERNATIVE THERAPY USE. Because many patients use these therapies, you need to collect data on the use of complementary and alternative therapies as part of your nursing assessment. This is important because most patients do not voluntarily tell their health care provider about their use of these therapies. However, they usually share this information when asked. Ask general, open-ended questions, while remaining nonjudgmental and respectful of the patient's response.

Examples of assessment questions include the following:

- Do you have any conditions that have not responded to conventional medicine? If so, have you tried any other approaches?
- Are you using any vitamin, mineral, dietary, or herbal supplements?
- Are you interested in obtaining information about complementary and alternative therapies?

Additional specific questions for assessing the use of herbs and dietary supplements are presented in the Complementary & Alternative Therapies box in Chapter 3 on p. 44.

PROMOTING SAFE USE OF THERAPIES. The American Nurses Association Code of Ethics states: "The nurse promotes, advocates for, and strives to protect the health, safety, and rights of the patient." A wide variety of therapies are considered complementary and alternative, and some of these therapies may be ineffective or even harmful. However, patients self-select use of these therapies, generally without consulting a health care professional. Safety concerns encompass the reliability of information, the safety and effectiveness of therapies, and the regulation of practitioners. Patients usually get their information from health food stores, friends, books, magazines, and the Internet. Encourage patients to seek professional assistance with these decisions.

There is a lack of regulation of providers of complementary and alternative therapies. For example, in most states massage therapists and acupuncturists are licensed by the state. However, this practice varies by state. Practitioners of some other therapies are more loosely regulated. Along with the challenge of obtaining accurate information, patients may be unable to assess the competency of practitioners. You can serve as a resource to guide patients in the safe use of therapies and in the safe choice of health care practitioners.

INCORPORATING THERAPIES IN PRACTICE. Nursing has a long history of providing therapies that have been considered complementary and alternative. These include massage, relaxation therapy, music therapy, humor, and other strategies to promote comfort, reduce stress, improve coping, and promote symptom relief (Table 6-7). Although these therapies are generally included within the scope of nursing practice, they are not specifically addressed in some state board of nursing practice acts.

TABLE 6-7 NURSES CAN USE COMPLEMENTARY AND ALTERNATIVE THERAPIES

If you have the training and experience, you can use the following:

• Acupressure	• Massage
• Animal-assisted therapy	• Meditation
• Aromatherapy	• Music
• Healing Touch	• Prayer
• Humor	• Reiki
• Imagery	• Relaxation breathing
• Journaling	• Therapeutic Touch

Some of these therapies require additional education, training, or supervision. Check with the board of nursing in your state to determine what therapies fall within the nursing domain. You are expected to obtain the necessary additional education and experience to be competent to use a selected therapy. In addition, institutional or workplace policies must be in place supporting the use of these therapies.

You are responsible for ensuring that the patient has given consent for a given therapy. The patient must be aware of the proposed benefit and any potential risks involved. Document the effectiveness of the intervention and evaluate the outcome.

SELF-CARE PRACTICE

Learning about complementary and alternative therapies can be one road to self-care. Initially, you may be eager to learn about complementary and alternative therapies so you can provide better patient care and be a holistic practitioner. At the same time, you may find that these therapies can enhance your own level of health and wellness. With the many different complementary and alternative therapies available, you should be able to find some that will promote your personal well-being. Examples of therapies that nurses commonly use for personal well-being include deep-breathing exercises, meditation, prayer, yoga, aromatherapy, massage, and music. It is essential that you, as the caregiver, first care for yourself before you can help the patients who need your care.

BRIDGE TO NCLEX EXAMINATION

The number of the question corresponds to the same-numbered outcome at the beginning of the chapter.

1. One characteristic of the integrative model of health care is
   a. increased cost.
   b. a focus on physical disease states.
   c. an integration of mind-body-spirit.
   d. the plan of care is directed by the health care provider.
2. The nurse is preparing to teach a patient about stress management. Which category of complementary and alternative therapies can guide the nurse in preparing this intervention?
   a. Natural products
   b. Energy therapies
   c. Mind-body medicine
   d. Manipulative and body-based practices
3. The nurse is teaching a patient about safe use of herbal therapies. Which statement indicates that the teaching has been effective?
   a. "I can increase the dose if I need to, since these pills are natural."
   b. "I don't have to tell my physician about this herb that I am taking."
   c. "I must remember to stop taking these herbs 2 to 3 weeks before I have surgery."
   d. "I can stop taking my blood pressure medication now that I am taking these herbs."
4. Which herbs can increase a patient's risk of bleeding *(select all that apply)*?
   a. Aloe
   b. Kava
   c. Garlic
   d. Ginger
   e. Feverfew
5. The nurse decides to incorporate complementary and alternative therapies into her practice. Which is the best source of information?
   a. Internet websites
   b. Board of nursing for her state
   c. Salesperson at the health food store
   d. Another nurse who claims his practice is holistic
6. The nurse is preparing to collect data on an older patient's use of complementary and alternative therapies. Which guidelines should the nurse follow?
   a. The patient's culture will probably dictate which therapies are used.
   b. Begin by asking general questions, and then move to more specific questions.
   c. Obtain this information from the medical record. It is not necessary to ask the patient.
   d. Older patients do not use complementary and alternative therapies because of age-related changes in pharmacokinetics.
7. The nurse is experiencing work-related stress and desires to develop a holistic plan of self-care. What is the best source of reliable information?
   a. A self-help book
   b. Internet websites
   c. Another nurse who does not seem stressed
   d. Professional nursing organizations such as AHNA

1. c, 2. c, 3. c, 4. c, d, e, 5. b, 6. b, 7. d.

evolve

For rationales to these answers and even more NCLEX review questions, visit *http://evolve.elsevier.com/Lewis/medsurg.*

REFERENCES

1. National Center for Complementary and Alternative Medicine: What is CAM? Retrieved from *http://nccam.nih.gov/health/whatiscam*.
2. American Holistic Nurses Association: What is holistic nursing? Retrieved from *www.ahna.org/home/FAQs*.
3. American Holistic Nurses Association: Mission statement. Retrieved from *www.ahna.org/AboutUs/MissionStatement*.
4. National Center for Complementary and Alternative Medicine: Facts at a glance. Retrieved from *www.nccam.nih.gov/about/ataglance*.
5. National Center for Complementary and Alternative Medicine: Statistics on Complementary and Alternative Medicine National Health Interview Survey. Retrieved from *http://nccam.nih.gov/news/camstats/NHIS.htm*.
6. American Holistic Nurses Association: Integrative healthcare. Retrieved from *www.ahna.org/Resources/IntegratedHealthcare*.
7. Natural Standard: Acupuncture. Retrieved from *www.naturalstandard.com*.

RESOURCES

American Holistic Nurses Association
www.ahna.org

Cochrane CAM Field
www.compmed.umm.edu/cochrane.asp

Dietary Supplements Labels Database
http://dietarysupplements.nlm.nih.gov/dietary

Evidence-Based Complementary and Alternative Medicine
www.hindawi.com/journals/ecam

HerbMed
www.herbmed.org

National Center for Complementary and Alternative Medicine
http://nccam.nih.gov

CHAPTER

7

I am an old man and have known a great many troubles,
but most of them never happened.
Mark Twain

Stress and Stress Management

Sharon L. Lewis

evolve WEBSITE

http://evolve.elsevier.com/Lewis/medsurg

- NCLEX Review Questions
- Key Points
- Pre-Test
- Answer Guidelines for Case Study on p. 97
- Rationales for Bridge to NCLEX Examination Questions
- Concept Map Creator
- Glossary
- Stress-Busting Kit for Nursing Students
- Content Updates

eTable

- eTable 7-1: Stages of the General Adaptation Syndrome

LEARNING OUTCOMES

1. Differentiate between the terms *stressor* and *stress.*
2. Explain the role of coping in managing stress.
3. Describe the role of the nervous and endocrine systems in the stress process.
4. Describe the effects of stress on the immune system.
5. Discuss the effects of stress on health.
6. Describe the coping and relaxation strategies that can be used by you or a patient experiencing stress.
7. Describe the nursing assessment and management of a patient experiencing stress.

KEY TERMS

coping, p. 92
emotion-focused coping, p. 92
imagery, p. 94
meditation, p. 94
problem-focused coping, p. 92
psychoneuroimmunology (PNI), p. 91
relaxation breathing, p. 93
stress, p. 88
stressors, p. 88

High levels of stress and anxiety are common among patients and their caregivers. How they deal with their stress is critical to their well-being. As a nurse, you have an important role in helping them manage stressful events.

Stress has a powerful effect on the mind, and therefore a significant effect on one's health and well-being. This chapter focuses on how stress can affect the mind and the body and how a person can effectively deal with stress.

DEFINITION OF STRESS

Stress is the inability to cope with perceived (real or imagined) demands or threats to one's mental, emotional, or spiritual well-being.[1] Because demands are perceived differently based on the person and situation, what is emotionally or psychologically stressful to one person may not be stressful to another. Individual responses to the same stressor vary greatly. *Perception* of the potential stressor influences the way an individual responds to that stressor (Fig. 7-1). This is demonstrated in the following examples.

- B.J., a 43-year-old woman, becomes depressed after a laparoscopic hysterectomy for fibroids. She is unwilling to participate in normal self-care activities. You are surprised by her response and think that this is fairly simple surgery and she should get on with her life. After further assessment, you discover that the removal of her uterus is a great psychologic stressor because she perceives it as a loss of her womanhood and femininity.
- K.R., a 52-year-old woman, has just been told by her physician of her new diagnosis of type 2 diabetes. After the physician's visit to her, you are prepared to provide emotional support. However, you are puzzled when she is smiling and breathing a sigh of relief. You think that this diagnosis should be stressful. However, K.R. tells you that she is so relieved because for weeks she has worried that her symptoms were related to terminal cancer.

Many different events or factors can be **stressors.** They can be physiologic or emotional/psychologic (see Fig. 7-1). The emotional/psychologic stressors can be positive or negative. For example, the birth of a baby is a positive stressor. Marital discord is a negative stressor.

The key aspect of stressors is that they require an individual to adapt. In addition, differences in the behavioral and physiologic adaptive responses to a stressor can be based on the duration of a stressor (acute or chronic) and intensity of a stressor (mild, moderate, or severe). For example, an

Reviewed by Margie Hesson, RN, MSN, Certified Holistic Stress Management Instructor, Instructor of Nursing, South Dakota State University, Rapid City, South Dakota.

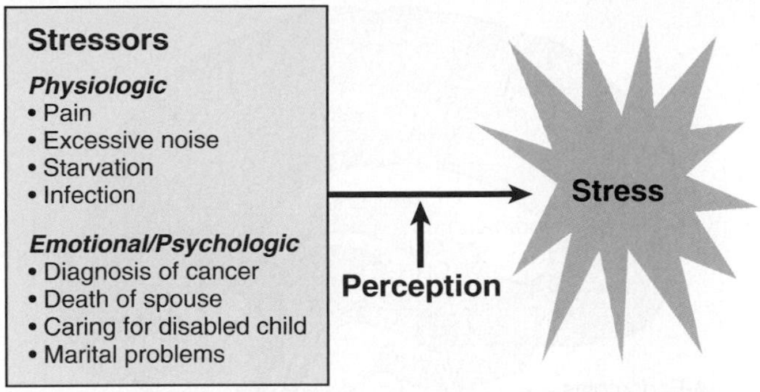

FIG. 7-1 Stressors can be physiologic or emotional/psychologic. Your perception of these stressors will determine whether they cause stress. Events or circumstances become stressful when you perceive them to be.

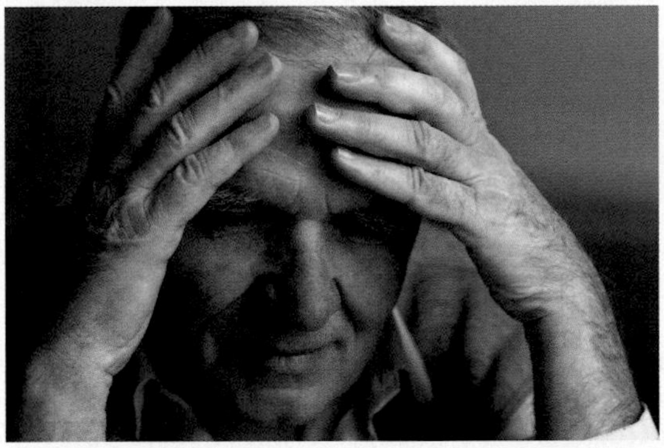

FIG. 7-2 During stressful situations, the demands seem to exceed the resources. (iStockphoto/Thinkstock)

TABLE 7-1 FACTORS AFFECTING PERSON'S RESPONSE TO STRESS

Internal	External
• Age • Health status • Personality characteristics • Previous experience with stressors • Genetic background • Resilience • Hardiness • Attitude • Optimistic outlook • Nutritional status • Sleep status	• Cultural and ethnic influences • Socioeconomic status • Social support • Religious or spiritual influences • Timing of stressors • Number of stressors already experiencing

PATHOPHYSIOLOGY MAP

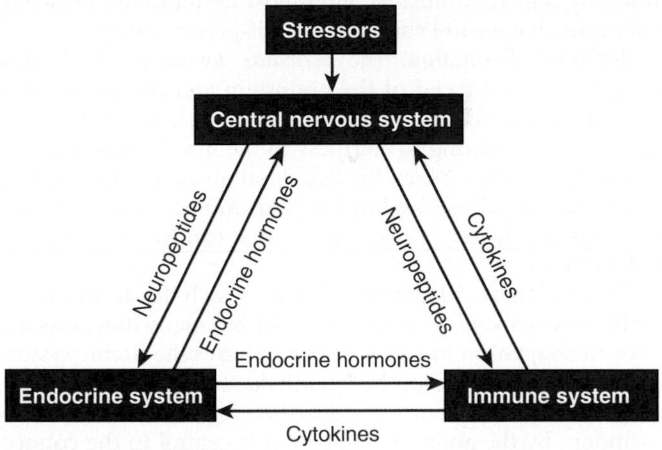

FIG. 7-3 Neurochemical links among the nervous, endocrine, and immune systems. The communication among these three systems is bidirectional.

individual dealing with the chronic stress of caring for a loved one may also be exposed to many acute episodic stressors (e.g., car accident, influenza). Therefore the type, duration, and intensity of a stressor are important variables that can influence an individual's adaptive response (Fig. 7-2).

FACTORS AFFECTING RESPONSE TO STRESS

Why do people respond so differently to stress? Why do some people cope better with stress than others? Interestingly, some individuals experience significant adverse life events but do not succumb to the effects of stress. Factors that affect an individual's response to stress include internal and external influences (Table 7-1). These factors indicate the importance of using a holistic approach when assessing the impact of stress on a person.

Four key personal characteristics that buffer the effects of stress are resilience, hardiness, attitude, and optimism. *Resilience* is being resourceful and flexible and having good problem-solving skills. Individuals who possess a high degree of resilience are not as likely to perceive an event as stressful or taxing.

Hardiness is a combination of three characteristics: commitment, control, and openness to change. Together they provide the courage and motivation needed to turn stressful circumstances from potential calamities into opportunities for personal growth.[2]

Attitude can also influence the effect of stress on a person. People with positive attitudes view situations differently from those with negative attitudes. A person's attitude also influences how he or she manages stress. To some extent, positive emotional attitudes can prevent disease and prolong life.[3]

Optimists are able to cope more effectively with stress. Optimism also reduces a person's chances of developing stress-related illnesses. When optimistic people do become ill, they tend to recover more quickly. Pessimists are likely to deny the problem, distance themselves from the stressful event, focus on stressful feelings, or allow the stressor to interfere with achieving a goal. People with a more pessimistic attitude tend to report poorer health than people with optimistic attitudes.[3]

In addition to personal characteristics, external factors play an important role in one's ability to cope with stress. Being surrounded by a strong social support system and receiving positive support from friends and family have a large impact on an individual's ability to cope with stressors.

PHYSIOLOGIC RESPONSE TO STRESS

The following section discusses the roles of the nervous, endocrine, and immune systems. These systems are interrelated, and that interrelationship is reflected in a person's physiologic response to stress (Fig. 7-3). Further, stress activation of these systems affects other body systems, such as the cardiovascular, respiratory, gastrointestinal, renal, and reproductive systems.

The complex process by which an event is perceived as a stressor and the body responds is not fully understood. A person's response to a stressor (real or imagined, and physiologic or emotional/psychologic) determines the impact that stress will have on the body.[4]

Hans Selye, a pioneer in stress research more than 70 years ago, showed that stressors from different sources produced a similar physical response. He termed this physical response to stress the *general adaptation syndrome* (GAS), which has three stages: alarm reaction, stage of resistance, and stage of exhaustion.[5] The GAS is presented in eTable 7-1 on the website for this chapter.

Nervous System

Cerebral Cortex. The cerebral cortex evaluates the emotional/psychologic event (stressor) in light of past experiences and future consequences, and thus plans a course of action. These functions are involved in the perception of a stressor.

Limbic System. The *limbic system* lies in the inner midportion of the brain near the base of the brain. The limbic system is an important mediator of emotions and behavior. When the limbic system is stimulated, emotions, feelings, and behaviors can occur that ensure survival and self-preservation.

Reticular Formation. The *reticular formation* is located between the lower end of the brainstem and the thalamus. It contains the *reticular activating system* (RAS), which sends impulses contributing to alertness to the limbic system and to the cerebral cortex. When the RAS is stimulated, it increases its output of impulses, leading to wakefulness. Stress usually increases the degree of wakefulness and can lead to sleep disturbances.

Hypothalamus. The hypothalamus, which lies at the base of the brain just above the pituitary gland, has many functions that assist in adaptation to stress. Stress activates the limbic system, which in turn stimulates the hypothalamus. Because the hypothalamus secretes neuropeptides that regulate the release of hormones by the anterior pituitary, it is central to the connection between the nervous and endocrine systems in responding to stress (Fig. 7-4).

The hypothalamus plays a primary role in the stress response by regulating the function of both the sympathetic and parasympathetic branches of the autonomic nervous system. When an individual perceives a stressor, the hypothalamus sends signals that initiate both the nervous and endocrine responses to the stressor. It does this primarily by sending signals via nerve fibers to stimulate the sympathetic nervous system (SNS) and by releasing corticotropin-releasing hormone (CRH), which stimulates the pituitary to release adrenocorticotropic hormone (ACTH) (see Chapter 48).

Endocrine System

Once the hypothalamus is activated in response to stress, the endocrine system becomes involved. The SNS stimulates the adrenal medulla to release epinephrine and norepinephrine (catecholamines). The effect of catecholamines and the SNS, including the response of the adrenal medulla, is referred to as the *sympathoadrenal response*. Epinephrine and norepinephrine prepare the body for the *fight-or-flight response* (Fig. 7-5).

Stress activates the hypothalamic-pituitary-adrenal (HPA) axis. In response to stress, the hypothalamus releases CRH, which stimulates the anterior pituitary to release proopiomelanocortin (POMC). Both ACTH (a hormone) and β-endorphin (a neuropeptide) are derived from POMC. Endorphins have analgesic-like effects and blunt pain perception during stress situations involving pain stimuli. ACTH, in turn, stimulates the

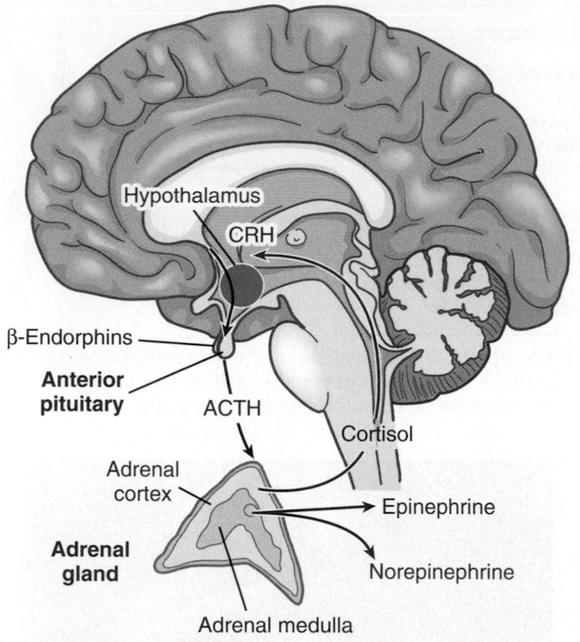

FIG. 7-4 Hypothalamic-pituitary-adrenal axis. *ACTH*, Adrenocorticotropic hormone; *CRH*, corticotropin-releasing hormone.

adrenal cortex to synthesize and secrete corticosteroids (e.g., cortisol) and, to a lesser degree, aldosterone.

Corticosteroids are essential for the stress response. Cortisol produces a number of physiologic effects, such as increasing blood glucose levels, potentiating the action of catecholamines on blood vessels, and inhibiting the inflammatory response. Corticosteroids play an important role in "turning off" or blunting aspects of the stress response, which if uncontrolled can become self-destructive. This is exemplified by corticosteroids' ability to suppress the release of proinflammatory mediators, such as the cytokines tumor necrosis factor (TNF) and interleukin-1 (IL-1). The persistent release of such mediators is believed to initiate organ dysfunction in conditions such as sepsis. Thus corticosteroids act not only to support the body's adaptive response to a stressor, but also to suppress an overzealous and potentially self-destructive response.

The stress response involves increases in (1) cardiac output (resulting from the increased heart rate and increased stroke volume), (2) blood glucose levels, (3) oxygen consumption, and (4) metabolic rate (see Fig. 7-5). In addition, dilation of skeletal muscle blood vessels increases blood supply to the large muscles and provides for quick movement. Increased cerebral blood flow increases mental alertness. The increased blood volume (from increased extracellular fluid and the shunting of blood away from the gastrointestinal system) helps maintain adequate circulation to vital organs in case of traumatic blood loss.

Summary of Stress Response

In summary, the fight-or-flight response is an important adaptive mechanism of the body to acute stress. This response to stressors is activated regardless of whether they are physiologic (e.g., acute pain) or emotional/psychologic (e.g., death of a child, loss of a home through fire, fear).

The acute stress response is a state of physiologic and psychologic arousal characterized by increased SNS activity that leads to increased heart and respiratory rate, increased blood

PATHOPHYSIOLOGY MAP

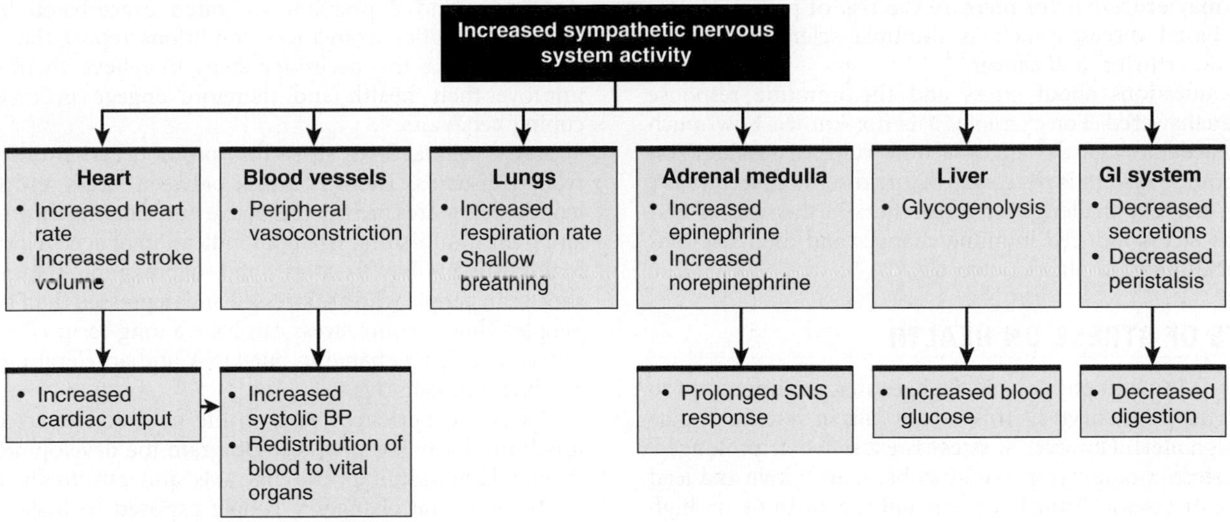

FIG. 7-5 "Fight-or-flight" reaction. Alarm reaction responses resulting from increased sympathetic nervous system *(SNS)* activity.

pressure, increased muscle tension, increased brain activity, and decreased skin temperature.

Immune System

Stress also has an impact on the immune system. **Psychoneuroimmunology (PNI)** is an interdisciplinary science that studies the interactions among psychologic, neurologic, and immune responses.[6] Because the brain is connected to the immune system by neuroanatomic and neuroendocrine pathways, stressors have the potential to lead to alterations in immune function (Fig. 7-6).

Nerve fibers extend from the nervous system and synapse on cells and tissues of the immune system (i.e., spleen, lymph nodes). In turn, the cells of the immune system have receptors for many neuropeptides and hormones, which permit them to respond to nervous and neuroendocrine signals. As a result, the mediation of stress by the central nervous system leads to corresponding changes in immune cell activity.

Both acute and chronic stress can cause immunosuppression. Stress affects immune function by (1) decreasing the number and function of natural killer cells; (2) decreasing lymphocyte proliferation; (3) altering production of *cytokines* (soluble factors secreted by white blood cells and other cells), such as interferon and interleukins; and (4) decreasing phagocytosis by neutrophils and monocytes.[7] (Natural killer cells, lymphocytes, and cytokines are discussed in Chapter 14.)

Importantly, the network that links the brain and immune system is bidirectional (see Fig. 7-3). Signals from these systems travel back and forth, allowing for communication among these systems. Consequently, not only do emotions modify the immune response, but products of immune cells send signals back to the brain and alter its activity. Many of the communication signals sent from the immune system to the brain are mediated by cytokines, which are central to the coordination of the immune response. For example, IL-1 (a cytokine made by monocytes) acts on the temperature regulatory center of the hypothalamus and initiates the febrile response to infectious pathogens (see Fig. 12-3).

PATHOPHYSIOLOGY MAP

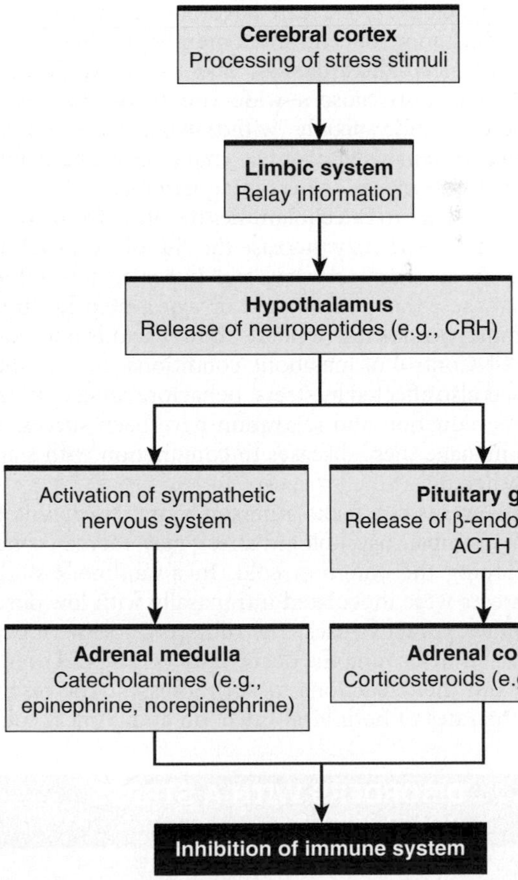

FIG. 7-6 The cerebral cortex processes stressful stimuli and relays the information via the limbic system to the hypothalamus. Corticotropin-releasing hormone *(CRH)* stimulates the release of adrenocorticotropic hormone *(ACTH)* from the pituitary gland. ACTH stimulates the adrenal cortex to release corticosteroids. The sympathetic nervous system is also stimulated, resulting in the release of epinephrine and norepinephrine from the adrenal medulla. The end result is the inhibition of the immune system.

The central nervous system is capable of influencing the function of the immune system. Stress-induced immunosuppression may exacerbate or increase the risk of progression of immune-based diseases such as multiple sclerosis, asthma, rheumatoid arthritis, and cancer.[7-9]

Many questions about stress and the immune response remain unanswered. For example, it is not known how much stress is needed to cause changes or how much of an alteration in the immune system is necessary before disease susceptibility occurs. A current challenge for researchers in the field of PNI is to study stress-induced immune changes and their relationship to health and to illness outcomes.

EFFECTS OF STRESS ON HEALTH

Acute stress leads to physiologic changes that are important to a person's adaptive survival. This is your "alarm system." It puts you on high alert. However, if stress is excessive or prolonged, these same physiologic responses can be maladaptive and lead to harm and disease. Your body was not meant to be on high alert all of the time. When a person sustains chronic, unrelieved stress, the body's defenses can no longer keep up with the demands. Therefore stress plays a role in the development or progression in the diseases of adaptation, or stress-related illnesses (Table 7-2).

Stress is linked to leading causes of death, including cancer, accidents, and suicides. Stress can have effects on cognitive function, including poor concentration, memory problems, distressing dreams, sleep disturbances, and impaired decision making. Stress can also cause a wide variety of changes in behavior. These include people withdrawing from others, becoming quiet or unusually talkative, changing eating habits, drinking alcohol excessively, or becoming irritable.[4,8-10]

Long-term exposure to catecholamines resulting from excessive activation of the SNS may increase the risk of cardiovascular diseases such as atherosclerosis and hypertension. Other conditions that are either precipitated or aggravated by stress include migraine headaches, irritable bowel syndrome, and peptic ulcers.[9,10] Control of metabolic conditions, such as diabetes mellitus, is also affected by stress. Behavioral interventions aimed at stress reduction and relaxation have been successful in helping to manage these diseases in conjunction with standard medical therapy.

Stressful life events can make a person more susceptible to infection. For example, psychologic stress may increase one's risk for developing the common cold. In a landmark study, healthy volunteers were inoculated intranasally with low doses of upper respiratory tract viruses. The subjects underwent psychologic testing to determine the occurrence of stressful events in their lives and their reactions to such stresses. The results showed that the rates of both viral infection and clinical colds increased with the degree of psychologic stress. In this study, social support buffered the harmful effects of stress.[11]

Obesity and depression are often exacerbated by stress. Those who suffer from these conditions report that they are unable to take the necessary steps to relieve their stress or improve their health and therefore engage in maladaptive coping behaviors.[12]

At the cellular level, stress may promote earlier onset of age-related diseases. There is a link between stress and telomere length. Telomeres are the protective end caps on chromosomes, and their diminishing size is an indication of age. Telomeres are highly susceptible to stress and depression. Telomeres are shorter in people who are stressed and depressed than in healthy people. Thus chronic stress can have a long-term effect on our overall health by changing our DNA and accelerating the rate at which our cells age.[13,14]

Adverse experiences early in life have an impact on brain functions. Early life stress can program the development of the hypothalamic-pituitary-adrenal axis and eventually result in neurobehavioral changes.[15] People exposed to major psychologic stressors in early life have elevated rates of morbidity and mortality from chronic diseases of aging. Children raised in poverty or mistreated by their parents have increased risk for vascular disease, autoimmune disorders, and premature death.[16]

Chronic stress is a major driver of chronic illness, which in turn is a major driver of escalating health care costs. It is critical that the entire health care community recognize the role of stress and unhealthy behaviors in causing and exacerbating chronic health conditions.[12]

TABLE 7-2 DISORDERS WITH A STRESS COMPONENT*

• Depression	• Hypertension
• Dyspepsia	• Insomnia
• Eating disorders	• Irritable bowel syndrome
• Erectile dysfunction	• Low back pain
• Fatigue	• Menstrual irregularities
• Fibromyalgia	• Peptic ulcer disease
• Headaches	• Sexual dysfunction

*List is not all inclusive.

COPING

Coping is a person's cognitive and behavioral efforts to manage stressors that seem to exceed available resources.[17] Coping can be either positive or negative. Positive coping includes activities such as exercise and spending time with friends and family. Negative coping may include substance abuse and denial.

The availability of coping resources affects an individual's ability to cope with stressful situations. *Coping resources* are characteristics or behaviors drawn on to manage stress. They include factors within the person or the environment, such as health status, belief systems, problem-solving skills, social skills, social support, and financial resources. Knowledge of a patient's coping resources can assist you in supporting existing resources and developing strategies to expand the patient's coping resources.

Coping strategies can be divided into two broad categories: emotion-focused coping and problem-focused coping. **Emotion-focused coping** involves managing the emotions that an individual feels when a stressful event occurs. Examples of emotion-focused coping include discussing feelings with a friend or taking a hot bath. **Problem-focused coping** involves attempts to resolve the problems causing the stress. Setting priorities or collecting information and seeking advice are examples of problem-focused coping.

Both strategies can be used to cope with stressors, and a combination of these strategies can be used to cope with the same stressor. Table 7-3 provides examples of emotion- and problem-focused coping when applied to the same stressful situation. Table 7-4 contains examples of coping strategies.

> *You cannot always choose your destiny in life, but you can choose how you cope with it.*
> *Norman Vincent Peale*

TABLE 7-3 PROBLEM- AND EMOTION-FOCUSED COPING

Stressor	Problem-Focused Coping	Emotion-Focused Coping
Failing an examination	Obtaining a tutor	Going for a run
Being diagnosed with diabetes	Attending diabetic education classes	Getting a massage
Receiving questionable mammogram results	Scheduling follow-up testing for ultrasound	Expressing feelings of anxiety to friends and nurse

TABLE 7-4 COPING STRATEGIES

Strategy	Description
Social support	• Self-help groups and professional help • Relationships with family and friends
Exercise	• Any form of movement, especially aerobic movement • Can be viewed as meditation in motion • Results in improved circulation, increased release of endorphins, and an enhanced sense of well-being
Journaling	• Allows an individual to express self in writing • Can write about personal events, thoughts, feelings, memories, and perceptions • Allows an individual to reduce stress, enhance coping, and increase self-awareness
Art therapy	• Allows an individual to nonverbally express and communicate feelings, emotions, and thoughts • Can reduce stress, promote relaxation, and help process experiences • Based on the belief that creative process is healing and life enhancing
Humor	• Can take the form of laughter, cartoons, funny movies, videos, riddles, comic books, and joke books • Humor carts set up in many clinical settings to be used by patients and families

When a situation is unchangeable or uncontrollable, emotion-focused coping may predominate. The primary purpose of emotion-focused coping is to help decrease negative emotions and create a feeling of well-being. Although it may not seem to be working toward a solution, emotion-focused coping is a valid and appropriate way to deal with different stressful situations.

If a problem can be changed or controlled, problem-focused coping is the most helpful coping strategy. Problem-focused coping strategies allow an individual to look at a challenge objectively, take action to address the problem, and thereby reduce the stress.

A key aspect of successful coping is *coping flexibility*, which involves the ability to change and adapt coping strategies over time and across different stressful conditions. Stressful circumstances are handled best when an individual uses coping flexibility because certain strategies work more effectively than others depending on the circumstances.

RELAXATION STRATEGIES

The *relaxation response* is a state of physiologic and psychologic rest. It is the opposite of the stress response. The relaxation response is characterized by decreased SNS activity, which leads to decreased heart and respiratory rate, decreased blood pressure, decreased muscle tension, decreased brain activity, and increased skin temperature.[18]

TABLE 7-5 RELAXATION BREATHING TECHNIQUES*

Breathing Assessment
- Begin by placing one hand gently on your abdomen below your waistline.
- Place the other hand on the center of your chest on the sternum.
- Without changing the normal breathing pattern, take several breaths. During inhalation notice which hand rises the most.
- When relaxation breathing is performed properly, the hand on the abdomen should rise more than the hand on the chest.

4 × 4 Technique
- Sit up straight with your back flush to the support of the chair and your feet flat on the floor.
- Rest your arms on your lap, thighs, or arms of the chair.
- Take in a deep breath through your nose to a count of four (1 … 2 … 3 … 4).
- Hold your breath to a count of four (1 … 2 … 3 … 4).
- Release your breath through your mouth to a count of four (1 … 2 … 3 … 4).
- Rest for a count of four (1 … 2 … 3 … 4).
- Repeat the cycle four times.

*evolve Video demonstrations of these techniques are available in the Stress-Busting Kit for Nursing Students on the website for this book.

The relaxation response can be elicited through a variety of relaxation strategies, including relaxation breathing, meditation, imagery, muscle relaxation, prayer, and physical exercise. The most common relaxation strategies are described here. Regular elicitation of the relaxation response has been proven to be an effective treatment for a wide range of stress-related disorders, including chronic pain, insomnia, and hypertension. Individuals who regularly engage in relaxation strategies are able to deal better with their stressors, increase their sense of control over stressors, and reduce their tension.[19]

Relaxation Breathing

The way one breathes affects every aspect of one's life. When a person is stressed, muscles tense and breathing becomes shallow and rapid. Therefore one of the simplest and most effective ways to stop the stress response is to breathe deeply and slowly. It is difficult to maintain tension when breathing in a slow, deep, and relaxed pattern.

Relaxation (abdominal) **breathing** can be performed while sitting, standing, or lying down. It is especially useful during a stressful or anxious situation to reduce stress. Relaxation breathing forms the basis for most relaxation strategies.

Before practicing relaxation breathing, it is important to assess one's normal breathing pattern (Table 7-5). Chest breathing, which involves the upper chest and shoulders, is inefficient. This type of breathing is often used during times of anxiety and distress. Relaxation breathing, which involves the diaphragm, is natural for newborns and sleeping adults. It is a more efficient type of breathing.

Relaxation breathing involves the primary use of the diaphragm and less use of the upper chest and shoulders to assist in each breath. In this type of breathing, the abdomen gently moves in and out during exhalation and inhalation. The breaths should be slow, steady, and deep.

One basic technique for relaxation breathing is as follows: (1) Inhale slowly and deeply, pushing the abdomen out, thinking about breathing in peace. (2) Exhale slowly, letting the abdomen come in and all the muscles relax. (3) Repeat these deep breaths 10 times without interruption. As with any breathing exercise, if a light-headed feeling arises, stop for 30 seconds and then start again.

A common method used to teach relaxation breathing is the 4 × 4 technique (see Table 7-5). Other breathing techniques are discussed in the Stress-Busting Kit for Nursing Students available on the website for this book.

Initially, relaxation breathing may feel unusual. With practice it becomes easier, and its relaxing benefits are soon obvious. You should personally learn to use relaxation breathing before teaching it to patients. Once learned, relaxation breathing can be easily taught to patients in a variety of settings, particularly when they are undergoing stressful and painful procedures.

Meditation

Meditation is a state of being with increased concentration and awareness. Meditation can be used to create a sustained period during which one focuses attention and increases self-awareness. Many seek out meditation in response to a deep human need for something transcendental or beyond everyday experiences. However, meditation can also be used to reduce stress.

Three basic ways to practice meditation are (1) concentration methods, (2) guided meditation, and (3) mindfulness practices. The *concentration technique* (e.g., Zen meditation) directs the mind to a single focus, such as the breath, an object, or a *mantra*. A *guided meditation* is similar to guided imagery (described below), where the mind and imagination are focused on a conscious goal. *Mindfulness practices* (e.g., transcendental meditation) are not restricted to any one object but rather attend to any and all sensations, perceptions, thoughts, and emotions as they arise moment to moment in the field of awareness.

Although meditation can be performed anywhere, it is best to practice meditation in a quiet place, free of distractions. Table 7-6 provides some basic guidelines on how to meditate. Meditation is often practiced while seated, and it is important to maintain a comfortable posture. Meditation can also be performed while walking and focusing on a single action such as the movement of the feet. In the beginning, individuals typically start with just 5 to 10 minutes of meditation at a time and often increase the time as the practice becomes more comfortable.

In people who meditate regularly, the brain is reoriented from a stressful fight-or-flight mode to one of acceptance, a shift that increases contentment.[20] Similarly, long-term meditation practices create structural differences in the lower brainstem, which could account for some of the cardiovascular and respiratory parasympathetic effects, as well as cognitive, emotional, and immunoreactive changes. Meditation has many positive health benefits, including reversal of coronary artery disease, decreased levels of cortisol, decreased cholesterol levels, increased airflow to the lungs, and increased immune functions.[21]

TABLE 7-6 GUIDE TO MEDITATION*

You can teach yourself the basics of meditation by following a few simple steps:

- Find a quiet place.
- Make sure there are no distractions.
- Sit in a comfortable position.
- Close your eyes.
- Shut out the world so your brain can stop processing information coming from your senses.
- Pick a word or phrase. Find a word or phrase that means something to you, whose sound or rhythm is soothing when repeated (e.g., one, peace, shalom, the Lord is my shepherd, Hail Mary full of grace).
- Breathe slowly and practice relaxation breathing.
- Say the word or phrase again and again.
- Try saying the word or phrase silently to yourself with every exhalation. The monotony will help you focus.
- Do not be concerned when other thoughts come to mind. Just acknowledge them and return calmly to your word or phrase.
- Continue for 10 to 20 minutes, but even 5 minutes can leave you feeling calm and refreshed.
- Rise slowly.

Practice once or twice daily.

*evolve Meditation exercises are available in the Stress-Busting Kit for Nursing Students on the website for this book.

Imagery

Imagery is the use of one's mind to generate images that have a calming effect on the body. It involves focusing the mind and incorporates all the senses to create physiologic and emotional changes. It is a simple relaxation technique that requires no equipment other than an active imagination. *Guided imagery* is a variation of imagery in which images are suggested by another person (either live or on a CD or MP3 file).

Imagery can be used in many clinical settings for stress reduction and pain relief. Benefits of imagery include anxiety reduction, decreased muscle tension, improved comfort during medical procedures, enhanced immune function, decreased recovery time after surgery, and reduction in sleeping problems. You can use imagery in your own life or use guided imagery with your patients. One of the uses of imagery is to create a safe and special place for mental retreat to elicit the relaxation response. Table 7-7 describes the steps involved in creating a special place.

When imagery is performed, it is best to find a comfortable position. Take slow, deep breaths. Focus should involve all senses (sight, hearing, touch, smell). For example, one can use an image such as Fig. 7-7, engaging all the senses as one focuses on the image.

Imagery can also be used to specifically target a disease, problem, or stressor. Table 7-8 describes some suggestions for using imagery in specific diseases or disorders.

TABLE 7-7 IMAGERY: CREATING YOUR SPECIAL PLACE*

- Begin by closing your eyes and taking several slow, deep breaths.
- Imagine a place where you feel completely comfortable and peaceful. It may be a real place or one you imagine; one from your past or some place you have always wanted to go.
- Allow this special place to take form, slowly. As it takes form, look around, to your left, to your right. Enjoy the scenery: the colors, the texture, the shapes.
- Listen carefully to the sounds of your place. What do you hear?
- Is there a gentle breeze or sunshine warming your face? Pick up or touch some favorite objects from your special place.
- Take in a deep breath through your nose, and notice the rich smells around you. Perhaps your favorite flower is in bloom, or you smell the scents of the ocean.
- Take another deep breath and relax. Enjoy the peace, comfort, and safety of your special place.
- This is your special place. You relax and feel thankful that you are here, in your special place.
- You can return to this place any time that you wish.

*evolve Imagery exercises are available in the Stress-Busting Kit for Nursing Students on the website for this book.

Imagery can also be used to enhance performance or process stressful or difficult tasks. For example, an athlete or musician can use imagery to achieve greater success. Imagery allows one to mentally rehearse the difficult or challenging situation. Imagery can help a fearful nurse start an IV line or perform a difficult procedure. It can also be used with a patient who is afraid to have a stressful procedure performed (e.g., radiation therapy).

Music for Relaxation

Music can help achieve relaxation and bring about healthy changes in emotional or physical states. Listening to relaxing music may divert one's focus from a stressful situation. In addition, healing vibrations from music can return the mind and body to a deeper level of balance.

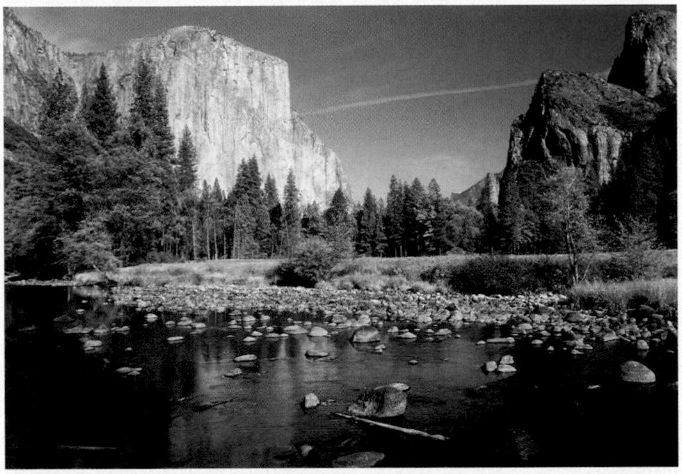

FIG. 7-7 In imagery, special places are created involving all the senses, such as a place where one can hear rustling water, smell flowers, feel the wind, and see a colorful landscape. (iStockphoto/Thinkstock)

TABLE 7-8 EXAMPLES OF IMAGERY

Imagery can be used to relieve stress and promote health and healing in conjunction with regular medical care. Special images can be created to alleviate symptoms or treat diseases or disorders. The image should be strong and vivid for the person, using many senses to create the image. Below are some examples that some people have found useful.

Disease or Disorder	Images
Infection	• White blood cells with flashing red sirens arrest and imprison harmful germs.
Cancer	• Shark gobbles up cancer cells. • Radiation or chemotherapy treatments enter the body like healing rays of light; they destroy cancer cells.
Coronary artery disease	• Water flows freely through a wide, open river.
Weakened immune system	• White blood cells rapidly multiply like millions of seeds bursting from ripe seed pod.
Asthma	• Tiny elastic rubber bands that constrict the airways pop open.
Depression	• Troubles and feelings of sadness are attached to big colorful helium balloons and are floating off into a clear blue sky.
Pain	• Pain is washed away by a cool calm river flowing through the entire body.

Adapted from Sobel DS, Ornstein R: *Healthy mind, healthy body,* New York, 1996, Patient Education Materials, Time Life.

Music has been used in many clinical settings. Music decreases anxiety and evokes the relaxation response. This relaxation helps people with insomnia go to sleep. In oncology patients it has succeeded in decreasing muscular tension, pain sensation, and emotional stress associated with cancer. In general, music affects the heart rate, blood pressure, gastrointestinal secretions and motility, muscle tone, sweat glands, and skin temperature.[22]

Music that contains approximately 60 to 80 beats/min is considered soothing. Low-pitched tones and music without words is recommended for relaxation. Mozart's music is a popular form of music used for relaxation. On the other hand, fast-tempo music can stimulate and uplift a person. Each person considers different types of music to be relaxing, so it is important to find the music that best matches the person's needs and circumstance. To achieve optimal relaxation, minimize all interruptions and assume a comfortable posture while listening to music.

Music can be incorporated into clinical practice. It is noninvasive, safe, inexpensive, and easy to use. First, it is important to establish the purpose and benefit of using music with patients in a given clinical setting. Then assess each individual patient's interest and preference in music. Create a listening environment, encouraging the patient to find a comfortable position. Headphones or earphones and an MP3 or CD player can be used. Music can be played for 20 to 30 minutes per day at least twice a day. Evaluate patients' response to the music, asking them how it sounds and how it makes them feel.

Massage

Massage is another important relaxation strategy. It involves the systematic manipulation of the soft tissue of the body to reduce tension and enhance health and healing. It also meets an essential human need: touch. Massage can be implemented as back rubs for patients. Massage is discussed in more detail in Chapter 6.

> *You may not be able to change the stressors in your life, but you can change your reaction or response to them.*
> *Florence Nightingale*

NURSING MANAGEMENT STRESS

NURSING ASSESSMENT

As a nurse, you are in a key position to assess stress in patients and their caregivers, to assist them in identifying high-risk periods for stress, and to implement stress management strategies that can prevent the negative consequences of stress on their health (Fig. 7-8). Assess the number of stressors, the duration of these stressors, and previous experience with similar demands. Also assess the personal meaning attached to the stressful situation to provide useful insight for planning stress management strategies with the patient. Also consider family responses to the demands on the patient.

The patient faces many potential stressors that can have health consequences. Be aware of situations that are likely to result in stress, and determine the patient's perception of these situations. In addition to the stressor itself, specific coping strategies have health consequences and therefore must be included in the assessment.

Although the manifestations of stress may vary from person to person, assess the patient for the signs and symptoms of the stress response, including an increased heart rate and blood pressure, hyperventilation, sweating, headache, musculoskeletal pain, gastrointestinal upset, loss of appetite, skin disorders, insomnia, and fatigue. In addition, the patient may exhibit some of the stress-related illnesses or diseases of adaptation (see Table 7-2).

Behavioral manifestations may include an inability to concentrate, accident proneness, impaired speech, anxiety, crying, frustration, and irritability. Work-related responses to stress may include absenteeism or tardiness at work, decreased productivity, and job dissatisfaction. Cognitive responses include self-reports of an inability to make decisions and forgetfulness. Some of these responses may also be apparent to significant others.

Another major source of stress relates to the patient's illness, which often also causes stress for the caregiver and other family members. Assess what aspects of the illness are the most stressful for the patient. These may include the patient's physical health, job responsibilities, finances, and children. This information is valuable because it gives you the patient's perspective of the stressors. Knowledge of stressors, the feelings these stressors invoke, and the psychologic sequelae they can produce will assist you in identifying potential and actual sources of stress and their effect on the patient.

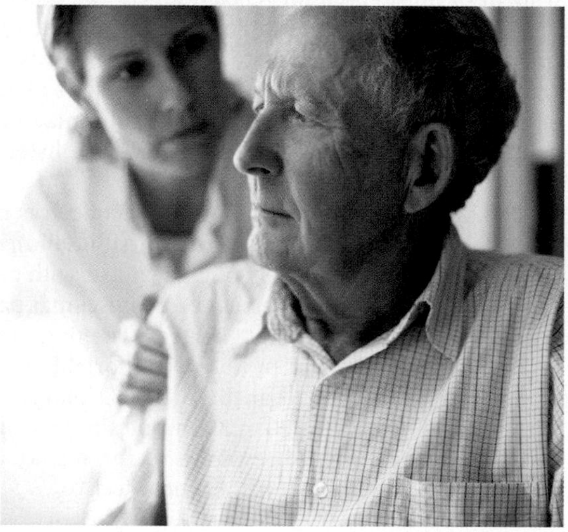

FIG. 7-8 As a nurse, you have an important role in helping patients deal with stress. (Hemera/Thinkstock)

COMPLEMENTARY & ALTERNATIVE THERAPIES

St. John's Wort

Scientific Evidence

- Although some studies of St. John's wort have reported benefits for depression, others have not.
- For treating major depression of moderate severity, a large study found that the herb was no more effective than a placebo.*
- For symptoms of minor depression, a study found that neither St. John's wort nor citalopram (Celexa), a prescription antidepressant, relieved symptoms better than a placebo.†

Nursing Implications

- Depression is a serious illness. Advise patients to consult with a health care provider before self-medicating with St. John's wort.
- St. John's wort is not a proven therapy for depression. If depression is not adequately treated, it can become severe. Anyone who may have depression should see a health care provider. Effective proven therapies are available.
- Serious interactions can occur with numerous herbs, supplements, over-the-counter drugs, or prescription drugs.
- St. John's wort interferes with the metabolism of drugs that use the cytochrome P450 enzyme system, including birth control pills, cyclosporine, carbamazepine, warfarin, midazolam, nifedipine, tricyclic antidepressants, simvastatin, and HIV drugs.
- Use of St. John's wort may lead to increased side effects when taken with other antidepressants.

*Hypericum Depression Trial Study Group: Effect of *Hypericum perforatum* (St. John's wort) in major depressive disorder: a randomized controlled trial, *JAMA* 287(14):1807, 2002.

†Rapaport MH, Nierenberg AA, Howland R, et al: The treatment of minor depression with St. John's wort or citalopram: failure to show benefit over placebo, *J Psych Res* 45:931, 2011.

NURSING IMPLEMENTATION

The first step in managing stress is to become aware of its presence. This includes identifying and expressing stressful feelings. Your role is to facilitate and enhance the patient's coping and adaptation. Nursing interventions depend on the severity of the stress experience. For example, a patient with multiple traumas expends energy in an attempt to physically survive. As a nurse, your efforts are directed to life-supporting interventions and to approaches aimed at reducing additional stressors for the patient. The patient with multiple traumas is much less likely to adapt or recover if faced with additional stressors such as sleep deprivation or an infection.

Coping resources and strategies that are used should be adaptive and not a source of additional stress for the patient. Coping resources and strategies were previously discussed in this chapter.

You can assume a primary role in implementing stress management strategies. Some personal tips for handling stress are presented in Table 7-9. These tips will benefit you personally and can be shared with patients. Ideas for how to incorporate stress management strategies into nursing practice are presented in Table 7-10. Although some may require additional training, many stress management strategies are within the scope of nursing practice. These include relaxation breathing, imagery, music for relaxation, exercise, massage, meditation, art therapy, and journaling. (Additional resources are listed at the

TABLE 7-9 PERSONAL TIPS FOR HANDLING STRESS

- Do not try to be superhuman.
- Learn to "let go" of things that are outside of your control.
- Learn acceptance of yourself.
- Exercise regularly.
- Share your feelings.
- Keep a sense of humor; laugh often.
- Learn relaxation breathing.
- Use imagery.
- Meditate or pray.
- Get adequate sleep
- Live a healthy lifestyle.
- Try to look at change as a positive challenge, not as a threat.
- Solve the little problems, since this can help you gain a feeling of control.
- Work to resolve conflicts with other people.
- If needed, get professional counseling.

end of the chapter and in the Stress-Busting Kit for Nursing Students on the website for this book.)

Before teaching stress management strategies to patients, you need to personally become familiar with them. Most relaxation strategies can be taught to patients in 10 to 15 minutes. To prepare for a relaxation training session, have the patient wear loose-fitting clothing, and ensure that the setting is private, comfortable, and free from distractions or noises. Choose a relaxation strategy to best suit the patient and the situation. Give directions calmly and slowly in short, simple sentences. End the session gradually so as to not disrupt the relaxation that was just elicited. Say a phrase such as, "I am going to count backward from five to one. With each number, you will feel more alert, but still feel at peace." After counting backward, instruct the patient to slowly open his or her eyes.

Effective stress management provides an individual a sense of control of the stressful situation. As stress management practices are incorporated into daily activities, the individual is able to increase his or her confidence and self-reliance and limit the emotional response to the stressful circumstances. Possessing a sense of control can deter the harmful effects from the stress response.

As a nurse, you are in an ideal situation to integrate stress management in clinical practice. You are also well equipped to develop and test the effectiveness of new approaches to manage stress and promote positive health outcomes. However, it is important to recognize when the patient or caregiver needs to be referred to a professional with advanced training in counseling.

TABLE 7-10 HOW TO IMPLEMENT STRESS MANAGEMENT IN PRACTICE

- Learn relaxation breathing. It is the easiest method of relaxation to use.
- Practice teaching relaxation breathing with peers, then patients.
- Pick coping strategies (see Table 7-4) and relaxation strategies that are appropriate for your clinical area.
- Practice using the strategy yourself. It becomes easier with time.
- Take advantage of opportunities to teach coping and relaxation strategies to patients.
- Anticipate setbacks. They provide feedback about what you are doing wrong. Do NOT quit!
- Attend seminars and workshops on stress management to learn more.

COMPLEMENTARY & ALTERNATIVE THERAPIES

Kava

Scientific Evidence

Although scientific studies provide some evidence that kava may be beneficial for the management of anxiety, the U.S. Food and Drug Administration (FDA) has issued a warning that use of kava supplements has been linked to a risk of severe liver damage.

Nursing Implications

- Kava has been reported to cause liver damage, including hepatitis and liver failure (which can cause death).
- It should be avoided by patients with liver problems and patients taking medications that affect the liver.
- Kava has been associated with several cases of abnormal muscle spasm or involuntary muscle movements. Kava may interact with several drugs, including drugs used for Parkinson's disease.
- Long-term or heavy use of kava may result in scaly, yellowed skin.
- Avoid driving and operating heavy machinery while taking kava because the herb has been reported to cause drowsiness.

Source: National Center for Complementary and Alternative Medicine: Kava. Retrieved from *http://nccam.nih.gov/health/kava.*

CASE STUDY

Stress-Induced Complaints

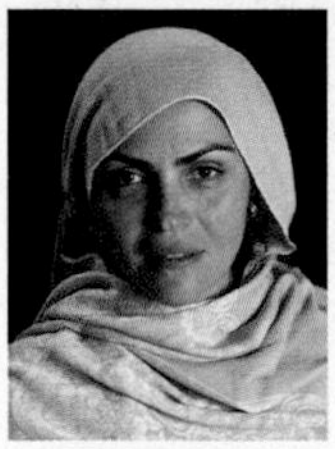
iStockphoto/Thinkstock

Patient Profile

K.F., a 43-year-old woman, recently moved to the United States from Turkey with her two teenage children. She has no family in the country and was recently divorced. She has taken a job as a waitress in a hectic restaurant and works as a seamstress out of her home in the evenings.

She has developed some unusual symptoms and comes to see the nurse practitioner at a community clinic. Although she states that she was in good health when she left Turkey, she now complains of fatigue, inability to sleep, and aches all over her body. Even when she is able to get some extra sleep, she still feels exhausted. Her co-worker told her she has fibromyalgia.

Discussion Questions

1. Consider K.F.'s situation and describe the stressors with which she is dealing. Describe the possible effects of these stressors on her health.
2. ***Priority Decision:*** What are the priority coping strategies that you should include in K.F.'s plan of care?
3. What limitations should be considered when discussing specific coping strategies?
4. What cultural considerations should be included in the plan of care?

evolve Answers available at *http://evolve.elsevier.com/Lewis/medsurg.*

BRIDGE TO NCLEX EXAMINATION

The number of the question corresponds to the same-numbered outcome at the beginning of the chapter.

1. Determination of whether an event is a stressor is based on a person's
   a. tolerance.
   b. perception.
   c. adaptation.
   d. stubbornness.
2. The nurse recognizes that a patient with newly diagnosed breast cancer is using an emotion-focused coping process when she
   a. joins a support group for women with breast cancer.
   b. considers the pros and cons of the various treatment options.
   c. delays treatment until her family can take a weekend trip together.
   d. tells the nurse that she has a good prognosis because the tumor is small.

3. The nurse would expect which findings in a patient as a result of the physiologic effect of stress on the reticular formation?
   a. An episode of diarrhea while awaiting painful dressing changes
   b. Refusal to communicate with nurses while awaiting a cardiac catheterization
   c. Inability to sleep the night before beginning to self-administer insulin injections
   d. Increased blood pressure, decreased urine output, and hyperglycemia after a car accident
4. The nurse uses knowledge of the effects of stress on the immune system by encouraging patients to
   a. sleep for 10 to 12 hours per day.
   b. avoid exposure to upper respiratory tract infections.
   c. receive regular immunizations when they are stressed.
   d. use emotion-focused rather than problem-focused coping strategies.
5. The nurse recognizes that a person who is subjected to chronic stress could be at higher risk for
   a. osteoporosis.
   b. colds and flu.
   c. low blood pressure.
   d. high serum cholesterol.
6. During a stressful circumstance that is uncontrollable, which type of coping strategy is the most effective?
   a. Avoidance
   b. Coping flexibility
   c. Emotion-focused coping
   d. Problem-focused coping
7. An appropriate nursing intervention for a hospitalized patient who states she cannot cope with her illness is
   a. controlling the environment to prevent sensory overload and promote sleep.
   b. encouraging the patient's family to offer emotional support by frequent visiting.
   c. arranging for the patient to phone family and friends to maintain emotional bonds.
   d. asking the patient to describe previous stressful situations and how she managed to resolve them.

1. b, 2. a, 3. c, 4. b, 5. b, 6. c, 7. d.

evolve

For rationales to these answers and even more NCLEX review questions, visit *http://evolve.elsevier.com/Lewis/medsurg.*

REFERENCES

1. Seward BL: *Managing stress: principles and strategies for health and well-being,* ed 7, Burlington, Mass, 2012, Jones & Bartlett.
2. Maddi SR: Hardiness: the courage to grow from stresses, *J Pos Psych* 1(3):160, 2006. (Classic)
3. Williams G: Attitude and stress: effects on the body. Retrieved from *http://ezinearticles.com/?Attitude-And-Stress,-Effects-On-The-Body&id=702403.*
4. National Institute of Mental Health: Fact sheet on stress. Retrieved from *www.nimh.nih.gov/health/publications/stress/fact-sheet-on-stress.shtml.*
5. Selye H: The stress concept: past, present, and future. In Cooper CL, editor: *Stress research: issues for the eighties,* New York, 1983, Wiley. (Classic)
6. Segerstrom SC: Resources, stress, and immunity: an ecological perspective on human psychoneuroimmunology, *Ann Behav Med* 40(1):114, 2010.
7. Heffner KL: Neuroendocrine effects of stress on immunity in the elderly: implications for inflammatory disease, *Immunol Allergy Clin North Am* 31(1):95, 2011.
8. Conti CM, Angelucci D, Ferri M, et al: Relationship between cancer and psychology: an updated history, *J Biol Regul Homeost Agents* 25(3):331, 2011.
9. Janusek LW, Cooper DT, Matthews HL: Stress, immunity, and health outcomes. In Rice VH, editor: *Handbook of stress, coping, and health,* Thousand Oaks, Calif, 2012, Sage.
10. Koenig JI, Walker CD, Romeo RD, et al: Effects of stress across the lifespan, *Stress* 14(5):475, 2011.
11. Cohen S, Tyrrell DA, Smith AP: Psychological stress and susceptibility to the common cold. *N Engl J Med* 325:606, 1991. (Classic)
12. American Psychological Association: Stress in America: our health at risk. Retrieved from *www.apa.org/news/press/releases/stress/2011/final-2011.pdf.*
13. Peres J: Telomere research offers insight on stress-disease connection, *J Natl Cancer Inst* 103(11):848, 2011.
14. Effros RB: Telomere/telomerase dynamics within the human immune system: effect of chronic infection and stress, *Exp Gerontol* 46(2-3):135, 2011.
15. Lai MC, Huang LT: Effects of early life stress on neuroendocrine and neurobehavior: mechanisms and implications, *Pediatr Neonatol* 52(3):122, 2011.
16. Miller GE, Chen E, Parker KJ: Psychological stress in childhood and susceptibility to the chronic diseases of aging: moving toward a model of behavioral and biological mechanisms, *Psychol Bull* 137(6):959, 2011.
17. Lazarus R, Folkman S: *Stress, appraisal, and coping,* New York, 1984, Springer. (Classic)
18. Benson H: *The relaxation response,* New York, 1975, Avon. (Classic)
19. Fjorback LO, Arendt M, Ornbøl E, et al: Mindfulness-based stress reduction and mindfulness-based cognitive therapy: a systematic review of randomized controlled trials, *Acta Psychiatr Scand* 124(2):102, 2011.
20. Fortney L, Taylor M: Meditation in medical practice: a review of the evidence and practice, *Prim Care* 37(1):81, 2010.
21. Young LA: Mindfulness meditation: a primer for rheumatologists, *Rheum Dis Clin North Am* 37(1):63, 2011.
22. Chan MF, Wong ZY, Thayala NV: The effectiveness of music listening in reducing depressive symptoms in adults: a systematic review, *Comp Therap Med* 19(6):332, 2011.

RESOURCES

Academy for Guided Imagery
www.academyforguidedimagery.com

American Institute of Stress
www.stress.org

American Music Therapy Association
www.musictherapy.org

Centre for Stress Management
www.managingstress.com/index.html

International Stress Management Association
www.isma.org.uk

Medline Plus: Stress Resources
www.nlm.nih.gov/medlineplus/stress.html

Stress Management Resources
www.mentalhealth.about.com/cs/stressmanagement

CHAPTER

8

The best bridge between despair and hope is a good night's sleep.
E. Joseph Cossman

Sleep and Sleep Disorders

Carol A. Landis and Margaret McLean Heitkemper

evolve WEBSITE

http://evolve.elsevier.com/Lewis/medsurg

- NCLEX Review Questions
- Key Points
- Pre-Test
- Answer Guidelines for Case Study on p. 111
- Rationales for Bridge to NCLEX Examination Questions
- Concept Map Creator
- Glossary
- Content Updates

eFigure
- eFig. 8-1: Stages of sleep

eTables
- eTable 8-1: Pittsburgh Sleep Quality Index
- eTable 8-2: Insomnia Severity Index (ISI)
- eTable 8-3: Epworth Sleepiness Scale
- eTable 8-4: Traditional Sleep Diary

LEARNING OUTCOMES

1. Define *sleep.*
2. Describe stages of sleep.
3. Explain the relationship of various diseases/disorders and sleep disorders.
4. Describe the etiology, clinical manifestations, and collaborative and nursing management of insomnia.
5. Describe the etiology, clinical manifestations, and collaborative and nursing management of narcolepsy.
6. Describe the etiology, clinical manifestations, collaborative care, and nursing management of obstructive sleep apnea.
7. Describe parasomnias, including sleepwalking, sleep terrors, and nightmares.
8. Select appropriate strategies for managing sleep problems associated with shift work sleep disorder.

KEY TERMS

SLEEP

Sleep is a state in which an individual lacks conscious awareness of environmental surroundings, but can be easily aroused. Sleep is distinct from unconscious states such as coma in which the individual cannot be aroused. Sleep is a basic, dynamic, highly organized, and complex behavior that is essential for healthy functioning and survival. Over a life span of 80 years, an individual who sleeps 7 hours each night will spend approximately 24 years sleeping. Sleep influences both behavioral and physiologic functions, including memory, mood, hormone secretion, glucose metabolism, immune function, and body temperature.

Most adults require 7 to 8 hours of sleep within a 24-hour period. Adequate sleep is defined as the amount of sleep one needs to be fully awake and alert the next day. *Insufficient sleep* refers to obtaining less than recommended amounts of sleep. *Fragmented sleep* refers to frequent arousals or actual awakenings that interrupt sleep continuity.

Sleep disturbance is a term used to indicate conditions of poor sleep quality. **Sleep disorders** are abnormalities unique to sleep. They can be classified as dyssomnias or parasomnias (Table 8-1). *Dyssomnia* is a term used to describe problems associated with initiating or maintaining sleep. Parasomnias are discussed later in this chapter on p. 110.

More than 70 million people in the United States have a sleep disorder, and many are unaware that they have a problem[1,2] (Fig. 8-1). On average most Americans report sleeping 6½ hours on workdays and 7½ hours on nonworkdays. Seventy percent of adults report habitually sleeping less than 7 hours a night.

Insufficient sleep is a serious problem with health consequences. In the 2011 National Sleep Foundation survey, 87% of Americans reported at least one sleep problem such as

Reviewed by Dana R. Epstein, RN, PhD, Adjunct Faculty, College of Nursing and Health Innovation, Arizona State University, Phoenix, Arizona; and Jo Ann Baker, RN, MSN, FNP-C, Department Chair, Nursing, Delaware Technical and Community College, Terry Campus, Dover, Delaware.

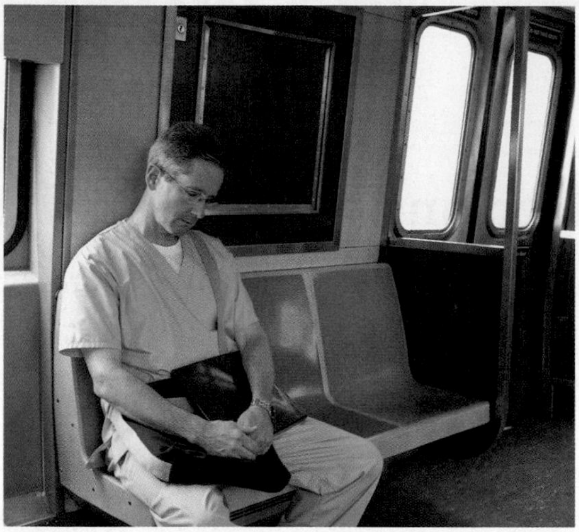

FIG. 8-1 Sleep disorders are common in our society. (Jupiterimages/Creatas/Thinkstock)

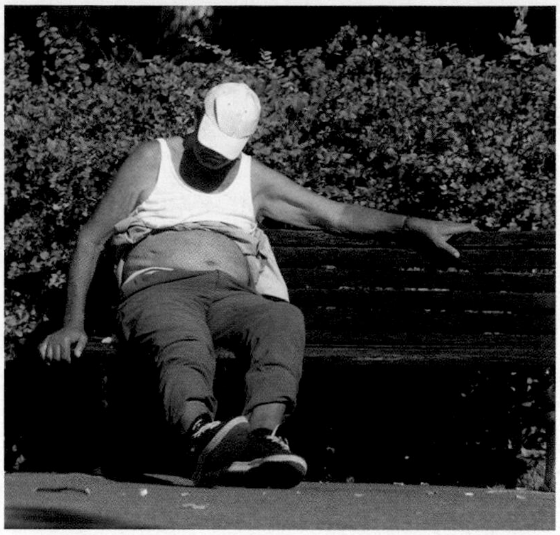

FIG. 8-2 Excessive daytime sleepiness can occur in people with sleep disorders. (iStockphoto/Thinkstock)

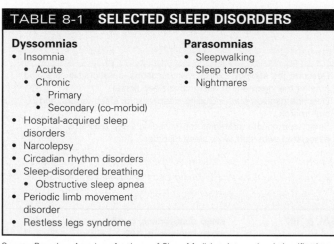

TABLE 8-1 SELECTED SLEEP DISORDERS

Dyssomnias	Parasomnias

• Insomnia
  • Acute
  • Chronic
    • Primary
    • Secondary (co-morbid)
• Hospital-acquired sleep disorders
• Narcolepsy
• Circadian rhythm disorders
• Sleep-disordered breathing
  • Obstructive sleep apnea
• Periodic limb movement disorder
• Restless legs syndrome
	• Sleepwalking
	• Sleep terrors
	• Nightmares

Source: Based on American Academy of Sleep Medicine: International classification of sleep disorders, 2nd ed: Diagnostic and coding manual, Westchester, Ill., The Academy, 2005. Retrieved from *www.esst.org/adds/ICSD.pdf.*

difficulty falling asleep, fragmented sleep, or snoring a few nights per week.[3] Daytime sleepiness can be so severe that it interferes with work and social functioning (Fig. 8-2). People with chronic illnesses are at the greatest risk for sleep disturbances.

Many sleep disorders go untreated because health care providers do not ask and patients do not talk about sleep problems. Untreated sleep disorders pose considerable health and economic consequences. Driving while drowsy is related to 100,000 accidents and 1500 traffic fatalities per year.[4] Each year, sleep disorders, sleep loss, and excessive daytime sleepiness cost the United States billions of dollars from the cost of health care, work-related accidents, and lost productivity.[1]

PHYSIOLOGIC SLEEP MECHANISMS

Sleep-Wake Cycle

The brain controls the cyclic changes between sleep and waking, but no single structure regulates these states. Rather, complex networks in the brainstem, hypothalamus, and thalamus interact to regulate the sleep and wake cycle.

Wake Behavior. Wake behavior is maintained by an integrated network of arousal systems from the brainstem and basal forebrain. A cluster of neuronal structures in the middle of the brainstem, called the reticular activating system (RAS), is associated with generalized cortical activation and behavioral arousal. Various neurotransmitters (glutamate, acetylcholine, norepinephrine, dopamine, histamine, serotonin) promote wake behavior.[5]

People with Alzheimer's disease have a loss of cholinergic neurons in the basal forebrain, which results in sleep disturbances. People with Parkinson's disease have degeneration of dopamine neurons in the substantia nigra, leading to excessive daytime sleepiness. Histamine neurons in the hypothalamus stimulate cortical activation and wake behavior. The sedating properties of many over-the-counter (OTC) medications result from inhibiting one of these arousal systems.

Orexin (also called hypocretin), a neuropeptide, is found in the lateral hypothalamus. Orexin activates arousal systems and simultaneously inhibits sleep active neurons. Decreased levels of orexin or its receptors lead to difficulties staying awake and the syndrome called *narcolepsy*. (Narcolepsy is discussed later in this chapter on pp. 106-107.)

Sleep Behavior. An area in the hypothalamus just above the optic chiasm contains many sleep-promoting neurons. These neurons act to inhibit the RAS and promote sleep.[5] Sleep is stimulated by a variety of sleep-promoting neurotransmitters and peptides, including γ-aminobutyric acid (GABA), galanin, melatonin, adenosine, somatostatin, growth hormone–releasing hormone, delta-sleep–inducing peptide, prostaglandins, and proinflammatory cytokines (interleukin-1, tumor necrosis factor, interleukin-6). Proinflammatory cytokines are important in mediating sleepiness and lethargy associated with infection. Peptides, such as cholecystokinin, released by the gastrointestinal tract after food ingestion may mediate the sleepiness *(postprandial sleepiness).*

Melatonin is an endogenous hormone produced by the pineal gland in the brain from the amino acid tryptophan. Melatonin secretion is tightly linked to the environmental light-dark cycle. Under normal day-night conditions, melatonin is released in the evening as it gets dark. Light exposure at night can suppress melatonin secretion.[6]

Circadian Rhythms. Many biologic rhythms of behavior and physiology fluctuate within a 24-hour period. Because the **circadian** (*circa dian,* about a day) **rhythms** are controlled by internal clock mechanisms, they persist when people are placed in environments free of external time cues. The suprachiasmatic nucleus (SCN) in the hypothalamus is the master clock of the body. The 24-hour cycle of sleep and wake is synchronized to the environmental light and dark periods through specific light detectors in the retina. Pathways from the retina reach the SCN, and pathways from the SCN innervate brain regions controlling wake and sleep behavior.[5]

Light is the strongest time cue for the sleep-wake rhythm. Thus light can be used as a therapy to shift the timing of the sleep-wake rhythm. For example, bright light used early in the morning will cause the sleep-wake rhythm to move to an earlier time; bright light used in the evening will cause the sleep-wake rhythm to move to a later time.

Sleep Architecture

Sleep architecture refers to the pattern of nighttime sleep recorded from physiologic measures of brain waves, eye movements, and muscle tone called *polysomnography* (PSG). Sleep consists of two basic states: rapid eye movement (REM) sleep and non–rapid eye movement (NREM) sleep (see eFig. 8-1 on the website for this chapter). During sleep, the body cycles between NREM and REM sleep. Once asleep, a person goes through four to six NREM and REM sleep cycles.[7]

NREM Sleep. In healthy adults the largest percentage of total sleep time, approximately 75% to 80%, is spent in NREM sleep. NREM sleep is subdivided into three stages:[8]

Stage 1 occurs in the beginning of sleep, with slow eye movements, and is a transition phase from wakefulness to sleep. During this period the person can be easily awakened.

Stage 2 encompasses most of the night's sleep. The heart rate slows down, and the body temperature drops. This stage is associated with specific electroencephalographic (EEG) wave forms that help to maintain sleep.

Stage 3 is deep sleep or slow-wave sleep (SWS). This stage is associated with large EEG wave forms, called delta waves, which are used as a measure of sleep intensity. SWS sleep declines as people age such that most adults over 60 years of age have little NREM stage 3 sleep.

REM Sleep. REM sleep accounts for 20% to 25% of sleep. REM sleep follows NREM sleep in a sleep cycle (see eFig. 8-1). In this stage brain waves resemble wakefulness and postural muscles are inhibited, leading to greatly reduced skeletal muscle tone. During REM sleep an individual cannot stand up and move around. REM sleep is the period when the most vivid dreaming occurs.

INSUFFICIENT SLEEP AND SLEEP DISORDERS

Insufficient sleep and sleep disorders are associated with changes in body function (Fig. 8-3) and health problems (Table 8-2). Impaired cognitive function and impaired performance on simple behavioral tasks occur within 24 hours of sleep loss. The effects of sleep loss are cumulative. Individuals who report less than 6 hours of sleep a night have a higher body mass index (BMI) and are more likely to be obese. The risk for developing glucose intolerance and diabetes is increased in individuals with a history of insufficient sleep.[9,10] Chronic loss of sleep places older adults at risk for depression, impaired daytime functioning, social isolation, and overall reduction in quality of life. In patients with chronic illnesses, especially cardiovascular disease and stroke, insomnia and sleep-disordered breathing are associated with increased morbidity and mortality.[11,12]

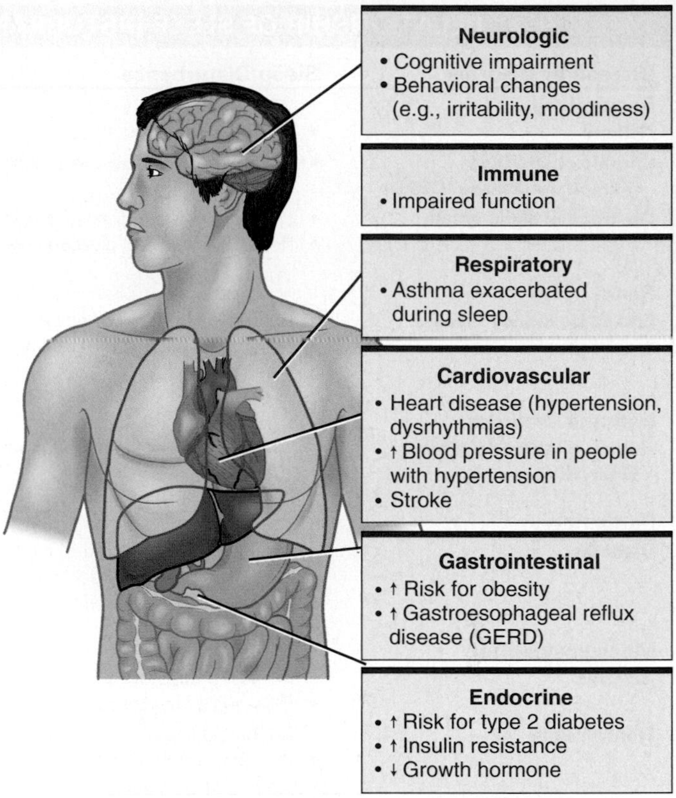

FIG. 8-3 Effects of sleep deprivation and sleep disorders on the body.

INSOMNIA

The most common sleep disorder is insomnia. **Insomnia** is characterized by difficulty falling asleep, difficulty staying asleep, waking up too early, or complaints of waking up feeling unrefreshed. Insomnia is a common problem; one in three adults experiences insomnia.

Acute insomnia refers to difficulties falling or remaining asleep at least 3 nights per week for less than a month. *Chronic insomnia* is defined by the same symptoms and a daytime complaint (e.g., fatigue, poor concentration, interference with social or family activities) that persist for 1 month or longer. Chronic insomnia occurs in 10% to 15% of Americans and is more common in women than men.[13] Chronic insomnia increases with age up to about age 65. Insomnia rates are higher in divorced, widowed, and separated individuals than in those who are married. Insomnia is more prevalent in individuals with low socioeconomic status and less education.[12,13]

Etiology and Pathophysiology

Behaviors, lifestyle, diet, physical and mental conditions, and medications contribute to insomnia. *Inadequate sleep hygiene* refers to those practices or behaviors that are inconsistent with good quality sleep. Intake of stimulants (e.g., caffeine, nicotine, methamphetamine), especially in the evening hours, predisposes a person to insomnia. Insomnia is a common side effect

TABLE 8-2 RELATIONSHIP OF SLEEP DISTURBANCES TO DISEASES AND DISORDERS

Disease or Disorder	Sleep Disturbance
Respiratory	
Asthma	• Exacerbated during sleep.
Chronic obstructive pulmonary disease (COPD)	• Associated with poor sleep quality, nocturnal oxygen desaturation, and coexisting sleep apnea.
Obstructive sleep apnea	• Linked with heart disease (hypertension, stroke, coronary artery disease, dysrhythmias). • Results in impaired glucose control similar to that which occurs in type 2 diabetes.
Renal	
End-stage kidney disease	• Disrupted nocturnal sleep with excessive daytime sleepiness. • Patients on dialysis have a high incidence of SDB and RLS, which are both significant predictors of mortality in these patients.
Immune Disorders	
Human immunodeficiency virus (HIV)	• Sleep disturbances and fatigue highly prevalent and associated with survival.
Endocrine	
Diabetes	• Insufficient sleep linked to increased risk for type 2 diabetes. • Sleep deprivation in healthy people increases insulin resistance. • Sleep duration and quality are predictors of Hb A1C levels, an important marker of blood glucose control.
Musculoskeletal	
Arthritis	• Increased rates of RLS and SDB. • Disease activity linked to sleep complaints.
Fibromyalgia	• Co-morbid insomnia, especially complaint of nonrestorative sleep. • Increased rates of PLMD and RLS. • Lower concentrations of sleep-dependent hormones (growth hormone, prolactin).
Chronic fatigue syndrome	• Co-morbid insomnia. • Increased rates of SDB.
Cardiovascular (CV)	• People with sleep apnea or sleep disorders are at increased risk for CV disorders, including hypertension, dysrhythmias, and coronary artery disease.
Heart failure (HF)	• Sleep disturbances (insomnia, PLMD, SDB) are common. • Cheyne-Stokes breathing and central apnea are signs of HF exacerbation related to fluid overload.
Hypertension	• Inadequate sleep in people with hypertension can lead to further elevations in BP.
Gastrointestinal	
Obesity	• Association between short sleep duration and excess body weight. Short sleep duration may result in metabolic changes that are linked to obesity. • Higher BMI in people who sleep <6 hours, compared with people who sleep >8 hours. • Risk factor for SDB.
Gastroesophageal reflux disease (GERD)	• Reflux of gastric contents into the esophagus occurs during sleep because of incompetent lower esophageal sphincter. • Swallowing is depressed during sleep.
Chronic liver disease	• Associated with excessive sleepiness, nocturnal arousal, and RLS.
Neurologic	
Parkinson's disease	• Associated with difficulty initiating or maintaining sleep, parasomnias, and excessive daytime sleepiness.
Alzheimer's disease	• Many have SDB (frequently sleep apnea). • Circadian rhythm alterations with nocturnal wandering, daytime sleepiness, and sleep disruption and awakening.
Pain (acute and chronic)	• Decreased quantity and quality of sleep. Poor sleep can intensify pain.
Cancer	• Higher rates of insomnia. • Chemotherapy for cancer treatment associated with fragmented sleep and fatigue.

Source: National Center on Sleep Disorders and National Heart, Lung, and Blood Institute: National Sleep Disorders Research Plan: section 4, sleep and health. Retrieved from *www.cdc.gov/sleep/about_sleep/chronic_disease.htm.*
BMI, Body mass index; *PLMD,* periodic limb movement disorder; *RLS,* restless legs syndrome; *SDB,* sleep-disordered breathing.

of many medications (e.g., antidepressants, antihypertensives, corticosteroids, psychostimulants, analgesics). Insomnia is exacerbated or perpetuated by drinking alcohol to help induce sleep, smoking close to bedtime, taking long naps in the afternoon, sleeping late in the morning, having nightmares, exercising near bedtime, and having jet lag.

Chronic insomnia is classified as primary or co-morbid. *Primary insomnia* is difficulty in initiating and maintaining sleep, resulting in poor daytime functioning that is not explained by other causes. The diagnosis of primary insomnia occurs after medical, neurologic, and psychiatric causes have been excluded.[14] The cause of primary insomnia is not known.

Certain individuals may be genetically predisposed or have psychologic traits that make them vulnerable to insomnia. Often individuals report that the onset occurred after a stressful life event (e.g., loss of loved one).

Co-morbid insomnia is common. It is associated with psychiatric illnesses, medical conditions (see Table 8-2), medications, or substance abuse. Patients with psychiatric or medical conditions are 2 times more likely to have insomnia than individuals without these conditions.[15]

Once chronic insomnia manifests, symptoms are likely to persist over time. Individuals may perpetuate disturbed sleep by keeping irregular sleep-wake schedules, using OTC medications or alcohol as sleep aids, and spending more time in bed trying to sleep. Increased attention to one's environment, worry or fear about not obtaining sufficient sleep, and poor sleep habits can lead to arousal that becomes associated with the bed and bedroom. This is called *conditioned arousal.*

Clinical Manifestations

Manifestations of insomnia include one or more of the following symptoms: (1) difficulty falling asleep *(long sleep latency),* (2) frequent awakenings *(fragmented sleep),* (3) prolonged nighttime awakenings or awakening too early and not being able to fall back to sleep, and (4) awakening feeling unrefreshed, called *nonrestorative sleep.* Daytime consequences of insomnia include feeling tired, having trouble concentrating at work or school, and having an altered mood. Falling asleep during the day or complaints of sleepiness are common. Behavioral manifestations of poor sleep include irritability, forgetfulness, confusion, and anxiety.

Diagnostic Studies

Self-Report. The diagnosis of insomnia is made based on subjective complaints and on an evaluation of a 1- or 2-week sleep diary completed by the patient. In ambulatory care settings the evaluation of insomnia requires a comprehensive sleep history to establish the type of insomnia and to screen for possible psychiatric, medical, or other sleep disorders that would require specific treatment. Questionnaires such as the Pittsburgh Sleep Quality Index (see eTable 8-1 on the website for this chapter), Insomnia Severity Index (see eTable 8-2), and Epworth Sleepiness Scale (see eTable 8-3) are commonly used to assess sleep quality.[16-18]

Actigraphy. Actigraphy is a relatively noninvasive method of monitoring rest and activity cycles. A small actigraph watch can be worn on the wrist to measure gross motor activity. The unit continuously records the patient's movements, producing data that are downloaded to a computer and analyzed.

Polysomnography. A clinical PSG study is not required to establish a diagnosis of insomnia. A PSG study is done only if there are symptoms or signs of another sleep disorder, such as sleep-disordered breathing (discussed later in the chapter). In a PSG study, electrodes simultaneously record physiologic measures that define the main stages of sleep and wakefulness.[7,8] These measures include (1) muscle tone recorded using an electromyogram (EMG), (2) eye movements recorded with an electro-oculogram (EOG), and (3) brain activity recorded through EEG. To determine additional characteristics of specific sleep disorders, other measures made during PSG include airflow at the nose and mouth, respiratory effort around the chest and abdomen, heart rate, noninvasive oxygen saturation, and EMG of the anterior tibialis muscles (used to detect periodic leg movements). Finally, a patient's gross body movements are monitored continuously by audiovisual means.

Collaborative Care

Insomnia treatments are oriented toward symptom management (Table 8-3). A key to management is to change behaviors that perpetuate insomnia. An important first step is to provide teaching about sleep along with behavioral strategies. **Sleep hygiene** is a variety of different practices that are important to have normal, quality nighttime sleep and daytime alertness (Table 8-4).

Cognitive-Behavioral Therapy for Insomnia. Although teaching about sleep hygiene practices is useful, individuals with chronic insomnia require more in-depth cognitive-behavioral therapy for insomnia (CBT-I).[14] CBT-I is based on structured treatment plans that could include relaxation training, guided imagery, cognitive strategies to address misconceptions about sleep, and behavioral strategies. Behavioral strategies for insomnia include instructions to (1) limit the amount of time an individual can stay in bed, (2) maintain a scheduled

TABLE 8-3 COLLABORATIVE CARE

Insomnia

Diagnostic	Collaborative Therapy
History • Self-report sleep log or diary • Sleep assessment (see Table 8-6) • Pittsburgh Sleep Quality Index (see eTable 8-1*) • Insomnia Severity Index (see eTable 8-2*) • Epworth Sleepiness Scale (see eTable 8-3*) Physical assessment • Polysomnography	Nondrug • Sleep hygiene (see Table 8-4) • Cognitive behavioral therapies for insomnia (CBT-I) Drugs (see Table 8-5) • Benzodiazepines • Benzodiazepine-receptor–like agents • Melatonin-receptor agonist • Antidepressants • Antihistamines Complementary and alternative therapies • Melatonin

*evolve Available on website for this chapter.

TABLE 8-4 PATIENT TEACHING GUIDE

Sleep Hygiene

Include the following instructions when teaching a patient who has a sleep disturbance or disorder.

- Don't go to bed unless you are sleepy.
- If you are not asleep after 20 minutes, get out of the bed.
- Adopt a regular pattern in terms of bedtime and awakening.
- Begin rituals (e.g., warm bath, light snack, reading) that help you relax each night before bed.
- Get a full night's sleep on a regular basis.
- Make your bedroom quiet, dark, and a little bit cool.
- Don't read, write, eat, watch TV, talk on the phone, or play cards in bed.
- Avoid caffeine, nicotine, and alcohol at least 4 to 6 hours before bedtime.
- Don't go to bed hungry, but don't eat a big meal near bedtime either.
- Avoid strenuous exercise within 6 hours of your bedtime.
- Avoid sleeping pills, or use them cautiously.
- Practice relaxation techniques (e.g., relaxation breathing) to help you cope with stress in your life (see Chapter 7).

Adapted from American Academy of Sleep Medicine: Sleep hygiene: the healthy habits of good sleep, 2010. Retrieved from *http://yoursleep.aasmnet.org/hygiene.aspx.*

TABLE 8-5 DRUG THERAPY

Insomnia

Benzodiazepines • diazepam (Valium) • flurazepam (Dalmane) • lorazepam (Ativan) • quazepam (Doral) • triazolam (Halcion)	**Melatonin-Receptor Agonist** • ramelteon (Rozerem) **Antidepressants** • amitriptyline (Elavil) • bupropion (Wellbutrin) • doxepin (Sinequan) • fluoxetine (Prozac) • trazodone (Desyrel)
Benzodiazepine-Receptor–like Agents • zolpidem (Ambien, Ambien CR, Intermezzo, Edluar, ZolpiMist) • zaleplon (Sonata) • eszopiclone (Lunesta)	**Antihistamines** • diphenhydramine (Benadryl, Nytol, Sominex)

time to get up in the morning, (3) go to bed only when an individual feels sleepy, and (4) get out of bed when unable to sleep. CBT-I also includes teaching about sleep hygiene practices (see Table 8-4). CBT-I requires individuals to change behavior, which sometimes is difficult.

Encourage individuals with insomnia not to watch television or read in bed. Time in bed is limited to the actual time that the individual can sleep. Teach the person with insomnia to avoid naps and consumption of large meals, alcohol, and stimulants, especially a few hours before bedtime. Naps are less likely to affect nighttime sleep if they are limited to 15 to 20 minutes, once per day, and scheduled 7 to 9 hours after morning awakening. Regular exercise (performed several hours before bedtime) may enhance sleep quality.

Drug Therapy. Hypnotic and anxiolytic medications are effective for improving sleep, but the benefits for improving daytime functioning are less certain. Few studies have evaluated the use of hypnotics for chronic insomnia, and their use in older adults is controversial.[19] Many individuals with insomnia become used to taking OTC or prescription medications to treat insomnia and risk becoming dependent on them, both psychologically and physically.[20] *Rebound insomnia* is common with abrupt withdrawal of some hypnotic medications. The resulting daytime fatigue can negatively influence the patient's efforts to use nondrug approaches. Classes of medications used to treat insomnia include benzodiazepines, benzodiazepine-receptor–like agents, melatonin-receptor agonists, and antidepressant and antihistamine medications (Table 8-5).

Benzodiazepines. Benzodiazepines such as diazepam (Valium) activate the γ-aminobutyric acid (GABA) receptors to promote sleep. The prolonged half-life of some of these agents (e.g., flurazepam [Dalmane]) can result in daytime sleepiness, amnesia, dizziness, and rebound insomnia. Tolerance to these agents develops, and there is risk for dependence. It is recommended that the use of benzodiazepines be limited to 2 to 3 weeks. All benzodiazepines have the potential for abuse. In addition, benzodiazepines interact with alcohol and other central nervous system (CNS) depressants. These agents are no longer recommended as first-line therapy for insomnia.

Benzodiazepine-Receptor–like Agents. Zolpidem (Ambien), zaleplon (Sonata), and eszopiclone (Lunesta) are the drugs of first choice for insomnia. Because they are benzodiazepine-receptor agonists, they work similarly to benzodiazepines.[20] These drugs are effective and safe for use from 6 months to a year. Food has the potential to delay onset of action and should not be taken with these agents. These agents have short half-lives, making their duration of action short. The extended-release formulation of zolpidem (Ambien CR) is used for problems of sleep onset and sleep maintenance. A dissolvable tablet form of zolpidem (Edluar) and an oral spray formulation (ZolpiMist) may be useful for individuals who have difficulty swallowing pills or are on restricted oral fluid intake.[20] Zolpidem tartrate (Intermezzo), a sublingual tablet, is used for patients with insomnia characterized by middle-of-the-night waking followed by difficulty returning to sleep.

Melatonin-Receptor Agonist. Ramelteon (Rozerem) is a melatonin-receptor agonist. It has a rapid onset that is effective for sleep onset but a short duration of action. Unlike benzodiazepines, ramelteon does not cause tolerance, but the drug is not always effective in improving sleep quality.[19]

Antidepressants. Trazodone (Desyrel) is an atypical antidepressant that has sedative properties. It is one of the most common agents prescribed in the United States to treat insomnia, especially in older adults. The insomnia dose of antidepressants like trazodone is much lower than the antidepressant dose. The administration of this drug to older adults is controversial. Daytime sleepiness is a common side effect. Tolerance can develop within a few weeks.

Doxepin (Sinequan) is another antidepressant used to treat insomnia. In very low doses doxepin inhibits histamine receptors in the brain. Doxepin improves sleep without next-day drowsiness in older and middle-aged adults with chronic primary insomnia.[21]

Antihistamines. Many individuals with insomnia self-medicate with OTC sleep aids. Most OTC agents include diphenhydramine (Benadryl, Nytol, Sominex). These agents are less effective than benzodiazepines, and tolerance develops quickly. In addition, antihistamines have anticholinergic side effects, including daytime sleepiness, impaired cognitive function, blurred vision, urinary retention, constipation, and risk of increased intraocular pressure. Agents with diphenhydramine are not intended for long-term use and should not be used by older adults.[11,19]

Complementary and Alternative Therapies. Many types of complementary therapies and herbal products are used as sleep aids. As noted earlier in the chapter, melatonin is a hormone produced by the pineal gland[22] (see Complementary & Alternative Therapies box). Melatonin is effective for improving sleep disturbance associated with jet lag. It also helps night shift

COMPLEMENTARY & ALTERNATIVE THERAPIES

Melatonin

Scientific Evidence

Overall, the scientific evidence suggests the benefits of melatonin in people who take it for jet lag. The majority of scientific evidence suggests that it may decrease the time it takes to fall asleep (sleep latency).

Nursing Implications

- Regarded as safe in recommended doses for short-term use.
- Avoid in patients using warfarin (Coumadin).
- Avoid in patients using central nervous system depressants.
- May cause a drop in blood pressure. Caution is advised in patients taking drugs that may also lower blood pressure.

Source: Based on a systematic review of scientific literature. Retrieved from *www.naturalstandard.com*.

workers sleep during the daytime. However, melatonin is not considered effective for improving nighttime sleep. Valerian is an herb that has been used for many years as a sleep aid and to relieve anxiety. Although valerian is safe, it is not effective in treating insomnia.[23]

NURSING MANAGEMENT INSOMNIA

NURSING ASSESSMENT

As a nurse, you are in a key position to assess sleep problems in patients and their caregivers. Sleep assessment is important in helping patients identify personal habits and environmental factors that contribute to poor sleep. Family caregivers may experience sleep disruptions due to the necessity of providing care to patients in the home. These sleep disruptions can increase the burden of caregiving.

Both self-report and objective data are used to assess sleep duration and quality. Many patients do not tell their health care provider about their sleep problems. Therefore all patients should be asked about their sleep on a regular basis. A sleep history includes characteristics of sleep such as the duration, the pattern of sleep, and daytime alertness. Before using any questionnaire, assess the patient's cognitive function, reading level (if a paper form is used), and language ability (Table 8-6). Also assess the diet. Question the patient about the intake of caffeine and other food stimulants (chocolate). Ask about alcohol consumption and whether it is used as a sleep aid.

Ask the patient about sleep aids. This includes both OTC and prescription medications. Note the drug dose, frequency of use, and any side effects (e.g., daytime drowsiness, dry mouth). Many individuals also consume herbal or dietary supplements that they believe improve sleep, including valerian, melatonin, hops, lavender, passion flower, kava, and skullcap. Inform the patient that many of these products are sold as dietary supplements and do not have U.S. Food and Drug Administration (FDA) approval or regulatory oversight. The exact components and concentrations of herbs and supplements often are unknown, and patients may experience adverse effects. Certain agents such as kava are associated with liver toxicity. Additional sleep aids include white noise devices or relaxation strategies.

Encourage individuals to keep a sleep diary for 2 weeks. In the diary they record when they go to sleep, when they wake up, and how long they were awake during the night (see eTable 8-4 on the website for this chapter). The number and duration of naps are also recorded. Standardized questionnaires such as the Epworth Sleepiness Scale (see eTable 8-3) may be used to assess daytime sleepiness.[18]

The patient's medical history can also provide important information about factors that contribute to poor sleep. For example, men with benign prostatic hyperplasia often report frequent awakenings during the night for voiding. Psychiatric problems (e.g., depression, anxiety, posttraumatic stress disorder [PTSD], drug abuse) are associated with sleep disturbances. Sleep disturbances often develop as a consequence or complication of a chronic or terminal condition (e.g., heart disease, dementia, cancer).[14]

Ask about work schedules and cross-country and international travel. Shift work contributes to reduced or poor-quality sleep. Work-related behaviors resulting from poor sleep may include poor performance, decreased productivity, and job absenteeism.

TABLE 8-6 NURSING ASSESSMENT

Sleep

Use the following questions to do an initial assessment regarding sleep.

1. What time do you normally go to bed at night? What time do you normally wake up in the morning?
2. Do you often have trouble falling asleep at night?
3. About how many times do you wake up at night?
4. If you do wake up during the night, do you usually have trouble falling back asleep?
5. Does your bed partner say or are you aware that you frequently snore, gasp for air, or stop breathing?
6. Does your bed partner say or are you aware that you kick or thrash about while asleep?
7. Are you aware that you ever walk, eat, punch, kick, or scream during sleep?
8. Are you sleepy or tired during much of the day?
9. Do you usually take one or more naps during the day?
10. Do you usually doze off without planning to during the day?
11. How much sleep do you need to feel alert and function well?
12. Are you currently taking any type of medication or other preparation to help you sleep?

Source: Bloom HG, Ahmed I, Alessi CA, et al: Evidence-based recommendations for the assessment and management of sleep disorders in older people, *J Am Geriatr Soc* 57:761, 2009.

NURSING DIAGNOSES

Specific nursing diagnoses related to sleep include insomnia, sleep deprivation, disturbed sleep pattern, and readiness for enhanced sleep.

NURSING IMPLEMENTATION

Nursing interventions depend on the severity and duration of the sleep problem, as well as individual characteristics. Optimally, healthy adults should have 7 to 8 hours of sleep a night. Individuals with longer (more than 9 hours) and shorter (less than 6 hours) sleep durations have increased morbidity and mortality risks. Those with short sleep duration have increased risk for weight gain, impaired glucose tolerance and diabetes, hypertension, cardiovascular disease, and stroke. Occasional difficulty getting to sleep or awakening during the night is not unusual. However, sleep disturbances longer than 1 month are problematic.

Although teaching about sleep hygiene practices (see Table 8-4) is beneficial, individuals with chronic insomnia require more in-depth intervention using CBT-I strategies. An important component of sleep hygiene is reducing dietary intake of substances containing caffeine (Table 8-7). Caffeine has a half-life of about 6 hours, perhaps as long as 9 hours, in older adults. Consuming caffeinated beverages after 12 o'clock should be avoided.

Suggest and implement changes in home and institutional environments to enhance sleep. Reducing light and noise levels enhances sleep. Awareness of time passing and watching the clock adds to anxieties about not falling asleep or returning to sleep. Keeping the bedroom dark and cool is conducive to good sleep.

Teach patients about sleeping medications. With the benzodiazepines, benzodiazepine receptor–like agents, and melatonin-receptor agonists, teach the patient to take the drug right before bedtime, be prepared to get a full night's sleep of at least 6 to 8 hours, and not plan activities the next morning that require

TABLE 8-7 CAFFEINE CONTENT OF SELECTED FOODS AND BEVERAGES

Food or Beverage	Caffeine (mg)
Coffee, brewed (8 oz)	95-200
Coffee, instant (8 oz)	27-173
Coffee, decaffeinated	5
Tea, leaf or bag (8 oz)	50
Celestial Seasoning herbal tea, all varieties	0
Diet Coke (12 oz)	47
Coca-Cola (12 oz)	35
Dr. Pepper (12 oz)	54
Pepsi-Cola (12 oz)	37
7-Up, Sprite, or Diet 7-Up (12 oz)	0
A&W Root Beer (12 oz)	0
Red Bull (12 oz)	80
Mountain Dew (12 oz)	55
Ben & Jerry's no-fat coffee fudge frozen yogurt (1 cup)	85
Dannon coffee yogurt (8 oz)	45
Hershey's special dark chocolate bar (1.5 oz)	31
Hershey bar (milk chocolate) (1.5 oz)	12
Hot chocolate (8 oz)	5

highly skilled psychomotor coordination. Advise patients not to take these medications with high-fat food (delays absorption), alcohol, or other CNS depressants.

Patient follow-up regarding medications is important. Ask about daytime sleepiness, nightmares, and any difficulties in activities of daily living.

SLEEP DISTURBANCES IN THE HOSPITAL

Hospitalization, especially in the intensive care unit (ICU), is associated with decreased total sleep time and decreased SWS and REM sleep.[24] Because of the nature of a critical illness and its treatment, sleep loss may be inevitable for patients in ICUs. Preexisting sleep disorders may be aggravated or triggered in the hospital. Patients with sleep apnea should use continuous positive airway pressure (CPAP) in the hospital. Sleep-disordered breathing is a major concern in the ICU.

Environmental sleep-disruptive factors, psychoactive medications, and acute and critical illness all contribute to poor sleep. Patient symptoms, including pain, dyspnea, and nausea, can also contribute to sleep loss in the acutely ill patient. Medications commonly used in acutely and critically ill patients can further contribute to sleep loss. Hospitalized patients are also at risk for poor sleep because of circadian rhythm disruptions and reduced melatonin levels. The hospital is a new environment and thus normal cues linked to sleep are absent.

Hospital and ICU noise (e.g., staff paging system, respirator alarms, bedside monitors, infusion alarms) and especially staff conversations near patients (e.g., in hallways) during both the day and night disturb sleep. Bright lights during the night also disrupt sleep and reduce melatonin levels. Patient care activities (e.g., dressing changes, blood draws, vital sign monitoring) disrupt sleep. Inactivity, boredom, and certain medications lead to napping during the day and evening that can affect nighttime sleep.

Decreased sleep duration and sleep loss influence pain perception.[25] Psychologic factors, such as anxiety and depression, also modify the sleep-pain relationship. Adequate pain management may improve total sleep time, but medications commonly used to relieve pain, especially opioids, also alter sleep and place an individual at risk for sleep-disordered breathing. Withdrawal of opioids is associated with rebound effects on sleep architecture.

You have an important role in creating an environment conducive to sleep. This includes the scheduling of medications and procedures. Reducing light and noise levels can promote opportunities for sleep. Hypnotic medications are often available on an as-needed basis. Ask patients if they would like medication to help them sleep.

NARCOLEPSY

Narcolepsy is a chronic neurologic disorder caused by the brain's inability to regulate sleep-wake cycles normally. At various times throughout the day, people with narcolepsy experience uncontrollable urges to sleep. As the urge becomes overwhelming, individuals fall asleep for periods lasting from a few seconds to several minutes. Patients with narcolepsy often go directly into REM sleep from wakefulness. This is a unique feature of narcolepsy. Patients with narcolepsy also experience fragmented and disturbed nighttime sleep.[26]

In both genders the onset of narcolepsy typically occurs in adolescence or early in the third decade. However, approximately 25% of the patients are not diagnosed until after 40 years of age. Head trauma, a sudden change in sleep-wake habits, and infection may trigger the onset of narcolepsy symptoms. Patients with narcolepsy are included in the Americans with Disabilities Act, which requires employers to provide reasonable accommodations for all employees with disabilities.

Narcolepsy has two categories: with and without cataplexy. **Cataplexy** is a brief and sudden loss of skeletal muscle tone or muscle weakness. It can manifest as a brief episode of muscle weakness or complete postural collapse and falling. Laughter, anger, or surprise often triggers episodes. Approximately 30% to 50% of patients with narcolepsy experience cataplexy.[27]

Etiology and Pathophysiology

The cause of narcolepsy remains unknown. It is associated with a deficiency of orexin (hypocretin), a neuropeptide linked to waking, from the destruction of orexin neurons. The reason for the loss of neurons is not well understood, but an autoimmune process is suspected.

Clinical Manifestations and Diagnostic Studies

Manifestations in some patients include brief episodes of sleep paralysis, hallucinations, cataplexy, and fragmented nighttime sleep. *Sleep paralysis* is a temporary (few seconds to minutes) paralysis of skeletal muscles (except respiratory and extraocular muscles) that occurs in the transition from REM sleep to waking. The loss of muscle tone, often triggered by strong emotions, usually lasts less than 2 minutes. During the period of muscle tone loss, the individual remains conscious.

With narcolepsy, unwanted episodes of REM sleep occur throughout the day. These sleep episodes are usually of short duration, but can last for more than 1 hour, and patients feel refreshed afterward. Patients may complain of feeling drowsy and being unable to remain awake while watching a movie, sitting in a classroom, reading, or performing other sedentary activities. As a result, they often show poor performance at work, have reduced quality of life, and experience poor interpersonal relationships.

TABLE 8-8 **DRUG THERAPY**

Narcolepsy

Wakefulness Promoting	Antidepressants
• dextroamphetamine (Dexedrine) • methamphetamine (Desoxyn) • methylphenidate (Concerta) • modafinil (Provigil)	***Tricyclic*** • atomoxetine (Strattera) • protriptyline (Vivactil) • desipramine (Norpramin)
Gabaminergic • sodium oxybate or γ-hydroxybutyrate (Xyrem)	***Selective Serotonin Reuptake Inhibitors (SSRIs)*** • fluoxetine (Prozac) • venlafaxine (Effexor)

Narcolepsy is diagnosed based on a history of sleepiness, PSG, and daytime *multiple sleep latency tests* (MSLTs). For the MSLT, patients undergo an overnight PSG evaluation followed by four or five naps scheduled every 2 hours during the next day. Short sleep latencies and onset of REM sleep in more than two MSLTs are diagnostic signs of narcolepsy.

Nursing and Collaborative Management

Management of narcolepsy is focused on symptom management (see Table 8-3). Provide teaching about sleep and sleep hygiene. Advise the patient with narcolepsy to take three or more short (15 minute) naps throughout the day and to avoid large or heavy meals and alcohol. You can play a key role in ensuring patient safety by teaching safety behaviors and encouraging adherence to the prescribed medication regimen.

Drug Therapy. Narcolepsy cannot be cured. However, excessive daytime sleepiness and cataplexy (the most disabling manifestation of the disorder) can be controlled in most patients with drug treatment. A nonamphetamine wake-promotion drug, modafinil (Provigil), is considered a first-line drug therapy for narcolepsy. Other agents, including amphetamine drugs such as dextroamphetamine (Dexedrine), methamphetamine (Desoxyn), and methylphenidate (Concerta), are used to manage daytime sleepiness[28] (Table 8-8). Tricyclic antidepressant drugs such as atomoxetine (Strattera), protriptyline (Vivactil), and desipramine (Norpramin) are effective in the management of cataplexy. High doses of selective serotonin reuptake inhibitors (SSRIs) such as fluoxetine (Prozac) and venlafaxine (Effexor) may be prescribed for management of cataplexy. Sodium oxybate, or γ-hydroxybutyrate (Xyrem), a metabolite of GABA, is also used in the treatment of narcolepsy.[28]

Behavioral Therapy. None of the current drug therapies cures narcolepsy or allows patients to consistently maintain a full, normal state of alertness. As a result, drug therapy needs to be combined with various behavioral strategies. The behavioral therapies for insomnia (discussed earlier in this chapter) are also used for patients with narcolepsy.

Safety precautions, especially when driving, are critically important for patients with narcolepsy. Excessive daytime sleepiness and cataplexy can result in serious injury or death if not treated. Individuals with untreated narcolepsy symptoms are involved in automobile accidents roughly 10 times more frequently than the general population. Among those receiving appropriate treatment, the accident rate is normal.[27,28]

Patient support groups are also useful for patients with narcolepsy and their family members. Social isolation can occur because of symptoms. Patients with narcolepsy can be stigmatized as being lazy and unproductive because of lack of understanding about this disorder.

CIRCADIAN RHYTHM DISORDERS

Circadian rhythm disorders can occur when the circadian time-keeping system loses synchrony with the environment. Lack of synchrony between the circadian time-keeping system and the environment disrupts the sleep-wake cycle and affects the patient's ability to have quality sleep. The two common symptoms are insomnia and excessive sleepiness. *Jet lag disorder* and *shift work sleep disorder* (see Special Sleep Needs of Nurses section on p. 110) are the most common types of circadian rhythm disorders.[29]

Jet lag disorder occurs when a person travels across multiple time zones. One's body time is not synchronized with environmental time. Most individuals crossing at least three time zones experience jet lag. The number of time zones crossed affects the severity of symptoms and the time it takes to recover. Resynchronization of the body's clock occurs at a rate of about 1 hr/day when traveling eastward and 1.5 hr/day when traveling westward. Melatonin is effective as a sleep aid to help synchronize the body's rhythm. Exposure to daylight assists synchronization of the body clock to environmental time.

Several strategies may help to reduce the risk of developing jet lag. Before travel the individual can start to get in harmony with the time schedule of the destination. When time at destination is brief (i.e., 2 days or less), keeping home-based sleep hours rather than adopting destination sleep hours may reduce sleepiness and jet lag symptoms.

SLEEP-DISORDERED BREATHING

The term **sleep-disordered breathing (SDB)** indicates abnormal respiratory patterns associated with sleep.[30] These include snoring, apnea, and hypopnea with increased respiratory effort leading to frequent arousals. SDB results in frequent sleep disruptions and alterations in sleep architecture. Obstructive sleep apnea is the most commonly diagnosed SDB problem.[31]

Obstructive Sleep Apnea

Obstructive sleep apnea (OSA), also called *obstructive sleep apnea–hypopnea syndrome* (OSAHS), is characterized by partial or complete upper airway obstruction during sleep. *Apnea* is the cessation of spontaneous respirations lasting longer than 10 seconds. *Hypopnea* is a condition characterized by shallow respirations (30% to 50% reduction in airflow). Airflow obstruction occurs because (1) narrowing of the air passages with relaxation of muscle tone during sleep leads to apnea and hypopnea or (2) the tongue and the soft palate fall backward and partially or completely obstruct the pharynx (Fig. 8-4).

Each obstruction may last from 10 to 90 seconds. During the apneic period the patient can experience *hypoxemia* (decreased PaO_2 or SpO_2) and *hypercapnia* (increased $PaCO_2$). These changes are ventilatory stimulants and cause brief arousals, but the patient may not fully awaken. The patient has a generalized startle response, snorts, and gasps, which cause the tongue and soft palate to move forward and the airway to open. Apnea and arousal cycles occur repeatedly, as many as 200 to 400 times during 6 to 8 hours of sleep.

Sleep apnea occurs in 2% to 10% of Americans but is considered to be underreported. The risk increases with obesity

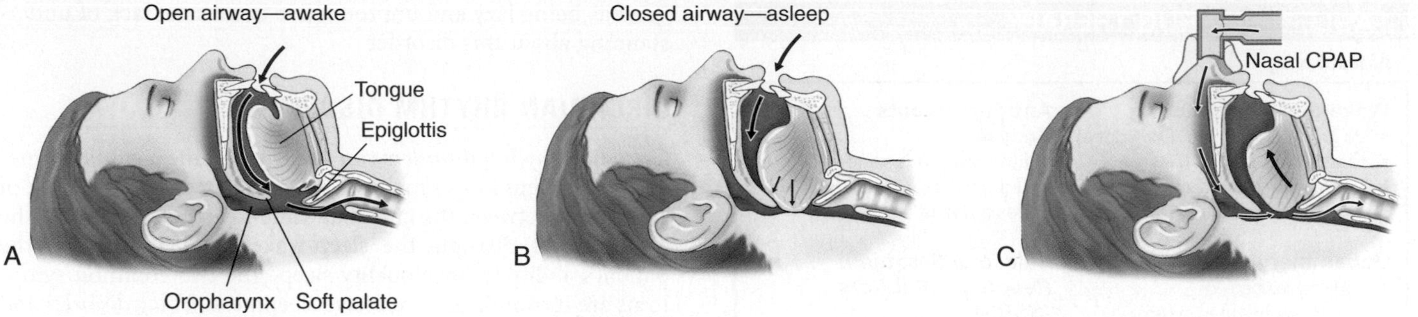

FIG. 8-4 How sleep apnea occurs. **A,** The patient predisposed to obstructive sleep apnea (OSA) has a small pharyngeal airway. **B,** During sleep, the pharyngeal muscles relax, allowing the airway to close. Lack of airflow results in repeated apneic episodes. **C,** Continuous positive airway pressure *(CPAP)* splints the airway open, preventing airflow obstruction.

INFORMATICS IN PRACTICE

Sleep Apnea Diagnosis and Monitoring

- Home respiratory monitoring is a cost-effective alternative for diagnosing sleep-related breathing disorders that allows patients the convenience of sleeping in their own home.
- Home respiratory monitoring is used as part of a comprehensive sleep evaluation and in patients likely to have moderate to severe obstructive sleep apnea but without heart failure, obstructive lung disease, or neuromuscular disease.
- Home respiratory monitoring is used to monitor the effectiveness of non-CPAP therapies for patients with sleep-related breathing disorders.
- Wireless monitors can detect changes in vital signs and pulse oximetry, raising an alarm if values fall outside of set parameters.
- Your patient may benefit from telehealth to diagnose and monitor for sleep apnea in the home.

CPAP, Continuous positive airway pressure.

(BMI greater than 28 kg/m^2), age greater than 65 years, neck circumference greater than 17 inches, craniofacial abnormalities that affect the upper airway, and acromegaly.[12,31] Smokers are more likely to have OSA. OSA is more common in men than in women until after menopause, when the prevalence of the disorder is equal.[13] Women with OSA have higher mortality rates than men with OSA. OSA patients with excessive daytime sleepiness have increased mortality.[31] Hypoxemia associated with OSA is greater in those patients with chronic obstructive pulmonary disease (COPD).[32]

Clinical Manifestations and Diagnostic Studies. Clinical manifestations of sleep apnea include frequent arousals during sleep, insomnia, excessive daytime sleepiness, and witnessed apneic episodes. The patient's bed partner may complain about the patient's loud snoring. Other symptoms include morning headaches (from hypercapnia or increased blood pressure that causes vasodilation of cerebral blood vessels), personality changes, and irritability.

Complications that can result from untreated sleep apnea include hypertension, right-sided heart failure from pulmonary hypertension caused by chronic nocturnal hypoxemia, and cardiac dysrhythmias. Chronic sleep loss predisposes the person to diminished ability to concentrate, impaired memory, failure to accomplish daily tasks, and interpersonal difficulties. The male patient may experience impotence. Driving accidents are more common in habitually sleepy people. Family life and the patient's ability to maintain employment are often compromised. As a result, the patient may experience severe depression. Cessation of breathing reported by the bed partner is usually a source of great anxiety because of the fear that breathing may not resume.

Assessment of the patient with OSA includes a thorough sleep and medical history. Symptoms of OSA, including daytime sleepiness, snoring, and witnessed apnea, are obvious characteristics of the disorder. Less obvious symptoms may include cardiovascular manifestations, muscle pain, and mood changes. Patients with OSA frequently have co-morbidities, including a history of stroke and cardiovascular disease.

PSG is used to make the diagnosis of sleep apnea. The patient's chest and abdominal movement, oral and nasal airflow, SpO_2, ocular movement, and heart rate and rhythm are monitored. A diagnosis of sleep apnea requires documentation of apneic events (no airflow with respiratory effort) or hypopnea (airflow diminished 30% to 50% with respiratory effort) of at least 10 seconds' duration. OSA is defined as more than five apnea/hypopnea events per hour accompanied by a 3% to 4% decrease in oxygen saturation. Severe apnea can be associated with apneic events of more than 30 to 50 per hour of sleep.[8]

Typically, PSG is done in a clinical sleep laboratory with technicians monitoring the patient. In some instances, portable sleep studies are conducted in the home setting. Overnight pulse oximetry assessment may be done to determine whether nocturnal oxygen supplementation is indicated.

NURSING AND COLLABORATIVE MANAGEMENT SLEEP APNEA

CONSERVATIVE TREATMENT

Mild sleep apnea (5 to 10 apnea/hypopnea events per hour) may respond to simple measures. Conservative treatment at home begins with sleeping on one's side rather than on the back. Elevating the head of the bed may eliminate OSA in some patients. Instruct the patient to avoid taking sedatives or consuming alcoholic beverages for 3 to 4 hours before sleep. Sleep medications often make OSA worse. OSA is a potentially life-threatening disorder. Because excessive weight worsens sleep apnea, referral to a weight loss program may be indicated. Weight loss and bariatric surgery reduce OSA.[33] Instruct the patient on the dangers of driving or using heavy equipment.

Symptoms may resolve in up to half of patients with OSA who use a special mouth guard, also called an oral appliance, during sleep to prevent airflow obstruction. Oral appliances bring the mandible and tongue forward to enlarge the airway

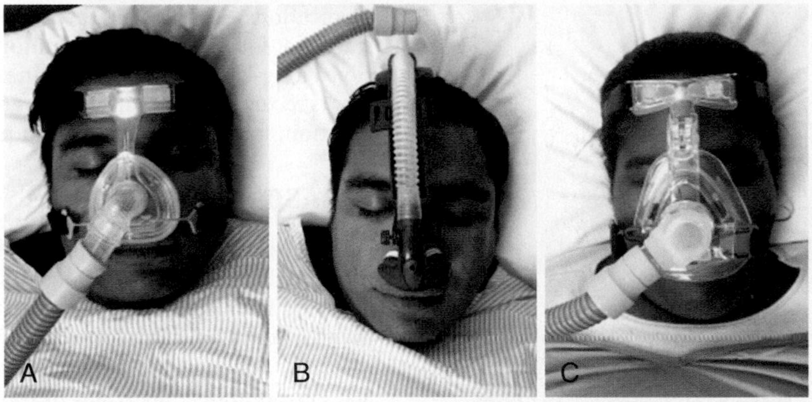

FIG. 8-5 Examples of positive airwave pressure devices for sleep apnea. **A,** Patient wearing a nasal mask and headgear (positive pressure only through nose). **B,** Patient wearing nasal pillows (positive pressure only through nose). **C,** Patient wearing a full face mask (positive pressure to both nose and mouth).

space, thereby preventing airway occlusion.[34] Some individuals find a support group beneficial, where they can express concerns and feelings and discuss strategies for resolving problems.

In patients with more severe symptoms (more than 15 apnea/hypopnea events per hour), continuous positive airway pressure (CPAP) by mask is the treatment of choice. With CPAP, the patient applies a nasal mask that is attached to a high-flow blower (Fig. 8-5). The blower is adjusted to maintain sufficient positive pressure (5 to 25 cm H_2O) in the airway during inspiration and expiration to prevent airway collapse. Some patients cannot adjust to wearing a mask over the nose or mouth or to exhaling against the high pressure. A technologically more sophisticated therapy, bilevel positive airway pressure (BiPAP), can deliver a higher inspiration pressure and a lower pressure during expiration. With BiPAP, the apnea can be relieved with a lower mean pressure and may be better tolerated.

CPAP reduces apnea episodes, daytime sleepiness, and fatigue. It improves quality of life ratings and returns cognitive functioning to normal.[35] Although CPAP is a highly effective treatment, compliance and adherence are poor. Approximately two thirds of patients using CPAP report side effects such as nasal stuffiness. First assess the patient's knowledge about OSA and CPAP, and involve the bed partner in teaching. Evaluate the patient for nasal resistance. Patient-centered selection of mask and device and exposure to CPAP before initiation of therapy are associated with successful adherence to CPAP treatment.[33] If necessary, facilitate referral for evaluation of equipment. For anxiety related to CPAP, the patient may be referred to a psychologist for desensitization therapy.

When patients with a history of OSA are hospitalized, be aware that the administration of opioid analgesics and sedating medications (benzodiazepines, barbiturates, hypnotics) may worsen OSA symptoms by depressing respiration. This will necessitate that the patient wear the CPAP or BiPAP when resting or sleeping. Many patients are able to use their own CPAP equipment, but hospital policy should be checked to be certain it can be used.

SURGICAL TREATMENT

If other measures fail, sleep apnea can be managed surgically. The two most common procedures are uvulopalatopharyngoplasty (UPPP or UP3) and genioglossal advancement and hyoid myotomy (GAHM). UPPP involves excision of the tonsillar pillars, uvula, and posterior soft palate to remove the obstructing tissue.[34] GAHM involves advancing the attachment of the muscular part of the tongue on the mandible. When GAHM is performed, UPPP is generally performed as well. Depending on the site of the obstruction, symptoms are relieved in up to 80% of patients. Radiofrequency ablation (RFA) alone or in combination with other surgical techniques is also used. RFA is the least invasive surgical intervention.[34]

Complications of airway obstruction or hemorrhage occur most often in the immediate postoperative period. Patients can usually be discharged home within 1 day after the procedure. Before going home the patient is taught what to expect during the postoperative recovery period. Tell patients that their throat will be sore. They may have a foul breath odor that may be reduced by rinsing with diluted mouthwash and then salt water after several days. Snoring may persist until the inflammation has subsided. Follow-up of patients after surgery is important. A repeat PSG is performed 3 to 4 months after surgery.

PERIODIC LIMB MOVEMENT DISORDER

Periodic limb movement disorder (PLMD) is characterized by involuntary, continual movement of the legs and/or arms that affects people only during sleep. PLMD rarely involves the arms. Sometimes abdominal, oral, and nasal movement accompanies PLMD. Movements typically occur for 0.5 to 10 seconds, in intervals separated by 5 to 90 seconds. PLMD causes poor-quality sleep, which may lead to excessive daytime sleepiness. PLMD occurs in 80% to 90% of individuals with restless legs syndrome (RLS).[36] (RLS is a disorder that is discussed in Chapter 59.)

PLMD is diagnosed using a detailed history from the patient and/or bed partner and doing a PSG. PLMD is treated by medications aimed at reducing or eliminating the limb movements or the arousals. Dopamine agonists (pramipexole [Mirapex] and ropinirole [Requip]) are preferred.

GERONTOLOGIC CONSIDERATIONS

SLEEP

With aging, the most notable changes are a decrease in the amount of deep sleep and an increase in arousals and awakenings. Older adults report greater problems getting to and main-

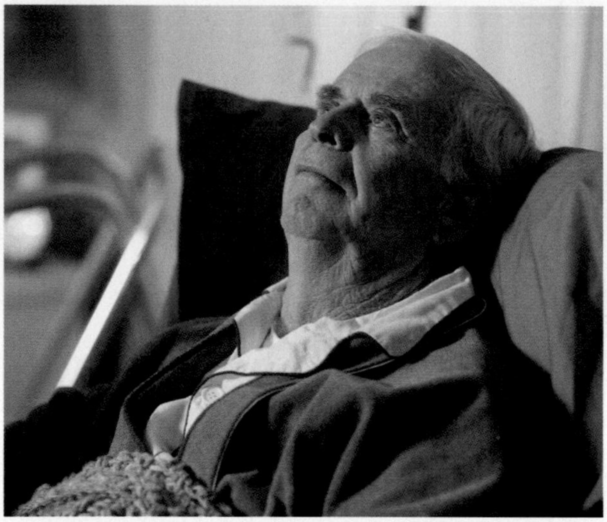

FIG. 8-6 Many older people have sleep problems. (Photodisc/Thinkstock)

taining sleep as compared with younger adults (Fig. 8-6). Older age is associated with overall shorter total sleep time, decreased sleep efficiency, and more awakenings.[37]

A common misconception is that older people need less sleep than younger people. In fact, the amount of sleep needed as a person ages remains relatively constant.[38]

Healthy older adults who do not complain of sleep disturbance often have fragmented sleep, nocturnal wakefulness, and reduced sleep efficiency when studied with PSG. Because older adults may attribute their disturbed sleep to normal aging, they may fail to report symptoms of sleep disorders to their health care providers.[37] Use a sleeping assessment (see Table 8-6) to detect sleep disturbances in older adults.

Multiple factors impair older adults' ability to obtain quality sleep. Insomnia symptoms in older adults frequently occur with depression, heart disease, body pain, and cognitive problems. Insomnia may have detrimental effects on cognitive function in healthy older adults. Older women report more trouble falling asleep and, especially, staying asleep. Other sleep disorders (e.g., sleep-disordered breathing) also increase with age and may manifest with insomnia symptoms.[37,38]

Awakening and getting out of bed during the night (e.g., to use the bathroom) increase the risk for falls. Older adults may use OTC medications or alcohol as a sleep aid. This practice can further increase the risk of falls at night. Chronic disturbed sleep in older adults can result in disorientation, delirium, impaired intellect, disturbed cognition, and increased risk of accidents and injury.[38]

Chronic conditions that are more common in older adults (COPD, diabetes, dementia, chronic pain, cancer) can affect sleep quality.[38] Medications used to treat these conditions can contribute to sleep problems. OTC medications also can lead to sleep disturbance. Cough and cold medications, especially those containing pseudoephedrine; caffeine-containing drugs; and drugs containing nicotine (e.g., nicotine gum, transdermal patches), are stimulants. Diphenhydramine, alone or in combination with other drugs, is sedating with anticholinergic effects. Any OTC medication labeled "PM" probably has diphenhydramine and should be used cautiously by older adults.[39]

Metabolism of most hypnotic drugs decreases with aging. Older adults have increased sensitivity to hypnotic and sedative medications. Thus drug therapies for sleep disturbances are started at lower doses and monitored carefully. Whenever possible, long-acting benzodiazepines should be avoided. Older adults receiving benzodiazepines are at increased risk of daytime sedation, falls, and cognitive and psychomotor impairment.

PARASOMNIAS

Parasomnias are unusual and often undesirable behaviors that occur while falling asleep, transitioning between sleep stages, or arousing from sleep. They are due to CNS activation and often involve complex behaviors. The parasomnia is generally goal directed, although the person is not aware or conscious of the act. Parasomnias may result in fragmented sleep and fatigue.

Sleepwalking and sleep terrors are arousal parasomnias that occur during NREM sleep. *Sleepwalking* behaviors can range from sitting up in bed, moving objects, and walking around the room to driving a car. During a sleepwalking event the individual may not speak and may have limited or no awareness of the event. On awakening, the individual does not remember the event. In the ICU a parasomnia may be misinterpreted as ICU psychosis. Sedated ICU patients can exhibit manifestations of a parasomnia.

Sleep terrors (night terrors) are characterized by a sudden awakening from sleep along with a loud cry and signs of panic. The person has marked increases in heart rate and respiration and diaphoresis. Factors in the ICU such as sleep disruption and deprivation, fever, stress, and exposure to noise and light can contribute to sleep terrors.

Nightmares are a parasomnia characterized by recurrent awakening with recall of a frightful or disturbing dream. These normally occur during the final third of sleep and in association with REM sleep. In critically ill patients nightmares are common and are most likely due to medications. Drug classes most likely to cause nightmares are sedative-hypnotics, β-adrenergic antagonists, dopamine agonists, and amphetamines.

SPECIAL SLEEP NEEDS OF NURSES

Nursing is one of several professions that necessitates night shift and rotating shift schedules. In many settings, nurses are asked to or volunteer to work a variety of day and night shifts, often alternating and rotating them. Unfortunately, nurses who do shift work often report less job satisfaction and more job-related stress. A large number of nurses who work the night shift report episodes of nodding off while driving home after work.[40]

Nurses on permanent night or rapidly rotating shifts are at increased risk of experiencing *shift work sleep disorder,* characterized by insomnia, sleepiness, and fatigue. Nurses on rotating shifts get the least amount of sleep. With repeated periods of inadequate sleep, the sleep debt grows. Poor sleep is the strongest predictor of chronic fatigue in nurses doing shift work. As a result, rotating and night shift schedules pose challenges for the individual nurse's health and patient safety.[40]

Shift work alters the synchrony between circadian rhythms and the environment, leading to sleep disruption. Nurses working the night shift are often too sleepy to be fully alert at work and too alert to sleep soundly the next day. Sustained alterations in circadian rhythms such as those imposed by rotating shift work have been linked to increased morbidity and mortality risks associated with cardiovascular problems. In addition, mood disorders such as anxiety are higher in nurses who work rotating shifts.

From a safety perspective, disturbed sleep and subsequent fatigue can result in errors and accidents for nurses as well as for their patients.[41] Fatigue diminishes or distorts perceptual skills, judgment, and decision-making capabilities. Lack of sleep reduces the ability to cope and handle stress and may result in physical, mental, and emotional exhaustion.

The problem of sleep disruption is critically important to nursing. Several strategies may help reduce the distress associated with rotating shift work. These include brief periods of on-site napping. Maintaining a consistent sleep-wake schedule even on days off is optimum but perhaps unrealistic. For night shift work, scheduling the sleep period just before going to work increases alertness and vigilance, improves reaction times, and decreases accidents during night shift work. Nurses who have control over their work schedules appear to experience less sleep disruption than those whose schedule is imposed. As a nurse, you need to manage the impact of sleep disruption through the use of sleep hygiene practices.

CASE STUDY

Insomnia

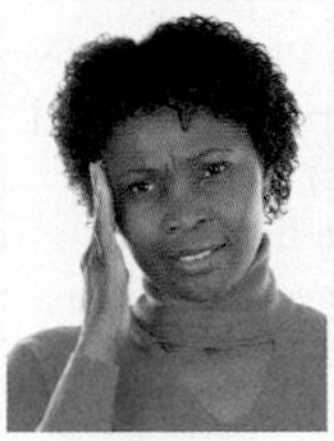

iStockphoto/Thinkstock

Patient Profile

G.P., a 49-year-old African American woman, is seen in the primary care clinic for complaints of chronic fatigue. She is postmenopausal based on self-report. In the past year, since the end of her periods, she has experienced daily hot flashes and sleep problems. She denies any other health problems. On a usual workday she drinks two cups of hot tea in the morning and one can of diet cola in the late afternoon. Currently she is taking OTC diphenhydramine for sleep. Her partner, who has accompanied her to the clinic, states that her snoring has gotten worse and it is interfering with his sleep.

Subjective Data

- Complains of hot flashes and nighttime sweating
- Complains of daytime tiredness and fatigue
- States she has trouble getting to sleep and staying asleep

Objective Data

Physical Examination

- Laboratory evaluations within normal limits
- Overweight (20% over ideal body weight for height)
- BP 155/92 mm Hg

Diagnostic Studies

- Nighttime polysomnography study reveals episodes of obstructive sleep apnea

Collaborative Care

- CPAP nightly
- Referred for weight reduction counseling
- Follow-up to rule out other potential sleep disturbances

Discussion Questions

1. What are G.P.'s risk factors for sleep apnea?
2. What specific sleep hygiene practices could G.P. use to improve the quality of her sleep?
3. How does CPAP work?
4. Based on the data above, what are the major health risks for G.P. from sleep apnea?
5. ***Priority Decision:*** What are the priority nursing interventions for G.P.? What collaborative care treatment ought to be added to the treatment plan?
6. ***Delegation Decision:*** For the interventions that you identified in the above question, which of the following personnel could be responsible for implementing them: RN, LPN, UAP?
7. ***Priority Decision:*** Based on the assessment data provided, what are the priority nursing diagnoses? Are there any collaborative problems?

evolve Answers available at *http://evolve.elsevier.com/Lewis/medsurg.*

BRIDGE TO NCLEX EXAMINATION

The number of the question corresponds to the same-numbered outcome at the beginning of the chapter.

1. Sleep is best described as a
   a. loosely organized state similar to coma.
   b. state in which pain sensitivity decreases.
   c. quiet state in which there is little brain activity.
   d. state in which an individual lacks conscious awareness of the environment.
2. Which statement is true regarding rapid eye movement (REM) sleep?
   a. The EEG pattern is quiescent.
   b. It occurs only once in the night.
   c. It is separated by distinct physiologic stages.
   d. The most vivid dreaming occurs during this phase.
3. Insufficient sleep is associated with *(select all that apply)*
   a. increased body mass index.
   b. increased insulin resistance.
   c. impaired cognitive functioning.
   d. increased immune responsiveness.
   e. increased daytime body temperature.
4. When teaching the patient with primary insomnia about sleep hygiene, the nurse should emphasize
   a. the importance of daytime naps.
   b. the need to exercise before bedtime.
   c. the need for long-term use of hypnotics.
   d. avoiding caffeine-containing beverages 6 to 9 hours before bedtime.
5. While caring for a patient with a history of narcolepsy with cataplexy, the nurse can delegate which activity to the unlicensed assistive personnel (UAP)?
   a. Teaching about the timing of medications
   b. Walking the patient to and from the bathroom
   c. Developing a plan of care with a family member
   d. Planning an appropriate diet that avoids caffeine-containing foods

6. A patient with sleep apnea would like to avoid using a nasal CPAP device if possible. To help him reach this goal, the nurse suggests that the patient
   a. lose excess weight.
   b. take a nap during the day.
   c. eat a high-protein snack at bedtime.
   d. use mild sedatives or alcohol at bedtime.
7. A patient on the surgical unit has a history of parasomnia (sleepwalking). What statement describes parasomnia?
   a. Hypnotic medications reduce the risk of sleepwalking.
   b. The patient is often unaware of the activity on awakening.
   c. The patient should be restrained at night to prevent personal harm.
   d. The potential for sleepwalking is reduced by exercise before sleep.
8. Strategies to reduce sleepiness during nighttime working include
   a. exercising before work.
   b. taking melatonin before working the night shift.
   c. sleeping for at least 2 hours immediately before work time.
   d. walking for 10 minutes every 4 hours during the night shift.

1. d, 2. d, 3. a, b, c, 4. d, 5. b, 6. a, 7. b, 8. c

evolve

For rationales to these answers and even more NCLEX review questions, visit *http://evolve.elsevier.com/Lewis/medsurg.*

REFERENCES

1. Redeker NS, McEnany GP: The nature of sleep disorders and their impact. In Redeker NS, McEnany GP, editors: *Sleep disorders and sleep promotion in nursing practice*, New York, 2011, Springer.
2. National Sleep Foundation: Can't sleep? Learn about insomnia. Retrieved from *www.sleepfoundation.org/site.*
3. National Sleep Foundation: 2011 sleep in America poll: communications technology and sleep. Retrieved from *www.sleepfoundation.org/2011poll.*
4. National Sleep Foundation: DrowsyDriving.org. Retrieved from *www.drowsydriving.org/tag/national-sleep-foundation.*
5. España RA, Scammell TE: Sleep neurobiology from a clinical perspective, *Sleep* 34:845, 2011.

*6. Rea MS, Brons JA, Figueiro MG: Measurements of light at night (LAN) for a sample of female school teachers, *Chronobiol Intern* 28:673, 2011.

7. Landis CA: Physiological and behavioral aspects of sleep. In Redeker NS, McEnany GP, editors: *Sleep disorders and sleep promotion in nursing practice*, New York, 2011, Springer.
8. Iber C, Ancoli-Israel S, Chesson A, et al: *The American Academy of Sleep Medicine: The AASM manual for the scoring of sleep and associated events: rules, terminology and technical specifications*, Westchester, Ill, 2007, The Academy. (Reference Manual)
9. Van Cauter E: Sleep disturbances and insulin resistance, *Diabetic Med* 28:1455, 2011.

*10. Anic GM, Titus-Ernstoff L, Newcomb PA, et al: Sleep duration and obesity in a population study, *Sleep Med* 11:47, 2010.

*11. Bloom HG, Ahmed I, Alessi CA, et al: Evidence-based recommendations for the assessment and management of sleep disorders in older people, *J Am Geriatr Soc* 57:761, 2009. (Classic)

12. Partinen M: Epidemiology of sleep disorders, *Handb Clin Neurol* 98:275, 2011.
13. Walsleben JA: Women and sleep, *Handb Clin Neurol* 98:639, 2011.
14. Jungquist C: Insomnia. In Redeker NS, McEnany GP, editors: *Sleep disorders and sleep promotion in nursing practice*, New York, 2011, Springer.
15. Budhiraja R, Roth T, Hudgel DW, et al: Prevalence and polysomnographic correlates of insomnia comorbid with medical disorders, *Sleep* 34:859, 2011.
16. Buysse DJ, Reynolds CF, Monk TH, et al: The Pittsburgh Sleep Quality Index: a new instrument for psychiatric practice and research, *Psychiatry Res* 28:193, 1989. (Classic)
17. Morin CM, Belleville G, Belanger L, et al: The Insomnia Severity Index: psychometric indicators to detect insomnia cases and evaluate treatment response, *Sleep* 34:601, 2011.
18. Johns MW: A new method for measuring daytime sleepiness: the Epworth Sleepiness Scale, *Sleep* 14:540, 1991. (Classic)
19. Sullivan SS: Insomnia pharmacology, *Med Clin North Am* 94:563, 2010.

*20. Roehrs TA, Randall S, Harris E, et al: Twelve months of nightly zolpidem does not lead to dose escalation: a prospective placebo-controlled study, *Sleep* 34:207, 2011.

*21. Krystal AD, Lankford A, Durrence HH, et al: Efficacy and safety of doxepin 3 and 6 mg in a 35-day sleep laboratory trial in adults with chronic primary insomnia, *Sleep* 34:1433, 2011.

22. Ferguson SA, Rajaratnam SM, Dawson D: Melatonin agonists and insomnia, *Expert Rev Neurother* 10:305, 2010.

*23. Taibi DM, Vitiello MV, Barsness S, et al: A randomized clinical trial of valerian fails to improve self-reported, polysomnographic, and actigraphic sleep in older women with insomnia, *Sleep Med* 10:319, 2008. (Classic)

24. Redeker NS, Hedges C, Booker KJ: Sleep in adult acute and critical care settings. In Redeker NS, McEnany GP, editors: *Sleep disorders and sleep promotion in nursing practice*, New York, 2011, Springer.
25. Landis CA: Sleep, pain, fibromyalgia, and chronic fatigue syndrome, *Handb Clin Neurol* 98:613, 2011.
26. Rodgers A: Narcolepsy. In Redeker NS, McEnany GP, editors: *Sleep disorders and sleep promotion in nursing practice*, New York, 2011, Springer.
27. National Institutes of Health: Narcolepsy fact sheet. Retrieved from *www.nhlbi.nih.gov/health/health-topics/topics/nar.*
28. Hiria N, Nishino S: Recent advances in the treatment of narcolepsy, *Curr Treatment Options Neurol* 13:437, 2011.
29. Dowling G, Mastick J: Circadian rhythm disorders. In Redeker NS, McEnany GP, editors: *Sleep disorders and sleep promotion in nursing practice*, New York, 2011, Springer.
30. Sawyer AM, Weaver TE: Sleep related-breathing disorders. In Redeker NS, McEnany GP, editors: *Sleep disorders and sleep promotion in nursing practice*, New York, 2011, Springer.

*31. Gooneratne NS, Richards KC, Joffe M, et al: Sleep disordered breathing with excessive daytime sleepiness is a risk factor for mortality in older adults, *Sleep* 34:435, 2011.

32. Tamisier R, Pepin JL, Levy P: Sleep and pulmonary disorders, *Handb Clin Neurol* 98:471, 2011.

*Evidence-based information for clinical practice.

33. Tomfohr LM, Ancoli-Israel S, Loredo JS, et al: Effects of continuous positive airway pressure on fatigue and sleepiness in patients with obstructive sleep apnea: data from a randomized controlled trial, *Sleep* 34:121, 2011.
34. Fleetham JA: Medical and surgical treatment of obstructive sleep apnea syndrome, including dental appliances, *Handb Clin Neurol* 98:441, 2011.
*35. Antic NA, Catcheside P, Buchan C, et al: The effect of CPAP in normalizing daytime sleepiness, quality of life, and neurocognitive function in patients with moderate to severe OSA, *Sleep* 34:111, 2011.
36. eMedicinehealth: Periodic limb movement disorder. Retrieved from *www.emedicinehealth.com/periodic_limb_movement_disorder/article_em.htm*.
37. Cole CS: Sleep and primary care in adults and older adults. In Redeker NS, McEnany GP, editors: *Sleep disorders and sleep promotion in nursing practice*, New York, 2011, Springer.
38. Klerman EB, Dijk DJ: Age-related reduction in the maximal capacity for sleep—implications for insomnia, *Curr Biol* 18:1118, 2008.
39. Cooke JR, Ancoli-Israel S: Normal and abnormal sleep in the elderly, *Handb Clin Neurol* 98:653, 2011.
*40. Scott LD, Hwang WT, Rogers AE, et al: The relationship between nurse work schedules, sleep duration, and drowsy driving, *Sleep* 30:1801, 2007.
*41. Scott LD, Hofmeister N, Rogness N, et al: An interventional approach for patient and nurse safety, *Nurs Res* 59:250, 2010.

RESOURCES

American Academy of Sleep Medicine
www.aasmnet.org
American Sleep Apnea Association
www.sleepapnea.org
Better Sleep Council
www.bettersleep.org
Narcolepsy Network
www.narcolepsynetwork.org
National Institutes of Health
http://health.nih.gov/topic/SleepDisorders
www.nhlbi.nih.gov/health/public/sleep/healthy_sleep.htm
National Sleep Foundation
www.sleepfoundation.org

CHAPTER

9

Pain

Pain is inevitable. Suffering is optional.
Anonymous

Lindsay L. Kindler and Rosemary C. Polomano

evolve WEBSITE

http://evolve.elsevier.com/Lewis/medsurg

- NCLEX Review Questions
- Key Points
- Pre-Test
- Answer Guidelines for Case Study on p. 137
- Rationales for Bridge to NCLEX Examination Questions
- Case Study
  - Patient With Pain
- Concept Map Creator
- Glossary
- Stress-Busting Kit for Nursing Students
- Content Updates

eFigures

- eFig. 9-1: Spinal dermatomes
- eFig. 9-2: Initial pain assessment tool
- eFig. 9-3: Wong-Baker FACES™ Pain Rating Scale
- eFig. 9-4: FACES Pain Scale—Revised (FPS-R)

LEARNING OUTCOMES

1. Define pain.
2. Describe the neural mechanisms of pain and pain modulation.
3. Differentiate between nociceptive and neuropathic types of pain.
4. Explain the physical and psychologic effects of unrelieved pain.
5. Interpret the subjective and objective data that are obtained from a comprehensive pain assessment.
6. Describe effective interdisciplinary pain management techniques.
7. Describe drug and nondrug methods of pain relief.
8. Explain your role and responsibility in pain management.
9. Discuss ethical and legal issues related to pain and pain management.
10. Evaluate the influence of one's own knowledge, beliefs, and attitudes about pain assessment and management.

KEY TERMS

analgesic ceiling, p. 123
breakthrough pain, p. 121
complex regional pain syndrome (CRPS), p. 119
equianalgesic dose, p. 129
modulation, p. 118
neuropathic pain, p. 119
nociception, p. 116
nociceptive pain, p. 119
pain, p. 115
patient-controlled analgesia (PCA), p. 131
transduction, p. 116
transmission, p. 117
trigger point, p. 132

Pain is a complex, multidimensional experience that can cause suffering and decreased quality of life. Pain is one of the major reasons that people seek health care. To effectively assess and manage patients with pain, you need to understand the physiologic and psychosocial dimensions of pain. This chapter presents evidence-based information to help you assess and manage pain successfully in collaboration with other health care providers.

MAGNITUDE OF PAIN PROBLEM

Every year, millions of people suffer from pain. Annually in the United States, at least 25 million people experience acute pain as a result of injury or surgery.[1] Common chronic pain conditions such as arthritis, migraine headache, and back pain affect approximately 116 million American adults.[2] Seventy percent of all cancer patients experience significant pain during their illness.[3] The financial impact of pain is staggering. In the United States, unrelieved pain and inadequate management of pain costs an estimated $560 billion to $635 billion each year in direct medical treatment costs and lost work productivity.[2]

Despite the high prevalence and costs of acute and chronic pain, inadequate pain management occurs. For example, approximately a third of patients enrolled in hospice reported pain at their last hospice visit.[4] Cancer pain is often undertreated.[5]

Consequences of untreated pain include unnecessary suffering, physical and psychosocial dysfunction, immunosup-

Reviewed by Judith A. Paice, RN, PhD, Director, Cancer Pain Program, Division Hematology-Oncology, Northwestern University, Feinberg School of Medicine, Chicago, Illinois; Debra B. Gordon, RN-BC, DNP, ACNS-BC, FAAN, Teaching Associate, Department of Anesthesiology and Pain Medicine, University of Washington, Seattle, Washington; Jo Ann Baker, RN, MSN, FNP-C, Department Chair, Nursing, Delaware Technical and Community College, Terry Campus, Dover, Delaware; Susan Turner, RN, MSN, FNP, Professor of Nursing, Gavilan College, Gilroy, California; and Linda Wilson, RN, PhD, CPAN, CAPA, BC, CNE, Assistant Dean for Special Projects, Simulation and CNE Accreditation, Drexel University, College of Nursing and Health Professions, Philadelphia, Pennsylvania.

TABLE 9-1 HARMFUL EFFECTS OF UNRELIEVED ACUTE PAIN

Response	Possible Consequences
Endocrine and Metabolic	
↑ Adrenocorticotropic hormone (ACTH)	Weight loss (from ↑ catabolism)
↑ Cortisol	↑ Respiratory rate
↑ Antidiuretic hormone (ADH)	↑ Heart rate
↑ Epinephrine and norepinephrine	Shock
↑ Renin, ↑ aldosterone	Glucose intolerance
↓ Insulin	Hyperglycemia
Gluconeogenesis	Fluid overload
Glycogenolysis	Hypertension
Muscle protein catabolism	Urinary retention, ↓ urine output
Cardiovascular	
↑ Heart rate	Hypertension
↑ Cardiac output	Unstable angina
↑ Peripheral vascular resistance	Myocardial infarction
↑ Myocardial oxygen consumption	Deep vein thrombosis
↑ Coagulation	
Respiratory	
↓ Tidal volume	Atelectasis
Hypoxemia	Pneumonia
↓ Cough, sputum retention	
Renal and Urologic	
↓ Urine output	Fluid imbalance
Urinary retention	Electrolyte disturbance
Gastrointestinal	
↓ Gastric and intestinal motility	Constipation
	Anorexia
	Paralytic ileus
Musculoskeletal	
Muscle spasm	Immobility
Impaired muscle function	Weakness and fatigue
Neurologic	
Impaired cognitive function	Confusion
	Impaired ability to think, reason, and make decisions
Immunologic	
↓ Immune response	Infection

pression, and sleep disturbances[2] (Table 9-1). The varied reasons for the undertreatment of pain are discussed in this chapter.

DEFINITIONS AND DIMENSIONS OF PAIN

In 1968 Margo McCaffery, a nurse and pioneer in pain management, defined **pain** as "whatever the person experiencing the pain says it is, existing whenever the person says it does."[6] The International Association for the Study of Pain (IASP) defines *pain* as "an unpleasant sensory and emotional experience associated with actual or potential tissue damage, or described in terms of such damage."[2]

Note that these definitions emphasize the subjective nature of pain, in which the patient's self-report is the most valid means of assessment. Although understanding the patient's experience and relying on his or her self-report is essential, this view is problematic for many patients. For example, patients who are comatose or who suffer from dementia, patients who are mentally disabled, and patients with expressive aphasia possess varying abilities to report pain. In these instances, you must incorporate nonverbal information such as behaviors into your pain assessment.

TABLE 9-2 DIMENSIONS OF PAIN

Dimension	Description
Physiologic	• Genetic, anatomic, and physical determinants of pain influence how painful stimuli are processed, recognized, and described.
Affective	• Emotional responses to pain include anger, fear, depression, and anxiety. • Negative emotions impair patient's quality of life.
Cognitive	• Beliefs, attitudes, memories, and meaning attributed to pain influence the ways in which a person responds to pain.
Behavioral	• Observable actions (e.g., grimacing, irritability) are used to express or control pain. • People unable to communicate may have behavioral changes (e.g., agitation, combativeness).
Sociocultural	• Age and gender influence nociceptive processes and responses to opioids. • Families and caregivers influence patient's response to pain through their beliefs, behaviors, and support. • Culture affects pain expression, medication use, and pain-related beliefs and coping methods.

GENDER DIFFERENCES

Pain

Men

- Men are less likely to report pain than women.
- Men report more control over pain.
- Men are less likely than women to use alternative treatments for pain.

Women

- Women experience more chronic pain than men.
- Even when they have the same condition as men, women have higher levels of pain. Women more frequently experience migraine headache, back pain, arthritis, fibromyalgia, irritable bowel syndrome, neuropathic pain, abdominal pain, and foot ache.
- Women are more likely to be diagnosed with a nonspecific, somatic diagnosis and less likely to receive analgesics for symptoms of chest and abdominal pain.

With pain defined as a human experience, successful pain assessment and treatment must incorporate multiple dimensions.[7] The biopsychosocial model of pain includes the physiologic, affective, cognitive, behavioral, and sociocultural dimensions of pain (Table 9-2).

The emotional distress of pain can cause *suffering,* which is the state of distress associated with loss. Suffering can result in a profound sense of insecurity and lack of control. When suffering occurs, people can experience spiritual distress. Achieving pain relief is an essential step in relieving suffering. In addition, the assessment of ways in which a person's spirituality influences and is influenced by pain is important.[8]

The meaning of the pain can be critical. For example, a woman in labor may experience severe pain but can manage it without analgesics because for her it is associated with a joyful event. Moreover, she may feel control over her pain because of the training she received in prenatal classes and the knowledge that the pain is time-limited. In contrast, a woman with chronic, undefined musculoskeletal pain may be plagued by thoughts that her pain is "not real," is uncontrollable, or is caused by her own actions. These perceptions will influence the ways in which a person responds to pain and must be incorporated into a comprehensive treatment plan.

Some people cope with pain by distracting themselves, whereas others convince themselves that the pain is permanent, untreatable, and overwhelming. People who believe that their pain is uncontrollable and overwhelming are more likely to have poor outcomes.[9]

Families and caregivers influence the patient's response to pain through their beliefs and behaviors. For example, families may discourage the patient from taking opioids because they fear the patient will become addicted.

Pain Mechanisms

Nociception is the physiologic process by which information about tissue damage is communicated to the central nervous system (CNS). It involves four processes: (1) transduction, (2) transmission, (3) perception, and (4) modulation (Fig. 9-1).

Transduction. **Transduction** involves the conversion of a noxious mechanical, thermal, or chemical stimulus into an electrical signal called an action potential. Noxious (tissue-damaging) stimuli, including thermal (e.g., sunburn), mechanical (e.g., surgical incision), or chemical (e.g., toxic substances) stimuli, cause the release of numerous chemicals such as hydrogen ions, substance P, and adenosine triphosphate (ATP) into the damaged tissues. Other chemicals are released from mast cells (e.g., serotonin, histamine, bradykinin, prostaglandins) and macrophages (e.g., interleukins, tumor necrosis factor [TNF]). These chemicals activate nociceptors, which are specialized receptors, or free nerve endings, that respond to painful stimuli. Activation of nociceptors results in an action potential that is carried from the nociceptors to the spinal cord primarily via small, rapidly conducting, myelinated A-delta fibers and slowly conducting unmyelinated C fibers.

In addition to stimulating nociceptors to fire, inflammation and the subsequent release of chemical mediators lower nociceptor thresholds. As a result, nociceptors may fire in response to stimuli that previously were insufficient to elicit a response. They may also fire in response to non-noxious stimuli, such as light touch. This increased susceptibility to nociceptor activation is called *peripheral sensitization.* Leukotrienes, prostaglandins, cytokines, and substance P are involved in peripheral sensitization. Cyclooxygenase (COX), an enzyme produced in the inflammatory response, also plays an important role in peripheral sensitization. A clinical example of this process is sunburn. This thermal injury causes inflammation that results in a sensation of pain when the affected skin is lightly touched. Peripheral sensitization also amplifies signal transmission, which in turn contributes to central sensitization (discussed under Dorsal Horn Processing). The pain produced from activation of peripheral nociceptors is called *nociceptive pain* (described later in the chapter on p. 119).

Therapies that alter either the local environment or sensitivity of the peripheral nociceptors can prevent transduction and initiation of an action potential. Decreasing the effects of chemicals released at the periphery is the basis of several drug approaches to pain relief. For example, nonsteroidal antiinflammatory drugs (NSAIDs), such as ibuprofen (Advil, Motrin) and naproxen (Naprosyn, Aleve), and corticosteroids, such as dexamethasone (Decadron), exert their analgesic effects by blocking pain-sensitizing chemicals. NSAIDs block the action of COX, thereby interfering with the production of prostaglandins. Corticosteroids reduce the production of both prostaglandins and leukotrienes (see Fig. 12-2).

Drugs that stabilize the neuronal membrane and inactivate peripheral sodium channels inhibit production of the nerve impulse. These medications include local anesthetics (e.g., injectable or topical lidocaine, bupivacaine [Sensorcaine], and

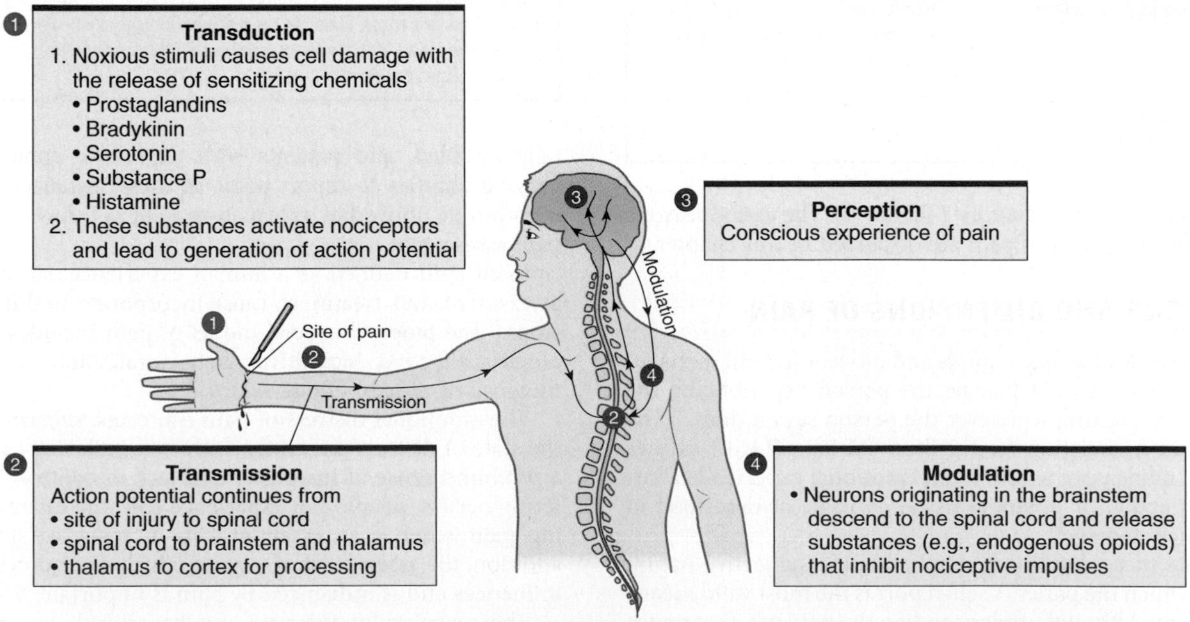
1
Transduction
1. Noxious stimuli causes cell damage with the release of sensitizing chemicals
• Prostaglandins
• Bradykinin
• Serotonin
• Substance P
• Histamine
2. These substances activate nociceptors and lead to generation of action potential
3
Perception
Conscious experience of pain
Modulation
Site of pain
Transmission
2
Transmission
Action potential continues from
• site of injury to spinal cord
• spinal cord to brainstem and thalamus
• thalamus to cortex for processing
4
Modulation
• Neurons originating in the brainstem descend to the spinal cord and release substances (e.g., endogenous opioids) that inhibit nociceptive impulses

FIG. 9-1 Nociceptive pain originates when the tissue is injured. *1,* Transduction occurs when there is release of chemical mediators. *2,* Transmission involves the conduct of the action potential from the periphery (injury site) to the spinal cord and then to the brainstem, thalamus, and cerebral cortex. *3,* Perception is the conscious awareness of pain. *4,* Modulation involves signals from the brain going back down the spinal cord to modify incoming impulses.

ropivacaine [Naropin]) and antiseizure drugs (e.g., carbamazepine [Tegretol] and lamotrigine [Lamictal]).

Transmission. Transmission is the process by which pain signals are relayed from the periphery to the spinal cord and then to the brain. The nerves that carry pain impulses from the periphery to the spinal cord are called primary afferent fibers. These include A-delta and C fibers, each of which is responsible for a different pain sensation. As previously mentioned, A-delta fibers are small, myelinated fibers that conduct pain rapidly and are responsible for the initial, sharp pain that accompanies tissue injury. C fibers are small, unmyelinated fibers that transmit painful stimuli more slowly and produce pain that is typically aching or throbbing in quality. Primary afferent fibers terminate in the dorsal horn of the spinal cord. Activity in the dorsal horn integrates and modulates pain inputs from the periphery.

The propagation of pain impulses from the site of transduction to the brain is shown in Fig. 9-1. Three segments are involved in nociceptive signal transmission: (1) transmission along the peripheral nerve fibers to the spinal cord, (2) dorsal horn processing, and (3) transmission to the thalamus and the cerebral cortex.

Transmission to Spinal Cord. The first-order neuron extends the entire distance from the periphery to the dorsal horn of the spinal cord with no synapses. For example, an afferent fiber from the great toe travels from the toe through the fifth lumbar nerve root into the spinal cord; it is one cell. Once generated, an action potential travels all the way to the spinal cord unless it is blocked by a sodium channel inhibitor (e.g., local anesthetic) or disrupted by a lesion such as a dorsal root entry zone lesion.

The manner in which nerve fibers enter the spinal cord is central to the notion of spinal dermatomes. *Dermatomes* are areas on the skin that are innervated primarily by a single spinal cord segment. The distinctive pattern of the rash caused by herpes zoster (shingles) across the back and trunk is determined by dermatomes (see Fig. 24-7). Different dermatomes and their innervations are illustrated in eFig. 9-1 (available on the website for this chapter) and Fig. 56-6.

Dorsal Horn Processing. Once a nociceptive signal arrives in the spinal cord, it is processed within the dorsal horn. Neurotransmitters released from the afferent fiber bind to receptors on nearby cell bodies and dendrites of cells. Some of these neurotransmitters (e.g., glutamate, aspartate, substance P) produce activation, whereas others (e.g., γ-aminobutyric acid [GABA], serotonin, norepinephrine) inhibit activation of nearby cells. In this area, exogenous and endogenous opioids also play an important role by binding to opioid receptors and blocking the release of neurotransmitters, particularly substance P. Endogenous opioids include enkephalin and β-endorphin. They are capable of producing analgesic effects similar to those of exogenous opioids such as morphine.

Increased sensitivity and hyperexcitability of neurons in the CNS is called *central sensitization.* Peripheral tissue damage or nerve injury can cause central sensitization, and continued nociceptive input from the periphery is necessary to maintain it. As a result of the increased excitability of neurons within the CNS, normal sensory inputs cause abnormal sensing and responses to painful and other stimuli. This explains why some people experience significant pain from touch or tactile stimulation in and around the areas of tissue or nerve injury. This is called *allodynia*. With central sensitization, the central processing circuits are altered. In some cases, central sensitization can be long-lasting due to changes in the synapse.[10]

With ongoing stimulation of slowly conducting unmyelinated C-fiber nociceptors, firing of specialized dorsal horn neurons gradually increases. These inputs create many problems, including the sprouting of wide dynamic range (WDR) neurons and induction of glutamate-dependent *N*-methyl-D-aspartate (NMDA) receptors. WDR neurons respond to both nociceptive and non-nociceptive inputs that are of varying levels of stimulus intensity. When these neuron dendrites sprout, they grow into areas where pain-receiving nerve cell bodies are located. This results in the capacity to transmit a broader range of stimuli-producing signals, which are then passed up the spinal cord and brain. This process is known as *windup* and depends on the activation of NMDA receptors. NMDA receptor antagonists, such as ketamine (Ketalar), potentially interrupt or block mechanisms that lead to or sustain central sensitization. Windup, like central sensitization and hyperalgesia (increased pain responses to noxious stimuli), is induced by C-fiber inputs. Windup is different, however, in that it can be short lasting, whereas central sensitization and hyperalgesia persist over time.[11]

It is important for you to understand that acute, unrelieved pain leads to chronic pain through the process of central sensitization. Acute tissue injury produces a cascade of events that involve the release of certain excitatory neurotransmitters (e.g., glutamate) and neuropsychologic responses. Even brief intervals of acute pain are capable of inducing long-term neuronal remodeling and sensitization *(plasticity),* chronic pain, and lasting psychologic distress.

Neuroplasticity refers to processes that allow neurons in the brain to compensate for injury and adjust their responses to new situations or changes in their environment.[12] Neuroplasticity contributes to adaptive mechanisms for reducing pain but also can result in maladaptive mechanisms that enhance pain. Genetic variability among individuals may have an important effect on the plasticity of the CNS.[12] Understanding this phenomenon helps explain individual differences in response to pain and why some patients develop chronic pain conditions whereas others do not. Clinically, central sensitization of the dorsal horn results in (1) hyperalgesia, (2) painful responses to normally innocuous stimuli (allodynia), (3) prolonged pain after the original noxious stimulus ends (called *persistent pain*), and (4) the extension of tenderness or increased pain sensitivity outside of an area of injury to include uninjured tissue (i.e., expansion of nociceptive receptive fields, or secondary hyperalgesia).[13]

Referred pain must be considered when interpreting the location of pain reported by the person with an injury or a disease involving visceral organs. The location of a stimulus may be distant from the pain location reported by the patient (Fig. 9-2). For example, pain from liver disease is frequently located in the right upper abdominal quadrant, but can also be referred to the anterior and posterior neck region and to a posterior flank area. If referred pain is not considered when evaluating a pain location report, diagnostic tests and therapy could be misdirected.

Transmission to Thalamus and Cortex. From the dorsal horn, nociceptive stimuli are communicated to the *third-order neuron,* primarily in the thalamus, and several other areas of the brain. Fibers of dorsal horn projection cells enter the brain through several pathways, including the spinothalamic tract and spinoreticular tract. Distinct thalamic nuclei receive nociceptive input from the spinal cord and have projections to several regions in the cerebral cortex, where the perception of pain is presumed to occur.

Therapeutic approaches that target pain transmission include opioid analgesics that bind to opioid receptors on primary afferent and dorsal horn neurons. These agents mimic the inhibitory effects of endogenous opioids. Another medication, baclofen (Lioresal), inhibits transmission by binding to GABA receptors, thus mimicking the inhibitory effects of GABA.

Perception. *Perception* occurs when pain is recognized, defined, and assigned meaning by the individual experiencing the pain. In the brain, nociceptive input is perceived as pain. There is no single, precise location where pain perception occurs. Instead, pain perception involves several brain structures. For example, it is believed that the reticular activating system (RAS) is responsible for warning the individual to attend to the pain stimulus; the somatosensory system is responsible for localization and characterization of pain; and the limbic system is responsible for the emotional and behavioral responses to pain. Cortical structures also are crucial to constructing the meaning of the pain.

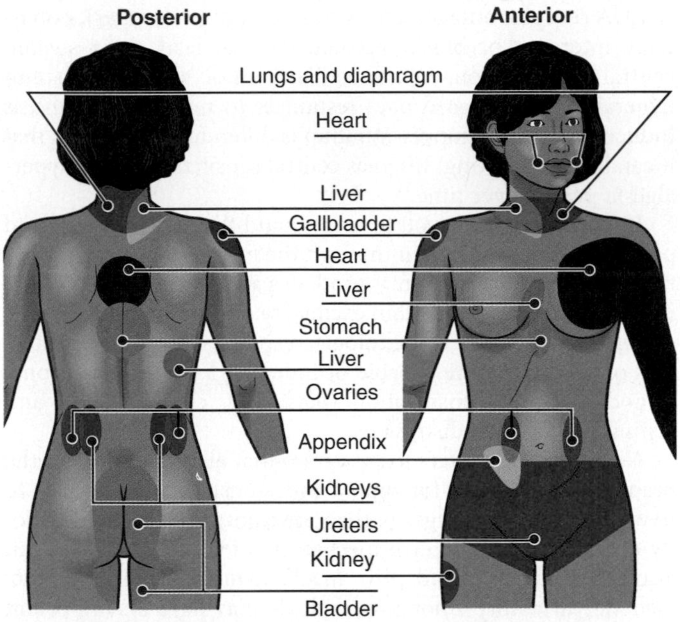

FIG. 9-2 Typical areas of referred pain.

Therefore behavioral strategies such as distraction and relaxation are effective pain-reducing therapies for many people. By directing attention away from the pain sensation, patients can reduce the sensory and affective components of pain. Opioids and other classes of analgesics such as some types of antiseizure drugs and antidepressants modify pain perception.

Modulation. Modulation involves the activation of descending pathways that exert inhibitory or facilitatory effects on the transmission of pain (see Fig. 9-1). Depending on the type and degree of modulation, nociceptive stimuli may or may not be perceived as pain. Modulation of pain signals can occur at the level of the periphery, spinal cord, brainstem, and cerebral cortex. Descending modulatory fibers release chemicals such as serotonin, norepinephrine, GABA, and endogenous opioids that can inhibit pain transmission.

Several antidepressants exert their effects through the modulatory systems. For example, tricyclic antidepressants (e.g., amitriptyline [Elavil]) and serotonin norepinephrine reuptake inhibitors (SNRIs) (e.g., venlafaxine [Effexor] and duloxetine [Cymbalta]) are used in the management of chronic nonmalignant and cancer pain. These agents interfere with the reuptake of serotonin and norepinephrine, thereby increasing their availability to inhibit noxious stimuli.

CLASSIFICATION OF PAIN

Pain can be categorized in several ways. Most commonly, pain is categorized as nociceptive or neuropathic based on underlying pathology (Table 9-3). Another useful scheme is to classify pain as acute or chronic (Table 9-4).

TABLE 9-3 COMPARISON OF NOCICEPTIVE AND NEUROPATHIC PAIN

	Nociceptive Pain	Neuropathic Pain*
Definition	Normal processing of stimulus that damages normal tissue or has the potential to do so if prolonged.	Abnormal processing of sensory input by the peripheral or central nervous system.
Treatment	Usually responsive to nonopioid and/or opioid drugs.	Treatment usually includes adjuvant analgesics.
Types	**Superficial Somatic Pain** Pain arising from skin, mucous membranes, subcutaneous tissue. Tends to be well localized. *Examples:* sunburn, skin contusions **Deep Somatic Pain** Pain arising from muscles, fasciae, bones, tendons. Localized or diffuse and radiating. *Examples:* arthritis, tendonitis, myofascial pain **Visceral Pain** Pain arising from visceral organs, such as the GI tract and bladder. Well or poorly localized. Often referred to cutaneous sites. *Examples:* appendicitis, pancreatitis, cancer affecting internal organs, irritable bowel and bladder syndromes	**Central Pain** Caused by primary lesion or dysfunction in the CNS. *Examples:* poststroke pain, pain associated with multiple sclerosis **Peripheral Neuropathies** Pain felt along the distribution of one or many peripheral nerves caused by damage to the nerve. *Examples:* diabetic neuropathy, alcohol-nutritional neuropathy, trigeminal neuralgia, postherpetic neuralgia **Deafferentation Pain** Pain resulting from a loss of afferent input. *Examples:* phantom limb pain, postmastectomy pain, spinal cord injury pain **Sympathetically Maintained Pain** Pain that persists secondary to sympathetic nervous system activity. *Examples:* phantom limb pain, complex regional pain syndrome

Adapted from National Institute of Neurological Disorders and Stroke: Complex regional pain syndrome fact sheet. Retrieved from *www.ninds.nih.gov/disorders/reflex_sympathetic_dystrophy/detail_reflex_sympathetic_dystrophy.htm.*

*Note: Some types of neuropathic pain (e.g., postherpetic neuralgia) are caused by more than one neuropathologic mechanism.

CNS, Central nervous system; *GI,* gastrointestinal.

Nociceptive Pain

Nociceptive pain is caused by damage to somatic or visceral tissue. *Somatic pain* often is further categorized as superficial or deep. *Superficial pain* arises from skin, mucous membranes, and subcutaneous tissues. It is often described as sharp, burning, or prickly. *Deep pain* is often characterized as deep, aching, or throbbing and originates in bone, joint, muscle, skin, or connective tissue.

Visceral pain comes from the activation of nociceptors in the internal organs and lining of the body cavities such as the thoracic and abdominal cavities. Visceral nociceptors respond to inflammation, stretching, and ischemia. Stretching of hollow viscera in the intestines and bladder that occurs from tumor involvement or obstruction can produce distention and intense cramping pain. Examples of visceral nociceptive pain include pain from a surgical incision, pancreatitis, and inflammatory bowel disease.

Neuropathic Pain

Neuropathic pain is caused by damage to peripheral nerves or structures in the CNS.[14] Typically described as numbing, hot, burning, shooting, stabbing, sharp, or electric shock–like, neuropathic pain can be sudden, intense, short lived, or lingering. Paroxysmal firing of injured nerves is responsible for shooting and electric shock–like sensations. Common causes of neuropathic pain include trauma, inflammation (e.g., secondary to a herniated disc inflaming the adjacent nerve and dorsal root ganglion), metabolic diseases (e.g., diabetes mellitus), alcoholism, infections of the nervous system (e.g., herpes zoster, human immunodeficiency virus), tumors, toxins, and neurologic diseases (e.g., multiple sclerosis).

Deafferentation pain results from loss of afferent input secondary to either peripheral nerve injury (e.g., amputation) or CNS damage, including a spinal cord injury. *Sympathetically maintained pain* is associated with dysregulation of the autonomic nervous system, and *central pain* is caused by CNS lesions or dysfunction. Painful peripheral polyneuropathies (pain felt along the distribution of multiple peripheral nerves) and painful mononeuropathies (pain felt along the distribution of a damaged nerve) arise from damage to peripheral nerves and generate pain that may be described as burning, paroxysmal, or shock-like. The patient may have associated positive or negative motor and sensory signs, including numbness, allodynia, or change in reflexes and motor strength. No single quality descriptor or sign or symptom is diagnostic for neuropathic pain. Examples of neuropathic pain include postherpetic neuralgia, phantom limb pain, diabetic neuropathies, and trigeminal neuralgia.

One particularly debilitating type of neuropathic pain is **complex regional pain syndrome (CRPS).** Typical features include dramatic changes in the color and temperature of the skin over the affected limb or body part, accompanied by intense burning pain, skin sensitivity, sweating, and swelling. CRPS type I is frequently triggered by tissue injury, surgery, or a vascular event such as stroke.[14] CRPS type II includes all these features in addition to a peripheral nerve lesion.

Neuropathic pain often is not well controlled by opioid analgesics alone. Treatment frequently necessitates a multimodal approach combining various adjuvant analgesics, including tricyclic antidepressants (e.g., nortriptyline [Pamelor], desipramine [Norpramin]), SNRIs (e.g., venlafaxine, duloxetine, bupropion [Wellbutrin, Zyban]), antiseizure drugs (e.g., gabapentin [Neurontin], pregabalin [Lyrica]), transdermal lidocaine, and α_2-adrenergic agonists (e.g., clonidine [Catapres]). NMDA receptor antagonists such as ketamine have shown promise in alleviating neuropathic pain refractory to other drugs.[14]

Acute and Chronic Pain

Acute pain and chronic pain differ in their cause, course, manifestations, and treatment (see Table 9-4). Examples of *acute pain* include postoperative pain, labor pain, pain from trauma (e.g., lacerations, fractures, sprains), pain from infection (e.g., dysuria from cystitis), and pain from acute ischemia. For acute pain, treatment includes analgesics for symptom control and treatment of the underlying cause (e.g., splinting for a fracture, antibiotic therapy for an infection). Normally, acute pain diminishes over time as healing occurs. However, acute pain that persists can ultimately lead to disabling chronic pain states. For example, pain associated with herpes zoster (shingles) subsides as the acute infection resolves, usually within a month. However, sometimes the pain persists and develops into a chronic pain state called *postherpetic neuralgia.*

Chronic pain, or *persistent pain,* lasts for longer periods, often defined as longer than 3 months or past the time when an expected acute pain or acute injury should subside. The severity and functional impact of chronic pain often are disproportionate to objective findings because of changes in the nervous

TABLE 9-4 DIFFERENCES BETWEEN ACUTE AND CHRONIC PAIN

	Acute Pain	Chronic Pain
Onset	Sudden.	Gradual or sudden.
Duration	<3 mo or as long as it takes for normal healing to occur.	>3 mo. May start as acute injury or event but continues past the normal time for recovery.
Severity	Mild to severe.	Mild to severe.
Cause of pain	Generally can identify a precipitating event (e.g., illness, surgery).	May not be known. Original cause of pain may differ from mechanisms that maintain the pain.
Course of pain	Decreases over time and goes away as recovery occurs.	Typically pain does not go away. Characterized by periods of increasing and decreasing pain.
Typical physical and behavioral manifestations	Manifestations vary but can reflect sympathetic nervous system activation: • ↑ Heart rate, respiratory rate, blood pressure • Diaphoresis, pallor • Anxiety, agitation, confusion • Urine retention	Predominantly behavioral manifestations: • Flat affect • ↓ Physical activity • Fatigue • Withdrawal from social interaction
Usual goals of treatment	Pain control with eventual elimination.	Pain control to the extent possible. Focus on enhancing function and quality of life.

TABLE 9-5 CORE PRINCIPLES OF PAIN ASSESSMENT

Principles	Nursing Implications
1. Patients have the right to appropriate assessment and management of pain.	• Assess pain in *all* patients.
2. Pain is always subjective.	• Patient's self-report of pain is the single most reliable indicator of pain. • Accept and respect this self-report unless there are clear reasons for doubt.
3. Physiologic and behavioral signs of pain (e.g., tachycardia, grimacing) are not reliable or specific for pain.	• Do not rely primarily on observations and objective signs of pain unless the patient is unable to self-report pain.
4. Pain is an unpleasant sensory and emotional experience.	• Address both physical and psychologic aspects of pain when assessing pain.
5. Assessment approaches, including tools, must be appropriate for the patient population.	• Special considerations are needed for assessing pain in patients with difficulty communicating. • Include family members in the assessment process (when appropriate).
6. Pain can exist even when no physical cause can be found.	• Do not attribute pain that does not have an identifiable cause to psychologic causes.
7. Different patients experience different levels of pain in response to comparable stimuli.	• A uniform pain threshold does not exist.
8. Patients with chronic pain may be more sensitive to pain and other stimuli.	• Pain tolerance varies among and within individuals depending on various factors (e.g., heredity, energy level, coping skills, prior experience with pain).
9. Unrelieved pain has adverse consequences. Acute pain that is not adequately controlled can result in physiologic changes that increase the likelihood of developing persistent pain.	• Encourage patients to report pain, especially patients who are reluctant to discuss pain, deny pain when it is probably present, or fail to follow through on prescribed treatments.

system not detectable with standard tests. Whereas acute pain functions as a signal, warning the person of potential or actual tissue damage, chronic pain does not appear to have an adaptive role. Chronic pain can be disabling and often is accompanied by anxiety and depression. As previously discussed, untreated acute pain leads to chronic pain through central sensitization and neuroplasticity. Consequently, it is imperative to treat acute pain aggressively and effectively to help prevent chronic pain.

PAIN ASSESSMENT

Assessment is an essential, though often overlooked, step in pain management. Regularly screen all patients for pain and, when present, perform a more thorough pain assessment. The key to accurate and effective pain assessment is to consider the core principles of pain assessment (Table 9-5).

The goals of a nursing pain assessment are to (1) describe the patient's pain experience in order to identify and implement appropriate pain management techniques and (2) identify the patient's goal for therapy and resources for self-management.

Elements of a Pain Assessment

Most components of a pain assessment involve direct interview or observation of the patient. Diagnostic studies and physical examination findings complete the initial assessment. Although the assessment differs according to the clinical setting, patient population, and point of care (i.e., whether the assessment is part of an initial workup or a reassessment of pain following therapy), the evaluation of pain should always be multidimensional (Table 9-6).

Before beginning any assessment, recognize that patients may use words other than "pain." For example, older adults may deny that they have pain but respond positively when asked if they have soreness or aching. Document the specific words that the patient uses to describe pain. Then consistently ask the patient about pain using those words.

Pain Pattern. Assessing pain *onset* involves determining when the pain started. Patients with acute pain resulting from injury, acute illness, or treatment (e.g., surgery) typically know exactly when their pain began. Those with chronic pain may be less able to identify when the pain started. Establish the *duration* of the pain (how long it has lasted). This information helps to determine whether the pain is acute or chronic and assists in identifying the cause of the pain. For example, a patient with advanced cancer who also has chronic low back pain from spinal stenosis reports a sudden, severe pain in the back that began 2 days ago. Knowing the onset and duration can lead to a diagnostic workup that may reveal new metastatic disease in the spine.

TABLE 9-6 NURSING ASSESSMENT

Pain

Subjective Data

Important Health Information

Health history: Pain history includes onset, location, intensity, quality, patterns, aggravating and alleviating factors, and expression of pain; coping strategies; past treatments and their effectiveness; review of health care utilization related to the pain problem (e.g., emergency department visits, treatment at pain clinics, visits to primary health care providers and specialists)

Medications: Use of any prescription or over-the-counter, illicit, or herbal products for pain relief; alcohol use

Functional Health Patterns

Health perception–health management: Social and work history; mental health history; smoking history; effects of pain on emotions, relationships, sleep, and activities; interviews with family members; records from psychiatric treatment related to the pain

Elimination: Constipation related to opioid drug use

Activity-exercise: Fatigue, limitations in activities, pain related to muscle use

Sexuality-reproductive: Decreased libido

Coping–stress tolerance: Psychologic evaluation using standardized measures to examine coping style, depression, anxiety

Objective Data

Physical examination, including evaluation of functional limitations

Psychosocial evaluation, including mood

Pain pattern also provides clues about the cause of the pain and directs its treatment. Many types of chronic pain (e.g., arthritis pain) increase and decrease over time. A patient may have pain all the time (constant, around-the-clock pain), as well as discrete periods of intermittent pain.

Breakthrough pain (BTP) is transient, moderate to severe pain that occurs in patients whose baseline persistent pain is otherwise mild to moderate and fairly well controlled. The average peak of BTP can be 3 to 5 minutes, and can last up to 30 minutes or even longer. BTP can either be predictable or unpredictable, and patients can have one to many episodes per day. Several transmucosal fentanyl products are specifically used to treat BTP.

End-of-dose failure is pain that occurs before the expected duration of a specific analgesic. It should not be confused with BTP. Pain that occurs at the end of the duration of an analgesic often leads to a prolonged increase in the baseline persistent pain. For example, in a patient on transdermal fentanyl (Duragesic patches) the typical duration of action is 72 hours. An increase in pain after 48 hours on the drug would be characterized as end-of-dose failure. End-of-dose failure signals the need for changes in the dose or scheduling of the analgesic. Episodic, procedural, or *incident pain* is a transient increase in pain that is caused by a specific activity or event that precipitates pain. Examples include dressing changes, movement, position changes, and procedures such as catheterization.

Location. Determining the *location* of pain assists in identifying possible causes and treatment. Some patients may be able to specify the precise location(s) of their pain, whereas others may describe general areas or comment that they "hurt all over." The location of the pain may also be referred from its origin to another site (see Fig. 9-2). For example, myocardial infarction can result in pain in the left shoulder. Pain may also radiate from its origin to another site. For example, angina pectoris can radiate from the chest to the jaw or down the left arm. This is referred to as radiating pain. *Sciatica* is pain that follows the course of the sciatic nerve. It may originate from joints or muscles around the back or from compression or damage to the sciatic nerve. The pain is projected along the course of the peripheral nerve, causing painful shooting sensations down the back of the thigh and inside of the leg to the foot.

Obtain information about the location of pain by asking the patient to (1) describe the site(s) of pain, (2) point to painful areas on the body, or (3) mark painful areas on a pain map (see eFig. 9-2, available on the website for this chapter). Because many patients have more than one site of pain, make certain that the patient describes every location.

Intensity. Assessing the severity, or *intensity*, of pain provides a reliable measure to determine the type of treatment and its effectiveness. Pain scales help the patient communicate pain intensity. Choice of a scale to use should be based on the patient's developmental needs and cognitive status. Most adults can rate the intensity of their pain using numeric scales (e.g., 0 = no pain, 10 = the worst pain) or verbal descriptor scales (e.g., none, a little, moderate, severe). These tools are sometimes easier for patients to use if they are oriented vertically or include a visual component. The Pain Thermometer Scale is an example of this type of scale[15] (Fig. 9-3). Other visual pain measures or scales include the Wong-Baker FACES Pain Rating Scale (see eFig. 9-3 on the website for this chapter) and the FACES Pain Scale–Revised (see eFig. 9-4 on the website for this chapter). These and other pain scales may be useful for patients with cognitive

Name ______________________ **Date** __________

Pain thermometer use

This tool is excellent for patients whose cognitive deficits are moderate to severe, or who have difficulty communicating verbally. Ask the patient to circle words next to the thermometer or to mark the area on the thermometer to indicate the intensity of current pain.

Pain thermometer scoring

Document the words circled or those corresponding to the area of the thermometer the patient marks to identify level of pain intensity. Evaluate the change in pain descriptors selected by the patient over time to determine the effectiveness of pain treatments. Alternately, the words can be scored from 0 to 5 for recording purposes.

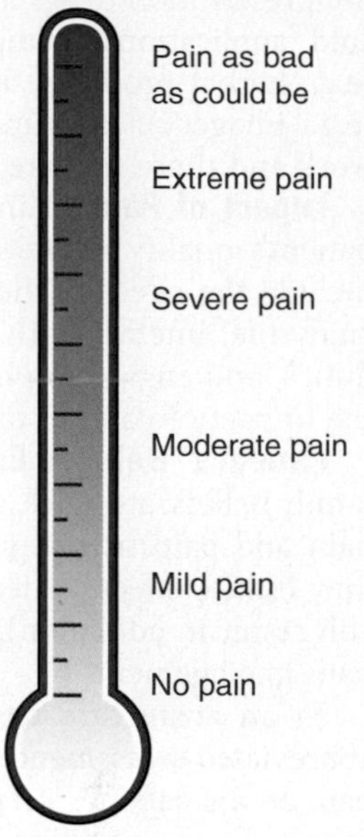

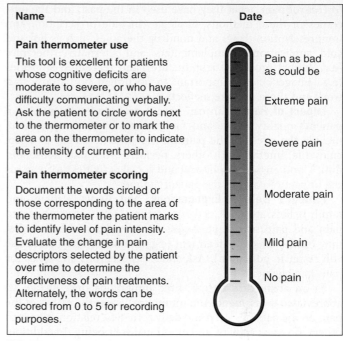

FIG. 9-3 Pain thermometer scale. Ask the patient to circle words next to the thermometer or to mark the area on the thermometer to indicate the intensity of pain. (Used with permission of Keela Herr, RN, PhD, AGSF, FAAN, The University of Iowa.)

or language barriers to describe their pain.[16] Pain assessment measures for cognitively impaired adults and nonverbal adults are addressed later in this chapter.

Although intensity is an important factor in determining analgesic approaches, do not dose patients with opioids solely based on reported pain scores.[17] Opioid "dosing by numbers" without taking into account a patient's sedation level and respiratory status can lead to unsafe practices and serious adverse events. Safer analgesic administration can be achieved by balancing an amount of pain relief with analgesic side effects. Adjustments in therapy can be made to promote better pain control and minimize adverse outcomes.

Quality. The pain *quality* refers to the nature or characteristics of the pain. For example, patients often describe neuropathic pain as burning, numbing, shooting, stabbing, electric shock–like, or itchy. Nociceptive pain may be described as sharp, aching, throbbing, dull, and cramping. Since the quality of pain relates to some degree to the classification of pain (e.g., neuropathic, nociceptive, or visceral), these descriptors can help to guide treatment options that best address the specific mechanism of pain.

Associated Symptoms. *Associated symptoms* such as anxiety, fatigue, and depression may exacerbate or be exacerbated by pain. Ask about activities and situations that increase or alleviate pain. For example, musculoskeletal pain may be increased or decreased with movement and ambulation. Resting or immobilizing a painful body part can decrease pain. Knowing what makes pain better or worse can help characterize the type of pain and be helpful in selecting treatments.

Management Strategies. As people experience and live with pain, they may cope differently and be more or less willing to try different strategies to manage it. Some strategies are successful, whereas others are not. To maximize the effectiveness of the pain treatment plan, ask patients what they are using now to control pain, what they have used in the past, and the outcomes of these methods. Strategies include prescription and nonprescription drugs and nondrug therapies such as hot and cold applications, complementary and alternative therapies (e.g., herbal products, acupuncture), and relaxation strategies (e.g., imagery). It is important to document both those that work and those that are ineffective.

Impact of Pain. Pain can have a profound influence on a patient's quality of life and functioning. In your assessment, include the effect of the pain on the patient's ability to sleep, enjoy life, interact with others, perform work and household duties, and engage in physical and social activities. Also assess the impact of pain on the patient's mood.

Patient's Beliefs, Expectations, and Goals. Patient and family beliefs, attitudes, and expectations influence responses to pain and pain treatment. Assess for attitudes and beliefs that may hinder effective treatment (e.g., the belief that opioid use will result in addiction). Ask about expectations and goals for pain management.

In an acute care setting, time limitations may dictate an abbreviated assessment. At a minimum, assess the effects of the pain on the patient's sleep and daily activities, relationships with others, physical activity, and emotional well-being. In addition, include the ways in which the patient describes the pain and the strategies used to cope with and control the pain.

Documentation

Document the pain assessment, since this is critical to ensure effective communication among team members. Many health care facilities and agencies have adopted specific tools to record an initial pain assessment, treatment, and reassessment. (An example of an initial pain assessment tool appears in eFig. 9-2 on the website for this chapter.) There also are many multidimensional pain assessment tools, such as the Brief Pain Inventory, the McGill Pain Questionnaire, the Memorial Pain Assessment Card, and the Neuropathic Pain Scale.

Reassessment

It is critical for you to reassess pain at appropriate intervals. The frequency and scope of reassessment are guided by factors such as pain severity, physical and psychosocial condition, type of intervention and risks of adverse effects, and institutional policy. For example, reassessment for a postoperative patient is done within 30 minutes of an IV dose of an analgesic. In a long-term care facility, residents with chronic pain are reassessed at least quarterly or with a change in condition or functional status.

PAIN TREATMENT

Basic Principles

All pain treatment plans are based on the following 10 principles and practice standards:

1. *Follow the principles of pain assessment* (see Table 9-5). Remember that pain is a subjective experience. The patient is not only the best judge of his or her own pain, but also the expert on the effectiveness of each pain treatment.
2. *Use a holistic approach to pain management.* The experience of pain affects all aspects of a person's life. Thus a holistic approach to assessment, treatment, and evaluation is required.[18]
3. *Every patient deserves adequate pain management.* Many patient populations, including ethnic minorities, older adults, and people with past or current substance abuse, are at risk for inadequate pain management. Be aware of your own biases and ensure that all patients are treated respectfully.
4. *Base the treatment plan on the patient's goals.* Discuss with the patient realistic goals for pain relief during the initial pain assessment. Although goals can be described in terms of pain intensity (e.g., the desire for average pain to decrease from "8/10" to "3/10"), with chronic pain conditions functional goal setting should be encouraged (e.g., a goal of performing certain daily activities, such as socializing and hobbies). Over the course of prolonged therapy, reassess these goals and progress made toward meeting them. The patient, in collaboration with the health care team, determines new goals. If the patient has unrealistic goals for therapy, such as wanting to be completely rid of all chronic arthritis pain, work with the patient to establish a more realistic goal.
5. *Use both drug and nondrug therapies.* Although drugs are often considered the mainstay of therapy, incorporate self-care activities and nondrug therapies to increase the overall effectiveness of therapy and to allow for the reduction of drug dosages to minimize adverse drug effects.[19]
6. *When appropriate, use a multimodal approach to analgesic therapy. Multimodal analgesia* is the use of two or more classes of analgesic medications to take advantage of the various mechanisms of action. This approach achieves superior pain relief, enhances patient satisfaction, and decreases adverse effects of individual drugs.[20]
7. *Address pain using an interdisciplinary approach.* The expertise and perspectives of an interdisciplinary team are often necessary to provide effective evaluation and therapies for patients with pain, especially chronic pain. Interdisciplinary teams frequently include psychology, physical and occupational therapy, pharmacy, spiritual care, and multiple medical specialties (e.g., neurology, palliative care, oncology, surgery, anesthesiology). Some pain teams also include massage therapists, music therapists, acupuncturists, and art therapists.
8. *Evaluate the effectiveness of all therapies to ensure that they are meeting the patient's goals.* Achievement of an effective treatment plan often requires trial and error. Adjustments in drug, dosage, or route are common to achieve maximal benefit while minimizing adverse effects. This trial-and-error process can become frustrating for the patient and caregivers. Reassure them that pain relief, if not pain cessation, is possible and that the health care team will continue to work with them to achieve adequate pain relief.
9. *Prevent and/or manage medication side effects.* Side effects are a major reason for treatment failure and nonadherence. Side effects are managed in one of several ways, as described in Table 9-7. You play a key role in monitoring for and treating side effects, and in teaching patients and caregivers how to minimize these effects.
10. *Incorporate patient and caregiver teaching throughout assessment and treatment.* Content should include information about the causes of the pain, pain assessment methods, treatment goals and options, expectations of pain management, proper use of drugs, side effect management, and nondrug and self-help pain relief measures. Document the teaching, and include evaluation of patient and caregiver comprehension.

TABLE 9-7 DRUG THERAPY

Managing Side Effects of Pain Medications

Side effects can be managed in one or more of the following methods.

- Decreasing the dose of analgesic by 10%-15%
- Changing to a different medication in the same class
- Adding a drug to counteract the adverse effect of the analgesic (e.g., using a stool softener for patients experiencing opioid-induced constipation)
- Using an administration route that minimizes drug concentrations (e.g., intraspinal administration of opioids used to minimize high drug levels that produce sedation, nausea, and vomiting)

Drug Therapy for Pain

Pain medications generally are divided into three categories: nonopioids, opioids, and adjuvant drugs. Treatment regimens may include medications from one or more of these groups. Mild pain often can be relieved using nonopioids alone. Moderate to severe pain usually requires an opioid. Certain types of pain, such as neuropathic pain, typically require adjuvant drug therapy alone or in combination with an opioid or another class of analgesics. Pain caused by specific medical conditions, such as cancer, may be treated with chemotherapy or radiation therapy as well as pain medications.

Nonopioids. Nonopioid analgesics include acetaminophen, aspirin and other salicylates, and NSAIDs (Table 9-8). These agents are characterized by the following: (1) their analgesic properties have an **analgesic ceiling;** that is, increasing the dose beyond an upper limit provides no greater analgesia; (2) they do not produce tolerance or physical dependence; and (3) many are available without a prescription. Monitor over-the-counter (OTC) analgesic use to avoid serious problems related to drug interactions, side effects, and overdose.

Nonopioids are effective for mild to moderate pain. They are often used in conjunction with opioids because they allow for effective pain relief using lower opioid doses (thereby causing fewer opioid side effects). This phenomenon is called the *opioid-sparing effect.*[21]

Aspirin is effective for mild pain, but its use is limited by its common side effects, including increased risk for bleeding, especially gastrointestinal (GI) bleeding. Other salicylates such as choline magnesium trisalicylate (Trilisate) cause fewer GI disturbances and bleeding abnormalities. Similar to aspirin, acetaminophen (Tylenol) has analgesic and antipyretic effects, but unlike aspirin, it has no antiplatelet or antiinflammatory effects. Although acetaminophen is well tolerated, it is metabolized by the liver. Hepatotoxicity may result from chronic dosing of more than 4 g/day, acute overdose, or use by patients with severe preexisting liver disease. The addition of acetaminophen to opioid therapy produces an opioid-sparing effect, lower pain scores, and fewer side effects, which is the reason for opioid-acetaminophen combinations such as Percocet and Lortab.[22] IV acetaminophen (OFIRMEV) is used for the treatment of acute mild to moderate pain and moderate to severe pain as an adjunct to opioid analgesics or part of a multimodal analgesic regimen, and reduction of fever. IV acetaminophen is administered over 15 minutes, and the daily dose should also not exceed 4 g/day.

NSAIDs represent a broad class of drugs with varying efficacy and side effects. All NSAIDs inhibit cyclooxygenase

TABLE 9-8 DRUG THERAPY

Selected Nonopioid Analgesics

Drug	Nursing Considerations
Nonsalicylate	
acetaminophen (Tylenol)	• Rectal suppository and injectable form (OFIRMEV) available; sustained-release preparations available; maximum daily dose of 3-4 g. • Doses >4 g/day may cause hepatotoxicity. • Acute overdose: acute liver failure. • Chronic overdose: liver toxicity.
Salicylates	
aspirin	• Rectal suppository and sustained-release preparations available. • Possibility of upper GI bleeding. • Used more commonly in low doses as a cardioprotective measure than for its analgesic properties.
choline magnesium trisalicylate (Trilisate)	• Unlike aspirin and NSAIDs, does not increase bleeding time.
Nonsteroidal Antiinflammatory Drugs (NSAIDs)	
ibuprofen (Motrin, Nuprin, Advil)	• Use lowest effective dose for shortest possible duration. • Increased risk of serious GI adverse events (bleeding, ulceration, perforation), especially in older adults. • May increase risk of serious cardiovascular thrombotic events, myocardial infarction, and stroke. • May increase risk of hypertension and renal insufficiency.
naproxen (Naprosyn, Aleve)	• Use lowest effective dose for shortest possible duration. • Increased risk of serious GI adverse events (bleeding, ulceration, perforation), especially in older adults. • Contraindicated for the treatment of perioperative pain in setting of coronary artery bypass graft (CABG) surgery.
ketorolac (Toradol)	• Limit treatment to 5 days. • May precipitate renal failure in dehydrated patients.
diclofenac K (Cataflam)	• Use lowest effective dose for shortest possible duration. • Available in oral, ophthalmic, topical preparations.
celecoxib (Celebrex)	• Causes fewer GI side effects (e.g., bleeding) than other NSAIDs but risk still present. Is more costly than other NSAIDs. • May increase risk of serious cardiovascular thrombotic events, myocardial infarction, and stroke. • Risks may increase with duration of use, preexisting cardiovascular disease, or risk factors for cardiovascular disease.

(COX), the enzyme that converts arachidonic acid into prostaglandins and related compounds. The enzyme has two forms: COX-1 and COX-2. COX-1 is found in almost all tissues and is responsible for several protective physiologic functions. In contrast, COX-2 is produced mainly at the sites of tissue injury, where it mediates inflammation (Fig. 9-4). Inhibition of COX-1 causes many of the untoward effects of NSAIDs, such as

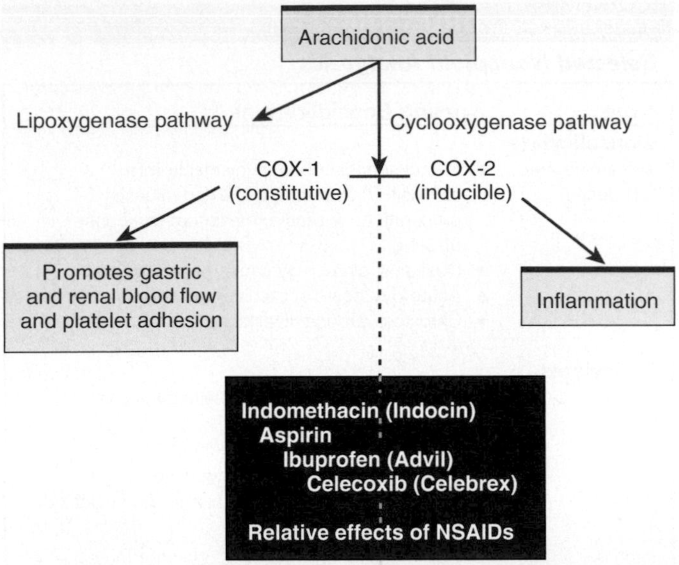

FIG. 9-4 Arachidonic acid is oxidized by two different pathways: lipoxygenase and cyclooxygenase. The cyclooxygenase pathway leads to two forms of the enzyme cyclooxygenase: COX-1 and COX-2. COX-1 is known as *constitutive* (always present), and COX-2 is known as *inducible* (its expression varies markedly depending on the stimulus). Nonsteroidal antiinflammatory drugs (NSAIDs) differ in their actions, with some having more effects on COX-1 and others more on COX-2. Indomethacin acts primarily on COX-1, whereas ibuprofen is equipotent on COX-1 and COX-2. Celecoxib primarily inhibits COX-2.

impairment of renal function, bleeding tendencies, GI irritation, and ulceration. Inhibition of COX-2 is associated with the therapeutic, antiinflammatory effects of NSAIDs. (Celecoxib [Celebrex] is a COX-2 inhibitor.) Older NSAIDs, such as ibuprofen, inhibit both forms of COX and are referred to as nonselective NSAIDs.

Patients vary greatly in their responses to a specific NSAID, so when one NSAID does not provide relief, another should be tried. NSAIDs are associated with many side effects, including GI problems ranging from dyspepsia to life-threatening ulceration and hemorrhage. NSAIDs can also cause cognitive impairment and hypersensitivity reactions with asthma-like symptoms.

Individuals at risk for NSAID-associated GI toxicity include those who have a recent history of peptic ulcer disease, patients who are older than 65, and those concurrently using corticosteroids or anticoagulants. If NSAIDs are used in patients at risk for GI bleeding, they should have concomitant therapy with a misoprostol (Cytotec) or a proton pump inhibitor (PPI) such as omeprazole (Prilosec). NSAIDs should not be administered concurrently with aspirin, since this increases the risk for GI bleeding.[23]

DRUG ALERT

Nonsteroidal Antiinflammatory Drugs (NSAIDs)

- NSAIDs (except aspirin) have been linked to a higher risk for cardiovascular events such as myocardial infarction, stroke, and heart failure.
- Patients who have just had heart surgery should not take NSAIDs.

Opioids. Opioids (Table 9-9) produce their effects by binding to receptors in the CNS. This results in (1) inhibition of the transmission of nociceptive input from the periphery to the spinal cord, (2) altered limbic system activity, and (3) activation of the descending inhibitory pathways that modulate transmission in the spinal cord. Thus opioids act on several nociceptive processes.

Types of Opioids. Opioids are categorized according to their physiologic action (i.e., agonist and antagonist) and binding at specific opioid receptors (e.g., mu, kappa, and delta). The most commonly administered subclass of opioids is the opioid pure agonists, or morphine-like opioids, which bind to mu receptors.

Opioid agonists are used for both acute and chronic pain. Although nociceptive pain appears to be more responsive to opioids than neuropathic pain, opioids are used to treat both types of pain. Pure opioid agonists include morphine, oxycodone (OxyContin), hydrocodone, codeine, methadone, hydromorphone (Dilaudid), oxymorphone (Opana, Opana ER), and levorphanol (Levo-Dromoran) (see Table 9-9). These drugs are effective for moderate to severe pain because they are potent, have no analgesic ceiling, and can be administered through several routes. When opioids are prescribed for moderate pain, they are usually combined with a nonopioid analgesic such as acetaminophen (e.g., codeine plus acetaminophen [Tylenol #3], or hydrocodone plus acetaminophen [Vicodin] or ibuprofen [Vicoprofen]). Addition of acetaminophen or NSAIDs limits the total daily dose that can be given.

Methadone is a unique mu opioid receptor agonist. When methadone is first administered, it has a relatively short analgesic action (4 to 6 hours) and can be titrated every few days, similar to other short-acting oral opioids. However, after 3 or 4 days of regular dosing, the drug's half-life can become prolonged (90 to 120 hours). Doses should not be increased more than once every 1 to 2 weeks to avoid accumulation. Overdose can result in respiratory depression, leading to death.

DRUG ALERT

Morphine

- Morphine may cause respiratory depression.
- If respirations are 12 or less breaths per minute, withhold medication and contact the health care provider.

DRUG ALERT

Methadone (Dolophine)

- Methadone may cause respiratory depression.

Mixed *agonist-antagonists* (e.g., nalbuphine [Nubain], pentazocine [Talwin], butorphanol [Stadol]) bind as agonists on kappa receptors and as weak antagonists or partial agonists on mu receptors. Because of this difference in binding, mixed agonist-antagonists produce less respiratory depression than drugs that act only at mu receptors. These drugs cause more dysphoria and agitation. In addition, opioid agonist-antagonists have an analgesic ceiling and can precipitate withdrawal if used by a patient who is physically dependent on mu agonist drugs. Partial opioid agonists (e.g., buprenorphine [Buprenex]) bind weakly to mu and kappa receptors, which decreases their analgesic efficacy. Agonist-antagonists and partial agonists currently have limited clinical application in pain management.

Mixed Mu Agonist Opioid and Dual Mechanism Agents. Some analgesics have two distinct actions, or dual mechanisms. Tramadol (Ultram) is a weak mu agonist and also inhibits the reuptake of norepinephrine and serotonin. It is effective in low back pain, osteoarthritis, fibromyalgia, diabetic peripheral neuropathic pain, polyneuropathy, and postherpetic neuralgia. The most common side effects are similar to those of other opioids, including nausea, constipation, dizziness, and sedation. As with other medications that increase serotonin and norepinephrine,

TABLE 9-9 DRUG THERAPY

Opioid Analgesics

Drug	Routes of Administration	Nursing Considerations
Mu Agonists		
morphine (Roxanol, MSIR, MS Contin, Avinza, Kadian, Epimorph, Oramorph SR)	PO (short-acting and sustained-release forms), rectal, IV, subcutaneous, epidural, intrathecal, sublingual	• Standard of comparison for opioid analgesics (Table 9-10). • Indicated for moderate to severe pain. • Can stimulate histamine release, leading to pruritus, with systemic administration. • Tablets for sustained-release preparations are to be swallowed whole, and must not be broken, chewed, dissolved, or crushed. • Preparations for neuraxial* administration must be preservative free.
hydromorphone (Dilaudid)	PO (short-acting and sustained-release forms), rectal, IV, subcutaneous, epidural, intrathecal	• Slightly shorter duration than morphine. • Indicated for moderate to severe pain. • Preparations for neuraxial* administration must be preservative free.
methadone (Dolophine)	PO, IV, IM	• High oral and rectal bioavailability. • Accumulates with repeated dosing. • Use with caution in older adults. • Risk of QT interval prolongation with high doses.
levorphanol (Levo-Dromoran)	PO, IV, IM, subcutaneous	• Accumulates with repeated dosing.
fentanyl (Sublimaze [IV], Duragesic [transdermal], Actiq [transmucosal]), buccal tablet (Fentora), sublingual (Abstral), buccal soluble film (Onsolis), nasal spray (Lazanda)	IV, epidural, intrathecal, transmucosal, transdermal	• Immediate onset after IV route; 7-8 min after IM route; 5-15 min after transmucosal route; up to 6 hr after transdermal route. • For procedures, IV fentanyl often combined with benzodiazepines for analgesia and sedation. • Very potent—dosage is in micrograms (mcg). • Transdermal fentanyl only indicated for chronic pain and should not be administered to opioid-naive patients.
oxymorphone (Opana, Opana ER)	IV, PO (short-acting and extended-release forms)	• Tablets for extended-release forms are to be swallowed whole, and must not be broken, chewed, dissolved, or crushed. • Use with caution in older and debilitated patients and patients with hepatic and renal impairment.
oxycodone (Roxicodone, OxyContin) oxycodone plus acetaminophen (Percocet, Endocet, Tylox) oxycodone plus aspirin (Percodan) oxycodone plus ibuprofen (Combunox)	PO (short-acting and sustained-release forms)	• Available as single entity and in combination with a nonopioid. • Can be used similarly to oral morphine for moderate to severe pain. • Often combined with a nonopioid for acute, moderate pain.
hydrocodone (with acetaminophen [Lortab, Vicodin, Zydone])	PO (short acting) Only available in combination with co-analgesics (acetaminophen, aspirin, or ibuprofen)	• Used for moderate or moderately severe pain. • Generally indicated for short-term management of acute pain (e.g., trauma, musculoskeletal).
codeine oral (with acetaminophen [Tylenol #3]), codeine injectable	PO, subcutaneous	• Associated with higher incidence of nausea and constipation than other mu agonists. • Many codeine preparations are combined with acetaminophen. • 5%-10% of European Americans lack the enzyme to metabolize codeine to morphine.
tramadol (Ultram)	PO, short acting and extended release	• Dual mechanism of action: mu opioid agonist and blocks reuptake of norepinephrine and serotonin. • Used for moderate pain.
tapentadol (Nucynta)	PO, short acting and extended release	• Dual mechanism of action: mu opioid agonist and blocks reuptake of norepinephrine and serotonin.
Mixed Agonist-Antagonists		
pentazocine (Talwin)	Formulated in combination with acetaminophen, aspirin, ibuprofen	• May cause psychotomimetic effects (e.g., hallucinations) and may precipitate withdrawal in opioid-dependent patients. • Not recommended for treatment of chronic pain and rarely for acute pain.
pentazocine plus naloxone (Talwin NX)	Abuse-deterrent preparation includes naloxone to discourage parenteral abuse	
butorphanol (Stadol)	Available in a nasal spray and injectable form Not available orally	• Psychotomimetic effects lower than with pentazocine. • May precipitate withdrawal in opioid-dependent patients. • Injectable used for acute pain. • Nasal spray indicated for migraine headaches.
Partial Agonists		
buprenorphine injectable (Buprenex) buprenorphine plus naloxone sublingual (Suboxone)	Sublingual and injectable forms	• Should not be chewed or swallowed. • Lower abuse potential than morphine. Does not produce psychotomimetic effects. • Buprenorphine plus naloxone used as a sublingual preparation to treat opioid dependence for easier withdrawal when necessary to taper from opioids. • May precipitate withdrawal in opioid-dependent patients. Not readily reversed by naloxone.

*Neuraxial anesthesia pertains to local anesthetics placed around the nerves of the central nervous system such as spinal and epidural anesthesia.

TABLE 9-10 OPIOID EQUIANALGESIC DOSES*

	Dose Equal to Parenteral Morphine 10 mg	
Drug	**Oral (mg)**	**Parenteral (IM, IV, Subcutaneous) (mg)**
Morphine	30	10
Codeine	200	120-130
Fentanyl	NA	0.1 (100 mcg)
Hydrocodone	30	NA
Hydromorphone	7.5	1.5
Levorphanol	4	2
Meperidine	300	75
Methadone	20	10
Oxycodone	15-30	NA
Oxymorphone	NA	1

*All equivalencies should be considered approximations. These amounts can be affected by many factors, including interpatient variability, type of pain, and tolerance. Monitor patients for effectiveness and adverse reactions and adjust the dose accordingly
NA, Not available.

this drug should be avoided in patients with a history of seizures because it lowers seizure threshold.

Tapentadol (Nucynta) is a centrally acting analgesic that works at mu receptors and inhibits norepinephrine reuptake.[24] It is approved for management of moderate to severe acute pain. For chronic moderate to severe pain, an extended-release formula is available. The side effects are similar to those of conventional opioids, except that this drug is associated with less nausea and constipation.

Opioids to Avoid. Some opioids should be avoided for pain relief because of limited efficacy and/or toxicities. Meperidine (Demerol) or pethidine is associated with neurotoxicity (e.g., seizures) caused by accumulation of its metabolite, normeperidine. Its use is limited for very short-term (i.e., less than 48 hours) treatment of acute pain when other opioid agonists are contraindicated.[25]

DRUG ALERT

Meperidine (Demerol)

The American Pain Society does not recommend the use of meperidine as an analgesic.

Side Effects of Opioids. Common side effects of opioids include constipation, nausea and vomiting, sedation, respiratory depression, and pruritus. With continued use, many side effects diminish; the exception is constipation. Less common side effects include urinary retention, myoclonus, dizziness, confusion, and hallucinations. *Constipation* is the most common side effect of opioids. Left untreated, constipation may increase the individual's pain and can lead to fecal impaction and paralytic ileus.

Because tolerance to opioid-induced constipation does not develop, a bowel regimen should be instituted at the beginning of opioid therapy and continued for as long as the person takes opioids. Although dietary roughage, fluids, and exercise should be encouraged, these measures alone may not be sufficient. Most patients should use a gentle stimulant laxative (e.g., senna) plus a stool softener (e.g., docusate sodium [Colace]). Other agents (e.g., milk of magnesia, bisacodyl [Dulcolax], polyethylene glycol [MiraLAX], or lactulose [Constulose]) can be added if necessary.

Methylnaltrexone (Relistor) is a peripheral opioid receptor antagonist used for opioid-induced constipation in patients with advanced disease (e.g., incurable cancer, heart failure, chronic obstructive pulmonary disease) when the response to traditional laxative therapy is insufficient. It is generally administered subcutaneously once a day every other day or less frequently, but not more frequently that once daily.

Nausea is often a problem in opioid-naive patients. The use of an antiemetic such as ondansetron (Zofran), metoclopramide (Reglan), transdermal scopolamine (Transderm Scōp), hydroxyzine (Vistaril), or a phenothiazine (e.g., prochlorperazine [Compazine]) can prevent or minimize nausea and vomiting until tolerance develops, usually within 1 week. Opioids delay gastric emptying (patient complains of gastric fullness), and this effect can be reduced by metoclopramide. If nausea and vomiting are severe and persistent, changing to a different opioid may be necessary.

Sedation is usually seen in opioid-naive patients being treated for acute pain. Hospitalized patients receiving opioid analgesics for acute pain should be monitored regularly, especially in the first few days after surgery. Be aware that the risk for unintended advancing sedation in postoperative patients is greatest within 4 hours after leaving the postanesthesia care unit. Opioid-induced sedation resolves with the development of tolerance. Persistent sedation with chronic opioid use can be effectively treated with psychostimulants such as caffeine, dextroamphetamine (Dexedrine), methylphenidate (Ritalin), or the anticataleptic drug modafinil (Provigil).

The risk of *respiratory depression* is also higher in opioid-naive, hospitalized patients who are treated for acute pain. Clinically significant respiratory depression is rare in opioid-tolerant patients and when opioids are titrated to analgesic effect. Patients most at risk for respiratory depression include those who are age 65 or older, have a history of snoring or witnessed apneic episodes, report excessive daytime sleepiness, have underlying cardiac or lung disease, are obese (body mass index greater than 30 kg/m^2), have a history of smoking (more than 20 pack-years), or are receiving other CNS depressants (e.g., sedatives, benzodiazepines, antihistamines). For postoperative patients the greatest risk for opioid-related respiratory adverse events is within the first 24 hours after surgery. Clinically significant respiratory depression cannot occur in patients who are fully awake. Frequently monitor both the sedation level and respiratory rate in patients receiving opioid analgesics. An extensive evidence-based, expert consensus report outlines the risks for unintended advancing sedation and respiratory depression with opioids and recommendations for monitoring to deliver quality and safe patient care.[20]

A sedation scale can be used for monitoring and providing appropriate interventions based on the level of sedation (Table 9-11).

SAFETY ALERT

- If the patient's respirations fall below 8 or 10 breaths/minute and the sedation level is 5 or greater, you should vigorously stimulate the patient and try to keep the patient awake.[20]
- If the patient becomes oversedated, administer oxygen.
- In this situation, the opioid dose should be reduced.

For patients who are excessively sedated or unresponsive, naloxone (Narcan), an opioid antagonist that rapidly reverses the effects of opioids, can be administered. Naloxone can be given IV or subcutaneously every 2 minutes. If the patient has been taking opioids regularly for more than a few days, use naloxone judiciously and titrate carefully because it can precipitate severe, agonizing pain; profound withdrawal symptoms;

TABLE 9-11 PASERO OPIOID-INDUCED SEDATION SCALE (POSS) WITH INTERVENTIONS

Level of Sedation	Nursing Intervention
S = Sleep, easy to arouse	• Acceptable • No action necessary • May increase opioid dose if needed
1 Awake and alert	• Acceptable • No action necessary • May increase opioid dose if needed
2 Slightly drowsy, easily aroused	• Acceptable • No action necessary • May increase opioid dose if needed
3 Frequently drowsy, arousable, drifts off to sleep during conversation	• Unacceptable • Monitor respiratory status and sedation level closely until sedation level is stable at less than 3 and respiratory status is satisfactory • Decrease opioid dose 25% to 50% or notify health care provider or anesthesiologist for orders • Consider administering a non-sedating, opioid-sparing nonopioid, such as acetaminophen or an NSAID, if not contraindicated
4 Somnolent, minimal or no response to verbal or physical stimulation	• Unacceptable • Stop opioid • Consider administering naloxone • Notify health care provider or anesthesiologist • Monitor respiratory status and sedation level closely until sedation level is stable at less than 3 and respiratory status is satisfactory

Adapted from Pasero C: Assessment of sedation during opioid administration for pain management, *Journal of PeriAnesthesia Nursing* 24:186, 2009.

hypertension; and pulmonary edema. Because naloxone's half-life is shorter than that of most opiates, monitor the patient's respiratory rate because it can drop again as soon as 20 minutes after naloxone administration.

Pruritus (itching) is another common side effect of opioids and occurs most frequently when opioids are administered via neuraxial (i.e., epidural, intrathecal) routes. Management of opioid-induced pruritus may include low-dose infusions of naloxone.

A rare but concerning problem with long-term and even short-term use of high-dose opioids is *opioid-induced hyperalgesia* (OIH). OIH is a state of nociceptive sensitization caused by exposure to opioids. It is characterized by a paradoxic response in which patients actually become more sensitive to certain painful stimuli and report increased pain with opioid use. The exact mechanism for this phenomenon is not clearly understood, but it may be due to neuroplasticity changes. This may explain why opioids tend to lose their effectiveness in certain patients over time.

Adjuvant Analgesic Therapy. These medications comprise classes of drugs that can be used alone or in conjunction with opioid and nonopioid analgesics. Generally, these agents were developed for other purposes (e.g., antiseizure drugs, antidepressants) and found later to be effective for pain. Commonly used analgesic adjuvants are listed in Table 9-12.

Corticosteroids. These drugs, which include dexamethasone, prednisone, and methylprednisolone (Medrol), are used for management of acute and chronic cancer pain, pain secondary to spinal cord compression, and inflammatory joint pain syndromes. Mechanisms of action are unknown but may be related to the ability of corticosteroids to decrease edema and inflammation. They also may decrease activation of an inflamed neuron. Because of this effect, corticosteroids are useful when injected epidurally for acute or subacute disc herniations.

Corticosteroids have many side effects, especially when given chronically in high doses. Adverse effects include hyperglycemia, fluid retention, dyspepsia and GI bleeding, impaired healing, muscle wasting, osteoporosis, adrenal suppression, and susceptibility to infection. Because they act through the same final pathway as NSAIDs, corticosteroids should not be given at the same time as NSAIDs.

Antidepressants. Tricyclic antidepressants (TCAs) enhance the descending inhibitory system by preventing the cellular reuptake of serotonin and norepinephrine. Higher levels of serotonin and norepinephrine in the synaptic cleft inhibit the transmission of nociceptive signals in the CNS. Other potential beneficial actions of TCAs include sodium channel modulation, α_1-adrenergic antagonist effects, and a weak NMDA receptor modulation. They appear to be effective for a variety of pain syndromes, especially neuropathic pain syndromes. However, side effects such as sedation, dry mouth, blurred vision, and weight gain limit their usefulness. Antidepressants that selectively inhibit reuptake of serotonin and norepinephrine (in particular the SNRIs) are effective for many neuropathic pain syndromes and have fewer side effects than the TCAs. These agents include venlafaxine, desvenlafaxine (Pristiq), duloxetine, milnacipran (Savella), and bupropion. A disadvantage to their use is higher cost compared with TCAs.

Antiseizure Drugs. Antiseizure drugs affect both peripheral nerves and the CNS in several ways, including sodium channel modulation, central calcium channel modulation, and changes in excitatory amino acids and other receptors. Agents such as gabapentin, lamotrigine, and pregabalin are valuable adjuvant agents in chronic pain therapy and are being increasingly used in the treatment of acute pain.

GABA Receptor Agonist. Baclofen, an analog of the inhibitory neurotransmitter GABA, can interfere with the transmission of nociceptive impulses and is mainly used for muscle spasms. It crosses the blood-brain barrier poorly and is much more effective for spasticity when delivered intrathecally.

α_2-Adrenergic Agonists. Clonidine and tizanidine (Zanaflex) are the most widely used α_2-adrenergic agonists. They are thought to work on the central inhibitory α-adrenergic receptors. These agents may also decrease norepinephrine release peripherally. They are used for chronic headache and neuropathic pain.

Local Anesthetics. For acute pain from surgery or trauma, local anesthetics such as bupivacaine and ropivacaine can be administered epidurally by continuous infusion, but also by intermittent or continuous infusion with regional nerve blocks. Topical applications of local anesthetics are used to interrupt transmission of pain signals to the brain. For example, 5% lidocaine patch (Lidoderm) is recommended as a first-line agent for the treatment of several types of neuropathic pain. In the treatment of chronic severe neuropathic pain that is refractory to other analgesics, oral therapy with mexiletine (Mexitil) may be tried. Systemic lidocaine administered in the form of an IV infusion is also sometimes used for neuropathic and postoperative visceral pain.

TABLE 9-12 **DRUG THERAPY**

Adjuvant Drugs Used for Pain

Drug	Specific Indication	Nursing Considerations
Corticosteroids	Inflammation	• Avoid high doses for long-term use.
Antidepressants		
Tricyclic Antidepressants		
amitriptyline (Elavil) doxepin (Sinequan) imipramine (Tofranil) nortriptyline (Pamelor) desipramine (Norpramin)	Neuropathic pain	• Side-effect profile differs for each agent and is often dose dependent. • Common side effects include anticholinergic effects (e.g., dry mouth) and sedation. • Monitor for anticholinergic side effects. • Titrate slowly over days to weeks to reach optimal therapeutic doses.
Serotonin Norepinephrine Reuptake Inhibitor (SNRI) Antidepressants		
venlafaxine (Effexor) duloxetine (Cymbalta) bupropion (Wellbutrin) milnacipran (Savella)	Neuropathic pain Multimodal therapy for acute pain (venlafaxine) Fibromyalgia (duloxetine)	• Side effects vary with each agent.
Antiseizure Drugs		
First generation: carbamazepine (Tegretol) phenytoin (Dilantin) *Second generation*: gabapentin (Neurontin) pregabalin (Lyrica) lamotrigine (Lamictal)	Neuropathic pain Multimodal therapy for acute pain (gabapentin, pregabalin) Fibromyalgia (pregabalin)	• Start with low doses, increase slowly. • Side effects vary with each agent.
GABA Receptor Agonist		
baclofen (Lioresal)	Neuropathic pain Muscle spasms	• Monitor for weakness, urinary dysfunction. • Avoid abrupt discontinuation because of CNS irritability.
α_2-Adrenergic Agonist		
clonidine (Duraclon) tizanidine (Zanaflex)	Particularly useful for neuropathic pain when administered intrathecally	• Side effects include sedation, orthostatic hypotension, dry mouth. • Often combined with anesthetics (e.g., bupivacaine [Sensorcaine]).
Anesthetics: Oral or Systemic		
mexiletine (Mexitil)	Diabetic neuropathy Neuropathic pain	• Monitor for side effects: high incidence of nausea, dizziness, perioral numbness, paresthesias, tremor, seizures (at high doses), dysrhythmias, and myocardial depression. • Avoid in patients with preexisting cardiac disease.
5% lidocaine–impregnated transdermal patch (Lidoderm patch)	Postherpetic neuralgia	• Local skin reactions (e.g., change in color, colored spots, irritation, itching, rash, burning) occur at the site of application; typically mild.
Anesthetics: Local		
lidocaine (L-M-X)	Topical local anesthetic cream applied to intact skin before venipuncture or lumbar puncture. Possible effective for postherpetic neuralgia	• Apply bubble layer to intact skin, wait at least 20-30 minutes before wiping and performing painful procedure. • Duration is approximately 60 minutes after removed from skin. • Available without prescription.
lidocaine 2.5% + prilocaine 2.5% (topical EMLA [eutectic mixture of local anesthetics])	Longer time to take effect than L-M-X	• Apply under an occlusive dressing (e.g., Tegaderm, DuoDerm) or on an anesthetic disk. • Side effects include mild erythema, edema, skin blanching.
capsaicin (Zostrix)	Pain associated with arthritis, postherpetic neuralgia, diabetic neuropathy	• Apply very sparingly onto affected area. Use gloves or wash hands with soap and water after application. • Monitor for side effects: skin irritation (burning, stinging) at application site and cough when inhaled.

CNS, Central nervous system.

Cannabinoids. Cannabinoid-derived medications show promise in the treatment of certain pain syndromes and symptoms. However, these preparations have sparked considerable controversy and confusion, mostly because cannabinoids are related to the cannabis plant, also known as marijuana. Synthetic cannabinoids (e.g., dronabinol [Marinol]) have been approved for medical use in Canada, the United Kingdom, and the United States. Smoking marijuana or cannabis rapidly increases plasma levels of tetrahydrocannabinol (THC), but the amount is highly dependent on composition of the marijuana cigarette and inhalation technique, so this form of use is associated with highly variable results in relief of pain and symptoms.[26] With commercially available oral preparations, the absorption and bioavailability are more reliable and predictable.

Cannabinoids exert their analgesic effects primarily through the cannabinoid-1 (CB1) and CB2 receptors. Activation of cannabinoid receptors modulates neurotransmission in the serotoninergic, dopaminergic, and glutamatergic systems, as well as other systems. Cannabinoids also enhance the endogenous opioid system. Other beneficial effects include alleviation of nausea and increased appetite. They may also have opioid-sparing effects, possibly reduce opioid tolerance, and even ameliorate symptoms of opioid withdrawal.[26] In Canada an oromucosal spray, nabiximols (Sativex), is available for adjunctive treatment of neuropathic pain and moderate to severe pain in cancer.[27]

Administration

Scheduling. Appropriate analgesic scheduling focuses on preventing or controlling pain, rather than providing analgesics only after the patient's pain has become severe. A patient should be premedicated before procedures and activities that are expected to produce pain. Similarly, a patient with constant pain should receive analgesics around the clock rather than on an "as needed" (PRN) basis. These strategies control pain before it starts and usually result in lower analgesic requirements. Fast-acting drugs should be used for incident or breakthrough pain, whereas long-acting analgesics are more effective for constant pain. Examples of fast-acting and sustained-release analgesics are described later in this section.

Titration. *Analgesic titration* is dose adjustment based on assessment of the adequacy of analgesic effect versus the side effects produced. The amount of analgesic needed to manage pain varies widely, and titration is an important strategy in addressing this variability. An analgesic can be titrated upward or downward, depending on the situation. For example, in a postoperative patient the dose of analgesic generally decreases over time as the acute pain resolves. On the other hand, opioids for chronic, severe cancer pain may be titrated upward many times over the course of therapy to maintain adequate pain control. The goal of titration is to use the smallest dose of analgesic that provides effective pain control with the fewest side effects.

Equianalgesic Dosing. The term **equianalgesic dose** refers to a dose of one analgesic that is approximately equivalent in pain-relieving effects to a given dose of another analgesic (see Table 9-10). This equivalence helps guide opioid dosing when changing routes or opioids when a particular drug is ineffective or causes intolerable side effects. Equianalgesic charts and conversion programs are widely available in clinical guidelines, in health care facility pain protocols, and on the Internet. They are useful tools, but you need to understand their limitations, since equianalgesic doses are estimates.[28] All changes in opioid therapy must be carefully monitored and adjusted for an individual patient.

Administration Routes. Opioids and other analgesic agents can be delivered via many routes. This flexibility allows the health care provider to (1) target a particular anatomic source of the pain, (2) achieve therapeutic blood levels rapidly when necessary, (3) avoid certain side effects through localized administration, and (4) provide analgesia when patients are unable to swallow. The following discussion highlights the uses and nursing considerations for analgesic agents delivered through a variety of routes.

Oral. Generally, oral administration is the route of choice for the person with a functioning GI system. Most pain medications are available in oral preparations, such as liquid and tablet. For opioids, larger oral doses are needed to achieve the equivalent analgesia of doses administered intramuscularly (IM) or IV (see Table 9-10). For example, 10 mg of parenteral morphine is equivalent to approximately 30 mg of oral morphine. The reason larger doses are required is related to the *first-pass effect* of hepatic metabolism. This means that oral opioids are absorbed from the GI tract into the portal circulation and shunted to the liver. Partial metabolism in the liver occurs before the drug enters the systemic circulation and becomes available to peripheral receptors or can cross the blood-brain barrier and access CNS opioid receptors, which is necessary to produce analgesia. Oral opioids are as effective as parenteral opioids if the dose administered is large enough to compensate for the first-pass metabolism.

Many opioids are available in short-acting (immediate-release) and long-acting (sustained-release or extended-release) oral preparations. Immediate-release products are effective in providing rapid, short-term pain relief. Sustained-release preparations generally are administered every 8 to 12 hours, although some preparations (e.g., Kadian, Avinza, Exalgo) may be dosed every 24 hours. Sustained- or extended-release preparations should not be crushed, broken, or chewed.

Transmucosal and Buccal Routes. Although morphine has historically been administered sublingually to people with cancer pain who have difficulty swallowing, little of the drug is actually absorbed from the sublingual tissue. Instead, most of the drug is dissolved in saliva and swallowed, making its metabolism the same as that of oral morphine.

Several transmucosal fentanyl products are used for the treatment of breakthrough pain including oral transmucosal fentanyl citrate (OTFC) (Actiq) with the fentanyl embedded in a flavored lozenge on a stick, absorbed by the buccal mucosa after being rubbed actively over it when administered as the lozenge (not sucked as a lollipop), fentanyl buccal tablet (FBT) (Fentora) in the form of a buccal tablet that disintegrates, fentanyl sublingual (Abstral), and fentanyl buccal soluble film (Onsolis) for application to the buccal membrane. Transmucosal absorption allows the drug to enter the bloodstream and travel directly to the CNS. Pain relief typically occurs 5 to 7 minutes after administration. These formulations of fentanyl should be used only for patients who are already receiving and are tolerant to opioid therapy.

An oromucosal spray delivery of cannabinoid extract (Sativex) is an adjunctive treatment for neuropathic pain and spasticity in patients with multiple sclerosis. It is not currently available in the United States.

Intranasal Route. Intranasal administration allows delivery of medication to highly vascular mucosa and avoids the first-pass effect. Butorphanol is indicated for acute headache and other intense, recurrent types of pain. A transmucosal fentanyl nasal spray (Lazanda) is available for the treatment of breakthrough pain.

Rectal. The rectal route is often overlooked but is particularly useful when the patient cannot take an analgesic by mouth, such as those patients with severe nausea and vomiting. Analgesics that are available as rectal suppositories include hydromorphone, oxymorphone, morphine, and acetaminophen. If rectal preparations are not available, many oral formulations can be given rectally if the patient is unable to take medications by mouth.

Transdermal Route. Fentanyl (Duragesic) is available as a transdermal patch system for application to nonhairy skin. This delivery system is useful for the patient who cannot tolerate oral analgesic drugs. Absorption from the patch is slow, and it takes 12 to 17 hours to reach full effect with the first application. Therefore transdermal fentanyl is not suitable for rapid dose titration but can be effective if the patient's pain is stable and the dose required to control it is known. Patches may need to be changed every 48 hours rather than the recommended 72 hours based on individual patient responses. Rashes caused by the adhesive of the patch may be reduced by preparing the skin 1 hour before placement with a weak corticosteroid cream. Bio-occlusive dressings are available if the patch keeps falling off because of sweating. A transdermal patient-controlled analgesia (PCA) system (iontophoretic transdermal system [ITS]) is available.

DRUG ALERT

Fentanyl Patches

- Fentanyl patches (Duragesic) may cause death from overdose.
- Signs of overdose include trouble breathing or shallow respirations; tiredness, extreme sleepiness, or sedation; inability to think, talk, or walk normally; and faintness, dizziness, or confusion.

An important distinction should be made between transdermal patches designed for systemic drug delivery (e.g., Duragesic) and those for topical or local delivery (e.g., Lidoderm).

A 5% lidocaine-impregnated transdermal patch (Lidoderm patch) is used for postherpetic neuralgia. The patch is placed directly on the intact skin in the area of postherpetic pain and left in place for up to 12 hours. Topical local anesthetics are generally well tolerated and cause few systemic side effects, even with chronic use.

Creams and lotions containing 10% trolamine salicylate (Aspercreme, Myoflex Creme) are available for joint and muscle pain. This aspirin-like substance is absorbed locally. This route of administration avoids GI irritation but not the other side effects of high-dose salicylates. Topical diclofenac solution and a diclofenac patch (Flector) have been shown to be effective for osteoarthritic pain of the knee.

Other topical analgesic agents, such as capsaicin (e.g., Zostrix) and lidocaine (L-M-X cream), also provide analgesia. Derived from red chili pepper, capsaicin acts on C fiber heat receptors. If used three or four times a day for 4 to 6 weeks, it will cause the C nociceptor fibers to become inactive. The result is neuronal resistance to painful stimuli. Capsaicin can control pain associated with diabetic neuropathy, arthritis, and possibly postherpetic neuralgia. L-M-X cream is useful for control of pain associated with venipunctures. Cover the targeted area of intact skin with a layer of L-M-X for at least 20 to 30 minutes before it is wiped off prior to beginning a painful procedure. An occlusive dressing is recommended but not required during this time.

Parenteral Routes. The parenteral routes include subcutaneous, IM, and IV administration. Single, repeated, or continuous dosing (subcutaneous or IV) is possible via parenteral routes. Although it is frequently used, the IM route is not recommended because injections cause significant pain and result in unreliable absorption. With chronic use, IM injections can result in abscesses and fibrosis. Onset of analgesia after subcutaneous administration is slow, and thus the subcutaneous route is rarely used for acute pain management. However, continuous subcutaneous infusions are effective for pain management at the end of life. This route is especially helpful for people with abnormal GI function and limited venous access. IV administration is the best route when immediate analgesia and rapid titration

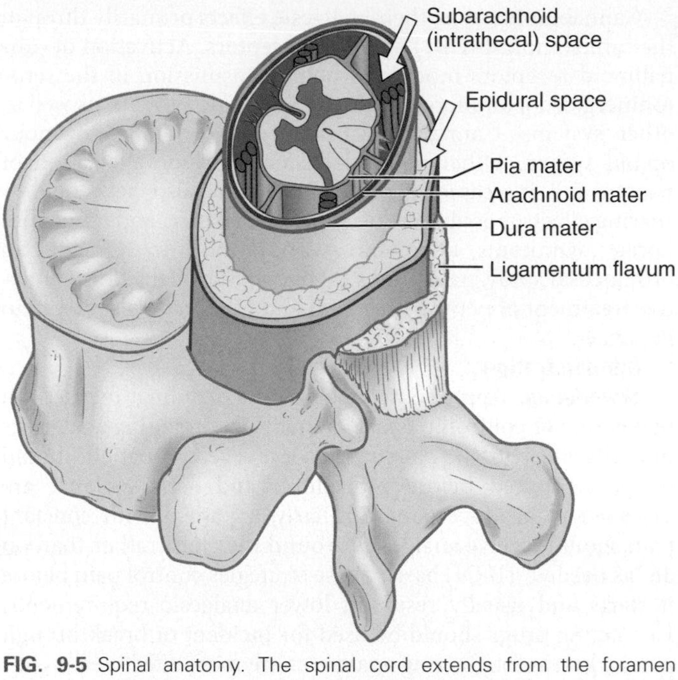

FIG. 9-5 Spinal anatomy. The spinal cord extends from the foramen magnum to the first or second lumbar vertebral space. The subarachnoid space (intrathecal space) is filled with cerebrospinal fluid that continuously circulates and bathes the spinal cord. The epidural space is a potential space filled with blood vessels, fat, and a network of nerve extensions.

are necessary. Continuous IV infusions provide excellent steady-state analgesia through stable blood levels.

Intraspinal Delivery. Intraspinal opioid therapy involves inserting a catheter into the subarachnoid space *(intrathecal delivery)* or the epidural space *(epidural delivery)* (Fig. 9-5). Analgesics are injected either by intermittent bolus doses or continuous infusion.

Percutaneously placed temporary catheters are used for short-term therapy (2 to 4 days), and surgically implanted catheters are used for long-term therapy. Although the lumbar region is the most common site of placement, epidural catheters may be placed at any point along the spinal column (cervical, thoracic, lumbar, or caudal). The tip of the epidural catheter is placed as close to the nerve supplying the painful dermatome as possible. For example, a thoracic catheter is placed for upper abdominal surgery, and a high lumbar catheter is used for lower abdominal surgery. Fluoroscopy is used to ensure correct placement of the catheter.

Intraspinally administered analgesics are highly potent because they are delivered close to the receptors in the spinal cord dorsal horn. Smaller doses of analgesics are needed than with other routes, including IV. For example, 1 mg of intrathecal morphine is approximately equivalent to 10 mg of epidural morphine, 100 mg of IV morphine, and 300 mg of oral morphine. Drugs that are delivered intraspinally include morphine, fentanyl, sufentanil (Sufenta), alfentanil (Alfenta), hydromorphone, ziconotide (Prialt) (a calcium channel receptor modulator for use in neuropathic pain syndromes), and clonidine. Nausea, itching, and urinary retention are common side effects of intraspinal opioids.

Complications of intraspinal analgesia include catheter displacement and migration, accidental infusions of neurotoxic agents, epidural hematomas, and infection. Clinical manifestations of catheter displacement or migration depend on catheter location and the drug being infused. A catheter that migrates out of the intrathecal or epidural space will cause a decrease in pain relief with no improvement with additional boluses or increases in the infusion rate. If an epidural catheter migrates into the subarachnoid space, increased side effects become quickly apparent. Somnolence, confusion, and increased anesthesia (if the infusate contains an anesthetic) occur. Check with institutional policy before aspirating cerebrospinal fluid to determine intrathecal catheter placement. Migration of a catheter into a blood vessel may cause an increase in side effects because of systemic drug distribution.

Many drugs and chemicals are highly neurotoxic when administered intraspinally. These include many preservatives such as alcohol and phenol, antibiotics, chemotherapy agents, potassium, and parenteral nutrition. To avoid inadvertent injection of IV drugs into an intraspinal catheter, the catheter should be clearly marked as an intraspinal access device, and only preservative-free drugs should be injected.

Infection is a rare but serious complication of intraspinal analgesia. Assess the skin around the exit site for inflammation, drainage, or pain. Manifestations of an intraspinal infection include diffuse back pain, pain or paresthesia during bolus injection, and unexplained sensory or motor deficits in the lower limbs. Fever may or may not be present. Acute bacterial infection (meningitis) is manifested by photophobia, neck stiffness, fever, headache, and altered mental status. Infection is avoided by providing regular, meticulous wound care and using sterile technique when caring for the catheter and injecting drugs.

Long-term epidural catheters may be placed for terminal cancer patients or patients with certain pain syndromes that are unresponsive to other treatments. If a long-term indwelling epidural catheter is used, bacterial filters are recommended.

Implantable Pumps. Intraspinal catheters can be surgically implanted for long-term pain relief. The surgical placement of an intrathecal catheter to a subcutaneously placed pump and reservoir allows for the delivery of drugs directly into the intrathecal space. The pump, which is normally placed in a pocket made in the subcutaneous tissue of the abdomen, may be programmable or fixed. Changes are made by either reprogramming the pump or changing the mixture or concentration of drug in the reservoir. The pump is refilled every 30 to 90 days depending on flow rate, mixture, and reservoir size.

Patient-Controlled Analgesia. A specific type of IV delivery system is **patient-controlled analgesia (PCA)**, or demand analgesia. It can also be connected to an epidural catheter (patient-controlled epidural analgesia). With PCA, a dose of opioid is delivered when the patient decides a dose is needed. PCA uses an infusion system in which the patient pushes a button to receive a bolus infusion of an analgesic. PCA is used widely for the management of acute pain, including postoperative pain and cancer pain.

Opioids such as morphine and hydromorphone are commonly administered via IV PCA therapy for both acute and chronic pain management. Fentanyl is less often used for acute pain. Sometimes IV PCA is administered with a continuous or background infusion called a *basal rate,* depending on the patient's opioid requirement. For acute pain (e.g., postoperative pain), basal rates are not recommended when initiating therapy in opioid-naive patients. The addition of a basal rate in opioid-naive patients and those at risk for adverse respiratory outcomes (e.g., older age, obstructive sleep apnea, pulmonary disease) may lead to serious respiratory events.[20]

Use of PCA begins with patient teaching. Help the patient understand the mechanics of getting a drug dose and how to titrate the drug to achieve good pain relief. Teach the patient to self-administer the analgesic before pain is severe. Assure the patient that he or she cannot "overdose" because the pump is programmed to deliver a maximum number of doses per hour. Pressing the button after the maximum dose is administered will not result in additional analgesic. If the maximum doses are inadequate to relieve pain, the pump can be reprogrammed to increase the amount or frequency of dosing. In addition, you can give bolus doses if they are included in the physician's orders. To make a smooth transition from infusion PCA to oral drugs, the patient should receive increasing doses of oral drug as the PCA analgesic is tapered.

Interventional Therapy

Therapeutic Nerve Blocks. Nerve blocks generally involve one-time or continuous infusion of local anesthetics into a particular area to produce pain relief. These techniques are also called *regional anesthesia.* Nerve blocks interrupt all afferent and efferent transmission to the area and thus are not specific to nociceptive pathways. They include local infiltration of anesthetics into a surgical area (e.g., chest incisions, inguinal hernia, joint) and injection of anesthetic into a specific nerve (e.g., occipital or pudendal nerve) or nerve plexus (e.g., brachial or celiac plexus). Nerve blocks often are used during and after surgery to manage pain. For longer-term relief of chronic pain syndromes, local anesthetics can be administered via a continuous infusion.

Adverse effects of nerve blocks are similar to those for local anesthetics delivered via other systemic routes and include systemic toxicity resulting in dysrhythmias, confusion, nausea and vomiting, blurred vision, tinnitus, and metallic taste. Temporary nerve blocks affect both motor function and sensation and typically last 2 to 24 hours, depending on the agent and the site of injection. Motor ability generally returns before sensation.

Neuroablative Techniques. *Neuroablative interventions* are performed for severe pain that is unresponsive to all other therapies. Neuroablative techniques destroy nerves, thereby interrupting pain transmission. Destruction is accomplished by surgical resection or thermocoagulation, including radiofrequency coagulation. Neuroablative interventions that destroy the sensory division of a peripheral or spinal nerve are classified as *neurectomies, rhizotomies,* and *sympathectomies.* Neurosurgical procedures that ablate the lateral spinothalamic tract are classified as *cordotomies* if the tract is interrupted in the spinal cord, or *tractotomies* if the interruption is in the medulla or the midbrain of the brainstem (Fig. 9-6). Both cordotomy and tractotomy can be performed with the aid of local anesthesia by a percutaneous technique under fluoroscopy.

Neuroaugmentation. *Neuroaugmentation* involves electrical stimulation of the brain and the spinal cord. Spinal cord stimulation (SCS) is performed much more often than brain stimulation. The most common use of SCS is for chronic back pain secondary to nerve damage that is unresponsive to other therapies. Other uses include complex regional pain syndrome (CRPS), spinal cord injury pain, and interstitial cystitis. Potential complications include those related to the surgery (bleeding and infection), migration of the generator (which usually is implanted in the subcutaneous tissues of the upper gluteal or pectoralis area), and nerve damage.[29]

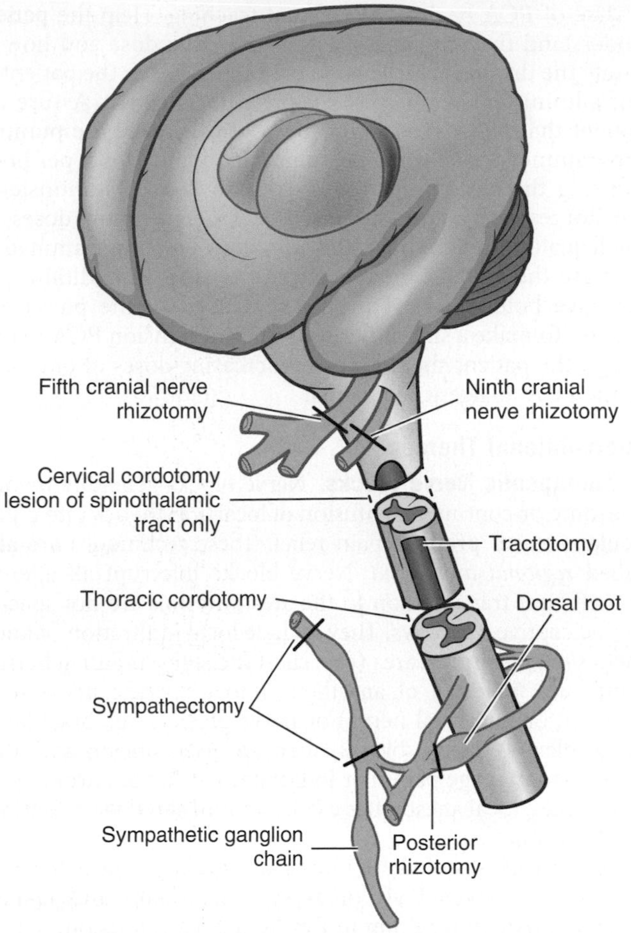

FIG. 9-6 Sites of neurosurgical procedures for pain relief.

Nondrug Therapies for Pain

Nondrug strategies play an important role in pain management (Table 9-13). They can reduce the dose of an analgesic required to relieve pain and thereby minimize side effects of drug therapy. Moreover, they increase the patient's sense of personal control about managing pain and bolster coping skills. Some strategies are believed to alter ascending nociceptive input or stimulate descending pain modulation mechanisms (see discussion on perception on p. 118). These nondrug therapies are especially important in the treatment of chronic pain.[30]

Physical Pain Relief Strategies

Massage. Massage is useful for both acute and chronic pain.[31] Many different massage techniques exist, including moving the hands or fingers over the skin slowly or briskly with long strokes or in circles (superficial massage) or applying firm pressure to the skin to maintain contact while massaging the underlying tissues (deep massage). Another type is trigger point massage. A **trigger point** is a circumscribed hypersensitive area within a tight band of muscle. It is caused by acute or chronic muscle strain and can often be felt as a tight knot under the skin. Trigger point massage is performed by applying either strong, sustained digital pressure; deep massage; or gentler massage with ice followed by muscle heating. (Massage is discussed in Chapter 6.)

Exercise. Exercise is an essential part of the treatment plan for patients with chronic pain, particularly those with musculoskeletal pain.[32] Many patients become physically deconditioned as a result of their pain, which in turn leads to more pain. Exercise acts via many mechanisms to relieve pain. It enhances circulation and cardiovascular fitness, reduces edema, increases muscle strength and flexibility, and enhances physical and psychosocial functioning. An exercise program should be tailored to the patient's physical needs and lifestyle. It may include aerobic exercise, stretching, and strengthening exercises. The program should be supervised by trained personnel (e.g., exercise physiologist, physical therapist).

TABLE 9-13 NONDRUG THERAPIES FOR PAIN

Physical Therapies	Cognitive Therapies

• Acupuncture
• Application of heat and cold (see Table 9-14)
• Exercise
• Massage
• Transcutaneous electrical nerve stimulation (TENS)
	• Distraction
	• Hypnosis
	• Imagery
	• Relaxation strategies (see Chapter 7)
	  • Relaxation breathing
	  • Imagery
	  • Meditation
	  • Art therapy
	  • Music therapy

Transcutaneous Electrical Nerve Stimulation. *Transcutaneous electrical nerve stimulation* (TENS) involves the delivery of an electric current through electrodes applied to the skin surface over the painful region, at trigger points, or over a peripheral nerve. A TENS system consists of two or more electrodes connected by lead wires to a small, battery-operated stimulator (Fig. 9-7). Usually a physical therapist is responsible for administering TENS therapy, although nurses can be trained in the technique.

TENS may be used for acute pain, including postoperative pain and pain associated with physical trauma. The effects of TENS on chronic pain are less clear, but it may be effective in these cases.[33]

Acupuncture. Acupuncture is a technique of Traditional Chinese Medicine in which very thin needles are inserted into the body at designated points. Acupuncture is used for many different kinds of pain. (Acupuncture is discussed in Chapter 6.)

Heat Therapy. Heat therapy is the application of either moist or dry heat to the skin. Heat therapy can be either superficial or deep. Superficial heat can be applied using an electric heating

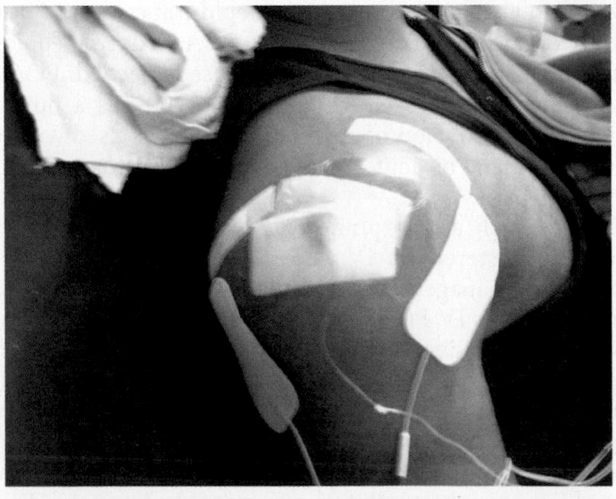

FIG. 9-7 Transcutaneous electrical nerve stimulation (TENS) treatment being given for treatment of pain after shoulder surgery.

TABLE 9-14 PATIENT & CAREGIVER TEACHING GUIDE

Heat and Cold Therapy

Include the following instructions when teaching the patient and caregiver about superficial heat or cold techniques.

Heat Therapy
- Do not use heat on an area that is being treated with radiation therapy, is bleeding, has decreased sensation, or has been injured in the past 24 hours.
- Do not use any menthol-containing products (e.g., Ben-Gay, Vicks, Icy Hot) with heat applications because this may cause burns.
- Cover the heat source with a towel or cloth before applying to the skin to prevent burns.

Cold Therapy
- Cover the cold source with a cloth or towel before applying to the skin to prevent tissue damage.
- Do not apply cold to areas that are being treated with radiation therapy, have open wounds, or have poor circulation.
- If it is not possible to apply the cold directly to the painful site, try applying it right above or below the painful site or on the opposite side of the body on the corresponding site (e.g., left elbow if the right elbow hurts).

pad (dry or moist), a hot pack, hot moist compresses, warm wax (paraffin), or a hot water bottle. To expose large areas of the body, patients can immerse themselves in a hot bath, shower, or whirlpool. Physical therapy departments provide deep-heat therapy through such techniques as short-wave diathermy, microwave diathermy, and ultrasound therapy. Patient teaching regarding heat therapy is described in Table 9-14.

Cold Therapy. Cold therapy involves the application of either moist or dry cold to the skin. Dry cold can be applied by means of an ice bag, moist cold by means of towels soaked in ice water, cold hydrocollator packs, or immersion in a bath or under running cold water. Icing with ice cubes or blocks of ice made to resemble Popsicles is another technique used for pain relief. Cold therapy is believed to be more effective than heat for a variety of painful conditions, including acute pain from trauma or surgery, acute flare-ups of arthritis, muscle spasms, and headache. Patient teaching regarding cold therapy is described in Table 9-14.

Cognitive Therapies. Techniques to alter the affective, cognitive, and behavioral components of pain include a variety of cognitive strategies and behavioral approaches. For example, patients can identify and challenge negative pain-related thoughts and replace them with more positive coping thoughts. Some of these techniques require little training and often are adopted independently by the patient. For others, a trained therapist is necessary.

Distraction. Distraction involves redirection of attention away from the pain and onto something else. It is a simple but powerful strategy to relieve pain. Distraction can be achieved by engaging the patient in any activity that can hold his or her attention (e.g., watching TV or a movie, conversing, listening to music, playing a game). It is important to match the activity with the patient's energy level and ability to concentrate.

Hypnosis. Hypnotherapy is a structured technique that enables a patient to achieve a state of heightened awareness and focused concentration that can be used to alter the patient's pain perception. Hypnosis should be administered and monitored only by specially trained clinicians.[34]

Relaxation Strategies. Relaxation strategies are varied, but their goal is to reach a state that is free from anxiety and muscle tension. Relaxation reduces stress, decreases acute anxiety, distracts from pain, alleviates muscle tension, combats fatigue, facilitates sleep, and enhances the effectiveness of other pain relief measures.[35] Relaxation strategies include relaxation breathing, music, imagery, meditation, and muscle relaxation. These strategies are described in Chapter 7.

NURSING AND COLLABORATIVE MANAGEMENT PAIN

You are an important member of the interdisciplinary pain management team. You provide input into the assessment and reassessment of pain. You help in planning and implementing treatments, including education, advocacy, and support of the patient and family. Because patients in any care setting can experience pain, you must be knowledgeable about current therapies and flexible in trying new approaches to pain management.

Together with the patient, develop a written agreement or treatment plan that describes the pain management. The plan should ensure that pain will be treated based on the patient's perception and report of pain. In addition, the plan should clearly outline the gradual tapering of the analgesic dose, with eventual substitution of parenteral analgesics with long-acting oral preparations, and possibly cessation of opioids.

Many nursing roles are described earlier in this chapter, including assessing pain, administering treatment, monitoring for side effects, and teaching patients and caregivers. However, the success of these actions depends on your ability to establish a trusting relationship with the patient and caregiver and to address their concerns regarding pain and its treatment.

EFFECTIVE COMMUNICATION

Because pain is a subjective experience, patients need to feel confident that their reporting of pain will be believed and will not be perceived as "complaining." The patient and the caregiver also need to know that you consider the pain significant and understand that pain may profoundly disrupt a person's life. Communicate concern and commit to helping the patient obtain pain relief and cope with any unrelieved pain. Support the patient and the caregiver through the period of trial and error that may be necessary to implement an effective therapeutic plan. It also is important to clarify responsibilities in pain relief. Help the patient understand the role of the health care team members, as well as the patient's roles and expectations.

In addition to addressing specific aspects of pain assessment and treatment, evaluate the impact that the pain has on the lives of the patient and the caregiver. Table 9-15 addresses teaching needs of patients and caregivers related to pain management.

CHALLENGES TO EFFECTIVE PAIN MANAGEMENT

Common challenges to effective pain management include misunderstandings about tolerance, physical dependence, and addiction. It is important for you to understand and be able to explain these concepts.

TOLERANCE. *Tolerance* occurs with chronic exposure to a variety of drugs. In the case of opioids, tolerance to analgesia is characterized by the need for an increased opioid dose to maintain the same degree of analgesia. Although the development of

TABLE 9-15 PATIENT & CAREGIVER TEACHING GUIDE

Pain Management

Include the following information in the teaching plan for the patient with pain and caregiver.

- Self-management techniques.
- Realistic goals for pain control.
- Negative consequences of unrelieved pain.
- Need to maintain a record of pain level and effectiveness of treatment.
- Pain should be treated with drugs and/or nondrug therapies before it becomes severe.
- Medication may stop working after it is taken for a period of time, and dosages may need to be adjusted.
- Potential side effects and complications associated with pain therapies can include nausea and vomiting, constipation, sedation and drowsiness, itching, urinary retention, and sweating.
- Need to report when pain is not relieved to tolerable levels.

tolerance to side effects (except constipation) is more predictable, the incidence of clinically significant analgesic opioid tolerance in chronic pain patients is unknown, since dosage needs may increase as the disease (e.g., cancer) progresses. It is essential to assess for increased analgesic needs in patients on long-term therapy. The health care team needs to evaluate and rule out other causes of increased analgesic needs, such as disease progression or infection.

If significant tolerance to opioids develops and it is believed that an opioid is losing its effectiveness, or intolerable side effects are associated with escalation of doses, the practice of *opioid rotation* may be considered. This involves switching from one opioid to another, assuming that the new opioid will be more effective at lower equianalgesic doses. However, very high opioid doses can result in opioid-induced hyperalgesia rather than pain relief. This means that increases in the dose can lead to higher pain levels.

PHYSICAL DEPENDENCE. Like tolerance, physical dependence is a normal physiologic response to ongoing exposure to drugs. It is manifested by a withdrawal syndrome when the drug is abruptly decreased. Manifestations of opioid withdrawal are listed in Table 9-16. When opioids are no longer needed to provide pain relief, a tapering schedule should be used in conjunction with careful monitoring. A typical tapering schedule is determined by calculating the 24-hour dose used by the patient and dividing by 2. Of this decreased amount, 25% is given every 6 hours. After 2 days the daily dose is reduced by an additional 25%; this reduction continues every 2 days until the 24-hour oral dose is 30 mg (morphine equivalent) per day. After 2 days on this minimum dose, the opioid is then discontinued.

PSEUDOADDICTION. Inadequate treatment of pain can lead to a phenomenon called *pseudoaddiction*.[36] This occurs when patients exhibit behaviors commonly associated with addiction (e.g., frequent requests for analgesic refills or higher dosages), but the behaviors resolve with adequate treatment of the patient's pain. These patients are often labeled as drug-seeking, which can result in a crisis of mistrust between the patient and the provider. This phenomenon can be avoided by effective communication strategies and optimal pain management.

ADDICTION. *Addiction* is a complex neurobiologic condition characterized by aberrant behaviors arising from a drive to obtain and take substances for reasons other than the prescribed therapeutic value (see Chapter 11). Tolerance and physical dependence are not indicators of addiction. Rather they are normal physiologic responses to chronic exposure to certain drugs, including opioids. Addiction rarely occurs in patients who receive opioids for pain control. If addiction is suspected, it needs to be investigated and diagnosed, if appropriate, but it should not be implied without evidence because this interferes with pain management. The hallmarks of addiction include (1) compulsive use, (2) loss of control of use, and (3) continued use despite risk of harm.

The risk of developing addiction is associated with certain factors, including younger age, personal or family history of substance abuse, and mood disorders. However, the risk of addiction should not prevent health care providers from using opioids to effectively treat moderate to severe acute and chronic pain. Professional organizations and government agencies have issued joint statements about the roles and responsibilities of health care professionals in the appropriate use of opioids for pain management.[37]

TABLE 9-16 MANIFESTATIONS OF OPIOID WITHDRAWAL SYNDROME

	Early Response (6-12 Hr)	Late Response (48-72 Hr)
Psychosocial	• Anxiety	• Excitation
Secretions	• Lacrimation • Rhinorrhea • Diaphoresis	• Diarrhea
Other	• Yawning • Piloerection • Shaking, chills • Dilated pupils • Anorexia • Tremor	• Restlessness • Fever • Nausea and vomiting • Abdominal cramping pain • Hypertension • Tachycardia • Insomnia

DELEGATION DECISIONS

Pain

Effective pain management should be a focus for all members of the nursing team.

Role of Registered Nurse (RN)

- Assess pain characteristics (pattern and onset, area or location, intensity, quality, associated symptoms, and management strategies).
- Develop treatment plan for patient's pain (including drug and nondrug therapies).
- Evaluate whether current treatment plan is effective.
- Teach patient and caregiver about treatment plan.
- Implement discharge teaching about pain management.

Role of Licensed Practical/Vocational Nurse (LPN/LVN)

- Administer ordered pain medications (consider the state nurse practice act and agency policy, since LPNs may not be able to give medications by all routes).
- Assess patient's pain.

Role of Unlicensed Assistive Personnel (UAP)

- Assist with screening for pain and notify RN if patient expresses pain.
- Take and report vital signs before and after pain medications are given.
- Note and report if patient is refusing to participate in ordered activities such as ambulation (since this may indicate inadequate pain management).

TABLE 9-17 PATIENT & CAREGIVER TEACHING GUIDE

Reducing Barriers to Pain Management

When teaching the patient and caregiver about pain management, discuss the following barriers.

Barrier	Nursing Considerations
Fear of addiction	• Explain that addiction is uncommon in patients taking opioids for pain.
Fear of tolerance	• Teach that tolerance is a normal physiologic response to chronic opioid therapy. If tolerance does develop, the drug may need to be changed (e.g., morphine in place of oxycodone). • Teach that there is no absolute upper limit to pure opioid agonists (e.g., morphine). Dosages can be increased, and patient should not save drugs for when the pain is worse. • Teach that tolerance develops more slowly to analgesic effects of opioids than to side effects (e.g., sedation, respiratory depression). Tolerance does not develop to constipation; thus, a regular bowel program should be started early.
Concern about side effects	• Teach methods to prevent and to treat common side effects. • Emphasize that side effects such as sedation and nausea decrease with time. • Explain that different drugs have unique side effects, and other pain drugs can be tried to reduce the specific side effect.
Fear of injections	• Explain that oral medicines are preferred. • Emphasize that even if oral route becomes unusable, transdermal or indwelling parenteral routes can be used rather than injections.
Desire to be "good" patient	• Explain that patients are partners in their care and that the partnership requires open communication of both the patient and the nurse. • Emphasize to patients that they have a responsibility to keep you informed about their pain.
Desire to be stoic	• Explain that although stoicism is a valued behavior in many cultures, failure to report pain can result in undertreatment and severe, unrelieved pain.
Forgetting to take analgesic	• Provide and teach use of pill containers. • Provide methods of record keeping for drug use. • Recruit caregivers to assist with the analgesic regimen.
Concern that pain indicates disease progression	• Explain that increased pain or the need for analgesics may reflect tolerance. • Emphasize that new pain may come from a non–life-threatening source (e.g., muscle spasm, urinary tract infection). • Institute drug and nondrug strategies to reduce anxiety. • Ensure that patient and caregivers have current, accurate, comprehensive information about the disease and prognosis. • Provide psychologic support.
Sense of fatalism	• Explain that pain can be managed in most patients. • Explain that most therapies require a period of trial and error. • Emphasize that side effects can be managed.
Ineffective medication	• Teach that there are multiple options within each category of medication (e.g., opioids, NSAIDs), and another medication from the same category may provide better relief. • Emphasize that finding the best treatment regimen often requires trial and error. • Incorporate nondrug approaches in treatment plan.

Adapted from Ersek M: Enhancing effective pain management by addressing patient barriers to analgesic use, *J Hospice Palliat Nurs* 1:87, 1999.
NSAIDs, Nonsteroidal antiinflammatory drugs.

In addition to the fears about addiction, physical dependence, and tolerance, other barriers hinder effective pain management. Table 9-17 lists some barriers and strategies to address them.

INSTITUTIONALIZING PAIN EDUCATION AND MANAGEMENT

Besides patient and caregiver barriers, other barriers to effective pain management include inadequate health care provider education and lack of organizational support. Traditionally, medical and nursing school curricula have spent little time teaching future physicians and nurses about pain and symptom management. The lack of emphasis on pain in medical and nursing schools has contributed to inadequate training of health care providers.

Progress has been made in overcoming these barriers. Medical and nursing schools now devote more time to addressing pain. Numerous professional organizations have published evidence-based guidelines for assessing and managing pain in many patient populations and clinical settings.

Researchers and health care providers have documented the central role that institutional commitment and practices have in changing clinical practice. Without institutional support, pain outcomes are unlikely to change. One major step in institutionalizing pain management is the development and adoption of The Joint Commission (TJC) guideline on pain.[37] TJC is the accrediting body for most health care facilities (hospitals, nursing homes, and health care clinics). Under these standards, health care facilities are required to (1) recognize the patient's right to appropriate assessment and management of pain; (2) identify pain in patients during their initial assessment and as needed, during ongoing, periodic reassessments; (3) educate health care providers about pain assessment and management and ensure competency; and, (4) educate patients and their families about pain management.

ETHICAL ISSUES IN PAIN MANAGEMENT

Fear of Hastening Death by Administering Analgesics

A common concern of health care professionals and caregivers is that providing sufficient drug to relieve pain will hasten or precipitate death of a terminally ill person. However, there is no scientific evidence that opioids can hasten death, even among patients at the very end of life. Moreover, as a nurse, you have a moral obligation to provide comfort and pain relief at the end of life. Even if there is a concern about the possibility of hastening death, the rule of double effect provides ethical justification. This rule states that if an unwanted consequence (i.e., hastened death) occurs as a result of an action taken to achieve a moral good (i.e., pain relief), the action is justified if the nurse's intent is to relieve pain and not to hasten death.[38]

Requests for Assisted Suicide

Unrelieved pain is one of the reasons that patients make requests for assisted suicide. Aggressive and adequate pain management may decrease the number of such requests. Assisted suicide is a complex issue that extends beyond pain and pain management. Currently Oregon, Washington, and Montana are the only states where assisted suicide is legal. To address the legal and ethical issues confronting nurses in this unique situation, the Oregon Nurses Association prepared a position paper on this topic.[39]

Use of Placebos in Pain Assessment and Treatment

Placebos are still sometimes used to assess and to treat pain. Using a placebo involves deceiving patients by making them believe that they are receiving an analgesic when in fact they are typically receiving an inert substance such as saline. The use of placebos to assess or treat pain is condemned by several professional organizations.[40]

GERONTOLOGIC CONSIDERATIONS

PAIN

Persistent pain is a common problem in older adults and is often associated with physical disability and psychosocial problems. The prevalence of chronic pain among community-dwelling older adults exceeds 50%, and among older nursing home patients it is approximately 80%. The most common painful conditions among older adults are musculoskeletal conditions such as osteoarthritis and low back pain. Chronic pain often results in depression, sleep disturbance, decreased mobility, increased health care utilization, and physical and social role dysfunction. Despite its high prevalence, pain in older adults is often inadequately assessed and treated.[41]

Several barriers to pain assessment in the older patient exist. Older adults and their health care providers often believe that pain is a normal, inevitable part of aging and that nothing can be done to relieve the pain. Older adults may not report pain for fear of being a "burden" or a "complainer." They may have greater fears of taking opioids than other age-groups. In addition, older patients are more likely to use words such as "aching," "soreness," or "discomfort" rather than "pain." For all these reasons, be persistent in asking older adults about pain. Carry out the assessment in an unhurried, supportive manner.

Another barrier to pain assessment in older adults is the increased prevalence of cognitive, sensory-perceptual, and motor problems that interfere with a person's ability to process information and to communicate. Examples include dementia and delirium, poststroke aphasia, and other communication barriers. Hearing and vision deficits may complicate assessment. Therefore pain assessment tools may need to be adapted for older adults. For example, it may be necessary to use a large-print pain intensity scale. Most older adults, even those with mild to moderate cognitive impairment, can use quantitative scales accurately and reliably.

In older patients with chronic pain, perform a thorough physical examination and history to identify causes of pain, possible therapies, and potential problems. Because depression and functional impairments are common among older adults with pain, they also must be assessed.

Treatment of pain in older adults is complicated by several factors. First, older adults metabolize drugs more slowly than younger people and thus are at greater risk for higher blood levels and adverse effects. The adage "start low and go slow" needs to be applied to analgesic therapy in this age-group. Second, the use of NSAIDs in older adults is associated with a high frequency of GI bleeding. Third, older adults often are taking many drugs for one or more chronic conditions. The addition of analgesics can result in dangerous drug interactions and increased side effects. Fourth, cognitive impairment and ataxia can be exacerbated by analgesics such as opioids, antidepressants, and antiseizure drugs. This requires that health care providers titrate drugs slowly and monitor carefully for side effects.

Treatment regimens for older adults must incorporate nondrug modalities. Exercise and patient teaching are important nondrug interventions for older adults with chronic pain. Also include family and caregivers in the treatment plan (see Table 9-17).

MANAGING PAIN IN SPECIAL POPULATIONS

Patients Unable to Self-Report Pain

Although patient self-report is the gold standard of pain assessment, many illnesses and conditions affect a patient's ability to report pain. These diagnoses and conditions include advanced dementia and other progressive neurologic diseases such as Parkinson's disease and multiple sclerosis, cerebrovascular disease, psychosis, and delirium. For these people, behavioral and physiologic changes may be the only indicators of pain. You must be astute at recognizing behavioral symptoms of pain.

A guide for assessing pain in nonverbal patients is presented in Table 9-18. Several scales have been developed to assess pain-related behaviors in nonverbal patients, particularly those with advanced dementia.[42,43] Several pain assessment tools for people with dementia are available at the City of Hope Pain and Palliative Care Resource Center website *(http://prc.coh.org)*.

TABLE 9-18 ASSESSING PAIN IN NONVERBAL PATIENTS

The following assessment techniques are recommended.

- Obtain a self-report when possible (never assume a person is unable to give verbal report).
- Investigate potential causes of pain.
- Observe patient behaviors that indicate pain (e.g., grimacing, frowning, rubbing a painful area, groaning, restlessness).
- Obtain surrogate reports of pain from professional and family caregivers.
- Try to use analgesics and reassess the patient to observe for a decrease in pain-related behaviors.

Source: Position statement from the American Society for Pain Management Nursing (ASPMN). Modified from Herr K, Coyne PJ, Key T, et al: Pain assessment in the nonverbal patient: position statement with clinical practice recommendations, *Pain Manag Nurs* 7:44, 2006.

Patients With Substance Abuse Problems

Health care providers are often reluctant to administer opioids to substance-abusing patients for fear of promoting or enhancing addictions. However, there is no evidence that providing opioid analgesia to these patients in any way worsens their addictive disease. In fact, the stress of unrelieved pain may contribute to relapse in the recovering patient or increased drug use in the patient who is actively abusing drugs.[44]

Guidelines for pain management in patients with addictive disease have been established by the American Society for Pain Management Nursing.[45] These guidelines reflect your role in a team approach in which patients with addictive disease and pain have the right to be treated with dignity, respect, and the same quality of pain assessment and management as all other patients.

If the patient acknowledges opioid use, it is important to determine the types and amounts of drugs used. It is best to avoid exposing the patient to the drug of abuse, and effective equianalgesic doses of other opioids may be determined if daily drug doses are known. If a history of drug abuse is unknown or if the patient does not acknowledge substance abuse, you should suspect abuse when normal doses of analgesics do not relieve the patient's pain.

Aggressive behavior patterns and signs of withdrawal may also occur. Withdrawal symptoms can exacerbate pain and lead to drug-seeking behavior or illicit drug use. Toxicology screens may be helpful in determining recently used drugs. Discussing these findings with the patient may help gain the patient's cooperation in pain control.

Severe pain should be treated with opioids, and at much higher doses than those used with drug-naive patients. The use of a single opioid is preferred. Avoid using a mixed opioid agonist-antagonist such as butorphanol or a partial agonist such as buprenorphine because these drugs may precipitate withdrawal symptoms. Nonopioid and adjuvant analgesics and nondrug pain relief measures may also be used as appropriate. To maintain opioid blood levels and prevent withdrawal symptoms, provide analgesics around the clock. Use supplemental doses to treat breakthrough pain. IV or PCA infusions may be considered for acute pain management.[38]

Pain management for people with addiction is challenging and requires an interdisciplinary team approach. When possible, the team includes pain management and addiction specialists. Team members need to be aware of their own attitudes about people with substance abuse problems, which may result in undertreatment of pain.

CASE STUDY

Pain

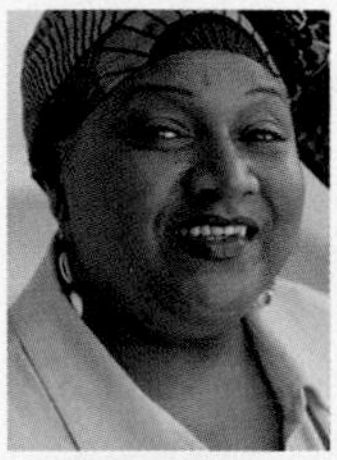

Ryan McVay/Photodisc/ Thinkstock

Patient Profile

K.C. is a 280-lb (127-kg) 68-year-old African American woman with diabetes who was admitted for an incision and drainage of a right abdominal abscess. She is being discharged on her second postoperative day. Her married daughter will assist with dressing changes at home.

Subjective Data

- Lives alone
- Desires 0 pain but will accept 1 or 2 on a scale of 0 to 10
- Reports incision area pain as a 2 or 3 between dressing changes and as a 6 during dressing changes
- States sharp pain persists 1 to 2 hours after dressing change
- Reports pain between dressing changes controlled by two Percocet tablets
- Has history of fibromyalgia and is complaining of pain "everywhere"

Objective Data

- Requires qid dressing changes after discharge
- For discharge, Percocet (two tablets q4hr for pain PRN) is prescribed

Discussion Questions

1. Describe the assessment data that are important for determining whether K.C. has adequate pain management.
2. How long should the daughter wait after the Percocet is given to begin the dressing change?
3. What additional pain therapies might you plan to help K.C. through the dressing change?
4. ***Priority Decision:*** What are the priority nursing interventions for K.C.?
5. What side effects might she experience because of her pain medication? How can these be managed?
6. ***Delegation Decision:*** To whom can you delegate teaching K.C. and her daughter the plan of care at home?
7. ***Priority Decision:*** Based on the data presented, what are the priority nursing diagnoses? Are there any collaborative problems?
8. ***Evidence-Based Practice:*** K.C.'s daughter asks you if any other strategies could be used to help decrease her mother's incisional pain and her overall fibromyalgia pain.

evolve Answers available at *http://evolve.elsevier.com/Lewis/medsurg.*

BRIDGE TO NCLEX EXAMINATION

The number of the question corresponds to the same-numbered outcome at the beginning of the chapter.

1. Pain is best described as
   a. a creation of a person's imagination.
   b. an unpleasant, subjective experience.
   c. a maladaptive response to a stimulus.
   d. a neurologic event resulting from activation of nociceptors.
2. A patient is receiving a PCA infusion after surgery to repair a hip fracture. She is sleeping soundly but awakens when the nurse speaks to her in a normal tone of voice. Her respirations are 8 breaths/minute. The most appropriate nursing action in this situation is to
   a. stop the PCA infusion.
   b. obtain an oxygen saturation level.
   c. continue to closely monitor the patient.
   d. administer naloxone and contact the physician.

3. Which words are most likely to be used to describe neuropathic pain *(select all that apply)?*
   a. Dull
   b. Mild
   c. Burning
   d. Shooting
   e. Shock-like
4. Unrelieved pain is
   a. expected after major surgery.
   b. expected in a person with cancer.
   c. dangerous and can lead to many physical and psychologic complications.
   d. an annoying sensation, but it is not as important as other physical care needs.
5. A cancer patient who reports ongoing, constant moderate pain with short periods of severe pain during dressing changes is
   a. probably exaggerating his pain.
   b. best treated by referral for surgical treatment of his pain.
   c. best treated by receiving both a long-acting and a short-acting opioid.
   d. best treated by regularly scheduled short-acting opioids plus acetaminophen.
6. An example of distraction to provide pain relief is
   a. TENS.
   b. music.
   c. exercise.
   d. biofeedback.
7. Appropriate nonopioid analgesics for mild pain include *(select all that apply)*
   a. oxycodone.
   b. ibuprofen (Advil).
   c. lorazepam (Ativan).
   d. acetaminophen (Tylenol).
   e. codeine with acetaminophen (Tylenol #3).
8. An important nursing responsibility related to pain is to
   a. leave the patient alone to rest.
   b. help the patient appear to not be in pain.
   c. believe what the patient says about the pain.
   d. assume responsibility for eliminating the patient's pain.
9. Providing opioids to a dying patient who is experiencing moderate to severe pain
   a. may cause addiction.
   b. will probably be ineffective.
   c. is an appropriate nursing action.
   d. will likely hasten the person's death.
10. A nurse believes that patients with the same type of tissue injury should have the same amount of pain. This statement reflects
    a. a belief that will contribute to appropriate pain management.
    b. an accurate statement about pain mechanisms and an expected goal of pain therapy.
    c. a belief that will have no effect on the type of care provided to people in pain.
    d. a lack of knowledge about pain mechanisms, which is likely to contribute to poor pain management.

1. b, 2. c, 3. c, d, e, 4. c, 5. c, 6. b, 7. b, d, 8. c, 9. c, 10. d.

evolve

For rationales to these answers and even more NCLEX review questions, visit *http://evolve.elsevier.com/Lewis/medsurg.*

REFERENCES

1. National Center of Health Statistics: *Health, United States, 2007, with chartbook on trends in the health of Americans*, Hyattsville, Md, 2007, US Government Printing Office.
2. Institute of Medicine Report from the Committee on Advancing Pain Research, Care, and Education: *Relieving pain in America: a blueprint for transforming prevention, care, education, and research*, Washington, DC, 2011, National Academies Press.
3. American Pain Foundation: Pain facts and figures. Retrieved from *www.painfoundation.org.*
4. Centers for Disease Control and Prevention, National Center for Health Statistics: *Health, United States, 2010, with chartbook on special feature on death and dying*, Hyattsville, Md, 2010, US Government Printing Office.
5. Christo PJ, Mazloomdoost D: Cancer pain and analgesia, *Ann NY Acad Sci* 1138:278, 2008.
6. McCaffery M: *Nursing practice theories related to cognition, bodily pain and man-environmental interactions*, Los Angeles, 1968, UCLA Students Store. (Classic)
7. Keefe FJ: Behavioral medicine: a voyage to the future, *Ann Behav Med* 41:141, 2011.

*8. Lucchetti G, Lucchetti AG, Badan-Neto AM, et al: Religiousness affects mental health, pain and quality of life in older people in an outpatient rehabilitation setting, *J Rehabil Med* 43:316, 2011.

*9. Riddle DL, Keefe FJ, Nay WT, et al: Pain coping skills training for patients with elevated pain catastrophizing who are scheduled for knee arthroplasty: a quasi-experimental study, *Arch Phys Med Rehabil* 92:859, 2011.

10. Tan AM, Waxman SG: Spinal cord injury, dendritic spine remodeling, and spinal memory mechanisms, *Exp Neurol* 235:142, 2012.
11. Cohen SP, Liao W, Gupta A, et al: Ketamine in pain management, *Adv Psychosom Med* 30:139, 2011.
12. Davis KD: Neuroimaging of pain: what does it tell us? *Curr Opin Support Palliat Care* 5:116, 2011.
13. Neziri AY, Haesler S, Petersen-Felix S, et al: Generalized expansion of nociceptive reflex receptive fields in chronic pain patients, *Pain* 151:798, 2010.
14. O'Connor AB, Dworkin RH: Treatment of neuropathic pain: an overview of recent guidelines, *Am J Med* 122:S22, 2009.
15. Herr K, Bjoro K, Decker S: Tools for assessment of pain in nonverbal older adults with dementia: a state-of-the-science review, *J Pain Symptom Manage* 31:170, 2006.

*16. McGuire DB, Reifsnyder J, Soeken K, et al: Assessing pain in nonresponsive hospice patients: development and preliminary testing of the multidimensional objective pain assessment tool (MOPAT), *J Palliat Med* 14:287, 2011.

*Evidence-based information for clinical practice.

*17. Gordon DB, Dahl J, Phillips P, et al: The use of "as-needed" range orders for opioid analgesic in the management of acute pain: a consensus statement of the American Society of Pain Management Nurses and the American Pain Society, *Pain Manag Nurs* 5:53, 2004. (Classic)
18. Kolcaba K: Evolution of the mid range theory of comfort for outcomes research, *Nurs Outlook* 49:86, 2001. (Classic)
19. Fouladbakhsh JM, Szczesny S, Jenuwine ES, et al: Nondrug therapies for pain management among rural older adults, *Pain Manag Nurs* 12:70, 2011.
20. Jarzyna D, Jungquist CR, Pasero C, et al: American Society for Pain Management Nursing guidelines on monitoring for opioid-induced sedation and respiratory depression, *Pain Manag Nurs* 12:118, 2011.
21. Sinatra RS, Jahr JS, Reynolds L, et al: Intravenous acetaminophen for pain after major orthopedic surgery: an expanded analysis, *Pain Pract* 12:357, 2011.
22. Lanza FL, Chan FK, Quigley EM: Guidelines for prevention of NSAID-related ulcer complications, *Am J Gastroenterol* 104:728, 2009.
23. Roth SH, Anderson S: The NSAID dilemma: managing osteoarthritis in high-risk patients, *Phys Sportsmed* 39:62, 2011.
24. Vadivelu N, Timchenko A, Huang Y, et al: Tapentadol extended-release for treatment of chronic pain: a review, *J Pain Res* 4:211, 2011.
25. Micromedex® Healthcare Series [Internet database]. Greenwood Village, Colo: Thomson Reuters (Healthcare) Inc. Updated periodically.
26. Abrams DI, Couey P, Shade SB, et al: Cannabinoid-opioid interaction in chronic pain, *Clin Pharmacol Ther* 90:844, 2011.
27. GW Pharmaceuticals: Sativex. Retrieved from *www.gwpharm.com/Sativex.aspx.*
28. Shaheen PE, Walsh D, Lasheen W, et al: Opioid equianalgesic tables: are they all equally dangerous? *J Pain Symptom Manage* 38:409, 2009.
29. Falowski S, Celii A, Sharan A: Spinal cord stimulation: an update, *Neurotherapeutics* 5:86, 2008.
*30. Reid MC, Papaleontiou M, Ong A, et al: Self-management strategies to reduce pain and improve function among older adults in community settings: a review of the evidence, *Pain Med* 9:409, 2008.
*31. Cherkin DC, Sherman KJ, Kahn J, et al: A comparison of the effects of two types of massage and usual care on chronic low back pain: a randomized, controlled trial, *Ann Intern Med* 155:1, 2011.
*32. Marinko LN, Chacko JM, Dalton D, et al: The effectiveness of therapeutic exercise for painful shoulder conditions: a meta analysis, *J Shoulder Elbow Surg* 20:1351, 2011.
*33. Wanich T, Gelber J, Rodeo S, et al: Percutaneous neuromodulation pain therapy following knee replacement, *J Knee Surg* 24:197, 2011.
*34. Bernardy K, Fuber N, Klose P, et al: Efficacy of hypnosis/guided imagery in fibromyalgia syndrome—a systematic review and meta-analysis of controlled trials, *BMC Musculoskelet Disord* 12:133, 2011.
35. Tracy MF, Chlan L: Nonpharmacological interventions to manage common symptoms in patients receiving mechanical ventilation, *Crit Care Nurse* 31:19, 2011.
36. Bell K, Salmon A: Pain, physical dependence and pseudoaddiction: redefining addiction for 'nice' people? *Int J Drug Policy* 20:170, 2009.
37. The Joint Commission: Standard on pain assessment and management. Retrieved from *www.jointcommission.org.*
38. Beauchamp T, Childress J: *Principles of biomedical ethics*, New York, 2009, Oxford University Press.
39. Oregon Nurses Association: ONA provides guidance on nurses' dilemma. Retrieved from *www.oregonrn.org/associations/3019/files/AssistedSuicide.pdf.*
40. American Society for Pain Management Nursing: Position statement on the use of placebos in pain management. Retrieved from *www.aspmn.org/pdfs/Use%20of%20Placebos.pdf.*
*41. Ersek M, Polissar N, Neradilek MB: Development of a composite pain measure for people with advanced dementia: exploratory analyses in self-reporting nursing home residents, *J Pain Symptom Manage* 41:566, 2011.
*42. Jordon A, Regnard C, O'Brien JT, et al: Pain and distress in advanced dementia: choosing the right tools for the job, *Palliat Med* 26:873, 2012.
*43. Paulson-Conger M, Leske J, Maidl C, et al: Comparison of two pain assessment tools in nonverbal critical care patients, *Pain Manag Nurs* 12:218, 2011.
44. Ling W, Mooney L, Hillhouse M: Prescription opioid abuse, pain, and addiction: clinical issues and implications, *Drug Alcohol Rev* 30:300, 2011.
45. American Society for Pain Management Nursing: Pain management in patients with addictive disease. Retrieved from *www.aspmn.org/Organization/documents/addictions_9pt.pdf.*

RESOURCES

American Academy of Pain Management
www.aapainmanage.org
American Academy of Pain Medicine (AAPM)
www.painmed.org
American Chronic Pain Association
www.theacpa.org
American Pain Society
www.ampainsoc.org
American Society for Pain Management Nursing
www.aspmn.org
City of Hope Pain and Palliative Care Resource Center
http://prc.coh.org
International Association for the Study of Pain (IASP)
www.iasp-pain.org
Pain Link
www2.edc.org/painlink

CHAPTER

10

Palliative Care at End of Life

Margaret McLean Heitkemper

You matter because you are you. You matter to the last moment of your life, and we will do all we can, not only to help you die peacefully, but also to live until you die.
Dame Cicely Saunders

evolve WEBSITE

http://evolve.elsevier.com/Lewis/medsurg

- NCLEX Review Questions
- Key Points
- Pre-Test
- Rationales for Bridge to NCLEX Examination Questions
- Case Study
  - Patient With Chronic Myelogenous Leukemia Including End-of-life Care
- Concept Map Creator
- Glossary
- Content Updates

LEARNING OUTCOMES

1. Discuss the purpose of palliative care.
2. Describe the purpose of and services provided by hospice.
3. Describe the physical and psychologic manifestations at the end of life.
4. Explain the process of grief and bereavement at the end of life.
5. Describe the nursing management for the dying patient.
6. Examine the cultural and spiritual issues related to end-of-life care.
7. Discuss ethical and legal issues in end-of-life care.
8. Explore the special needs of family caregivers in end-of-life care.
9. Discuss the special needs of the nurse who cares for dying patients and their families.

KEY TERMS

advance directives, p. 146
bereavement, p. 143
brain death, p. 142
Cheyne-Stokes respiration, p. 142
death, p. 142
death rattle, p. 142
end of life, p. 142
grief, p. 143
hospice, p. 141
palliative care, p. 140
spirituality, p. 144

PALLIATIVE CARE

Palliative care is any form of care or treatment that focuses on reducing the severity of disease symptoms, rather than trying to delay or reverse the progression of the disease itself or provide a cure. The overall goals of palliative care are to (1) prevent and relieve suffering and (2) improve quality of life for patients with serious, life-limiting illnesses (Fig. 10-1). Specific goals of palliative care are listed in Table 10-1.

Palliative care originated as end-of-life (EOL) care in the 1960s. Initially this care focused on providing the relief of symptoms and emotional support to the patient, family, and significant others during the terminal phase of a serious life-limiting disease. Now that phase of palliative care is called palliative care at end-of-life, which is the focus of this chapter. Since its beginning, the scope of palliative care has greatly expanded. Now palliative care focuses on maintaining and improving the quality of life for all patients and their families during any stage of a life-limiting illness, whether acute, chronic, or terminal.

According to the World Health Organization (WHO), palliative care is an approach that improves the quality of life of patients and their families who face problems associated with life-threatening illness. Palliative care aims to prevent and relieve suffering by early identification, assessment, and treatment of pain and other types of physical, psychologic, emotional, and spiritual distress.[1] Ideally, all patients receiving curative or restorative health care should receive palliative care concurrently. Palliative care extends into the period of EOL care; bereavement care follows the patient's death[2] (Fig. 10-2).

To optimize the benefits of palliative care, it should be initiated after a person receives a diagnosis of a life-limiting

TABLE 10-1 GOALS OF PALLIATIVE CARE

- Provide relief from symptoms, including pain.
- Regard dying as a normal process.
- Affirm life and neither hasten nor postpone death.
- Support holistic patient care and enhance quality of life.
- Offer support to patients to live as actively as possible until death.
- Offer support to the family during the patient's illness and in their own bereavement.

Adapted from World Health Organization: WHO definition of palliative care. Retrieved from *www.who.int/cancer/palliative/definition/en.*

Reviewed by Lynn F. Reinke, PhD, ARNP, Research Investigator/Pulmonary Nurse Practitioner, VA Puget Sound Health Care System, Health Services R&D, Seattle, Washington; and Arlene H. Morris, RN, EdD, CNE, Distinguished Teaching Associate Professor of Nursing, Auburn University Montgomery, Montgomery, Alabama.

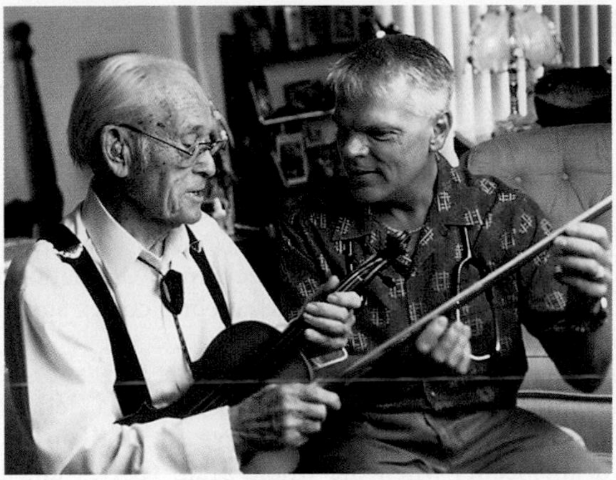

FIG. 10-1 One goal of palliative care is to improve the quality of the patient's remaining life.

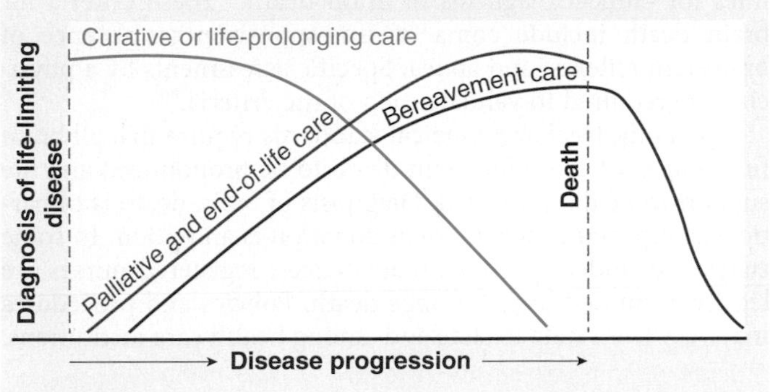

FIG. 10-2 Integrated model of curative care, palliative and end-of-life care, and bereavement care.

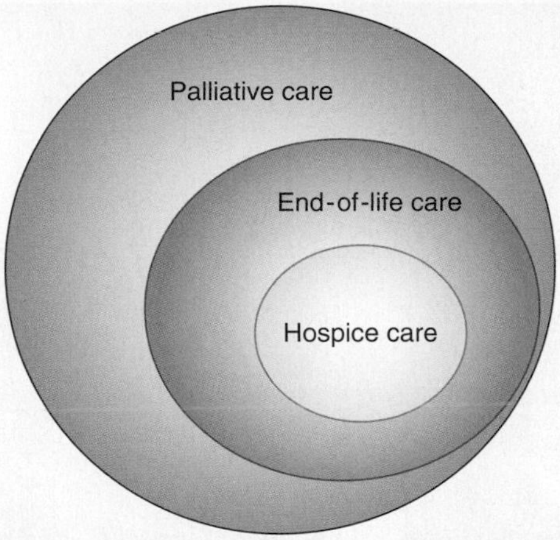

FIG. 10-3 Relationship of palliative care, end-of-life care, and hospice care.

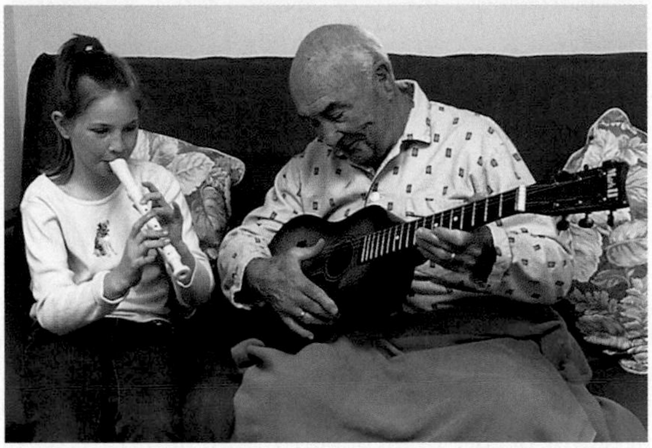

FIG. 10-4 Hospice care is designed to provide compassion, concern, and support for the dying.

illness, such as cancer, heart failure, chronic obstructive pulmonary disease, dementia, or end-stage kidney disease. Ideally, the palliative care team is an interdisciplinary collaboration involving physicians, social workers, pharmacists, nurses, chaplains, and other health care professionals. Communication among the patient, family, and palliative health care team is important to provide optimal care. Patients receive palliative care services in the home and in long-term and acute care facilities. More recently, emergency departments and intensive care units (ICUs) have integrated palliative care into the delivery of care. Many institutions have established interdisciplinary palliative and hospice care teams.[3]

HOSPICE CARE

Palliative care often includes hospice care before or at the end of life (Fig. 10-3). **Hospice** is not a place but a concept of care that provides compassion, concern, and support for the dying (Fig. 10-4). Hospice exists to provide support and care for persons in the last phases of a terminal disease so that they might live as fully and as comfortable as possible. Hospice programs provide care with an emphasis on symptom management, advance care planning, spiritual care, and family support.[4]

The major difference between palliative care and hospice care is that palliative care allows a person to simultaneously receive curative and palliative treatments. Hospice care is provided once a person decides to forgo curative treatments.

Approximately 1.5 million patients every year receive services through hospice programs. About 42% of the patients who die in the United States are under the care of a hospice program.[5] More than a third of all hospice patients are 85 years of age or older, and 83% are over 65. Of these patients, the most common diagnosis is cancer. Eighty percent of patients using hospice services are white.[5] Currently the median length of stay in a hospice program is 21 days.

Hospice programs are organized under a variety of models. Some are hospital-based programs, others are part of existing home health care agencies, and others are freestanding or community-based programs. However, regardless of their organization, all hospices emphasize palliative rather than curative care, and quality rather than quantity of life.

Hospice care is provided in a variety of locations, including the home, inpatient settings, and long-term care facilities. Hospice care can be on a part-time, intermittent, on-call, regularly scheduled, or continuous basis. Hospice services are available 24 hours a day, 7 days a week to provide help to patients and families in their homes. The inpatient hospice settings have been deinstitutionalized to make the atmosphere as relaxed and homelike as possible (Fig. 10-5). Staff and volunteers are available for the patient and the family.

A medically supervised interdisciplinary team of professionals and volunteers provides holistic hospice services. The hospice nurse plays a pivotal role in coordination of the hospice team.[6] Hospice nurses work collaboratively with hospice physicians, pharmacists, dietitians, physical therapists, social workers, cer-

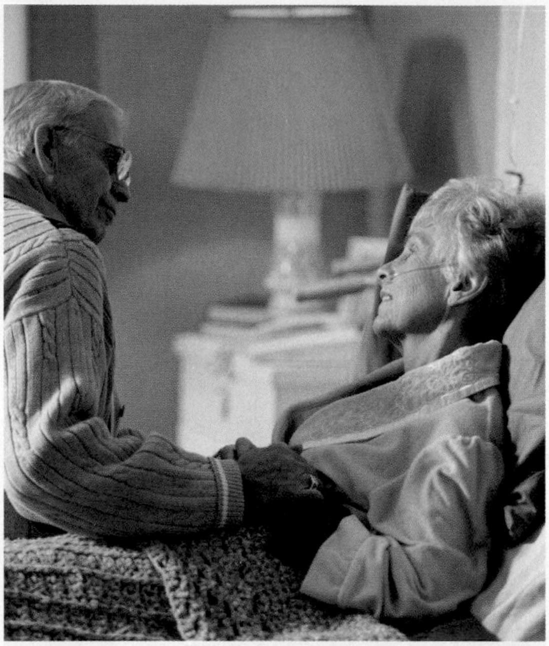

FIG. 10-5 Inpatient hospice settings have been deinstitutionalized to make the atmosphere as relaxed and homelike as possible. (Photodisc/Thinkstock)

tified nursing assistants, chaplains and other clergy, and volunteers to provide care and support to the patient and the family. Hospice nurses are educated in pain control and symptom management, spiritual assessment, and assessment and management of family needs. To meet patient and family needs, hospice nurses need excellent teaching skills, compassion, flexibility, cultural competence, and adaptability.

The decision to begin hospice care is difficult for several reasons. Frequently patients, families, physicians, and other health care providers lack information about hospice care. Some cultural/ethnic groups may underutilize hospice because of lack of awareness of hospice services, desire to continue with potentially curative therapies, and concerns about lack of minority hospice workers.[7] Physicians may be reluctant to give referrals because they sometimes view a patient's decline as their personal failure. Some patients or family members see it as giving up.

Admission to a hospice program has two criteria. The first criterion is that the patient must desire the services and agree in writing that only hospice care (and not curative care) can be used to treat the terminal illness. Patients in hospice programs can withdraw from the program at any time (e.g., if their condition unexpectedly improves). Patients can receive care for other health problems that begin after starting hospice.

The second criterion is that the patient must be considered eligible for hospice. Medicare, Medicaid, and other insurers require that two physicians certify that the patient's prognosis is terminal, with less than 6 months to live. It is important to realize that the physician who certified that a hospice patient is terminal does not "guarantee" death within 6 months. Indeed, if a patient in hospice survives beyond 6 months, Medicare and other reimbursement organizations will continue to reimburse for more extended periods of treatment if the patient still meets enrollment criteria. After this initial certification, only one physician (e.g., the hospice medical director) is needed to recertify the patient.

DEATH

Death occurs when all vital organs and body systems cease to function. It is the irreversible cessation of cardiovascular, respiratory, and brain function.

Brain death is an irreversible loss of all brain functions, including those of the brainstem. Brain death is a clinical diagnosis, and it can be made in patients whose hearts continue to beat and who are maintained on mechanical ventilation in the ICU.[8] Brain death occurs when the cerebral cortex stops functioning or is irreversibly destroyed.

Since the development of technology that assists in supporting life, controversies have arisen over the exact definition of death. Questions and discussions have focused on whether brain death occurs when the whole brain (cortex and brainstem) ceases activity or when function of the cortex alone stops. In 1995 the Quality Standards Subcommittee of the American Academy of Neurology recommended diagnostic criteria guidelines for clinical diagnosis of brain death.[9] These criteria for brain death include coma or unresponsiveness, absence of brainstem reflexes, and apnea. Specific assessments by a physician are required to validate each of the criteria.[8,9]

Currently, legal and medical standards require that all brain function must cease for brain death to be pronounced and life support to be disconnected. Diagnosis of brain death is of particular importance when organ donation is an option. In some states and under specific circumstances, registered nurses are legally permitted to pronounce death. Policies and procedures may vary from state to state and among health care institutions.

END-OF-LIFE CARE

End of life generally refers to the final phase of a patient's illness when death is imminent. The time from diagnosis of a terminal illness to death varies considerably, depending on the patient's diagnosis and extent of disease.

The Institute of Medicine defines *end of life* as the period during which an individual copes with declining health from a terminal illness or from the frailties associated with advanced age, even if death is not clearly imminent.[10] In some cases it is obvious to health care providers that the patient is at the end of life, but in other cases they may be uncertain if the end is close at hand. This uncertainty adds to the challenge of answering common questions the patient and family may ask, such as "How much time is left?"

End-of-life care (EOL care) is the term used for issues and services related to death and dying. EOL care focuses on physical and psychosocial needs for the patient and the patient's family. The goals for EOL care are to (1) provide comfort and supportive care during the dying process, (2) improve the quality of the patient's remaining life, (3) help ensure a dignified death, and (4) provide emotional support to the family.

Physical Manifestations at End of Life

As death approaches, metabolism is reduced and the body gradually slows down until all functions end. Respiratory changes are common at the end of life. Respirations may be rapid or slow, shallow, and irregular. Breath sounds may become wet and noisy, both audibly and on auscultation. Noisy, wet-sounding respirations, termed the **death rattle,** are caused by mouth breathing and accumulation of mucus in the airways. **Cheyne-Stokes respiration** is a pattern of breathing characterized by

TABLE 10-2 PHYSICAL MANIFESTATIONS AT END OF LIFE

System	Manifestations
Sensory system	
Hearing	• Usually last sense to disappear
Touch	• Decreased sensation • Decreased perception of pain and touch
Taste and smell	• Decreased with disease progression
Sight	• Blurring of vision • Sinking and glazing of eyes • Blink reflex absent • Eyelids remain half-open
Cardiovascular system	• Increased heart rate; later slowing and weakening of pulse • Irregular rhythm • Decreased blood pressure • Delayed absorption of drugs administered intramuscularly or subcutaneously
Respiratory system	• Increased respiratory rate • Cheyne-Stokes respiration (pattern of respiration characterized by alternating periods of apnea and deep, rapid breathing) • Inability to cough or clear secretions resulting in grunting, gurgling, or noisy congested breathing (death rattle) • Irregular breathing, gradually slowing down to terminal gasps (may be described as guppy breathing)
Urinary system	• Gradual decrease in urine output • Incontinence of urine • Inability to urinate
Gastrointestinal system	• Slowing or cessation of GI function (may be enhanced by pain-relieving drugs) • Accumulation of gas • Distention and nausea • Loss of sphincter control, producing incontinence • Bowel movement before imminent death or at time of death
Musculoskeletal system	• Gradual loss of ability to move • Sagging of jaw resulting from loss of facial muscle tone • Difficulty speaking • Swallowing becoming more difficult • Difficulty maintaining body posture and alignment • Loss of gag reflex • Jerking seen in patients on large amounts of opioids
Integumentary system	• Mottling on hands, feet, arms, and legs • Cold, clammy skin • Cyanosis of nose, nail beds, knees • "Waxlike" skin when very near death

alternating periods of apnea and deep, rapid breathing. When respirations cease, the heart stops beating within a few minutes. The physical manifestations of approaching death are listed in Table 10-2.

Psychosocial Manifestations at End of Life

A variety of feelings and emotions can affect the dying patient and family at the end of life (Table 10-3). Most patients and families struggle with a terminal diagnosis and the realization that there is no cure. The patient and the family may feel overwhelmed, fearful, powerless, and fatigued. The family's response depends in part on the type and length of the illness and their relationship with the person.

TABLE 10-3 PSYCHOSOCIAL MANIFESTATIONS AT END OF LIFE

• Altered decision making	• Life review
• Anxiety about unfinished business	• Peacefulness
• Decreased socialization	• Restlessness
• Fear of loneliness	• Saying goodbyes
• Fear of meaninglessness of one's life	• Unusual communication
• Fear of pain	• Vision-like experiences
• Helplessness	• Withdrawal

TABLE 10-4 KÜBLER-ROSS MODEL OF GRIEF

Stage	What Person May Say	Characteristics
Denial	No, not me. It cannot be true.	Denies the loss has taken place and may withdraw. This response may last minutes to months.
Anger	Why me?	May be angry at the person who inflicted the hurt (even after death) or at the world for letting it happen. May be angry with self for letting an event (e.g., car accident) take place, even if nothing could have stopped it.
Bargaining	Yes me, but…	May make bargains with God, asking "If I do this, will you take away the loss?"
Depression	Yes me, and I am sad	Feels numb, although anger and sadness may remain underneath.
Acceptance	Yes me, but it is okay	Anger, sadness, and mourning have tapered off. Accepts the reality of the loss.

Adapted from Kübler-Ross E: *On death and dying,* New York, 1969, Macmillan. (Classic)

The patient's needs and wishes must be respected. Patients need time to think and express their feelings. Response time to questions may be sluggish because of fatigue, weakness, and confusion.

Bereavement and Grief

Although the terms are often used interchangeably, *bereavement* refers to the state of loss, and *grief* refers to the reaction to loss. **Bereavement** is the period following the death of a loved one during which grief is experienced and mourning occurs. The time spent in bereavement depends on a number of factors, including how attached one was to the person who died and how much time was spent anticipating the loss.

Grief is a normal reaction to loss. Grief occurs in response to the real loss of a loved one and the loss of what might have been. Grief is dynamic and includes both psychologic and physiologic responses following a loss. Psychologic responses include anger, guilt, anxiety, sadness, depression, and despair. Physiologic reactions include sleeping problems, changes in appetite, physical problems, and illness.

Grief is a powerful emotional state that affects all aspects of a person's life. It is a complex and intense emotional experience. In the Kübler-Ross model of grief, there are five stages[11,12] (Table 10-4). Not every person experiences all the stages of grieving, and they are not always progressive in order. It is common to reach a stage and then go backward. For example, a person may have reached the stage of bargaining, and then revert back to the denial or anger stage.

Another model of grief is the grief wheel (Fig. 10-6). After a person experiences the loss, he or she feels *shock* (numbness, denial, inability to think straight). Then comes the *protest* stage where a person experiences anger, guilt, sadness, fear, and searching. Then comes the *disorganization* stage where a person feels despair, apathy, anxiety, and confusion. The next stage is *reorganization* where a person gradually returns to normal functioning, but he or she feels different. The final stage is the *new normal.* Eventually the destabilization experienced in grief resolves and a normal state can began. However, because of the loss, the normal state is not the same as before. The challenge is to accept the new normal. Trying to go back to the "old" normal (which is not there anymore) is what causes a great deal of anxiety and stress.

The manner in which a person grieves depends on factors such as the relationship with the person who has died (e.g., spouse, parent), physical and emotional coping resources, concurrent life stresses, cultural beliefs, and personality. Additional factors that affect the grief response include mental and physical health, economic resources, religious influences or spiritual beliefs, family relationships, social support, and time spent preparing for the death. Issues that occurred before the death (e.g., marital problems) may affect the grief response.[13]

The grief experience for the caregiver of the patient with a chronic illness often begins long before the actual death event. This is called *anticipatory grief.* Patients at the end of life can also experience anticipatory grief.

Working in a positive way through the grief process helps to adapt to the loss.[14] Grief that assists the person in accepting the reality of death is called *adaptive grief,* which is a healthy response. It may be associated with grieving before a death actually occurs or when the inevitability of the death is known. Indicators of adaptive grief include the ability to see some good resulting from the death and positive memories of the deceased person.

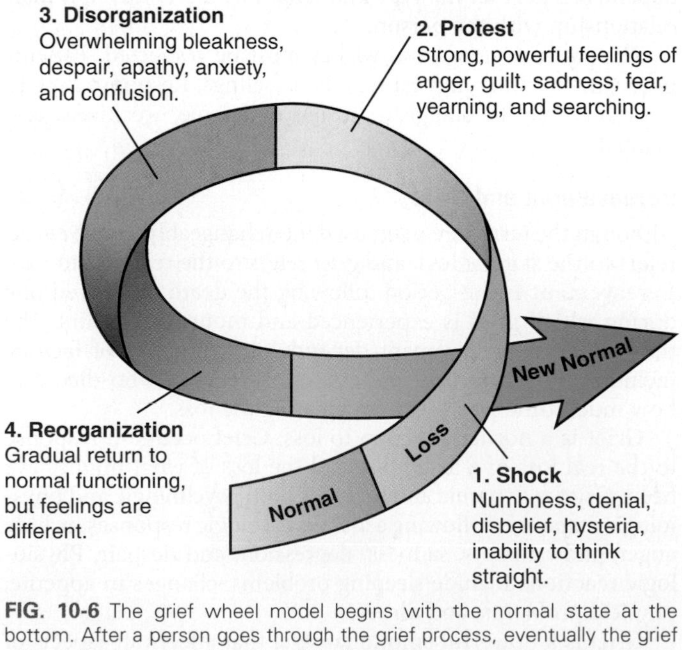
3. Disorganization
Overwhelming bleakness, despair, apathy, anxiety, and confusion.
2. Protest
Strong, powerful feelings of anger, guilt, sadness, fear, yearning, and searching.
New Normal
Loss
Normal
4. Reorganization
Gradual return to normal functioning, but feelings are different.
1. Shock
Numbness, denial, disbelief, hysteria, inability to think straight.

FIG. 10-6 The grief wheel model begins with the normal state at the bottom. After a person goes through the grief process, eventually the grief will resolve. However, because of the loss, the normal state is not the same as before. The challenge is to accept the "new normal." (Adapted from Powell TJ: *Stress-free living,* Dorling Kindersley Ltd 2000. © Dorling Kindersley Ltd.)

Dysfunctional reactions to loss can occur, and the physical and psychologic impact of the loved one's death may persist for years. *Prolonged grief disorder,* formerly called *complicated grief,* is a term used to describe prolonged and intense mourning. Prolonged grief disorder can include symptoms such as recurrent and severe distressing emotions and intrusive thoughts related to the loss of a loved one, self-neglect, and denial of the loss for longer than 6 months. Bereaved individuals with prolonged grief disorder may feel "stuck" and unable to move forward after the death of a loved one. It is estimated that one in five bereaved individuals experiences prolonged grief disorder. Those who experience prolonged grief disorder are at great risk for illness and have work and social impairments. Some studies suggest that prolonged grief disorder is less likely to occur after deaths in hospice compared with those in acute care settings.[15]

Bereavement and grief counseling is an important aspect of palliative care. The goal of a bereavement program is to provide support and to assist survivors in the transition to a life without the deceased person. Incorporate grief support into the plan of care for the family and significant others during the patient's illness and after the death.

Priority interventions for grief must focus on providing an environment that allows the patient and the family to express their feelings such as anger, fear, and guilt. Discussion of feelings helps both the patient and the family work toward resolution of the grief process. Respect for the patient's privacy and need or desire to talk (or not to talk) is important. Honesty in answering questions and giving information is essential.

Spiritual Needs

Assessment of spiritual needs in EOL care is a key consideration (Table 10-5). Spiritual needs do not necessarily equate to religion. **Spirituality** is defined as those beliefs, values, and practices that relate to the search for existential meaning and purpose and that may or may not include a belief in a higher power.[16] A person may not be part of a particular religion but have a deep spirituality. Many times at the end of life, patients question their beliefs about a higher power, their journey through life, religion, and an afterlife (Fig. 10-7). Some patients may choose to pursue

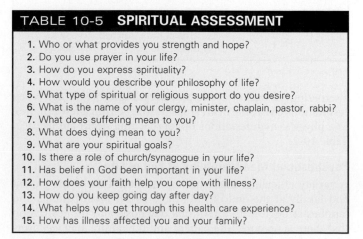

TABLE 10-5 SPIRITUAL ASSESSMENT

1. Who or what provides you strength and hope?
2. Do you use prayer in your life?
3. How do you express spirituality?
4. How would you describe your philosophy of life?
5. What type of spiritual or religious support do you desire?
6. What is the name of your clergy, minister, chaplain, pastor, rabbi?
7. What does suffering mean to you?
8. What does dying mean to you?
9. What are your spiritual goals?
10. Is there a role of church/synagogue in your life?
11. Has belief in God been important in your life?
12. How does your faith help you cope with illness?
13. How do you keep going day after day?
14. What helps you get through this health care experience?
15. How has illness affected you and your family?

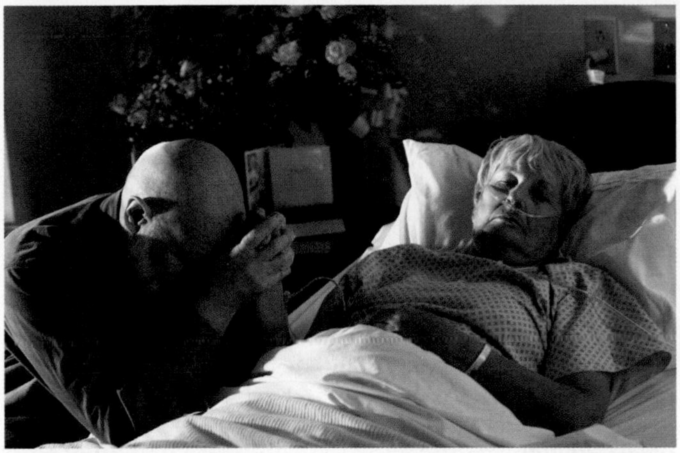

FIG. 10-7 Spiritual needs are an important consideration in end-of-life care. (Photodisc/Thinkstock)

a spiritual path. Some may not. Respect an individual's choice. Assess the patient's and the family's preferences related to spiritual guidance or pastoral care services and make appropriate referrals.[16]

Deep-seated spiritual beliefs may surface for some patients when they deal with their terminal diagnosis and related issues. Spiritual distress may occur.[17] Characteristics of spiritual distress include anger toward God or a higher being, change in behavior and mood, desire for spiritual assistance, or displaced anger toward clergy.[16]

Spirituality has been associated with decreased despair in patients at the end of life. Some dying patients are secure in their faith about the future. It is common to observe patients relinquishing material possessions of life and focusing on values that they believe will lead them on to another place. Many turn to religion because it may provide order to the world even in the presence of physical decline, social losses, suffering, and impending death. Religion may offer an existential meaning that offers a sense of peace and recognition of one's place in the broader cosmic context.[17]

> *The loss of a loved person is one of the most intensely painful experiences any human being can suffer.*
> *John Bowlby*

CULTURALLY COMPETENT CARE

END OF LIFE

Culture and ethnicity should be considered throughout the EOL process. Cultural beliefs affect a person's understanding of and reaction to death or loss. In some cultural/ethnic groups, death and dying are private matters shared only with significant others. Often feelings are repressed or internalized. People who believe in "toughing it out" or "being strong" may not express themselves when they are experiencing a loss. Some cultural groups, such as African Americans and Hispanic/Latinos, may easily express their feelings and emotions. Kinship tends to be strong in the Hispanic culture, and both immediate and extended family provide support for one another. Expressing feelings of loss is encouraged and accepted easily.[18,19]

If palliative or hospice care is recommended, some cultural/ethnic groups are less likely to use these resources. For example, African Americans use hospice care less often because they value "toughness" in times of hardship and rely on God.[18] For Hispanics, often spouses and daughters need to be involved in decisions regarding palliative care and hospice.[20]Consider patient attitudes toward death and suffering and preferences for information. The decision to use palliative care or hospice services may be perceived as "giving up" or receiving second-rate care. Such attitudes are best approached through clear, open discussions with the patient and the family about the philosophy and services of palliative and hospice organizations.[18-21] Culture and ethnicity affect decision making with regard to life support and withholding and withdrawing of treatments.[22] In some cultures, such as the Filipino American culture, it may be appropriate to first discuss a terminal diagnosis with the family before informing the patient.

Rituals associated with dying are part of all cultures.[18] In certain cultures the family may want to keep constant vigil in the room of a dying patient or in the waiting area. For example, some Jewish Americans believe that the spirit should not be alone when it leaves the body at the time of death. Therefore someone who is terminally ill should never be left alone. The Jewish culture believes all body tissues must be buried with the individual. Once a death has occurred, some cultures, such as the Puerto Rican American culture, may want to kiss and touch the body to say goodbye.

Families with non–English-speaking members are at risk for receiving less information about their family member's critical illness and prognosis.[23] Cultural variations also exist in symptom expression (e.g., pain expression) and use of health care services. Providing culturally competent care requires assessment of nonverbal cues such as grimaces, body position, and decreased or guarded movements. Issues related to pain assessment and management are discussed in Chapter 9.

Differences among cultural beliefs and values in relation to death and dying are innumerable. Nursing assessment of beliefs and preferences should be made on an individual basis to avoid stereotyping individuals with different cultural belief systems. This includes assessing and documenting the patient's cultural background, concerns, health practices, and attitudes about suffering. Early in the assessment, ask the patient and family to describe their desires for care before death and care of the body after death. Use open-ended questions related to the patient's perspectives on his or her illness and the patient's expectations of care. Use this assessment to guide the patient's plan of care and evaluation. You can also suggest or plan grief and bereavement counseling for the family. At the same time, accommodations need to be made related to the patient's language, diet, and cultural beliefs and practices. When appropriate, access medical interpreter services so that the patient's wishes are known. (Culturally competent care is discussed in Chapter 2.)

LEGAL AND ETHICAL ISSUES AFFECTING END-OF-LIFE CARE

Patients and families struggle with many decisions during the terminal illness and dying experience. Many people decide that the outcomes related to their care should be based on their own wishes and values. It is important to provide information to assist patients with these decisions. The decisions may involve the choice for (1) organ and tissue donations, (2) advance directives (e.g., medical power of attorney, living wills), (3) resuscitation, (4) mechanical ventilation, and (5) feeding tube placement.

Organ and Tissue Donation

Persons who are legally competent may choose organ donation. Any body part or the entire body may be donated. The decision to donate organs or to provide anatomic gifts may be made by a person before death or by immediate family after death. Family permission must be obtained at the time of donation.[24]

Some people carry donor cards. Some states allow organ donation to be marked on drivers' licenses. The names of agencies that handle organ donation vary by state and community. Common names for such an agency might be the organ bank, organ-sharing network, and organ-sharing alliance. Both organ and tissue donations follow specific legal guidelines. Legal requirements and facility policies for organ or tissue donation must be followed. The physician must be notified immediately when organ donation is intended because some tissues must be used within hours after death.

Advance Care Planning and Advance Directives

Advance care planning is a process that involves having patients (1) think through their values and goals for treatment, (2) talk about their values and goals with others, and (3) document them. **Advance directives** are the written documents that provide information about the patient's wishes and his or her designated spokesperson (Table 10-6).

The first advance directive was known by laypersons as a *living will.* Most states have replaced the idea of living wills with *natural death acts,* which may include *directives to physicians* (DTPs), *durable power of attorney for health care* (DPAHC), and *medical power of attorney* (MPOA). Under the natural death acts, an individual can tell the physician exactly what treatment is or is not desired. Each state has its own unique requirements. Keep in mind that patients often change their minds about desired treatments as their disease state progresses. Therefore it is important to reassess a patient's advance directives. For cognitively impaired older adults, consider the person's values and manner of life to make health care decisions consistent with decisions they made when they were cognitively intact.

Copies of state-specific forms can be obtained from local medical associations and on the Internet. However, a person may write his or her wishes without special forms. Verbal directives may be given to physicians with specific instructions in the presence of two witnesses. Attorneys and notaries may not be required. If the person is not capable of communicating his or her wishes, the surrogate decision maker (most often family or significant other) determines the measures that will or will not be taken. The physician and the nurse can discuss the options that are available with the family. Then it is important to document the family's decision.

Resuscitation

Cardiopulmonary resuscitation (CPR) has become common practice in health care. Patients who have respiratory or cardiac arrest are given CPR unless a *do-not-resuscitate (DNR) order* is given by the physician. A DNR order is a written medical order that documents a patient's wishes regarding resuscitation and, more important, the patient's desire to avoid CPR.[25]

The patient or the patient's family has the right to decide whether CPR will be used. It is no longer the sole decision of the physician. The American Nurses Association (ANA) supports the patient's right to self-determination and believes that nurses have a primary role in supporting the patient and family's decisions.[26]

A physician's order should be written concerning the patient's or family's wishes for the use of CPR. Several different types of CPR decisions can be made. Complete and total heroic measures, which may include CPR, drugs, and mechanical ventilation, can be referred to as a *full code.* Some people choose variations of the full code. A *chemical code* involves the

TABLE 10-6 COMMON DOCUMENTS USED IN END-OF-LIFE CARE

Document	Description	Special Considerations
Advance directive	General term used to describe documents that give instructions about future medical care and treatments and who should make the decisions in the event the person is unable to communicate.	• Should comply with guidelines established by state of residence.
Directive to physicians	Written document specifying the patient's wish to be allowed to die without heroic or extraordinary measures.	• Indicates specific measures to be used or withheld.
Do not resuscitate (DNR)	Written physician's order instructing health care providers not to attempt CPR. DNR order often requested by family. Must be signed by a physician to be valid.	• Must indicate any specific measures to be used or withheld.
Durable power of attorney for health care	Term used by some states to describe a document used for listing the person(s) to make health care decisions should a patient become unable to make informed decisions for self.	• May be the same as medical power of attorney. • Indicates specific measures to be used or withheld.
Living will	Lay term used to describe any documents that give instructions about future medical care and treatments or the wish to be allowed to die without heroic or extraordinary measures should the patient be unable to communicate for self.	• Must identify specific treatments that a person wants or does not want at end of life.
Medical power of attorney	Term used by some states to describe a document used for listing the person(s) to make health care decisions should a patient become unable to make informed decisions for self.	• May be the same as durable power of attorney for health care, health care proxy, or appointment of a health care agent or surrogate. Specifies measures to be used or withheld. • Person appointed may be called a health care agent, surrogate, attorney-in-fact, or proxy.

CPR, Cardiopulmonary resuscitation.

use of drugs for resuscitation without the use of CPR. A "no code," or a DNR order, allows the person to die with comfort measures only and without the interference of technology. Some states have implemented a form called *out-of-hospital DNR* for use by terminally ill patients who wish to have no heroic measures used to prolong life after they leave an acute care facility.[27,28]

Allow natural death (AND) is a term being used to replace "no code" or DNR.[28] This term more accurately conveys what actually happens. It is also sometimes referred to as *"comfort measures only"* status, meaning that all comfort measures associated with pain control and symptom management are carried out, but the natural physiologic progression to death is not delayed or interrupted.

Withholding or withdrawing treatments must be included in an advance directive. The directive must clearly state what is to be done and what is not to be done. The ANA position statement on foregoing nutrition and hydration states that the decision to withhold artificial nutrition and hydration should be made by the patient or surrogate with the health care team.[26] For patients who are no longer receiving artificial nutrition and hydration, it is important to continue to provide expert nursing care.

Euthanasia is the deliberate act of hastening death. The ANA statement on active euthanasia states that the nurse should not participate in active euthanasia because such an act is in direct violation of the Code for Nurses, the ethical traditions and goals of the profession, and its covenant with society. As a nurse, you have an obligation to provide timely, humane, comprehensive, and compassionate EOL care.

You need to be aware of legal issues and the patient's wishes. Advance directives and organ donor information should be located in the medical record and identified on the patient's record and/or the nursing care plan. All caregivers responsible for the patient need to know the patient's wishes. Additionally, you are responsible for becoming familiar with state, local, and agency procedures in EOL care documentation.

ETHICAL/LEGAL DILEMMAS

End-of-Life Care

Situation

A.P., a terminally ill 50-year-old woman with metastatic breast cancer, has developed severe bone pain that is not adequately controlled by her present dose of IV morphine. She moans at rest and verbalizes severe pain from any movement to reposition her. At the team conference the nurses discuss the need for more effective pain control, but are concerned that additional pain medicine could hasten her death.

Ethical/Legal Points for Consideration

- Adequate pain relief is an important outcome for all patients, especially patients who are terminally ill. The *principle of beneficence* means that care is provided to benefit patients. The goal of adequate pain control in the terminally ill to alleviate suffering is based on the *principle of nonmaleficence:* preventing or reducing harm to the patient. The secondary effect of hastening the patient's death is ethically justified; this is known as the concept of *double effect.*
- Legally, the *standard of care* is used to define the nursing acts that are required for safe and competent nursing practice. When the actual nursing care falls below the standard of care, it is considered negligent and unsafe, and the nurse is at risk for being found incompetent.
- In a court of law the standard of care in nursing is determined by nursing experts and evidence-based practices. The increasing use of technology to access the latest scientific findings is changing the standard of nursing care to a national, if not global, standard defined by research findings and nationally recognized expert testimony.
- In this situation the standard of care is that the patient will experience pain relief. Failure of the nurse to act assertively to achieve pain relief for the patient and failure to effectively use resources to obtain that pain relief will be considered below the standard of care and unsafe and incompetent practice.

Discussion Questions

1. What types of discussions need to occur among the health care team, patient, and family as the terminally ill patient approaches this phase of care?
2. Distinguish between promotion of comfort and relief of pain in dying patients, and between assisted suicide and euthanasia. (Use the American Nurses Association position statements at *www.ana.org.*)

NURSING MANAGEMENT END OF LIFE

Nurses spend more time with patients near the end of life than any other health care professionals. Nursing care of terminally ill and dying patients is holistic and encompasses all psychosocial and physical needs. Respect, dignity, and comfort are important for the patient and the family. In addition, you need to recognize your own needs when dealing with grief and dying.

NURSING ASSESSMENT

Assessment of the terminally ill or dying patient varies with the patient's condition. Be sensitive and do not impose repeated, unnecessary assessments on the dying patient. When possible, use health history data that are available in the medical record rather than tiring the patient with an interview.

Document the specific event or change that brought the patient into the health care setting. Record the patient's medical diagnoses, medication profile, and allergies.

If the patient is alert, do a brief review of the body systems to detect important signs and symptoms. Assess for discomfort, pain, nausea, and dyspnea so that prompt interventions can be implemented. In addition, evaluate and manage co-morbidities or acute episodes of problems such as diabetes mellitus or headache. Elicit information about the patient's abilities, food and fluid intake, patterns of sleep and rest, and response to the stress of terminal illness. Assess the patient's ability to cope with the diagnosis and prognosis of the illness. Also determine the family's capacity to manage the needed care and to cope with the illness and its consequences.

The physical assessment is abbreviated and focuses on changes that accompany terminal illness and the specific disease process.[29] The frequency of assessment depends on the patient's stability, but assessment is done at least every 8 hours in the institutional setting. For patients cared for in their homes by hospice programs, assessment may occur weekly. As changes occur, assessment and documentation may need to be done more frequently. If the patient is in the final hours of life, the physical assessment may be limited to essential data.

Key elements of a social assessment include determining the relationships and patterns of communication among the family. If multiple family members are present, listen to varying concerns from different members. Differences in expectations and interpersonal conflict can result in family disruptions after the death of the loved one. Social assessment also includes evaluating the goals of the patient and the family.

As death approaches, monitor the patient for multiple systems that often are failing during the EOL period. This requires vigilance and attention to physical changes that are often subtle. Neurologic assessment is especially important and includes level of consciousness, presence of reflexes, and pupil responses. Evaluation of vital signs, skin color, and temperature indicates changes in circulation. Monitor and describe respiratory status, character and pattern of respirations, and characteristics of breath sounds. Monitor nutritional and fluid intake, urine output, and bowel function, since this provides assessment data for renal and gastrointestinal functioning. Assess skin condition on an ongoing basis because skin becomes fragile and may easily break down.

PLANNING

Planning and coordinating care at EOL must focus on the needs of the patient, family, and significant others. In some cases a family conference may be helpful to develop a coordinated plan of care.

Develop a comprehensive plan to support, teach, and evaluate patients and families. Nursing care goals during the last stages of life involve comfort measures and care of the patient's emotional and physical needs. These goals may also include determining where the patient would like to die and whether this is possible. For example, the patient may want to die at home, but the family may object.

The last hours or days of the patient experiencing brain death are frequently spent in the ICU. Planning for EOL care may be particularly challenging in the ICU environment. At this time, some families are approached about organ donation. Consultation from palliative care specialists may help the family plan and cope with EOL issues.

NURSING IMPLEMENTATION

Psychosocial care and physical care are interrelated for both the dying patient and family. Teaching them is an important part of EOL care. Families need ongoing information on the disease, the dying process, and any care that will be provided. They need information on how to cope with the many issues during this period of their lives. Denial and grieving may be barriers to learning and understanding at the end of life for both the patient and family.

PSYCHOSOCIAL CARE. As death approaches, respond appropriately to the patient's psychosocial manifestations at the end of life (Table 10-7).

Anxiety and Depression. Patients often exhibit signs of anxiety and depression during the EOL period. Anxiety is an uneasy feeling whose cause is not easily identified. Anxiety is frequently related to fear.

Causes of anxiety and depression may include uncontrolled pain and dyspnea, psychosocial factors related to the disease process or impending death, altered physiologic states, and drugs used in high dosages. Encouragement, support, and teaching decrease some of the anxiety and depression. Management of anxiety and depression may include both medications and nonpharmacologic interventions. Relaxation strategies such as relaxation breathing, muscle relaxation, music, and imagery may be useful (see Chapter 7).

Anger. Anger is a common and normal response to grief. A grieving person cannot be forced to accept the loss. The surviving family members may be angry with the dying loved one who is leaving them. Encourage the expression of feelings, but at the same time realize how difficult it is to come to terms with loss. As a nurse, you may be the target of the anger. You need to understand what is happening and not react on a personal level.

TABLE 10-7 NURSING ASSESSMENT

Psychosocial Care at End of Life

Characteristic	Nursing Management
Withdrawal	
Patient near death may seem withdrawn from the physical environment, maintaining the ability to hear but unable to respond.	Converse as though the patient were alert, using a soft voice and gentle touch.
Unusual Communication	
This may indicate that an unresolved issue is preventing the dying person from letting go. Patient may become restless and agitated or perform repetitive tasks (may also indicate terminal delirium).	Encourage the family to talk with and reassure the dying person.
Vision-like Experiences	
Patient may talk to persons who are not there or see places and objects not visible. Vision-like experiences assist the dying person in coming to terms with meaning in life and transition from it.	Affirm the dying person's experience as a part of transition from this life.
Saying Goodbyes	
It is important for the patient and family to acknowledge their sadness, mutually forgive one another, and say goodbye.	Encourage the dying person and family to verbalize their feelings of sadness, loss, forgiveness; to touch, hug, cry. Allow the patient and family privacy to express their feelings and comfort one another.
Spiritual Needs	
Patient or family may request spiritual support such as the presence of a chaplain.	Encourage visit by appropriate spiritual care service provider, chaplain, or family member. Allow patient to express his or her spiritual needs.

Hopelessness and Powerlessness. Feelings of hopelessness and powerlessness are common at the EOL. Encourage realistic hope within the limits of the situation. Allow the patient and the family to deal with what is within their control, and help them to recognize what is beyond their control. When possible, support the patient's involvement in decision making about care to foster a sense of control and autonomy.

Fear. Fear is a typical feeling associated with dying. Four specific fears associated with dying are fear of pain, fear of shortness of breath, fear of loneliness and abandonment, and fear of meaninglessness.

Fear of Pain. Many people assume that pain always accompanies death. Physiologically, there is no absolute indication that death is always painful. Psychologically, pain may occur based on the anxieties and separations related to dying. Terminally ill patients who do experience physical pain should have pain-relieving drugs available. Assure the patient and the family that

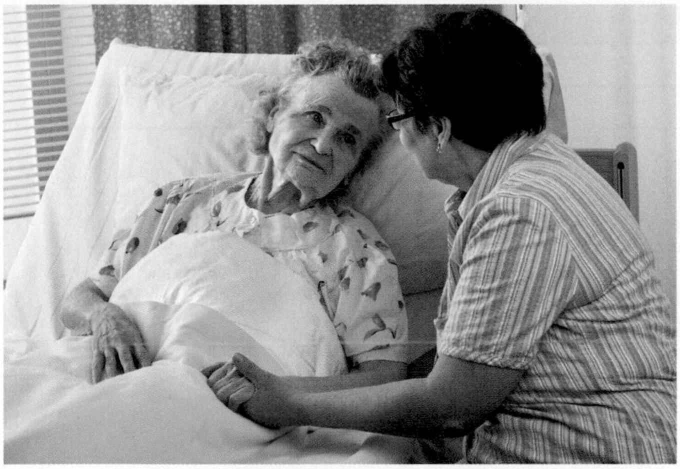

FIG. 10-8 Dying patients typically want someone whom they know and trust to stay with them. (iStockphoto/Thinkstock)

drugs will be given promptly when needed and that side effects of drugs can and will be managed. Patients can participate in their own pain relief by discussing pain relief measures and their effects. Most patients want their pain relieved without the side effects of grogginess or sleepiness. Pain relief measures do not need to deprive the patient of the ability to interact with others.[30]

Fear of Shortness of Breath. Respiratory distress and dyspnea are common near the end of life. The sensation of air hunger results in anxiety for the patient and family. Current therapies include opioids, bronchodilators, and oxygen, depending on the cause of the dyspnea. Anxiety-reducing agents (e.g., anxiolytics) may help produce relaxation.

Fear of Loneliness and Abandonment. Most terminally ill and dying people fear loneliness and do not want to be alone. Many dying patients are afraid that loved ones who are unable to cope with the patient's imminent death will abandon them. The simple presence of someone provides support and comfort (Fig. 10-8). Holding hands, touching, and listening are important nursing interventions. Providing companionship allows the dying person a sense of security.

Fear of Meaninglessness. Fear of meaninglessness leads people to review their lives. They review their intentions during life, examining actions and expressing regrets about what might have been. *Life review* helps patients recognize the value of their lives. Assist patients and their families in identifying the positive qualities of the patient's life. Practical ways of helping may include looking at photo albums or collections of important mementos. Sharing thoughts and feelings may enhance spirituality and provide comfort for the patient at this time. Respect and accept the practices and rituals associated with the patient's life review while remaining nonjudgmental.[30]

> *What we leave behind is not what is engraved in stone monuments, but what is woven into the lives of others.*
> *Pericles (fifth-century Greek statesman)*

Communication. Communication among health care providers, patient, and family is essential at the end of life. Empathy and active listening are essential components of communication in EOL care. *Empathy* is the identification with and understanding of another's situation, feelings, or motives. *Active listening* is paying attention to what is said, observing the patient's nonverbal cues, and not interrupting.

There may be silence. Frequently silence is related to the overwhelming feelings experienced at the end of life. Silence can also allow time to gather thoughts. Listening to the silence sends a message of acceptance and comfort. Communication also needs to consider the patient's ethnic, cultural, and religious backgrounds.

Patients and family members may have difficulties expressing themselves emotionally. Allow time for them to express their feelings and thoughts. Make time to listen and interact in a sensitive way to enhance the relationship among you, the patient, and the family. A family conference is one way to create a more conducive environment for communication.

Unusual communication by the patient may take place at the end of life. The patient's speech may become confused, disoriented, or garbled. Patients may speak to or about family members or others who have predeceased them, give instructions to those who will survive them, or speak of projects yet to be completed. Active, careful listening allows for the identification of specific patterns in the dying person's communication and decreases the risk for inappropriate labeling of behaviors.

PHYSICAL CARE. Nursing management related to physical care at the end of life focuses on symptom management and comfort rather than treatment for curing a disease or disorder (Table 10-8). The priority is meeting the patient's physiologic and safety needs. Physical care focuses on the needs for oxygen, nutrition, pain relief, mobility, elimination, and skin care. People who are dying deserve and require the same physical care as people who are expected to recover.

Postmortem Care. After the patient is pronounced dead, prepare or delegate preparation of the body for immediate viewing by the family with consideration for cultural customs and in accord with state law and agency policies and procedures. In some cultures and in some types of death, it may be important to allow the family to prepare or assist in preparing the body. In general, close the patient's eyes, replace dentures, wash the body as needed (placing pads under the perineum to absorb urine and feces), and remove tubes and dressings (if appropriate). The body is straightened, leaving the pillow to support the head and prevent pooling of blood and discoloration of the face. Allow the family privacy and as much time as they need with the deceased person. In the case of an unexpected or unanticipated death, preparation of the body for viewing or release to a funeral home depends on state law and agency policies and procedures.

SPECIAL NEEDS OF CAREGIVERS AND NURSES IN END-OF-LIFE CARE

Special Needs of Family Caregivers

Family caregivers are important in meeting the patient's physical and psychosocial needs. The role of caregivers includes working and communicating with the patient and other family members, supporting the patient's concerns, and helping the patient resolve any unfinished business. Families often face emotional, physical, and economic consequences as a result of caring for a family member who is dying. The caregiver's responsibilities do not end when the person is admitted to an acute care, inpatient hospice, or long-term care facility.

TABLE 10-8 NURSING MANAGEMENT

Physical Care at End of Life

Characteristic	Nursing Management
Pain	
• Pain may be a major symptom associated with terminal illness and the one most feared. • Pain can be acute or chronic. • Physical and emotional irritations can aggravate pain.	• Assess pain thoroughly and regularly to determine the quality, intensity, location, and contributing factors. • Minimize possible irritants such as skin irritations from wetness, heat or cold, and pressure. • Administer medications around the clock in a timely manner and on a regular basis to provide constant relief rather than waiting until the pain is unbearable and then trying to relieve it. • Provide complementary and alternative therapies such as guided imagery, massage, and relaxation techniques as needed (see Chapters 6 and 7). • Evaluate effectiveness of pain relief measures frequently to ensure that the patient is on a correct, adequate drug regimen. • Do not delay or deny pain relief measures to a terminally ill patient.
Delirium	
• A state characterized by confusion, disorientation, restlessness, clouding of consciousness, incoherence, fear, anxiety, excitement, and often hallucinations. • May be misidentified as depression, psychosis, anger, or anxiety. • Use of opioids or corticosteroids may cause delirium. • Underlying disease process may contribute to delirium. • Generally considered a reversible process.	• Perform a thorough assessment for reversible causes of delirium, including pain, constipation, and urinary retention. • Provide a room that is quiet, well lit, and familiar to reduce the effects of delirium. • Reorient the dying person to person, place, and time with each encounter. • Administer ordered benzodiazepines and sedatives as needed. • Stay physically close to frightened patient. Reassure in a calm, soft voice with touch and slow strokes of the skin. • Provide family with emotional support and encouragement in their efforts to cope with the behaviors associated with delirium. • Encourage the family to participate in care of the patient.
Restlessness	
• May occur as death approaches and cerebral metabolism slows.	• Assess for spiritual distress as a cause of restlessness and agitation. • Do not restrain. • Use soothing music; slow, soft touch and voice. • Limit the number of persons at the bedside.
Dysphagia	
• May occur because of extreme weakness and changes in level of consciousness.	• Identify the least invasive alternative routes of administration for drugs needed for symptom management. • Suction orally as needed.
Weakness and Fatigue	
• Expected at the end of life. • Metabolic demands related to disease process contribute to weakness and fatigue.	• Assess the patient's tolerance for activities. • Time nursing interventions to conserve energy. • Help the patient identify and complete valued or desired activities. • Provide support as needed to maintain positions in bed or chair. • Provide frequent rest periods.
Dehydration	
• May occur during the last days of life. • Hunger and thirst are rare in the last days of life. • As the end of life approaches, patients tend to take in less food and fluid.	• Assess mucous membranes frequently to prevent excessive dryness, which can lead to discomfort. • Maintain complete, regular oral care to provide for comfort and hydration of mucous membranes. • Do not force the patient to eat or drink. • Encourage consumption of ice chips and sips of fluids or use moist cloths to provide moisture to the mouth. • Use moist cloths and swabs for unconscious patients to avoid aspiration. • Apply lubricant to the lips and oral mucous membranes as needed. • Reassure family that cessation of food and fluid intake is a natural part of the process of dying.
Dyspnea	
• Subjective symptom. • Accompanied by fear of suffocation and anxiety. • Underlying disease process can exacerbate dyspnea. • Coughing and expectorating secretions become difficult.	• Assess respiratory status regularly. • Elevate the head and/or position patient on side to improve chest expansion. • Use a fan or air conditioner to facilitate movement of cool air. • Administer supplemental oxygen as ordered. • Suction PRN to remove accumulation of mucus from the airways. Suction cautiously in the terminal phase.

TABLE 10-8 NURSING MANAGEMENT—cont'd

Physical Care at End of Life

Characteristic	Nursing Management
Myoclonus	
• Mild to severe jerking or twitching sometimes associated with use of high dose of opioids. • Patient may complain of involuntary twitching of extremities.	• Assess for initial onset, duration, and any discomfort or distress experienced by patient. • If myoclonus is distressing or becoming more severe, discuss possible drug therapy modifications with the health care provider. • Changes in opioid medication may alleviate or decrease myoclonus.
Skin Breakdown	
• Skin integrity is difficult to maintain at the end of life. • Immobility, urinary and bowel incontinence, dry skin, nutritional deficits, anemia, friction, and shearing forces lead to a high risk for skin breakdown. • Disease and other processes may impair skin integrity. • As death approaches, circulation to the extremities decreases and they become cool, mottled, and cyanotic.	• Assess the skin for signs of breakdown. • Implement protocols to prevent skin breakdown by controlling drainage and odor and keeping the skin and any wound areas clean. • Perform wound assessments as needed. • Follow appropriate nursing management protocol for dressing wounds. • Follow appropriate nursing management protocol for a patient who is immobile, but consider realistic outcomes of skin integrity vs. maintenance of comfort. • Follow appropriate nursing management to prevent skin irritations and breakdown from urinary and bowel incontinence. • Use blankets to cover for warmth; never apply heat. • Prevent the effects of shearing forces.
Bowel Patterns	
• Constipation can be caused by immobility, use of opioid medications, lack of fiber in the diet, and dehydration. • Diarrhea may occur as muscles relax or from a fecal impaction related to the use of opioids and immobility.	• Assess bowel function. • Assess for and remove fecal impactions. • Encourage movement and physical activities as tolerated. • Encourage fiber in the diet if appropriate. • Encourage fluids if appropriate. • Use suppositories, stool softeners, laxatives, or enemas if ordered.
Urinary Incontinence	
• May result from disease progression or changes in the level of consciousness. • As death becomes imminent, the perineal muscles relax.	• Assess urinary function. • Use absorbent pads for urinary incontinence. • Follow appropriate nursing protocol for the consideration and use of indwelling or external catheters. • Follow appropriate nursing management to prevent skin irritations and breakdown from urinary incontinence.
Anorexia, Nausea, and Vomiting	
• May be caused by complications of disease process. • Drugs contribute to nausea. • Constipation, impaction, and bowel obstruction can cause anorexia, nausea, and vomiting.	• Assess the patient for complaints of nausea or vomiting. • Assess possible contributing causes of nausea or vomiting. • Have family provide the patient's favorite foods. • Discuss modifications to the drug regimen with the health care provider. • Provide antiemetics before meals if ordered. • Offer and provide frequent meals with small portions of favorite foods. • Offer culturally appropriate foods. • Provide frequent mouth care, especially after vomiting.

An understanding of the grieving process as it affects both the patient and family is important. Being present during a family member's dying process can be highly stressful. Recognize signs and behaviors among family members who may be at risk for abnormal grief reactions, and be prepared to intervene if necessary. Warning signs may include dependency and negative feelings about the dying person, inability to express feelings, sleep disturbances, a history of depression, difficult reactions to previous losses, perceived lack of social or family support, low self-esteem, multiple previous bereavements, alcoholism, or substance abuse. Caregivers with concurrent life crises (e.g., divorce) will be especially at risk.

Family caregivers and other family members need encouragement to continue their usual activities as much as possible. They need to discuss their activities and maintain some control over their lives.

Inform caregivers about appropriate resources for support, including respite care. Resources such as community counseling and local support may assist some people in working through their grief. Encourage caregivers to build a support system of extended family, friends, faith community, and clergy. The caregivers should have people to call on at any time to express any feelings they are experiencing. (The stressors and special needs of family caregivers are discussed in Chapter 4 on pp. 51-52.)

Special Needs of Nurses

Many nurses who care for dying patients do so because they are passionate about providing high-quality EOL care. Caring for patients and their families at the end of life is challenging and rewarding, but also intense and emotionally charged. A bond or connection may develop between you and the patient or family. Be aware of how grief personally affects you. When you provide care for terminally ill or dying patients, you are not immune to feelings of loss. It is common to feel helpless and powerless when dealing with death. Express feelings of sorrow, guilt, and frustration.

Interventions are available that may help ease your physical and emotional stress. Be aware of what you can and cannot control. Recognizing personal feelings allows openness in exchanging feelings with the patient and the family. Realizing that it is okay to cry with the patient or family during the end of life may be important for your well-being.

To meet your personal needs, focus on interventions that will help decrease your stress. Get involved in hobbies or other interests, schedule time for yourself, maintain a peer support system, and develop a support system beyond the workplace.[31] Hospice agencies can help you cope through professionally assisted groups, informal discussion sessions, and flexible time schedules.

BRIDGE TO NCLEX EXAMINATION

The number of the question corresponds to the same-numbered outcome at the beginning of the chapter.

1. An 80-year-old female patient is receiving palliative care for heart failure. Primary purpose(s) of her receiving palliative care is (are) to *(select all that apply)*
   a. improve her quality of life.
   b. assess her coping ability with disease.
   c. have time to teach patient and family about disease.
   d. focus on reducing the severity of disease symptoms.
   e. provide care that the family is unwilling or unable to give.
2. The primary purpose of hospice is to
   a. allow patients to die at home.
   b. provide better quality of care than the family can.
   c. coordinate care for dying patients and their families.
   d. provide comfort and support for dying patients and their families.
3. A 67-year-old woman was recently diagnosed with inoperable pancreatic cancer. Before the diagnosis she was very active in her neighborhood association. Her husband is concerned because his wife is staying at home and missing her usual community activities. Which common EOL psychologic manifestation is she most likely demonstrating?
   a. Peacefulness
   b. Decreased socialization
   c. Decreased decision making
   d. Anxiety about unfinished business
4. For the past 5 years Tom has repeatedly asked his mother to donate his deceased father's belongings to charity, but his mother has refused. She sits in the bedroom closet, crying and talking to her long-dead husband. What type of grief is Tom's mother experiencing?
   a. Adaptive grief
   b. Disruptive grief
   c. Anticipatory grief
   d. Prolonged grief disorder
5. The home health nurse visits a 40-year-old patient with metastatic breast cancer who is receiving palliative care. The patient is experiencing pain at a level of 7 (on a 10-point scale). In prioritizing activities for the visit, the nurse would do which first?
   a. Auscultate for breath sounds.
   b. Administer PRN pain medication.
   c. Check pressure points for skin breakdown.
   d. Ask family about patient's food and fluid intake.
6. While caring for his dying wife, the husband states that his wife is a devout Roman Catholic but he is a Baptist. Who is considered the most reliable source for spiritual preferences concerning EOL care for the dying wife?
   a. A priest
   b. Dying wife
   c. Hospice staff
   d. Husband of dying wife
7. The family attorney informed a patient's adult children and wife that the patient did not have an advance directive after he suffered a serious stroke. Who is responsible for making the decision about EOL measures when the patient cannot communicate his or her specific wishes?
   a. Notary and attorney
   b. Physician and family
   c. Wife and adult children
   d. Physician and nursing staff
8. The children caregivers of an elderly patient whose death is imminent have not left the bedside for the past 36 hours. In the nurse's assessment of the family, what findings indicate the potential for an abnormal grief reaction to occur *(select all that apply)*?
   a. Family cannot express their feelings to one another.
   b. Dying patient is becoming more restless and agitated.
   c. A family member is going through a difficult divorce.
   d. Family talks with and reassures the patient at frequent intervals.
   e. Siblings who were estranged from each other have now reunited.
9. A nurse has been working full time with terminally ill patients for 3 years. He has been experiencing irritability and mixed emotions when expressing sadness since four of his patients died on the same day. To optimize the quality of his nursing care, he should examine his own
   a. full-time work schedule.
   b. past feelings toward death.
   c. patterns for dealing with grief.
   d. demands for involvement in patient care.

1. a, d, 2. d, 3. b, 4. d, 5. b, 6. b, 7. c, 8. a, c, 9. c.

evolve

For rationales to these answers and even more NCLEX review questions, visit *http://evolve.elsevier.com/Lewis/medsurg.*

REFERENCES

1. World Health Organization: Palliative care. Retrieved from *www.who.int/cancer/palliative/en.*
2. Hospice Foundation of America: What is hospice? Retrieved from *www.hospicefoundation.org/hospiceinfo.*
3. National Consensus Project for Quality Palliative Care: Clinical practice guidelines for palliative care, ed 2. Retrieved from *www.nationalconsensusproject.org/guideline.pdf.*
4. American Cancer Society: Hospice care. Retrieved from *www.cancer.org/Treatment/FindingandPayingforTreatment/ChoosingYourTreatmentTeam/HospiceCare/hospice-care-what-is-hospice-care.*
5. National Hospice and Palliative Care Organization: Hospice care in America. Retrieved from *www.nhpco.org/files/public/statistics_research/hospice_facts_figures_oct-2010.pdf.*
6. Hospice and Palliative Nurses Association Care. HPNA Position statement: Value of the professional nurse in palliative care. Copyright by the Hospice and Palliative Nurses Association, Pittsburgh, 2011. Retrieved from *www.hpna.org.*

*7. Johnson KS, Kuchibhatia M, Tulsky JA: Racial differences in self-reported exposure to information about hospice care. *J Palliat Med* 12(10):921, 2009.

8. Teitelbaum J, Shemi SD: Neurologic determination of death, *Neurol Clin* 29:787, 2011.

*9. American Academy of Neurology: Practice parameters: determining brain death in adults. Retrieved from *www.aan.com/professionals/practice/guidelines/pda/Brain_death_adults.pdf.*

10. Field M, Cassel C: *Approaching death: improving care at the end of life*, Washington, DC. 1997, National Academy Press. (Classic)
11. Kübler-Ross E: *On death and dying*, New York, 1969, Macmillan. (Classic)
12. Kübler-Ross E, Kessler D: The five stages of grief. Retrieved from *www.grief.com/the-five-stages-of-grief*
13. A guide to grief: bereavement, mourning, and grief. Retrieved from *www.hospicenet.org/html/grief_guide.html.*
14. Anderson WG, Arnold RM, Angus DC, et al: Posttraumatic stress and complicated grief in family of patients in the intensive care unit, *J Gen Intern Med* 23:1871, 2008.
15. Kacel E, Gao X, Prigerson HG: Understanding bereavement: what every oncology practitioner should know, *J Support Oncol* 9:172, 2011.
16. Selman L, Harding R, Gysels M, et al: The measurement of spirituality in palliative care and the content of tools validated cross-culturally: a systematic review, *J Pain Symptom Manage* 41:728, 2011.
17. Bruce A, Schreiber R, Petrovskaya O, et al: Longing for ground in a ground(less) world: a qualitative inquiry of existential suffering, *BMS Nurs* 27:2, 2011.
18. Zhang AY, Zyzanski SJ, Siminoff LA: Differential patient-caregiver opinions of treatment and care for advanced lung cancer patient, *Soc Sci Med* 70:115, 2010.
19. Liaschenko J, Peden-McAlpine C, Andrews GJ: Institutional geographics in dying: nurses' actions and observations on dying spaces inside and outside intensive care units, *Health Place* 17:814, 2011.
20. Kelley AS, Wenger NS, Sarkisian CA: Opinions: End of life care preferences and planning among older Latinos, *J Am Geriatr Soc* 58:1109, 2010.
21. Sharma RK, Hughes MT, Nolan MT, et al: Family understanding of seriously-ill patient preferences for family involvement in healthcare decision making, *J Gen Intern Med* 26:881, 2011.
22. Carr D: Racial differences in end-of-life planning: why don't Blacks and Latinos prepare for the inevitable? *Omega (Westport)* 63:1, 2011.
23. Thornton JD, Pham K, Engelberg RA, et al: Families with limited English proficiency receive less information and support in interpreted intensive care unit family conferences, *Crit Care Med* 37:89, 2009.
24. DeWispelaere J, Stirton L: Advance commitment: an alternative approach to the family veto problem in organ procurement, *J Med Ethics* 36:180, 2010.
25. Billings JA, Krakauer EL: On patient autonomy and physician responsibility in end of life care, *Arch Intern Med* 171:849, 2011.
26. American Nurses Association: ANA position statements. Retrieved from *http://nursingworld.org/MainMenuCategories/HealthcareandPolicyIssues/ANAPositionStatements/EthicsandHumanRights.aspx.*
27. Iowa Department of Public Health: Out of hospital DNR. Retrieved from *www.idph.state.ia.us/ems/dnr.asp.*
28. Walker KA, Peltier H, Mayo RL, et al: Impact of writing "comfort measures only" orders in a community teaching hospital, *J Palliat Med* 13:241, 2010.
29. Adams JA, Bailey DE, Anderson RA, et al: Nursing roles and strategies in end-of-life decision making in acute care: a systematic review of the literature, *Nurs Res Pract* 2011:527834, 2011. Published online doi:10.1155/2011/527834.
30. Prince-Paul M, Exline JJ: Personal relationships and communication messages at the end of life, *Nurs Clin North Am* 45:449, 2010.
31. Sinclair S: Impact of death and dying on the personal lives and practices of palliative and hospice care professionals, *CMAJ* 183:180, 2011.

*Evidence-based information for clinical practice.

RESOURCES

End-of-Life Nursing Education Consortium (ELNEC), American Association of Colleges of Nursing
www.aacn.nche.edu/ELNEC

Hospice and Palliative Nurses Association
www.hpna.org

National Hospice and Palliative Care Organization
www.nhpco.org

CHAPTER

11 Substance Abuse

Mariann M. Harding

If you are on the wrong road, progress means doing an about-turn and walking back to the right road.
C. S. Lewis

evolve WEBSITE

http://evolve.elsevier.com/Lewis/medsurg
- NCLEX Review Questions
- Key Points
- Pre-Test
- Answer Guidelines for Case Study on p. 167
- Rationales for Bridge to NCLEX Examination Questions
- Nursing Care Plan (Customizable)
  - NCP 11-1: Patient in Alcohol Withdrawal
- Concept Map Creator
- Glossary
- Content Updates

eTable
- eTable 11-1: Clinical Institute Withdrawal Assessment of Alcohol Scale, Revised (CIWA-Ar)

LEARNING OUTCOMES

1. Apply the terms *addiction, addictive behavior, substance misuse, substance abuse, dependence, tolerance, withdrawal, craving,* and *abstinence* to clinical situations.
2. Relate the effects of substance abuse to its resulting major health complications.
3. Differentiate among the effects of the use of stimulants, depressants, and cannabis.
4. Explain your role in promoting the cessation of smoking and tobacco use.
5. Summarize the nursing management and collaborative care of patients who experience intoxication, overdose, or withdrawal from stimulants and depressants.
6. Describe the incidence and effects of substance abuse and dependence in the older adult.

KEY TERMS

Substance abuse and addiction are serious problems affecting the health care system and society today. Addiction to chemical substances usually includes dependence on psychoactive agents that result in pleasure or modify thinking and perception. These include substances that are legal for adult use such as alcohol and tobacco, and illicit drugs including marijuana/hashish, cocaine, heroin, hallucinogens, inhalants, and prescription medications used nonmedically. In 2010 an estimated 22.6 million Americans ages 12 or older, or 8.9% of the population, were using illicit drugs monthly.[1] Americans' abuse and misuse of prescription medications such as analgesics, sedative-hypnotics, tranquilizers, and amphetamines have increased and can create harmful effects that are more deadly than the abuse of illicit drugs.[2]

The *Diagnostic and Statistical Manual of Mental Disorders IV* states that **substance abuse** and **dependence** (defined in Table 11-1) are specific psychiatric diagnoses.[3] Abused substances are discussed in detail in psychiatric and pharmacologic books and resources. Long-term management of patients who abuse substances is most often provided in specialized treatment facilities that provide both drug and behavior therapies.

Individuals who abuse substances use the health care system more than those who do not.[4] Almost every drug of abuse harms some tissue or organ in addition to the brain. Some health problems are caused by the effects of specific drugs, such as liver damage related to alcohol use or chronic obstructive pulmonary disease (COPD) related to smoking. Other health problems result from behaviors associated with substance abuse, such as injecting drugs or neglecting nutrition and hygiene. Common health complications related to substance abuse are identified in Table 11-2.

This chapter focuses on the role of the medical-surgical nurse in identifying and managing the substance-abusing patient in acute care settings. All nurses care for patients dependent on substances, whether they are identified as dependent or not, simply because of the prevalence of substance abuse and its association with health problems.

Reviewed by Carol Capitano, RN, PhD(C), College of Nursing, University of New Mexico, Albuquerque, New Mexico.

TABLE 11-1 TERMINOLOGY OF SUBSTANCE ABUSE

Term	Definition
Abstinence	Avoidance of substance use.
Addiction	Compulsive, uncontrollable dependence on a substance, behavior, or practice to such a degree that cessation causes severe emotional, mental, or physiologic reactions.
Addictive behavior	Behavior associated with maintaining an addiction.
Craving	Subjective need for a substance, usually experienced after decreased use or abstinence. Cue-induced craving occurs in the presence of experiences previously associated with drug taking.
Dependence	Reliance on a substance to the degree that its absence will cause impairment in function.
• Physical	Altered physiologic state from prolonged substance use; regular use is necessary to prevent withdrawal.
• Psychologic	Compulsive need to experience pleasurable response from the substance.
Overdose	Ingestion of excessive dose of one drug or a combination of similarly acting drugs. Leads to toxic reactions, including respiratory and circulatory arrest.
Relapse	Return to substance use after a period of abstinence.
Substance	Drug, chemical, or biologic entity that is self-administered. The words *"drug," "substance,"* and *"chemical"* are often used interchangeably.
Substance abuse	Overindulgence in a substance that has a negative impact on an individual's psychologic, physiologic, and/or social functioning.
Substance misuse	Use of a drug for purposes other than those for which it is intended.
Tolerance	Decreased effect of a substance that results from repeated exposure. It is possible to develop cross-tolerance to other substances in the same category.
Withdrawal	Combination of physiologic and psychologic responses that occur when there is abrupt cessation or reduced intake of a substance on which an individual is dependent.

TABLE 11-2 COMMON HEALTH PROBLEMS RELATED TO SUBSTANCE ABUSE

Substance	Health Problems*
Nicotine and smoking	• Chronic obstructive pulmonary disease (COPD) • Cancers of lung, mouth, larynx, esophagus, stomach, pancreas, bladder, prostate, cervix • Coronary artery disease, peripheral artery disease • Peptic ulcer disease, GERD
Cocaine	• Nasal sores, septal necrosis or perforation • Chronic sinusitis • Cardiac dysrhythmias, myocardial ischemia and infarction • Stroke • Psychosis
Amphetamines	• Cardiac dysrhythmias, myocardial ischemia and infarction • Death of brain cells • Mood disturbances, violent behavior, psychoses
Caffeine	• Gastrointestinal irritation, peptic ulcer disease, GERD • Anxiety, insomnia
Alcohol	• See Table 11-7 on p. 160
Sedative-hypnotics	• Possible memory impairment • Respiratory depression • Risk for falls and fractures
Opioids	• Sexual dysfunction • Gastric ulcers • Glomerulonephritis
Cannabis	• Bronchitis, chronic sinusitis • Cardiac dysrhythmias, myocardial ischemia and palpitations • Memory impairment • Impaired immune function
Behaviors	**Health Problems**
Injecting drugs	• Blood clots, phlebitis, skin infections • Hepatitis B and C • HIV/AIDS • Other infections: endocarditis, tuberculosis, pneumonia, meningitis, tetanus, bone and joint infections, lung abscesses
Snorting drugs	• Nasal sores, septal necrosis or perforation • Chronic sinusitis
Risky sexual behavior	• HIV/AIDS • Hepatitis B and C • Other sexually transmitted infections
Personal neglect	• Malnutrition, impaired immunity • Accidental injuries

Source: National Institute on Drug Abuse: Addiction and health. In NIDA: *Drugs, brains, and behavior—the science of addiction,* NIH pub no 07-5605, Rockwell, Md, 2008, National Institutes of Health, US Department of Health and Human Services. Retrieved from *www.nida.nih.gov/scienceofaddiction/health.html.*

*The health problems related to substance abuse are discussed in the appropriate chapters throughout the text where they are identified as risk factors for these problems.

GERD, Gastroesophageal reflux disease.

COMMON DRUGS OF ABUSE

NICOTINE

The addictive behavior that you are most likely to encounter is tobacco use. Nicotine is a stimulant substance in tobacco and is the most rapidly addictive of commonly abused drugs. Cigarette smoking is the predominant form of tobacco abuse in the United States. Tobacco use is the leading cause of preventable illness and death in the United States, claiming 443,000 lives a year.[5]

Effects of Use and Complications

The effects of nicotine are identical to those of other highly addictive stimulant drugs, including cocaine. Although users report that nicotine causes a depressant effect with relaxation and relief of anxiety, these effects are thought to occur when withdrawal is relieved with more nicotine.

Smoking is the most harmful method of nicotine use and can injure nearly every organ in the body. Smoking causes chronic lung disease, cardiovascular disease, and many cancers, and it is associated with cataracts, pneumonia, periodontitis, and abdominal aortic aneurysm[6] (see Table 11-2). The chronic respiratory irritation caused by exposure to cigarette smoke is a key risk factor in the development of COPD and lung cancer (carcinogens in tobacco are also involved). The toxic gases inhaled in cigarette smoke constrict the bronchi, paralyze the cilia, thicken the mucus-secreting membranes, dilate the distal airways, and destroy the alveolar walls.

Carbon monoxide is a component of cigarette smoke. Its effects, combined with those of nicotine, increase the risk for coronary artery disease. Carbon monoxide has a high affinity for hemoglobin and combines with it more readily than oxygen, reducing the oxygen-carrying capacity of the blood. Smokers inhale less oxygen when smoking, further decreasing the available oxygen. Together with the increased myocardial oxygen consumption that nicotine causes, carbon monoxide significantly decreases the oxygen available to the myocardium. The result is a cycle of increases in heart rate and myocardial oxygen consumption that can lead to myocardial ischemia.

Children whose parents smoke have a higher rate of respiratory illnesses and sudden infant death syndrome. In adults, secondhand smoking is associated with decreased pulmonary function, increased risk for lung cancer, and increased mortality rates from coronary artery disease.

Women appear to be at greater risk than men for smoking-related diseases. Smoking in women is associated with increased menstrual bleeding and dysmenorrhea, early menopause, and infertility. Lung cancer related to smoking has surpassed breast cancer as the leading cause of cancer deaths among women.[7]

Although those who use smokeless tobacco (snuff, plug, and leaf) have less risk of lung disease than smokers, the use of smokeless tobacco is not without complications. Holding tobacco in the mouth increases the risk of cancer of the mouth, the cheek, the tongue, and gingiva nearly 50-fold. Smokeless tobacco users also experience the systemic effects of nicotine on the cardiovascular system, thus increasing the risk for cardiovascular disease.[6]

All users of nicotine in any form may develop complications directly related to the effects of nicotine itself, including an increased risk for peripheral artery disease, delayed wound healing, peptic ulcer disease, and gastroesophageal reflux disease (GERD).[6]

NURSING AND COLLABORATIVE CARE TOBACCO USE

TOBACCO CESSATION

As a nurse, you have a professional responsibility to help individuals stop smoking or using tobacco. The Joint Commission mandates that every health professional is responsible for identifying tobacco users and providing them with information on ways to stop the use of tobacco. Hospitalization offers an ideal opportunity to provide cessation assistance because hospitals are tobacco-free environments, and patients may be more motivated to quit because of their illness. Patients who receive even brief advice and intervention from you are more likely to quit than those who receive no intervention.

Because many health care facilities are tobacco-free environments, an admitted patient who is addicted to nicotine may experience withdrawal symptoms since they are unable to smoke. These symptoms are the same as for the person who stops using tobacco "cold turkey." Ask each patient about his or her tobacco status. Unless contraindicated, offer nicotine replacement therapy to those who desire it to control with-

TABLE 11-3 CLINICAL PRACTICE GUIDELINE

Treating Tobacco Use and Dependence

The Five *As* for Individuals Who Desire to Quit	The Five *Rs* for Individuals Unwilling to Quit
1. **Ask:** Identify all tobacco users at every contact.	1. **Relevance:** Ask the patient to indicate why quitting is personally relevant (e.g., family, health).
2. **Advise:** Strongly urge all tobacco users to quit.	2. **Risks:** Ask the patient to identify negative consequences of tobacco use (e.g., cough, shortness of breath).
3. **Assess:** Determine willingness to make a quit attempt.	3. **Rewards:** Ask the patient to identify potential benefits of stopping tobacco use (e.g., saving money, feeling better).
4. **Assist:** Aid the patient in developing a plan to quit.	4. **Roadblocks:** Ask patient to identify barriers or impediments to quitting (e.g., weight gain, partner smokes).
5. **Arrange:** Schedule follow-up contact.	5. **Repetition:** Repeat process every clinic visit.

Source: Agency for Healthcare Research and Quality: *AHCPR supported clinical practice guideline: treating tobacco use and dependence: 2008 update,* Washington, DC, 2008, US Public Health Service.

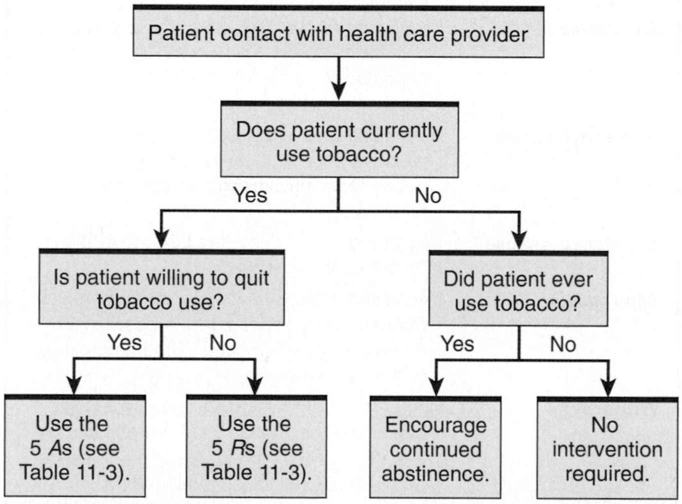

FIG. 11-1 Clinical practice guidelines: treating tobacco use and dependence.

TABLE 11-4 INPATIENT TOBACCO CESSATION INTERVENTIONS

Take the following steps for every hospitalized patient.

- Ask each patient on admission if he or she uses tobacco and document tobacco use status.
- For current tobacco users, list tobacco use status on the admission problem list and as a discharge diagnosis.
- Use counseling and medication to help all tobacco users maintain abstinence and to treat withdrawal symptoms.
- Provide advice and assistance on how to quit during hospitalization and remain abstinent after discharge.
- Arrange for follow-up regarding smoking status. Supportive contact should be provided for at least a month after discharge.

Source: Agency for Healthcare Research and Quality: *AHCPR supported clinical practice guideline: treating tobacco use and dependence: 2008 update,* Washington, DC, 2008, US Public Health Service.

drawal symptoms during their hospitalization. These symptoms include craving, restlessness, depression, headache, hyperirritability, drowsiness or insomnia, decreased BP and heart rate, and increased appetite.

With each patient encounter, encourage the patient to quit and offer specific smoking cessation interventions. The Agency for Healthcare Research and Quality has issued clinical practice guidelines for clinicians, including nurses, to use to motivate users to quit[8] (Tables 11-3 and 11-4 and Fig. 11-1). Use these brief clinical interventions, called the "five *A*s," with each patient encounter. These interventions are designed to identify tobacco users, encourage them to quit, determine their willingness to quit, assist them in quitting, and arrange for follow-up to prevent relapse.

If a tobacco user is unwilling to quit, *motivational interventions* based on the principles of motivational interviewing have been shown to increase future quit attempts. The content areas that should be addressed in a motivational counseling intervention can be captured by the "five *R*s": relevance, risks, rewards, roadblocks, and repetition. A patient teaching guide (Table 11-5) expands on the fourth "A" strategy, "Assist: aid the patient in quitting."

The patient is most likely to achieve long-term tobacco cessation with a combination of nicotine replacement products,

TABLE 11-5 PATIENT TEACHING GUIDE

Smoking and Tobacco Use Cessation

The following interventions are methods that work for quitting tobacco use. Tobacco users have the best chance of quitting if they use more than one method.

Develop a Quit Plan

- Set a quit date, ideally within 2 weeks.
- Talk to your health care provider about getting help to quit.
- Tell family, friends, and co-workers about quitting and request understanding and support.
- Anticipate withdrawal symptoms and challenges when quitting.
- Before quitting, avoid smoking in places where you spend a lot of time (work, car, home).
- Throw away all tobacco products from your home, car, and work.
- Do not take even a single puff or dip after the quit date. Total abstinence is essential.

Use Approved Nicotine Replacement Systems

- Use a nicotine replacement agent unless you are a pregnant or nursing woman (see Table 11-6).
- Do not use other forms of tobacco when using nicotine replacement systems.

Dealing With Urges to Use Tobacco

- Identify situations that may cause you to want to smoke or use other tobacco, such as being around other smokers, being under time pressure, getting into an argument, feeling sad or frustrated, and drinking alcohol.
- Avoid difficult situations while you are trying to quit. Try to lower your stress level.
- Exercise can help, such as walking, jogging, or bicycling.
- Distract yourself from thoughts of smoking and the urge to use tobacco by talking to someone, getting busy with a task, or reading a book.
- Drink a lot of water.
- Take a shower or soak in the tub.

Support and Encouragement

- If you have tried to stop using tobacco before, identify what helped and what hurt in previous quit attempts.
- Joining a quit-tobacco support group will increase your chances of stopping permanently.
- If you get the urge for tobacco, call someone to help talk you out of it—preferably an ex-user.
- Do not be afraid to talk about how you feel while quitting, especially fears of not being able to quit for good. Ask your spouse or partner, friends, and co-workers to support you. Self-help materials and hot lines are also available:
  - American Lung Association: 800-586-4872; *www.lungusa.org*
  - American Cancer Society: 800-227-2345; *www.cancer.org*
  - National Cancer Institute: 877-448-7848 or 800-784-8669; *www.smokefree.gov*
  - Make Smoking History, Massachusetts Department of Public Health: 800-784-8669; *http://makesmokinghistory.org*

Avoiding Relapse

Most relapses occur within the first 3 months after quitting. Do not be discouraged if you start using tobacco again. Remember, most people try several times before they finally quit. Explore different ways to break habits. You may have to deal with some of the following triggers that cause relapse.

- *Change your environment.* Get rid of cigarettes, tobacco (in any form), and ashtrays in your home, car, and place of work. Get rid of the smell of cigarettes in your car and home.
- *Alcohol.* Consider limiting or stopping alcohol use while you are quitting tobacco.
- *Other smokers at home.* Encourage housemates to quit with you. Work out a plan to cope with others who smoke, and avoid being around them.
- *Weight gain.* Tackle one problem at a time. Work on quitting tobacco first. You will not necessarily gain weight, and increased appetite is often temporary.
- *Negative mood or depression.* If these symptoms persist, talk to your health care provider. You may need treatment for depression.
- *Withdrawal symptoms.* Your body will go through many changes when you quit tobacco. You may have a dry mouth, cough, or scratchy throat, and you may feel irritable. The nicotine patch or gum may help with cravings (see Table 11-6).
- *Thoughts.* Get your mind off tobacco. Exercise and do things you enjoy.
- *Keep a list.* Keep a list of "slips" and near-slips, what caused them, and what you can learn from them.
- *Focus on the benefits of quitting:*
  1. At 20 minutes after you quit, blood pressure decreases, pulse rate drops, and the body temperature of your hands and feet increases.
  2. At 12 hours, the carbon monoxide level in your blood drops to normal, and the oxygen level in your blood increases to normal.
  3. At 24 hours, your chance of a heart attack decreases.
  4. At 48 hours, nerve endings start regrowing, and the ability to smell and taste is enhanced.
  5. At 2 weeks to 3 months, your circulation improves; walking becomes easier; lung function increases; and coughing, sinus congestion, fatigue, and shortness of breath decrease.
  6. At 1 year, your risk of heart disease decreases to half that of a smoker.
  7. By 10 to 15 years, your risk of stroke, lung and other cancers, and early death returns to nearly the level of people who have never smoked.

Sources: Agency for Healthcare Research and Quality: *Help for smokers and other tobacco users: consumer guide,* Washington, DC, May 2008, US Public Health Service. Retrieved from *www.ahrq.gov/consumer/tobacco/helpsmokers.htm*; and American Lung Association: Freedom from smoking online. Retrieved from *www.lungusa.org.*

TABLE 11-6 **DRUG THERAPY**

Smoking Cessation*

Agents	Common Side Effects	Considerations
Nicotine Replacement Agents		
Nicotine Gum (OTC) Nicorette 2 mg, 4 mg • Use 12 wk or more • Use 9-12 pieces/day • Maximum dose: 30 pieces of 2 mg, 20 pieces of 4 mg	Hiccups, mouth ulcers, indigestion, jaw pain	Specific 30-min chewing regimen with periods of holding the gum between cheek and teeth. Avoid food and drink 15 min before and during use.
Nicotine Lozenge (OTC) Commit 2 mg, 4 mg • Use 8-12 wk or more • Use 1 lozenge q1-2hr tapering to 1 lozenge q4-8hr in 12 wk	Nausea and indigestion, hiccups, headache, cough, mouth soreness, flatulence	Dissolves in the mouth in 20-30 min. Chewing and swallowing the lozenge increases GI side effects. Avoid food and drink during use.
Nicotine Patch (OTC) NicoDerm CQ, Habitrol, Nicotine transdermal system • 18- or 24-hr doses • Use ≥8 wk	Transient itching, burning, and redness at patch site. Sleep disturbances with 24-hr patch	Provides steady level of nicotine and is easy to use. Cannot be used by those with adhesive allergies.
Nicotine Nasal Spray Nicotrol NS • Use up to 6 mo	Nose and throat irritation, sneezing, rhinitis, watery eyes, cough	Requires a prescription. Provides fastest nicotine delivery and highest nicotine levels. Most irritating product.
Nicotine Inhaler Nicotrol nicotine inhalation system • Delivers 4 mg • Use up to 6 mo	Cough. Nose, mouth, and throat irritation. Heartburn and nausea	Requires a prescription. Simulates smoking with mouthpiece and nicotine cartridge. May not be advisable for those with asthma or pulmonary disease.
Non-Nicotine Agents		
Bupropion (Zyban) • 150 mg/day for 3 days, then 150 mg bid • Use 12 wk; can use up to 6 mo or longer	Insomnia, dry mouth, irritability, anorexia	Contraindicated with history of seizures or eating disorders. Promotes weight loss. First choice for smokers with depression.
Varenicline (Chantix)† • 0.5 mg/day for 3 days, 0.5 mg bid for 4 days, then 1 mg bid • Use 12 wk; additional 12 wk recommended for those who stop smoking to increase chance of long-term abstinence	Nausea, sleep disturbances, constipation, flatulence, vomiting, headache	If taken concurrently with nicotine replacement therapy, incidence of nausea, headache, vomiting, dizziness, dyspepsia, and fatigue is increased, but nicotine pharmacokinetics not affected.
Nortriptyline (Aventyl)‡ • 25-75 mg/day • Use 12 wk, longer if depressed	Dry mouth, drowsiness, dizziness	Must have stable ECG. Do not use immediately after MI.
Clonidine (Catapres)‡ • 0.1 mg q6hr PRN for craving	Dry mouth, drowsiness, constipation, hypotension	Used to control craving. Change position slowly to prevent postural hypotension.

*OTC nicotine replacement agents are also available in generic forms. Additional information and patient instructions are available from the American Lung Association at *www.lungusa.org*.
†See the Drug Alert for varenicline on p. 157.
‡Nortriptyline and clonidine are not approved by the U.S. Food and Drug Administration for treatment of smoking cessation but have been used successfully for this purpose.

medications, behavioral approaches, and support.[9] Support the patient by providing the resources needed to continue or start a quit attempt.

A variety of nicotine replacement products can be used to reduce the craving and withdrawal symptoms associated with tobacco cessation (Table 11-6). These agents enable a smoker to reduce nicotine previously obtained from cigarettes with a system that delivers the drug more slowly and eliminates the carcinogens and gases associated with tobacco smoke. Nicotine replacement therapy is generally not recommended for pregnant women and people who have experienced an acute myocardial infarction within 2 weeks, have unstable angina, or have life-threatening dysrhythmias.

Varenicline (Chantix) is a drug used to aid smoking cessation. Varenicline is unique in that it has both agonist and antagonist actions at nicotinic receptors. Its agonist activity at one subtype of nicotinic receptors provides some nicotine effects to ease the withdrawal symptoms. It also prevents stimulation of the dopamine system by blocking another subtype of nicotinic receptors. Thus it eases withdrawal symptoms while blocking the effects of nicotine if a person resumes smoking.

Non-nicotine drugs may also be used in smoking cessation. Bupropion (Zyban) is an antidepressant approved as an aid to quit smoking. It reduces the urge to smoke, reduces some symptoms of withdrawal, and helps prevent weight gain associated with smoking cessation. Nortriptyline (Aventyl) and clonidine (Catapres) are not approved by the U.S. Food and Drug Administration (FDA) for use in smoking cessation, but are used in some cases to reduce withdrawal symptoms and promote cessation.[10]

DRUG ALERT: Varenicline (Chantix) and Bupropion (Zyban)
- Serious neuropsychiatric symptoms such as changes in behavior, hostility, agitation, depressed mood, suicidal thoughts and behavior, and attempted suicide can occur.
- Advise patients to stop taking these drugs and contact a health care provider immediately if they experience any of these symptoms.

Participation in tobacco cessation programs is recommended in conjunction with nicotine replacement therapy. You should be aware of community resources that assist individuals who are motivated to quit. Local chapters of the American Lung Association and the American Cancer Society have information on available programs. Cessation programs may involve hypnosis, acupuncture, behavioral interventions, aversion therapy, group support programs, individual therapy, and self-help options. Behavioral approaches teach patients to avoid high-risk situations for smoking relapse, such as those that promote *cue-induced craving.* Cessation programs also promote development of other coping skills, such as cigarette refusal skills, assertiveness, alternative activities to cope with stress, and use of peer support systems.

Women are less successful than men in quitting smoking. Some of the reasons include concern about weight gain, less responsiveness to nicotine replacement therapy, influences of the menstrual cycle, and inadequate emotional support from others. Smoking-associated environmental cues may be more influential in smoking behavior in women than in men. The identification of gender differences in smoking cessation suggests that women who use nicotine replacement do better with nicotine inhalers than the nicotine patch and that women can increase their chances for quitting by timing their attempt to coincide with the first half of their menstrual cycles.[7]

ALCOHOL

Almost half of Americans ages 12 and older consume alcohol (Fig. 11-2). Although most people use alcohol in moderation, it is estimated that alcoholism, or alcohol dependence, affects 7% of the population.[1] Alcoholism is currently viewed as a chronic, progressive, potentially fatal disease if untreated. Alcohol dependence generally occurs over a period of years and may be preceded by heavy social drinking.

Effects of Use and Complications

Alcohol affects almost all cells of the body and has complex effects on the neurons in the central nervous system (CNS). Alcohol, like other addictive substances, causes increased levels of dopamine in the brain, but it also depresses all areas and functions of the CNS.[11] Alcohol is absorbed directly from the stomach and small intestine. In a moderate drinker the metabolism of alcohol by the liver and the stomach occurs at a relatively constant rate of approximately one drink (7 g of alcohol) per hour. One drink is equal to 12 oz of beer, 5 oz of wine, or 1 oz of distilled spirits. Because women have significantly lower rates of stomach metabolism, they have higher blood alcohol levels than men do after the same amount of alcohol intake.[12]

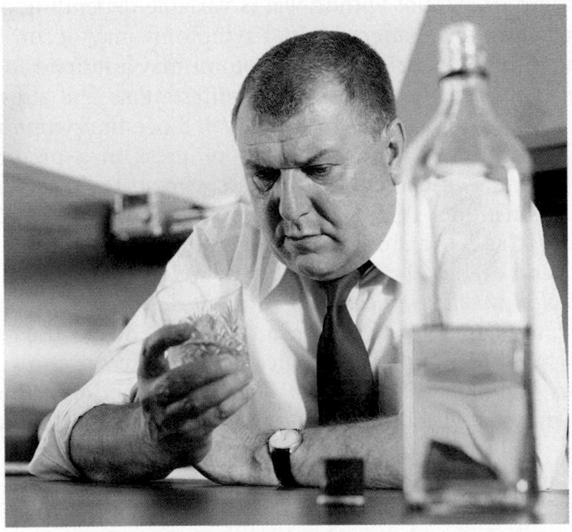

FIG. 11-2 Alcohol is often used to cope with the stresses of life. (Digital Vision/Thinkstock)

The effects of alcohol are related to the concentration of alcohol and individual susceptibility to the drug. The concentration of alcohol in the body can be determined by assessing the blood alcohol concentration (BAC). For the person who is not dependent on alcohol, the BAC is generally predictable of alcohol's effects. The relationship between BAC and behavior is different in a person who has developed tolerance to alcohol and its effects. This tolerant individual is usually able to drink large amounts without obvious impairment and perform complex tasks without problems at BAC levels several times higher than levels that would produce obvious impairment in the nontolerant drinker.[12] In the United States the legal limit for intoxication is 0.08 mg% BAC as measured by a breath device, urinalysis, or blood test.

Individuals who abuse alcohol have many health problems (Table 11-7), which frequently are the reasons they seek health care. One serious complication of chronic alcohol abuse is **Wernicke's encephalopathy,** an inflammatory, hemorrhagic, degenerative condition of the brain. Wernicke's encephalopathy is caused by a thiamine deficiency resulting from poor diet and alcohol-induced suppression of thiamine absorption. This syndrome is readily reversible with administration of thiamine. Untreated or progressive Wernicke's encephalopathy may lead to **Korsakoff's psychosis,** an irreversible form of amnesia characterized by loss of short-term memory and an inability to learn.

Complications may also arise from the interaction of alcohol with commonly prescribed or over-the-counter (OTC) drugs. Drugs that interact with alcohol in an additive manner include antihypertensives, antihistamines, and antianginals. Alcohol taken with aspirin may cause or exacerbate GI bleeding. Alcohol taken with acetaminophen may increase the risk of liver damage. Potentiation and cross-tolerance with other CNS depressants also may occur. *Potentiation* occurs when an additional CNS depressant is taken with alcohol, increasing the effect. *Cross-tolerance,* requiring an increased dose for effect, occurs when an alcohol-dependent individual is alcohol free and receives other CNS depressants.

NURSING AND COLLABORATIVE CARE ALCOHOL DEPENDENCE

ALCOHOL INTOXICATION

Acute alcohol toxicity may occur with binge drinking or the use of alcohol with other CNS depressants. It manifests as an emergency primarily because of the narrow range between the intoxicating, the anesthetic, and the lethal doses of alcohol. Alcohol-induced CNS depression leads to respiratory and circulatory failure.

Obtain as accurate a history as possible and assess for injuries, trauma, diseases, and hypoglycemia. No antidote for alcohol is available. Implement supportive care measures to maintain airway, breathing, and circulation (the ABCs) until detoxification is complete and the alcohol is metabolized. Fre-

TABLE 11-7 EFFECTS OF CHRONIC ALCOHOL ABUSE

Body System	Effects
Central nervous system	Alcoholic dementia. Wernicke's syndrome (confusion, nystagmus, paralysis of ocular muscles, ataxia). Korsakoff's psychosis (confabulation, amnesic disorder). Impairment of cognitive function, psychomotor skills, abstract thinking, and memory. Depression, attention deficit, labile moods, seizures, sleep disturbances.
Peripheral nervous system	Peripheral neuropathy, including pain, paresthesias, weakness.
Immune system	Increased risk for tuberculosis and viral infections. Increased risk for cancer of oral cavity, pharynx, esophagus, liver, colon, rectum, and possibly breast.
Hematologic system	Bone marrow depression, anemia, leukopenia, thrombocytopenia, blood clotting abnormalities.
Musculoskeletal system	Painful, tender swelling of large muscle groups. Painless progressive muscle weakness and wasting; osteoporosis.
Cardiovascular system	Elevated pulse and blood pressure. Decreased exercise tolerance. Cardiomyopathy (irreversible). Increased risk for hemorrhagic stroke, coronary artery disease, hypertension, sudden cardiac death.
Hepatic system	Steatosis* (nausea, vomiting, hepatomegaly). Alcoholic hepatitis* (anorexia, nausea, vomiting, fever, chills, abdominal pain). Cirrhosis, hepatocellular cancer.
Gastrointestinal system	Gastritis, gastroesophageal reflux disease (GERD), peptic ulcer, esophagitis, esophageal varices, enteritis, colitis, Mallory-Weiss tear, chronic pancreatitis.
Nutrition	Decreased appetite, indigestion, malabsorption, vitamin deficiencies (especially thiamine).
Urinary system	Diuretic effect from inhibition of antidiuretic hormone.
Endocrine and reproductive systems	Altered gonadal function, testicular atrophy, decreased beard growth, decreased libido, diminished sperm count, gynecomastia, glucose intolerance.
Integumentary system	Palmar erythema, spider angiomas, rosacea, rhinophyma.

*In the early stages of the disease this is reversible if the person quits drinking.

quently monitor vital signs and level of consciousness. Treat alcohol-induced hypotension with IV fluids. Do not give stimulants to an intoxicated patient. In addition, do not give other depressants because of their additive effects.

Patients experiencing hypoglycemia are given glucose-containing IV solutions. Glucose administration may precipitate Wernicke's encephalopathy in a previously unaffected patient. To identify Wernicke's encephalopathy in the patient with chronic alcoholism, assess the patient for eye abnormalities (e.g., nystagmus, paralysis of the lateral rectus muscles), ataxia, and confusion.

Because the intoxicated patient may have symptoms similar to those of encephalopathy and because untreated encephalopathy may progress to Korsakoff's psychosis, administer IV thiamine before or with IV glucose solutions to all intoxicated patients. Many patients also have decreased serum magnesium levels and other signs of malnutrition, so health care providers frequently add multivitamins and magnesium to the IV fluids.

TABLE 11-8 CLINICAL MANIFESTATIONS AND TREATMENT OF ALCOHOL WITHDRAWAL

Clinical Manifestations	Drug Treatment
Minor Withdrawal Syndrome	
Tremulousness, anxiety ↑ Heart rate ↑ Blood pressure Sweating Nausea Hyperreflexia Insomnia ↑ Hyperactivity without seizures	Benzodiazepines (such as chlordiazepoxide [Librium], lorazepam [Ativan], or diazepam [Valium]) to stabilize vital signs, reduce anxiety, and prevent seizures and delirium Thiamine (prevents Wernicke's encephalopathy) Multivitamins (folic acid, B vitamins) Magnesium sulfate (if serum magnesium is low) IV glucose solution
Major Withdrawal Syndrome	
Visual or auditory hallucinations Gross tremors Seizures Alcohol withdrawal delirium	Continued use of benzodiazepines Carbamazepine (Tegretol) or phenytoin (Dilantin) to treat seizures Antipsychotic agents (e.g., chlorpromazine [Thorazine], haloperidol [Haldol]) if psychosis persists after benzodiazepine administration

Agitation and anxiety are common. Stay with the patient as much as possible, orienting to reality as necessary. Assess the patient for increasing belligerence and a potential for violence. Because the patient is also at risk for injury because of lack of coordination and impaired judgment, use protective measures. It is critical to continue assessment and interventions until the BAC has fallen to at least 100 mg/dL (0.10 mg%) and until any associated disorders or injuries have been ruled out.

ALCOHOL WITHDRAWAL SYNDROME

A patient with alcohol dependence who is hospitalized for any condition can develop *alcohol withdrawal syndrome* when the ingestion of alcohol is abruptly stopped. The onset of signs and symptoms of alcohol withdrawal is variable depending on the patient's drinking pattern. Initial symptoms may occur 4 to 6 hours after the last drink, and symptoms may last up to 14 days. Table 11-8 presents the clinical manifestations and suggested drug treatment for alcohol withdrawal. Since the symptoms of alcohol withdrawal do not always progress in a predictable manner, use a clinical withdrawal assessment tool, such as the Clinical Institute Withdrawal Assessment of Alcohol Scale, Revised (CIWA-Ar), to determine treatment (see Table 11-9 on p. 162 and eTable 11-1 on the website for this chapter).

Alcohol withdrawal delirium is a serious complication that can occur from 30 to 120 hours after the last drink. The greater the patient's dependence on alcohol, the greater the risk of serious withdrawal symptoms. Delirium components include disorientation, visual or auditory hallucinations, and increased hyperactivity without seizures. Death may result from hyperthermia, peripheral vascular collapse, or cardiac failure.[13]

Anticipating withdrawal syndrome in patients is important because alcohol withdrawal delirium can usually be prevented or controlled by administration of benzodiazepines such as

NURSING CARE PLAN 11-1

Patient in Alcohol Withdrawal

NURSING DIAGNOSIS **Acute confusion** *related to* alcohol abuse and delirium *as evidenced by* increased agitation, hallucinations, fluctuations in level of consciousness and psychomotor activity, disorientation, or misperceptions.

PATIENT GOALS
1. Demonstrates decrease in alcohol withdrawal severity.
2. Experiences no injury or complications of acute alcohol withdrawal.
3. Experiences no hallucinations.
4. Experiences no seizures.

Outcomes (NOC)

Substance Withdrawal Severity
- Substance cravings ___
- Agitation ___
- Hyperreflexia ___
- Tremors ___
- Change in vital signs ___
- Disorientation ___
- Altered level of consciousness ___
- Difficulty interpreting environmental stimuli ___
- Misinterpretation of cues ___
- Sleeplessness ___
- Hallucinations ___
- Seizures ___

Measurement Scale
1 = Severe
2 = Substantial
3 = Moderate
4 = Mild
5 = None

Distorted Thought Self-Control
- Asks for validation of reality ___
- Reports decrease in hallucinations or delusions ___
- Perceives environment accurately ___
- Exhibits logical thought flow patterns ___
- Exhibits reality-based thinking ___
- Exhibits appropriate thought content ___

Measurement Scale
1 = Never demonstrated
2 = Rarely demonstrated
3 = Sometimes demonstrated
4 = Often demonstrated
5 = Consistently demonstrated

Interventions (NIC) and *Rationales*

Substance Use Treatment: Alcohol Withdrawal
- Monitor vital signs during withdrawal *to identify extreme autonomic nervous system response.*
- Administer antiseizure drugs or sedatives *to prevent alcohol withdrawal delirium and relieve other symptoms during withdrawal.*
- Administer vitamin therapy *to prevent Wernicke's syndrome.*
- Address hallucinations in a therapeutic manner *to provide reality orientation.*
- Determine CIWA-Ar score every 4 hours until it is less than 8 for 24 hours *to assess need for medications.*
- Provide emotional support to patient/family *to decrease anxiety.*

Seizure Precautions
- Keep suction, Ambu-bag, and oral or nasopharyngeal airway at bedside *to establish respiratory function after seizure activity.*
- Use padded side rails and keep side rails up *to prevent injury during seizure activity.*

Delirium Management
- Monitor neurologic status on an ongoing basis *to determine appropriate interventions.*
- Verbally acknowledge the patient's fears and feelings to *decrease anxiety.*
- Provide patient with information about what is happening and what can be expected to occur in the future *to assist in reality orientation.*
- Maintain a well-lit environment that reduces sharp contrasts and shadows *to reduce external stimuli.*
- Remove stimuli, when possible, that create misperception in a particular patient (e.g., pictures on the wall or television) *to reduce misinterpretation of environment.*
- Inform patient of person, place, and time *to promote orientation.*
- Use environmental cues (e.g., signs, pictures, clocks, calendars, and color coding of environment) *to stimulate memory, reorient, and promote appropriate behavior.*

NURSING DIAGNOSIS **Ineffective self-health management** *related to* inadequate coping mechanisms and resources *as evidenced by* abuse of alcohol

PATIENT GOALS
1. Acknowledges a substance abuse problem
2. Commits to alcohol cessation
3. Identifies positive coping mechanisms and resources to use during alcohol abstinence

Outcomes (NOC)

Alcohol Abuse Cessation Behavior
- Expresses willingness to stop alcohol use ___
- Develops effective strategies to eliminate alcohol use ___
- Commits to alcohol elimination strategies ___
- Uses strategies to cope with withdrawal symptoms ___
- Uses effective coping mechanisms ___
- Adjusts lifestyle to promote alcohol elimination ___
- Obtains assistance from health professional ___
- Uses available support groups ___
- Eliminates alcohol use ___

Measurement Scale
1 = Never demonstrated
2 = Rarely demonstrated
3 = Sometimes demonstrated
4 = Often demonstrated
5 = Consistently demonstrated

Interventions (NIC) and *Rationales*

Substance Use Treatment
- Encourage patient to take control over own behavior *to change undesired behaviors.*
- Discuss with patient the impact of substance use on medical condition or general health *to promote acknowledgment of consequences of use.*
- Identify constructive goals with patient *to provide alternatives to the use of substances to reduce stress.*
- Assist patient to learn alternative methods of coping with stress or emotional distress *to reduce substance use.*
- Identify support groups in the community for long-term substance abuse treatment *to promote continued abstinence.*

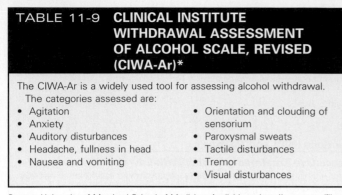

TABLE 11-9 CLINICAL INSTITUTE WITHDRAWAL ASSESSMENT OF ALCOHOL SCALE, REVISED (CIWA-Ar)*

The CIWA-Ar is a widely used tool for assessing alcohol withdrawal. The categories assessed are:

- Agitation
- Anxiety
- Auditory disturbances
- Headache, fullness in head
- Nausea and vomiting
- Orientation and clouding of sensorium
- Paroxysmal sweats
- Tactile disturbances
- Tremor
- Visual disturbances

Source: University of Maryland School of Medicine. Available at *http://umem.org/files/uploads/1104212257_CIWA-Ar.pdf*.
*evolve The complete CIWA-Ar and instructions for how to use it are presented in eTable 11-1 (available on the website for this chapter).

chlordiazepoxide (Librium) or lorazepam (Ativan).[13] A quiet, calm environment is important to prevent exacerbation of symptoms. Avoid the use of restraints and IV lines whenever possible. Supportive care is needed to ensure adequate rest and nutrition. The nursing care for a patient in alcohol withdrawal is presented in NCP 11-1 on p. 161.

OTHER DRUGS OF ABUSE

STIMULANTS

Frequently abused stimulants include cocaine and amphetamines. The use of cocaine is illegal, but amphetamines may be prescribed for the treatment of narcolepsy, attention deficit disorders, and weight control. All stimulants work in part by increasing the amount of dopamine in the brain, producing euphoria, alertness, and rapid dependence (see Table 11-10). Cocaine and amphetamines also stimulate the peripheral nervous and cardiovascular systems, thus creating adrenalin-like effects.[11]

Caffeine is the most widely used psychoactive substance in the world, but it is very weak when compared with the other stimulants. It is not regulated, and its use is safe in most people. Recently, more problems with caffeine have occurred because of high doses in popular “power” drinks. Caffeine dependence in a hospitalized patient can result in withdrawal headaches after general anesthesia or during restrictions on usual coffee or tea intake.

NURSING AND COLLABORATIVE CARE STIMULANT ABUSE

OVERDOSE

Almost 500,000 people are treated each year for cocaine and amphetamine use.[1] At high levels of overdose, the patient experiences restlessness, paranoia, agitated delirium, confusion, and repetitive stereotyped behaviors. Death is often related to stroke, dysrhythmias, or myocardial infarction.[14]

Emergency management of cocaine and amphetamine toxicity depends on the clinical manifestations at the time of treatment (Table 11-11). Therapy may be complicated by the possibility that the patient has combined the use of stimulants with heroin, alcohol, or phencyclidine hydrochloride (PCP). A specific antidote for cocaine and amphetamine toxicity is not available.

WITHDRAWAL

It is unusual for an individual dependent on stimulants to be hospitalized for management of withdrawal symptoms. However, you may identify withdrawal symptoms in a patient dependent on cocaine or amphetamines who is hospitalized for other health problems. Withdrawal from cocaine and amphetamines usually causes few physical symptoms, but fatigue, prolonged sleep, and depression occur in some individuals (see Table 11-10). Craving for the drug is intense during the first hours to days of drug cessation and may continue for weeks. Treatment is supportive.

DEPRESSANTS

Commonly abused depressants include sedative-hypnotics and opioids. With the exception of alcohol and some federally regulated drugs, most CNS depressants are medically useful. These drugs are widely recognized for their rapid development of tolerance and dependence and for medical emergencies involving overdose and withdrawal.

Sedative-Hypnotics

Commonly abused sedative-hypnotic agents include barbiturates, benzodiazepines, and barbiturate-like drugs. Barbiturates are preferred as recreational drugs because they more frequently produce euphoric effects. Sedative-hypnotic drugs depress the CNS, causing sedation at low doses and sleep at high doses. Excessive amounts produce an initial euphoria and an intoxication that resembles that of alcohol. The effects of sedative-hypnotics are presented in Table 11-10.

Tolerance develops rapidly to the effects of the drug, requiring higher doses to achieve euphoria. Tolerance may not develop to the brainstem-depressant effects. As a result, an increased dose may trigger hypotension and respiratory depression, resulting in death.[15]

Health problems resulting from the use of sedative-hypnotics are identified in Table 11-2. Complications associated with IV use of the drugs (e.g., blood-borne infections) also occur. An overdose of sedative-hypnotics can cause death from respiratory depression and arrest.

Opioids

Commonly abused opioids are identified in Table 11-10. Individuals dependent on opioids include those who use illegal drugs sold on the street and those who misuse prescription opioids. Heroin is a commonly used street drug. Misusing medications such as oxycodone (OxyContin) and acetaminophen plus hydrocodone (Vicodin) can result in the same harmful consequences as abusing heroin (Fig. 11-3). By acting on opiate receptors and neurotransmitter systems in the CNS, opioids cause CNS depression and have a major effect on the brain reward system. Cross-tolerance among the opioids is common. Cross-tolerance to other CNS depressants does not occur. However, additive effects of other CNS depressants may cause increased CNS depression.

Opioids are usually injected IV, increasing the user’s risk for human immunodeficiency virus (HIV) infection, hepatitis B virus (HBV) infection, and hepatitis C virus (HCV) infection. In addition, drug abuse by any route increases the risk of contracting HIV because of risky sexual behaviors in exchange for drugs or money or because of lack of inhibition. Like all depressants, opioids can cause death from CNS and respiratory

TABLE 11-10 COMMONLY ABUSED ADDICTIVE SUBSTANCES

Substance	Physiologic and Psychologic Effects	Manifestations of Withdrawal	Treatment of Withdrawal
Stimulants			
Cocaine and Amphetamines			
Cocaine (street names: crack, snow, nose candy, coke, flake) dextroamphetamine (Dexedrine) methamphetamine (Desoxyn) methylphenidate (Ritalin) phentermine (Adipex-P)	*Early:* euphoria, grandiosity, excitation, restlessness, insomnia; tachycardia, hypertension, angina, dysrhythmias; dyspnea, tachypnea; sexual arousal, delayed orgasm; anorexia *Long-term:* depression, hallucinations, tremors, myocardial infarction, heart failure, cardiomyopathy; lung congestion; rhinorrhea; loss of interest in sexual activity	Severe craving, severely depressed mood, exhaustion, prolonged sleep, vivid dreams, apathy, irritability, disorientation	No specific drug therapy is effective in treating withdrawal. Supportive care includes taking measures to decrease agitation and restlessness in the early phase and allowing the patient to sleep and eat as needed in later phases. Refer to psychotherapy or behavioral therapy once stable.
Depressants			
Sedative-Hypnotics			
Barbiturates: secobarbital (Seconal), pentobarbital (Nembutal), amobarbital (Amytal) *Benzodiazepines:* diazepam (Valium), chlordiazepoxide (Librium), alprazolam (Xanax) *Nonbarbiturates-nonbenzodiazepines:* methaqualone (Quaalude), chloral hydrate (Somnote)	Initial relaxation, emotional lability, decreased inhibitions, drowsiness, lack of coordination, impaired judgment, slurred speech, hypotension, bradycardia, bradypnea, constricted pupils	*Early:* Weakness, restlessness, insomnia, hyperthermia, orthostatic hypotension, confusion, disorientation *Days 3-5:* Major convulsive episodes, psychotic delirium, exhaustion, cardiovascular collapse, death	Stabilize on phenobarbital or a long-acting benzodiazepine. Gradually taper dose after stabilization. Supportive care includes measures to ensure patient safety and comfort, frequent assessment of neurologic status and vital signs, and provision of reassurance and orientation. Motivate the patient to engage in long-term treatment and refer to psychotherapy or behavioral therapy once stable.
Opioids			
Heroin (street names: brown sugar, dope, horse, junk, mud, smack), morphine, opium, codeine, fentanyl (Sublimaze), meperidine (Demerol), hydromorphone (Dilaudid), pentazocine (Talwin), oxycodone (OxyContin), methadone (Dolophine)	Analgesia, euphoria, drowsiness, detachment from environment, relaxation, constricted pupils, constipation, nausea, decreased respiratory rate, slurred speech, impaired judgment, decreased sexual and aggressive drives	Watery eyes, dilated pupils, runny nose, yawning, tremors, muscle and joint pain, chills, fever, diaphoresis, insomnia, tachycardia, hypertension, nausea, vomiting, diarrhea, abdominal cramps, food cravings	Methadone in decreasing doses is used during detoxification to decrease symptoms. Symptom management includes bismuth subsalicylate (Kaopectate) for diarrhea, acetaminophen (Tylenol) for muscle aches, and clonidine (Catapres) for generalized symptoms. Once stable, continued use of opioid agonists (methadone), opioid antagonists (naltrexone [ReVia]), or mixed opioid agonists-antagonists (buprenorphine [Subutex, Suboxone]) is recommended under outpatient supervision.
Cannabis			
Marijuana (street names: pot, reefer, weed, herb), hashish (street names: hash, hemp)	Euphoria, sedation, hallucinations	Flulike illness, disturbed sleep, irritability, anxiety, insomnia, tremor, anorexia	No specific drug therapy is effective in treating withdrawal. Supportive care includes measures to ensure patient comfort, including analgesics and hydration. Benzodiazepines are used for symptomatic relief. Refer to psychotherapy or behavioral therapy once stable.

depression. Other complications associated with opioid use are presented in Table 11-2.

NURSING AND COLLABORATIVE CARE DEPRESSANT ABUSE

OVERDOSE

Unintentional overdose frequently occurs with recreational use of depressants because of the unpredictability in potency and purity. If the patient has ingested multiple substances, a complex and potentially confusing clinical picture can result. Serum and urine drug screens may be helpful in identifying the type and amounts of drugs present in the body. The first priority of care in overdose is always the patient's ABCs. Continuous monitoring of neurologic status, including level of consciousness, and respiratory and cardiovascular function is critical until the patient is stable.[15] Emergency management of depressant drug overdose is presented in Table 11-12.

SEDATIVE-HYPNOTICS. Overdoses of benzodiazepines are treated with flumazenil (Romazicon), a specific benzodiazepine antagonist. Flumazenil is used with caution because it can cause seizures in patients with physical dependence on benzodiaze-

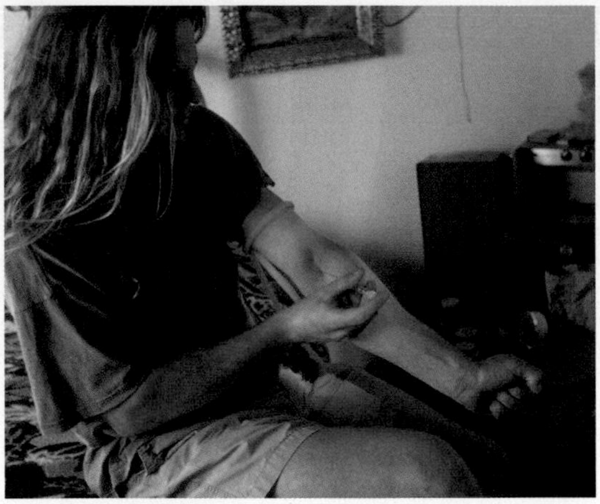

FIG. 11-3 Use of oxycodone injections has increased rapidly. (Doug Menuez/Photodisc/Thinkstock)

pines. Because flumazenil may have a shorter duration of action than some benzodiazepines, doses may need to be repeated until the benzodiazepine is metabolized.

There are no known antagonists to counteract the effects of barbiturates or other sedative-hypnotic drugs. The patient who has overdosed on sedative-hypnotics other than benzodiazepines must be treated aggressively. Dialysis may be required to decrease the drug level and to prevent irreversible CNS depressant effects and death. Gastric lavage and administration of activated charcoal may be instituted if the drug was taken orally within the previous hour. CNS stimulants are avoided, since their use is associated with higher mortality rates.

OPIOIDS. A patient with an opioid overdose can be seen at the emergency department in a coma and respiratory arrest. A toxicologic blood or urine screen may be helpful to identify the specific drug, but treatment is not delayed for toxicology results. Death can occur if the overdose is not treated. An opioid antagonist such as naloxone (Narcan) should be given as soon as life support is instituted. Monitor the patient closely because naloxone has a shorter duration of action than most opioids. The patient may have a mixed drug ingestion that does not respond to opioid antagonists.

TABLE 11-11 EMERGENCY MANAGEMENT

Cocaine and Amphetamine Toxicity

Assessment Findings	Interventions
Cardiovascular • Palpitations • Tachycardia • Hypertension • Dysrhythmias • Myocardial ischemia or infarction **Central Nervous System** • Feeling of impending doom • Euphoria • Agitation • Combativeness • Seizures • Hallucinations • Confusion • Paranoia • Fever **Other** • Track marks • Consumption of bags of cocaine	• Ensure patent airway. • Anticipate need for intubation if respiratory distress evident. • Establish IV access and initiate fluid replacement as appropriate. • Obtain a 12-lead ECG and initiate ECG monitoring. • Treat ventricular dysrhythmias as appropriate with lidocaine, bretylium (Bretylol), or procainamide (Pronestyl). • Hypertension and chest pain may require administration of nitroprusside (Nipride) or phentolamine (Regitine). • Aspirin may be administered to lower the risk of myocardial infarction. • Administer IV diazepam (Valium) or lorazepam (Ativan) for seizures. • Administer IV antipsychotic drugs for psychosis and hallucinations. • Naloxone (Narcan) IV should be given if CNS depression is present and concurrent opioid use is suspected. • Monitor vital signs and level of consciousness. • Initiate cooling measures for hyperthermia.

TABLE 11-12 EMERGENCY MANAGEMENT

Depressant Drug Overdose

Assessment Findings	Interventions
• Aggressive behavior • Agitation • Confusion • Lethargy • Stupor • Hallucinations • Depression • Slurred speech • Pinpoint pupils • Nystagmus • Seizures • Needle tracks • Cold, clammy skin • Rapid, weak pulse • Slow or rapid shallow respirations • Decreased oxygen saturation • Hypotension • Dysrhythmias • ECG changes • Cardiac or respiratory arrest	• Ensure patent airway. • Anticipate intubation if respiratory distress evident. • Establish IV access. • Obtain temperature. • Obtain 12-lead ECG and initiate continuous ECG monitoring. • Obtain information about substance (name, route, when taken, amount). • Obtain specific drug levels or comprehensive toxicology screen. • Obtain a health history, including drug use and allergies. • Administer antidotes as appropriate. • Perform gastric lavage if necessary. • Administer activated charcoal and cathartics as appropriate. • Monitor vital signs, level of consciousness, and oxygen saturation.

WITHDRAWAL

SEDATIVE-HYPNOTICS. Withdrawal from sedative-hypnotics can be life threatening. The manifestations are nearly identical to those of alcohol withdrawal (see Table 11-8). Because the patient may experience delirium, seizures, and respiratory and cardiac arrest within 24 hours after the last dose, close monitoring in an inpatient setting is often required[16] (see Table 11-10). Mild to moderate symptoms can persist for 2 to 3 weeks after a 3- to 5-day period of acute symptoms.

OPIOIDS. Withdrawal from opioids occurs with decreased amounts or cessation of the drug after prolonged moderate to heavy use. The administration of an opioid antagonist, such as naloxone, will also cause withdrawal symptoms in dependent individuals. Symptoms of withdrawal are not usually life threatening but can be severe, depending on the potency of the abused opioid, route of administration, and duration of use (see Table 11-10). Treatment is based on symptoms and may require the use of medications. Methadone (Dolophine) in decreasing doses is the drug used most often during detoxification to decrease symptoms.

CANNABIS

Cannabis, called marijuana or hashish, is the most widely used illicit drug in North America.[1] Patterns of use are similar to those of alcohol in that there is occasional use, misuse resulting in temporary problems, and abuse or dependence associated with a high potential for future problems.

The key active ingredient in cannabis responsible for most of the psychoactive effects is tetrahydrocannabinol (THC). Two THC preparations, dronabinol (Marinol) and nabilone (Cesamet), are available by prescription to control nausea and vomiting resulting from cancer chemotherapy. Dronabinol may also be used to stimulate the appetite in patients with acquired immunodeficiency syndrome (AIDS). Some states have legalized marijuana use for specified health problems. At low to moderate doses, THC produces fewer physiologic and psychologic alterations than do other classes of psychoactive drugs, including alcohol. Health problems caused by heavy use are identified in Table 11-2.

In the patient with acute marijuana intoxication, perform a physical examination and a thorough history. An individual with marijuana intoxication is seldom hospitalized. Panic, flashbacks, and toxic reactions related to the use of marijuana are managed by providing a quiet environment and supporting and reassuring the patient by explaining what is happening. The patient needs to understand that the level of intoxication may fluctuate over several days as metabolites are released.

You may identify withdrawal symptoms in a patient dependent on cannabis who is hospitalized for other health problems. Withdrawal usually causes few physical symptoms, but some patients have flu-like illness, disturbed sleep, and tremors[17] (see Table 11-10). Treatment is supportive.

NURSING MANAGEMENT SUBSTANCE ABUSE

NURSING ASSESSMENT

Any patient with substance dependence who is hospitalized for any condition can develop withdrawal syndrome when the ingestion of the substance is abruptly stopped. Early recognition and identification of withdrawal syndrome are crucial to successful treatment outcomes for any health problem. Hospitalization also provides a chance to address substance use, and for many patients, controlling their health problems requires addressing their substance use.

Question every patient about the use of all substances, including prescribed medications, OTC drugs, caffeine, tobacco, and recreational drugs. Screen for alcohol use using a validated screening questionnaire. Although a variety of screening tools are available, one culturally sensitive tool that is easily used by nurses to identify alcohol dependence is the Alcohol Use Disorders Identification Test (AUDIT) (Table 11-13). A score of 8 points or less is considered nonalcoholic, whereas 9 points or above indicates alcoholism. Another frequently used instrument is the Drug Abuse Screening Test (DAST-10) questionnaire (Table 11-14).

Take a history in a setting that ensures privacy and avoids interruption. To obtain accurate information, use open and nonjudgmental communication with the patient. Ask questions in a way that lets the patient know that you find a behavior normal or at least understandable. You might say, "Given your situation, I wonder if you have been using anything to help relieve your stress." You may also collect a history from any available collateral sources (e.g., spouse) because patients often underreport or minimize their alcohol and drug use.

Reassure the patient that all information will remain confidential and will be used only to provide safe care. The substance-abusing patient may be afraid of losing control of drug administration and may be concerned that substance use will be reported to legal authorities. Inform the patient that federal privacy laws prohibit nurses and other health care providers from disclosing any treatment of substance abuse without the patient's specific written consent.

TABLE 11-13 ALCOHOL USE DISORDERS IDENTIFICATION TEST (AUDIT)

Please answer each question by checking one of the circles in the second column.		**Score**
1. How often do you have a drink containing alcohol?	o Never	(0)
	o Monthly or less	(1)
	o 2-4 times per month	(2)
	o 2-4 times per week	(3)
	o 4+ times per week	(4)
2. How many drinks containing alcohol do you have on a typical day when you are drinking?	o 1 or 2	(0)
	o 3 or 4	(1)
	o 5 or 6	(2)
	o 7 to 9	(3)
	o 10 or more	(4)
3. How often do you have six or more drinks on one occasion?	o Never	(0)
	o Less than monthly	(1)
	o Monthly	(2)
	o Weekly	(3)
	o Daily or almost daily	(4)
4. How often during the last year have you found that you were not able to stop drinking once you had started?	o Never	(0)
	o Less than monthly	(1)
	o Monthly	(2)
	o Weekly	(3)
	o Daily or almost daily	(4)
5. How often in the last year have you failed to do what was normally expected of you because you were drinking?	o Never	(0)
	o Less than monthly	(1)
	o Monthly	(2)
	o Weekly	(3)
	o Daily or almost daily	(4)
6. How often during the last year have you needed a first drink in the morning to get yourself going after a heavy drinking session?	o Never	(0)
	o Less than monthly	(1)
	o Monthly	(2)
	o Weekly	(3)
	o Daily or almost daily	(4)
7. How often during the last year have you had a feeling of guilt or remorse about drinking?	o Never	(0)
	o Less than monthly	(1)
	o Monthly	(2)
	o Weekly	(3)
	o Daily or almost daily	(4)
8. How often during the last year have you been unable to remember what happened the night before because you had been drinking?	o Never	(0)
	o Less than monthly	(1)
	o Monthly	(2)
	o Weekly	(3)
	o Daily or almost daily	(4)
9. Have you or someone else been injured as a result of your drinking?	o No	(0)
	o Yes, but not in the last year	(2)
	o Yes, during the last year	(4)
10. Has a relative, friend, or other health worker been concerned about your drinking or suggested that you cut down?	o No	(0)
	o Yes, but not in the last year	(2)
	o Yes, during the last year	(4)

Scoring for AUDIT: Questions 1 through 8 are scored 0, 1, 2, 3, or 4. Questions 9 and 10 are scored 0, 2, or 4 only. The minimum score (nondrinkers) is 0 and the maximum possible score is 40. A score of 9 or more indicates hazardous or harmful alcohol consumption.

Source: Saunders JB, Aasland OG, Babor TF, et al: Development of the Alcohol Use Disorders Identification Test (AUDIT), WHO collaborative project on early detection of people with harmful alcohol consumption, II, *Addiction* 88:791, 1993. Retrieved from *http://pubs.niaaa.nih.gov/publications/Practitioner/CliniciansGuide2005/clinicians_guide11.htm.*

TABLE 11-14 DRUG ABUSE SCREENING TEST (DAST-10)

In the last 12 months:

1. Have you used drugs other than those required for medical reasons?	No	Yes
2. Do you abuse more than one drug at a time?	No	Yes
3. Are you always able to stop using drugs when you want to?	No	Yes
4. Have you had "blackouts" or "flashbacks" as a result of drug use?	No	Yes
5. Do you ever feel bad or guilty about your drug use?	No	Yes
6. Does your spouse (or parents) ever complain about your involvement with drugs?	No	Yes
7. Have you neglected your family because of your use of drugs?	No	Yes
8. Have you engaged in illegal activities in order to obtain drugs?	No	Yes
9. Have you ever experienced withdrawal symptoms or felt sick when you stopped taking drugs?	No	Yes
10. Have you had medical problems as a result of your drug use?	No	Yes

TABLE 11-15 SIGNS SUGGESTING SUBSTANCE ABUSE

- Fatigue
- Insomnia
- Headaches
- Seizure disorder
- Changes in mood
- Anorexia, weight loss
- Vague physical complaints
- Overabundant use of mouthwash or toiletries
- Appearing older than stated age, unkempt appearance
- Leisure activities that involve alcohol and/or other drugs
- Sexual dysfunction, decreased libido, erectile dysfunction
- Trauma secondary to falls, auto accidents, fights, or burns
- Driving while intoxicated (more than one citation suggests dependence)
- Failure of standard doses of sedatives to have a therapeutic effect
- Financial problems, including those related to spending for substances
- Defensive or evasive answers to questions about substance use and its importance in the person's life
- Problems in areas of life function (e.g., frequent job changes; marital conflict, separation, or divorce; work-related accidents, tardiness, absenteeism; legal problems; social isolation, estrangement from friends or family)

During your assessment, observe for patient behaviors that influence history taking such as denial, avoidance, underreporting or minimizing of substance use, or provision of inaccurate information. Possible behaviors and physical complaints suggesting substance dependence are listed in Table 11-15, but these behaviors are not all-inclusive. Even if a patient denies addiction or dependence, if there is any indication of alcohol or other CNS depressant use when a patient is hospitalized, always ask when the patient last used the substance. This information will help you anticipate drug interactions or the time of possible onset of withdrawal symptoms if the patient is indeed dependent on a substance.

Problems associated with substance abuse are often revealed through physical assessment, including assessment of the patient's general appearance and nutritional status and examination of the abdomen; the skin; and the cardiovascular, respiratory, and neurologic systems. Urine and blood drug screenings may be performed in some situations to determine drug use. A complete blood count, serum electrolytes, blood urea nitrogen, creatinine, and hepatic function tests may be done to evaluate for electrolyte imbalances or kidney or liver dysfunction.

NURSING DIAGNOSES

Nursing diagnoses for an individual with substance abuse may include, but are not limited to, those presented in NCP 11-1.

PLANNING

The overall goals are that the patient with a substance abuse problem will (1) have normal physiologic functioning, (2) acknowledge a substance abuse problem, (3) explain the psychologic and physiologic effects of substance use, (4) abstain from the use of addicting substances, and (5) cooperate with a proposed treatment plan.

NURSING IMPLEMENTATION

HEALTH PROMOTION. Your role in health promotion includes prevention and early detection of substance abuse. Teaching about the effects and negative outcomes of substance abuse is essential in preventing this problem. When individuals have substance abuse problems, it is critical to motivate them to enter treatment programs.

ACUTE INTERVENTION. Acute intoxication, overdose, and withdrawal may be seen in acute care situations. Intoxication and overdose may require physiologic support until detoxification can occur. During detoxification the patient is treated to diminish or remove drugs or their effects from the body. Treatments may involve administration of antagonistic drugs, promotion of metabolism and elimination of the drug, or intensive supportive care until the drug is naturally eliminated. Be aware that intoxication and overdose could occur in a hospitalized patient dependent on substances if visitors provide the substances.

You are in a unique position to motivate and facilitate behavior change in people who are abusing substances. When patients seek care for health problems related to substance abuse or when hospitalization interferes with the patient's usual pattern of substance use, the patient's awareness of a substance abuse problem is increased. Intervention by nurses at this time can be a crucial factor in promoting behavior change. Take an active role in performing motivational interviewing and providing counseling aimed at promoting cessation. Document all the interventions in the patient's chart.

AMBULATORY AND HOME CARE. Before treatment and rehabilitation for substance abuse are considered, acute health problems must be resolved. Many of the patients with substance abuse problems that you encounter in hospitals and primary care centers seek care for health problems associated with substance abuse, not for their addiction itself. When you are working in a medical-surgical setting, you usually will not be involved in long-term treatment of patients with substance abuse problems. However, it is your responsibility to identify the problem, motivate the patient to change behavior, and be prepared to refer the patient to inpatient and outpatient programs in the community that provide treatment and rehabilitation. Failure to confront the patient's substance abuse problem, thus enabling the behavior, is a breach of your professional responsibility.

GERONTOLOGIC CONSIDERATIONS

SUBSTANCE ABUSE

Health care providers are much less likely to recognize substance misuse, abuse, and dependence in older adults than in younger adults. Older adults do not fit the image of abusers. In addition, their patterns of misuse of prescription psychoactive agents and alcohol are less commonly seen than those of younger populations. Because the effects of alcohol and drug use can be mistaken for medical conditions common among older adults, such as insomnia, depression, poor nutrition, heart failure, and frequent falls, the substance abuse problem is often not diagnosed and not treated.[18]

Older adults' misuse and abuse of psychoactive agents, either alone or in combination, may cause confusion, disorientation, delirium, memory loss, and neuromuscular impairment. Physiologic changes that accompany aging, such as decreased circulation, metabolism, and excretion, may lead to intoxication at levels that may not have been a problem at a younger age. Withdrawal symptoms that occur in the older adult when alcohol, opioids, or sedative-hypnotics are abruptly stopped may be more severe than in younger individuals. Always consider that behavior changes in older adults may be caused by substance use or withdrawal.

Identification of substance misuse, abuse, and dependence in older adults presents a challenge. Family members are important sources of information. As with all patients, it is important for you to discuss all drug and alcohol use with older adult patients, including OTC, herbal, and homeopathic drug use. Assess the patient's knowledge of medications that are currently being taken.

The older adult may not exhibit the social, legal, and occupational consequences of substance abuse identified by common screening questionnaires. However, the Short Michigan Alcoholism Screening Test–Geriatric Version (SMAST-G) has been developed as a short-form alcoholism-screening instrument for older adults.[19] This tool, available at *http://consultgerirn.org,* can identify those at risk for negative outcomes of alcohol use. The AUDIT and DAST-10 questionnaires (discussed previously) can also be used with or instead of the SMAST-G to identify alcohol and drug abuse or dependence in older adults.

Smoking and other tobacco use is also an issue in older adults. Older adults who have been chronic smokers for decades may feel unable to stop, or they may believe there is no benefit to stopping at an advanced age. However, smoking contributes to and exacerbates many chronic illnesses found in the older adult population. Smoking cessation at any age is beneficial. The clinical practice guideline for treating tobacco use and dependence discussed earlier is appropriate for helping older adults with smoking cessation (see Tables 11-3 to 11-6).

Patient teaching for the older adult includes teaching about the desired effects, possible side effects, and appropriate use of prescribed and OTC drugs. Advise patients not to drink alcohol when using prescribed and OTC drugs. If no medical condition or possible drug interactions preclude the use of alcohol, advise older patients to limit their alcohol intake to one drink per day. When you suspect alcohol or substance dependence in the older patient, refer the patient for treatment. It is a mistaken belief that older people have little to gain from alcohol and drug dependence treatment. The rewards of treatment can lead to greater quality and quantity of life for older adults.

CASE STUDY

Substance Misuse and Abuse

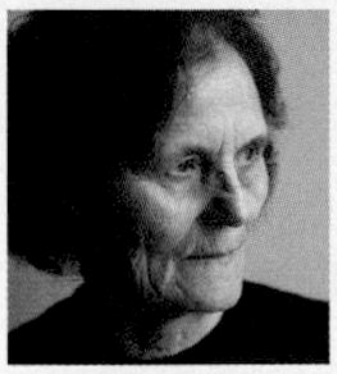

iStockphoto/Thinkstock

Patient Profile

C.M., a 78-year-old white woman, is admitted to the emergency department after falling and injuring her right hip. She has been widowed for 4 years and lives alone. Recently her best friend died. Her only family is a daughter who lives out of town. When contacted by phone, the daughter tells the nurse that her mother has appeared more disoriented and confused over the past few months when she has talked to her on the phone.

Subjective Data

- Is complaining of severe pain in her right hip
- Admits she had some wine in the late afternoon to stimulate her appetite
- Has experienced several falls in the past 2 months
- Reports that she fell after taking her sleeping pill prescribed by her physician because she does not sleep well
- Speech is hesitant and slurred
- Says she smokes about one-half pack of cigarettes a day

Objective Data

Physical Examination

- Oriented to person and place, but not time
- BP 162/94, pulse 92, respirations 24
- Severe pain and tenderness in the right hip region
- Tremors of hands

Diagnostic Tests

- X-ray reveals a subtrochanteric fracture of the right femur requiring surgical repair
- Blood alcohol concentration (BAC) 120 mg/dL (0.12 mg%)
- Complete blood count: hemoglobin 10.6 g/dL, hematocrit 33%

Discussion Questions

1. What other information is needed to assess C.M.'s condition?
2. How should questions regarding substance use be addressed?
3. What factors may contribute to C.M.'s use of psychoactive substances?
4. ***Priority Decision:*** What are the priority nursing interventions during C.M.'s preoperative period?
5. What possible complications and other health problems may become apparent during C.M.'s postoperative recovery?
6. ***Priority Decision:*** What are the priority nursing interventions after C.M.'s surgery?
7. ***Delegation Decision:*** How would you use the following nursing personnel on the postoperative unit to carry out the priority interventions that you identified in question 6: registered nurse (RN), licensed practical nurse (LPN), unlicensed assistive personnel (UAP)?
8. ***Priority Decision:*** Based on the assessment data presented, what are the priority nursing diagnoses? Are there any collaborative problems?

evolve Answers available at *http://evolve.elsevier.com/Lewis/medsurg.*

BRIDGE TO NCLEX EXAMINATION

The number of the question corresponds to the same-numbered outcome at the beginning of the chapter.

1. A person who injects heroin to experience the euphoria that it causes is demonstrating
   - **a.** abuse.
   - **b.** addiction.
   - **c.** tolerance.
   - **d.** addictive behavior.
2. When admitting a patient, the nurse must assess the patient for substance use based on the knowledge that long-term use of addictive substances leads to
   - **a.** the development of coexisting psychiatric illnesses.
   - **b.** a higher risk for complications from underlying health problems.
   - **c.** increased availability of dopamine, resulting in decreased sleep requirements.
   - **d.** potentiation of effects of similar drugs taken when the individual is drug free.
3. The nurse would suspect cocaine overdose in the patient who is experiencing
   - **a.** craving, restlessness, and irritability.
   - **b.** agitation, cardiac dysrhythmias, and seizures.
   - **c.** diarrhea, nausea and vomiting, and confusion.
   - **d.** slow, shallow respirations; hyporeflexia; and blurred vision.
4. The most appropriate nursing intervention for a patient who is being treated for an acute exacerbation of chronic obstructive pulmonary disease who is not interested in quitting smoking is to
   - **a.** accept the patient's decision and not intervene until the patient expresses a desire to quit.
   - **b.** realize that some smokers will never quit, and trying to assist them increases the patient's' frustration.
   - **c.** motivate the patient to quit by describing how continued smoking will worsen the breathing problems.
   - **d.** ask the patient to identify the relevance, risks, and benefits of quitting and what barriers to quitting are present.
5. While caring for a patient who is experiencing alcohol withdrawal, the nurse should *(select all that apply)*
   - **a.** monitor neurologic status on a routine basis.
   - **b.** provide a quiet, nonstimulating, dimly lit environment.
   - **c.** pad the side rails and place suction equipment at the bedside.
   - **d.** orient the patient to environment and person with each contact.
   - **e.** administer antiseizure drugs and sedatives to relieve symptoms during withdrawal.
6. Substance abuse problems in older adults are usually related to
   - **a.** use of drugs and alcohol as a social activity.
   - **b.** misuse of prescribed and over-the-counter drugs and alcohol.
   - **c.** continuing the use of illegal drugs initiated during middle age.
   - **d.** a pattern of binge drinking for weeks or months with periods of sobriety.

1. d, 2. b, 3. b, 4. d, 5. a, c, d, e, 6. b

evolve

For rationales to these answers and even more NCLEX review questions, visit *http://evolve.elsevier.com/Lewis/medsurg.*

REFERENCES

1. Substance Abuse and Mental Health Services Administration: Results from the 2010 national survey on drug use and health. Retrieved from *http://oas.samhsa.gov.*
2. National Institute on Drug Abuse: Prescription drugs: abuse and addiction. Retrieved from *www.nida.nih.gov/PDF/RRPrescription.pdf.*
3. American Psychiatric Association: *The diagnostic and statistical manual of mental disorders (DSM-IV-TR)*, ed 4, Arlington, Va, 2000, The Association. (Classic)
4. Robin C, O'Connell E, Samnaliev M: Overview of substance abuse and healthcare costs. Retrieved from *http://saprp.org/knowledgeassets/knowledge_detail.cfm?KAID=21.*
5. Centers for Disease Control and Prevention: Adult smoking in the U.S. Retrieved from *www.cdc.gov/VitalSigns/pdf/2011-09-vitalsigns.pdf.*
6. US Department of Health and Human Services: How tobacco smoke causes disease: the biology and behavioral basis for smoking-attributable disease: a report of the Surgeon General. Retrieved from *www.surgeongeneral.gov/library/tobaccosmoke/index.html.*
7. American Cancer Society: Women and smoking. Retrieved from *www.cancer.org/Cancer/CancerCauses/TobaccoCancer/WomenandSmoking/index.*
8. Agency for Healthcare Research and Quality: Treating tobacco use and dependence: 2008 update. Retrieved from *www.ncbi.nlm.nih.gov/books/bv.fcgi?rid=hstat2.chapter.28163.*

*9. Reynolds S: Combination therapy most effective for helping smokers quit, *NIDA Notes* 23:7, 2011.

*10. Raupach T, van Schayck C: Pharmacotherapy for smoking cessation: current advances and research topics, *CNS Drugs* 25:371, 2011.

11. National Institute on Drug Abuse: Drugs, brains, and behavior: the science of addiction. Retrieved from *www.nida.nih.gov/scienceofaddiction/brain.html.*
12. Keltner NL, Bostrom CE, McGuinness T: *Psychiatric nursing*, ed 7, St Louis, 2010, Mosby.

*Evidence-based information for clinical practice.

*13. Tovar R: Diagnosis and treatment of alcohol withdrawal, *JCOM* 18:361, 2011.
14. Wood DM, Dargan PI: Putting cocaine use and cocaine-associated cardiac arrhythmias into epidemiological and clinical perspective, *Br J Clin Pharmacol* 69:443, 2010.
15. Lehne RA: *Pharmacology for nursing care*, ed 7, St Louis, 2010, Saunders.
16. Tetrault JM, O'Connor PG: Substance abuse and withdrawal in the critical care setting, *Crit Care Clin* 24:767, 2008.
17. Maldonado JR: An approach to the patient with substance use and abuse, *Med Clin North Am* 94:1169, 2010.
18. Frances RJ: Geriatric addictions, *Am J Geriatr Psychiatry* 19: 681, 2011.
19. Naegle M: Alcohol use screening and assessment for older adults. Retrieved from *http://consultgerirn.org/uploads/File/trythis/try_this_17.pdf.*

RESOURCES

American Lung Association
www.lungusa.org

American Psychiatric Nurses Association
www.apna.org

American Society of Addiction Medicine
www.asam.org

National Council on Alcoholism and Drug Dependence, Inc.
www.ncadd.org

National Institute on Drug Abuse
www.nida.nih.gov

Substance Abuse and Mental Health Services Administration
http://www.samhsa.gov/

Tobacco Information and Prevention Source (TIPS)
www.cdc.gov/tobacco

MANAGING MULTIPLE PATIENTS

Introduction

You are assigned to care for the following five patients on a medical-surgical unit. Your team consists of yourself, a new LPN still on orientation, and an unlicensed assistive personnel (UAP).

Patients

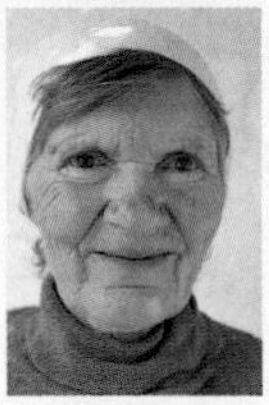

iStockphoto/Thinkstock

A.Z. is a 75-year-old woman who came to the United States from Russia 10 years ago with her daughter, her son-in-law, and their five children. She speaks minimal English, relying on her oldest granddaughter to translate. A.Z., who has a history of diabetes mellitus, was admitted to the hospital yesterday with a diagnosis of heart failure.

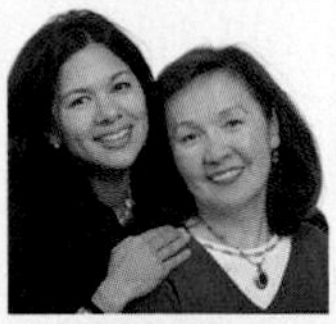

Thomas M. Perkins/Shutterstock.com

M.L. is a 60-year-old Asian woman who was admitted to the hospital with a diagnosis of exacerbation of chronic obstructive pulmonary disease (COPD). She is receiving oxygen at 2 L/min via nasal cannula and her condition is currently stable.

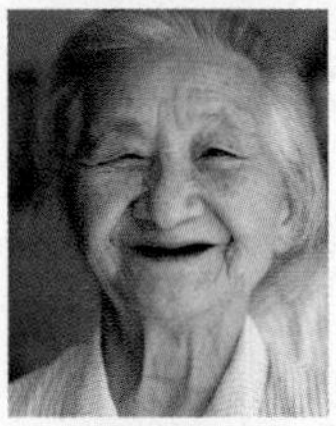

iStockphoto/Thinkstock

L.X. is a 79-year-old Chinese woman who was admitted through the emergency department with a chief complaint of shortness of breath. She was diagnosed with community-acquired pneumonia, which is being treated with IV antibiotics.

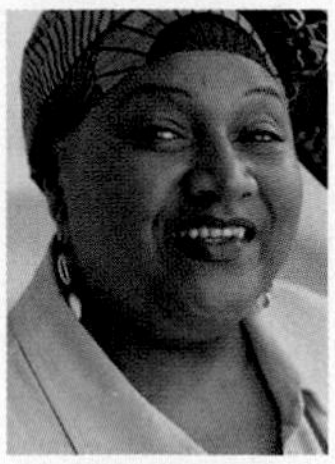

Ryan McVay/Photodisc/Thinkstock

K.C. is a 280-lb (127-kg) 68-year-old African American woman with diabetes who was admitted for an incision and drainage of a right abdominal abscess. She is being discharged on her second postoperative day. Her married daughter will assist with dressing changes at home.

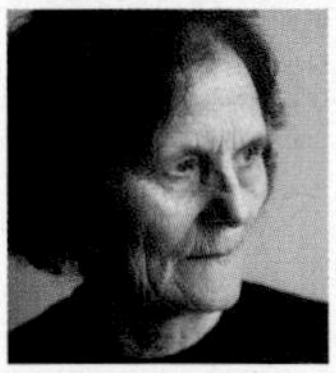

iStockphoto/Thinkstock

C.M. is a 78-year-old white woman who was admitted from the emergency department after falling and fracturing her right hip. She is in Buck's traction and is scheduled to undergo surgical repair later this morning. She has a history of substance abuse and her blood alcohol content (BAC) was 120 mg/dL (0.12 mg%) on admission. The night nurse reports that she has been somewhat confused and restless overnight.

Management Discussion Questions

1. ***Priority Decision:*** After receiving report, which patient should you see first? Provide rationale.
2. ***Delegation Decision:*** Which morning task(s) could you delegate to the LPN *(select all that apply)?*
   a. Obtain a capillary blood glucose reading on K.C.
   b. Assess L.X.'s IV site for signs of phlebitis or infiltration.
   c. Access the hospital's available translation services for A.Z.
   d. Titrate M.L.'s oxygen to obtain a pulse oximetry reading of 95%, as ordered by the health care provider.
3. ***Priority and Delegation Decision:*** When you and the LPN enter A.Z.'s room, you find the patient sitting up in bed with labored respirations. Although you cannot understand what she is saying, you note that she is unable to say more than two words without stopping for a breath. Which initial action would be the most appropriate?
   a. Ask the LPN to get A.Z.'s vital signs while you auscultate her lung sounds.
   b. Administer A.Z.'s cardiac and respiratory medications and reassess her in 30 minutes.
   c. Have the LPN find A.Z.'s granddaughter so that she can translate what A.Z. is trying to tell you.
   d. Ask the LPN to stay with A.Z. while you go to the nurse's station to call A.Z.'s health care provider.

Case Study Progression

A.Z.'s assessment reveals bibasilar crackles, 2+ dependent pitting edema, BP 175/84, pulse 96, RR 32, temp 36.8°C, and pulse oximetry 88% on room air. You administer oxygen at 2 L/min via nasal cannula and obtain an order from A.Z.'s health care provider for furosemide 40 mg IV stat. After administering the diuretic, A.Z.'s granddaughter arrives and you discuss her grandmother's condition. She tells you that her grandmother asked her to bring in potato chips and soda yesterday. She did not think her grandmother should be eating salt, but A.Z. insisted that the dietitian said that she could eat them.

4. On further investigation, the dietitian tells you that a translator was not available when she saw A.Z. yesterday. Because the dietitian did not understand what the patient was saying, she could not respond to any of her questions. She planned to visit A.Z. today when the granddaughter is present. Being a culturally competent nurse, you realize that A.Z. most likely interpreted the dietitian's silence as
   a. agreement with what A.Z. was asking.
   b. demonstrating a lack of respect for A.Z.'s wishes.
   c. a lack of understanding by the dietitian as to what she was asking.
   d. a need for the dietitian to get more information before answering her questions.
5. Which assessment findings might suggest elder mistreatment by L.X.'s son, with whom she lives *(select all that apply)?*
   a. Two sacral ulcers
   b. Asking when her son is coming to visit
   c. Multiple small bruises on her forearms and shins
   d. Matted hair, poor oral hygiene, overgrown toenails
6. Knowing that C.M.'s reported restlessness overnight may indicate acute alcohol withdrawal, you perform a more thorough assessment. Your assessment reveals a score of 11 on the Clinical Institute Withdrawal Assessment for Alcohol Scale. To prevent alcohol delirium, you plan to administer
   a. IV thiamine.
   b. morphine sulfate.
   c. naloxone (Narcan).
   d. lorazepam (Ativan).
7. ***Management Decision:*** The UAP informs you that the LPN is not following hospital protocol when caring for patients at risk for falling. What is your most appropriate action?
   a. Notify the unit manager as soon as possible.
   b. Ask the UAP to explain hospital protocol to the LPN.
   c. Write up the LPN's actions so they are included in her evaluation.
   d. Talk to the LPN about the importance of following hospital protocol to prevent injury in patients at risk for falling.

evolve Answers available at *http://evolve.elsevier.com/Lewis/medsurg.*

SECTION 2

Pathophysiologic Mechanisms of Disease

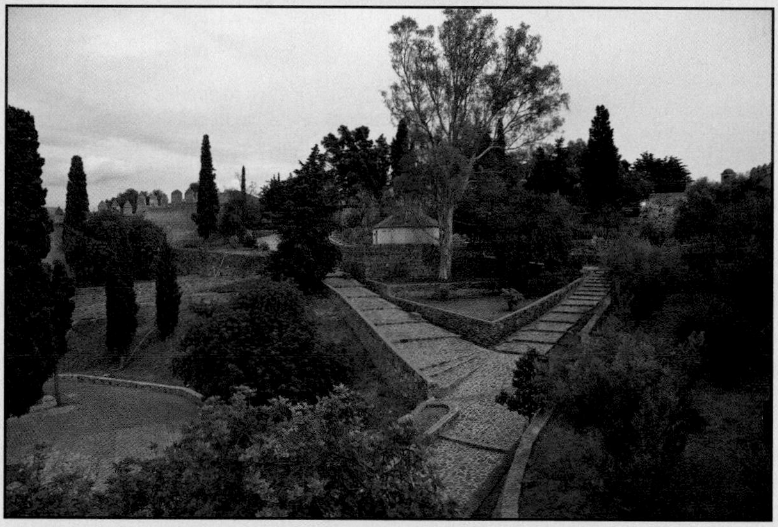

iStockphoto/Thinkstock

When you arrive at a fork in the road, take it.
Yogi Berra

CHAPTER 12

Unless someone like you cares a whole awful lot,
nothing is going to get better. It's not.
Dr. Seuss

Inflammation and Wound Healing

Sharon L. Lewis

evolve WEBSITE

http://evolve.elsevier.com/Lewis/medsurg

- NCLEX Review Questions
- Key Points
- Pre-Test
- Answer Guidelines for Case Study on p. 188
- Rationales for Bridge to NCLEX Examination Questions
- Case Study
  - Patient With Pressure Ulcers
- Nursing Care Plans (Customizable)
  - eNCP 12-1: Patient With a Fever
  - eNCP 12-2: Patient With a Pressure Ulcer
- Concept Map Creator
- Glossary
- Content Updates

eFigures

- eFig. 12-1: Margination, diapedesis, and chemotaxis of white blood cells
- eFig. 12-2: Sequential activation and biologic effects of the complement system
- eFig. 12-3: Granulating wound

eTables

- eTable 12-1: Wound Classification by Etiology
- eTable 12-2: Wound Classification Systems
- eTable 12-3: Braden Scale for Predicting Pressure Sore Risk
- eTable 12-4: Pressure Ulcer Scale for Healing (PUSH)

LEARNING OUTCOMES

1. Describe the inflammatory response, including vascular and cellular responses and exudate formation.
2. Explain local and systemic manifestations of inflammation and their physiologic bases.
3. Describe the drug therapy, nutrition therapy, and nursing management of inflammation.
4. Differentiate among healing by primary, secondary, and tertiary intention.
5. Describe the factors that delay wound healing and common complications of wound healing.
6. Describe the nursing and collaborative management of wound healing.
7. Explain the etiology and clinical manifestations of pressure ulcers.
8. Apply a patient risk assessment for pressure ulcers to measures used to prevent the development of pressure ulcers.
9. Discuss nursing and collaborative management of a patient with pressure ulcers.

KEY TERMS

adhesions, Table 12-8, p. 180
dehiscence, Table 12-8, p. 180
evisceration, Table 12-8, p. 180
fibroblasts, p. 178
hypertrophic scars, Table 12-8, p. 180
inflammatory response, p. 172
pressure ulcer, p. 184
regeneration, p. 177
repair, p. 177
shearing force, p. 184

This chapter focuses on inflammation and wound healing. Pressure ulcer prevention and treatment are also described.

INFLAMMATORY RESPONSE

The **inflammatory response** is a sequential reaction to cell injury. It neutralizes and dilutes the inflammatory agent, removes necrotic materials, and establishes an environment suitable for healing and repair. The term *inflammation* is often but incorrectly used as a synonym for the term *infection.* Inflammation is always present with infection, but infection is not always present with inflammation. However, a person who is neutropenic may not be able to mount an inflammatory response. An infection involves invasion of tissues or cells by microorganisms such as bacteria, fungi, and viruses. In contrast, inflammation can also be caused by heat, radiation, trauma, chemicals, allergens, and an autoimmune reaction.

The mechanism of inflammation is basically the same regardless of the injuring agent. The intensity of the response depends on the extent and severity of injury and on the injured person's reactive capacity. The inflammatory response can be divided into a vascular response, a cellular response, formation of exudate, and healing. Fig. 12-1 illustrates the vascular and cellular response to injury.

Reviewed by Trevah A. Panek, RN, MSN, CCRN, Assistant Professor of Nursing, Saint Francis University, Loretto, Pennsylvania; and Clemma K. Snider, RN, MSN, Assistant Professor, Associate Degree Nursing, Eastern Kentucky University, Richmond, Kentucky.

PATHOPHYSIOLOGY MAP

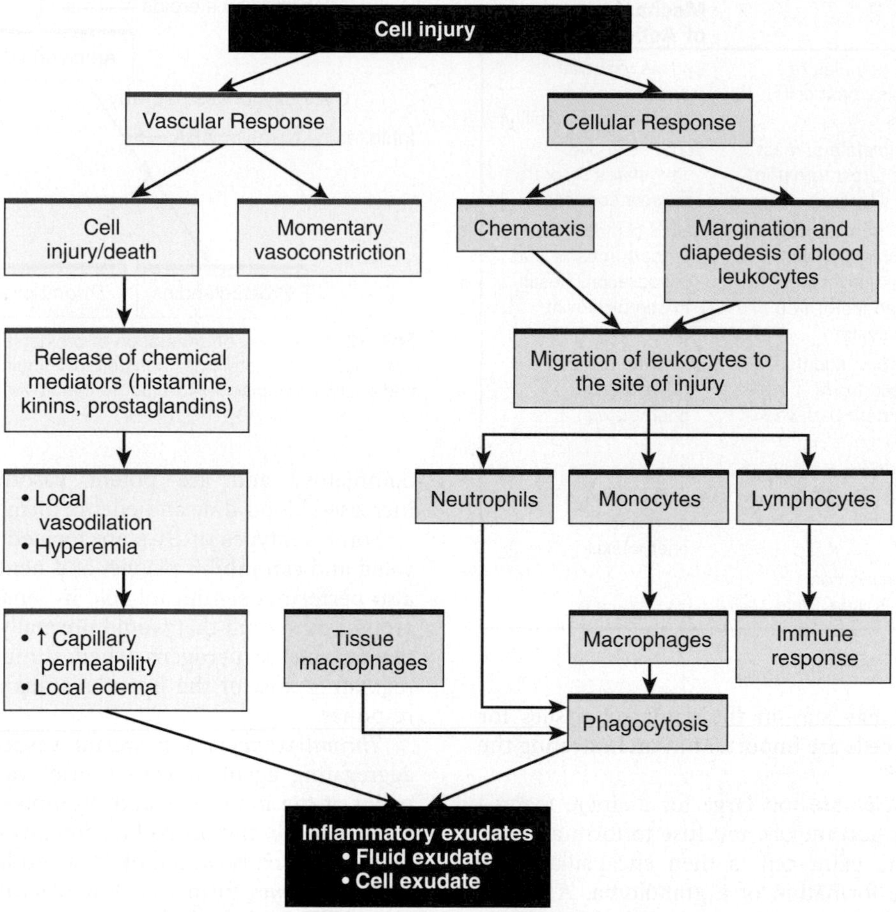

FIG. 12-1 Vascular and cellular responses to tissue injury.

Vascular Response

After cell injury, local arterioles briefly undergo transient vasoconstriction. After release of histamine and other chemicals by the injured cells, the vessels dilate. Chemical mediators cause increased capillary permeability and facilitate fluid movement from capillaries into tissue spaces. Initially composed of serous fluid, this inflammatory exudate later contains plasma proteins, primarily albumin. These proteins exert oncotic pressure that further draws fluid from blood vessels. Both vasodilation and increased capillary permeability are responsible for redness, heat, and swelling at the site of injury.

As the plasma protein fibrinogen leaves the blood, it is activated to fibrin by the products of the injured cells. Fibrin strengthens a blood clot formed by platelets. In tissue the clot functions to trap bacteria, prevent their spread, and serve as a framework for the healing process. Platelets release growth factors that start the healing process.

Cellular Response

Neutrophils and monocytes move from circulation to the site of injury (see Fig. 12-1). *Chemotaxis* is the directional migration of white blood cells (WBCs) to the site of injury, resulting in an accumulation of neutrophils and monocytes at the site. (eFig. 12-1 showing chemotaxis is available on the website for this chapter.)

Neutrophils. Neutrophils are the first leukocytes to arrive at the injury site (usually within 6 to 12 hours). They phagocytize (engulf) bacteria, other foreign material, and damaged cells. With their short life span (24 to 48 hours), dead neutrophils soon accumulate. In time a mixture of dead neutrophils, digested bacteria, and other cell debris accumulates as a creamy substance termed *pus*.

To keep up with the demand for neutrophils, the bone marrow releases more neutrophils into circulation. This results in an elevated WBC count, especially the neutrophil count. Sometimes the demand for neutrophils increases to the extent that the bone marrow releases immature forms of neutrophils *(bands)* into circulation. (Mature neutrophils are called segmented neutrophils.) The finding of increased numbers of band neutrophils in circulation is called a *shift to the left,* which is commonly found in patients with acute bacterial infections. (See Chapter 30 for a discussion of neutrophils.)

Monocytes. Monocytes are the second type of phagocytic cells that migrate from circulating blood. They usually arrive at the site within 3 to 7 days after the onset of inflammation. On entering the tissue spaces, monocytes transform into macrophages. Together with the tissue macrophages, these newly arrived macrophages assist in phagocytosis of the inflammatory debris. The macrophage role is important in cleaning the area before healing can occur. Macrophages have a long life span;

TABLE 12-1 MEDIATORS OF INFLAMMATION

Mediator	Source	Mechanisms of Action
Histamine	Stored in granules of basophils, mast cells, platelets	Causes vasodilation and increased capillary permeability.
Serotonin	Stored in platelets, mast cells, enterochromaffin cells of GI tract	Same as above. Stimulates smooth muscle contraction.
Kinins (e.g., bradykinin)	Produced from precursor factor kininogen as a result of activation of Hageman factor (XII) of clotting system	Cause contraction of smooth muscle and vasodilation. Result in stimulation of pain.
Complement components (C3a, C4a, C5a)	Anaphylatoxic agents generated from complement pathway activation	Stimulate histamine release and chemotaxis.
Prostaglandins (PGs) and leukotrienes (LTs)	Produced from arachidonic acid (see Fig. 12-2)	PGs cause vasodilation. LTs stimulate chemotaxis.
Cytokines	For information on cytokines, see Table 14-3	

they can multiply and may stay in the damaged tissues for weeks. These long-lived cells are important in orchestrating the healing process.

In cases where particles are too large for a single macrophage, the macrophages accumulate and fuse to form a *multinucleated giant cell.* The giant cell is then encapsulated by collagen, leading to the formation of a granuloma. A classic example of this process occurs in tuberculosis of the lung. While the *Mycobacterium* bacillus is walled off, a chronic state of inflammation exists. The granuloma formed is a cavity of necrotic tissue.

Lymphocytes. Lymphocytes arrive later at the site of injury. Their primary role is related to humoral and cell-mediated immunity (see Chapter 14).

Chemical Mediators

Mediators of the inflammatory response are presented in Table 12-1.

Complement System. The complement system is an enzyme cascade (C1 to C9) consisting of pathways to mediate inflammation and destroy invading pathogens. (eFig. 12-2 showing the complement cascade is available on the website for this chapter.) Major functions of the complement system are enhanced phagocytosis, increased vascular permeability, chemotaxis, and cellular lysis. All of these activities are important mediators of the inflammatory response and healing.

Cell lysis occurs when the final components create holes in the cell membranes and cause targeted cell death by membrane rupture. In autoimmune disorders, healthy tissue can be damaged by complement activation and the resulting inflammatory response. Examples of this include rheumatoid arthritis and systemic lupus erythematosus.

Prostaglandins and Leukotrienes. When cells are activated by injury, the arachidonic acid in the cell membrane is rapidly converted to produce prostaglandins (PGs), thromboxane, and leukotrienes (Fig. 12-2). PGs are generally considered proinflammatory and are potent vasodilators contributing to increased blood flow and edema formation.

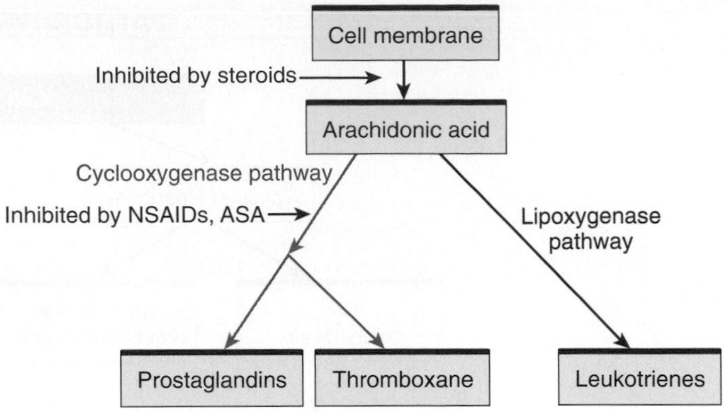

FIG. 12-2 Pathway of generation of prostaglandins, thromboxane, and leukotrienes. Corticosteroids, nonsteroidal antiinflammatory drugs *(NSAIDs)*, and acetylsalicylic acid *(ASA)* act to inhibit various steps in this pathway.

Some subtypes of PGs are formed when platelets are activated and can inhibit platelet and neutrophil aggregation. PGs also perform a significant role in sensitizing pain receptors to arousal by stimuli that would normally be painless. PGs have a pivotal role as pyrogens when stimulating the temperature-regulating area of the hypothalamus and producing a febrile response.

Thromboxane is a powerful vasoconstrictor and platelet-aggregating agent. It causes brief vasoconstriction and skin pallor at the injury site and promotes clot formation. It has a short half-life, and the pallor soon gives way to vasodilation and redness, which is caused by PGs and histamine.

Leukotrienes form the slow-reacting substance of anaphylaxis (SRS-A), which constricts smooth muscles of bronchi, causing narrowing of the airway, and increases capillary permeability, leading to airway edema.

Exudate Formation

Exudate consists of fluid and leukocytes that move from the circulation to the site of injury. The nature and quantity of exudate depend on the type and severity of the injury and the tissues involved (Table 12-2).

Clinical Manifestations

The *local response* to inflammation includes the manifestations of redness, heat, pain, swelling, and loss of function (Table 12-3). *Systemic* manifestations of inflammation include an increased WBC count with a shift to the left, malaise, nausea and anorexia, increased pulse and respiratory rate, and fever.

Leukocytosis results from the increased release of WBCs from the bone marrow. Although the causes of other systemic manifestations are poorly understood, they may be related to complement activation and the release of *cytokines* (soluble factors secreted by WBCs and other types of cells that act as intercellular and intracellular messengers). Some of these cytokines (e.g., interleukins [ILs], tumor necrosis factor [TNF]) are important in causing the systemic manifestations of inflammation, as well as inducing fever. An increase in pulse and respiration follows the rise in metabolism as a result of an increase in body temperature. (Cytokines are discussed in Chapter 14.)

Fever. The onset of fever is triggered by the release of cytokines, which cause fever by initiating metabolic changes in the

TABLE 12-2 TYPES OF INFLAMMATORY EXUDATE

Type	Description	Examples
Serous	Results from outpouring of fluid. Seen in early stages of inflammation or when injury is mild.	Skin blisters, pleural effusion
Serosanguineous	Found during the midpoint in healing after surgery or tissue injury. Composed of RBCs and serous fluid, which is semiclear pink and may have red streaks.	Surgical drain fluid
Fibrinous	Occurs with increasing vascular permeability and fibrinogen leakage into interstitial spaces. Excessive amounts of fibrin that coats tissue surfaces may cause them to adhere.	Adhesions, gelatinous ribbons seen in surgical drain tubing. Frequently covers fluid-exuding wounds such as venous ulcers
Hemorrhagic	Results from rupture or necrosis of blood vessel walls.	Hematoma, bleeding after surgery or tissue trauma
Purulent (pus)	Consists of WBCs, microorganisms (dead and alive), liquefied dead cells, and other debris.	Furuncle (boil), abscess, cellulitis (diffuse inflammation in connective tissue)
Catarrhal	Found in tissues where cells produce mucus. Mucus production is accelerated by inflammatory response.	Runny nose associated with upper respiratory tract infection

TABLE 12-3 LOCAL MANIFESTATIONS OF INFLAMMATION

Manifestations	Cause
Redness (rubor)	Hyperemia from vasodilation.
Heat (calor)	Increased metabolism at inflammatory site.
Pain (dolor)	Change in pH. Nerve stimulation by chemicals (e.g., histamine, prostaglandins). Pressure from fluid exudate.
Swelling (tumor)	Fluid shift to interstitial spaces. Fluid exudate accumulation.
Loss of function (functio laesa)	Swelling and pain.

temperature-regulating center in the hypothalamus (Fig. 12-3). The synthesis of PGs is the most critical metabolic change. PGs act directly to increase the thermostatic set point. The hypothalamus then activates the autonomic nervous system to stimulate increased muscle tone and shivering and decreased perspiration and blood flow to the periphery. Epinephrine released from the adrenal medulla increases the metabolic rate. The net result is fever.

With the physiologic thermostat fixed at a higher-than-normal temperature, the rate of heat production is increased until the body temperature reaches the new set point. As the set point is raised, the hypothalamus signals an increase in heat

PATHOPHYSIOLOGY MAP

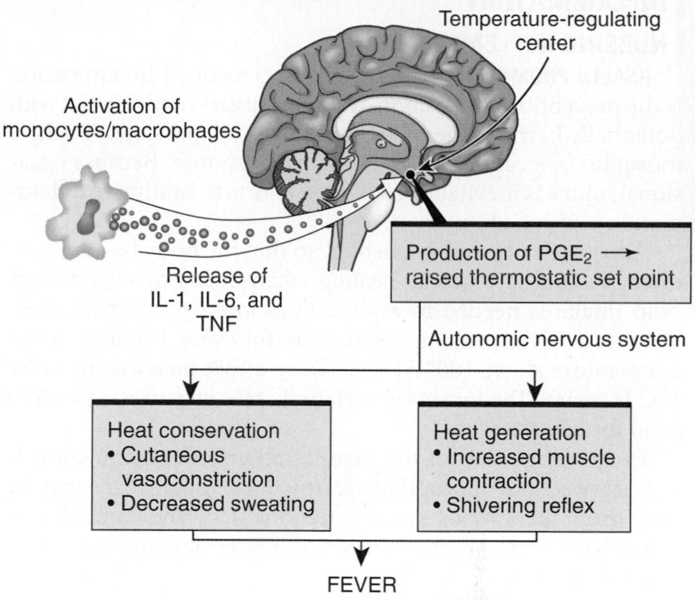

FIG. 12-3 Production of fever. When monocytes/macrophages are activated, they secrete cytokines such as interleukin-1 *(IL-1)*, interleukin-6 *(IL-6)*, and tumor necrosis factor *(TNF)*, which reach the hypothalamic temperature-regulating center. These cytokines promote the synthesis and secretion of prostaglandin E_2 *(PGE_2)* in the anterior hypothalamus. PGE_2 increases the thermostatic set point, and the autonomic nervous system is stimulated, resulting in shivering, muscle contraction, and peripheral vasoconstriction.

production and conservation to raise the body temperature to the new level. At this point the individual feels chilled and shivers. The shivering response is the body's method of raising the body's temperature until the new set point is attained. This seeming paradox is dramatic: the body is hot, yet an individual piles on blankets and may go to bed to get warm. When the body temperature reaches the set point, the chills and warmth-seeking behavior cease.

The released cytokines and the fever they trigger activate the body's defense mechanisms. Beneficial aspects of fever include increased killing of microorganisms, increased phagocytosis by neutrophils, and increased proliferation of T cells. Higher body temperatures may also enhance the activity of interferon, the body's natural virus-fighting substance[1] (see Chapter 14).

Types of Inflammation

The basic types of inflammation are acute, subacute, and chronic. In *acute inflammation* the healing occurs in 2 to 3 weeks and usually leaves no residual damage. Neutrophils are the predominant cell type at the site of inflammation. A *subacute inflammation* has the features of the acute process but lasts longer. For example, infective endocarditis is a smoldering infection with acute inflammation, but it persists for weeks or months (see Chapter 37).

Chronic inflammation lasts for weeks, months, or even years. The injurious agent persists or repeatedly injures tissue. The predominant cell types present at the site of inflammation are lymphocytes and macrophages. Examples of chronic inflammation include rheumatoid arthritis and osteomyelitis. The prolongation and chronicity of any inflammation may be the result of an alteration in the immune response (e.g., autoimmune disease) and can lead to physical deterioration.

NURSING AND COLLABORATIVE MANAGEMENT INFLAMMATION

NURSING IMPLEMENTATION

HEALTH PROMOTION. The best management of inflammation is the prevention of infection, trauma, surgery, and contact with potentially harmful agents. This is not always possible. A simple mosquito bite causes an inflammatory response. Because occasional injury is inevitable, concerted efforts to minimize inflammation and infection are needed.

Adequate nutrition is essential so that the body has the necessary factors to promote healing when injury occurs. A high fluid intake is needed to replace fluid loss from perspiration. There is a 7% increase in metabolism for every 1° F increase in temperature above 100° F (37.8° C), or a 13% increase for every 1° C increase. The increased metabolic rate increases a patient's need for calories.

Early recognition of the manifestations of inflammation is necessary so that appropriate treatment can begin. This may be rest, drug therapy, or specific treatment of the injured site. Immediate treatment may prevent the extension and complications of inflammation.

ACUTE INTERVENTION

Observation and Vital Signs. The ability to recognize the clinical manifestations of inflammation is important. In the individual who is immunosuppressed (e.g., taking corticosteroids or receiving chemotherapy), the classic manifestations of inflammation may be masked. In this individual, early symptoms of inflammation may be malaise or "just not feeling well."

Vital signs are important to note with any inflammation, especially when an infectious process is present. With infection, the temperature may rise, and pulse and respiration rates may increase.

Fever. An important aspect of fever management is determining its cause. Although fever is usually regarded as harmful, an increase in body temperature is an important host defense mechanism. In the seventeenth century, Thomas Sydenham[1] noted that "fever is a mighty engine which nature brings into the world for the conquest of her enemies."

Steps are frequently taken to lower body temperature to relieve the anxiety of the patient and health care professionals. Because mild to moderate fever usually does little harm, imposes no great discomfort, and may benefit host defense mechanisms, antipyretic drugs are rarely essential to patient welfare. Moderate fevers (up to 103° F [39.4° C]) usually produce few problems in most patients. However, if the patient is very young or very old, is extremely uncomfortable, or has a significant medical problem (e.g., severe cardiopulmonary disease, brain injury), the use of antipyretics should be considered. Fever in the immunosuppressed patient should be treated immediately with antibiotic therapy because infections can rapidly progress to septicemia. (Neutropenia is discussed in Chapter 31 on p. 660.)

Fever (especially if greater than 104° F [40° C]) can damage body cells, and delirium and seizures can occur. At temperatures greater than 105.8° F (41° C), regulation by the hypothalamic temperature control center becomes impaired. Damage can occur to many cells, including those in the brain.

Older adults have a blunted febrile response to infection. The body temperature may not rise to the level expected for a younger adult, or the rise may be delayed in its onset. The blunted response can delay diagnosis and treatment. By the time fever (as defined for younger adults) is present, the illness may be more severe. Patients who are taking nonsteroidal antiinflammatory drugs (NSAIDs) on a regular basis (e.g., for treatment of rheumatoid arthritis) may also have a blunted febrile response.

Although sponge baths increase evaporative heat loss, they may not decrease the body temperature unless antipyretic drugs have been given to lower the set point. Otherwise, the body will initiate compensatory mechanisms (e.g., shivering) to restore body heat. The same principle applies to the use of cooling blanket, which are most effective in lowering body temperature when the set point has also been lowered.

A nursing care plan for the patient with a fever (eNursing Care Plan 12-1) is available on the website for this chapter.

Drug Therapy. Drugs are used to decrease the inflammatory response and lower the body temperature (Table 12-4). Aspirin blocks PG synthesis in the hypothalamus and elsewhere in the body. Acetaminophen acts on the heat-regulating center in the hypothalamus. Some NSAIDs (e.g., ibuprofen [Motrin, Advil]) have antipyretic effects. Corticosteroids are antipyretic through the dual mechanisms of preventing both cytokine production and PG synthesis. The action of these drugs results in dilation of superficial blood vessels, increased skin temperature, and sweating.

Antipyretics should be given around the clock to prevent acute swings in temperature. Chills may be evoked or perpetuated by the intermittent administration of antipyretics. These agents cause a sharp decrease in temperature. When the antipyretic wears off, the body may initiate a compensatory involuntary muscular contraction (i.e., chill) to raise the body

TABLE 12-4 DRUG THERAPY

Inflammation and Healing

Drug	Mechanism of Action
Antipyretic Drugs	
Salicylates (aspirin)	Inhibit synthesis of PGs (see Fig. 12-2). Lower temperature by action on heat-regulating center in hypothalamus, resulting in peripheral vasodilation and heat loss
acetaminophen (Tylenol)	Inhibits synthesis of PGs. Lowers temperature by action on heat-regulating center in hypothalamus
NSAIDs (e.g., ibuprofen [Motrin, Advil])	Inhibit synthesis of PGs
Antiinflammatory Drugs	
Salicylates (aspirin)	Inhibit synthesis of PGs, reduce capillary permeability
Corticosteroids (e.g., prednisone)	Interfere with tissue granulation, induce immunosuppressive effects (decreased synthesis of lymphocytes), prevent liberation of lysosomes
NSAIDs (e.g., ibuprofen, piroxicam [Feldene])	Inhibit synthesis of PGs
Vitamins	
Vitamin A	Accelerates epithelialization
Vitamin B complex	Acts as coenzymes
Vitamin C	Assists in synthesis of collagen and new capillaries
Vitamin D	Facilitates calcium absorption

PGs, Prostaglandins.

temperature back up to its previous level. This unpleasant side effect of antipyretic drugs can be prevented by administering these agents regularly at 2- to 4-hour intervals.

Antihistamine drugs may also be used to inhibit the action of histamine. (Antihistamines are discussed in Chapters 14 and 27.)

RICE. **R**est, **i**ce, **c**ompression, and **e**levation (RICE) is a key concept in treating soft tissue injuries and related inflammation.

Rest. Rest helps the body use its nutrients and O_2 for the healing process. The repair process is facilitated by allowing fibrin and collagen to form across the wound edges with little disruption.

Cold and Heat. Cold application is usually appropriate at the time of the initial trauma to promote vasoconstriction and decrease swelling, pain, and congestion from increased metabolism in the area of inflammation. Heat may be used later (e.g., after 24 to 48 hours) to promote healing by increasing the circulation to the inflamed site and subsequent removal of debris. Heat is also used to localize the inflammatory agents. Warm, moist heat may help debride the wound site if necrotic material is present.

Compression and Immobilization. Compression counters the vasodilation effects and development of edema. Compression by direct pressure over a laceration occludes blood vessels and stops bleeding. Compression bandages provide support to injured joints that have tendons and muscles unable to provide support on their own. Assess distal pulses and capillary refill before and after application of compression to evaluate whether compression has compromised circulation (e.g., pale color of skin, loss of feeling).

Immobilization of the inflamed or injured area promotes healing by decreasing the tissues' metabolic needs. Immobilization with a cast or splint supports fractured bones and prevents further tissue injury by sharp bone fragments that could sever nerves or blood vessels (causing hemorrhage). As with compression, evaluate the patient's circulation after application and at regular intervals. Swelling can occur within the closed space of a cast and compromise circulation.

Elevation. Elevating the injured extremity above the level of the heart reduces the edema at the inflammatory site by increasing venous and lymphatic return. Elevation also helps reduce pain associated with blood engorgement at the injury site. Elevation may be contraindicated in patients with significantly reduced arterial circulation.

HEALING PROCESS

The final phase of the inflammatory response is healing. Healing includes two major components: regeneration and repair.

Regeneration

Regeneration is the replacement of lost cells and tissues with cells of the same type. The ability of cells to regenerate depends on the cell type (Table 12-5).

Repair

Repair is healing as a result of lost cells being replaced by connective tissue. Repair is the more common type of healing and usually results in scar formation. Repair is a more complex process than regeneration. Most injuries heal by connective tissue repair. Repair healing occurs by primary, secondary, or tertiary intention (Fig. 12-4).

TABLE 12-5 REGENERATIVE ABILITY OF DIFFERENT TYPES OF TISSUES

Tissues	Cell Type	Description
Skin, lymphoid organs, bone marrow, and mucous membranes	Labile cells	Cells divide constantly. Injury to these organs is followed by rapid regeneration.
Liver, pancreas, kidney, and bone cells	Stable cells	Retain their ability to regenerate but do so only if the organ is injured. Regeneration is slow.
Neurons of the central nervous system (CNS) and skeletal and cardiac muscle cells	Permanent cells	Do not divide. Damage to CNS neurons or skeletal or heart muscle can lead to permanent loss. Healing of skeletal and cardiac muscle will occur by repair with scar tissue. If neurons in the CNS are destroyed, the tissue is generally replaced by glial cells. However, neurogenesis may occur from stem cells (see Chapter 56).

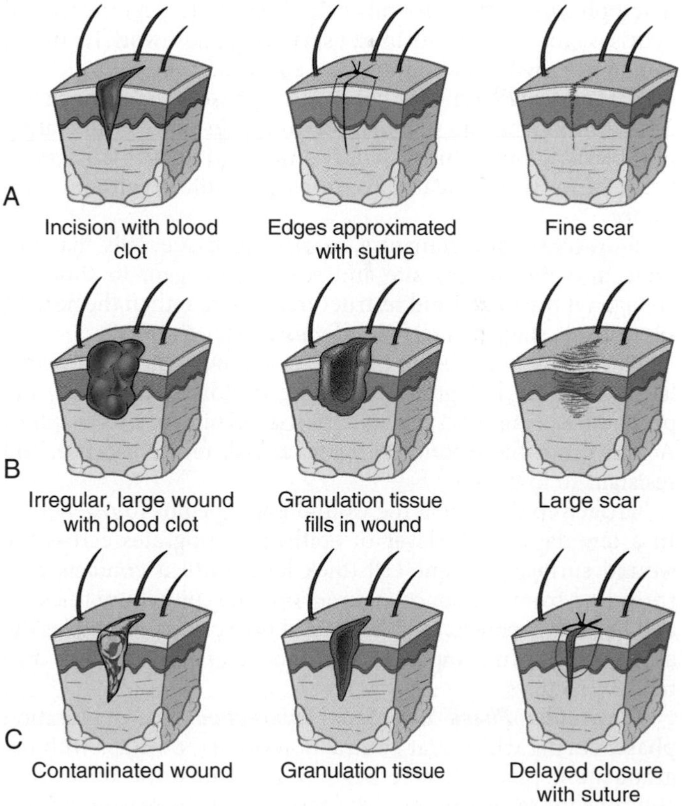

FIG. 12-4 Types of wound healing. **A,** Primary intention. **B,** Secondary intention. **C,** Tertiary intention.

Primary Intention. *Primary intention* healing takes place when wound margins are neatly approximated, as in a surgical incision or a paper cut. A continuum of processes is associated with primary healing (Table 12-6). These processes include three phases.

Initial Phase. In the *initial* (inflammatory) phase, the edges of the incision are first aligned and sutured (or stapled) in place. The incision area fills with blood from the cut blood vessels, blood clots form, and platelets release growth factors to begin

TABLE 12-6 PHASES IN PRIMARY INTENTION HEALING

Phase	Duration	Description
Initial	3-5 days	Approximation of incision edges. Migration of epithelial cells. Clot serving as meshwork for starting capillary growth.
Granulation	5 days to 4 wk	Migration of fibroblasts. Secretion of collagen. Abundance of capillary buds. Wound fragile.
Maturation and scar contraction	7 days to several months	Remodeling of collagen. Strengthening of scar.

the healing process. This forms a matrix for WBC migration. An acute inflammatory reaction occurs.

The area of injury is composed of fibrin clots, erythrocytes, neutrophils (both dead and dying), and other debris. Macrophages ingest and digest cellular debris, fibrin fragments, and red blood cells (RBCs). Extracellular enzymes derived from macrophages and neutrophils help digest fibrin. As the wound debris is removed, the fibrin clot serves as a meshwork for future capillary growth and migration of epithelial cells.

Granulation Phase. The *granulation* phase is the second step. The components of granulation tissue include proliferating fibroblasts; proliferating capillary sprouts *(angioblasts);* various types of WBCs; exudate; and loose, semifluid, ground substance.

Fibroblasts are immature connective tissue cells that migrate into the healing site and secrete collagen. In time the collagen is organized and restructured to strengthen the healing site. At this stage it is termed *fibrous* or *scar tissue.*

During the granulation phase, the wound is pink and vascular. Numerous red granules (young budding capillaries) are present (see eFig. 12-3 available on the website for this chapter). At this point the wound is friable, at risk for dehiscence, and resistant to infection.

Surface epithelium at the wound edges begins to regenerate. In a few days a thin layer of epithelium migrates across the wound surface in a one-cell-thick layer until it contacts cells spreading from the opposite direction. The epithelium thickens and begins to mature, and the wound now closely resembles the adjacent skin. In a superficial wound, re-epithelialization may take 3 to 5 days.

Maturation Phase and Scar Contraction. The maturation phase, during which scar contraction occurs, overlaps with the granulation phase. It may begin 7 days after the injury and continue for several months or years. This is the reason abdominal surgery discharge instructions limit lifting for up to 6 weeks.

Collagen fibers are further organized, and the remodeling process occurs. Fibroblasts disappear as the wound becomes stronger. The active movement of the myofibroblasts causes contraction of the healing area, helping to close the defect and bring the skin edges closer together. A mature scar is then formed. In contrast to granulation tissue, a mature scar is virtually avascular and pale. The scar may be more painful at this phase than in the granulation phase.

Secondary Intention. Wounds that occur from trauma, ulceration, and infection have large amounts of exudate and wide, irregular wound margins with extensive tissue loss. These wounds may have edges that cannot be *approximated* (brought together). The inflammatory reaction may be greater than in primary healing. This results in more debris, cells, and exudate. The debris may have to be cleaned away *(debrided)* before healing can take place.

The process of healing by secondary intention is essentially the same as healing by primary intention. The major differences are the greater defect and the gaping wound edges. Healing and granulation take place from the edges inward and from the bottom of the wound upward until the defect is filled. There is more granulation tissue, and the result is a much larger scar.

Tertiary Intention. *Tertiary intention* (delayed primary intention) healing occurs with delayed suturing of a wound in which two layers of granulation tissue are sutured together. This occurs when a contaminated wound is left open and sutured closed after the infection is controlled. It also occurs when a primary wound becomes infected, is opened, is allowed to granulate, and is then sutured. Tertiary intention usually results in a larger and deeper scar than primary or secondary intention.

Wound Classification

Identifying the etiology of a wound is essential to classifying the wound properly. Wounds can be classified by their cause (surgical or nonsurgical; acute or chronic) or depth of tissue affected (superficial, partial thickness, or full thickness). A *superficial wound* involves only the epidermis. *Partial-thickness* wounds extend into the dermis. *Full-thickness* wounds have the deepest layer of tissue destruction because they involve the subcutaneous tissue and sometimes even extend into the fascia and underlying structures such as the muscle, tendon, or bone (see Fig. 25-3). (Wound classification systems are described in eTables 12-1 and 12-2, available on the website for this chapter.)

Another system used to classify open wounds is based on the color of the wound (red, yellow, black) rather than on the depth of tissue destruction (Table 12-7). The red-yellow-black classification can be applied to any wound allowed to heal by secondary intention, including surgically induced wounds left to heal without skin closure because of a risk for infection. A wound may have two or three colors at the same time. In this situation the wound is classified according to the least-desirable color present.

Complications of Healing

The shape and location of the wound determine how well the wound will heal. Certain factors can interfere with wound healing and lead to complications (Table 12-8 on p. 180).

NURSING AND COLLABORATIVE MANAGEMENT WOUND HEALING

NURSING ASSESSMENT

Observe and record the characteristics of the wound. Thoroughly assess the wound on admission (or first clinic visit) and on a regular basis thereafter. Deterioration in the wound will require you to assess and document changes more frequently. Various methods exist for measuring wounds. One method is presented in Fig. 12-9 on p. 181.

Record the consistency, color, and odor of any drainage and report if abnormal for the situation. *Staphylococcus* and *Pseudomonas* are common organisms that cause purulent, draining wounds.

TABLE 12-7 RED-YELLOW-BLACK CONCEPT OF WOUND CARE

	Red Wound	Yellow Wound	Black Wound
	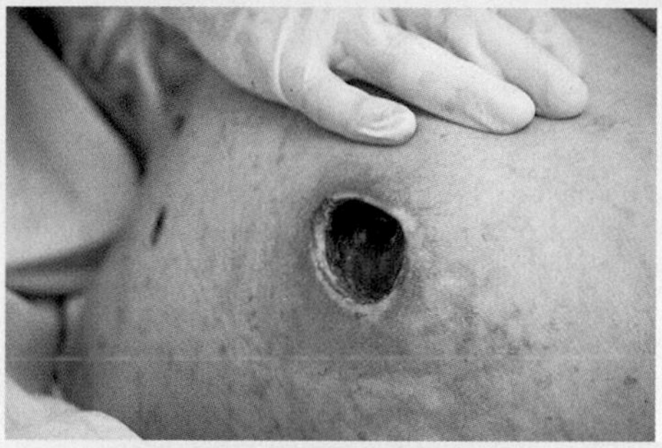	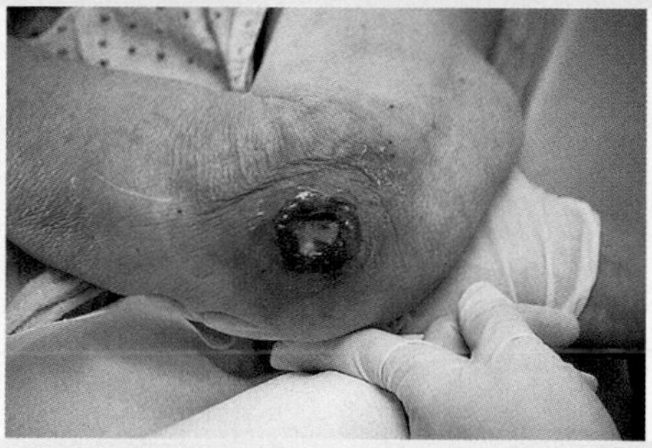	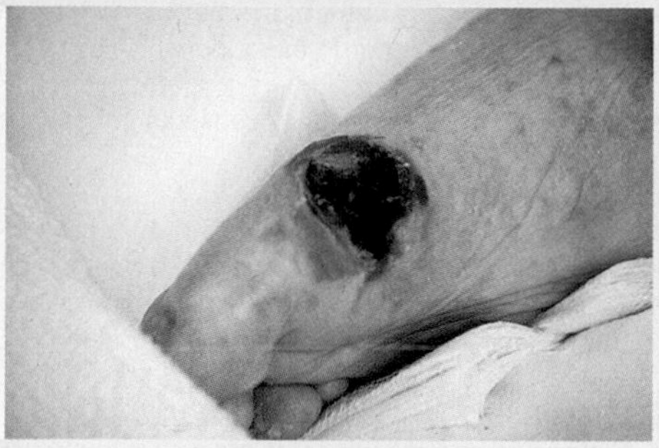
Description and Characteristics	Can be a superficial or deep wound if it is clean and pink in appearance, possible presence of serosanguineous drainage, pink to bright or dark red healing, or chronic wound with granulating tissue.	Presence of slough or soft necrotic tissue. Liquid to semiliquid slough with exudate ranging from creamy ivory to yellow-green.	Black, gray, or brown adherent necrotic tissue called eschar. Possible presence of purulent drainage. Risk of wound infection increases in proportion to amount of necrotic tissue present.
Examples	Skin tears, pressure ulcers (stage II), partial-thickness or second-degree burns, and wounds created by trauma or surgery that are allowed to heal by secondary intention.	Wounds with nonviable necrotic tissue, which creates an ideal situation for bacterial growth and therefore must be removed.	Full-thickness or third-degree burns, pressure ulcers (stages III and IV), and gangrenous ulcers.
Purpose of Treatment	Protection and gentle atraumatic cleansing.	Wound cleansing to remove nonviable tissue and absorb excess drainage.	Debridement of eschar and nonviable tissue.
Dressings and Therapy	Transparent film dressing (e.g., Tegaderm, OpSite), hydrocolloid dressing (e.g., DuoDerm), hydrogels (e.g., Tegagel), gauze dressing with antimicrobial ointment or solution, Telfa dressing with antibiotic ointment.	Absorptive dressing, hydrocolloidal dressing, hydrogel covered with gauze, wound irrigations, hydrotherapy, moist gauze dressing with or without antibiotic or antimicrobial agent.	Topical debridement (enzyme, surgical, chemical) (see Table 12-11), hydrotherapy, moist gauze dressing, hydrogel covered with gauze, absorptive dressing covered with gauze.

In healthy people, wounds heal at a normal, predictable rate. Identify factors that may delay wound healing and contribute to chronic nonhealing wounds (Table 12-9, p. 181).

Chronic wounds are those that do not heal within the normal time (approximately 3 months). If a wound fails to heal in a timely manner, assess and identify factors that may delay healing. Refer the patient to a health care provider specializing in wound management. Time does not heal all wounds. While caring for patients during the healing process, you need to continually assess for complications (e.g., infection) associated with healing[2] (see Table 12-8).

NURSING IMPLEMENTATION

The type of wound management and dressings required depend on the type, extent, and characteristics of the wound and the phase of healing. The purposes of wound management include (1) cleaning a wound to remove any dirt and debris from the wound bed, (2) treating infection to prepare the wound for healing, and (3) protecting a clean wound from trauma so it can heal normally.

Superficial skin injuries may only need cleansing. Adhesive strips (e.g., Steri-Strips, butterflies), sutures (stitches), or tissue adhesives (fibrin sealants) are used to close wounds. Adhesive strips may be used instead of *sutures* in some injuries because they decrease *scarring* and are easier to care for. Sutures are used to close wounds because suture material provides the mechanical support necessary to sustain closure. A wide variety of suturing materials are available. In contrast, tissue adhesives are a biologic adhesive that can be used by themselves or in conjunction with sutures or tape.

If the wound is contaminated, it must be converted into a clean wound before healing can occur normally. Debridement of a wound that has multiple fragments or devitalized tissue may be necessary. If the source of inflammation is an internal organ (e.g., appendix, ruptured spleen), surgical removal of the organ is the treatment of choice.

For wounds that heal by primary intention, it is common to cover the incision with a dry, sterile dressing that is removed as soon as the drainage stops or in 2 to 3 days. Medicated sprays that form a transparent film on the skin may be used for dressings on a clean incision or injury. Transparent film dressings are also commonly used. Sometimes a surgeon will leave a surgical wound uncovered.

Sometimes drains are inserted into the wound to facilitate removal of fluid. The Jackson-Pratt drain is a suction drainage device consisting of a flexible plastic bulb connected to an internal plastic drainage tube (Fig. 12-10).

Topical antimicrobials and antibactericidals (e.g., povidone-iodine [Betadine], Dakin's solution [sodium hypochlorite],

TABLE 12-8 COMPLICATIONS OF WOUND HEALING

Adhesions
- Bands of scar tissue that form between or around organs.
- Adhesions may occur in the abdominal cavity or between the lungs and the pleura.
- Adhesions in abdomen may cause an intestinal obstruction.

Contractions
- Wound contraction is a normal part of healing.
- Complications occur when excessive contraction results in deformity.
- Shortening of muscle or scar tissue, especially over joints, results from excessive fibrous tissue formation (see Fig. 25-14).

Dehiscence
- Separation and disruption of previously joined wound edges (Fig. 12-5).
- Usually occurs when a primary healing site bursts open.
- May be caused by the following:
  - Infection causing an inflammatory process
  - Granulation tissue not strong enough to withstand forces imposed on wound
  - Obesity placing individuals at high risk for dehiscence because adipose tissue has less blood supply and may slow healing
  - Pocket of fluid (seroma, hematoma) developing between tissue layers and preventing the edges of the wound from coming together

Evisceration
- Occurs when wound edges separate to the extent that intestines protrude through wound.

Excess Granulation Tissue ("Proud Flesh")
- Excess granulation tissue may protrude above surface of healing wound.
- If the granulation tissue is cauterized or cut off, healing continues in normal manner.

Fistula Formation
- An abnormal passage between organs or a hollow organ and skin (abdominal or perianal fistula).

Infection (Fig. 12-6)
- ↑ Risk of infection when wound contains necrotic tissue or blood supply is ↓, patient's immune function is ↓ (e.g., from immunosuppressive drugs such as corticosteroids), undernutrition, multiple stressors, and hyperglycemia in diabetes.

Hemorrhage
- Bleeding is normal immediately after tissue injury and ceases with clot formation.
- Hemorrhage occurs as abnormal internal or external blood loss caused by suture failure, clotting abnormalities, dislodged clot, infection, or erosion of a blood vessel by a foreign object (tubing, drains) or infection process.

Hypertrophic Scars
- Inappropriately large, raised red and hard scars (Fig. 12-7).
- Occur when an overabundance of collagen is produced during healing.

Keloid Formation
- Great protrusion of scar tissue that extends beyond wound edges and may form tumor-like masses of scar tissue (Fig. 12-8).
- Permanent without any tendency to subside.
- Patients often complain of tenderness, pain, and hyperparesthesia, especially in early stages.
- Thought to be a hereditary condition occurring most often in dark-skinned people, particularly African Americans.

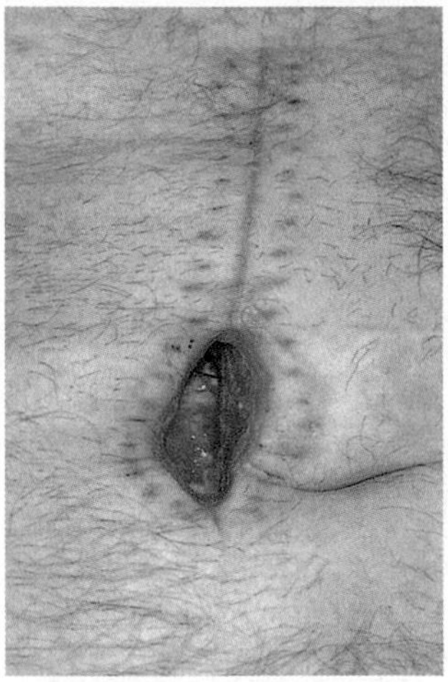

FIG. 12-5 Dehiscence following a cholecystectomy.

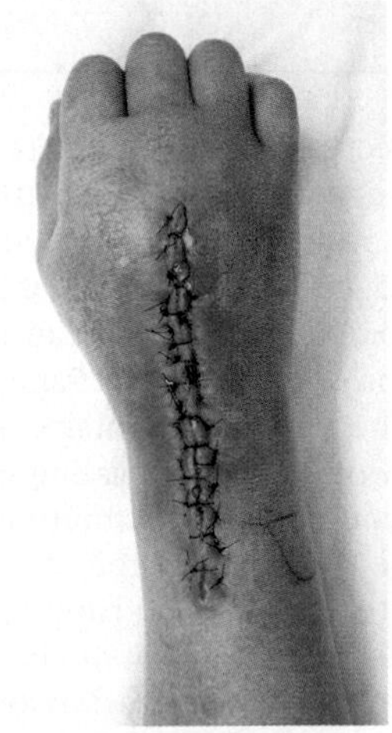

FIG. 12-6 Postoperative deep wound infection following wrist surgery.

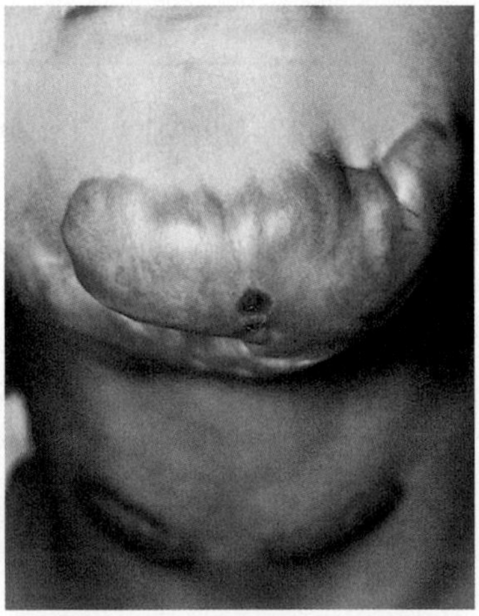

FIG. 12-7 Hypertrophic scarring.

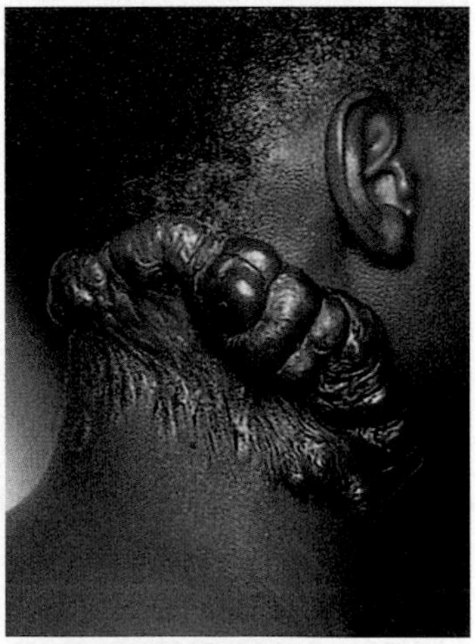

FIG. 12-8 Keloid scarring.

hydrogen peroxide [H_2O_2], and chlorhexidine [Hibiclens]) should be used with caution in wound care because they can damage the new epithelium of healing tissue and delay healing. Therefore they should never be used in a clean granulating wound.

RED, YELLOW, AND BLACK WOUNDS. The management of wounds that heal by secondary intention depends on the cause of the injury and type of tissue in the wound. The red-yellow-black concept of wound care presented in Table 12-7 provides a method of dressing selection based on the wound tissue color. Examples of types of wound dressings are presented in Table 12-10, p. 182.

Red Wounds. In red wounds the purpose of treatment is protection of the wound and gentle cleansing (if indicated). Clean wounds that are granulating and re-epithelializing should be kept slightly moist and protected from further trauma until they

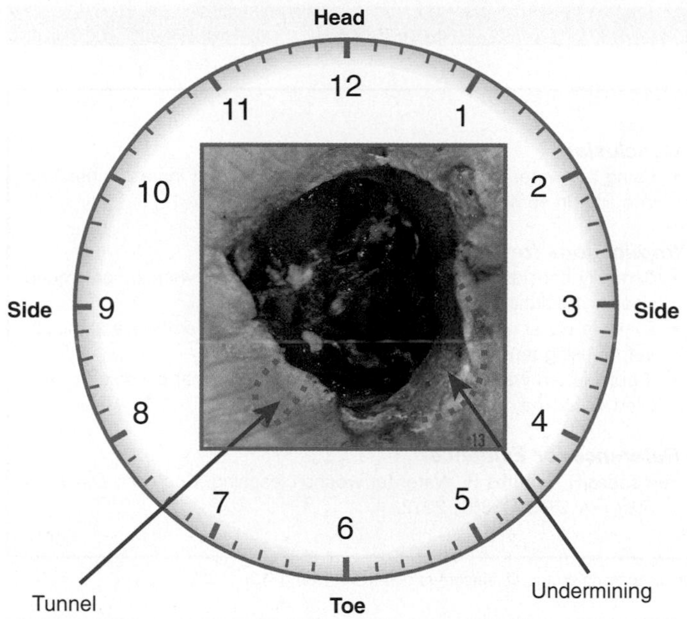

FIG. 12-9 Wound measurements are made in centimeters. The first measurement is oriented from head to toe, the second is from side to side, and the third is the depth (if any). If there is any tunneling (when cotton-tipped applicator is placed in wound, there is movement) or undermining (when cotton-tipped applicator is placed in wound, there is a "lip" around the wound), this is charted in respect to a clock, with 12 o'clock being toward the patient's head. This wound would be charted as a full-thickness, red wound, 7 × 5 × 3 cm, with a 3-cm tunnel at 7 o'clock and 2 cm undermining from 3 o'clock to 5 o'clock.

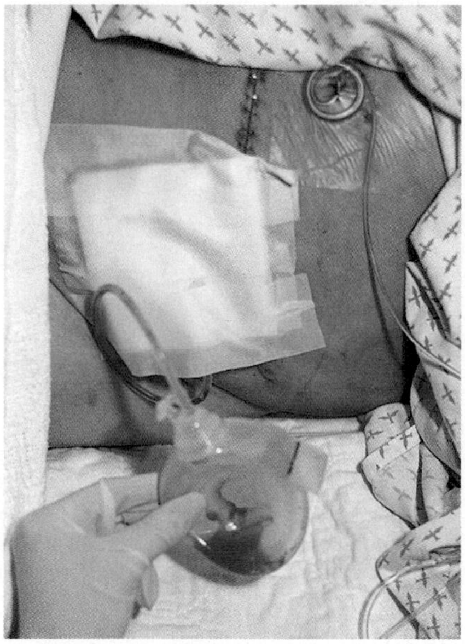

FIG. 12-10 Jackson-Pratt drainage device.

heal naturally. Do not let a wound dry out. Dryness is an enemy of wound healing. "Airing out" a wound is a great mistake. Wounds need a moist environment to heal.

A dressing material that keeps the wound surface clean and slightly moist is optimal to promote epithelialization. Transparent film or adhesive semipermeable dressings (e.g., OpSite, Tegaderm) are occlusive dressings that are permeable to oxygen. The wound is then usually covered with a sterile dressing. Unnecessary manipulation during dressing changes may destroy new granulation tissue and break down fibrin formation.

TABLE 12-9 FACTORS DELAYING WOUND HEALING

Factor	Effect on Wound Healing
Nutritional deficiencies	
• Vitamin C	Delays formation of collagen fibers and capillary development
• Protein	Decreases supply of amino acids for tissue repair
• Zinc	Impairs epithelialization
Inadequate blood supply	Decreases supply of nutrients to injured area, decreases removal of exudative debris, inhibits inflammatory response
Corticosteroid drugs	Impair phagocytosis by WBCs, inhibit fibroblast proliferation and function, depress formation of granulation tissue, inhibit wound contraction
Infection	Increases inflammatory response and tissue destruction
Smoking	Nicotine, a potent vasoconstrictor, impedes blood flow to healing areas
Mechanical friction on wound	Destroys granulation tissue, prevents apposition of wound edges
Advanced age	Slows collagen synthesis by fibroblasts, impairs circulation, requires longer time for epithelialization of skin, alters phagocytic and immune responses
Obesity	Decreases blood supply in fatty tissue
Diabetes mellitus	Decreases collagen synthesis, retards early capillary growth, impairs phagocytosis (result of hyperglycemia), reduces supply of O_2 and nutrients secondary to vascular disease
Poor general health	Causes generalized absence of factors necessary to promote wound healing
Anemia	Supplies less O_2 at tissue level

Yellow Wounds. A type of dressing used in yellow wounds is an absorption dressing that absorbs exudate and cleanses the wound surface. Absorption dressings work by drawing excess drainage from the wound surface. The amount of wound secretions determines the number of dressing changes.

Hydrocolloid dressings such as DuoDerm are also used to treat yellow wounds. The inner part of these dressings interacts with the exudate, forming a hydrated gel over the wound. When the dressing is removed, the gel separates and stays over the wound. The wound must be cleansed gently to prevent damage to newly formed tissue. These types of dressings are designed to be left in place for up to 7 days or until leakage occurs around the dressing.

Black Wounds. The immediate treatment is debridement of the nonviable, eschar tissue. The debridement method used depends on the amount of debris and the condition of the wound tissue (Table 12-11, p. 183).

NEGATIVE-PRESSURE WOUND THERAPY. Negative-pressure wound therapy *(vacuum-assisted wound closure)* is a type of therapy that uses suction to remove drainage and speed wound healing.[3] In this therapy the wound is cleaned, and a gauze or foam dressing is cut to the dimensions of the wound. A large occlusive dressing is applied, and a small hole is made over the gauze or foam dressing where the tubing is attached (Fig. 12-11, p. 183). The tubing is connected to a pump, which creates a negative pressure in the wound bed.

EVIDENCE-BASED PRACTICE

Translating Research Into Practice

What Is the Effect of Tap Water on Wound Cleansing?

Clinical Question

In patients with an infected wound (P), what is the effect of tap water (I) versus normal saline or no cleansing (C) on infection and healing rates (O)?

Best Available Evidence

Randomized controlled trials (RCTs) and quasi-randomized controlled trials

Critical Appraisal and Synthesis of Evidence

- Ten trials (*n* = 35 to 705/trial) with people who had acute infected wounds. Seven trials compared infection and healing rates with water versus normal saline. Three trials compared wound cleansing with various solutions versus no cleansing at all.
- No significant differences were found in infection rate and healing in wounds cleansed with tap water versus not cleansed at all.
- Tap water was more effective than saline in reducing wound infection rate.

Conclusion

- Using tap water to cleanse acute wounds does not increase infection rate and, in some cases, it may reduce infection.

Implications for Nursing Practice

- Carefully consider the option of using tap water when other wound cleansing solutions are not accessible.
- Evaluate water quality, type of wound, and the patient's overall health before using tap water.
- If potable tap water is not available, boiled water that is cooled or distilled water may be used in wound cleansing.

Reference for Evidence

Fernandez R, Griffiths R: Water for wound cleansing, *Cochrane Database Syst Rev* 2:CD003861, 2012.

P, Patient population of interest; *I*, intervention or area of interest; *C*, comparison of interest or comparison group; *O*, outcomes of interest (see p. 12).

TABLE 12-10 TYPES OF WOUND DRESSINGS

Type	Description	Uses	Examples
Gauzes and nonwovens	Provide absorption of exudates. Support debridement if applied and kept moist.	Maintaining moist wound surface. Cleansing, packing, and covering a variety of wounds.	Numerous products available (e.g., Curity, Kling, Kerlix)
Nonadherent dressings	Woven or nonwoven dressings. May be impregnated with saline, petrolatum, or antimicrobials. Are minimally absorbent.	Minor wounds or as a second dressing.	Adaptic, Vaseline gauze, Xeroform
Semipermeable transparent films	Semipermeable membrane of polyurethane with acrylic adhesive. Transparency allows visualization of the wound. Minimally absorbent.	Dry, uninfected wounds or wounds with minimal drainage.	Bioclusive, Blisterfilm, OpSite, Polyskin, Suresite, Tegaderm, Transeal
Hydrocolloids	Gelatin, pectin, or carboxymethylcellulose bonded to a film or sheet. Produce a flat occlusive dressing that forms a gel on wound surface. Occlusion does not interfere with wound healing. Support debridement and prevent secondary infections.	Wounds with moderate to heavy drainage.	Aquacel, Combiderm, Comfeel, DuoDerm, Tegasorb
Foams	Sheets and other shapes of foamed polyurethane or silicone. Able to hold large amounts of exudate. Some come with adhesive backings; others require gauze wrapping.	Wounds with moderate to heavy drainage. Often used on new wounds.	Allevyn, Curafoam, Hydrasorb, Lyofoam, PolyMem
Hydrogels	Available in gels, gel-covered gauze, or sheets. Donate moisture to a dry wound and maintain a moist environment. Can rehydrate wound tissue. Debridement because of moisturizing effects. Require a secondary dressing.	Wounds with minimal drainage. Necrotic wounds.	Aquaform, Curasol, GranuGel, IntraSite, Nu-Gel, Purilon, Tegagel
Alginates	Derived from seaweed. Form a nonsticky gel on contact with draining wound. Easy to use over irregular-shaped wounds. Generally require a secondary dressing.	Wounds with moderate to heavy exudates (e.g., pressure ulcers, infected wounds).	AlgiSite, Algosteril, Kaltostat, Melgisorb, SeaSorb, Sorbsan
Antimicrobials	Wound covers that deliver agents such as silver and iodine, and polyhexamethylene biguanide (PHMB), which have antibacterial properties. Bacteria are not able to develop resistance to metals. Available as sponges, impregnated woven gauzes, film dressings, absorptive products, nylon fabric, nonadherent barriers, or a combination of materials.	Partial- and full-thickness wounds, over surgical incisions, or around tracheostomies.	Acticoat, Curity AMD, Iodoflex, Iodosorb, SilverDerm, Silverlon

For more information, see *http://search.woundsource.com*.

Although the exact mechanism for promoting healing is not known, it is thought that this therapy pulls excess fluid from the wound, reduces bacterial load, and encourages blood flow into the wound base. Monitor the patient's serum protein levels and fluid and electrolyte balance because of losses from the wound. Additionally, monitor the patient's coagulation studies (platelet count, prothrombin time [PT], partial thromboplastin time [PTT]).

HYPERBARIC OXYGEN THERAPY. Hyperbaric O_2 therapy (HBOT) is the delivery of O_2 at increased atmospheric pressures. It can be given systemically with the patient placed in an enclosed chamber where 100% O_2 is administered at 1.5 to 3 times the normal atmospheric pressure. HBOT allows O_2 to diffuse into the serum, rather than RBCs, and be transported to the tissues. By increasing the O_2 content in the serum, HBOT moves the O_2 past narrowed arteries and capillaries where RBCs cannot go.[4]

In addition, elevated O_2 levels stimulate *angiogenesis* (the production of new blood vessels), kill anaerobic bacteria, and increase the killing power of WBCs and certain antibiotics (e.g.,

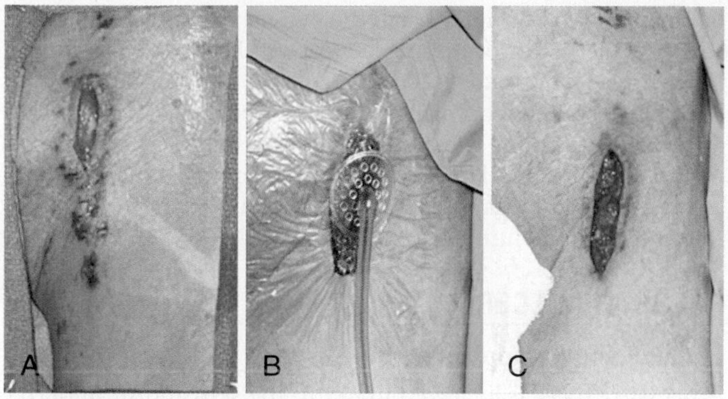

FIG. 12-11 Negative-pressure wound therapy. **A,** Femoral wound that is not healing. **B,** Negative-pressure wound therapy in place. **C,** Granulation tissue formation after therapy.

DELEGATION DECISIONS

Wound Care

In general, wound care for complex or nonhealing wounds should be managed by the registered nurse (RN). State nurse practice acts vary in the wound care actions allowed by licensed practical/vocational nurses (LPN/LVNs) and unlicensed assistive personnel (UAP).

Role of Registered Nurse (RN)

- Assess patients for pressure ulcer risk and develop a plan of care to prevent the development of pressure ulcers.
- Assess patients for factors that might delay wound healing and develop a plan of care to address these factors.
- Assess and document initial wound appearance, including wound size, depth, color, and drainage.
- Plan nursing actions to assist with wound healing, including wound care, positioning, and nutritional interventions.
- Choose dressings and therapies for wound treatment (in conjunction with the health care provider and/or wound care specialist).
- Implement wound care for complex or new wounds, including negative-pressure wound therapy and hyperbaric O_2 therapy.
- Evaluate whether wound care is effective in promoting wound healing.
- Provide teaching to patient and caregivers about home wound care and pressure ulcer prevention.

Role of Licensed Practical/Vocational Nurse (LPN/LVN)

- Perform sterile dressing changes on acute and chronic wounds.
- Apply ordered topical antimicrobials and antibactericidals to wounds.
- Apply prescribed dressings or medications for wound debridement.
- Collect and record data about wound appearance.
- Reinforce teaching that was provided by the RN.

Role of Unlicensed Assistive Personnel (UAP)

- Perform dressing changes for chronic wounds using clean technique (need to consider state nurse practice act and agency policy).
- Empty wound drainage containers and document drainage on intake and output record.
- Report changes in wound appearance or drainage to RN.

fluoroquinolones, aminoglycosides). HBOT accelerates granulation tissue formation and wound healing.

An alternative approach is to topically administer hyperbaric O_2 by creating a chamber around the injured limb. Most systemic treatments last from 90 to 120 minutes, and the number of treatments may vary from 10 to 60 depending on the condition being treated. The topical treatments can last 20 minutes twice daily or 4 to 6 hours daily. The number of treatments is highly variable.

TABLE 12-11 TYPES OF DEBRIDEMENT

Type	Description
Surgical debridement	• Quick method of debridement to prevent, control, or remove infection. • Used when large amounts of nonviable tissue are present. • Prepares wound bed for healing, skin grafting, or flaps.
Mechanical debridement	• Three methods: • *Wet-to-dry dressings* in which open-mesh gauze is moistened with normal saline, packed on or into wound surface, and allowed to dry. Wound debris adheres to dressing and then dressing is removed. • *Wound irrigation.* Make certain bacteria are not accidentally driven into wound with high irrigation pressure. • *Whirlpool.* Should not be used in a clean granulating wound. Used when minimal debris is present. Nonselective and will also debride some healthy tissue.
Autolytic debridement	• Semiocclusive or occlusive dressings (see Table 12-10) used to soften dry eschar by autolysis. • Assess area around wound for maceration when using these dressings. • Malodorous.
Enzymatic debridement	• Drugs applied topically to dissolve necrotic tissue and then covered with moist dressing (e.g., saline-moistened gauze). • Examples of these drugs include collagenase and papain and urea (e.g., Panafil, Gladase). • Process can be slow, and thick eschar may need to be scored with scalpel.

DRUG THERAPY. Platelet-derived growth factor is released from the platelets and stimulates cell proliferation and migration. Becaplermin (Regranex), a recombinant human platelet–derived growth factor gel, actively stimulates wound healing. This product should be used only when the wound is free of devitalized tissue and infection. It should not be used if cancer is suspected in the wound.

NUTRITIONAL THERAPY. Special nutritional measures facilitate wound healing. A high fluid intake is needed to replace fluid loss from perspiration and exudate formation. An increased metabolic rate intensifies water loss. Individuals at risk for wound healing problems are those with malabsorption problems (e.g., Crohn's disease, gastrointestinal [GI] surgery, liver disease), deficient intake or high energy demands (e.g., malignancy, major trauma or surgery, sepsis, fever), and diabetes.

Undernutrition puts a person at risk for poor healing. A diet high in protein, carbohydrate, and vitamins with moderate fat intake is necessary to promote healing. Protein is needed to correct the negative nitrogen balance resulting from the increased metabolic rate. Protein is also necessary for synthesis of immune factors, leukocytes, fibroblasts, and collagen, which are the building blocks for healing. Carbohydrate is needed for the increased metabolic energy required in inflammation and healing. If there is a carbohydrate deficit, the body will break down protein for the needed energy. Fats are also a necessary component in the diet to help in the synthesis of fatty acids and triglycerides, which are part of the cellular membrane.

Vitamin C is needed for capillary synthesis and collagen production by fibroblasts. The B-complex vitamins are necessary as coenzymes for many metabolic reactions. If a vitamin B deficiency develops, a disruption of protein, fat, and carbohydrate metabolism will occur. Vitamin A is also needed in healing because it aids in the process of epithelialization. It increases collagen synthesis and tensile strength of the healing wound.

If the patient is unable to eat, enteral feedings and supplements should be the first choice if the GI tract is functional. Parenteral nutrition is indicated when enteral feedings are contraindicated or not tolerated. (Enteral and parenteral nutrition is discussed in Chapter 40.)

INFECTION PREVENTION AND CONTROL. You and the patient must scrupulously follow aseptic procedures for keeping the wound free from infection. Do not allow the patient to touch a recently injured area. The patient's environment should be as free as possible from contamination from items introduced by roommates and visitors. Antibiotics may be administered prophylactically to some patients.

If an infection develops, a culture and sensitivity test should be done to determine the organism and the most effective antibiotic for that specific organism. The culture should be taken before the first dose of antibiotic is given. Cultures can be obtained by needle aspiration, tissue culture, or swab technique. Physicians will obtain needle and tissue punch biopsy samples. As a nurse, you can obtain cultures using the swab technique.

Concurrent swab specimens are obtained from wounds using (1) wound exudates, (2) Z-technique, and (3) Levine's technique. The first technique samples visible wound exudates from the wound bed before cleansing. The Z-technique involves rotating a culture swab over the cleansed wound bed surface in a 10-point Z-track fashion. Levine's technique involves rotating a culture swab over a cleansed 1-cm^2 area near the center of the wound using sufficient pressure to extract wound fluid from deep tissue layers. Finally, a specimen of viable wound tissue is removed from the center of the wound using sterile technique. When collecting samples, do not take the specimen from exudate or eschar and do not use cotton-tipped swabs.

PSYCHOLOGIC IMPLICATIONS. The patient may be distressed at the thought or sight of an incision or wound because of fear of scarring or disfigurement. Drainage and odor from a wound often cause increased alarm. The patient needs to understand the healing process and the normal changes that occur as the wound heals. When changing a dressing, avoid inappropriate facial expressions that might alert the patient to problems with the wound or raise doubts about your ability to care for it. Wrinkling your nose may convey disgust to the patient. Be careful not to focus on the wound to the extent that the patient is not treated as a total person.

PATIENT TEACHING. Because patients are being discharged earlier after surgery and many have surgery as outpatients, it is important that the patient, the family, or both know how to care for the wound and perform dressing changes. Wound healing may not be complete for 4 to 6 weeks or longer. Adequate rest and good nutrition should be continued throughout this time. Physical and emotional stress should be minimal. Observing the wound for complications such as contractures, adhesions, and secondary infection is important. The patient should understand the signs and symptoms of infection. The patient should note changes in wound color and the amount of drainage. Teach the patient to notify the health care provider of any signs of abnormal wound healing.

Drugs are often taken for a time after recovery from the acute infection. Review drug-specific side effects and adverse effects with the patient, as well as methods to prevent side effects (e.g., taking with food or not). Teach the patient to contact the health care provider if any of these effects occur. Inform the patient of the need to continue the drugs for the specified time. For example, a patient who is instructed to take an antibiotic for 10 days may stop taking the drug after 5 days because of decreased or absent symptoms. However, the organism may not be entirely eliminated, and it may also become resistant to the antibiotic if the drug is not continued.

PRESSURE ULCERS

Etiology and Pathophysiology

A **pressure ulcer** is localized injury to the skin and/or underlying tissue (usually over a bony prominence) as a result of pressure or pressure in combination with shear and/or friction.

Pressure ulcers generally fall under the category of healing by secondary intention. The most common site for pressure ulcers is the sacrum, with heels being second. Factors that influence the development of pressure ulcers include the amount of pressure (intensity), the length of time the pressure is exerted on the skin (duration), and the ability of the patient's tissue to tolerate the externally applied pressure. Besides pressure, other factors that contribute to pressure ulcer formation include **shearing force** (pressure exerted on the skin when it adheres to the bed and the skin layers slide in the direction of body movement [e.g., when pulling patient up in bed]), *friction* (two surfaces rubbing against each other), and *excessive moisture.*

Factors that put a patient at risk for the development of pressure ulcers are presented in Table 12-12. Individuals at risk include those who are older, incontinent, bed- or wheelchair-bound, or recovering from spinal cord injuries.

Clinical Manifestations

The clinical manifestations of pressure ulcers depend on the extent of the tissue involved. Pressure ulcers are graded or staged according to their deepest level of tissue damage. Table 12-13 illustrates the pressure ulcer stages based on the National Pressure Ulcer Advisory Panel (NPUAP) guidelines. A pressure ulcer may be unstageable (see Table 12-13).

If the pressure ulcer becomes infected, the patient may display signs of infection (e.g., leukocytosis, fever). In addition, the pressure ulcer may increase in size, odor, and drainage; have necrotic tissue; and be indurated, warm, and painful. Untreated ulcers may lead to cellulitis, chronic infection, sepsis, and possibly death. The most common complication of a pressure ulcer is recurrence. Therefore it is important to note the location of previously healed pressure ulcers on a patient's initial admission assessment.

TABLE 12-12 RISK FACTORS FOR PRESSURE ULCERS

- Advanced age
- Anemia
- Contractures
- Diabetes mellitus
- Elevated body temperature
- Immobility
- Impaired circulation
- Incontinence
- Low diastolic blood pressure (<60 mm Hg)
- Mental deterioration
- Neurologic disorders
- Obesity
- Pain
- Prolonged surgery
- Vascular disease

NURSING AND COLLABORATIVE MANAGEMENT PRESSURE ULCERS

In 1859 Florence Nightingale wrote, "If he has a bedsore, it's generally not the fault of the disease, but of the nursing."[5] Her comment emphasizes the critical role that nurses have in prevention and treatment of pressure ulcers.

Nursing and collaborative management are discussed together because the activities are interrelated. In addition to the nurse, other members of the health team, such as the wound care specialist, plastic surgeon, dietitian, physical therapist, and occupational therapist, can provide valuable input into the complex treatment necessary to prevent and treat pressure ulcers.

TABLE 12-13 STAGING OF PRESSURE ULCERS

Suspected Deep Tissue Injury

Purple or maroon localized area of discolored intact skin or blood-filled blister caused by damage of underlying soft tissue from pressure and/or shear. The area may be painful, firm, mushy, boggy, warmer, or cooler compared with adjacent tissue.

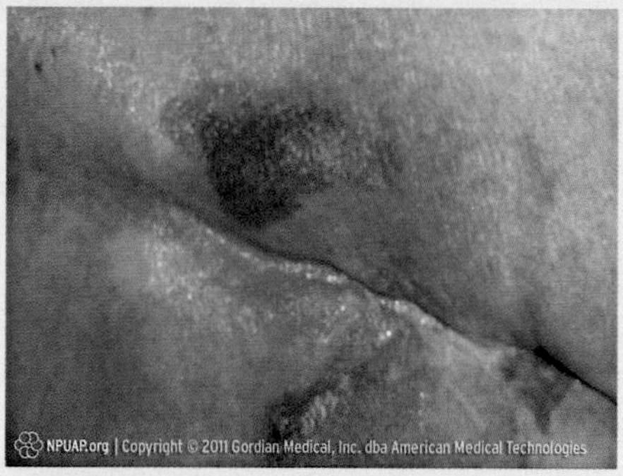

Stage III

Full-thickness tissue loss. Subcutaneous fat may be visible, but bone, tendon, and muscle are not exposed. Slough may be present but does not obscure the depth of tissue loss. May include undermining and tunneling.

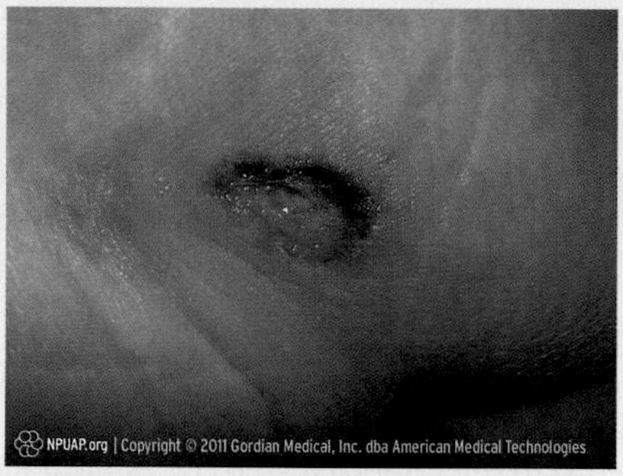

Stage I

Intact skin with nonblanchable redness of a localized area, usually over a bony prominence. Darkly pigmented skin may not have visible blanching. Its color may differ from the surrounding area.

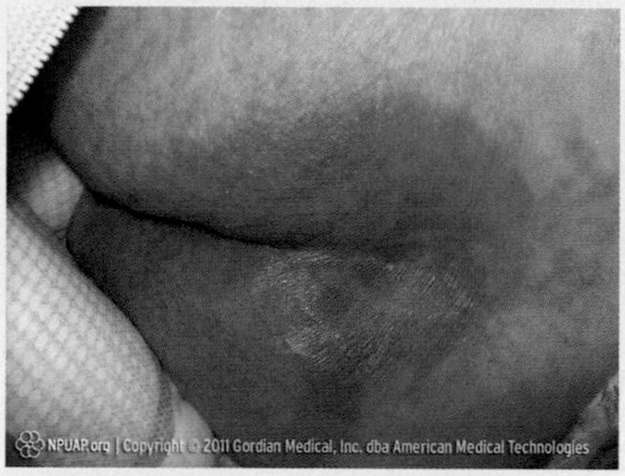

Stage IV

Full-thickness tissue loss with exposed bone, tendon, or muscle. Slough or eschar may be present on some parts of the wound bed. Often includes undermining and tunneling.

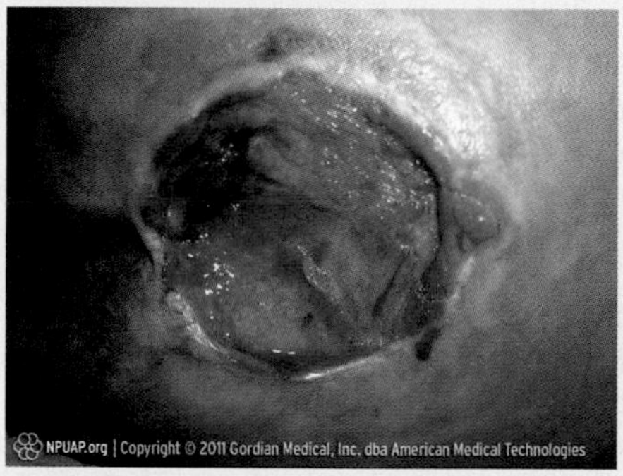

Stage II

Partial-thickness loss of dermis manifesting as a shallow open ulcer with a red-pink wound bed, without slough. May also manifest as an intact or open/ruptured serum-filled blister.

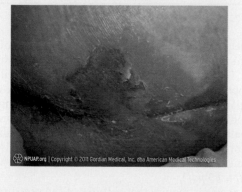

Unstageable Ulcer

Full-thickness tissue loss in which the base of the ulcer is covered by slough (yellow, tan, gray, green, or brown) and/or eschar (tan, brown, or black) in the wound bed.

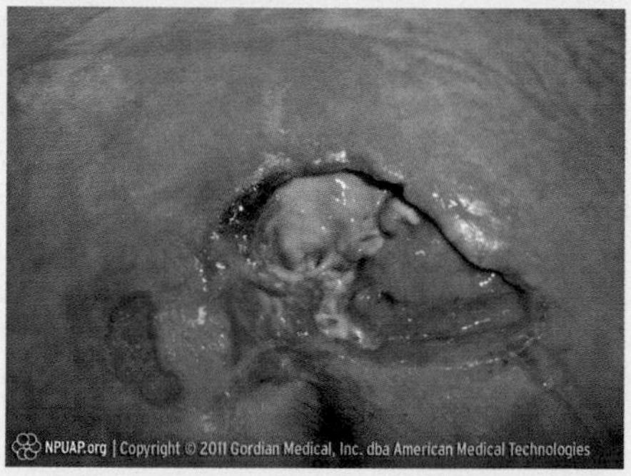

The true depth and stage of the ulcer cannot be determined until enough slough and eschar are removed. Stable (dry, adherent, intact without erythema or fluctuance) eschar on the heels provides a natural biologic cover and should not be removed.

Photos used with permission of the National Pressure Ulcer Advisory Panel.

NURSING ASSESSMENT

Assess patients for pressure ulcer risk initially on admission and at periodic intervals based on the patient's condition.

SAFETY ALERT
- In acute care, reassess patients for pressure ulcers every 24 hours.
- In long-term care, reassess residents weekly for the first 4 weeks after admission and then at least monthly or quarterly.
- In home care, reassess patients at every nurse visit.

Risk assessment should be done using a validated assessment tool such as the Braden Scale (available at *www.bradenscale.com* or in eTable 12-3 on the website for this chapter). Knowing the level of risk can help determine how aggressive preventive measures should be.

Conduct a thorough head-to-toe assessment on admission to identify and document a pressure ulcer. Thereafter conduct periodic reassessment of the skin and wounds. Identification of skin changes may be difficult in patients with dark skin. Table 12-14 presents techniques to help assess darker skin.

Subjective and objective data that should be obtained from a person with or at risk for a pressure ulcer are presented in Table 12-15.

NURSING DIAGNOSES

Nursing diagnoses for the patient with a pressure ulcer may include, but are not limited to, the following:
- Impaired skin integrity *related to* mechanical factors and physical immobilization
- Impaired tissue integrity *related to* impaired circulation and imbalanced nutritional state

PLANNING

The overall goals are that the patient with a pressure ulcer will (1) have no deterioration of the ulcer, (2) reduce or eliminate the factors that lead to pressure ulcers, (3) not develop an infection in the pressure ulcer, (4) have healing of pressure ulcers, and (5) have no recurrence.

NURSING IMPLEMENTATION

HEALTH PROMOTION. A primary nursing responsibility is the identification of patients at risk for developing pressure ulcers (see Tables 12-12 and 12-15) and implementation of pressure ulcer prevention strategies for those who are at risk. Prevention remains the best treatment for pressure ulcers.[6,7]

SAFETY ALERT
- Reposition patients frequently to prevent pressure ulcers (usually every 2 hours).
- Use devices to reduce pressure and shearing force (e.g., low-air-loss mattresses, foam mattresses, wheelchair cushions, padded commode seats, boots [foam, air], lift sheets) as appropriate.
- These devices do not replace the need for frequent repositioning.

ACUTE INTERVENTION. Care of a patient with a pressure ulcer requires local care of the wound and support measures of the whole person, such as adequate nutrition, pain management, control of other medical conditions, and pressure relief. Both conservative and surgical strategies are used in the treatment of pressure ulcers, depending on the stage and condition of the ulcer.

Once a pressure ulcer has developed, initiate interventions based on the ulcer characteristics (e.g., stage, size, location, amount of exudate, type of wound, presence of infection or pain) and the patient's general status (e.g., nutritional state, age, cardiovascular status, level of mobility). Carefully document the size of the pressure ulcer. A wound-measuring card or tape can be used to note the ulcer's maximum length and width in centimeters. To find the depth of the ulcer, take a sterile cotton-tipped applicator and soak it with saline. Gently place it into the deepest part of the ulcer, and then measure the length of the portion of the applicator that probed the ulcer. Documentation of the healing wound can be done using several available pressure ulcer healing tools such as the NPUAP Pressure Ulcer Scale for Healing (PUSH) tool[8] (eTable 12-4; available at *www.npuap.org/PDF/push3.pdf*).

Some agencies require that pictures of the pressure ulcer be taken initially and at regular intervals during the course of treatment. The informatics box on p. 187 has suggestions for digital imaging.

TABLE 12-14 ASSESSING PATIENTS WITH DARK SKIN

- Look for changes in skin color, such as skin that is darker (purplish, brownish, bluish) than surrounding skin.
- Use natural or halogen light source to accurately assess the skin color. Fluorescent light casts blue color, which can make skin assessment difficult.
- Assess the area for the skin temperature using your hand. The area may feel initially warm, then cooler.
- Touch the skin to feel its consistency. Boggy or edematous feel may indicate a stage I pressure ulcer.
- Ask the patient if he or she has any pain or itchy sensation.

TABLE 12-15 NURSING ASSESSMENT

Pressure Ulcers

Subjective Data

Important Health Information

Past health history: Stroke, spinal cord injury; prolonged bed rest or immobility; circulatory impairment; poor nutrition; altered level of consciousness; prior history of pressure ulcer; immunologic abnormalities; advanced age; diabetes; anemia; trauma

Medications: Use of opioids, hypnotics, systemic corticosteroids

Surgery or other treatments: Recent surgery

Functional Health Patterns

Nutritional-metabolic: Obesity, emaciation; decreased fluid, calorie, or protein intake; vitamin or mineral deficiencies; clinically significant malnutrition as indicated by low serum albumin, decreased total lymphocyte count, and decreased body weight (15% less than ideal body weight)

Elimination: Incontinence of urine, feces, or both

Activity-exercise: Weakness, debilitation, inability to turn and position body; contractures

Cognitive-perceptual: Pain or altered cutaneous sensation in pressure ulcer area; decreased awareness of pressure on body areas; capacity to follow treatment plan

Objective Data

General

Fever

Integumentary

Diaphoresis, edema, and discoloration, especially over bony areas such as sacrum, hips, elbows, heels, knees, ankles, shoulders, and ear rims, progressing to increased tissue damage characteristic of ulcer stages*

Possible Diagnostic Findings

Leukocytosis, positive cultures for microorganisms from pressure ulcer

*See Table 12-13.

EVIDENCE-BASED PRACTICE

Applying the Evidence

You are caring for S.W., an obese 86-year-old woman with a history of diabetes, hypertension, and chronic kidney disease. S.W. spends most of her time in bed or a wheelchair and now has a stage I pressure ulcer on her sacral area. You are doing discharge teaching with her daughter, who is her primary caregiver. You explain the importance of preventing further skin breakdown and that she needs to reposition her mother every 2 to 3 hours during the night. S.W.'s daughter tells you that she will reposition her mother during the night if her mother wakes up to use the commode. Otherwise, she needs her sleep because she watches her two young grandchildren during the day.

Best Available Evidence	Clinician Expertise	Patient Preferences and Values
Repositioning remains the primary method of reducing risk for pressure ulcers. Pressure-reducing devices (e.g., foam mattress, padded commode seats) can also be used but should not be a substitute for repositioning.	You know that patients with pressure ulcers should be repositioned at least every 2 hours while in bed and every hour when in a chair. You also know that stage I pressure ulcers can rapidly deteriorate to stage II if proper care is not taken.	S.W.'s caregiver expresses the need to have a certain amount of uninterrupted sleep to maintain multiple family responsibilities. States she will reposition her mother at least every 2 hours while she is in bed during the day and every hour when she is in a wheelchair. S.W.'s caregiver states she will purchase a foam mattress, wheelchair cushion, and padded commode seat to help prevent further skin issues.

Your Decision and Action

You discuss the importance of repositioning as the primary method to prevent pressure ulcers and decrease the progression of existing pressure ulcers to more serious ones. S.W.'s daughter reiterates that she will not reposition her mother every 2 hours during the night. You can understand her decision and document this discussion in the patient's discharge teaching record.

Reference for Evidence

European Pressure Ulcer Advisory Panel and National Pressure Ulcer Advisory Panel: *Pressure ulcer treatment: quick reference guide*, Washington, DC, 2009, National Pressure Ulcer Advisory Panel. Retrieved from *www.npuap.org/wp-content/uploads/2012/03/Final_Quick_Treatment_for_web_2010.pdf.*

INFORMATICS IN PRACTICE

Digital Images

To monitor wound progress, use digital photography. For the best images:

- Include a ruler with date, length, width, and depth of the wound in each photo.
- Position the patient the same way for each photo.
- Take the photo from the same angle each time. Pointing perpendicularly at the wound is best.
- Use natural light, without flash, whenever possible.
- Show the wound on a solid background, avoiding shiny underpads.

TABLE 12-16 PATIENT & CAREGIVER TEACHING GUIDE

Pressure Ulcer

When teaching the patient and caregiver to prevent and care for pressure ulcers do the following.

1. Identify and explain risk factors and etiology of pressure ulcers to patient and caregiver.
2. Assess all at-risk patients at time of first hospital and/or home visit or whenever the patient's condition changes. Thereafter assess at regular intervals based on care setting (every 24 hours for acute care or every visit in home care).
3. Teach the caregiver techniques for incontinence. If incontinence occurs, cleanse skin at time of soiling and use absorbent pads or briefs.
4. Demonstrate correct positioning to decrease risk of skin breakdown. Instruct caregiver to reposition a bed-bound patient at least every 2 hours, a chair-bound patient every hour. NEVER position the patient directly on the pressure ulcer.
5. Assess resources (i.e., caregiver's availability and skill, finances, equipment) of patients requiring pressure ulcer care at home. When selecting ulcer care dressing, consider cost and amount of caregiver time required.
6. Teach patient and/or caregiver to place clean dressings over sterile dressings using "no touch" technique when changing dressings. Instruct caregiver on disposal of contaminated dressings.
7. Teach patient and caregiver to inspect skin daily. Tell them to report any significant changes to the health care provider.
8. Teach patient and caregiver the importance of good nutrition to enhance ulcer healing.
9. Evaluate program effectiveness.

Local care of the pressure ulcer may involve debridement, wound cleaning, application of a dressing, and relief of pressure. It is important to select the appropriate pressure-relieving technique (e.g., pad, overlay, mattress, specialty bed) to relieve pressure and keep the patient off of the pressure ulcer. Whenever possible, do not turn the patient onto a body surface that is still reddened. Massage is contraindicated in the presence of acute inflammation and where there is the possibility of damaged blood vessels or fragile skin.[7]

Sliding down in bed causes friction and sheer. Encourage patients to reposition themselves by lifting rather than sliding and to use a trapeze if indicated. Lift sheets may be used to move patients up in bed or to transfer them.[9]

A pressure ulcer that has necrotic tissue or eschar (except for dry, stable necrotic feet or heels) must have the tissue removed by surgical, mechanical, enzymatic, or autolytic debridement methods. Once the pressure ulcer has been successfully debrided and has a clean granulating base, the goal is to provide an appropriate wound environment that supports moist wound healing and prevents disruption of the newly formed granulation tissue. Reconstruction of the pressure ulcer site by operative repair, including skin grafting, skin flaps, musculocutaneous flaps, or free flaps, may be necessary.

Clean pressure ulcers with noncytotoxic solutions that do not kill or damage cells, especially fibroblasts. Solutions such as Dakin's solution (sodium hypochlorite solution), acetic acid, povidone-iodine, and hydrogen peroxide are cytotoxic and therefore should not be used to clean pressure ulcers. It is also important to use enough irrigation pressure to adequately clean the pressure ulcer (4 to 15 psi) without causing trauma or damage to the wound. To obtain this pressure, use a 30-mL syringe and a 19-gauge needle.

After the pressure ulcer has been cleansed, cover it with an appropriate dressing. The current trend is to keep a pressure ulcer slightly moist, rather than dry, to enhance re-epithelialization. Some factors to consider when selecting a dressing are maintenance of a moist environment, prevention of the wound from drying out, ability to absorb the wound drainage, location of the wound, amount of caregiver time required to change the dressing, cost of the dressing, presence of infection, clean versus sterile dressings, and care delivery setting. A wet-to-dry dressing should never be used on a clean granulating pressure ulcer. This type of dressing should be used only for mechanical debridement of the wound. (Dressings are discussed in Table 12-10.)

Stages II through IV pressure ulcers are considered contaminated or colonized with bacteria. Remember that in people who have chronic wounds or are immunocompromised, the clinical signs of infection (purulent exudate, odor, erythema, warmth, tenderness, edema, pain, fever, and elevated WBC count) may not be present even though the pressure ulcer is infected.[10]

The maintenance of adequate nutrition is an important nursing responsibility for the patient with a pressure ulcer. Often, the patient is debilitated and has a poor appetite secondary to inactivity. Oral feedings must be adequate in calories, protein, fluids, vitamins, and minerals to meet the patient's nutritional requirements. The caloric intake needed to correct and maintain nutritional balance may be 30 to 35 calories/kg/day and 1.25 to 1.50 g of protein/kg/day.

Enteral feedings can be used to supplement the oral feedings. When oral and enteral feedings are inadequate, parenteral nutrition consisting of amino acid and glucose solutions is used. (Parenteral and enteral nutrition is discussed in Chapter 40.)

AMBULATORY AND HOME CARE. Pressure ulcers affect the quality of life of patients and their caregivers. Because pressure ulcers commonly recur, teaching prevention techniques to both the patient and the caregiver is extremely important (Table 12-16, p. 187). A sixth-grade-level version of the patient guide to pressure ulcer prevention is available for use in patient teaching *(www.npuap.org/PU_Prev_Points.pdf)*. The caregiver needs to know the etiology of pressure ulcers, prevention techniques, early signs, nutritional support, and care techniques for actual pressure ulcers. Because the patient with a pressure ulcer often requires extensive care for other health problems, it is important that the nurse support the caregiver with the added responsibility for pressure ulcer treatment. eNursing Care Plan 12-2 (available on the website for this chapter) outlines the care for the patient with a pressure ulcer.

EVALUATION

The expected outcomes are that the patient with a pressure ulcer will have

- Healing of pressure ulcer(s)
- Intact skin with no further breakdown

CASE STUDY

Inflammation and Infection

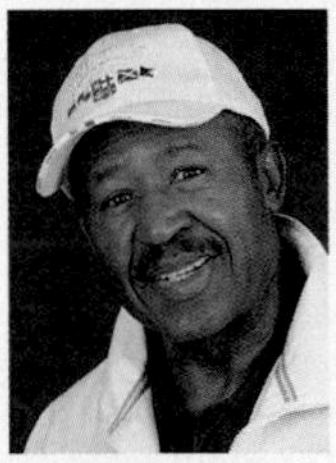

iStockphoto/Thinkstock

Patient Profile

G.N., a 58-year-old African American man, was admitted to the hospital emergency department with partial-thickness burns that involved his face, neck, and upper trunk. He also had a lacerated right leg. His injuries occurred about 36 hours earlier when he fell out of a tree onto his gas grill (which was lit) while trying to get his cat.

Subjective Data

- Complains of slightly hoarse voice and irritated throat
- States that he tried to treat himself because he does not have health insurance
- Has been coughing up sooty sputum
- Complains of severe pain in left hip

Objective Data

Physical Examination

- Leg wound is gaping and has drainage: temperature 101.1° F (38.4° C).
- X-rays reveal a fractured right tibia and fractured left hip.

Laboratory Studies

- WBC count 26,400/μL (26.4×10^9/L) with 80% neutrophils (10% bands)

Collaborative Care

- Surgery is performed to repair the left hip.

Discussion Questions

1. What clinical manifestations of inflammation did G.N. exhibit, and what are their pathophysiologic mechanisms?
2. What type of exudate formation did he develop?
3. What is the basis for the development of the temperature?
4. What is the significance of his WBC count and differential?
5. Because his wound was deep, primary tissue healing was not possible. How would you expect healing to take place? What complications could he develop?
6. What risk factors does G.N. have to develop a pressure ulcer?
7. ***Priority Decision:*** Based on the assessment data provided, what are the priority nursing diagnoses? Are there any collaborative problems?
8. ***Delegation Decision:*** What nursing activities related to wound care can be delegated to unlicensed assistive personnel (UAP)?

evolve Answers available at *http://evolve.elsevier.com/Lewis/medsurg.*

BRIDGE TO NCLEX EXAMINATION

The number of the question corresponds to the same-numbered outcome at the beginning of the chapter.

1. A patient 1 day postoperative after abdominal surgery has incisional pain, 99.5° F temperature, slight erythema at the incision margins, and 30 mL serosanguineous drainage in the Jackson-Pratt drain. Based on this assessment, what conclusion would the nurse make?
   a. The abdominal incision shows signs of an infection.
   b. The patient is having a normal inflammatory response.
   c. The abdominal incision shows signs of impending dehiscence.
   d. The patient's physician needs to be notified about her condition.
2. The nurse assessing a patient with a chronic leg wound finds local signs of erythema and pain at the wound site. What would the nurse anticipate being ordered to assess the patient's systemic response?
   a. Serum protein analysis
   b. WBC count and differential
   c. Punch biopsy of center of wound
   d. Culture and sensitivity of the wound

3. A patient in the unit has a 103.7° F temperature. Which intervention would be most effective in restoring normal body temperature?
   a. Use a cooling blanket while the patient is febrile.
   b. Administer antipyretics on an around-the-clock schedule.
   c. Provide increased fluids and have the UAP give sponge baths.
   d. Give prescribed antibiotics and provide warm blankets for comfort.
4. A nurse is caring for a patient who has a pressure ulcer that is treated with debridement, irrigations, and moist gauze dressings. How should the nurse anticipate healing to occur?
   a. Tertiary intention
   b. Secondary intention
   c. Regeneration of cells
   d. Remodeling of tissues
5. A nurse is caring for a patient with diabetes who is scheduled for amputation of his necrotic left great toe. The patient's WBC count is $15.0 \times 10^6/\mu L$, and he has coolness of the lower extremities, weighs 75 lb more than his ideal body weight, and smokes two packs of cigarettes per day. Which priority nursing diagnosis addresses the primary factor affecting the patient's ability to heal?
   a. Imbalanced nutrition: more than body requirements *related to* high-fat foods
   b. Impaired tissue integrity *related to* decreased blood flow secondary to diabetes and smoking
   c. Ineffective peripheral tissue perfusion *related to* narrowed blood vessels secondary to diabetes and smoking
   d. Ineffective individual coping *related to* indifference and denial of the long-term effects of diabetes and smoking
6. Which one of the orders should a nurse question in the plan of care for a patient with a stage III pressure ulcer?
   a. Pack the ulcer with foam dressing.
   b. Turn and position the patient every 2 hours.
   c. Clean the ulcer every shift with Dakin's solution.
   d. Assess for pain and medicate before dressing change.
7. An 85-year-old patient is assessed to have a score of 16 on the Braden Scale. Based on this information, how should the nurse plan for this patient's care?
   a. Implement a q2hr turning schedule with skin assessment.
   b. Place DuoDerm on the patient's sacrum to prevent breakdown.
   c. Elevate the head of bed to 90 degrees when the patient is supine.
   d. Continue with weekly skin assessments with no special precautions.
8. A 65-year-old stroke patient with limited mobility has a purple area of suspected deep tissue injury on the left greater trochanter. Which nursing diagnoses is/are most appropriate *(select all that apply)?*
   a. Acute pain *related to* tissue damage and inflammation
   b. Impaired skin integrity *related to* immobility and decreased sensation
   c. Impaired tissue integrity *related to* inadequate circulation secondary to pressure
   d. Risk for infection *related to* loss of tissue integrity and undernutrition secondary to stroke
9. An 82-year-old man is being cared for at home by his family. A pressure ulcer on his right buttock measures 1 × 2 × 0.8 cm in depth, and pink subcutaneous tissue is completely visible on the wound bed. Which stage would the nurse document on the wound assessment form?
   a. Stage I
   b. Stage II
   c. Stage III
   d. Stage IV

1. b, 2. b, 3. b, 4. b, 5. b, 6. c, 7. a, 8. b, c, 9. c

evolve

For rationales to these answers and even more NCLEX review questions, visit *http://evolve.elsevier.com/Lewis/medsurg.*

REFERENCES

1. Atkins E: Fever: its history, cause, and function, *Yale J Biol Med* 55:283, 1982. (Classic)
2. Reddy M, Gill SS, Wu W, et al: Does this patient have an infection of a chronic wound? *JAMA* 307(6):605, 2012.
3. Martindell D: The safe use of negative-pressure wound therapy, *Am J Nurs* 112:59, 2012.
4. Kranke P, Bennett MH, Martyn-St James M, et al: Hyperbaric oxygen therapy for chronic wounds, *Cochrane Database Syst Rev* 4:CD004123, 2012.
5. Nightingale F: *Notes on nursing,* Philadelphia, 1859, Lippincott. (Classic)
6. Lynch S, Vickery P: Steps to reduce hospital-acquired pressure ulcers, *Nursing* 40:61, 2010.
7. European Pressure Ulcer Advisory Panel and National Pressure Ulcer Advisory Panel: *Pressure ulcer prevention: quick reference guide,* Washington, DC, 2009, National Pressure Ulcer Advisory Panel. Retrieved from *www.npuap.org/wp-content/uploads/2012/03/Final_Quick_Prevention_for_web_2010.pdf.*
8. National Pressure Ulcer Advisory Panel: PUSH tool. Retrieved from *www.npuap.org/resources/educational-and-clinical-resources/push-tool/push-tool.*
9. Blaney WD: Taking steps to prevent pressure ulcers, *Nursing* 40:45, 2010.
10. Pham B, Stern A, Chen W: Preventing pressure ulcers in long-term care: a cost-effective analysis, *Arch Intern Med* 171:1839, 2011.

RESOURCES

Braden Scale for Predicting Pressure Sore Risk
www.bradenscale.com/images/bradenscale.pdf

National Pressure Ulcer Advisory Panel
www.npuap.org

Wound Ostomy and Continence Nurses Society
www.wocn.org

CHAPTER 13

The laws of genetics apply even if you refuse to learn them.
Allison Plowden

Genetics and Genomics

Sharon L. Lewis

evolve WEBSITE

http://evolve.elsevier.com/Lewis/medsurg

- NCLEX Review Questions
- Key Points
- Pre-Test
- Rationales for Bridge to NCLEX Examination Questions
- Concept Map Creator
- Glossary
- Content Updates

eFigure

- eFig. 13-1: Transcription and translation

LEARNING OUTCOMES

1. Differentiate the common terms related to genetics and genetic disorders: *autosomal, carrier, heterozygous, homozygous, mutation, recessive,* and *X-linked gene.*
2. Differentiate between the two common causes of genetic mutations.
3. Compare and contrast the three most common inheritance patterns of genetic disorders.
4. Describe the most common classifications of genetic disorders.
5. Explore the complex ethical and social implications of genetic testing.
6. Analyze the role of pharmacogenetics in developing personalized drug therapy.
7. Discuss your role in assisting the patient and family in dealing with genetic issues.

KEY TERMS

genetics, p. 190
genomics, p. 190
hereditary, Table 13-1, p. 191
heterozygous, Table 13-1, p. 191
homozygous, Table 13-1, p. 191
mutation, Table 13-1, p. 191
pharmacogenetics, p. 198
pharmacogenomics, p. 198

GENETICS AND GENOMICS

In the 1860s an Austrian monk named Gregor Mendel, while experimenting with pea plants, discovered how traits are transmitted from parents to offspring. This discovery laid the foundation for modern **genetics,** the study of genes and their role in inheritance. Genetics determines the way that certain traits or conditions are passed down from one generation to another. **Genomics** is the study of all of a person's genes (the *genome*), including interactions of these genes with each other and with the person's environment. (Common terms used in genetics and genomics are defined in Table 13-1.) Genomics includes the study of complex diseases such as heart disease, asthma, diabetes mellitus, and cancer because these diseases are typically caused by a combination of genetic and environmental factors rather than by a single gene.

A person's genes can have a profound impact on health and disease. More than 4000 diseases are thought to be related to altered genes. Genomic factors play a role in 9 of the 10 leading causes of death in the United States, including heart disease, cancer, diabetes, stroke, and Alzheimer's disease.[1]

Genomics may help us understand why some people who eat healthy diets and exercise regularly still die at a young age of cancer, whereas some people eat unhealthy diets and never exercise, and yet live to an old age.

The identification of a genetic basis for many human diseases has the potential to strongly influence the care of patients at risk for or diagnosed with a disease that has a genetic link. You need to know the basic principles of genetics, be familiar with the impact that genetics and genomics have on health and disease, and be prepared to assist the patient and family with genetic issues.

Basic Principles of Genetics

Genes. *Genes* are the basic units of heredity. There are approximately 20,000 to 25,000 genes in each person's genetic makeup, or *genome.* Genes encode (carry the instructions) for proteins that direct the activities of cells and functions of the

Reviewed by Mindy B. Tinkle, RN, PhD, WHNP-BC, Associate Professor and Chair, Research and PhD Studies, University of New Mexico, College of Nursing, Albuquerque, New Mexico; Laura Mallett, RN, MSN, Assistant Lecturer, University of Wyoming, Fay W. Whitney School of Nursing, Laramie, Wyoming; and Bernice Coleman, PhD, ACNP-BC, FAHA, Nurse Practitioner, Heart Transplantation and Ventricular Assist Device Programs, Cedars Sinai Medical Center, Los Angeles, California.

TABLE 13-1 GLOSSARY OF GENETIC AND GENOMIC TERMS

Term	Definition
Allele	An alternative form of a gene. Each person receives two alleles of a gene, one from each biologic parent. Different alleles produce variations in inherited traits such as eye color and blood type.
Autosome	Any chromosome that is not a sex chromosome. Humans have 22 pairs of autosomes.
Carrier	Individual who carries a copy of a mutated gene for a recessive disorder.
Chromosome	A compact structure containing DNA and proteins present in nearly all cells of the body. Normally each cell has 46 chromosomes in 23 pairs. Each biologic parent contributes one of each pair of chromosomes.
Codominance	Two dominant versions of a trait that are both expressed in the same individual.
Congenital disorder	Condition present at birth.
Dominant allele	Gene that is expressed in the phenotype of a heterozygous individual.
Familial disorder	Condition that affects more than one person in a family.
Gene	The basic unit of heredity information located on a specific part of a chromosome. Genes direct cells to make proteins and guide almost every aspect of operation and repair of cells.
Genetic risk factor	A change in a gene that increases a person's risk of developing a disease.
Genetics	Study of genes and their role in inheritance.
Genome	All the DNA contained in an individual.
Genome-wide association study (GWAS)	A study approach that involves scanning complete sets of DNA (genomes) of many individuals to find genetic variations associated with a particular disease.
Genomics	Study of how genes interact and influence people's biologic and physical characteristics.
Genotype	Genetic identity of an individual. This identity does not show as outward characteristics.
Hereditary	Transmission of a disease, condition, or trait from parent to children.
Heterozygous	Having two different alleles for one given gene, one inherited from each parent.
Homozygous	Having two identical alleles for one given gene, one inherited from each parent.
Locus	Position of a gene on a chromosome.
Mutation	A change in DNA or a gene. Sometimes these changes are passed from parent to children.
Oncogene	Gene that is able to initiate and contribute to the conversion of normal cells to cancer cells.
Pedigree	Family tree that contains the genetic characteristics and disorders of that particular family.
Pharmacogenetics	Study of variability of responses to drugs related to variations in single genes.
Pharmacogenomics	Study of variability of responses to drugs related to variations in and interactions of multiple genes.
Phenotype	Observable traits or characteristics of an individual (e.g., hair color).
Protooncogene	Normal cellular genes that are important regulators of normal cellular processes. Mutations can activate them to become oncogenes.
Recessive allele	Allele that has no noticeable effect on the phenotype in a heterozygous individual.
Trait	Physical characteristic that one inherits, such as hair or eye color.
X-linked gene	Gene located on the X chromosome. In general, sex-linked disorders are only seen in males.

body. Genes control how a cell functions, including how quickly it grows, how often it divides, and how long it lives. To control these functions, genes produce proteins that perform specific tasks and act as messengers for the cell. Therefore it is essential that each gene have the correct instructions or "code" for making its protein so that the protein can perform the proper function for the cell.[2]

Genes are arranged in a specific linear formation along a chromosome (Fig. 13-1). Each gene has a specific location on a chromosome, termed a *locus.* An *allele* is one of two or more alternative forms of a gene that occupy corresponding loci on *homologous chromosomes* (a pair of chromosomes having corresponding deoxyribonucleic acid [DNA] sequences, with one coming from the mother and the other from the father). Each allele codes for a specific inherited characteristic.

When there are two different alleles, the allele that is fully expressed is the *dominant allele.* The other allele that lacks the ability to express itself in the presence of a dominant allele is the *recessive allele.* Physical traits expressed by an individual are termed the *phenotype,* and the actual genetic makeup of the individual is termed the *genotype.*

Chromosomes. *Chromosomes* are contained in the nucleus of a cell and occur in pairs. Humans have 23 pairs of chromosomes; 22 of the 23 pairs of chromosomes are *homologous* and are termed *autosomes.* Autosomes are the same in both males and females. The sex chromosomes make up the twenty-third pair of chromosomes. A female has two X chromosomes, and a male has one X and one Y chromosome. One chromosome of each pair is inherited from the mother and one from the father. One half of each child's chromosomes (and therefore the genetic makeup) comes from his or her father and one half from his or her mother.

DNA. Genes are made up of a nucleic acid called *deoxyribonucleic acid* (DNA). DNA stores genetic information and encodes the instructions for synthesizing specific proteins needed to maintain life. DNA also dictates the rate at which proteins are made. Every somatic cell in a person's body has the same DNA.

The information in DNA is stored as a code made up of four nitrogenous bases: adenine (A), guanine (G), cytosine (C), and thymine (T). Human DNA consists of about 3 billion bases, and more than 99% of those bases are the same in all people. The

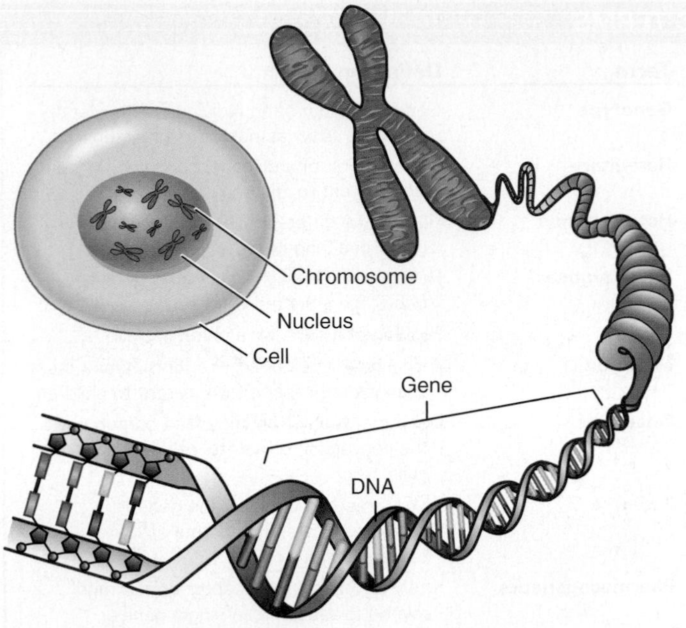

FIG. 13-1 The long, stringy DNA that makes up genes is spooled within chromosomes inside the nucleus of a cell. (Note that a gene would actually be a much longer stretch of DNA than what is shown here.)

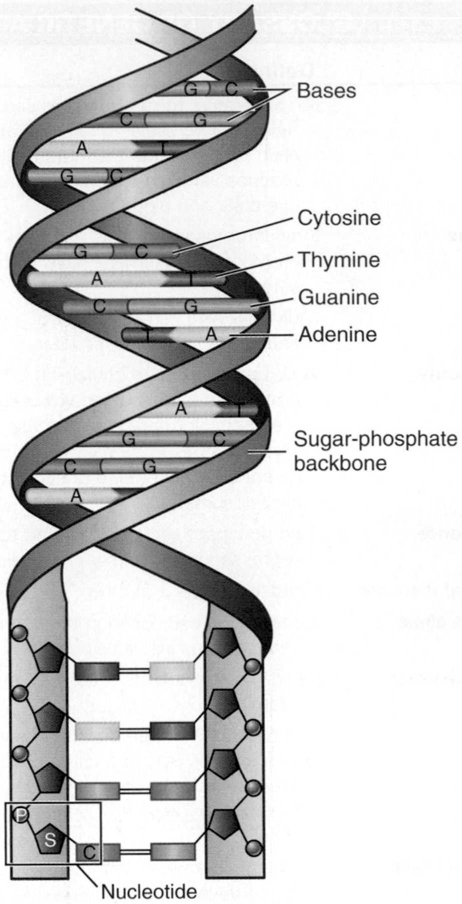

FIG. 13-2 DNA consists of two long, twisted chains made up of nucleotides. Each nucleotide contains one base, one phosphate molecule *(P)*, and the sugar molecule deoxyribose *(S)*. The bases in DNA nucleotides are adenine *(A)*, thymine *(T)*, cytosine *(C)*, and guanine *(G)*.

order (or sequence) of these bases determines the information for building and maintaining an organism. This is similar to the way letters of the alphabet are used to create words and sentences.

DNA bases pair up with each other, A with T and C with G, to form units called *base pairs*. Each base is also attached to a sugar molecule and a phosphate molecule (Fig. 13-2). Together, a base, sugar, and phosphate are called a *nucleotide*. Nucleotides are arranged in two long strands that form a spiral called a *double helix*. The structure of the double helix is somewhat like a ladder, with the base pairs forming the ladder's rungs and the sugar and phosphate molecules forming the ladder's vertical sidepieces.

DNA can *replicate* (make copies of itself). Each strand of DNA in the double helix can serve as a pattern for duplicating the sequence of bases. When cells divide, each new cell needs to have an exact copy of the DNA that was in the parent (original) cell.

If the chromosomes in one of your cells were uncoiled and placed end-to-end, the DNA would be about 6 feet long. If all of the DNA in your body were connected, it would stretch about 67 billion miles.[3]

RNA. *Ribonucleic acid* (RNA) is similar to DNA, but with some significant differences. Like DNA, RNA contains the nitrogenous bases adenine, guanine, and cytosine. However, RNA lacks the nitrogenous base thymine and instead contains uracil. RNA is single stranded and contains ribose instead of deoxyribose sugar. RNA transfers the genetic information obtained from DNA to the proper location for protein synthesis.

Protein Synthesis. Protein synthesis, or the making of proteins, occurs in two steps: *transcription* and *translation*. (Transcription and translation are shown in eFig. 13-1 on the website for this chapter.) Transcription is the process by which messenger RNA (mRNA) is synthesized from single-stranded DNA. The mRNA becomes attached to a ribosome, where translation occurs. At this point another specialized type of RNA, transfer RNA (tRNA), arranges the amino acids in the correct sequence to assemble the protein. Once the protein is completed, it is released from the ribosome and is able to perform its specific function in the cell.

Mitosis. *Mitosis* is a type of cell division that results in the formation of genetically identical daughter cells. Before cell division the chromosomes duplicate, and each new cell (called daughter cells) receives an exact replica of the chromosomes from the original cell (called the parent cell).

Meiosis. *Meiosis* occurs only in sexual reproductive cells. In meiosis the number of chromosomes is reduced, resulting in half of the usual number of chromosomes. Therefore oocytes and sperm contain only a single copy of each chromosome, whereas all other body cells contain duplicates of each chromosome.

Genetic Mutations

A *mutation* is any change in the usual DNA sequence. Subtle variations in DNA are called *polymorphisms* (meaning *many forms*). Many of these *gene* polymorphisms account for slight variations among people such as hair and eye color. However, some gene variations may result in disease or an increased risk for disease. These gene variations or changes are referred to as *mutations*.

A genetic mutation is like a spelling error in a gene's sequence. For example, in people with sickle cell disease, a substitution of a single base (adenine is replaced by thymine) in a single gene

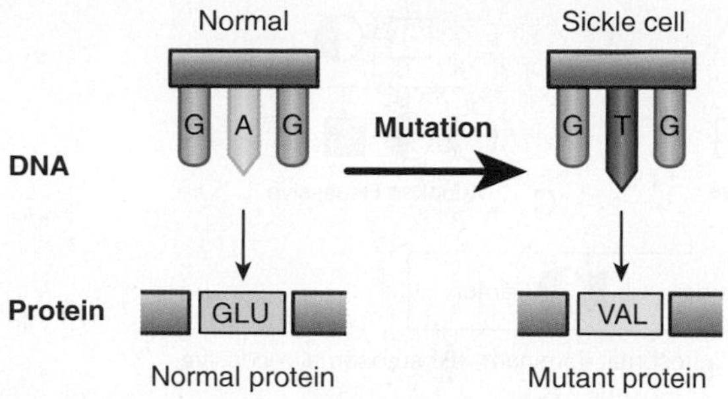

FIG. 13-3 In sickle cell disease a single gene mutation leads to mutant (incorrect) protein. The substitution of valine *(VAL)* for glutamic acid on the β-globin chain of hemoglobin produces abnormal hemoglobin, hemoglobin S (Hb S). In response to low O_2 levels, the erythrocytes with Hb S stiffen and elongate, taking on a sickle shape (see Fig. 31-3).

(β-globin gene) causes the disease (Fig. 13-3). Mutations range in size from a single DNA base (building block) to a large segment of a chromosome.

The change in gene structure may alter the type and/or amount of protein produced. The protein may not work at all, or it may work incorrectly. In some cases, genetic mutations do not have an obvious effect on the people who have them.

Types of Mutations. Genetic mutations occur in two ways. They can be inherited from a parent (germline mutation) or acquired (somatic mutation) during a person's lifetime.

Germline mutations are passed from parent to child. These mutations are present in the oocyte and sperm cells. This type of mutation is present throughout a person's life in virtually every cell in the body.

Acquired (somatic) mutations occur in the DNA of a cell at some time during a person's life. An acquired mutation is passed on to all cells that develop from that single cell. These mutations in somatic cells cannot be passed on to the next generation. Acquired mutations can occur if (1) a mistake is made as DNA replicates during cell division or (2) environmental factors alter the DNA.

Mutations can occur when a cell is dividing. Considering that 3 billion base pairs are replicated in each cell division, DNA replication is very accurate. However, during replication occasionally mistakes such as deletions, insertions, or duplication of DNA material can occur. Although DNA repair enzymes can correct replication errors, mistakes can go uncorrected.[4]

In addition to cell division, DNA damage can also occur from environmental factors. For example, ultraviolet (UV) radiation can cause DNA damage, leading to skin cancer. Toxins in cigarettes can lead to lung cancer. Many chemotherapy drugs used to treat cancer target the DNA of both cancer cells and healthy cells. In the process these drugs increase a person's risk of developing secondary cancers (see Chapter 16).

Cells have built-in mechanisms that catch and repair most of the changes that occur during DNA replication or from environmental damage. However, as we age, our DNA repair does not work as effectively and we accumulate changes in our DNA.

Inheritance Patterns

Genetic disorders can be categorized into autosomal dominant, autosomal recessive, or X-linked (sex-linked) recessive disorders (Table 13-2). If the mutant gene is located on an autosome, the genetic disorder is called *autosomal.* If the mutant gene is on the X chromosome, the genetic disorder is called *X-linked.*

TABLE 13-2 COMPARISON OF GENETIC DISORDERS

Characteristics	Examples
Autosomal Dominant	
Males and females are affected* equally.	Breast and ovarian cancer related to *BRCA* genes
More common than recessive disorders and usually less severe.	Familial hypercholesterolemia
Affected individuals show variable expression.	Hereditary nonpolyposis colorectal cancer
Affected individuals may have an affected parent.	Huntington's disease
Children of a heterozygous (affected) parent have a 50% chance of being affected.	Neurofibromatosis
Individuals are affected in successive generations.	Marfan's syndrome
Autosomal Recessive	
Males and females are affected equally.	Cystic fibrosis
Heterozygotes are carriers and usually asymptomatic.	Phenylketonuria
Affected individuals may have unaffected† parents who are heterozygous for trait.	Sickle cell disease
Children of two heterozygous parents have 25% chance of being affected and 50% chance of being carriers (see Fig. 13-9).	Tay-Sachs disease
Frequently there is a no family history of disease.	Thalassemia
X-Linked Recessive	
Most affected individuals have unaffected parents.	Duchenne muscular dystrophy
Affected individuals are usually males.	Hemophilia
Daughters of affected male are carriers.	Wiskott-Aldrich syndrome
Sons of affected male are unaffected (unless mother is a carrier).	

*Have the disease.
†Do not have the disease.

Family pedigrees for autosomal recessive and dominant disorders and X-linked recessive disorders are shown in Figs. 13-4 and 13-5.

Autosomal dominant disorders are caused by a mutation of a single gene pair (heterozygous) on a chromosome. A dominant allele prevails over a normal allele. Autosomal dominant disorders show variable expression. *Variable expression* means that the symptoms expressed by the individuals with the mutated gene vary from person to person even though they have the same mutated gene. Although autosomal dominant disorders have a high probability of occurring in families, sometimes these disorders cause a new mutation or skip a generation. This is termed *incomplete penetrance.*

Autosomal recessive disorders are caused by mutations of two gene pairs (homozygous) on a chromosome. A person who inherits one copy of the recessive allele does not develop the disease because the normal allele predominates. However, this person is a *carrier.*

X-linked recessive disorders are caused by a mutation on the X chromosome. Usually only men are affected by this disorder because women who carry the mutated gene on one X chromosome have another X chromosome to compensate for the mutation. However, women who carry the mutated gene can transmit it to their offspring. It is possible for women to have X-linked recessive disorders, and this can occur when an affected male mates with an unaffected female carrier. This points to the

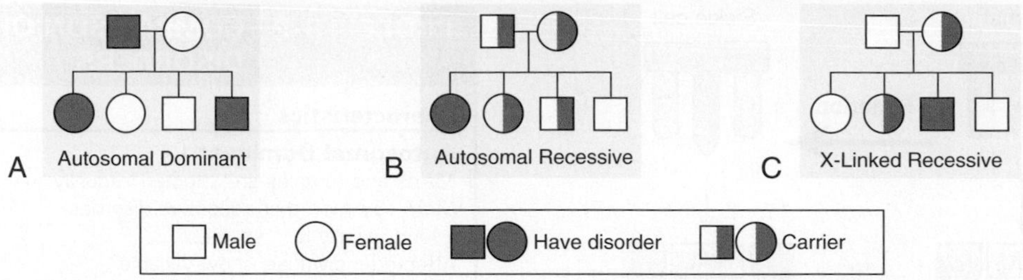

FIG. 13-4 Examples of family pedigrees showing inheritance of **(A)** autosomal dominant, **(B)** autosomal recessive, and **(C)** X-linked recessive disorders.

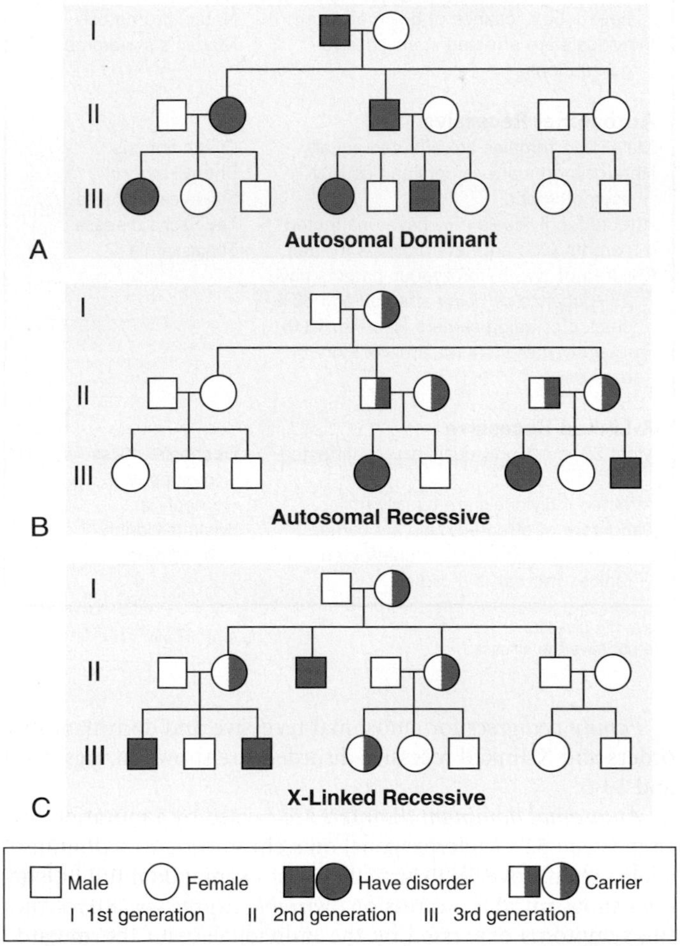

FIG. 13-5 Family pedigrees showing three generations. **A,** Family pedigree suggestive of an autosomal dominant disorder. **B,** Family pedigree suggestive of an autosomal recessive disorder. **C,** Family pedigree suggestive of an X-linked recessive disorder.

importance of testing the carrier status of the female partner of affected males. *X-linked dominant disorders* do exist but are rare.

Multifactorial inherited conditions are caused by a combination of genetic and environmental factors. These disorders run in families but do not show the same inherited characteristics as the single gene mutation conditions. Multifactorial conditions include diabetes mellitus, obesity, hypertension, cancer, and coronary artery disease.

Human Genome Project

The Human Genome Project (HGP), which was completed in 2003, mapped the entire human genome.[5] Analysis of the data will continue for many years. The knowledge gained through the HGP will (1) help improve the diagnosis of diseases, (2) allow for earlier detection of genetic predisposition to diseases, and (3) play a critical role in determining risk assessment for genetic-related diseases. In addition, the results of the HGP assist in matching organ donors with transplant recipients.

GENETIC DISORDERS

A *genetic disorder* is caused in whole or in part by an alteration in the DNA sequence. As discussed in the section on genetic mutations (pp. 192-193), genetic disorders can be inherited (person born with altered genetic code) or they can be acquired (e.g., replication errors, damage to DNA from toxins). Genetic disorders can be caused by (1) a mutation in one gene (single gene disorder); (2) mutations in multiple genes (multifactorial inheritance disorder), which are often related to environmental factors; or (3) damage to chromosomes (changes in the number or structure of entire chromosomes).

Classification of Genetic Disorders

Single Gene Disorders. Some genetic disorders result from a single gene mutation (Fig. 13-6, *A*). Examples of these diseases include cystic fibrosis, sickle cell disease, and polycystic kidney disease. The pattern of inheritance for single gene disorders can be autosomal dominant, autosomal recessive, or X-linked. Single gene disorders are relatively rare compared with more commonly occurring multifactorial genetic disorders such as diabetes mellitus and heart disease.

Multifactorial Genetic Disorders. Multifactorial genetic disorders are complex diseases that result from small inherited variations in genes, often acting together with environmental factors (Fig. 13-6, *B*). Heart disease, diabetes, and most cancers are examples of such disorders.

Although many common diseases are usually caused by inheritance of mutations in multiple genes, such diseases can also be caused by rare hereditary mutations in a single gene. In these cases, genetic mutations that cause or strongly predispose a person to these diseases run in a family. These mutations can significantly increase each family member's risk of developing the disease. One example is breast cancer, where inheritance of a mutated *BRCA1* or *BRCA2* gene confers significant risk of developing the disease.

Epigenetics. Environmental factors can alter the way our genes are expressed (i.e., which genes are "switched" on or off). Identical twins, who have the same genetic makeup, do not always develop the same diseases or at the same rate.[6]

Genetic and environmental factors interact to influence a person's predisposition to different diseases. *Epigenetics* is the study of changes in gene function that do not involve a change

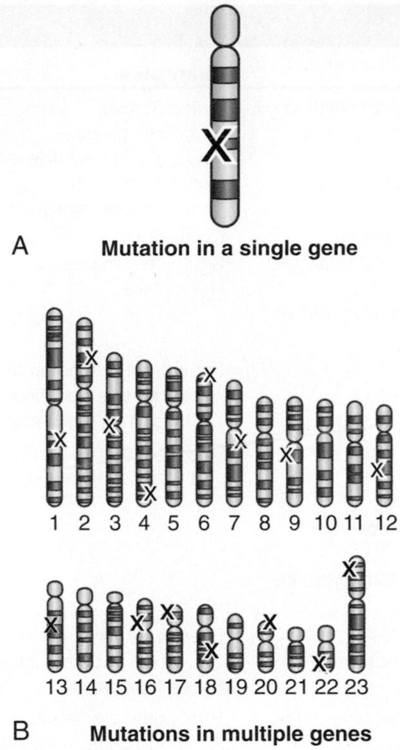

FIG. 13-6 **A,** Genetic disorders can be caused by a mutation in a single gene (e.g., sickle cell disease, cystic fibrosis, hemophilia). **B,** Most genetic disorders are multifactorial genetic disorders caused by a combination of mutations in multiple genes, often interacting with environmental factors. Examples include cancer, diabetes mellitus, obesity, and hypertension.

in DNA sequence. Epigenetics focuses on how and when particular genes are expressed. The expression of genes can be affected both positively and negatively by environmental factors, such as exercise, diet, chemicals, toxins, or smoking. Epigenetic changes can be inherited.

Chromosome Disorders. *Chromosome disorders* are caused by structural changes within chromosomes or by an excess or deficiency of the genes that are located on chromosomes. For example, Down syndrome is caused by an extra copy of chromosome 21 (called trisomy 21), so there are three copies of this chromosome instead of two. In Down syndrome there is no individual abnormal gene on the chromosome.

Chronic myelocytic leukemia can be caused by a chromosomal translocation, in which portions of two chromosomes (chromosomes 9 and 22) are exchanged. This translocation is called the Philadelphia chromosome.

Throughout the book, genetic disorders are highlighted in Genetics in Clinical Practice boxes, Genetic Risk Alert boxes (in the assessment chapters), and Genetic Links content (in the management chapters).

GENETIC TESTING

Genetic testing includes any procedure done to analyze chromosomes, genes, or any gene product that can determine whether a mutation or predisposition to a condition exists. Genetic tests have been developed for more than 2000 diseases. Samples from a person's blood, skin, hair, or saliva can be used to obtain samples for genetic testing. Tissues and cells can also be obtained prenatally.

GENETICS IN CLINICAL PRACTICE

Genetics in Clinical Practice Boxes Throughout Book

GENETIC DISORDER	CHAPTER	PAGE
α_1-Antitrypsin (AAT) Deficiency	29	582
Alzheimer's Disease (AD)	60	1446
Ankylosing Spondylitis	65	1580
Breast Cancer	52	1244
Cystic Fibrosis (CF)	29	602
Duchenne and Becker Muscular Dystrophy (MD)	64	1545
Familial Adenomatous Polyposis (FAP)	43	985
Familial Hypercholesterolemia	34	733
Genetic Information Nondiscrimination Act (GINA)	13	196
Hemochromatosis	31	648
Hemophilia A and B	31	655
Hereditary Nonpolyposis Colorectal Cancer (HNPCC) or Lynch Syndrome	43	986
Huntington's Disease	59	1440
Ovarian Cancer	54	1295
Polycystic Kidney Disease (PKD)	46	1083
Sickle Cell Disease	31	645
Types 1 and 2 Diabetes Mellitus	49	1155

Genetic testing has been very useful in health care (Table 13-3). Most tests assess single genes and are used to diagnose genetic disorders such as cystic fibrosis or Duchenne muscular dystrophy.[7] Some genetic tests look at rare inherited mutations of otherwise protective genes, such as *BRCA1* and *BRCA2,* which are responsible for some types of hereditary breast and ovarian cancers.

The results of these tests are used in diagnosing an illness or risk for a disorder, and provide the basis for appropriate treatments. Other genetic tests identify people at high risk for conditions that may be preventable. For example, monitoring for and removing polyps or the entire colon in those inheriting a gene for familial adenomatous polyposis (FAP) has saved many lives. (FAP is discussed in Chapter 43 on p. 985.)

Genetic testing of individuals may raise both ethical and social issues. People considering genetic testing should be aware that test results in their medical records might not be kept private. However, the Genetic Information Nondiscrimination Act (GINA) protects people from discrimination by employers and health insurance companies.

If an individual has genetic testing, it may uncover information that may also affect a family member who was not tested. These individuals are frequently not a part of the decision-making process to undergo testing. Similarly, if a whole family is tested, the results may indicate that the biologic relationship is not what the family believed it to be. Some tests are used to help guide health care providers' recommendations for treatment in consultation with the patient (e.g., *BRCA* testing). Other tests allow families to make the decision about not having children with devastating diseases (e.g., cystic fibrosis) or identify people at high risk for conditions that may be prevented by monitoring or having prophylactic surgery (e.g., familial adenomatous polyposis [FAP]).

Currently, many genetic tests are available from testing laboratories. In most cases insurance companies will not cover the cost of genetic testing. For more information about genetic testing, see *www.cdc.gov/dls/moleculartesting.*

TABLE 13-3 USE OF GENETIC TESTS*

Type of Test	Description	Examples
Diagnostic testing	• Used to diagnose, rule out, or confirm a specific genetic or chromosomal condition. • Used to confirm findings when patient's signs and symptoms suggest a genetic disorder. • Can be performed at any time during a person's life, but is not available for all genes or all genetic conditions.	Cystic fibrosis Sickle cell disease Polycystic kidney disease Hemophilia Familial hypercholesterolemia
Carrier screening	• Can be used to identify unaffected individuals who carry one copy of a gene. • Offered to individuals who have a family history of a genetic disorder and to people in ethnic groups with an increased risk of specific genetic conditions. • If both parents are tested, the test can provide information about a couple's risk of having a child with a genetic condition.	Cystic fibrosis Sickle cell disease Hemophilia
Preimplantation genetic diagnosis (PGD)	• Fertilized embryos tested before implantation and pregnancy. • Allows embryos free of particular disorders to be placed into the uterus. • Embryos that test positive for genetic disorders can be destroyed.	For individuals known to have or be a carrier for a genetic mutation (e.g., Huntington's disease)
Prenatal diagnostic testing	• Fluid obtained from amniocentesis or tissue from chorionic villus used to obtain fetal cells. • Used to detect changes in genes or chromosomes of fetus before birth. • Type of testing offered to couples with an increased risk of having a baby with a genetic or chromosomal disorder. • Can decrease a couple's uncertainty or help them decide whether to terminate the pregnancy.	Down syndrome or other genetic alterations in fetuses
Newborn screening	• Most widespread use of genetic testing. • Early intervention to treat these disorders can eliminate or reduce symptoms that might otherwise cause a lifetime of disability.	Phenylketonuria Congenital hypothyroidism Cystic fibrosis
Presymptomatic testing	• Used to detect genetic mutations associated with disorders that appear later in life. • Can be helpful to people who have a family member with a genetic disorder, but who have no features of the disorder themselves at the time of testing. • Results can provide information about a person's risk of developing a specific disorder and help with making decisions about treatment.	Huntington's disease Adult polycystic kidney disease Hemochromatosis Familial adenomatous polyposis Hereditary nonpolyposis colorectal cancer syndrome
Predictive testing	• Can identify mutations that increase a person's risk of developing disorders. • If results are positive, person can have prophylactic measures (e.g., mastectomy, oophorectomy) to prevent development of cancer.	Breast cancer Ovarian cancer
Forensic testing	• Done to identify an individual for legal purposes.	Identify crime or victims in catastrophic situations Rule out or implicate a crime suspect
Parental testing	• Establish biologic relationships between people.	Paternity testing
Pharmacogenetic testing	• Identifies genetic variations that influence a person's response to drugs. • Results provide information to help select drug therapy that is best for the person.	warfarin (Coumadin) dose

*The laboratory performing the tests must, by law, keep your personal information and test results confidential.

GENETICS IN CLINICAL PRACTICE

Genetic Information Nondiscrimination Act (GINA)

What Is GINA?

The Genetic Information Nondiscrimination Act (GINA) prohibits discrimination in health care coverage and employment based on genetic information.

Why Was GINA Needed?

- Decreases concerns about discrimination that might prevent people from getting genetic tests.
- Enables people to take part in research studies without fear that their DNA information might be used against them in the workplace or prevent them from getting health insurance.

What Is a Genetic Test?

- An analysis of human genes (DNA, RNA), chromosomes, proteins, or metabolites that detects genotypes, mutations, or chromosomal changes.

What Is Genetic Information?

- Any information about a person's genetic tests, family members' genetic tests, and family history of a genetic disease or disorder.
- Referral of a person or family for, or use of, genetic services and participation in clinical research that involves genetic services.

What Does GINA Do?

- Prevents health insurers from denying health insurance coverage, adjusting premiums, and discriminating against a person based solely on his or her genetic or family history information.
- Prevents health insurers from requesting that a person have a genetic test.
- Prohibits most employers from using genetic information for hiring, firing, or promotion decisions, and for any decisions regarding terms of employment.
- GINA's health coverage nondiscrimination protection does not extend to life insurance, disability insurance, and long-term care insurance.

For more information see

- *www.genome.gov/Pages/PolicyEthics/GeneticDiscrimination/GINAInfoDoc.pdf*
- Frequently Asked Questions about GINA at *www.dnapolicy.org/gina/faqs.html*

Interpreting Genetic Test Results

The results of genetic tests are not always straightforward, which often makes them challenging to interpret and explain. When interpreting test results, health care professionals need to consider a person's medical history, family history, and the type of genetic test that was done.

A *positive test* result means that the laboratory found a change in a particular gene, chromosome, or protein that was being tested. Depending on the purpose of the test, this result may confirm a diagnosis (e.g., Huntington's disease), indicate that a person is a carrier of a particular genetic mutation (e.g., cystic fibrosis), identify an increased risk of developing a disease (e.g., breast cancer), or suggest a need for further testing. A positive result of a predictive or presymptomatic genetic test usually cannot establish the absolute risk of developing a disorder. In addition, a positive test cannot predict the course or severity of a condition.

In some situations it is difficult to interpret a positive result because some people who have the genetic mutation being tested never develop the disease. For example, having the apolipoprotein E-4 *(Apo E-4)* allele increases the risk of developing Alzheimer's disease. However, many people who test positive for *Apo E-4* never develop Alzheimer's disease (see Chapter 60).

A *negative test* result means that the laboratory did not find an altered form of the gene, chromosome, or protein under consideration. This result can indicate that a person is not affected by a particular disorder, is not a carrier of a specific genetic mutation, or does not have an increased risk of developing a certain disease. However, it is possible that the test missed a disease-causing genetic alteration, since many tests cannot detect all the genetic changes that cause a particular disorder. Further testing may be required to confirm a negative result.

ETHICAL/LEGAL DILEMMAS

Genetic Testing

Situation

A 30-year-old woman informs you that she is 3 months' pregnant. She has two children with her current husband. This pregnancy was unplanned, and her youngest child has cystic fibrosis (CF). She expresses concern regarding the possibility of having another child with CF. She mentions that she would like to have genetic testing on her fetus. Her husband asks you what the likelihood is of having another child with CF.

Ethical/Legal Points for Consideration

- With genetic testing, the patient and her family can find out whether their child will have CF. The woman and her husband can then make an informed decision.
- Genetic counseling is recommended before and after obtaining genetic testing because of the complexity of the information and the emotional issues involved with implications and options.
- Knowing that CF is an autosomal recessive condition, you can use Punnett squares (see Fig. 13-9) or a family pedigree (see Figs. 13-4 and 13-5) to show the woman and her husband the probability of having another child with CF.

Discussion Questions

1. What information would you give the patient and her husband regarding genetic testing in order for them to make an informed decision?
2. What options are available for this couple?
3. How would you assist this couple as they are considering terminating the pregnancy if the results of the genetic testing reveal that the fetus will have CF?

Direct-to-Consumer Genetic Tests

Direct-to-consumer genetic tests (at-home testing) are marketed directly to people (consumers) via television, print advertisements, or the Internet. The test kit is mailed to the person instead of being ordered through a health care provider's office. The test typically involves collecting a DNA sample at home, often by swabbing the inside of the cheek, and mailing the sample back to the laboratory. In some cases the person must visit a health clinic to have blood drawn.

Consumers are notified of their results by mail or over the telephone, or the results are posted online. In some cases a genetic counselor or other health care provider is available to explain the results and answer questions. The price for at-home genetic testing ranges from several hundred dollars to more than $1000.

Direct-to-consumer genetic tests have significant risks and limitations. Consumers are vulnerable to being misled by the results of unproven or invalid tests. Without guidance from a health care provider, they may make important decisions about disease treatment or prevention based on inaccurate, incomplete, or misunderstood information about their health. Consumers may also experience an invasion of genetic privacy if testing companies use their genetic information in an unauthorized way.

If your patients are considering using these kinds of genetic tests, let them know that they first need to discuss the issue with their health care provider or a genetic counselor. Patient teaching related to genetic testing is presented in Table 13-4.

Genetic Technology

DNA Finger Printing. DNA (genetic) finger printing begins by extracting DNA from the cells in a sample of blood, saliva, semen, or other appropriate fluid or tissue. *Polymerase chain reaction* (PCR) is a quick, easy method to provide unlimited copies of a DNA or RNA sequence using only a small amount of sample. PCR involves the artificial replication of a DNA or RNA sequence. The DNA or RNA strands can be separated to form new templates that are used for replication.[8]

PCR is a key element in *genetic finger printing.* It is an essential technique to finding mutations in genes. It is also used extensively in forensic medicine to identify DNA of criminal suspects by using samples from blood, hair, saliva, and semen. PCR has also been used in finding evidence to free innocent prisoners and in paternity testing.

PCR can also be used as a confirmatory test in HIV testing. This is especially important when an infant of a mother who is HIV-antibody positive also tests HIV positive. In this situation it is not known whether the antibodies from the infant's blood are from the baby or the mother. PCR techniques can be used on the baby's lymphocytes to determine whether the baby is infected with HIV.

DNA Microarray (DNA Chip). Although all of a person's somatic cells contain identical genetic material, the same genes are not active in every cell. Studying which genes are active and which are inactive in different cell types helps to understand (1) how these cells function normally and (2) how they are affected when various genes do not perform properly.

Gene expression profiling uses a technology called *DNA microarrays* (DNA chips). This technology is used to measure the expression levels of large numbers of genes simultaneously or to genotype multiple regions of a genome. The chips are laid

TABLE 13-4 PATIENT & FAMILY TEACHING GUIDE

Genetic Testing

Genetic Counselors

- Individuals who are considering genetic testing should meet with a genetic counselor who is specially trained in medical genetics and counseling.
- Counseling is advised to help you understand the purpose of genetic testing, considerations before testing, and the emotional and medical impact of the test results.
- Genetic counseling can help you understand the pros and cons of genetic testing before making a decision to undergo a genetic test.

General Information

The following includes some important general information about genetic testing.

- Genetic testing can be expensive and may not be included in your medical insurance policy.
- Genetic testing may determine whether you are predisposed to developing an inherited disease.
- A particular genetic test will only tell you whether there is a specific genetic variant or mutation. Positive tests do not mean you will develop that disease or disorder. Neither can the results tell you when you will develop the disease.
- If a genetic test demonstrates a genetic predisposition to an inherited disorder, the news can be depressing.
- Knowledge of a genetic predisposition to a disease may give you the motivation to take preventive measures (e.g., taking drugs for familial hypercholesterolemia) or make lifestyle changes to lower the risk of a disease (e.g., exercising to decrease the risk of type 2 diabetes).
- If a genetic test reveals a strongly negative result, you probably will not develop that disease.
- If a genetic test reveals you are at risk for a specific genetic disorder, there is the possibility that other family members may also be at risk.
- If a genetic test reveals you are at risk for developing an inherited disease, whether or not you decide to share that information with family members is both a personal and an ethical decision that you will have to make.
- Genetic testing may provide important information that you can use when making decisions about having children.

out by robots that can position DNA fragments so precisely that more than 20,000 of them can fit on one microscope slide.

Then fluorescent-tagged molecules are washed over the DNA fragments. Some molecules (with green fluorescent tags) bind to their complementary sequence. These molecules can be identified because they glow under fluorescent light when scanned using automated equipment. Complete patterns of gene activity can be captured with this technology.

Genome-Wide Association Study (GWAS)

Genome-wide association study (GWAS) is an approach that involves rapidly scanning complete sets of DNA, or genomes, of many individuals to find genetic variations associated with the development or progression of a particular disease.

Until recently, researchers looked at single genes and the proteins that they encode. With GWAS, researchers study large numbers of genes and proteins, including how they act and interact. This provides a more complete picture of what goes on in a person. After the genetic associations are identified, researchers may be able to learn how to stop or jump-start genes on demand, change the course of a disease, or prevent it from ever happening.[4,8] GWAS is particularly useful in finding genetic variations that contribute to multifactorial inherited disorders such as asthma, cancer, diabetes, and heart disease.

To carry out a GWAS, researchers use two groups of participants: people with the disease being studied and similar people without the disease. Each person's complete set of DNA, or genome, is then purified from the blood or cells, placed on tiny chips, and scanned on automated laboratory machines. The machines quickly survey each participant's genome for strategically selected markers of genetic variation.

If certain genetic variations are found to be significantly more common in people with the disease compared to people without the disease, the variations are said to be "associated" with the disease. The associated genetic variations can serve as powerful pointers to the region of the human genome where the disease-causing problem resides.

The potential impact of GWAS is substantial, since it lays the groundwork for personalized medicine, in which the current one-size-fits-all approach to health care gives way to more customized strategies. Tools such as GWAS can provide patients with individualized information about their risks of developing certain diseases. The information will help health care professionals tailor prevention programs to each person's unique genetic makeup.

PHARMACOGENETICS AND PHARMACOGENOMICS

Patients vary widely in their response to drugs. Although the reasons for this are complex, genetic factors may account for a large percentage of patient variability in response to individual drugs. **Pharmacogenetics** is the study of genetic variability of drug responses related to variations in single genes. **Pharmacogenomics** is similar to pharmacogenetics except that it involves multiple genes associated with variability in drug response. These two terms are frequently used interchangeably in describing the relationship between pharmacology and genetic variability in determining an individual's response to drugs.

Pharmacogenetic and pharmacogenomic studies can potentially lead to drugs that can be tailor-made or adapted to each person's particular genetic makeup.[9] Table 13-5 has examples of pharmacogenetics.

One important area of study has been focused on the cytochrome P450 (CYP450) family of major enzymes, which are important in *drug metabolism*. Alterations in the *CYP450* gene can affect how the liver breaks down certain drugs, such as warfarin (Coumadin). People with a less active form of the enzyme (who metabolize the drug slowly) might get too much of the drug, whereas people with a more active form of the enzyme (who metabolize the drug quickly) might get too little of the drug. Too much warfarin can lead to internal bleeding, whereas too little warfarin may still allow blood clots to form. Pharmacogenetic testing can assist health care providers in prescribing the right amount of a medicine based on a patient's particular genetic makeup (Fig. 13-7).

Currently a genetic test for identifying *CYP450* polymorphisms is available that has been approved by the U.S. Food and Drug Administration (FDA). In addition to maximizing the safety and effectiveness of drugs, this type of genetic testing can lead to individualized drug therapy.

Health care providers are starting to use pharmacogenomic information to prescribe drugs, but at this time such tests are

TABLE 13-5 **EXAMPLES OF PHARMACOGENETICS**

Drug	Role of Pharmacogenetics
trastuzumab (Herceptin)	• In breast cancer, drug only works for women whose tumors have genes that lead to the overproduction of a protein called HER-2. • Drug is a monoclonal antibody to HER-2. After the antibody attaches to the antigen, it kills the cells. • Genetic testing provides information on which patients are good candidates for treatment with drug. • Drug does not work for patients whose tumor genes do not express HER-2.
crizotinib (Xalkori)	• Drug used to treat patients with late-stage (locally advanced or metastatic), non–small cell lung cancers (NSCLC) who express the abnormal anaplastic lymphoma kinase *(ALK)* gene. • *ALK* gene abnormality causes cancer development and growth. • Crizotinib works by blocking certain proteins called kinases, including the protein produced by the abnormal *ALK* gene. • Drug was approved for use with a companion genetic diagnostic test that determines whether a patient with NSCLC has the abnormal *ALK* gene.
vemurafenib (Zelboraf)	• Approved for patients with late-stage (metastatic) or unresectable melanoma. • Indicated for the treatment of patients with melanoma whose tumors express a gene mutation called *BRAF V600E*. • To be considered for treatment, patients must first have genetic testing to determine whether melanoma cells have the *BRAF V600E* mutation.
warfarin (Coumadin)	• Genetic variants in the genes *VKORC1* and cytochrome P450 2C9 *(CYP2C9)* have a significant impact on people's sensitivity to warfarin. • Individuals with particular variations in these genes require a lower warfarin dose to maintain therapeutic levels of anticoagulation. • Individuals with other variations require higher doses. • Together these genetic variations explain about 50% of the required dose difference between individuals. • Testing for patient's *CYP2C9* and *VKORC1* genotype information can assist in selecting the starting dose.
abacavir (Ziagen)	• Some people are at greater risk for serious allergic reactions when first starting treatment with this drug. • Genetic testing for *HLA-B*5701* before taking the drug can identify people who carry a genetic marker that is associated with life-threatening hypersensitivity reactions.
clopidogrel (Plavix)	• For clopidogrel to work, cytochrome P450 enzymes in the liver (particularly CYP2C19) must convert the drug to its active form. • About 2% to 14% of the population are poor metabolizers, and these patients may not receive the full benefits of the drug. • Genetic tests are available to identify genetic differences in CYP2C19 function.

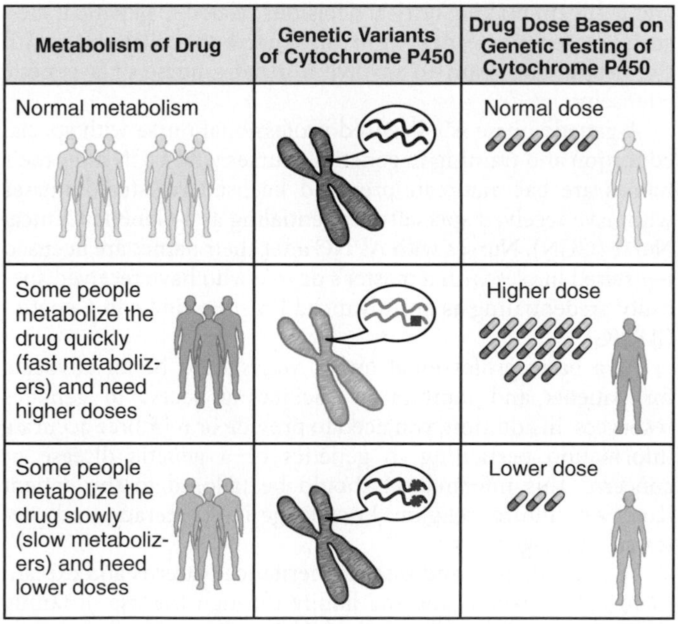

Metabolism of Drug
Genetic Variants of Cytochrome P450
Drug Dose Based on Genetic Testing of Cytochrome P450
Normal metabolism
Normal dose
Some people metabolize the drug quickly (fast metabolizers) and need higher doses
Higher dose
Some people metabolize the drug slowly (slow metabolizers) and need lower doses
Lower dose

FIG. 13-7 Individuals respond differently to the drug warfarin (Coumadin). The diversity of responses is partially due to genetic variants in one of the cytochrome *P450* genes.

routine for only a few diseases or disorders (examples are presented in Table 13-5). However, given the field's rapid growth, pharmacogenomics may soon lead to personalized medicine and individualized drug therapy to manage heart disease, cancer, asthma, depression, and many other common diseases.

GENE THERAPY

Gene therapy is an experimental technique that uses genes to treat or prevent disease. Gene therapy is an approach to treating potentially lethal and disabling diseases that are caused by single gene deficiencies. With specialized techniques, gene expression can be manipulated to correct the problem in the particular patient, although the correction will not be passed along to offspring of that person. Approaches to gene therapy include:[10]

- Replacing a mutated gene with a healthy copy of the gene
- Inactivating, or "knocking out," a mutated gene that is functioning improperly
- Introducing a new gene into the body to help fight a disease

A gene that is inserted directly into a cell usually does not function. A carrier molecule called a *vector* must be used to deliver the therapeutic gene to the patient's target cells. Currently, the most common vector is a virus that has been genetically altered to carry normal human DNA. The vector can be injected or given IV directly into specific tissue. The vector unloads its genetic material containing the therapeutic human gene into the target cell. If the treatment is successful, the new gene will make a functional protein and restore the target cell to a normal state. A diagram of gene therapy is depicted in Fig. 13-8.

Although gene therapy is a promising treatment option for a number of diseases (including inherited disorders, some types of cancer, and certain viral infections), the technique remains risky and is still under study to make sure that it will be safe

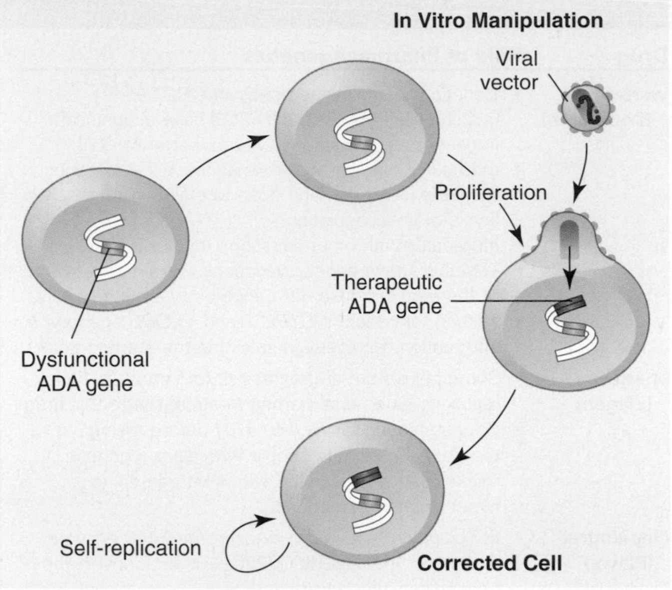

FIG. 13-8 Gene therapy for adenosine deaminase *(ADA)* deficiency attempts to correct this immunodeficiency state. The viral vector containing the therapeutic ADA gene is inserted into the patient's lymphocytes. These cells can then make the ADA enzyme.

and effective. Gene therapy is currently only being tested for the treatment of diseases that have no other cures.[10]

STEM CELL THERAPY

Stem cells are the subject of much discussion because they may offer treatment for many diseases. The use of stem cells may allow for the regeneration of lost tissue and restoration of function in various diseases.

Stem cells are unspecialized cells in the body that have the ability to (1) remain in their unspecialized state and divide or (2) differentiate and develop into specialized cells such as a brain cell or a muscle cell. In some body organs such as the gastrointestinal (GI) tract and bone marrow, stem cells divide to repair and replace damaged or old tissues. In other organs such as the pancreas and the heart, stem cells divide only under special conditions.

Stem cells can be divided into two types: embryonic and adult, or somatic. *Embryonic stem cells* come from the embryo at a very early stage in development (4 to 5 days old) and have the ability to become any one of the hundreds of types of cells in the human body. These stem cells can be stimulated to differentiate into any type of tissue (skin, liver, kidney, blood, etc.) found in an adult human.

Adult stem cells are undifferentiated cells that are found in small numbers in many adult organs and tissues, including brain, bone marrow, peripheral blood, blood vessels, skeletal muscle, skin, teeth, heart, GI tract, liver, ovarian epithelium, and testes. They are thought to reside in a specific area of each tissue called a *stem cell niche*. Adult stem cells are more limited than embryonic stem cells in their potential (e.g., stem cells from liver may only develop into more liver cells).

The primary roles of adult stem cells in the body are to maintain and repair tissues in which they are found. They are usually thought of as multipotent cells, giving rise to a closely related family of cells within the tissue. For example, skin stem cells produce new skin cells. Hematopoietic stem cells found within the bone marrow are capable of forming all of the various blood cells. These cells are prolific by design and are already being used for bone marrow transplants (see Chapter 16).

Medical researchers are investigating the use of stem cells to repair or replace damaged body tissues, similar to whole organ transplants. Currently not enough donated organs are available to meet the demand for transplants. In organ transplants, when tissues from a donor are placed into a patient's body, the patient's immune system may react and reject the donated tissue as "foreign." However, using stem cells presents less risk of this immune rejection, and the therapy may be more successful.

In addition, stem cells could be directed to differentiate into specific cell types. They would then become a renewable source of replacement cells and tissues to treat conditions such as Alzheimer's disease, spinal cord injury, stroke, burns, heart disease, diabetes, osteoarthritis, and rheumatoid arthritis. It may become possible to generate healthy heart muscle cells in the laboratory and then transplant those cells into patients with chronic heart disease. Whether these cells can generate heart muscle cells or stimulate the growth of new blood vessels is under investigation.[11]

NURSING MANAGEMENT GENETICS AND GENOMICS

You need to be knowledgeable about the fundamentals of genetics and genomics.[12,13] By understanding the profound influence that genetics has on health and illness, you can assist the patient and family in making critical decisions related to genetic issues, such as genetic testing. You also need to collaborate with the health care team to involve a genetic nurse or a genetic counselor.

A genetic nurse is a licensed professional nurse with special education and training in genetics. Nurses with GCN after their names are baccalaureate-prepared licensed registered nurses who have received specialty credentialing as a Genetic Clinical Nurse (GCN). Nurses with APNG after their names are licensed registered nurses with a master's degree who have received specialty credentialing as an Advanced Practice Nurse in Genetics (APNG).

As a basic professional nurse, you should be an advocate for patients and families by facilitating access to genetics resources. In addition, you need to provide or reinforce accurate information pertaining to genetics or a genetic disease or concern. This information should be tailored to the patient based on culture, religion, knowledge level, literacy, and preferred language.[14]

You can identify and assess inheritance patterns and explain them to the patient and the family through the use of family pedigrees (see Figs. 13-4 and 13-5) and Punnett squares (Fig. 13-9). Maintain the patient's confidentiality and respect the patient's values and beliefs because genetic information may have major health and social implications.

Genetic testing may raise many psychologic and emotional issues. Knowledge of carrier status of a genetic disorder may influence a person's decisions for a career, marriage, and childbearing. It may also affect significant others in grappling with serious life and health care issues. For example, how should a wife deal with a husband who has tested positive for Hunting-

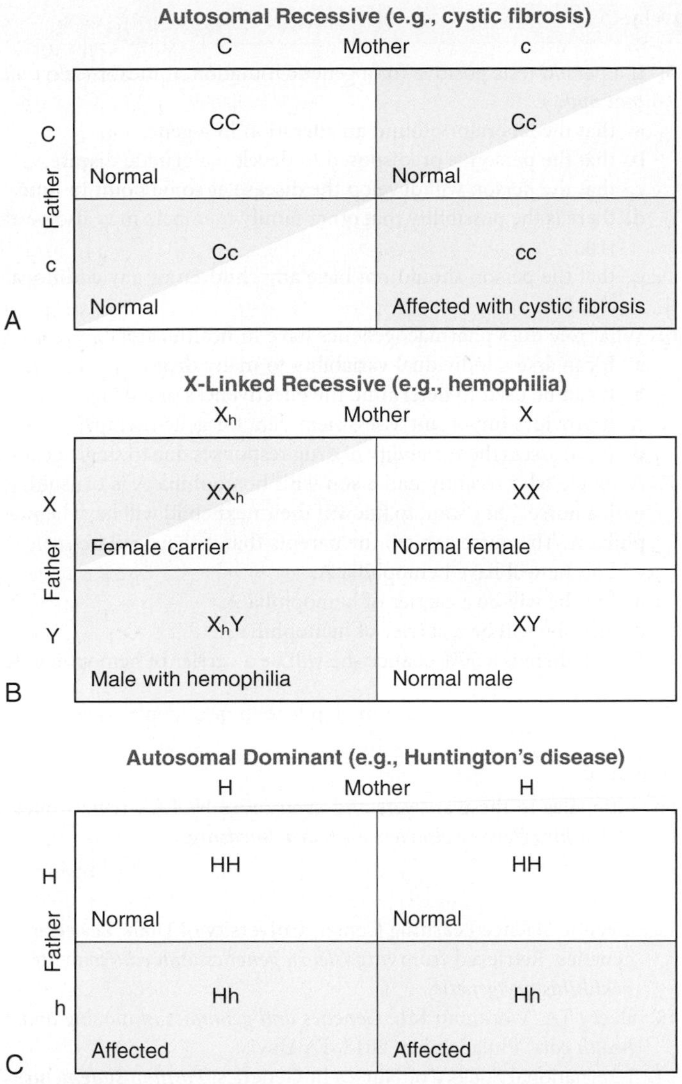

FIG. 13-9 Punnett squares illustrate inheritance possibilities. **A,** If the mother and father are both carriers for cystic fibrosis, there is a 25% chance that offspring will have cystic fibrosis. **B,** If the mother is a carrier for the hemophilia gene and the father has a normal genotype, there is a 50% chance that any male offspring will have hemophilia. There is a 50% chance that any female offspring will be a carrier. **C,** If the mother has a normal genotype and the father has Huntington's disease, there is a 50% chance that offspring will have the disease.

ton's disease and shows early signs of cognitive impairment but does not yet show any other neurologic manifestations of the disease? Should their children be tested for the disease? A 43-year-old woman who has a family history of breast cancer and is now diagnosed with breast cancer wants to know if she and her two teenage daughters should have *BRCA* testing. What do you tell her?

Furthermore, there are ethical concerns. Who should know the results of a genetic test? Who should protect the privacy of individuals' test results and prevent individuals from possible discrimination? Genetic information should not be misused to label individuals or particular ethnic groups. Close attention must be paid to better understand the psychosocial needs of individuals and societal responses and health care policy related to genetic testing.

People may be reluctant to share or disclose information about family history or genetic test results. They fear they are vulnerable to discrimination based on their DNA. Inform your patients about the Genetic Information Nondiscrimination Act (GINA), which protects them from discrimination by employers and health care insurance companies (see Genetics in Clinical Practice Box on p. 196).

Resources on genetics for nurses and nurse educators are available in the list of resources at the end of this chapter.

NURSING ASSESSMENT FAMILY HISTORY

Family history is one of the strongest influences on a person's risk of developing genetic-related disorders such as heart disease, stroke, diabetes, or cancer. Even though a person cannot change his or her genetic makeup, knowing the family history can help in the prevention or early diagnosis and treatment of a disorder. For example, it is important to monitor cholesterol levels in a person with a family history of familial hypercholesterolemia.

The key features of a family history that may increase a person's risk for genetic-related diseases are

- Disease in more than one close relative
- Disease that does not usually affect a certain gender (e.g., breast cancer in a male)
- Diseases that occur at an earlier age than expected (e.g., myocardial infarction before age 35)
- Certain combinations of diseases within a family (e.g., breast and ovarian cancer, heart disease and diabetes)

If a family has one or more of these features, the family history may hold important clues about a person's risk for a genetic disease. People with a family history of disease may have the most to gain from lifestyle changes and screening tests. People cannot change their genes, but they can change unhealthy behaviors (e.g., smoking, poor eating habits). They can also get screening tests to detect diseases and disease risk factors (e.g., elevated cholesterol, hypertension) that can be treated.

Genetic Risk Alert boxes in the assessment chapters in this book highlight a patient's risks related to genetic diseases and disorders. Use the information in these boxes when obtaining a nursing history.

Family health history is a written or graphic record of the diseases and health conditions present in one's family (see Chapter 3). A useful family health history shows three generations of a person's biologic relatives, the age of diagnosis of a disease, and the age and cause of death of deceased family members. A family health history is a useful tool for understanding health risks and preventing disease in individuals and their close relatives.

Talk with your own family members about your family's health history. Record this information and update it periodically so you and your family members will have organized and accurate information ready to share with your health care provider. Family health history information may help health care providers determine which tests and screenings are recommended to help you and your family know their health risk.

To help individuals collect and organize their family history information, the Centers for Disease Control and Prevention (CDC) has collaborated with the U.S. Surgeon General and other federal agencies to develop a Web-based tool called *My Family Health Portrait (https://familyhistory.hhs.gov/fhh-web/home.action).*

BRIDGE TO NCLEX EXAMINATION

The number of the question corresponds to the same-numbered outcome at the beginning of the chapter.

1. If a person is heterozygous for a given gene, it means that the person
   a. is a carrier for a genetic disorder.
   b. is affected by the genetic disorder.
   c. has two identical alleles for the gene.
   d. has two different alleles for the gene.
2. Common causes of genetic mutations include *(select all that apply)*
   a. DNA damage from toxins.
   b. DNA damage from UV radiation.
   c. inheritance of altered genes from father.
   d. inheritance of altered genes from mother.
   e. inheritance of somatic mutations from either parent.
3. A father who has an X-linked recessive disorder and a wife with a normal genotype will
   a. pass the carrier state to his male children.
   b. pass the carrier state to all of his children.
   c. pass the carrier state to his female children.
   d. not pass on the genetic mutation to any of his children.
4. What characterizes multifactorial genetic disorders?
   a. Genetic testing available for most disorders
   b. Commonly caused by single gene alterations
   c. Many family members report having the disorder
   d. Caused by complex interactions of genetic and environmental factors
5. If a person tests positive for a genetic mutation, it means *(select all that apply)*
   a. that the laboratory found an alteration in a gene.
   b. that the person is predisposed to develop a genetic disease.
   c. that the person will develop the disease at some point in time.
   d. there is the possibility that other family members may also be at risk.
   e. that the person should not have any children or any additional children.
6. What role does pharmacogenetics have in health care?
   a. It can assess individual variability to many drugs.
   b. It can be used to determine the effectiveness of a drug.
   c. It provides important assessment data for gene therapy.
   d. It can assess the variability of drug responses due to single genes.
7. A couple who recently had a son with hemophilia A is consulting with a nurse. They want to know if their next child will have hemophilia A. The nurse can tell the parents that if their child is a
   a. boy, he will have hemophilia A.
   b. boy, he will be a carrier of hemophilia A.
   c. girl, she will be a carrier of hemophilia A.
   d. girl, there is a 50% chance she will be a carrier of hemophilia A.

1. d, 2. a, b, c, d, 3. c, 4. d, 5. a, d, 6. d, 7. d

evolve

For rationales to these answers and even more NCLEX review questions, visit *http://evolve.elsevier.com/Lewis/medsurg.*

REFERENCES

1. US Department of Health and Human Services: Genomics. Retrieved from *www.healthypeople.gov/2020/topicsobjectives2020/overview.aspx?topicid=15.*
2. Patton K, Thibodeau GA: *Anatomy and physiology*, ed 8, St Louis, 2013, Mosby.
3. The New Genetics, National Institute of General Medical Sciences, National Institutes of Health, US Department of Health and Human Services. Retrieved from *http://publications.nigms.nih.gov/thenewgenetics/thenewgenetics.pdf.*
4. Jorde LB, Carey JC, Bamshad MJ: *Medical genetics*, ed 4, St Louis, 2010, Mosby.
5. US Department of Energy: Human Genome Project information. Retrieved from *www.ornl.gov/sci/techresources/Human_Genome/home.shtml.*
6. Bell JT, Spector TD: A twin approach to unraveling epigenetics, *Trends Genet* 27(3):116, 2011.
7. National Center for Biotechnology Information: GeneTests. Retrieved from *www.ncbi.nlm.nih.gov/sites/GeneTests.*
8. Ellard S, Turnpenny P: *Emery's elements of medical genetics*, St Louis, 2012, Mosby.
9. Mayo Clinic staff: Personalized medicine and pharmacogenetics. Retrieved from *www.mayoclinic.com/health/personalized-medicine/CA00078.*
10. Lister Hill National Center for Biomedical Communications: Gene therapy. Retrieved from *http://ghr.nlm.nih.gov/handbook/therapy.pdf.*
11. National Institutes of Health: Stem cell basics. Retrieved from *stemcells.nih.gov.*
12. Genetic Science Learning Center, University of Utah: Learning genetics. Retrieved from *http://learn.genetics.utah.edu/content/health/history/genetic.*
13. Beery TA, Workman ML: *Genetics and genomics in nursing and health care*, Philadelphia, 2012, FA Davis.
14. International Society of Nurses in Genetics: *Position statements: Genetic counseling for vulnerable populations: The role of nursing.* Retrieved from *www.isong.org.*

RESOURCES

American Society of Human Genetics (ASHG)
www.ashg.org

Essential Nursing Competencies and Curricula Guidelines for Genetics and Genomics
www.genome.gov/17517146

GeneTests
www.ncbi.nlm.nih.gov/sites/GeneTests

Genetics Home Reference, National Library of Medicine
http://ghr.nlm.nih.gov

International Society of Nurses in Genetics (ISONG)
www.isong.org

National Coalition for Health Professional Education in Genetics (NCHPEG)
www.nchpeg.org

National Human Genome Research Institute
www.genome.gov

Nursing Competencies Relating to Genetics
www.genome.gov/27527634

Understanding Gene Testing
www.accessexcellence.org/AE/AEPC/NIH

CHAPTER

14

Altered Immune Responses and Transplantation

Sharon L. Lewis

A cloudy day is no match for a sunny disposition.
William Arthur Ward

evolve WEBSITE

http://evolve.elsevier.com/Lewis/medsurg

- NCLEX Review Questions
- Key Points
- Pre-Test
- Rationales for Bridge to NCLEX Examination Questions
- Concept Map Creator
- Glossary
- Animations
  - Function of B Cells
  - Function of T Cytotoxic Cells
- Content Updates

eFigures

- eFig. 14-1: Production of interferon
- eFig. 14-2: Monoclonal antibodies

eTables

- eTable 14-1: Mediators of Inflammation
- eTable 14-2: Technologies in Immunology

LEARNING OUTCOMES

1. Describe the functions and components of the immune system.
2. Compare and contrast humoral and cell-mediated immunity, including lymphocytes involved, types of reactions, and effects on antigens.
3. Characterize the five types of immunoglobulins.
4. Differentiate among the four types of hypersensitivity reactions in terms of immunologic mechanisms and resulting alterations.
5. Identify the clinical manifestations and emergency management of a systemic anaphylactic reaction.
6. Describe the assessment and collaborative care of a patient with chronic allergies.
7. Explain the relationship between the human leukocyte antigen system and certain diseases.
8. Describe the etiologic factors, clinical manifestations, and treatment modalities of autoimmune diseases.
9. Describe the etiologic factors and categories of immunodeficiency disorders.
10. Differentiate among the types of rejections following transplantation.
11. Identify the types and side effects of immunosuppressive therapy.

KEY TERMS

anergy, p. 209
antigen, p. 203
autoimmunity, p. 217
cell-mediated immunity, p. 208
cytokines, p. 206
human leukocyte antigen (HLA), p. 219
humoral immunity, p. 207
hypersensitivity reactions, p. 209
immunocompetence, p. 209
immunodeficiency, p. 218
immunosuppressive therapy, p. 221

This chapter discusses the normal immune response and the altered immune responses of hypersensitivity (including allergies), autoimmunity, and immunodeficiency. Histocompatibility, organ transplantation, and immunosuppressive therapy are also presented.

NORMAL IMMUNE RESPONSE

Immunity is the body's ability to resist disease. Immune responses serve the following three functions:

1. *Defense:* The body protects against invasions by microorganisms and prevents the development of infection by attacking foreign antigens and pathogens.
2. *Homeostasis:* Damaged cellular substances are digested and removed. Through this mechanism, the body's different cell types remain uniform and unchanged.
3. *Surveillance:* Mutations continually arise in the body but are normally recognized as foreign cells and destroyed.

Antigens

An **antigen** is a substance that elicits an immune response. Most antigens are composed of protein. However, other substances such as large polysaccharides, lipoproteins, and nucleic acids can act as antigens. All of the body's cells have antigens on their surface that are unique to that person and enable the body to recognize itself. The immune system normally

Reviewed by Bernice Coleman, PhD, ACNP-BC, FAHA, Nurse Practitioner, Heart Transplantation and Ventricular Assist Device Programs, Cedars Sinai Medical Center, Los Angeles, California; Devorah Overbay, RN, MSN, CNS, Assistant Nursing Professor and NCLEX Education Specialist ATI Testing, George Fox University, Department of Nursing, Newberg, Oregon; and Laura Mallett, RN, MSN, Assistant Lecturer, University of Wyoming, Fay W. Whitney School of Nursing, Laramie, Wyoming.

becomes "tolerant" to the body's own molecules. Therefore it is nonresponsive to "self" antigens.

Types of Immunity

Immunity is classified as innate or acquired.

Innate Immunity. *Innate immunity* is present at birth, and its primary role is first-line defense against pathogens. This type of immunity involves a nonspecific response, and neutrophils and monocytes are the primary white blood cells (WBCs) involved. Innate immunity is not antigen specific so it can respond within minutes to an invading microorganism without prior exposure to that organism.

Acquired Immunity. *Acquired immunity* is the development of immunity, either actively or passively (Table 14-1).

Active Acquired Immunity. *Active acquired immunity* results from the invasion of the body by foreign substances such as microorganisms and subsequent development of antibodies and sensitized lymphocytes. With each reinvasion of the microorganisms, the body responds more rapidly and vigorously to fight off the invader. Active acquired immunity may result naturally from a disease or artificially through immunization with a less virulent antigen. Because antibodies are synthesized, immunity takes time to develop but is long lasting.

Passive Acquired Immunity. *Passive acquired immunity* implies that the host receives antibodies to an antigen rather than synthesizing them. This may take place naturally through the transfer of immunoglobulins across the placental membrane from mother to fetus. Artificial passive acquired immunity occurs through injection with gamma globulin (serum antibodies). The benefit of this immunity is its immediate effect. Unfortunately, passive immunity is short lived because the person does not synthesize the antibodies and consequently does not retain memory cells for the antigen.

Lymphoid Organs

The lymphoid system is composed of central (or primary) and peripheral lymphoid organs. The *central lymphoid organs* are the thymus gland and bone marrow. The *peripheral lymphoid organs* are the lymph nodes; tonsils; spleen; and gut-, genital-, bronchial-, and skin-associated lymphoid tissues (Fig. 14-1).

Lymphocytes are produced in the bone marrow and eventually migrate to the peripheral organs. The thymus is involved in the differentiation and maturation of T lymphocytes and is therefore essential for a cell-mediated immune response. During childhood the thymus is large. It shrinks with age, and in the older person the thymus is a collection of reticular fibers, lymphocytes, and connective tissue.

When antigens are introduced into the body, they may be carried by the bloodstream or lymph channels to regional lymph nodes. The antigens interact with B and T lymphocytes and macrophages in the lymph nodes. The two important functions of lymph nodes are (1) filtration of foreign material brought to the site and (2) circulation of lymphocytes.

The tonsils are an example of lymphoid tissue. The spleen, a peripheral lymph organ, is important as the primary site for filtering foreign antigens from the blood. It consists of two kinds of tissue: white pulp containing B and T lymphocytes and red pulp containing erythrocytes. Macrophages line the pulp and sinuses of the spleen.

Lymphoid tissue is found in the submucosa of the gastrointestinal (GI) (gut-associated), genitourinary (genital-associated), and respiratory (bronchial-associated) tracts. This tissue protects the body surface from external microorganisms.

The skin-associated lymph tissue primarily consists of lymphocytes and Langerhans' cells (a type of dendritic cell) found in the epidermis of skin. When Langerhans' cells are depleted, the skin can neither initiate an immune response nor support a skin-localized delayed hypersensitivity reaction.

Cells Involved in Immune Response

Mononuclear Phagocytes. The *mononuclear phagocyte system* includes monocytes in the blood and macrophages found

TABLE 14-1 TYPES OF ACQUIRED SPECIFIC IMMUNITY

Type	Natural	Artificial
Active	Natural contact with antigen through clinical infection (e.g., recovery from chickenpox, measles, mumps)	Immunization with antigen (e.g., immunization with live or killed vaccines)
Passive	Transplacental and colostrum transfer from mother to child (e.g., maternal immunoglobulins in neonate)	Injection of serum from immune human (e.g., injection of human gamma globulin)

HEALTHY PEOPLE

Health Impact of Immunization

- Can help control the spread of infections within communities.
- Can prevent disability and death from infectious disease for individuals.
- Reduces and can possibly eliminate polio, measles, and other diseases with widespread use.
- Decreased incidence of infectious diseases (e.g., influenza, pneumonia) when more people are vaccinated against these diseases.

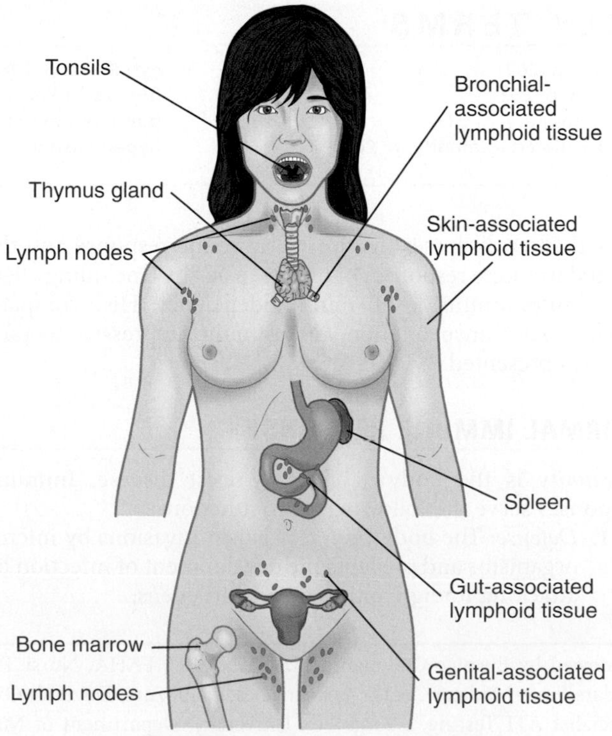

FIG. 14-1 Organs of the immune system.

throughout the body. Mononuclear phagocytes have a critical role in the immune system. They are responsible for capturing, processing, and presenting the antigen to the lymphocytes. This stimulates a humoral or cell-mediated immune response. Capturing is accomplished through phagocytosis. The macrophage-bound antigen, which is highly immunogenic, is presented to circulating T or B lymphocytes and thus triggers an immune response (Fig. 14-2).

Lymphocytes. Lymphocytes are produced in the bone marrow (Fig. 14-3). They then differentiate into B and T lymphocytes.[1]

B Lymphocytes. In the early research on *B lymphocytes* (bursa-equivalent lymphocytes) in birds, it was discovered that they mature under the influence of the bursa of Fabricius, hence the name *B cells.* However, this lymphoid organ does not exist in humans. The bursa-equivalent tissue in humans is the bone marrow. B cells differentiate into *plasma cells* when activated. Plasma cells produce antibodies (immunoglobulins) (Table 14-2).

T Lymphocytes. Cells that migrate from the bone marrow to the thymus differentiate into *T lymphocytes* (thymus-dependent cells). The thymus secretes hormones, including thymosin, that stimulate the maturation and differentiation of T lymphocytes. T cells make up 70% to 80% of the circulating lymphocytes and are primarily responsible for immunity to intracellular viruses, tumor cells, and fungi. T cells live from a few months to the life span of an individual and account for long-term immunity.

T lymphocytes can be categorized into T cytotoxic and T helper cells. Antigenic characteristics of WBCs have now been classified using monoclonal antibodies. These antigens are classified as *clusters of differentiation,* or *CD antigens.* Many types of WBCs, especially lymphocytes, are referred to by their CD designations. All mature T cells have the CD3 antigen.

T Cytotoxic Cells. T cytotoxic (CD8) cells are involved in attacking antigens on the cell membrane of foreign pathogens and releasing cytolytic substances that destroy the pathogen. These cells have antigen specificity and are sensitized by exposure to the antigen. Much like B lymphocytes, some sensitized T cells do not attack the antigen but remain as memory T cells. As in the humoral immune response, a second exposure to the antigen results in a more intense and rapid cell-mediated immune response.

T Helper Cells. T helper (CD4) cells are involved in the regulation of cell-mediated immunity and the humoral antibody response. T helper cells differentiate into subsets of cells that produce distinct types of cytokines (discussed in a later section). These subsets are called T_H1 cells and T_H2 cells. T_H1 cells stimulate phagocyte-mediated ingestion and killing of microbes, the key component of cell-mediated immunity. T_H2 cells stimulate eosinophil-mediated immunity, which is effective against parasites and is involved in allergic responses.

Natural Killer Cells. Natural killer (NK) cells are also involved in cell-mediated immunity. These cells are not T or B cells but are large lymphocytes with numerous granules in the cyto-

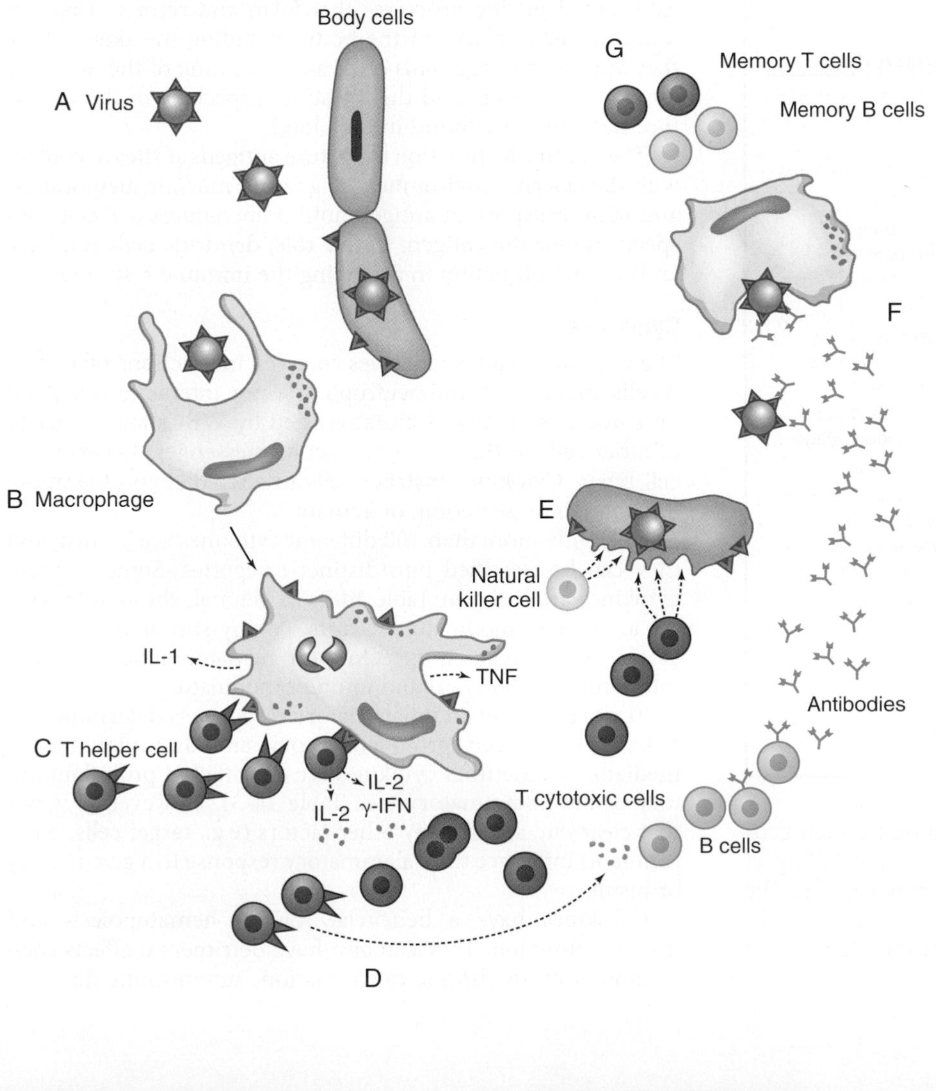

FIG. 14-2 The immune response to a virus. **A,** A virus invades the body through a break in the skin or another portal of entry. The virus must make its way inside a cell to replicate itself. **B,** A macrophage recognizes the antigens on the surface of the virus. The macrophage digests the virus and displays pieces of the virus (antigens) on its surface. **C,** A T helper cell recognizes the antigen displayed and binds to the macrophage. This binding stimulates the production of cytokines (interleukin-1 *[IL-1]* and tumor necrosis factor *[TNF]*) by the macrophage and interleukin-2 *(IL-2)* and γ-interferon *(γ-IFN)* by the T cell. These cytokines are intracellular messengers that provide communication among the cells. **D,** IL-2 instructs other T helper cells and T cytotoxic cells to proliferate (multiply). T helper cells release cytokines, causing B cells to multiply and produce antibodies. **E,** T cytotoxic cells and natural killer cells destroy infected body cells. **F,** The antibodies bind to the virus and mark it for macrophage destruction. **G,** Memory B and T cells remain behind to respond quickly if the same virus attacks again.

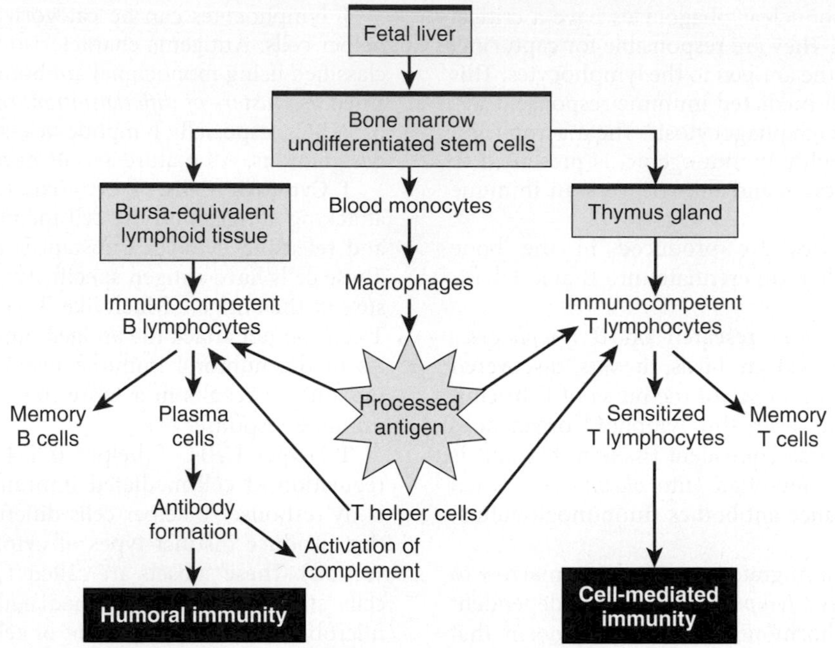

FIG. 14-3 Relationships and functions of macrophages, B lymphocytes, and T lymphocytes in an immune response.

TABLE 14-2 CHARACTERISTICS OF IMMUNOGLOBULINS

Class	Serum Concentration	Location	Characteristics
IgG	76%	Plasma, interstitial fluid	Is only immunoglobulin that crosses placenta Is responsible for secondary immune response
IgA	15%	Body secretions, including tears, saliva, breast milk, colostrum	Lines mucous membranes and protects body surfaces
IgM	8%	Plasma	Is responsible for primary immune response Forms antibodies to ABO blood antigens
IgD	1%	Plasma	Is present on lymphocyte surface Assists in the differentiation of B lymphocytes
IgE	0.002%	Plasma, interstitial fluids	Causes symptoms of allergic reactions Fixes to mast cells and basophils Assists in defense against parasitic infections

plasm. NK cells do not require prior sensitization for their generation. These cells are involved in recognition and killing of virus-infected cells, tumor cells, and transplanted grafts. The mechanism of recognition is not fully understood. NK cells have a significant role in immune surveillance for malignant cell changes.

Dendritic Cells. *Dendritic cells* make up a system of cells that are important to the immune system, especially the cell-mediated immune response. They have an atypical shape with extensive dendritic processes that form and retract. They are found in many places in the body, including the skin (where they are called Langerhans cells) and the lining of the nose, the lungs, the stomach, and the intestine. Especially in the immature state, they are found in the blood.[2]

They primarily function to capture antigens at sites of contact with the external environment (e.g., skin, mucous membranes) and then transport an antigen until it encounters a T cell with specificity for the antigen. In this role, dendritic cells can have an important function in activating the immune response.

Cytokines

The immune response involves complex interactions of T cells, B cells, monocytes, and neutrophils. These interactions depend on **cytokines** (soluble factors secreted by WBCs and a variety of other cells in the body) that act as messengers between the cell types. Cytokines instruct cells to alter their proliferation, differentiation, secretion, or activity.

Currently more than 100 different cytokines are known, and they can be classified into distinct categories. Some of these cytokines are listed in Table 14-3. In general, the interleukins act as immunomodulatory factors, colony-stimulating factors act as growth-regulating factors for hematopoietic cells, and interferons are antiviral and immunomodulatory.

The net effect of an inflammatory response is determined by a balance between proinflammatory and antiinflammatory mediators. Sometimes cytokines are classified as proinflammatory or antiinflammatory (see Table 14-3). However, it is not that clear-cut, since many other factors (e.g., target cells, environment) influence the inflammatory response to a given injury or insult.

Cytokines have a beneficial role in hematopoiesis and immune function. They can also have detrimental effects such as those seen in chronic inflammation, autoimmune diseases,

TABLE 14-3 TYPES AND FUNCTIONS OF CYTOKINES*

Type	Primary Functions
Interleukins (ILs)	
IL-1	Proinflammatory mediator. Promotes maturation and clonal expansion of B cells, enhances activity of NK cells, activates T cells, activates macrophages.
IL-2	Induces proliferation and differentiation of T cells; activation of T cells, NK cells, and macrophages. Stimulates release of other cytokines (α-IFN, TNF, IL-1, IL-6).
IL-3 (multicolony colony-stimulating factor)	Hematopoietic growth factor for hematopoietic precursor cells.
IL-4	Antiinflammatory mediator. B-cell growth factor, stimulates proliferation and differentiation of B cells. Induces differentiation into T_H2 cells. Stimulates growth of mast cells.
IL-5	B cell growth and differentiation. Promotes growth and differentiation of eosinophils.
IL-6	Proinflammatory mediator: T- and B-cell growth factor, promotes differentiation of B cells into plasma cells, stimulates antibody secretion, induces fever, synergistic effects with IL-1 and TNF.
IL-7	Promotes growth of T and B cells.
IL-8	Chemotaxis of neutrophils and T cells, stimulates superoxide and granule release.
IL-9	Enhances T cell survival, mast cell activation.
IL-10	Antiinflammatory mediator, inhibits cytokine production by T cells and NK cells, promotes B cell proliferation and antibody responses, potent suppressor of macrophage function.
Interferons (IFNs)	
α-IFN β-IFN	Inhibit viral replication, activate NK cells and macrophages, antiproliferative effects on tumor cells.
γ-IFN	Proinflammatory mediator: activates macrophages, neutrophils, and NK cells; promotes B cell differentiation. Inhibits viral replication.
Tumor Necrosis Factor (TNF)	Proinflammatory mediator; activates macrophages and granulocytes; promotes the immune and inflammatory responses; kills tumor cells; responsible for weight loss associated with chronic inflammation and cancer.
Colony-Stimulating Factors (CSFs)	
Granulocyte colony-stimulating factor (G-CSF)	Stimulates proliferation and differentiation of neutrophils, enhances functional activity of mature PMNs.
Granulocyte-macrophage colony-stimulating factor (GM-CSF)	Stimulates proliferation and differentiation of PMNs and monocytes.
Macrophage colony-stimulating factor (M-CSF)	Promotes proliferation, differentiation, and activation of monocytes and macrophages.
Erythropoietin	Stimulates erythroid progenitor cells in bone marrow to produce red blood cells.

*A more comprehensive presentation of cytokines is available at *www.rndsystems.com/molecule_group.aspx?g=704&;r=4.*
NK, Natural killer; *PMNs,* polymorphonuclear neutrophils.

and sepsis. Cytokines such as erythropoietin (see Chapter 47), colony-stimulating factors (see Table 16-14), interferons (see Table 16-13), and interleukin-2 (see Table 16-13) are used clinically to (1) stimulate hematopoiesis, (2) stimulate the bone marrow to make WBCs, and (3) treat various malignancies. In addition, inhibitors of cytokines such as soluble tumor necrosis factor receptor antagonist and interleukin-1 are used as antiinflammatory agents. (Clinical uses of cytokines are listed in Table 14-4.)

Interferon helps the body's natural defenses attack tumors and viruses. Three types of interferon have now been identified (see Table 14-3). In addition to their direct antiviral properties, interferons have immunoregulatory functions. These include enhancement of NK cell production and activation, and inhibition of tumor cell growth.

Interferon is not directly antiviral but produces an antiviral effect in cells by reacting with them and inducing the formation of a second protein termed *antiviral protein* (Fig. 14-4). This protein mediates the antiviral action of interferon by altering the cell's protein synthesis and preventing new viruses from becoming assembled.

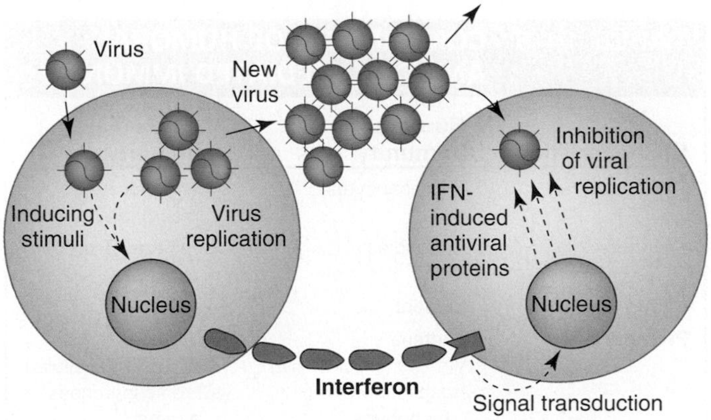

FIG. 14-4 Mechanism of action of interferon *(IFN).* When a virus attacks a cell, the cell begins to synthesize viral DNA and interferon. Interferon serves as an intercellular messenger and induces the production of antiviral proteins. Then the virus is not able to replicate in the cell.

Comparison of Humoral and Cell-Mediated Immunity

Humans need both humoral and cell-mediated immunity to remain healthy. Each type of immunity has unique properties, different methods of action, and reactions against particular antigens. Table 14-5 compares humoral and cell-mediated immunity.

Humoral Immunity. Humoral immunity consists of antibody-mediated immunity. The term *humoral* comes from the Greek word *humor,* which means body fluid. Since antibodies are produced by plasma cells (differentiated B cells) and found in plasma, the term *humoral immunity* is used. Production of antibodies is an essential component in a humoral immune response. Each of the five classes of immunoglobulins (Igs)—that is, IgG, IgA, IgM, IgD, and IgE—has specific characteristics (see Table 14-2).

TABLE 14-4 CLINICAL USES OF CYTOKINES

Cytokine	Clinical Uses
α-Interferon (Roferon-A, Intron A)*	Hairy cell leukemia, chronic myelogenous leukemia, malignant melanoma, renal cell carcinoma, ovarian cancer, multiple myeloma, Kaposi sarcoma, hepatitis B and C
β-Interferon (Betaseron, Avonex, Rebif)	Multiple sclerosis
Colony-Stimulating Factors	
G-CSF	
• filgrastim (Neupogen) • pegfilgrastim (Neulasta)	Chemotherapy-induced neutropenia
GM-CSF	
• sargramostim (Leukine)	Neutropenia, myeloid recovery after bone marrow transplantation
Soluble TNF Receptor	
etanercept (Enbrel)	Rheumatoid arthritis
Interleukin-2	
aldesleukin (Proleukin)	Metastatic renal cell carcinoma, metastatic melanoma
Interleukin 11 (platelet growth factor)	
oprelvekin (Neumega)	Prevention of thrombocytopenia after chemotherapy
Erythropoietin	
epoetin alfa (Epogen, Procrit) darbepoetin alfa (Aranesp)	Anemia of chronic cancer, anemia related to chemotherapy, anemia of chronic kidney disease
IL-1 Receptor Antagonist	
anakinra (Kineret)	Rheumatoid arthritis

*eFig. 14-1 on the website for this chapter shows how interferon is commercially made.
G-CSF, Granulocyte colony-stimulating factor; *GM-CSF,* granulocyte-macrophage colony-stimulating factor; *IL,* interleukin; *TNF,* tumor necrosis factor.

TABLE 14-5 COMPARISON OF HUMORAL AND CELL-MEDIATED IMMUNITY

Characteristics	Humoral Immunity	Cell-Mediated Immunity
Cells involved	B lymphocytes	T lymphocytes, macrophages
Products	Antibodies	Sensitized T cells, cytokines
Memory cells	Present	Present
Protection	Bacteria Viruses (extracellular) Respiratory and GI pathogens	Fungus Viruses (intracellular) Chronic infectious agents Tumor cells
Examples	Anaphylactic shock Atopic diseases Transfusion reaction Bacterial infections	Tuberculosis Fungal infections Contact dermatitis Graft rejection Destruction of cancer cells

When a pathogen (especially bacteria) enters the body, it may encounter a B lymphocyte that is specific for antigens located on that bacterial cell wall. In addition, a monocyte or macrophage may phagocytize the bacteria and present its antigens to a B lymphocyte. The B lymphocyte recognizes the antigen because it has receptors on its cell surface specific for

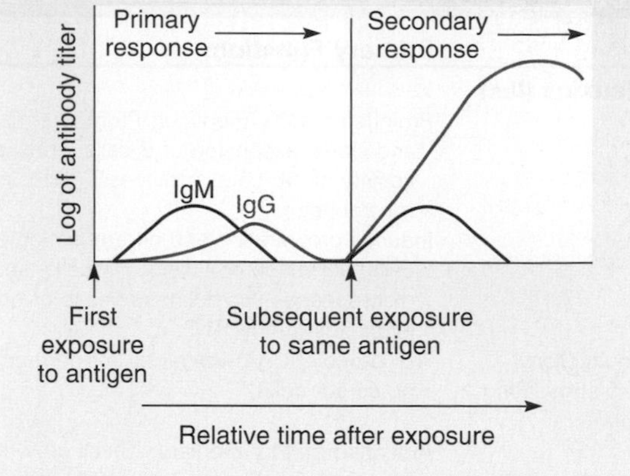

FIG. 14-5 Primary and secondary immune responses. The introduction of antigen induces a response dominated by two classes of immunoglobulins, IgM and IgG. IgM predominates in the primary response, with some IgG appearing later. After the host's immune system is primed, another challenge with the same antigen induces the secondary response, in which some IgM and large amounts of IgG are produced.

that antigen. When the antigen comes in contact with the cell surface receptor, the B cell becomes activated, and most B cells differentiate into plasma cells (see Fig. 14-3). The mature plasma cell secretes immunoglobulins. Some stimulated B lymphocytes remain as memory cells.

The primary immune response becomes evident 4 to 8 days after the initial exposure to the antigen (Fig. 14-5). IgM is the first type of antibody formed. Because of the large size of the IgM molecule, this immunoglobulin is confined to the intravascular space. As the immune response progresses, IgG is produced, and it can move from intravascular to extravascular spaces.

When the individual is exposed to the antigen the second time, a secondary antibody response occurs. This response occurs faster (1 to 3 days), is stronger, and lasts for a longer time than a primary response. Memory cells account for the memory of the first exposure to the antigen and the more rapid production of antibodies. IgG is the primary antibody found in a secondary immune response.

IgG crosses the placental membrane and provides the newborn with passive acquired immunity for at least 3 months. Infants may also get some passive immunity from IgA in breast milk and colostrum.

Cell-Mediated Immunity. Immune responses that are initiated through specific antigen recognition by T cells are termed **cell-mediated immunity.** Several cell types and factors are involved in cell-mediated immunity. The cell types involved include T lymphocytes, macrophages, and NK cells. Cell-mediated immunity is of primary importance in (1) immunity against pathogens that survive inside of cells, including viruses and some bacteria (e.g., mycobacteria); (2) fungal infections; (3) rejection of transplanted tissues; (4) contact hypersensitivity reactions; and (5) tumor immunity.

GERONTOLOGIC CONSIDERATIONS

EFFECTS OF AGING ON THE IMMUNE SYSTEM

With advancing age, there is a decline in the function of the immune response (Table 14-6). The primary clinical evidence of *immunosenescence* is the high incidence of malignancies in

TABLE 14-6 GERONTOLOGIC ASSESSMENT DIFFERENCES

Effects of Aging on the Immune System

- Thymic involution
- ↓ Cell-mediated immunity
- ↓ Delayed hypersensitivity reaction
- ↓ IL-1 and IL-2 synthesis
- ↓ Expression of IL-2 receptors
- ↓ Proliferative response of T and B cells
- ↓ Primary and secondary antibody responses
- ↑ Autoantibodies

IL, Interleukin.

older adults. Older people are also more susceptible to infections (e.g., influenza, pneumonia) from pathogens that they were relatively immunocompetent against earlier in life. Bacterial pneumonia is the leading cause of death from infections in older adults. The antibody response to immunizations (e.g., flu vaccine) in older adults is considerably lower than in younger adults.

The bone marrow remains relatively unaffected by increasing age. Immunoglobulin levels decrease with age and therefore lead to a suppressed humoral immune response in older adults. Thymic involution (shrinking) occurs with aging, along with decreased numbers of T cells. These changes in the thymus gland are a primary cause of immunosenescence. Both T and B cells show deficiencies in activation, transit time through the cell cycle, and subsequent differentiation. However, the most significant alterations involve T cells. As thymic output of T cells diminishes, the differentiation of T cells increases. Consequently, there is an accumulation of memory cells rather than new precursor cells responsive to previously unencountered antigens.

The delayed hypersensitivity reaction, as determined by skin testing with injected antigens, is frequently decreased or absent in older adults. This altered response reflects **anergy** (an immunodeficient condition characterized by lack of or diminished reaction to an antigen or a group of antigens).

ALTERED IMMUNE RESPONSE

Immunocompetence exists when the body's immune system can identify and inactivate or destroy foreign substances. When the immune system is incompetent or underresponsive, severe infections, immunodeficiency diseases, and malignancies may occur. When the immune system overreacts, hypersensitivity disorders such as allergies and autoimmune diseases may develop.

Hypersensitivity Reactions

Sometimes the immune response is overreactive against foreign antigens or reacts against its own tissue, resulting in tissue damage. These responses are termed **hypersensitivity reactions.** *Autoimmune diseases,* a type of hypersensitivity response, occur when the body fails to recognize self-proteins and reacts against self-antigens.

Hypersensitivity reactions can be classified according to the source of the antigen, the time sequence (immediate or delayed), or the basic immunologic mechanisms causing the injury. Four types of hypersensitivity reactions exist (Table 14-7). Types I, II, and III are immediate and are examples of humoral immunity. Type IV is a delayed hypersensitivity reaction and is related to cell-mediated immunity.

Type I: IgE-Mediated Reactions. *Anaphylactic reactions* are type I reactions that occur only in susceptible people who are highly sensitized to specific allergens. IgE antibodies, produced in response to the allergen, have a characteristic property of attaching to mast cells and basophils (Fig. 14-6; see Fig. 29-2). Within these cells are granules containing potent chemical mediators (histamine, serotonin, leukotrienes, eosinophil chemotactic factor of anaphylaxis [ECF-A], kinins, and bradyki-

TABLE 14-7 TYPES OF HYPERSENSITIVITY REACTIONS

Type I: IgE-Mediated	Type II: Cytotoxic	Type III: Immune-Complex	Type IV: Delayed Hypersensitivity
Antigen			
Exogenous pollen, food, drugs, dust	Cell surface of RBCs Cell basement membrane	Extracellular fungal, viral, bacterial	Intracellular or extracellular
Antibody Involved			
IgE	IgG, IgM	IgG, IgM	None
Complement Involved			
No	Yes	Yes	No
Mediators of Injury			
Histamine Mast cells Leukotrienes Prostaglandins	Complement lysis Macrophages in tissues	Neutrophils Complement lysis Monocytes, macrophages Lysosomal enzymes	Cytokines T cytotoxic cells
Examples			
Allergic rhinitis Asthma	Transfusion reaction Goodpasture syndrome Immune thrombocytopenic purpura Graves' disease	Systemic lupus erythematosus Rheumatoid arthritis	Contact dermatitis to poison ivy
Skin Test			
Wheal and flare	None	Erythema and edema in 3-8 hr	Erythema and edema in 24-48 hr (e.g., TB test)

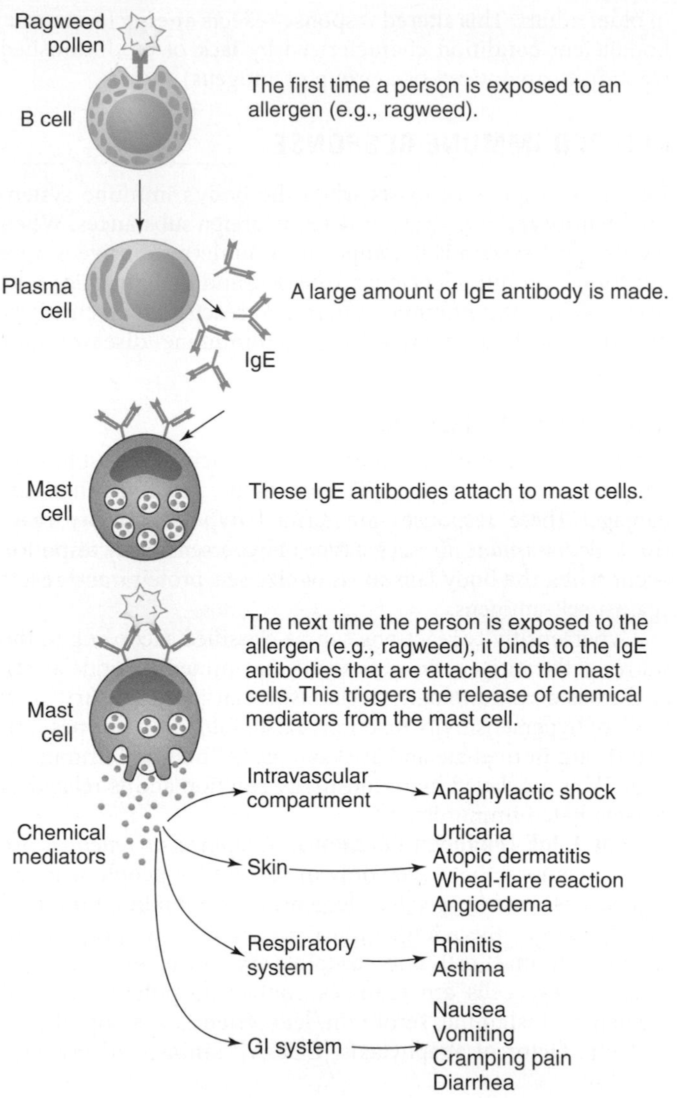

FIG. 14-6 Steps in a type I allergic reaction.

nin). (Chemical mediators of inflammation are discussed in Chapter 12 and Table 12-1.)

On the first exposure to the allergen, IgE antibodies are produced and bind to mast cells and basophils. On any subsequent exposures, the allergen links with the IgE bound to mast cells or basophils and triggers degranulation of the cells and the release of chemical mediators from the granules. In this process the mediators that are released attack target tissues, causing clinical allergy symptoms. These effects include smooth muscle contraction, increased vascular permeability, vasodilation, hypotension, increased secretion of mucus, and itching. Fortunately, the mediators are short acting and their effects are reversible. (The mediators and their effects are summarized in Table 14-8.)

A genetic predisposition to the development of allergic diseases exists. The capacity to become sensitized to an allergen, rather than the specific allergic disorder, appears to be the inherited trait. For example, a father with asthma may have a son who has allergic rhinitis.

The clinical manifestations of an anaphylactic reaction depend on whether the mediators remain local or become systemic, or whether they affect particular organs. When the

TABLE 14-8 MEDIATORS OF ALLERGIC RESPONSE*
• Histamine • Leukotrienes† • Prostaglandins • Platelet-activating factor • Kinins • Serotonin • Anaphylatoxins (C3a, C4a, C5a from complement activation)

*eTable 14-1 is an enhanced version of this table explaining biologic activity and clinical outcomes of these mediators.
†See Chapter 12, Fig. 12-2.

mediators remain localized, a cutaneous response termed the *wheal-and-flare reaction* occurs. This reaction is characterized by a pale wheal containing edematous fluid surrounded by a red flare from the hyperemia. The reaction occurs in minutes or hours and is usually not dangerous. A classic example of a wheal-and-flare reaction is the mosquito bite. The wheal-and-flare reaction serves a diagnostic purpose as a means of demonstrating allergic reactions to specific allergens during skin tests.

Common allergic reactions include anaphylaxis and atopic reactions.

Anaphylaxis. *Anaphylaxis* can occur when mediators are released systemically (e.g., after injection of a drug, after an insect sting). The reaction occurs within minutes and can be life threatening because of bronchial constriction and subsequent airway obstruction and vascular collapse. The target organs affected are seen in Fig. 14-7. Initial symptoms include edema and itching at the site of exposure to the allergen. Shock can occur rapidly and is manifested by rapid, weak pulse; hypotension; dilated pupils; dyspnea; and possibly cyanosis. This is compounded by bronchial edema and angioedema. Death will occur if emergency treatment is not initiated. Some of the important allergens that can cause anaphylactic shock in hypersensitive people are listed in Table 14-9.

Atopic Reactions. An estimated 20% of the population is *atopic,* having an inherited tendency to become sensitive to environmental allergens. The atopic diseases that can result are allergic rhinitis, asthma, atopic dermatitis, urticaria, and angioedema.

Allergic rhinitis, or hay fever, is the most common type I hypersensitivity reaction. It may occur year-round (perennial allergic rhinitis), or it may be seasonal (seasonal allergic rhinitis). Airborne substances such as pollens, dust, and molds are the primary causes of allergic rhinitis. Perennial allergic rhinitis may be caused by dust, molds, and animal dander. Seasonal allergic rhinitis is commonly caused by pollens from trees, weeds, or grasses. The target areas affected are the conjunctiva of the eyes and the mucosa of the upper respiratory tract. Symptoms include nasal discharge; sneezing; lacrimation; mucosal swelling with airway obstruction; and pruritus around the eyes, nose, throat, and mouth. (Treatment of allergic rhinitis is discussed in Chapter 27 on p. 500.)

Many patients with *asthma* have an allergic component to their disease. These patients frequently have a history of atopic disorders (e.g., infantile eczema, allergic rhinitis, food intolerances). Inflammatory mediators produce bronchial smooth muscle constriction, excessive secretion of viscoid mucus, edema of the mucous membranes of the bronchi, and decreased

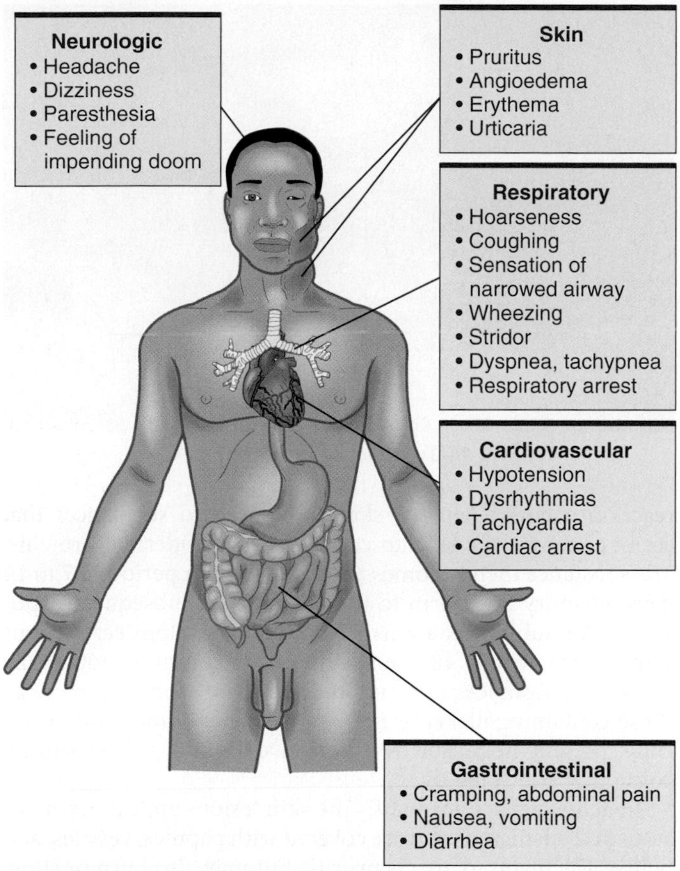

FIG. 14-7 Clinical manifestations of a systemic anaphylactic reaction.

TABLE 14-9 ALLERGENS CAUSING ANAPHYLACTIC SHOCK

Drugs	**Treatment Measures**
• Penicillins • Sulfonamides • Insulins • Aspirin • Tetracycline • Local anesthetics • Chemotherapeutic agents • Cephalosporins • Nonsteroidal antiinflammatory drugs	• Blood products (whole blood and components) • Iodine-contrast media for IVP or angiogram test • Allergenic extracts in hyposensitization therapy **Insect Venoms** • Wasps, hornets, yellow jackets, bumblebees, ants
Foods	**Animal Sera**
• Eggs, milk, nuts, peanuts, shellfish, fish, chocolate, strawberries	• Tetanus antitoxin • Rabies antitoxin • Diphtheria antitoxin • Snake venom antitoxin

IVP, Intravenous pyelogram.

lung compliance. Because of these physiologic alterations, patients manifest dyspnea, wheezing, coughing, tightness in the chest, and thick sputum. (Pathophysiology and management of asthma are discussed in Chapter 29.)

Atopic dermatitis is a chronic, inherited skin disorder characterized by exacerbations and remissions. It is caused by several environmental allergens that are difficult to identify. Although patients with atopic dermatitis have elevated IgE levels and positive skin tests, the histopathologic features do not represent the typical, localized wheal-and-flare type I reactions.

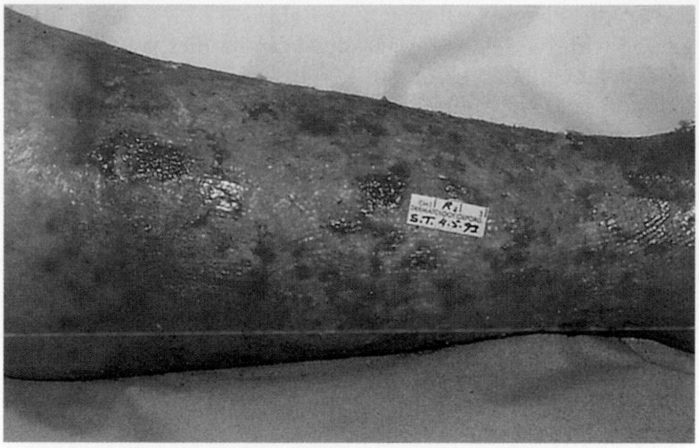

FIG. 14-8 Atopic dermatitis of the lower leg.

The skin lesions are more generalized and involve vasodilation of blood vessels, resulting in interstitial edema with vesicle formation (Fig. 14-8). (Dermatitis is discussed in Chapter 24.)

Urticaria (hives) is a cutaneous reaction against systemic allergens occurring in atopic people. It is characterized by transient wheals (pink, raised, edematous, pruritic areas) that vary in size and shape and may occur all over the body. Urticaria develops rapidly after exposure to an allergen and may last minutes or hours. Histamine causes localized vasodilation (erythema), transudation of fluid (wheal), and flaring. Flaring is due to dilated blood vessels on the edge of the wheal. Histamine is responsible for the pruritus associated with the lesions. (Urticaria is discussed in Chapter 24.)

Angioedema is a localized cutaneous lesion similar to urticaria but involving deeper layers of the skin and the submucosa. The principal areas of involvement include the eyelids, lips, tongue, larynx, hands, feet, GI tract, and genitalia. Swelling usually begins in the face and then progresses to the airways and other parts of the body. Dilation and engorgement of the capillaries secondary to the release of histamine cause the diffuse swelling. Welts are not apparent as in urticaria. The outer skin appears normal or has a reddish hue. The lesions may burn, sting, or itch, and can cause acute abdominal pain if in the GI tract. The swelling may occur suddenly or over several hours and usually lasts for 24 hours.

Type II: Cytotoxic and Cytolytic Reactions. Cytotoxic and cytolytic reactions are type II hypersensitivity reactions involving the direct binding of IgG or IgM antibodies to an antigen on the cell surface. Antigen-antibody complexes activate the complement system, which mediates the reaction. Cellular tissue is destroyed in one of two ways: (1) activation of the complement system resulting in cytolysis or (2) enhanced phagocytosis.

Target cells frequently destroyed in type II reactions are erythrocytes, platelets, and leukocytes. Some of the antigens involved are the ABO blood group, Rh factor, and drugs. Pathophysiologic disorders characteristic of type II reactions include ABO incompatibility transfusion reaction, Rh incompatibility transfusion reaction, autoimmune and drug-related hemolytic anemias, leukopenias, thrombocytopenias, erythroblastosis fetalis (hemolytic disease of the newborn), and Goodpasture syndrome. The tissue damage usually occurs rapidly.

Hemolytic Transfusion Reactions. A classic type II reaction occurs when a recipient receives ABO-incompatible blood from a donor. Naturally acquired antibodies to antigens of the ABO blood group are in the recipient's serum but are not present on the erythrocyte membranes (see Table 30-8). For example, a person with type A blood has anti-B antibodies, a person with type B blood has anti-A antibodies, a person with type AB blood has no antibodies, and a person with type O blood has both anti-A and anti-B antibodies.

If the recipient is transfused with incompatible blood, antibodies immediately coat the foreign erythrocytes, causing *agglutination* (clumping). The clumping of cells blocks small blood vessels in the body, uses existing clotting factors, and depletes them, leading to bleeding. Within hours, neutrophils and macrophages phagocytize the agglutinated cells. The complement system is activated (see eFig. 12-2), and cell lysis occurs, which causes the release of hemoglobin into the urine and plasma. In addition, a cytotoxic reaction causes vascular spasms in the kidney that further block the renal tubules. Acute kidney injury can result from the hemoglobinuria. (Blood transfusions are discussed in Chapter 31.)

Goodpasture Syndrome. *Goodpasture syndrome* is a disorder involving the lungs and kidneys. An antibody-mediated autoimmune reaction occurs involving the glomerular and alveolar basement membranes. The circulating antibodies combine with tissue antigen to activate the complement system, which causes deposits of IgG to form along the basement membranes of the lungs or kidneys. This reaction may result in pulmonary hemorrhage and glomerulonephritis. (Goodpasture syndrome is discussed in Chapter 46.)

Type III: Immune-Complex Reactions. Tissue damage in immune-complex reactions, which are type III reactions, occurs secondary to antigen-antibody complexes. Soluble antigens combine with immunoglobulins of the IgG and IgM classes to form complexes that are too small to be effectively removed by the mononuclear phagocyte system. Therefore the complexes deposit in tissue or small blood vessels. They cause activation of the complement system and release of chemotactic factors that lead to inflammation and destruction of the involved tissue.

Type III reactions may be local or systemic and immediate or delayed. The clinical manifestations depend on the number of complexes and the location in the body. Common sites for deposit are the kidneys, skin, joints, blood vessels, and lungs. Severe type III reactions are associated with autoimmune disorders such as systemic lupus erythematosus, acute glomerulonephritis, and rheumatoid arthritis. (Systemic lupus erythematosus and rheumatoid arthritis are discussed in Chapter 65, and acute glomerulonephritis is discussed in Chapter 46.)

Type IV: Delayed Hypersensitivity Reactions. A *delayed hypersensitivity reaction*—a type IV reaction—is also called a *cell-mediated immune response.* Although cell-mediated responses are usually protective mechanisms, tissue damage occurs in delayed hypersensitivity reactions.

The tissue damage in a type IV reaction does not occur in the presence of antibodies or complement. Rather, sensitized T lymphocytes attack antigens or release cytokines. Some of these cytokines attract macrophages into the area. The macrophages and enzymes released by them are responsible for most of the tissue destruction. In the delayed hypersensitivity reaction, it takes 24 to 48 hours for a response to occur.

Clinical examples of a delayed hypersensitivity reaction include contact dermatitis (Fig. 14-9); hypersensitivity reactions to bacterial, fungal, and viral infections; and transplant rejections. Some drug sensitivity reactions also fit this category.

Contact Dermatitis. *Allergic contact dermatitis* is an example of a delayed hypersensitivity reaction involving the skin. The reaction occurs when the skin is exposed to substances that easily penetrate the skin to combine with epidermal proteins. The substance then becomes antigenic. Over a period of 7 to 14 days, memory cells form to the antigen. On subsequent exposure to the substance, a sensitized person develops eczematous skin lesions within 48 hours. The most common potentially antigenic substances encountered are metal compounds (e.g., those containing nickel or mercury); rubber compounds; catechols present in poison ivy, poison oak, and poison sumac; cosmetics; and some dyes.

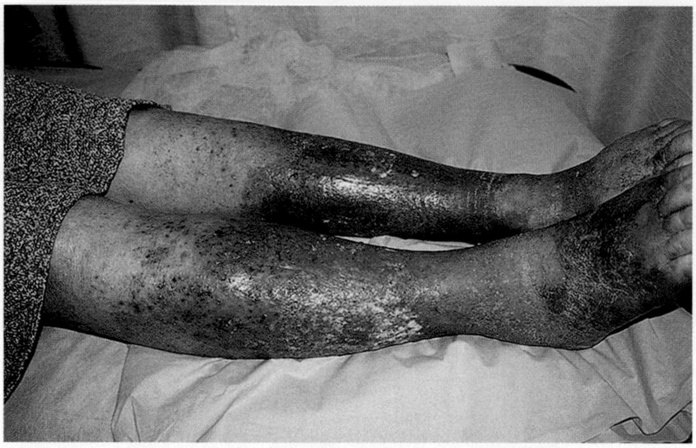

FIG. 14-9 Contact dermatitis to rubber.

In acute contact dermatitis the skin lesions appear erythematous and edematous and are covered with papules, vesicles, and bullae. The involved area is pruritic but may also burn or sting. When contact dermatitis becomes chronic, the lesions resemble atopic dermatitis because they are thickened, scaly, and lichenified. The main difference between contact dermatitis and atopic dermatitis is that contact dermatitis is localized and restricted to the area exposed to the allergens, whereas atopic dermatitis is usually widespread.

Microbial Hypersensitivity Reactions. The classic example of a microbial cell-mediated immune reaction is the body's defense against the tubercle bacillus. Tuberculosis results from invasion of lung tissue by the highly resistant tubercle bacillus. The organism itself does not directly damage the lung tissue. However, antigenic material released from the tubercle bacilli reacts with T lymphocytes, initiating a cell-mediated immune response. The resulting response causes extensive caseous necrosis of the lung.

After the initial cell-mediated reaction, memory cells persist, so subsequent contact with the tubercle bacillus or an extract of purified protein from the organism causes a delayed hypersensitivity reaction. This is the basis for the purified protein derivative (PPD) tuberculosis skin test, which is read 48 to 72 hours after the PPD is injected intradermally. (Tuberculosis is discussed in Chapter 28.)

ALLERGIC DISORDERS

Although an alteration of the immune system may be manifested in many ways, allergies, or type I hypersensitivity reactions, are seen most frequently.

Assessment

For a thorough assessment of a patient with allergies, a comprehensive patient history, physical examination, diagnostic workup, and skin testing for allergens should be done. Obtain information from the patient about family allergies, past and present allergies, and social and environmental factors.

Family history, including information about atopic reactions in relatives, is especially important in identifying at-risk patients. Assess the specific disorder, clinical manifestations, and treatments prescribed.

Note past and present allergies. Identifying the allergens that may have triggered a reaction is essential to control allergic reactions. The time of year when an allergic reaction occurs can be a clue to a seasonal allergen. Also obtain information about any over-the-counter or prescription medications used to treat the allergies.

In addition to identifying the allergen, also obtain information about the clinical manifestations and course of allergic reaction. For women patients, assessment of symptoms during pregnancy, menstruation, or menopause may be important.

Social and environmental factors, especially the physical environment, are important. Questions about pets, trees and plants on the property, pollutants in the air, floor coverings, houseplants, and cooling and heating systems in the home and workplace can provide valuable information about allergens. In addition, a daily or weekly food diary with a description of any untoward reactions is important. Of particular interest is a screening for any reaction to medication. Finally, ask about the patient's lifestyle and stress level in connection with the appearance of allergic symptoms.

Do a comprehensive head-to-toe physical examination, with particular attention focused on the site of the allergic manifestations. Obtain a comprehensive assessment that includes subjective and objective data (Table 14-10).

TABLE 14-10 NURSING ASSESSMENT

Allergies

Subjective Data

Important Health Information

Past health history: Recurrent respiratory problems, seasonal exacerbations; unusual reactions to insect bites or stings; past and present allergies

Medications: Unusual reactions to any medications; use of over-the-counter drugs, use of medications for allergies

Functional Health Patterns

Health perception–health management: Family history of allergies; malaise

Nutritional-metabolic: Food intolerances; vomiting

Elimination: Abdominal cramps, diarrhea

Activity-exercise: Fatigue; hoarseness, cough, dyspnea

Cognitive-perceptual: Itching, burning, stinging of eyes, nose, throat, or skin; chest tightness

Role-relationship: Altered home and work environment, presence of pets

Objective Data

Integumentary

Rashes, including urticaria, wheal and flare, papules, vesicles, bullae; dryness, scaliness, scratches, irritation

Eyes, Ears, Nose, and Throat

Eyes: Conjunctivitis; lacrimation; rubbing or excessive blinking; dark circles under the eyes ("allergic shiner")

Ears: Diminished hearing; immobile or scarred tympanic membranes; recurrent ear infections

Nose: Nasal polyps; nasal voice; nose twitching; itchy nose; rhinitis; pale, boggy mucous membranes; sniffling; repeated sneezing; swollen nasal passages; recurrent, unexplained nosebleeds; crease across the bridge of nose ("allergic salute")

Throat: Continual throat clearing; swollen lips or tongue; red throat; palpable neck lymph nodes

Respiratory

Wheezing, stridor; thick sputum

Possible Diagnostic Findings

Eosinophilia of serum, sputum, or nasal and bronchial secretions; ↑ serum IgE levels; positive skin tests; abnormal chest and sinus x-rays

Diagnostic Studies

Many specialized immunologic techniques can be performed to detect abnormalities of lymphocytes, eosinophils, and immunoglobulins. A complete blood count (CBC) with WBC differential is done, with an absolute lymphocyte count and eosinophil count. Immunodeficiency is diagnosed if the lymphocyte count is below 1200/μL (1.2×10^9/L). T cell and B cell quantification is used to diagnose specific immunodeficiency syndromes. The eosinophil count is elevated in type I hypersensitivity reactions involving IgE. The serum IgE level is also generally elevated in type I hypersensitivity reactions and serves as a diagnostic indicator of atopic diseases.

Sputum and nasal and bronchial secretions may also be tested for the presence of eosinophils. If asthma is suspected, pulmonary function tests for vital capacity, forced expiratory volume, and maximum midexpiratory flow rates are helpful.

Allergy skin testing is the preferred method, but in some cases blood testing may be ordered. Allergy blood tests for IgE antibodies to specific allergens can be done using an enzyme-linked immunosorbent assay (ELISA). Allergy blood testing is recommended if a person (1) is using a drug that interferes with skin test results (e.g., antihistamines, corticosteroids) and cannot stop taking it for a few days, (2) cannot tolerate the many needle scratches required for skin testing, or (3) has a skin disorder (e.g., severe eczema, dermatitis, psoriasis).

Skin Tests. Skin testing is used to identify the specific allergens that are causing the allergy symptoms. With the use of empiric allergy medications as the treatment of choice for most allergic rhinitis, it has become common practice to omit skin testing for specific allergens in these patients. However, diagnosing an allergy to a specific antigen enables the patient to avoid an allergen and makes him or her a candidate for immunotherapy. Unfortunately, skin testing cannot be done on patients who cannot be removed from medications that suppress the histamine response or patients with food allergies.

Procedure. Skin testing may be done by three different methods: (1) a scratch or prick test, (2) an intradermal test, or (3) a patch test. The areas of the body usually used in skin testing are the arms and the back. Allergen extracts are applied to the skin in rows with a corresponding control site opposite the test site. Saline or another diluent is applied to the control site. In the *scratch test* a drop of allergen is placed on the skin, and then a pricking device is used so the allergen can enter the skin. In the *intradermal test* the allergen extract is injected under the skin, similar to a PPD test for TB. In the *patch test* an allergen is applied to a patch that is placed on the skin (see Fig. 23-10).

Results. In the scratch and intradermal tests the reaction occurs in 5 to 10 minutes. In the patch test the patches need to be worn for 48 to 72 hours. If the person is hypersensitive to the allergen, a positive reaction will occur within minutes after insertion in the skin and may last for 8 to 12 hours. A positive reaction is manifested by a local wheal-and-flare response.

The size of the positive reaction does not always correlate with the severity of allergy symptoms. False-positive and false-negative results may occur. Negative results from skin testing do not necessarily mean the person does not have an allergic disorder, and positive results do not necessarily mean that the allergen was causing the clinical manifestations. Positive results imply that the person is sensitized to that allergen. Therefore correlating skin test results with the patient's history is important.

Precautions. A highly sensitive person is always at risk for developing an anaphylactic reaction to skin tests. Therefore a patient should never be left alone during the testing period. Sometimes skin testing is completely contraindicated and blood allergy testing is used. If a severe reaction does occur with a skin test, the extract is immediately removed and antiinflammatory topical cream is applied to the site. For intradermal testing, the arm is used so that a tourniquet can be applied during a severe reaction. A subcutaneous injection of epinephrine may also be necessary.

Collaborative Care

After an allergic disorder is diagnosed, treatment is aimed at reducing exposure to the offending allergen, treating the symptoms, and, if necessary, desensitizing the person through immunotherapy.

Anaphylaxis. Anaphylactic reactions occur suddenly in hypersensitive patients after exposure to the offending allergen. They may occur after parenteral injection of drugs (especially antibiotics) or blood products, and after insect stings. The cardinal principle in management is speed in (1) recognition of signs and symptoms of an anaphylactic reaction, (2) maintenance of a patent airway, (3) prevention of spread of the allergen by using a tourniquet, (4) administration of drugs, and (5) treatment for shock. Table 14-11 summarizes the emergency treatment of anaphylactic shock.

Severe cases of anaphylaxis may result in hypovolemic shock because of the loss of intravascular fluid into interstitial spaces that occurs secondary to increased capillary permeability. Peripheral vasoconstriction and stimulation of the sympathetic nervous system occur to compensate for the fluid shift. However, unless shock is treated early, the body will no longer be able to compensate, and irreversible tissue damage will occur, leading to death. (Hypovolemic shock is discussed in Chapter 67.)

All health care workers must be prepared for the rare but life-threatening anaphylactic reaction, which requires immediate medical and nursing interventions. It is extremely important to list all of a patient's allergies on the chart, the nursing care plan, and the medication record.

Chronic Allergies. Most allergic reactions are chronic and are characterized by remissions and exacerbations of symptoms. Treatment focuses on identification and control of allergens, relief of symptoms through drug therapy, and hyposensitization of a patient to an offending allergen.

Allergen Recognition and Control. You play an important role in helping the patient make lifestyle adjustments so that there is minimal exposure to offending allergens. Reinforce that, even with drug therapy and immunotherapy, the patient will never be totally desensitized or completely symptom free. Help the patient initiate various preventive measures to control the allergic symptoms.

Of primary importance is the need to identify the offending allergen. Sometimes this is done through skin testing. In the case of food allergies an elimination diet is sometimes valuable. If an allergic reaction occurs, all foods eaten shortly before the reaction should be eliminated and gradually reintroduced one at a time until the offending food is detected.

Many allergic reactions, especially asthma and urticaria, may be aggravated by fatigue and emotional stress. Assist the patient in planning a stress management program. Relaxation techniques can be practiced when the patient comes for frequent immunotherapy treatments.

Sometimes control of allergic symptoms requires environmental control, including changing an occupation, moving to a different climate, or giving up a favorite pet. In the case of airborne allergens, sleeping in an air-conditioned room, damp dusting daily, covering mattresses and pillows with hypoallergenic covers, and wearing a mask outdoors may be helpful.

If the allergen is a drug, instruct the patient to avoid the drug. The patient also has the responsibility to make his or her allergies well known to all health care providers. The patient should wear a Medic Alert bracelet listing the particular drug allergy and have the offending drug listed on all medical and dental records.

TABLE 14-11 EMERGENCY MANAGEMENT

Anaphylactic Shock

Etiology
- Injection of, inhalation of, ingestion of, or topical exposure to substance that produces profound allergic response (See Table 14-9 for more complete listing.)

Assessment Findings

See Fig. 14-7.

Interventions

Initial
- Ensure patent airway.
- Administer high-flow O_2 via non-rebreather mask.
- Remove insect stinger if present.
- Establish IV access.
- epinephrine 1 : 1000, 0.01 mL/kg (0.3-0.5 mL) IM into midanterior lateral thigh; repeat every 5-15 min.*
- Nebulized albuterol (Proventil).
- Diphenhydramine (Benadryl) IM or IV.
- Corticosteroids: methylprednisolone (Solu-Medrol) IV.

Hypotension
- Place recumbent and elevate legs.
- epinephrine 1 : 10,000, 0.1 mL/kg IV every 2-5 min.
- Maintain blood pressure with fluids, volume expanders, vasopressors (e.g., dopamine [Intropin]).

Ongoing Monitoring
- Monitor vital signs, respiratory effort, O_2 saturation, level of consciousness, and cardiac rhythm.
- Anticipate intubation with severe respiratory distress.
- Anticipate cricothyrotomy or tracheostomy with severe laryngeal edema.

*Patients receiving β-blockers may be resistant to treatment with epinephrine and can develop refractory hypotension and bradycardia. Glucagon should be administered in this setting because it has inotropic and chronotropic effects that are not mediated through β-receptors.

For a patient allergic to insect stings, commercial bee-sting kits containing preinjectable epinephrine and a tourniquet are available. Instruct the patient and the family about the technique of applying the tourniquet and self-injecting the subcutaneous epinephrine. This patient also should wear a Medic Alert bracelet and carry a bee-sting kit whenever going outdoors.

Drug Therapy. The major categories of drugs used for symptomatic relief of chronic allergic disorders include antihistamines, sympathomimetic/decongestant drugs, corticosteroids, antipruritic drugs, and mast cell–stabilizing drugs. Many of these drugs can be obtained over the counter and are often misused by patients.

Antihistamines. Antihistamines are the best drugs for treatment of allergic rhinitis and urticaria (see Chapter 27, Table 27-2). They are less effective for severe allergic reactions. They act by competing with histamine for H_1-receptor sites and thus blocking the effect of histamine. Best results are achieved if they are taken as soon as allergy symptoms appear. Antihistamines can be used effectively to treat edema and pruritus but are relatively ineffective in preventing bronchoconstriction. With seasonal rhinitis, antihistamines should be taken during peak pollen seasons. (Antihistamines are discussed in Chapter 27.)

Sympathomimetic/Decongestant Drugs. The major sympathomimetic drug is epinephrine (Adrenalin), which is the drug of choice to treat an anaphylactic reaction. Epinephrine is produced by the adrenal medulla and stimulates α- and β-adrenergic receptors. Stimulation of the α-adrenergic receptors causes vasoconstriction of peripheral blood vessels. β-Receptor stimulation relaxes bronchial smooth muscles. Epinephrine also acts directly on mast cells to stabilize them against further degranulation. The action of epinephrine lasts only a few minutes. For the treatment of anaphylaxis, the drug must be given parenterally (intramuscular [IM], IV).

Several specific, minor sympathomimetic drugs differ from epinephrine because they can be taken orally or nasally and last for several hours. Included in this category are phenylephrine (Neo-Synephrine) and pseudoephedrine (Sudafed). The minor sympathomimetic drugs are used primarily to treat allergic rhinitis.

Corticosteroids. Nasal corticosteroid sprays are effective in relieving the symptoms of allergic rhinitis (see Chapter 27 and Table 27-2). Occasionally patients have such severe manifestations of allergies that they are truly incapacitated. In these situations a brief course of oral corticosteroids can be used.

Antipruritic Drugs. Topically applied antipruritic drugs are most effective when the skin is not broken. These drugs protect the skin and provide relief from itching. Common over-the-counter drugs include calamine lotion, coal tar solutions, and camphor. Menthol and phenol may be added to other lotions to produce an antipruritic effect. Some more potent drugs that require a prescription include methdilazine (Tacaryl) and trimeprazine (Temaril). These drugs should be used with great caution because of the associated risk of agranulocytosis.

Mast Cell–Stabilizing Drug. Cromolyn (Intal, NasalCrom) is a mast cell–stabilizing agent that inhibits the release of histamines, leukotrienes, and other agents from the mast cell after antigen-IgE interaction. It is available as an inhalant nebulizer solution or a nasal spray. Cromolyn is used in the management of allergic rhinitis (see Chapter 27).

Leukotriene Receptor Antagonists. Leukotriene receptor antagonists (LTRAs) block leukotriene, one of the major mediators of the allergic inflammatory process (see Table 27-2). These medications can be taken orally. They may be used in the treatment of allergic rhinitis and asthma.

Immunotherapy. Immunotherapy is the recommended treatment for control of allergic symptoms when the allergen cannot be avoided and drug therapy is not effective.[3] Relatively few patients with allergies have symptoms so intolerable that they require allergy immunotherapy. (In individuals with anaphylactic reactions to insect venom, immunotherapy is definitely indicated.)

Immunotherapy involves administration of small titers of an allergen extract in increasing strengths until hyposensitivity to the specific allergen is achieved. For best results, teach the patient to avoid the offending allergen whenever possible because complete desensitization is impossible. Unfortunately, not all allergy-related conditions respond to immunotherapy. Food allergies cannot be safely treated with this therapy, and eczema may worsen with immunotherapy.

Mechanism of Action. The IgE level is elevated in atopic individuals. When IgE combines with an allergen in a hypersensitive person, a reaction occurs, releasing histamine in various body tissues. Allergens more readily combine with IgG than with other immunoglobulins. Therefore immunotherapy involves injecting allergen extracts that will stimulate increased IgG levels. The binding of IgG to allergen-reactive sites interferes with allergen binding to mast cell–bound IgE, preventing mast cell degranulation, and thus reduces the number of reactions that cause tissue damage. The goal of long-term immunotherapy is to keep "blocking" IgG levels high. In addition, allergen-specific T suppressor cells develop in individuals receiving immunotherapy.

Method of Administration. The allergens included in immunotherapy are chosen based on the results of skin testing with a panel of allergens.

Subcutaneous Immunotherapy. *Subcutaneous immunotherapy* involves the subcutaneous injection of titrated amounts of allergen extracts biweekly or weekly. The dose is small at first and is increased slowly until a maintenance dosage is reached. Generally it takes 1 to 2 years of immunotherapy to reach the maximal therapeutic effect. Therapy may be continued for about 5 years. After that, discontinuing therapy is considered. In many patients a decrease in symptoms is sustained after the treatment is discontinued. For patients with severe allergies or sensitivity to insect stings, maintenance therapy is continued indefinitely. Best results are achieved when immunotherapy is administered throughout the year.

Sublingual Immunotherapy. *Sublingual immunotherapy* involves allergen extracts taken under the tongue. This method of immunotherapy has a lower risk of severe adverse reaction than the traditional subcutaneous administration. Today in Europe, sublingual immunotherapy accounts for 40% of allergy treatment. In the United States, although some allergists are using sublingual immunotherapy, it is considered an investigational therapy. Most insurance plans do not cover sublingual immunotherapy. It is considered a U.S. Food and Drug Administration (FDA) "off-label" use. An advantage of this form of immunotherapy is that patients can do it at home.[3]

NURSING MANAGEMENT IMMUNOTHERAPY

You will often be the person responsible for administering subcutaneous immunotherapy. Always anticipate adverse reactions, especially when using a new-strength dose, after a previous reaction, or after a missed dose. Early manifestations of a systemic reaction include pruritus, urticaria, sneezing, laryngeal edema, and hypotension. Emergency measures for anaphylactic shock should be initiated immediately. Describe a local reaction according to the degree of redness and swelling at the injection site. If the area is greater than the size of a quarter in an adult, report the reaction to the health care provider so that the allergen dosage may be decreased.

Immunotherapy always carries the risk of a severe anaphylactic reaction. Therefore a health care provider, emergency equipment, and essential drugs should be available whenever injections are given.

Record keeping must be accurate and can be invaluable in preventing an adverse reaction to the allergen extract. Before giving an injection, check the patient's name against the name on the vial. Next, determine the vial strength, amount of last dose, date of last dose, and any reaction information.

Always administer the allergen extract in an extremity away from a joint so that a tourniquet can be applied for a severe reaction. Rotate the site for each injection. Aspirate for blood before giving an injection to ensure that the allergen extract is not injected into a blood vessel. An injection directly into the bloodstream can potentiate an anaphylactic reaction. After giving the injection, carefully observe the patient for 20 minutes, since systemic reactions are most likely to occur immediately. However, warn the patient that a delayed reaction can occur as long as 24 hours later.

Latex Allergies

Allergies to latex products have become an increasing problem, affecting both patients and health care professionals. The increase in allergic reactions has coincided with the sharp increase in glove use. It is estimated that 5% to 18% of health care workers regularly exposed to latex are sensitized. The more frequent and prolonged the exposure to latex, the greater the likelihood of developing a latex allergy.[4]

In addition to gloves, many latex-containing products are used in health care, such as blood pressure cuffs, stethoscopes, tourniquets, IV tubing, syringes, electrode pads, O_2 masks, tracheal tubes, colostomy and ileostomy pouches, urinary catheters, anesthetic masks, and adhesive tape. Latex proteins can become aerosolized through powder on gloves and can result in serious reactions when inhaled by sensitized individuals. It is recommended that all health care facilities use powder-free gloves to avoid respiratory exposure to latex proteins.

Types of Latex Allergies. Two types of latex allergies can occur: type IV allergic contact dermatitis and type I allergic reactions. *Type IV contact dermatitis* is caused by the chemicals used in the manufacturing process of latex gloves. It is a delayed reaction that occurs within 6 to 48 hours. Typically the person first has dryness, pruritus, fissuring, and cracking of the skin, followed by redness, swelling, and crusting at 24 to 48 hours. Chronic exposure can lead to lichenification, scaling, and hyperpigmentation. The dermatitis may extend beyond the area of physical contact with the allergen.

A *type I allergic reaction* is a response to the natural rubber latex proteins and occurs within minutes of contact with the proteins. The manifestations of these allergic reactions can vary from skin redness, urticaria, rhinitis, conjunctivitis, or asthma to full-blown anaphylactic shock. Systemic reactions to latex may result from exposure to latex protein via various routes, including the skin, mucous membranes, inhalation, and blood.[5]

Latex-Food Syndrome. Because some proteins in rubber are similar to food proteins, some foods may cause an allergic reaction in people who are allergic to latex. This is called *latex-food syndrome*. The most common of these foods are banana, avocado, chestnut, kiwi, tomato, water chestnut, guava, hazelnut, potato, peach, grape, and apricot. In people with latex allergy, most have a positive allergy test to at least one related food.

NURSING AND COLLABORATIVE MANAGEMENT LATEX ALLERGIES

Identifying patients and health care workers sensitive to latex is crucial to prevent adverse reactions. Obtain a thorough health history and history of any allergies, especially for patients with any complaints of latex contact symptoms. Not all latex-sensitive individuals can be identified, even with a careful and thorough history. The greatest risk factor is long-term multiple exposures to latex products (e.g., health care personnel, individuals who have had multiple surgeries, rubber industry workers). Additional risk factors include a patient history of hay fever, asthma, and allergies to certain foods (listed earlier).

Use latex precaution protocols for those patients identified as having a positive latex allergy test or a history of signs and symptoms related to latex exposure.[6] Many health care facilities have created latex-free product carts that can be used for patients with latex allergies. The National Institute for Occupational Safety and Health (NIOSH) has published recommendations for preventing allergic reactions to latex in the workplace (Table 14-12).

Because of the potential for severe symptoms of food allergy, teach patients to avoid those foods. Other recommendations for people with latex and food allergies include wearing a Medic Alert bracelet or necklace and carrying an injectable epinephrine pen.

Multiple Chemical Sensitivity

Multiple chemical sensitivity (MCS) is a chronic condition characterized by symptoms that the affected person attributes to low-level chemical exposure. Commonly accused substances

TABLE 14-12 GUIDELINES FOR PREVENTING ALLERGIC LATEX REACTIONS

- Use nonlatex gloves for activities that are not likely to involve contact with infectious materials (e.g., food preparation, housekeeping).
- Use powder-free gloves with reduced protein content.
- Do not use oil-based hand creams or lotions when wearing gloves.
- After removing gloves, wash hands with mild soap and dry thoroughly.
- Frequently clean work areas that are contaminated with latex-containing dust.
- Know the symptoms of latex allergy, including skin rash; hives; flushing; itching; nasal, eye, or sinus symptoms; asthma; and shock.
- If symptoms of latex allergy develop, avoid direct contact with latex gloves and products.
- Wear a Medic Alert bracelet and carry an epinephrine pen (e.g., EpiPen).

Source: National Institute for Occupational Safety and Health (NIOSH) *(www.cdc.gov/niosh)*.

include smoke, pesticides, plastics, synthetic fabrics, scented products, petroleum products, and paint fumes. Women between the ages of 30 and 50 are more likely to develop the symptoms. Symptoms have also been reported among military personnel, particularly Gulf War veterans. MCS is a controversial diagnosis and is not recognized as a chemical-caused illness by the American Medical Association or other authorities.[7,8]

The symptoms that people report are wide ranging and not specific. They include headache, fatigue, dizziness, nausea, congestion, itching, sneezing, sore throat, chest pain, breathing problems, muscle pain or stiffness, skin rash, diarrhea, bloating, gas, confusion, difficulty concentrating, memory problems, and mood changes. These symptoms are usually subjective, and there is no evidence of a pathologic condition or physiologic dysfunction.

Diagnosis is usually made based on a patient's health history. There is no established test to diagnose MCS. The most effective treatment for MCS is to avoid the chemicals that may trigger the symptoms and create a chemical-free and odor-free home and workplace. Antidepressants, including selective serotonin reuptake inhibitors (SSRIs) (e.g., citalopram [Celexa]), have been used for treatment. Drugs for anxiety and sleep have also been used.

AUTOIMMUNITY

Autoimmunity is an immune response against self in which the immune system no longer differentiates self from nonself. For some unknown reason, immune cells that are normally unresponsive (tolerant to self-antigens) are activated. In autoimmunity, autoantibodies and autosensitized T cells cause pathophysiologic tissue damage.

The cause of autoimmune diseases is still unknown. Age is thought to play some role because the number of circulating autoantibodies increases in people over age 50. However, the principal factors in the development of autoimmunity are (1) the inheritance of susceptibility genes, which may contribute to the failure of self-tolerance; and (2) initiation of autoreactivity by triggers, such as infections, which may activate self-reactive lymphocytes.

Autoimmune diseases tend to cluster, so that a given person may have more than one autoimmune disease (e.g., rheumatoid arthritis, Addison's disease), or the same or related autoimmune diseases may be found in other members of the same family. This observation has led to the concept of genetic predisposition to autoimmune disease. Most of the genetic research in this area correlates certain human leukocyte antigen (HLA) types with an autoimmune condition. (HLAs and disease association are discussed later in this chapter on p. 219.)

Even in a genetically predisposed person, some trigger is required for the initiation of autoreactivity. This may include infectious agents such as a virus. Viral infections can cause an alteration of cells or tissues that are not normally antigenic. The virally induced changes can make the cells or tissues antigenic. Viruses may be involved in the development of diseases such as type 1 diabetes mellitus.[9] Rheumatic fever and rheumatic heart disease are autoimmune responses triggered by streptococcal infection and mediated by antibodies against group A β-hemolytic streptococci that cross-react with heart muscles and valves and synovial membranes.

Drugs can also be precipitating factors in autoimmune disease. Hemolytic anemia can result from methyldopa (Aldomet) administration. Procainamide (Pronestyl) can induce the formation of antinuclear antibodies and cause a lupus-like syndrome.

Gender and hormones also have a role in autoimmune disease. More women than men have autoimmune disease. During pregnancy, many autoimmune diseases get better. After delivery, the woman with an autoimmune disease frequently has an exacerbation.

TABLE 14-13 EXAMPLES OF AUTOIMMUNE DISEASES*

Systemic Diseases	***Endocrine System***
• Mixed connective tissue disease	• Addison's disease
• Progressive systemic sclerosis (scleroderma)	• Graves' disease
• Rheumatoid arthritis	• Hypothyroidism
• Systemic lupus erythematosus	• Thyroiditis
	• Type 1 diabetes mellitus
Organ-Specific Diseases	***Gastrointestinal System***
Blood	• Celiac disease
• Autoimmune hemolytic anemia	• Pernicious anemia
• Immune thrombocytopenic purpura	• Ulcerative colitis
• Hemochromatosis	***Kidney***
Central Nervous System	• Glomerulonephritis
• Guillain-Barré syndrome	• Goodpasture syndrome
• Multiple sclerosis	***Liver***
Muscle	• Autoimmune hepatitis
• Myasthenia gravis	• Primary biliary cirrhosis
Heart	***Eye***
• Rheumatic fever	• Uveitis

* These diseases are discussed in various chapters throughout the book.

Autoimmune Diseases

Generally, autoimmune diseases are grouped according to organ-specific and systemic diseases (Table 14-13). Systemic lupus erythematosus (SLE) is a classic example of a systemic autoimmune disease characterized by damage to multiple organs. It occurs most frequently in women ages 20 to 40 years. The cause is unknown, but there appears to be a loss of self-tolerance for the body's own DNA antigens.

In SLE, tissue injury appears to be the result of the formation of antinuclear antibodies. For some reason (possibly a viral infection), the cell membrane is damaged and deoxyribonucleic acid (DNA) is released into the systemic circulation, where it is viewed as nonself. This DNA is normally sequestered inside the nucleus of cells. On release into the circulation, the DNA antigen reacts with an antibody. Some antibodies are involved in immune complex formation, and others may cause damage directly. Once the complexes are deposited, the complement system is activated and further damages the tissue, especially the renal glomerulus. (SLE is discussed in Chapter 65.)

Apheresis

Apheresis has been effectively used to treat autoimmune diseases and other diseases and disorders. *Apheresis* is a procedure to separate components of the blood followed by the removal of one or more of these components. Compound words are often used to describe any particular apheresis procedure, depending on the blood components being collected. *Plateletpheresis* is the removal of platelets, usually for collection from normal individuals to infuse into patients with low platelet counts (e.g., patients taking chemotherapy who develop thrombocytopenia). *Leukocytapheresis* is a general term indicating the removal of WBCs and is used in chronic myelogenous leukemia to remove high numbers of leukemic cells.

Apheresis is also used in peripheral stem cell transplantation to collect stem cells from peripheral blood. These stem cells can then be used to repopulate a person's bone marrow after high-dose chemotherapy (see section on hematopoietic stem cell transplants in Chapter 16).

Plasmapheresis. *Plasmapheresis* is the removal of plasma containing components causing or thought to cause disease. It can also be used to obtain plasma from healthy donors to administer to patients as replacement therapy.

When plasma is removed, it is replaced by substitute fluids such as saline, fresh-frozen plasma, or albumin. Thus the term *plasma exchange* more accurately describes this procedure.

Plasmapheresis has been used to treat autoimmune diseases such as SLE, glomerulonephritis, Goodpasture syndrome, myasthenia gravis, thrombocytopenic purpura, rheumatoid arthritis, and Guillain-Barré syndrome. Many disorders for which plasmapheresis is used are characterized by circulating autoantibodies (usually of the IgG class) and antigen-antibody complexes. The rationale for performing therapeutic plasmapheresis in autoimmune disorders is to remove pathologic substances present in plasma. Immunosuppressive therapy has been used to prevent recovery of IgG production, and plasmapheresis has been used to prevent antibody rebound.

In addition to removing antibodies and antigen-antibody complexes, plasmapheresis may also remove inflammatory mediators (e.g., complement) that are responsible for tissue damage. In the treatment of SLE, plasmapheresis is usually reserved for the patient having an acute attack who is unresponsive to conventional therapy.

Plasmapheresis involves the removal of whole blood through an IV device, and then the blood circulates through the apheresis machine. Inside the machine the blood is divided into plasma and its cellular components by centrifugation or membrane filtration. The plasma is generally replaced with normal saline, lactated Ringer's solution, fresh-frozen plasma, plasma protein fractions, or albumin. When blood is manually removed, only 500 mL can be taken at one time. However, with the use of apheresis procedures, more than 4 L of plasma can be pheresed in 2 to 3 hours.

As with administration of other blood products, be aware of side effects associated with plasmapheresis. The most common complications are hypotension and citrate toxicity. Hypotension is usually the result of a vasovagal reaction or transient volume changes. Citrate is used as an anticoagulant and may cause hypocalcemia, which may manifest as headache, paresthesias, and dizziness.

IMMUNODEFICIENCY DISORDERS

When the immune system does not adequately protect the body, **immunodeficiency** exists. Immunodeficiency disorders involve an impairment of one or more immune mechanisms, which include (1) phagocytosis, (2) humoral response, (3) cell-mediated response, (4) complement, and (5) a combined humoral and cell-mediated deficiency. Immunodeficiency disorders are *primary* if the immune cells are improperly developed or absent and *secondary* if the deficiency is caused by illnesses or treatment. Primary immunodeficiency disorders are rare and often serious, whereas secondary disorders are more common and less severe.

Primary Immunodeficiency Disorders

The basic categories of primary immunodeficiency disorders are (1) phagocytic defects, (2) B cell deficiency, (3) T cell deficiency, and (4) a combined B cell and T cell deficiency (Table 14-14).

Secondary Immunodeficiency Disorders

Some of the important factors that may cause secondary immunodeficiency disorders are listed in Table 14-15. Drug-induced immunosuppression is the most common. Immunosuppressive therapy is prescribed for patients to treat autoimmune disorders and to prevent transplant rejection. In addition, immunosuppression is a serious side effect of drugs used in cancer chemotherapy. Generalized leukopenia often results, leading to a decreased humoral and cell-mediated response. Therefore secondary infections are common in immunosuppressed patients.

TABLE 14-14 PRIMARY IMMUNODEFICIENCY DISORDERS

Disorder	Affected Cells	Genetic Basis
Chronic granulomatous disease	PMNs, monocytes	X-linked
Job syndrome	PMNs, monocytes	—
Bruton's X-linked agammaglobulinemia	B	X-linked
Common variable hypogammaglobulinemia	B	—
Selective IgA, IgM, or IgG deficiency	B	Some X-linked
DiGeorge syndrome (thymic hypoplasia)	T	—
Severe combined immunodeficiency disease	Stem, B, T	X-linked or autosomal recessive
Ataxia-telangiectasia	B, T	Autosomal recessive
Wiskott-Aldrich syndrome	B, T	X-linked
Graft-versus-host disease	B, T	—

PMNs, Polymorphonuclear neutrophils.

TABLE 14-15 CAUSES OF SECONDARY IMMUNODEFICIENCY

Drug-Induced Immunodeficiency
- Chemotherapy drugs
- Corticosteroids

Age
- Infants
- Older adults

Malnutrition
- Dietary deficiency
- Cachexia

Therapies
- Radiation
- Surgery
- Anesthesia

Diseases or Disorders
- Acquired immunodeficiency syndrome (AIDS)
- Cirrhosis
- Chronic kidney disease
- Diabetes mellitus
- Hodgkin's lymphoma
- Malignancies
- Systemic lupus erythematosus
- Burns
- Trauma
- Severe infection

Stress
- Chronic stress
- Trauma (physical or emotional)

Malnutrition alters cell-mediated immune responses. When protein is deficient over a prolonged period, the thymus gland atrophies and lymphoid tissue decreases. In addition, an increased susceptibility to infections always exists.

Hodgkin's lymphoma greatly impairs the cell-mediated immune response, and patients may die from severe viral or fungal infections. (Hodgkin's lymphoma is discussed in Chapter 31.) Viruses, especially rubella, may cause immunodeficiency by direct cytotoxic damage to lymphoid cells. Systemic infections can place such a demand on the immune system that resistance to a secondary or subsequent infection is impaired.

Radiation can destroy lymphocytes either directly or through depletion of stem cells. As the radiation dose is increased, more bone marrow atrophies, leading to severe pancytopenia and suppression of immune function. Splenectomy in children is especially dangerous and may lead to septicemia simply from respiratory tract infections.

Stress may alter the immune response. This response involves interrelationships among the nervous, endocrine, and immune systems (see Chapter 7).

HUMAN LEUKOCYTE ANTIGEN SYSTEM

The antigens responsible for rejection of genetically unlike tissues are called the *major histocompatibility antigens*. These antigens are products of histocompatibility genes. In humans they are called the **human leukocyte antigen (HLA)** system. The genes for the HLA antigens are linked and occur together on the sixth chromosome. HLAs are present on all nucleated cells and platelets. The HLA system is primarily used in matching organs and tissues for transplantation.

An important characteristic of HLA genes is that they are highly polymorphic (variable). Each HLA locus can have many different possible alleles, and thus many combinations exist. Each person has two alleles for each locus, one inherited from each parent. Both alleles of a locus are expressed independently (i.e., they are codominant). The proteins encoded by certain genes are known as *antigens*. The entire set of A, B, C, D, and DR genes (the HLA genes) located on one chromosome is termed a *haplotype*. A complete set is inherited as a unit (haplotype). One haplotype is inherited from each parent (Fig. 14-10). This means that a person has HLA genes that are one-half identical to those of each parent. The HLA genes have a 25% chance of being identical to the HLA genes of a sibling.

In organ transplantation A, B, and DR are primarily used for compatibility matching. The specific allele at each locus is identified by a number. For example, a person could have an HLA of A2, A6, B7, B27, DR4, and DR7. Currently more than 8000 HLA alleles have been identified for the various HLA genes.[10]

Human Leukocyte Antigen and Disease Associations

The early interest in HLAs was stimulated by the role of HLAs in matching donors and recipients of organ transplants. Since that time the interest in the association between HLAs and disease has grown.

A number of diseases show significant associations with specific HLA alleles. People who have these alleles are much more likely to develop the associated disease than those who do not have the allele. However, the possession of a particular HLA allele does not mean that the person will necessarily develop the associated disease—only that the relative risk is greater than in the general population.

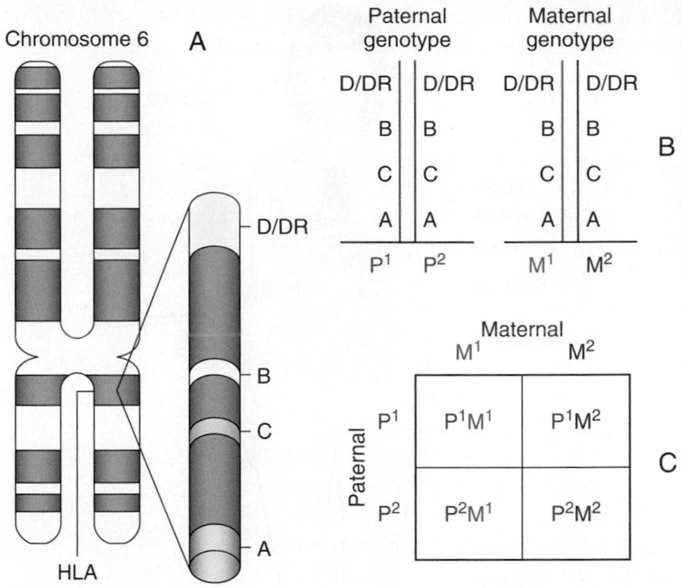

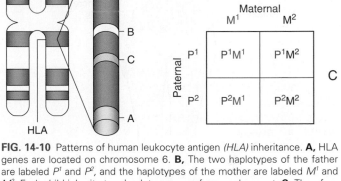

FIG. 14-10 Patterns of human leukocyte antigen *(HLA)* inheritance. **A,** HLA genes are located on chromosome 6. **B,** The two haplotypes of the father are labeled P^1 and P^2, and the haplotypes of the mother are labeled M^1 and M^2. Each child inherits two haplotypes, one from each parent. **C,** Therefore only four combinations—P^1M^1, P^1M^2, P^2M^1, and P^2M^2—are possible, and 25% of the offspring will have identical HLA haplotypes.

Most of the HLA-associated diseases are classified as autoimmune disorders. Examples of HLA types and disease associations include (1) HLA-B27 and ankylosing spondylitis, (2) HLA-DR2 and HLA-DR3 and SLE, (3) HLA-DR3 and HLA-DR4 and diabetes mellitus, and (5) HLA-DR2 and narcolepsy.

The discovery of HLA associations with certain diseases is a major breakthrough in understanding the genetic bases of these diseases. It is now known that at least part of the genetic bases of HLA-associated diseases lies in the HLA region, but the actual mechanisms involved in these associations are still unknown. However, most individuals who inherit a specific HLA type (e.g., HLA-DR3) that is associated with a disease will never develop that disease.

Currently the association between HLAs and certain diseases is of minimal practical clinical importance. Nevertheless, there is promise for the development of clinical applications in the future. For example, with certain autoimmune diseases, it may be possible to identify members of a family at greatest risk for developing the same or a related autoimmune disease. These people would need close medical supervision, implementation of preventive measures (if possible), and early diagnosis and treatment to prevent chronic complications.

ORGAN TRANSPLANTATION

Transplantation success has improved with advances in surgical technique, advances in histocompatibility testing, and more effective immunosuppressants. Common tissue transplants include corneas, skin, bone marrow, heart valves, bone, and connective tissues (Fig. 14-11). Cornea transplants can prevent or correct blindness. Skin grafts are used in managing burn patients. Bone marrow is donated to help patients with leukemias and other malignancies.

Transplanted organs currently come from many different body systems. These organs include the heart, lung, liver, kid-

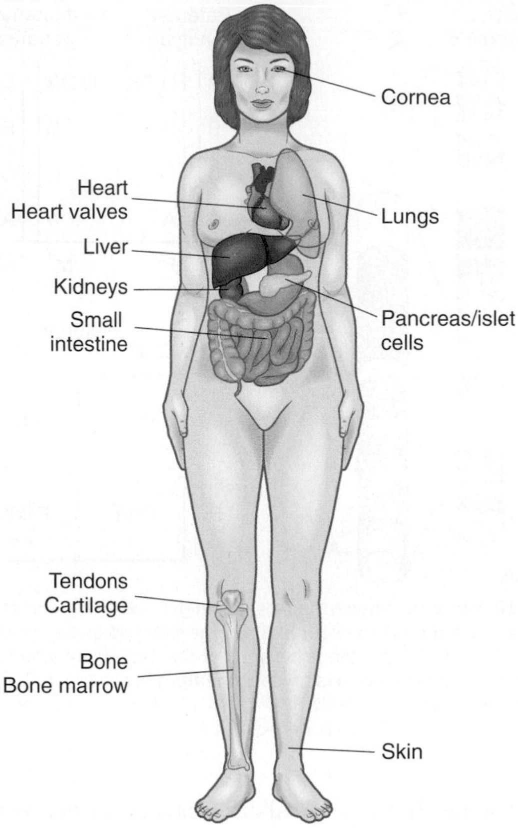

FIG. 14-11 Tissues and organs that can be transplanted.

ney, pancreas, and intestine. Certain organs can be transplanted together, such as kidney and pancreas, kidney and liver, and kidney and heart. For example, many diabetic patients who receive a pancreas transplant also receive a kidney transplant because the diabetes has not only impaired the pancreas, but also led to renal failure.

Some organs can be transplanted in parts or segments instead of transplanting an entire organ. Liver and lung lobes (rather than the whole organ) may be transplanted, or an intestine may be used in segments, thus allowing for one person's organ donation to benefit many recipients. This technique also enables living donors to donate part of an organ (or one of their organs in the case of kidneys).

Organ donations are taken from two sources: deceased (cadaver) and living donors. Most organs and tissues currently come from deceased donors. However, because of the shortage of organs from deceased donors, the use of both related and living unrelated donor organs is increasing.[11]

Individuals can make a decision to become a donor when they sign a donor card, the back of their driver's license, or a donor registry (depending on the state) and indicate their wish to donate organs. However, on their death or imminent death, ultimately the person's legal next of kin must consent to the donation regardless of whether the donor card is signed. That is why it is extremely important for people to notify their next of kin about their willingness to donate organs or tissues at the time of death.

Currently more than 115,000 people are on the organ procurement and transplantation network's national waiting list, which is maintained by the United Network for Organ Sharing (UNOS). However, fewer than 30,000 people receive transplants annually. The organs in highest demand are kidneys, hearts, and livers. These are also the most commonly transplanted organs.[12]

Organ and tissue donations are regulated by the Uniform Anatomical Gift Act to allow for fair and consistent transplantation laws among all states.[13] Patients are matched to available donors based on a number of factors: ABO blood and HLA typing, medical urgency, time on the waiting list, and geographic location.

Tissue Typing

The recipient usually receives a transplant from an ABO blood group–compatible donor (see Table 30-8). The donor and recipient do not need to share the same Rh factor.

HLA Typing. HLA typing is done on potential donors and recipients. Currently only the A, B, and DR antigens are thought to be clinically significant for transplantation. Because each locus has two alleles that encode for antigens, a total of six antigens are identified. In transplantation an attempt is made to match as many antigens as possible between the HLA-A, HLA-B, and HLA-DR loci. Antigen matches of five and six antigens and certain four-antigen matches have been found to have better clinical outcomes (i.e., the patient is less likely to reject the transplanted organ), especially in kidney and bone marrow transplants.

The degree of HLA matching required or deemed suitable for successful solid organ transplantation depends on the type of organ. Certain organ and tissue transplants require a closer histocompatibility match than other organs. For example, a cornea transplant can be accepted by nearly any individual because corneas are avascular and therefore no antibodies reach the cornea to cause rejection. In kidney and bone marrow transplantation, HLA matching is very important, since these transplants are at high risk for graft rejection. On the other hand, for liver transplants, HLA mismatches have little impact on graft survival. For heart and lung transplants, they fall somewhere in between, but minimizing HLA mismatches significantly improves survival. In addition, for liver, lung, and heart transplants, few donors are available and it is difficult to get good HLA matches.

Transporting and storing donated organs can take time. The "best" match may live many miles from the "ideal" recipient. The need to have the "best" matches has to be balanced against the time it takes to harvest and transport a donated organ and then transplant it.

Panel of Reactive Antibodies. A *panel of reactive antibodies (PRA)* indicates the recipient's sensitivity to various HLAs before receiving a transplant. To detect preformed antibodies to HLA, the recipient's serum is mixed with a randomly selected panel of donor lymphocytes to determine reactivity. The potential recipient may have been exposed to HLA antigens by means of previous blood transfusions, pregnancy, or a previous organ transplant.

For the PRA, the results are calculated in percentages. A high PRA indicates that the person has a large number of cytotoxic antibodies and is highly sensitized, which means there is a poor chance of finding a crossmatch-negative donor. In patients awaiting transplantation, a PRA panel is usually done on a regular basis. Plasmapheresis and IV immune globulin have been used to lower the number of preformed HLA antibodies in highly sensitized patients.

Crossmatch. A *crossmatch* uses serum from the recipient mixed with donor lymphocytes to test for any preformed anti-

HLA antibodies to the potential donor organ. The crossmatch can be used as a screening test when multiple possible living donors are being considered or once a cadaver donor is selected. A final crossmatch is done just before transplant.

A positive crossmatch indicates that the recipient has cytotoxic antibodies to the donor and is an absolute contraindication to transplantation. If transplanted, the organ would undergo hyperacute rejection. A negative crossmatch indicates that no preformed antibodies are present and it is safe to proceed with transplantation. Crossmatching, which is especially important for kidney transplants, may not be done for lung, liver, and heart transplants.

Transplant Rejection

Rejection is one of the major problems following organ transplantation. Rejection of organs occurs as a normal immune response to foreign tissue. The rejection can be prevented by using immunosuppression therapy, performing ABO and HLA matching, and ensuring that the crossmatch is negative. Unfortunately, many different HLAs exist, and a perfect match is nearly impossible unless the tissue is from oneself, an identical twin, or in some cases a sibling. Rejection can be hyperacute, acute, or chronic. Prevention, early diagnosis, and treatment of rejection are essential for long-term graft function.

Hyperacute Rejection. *Hyperacute rejection* occurs minutes to hours after transplantation because the blood vessels are rapidly destroyed. It occurs because the person had preexisting antibodies against the transplanted tissue or organ. There is no treatment for hyperacute rejection, and the transplanted organ is removed.

Fortunately hyperacute rejection is a rare event because the final crossmatch just before transplant usually determines whether the recipient is sensitized to any of the donor HLAs. On occasion, for unclear reasons, the final crossmatch does not detect these preformed antibodies, and hyperacute rejection occurs.

Acute Rejection. *Acute rejection* most commonly manifests in the first 6 months after transplantation. This type of rejection is usually mediated by the recipient's lymphocytes, which have been activated against the donated (foreign) tissue or organ (Fig. 14-12). In addition to cell-mediated rejection, another type of acute rejection occurs when the recipient develops antibodies to the transplanted organ.

It is not uncommon to have at least one rejection episode, especially with organs from deceased donors. These episodes are usually reversible with additional immunosuppressive therapy, which may include increased corticosteroid doses or polyclonal or monoclonal antibodies. Unfortunately, immunosuppressants increase the risk for infection. To combat acute rejection, all patients with transplants require long-term use of immunosuppressants, putting them at a high risk for infection, especially in the first few months after transplant when the immunosuppressive doses are highest.

Chronic Rejection. *Chronic rejection* is a process that occurs over months or years and is irreversible. Chronic rejection can occur for unknown reasons or from repeated episodes of acute rejection. The transplanted organ is infiltrated with large numbers of T and B cells characteristic of an ongoing, low-grade, immune-mediated injury. Chronic rejection results in fibrosis and scarring. In heart transplants it manifests as accelerated coronary artery disease. In lung transplants it manifests as bronchiolitis obliterans. In liver transplants it is characterized by loss of bile ducts. In kidney transplants it manifests as fibrosis and glomerulopathy.

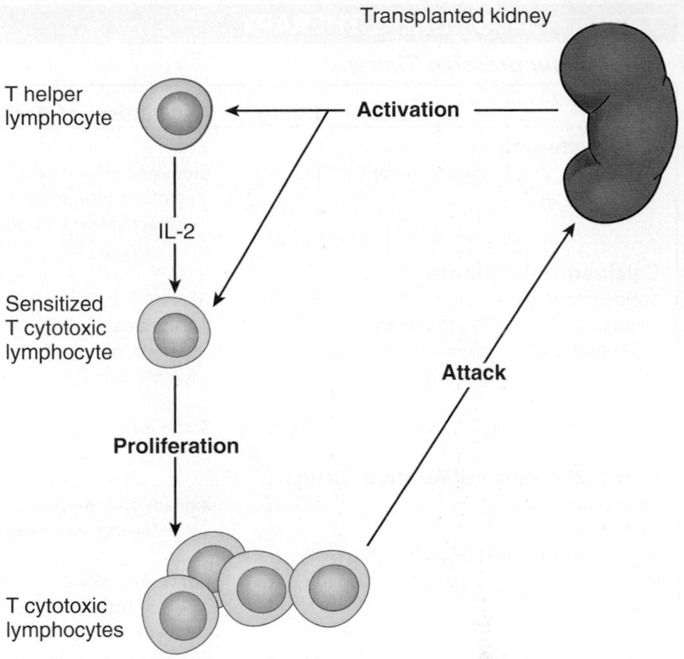

FIG. 14-12 Mechanism of action of T cytotoxic lymphocyte activation and attack of transplanted tissue. The transplanted organ (e.g., kidney) is recognized as foreign and activates the immune system. T helper cells are activated to produce interleukin-2 *(IL-2)*, and T cytotoxic lymphocytes are sensitized. After the T cytotoxic cells proliferate, they attack the transplanted organ.

There is no definitive therapy for this type of rejection. Treatment is primarily supportive. This type of rejection is difficult to manage and is not associated with the optimistic prognosis of acute rejection.

Immunosuppressive Therapy

Immunosuppressive therapy requires a balance. On one hand, the immune response needs to be suppressed to prevent rejection of the transplanted organ. On the other hand, an adequate immune response needs to be maintained to prevent overwhelming infection and the development of malignancies.[14]

Many of the drugs used to achieve immunosuppression have significant side effects. Because transplant recipients must take immunosuppressants for life, the risk of toxicity continues for the rest of their lives.[15]

Immunosuppressant drugs are listed in Table 14-16. With use of a combination of agents that work during different phases of the immune response (Fig. 14-13), lower doses of each drug can be given to produce effective immunosuppression while minimizing side effects.

The major immunosuppressive agents are (1) calcineurin inhibitors, including cyclosporine (Sandimmune, Neoral, Gengraf) and tacrolimus (Prograf, FK506); (2) corticosteroids (prednisone, methylprednisolone [Solu-Medrol] IV); (3) mycophenolate mofetil (CellCept); and (4) sirolimus (Rapamune). Azathioprine (Imuran) and cyclophosphamide (Cytoxan) can also be used. Antilymphocyte globulin (ALG) and muromonab-CD3 (Orthoclone OKT3) are IV medications used for short periods to prevent early rejection or reverse acute rejection.

Immunosuppression protocols are highly variable among transplant centers, with different combinations of medications

TABLE 14-16 **DRUG THERAPY**

Immunosuppressive Therapy

Agent	Route	Mechanism of Action	Side Effects
Corticosteroids			
prednisone, methylprednisolone (Solu-Medrol)	PO, IV	Suppress inflammatory response. Inhibit cytokine production (IL-1, IL-6, TNF) and T cell activation and proliferation.	Peptic ulcers, hypertension, osteoporosis, Na^+ and H_2O retention, muscle weakness, easy bruising, delayed healing, hyperglycemia, ↑ risk for infection.
Calcineurin Inhibitors			
cyclosporine (Sandimmune,* Neoral,* Gengraf*) (Neoral and Gengraf are microemulsions with better absorption than Sandimmune.)	PO, IV	Acts on T helper cells to prevent production and release of IL-2 and γ-interferon. Inhibits production of T cytotoxic lymphocytes and B cells.	Nephrotoxicity, ↑ risk for infection, neurotoxicity (tremors, seizures), hepatotoxicity, lymphoma, hypertension, tremors, hirsutism, leukopenia, gingival hyperplasia.
tacrolimus (Prograf, FK506)	PO, IV	Same as cyclosporine but more effective.	Same as cyclosporine.
Cytotoxic (Antiproliferative) Drugs			
mycophenolate mofetil (CellCept) mycophenolate acid (Myfortic)	PO, IV	Inhibits purine synthesis. Suppresses proliferation of T and B cells.	Diarrhea, nausea and vomiting, severe neutropenia, thrombocytopenia, ↑ risk for infection, ↑ incidence of malignancies.
cyclophosphamide (Cytoxan, Neosar)	PO, IV	Cross-links DNA, leading to cell injury and death. Results in decrease in number and activity of T and B cells.	Neutropenia, hemorrhagic cystitis.
azathioprine (Imuran)	PO, IV	Blocks purine synthesis. Suppresses cell-mediated and humoral immune responses by inhibiting proliferation of T and B cells.	Bone marrow suppression: neutropenia, anemia, thrombocytopenia.
sirolimus (Rapamune)	PO	Binds to mammalian target of rapamycin (mTOR), thereby suppressing T cell activation and proliferation.	↑ Risk for infection, leukopenia, anemia, thrombocytopenia, hyperlipidemia, hypercholesterolemia, arthralgias, diarrhea. ↑ incidence of malignancies. Not used in liver and lung transplants.
everolimus (Zortress)	PO	Same as above	Peripheral edema, constipation, hypertension, nausea, anemia, urinary tract infection, hyperlipidemia.
Monoclonal Antibodies			
muromonab-CD3 (Orthoclone OKT3)	IV push	Monoclonal antibody that binds to CD3 receptors on T cells, causing cell lysis. Inhibits function of cytotoxic T cells.	Fever, chills, dyspnea, chest pain, nausea and vomiting. Anaphylactic reactions include pulmonary edema, cardiac or respiratory arrest.
daclizumab (Zenapax)	IV	Monoclonal antibody that acts as IL-2 receptor antagonist by inhibiting the binding of IL-2. Inhibits T cell activation and proliferation.	Can cause acute hypersensitivity reaction, including anaphylaxis.
basiliximab (Simulect)	IV	Same as daclizumab.	Same as daclizumab.
Polyclonal Antibody			
Lymphocyte immune globulin (Atgam)	IV	Prepared by immunizing horse with human T cells. Polyclonal antibodies directed against T cells, thus depleting them.	Serum sickness (fever, chills, muscle and joint pain), tachycardia, back pain, shortness of breath, hypotension, anaphylaxis, leukopenia, thrombocytopenia, rash, ↑ risk for infection.
Other			
belatacept (Nulojix)	IV	Prevents the activation of T cells.	Anemia, constipation, urinary tract infection, peripheral edema.

*Not bioequivalent and cannot be interchanged.
IL, Interleukin; *TNF,* tumor necrosis factor.

being used. Most patients are initially on triple therapy. The standard triple therapy usually includes a calcineurin inhibitor, a corticosteroid, and mycophenolate mofetil.

The doses of immunosuppressant drugs are reduced over time after the transplant. Patients taking corticosteroids may be weaned off after a few years. The trend in many transplant centers is to use immunosuppression protocols that do not contain corticosteroids because of their many side effects.

Calcineurin Inhibitors. This group of drugs, including tacrolimus and cyclosporine, is the foundation of most immunosuppression regimens. As the most effective immunosuppressants, these drugs prevent a cell-mediated attack against the transplanted organ (see Fig. 14-13). These drugs do not cause bone marrow suppression or alterations of the normal inflammatory response. They are generally used in combination with corticosteroids, mycophenolate mofetil, and sirolimus. Tacrolimus is the most widely used calcineurin inhibitor.[15]

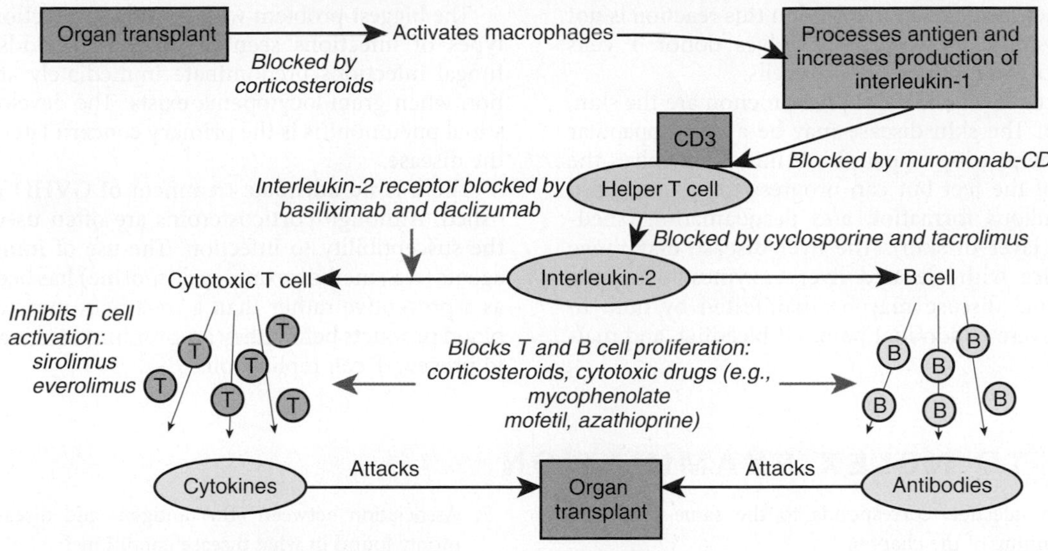

FIG. 14-13 Sites of action for immunosuppressive agents.

Many of the side effects of calcineurin inhibitors are dose related. These drugs are potentially nephrotoxic. Drug levels are monitored closely to prevent toxicity.

DRUG ALERT: Tacrolimus and Cyclosporine

- A substance in grapefruit and grapefruit juice prevents metabolism of these drugs.
- Consuming grapefruit or grapefruit juice while using these drugs could increase their toxicity.

Sirolimus. Sirolimus is an immunosuppressive agent approved for use in renal transplant recipients. It is used in combination with corticosteroids and cyclosporine. It is also used in combination with tacrolimus.

Mycophenolate Mofetil. Mycophenolate mofetil is a lymphocyte-specific inhibitor of purine synthesis with suppressive effects on both T and B lymphocytes. This drug appears to be most effective when used in combination with tacrolimus or cyclosporine. Its effects are additive because it acts later in the lymphocyte activation pathway by a different mechanism. It has also been shown to decrease the incidence of late graft loss. The major limitation of this drug is its GI toxicities, including nausea, vomiting, and diarrhea. In many cases the side effects can be diminished by lowering the dose or giving smaller doses more frequently.

DRUG ALERT: Mycophenolate Mofetil

- When given IV, it must be reconstituted in D_5W and no other solution.
- Do not give as IV bolus. Give over 2 or more hours.

Monoclonal Antibodies. Monoclonal antibodies are used for preventing and treating acute rejection episodes. (eFig. 14-2, showing how monoclonal antibodies are made, is available on the website for this chapter.) Muromonab-CD3 was the first of these monoclonal antibodies to be used in clinical transplantation. It is a mouse monoclonal antibody that binds with the CD3 antigen found on the surface of human thymocytes and mature T cells. It is an anti-antigen receptor antibody that interferes with the function of the T lymphocyte, the pivotal cell in the response to graft rejection. It is administered via IV bolus. All T cells are affected, rather than just the subset active in graft rejection. Within minutes after the initial infusion of muromonab-CD3, the number of circulating T cells decreases significantly.

A flulike syndrome occurs during the first few days of treatment because of cytokine release. Side effects include fever, rigors, headache, myalgias, and various GI disturbances. To reduce the expected side effects of muromonab-CD3, give patients acetaminophen (Tylenol), diphenhydramine (Benadryl), and IV methylprednisolone before administering the dose.

Newer generation monoclonal antibodies include daclizumab (Zenapax) and basiliximab (Simulect). These monoclonal antibodies are a hybrid of mouse and human antibodies and have fewer side effects than muromonab-CD3 because they have been "humanized."

Polyclonal Antibody. Lymphocyte immune globulin (Atgam) is used as induction therapy or to treat acute rejection. The purpose of induction therapy is to severely immunosuppress an individual immediately after transplantation to prevent early rejection. The drug is made by immunizing horses with human lymphocytes. The antibody made against the human lymphocytes is then purified and administered IV.

Allergic reactions to the foreign proteins from the host animal, manifested by fever, arthralgias, and tachycardia, are common but usually not severe enough to preclude use. These side effects can be attenuated by administering the preparation slowly, over 4 to 6 hours, and premedicating patients with acetaminophen, diphenhydramine, and methylprednisolone. The main toxicities of polyclonal antibodies are lymphopenia and thrombocytopenia caused by antibody contaminants that are not completely removed during preparation of the antibodies.

GRAFT-VERSUS-HOST DISEASE

Graft-versus-host disease (GVHD) occurs when an immunoincompetent (immunodeficient) patient receives immunocompetent cells.[16] A GVHD response may result from the infusion of any blood product containing viable lymphocytes, as in therapeutic blood transfusions, and from the transplantation of fetal thymus, fetal liver, or bone marrow. In most transplantation situations the biggest concern is the patient's (host's) rejection of the organ or transplant. However, in GVHD disease, the graft (donated tissue) rejects the host (recipient) tissue.

The GVHD response may begin 7 to 30 days after transplantation. Once the reaction is started, little can be done to modify its course. The exact mechanism involved in this reaction is not completely understood. However, it involves donor T cells attacking and destroying vulnerable host cells.

The target organs for the GVHD phenomenon are the skin, liver, and GI tract. The skin disease may be a maculopapular rash, which may be pruritic or painful. It initially involves the palms and soles of the feet but can progress to a generalized erythema with bullous formation and desquamation (shedding of the outer layer of skin). The liver disease may range from mild jaundice with elevated liver enzymes to hepatic coma. The intestinal disease may be manifested by mild to severe diarrhea, severe abdominal pain, GI bleeding, and malabsorption.

The biggest problem with GVHD is infection, with different types of infections seen in different periods. Bacterial and fungal infections predominate immediately after transplantation when granulocytopenia exists. The development of interstitial pneumonitis is the primary concern later in the course of the disease.

There is no adequate treatment of GVHD once it is established. Although corticosteroids are often used, they enhance the susceptibility to infection. The use of immunosuppressive agents (e.g., methotrexate, cyclosporine) has been most effective as a preventive rather than a treatment measure. Radiation of blood products before they are administered is another measure to prevent T cell replication.

BRIDGE TO NCLEX EXAMINATION

The number of the question corresponds to the same-numbered outcome at the beginning of the chapter.

1. The function of monocytes in immunity is related to their ability to
   - a. stimulate the production of T and B lymphocytes.
   - b. produce antibodies on exposure to foreign substances.
   - c. bind antigens and stimulate natural killer cell activation.
   - d. capture antigens by phagocytosis and present them to lymphocytes.
2. One function of cell-mediated immunity is
   - a. formation of antibodies.
   - b. activation of the complement system.
   - c. surveillance for malignant cell changes.
   - d. opsonization of antigens to allow phagocytosis by neutrophils.
3. The reason newborns are protected for the first 6 months of life from bacterial infections is because of the maternal transmission of
   - a. IgG.
   - b. IgA.
   - c. IgM.
   - d. IgE.
4. In a type I hypersensitivity reaction the primary immunologic disorder appears to be
   - a. binding of IgG to an antigen on a cell surface.
   - b. deposit of antigen-antibody complexes in small vessels.
   - c. release of cytokines used to interact with specific antigens.
   - d. release of chemical mediators from IgE-bound mast cells and basophils.
5. The nurse is alerted to possible anaphylactic shock immediately after a patient has received intramuscular penicillin by the development of
   - a. edema and itching at the injection site.
   - b. sneezing and itching of the nose and eyes.
   - c. a wheal-and-flare reaction at the injection site.
   - d. chest tightness and production of thick sputum.
6. The nurse advises a friend who asks him to administer his allergy shots that
   - a. it is illegal for nurses to administer injections outside of a medical setting.
   - b. he is qualified to do it if the friend has epinephrine in an injectable syringe provided with his extract.
   - c. avoiding the allergens is a more effective way of controlling allergies, and allergy shots are not usually effective.
   - d. immunotherapy should only be administered in a setting where emergency equipment and drugs are available.
7. Association between HLA antigens and diseases is most commonly found in what disease conditions?
   - a. Malignancies
   - b. Infectious diseases
   - c. Neurologic diseases
   - d. Autoimmune disorders
8. A patient is undergoing plasmapheresis for treatment of systemic lupus erythematosus. The nurse explains that plasmapheresis is used in her treatment to
   - a. remove T lymphocytes in her blood that are producing antinuclear antibodies.
   - b. remove normal particles in her blood that are being damaged by autoantibodies.
   - c. exchange her plasma that contains antinuclear antibodies with a substitute fluid.
   - d. replace viral-damaged cellular components of her blood with replacement whole blood.
9. The most common cause of secondary immunodeficiencies is
   - a. drugs.
   - b. stress.
   - c. malnutrition.
   - d. human immunodeficiency virus.
10. What accurately describes rejection following transplantation?
    - a. Hyperacute rejection can be treated with OKT3.
    - b. Acute rejection can be treated with sirolimus or tacrolimus.
    - c. Chronic rejection can be treated with tacrolimus or cyclosporine.
    - d. Hyperacute reaction can usually be avoided if crossmatching is done before the transplantation.
11. In a person having an acute rejection of a transplanted kidney, what would help the nurse understand the course of events *(select all that apply)*?
    - a. A new transplant should be considered.
    - b. Acute rejection can be treated with OKT3.
    - c. Acute rejection usually leads to chronic rejection.
    - d. Corticosteroids are the most successful drugs used to treat acute rejection.
    - e. Acute rejection is common after a transplant and can be treated with drug therapy.

1. d, 2. c, 3. a, 4. d, 5. a, 6. d, 7. d, 8. c, 9. a, 10. d, 11. b, e

evolve

For rationales to these answers and even more NCLEX review questions, visit *http://evolve.elsevier.com/Lewis/medsurg.*

REFERENCES

1. Kaufman C: The secret lives of lymphocytes, *Nursing* 41:50, 2011.
2. Abbas A, Lichtman A, Pillai S: *Cellular and molecular immunology*, ed 7, Philadelphia, 2012, Saunders.
3. Frati F, Incorvaia C, Lombardi C, et al: Allergen immunotherapy: 100 years, but it does not look like, *Eur Ann Allergy Clin Immunol* 44(3):99, 2012.
4. Mota AN, Turrini RN: Perioperative latex hypersensitivity reactions: an integrative literature review, *Rev Lat Am Enfermagem* 20(2):411, 2012.
5. Wade J: Care of the type 1 latex allergy patient, *Aust Nurs J* 19(9):30, 2012.
6. American Academy of Allergy, Asthma, and Immunology: Latex allergies: tips to remember. Retrieved from *www.aaaai.org/conditions-and-treatments/Library/At-a-Glance/Latex-Allergy.aspx*.
7. Multiple chemical sensitivity. Retrieved from *www.webmd.com/allergies/multiple-chemical-sensitivity*.
8. National Institute of Environmental Health Sciences: Allergies/multiple chemical sensitivity. Retrieved from *www.niehs.nih.gov/research/resources/library/consumer/conditions*.
9. National Institute of Diabetes and Digestive and Kidney Diseases: Autoimmunity and viral etiology of type 1 diabetes. Retrieved from *www2.niddk.nih.gov/Research/ScientificAreas/Diabetes/Type1Diabetes*.
10. HLA nomenclature. Retrieved from *www.hla.alleles.org/alleles/index.html*.
11. Lennerling A, Forsberg A: Donors self-reported experiences of live kidney donation: a prospective study, *J Ren Care* 38(4):207, 2012.
12. United Network of Organ Sharing (UNOS). Retrieved from *www.unos.org*.
13. Uniform Anatomical Gift Act. Retrieved from *http://uniformlaws.org/ActSummary.aspx?title=Anatomical%20Gift%20Act%20 (2006)*.
14. Engels EA, Pfeiffer RM, Fraumeni JF, et al: Spectrum of cancer risk among US solid organ transplant recipients, *JAMA* 306:1891, 2011.
15. Schroeder KS: Pharmacology of immunosuppressive medications in solid organ transplantation. In Lovasik D: Transplant, *Crit Care Nurs Clin North Am* 23:405, 2011.
16. Blazar BR, Murphy WJ, Abedi M: Advances in graft-versus-host disease biology and therapy, *Nat Rev Immunol* 12(6):443, 2012.

RESOURCE

National Institute of Allergy and Infectious Diseases (NIAID)
www.niaid.nih.gov

CHAPTER

15

Thought is an infection. In the case of certain thoughts, it becomes an epidemic.
Wallace Stevens

Infection and Human Immunodeficiency Virus Infection

Jeffrey Kwong and Lucy Bradley-Springer

evolve WEBSITE

http://evolve.elsevier.com/Lewis/medsurg

- NCLEX Review Questions
- Key Points
- Pre-Test
- Answer Guidelines for Case Study on p. 244
- Rationales for Bridge to NCLEX Examination Questions
- Case Study
  - Patient With Human Immunodeficiency Virus (HIV) Infection and Acquired Immunodeficiency Syndrome (AIDS)
- Concept Map Creator
- Glossary
- Content Updates

eTables

- eTable 15-1: Centers for Disease Control and Prevention (CDC) Guidelines for Isolation Precautions
- eTable 15-2: Treatment of Common Opportunistic Diseases Associated With HIV Infection
- eTable 15-3: Drug Therapy: Side Effects of Antiretroviral Agents Used in Human Immunodeficiency Virus (HIV) Infection
- eTable 15-4: Patient Teaching Guide: Proper Use and Placement of Male Condom
- eTable 15-5: Patient Teaching Guide: Proper Use and Placement of Female Condom
- eTable 15-6: Patient Teaching Guide: Proper Use of Drug-Using Equipment
- eTable 15-7: Nursing Interventions in HIV Infection

LEARNING OUTCOMES

1. Evaluate the impact of emerging and reemerging infections on health care.
2. Identify ways to decrease the development of resistance to antibiotics.
3. Explain the ways human immunodeficiency virus (HIV) is transmitted and the factors that affect transmission.
4. Describe the pathophysiology of HIV infection.
5. Chart the spectrum of untreated HIV infection.
6. Identify the diagnostic criteria for acquired immunodeficiency syndrome (AIDS).
7. Describe methods used to test for HIV infection.
8. Discuss the collaborative management of HIV infection.
9. Summarize the characteristics of opportunistic diseases associated with AIDS.
10. Describe the potential complications associated with long-term treatment of HIV infection.
11. Compare and contrast HIV prevention methods.
12. Describe the nursing management of HIV-infected patients and HIV-at-risk patients.

KEY TERMS

acquired immunodeficiency syndrome (AIDS), p. 234
antiretroviral therapy (ART), p. 237
emerging infection, p. 228
human immunodeficiency virus (HIV), p. 231
integrase, p. 232
opportunistic diseases, p. 233
postexposure prophylaxis (PEP), p. 241
protease, p. 232
retroviruses, p. 232
reverse transcriptase, p. 232
seroconversion, p. 234
viral load, p. 234
viremia, p. 232
window period, p. 235

This chapter presents a brief overview of infections (both emerging and health care–associated infections). In addition, this chapter provides a comprehensive discussion of human immunodeficiency (HIV) infection focusing on transmission, pathophysiology, collaborative care, and nursing management.

INFECTIONS

Infections, such as lower respiratory tract infections, malaria, HIV, and tuberculosis (TB), are responsible for a significant number of deaths worldwide.[1] Infection occurs when a *pathogen* (a microorganism that causes disease) invades the body, begins to multiply, and produces disease, usually causing harm to the host. The signs and symptoms of infection are a result of specific pathogen activity, which triggers inflammation and other immune responses.[2]

Infections can be divided into localized, disseminated, and systemic disease. A *localized* infection is limited to a small area. A *disseminated* infection has spread to areas of the body beyond the initial site of infection. *Systemic* infections have spread extensively throughout the body, often via the blood.

Reviewed by Danette Y. Wall, ACRN, MSN, MBA/HCM, ISO9001 Lead Auditor, Regional Nurse, Department of Veterans Affairs–Veterans Health Administration, Tampa, Florida.

TYPES OF PATHOGENS

The many different kinds of pathogens can be classified into several groups, including bacteria, viruses, fungi, protozoa, and prions.[3] *Bacteria* are one-celled organisms that are common throughout nature. Many bacteria are normal flora. They live harmoniously in or on the human body without causing disease under normal circumstances. Normal flora protect the human body by preventing the overgrowth of other microorganisms. For example, *Escherichia coli* is a bacteria that is part of the normal flora in the large intestine.

Bacteria cause disease in two ways: by entering the body and growing inside human cells (e.g., TB) or by secreting toxins that damage cells (e.g., *Staphylococcus aureus*). Bacteria are divided into categories based on the shape of their cells. *Cocci*, such as streptococci and staphylococci, are round. *Bacilli* are rod shaped and include tetanus and TB. *Curved rods* include *Vibrio* bacteria, one of which causes cholera. *Spirochetes* are spiral shaped and include the organisms that cause leprosy and syphilis. Table 15-1 lists common pathogenic bacteria and the diseases that they cause.

Viruses, unlike bacteria, do not have a cellular structure. They are simple infectious particles that consist of a small amount of genetic material (either ribonucleic acid [RNA] or deoxyribonucleic acid [DNA]) and a protein envelope. Viruses can reproduce only after releasing their genetic material into the cell of another living organism. Examples of diseases caused by viruses are shown in Table 15-2.

Fungi are organisms similar to plants, but they lack chlorophyll. *Mycosis* is any disease caused by a fungus. Pathogenic fungi cause infections that are usually localized but can become disseminated in an immunocompromised person. Tinea pedis

TABLE 15-1 DISEASE-CAUSING BACTERIA

Bacteria	Diseases Caused
Clostridia	
• *Clostridium botulinum*	Food poisoning with progressive muscle paralysis
• *Clostridium tetani*	Tetanus (lockjaw)
Corynebacterium diphtheriae	Diphtheria
Escherichia coli	Urinary tract infections, peritonitis, hemolytic-uremic syndrome
Haemophilus	
• *Haemophilus influenzae*	Nasopharyngitis, meningitis, pneumonia
• *Haemophilus pertussis*	Pertussis (whooping cough)
Helicobacter pylori	Peptic ulcers, gastritis
Klebsiella-Enterobacter organisms	Urinary tract infections, peritonitis, pneumonia
Legionella pneumophila	Pneumonia (Legionnaires' disease)
Mycobacteria	
• *Mycobacterium leprae*	Hansen's disease (leprosy)
• *Mycobacterium tuberculosis*	Tuberculosis
Neisseriae	
• *Neisseria gonorrhoeae*	Gonorrhea, pelvic inflammatory disease
• *Neisseria meningitidis*	Meningococcemia, meningitis
Proteus species	Urinary tract infections, peritonitis
Pseudomonas aeruginosa	Urinary tract infections, meningitis
Salmonella	
• *Salmonella typhi*	Typhoid fever
• Other *Salmonella* organisms	Food poisoning, gastroenteritis
Shigella	Shigellosis; diarrhea, abdominal pain, and fever (dysentery)
Staphylococcus aureus	Skin infections, pneumonia, urinary tract infections, acute osteomyelitis, toxic shock syndrome
Streptococci	
• *Streptococcus faecalis*	Genitourinary infection, infection of surgical wounds
• *Streptococcus pneumoniae*	Pneumococcal pneumonia
• *Streptococcus pyogenes* (group A β-hemolytic streptococci)	Pharyngitis, scarlet fever, rheumatic fever, acute glomerulonephritis, erysipelas, pneumonia
• *S. pyogenes* (group B β-hemolytic streptococci)	Urinary tract infections
• *Streptococcus viridans*	Bacterial endocarditis
Treponema pallidum	Syphilis

TABLE 15-2 DISEASE-CAUSING VIRUSES

Virus	Diseases Caused
Adenoviruses	Upper respiratory tract infection, pneumonia
Arbovirus	Syndrome of fever, malaise, headache, myalgia; aseptic meningitis; encephalitis
Coronavirus	Upper respiratory tract infection
Coxsackieviruses A and B	Upper respiratory tract infection, gastroenteritis, acute myocarditis, aseptic meningitis
Echoviruses	Upper respiratory tract infection, gastroenteritis, aseptic meningitis
Hepatitis A, B, C	Viral hepatitis
Herpesviruses	
• Cytomegalovirus (CMV)	Gastroenteritis; pneumonia and retinal damage in immunosuppressed individuals, infectious mononucleosis–like syndrome
• Epstein-Barr	Mononucleosis, Burkitt's lymphoma (possibly)
• Herpes simplex type 1	Herpes labialis ("fever blisters"), genital herpes infection
• Herpes simplex type 2	Genital herpes infection
• Varicella-zoster	Chickenpox, shingles
Human immunodeficiency virus (HIV)	HIV infection, AIDS
Influenza A and B	Upper respiratory tract infection, H1N1 (swine) flu, avian (bird) flu
Mumps	Parotitis, orchitis in postpubertal males
Papillomavirus	Warts
Parainfluenza 1-4	Upper respiratory tract infection
Parvovirus	Gastroenteritis
Poliovirus	Poliomyelitis
Pox viruses	Smallpox
Reoviruses 1, 2, 3	Upper respiratory tract infection
Respiratory syncytial virus	Gastroenteritis, respiratory tract infection
Rhabdovirus	Rabies
Rhinovirus	Upper respiratory tract infection, pneumonia
Rotaviruses	Gastroenteritis
Rubella	German measles
Rubeola	Measles
West Nile virus	Flulike symptoms, meningitis, encephalitis

TABLE 15-3 DISEASE-CAUSING FUNGI

Fungi	Diseases Caused	Organs Affected
Aspergillus fumigatus	Aspergillosis Otomycosis	Lungs* Ears
Blastomyces dermatitidis	Blastomycosis	Lungs, various organs
Candida albicans	Candidiasis Vaginitis Thrush	Intestines Vagina Skin,† mouth
Coccidioides immitis	Coccidioidomycosis	Lungs*
Pneumocystis jiroveci	Pneumocystis pneumonia (PCP)	Lungs*
Sporothrix schenckii	Sporotrichosis	Skin, lymph vessels
Trichophyton	Tinea pedis	Skin†
Microsporum	Tinea capitis	Skin†
Epidermophyton	Tinea corporis	Skin†

*See Table 28-14: Fungal Infections of the Lung.
†See Table 24-6: Common Fungal Infections of the Skin.

(athlete's foot) and tinea corporis (ringworm) are two common mycotic infections. Some fungi are normal flora in the body, but when overgrowth occurs, disease can result. Overgrowth of *Candida albicans,* for example, can cause candidiasis in the mouth (thrush), esophagus, intestines, and vagina. Other fungi and their respective mycotic infections are listed in Table 15-3.

Protozoa are single-cell, animal-like microorganisms. Protozoa normally live in soil and bodies of water. When introduced into the human body, they can cause infection. Amebic dysentery and giardiasis are caused by protozoal parasites. Malaria is caused by a sporozoa called *Plasmodium malariae.*

Prions are infectious particles that contain abnormally shaped proteins. Not all prions cause disease, but those that do typically affect the nervous system. They can cause a group of illnesses called transmissible spongiform encephalopathies (TSEs). Some of the more common TSEs are Creutzfeldt-Jakob disease and bovine spongiform encephalopathy in cattle (also known as mad cow disease).[4]

EMERGING INFECTIONS

An **emerging infection** is an infectious disease that has recently increased in incidence or that threatens to increase in the immediate future. Examples of emerging infections are described in Table 15-4. Emerging infectious diseases can originate from unknown sources or from contact with animals, changes in known diseases, or biologic warfare. For example, severe acute respiratory syndrome (SARS) and the West Nile virus come from animal sources. Others emerged when a previously treatable organism (e.g., *S. aureus*) developed resistance to antibiotics.

The battle against infection is not new, but modern technologies have changed the rules of the game. Global travel, population density, encroachment into new environments, misuse of antibiotics, and bioterrorism have increased the risk for widespread distribution of emerging infections.[5]

Not too long ago many believed that science had conquered infectious disease. However, newly recognized infectious diseases have emerged in recent decades. These include HIV, Lyme disease, hepatitis C, SARS, Ebola virus, and influenza A (H1N1) virus. Some diseases once thought to be under control, such as TB, measles, and pertussis, have reemerged.[6]

TABLE 15-4 EMERGING INFECTIONS

Microorganism	Related Disease
Bacteria	
Borrelia burgdorferi	Lyme disease
Campylobacter jejuni	Diarrhea
Escherichia coli O157:H7	Hemorrhagic colitis, hemolytic-uremic syndrome
Helicobacter pylori	Peptic ulcer disease
Legionella pneumophila	Pneumonia (Legionnaires' disease)
Vibrio cholerae 0139	New strain associated with epidemic cholera
Virus	
Ebola virus	Ebola hemorrhagic fever
H1N1	H1N1 (swine) flu
Hantavirus	Hemorrhagic fever associated with severe pulmonary syndrome
Hepatitis C virus	Parenterally transmitted hepatitis
Hepatitis E virus	Enterically transmitted hepatitis
Human immunodeficiency virus (HIV)	HIV infection and AIDS
Human herpesvirus 6 (HHV-6)	Roseola subitum
Human herpesvirus 8 (HHV-8)	Associated with Kaposi sarcoma in immunosuppressed patients, including people with HIV infection
West Nile virus	West Nile fever
Parasite	
Cryptosporidium parvum	Acute and chronic diarrhea

Studies in *zoonosis* (the science of transmission of diseases from animals to humans) have shown that many known infectious diseases come from animal and insect vectors. The SARS outbreak in China in 2003, for instance, was linked to the civet cat, a small carnivorous mammal found throughout much of Asia and Africa. (SARS is discussed in Chapter 68.)

West Nile virus is carried and transmitted by mosquitoes. Mosquitoes acquire the virus as they draw blood from infected animals and people. The virus does not cause illness in the mosquito, but can be transferred to uninfected animals and humans as the mosquito continues to feed. Bird deaths are an early warning sign of a West Nile virus outbreak, which can spread quickly if action is not taken in a timely manner. (West Nile virus is discussed in Chapter 57.)

Influenza viruses are examples of how disease can spread between animals and humans. Variants of influenza A viruses were responsible for influenza epidemics. These include the 2009 influenza A (H1N1) outbreak that was traced back to pigs, hence the name *swine flu.* In 1997 and 2003 outbreaks of the influenza A (H5N1) strain of avian flu resulted from transmission of influenza virus from chickens to humans.[7]

Ebola virus has presented an ongoing challenge to public health since it was first seen in 1976. Ebola virus causes severe hemorrhagic fever and is usually lethal. Therapeutic and preventive measures are extremely limited. The natural reservoir and path of transmission are unknown, which makes it impossible to effectively combat Ebola virus and the disease it causes.[8]

Reemerging Infections

Vaccines and proper medications have led to the near eradication of some infections (e.g., smallpox and polio), but infective

TABLE 15-5 REEMERGING INFECTIONS

Microorganism	Infection	Description
Bacteria		
Corynebacterium diphtheriae	Diphtheria	Localized infection of mucous membranes or skin.
Bordetella pertussis	Pertussis	Acute, highly contagious respiratory disease characterized by loud whooping inspiration. Also known as whooping cough.
Yersinia pestis	Plague	*Bubonic:* swollen glands, fever, chills, headache, and extreme exhaustion. *Pneumonic:* overwhelming pneumonia with high fever, cough, bloody sputum, and chills.
Mycobacterium tuberculosis	Tuberculosis	Chronic infection transmitted by inhalation of infected droplets (see Chapter 28).
Virus		
Dengue viruses (flaviviruses)	Dengue fever	Acute infection transmitted by mosquitoes and occurring mainly in tropical and subtropical regions.
Parasite		
Giardia	Giardiasis	Diarrheal illness that usually originates in water contaminated with fecal matter. Also known as traveler's diarrhea.

agents can reemerge if conditions are right. Table 15-5 presents some diseases that have shown resurgence in recent decades.

For example, the incidence of TB began to steadily decrease in the mid-1950s, but in 1984 TB cases began to rise. The growing HIV epidemic in the 1970s and 1980s contributed to the increase in TB as people with depressed immune systems developed new cases of TB or reactivated dormant TB infections. The emergence of multidrug-resistant forms of TB (MDR-TB) also contributed to the increase. Local and federal governments took measures to address the problem, and the rates of TB are now slowly declining again.[9] (TB is discussed in Chapter 28.)

International travel has created a new obstacle for the local eradication of diseases. For example, measles is no longer considered endemic in the United States, but it remains a leading cause of morbidity in developing countries, and outbreaks have occurred in the United States, typically in areas with low vaccination rates. Some measles cases in the United States have been found in people who have recently traveled to measles-endemic areas.[10]

Antibiotic-Resistant Organisms

Resistance occurs when pathogenic organisms change in ways that decrease the ability of a drug (or a family of drugs) to treat disease.[3] Microorganisms can become resistant to classic treatments (e.g., penicillin), as well as to newer antibiotics and antiviral agents. Microorganisms are highly adaptable. They have evolved genetic and biochemical mechanisms to defend against antimicrobial actions. Genetic mechanisms include mutation and acquisition of new DNA or RNA. Biochemically, bacteria can resist antibiotics by producing enzymes that destroy or

TABLE 15-6 ANTIBIOTIC-RESISTANT ORGANISMS AND TREATMENT

Bacteria	Resistant To	Preferred Treatment
Staphylococcus aureus	methicillin*	vancomycin (Vancocin)
Staphylococcus epidermidis	methicillin*	vancomycin
Enterococcus faecalis	vancomycin streptomycin gentamicin (Garamycin)	penicillin G or ampicillin
Enterococcus faecium	vancomycin streptomycin gentamicin	penicillin G or ampicillin
Streptococcus pneumoniae	penicillin G	ceftriaxone (Rocephin) cefotaxime (Claforan)
Klebsiella pneumoniae	Third-generation cephalosporins (e.g., ceftazidime [Ceptaz, Fortaz])	imipenem and cilastatin (Primaxin) meropenem (Merrem IV)

*This drug is no longer available in the United States.

inactivate the drugs. Drug target sites are then altered so that the antibiotic cannot bind to or enter the bacteria. If the drug cannot enter the cell, it cannot kill the bacteria. Table 15-6 describes the most common antibiotic-resistant bacteria.

Methicillin-resistant *S. aureus* (MRSA), vancomycin-resistant enterococci (VRE), and penicillin-resistant *Streptococcus pneumoniae* are examples of emerging strains of antibiotic-resistant organisms. These drug-resistant bacteria were initially seen primarily in health care settings, but are becoming more prevalent in the community. For example, MRSA, a form of *S. aureus* that does not respond to methicillin- or penicillin-based therapies, was initially considered a health care–associated infection (HA-MRSA). However, over the past decade a variant strain of MRSA that is primarily acquired in the community (community-acquired MRSA [CA-MRSA]) has emerged.[11] This strain of MRSA is more *virulent* (able to cause disease or infection) compared with HA-MRSA. CA-MRSA has been known to cause rapidly forming skin infections and systemic diseases, including pneumonia and sepsis. Rates of CA-MRSA infections appear to be on the rise. Conversely, there has been a reduction in HA-MRSA with the implementation of strict hygiene measures in health care settings.

VRE is another antibiotic-resistant bacteria that has become a concern for patients and health care workers. VRE is more virulent than MRSA and can remain viable on environmental surfaces for weeks.[12] Although antibiotic-resistant bacteria can infect anyone, patients who are hospitalized and those with immunosuppression are more likely to be exposed to these bacteria and to develop infection.

Health care providers have contributed to the development of drug-resistant organisms by (1) administering antibiotics for viral infections, (2) succumbing to pressures from patients to prescribe unnecessary antibiotic therapy, (3) using inadequate drug regimens to treat infections, or (4) using broad-spectrum or combination agents for infections that should be treated with first-line medications. Patients can also contribute to resistance development by (1) skipping doses, (2) not taking antibiotics for the full duration of prescribed therapy, or (3) saving unused antibiotics "in case I need them later." In addition, limited

TABLE 15-7 PATIENT & CAREGIVER TEACHING GUIDE

Decrease Risk for Antibiotic-Resistant Infection

Include the following instructions when teaching patients or their caregivers how to decrease the risk for antibiotic-resistant infection.

1. Do Not Take Antibiotics to Prevent Illness (unless prescribed)

Doing this increases your risk for developing resistant infection. Exceptions include taking antibiotics as prescribed before certain surgeries and dental work or in the presence of immune dysfunction.

2. Wash Your Hands Frequently

Hand washing is the single most important thing you can do to prevent infection.

3. Follow Directions When Taking Antibiotics

Not taking your antibiotic as prescribed or skipping doses can allow antibiotic-resistant bacteria to develop.

4. Do Not Request an Antibiotic for Flu or Colds

If your health care provider says that you do not need an antibiotic, chances are you do not. Antibiotics are effective against bacterial infections but not viruses, which cause colds and flu.

5. Finish Your Antibiotic

Do not stop taking your antibiotic when you feel better. If you stop taking your antibiotic early, the hardiest bacteria survive and multiply. Eventually you could develop an infection resistant to many antibiotics. You should never have leftover antibiotics.

6. Do Not Take Leftover Antibiotics

Do not save unfinished antibiotics for later use or borrow leftover drugs from family or friends. This is dangerous because (1) the leftover antibiotic may not be appropriate for you, (2) your illness may not be a bacterial infection, (3) old antibiotics can lose their effectiveness and in some cases can even be fatal, and (4) there will not be enough doses in a leftover bottle to provide full treatment.

resources and access to medications make it difficult for some patients to get adequate treatment for infections. Teaching patients and their families the proper use of antibiotics (Table 15-7) is crucial to treatment success and prevention of drug-resistant pathogens. The Centers for Disease Control and Prevention (CDC), the Infectious Diseases Society of America, and many health care organizations have been campaigning for greater vigilance in minimizing the misuse of antibiotics in reaction to this growing concern.

HEALTH CARE–ASSOCIATED INFECTIONS

Health care–associated infections (HAIs), formerly referred to as *nosocomial infections,* are infections that are acquired as a result of exposure to a microorganism in a health care setting. Approximately 2 million HAIs and 99,000 HAI-associated deaths occur in the United States each year. Antibiotic-resistant organisms cause half of these infections.[13] Up to 10% of hospitalized patients will acquire an HAI. Surgical and immunocompromised patients are at highest risk. Any organism can cause HAIs, but certain bacteria, including *E. coli, S. aureus, Enterobacter aerogenes,* and various types of streptococci, are the more common culprits. Some bacteria that do not normally cause disease can cause infections in high-risk patients as a result of illness or treatment of illness.[14]

TABLE 15-8 OSHA REQUIREMENTS FOR PERSONAL PROTECTIVE EQUIPMENT

The following equipment is used to minimize exposure to blood-borne pathogens.

Equipment	Indications for Use
Gloves	• Must be used when the employee can reasonably anticipate having contact with blood or other potentially infectious materials, when performing vascular access procedures, and when handling or touching contaminated items or surfaces. • Gloves must be replaced if torn, punctured, or contaminated or their ability to function as a barrier is compromised.
Clothing (gowns, aprons, caps, boots)	• Must be used when occupational exposure is anticipated. • The type and characteristics depend on the task and degree of exposure anticipated.
Face protection (mask and glasses with solid side shields or a chin-length face shield)	• Must be used when splashes, sprays, spatters, or droplets of blood or other potentially infectious materials pose a hazard to the eyes, nose, or mouth.

Source: Occupational Safety and Health Administration: Bloodborne pathogens and needlestick prevention. Retrieved from *www.osha.gov/SLTC/bloodbornepathogens.*
NOTE: Employers must provide, make accessible, and require the use of personal protective equipment (PPE) at no cost to the employee. PPE also must be provided in appropriate sizes. Hypoallergenic gloves or similar alternatives must be made available to employees who have an allergic sensitivity to gloves.
OSHA, Occupational Safety and Health Administration.

Approximately one third of HAIs are preventable. Health care providers often transmit HAIs from patient to patient through direct contact. Hand washing (or using an alcohol-based hand sanitizer) between patients and procedures and the appropriate use of protective equipment such as gloves remain the first lines of defense to prevent the spread of HAIs. Isolated infections can also be caused when bacteria that normally stay in one area of the body are introduced into another area. Therefore care must be taken to change gloves and wash hands when moving from one task to another, even when working with the same patient.[15] The Occupational Safety and Health Administration (OSHA) and the CDC recommend that precautions be followed to control the spread of disease, especially of antibiotic-resistant organisms (Table 15-8).

GERONTOLOGIC CONSIDERATIONS

INFECTIONS IN OLDER ADULTS

For older adults the rate of HAIs is two or three times higher than for younger patients.[13,16] Individuals in long-term care facilities are at special risk for HAI. Age-related changes (e.g., impaired immune function, co-morbidities such as diabetes, physical disabilities) can contribute to higher infection rates.[17]

Infections common in older adults include pneumonia, urinary tract infections, skin infections, and TB. Urinary tract infections are more common in older adults who reside in long-term care facilities. Patients with indwelling catheters are at particular risk. Infections in older adults often have atypical manifestations, such as cognitive and behavioral changes, before the emergence of fever, pain, or alterations in laboratory values.

Suspicion of disease should typically begin if a patient demonstrates changes in the ability to perform daily activities or in cognitive function. In addition, underlying diseases, increased frequency of drug reactions, and institutionalization can all complicate the management of the older adult with infection.

SAFETY ALERT

- Do not rely on the presence of fever to indicate infection in older adults because many have lower core body temperatures and decreased immune responses.

INFECTION PREVENTION AND CONTROL

Occupational Safety and Health Administration (OSHA) Guidelines

OSHA is a federal agency that protects workers from injury and illness in places of employment and supports activities that minimize or eliminate exposure to infectious materials in the workplace. OSHA mandates that any employer whose employees could be exposed to potentially infectious materials implement standard policies and procedures for protection of those employees. Employees must be provided with appropriate personal protective equipment (PPE) and safety equipment. These include gloves, gowns, facial protection, and disposal systems for sharps (see Table 15-8). Appropriate PPE varies depending on the situation, and as a nurse, you need to use sound judgment when deciding when and how to use protective equipment.

Infection Precautions

If a patient is admitted with or develops an infection that is considered a risk to others, infection precautions may be needed. The CDC has established guidelines with two levels of precautions: (1) *standard precautions*, designed for the care of all patients in hospitals and health care facilities; and (2) *transmission-based precautions,* designed for specific diseases.[15] The purpose of these precautions is to prevent the transmission of organisms from patients to health care providers, from health care providers to patients, from patients to other patients, and from providers and patients to people outside of the hospital. (CDC guidelines for isolation precautions are summarized in eTable 15-1 on the website for this chapter.)

The *standard precautions* system applies to (1) blood; (2) all body fluids, secretions, and excretions; (3) nonintact skin; and (4) mucous membranes. Standard precautions are designed to reduce the risk of transmission of microorganisms in hospitals. Standard precautions should be applied to all patients regardless of diagnosis or presumed infection status. The CDC's standard precautions incorporate all of the OSHA blood-borne pathogens standard requirements.

Transmission-based precautions are used for patients known to be or suspected of being infected with highly transmissible or epidemiologically important pathogens that require additional precautions to interrupt transmission and prevent infection. Transmission-based precautions include airborne precautions, droplet precautions, and contact precautions. *Airborne precautions* are used if the organism can cause infection over long distances when suspended in the air (e.g., TB, rubeola). *Droplet precautions* are used to minimize contact with pathogens that are spread through the air at close contact and that affect the respiratory system or mucous membranes (e.g., influenza, pertussis). *Contact precautions* are used to minimize the spread of pathogens that are acquired from direct or indirect contact, especially multidrug-resistant organisms (e.g., MRSA, VRE). Transmission-based precautions may be combined for diseases that have multiple routes of transmission. Whether used alone or in combination, transmission-based precautions should always be used in conjunction with standard precautions.

HUMAN IMMUNODEFICIENCY VIRUS INFECTION

Human immunodeficiency virus (HIV) infection is caused by HIV, which is a retrovirus that causes immunosuppression. The viral infection causes the person to be susceptible to infections that would normally be controlled through immune responses. The term *HIV disease* is used interchangeably with HIV infection. With advances in treatment, HIV is managed as a chronic disease, since people are living longer.

Significance of Problem

HIV has caused a global pandemic and affected millions. In the past 30 years, important advances have been made in HIV prevention, testing, and treatment. In developed countries the result has been decreases in the number of HIV-related deaths, improved quality of life, and a significant decrease in the number of children born with HIV.[18]

More than 1 million people are currently living with HIV in the United States, with an estimated 50,000 new infections occurring annually. With the availability of effective treatment, people with HIV infection can live for a longer time, resulting in a dramatic drop in the number of deaths attributable to HIV.[19-21]

In North America HIV has been most prevalent among men who have sex with men. However, increasing numbers of new HIV infections are occurring in women, people of color, people who live in poverty, and adolescents. For the most part, HIV remains a disease of marginalized individuals: those who are disenfranchised by virtue of gender, race, sexual orientation, poverty, drug use, or lack of access to health care.[21,22]

Transmission of HIV

HIV can be transmitted as a result of contact with infected blood, semen, vaginal secretions, or breast milk. Transmission of HIV occurs through sexual intercourse with an infected partner; exposure to HIV-infected blood or blood products; and perinatal transmission during pregnancy, at delivery, or through breastfeeding.[19]

HIV-infected individuals can transmit HIV to others within a few days after becoming infected. The ability to transmit HIV continues for life. Transmission of HIV is subject to the same requirements as other microorganisms (i.e., a large enough amount of the virus must enter the body of a susceptible host).

Variables that influence whether infection will be established after an exposure include (1) duration and frequency of contact with the organism; (2) volume, virulence, and concentration of the organism; and (3) host immune status. The concentration of virus is an important variable. Large amounts of HIV can be found in the blood, and to a lesser extent in the semen, during the first 6 months of infection and again during the late stages of the disease (Fig. 15-1). Although unprotected sexual intercourse or blood exposure to an infected individual during these

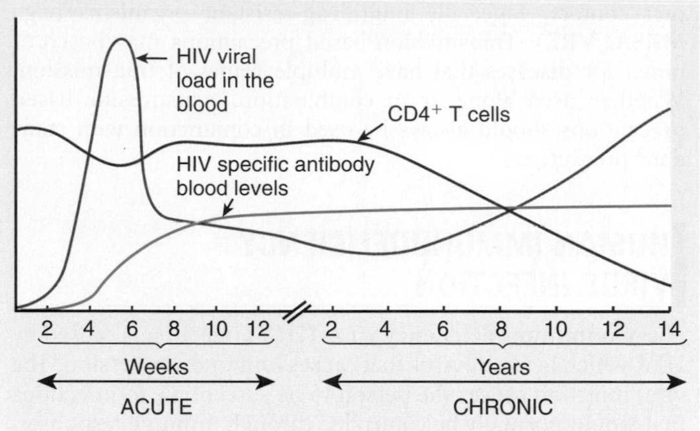

FIG. 15-1 Viral load in the blood in relationship to number of $CD4^+$ T cells over the spectrum of untreated HIV infection.

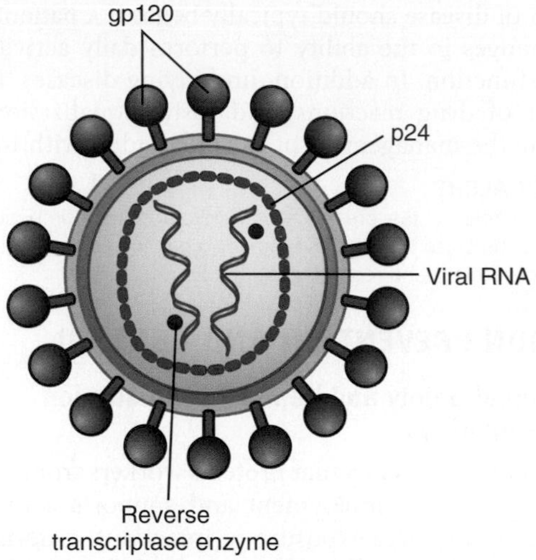

FIG. 15-2 HIV is surrounded by an envelope made up of proteins (including gp120) and contains a core of viral RNA and proteins.

periods is more risky, HIV can be transmitted during all phases of the disease.

HIV is not spread casually. The virus cannot be transmitted through hugging, dry kissing, shaking hands, sharing eating utensils, using toilet seats, or casual encounters in any setting.[19] It is not spread by tears, saliva, urine, emesis, sputum, feces, sweat, respiratory droplets, or enteric routes. Health care workers have a low risk of acquiring HIV at work, even after a needle-stick injury.[23]

Sexual Transmission. The most common mode of HIV transmission is unprotected sexual contact with an HIV-infected partner. Sexual activity involves contact with semen, vaginal secretions, and/or blood, all of which have lymphocytes that may contain HIV. During any form of sexual intercourse (anal, vaginal, or oral), the risk of infection is greater for the partner who receives the semen, although infection can also be transmitted to the inserting partner. This occurs because the receiver has prolonged contact with infected fluids, and it helps explain why it is easier to infect women than men during heterosexual intercourse. Sexual activities that cause trauma to local tissues can increase the risk of transmission. In addition, genital lesions from other sexually transmitted infections (e.g., herpes, syphilis) significantly increase the likelihood of transmission.

Contact With Blood and Blood Products. HIV can be transmitted during exposure to blood through drug-using equipment. Used equipment may be contaminated with HIV and other blood-borne organisms, and sharing that equipment can result in disease transmission.

In North America, transfusion of infected blood and blood products has caused only 1% of adult AIDS cases.[22] Routine screening of blood donors to identify at-risk individuals and testing donated blood for the presence of HIV have improved the safety of the blood supply. In countries that routinely test donated blood, HIV infection as a result of blood transfusions or hemophilia clotting factors is now unlikely.

Puncture wounds are the most common means of work-related HIV transmission. The risk of infection after a needle-stick exposure to HIV-infected blood is 0.3% to 0.4% (or 3 to 4 out of 1000).[23] The risk is higher if the exposure involves blood from a patient with a high level of circulating HIV, a deep puncture wound, a needle with a hollow bore and visible blood, a device used for venous or arterial access, or a patient who dies within 60 days. Splash exposures of blood on skin with an open lesion present some risk, but it is much lower than from a puncture wound.

Perinatal Transmission. Perinatal transmission from an HIV-infected mother to her infant can occur during pregnancy, delivery, or breastfeeding. On average, 25% of infants born to women with untreated HIV infection are born with HIV. Fortunately, the risk of transmission can be reduced to less than 2% in settings where pregnant women are routinely tested for HIV infection and, if found to be infected, treated with antiretroviral therapy (ART).[24]

Pathophysiology

HIV is an RNA virus. RNA viruses are called **retroviruses** because they replicate in a "backward" manner (going from RNA to DNA). Like all viruses, HIV cannot replicate unless it is inside a living cell. HIV enters a cell when the gp120 "knobs" (Fig. 15-2) on the viral envelope bind to specific CD4 and chemokine receptor sites on the cell's surface *(fusion)* (Fig. 15-3). Chemokine receptors are proteins normally found in cell membranes that respond to chemokines outside the cell and trigger a response inside the cell. HIV uses the chemokine receptors CXCR4 and CCR5 as co-receptors (CD4 is the main receptor) to support binding and entry into the $CD4^+$ T cell.[25]

Once bound, viral RNA enters the $CD4^+$ T cell, where it is transcribed into a single strand of viral DNA with the assistance of **reverse transcriptase,** an enzyme made by retroviruses. This strand copies itself, becoming double-stranded viral DNA, which then enters the cell's nucleus and, using another enzyme called **integrase,** splices itself into the human genome, becoming a permanent part of the cell's genetic structure. This action has two consequences: (1) because all genetic material is replicated during cell division, all daughter cells are also infected and (2) viral DNA in the genome directs the cell to make new HIV. HIV production in the cell starts with long strands of HIV RNA. These are cut into appropriate lengths in the presence of the enzyme **protease** during the budding sequence.[25]

Initial infection with HIV results in **viremia** (large amounts of virus in the blood). This is followed within a few weeks by a prolonged period in which HIV levels in the blood remain low even without treatment (see Fig. 15-1). During this time, which may last for more than 10 years, clinical symptoms can be

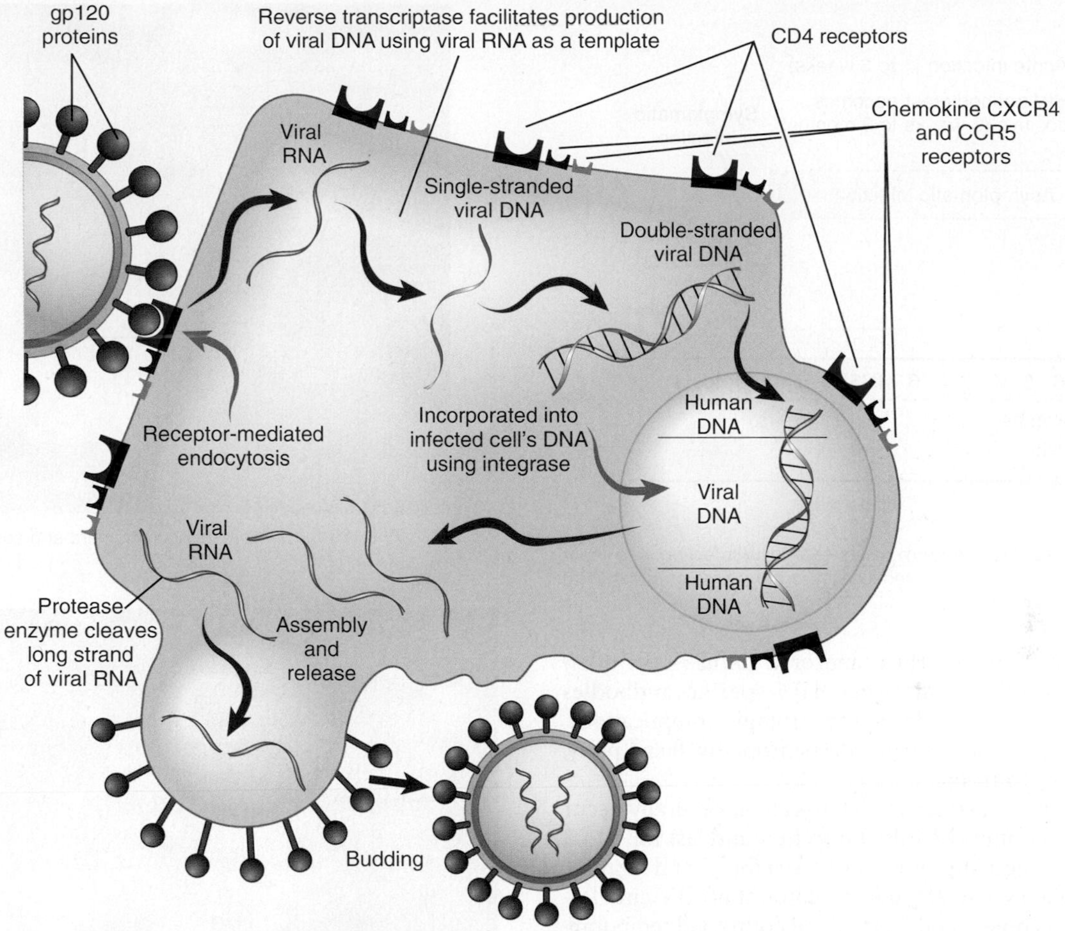

FIG. 15-3 HIV has gp120 glycoproteins that attach to CD4 and chemokine CXCR4 and CCR5 receptors on the surface of $CD4^+$ T cells. Viral RNA then enters the cell, produces viral DNA in the presence of reverse transcriptase, and incorporates itself into the cellular genome in the presence of integrase, causing permanent cellular infection and the production of new virions. New viral RNA develops initially in long strands that are cut in the presence of protease and leave the cell through a budding process that ultimately contributes to cellular destruction.

limited. Even without symptoms, HIV replication occurs at a rapid and constant rate in the blood and lymph tissues. A major consequence of rapid replication is that errors can occur in the copying process, causing mutations that can contribute to resistance to ART and limit treatment options.

In the initial stages of HIV infection, B cells and T cells respond and function normally. B cells make HIV-specific antibodies that are effective in reducing viral loads in the blood. Activated T cells mount a cellular immune response to viruses trapped in the lymph nodes.[25]

HIV infects human cells with CD4 receptors on their surfaces, including lymphocytes, monocytes/macrophages, astrocytes, and oligodendrocytes. However, immune dysfunction in HIV infection is predominantly the result of damage to and destruction of $CD4^+$ T cells (also known as T helper cells or $CD4^+$ T lymphocytes). These cells are targeted because they have more CD4 receptors on their surfaces than the other CD4 receptor–bearing cells. $CD4^+$ T cells play a key role in the immune system's ability to recognize and defend against pathogens.

Adults without immune dysfunction normally have 800 to 1200 $CD4^+$ T cells per microliter (μL) of blood. The normal life span of a $CD4^+$ T cell is about 100 days, but HIV-infected $CD4^+$ T cells die after an average of only 2 days.

HIV destroys about 1 billion $CD4^+$ T cells every day. The body can produce new $CD4^+$ T cells to replace the destroyed cells for many years. However, eventually the ability of HIV to destroy $CD4^+$ T cells exceeds the body's ability to replace the cells. The decline in the $CD4^+$ T cell count impairs immune function. Generally, the immune system remains healthy with more than 500 $CD4^+$ T cells/μL. Immune problems start to occur when the count drops below 500 $CD4^+$ T cells/μL. Severe problems develop with fewer than 200 $CD4^+$ T cells/μL. With HIV, a point is eventually reached where so many $CD4^+$ T cells have been destroyed that not enough are left to regulate immune responses (see Fig. 15-1). This allows **opportunistic diseases** (infections and cancers that occur in immunosuppressed patients) to develop. Opportunistic diseases are the main cause of disease, disability, and death in patients with HIV infection.

Clinical Manifestations and Complications

The typical course of untreated HIV infection follows the pattern shown in Fig. 15-4. It is important to remember that (1) disease progression is highly individualized, (2) treatment can significantly alter this pattern, and (3) an individual's prognosis is unpredictable.

Acute Infection. A mononucleosis-like syndrome of fever, swollen lymph glands, sore throat, headache, malaise, nausea,

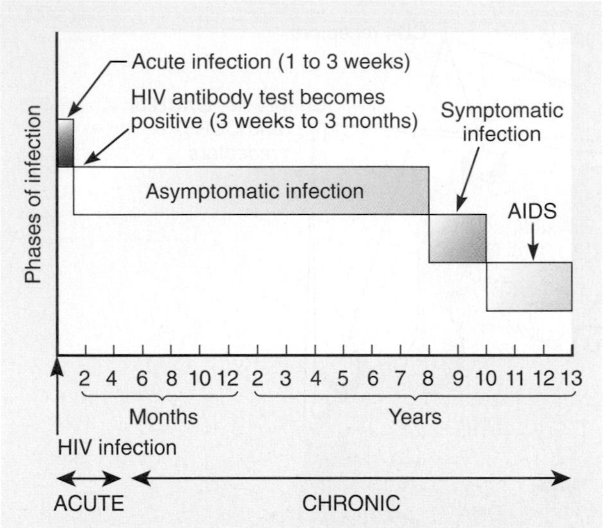

FIG. 15-4 Timeline for the spectrum of untreated HIV infection. The timeline represents the course of untreated illness from the time of infection to clinical manifestations of disease.

muscle and joint pain, diarrhea, and/or a diffuse rash often accompanies **seroconversion** (when HIV-specific antibodies develop). Some people also develop neurologic complications, such as aseptic meningitis, peripheral neuropathy, facial palsy, or Guillain-Barré syndrome.

These symptoms, called *acute HIV infection,* generally occur within 2 to 4 weeks after the initial infection and last for 1 to 3 weeks, although some symptoms may persist for several months. During this time a high **viral load** (the amount of HIV circulating in the blood) is noted, and CD4$^+$ T cell counts fall temporarily but quickly return to baseline or near-baseline levels (see Fig. 15-1). Many people, including health care providers, mistake acute HIV symptoms for a bad case of the flu.[26]

Chronic HIV Infection

Asymptomatic Infection. The interval between untreated HIV infection and a diagnosis of AIDS is about 10 years. During this time, CD4$^+$ T cell counts remain above 500 cells/μL (normal or only slightly decreased), and the viral load in the blood is low. This phase has been referred to as *asymptomatic infection,* although fatigue, headache, low-grade fever, night sweats, *persistent generalized lymphadenopathy* (PGL), and other symptoms may be present.[27]

Because most of the symptoms during early infection are vague and nonspecific for HIV, people may not be aware that they are infected. During this time, infected people continue their usual activities, which may include high-risk sexual and drug-using behaviors. This is a public health problem because infected individuals can transmit HIV to others even though they have no symptoms. Personal health is also affected because people who do not know that they are infected have little reason to seek treatment and are less likely to make behavior changes that could improve the quality and length of their lives.

Symptomatic Infection. As the CD4$^+$ T cell count drops to 200 to 500 cells/μL and the viral load increases, HIV advances to a more active stage. Symptoms seen in earlier phases become worse, leading to persistent fever, frequent drenching night sweats, chronic diarrhea, recurrent headaches, and fatigue severe enough to interrupt normal routines. Other problems may include localized infections, lymphadenopathy, and nervous system manifestations.[27]

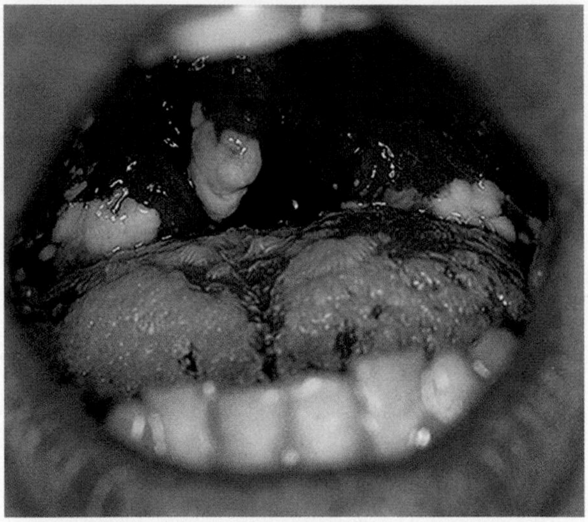

FIG. 15-5 Oral thrush involving hard and soft palate.

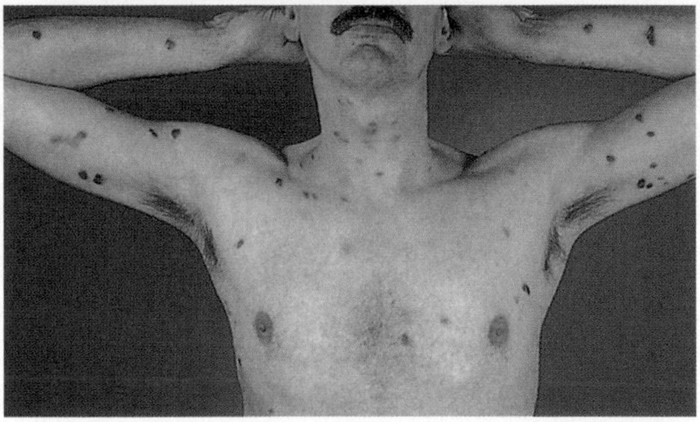

FIG. 15-6 Kaposi sarcoma (KS). The malignant vascular lesions of KS can appear anywhere on the skin surface or on internal organs. Lesions vary in size from pinpoint to large and may appear in a variety of shades.

The most common infection associated with this phase of HIV infection is oropharyngeal candidiasis, or thrush (Fig. 15-5). *Candida* organisms rarely cause problems in healthy adults, but are more common in HIV-infected people. Other infections that can occur at this time include shingles (caused by the varicella-zoster virus); persistent vaginal candidal infections; outbreaks of oral or genital herpes; bacterial infections; and Kaposi sarcoma (KS), which is caused by human herpesvirus 8 (Fig. 15-6). *Oral hairy leukoplakia,* an Epstein-Barr virus infection that causes painless, white, raised lesions on the lateral aspect of the tongue (Fig. 15-7), is another indicator of disease progression.[28]

AIDS. A diagnosis of **acquired immunodeficiency syndrome (AIDS)** is made when an HIV-infected patient meets criteria established by the CDC.[29] These criteria occur when the immune system becomes severely compromised (Table 15-9). As the viral load increases, the absolute number and percentage of T cells decrease and the risk of developing opportunistic diseases increases.

Opportunistic diseases generally do not occur in the presence of a functioning immune system. Many infections, a variety of malignancies, wasting, and HIV-related dementia can occur in patients with immune impairment (Table 15-10).

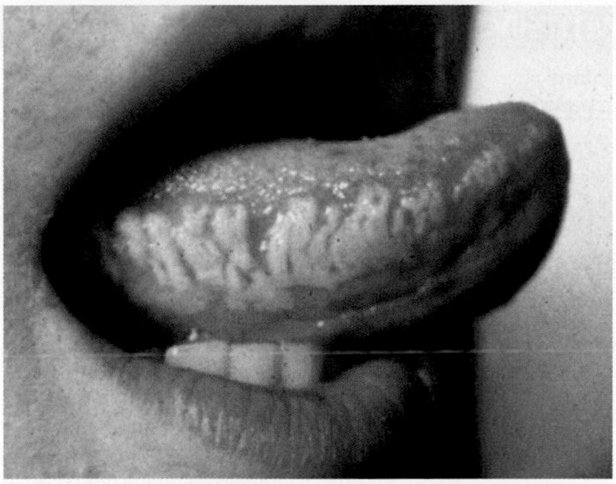

FIG. 15-7 Oral hairy leukoplakia on the lateral aspect of the tongue.

TABLE 15-9 DIAGNOSTIC CRITERIA FOR AIDS

AIDS is diagnosed when an individual with HIV develops at least one of the following conditions:

1. $CD4^+$ T cell count drops below 200 cells/μL.
2. One of the following opportunistic infections (OIs):
   - *Fungal*: candidiasis of bronchi, trachea, lungs, or esophagus; *Pneumocystis jiroveci* pneumonia (PCP); disseminated or extrapulmonary coccidioidomycosis; disseminated or extrapulmonary histoplasmosis
   - *Viral*: cytomegalovirus (CMV) disease other than liver, spleen, or nodes; CMV retinitis (with loss of vision); herpes simplex with chronic ulcer(s) or bronchitis, pneumonitis, or esophagitis; progressive multifocal leukoencephalopathy (PML); extrapulmonary cryptococcosis
   - *Protozoal*: toxoplasmosis of the brain, chronic intestinal isosporiasis, chronic intestinal cryptosporidiosis
   - *Bacterial: Mycobacterium tuberculosis* (any site); any disseminated or extrapulmonary mycobacteria, including *Mycobacterium avium* complex (MAC) or *Mycobacterium kansasii;* recurrent pneumonia; recurrent *Salmonella* septicemia
3. One of the following opportunistic cancers:
   - Invasive cervical cancer
   - Kaposi sarcoma (KS)
   - Burkitt's lymphoma
   - Immunoblastic lymphoma
   - Primary lymphoma of the brain
4. Wasting syndrome. *Wasting* is defined as a loss of 10% or more of ideal body mass.
5. AIDS dementia complex (ADC).

Modified from Centers for Disease Control and Prevention: 1993 Revised classification system for HIV infection and expanded surveillance case definition for AIDS among adolescents and adults, 1993. Retrieved from *www.cdc.gov/mmwr/preview/mmwrhtml/rr5710a1.htm?s_cid=rr5710a1_e*.

Organisms that do not cause severe disease in people with functioning immune systems can cause debilitating, disseminated, and life-threatening infections during this stage. Several opportunistic diseases may occur at the same time, compounding the difficulties of diagnosis and treatment. Advances in HIV treatment have decreased the occurrence of opportunistic diseases.

Diagnostic Studies

Diagnosis of HIV Infection. Diagnosis of HIV infection is made by testing for HIV antibodies and/or antigen in the blood. HIV-antibody tests detect HIV-specific antibodies, but typically it takes several weeks after the infection before antibodies can be detected on a screening test (see Fig. 15-1). This delay is known as the **window period.**

Standard antibody tests can be completed on blood or oral fluid specimens. They are sent to a laboratory, and results are reported back to the provider anywhere from a day to a week later. *Rapid* HIV-antibody tests are done in the office, and results can be shared with patients before they leave the office. They can also be done at home using a self-administered HIV test kit. A positive antibody test should be followed by a confirming test (usually the Western blot) (Table 15-11).

Laboratory Studies in HIV Infection. The progression of HIV infection is monitored by two important laboratory assessments: $CD4^+$ T cell counts and viral load. $CD4^+$ T cell counts provide a marker of immune function. As the disease progresses, the number of $CD4^+$ T cells usually decreases (see Fig. 15-1). The normal range for $CD4^+$ T cells is 800 to 1200 cells/μL. Laboratory tests that measure viral levels provide an assessment of disease progression. The lower the viral load, the less active the disease. In HIV, viral loads are reported as real numbers (e.g., 1260 copies/μL) or as undetectable. "Undetectable" indicates that the viral load is lower than the test is able to report. "Undetectable" does *not* mean that the virus has been eliminated from the body or that the individual can no longer transmit HIV to others.

Abnormal blood test results are common in HIV infection and may be caused by HIV, opportunistic diseases, or complications of therapy. Decreased white blood cell (WBC) counts, especially below-normal numbers of lymphocytes (lymphopenia) and neutrophils (neutropenia), are often seen. Low platelet counts (thrombocytopenia) may be caused by HIV, antiplatelet antibodies, or drug therapy. Anemia is associated with the chronic disease process and with adverse effects of ART. Altered liver function, caused by HIV infection, drug therapy, or co-infection with a hepatitis virus, is common. Early identification of co-infection with hepatitis B virus (HBV) or hepatitis C virus (HCV) is extremely important because these infections have a more serious course in patients with HIV, may ultimately limit options for ART, and can cause liver-related morbidity and mortality.[27]

Two types of resistance tests can determine if a patient's HIV is resistant to drugs used for ART. The *genotype assay* detects drug-resistant viral mutations that are present in reverse transcriptase and protease genes. The *phenotype assay* measures the growth of HIV in various concentrations of antiretroviral drugs (much like bacteria-antibiotic sensitivity tests). These assays help determine new drug combinations for patients who are not responding to therapy.

Collaborative Care

Collaborative care of the HIV-infected patient focuses on (1) monitoring HIV disease progression and immune function, (2) initiating and monitoring ART, (3) preventing the development of opportunistic diseases, (4) detecting and treating opportunistic diseases, (5) managing symptoms, (6) preventing or decreasing complications of treatment, and (7) preventing further transmission of HIV. To accomplish these objectives, ongoing assessment, clinician-patient interactions, and patient teaching and support are required.

The initial patient visit provides an opportunity to gather baseline data and to start establishing rapport. A complete history and physical examination, including an immunization history and psychosocial and dietary evaluations, should be

TABLE 15-10 OPPORTUNISTIC DISEASES ASSOCIATED WITH HIV INFECTION*

Organism or Disease	Clinical Manifestations
Candida albicans	Thrush (see Fig. 15-5), esophagitis, vaginitis; whitish yellow patches in mouth, esophagus, GI tract, vagina
Coccidioides immitis	Pneumonia and fever, weight loss, cough
CNS lymphoma	Cognitive dysfunction, motor impairment, aphasia, seizures, personality changes, headache
Cryptococcus neoformans	Meningitis, cognitive impairment, motor dysfunction, fever, seizures, headache
Cryptosporidium muris	Gastroenteritis, watery diarrhea, abdominal pain, weight loss
Cytomegalovirus (CMV)	*Retinitis:* retinal lesions, blurred vision, loss of vision *Esophagitis, stomatitis:* difficulty swallowing; colitis or gastritis: bloody diarrhea, pain, weight loss *Pneumonitis:* respiratory symptoms *Neurologic disease:* CNS manifestations
Hepatitis B virus (HBV)	Jaundice, fatigue, abdominal pain, loss of appetite, nausea, vomiting, joint pain; 30% may have no signs or symptoms
Hepatitis C virus (HCV)	Jaundice, fatigue, abdominal pain, loss of appetite, nausea, vomiting, dark urine; 80% may have no signs or symptoms
Herpes simplex	*HSV-1 (type 1):* orolabial and mucocutaneous vesicular and ulcerative lesions; keratitis; visual disturbances; encephalitis; CNS manifestations *HSV-2 (type 2):* genital and perianal vesicular and ulcerative lesions
Histoplasma capsulatum	*Pneumonia:* fever, cough, weight loss *Meningitis:* CNS manifestations, disseminated disease
Influenza virus	Fever (usually high), headache, extreme tiredness, dry cough, sore throat, runny or stuffy nose, muscle aches; nausea, vomiting, and diarrhea can occur
JC papovavirus	Progressive multifocal leukoencephalopathy (PML), CNS manifestations, mental and motor declines
Kaposi sarcoma (KS) caused by human herpesvirus 8 (HHV-8)	Vascular lesions on the skin (see Fig. 15-6), mucous membranes, and viscera with wide range of presentation: firm, flat, raised, or nodular; pinpoint to several cm in size; hyperpigmented, multicentric; can cause lymphedema and disfigurement, particularly when confluent; usually not serious unless occurring in the respiratory or gastrointestinal system
***Mycobacterium avium* complex (MAC)**	Gastroenteritis, watery diarrhea, weight loss
***Mycobacterium tuberculosis* (MTB, TB)**	Respiratory and disseminated disease; productive cough, fever, night sweats, weight loss
***Pneumocystis jiroveci* pneumonia (PCP)**	Pneumonia, nonproductive cough, hypoxemia, progressive shortness of breath, fever, night sweats, fatigue
Toxoplasma gondii	Encephalitis, cognitive dysfunction, motor impairment, fever, altered mental status, headache, seizures, sensory abnormalities
Varicella zoster virus (VZV)	*Shingles:* erythematous maculopapular rash along dermatomal planes, pain, pruritus *Ocular:* progressive outer retinal necrosis (PORN)

*Treatment of opportunistic diseases is presented in eTable 15-2 on the website for this chapter.

TABLE 15-11 HIV-ANTIBODY TESTS

1. A highly sensitive enzyme immunoassay (EIA) is done to detect serum antibodies that bind to HIV antigens on test plates. Blood samples that are negative on this test are reported as negative.
   - If the patient reports recent risky behaviors, encourage retesting at 3 wk, 6 wk, and 3 mo.
2. If the blood is EIA-antibody positive, repeat the test.
3. If the blood is repeatedly EIA-antibody positive, a more specific confirming test, such as the Western blot (WB) or immunofluorescence assay (IFA), is done.
4. Blood that is reactive in all of the first three steps is reported as HIV-antibody positive.
5. If the results are indeterminate, the following steps are taken:
   - If in-depth risk assessment reveals that the individual does not have a history of high-risk activities, reassure the patient that HIV infection is extremely unlikely and suggest retesting in 3 mo.
   - If in-depth risk assessment reveals that the individual does have a history of high-risk activities, consider tests that detect HIV antigen.

Rapid HIV-Antibody Testing

1. Rapid testing is strongly recommended by the Centers for Disease Control and Prevention. Results are highly accurate, and it can be done in a variety of settings (mobile health units, physicians' offices, or even in the privacy of an individual's home). Results are typically available within 20 min.
2. In-home use HIV test kits are available. Testing is done on an oral fluid sample.
3. Rapid tests are screening tests for antibodies, not for antigen.
4. Negative rapid tests should be followed by a risk assessment to determine the need for repeat tests.
5. Positive rapid tests can be disclosed to the patient, but need to be confirmed with the more specific WB or IFA (as above). This step necessitates a blood draw and a return appointment to get results.

Combined Antibody/Antigen Testing

1. The combined antibody/antigen test allows for diagnosis of HIV infection, especially during the window period when antibody may be undetectable but viral loads are generally high.

conducted. Findings from the history, assessment, and laboratory tests help to determine patient needs. This is also a good time to complete the case reports required by the state health department. Patient teaching about the spectrum of HIV disease, treatment, prevention of transmission to others, improvements in health, and family planning can be initiated at this meeting. Use patient input to develop a plan of care and determine the need for referrals. Remember that a newly diagnosed patient may not be able to retain or understand information. Be prepared to repeat and clarify information over the course of several months.

Drug Therapy for HIV Infection. The goals of drug therapy in HIV infection are to (1) decrease the viral load, (2) maintain or increase CD4$^+$ T cell counts, (3) prevent HIV-related symptoms and opportunistic diseases, (4) delay disease progression, and (5) prevent HIV transmission. HIV cannot be cured, but **antiretroviral therapy (ART)** can delay disease progression by decreasing viral replication. When taken consistently and correctly, ART can reduce viral loads by 90% to 99%, which makes adherence to treatment regimens extremely important.

Drugs used to treat HIV work at various points in the HIV replication cycle (Table 15-12). The major advantage of using drugs from different classes is that combination therapy can inhibit viral replication in several different ways, making it more difficult for the virus to recover and decreasing the likelihood of drug resistance. A major problem with most drugs used in ART is that resistance develops rapidly when they are used alone *(monotherapy)* or taken in inadequate doses.[27,28] For that reason, combinations of three or more drugs should be used.

Many antiretroviral drugs have dangerous and potentially lethal interactions with other commonly used drugs, including over-the-counter drugs and herbal therapies. For example, St. John's wort, an herb used to alleviate depression, can interfere with ART. Encourage patients to discuss the use of all over-the-counter and herbal products with their health care providers.

TABLE 15-12 DRUG THERAPY

HIV Infection

Drug Classification	Mechanism of Action	Examples*
Entry Inhibitors	Prevent binding of HIV to cells, thus preventing entry of HIV into cells where replication would occur	enfuvirtide (Fuzeon) maraviroc (Selzentry)
Reverse Transcriptase Inhibitors		
Nucleoside Reverse Transcriptase Inhibitors (NRTIs)	Insert a piece of DNA into the developing HIV DNA chain, blocking further development of the chain and leaving the production of the new strand of HIV DNA incomplete	zidovudine (AZT, ZDV, Retrovir) didanosine (ddI, Videx, Videx-EC [time-released]) stavudine (d4T, Zerit) lamivudine (3TC, Epivir) abacavir (Ziagen) emtricitabine (FTC, Emtriva)
Nonnucleoside Reverse Transcriptase Inhibitors (NNRTIs)	Inhibit the action of reverse transcriptase	nevirapine (Viramune) delavirdine (Rescriptor) efavirenz (Sustiva) etravirine (Intelence) rilpivirine (Edurant)
Nucleotide Reverse Transcriptase Inhibitor (NtRTI)	Combines with reverse transcriptase enzyme to block the process needed to convert HIV RNA into HIV DNA	tenofovir (Viread)
Integrase Inhibitors	Bind with integrase enzyme and prevent HIV from incorporating its genetic material into the host cell	raltegravir (Isentress) elvitegravir† dolutegravir (Tivicay)
Protease Inhibitors (PIs)	Prevent the protease enzyme from cutting HIV proteins into the proper lengths needed to allow viable virions to assemble and bud out from the cell membrane	saquinavir (Fortovase, Invirase) indinavir (Crixivan) ritonavir (Norvir)‡ nelfinavir (Viracept) atazanavir (Reyataz) fosamprenavir (Lexiva) tipranavir (Aptivus) darunavir (Prezista) lopinavir + ritonavir (Kaletra)
Fixed-Dose Combination Products	More than one drug combined into a single tablet. Drugs may be from the same or different classes.	Atripla (tenofovir DF + emtricitabine + efavirenz) Combivir (lamivudine + zidovudine) Complera (tenofovir DF + emtricitabine + rilpivirine) Epzicom (abacavir + lamivudine) Trizivir (abacavir + lamivudine + zidovudine) Truvada (tenofovir DF + emtricitabine) Stribild (tenofovir DF + emtricitabine + elvitegravir + cobicistat§)

*Side effects of these drugs are listed in eTable 15-3 available on the website for this chapter.
†Part of the combination pill Stribild (see below)
‡Most often used in low doses with other PIs to boost effect.
§Cobicistat is a pharmacologic booster that enhances the potency of some HIV antiretrovirals. It has no direct effects against HIV.
DF, Disoproxil fumarate.

DRUG ALERT: Efavirenz (Sustiva)

- In pregnant patients, efavirenz can be used after the first 8 weeks of pregnancy.
- Once-a-day doses should be taken at bed time (at least initially) to help patients cope with side effects, including dizziness and confusion.
- Inform patients that many people who use the drug have reported vivid and sometimes bizarre dreams.

Drug Therapy for Opportunistic Diseases. Management of HIV is complicated by the many opportunistic diseases that can develop as the immune system deteriorates (see Table 15-10). Prevention is the preferred approach to opportunistic diseases. A number of opportunistic diseases associated with HIV can be delayed or prevented with adequate ART, vaccines (including hepatitis B, influenza, and pneumococcal), and disease-specific prevention measures. Although it is usually not possible to eradicate opportunistic diseases once they occur, prophylactic medications can significantly decrease morbidity and mortality rates.[30] Advances in the prevention, diagnosis, and treatment of opportunistic diseases have contributed significantly to increased life expectancy. (Drug therapy for opportunistic infections is presented in eTable 15-2 on the website for this chapter.)

Preventing Transmission of HIV. Preexposure prophylaxis (PrEP) is a comprehensive HIV prevention strategy to reduce the risk of sexually acquired HIV infection in adults at high risk.[31] PrEP includes safe sex practices, risk reduction counseling, and regular HIV testing. In addition, emtricitabine and tenofovir (Truvada) can be used for PrEP.

Truvada is the first drug approved to reduce the risk of HIV infection in uninfected individuals who are at high risk of HIV infection and who may engage in sexual activity with HIV-infected partners. Truvada is also currently used in combination with other antiretroviral agents for the treatment of HIV-infected people. Guidelines for PrEP for HIV prevention are available at *www.cdc.gov/hiv/prep/pdf/PrEPfactsheet.pdf.*

NURSING MANAGEMENT HIV INFECTION

NURSING ASSESSMENT

Nursing assessment for individuals not known to be infected with HIV should focus on behaviors that put the person at risk for HIV and other sexually transmitted and blood-borne infections. Assess patients for risky behaviors on a regular basis. Do not assume that someone is without risk because he or she is too old or too young, is married, or sings in the church choir.

Help individuals assess risk by asking some basic questions: (1) Have you ever had a blood transfusion or used clotting factors? If so, was it before 1985? (2) Have you ever shared drug-using equipment with another person? (3) Have you ever had a sexual experience in which your penis, vagina, rectum, or mouth came into contact with another person's penis, vagina, rectum, or mouth? and (4) Have you ever had a sexually transmitted infection? These questions provide the minimum information needed to initiate a risk assessment. A positive response to any of these questions should be followed by an in-depth exploration of issues related to the identified risk.

Specific assessments are needed for an individual who has been diagnosed with HIV infection. Subjective and objective data that should be obtained are presented in Table 15-13. Repeated nursing assessments over time are essential because people's circumstances change. Early recognition and treatment can slow the progression of HIV infection and prevent new infections. A complete history and thorough systems review can help identify and address problems in a timely manner.

PLANNING

Nursing interventions can help the patient (1) adhere to drug regimens; (2) adopt a healthy lifestyle that includes avoiding exposure to other sexually transmitted infections and blood-borne diseases; (3) protect others from HIV; (4) maintain or develop healthy and supportive relationships; (5) maintain activities and productivity; (6) explore spiritual issues; (7) come to terms with issues related to disease, disability, and death; and (8) cope with symptoms caused by HIV and its treatments.

NURSING IMPLEMENTATION

The complexity of HIV disease is related to its chronic nature. As with most chronic and infectious diseases, primary preven-

ETHICAL/LEGAL DILEMMAS

Individual Versus Public Health Protection

Situation

A nurse in a community clinic is having a follow-up visit with V.T., a 38-year-old woman, who was found to have HIV during her annual examination 2 wk ago. During the visit, V.T. discloses that she has been verbally and physically abused by her partner. V.T. also indicates that she had not yet told her partner about the HIV diagnosis because she is afraid that he will hurt her. She has not used any protection during sex with him since she learned of her test results because she suspects he infected her.

Ethical/Legal Points for Consideration

- You face a conflict between preventing further harm to V.T. (possible increase in intimate partner violence), providing care to her partner (his need for an HIV test, diagnosis, and treatment), and protecting the public health (potential spread of HIV infection to her partner or from her partner to others in the community). Patient teaching and support are paramount because your primary obligation is to the patient.
- Because relevant law varies from state to state, your first step is to be familiar with your state law concerning mandated reporting for domestic partner abuse and infectious diseases.
- Laws regarding protection of privacy in HIV testing are federal and apply everywhere.
- In many states, reporting domestic abuse is mandatory only when the abuse is actually witnessed by the reporter or when the immediate effects of the abuse (e.g., wounds, contusions, broken bones) are witnessed.
- You should be familiar with crisis counseling services for V.T. and offer her the following advice: collect and stash a set of car keys or taxi money in a safe place, keep a bag packed and hidden or even stored in a locker somewhere accessible, develop a code phrase to use with a friend or family member to call for help, keep a cell phone charged and hidden with the money.

Discussion Questions

1. Within the parameters of your state's requirements for reportable conditions, how can you protect the patient's confidentiality to prevent further intimate partner violence?
2. What services are offered by your state to notify a partner without disclosing the source patient's name? How would V.T. access those services in your state?
3. How can you protect the partner from possible infection while also protecting V.T. from further violence?
4. How can you best address the issue of intimate partner violence? What resources would V.T. have in your community?
5. Discuss the benefits of universal, voluntary testing in light of V.T.'s case.

tion and health promotion are the most effective health care strategies. When prevention fails, disease results. Table 15-14 presents a synopsis of nursing goals, assessments, and interventions at each stage of HIV infection.

HEALTH PROMOTION. Even with recent successes in HIV treatment, prevention is the only way to eventually control the epidemic. In addition, health promotion encourages early detection of the disease so that, if primary prevention has failed, early intervention can be initiated.

Prevention of HIV Infection. HIV infection is preventable. Avoiding or modifying risky behaviors is the most effective prevention tool.[32] Nursing interventions to prevent disease transmission are based on an assessment of the individual's risky behaviors. Although changing behaviors is difficult, encourage the patient to adopt safer, healthier, and less risky behaviors. Provide culturally sensitive, language appropriate, and age-specific teaching and behavior change counseling. Nurses who are comfortable with and know how to talk about

HEALTHY PEOPLE

Prevention and Early Detection of HIV

- Increase safe sexual practices, including condom use.
- Decrease equipment sharing among IV drug users.
- Increase clinician skills to assess for risk factors for HIV infection, recommend HIV testing, and provide counseling for behavior change.
- Make voluntary HIV testing a routine part of health care.
- Increase access to new HIV testing technologies, especially rapid testing.
- Increase access to HIV testing facilities in traditional health care settings, as well as in alternative sites such as drug and alcohol treatment facilities and community-based organizations.
- Increase risk assessment and individualized behavior change messages to people with HIV to prevent new infections.
- Decrease perinatal HIV infection by offering voluntary HIV testing as a part of routine prenatal care.
- Provide counseling and appropriate HIV therapy to those who are infected.

TABLE 15-13 NURSING ASSESSMENT

HIV-Infected Patient

Subjective Data

Important Health Information

Past health history: Route of infection; hepatitis; other sexually transmitted infections; tuberculosis; frequent viral, fungal, and/or bacterial infections

Medications: Use of immunosuppressive drugs

Functional Health Patterns

Health perception–health management: Perception of illness; alcohol and drug use; malaise

Nutritional-metabolic: Weight loss, anorexia, nausea, vomiting; lesions, bleeding, or ulcerations of lips, mouth, gums, tongue, or throat; sensitivity to acidic, salty, or spicy foods; difficulty swallowing; abdominal cramping; skin rashes, lesions, or color changes; wounds that don't heal

Elimination: Persistent diarrhea, change in character of stools; painful urination, low back pain

Activity-exercise: Chronic fatigue, muscle weakness, difficulty walking; cough, shortness of breath

Sleep-rest: Insomnia, night sweats, fatigue

Cognitive-perceptual: Headaches, stiff neck, chest pain, rectal pain, retrosternal pain; blurred vision, photophobia, diplopia, loss of vision; hearing impairment; confusion, forgetfulness, attention deficit, changes in mental status, memory loss, personality changes; paresthesias, hypersensitivity in feet, pruritus

Role-relationship: Support system(s), career or job, financial resources

Sexuality-reproductive: Lesions on genitalia (internal or external), pruritus or burning in vagina, penis, or anus; painful sexual intercourse, rectal pain or bleeding, changes in menstruation, vaginal or penile discharge; use of birth control measures, pregnancies, desire for future children

Coping–stress tolerance: Stress levels, previous losses, coping patterns, self-concept; social withdrawal

Objective Data

General

Lethargy, persistent fever, lymphadenopathy, peripheral wasting, fat deposits in truncal areas and upper back

Integumentary

Decreased skin turgor, dry skin, diaphoresis; pallor, cyanosis; lesions, eruptions, discolorations, bruises of skin or mucous membranes; vaginal or perianal excoriation; alopecia; delayed wound healing

Eyes

Presence of exudates, retinal lesions or hemorrhage, papilledema

Respiratory

Tachypnea, dyspnea, intercostal retractions; crackles, wheezing, productive or nonproductive cough

Cardiovascular

Pericardial friction rub, murmur, bradycardia, tachycardia

Gastrointestinal

Mouth lesions, including blisters (HSV), white-gray patches (*Candida* infection), painless white lesions on lateral aspect of the tongue (hairy leukoplakia), discolorations (KS); gingivitis, tooth decay or loosening; redness or white patchy lesions of throat; vomiting, diarrhea, incontinence; rectal lesions; hyperactive bowel sounds, abdominal masses, hepatosplenomegaly

Musculoskeletal

Muscle wasting, weakness

Neurologic

Ataxia, tremors, lack of coordination; sensory loss; slurred speech, aphasia; memory loss, peripheral neuropathy, apathy, agitation, depression, inappropriate behavior; decreasing levels of consciousness, seizures, paralysis, coma

Reproductive

Genital lesions or discharge, abdominal tenderness secondary to pelvic inflammatory disease (PID)

Possible Diagnostic Findings

Positive HIV antibody assay (EIA, confirmed by WB or IFA); detectable viral load; ↓ $CD4^+$ T cell count, ↓ WBC count, lymphopenia, anemia, thrombocytopenia; electrolyte imbalances; abnormal liver function tests; ↑ cholesterol, triglycerides, and blood glucose

EIA, Enzyme immunoassay; *HSV,* herpes simplex virus; *IFA,* immunofluorescence assay; *KS,* Kaposi sarcoma; *WB,* Western blot; *WBC,* white blood cell.

TABLE 15-14 PATIENT & CAREGIVER TEACHING GUIDE

Antiretroviral Drugs

Resistance to antiretroviral drugs is a major problem in treating HIV infection. Include the following instructions when teaching the patient and/or caregiver to decrease the risk of developing resistance.

1. Discuss options with your health care provider to find the best regimen for you. Your provider should order at least three different antiretroviral drugs from at least two different drug groups.
2. Know the drugs you are taking and how to take them (some have to be taken with food, some must be taken on an empty stomach, some cannot be taken together). If you do not understand, ask. Have your nurse write the instructions clearly for you.
3. Take the full dose prescribed, and take it on schedule. If you cannot take the drug because of side effects or other problems, report it to your health care provider immediately.
4. Take all of your medications as prescribed. Do not quit taking one drug while continuing the others. If you cannot tolerate even one of your drugs, talk to your health care provider, who will recommend a way to deal with the side effects or a new set of drugs.
5. Many antiretroviral drugs interact with other drugs, including a number of common drugs you can buy without a prescription. Be sure your health care provider and pharmacist know all of the drugs that you are taking, and do not take any new drugs without checking for possible interactions.
6. The goals of antiretroviral therapy are to decrease the amount of virus in your blood (your viral load) and to keep your CD4$^+$ T cell count high. The best results reduce your viral load below detectable levels and keep your CD4$^+$ T cell count high. Most health care providers do routine laboratory work every 3 to 6 mo whether you are taking antiretroviral agents or not.
7. Two to 4 wk after you start on drug therapy (or change your therapy), your health care provider will test your viral load to find out how the drugs are working.
   - Your viral load is reported in absolute numbers or in logarithms (a mathematical concept). All you need to know is that you want to see the viral load drop. If reports are in logarithms, you want to see a drop of at least 1 unit, which means that 90% of your viral load has been eliminated. If your viral load drops by 2 units, your viral load will have decreased by 95%. If your viral load drops by 3 units, your viral load will have decreased by 99%.
   - Your CD4$^+$ T cell count is reported in absolute numbers or percentages. It is best for your CD4$^+$ T cell count to be above 500 to 600 cells/μL. If reported in percentages, you would like your CD4$^+$ T cell value to be above 14%.
8. An undetectable viral load means that the amount of virus is extremely low and HIV cannot be found in the blood using current testing technology. It does not mean that the virus is gone because the virus can be in lymph nodes and organs that blood tests cannot detect. It also does not mean that you are no longer able to transmit HIV to others. You will need to continue protecting all of your sexual and drug-using partners from HIV.

sensitive topics such as sexuality and drug use are best prepared to provide prevention teaching.

A wide variety of activities can reduce the risk of HIV infection. Individuals will choose the methods that best fit their needs and circumstances. Prevention techniques can be divided into *safe sexual activities* (those that eliminate risk) and *risk-reducing sexual activities* (those that decrease, but do not eliminate, risk).

The goal is to develop safer, healthier, and less risky behaviors. The more consistently and correctly prevention methods are used, the more effective they are in preventing HIV infection. It is also a good idea to use a combination of prevention

EVIDENCE-BASED PRACTICE

Applying the Evidence

As a nurse in an HIV clinic, you are counseling P.S., a 25-year-old gay man, and his partner. P.S. is on antiretroviral therapy. His viral load is very low, and his CD4$^+$ T cell count is normal. He tells you that since the medications are working, he and his partner (who is not infected with HIV) have decided to forgo the use of condoms. They tell you that they are in a committed relationship and have no other partners. You spend time explaining to both of them the risks of unprotected sex: his partner may get infected with HIV even with a low viral load (although the risk is decreased).

Best Available Evidence	Clinician Expertise	Patient Preferences and Values
One of the best ways to prevent HIV transmission from an infected person to an uninfected person is by using condoms.	You know that risk-reducing sexual activities in this situation include the continued use of condoms. However, you also know that a very low viral load decreases the risk of HIV transmission.	After listening, the patient tells you that he and his partner do not like using condoms. They both understand the risks and believe that while the medications are working, the risk is low and worth it.

Your Decision and Action

As his nurse, you respect his decision. You remind him of the importance of maintaining his medication regimen and attending his appointments at the clinic. You explain that this will be even more important now to keep P.S.'s infection under control.

Reference for Evidence

Cohen MS, McCauley M, Gamble RT: HIV treatment as prevention and HPTN 052, *Curr Opin HIV AIDS* 7(2):99, 2012.

methods (e.g., using condoms and decreasing the number of sex partners) to increase the prevention effect.

Decreasing Risks Related to Sexual Intercourse. *Safe sexual activities* eliminate the risk of exposure to HIV in semen and vaginal secretions.[33] Abstaining from all sexual activity is an effective way to accomplish this goal, but there are safe options for those who cannot or do not wish to abstain. Limiting sexual behavior to activities in which the mouth, penis, vagina, or rectum does not come into contact with a partner's mouth, penis, vagina, or rectum eliminates contact with blood, semen, or vaginal secretions. Safe activities include masturbation, mutual masturbation ("hand job"), and other activities that meet the "no contact" requirements. *Insertive sex* between partners who are not infected with HIV and not at risk of becoming infected with HIV is also considered safe.

Risk-reducing sexual activities decrease the risk of contact with HIV through the use of barriers. Barriers should be used when engaging in insertive sexual activity (oral, vaginal, or anal) with a partner who has HIV or whose HIV status is not known. The most commonly used barrier is the male condom. The *efficacy* (protection provided under ideal circumstances) of male condoms is essentially 100%. Their *effectiveness* (protection provided in actual or "real life" circumstances) is better than 90%. Male condoms can be used for protection during anal, vaginal, and oral intercourse. (The proper use and placement of the male condom are presented in eTable 15-4 on the website for this chapter.)

Female condoms provide an alternative to male condoms. Female condom efficacy is also close to 100%, and effectiveness

INFORMATICS IN PRACTICE

Use of Internet and Mobile Devices to Manage HIV

- The Internet offers resources and support for patients that can assist them in coping with their illness and educate them about signs and symptoms of serious illness.
- By monitoring their health and quickly spotting warning signs of serious illnesses, patients are able to alert their physicians and receive earlier treatment.
- These systems can help the patient manage antiretroviral therapy by sending medication reminders by text or e-mail.

is 94% to 97% against HIV and other sexually transmitted infections. (The proper use and placement of the female condom are presented in eTable 15-5 on the website for this chapter.) In addition, squares of latex (known as dental dams) can be used to cover the external female genitalia during oral sexual activity.

Decreasing Risks Related to Drug Use. Drug use, including alcohol and tobacco, is harmful. It can cause immunosuppression, poor nutrition, and a host of psychosocial problems, but drug use does not cause HIV infection. The major risk for HIV related to using drugs involves sharing equipment or having unsafe sexual experiences while under the influence of drugs. Basic risk reduction rules are (1) do not use drugs; (2) if you use drugs, do not share equipment; and (3) do not have sexual intercourse when under the influence of any drug (including alcohol) that impairs decision making.[34]

The safest method is to abstain from drugs, but this may not be a viable option for users who are not prepared to quit or have no access to drug treatment services. The risk of HIV for these individuals can be eliminated if they do not share equipment. Injecting equipment ("works") includes needles, syringes, cookers (spoons or bottle caps used to mix the drug), cotton, and rinse water. Equipment used to snort (straws) or smoke (pipes) drugs can also be contaminated with blood and should not be shared.

Access to sterile equipment is an important risk elimination tactic. Some communities have needle and syringe exchange programs (NSEPs) that provide sterile equipment in exchange for used equipment. Opposition to these programs is related to the fear that access to injecting supplies will increase drug use. However, studies have shown that, in communities with NSEPs, drug use does not increase, rates of HIV and other blood-borne infections are controlled, and an overall cost benefit results.[35] Cleaning equipment before use can also reduce risk by decreasing the chance of blood contact. (The proper use of drug equipment is presented in eTable 15-6 on the website for this chapter.)

Decreasing Risks of Perinatal Transmission. The best way to prevent HIV infection in infants is to prevent HIV infection in women. Women who are already infected with HIV should be asked about their reproductive desires. Those who choose not to have children need to have family planning methods discussed in detail. Should they become pregnant, abortion may be desired and should be discussed in conjunction with other options, including the possibility of maintaining the pregnancy and using ART to decrease the risk of transmission. If HIV-infected pregnant women are appropriately treated during pregnancy, the rate of perinatal transmission can be decreased from 25% to less than 2%.[24] ART has significantly decreased the risk for infants born to HIV-infected women, and more of these women are now becoming mothers. The current standard of care is for all women who are pregnant or contemplating pregnancy to be counseled about HIV, routinely offered access to voluntary HIV-antibody testing, and, if infected, offered optimal ART.[24]

Decreasing Risks at Work. The risk of infection from occupational exposure to HIV is small but real. OSHA requires employers to protect workers from exposure to blood and other potentially infectious materials (see Table 15-8). Precautions and safety devices decrease the risk of direct contact with blood and body fluids. Should exposure to HIV-infected fluids occur, **postexposure prophylaxis (PEP)** with combination ART can significantly decrease the risk of infection.[23] The need for timely treatment and counseling makes it even more critical for nurses to report all blood exposures.

HIV Testing. An estimated 21% of people living with HIV in the United States are not aware that they are infected. People who do not know they are infected are more likely to transmit the infection to others.[36,37] The CDC recommends universal, voluntary testing for all people ages 13 to 64 regardless of the patient's risk or perceived risk. The CDC recommends an "opt out" process in which the patient is given the opportunity to decline a test, but it is offered as "routine." The goal is to normalize the test, decrease the stigma related to HIV testing, find hidden cases, get infected individuals into care, and prevent new cases of infection.[38]

ACUTE INTERVENTION

Early Intervention. Early intervention after detection of HIV infection can promote health and limit disability. The nursing assessment in HIV disease should focus on early detection of symptoms, opportunistic diseases, and psychosocial problems[39] (see Tables 15-13 and eTable 15-7).

Initial Response to Diagnosis of HIV. Reactions to an HIV diagnosis are similar to the reactions of people who are diagnosed with any life-threatening, debilitating, or chronic illness. They include anxiety, panic, fear, depression, denial, hopelessness, anger, and guilt.[40] Unfortunately, all these emotions are overlaid with the stigma and discrimination that continue to pervade societal reactions to HIV. Many of these reactions are also seen in the patient's family members, friends, and caregivers. As time passes, patients and their loved ones will be confronted with complex treatment decisions; feelings of loss, anger, powerlessness, depression, and grief; social isolation; the possibility of death; and/or thoughts of suicide.

Antiretroviral Therapy. ART can significantly slow the clinical progression of HIV.[28] However, treatment regimens can be complex, the drugs have side effects, ART does not work for everyone, and it is expensive. These factors can contribute to problems with adherence to treatment, a dangerous situation because of the high risk of developing drug resistance.

As a nurse, you are often the person who works most closely with patients who are trying to cope with these issues. Interventions include teaching about (1) advantages and disadvantages of new treatments, (2) dangers of poor adherence to therapeutic regimens, (3) how and when to take each drug, (4) drug interactions to avoid, and (5) side effects that must be reported to the health care provider. Table 15-14 provides guidance for patient teaching in these areas.

Guidelines on when and how to initiate ART are based on the degree of immune suppression.[28] Issues to consider when selecting an initial drug regimen include the ability of the patient's HIV to resist specific drugs (assessed by the resistance tests discussed on p. 235), potential medication side effects, existing co-morbidities, and dosing schedules. This is a critical

TABLE 15-15 PATIENT & CAREGIVER TEACHING GUIDE

Improving Adherence to Antiretroviral Therapy

The following are strategies that you can use to improve a patient's adherence to using antiretroviral therapy:

- Determine whether the patient understands the importance of adherence and is ready to start therapy.
- Provide teaching on medication dosing.
- Review potential side effects of drugs.
- Assure the patient that side effects can be treated. If not, medication regimens can be changed.
- Use teaching and memory aids, including pictures, pillboxes, and calendars.
- Engage family and friends in the teaching process. Solicit their support to help the patient take treatment.
- Simplify regimens, dosing, and food requirements as much as possible.
- Use a team of nurses, physicians, pharmacists, case managers, and mental health and peer counselors to support the patient.
- Help the patient integrate the medication regimen into his or her typical life activities and work schedules.

Modified from Centers for Disease Control and Prevention: Guidelines for the use of antiretroviral agents in HIV-1-infected adults and adolescents, 2012. Retrieved from *http://aidsinfo.nih.gov*.

decision because the first treatment regimen is generally the patient's best chance for success. However, the most important consideration for initiating therapy is patient readiness.[39]

Adherence to ART is a critical component of successful drug therapy for people with HIV infection. Nurses are uniquely prepared to provide assistance with adherence to the drug regimen[39,41] (Table 15-15). Taking drugs as prescribed (right dose and time) is important for all drug therapy, but with HIV infection, missing even a few doses can lead to drug resistance. Patients can be helped to adhere to difficult treatment regimens with electronic reminders, beepers, timers on pillboxes, and calendars. Group support and individual counseling can also help, but the best approach is to learn about the patient's life and assist with problem solving related to taking medications within the confines of that life.

Delaying Disease Progression. HIV disease progression may be delayed by promoting a healthy immune system, whether the patient chooses to use ART or not. Useful interventions for HIV-infected patients include (1) getting nutritional support to maintain lean body mass and ensure appropriate levels of vitamins and micronutrients; (2) moderating or eliminating alcohol, tobacco, and drug use; (3) keeping up to date with recommended vaccines; (4) getting adequate rest and exercise; (5) reducing stress; (6) avoiding exposure to new infectious agents; (7) accessing mental health counseling; (8) getting involved in support groups and community activities; and (9) developing a consistent relationship with health care providers, including attendance at regular appointments.

Teach patients to recognize symptoms that may indicate disease progression and/or drug side effects so that prompt medical care can be initiated. Table 15-16 provides an overview of symptoms that patients should report.

Acute Exacerbations. Chronic diseases are characterized by acute exacerbations of recurring problems. This is especially true in HIV disease where infections, cancers, debility, and psychosocial or economic issues may interact to overwhelm the patient's ability to cope. Nursing care becomes more complex as the patient's immune system deteriorates and new problems arise to compound existing difficulties.[39] When opportunistic diseases or difficult treatment side effects develop, symptom management, teaching, and emotional support are needed.

Nursing care can help prevent the many opportunistic diseases associated with HIV infection. The best way to prevent opportunistic disease is to ensure that the patient is adhering to an effective ART regimen and, if appropriate, taking prophylactic medications for opportunistic infections. Should an opportunistic disease occur, nursing care can be an essential part of helping the patient adhere to medications and providing supportive care specific to the opportunistic disease. For example, if the patient has *Pneumocystis jiroveci* pneumonia (PCP) (Fig. 15-8), nursing interventions can ensure adequate oxygenation. If the patient has cryptococcal meningitis, an important nursing concern is maintaining a safe environment for a confused patient.

TABLE 15-16 PATIENT & CAREGIVER TEACHING GUIDE

Signs and Symptoms HIV Patients Need to Report

Teach the patient with HIV infection and the caregiver to report the following signs and symptoms.

Report Immediately

- Any change in level of consciousness: lethargic, hard to arouse, unable to be aroused, unresponsive, unconscious
- Headache accompanied by nausea and vomiting, changes in vision, changes in ability to perform coordinated activities, or after any head trauma
- Vision changes: blurry or black areas in vision field, new floaters, double vision
- Persistent shortness of breath related to activity and not relieved by a short rest period
- Nausea and vomiting accompanied by abdominal pain
- Vomiting blood
- Dehydration: unable to eat or drink because of nausea, diarrhea, or mouth lesions; severe diarrhea or vomiting; dizziness when standing
- Yellow discoloration of the skin
- Any bleeding from the rectum that is not related to hemorrhoids or trauma (e.g., from anal sexual intercourse)
- Pain in the flank with fever and inability to urinate for more than 6 hr
- Blood in the urine
- New onset of weakness in any part of the body, new onset of numbness that is not obviously related to pressure, new onset of difficulty speaking
- Chest pain not obviously related to cough
- Seizures
- New rash accompanied by fever
- New oral lesions accompanied by fever
- Severe depression, anxiety, hallucinations, delusions, or thoughts of causing danger to self or others

Report the Following Signs and Symptoms Within 24 Hr

- New or different headache; constant headache not relieved by over-the-counter medication
- Headache accompanied by fever, nasal congestion, or cough
- Burning, itching, or discharge from the eyes
- New or productive cough
- Vomiting 2-3 times a day
- Vomiting accompanied by fever
- New, significant, or watery diarrhea (more than 6 times a day)
- Painful urination, bloody urine, urethral discharge
- Significant new rash (widespread; painful; or following a path down the leg or arm, around the chest, or on the face)
- Difficulty eating or drinking because of mouth lesions
- Vaginal discharge, pain, or itching

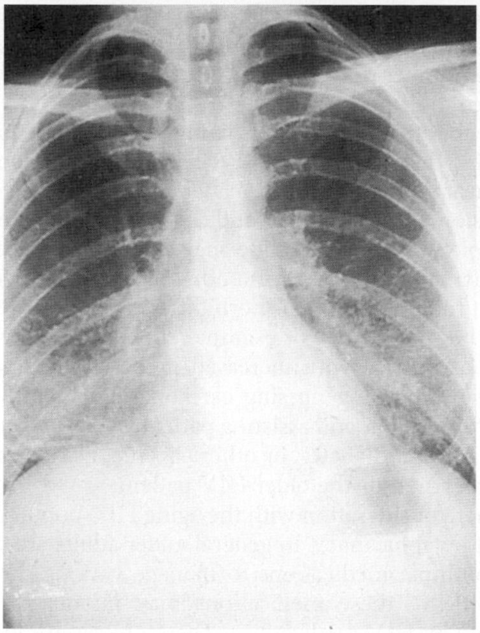

FIG. 15-8 Chest x-ray showing interstitial infiltrates as the result of *Pneumocystis jiroveci* pneumonia.

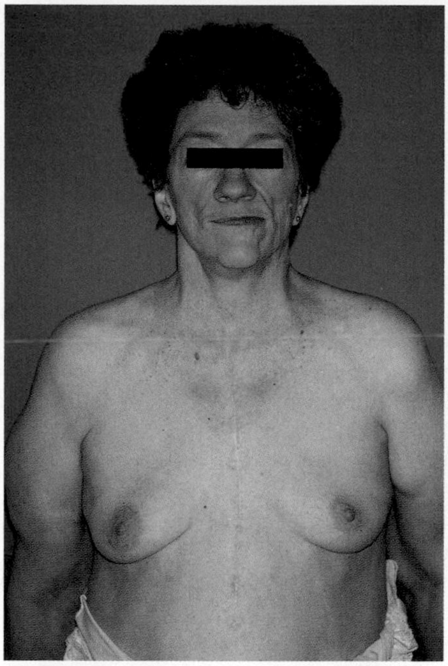

FIG. 15-9 Lipodystrophy manifestations.

AMBULATORY AND HOME CARE. HIV infection has no cure, continues for life, causes physical disability, and contributes to impaired health. In many cases it can lead to death. HIV infection affects the entire range of a person's life from physical health to social, emotional, economic, and spiritual well-being.

Stigma of HIV. HIV-infected patients share problems experienced by all individuals with chronic diseases, but these problems are exacerbated by negative social constructs surrounding HIV.[42] HIV-infected people may be thought to lack control over urges to have sex or use drugs. Some people then conclude that people with HIV brought the disease on themselves and deserve to be sick. Behaviors associated with HIV infection are viewed by some as immoral (e.g., homosexuality, having many sexual partners) and are sometimes illegal (e.g., using drugs, sex work). The fact that infected individuals can transmit HIV to others creates fear, which leads to stigma and discrimination in all facets of life.

In the United States, HIV-infected people have lost jobs, homes, and insurance, although these forms of discrimination are prohibited by the Americans with Disabilities Act (ADA).[43] HIV-related stigma is a global problem that is often more severe for women. Discrimination can lead to social isolation, dependence, frustration, low self-image, loss of control, and economic pressures.

Disease and Drug Side Effects. Physical problems related to HIV or its treatment can interfere with the patient's ability to maintain a desired lifestyle. HIV-infected patients frequently experience anxiety, fear, depression, diarrhea, peripheral neuropathy, pain, nausea, vomiting, and fatigue. Nursing interventions for these symptoms are similar to what they would be for the patient who does not have HIV infection. For example, nursing management of diarrhea includes helping patients collect specimens, recommending dietary changes, encouraging fluid and electrolyte replacement, instructing the patient about skin care, and managing skin breakdown around the perianal area. Nursing approaches for fatigue in HIV include teaching patients to assess fatigue patterns; determine contributing factors; set activity priorities; conserve energy; schedule rest periods; exercise regularly; and avoid substances such as caffeine, nicotine, alcohol, and other drugs that may disturb sleep.

Some HIV-infected patients, especially those who have been infected and on ART for a long time, develop a set of metabolic disorders that include changes in body shape (fat deposits in the abdomen, upper back, and breasts along with fat loss in the arms, legs, and face) because of lipodystrophy (Fig. 15-9), hyperlipidemia (elevated triglycerides, elevated low-density lipoproteins, and decreased high-density lipoproteins), insulin resistance and hyperglycemia, bone disease (osteoporosis, osteopenia, avascular necrosis), lactic acidosis, renal disease, and cardiovascular disease.[31]

It is still not clear why these disorders develop, but it is probably a combination of factors such as long-term infection with HIV, side effects of ART, genetic predisposition, and chronic stress. Management of metabolic disorders focuses on detecting problems early, dealing with symptoms, and helping the patient cope with emerging problems and changes to treatment regimens. It is important to recognize and treat these problems early, especially because cardiovascular disease and lactic acidosis are potentially fatal complications.

A frequent first intervention is to change ART medications because some drugs are more often associated with these disorders. Lipid abnormalities are generally treated with lipid-lowering drugs (see Table 34-5), dietary changes, and exercise. Insulin resistance is treated with hypoglycemic drugs and weight loss. Bone disease may be improved with exercise, dietary changes, and calcium and vitamin D supplements.

End-of-Life Care. Despite new developments in the treatment of HIV infection, many patients eventually experience disease progression, disability, and death. Sometimes these occur because treatments do not work for the patient. Sometimes the patient's HIV becomes resistant to all available drug therapies. In addition, ART is now allowing people living with HIV to live longer and to develop diseases of aging, such as cardiovascular and endocrine problems that lead to death.

Nursing care during the terminal phase of any disease should focus on keeping the patient comfortable, facilitating emotional and spiritual acceptance of the finite nature of life, helping the patient's significant others deal with grief and loss, and maintaining a safe environment. As a nurse, you are the pivotal care provider during this phase of illness, whether at home, through hospice, or in a health care facility.[39] (End-of-life care is discussed in Chapter 10.)

EVALUATION

The expected outcomes are that the patient at risk for HIV infection will

- Analyze personal risk factors
- Develop and implement a personal plan to decrease risks
- Get tested for HIV

The expected outcomes are that the patient with HIV infection will

- Describe basic aspects of the effects of HIV on the immune system
- Compare and contrast various treatment options for HIV disease
- Work with a team of health care providers to achieve optimal health
- Prevent transmission of HIV to others

GERONTOLOGIC CONSIDERATIONS

HIV INFECTION

The number of older adults who have HIV disease is increasing because (1) HIV treatment has been effective in reducing the number of deaths from HIV-related opportunistic infections and (2) people 60 and older are being infected at increasing rates. The number of people over the age of 60 living with HIV is expected to grow.

Remember that older people living with HIV are susceptible to the same diseases as non-HIV-infected older people. These include heart disease, cancer, diabetes, bone disease, arthritis, hypertension, kidney disease, and cognitive impairment. However, people with HIV infection may experience these diseases at an earlier age (compared with non-HIV-infected people) and may be at higher risk of co-morbidities related to the medications used to treat HIV. For example, some of the HIV medications are associated with increased lipids and altered insulin metabolism. Focusing nursing care on early identification of these complications, and assisting patients in reducing their risk for heart disease, diabetes, or other chronic disease, are critical aspects of caring for the older HIV patient.

Another consideration with the aging HIV population is the impact of polypharmacy. In general, older adults are often prescribed multiple medications to manage various chronic diseases. Some of these medications may interact with or be potentiated by HIV medications. Therefore careful monitoring and assessment of possible drug interactions is important when providing care to this population.

Older adults may be ashamed and hesitate to tell anyone that they have an HIV infection. This may make it difficult for them to get the appropriate health care and support. As a nurse, you need to recognize that HIV is a chronic disease that will affect more and more older adults and be prepared to help the older person who is living with HIV infection.

CASE STUDY

HIV Infection

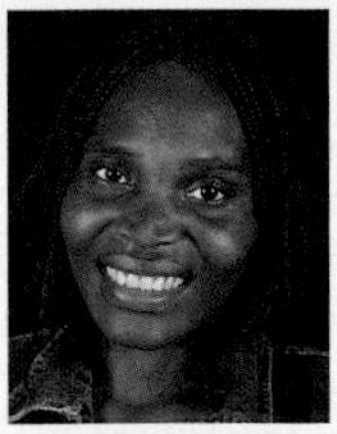

iStockphoto/Thinkstock

Patient Profile

J.N., a 35-year-old African American woman, was admitted to the hospital in respiratory distress. AIDS and *Pneumocystis jiroveci* pneumonia (PCP) were both diagnosed 2 days ago.

Subjective Data

- Seen by a physician 6 years ago for pain behind the sternum and difficulty swallowing, diagnosed as esophageal candidiasis; positive HIV-antibody test at that time
- Has consistently refused ART because, "We can't afford it"
- Married to Jim, a former IV drug user, for 15 years until his recent death from AIDS-related complications
- Has two children, ages 8 and 10; neither has been tested for HIV infection
- Experiences fatigue and frequent oral and vaginal candidiasis outbreaks
- Expresses concern about the welfare of her children, who are at home with her sister, and says, "Maybe I should take better care of myself for them"

Objective Data

Physical Examination

- 5 ft 6 in tall, 100 lb, temperature 100.4° F (38° C), O_2 saturation 92% on 3 L of O_2 via nasal cannula

Laboratory Studies

- $CD4^+$ T cell count 185 cells/μL
- Viral load 55,328 copies/μL
- Hematocrit 30%

Collaborative Care

- Trimethoprim/sulfamethoxazole
- Combination antiretroviral therapy: tenofovir and emtricitabine (Truvada), darunavir (Prezista), ritonavir (Norvir)

Discussion Questions

1. Why did J.N.'s initial medical problem (esophageal candidiasis) lead to an HIV test?
2. Why was trimethoprim/sulfamethoxazole ordered, and what are its common side effects?
3. What diagnostic criteria for AIDS are present in J.N.?
4. Is there a potential advantage to J.N.'s refusal to take antiretroviral drugs in the past? If so, why or why not?
5. Women often put their children's welfare first. What barriers could this cause for J.N.'s treatment? How can these problems be resolved?
6. ***Priority Decision:*** What priority teaching needs should be covered before J.N. is discharged from the hospital to return home? What referrals need to be made?
7. How can J.N. be helped to adhere to her medication schedule?
8. ***Priority Decision:*** What are the priority nursing interventions? What plans need to be made for continued nursing care after discharge?
9. ***Evidence-Based Practice:*** J.N. asks you if her kids should be tested. She is afraid of what the results may be. How should you respond?

evolve Answers available at *http://evolve.elsevier.com/Lewis/medsurg.*

BRIDGE TO NCLEX EXAMINATION

The number of the question corresponds to the same-numbered outcome at the beginning of the chapter.

1. Emerging infections can affect health care by *(select all that apply)*
   a. revealing antibiotic resistance.
   b. generating scientific discoveries.
   c. creating a strain on limited resources.
   d. challenging established medical traditions.
   e. limiting travel options for nursing personnel.
2. Which antibiotic-resistant organisms cannot be killed by normal hand soap?
   a. Vancomycin-resistant enterococci
   b. Methicillin-resistant *Staphylococcus aureus*
   c. Penicillin-resistant *Streptococcus pneumoniae*
   d. β-Lactamase–producing *Klebsiella pneumoniae*
3. Transmission of HIV from an infected individual to another most commonly occurs as a result of
   a. unprotected anal or vaginal sexual intercourse.
   b. low levels of virus in the blood and high levels of $CD4^+$ T cells.
   c. transmission from mother to infant during labor and delivery and breastfeeding.
   d. sharing of drug-using equipment, including needles, syringes, pipes, and straws.
4. During HIV infection
   a. the virus replicates mainly in B-cells before spreading to $CD4^+$ T cells.
   b. infection of monocytes may occur, but antibodies quickly destroy these cells.
   c. the immune system is impaired predominantly by the eventual widespread destruction of $CD4^+$ T cells.
   d. a long period of dormancy develops during which HIV cannot be found in the blood and there is little viral replication.
5. Which statements accurately describe HIV infection *(select all that apply)?*
   a. Untreated HIV infection has a predictable pattern of progression.
   b. Late chronic HIV infection is called acquired immunodeficiency syndrome (AIDS).
   c. Untreated HIV infection can remain in the early chronic stage for a decade or more.
   d. Untreated HIV infection usually remains in the early chronic stage for 1 year or less.
   e. Opportunistic diseases occur more often when the $CD4^+$ T cell count is high and the viral load is low.
6. A diagnosis of AIDS is made when an HIV-infected patient has
   a. a $CD4^+$ T cell count below 200/μL.
   b. a high level of HIV in the blood and saliva.
   c. lipodystrophy with metabolic abnormalities.
   d. oral hairy leukoplakia, an infection caused by Epstein-Barr virus.
7. Screening for HIV infection generally involves
   a. laboratory analysis of blood to detect HIV antigen.
   b. electrophoretic analysis for HIV antigen in plasma.
   c. laboratory analysis of blood to detect HIV antibodies.
   d. analysis of lymph tissues for the presence of HIV RNA.
8. Antiretroviral drugs are used to
   a. cure acute HIV infection.
   b. decrease viral RNA levels.
   c. treat opportunistic diseases.
   d. decrease pain and symptoms in terminal disease.
9. Opportunistic diseases in HIV infection
   a. are usually benign.
   b. are generally slow to develop and progress.
   c. occur in the presence of immunosuppression.
   d. are curable with appropriate drug interventions.
10. Which statement about metabolic side effects of ART is true *(select all that apply)?*
   a. These are annoying symptoms that are ultimately harmless.
   b. ART-related body changes include central fat accumulation and peripheral wasting.
   c. Lipid abnormalities include increases in triglycerides and decreases in high-density cholesterol.
   d. Insulin resistance and hyperlipidemia can be treated with drugs to control glucose and cholesterol.
   e. Compared to uninfected people, insulin resistance and hyperlipidemia are more difficult to treat in HIV-infected patients.
11. Which strategy can the nurse teach the patient to eliminate the risk of HIV transmission?
   a. Using sterile equipment to inject drugs
   b. Cleaning equipment used to inject drugs
   c. Taking zidovudine (AZT, ZDV, Retrovir) during pregnancy
   d. Using latex or polyurethane barriers to cover genitalia during sexual contact
12. What is the most appropriate nursing intervention to help an HIV-infected patient adhere to a treatment regimen?
   a. "Set up" a drug pillbox for the patient every week.
   b. Give the patient a video and a brochure to view and read at home.
   c. Tell the patient that the side effects of the drugs are bad but that they go away after a while.
   d. Assess the patient's routines and find adherence cues that fit into the patient's life circumstances.

1. a, b, c, d, 2. a, 3. a, 4. c, 5. a, b, c, 6. a, 7. c, 8. b, 9. c, 10. b, c, d, 11. a, 12. d

evolve

For rationales to these answers and even more NCLEX review questions, visit *http://evolve.elsevier.com/Lewis/medsurg.*

REFERENCES

1. World Health Organization: The top 10 causes of death. Retrieved from *www.who.int/mediacentre/factsheets.*
2. Huether SE, McCance K: *Understanding pathophysiology*, ed 5, St Louis, 2012, Mosby.
3. Pommerville JC: *Alcamo's fundamentals of microbiology*, ed 9, Sudsbury, Mass, 2011, Jones & Bartlett.
4. Centers for Disease Control and Prevention: Prion diseases. Retrieved from *www.cdc.gov/ncidod/dvrd/prions.*
5. United Nations Environmental Program: Environmental change and new infectious diseases. Retrieved from *www.grida.no.*
6. Hall-Baker PA, Groseclose SL, Jajosky RA, et al: Summary of notifiable diseases—United States 2009, *MMWR* 58:53, 2011.
7. World Health Organization: Disease outbreak news. Retrieved from *www.who.int.*
8. Centers for Disease Control and Prevention: Questions and answers about Ebola hemorrhagic fever, 2009. Retrieved from *www.cdc.gov/ncidod.*

9. Centers for Disease Control and Prevention: Reported cases of tuberculosis: United States, 2010. Retrieved from *www.cdc.gov/tb.*
10. Centers for Disease Control and Prevention: Measles update travel notice. Retrieved from *wwwnc.cdc.gov/travel.*
11. Mostofsky E, Lipsitch M, Regev-Yochay G: Is methicillin-resistant *Staphylococcus aureus* replacing methicillin-sensitive *S. aureus*? *J Antimicrob Chemother* 66(10):2199, 2011.
12. Calfee DP: Methicillin-resistant *Staphylococcus aureus* and vancomycin-resistant enterococci, and other gram-positives in healthcare, *Curr Opin Infect Dis*;25(4):385, 2012.
13. Centers for Disease Control and Prevention: Healthcare-associated infections: the burden. Retrieved from *www.cdc.gov/HAI.*
14. US Department of Health and Human Services Agency for Healthcare Research & Quality: Healthcare-associated infections. Retrieved from *www.ahrq.gov.*
*15. Centers for Disease Control and Prevention: Guidelines for isolation precautions: preventing transmission of infectious agents in healthcare settings, 2007. Retrieved from *www.cdc.gov/hicpac.*
*16. Centers for Disease Control and Prevention: Top CDC recommendations to prevent healthcare-associated infections. Retrieved from *www.cdc.gov/HAI.*
17. Mattison M, Marcantonio ER: Hospital care of the older adult. Retrieved from *www.uptodate.com.*
18. DeCock DM, Jaffe HW, Curran JW: Reflections on 30 years of AIDS, *Emerg Infect Dis* 17(6):1044, 2011.
19. Centers for Disease Control and Prevention: Basic information about HIV and AIDS. Retrieved from *www.cdc.gov/hiv.*
20. Prejean J, Song R, Hernandez A, et al: Estimated HIV incidence in the United States, 2006-2009, *PLOS ONE* 6(8):e17502, 2011.
21. Centers for Disease Control and Prevention: HIV surveillance report 2010, 22. Retrieved from *www.cdc.gov/hiv/surveillance/resources/reports.*
22. World Health Organization: HIV/AIDS data and statistics. *www.who.int/hiv/data/en.*
*23. Centers for Disease Control and Prevention: Updated US Public Health Service guidelines for the management of occupational exposures to HIV and recommendations for postexposure prophylaxis, 2005. Retrieved from *www.aidsinfo.nih.gov.*
*24. Centers for Disease Control and Prevention: US Public Health Service Task Force recommendations for use of antiretroviral drugs in pregnant HIV-1-infected women for maternal health and interventions to reduce perinatal HIV transmission in the United States—July 31, 2012. Retrieved from *www.aidsinfo.nih.gov.*
25. The HIV life cycle: fact sheet 106, New Mexico AIDS InfoNet, 2012. Retrieved from *www.aidsinfo.nih.gov.*
26. Cohen MS, Shaw GM, McMichael AJ, et al: Acute HIV-1 infection, *N Engl J Med* 364:1943, 2011.
27. Longo DL, Fauci AS, Kasper DL, et al: *Harrison's principles of internal medicine*, ed 18, New York, 2012, McGraw Hill.
*28. Centers for Disease Control and Prevention: Guidelines for the prevention and treatment of opportunistic infections in HIV-infected adults and adolescents, *MMWR* 58(RR-4), 2009. Retrieved from *www.aidsinfo.nih.gov.*
29. Centers for Disease Control and Prevention: Revised surveillance case definitions for HIV infection among adults, adolescents and children <18 months and for HIV infection and AIDS among children aged 18 months to <13 years—United States, 2008. Retrieved from *www.cdc.gov/mmwr.*
30. Luetkemeyer AF, Havlir DV, Currier JS: Complications of HIV disease and antiretroviral therapy, *Top Antivir Med* 20(2):48, 2012.
31. Buchbinder SP, Liu A: Pre-exposure prophylaxis and the promise of combination prevention approaches, *AIDS Behav* 25:S72, 2011.
*32. Centers for Disease Control and Prevention: Sexually transmitted diseases treatment guidelines, 2010. Retrieved from *www.cdc.gov/std/treatment/2010/default.htm.*
33. Fisher JD, Smith LR, Lenz EM: Secondary prevention of HIV in the United States: past, current, and future perspectives, *JAIDS* 55:106, 2010.
34. Drug use and HIV: fact sheet 154, New Mexico AIDS InfoNet, 2011. Retrieved from *www.aidsinfonet.org.*
35. Arkin E: Studies confirm effectiveness of harm reduction for people who inject drugs, *HIV AIDS Policy Law Rev* 15:29, 2011.
36. Gardner EM, McLees MP, Steiner JF, et al: The spectrum of engagement in HIV care and its relevance to test-and-treat strategies for prevention of HIV infection, *CID* 52:793, 2011.
37. Hunter E, Perry M, Leen C, et al: HIV testing: getting the message across—a survey of knowledge, attitudes, practice of non-HIV specialist physicians, *Postmed Grad J* 88(1036):59, 2012.
*38. Centers for Disease Control and Prevention: Revised guidelines for HIV testing of adults, adolescents, and pregnant women in health-care settings—September 22, 2006. Retrieved from *www.aidsinfo.nih.gov.*
39. Smith B: *ANAC's core curriculum HIV/AIDS nursing*, ed 3, Sudbury, Mass, 2010, Jones & Bartlett.
40. Nachega JB, Morroni C, Zuniga JM, et al: HIV-related stigma, isolation, and serostatus disclosure: a global survey of 2035 HIV-infected adults, *J Int Assoc Physicians AIDS Care* 3:172, 2012.
41. Enriquez M, McKinsey DS: Strategies to improve HIV treatment adherence in developed countries: clinical management at the individual level, *HIV/AIDS* 3:45, 2011.
42. Holzemer WL, Human S, Arudo J, et al: Exploring HIV stigma and quality of life for persons living with HIV infection, *J Assoc Nurses AIDS Care* 20:161, 2009. (Classic)
43. Americans with Disabilities Act, 42 U.S.C. §1201 et seq (1992 and 1994).

*Evidence-based information for clinical practice.

RESOURCES

AIDS Education and Training Centers National Resource Center
www.aidsetc.org
AIDS Info
http://aidsinfo.nih.gov
AIDS InfoNet
www.aidsinfonet.org
Association of Nurses in AIDS Care (ANAC)
www.nursesinaidscare.org
Centers for Disease Control and Prevention HIV/AIDS Information
www.cdc.gov/hiv
Journal of the Association of Nurses in AIDS Care
www.janacnet.org
National Association of People with AIDS (NAPWA)
www.napwa.org
National Minority AIDS Council (NMAC)
www.nmac.org
National Native American AIDS Prevention Center (NNAAPC)
www.nnaapc.org
Office of National AIDS Policy
www.whitehouse.gov/administration/eop/onap

CHAPTER

16

Never, never, never give up.
Winston Churchill

Cancer

Jormain Cady and Joyce A. Jackowski

evolve WEBSITE

http://evolve.elsevier.com/Lewis/medsurg

- NCLEX Review Questions
- Key Points
- Pre-Test
- Rationales for Bridge to NCLEX Examination questions
- Concept Map Creator
- Glossary
- Content Updates

eFigure

- eFig. 16-1: Normal cell differentiation

eTables

- eTable 16-1: Karnofsky Functional Performance Scale
- eTable 16-2: Katz Index of Independence in Activities of Daily Living
- eTable 16-3: Screening Guidelines for Early Detection of Cancer in Asymptomatic People
- eTable 16-4: Four *R*s of Radiobiology
- eTable 16-5: Uses of Radiation Therapy
- eTable 16-6: Precautions to Minimize Risks From Neutropenia
- eTable 16-7: Drug Therapy: Biologic and Targeted Therapy (Enhanced)

LEARNING OUTCOMES

1. Describe the prevalence, incidence, survival, and mortality rates of cancer in the United States.
2. Describe the processes involved in the biology of cancer.
3. Differentiate the three phases of cancer development.
4. Describe the role of the immune system related to cancer.
5. Differentiate among the various classifications of drugs used to treat cancer.
6. Discuss the role of the nurse in the prevention, detection, and diagnosis of cancer.
7. Explain the use of surgery, chemotherapy, radiation therapy, and biologic and targeted therapies in the treatment of cancer.
8. Identify the classifications of chemotherapy agents and methods of administration.
9. Differentiate between teletherapy (external beam radiation) and brachytherapy (internal radiation).
10. Describe the effects of radiation therapy and chemotherapy on normal tissues.
11. Identify the types and effects of biologic and targeted therapy agents.
12. Describe the nursing management of patients receiving chemotherapy, radiation therapy, and biologic and targeted therapy.
13. Describe nutritional therapy for patients with cancer.
14. Identify the various complications associated with advanced cancer.
15. Describe the psychologic support interventions for cancer patients, cancer survivors, and their caregivers.

KEY TERMS

biologic therapy, p. 271
bone marrow transplantation (BMT), p. 274
brachytherapy, p. 264
cancer, p. 247
carcinogens, p. 250
carcinoma in situ (CIS), p. 254
chemotherapy, p. 258
hematopoietic stem cell transplantation (HSCT), p. 274
histologic grading, p. 254
immunologic surveillance, p. 252
malignant neoplasms, p. 253
metastasis, p. 251
nadir, p. 265
oncogenes, p. 249
peripheral stem cell transplantation (PSCT), p. 274
protooncogenes, p. 249
radiation, p. 262
staging, p. 254
targeted therapy, p. 271
teletherapy, p. 263
tumor angiogenesis, p. 251
tumor-associated antigens (TAAs), p. 252
vesicants, p. 261

Cancer is a group of more than 200 diseases characterized by uncontrolled and unregulated growth of cells. Although cancer is often considered a disease of aging, with the majority of cases (77%) diagnosed in those over age 55 years, it occurs in people of all ages. An estimated 1,660,290 people in the United States are diagnosed annually with invasive carcinoma (excluding basal and squamous cell skin cancers).[1]

Overall the incidence of cancer has been declining since the 1990s. The mortality rate for the most common cancers (prostate, breast, lung, and colorectal) is also declining.[2] The incidences of many cancers, such as colorectal, lung, breast, and oropharyngeal cancers, have declined largely as a result of preventive efforts. However, the incidence of other types of cancers, such as leukemia, liver cancer, and skin cancers, has

Reviewed by Shelley Fess, RN, MS, AOCN, CRNI, Assistant Professor in Nursing, Monroe Community College, Rochester, New York.

TABLE 16-1 CANCER INCIDENCE BY SITE AND GENDER*

Male		Female	
Type	**%**	**Type**	**%**
Prostate	28	Breast	29
Lung	14	Lung	14
Colon/rectum	9	Colon/rectum	9
Urinary bladder	6	Uterus	6
Melanoma	5	Thyroid	6
Kidney and renal pelvis	5	Non-Hodgkin's lymphoma	4
Non-Hodgkin's lymphoma	4	Melanoma	4
Oropharynx	3	Ovary	3

Source: American Cancer Society: *Cancer facts and figures*, Atlanta, 2012, The Society. Retrieved from *www.cancer.org/acs/groups/content/@epidemiologysurveilance/documents/document/acspc-036845.pdf*.
*Numbers are estimates excluding basal and squamous cell skin cancers and carcinoma in situ.

TABLE 16-2 CANCER DEATHS BY SITE AND GENDER*

Male		Female	
Type	**%**	**Type**	**%**
Lung and bronchus	28	Lung and bronchus	26
Prostate	10	Breast	14
Colon/rectum	9	Colon/rectum	9
Pancreas	6	Pancreas	7
Liver and intrahepatic bile ducts	5	Ovary	5
		Leukemia	4
Leukemia	4	Non-Hodgkin's lymphoma	3
Esophagus	4	Uterus	3
Urinary bladder	3	Liver and intrahepatic bile ducts	2
Non-Hodgkin's lymphoma	3	Brain and other nervous system	2
Kidney and renal pelvis	3		

Source: American Cancer Society: *Cancer facts and figures*, Atlanta, 2012, The Society. Retrieved from *www.cancer.org/acs/groups/content/@epidemiologysurveilance/documents/document/acspc-031941.pdf*.
*Numbers are estimates based on 2008 statistics.

been on the rise. Notably, the incidence of melanoma rose faster than that for any other malignancy in the United States.[1]

Cancer incidence overall is higher in men than women. Gender differences in incidence and in death rates for specific cancers are presented in Tables 16-1 and 16-2 and the Gender Differences box. Although mortality rates from all cancers combined are on the decline, cancer is still the second most common cause of death in the United States (heart disease is the most common). However, in people less than 85 years of age, cancer is the leading cause of death. Annually about 580,350 Americans are expected to die as a result of cancer, which is more than 1500 people per day.[1]

Considerable progress has been made in controlling cancer for long periods. More than 13.7 million Americans are alive today who have a history of cancer. The overall 5-year survival rate is now 68% (19% increase over the past 30 years).[1] This statistic represents Americans living with cancer, including those who are disease free, in remission, or undergoing treatment. (Cancer survivors are discussed in this chapter on p. 281.)

Statistics are helpful in describing the scope of cancer as a public health problem, but they cannot describe the combined physiologic, psychologic, and social impact of cancer on individual patients and their caregivers and families. Considerable apprehension is associated with a cancer diagnosis, proportionately more than with other chronic diseases such as heart disease. Despite advances in treatment and care, a great deal of anxiety and fear continue to be associated with a diagnosis of cancer. Education of health care professionals and the public is essential to promote realistic attitudes about cancer and cancer treatment.

GENDER DIFFERENCES
Cancer

Men
- More men than women die from cancer-related deaths each year.
- Mortality rate from lung cancer is higher in men than in women.
- Esophageal cancer is more prevalent in men than in women.
- Cancer with the highest incidence among men is prostate cancer.
- Men are more likely to develop liver cancer than women.
- Head and neck cancer occurs more frequently in men than in women.
- Bladder cancer is at least three times more common in men than in women.

Women
- Cancer with the highest death rate among women is lung cancer.
- Nonsmoking women are at a greater risk than nonsmoking men of developing lung cancer.
- Cancer with the highest incidence among women is breast cancer.
- Thyroid cancer is more prevalent in women than in men.
- Women are less likely to have colon cancer screenings than men.

INFORMATICS IN PRACTICE
Managing Cancer Patients' Symptoms

- When patients arrive at some clinics, they are handed a tablet computer. While in the waiting room or chemotherapy infusion unit, with the touch of a finger they select the symptoms they have been experiencing.
- Health care providers can review the information and provide care aimed at managing the patient's specific symptoms.
- After the visit, the notes are stored in the patient's electronic health record. This system can assist with quality of care by determining if standards of care were followed.

You are in a strategic position to lead efforts at changing attitudes about cancer. Furthermore, you can also (1) assist individuals in decreasing their risk of cancer development, (2) help patients comply with cancer management regimens, and (3) support patients and their families as they cope with the effects of cancer and related treatment. You need to be knowledgeable about specific types of cancer, treatment options, management of side effects of therapy, and supportive therapies for cancer.

BIOLOGY OF CANCER

Two major dysfunctions in the process of cancer development are defective cell proliferation (growth) and defective cell differentiation.

Defect in Cell Proliferation

Normally, most tissues contain a population of undifferentiated cells known as stem cells. These stem cells ultimately differentiate and become mature, functioning cells of that tissue and only that tissue.

Cell proliferation originates in the stem cell and begins when the stem cell enters the cell cycle (Fig. 16-1). The time from

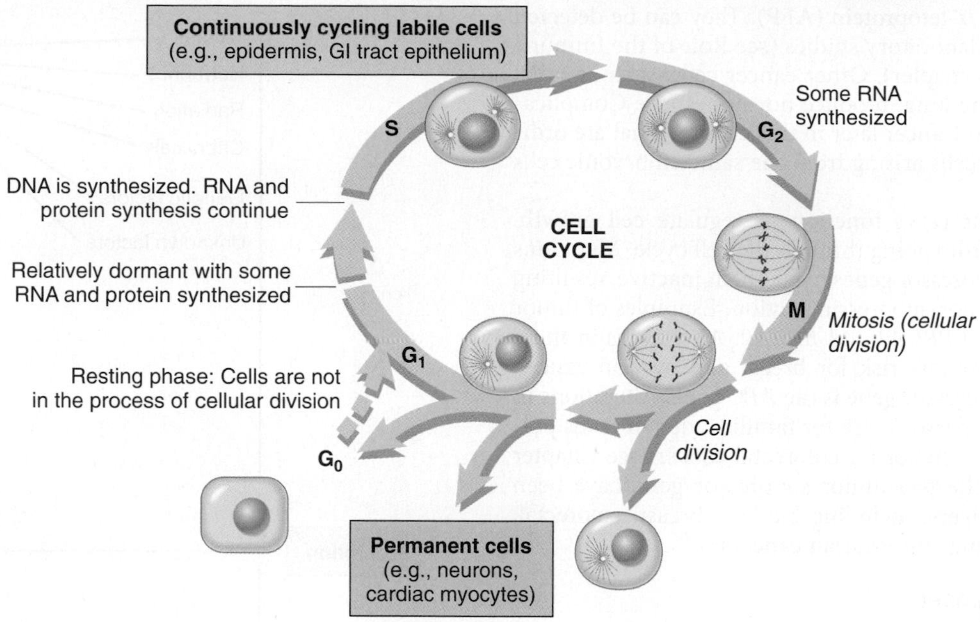

FIG. 16-1 Cell life cycle and metabolic activity. Generation time is the period from *M* phase to *M* phase. Cells not in the cycle but capable of division are in the resting phase *(G_0)*.

when a cell enters the cell cycle to when the cell divides into two identical cells is called the *generation time of the cell.* A mature cell continues to function until it degenerates and dies.

All of the body's cells are controlled by an intracellular mechanism that determines when cell proliferation is necessary. Under normal conditions, a state of dynamic equilibrium is constantly maintained (i.e., cell proliferation equals cell degeneration or death). Normally the process of cell division and proliferation is activated only in the presence of cell degeneration or death. Cell proliferation also occurs if the body has a physiologic need for more cells. For example, a normal increase in white blood cell (WBC) count occurs in the presence of infection.

Another mechanism for proliferation control in normal cells is *contact inhibition.* Normal cells respect the boundaries and territory of the cells surrounding them. They will not invade a territory that is not their own. The neighboring cells are thought to inhibit cell growth through the physical contact of the surrounding cell membranes. Cancer cells grown in tissue culture are characterized by loss of contact inhibition. These cells have no regard for cell boundaries and grow on top of one another and also on top of or between normal cells.

The rate of normal cell proliferation (from the time of cell birth to the time of cell death) differs in each body tissue. In some tissues, such as bone marrow, hair follicles, and epithelial lining of the gastrointestinal (GI) tract, the rate of cell proliferation is rapid. In other tissues, such as myocardium and cartilage, cell proliferation does not occur or is slow.

A common misconception regarding the characteristics of cancer cells is that the rate of proliferation is more rapid than that of normal body cells. Cancer cells usually proliferate at the same rate as the normal cells of the tissue from which they arise. However, cancer cells respond differently than normal cells to the intracellular signals that regulate the state of dynamic equilibrium. The difference is that proliferation of the cancer cells is indiscriminate and continuous. Sometimes they produce more than two cells at the time of mitosis. In this way, there is continuous growth of a tumor mass: $1 \times 2 \times 4 \times 8 \times 16$ and so on. This is termed the *pyramid effect.* The time required for a tumor mass to double in size is known as its *doubling time.*

Defect in Cell Differentiation

Cell differentiation is normally an orderly process that progresses from a state of immaturity to a state of maturity. Because all body cells are derived from the fertilized ova, all cells have the potential to perform all body functions. As cells differentiate, this potential is repressed, and the mature cell is capable of performing only specific functions (see eFig. 16-1 on the website for this chapter). With cell differentiation, there is a stable and orderly phasing out of cell potential. Under normal conditions the differentiated cell is stable and will not *dedifferentiate* (i.e., revert to a previous undifferentiated state).

Genetic Link

Cancer involves the malfunction of genes that control differentiation and proliferation. Two types of normal genes that can be affected by mutation are *protooncogenes* and *tumor suppressor genes.* **Protooncogenes** are normal cell genes that are important regulators of normal cell processes. Protooncogenes promote growth, whereas tumor suppressor genes suppress growth. Mutations that alter the expression of protooncogenes can activate them to function as **oncogenes** (tumor-inducing genes).

The protooncogene has been described as the genetic lock that keeps the cell in its mature functioning state. When this lock is "unlocked," as may occur through exposure to *carcinogens* (agents that cause cancer) or oncogenic viruses, genetic alterations and mutations occur. The abilities and properties that the cell had in fetal development are again expressed. Oncogenes can change a normal cell to a malignant one. This cell regains a fetal appearance and function. For example, some cancer cells produce new proteins, such as those characteristic of the embryonic and fetal periods of life. These proteins, located on the cell membrane, include carcinoembryonic antigen (CEA) and α-fetoprotein (AFP). They can be detected in human blood by laboratory studies (see Role of the Immune System later in this chapter). Other cancer cells, such as small cell carcinoma of the lung, produce hormones (see Complications Resulting from Cancer later in this chapter) that are ordinarily produced by cells arising from the same embryonic cells as the tumor cells.

Tumor suppressor genes function to regulate cell growth. They prevent cells from going through the cell cycle. Mutations that alter tumor suppressor genes make them inactive, resulting in a loss of their tumor-suppressing action. Examples of tumor suppressor genes are *BRCA1* and *BRCA2*. Alterations in these genes increase a person's risk for breast and ovarian cancer. Another tumor suppressor gene is the *APC* gene. Alterations in this gene increase a person's risk for familial adenomatous polyposis, which is a precursor for colorectal cancer (see Chapter 43). Mutations in the *p53* tumor suppressor gene have been found in many cancers, including bladder, breast, colorectal, esophageal, liver, lung, and ovarian cancers.

Development of Cancer

The following is a theoretical model of the development of cancer. The cause and development of each type of cancer are likely to be multifactorial. A common misbelief is that the development of cancer is a rapid, haphazard event. However, cancer is usually an orderly process that occurs over time and has several stages: initiation, promotion, and progression[2] (Fig. 16-2).

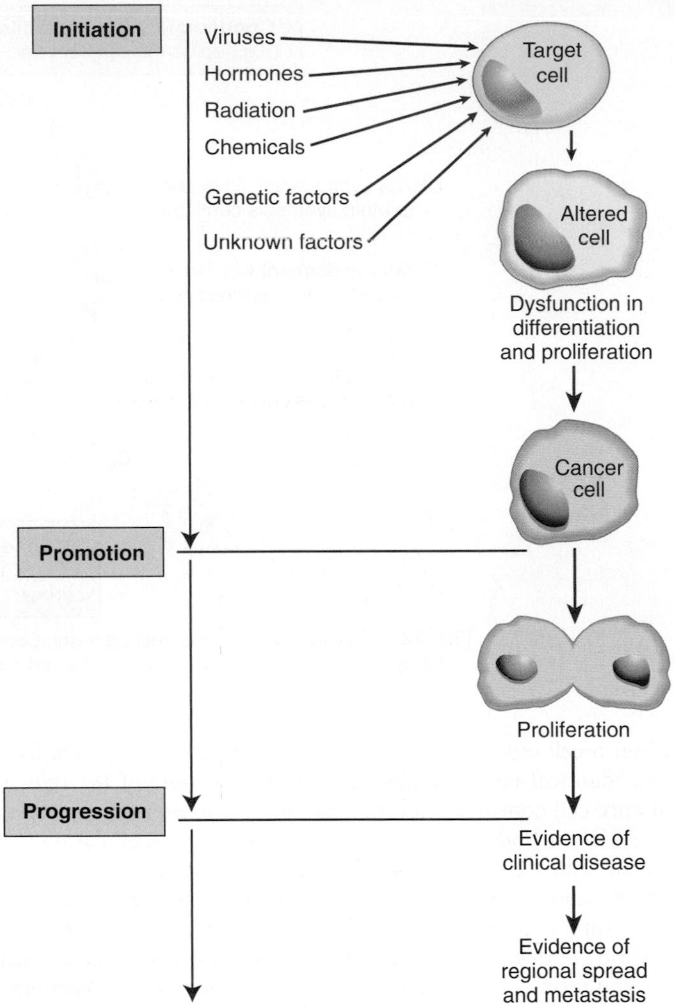

FIG. 16-2 Process of cancer development.

Initiation. Cancer cells arise from normal cells as a result of changes in genes. The first stage, *initiation*, involves a mutation in the cell's genetic structure. A *mutation* is any change in the usual DNA sequence.

Genetic Link

Gene mutations can occur in two different ways: *inherited* from a parent (passed from one generation to the next) or *acquired* during a person's lifetime. (Mutations are discussed in Chapter 13.)

About 5% of all cancers or the predisposition to the cancer is inherited from one's parents. These genetic alterations lead to a high risk of developing a specific type of cancer. However, most cancers do not result from inherited genes but are acquired from damage to genes occurring during one's lifetime.[1] An acquired mutation is passed on to all cells that develop from that single cell. The damaged cell may die or repair itself. However, if cell death or repair does not occur before cell division, the cell will replicate into daughter cells, each with the same genetic alteration.

Carcinogens. Many carcinogens (cancer-causing agents capable of producing cell alterations) are detoxified by protective enzymes and are harmlessly excreted. If this protective mechanism fails, carcinogens can enter the cell's nucleus and alter deoxyribonucleic acid (DNA). Carcinogens may be chemical, radiation, or viral.

Chemical Carcinogens. Chemicals were identified as cancer-causing agents in the latter part of the eighteenth century when Percival Pott noted that chimney sweeps had a higher incidence of cancer of the scrotum associated with exposure to soot residue in chimneys. As the years passed, many chemical agents have been identified as carcinogens. People exposed to certain chemicals over time have a greater incidence of certain cancers than others. The long latency period from the time of exposure to the development of cancer makes it difficult to identify cancer-causing chemicals.

Certain drugs have also been identified as carcinogens. Drugs that are capable of interacting with DNA (e.g., alkylating agents) and immunosuppressive agents have the potential to cause cancer. The use of alkylating agents (e.g., cyclophosphamide [Cytoxan]), either alone or in combination with radiation therapy, has been associated with an increased incidence of acute myelogenous leukemia in people treated for Hodgkin's lymphoma, non-Hodgkin's lymphoma, and multiple myeloma. These *secondary leukemias* are resistant to chemotherapy. Secondary leukemia has also been observed in people who have undergone transplant surgery and taken immunosuppressive drugs.

Radiation. Radiation can cause cancer in almost any body tissue. When cells are exposed to a source of radiation, damage occurs to DNA. Certain malignancies have been correlated with radiation as a carcinogenic agent:

- Leukemia, lymphoma, thyroid cancer, and other cancers increased in incidence in the general population of Hiroshima and Nagasaki after the atomic bomb explosions.
- A higher incidence of bone cancer occurs in people exposed to radiation in certain occupations, such as radiologists, radiation chemists, and uranium miners.

Ultraviolet (UV) radiation has long been associated with melanoma and squamous and basal cell carcinoma of the skin. Skin cancer is the most common type of cancer among whites in the United States. Of great concern is the increase in the incidence of melanoma. Although the cause of melanoma is probably multifactorial, UV radiation secondary to sunlight exposure is linked to the development of melanoma.

Viral Carcinogens. Certain DNA and ribonucleic acid (RNA) viruses, termed *oncogenic,* can transform the cells they infect and induce malignant transformation. Viruses have been identified as causative agents of cancer in animals and humans. Burkitt's lymphoma has consistently shown evidence of Epstein-Barr virus (EBV) in vitro. People with acquired immunodeficiency syndrome (AIDS), which is caused by human immunodeficiency virus (HIV), have a high incidence of Kaposi sarcoma (see Chapter 15). Other viruses that have been linked to the development of cancer include hepatitis B virus, which is associated with hepatocellular carcinoma; and human papillomavirus, which is believed to induce lesions that progress to squamous cell carcinomas, such as cervical, anal, and head and neck cancers.[3]

Promotion. A single alteration of the genetic structure of the cell is not sufficient to result in cancer. However, the odds of cancer development are increased with the presence of promoting agents. *Promotion,* the second stage in the development of cancer, is characterized by the reversible proliferation of the altered cells. An increase in the altered cell population further increases the likelihood of additional mutations.

An important distinction between initiation and promotion is that the activity of promoters is reversible. This is a key concept in cancer prevention. Promoting factors include such agents as dietary fat, obesity, cigarette smoking, and alcohol consumption. Changing a person's lifestyle to modify these risk factors can reduce the chance of cancer development. Approximately half of cancer-related deaths in the United States are related to tobacco use, unhealthy diet, physical inactivity, and obesity.[1]

Several promoting agents have activity against specific types of body tissues. Therefore these agents tend to promote specific kinds of cancer. For example, cigarette smoke is a promoting agent in bronchogenic carcinoma and, in conjunction with alcohol intake, promotes esophageal and bladder cancers.

Some carcinogens, termed *complete carcinogens,* are capable of both initiating and promoting the development of cancer. Cigarette smoke is an example of a complete carcinogen capable of initiating and promoting cancer.

A period of time, ranging from 1 to 40 years, elapses between the initial genetic alteration and the actual clinical evidence of cancer. This period, called the *latent* period, includes both the initiation and the promotion stages in the natural history of cancer. The variation in the length of time that elapses before the cancer becomes clinically evident is associated with the mitotic rate of the tissue of origin and environmental factors. In most cancers the process of developing cancer is years or even decades in length.

For the disease process to become clinically evident, the cells must reach a critical mass. A tumor that is 1.0 cm (0.4 inch) (the size usually detectable by palpation) contains 1 billion cancer cells. A 0.5-cm tumor is the smallest that can be detected by current diagnostic measures, such as magnetic resonance imaging (MRI).

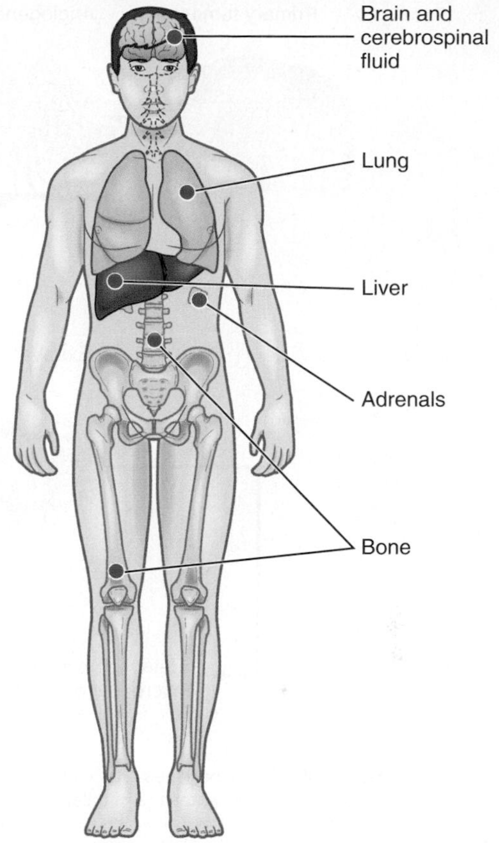

FIG. 16-3 Main sites of metastasis.

Progression. *Progression* is the final stage in the natural history of a cancer. This stage is characterized by increased growth rate of the tumor, increased invasiveness, and **metastasis**—spread of the cancer to a distant site. Certain cancers seem to have an affinity for a particular tissue or organ as a site of metastasis (e.g., colon cancer often spreads to the liver). Other cancers (e.g., melanoma) are unpredictable in their pattern of metastasis. The most frequent sites of metastasis are lungs, liver, bone, brain, and adrenal glands (Fig. 16-3).

Metastasis is a multistep process beginning with the rapid growth of the primary tumor (Fig. 16-4). As the tumor increases in size, development of its own blood supply is critical to its survival and growth. The process of the formation of blood vessels within the tumor itself is termed **tumor angiogenesis** and is facilitated by tumor angiogenesis factors produced by the cancer cells.

Tumor cells are able to detach from the primary tumor, invade the tissue surrounding the tumor, and penetrate the walls of lymph or vascular vessels for metastasis to a distant site. Once free from the primary tumor, metastatic tumor cells frequently travel to distant organ sites via lymphatic and hematogenous routes.

Hematogenous metastasis involves several steps beginning with primary tumor cells penetrating blood vessels. These tumor cells then enter the circulation, travel through the body, and adhere to and penetrate small blood vessels of distant organs. Most tumor cells do not survive this process and are destroyed by mechanical mechanisms (e.g., turbulence of blood flow) and cells of the immune system. However, the formation of a combination of tumor cells, platelets, and fibrin deposits may protect some tumor cells from destruction in blood vessels.

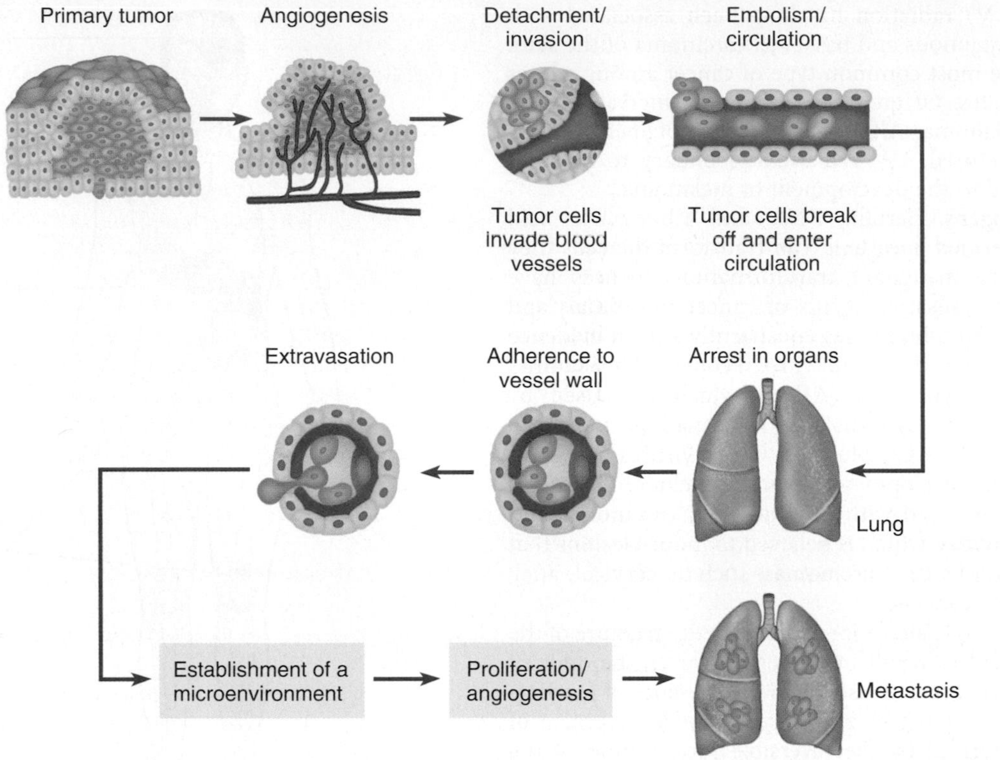

FIG. 16-4 The pathogenesis of cancer metastasis. To produce metastases, tumor cells must detach from the primary tumor and enter the circulation, survive in the circulation to arrest in the capillary bed, adhere to capillary basement membrane, gain entrance into the organ parenchyma, respond to growth factors, proliferate and induce angiogenesis, and evade host defenses.

In the lymphatic system, tumor cells may be "trapped" in the first lymph node confronted or they may bypass regional lymph nodes and travel to more distant lymph nodes, a phenomenon termed *skip metastasis*. This phenomenon is exhibited in malignancies such as esophageal cancers. It also raises questions about the effectiveness of dissection of regional lymph nodes for the prevention of distant metastases.[4]

Tumor cells that do survive the process of metastasis must create an environment in the distant organ site that is conducive to their growth and development. Growth and development are facilitated by the tumor cells' ability to evade cells of the immune system and to produce a vascular supply within the metastatic site similar to that developed in the primary tumor site. Vascularization is critical to the supply of nutrients to the metastatic tumor and to the removal of waste products. Vascularization of the metastatic site is also facilitated by tumor angiogenesis factors produced by the cancer cells.

Role of the Immune System

This section is limited to a discussion of the role of the immune system in the recognition and destruction of tumor cells. (For a detailed discussion of immune system function, see Chapter 14.)

The immune system has the potential to distinguish cells that are normal (self) from abnormal (nonself) cells. For example, cells of transplanted organs can be recognized by the immune system as *nonself* and thus elicit an immune response. This response can ultimately result in the rejection of the organ. Similarly, cancer cells can be perceived as nonself and elicit an immune response resulting in their rejection and destruction. However, unlike transplanted cells, cancer cells arise from normal human cells and, although they are mutated and thus different, the immune response that is mounted against cancer cells may be inadequate to effectively kill them.

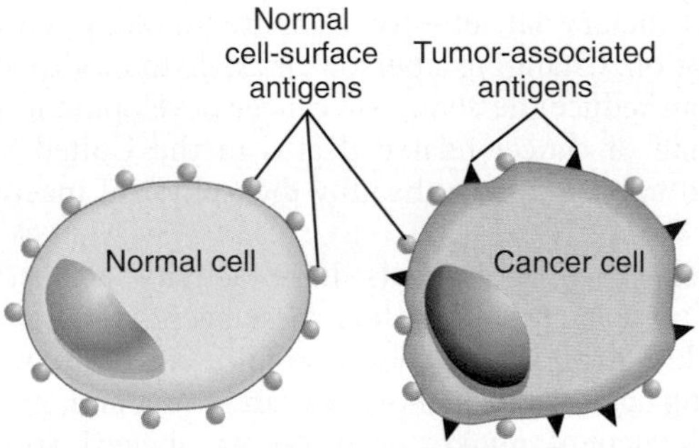

FIG. 16-5 Tumor-associated antigens appear on the cell surface of malignant cells.

Cancer cells may display altered cell-surface antigens as a result of malignant transformation. These antigens are termed **tumor-associated antigens (TAAs)** (Fig. 16-5). It is believed that one of the functions of the immune system is to respond to TAAs. The immune system's response to antigens of the malignant cells is termed **immunologic surveillance.** In this process lymphocytes continuously check cell-surface antigens and detect and destroy cells with abnormal or altered antigenic determinants. Under most circumstances, immune surveillance prevents these transformed cells from developing into clinically detectable tumors.

Immune response to malignant cells involves cytotoxic T cells, natural killer (NK) cells, macrophages, and B cells. *Cytotoxic T cells* play a dominant role in resisting tumor growth.

These cells are capable of killing tumor cells. T cells are also important in the production of cytokines (e.g., interleukin-2 [IL-2] and γ-interferon), which stimulate T cells, NK cells, B cells, and macrophages.

Natural killer (NK) cells are able to directly lyse tumor cells spontaneously without any prior sensitization. These cells are stimulated by γ-interferon and IL-2 (released from T cells), resulting in increased cytotoxic activity.

Monocytes and *macrophages* have several important roles in tumor immunity. Macrophages can be activated by γ-interferon (produced by T cells) to become nonspecifically lytic for tumor cells. Macrophages also secrete cytokines, including interleukin-1 (IL-1), tumor necrosis factor (TNF), and colony-stimulating factors (CSFs). The release of IL-1, coupled with the presentation of the processed antigen, stimulates T lymphocyte activation and production. α-Interferon augments the killing ability of NK cells. TNF causes hemorrhagic necrosis of tumors and exerts cytocidal or cytostatic actions against tumor cells. CSFs regulate the production of various blood cells in the bone marrow and stimulate the function of various WBCs.

B cells can produce specific antibodies that bind to tumor cells. These antibodies are often detectable in the patient's serum and saliva.

Escape Mechanisms From Immunologic Surveillance. The process by which cancer cells evade the immune system is termed *immunologic escape*. Theorized mechanisms by which cancer cells can escape immunologic surveillance include (1) suppression of factors that stimulate T cells to react to cancer cells; (2) weak surface antigens allowing cancer cells to "sneak through" immunologic surveillance; (3) the development of tolerance of the immune system to some tumor antigens; (4) suppression of the immune response by products secreted by cancer cells; (5) the induction of suppressor T cells by the tumor; and (6) blocking antibodies that bind TAAs, thus preventing their recognition by T cells (Fig. 16-6).

Oncofetal Antigens and Tumor Markers. *Oncofetal antigens* are a type of tumor antigen. They are found on both the surfaces and the inside of cancer cells and fetal cells. These antigens are an expression of the shift of cancerous cells to a more immature metabolic pathway, an expression usually associated with embryonic or fetal periods of life. The reappearance of fetal antigens in malignant disease is not well understood, but it is believed to occur as a result of the cell regaining its embryonic capability to differentiate into many different cell types.

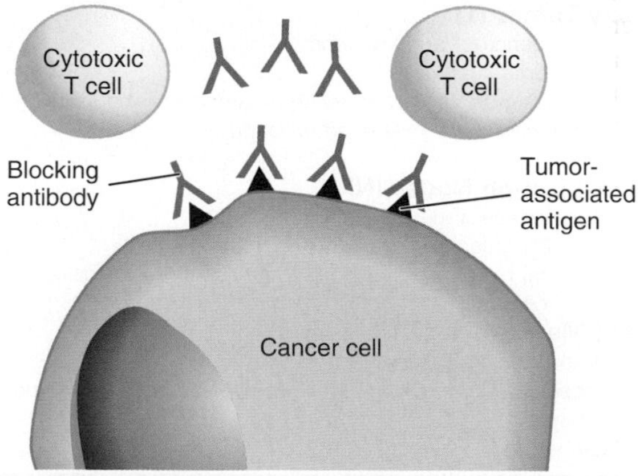

FIG. 16-6 Blocking antibodies prevent T cells from interacting with tumor-associated antigens and from destroying the malignant cell.

Examples of oncofetal antigens are carcinoembryonic antigen (CEA) and α-fetoprotein (AFP). CEA is found on the surfaces of cancer cells derived from the GI tract and from normal cells from the fetal gut, liver, and pancreas. Normally, it disappears during the last 3 months of fetal life. CEA was originally isolated from colorectal cancer cells. However, elevated CEA levels have also been found in nonmalignant conditions (e.g., cirrhosis of the liver, ulcerative colitis, heavy smoking).

These oncofetal antigens can be used as *tumor markers* that may be clinically useful to monitor the effect of therapy and indicate tumor recurrence. However, oncofetal antigens are not 100% specific for tumor recurrence. Tumor markers are affected by various factors that need to be accounted for when reviewing these results. For example, the persistence of elevated preoperative CEA titers after surgery indicates that the tumor is not completely removed. A rise in CEA levels after chemotherapy or radiation therapy may indicate recurrence or spread of the cancer and may be affected by chronic lung or liver disease and smoking.

AFP is produced by malignant liver cells and fetal liver cells. AFP levels have also been found to be elevated in some cases of testicular carcinoma, viral hepatitis, and nonmalignant liver disorders. AFP has diagnostic value in primary cancer of the liver (hepatocellular cancer), but it is also produced when metastatic liver growth occurs. The detection of AFP is of value in tumor detection and determination of tumor progression.

Other examples of oncofetal antigens are CA-125 (found in ovarian carcinoma), CA-19-9 (found in pancreatic and gallbladder cancer), prostate-specific antigen (PSA) (found in prostate cancer), and CA-15-3 and CA-27-29 (found in breast cancer). Molecular markers for specific tumors include kRAS (expression of oncogene in colon cancer), epidermal growth factor receptor (EGFR) often overexpressed in lung cancer, and human epidermal growth factor receptor 2 (HER-2) expression in breast cancer.

BENIGN VERSUS MALIGNANT NEOPLASMS

Tumors can be classified as benign or malignant. In general, *benign neoplasms* are well differentiated, and **malignant neoplasms** range from well differentiated to undifferentiated. The ability of malignant tumor cells to invade and metastasize is the major difference between benign and malignant neoplasms. Other differences are presented in Table 16-3.

CLASSIFICATION OF CANCER

Tumors can be classified according to anatomic site, histology (grading), and extent of disease (staging). Tumor classification

TABLE 16-3 COMPARISON OF BENIGN AND MALIGNANT NEOPLASMS

Characteristic	Benign	Malignant
Encapsulated	Usually	Rarely
Differentiated	Normally	Poorly
Metastasis	Absent	Capable
Recurrence	Rare	Possible
Vascularity	Slight	Moderate to marked
Mode of growth	Expansive	Infiltrative and expansive
Cell characteristics	Fairly normal, similar to parent cells	Cells abnormal, become more unlike parent cells

systems are intended to stratify risk. Classification systems provide a standardized way to (1) communicate the status of the cancer to all members of the health care team, (2) assist in determining the most effective treatment plan, (3) evaluate the treatment plan, (4) predict prognosis, and (5) compare like groups for statistical purposes.

Anatomic Site Classification

In the *anatomic classification* of tumors, the tumor is identified by the tissue of origin, the anatomic site, and the behavior of the tumor (i.e., benign or malignant) (Table 16-4). *Carcinomas* originate from embryonal *ectoderm* (skin and glands) and *endoderm* (mucous membrane linings of the respiratory tract, GI tract, and genitourinary [GU] tract) (see eFig. 16-1 on the website for this chapter). *Sarcomas* originate from embryonal *mesoderm* (connective tissue, muscle, bone, and fat). Lymphomas and leukemias originate from the hematopoietic system.

Histologic Classification

In **histologic grading** of tumors, the appearance of cells and the degree of differentiation are evaluated pathologically. For many tumor types, four grades are used to evaluate abnormal cells based on the degree to which the cells resemble the tissue of origin. Tumors that are poorly differentiated (undifferentiated) have a worse prognosis than those that are closer in appearance to the normal tissue of origin (well differentiated):

Grade I: Cells differ slightly from normal cells (mild dysplasia) and are well differentiated (low grade).
Grade II: Cells are more abnormal (moderate dysplasia) and moderately differentiated (intermediate grade).
Grade III: Cells are very abnormal (severe dysplasia) and poorly differentiated (high grade).
Grade IV: Cells are immature and primitive *(anaplasia)* and undifferentiated; cell of origin is difficult to determine (high grade).
Grade X: Grade cannot be assessed.

TABLE 16-4 ANATOMIC CLASSIFICATION OF TUMORS

Site	Benign	Malignant
Epithelial Tissue Tumors*	**-oma**	**-carcinoma**
Surface epithelium	Papilloma	Carcinoma
Glandular epithelium	Adenoma	Adenocarcinoma
Connective Tissue Tumors†	**-oma**	**-sarcoma**
Fibrous tissue	Fibroma	Fibrosarcoma
Cartilage	Chondroma	Chondrosarcoma
Striated muscle	Rhabdomyoma	Rhabdomyosarcoma
Bone	Osteoma	Osteosarcoma
Nervous Tissue Tumors	**-oma**	**-oma**
Meninges	Meningioma	Meningeal sarcoma
Nerve cells	Ganglioneuroma	Neuroblastoma
Hematopoietic Tissue Tumors		
Lymphoid tissue	—	Hodgkin's lymphoma, non-Hodgkin's lymphoma
Plasma cells	—	Multiple myeloma
Bone marrow	—	Lymphocytic and myelogenous leukemia

*Body surfaces, lining of body cavities, and glandular structures.
†Supporting tissue, fibrotic tissue, and blood vessels.

Extent of Disease Classification

Classifying the extent and spread of disease is termed **staging**. This classification system is based on the anatomic extent of disease rather than on cell appearance. Although there are similarities in the staging of various cancers, there are many differences for specific types of cancer.

Clinical Staging. The clinical staging classification system determines the anatomic extent of the malignant disease process by stages:

Stage 0: cancer in situ
Stage I: tumor limited to the tissue of origin; localized tumor growth
Stage II: limited local spread
Stage III: extensive local and regional spread
Stage IV: metastasis

Clinical staging has been used as a basis for staging a variety of tumor types, including cancer of the cervix (see Table 54-11) and Hodgkin's lymphoma (see Fig. 31-14). Other malignant diseases (e.g., leukemia) do not use this staging approach.

TNM Classification System. The *TNM classification system* (Table 16-5) is used to determine the anatomic extent of the disease involvement according to three parameters: tumor size and invasiveness (T), presence or absence of regional spread to the lymph nodes (N), and metastasis to distant organ sites (M). (Examples of the TNM classification system can be found in Tables 28-17 and 52-6.) TNM staging cannot be applied to all malignancies. For example, the leukemias are not solid tumors and therefore cannot be staged using these guidelines. **Carcinoma in situ (CIS)** refers to a neoplasm whose cells are localized and show no tendency to invade or metastasize to other tissues. CIS has its own designation in the system (T_{is}), since it has all the histologic characteristics of cancer except invasion—a primary feature of the TNM staging system.

Staging of the disease can be performed initially and at several evaluation points. Clinical staging is done at the completion of the diagnostic workup to guide effective treatment selection. Examples of diagnostic studies that may be performed to assess for extent of disease include radiologic studies, such as bone and liver scans; ultrasonography; and computed tomography (CT), MRI, and positron emission tomography (PET) scans.

Surgical staging refers to the extent of the disease as determined by surgical excision, exploration, and/or lymph node

TABLE 16-5 TNM CLASSIFICATION SYSTEM

Primary Tumor (T)	
T_0	No evidence of primary tumor
T_{is}	Carcinoma in situ
T_{1-4}	Ascending degrees of increase in tumor size and involvement
T_x	Tumor cannot be measured or found
Regional Lymph Nodes (N)	
N_0	No evidence of disease in lymph nodes
N_{1-4}	Ascending degrees of nodal involvement
N_x	Regional lymph nodes unable to be assessed clinically
Distant Metastases (M)	
M_0	No evidence of distant metastases
M_{1-4}	Ascending degrees of metastatic involvement, including distant nodes
M_x	Cannot be determined

NOTE: For examples of TNM classification system applied to diseases, see Fig. 31-14 and Table 28-17.

sampling. For example, a laparotomy and a splenectomy may be performed in staging of Hodgkin's lymphoma. During a staging laparotomy, lymph node biopsies may be done, and margins of any masses may be marked with metal clips for use during radiation therapy. However, exploratory surgical staging is being used less frequently as noninvasive diagnostic technology becomes increasingly sophisticated.

After the extent of the disease is determined, the stage classification is not changed. The original description of the extent of the tumor remains part of the record. If additional treatment is needed, or if treatment fails, retreatment staging is done to determine the extent of the disease process before retreatment. "Restaging" classification (rTNM) is differentiated from the stage at diagnosis, since the clinical significance may be quite different.

In addition to tumor classification systems, other rating scales can be used to describe and document the status of patients with cancer at the time of diagnosis, treatment, and retreatment and at each follow-up examination. For example, the Karnofsky Functional Performance Scale and the Katz Index of Independence in Activities of Daily Living describe patient performance in terms of function. (These scales are presented in eTables 16-1 and 16-2 available on the website for this chapter.)

PREVENTION AND EARLY DETECTION OF CANCER

As a nurse, you have an essential role in the prevention and early detection of cancer. Eliminating risk factors reduces the incidence of cancer. For example, rates of smoking-related cancers (e.g., lung and head and neck cancers) have declined following reduction in smoking rates.[1] Early detection and prompt treatment are responsible for increased survival rates in patients with cancer. Colonoscopy is important in reducing colon cancer mortality both by early detection of colon cancers and by prevention (e.g., excision of adenomatous polyps).[5]

Teach patients and the public about cancer prevention and early detection, including the following:

- Reduce or avoid exposure to known or suspected carcinogens and cancer-promoting agents, including cigarette smoke and sun exposure.
- Eat a balanced diet that includes vegetables and fresh fruits (see Fig. 40-1 and Table 40-1), whole grains, and adequate amounts of fiber. Reduce dietary fat and preservatives, including smoked and salt-cured meats containing high nitrite concentrations.
- Limit alcohol intake.
- Participate in regular exercise (i.e., 30 minutes or more of moderate physical activity five times weekly).
- Maintain a healthy weight.
- Obtain adequate, consistent periods of rest (at least 6 to 8 hours per night).
- Eliminate, reduce, or change the perception of stressors and enhance the ability to effectively cope with stressors (see Chapter 7).
- Have a regular physical examination that includes a health history. Be familiar with your own family history and your risk factors for cancer.
- Learn and follow the American Cancer Society's recommended cancer screening guidelines for breast, colon, cervical, and prostate cancer. (See eTable 16-3 on the website for this chapter.)

TABLE 16-6 SEVEN WARNING SIGNS OF CANCER

C hange in bowel or bladder habits
A sore that does not heal
U nusual bleeding or discharge from any body orifice
T hickening or a lump in the breast or elsewhere
I ndigestion or difficulty in swallowing
O bvious change in a wart or mole
N agging cough or hoarseness

HEALTHY PEOPLE

Prevention and Early Detection of Cancer

- Limit alcohol use.
- Get regular physical activity.
- Maintain a normal body weight.
- Obtain regular colorectal screenings.
- Avoid cigarette smoking and other tobacco use.
- Get regular mammography screening and Pap tests.
- Use sunscreen with a sun protection factor of 15 or higher.
- Practice healthy dietary habits, such as reduced fat consumption and increased fruit and vegetable consumption.

- Learn and practice self-examination (e.g., breast or testicular self-examination).
- Know the seven warning signs of cancer, and inform the health care provider if they are present (Table 16-6). (These actually detect fairly advanced disease.)
- Seek immediate medical care if you notice a change in what is normal for you and if cancer is suspected.

The goals of public education are to (1) motivate people to recognize and modify behaviors that may negatively affect health and (2) encourage awareness of and participation in health-promoting behaviors. When you teach about cancer, try to minimize the fear that surrounds the diagnosis.

Diagnosis of Cancer

When a patient has a possible diagnosis of cancer, it is a stressful time for the patient and the family. Patients may undergo several days to weeks of diagnostic studies. During this time, fear of the unknown may be more stressful than the actual diagnosis of cancer. Patients may also be overwhelmed or confused by the need for multiple diagnostic studies and consultations. Help to coordinate care between multiple specialists and explain the purpose of required tests and any special preparation needed for them.

While patients are waiting for the results of diagnostic studies, be available to actively listen to their concerns. Their anxiety may arise from myths and misconceptions about cancer (e.g., cancer is a "death sentence," cancer treatment is worse than the illness). Correcting those misconceptions can help to minimize their anxiety.

Learn to recognize your own discomfort during difficult conversations. Avoid communication patterns that may hinder exploration of feelings and meaning, such as providing false reassurances (e.g., "It's probably nothing"), redirecting the discussion (e.g., "Let's discuss that later"), generalizing (e.g., "Everyone feels this way"), and using overly technical language as a means of distancing yourself from the patient. These self-protective strategies deny patients the opportunity to share the meaning of their experience. In addition, they can jeopardize your ability to build a trusting relationship with your patients.

During this time of high anxiety, the patient may need repeated explanations of the diagnostic workup. Include as much information as needed by the patient and the family. Give clear, understandable explanations and reinforce them as needed. Written information is helpful for reinforcement of verbal information.

A diagnostic plan for the person suspected of having cancer includes the health history (including a history of present illness), identification of risk factors, the physical examination, and specific diagnostic studies. For many people, cancer is initially diagnosed after the findings of an abnormal screening test (e.g., mass on mammogram). For others, they are alerted to the presence of cancer by a presenting symptom or cluster of symptoms (e.g., cough and hemoptysis, anorexia and weight loss).

Concentrate on risk factors for malignancy such as family or personal history of cancer, exposure to or use of known carcinogens (e.g., cigarette smoking, occupational pollutants or chemicals, radiation exposure), diseases characterized by chronic inflammation or immunosuppression (e.g., ulcerative colitis), and drug ingestion (e.g., hormone therapy, previous anticancer therapies). Also assess factors that may warrant additional supportive care during therapy, including alcohol or recreational drug use, living situation, social support, and coping strategies for perceived stressors.

Diagnostic studies depend on the suspected primary or metastatic site(s) of the cancer. (Specific procedures as they relate to each body system are discussed in the respective assessment chapters.) Examples of diagnostic studies include the following:

- Cytology studies (e.g., Papanicolaou [Pap] test, bronchial washings)
- Tissue biopsy
- Chest x-ray
- Complete blood count, chemistry profile
- Liver function studies (e.g., aspartate aminotransferase [AST])
- Endoscopic examination: upper GI, sigmoidoscopy, or colonoscopy (including guaiac test for occult blood)
- Radiographic studies (e.g., mammography, ultrasound, CT scan, MRI)
- Radioisotope scans (e.g., bone, lung, liver, brain)
- PET scan (Fig. 16-7)
- Tumor markers (e.g., CEA, AFP, PSA, CA-125)
- Genetic markers (e.g., *BRCA1, BRCA2*)
- Molecular receptor status (e.g., estrogen and progesterone receptors)
- Bone marrow examination (if a hematolymphoid malignancy is suspected or to document metastatic disease)

Biopsy. A *biopsy* is the removal of a tissue sample for pathologic analysis. Various methods are used to obtain a biopsy depending on the location and size of the suspected tumor. *Percutaneous biopsy* is commonly performed for tissue that can be safely reached through the skin. *Endoscopic biopsy* may be used for lung or other intraluminal lesions (esophageal, colon, bladder). When a tumor is not easily accessible, a *surgical procedure* (laparotomy, thoracotomy, craniotomy) is often necessary to obtain a piece of the tumor tissue. Many radiographic techniques may be used in conjunction with the biopsy procedure (e.g., CT, MRI, ultrasound-guided biopsy, stereotactic biopsy, fluoroscopic-assisted biopsy) to improve tissue localization.

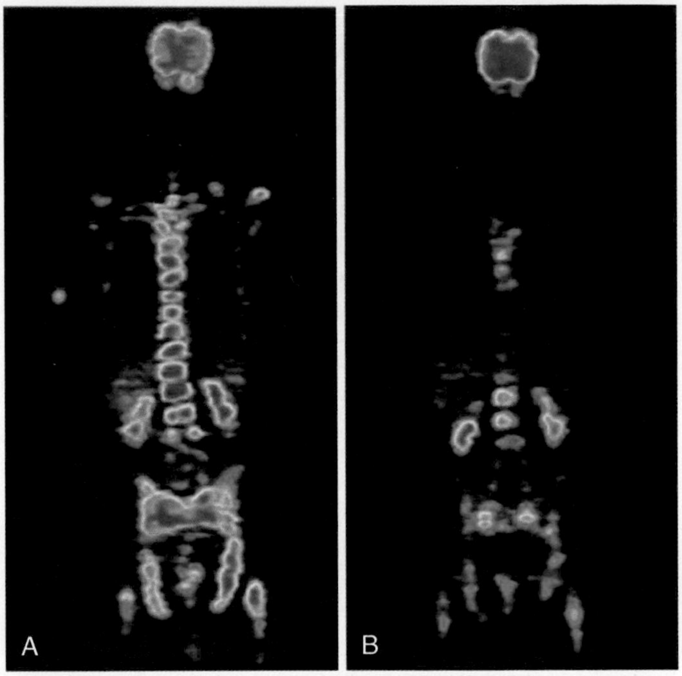

FIG. 16-7 Positron emission tomography (PET) scan before treatment **(A)** indicating metastasis throughout the body. PET scan after treatment **(B)** indicates the effects of therapy. More radioactive material accumulates in areas that have higher levels of activity. This often corresponds to areas of disease and shows up as brighter spots on the PET scan.

Various types and sizes of biopsy needles are available and are selected according to the type of tissue to be sampled. *Fine-needle aspiration* (FNA) may be accomplished with a small-gauge aspiration needle that provides cells from the mass for cytologic examination. *Large-core biopsy* cutting needles deliver an actual piece of tissue (core) that can be analyzed with the advantage of preserving the histologic architecture of the tissue specimen. *Excisional biopsy* involves the surgical removal of the entire lesion, lymph node, nodule, or mass. Therefore it is therapeutic as well as diagnostic. If an excisional biopsy is not feasible, an *incisional biopsy* (partial excision) may be performed with a scalpel or dermal punch.

Pathologic evaluation of a tissue sample is the only definitive means to diagnose a malignancy. The pathologist examines the tissue to determine whether it is benign or malignant, the anatomic tissue from which the tumor arises *(histology)*, and the degree of cell differentiation *(histologic grade)*. Other information that can be obtained includes the extent of malignant involvement (size of tumor and depth), evidence of invasiveness (extracapsular, lymphatic), adequacy of surgical excision (positive or negative surgical margin status), nuclear grade (mitotic rate), and special staining techniques that may provide insight into responsiveness of the tumor to treatment or disease behavior (receptor status, tumor markers).

COLLABORATIVE CARE

Treatment Goals

The goals of cancer treatment are cure, control, and palliation (Fig. 16-8). Primary factors that determine what therapy is used are the tumor histology and staging outcomes. Other important factors are the patient's physiologic status (e.g., presence of

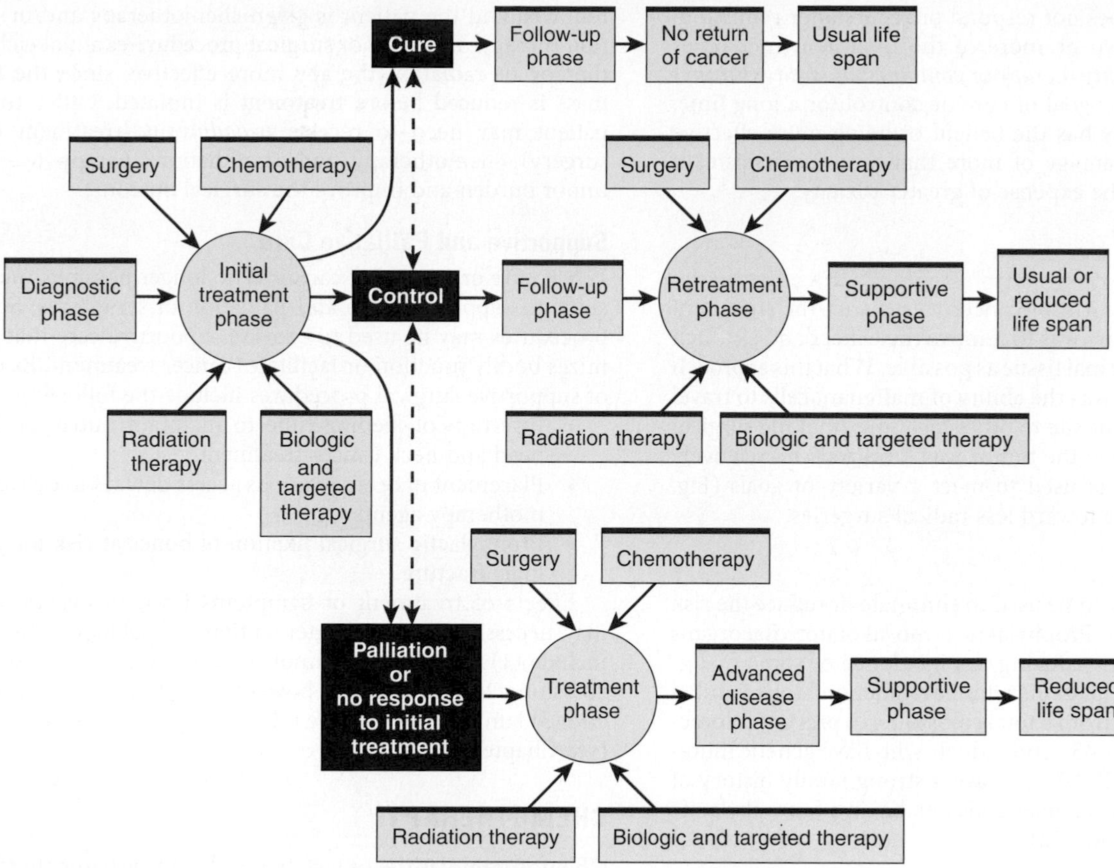

FIG. 16-8 Goals of cancer treatment.

co-morbid illnesses), psychologic status, and personal desires (e.g., active treatment versus palliation of symptoms). These factors influence the modalities chosen for treatment (i.e., surgery, radiation therapy, chemotherapy, biologic and targeted therapy), how therapies are sequenced, and the length of time the treatment is prescribed.

A variety of evidence-based cancer treatment guidelines have been developed to guide the appropriate treatment recommendations for individual patients. Some examples include guidelines of the American Society of Clinical Oncology (ASCO) *(www.asco.org)* and the National Comprehensive Cancer Network (NCCN) *(www.nccn.org)*.

Cure. When caring for the patient and family with cancer, know the treatment goals to appropriately communicate with, teach, and support the patient. When *cure* is the goal, treatment is expected to have the greatest chance of disease eradication. Curative cancer therapy differs according to the particular cancer being treated and may involve local therapies (i.e., surgery or radiation) alone or in combination, with or without periods of adjunctive systemic therapy (i.e., chemotherapy). For example, basal cell carcinoma of the skin is usually cured by surgical removal of the lesion and/or several weeks of radiation therapy. In the treatment plan for acute promyelocytic leukemia (which has curative potential), several chemotherapy drugs are given on a scheduled basis over many months to several years. Testicular cancer can be cured with a combination of surgery, chemotherapy, and radiation.

Although there is no benchmark that ensures "cure" for most malignancies, in general the risk for recurrent disease is highest after treatment completion, and gradually decreases the longer the patient remains disease free following treatment. Cancers with a higher mitotic rate (e.g., testicular cancer) are less likely to recur than cancers with slower mitotic rates (e.g., postmenopausal breast cancer). Therefore the timeframe to consider a person "cured" may differ according to the tumor and its characteristics.

Control. *Control* is the goal of the treatment plan for many cancers that cannot be completely eradicated, but are responsive to anticancer therapies. As with other chronic illnesses (e.g., diabetes mellitus, heart failure), cancer can be maintained for long periods with therapy. Examples include multiple myeloma and chronic lymphocytic leukemia (see Chapter 31). Patients may undergo an initial course of treatment followed by maintenance therapy for as long as the disease is responding. Patients are monitored closely for early signs and symptoms of disease recurrence or progression and the cumulative effects of therapy. Evidence of tumor resistance (such as disease progression) may warrant changing to an alternative therapy.

Palliation. *Palliation* is the treatment goal when relief or control of symptoms and the maintenance of a satisfactory quality of life are the primary objectives. An example of treatment in which palliation is the primary goal includes using radiation therapy or chemotherapy to reduce tumor size and relieve subsequent symptoms such as the pain of bone metastasis.

The goals of cure, control, and palliation are achieved through the use of four treatment modalities for cancer: surgery, radiation therapy, chemotherapy, and biologic and targeted therapy. Each can be used alone or in any combination during initial treatment or as maintenance therapy, as well as in retreatment if the disease does not respond or recurs after remission. For many cancers, two or more of the treatment modalities (known as *multimodality therapy* or *combined modality therapy*) are used to achieve the goal of cure or control for a long time. Multimodality therapy has the benefit of being more effective (because it takes advantage of more than one mechanism of action), but often at the expense of greater toxicity.

SURGICAL THERAPY

Surgery is the oldest form of cancer treatment. The treatment of choice for many years was to remove the cancer and as much of the surrounding normal tissue as possible. What this approach did not fully consider was the ability of malignant cells to travel from the original tumor site to other locations, making surgical cure possible only when the tumor was localized and relatively small. Today surgery is used to meet a variety of goals (Fig. 16-9), and the trend is toward less radical surgeries.

Prevention

Surgical intervention can be used to eliminate or reduce the risk of cancer development. Prophylactic removal of nonvital organs has been successful in reducing the incidence of some malignancies. For example, patients who have adenomatous familial polyposis may benefit from a total colostomy to prevent colorectal cancer (see Chapter 43). Individuals who have genetic mutations of *BRCA1* or *BRCA2* and have a strong family history of early-onset breast cancer may consider having a prophylactic mastectomy (see Chapter 52).

Cure or Control

When the goal is cure or control, the objective is to remove all or as much resectable tumor as possible while sparing normal tissue. Examples of surgical procedures used for cure or control of cancer include radical neck dissection, mastectomy, orchiectomy, thyroidectomy, nephrectomy, hysterectomy, and oophorectomy.

A *debulking* or *cytoreductive procedure* may be used if the tumor cannot be completely removed (e.g., a tumor attached to a vital organ). When this occurs, as much tumor as possible is removed and the patient is given chemotherapy and/or radiation therapy. This type of surgical procedure can make chemotherapy or radiation therapy more effective, since the tumor mass is reduced before treatment is initiated. Other times, a patient may need to receive *neoadjuvant* (treatment before surgery) chemotherapy and/or radiation therapy to reduce tumor burden and improve the surgical outcome.

Supportive and Palliative Care

When cure or control of cancer is no longer possible, the focus shifts to supportive care and palliation of symptoms. Surgical procedures may be used to provide supportive care that maximizes bodily function or facilitates cancer treatment. Examples of supportive surgical procedures include the following:

- Insertion of feeding tube to maintain nutrition during head and neck cancer treatment
- Placement of central venous access devices to deliver chemotherapy agents
- Prophylactic surgical fixation of bones at risk for pathologic fracture

Effects of treatment or symptoms from metastatic cancer may necessitate surgical intervention for palliation. Examples include (1) debulking of tumor to relieve pain or pressure, (2) colostomy for the relief of a bowel obstruction (see Chapter 43), and (3) laminectomy for the relief of a spinal cord compression (see Chapter 61).

CHEMOTHERAPY

Chemotherapy is the use of chemicals as a systemic therapy for cancer. In the 1940s nitrogen mustard, a chemical warfare agent used in World Wars I and II, was used in the treatment of lymphoma and acute leukemia. In the 1970s chemotherapy was established as an effective treatment modality for cancer. Chemotherapy is now a mainstay of cancer treatment for most solid tumors and hematologic malignancies (e.g., leukemias, lymphomas). Chemotherapy can offer cure for some cancers, control other cancers for long periods, and in some instances offer palliative relief of symptoms when cure or control is no longer possible (Fig. 16-10).

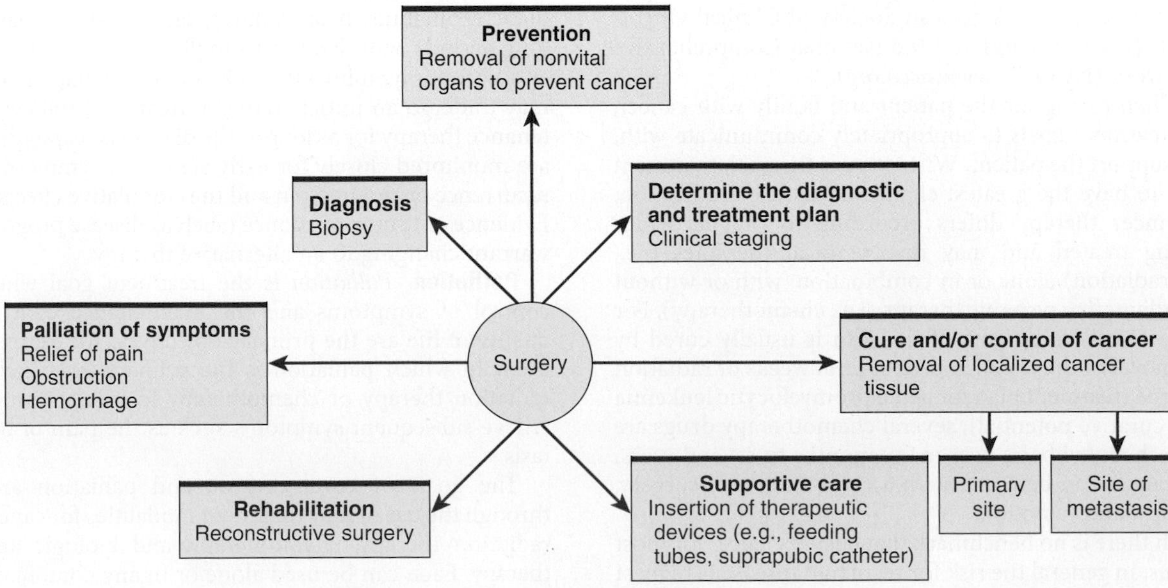

FIG. 16-9 Role of surgery in the treatment of cancer.

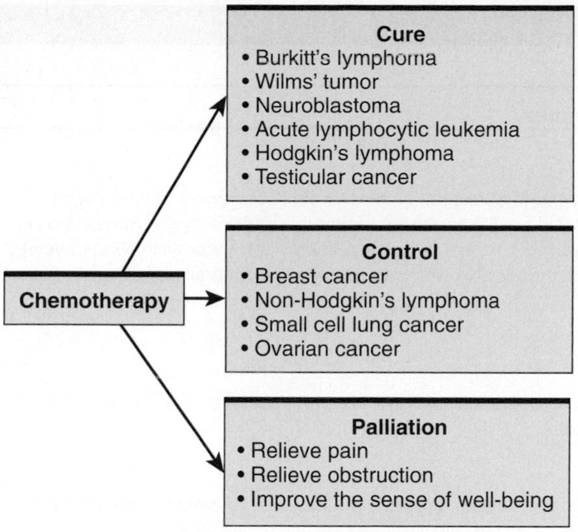

FIG. 16-10 Goals of chemotherapy.

Effect on Cells

The goal of chemotherapy is to eliminate or reduce the number of malignant cells in the primary tumor and metastatic tumor site(s). All cells (cancer cells and normal cells) enter the cell cycle for replication and proliferation (see Fig. 16-1). The effects of the chemotherapy drugs are described in relation to the cell cycle.

The two major categories of chemotherapy drugs are cell cycle phase–nonspecific and cell cycle phase–specific drugs. *Cell cycle phase–nonspecific chemotherapy drugs* have their effect on the cells during all phases of the cell cycle, including the process of cell replication and proliferation and the resting phase (G_0). *Cell cycle phase–specific chemotherapy drugs* exert their most significant effects during specific phases of the cell cycle (i.e., when cells are in the process of cell replication or proliferation during G_1, S, G_2, or M). Cell cycle phase–specific and cell cycle phase–nonspecific agents are often administered in combination to maximize effectiveness by using agents that function by differing mechanisms and throughout the cell cycle.

When cancer first begins to develop, most of the cells are actively dividing. As the tumor increases in size, more cells become inactive and convert to a resting state (G_0). Because most chemotherapy agents are most effective against dividing cells, cells can escape death by staying in the G_0 phase. A major challenge is to overcome the effect of resistant resting and non-cycling cells.

Classification of Chemotherapy Drugs

Chemotherapy drugs are classified in general groups according to their molecular structure and mechanisms of action (Table 16-7). Each drug in a particular classification has many similarities. However, there are major differences in how the drugs work and the unique side effects associated with drugs in each class.

TABLE 16-7 DRUG THERAPY

Chemotherapy Drugs

Mechanisms of Action	Examples
Alkylating Agents	
Cell Cycle Phase–Nonspecific Agents	
Damage DNA by causing breaks in the double-stranded helix. If repair does not occur, cells will die immediately (cytocidal) or when they attempt to divide (cytostatic).	bendamustine (Treanda), busulfan (Myleran), chlorambucil (Leukeran), cyclophosphamide (Cytoxan, Neosar), dacarbazine (DTIC-Dome), ifosfamide (Ifex), mechlorethamine (Mustargen), melphalan (Alkeran), temozolomide (Temodar), thiotepa (Thioplex)
Nitrosoureas	
Cell Cycle Phase–Nonspecific Agents	
Like alkylating agents, break DNA helix, interfering with DNA replication. Cross blood-brain barrier.	carmustine (BiCNU, Gliadel), lomustine (CeeNU), streptozocin (Zanosar)
Platinum Drugs	
Cell Cycle Phase–Nonspecific Agents	
Bind to DNA and RNA, miscoding information and/or inhibiting DNA replication, and cells die.	carboplatin (Paraplatin), cisplatin (Platinol-AQ), oxaliplatin (Eloxatin)
Antimetabolites	
Cell Cycle Phase–Specific Agents	
Mimic naturally occurring substances, thus interfering with enzyme function or DNA synthesis. Primarily act during S phase. Purine and pyrimidine are building blocks of nucleic acids needed for DNA and RNA synthesis.	
• Interfere with purine metabolism.	cladribine (Leustatin), clofarabine (Clolar), fludarabine (Fludara), mercaptopurine (Purinethol), nelarabine (Arranon), pentostatin (Nipent), thioguanine
• Interfere with pyrimidine metabolism.	capecitabine (Xeloda); cytarabine (ara-C [Cytosar-U, DepoCyt]), floxuridine (FUDR), 5-fluorouracil (5-FU [Adrucil]), gemcitabine (Gemzar)
• Interfere with folic acid metabolism.	methotrexate (Rheumatrex, Trexall), pemetrexed (Alimta)
• Interfere with DNA synthesis.	hydroxyurea (Hydrea, Droxia)

NOTE: Many of these drugs are irritants or vesicants that require special attention during administration to avoid extravasation. It is important to know this information about a drug before administering it.

Continued

TABLE 16-7 DRUG THERAPY—cont'd

Chemotherapy Drugs

Mechanisms of Action	Examples
Antitumor Antibiotics	
Cell Cycle Phase–Nonspecific Agents	
Bind directly to DNA, thus inhibiting the synthesis of DNA and interfering with transcription of RNA.	bleomycin (Blenoxane), dactinomycin (Cosmegen), daunorubicin (Cerubidine, DaunoXome), doxorubicin (Adriamycin, Rubex, Doxil), epirubicin (Ellence), idarubicin (Idamycin), mitomycin (Mutamycin), mitoxantrone (Novantrone), plicamycin (Mithracin), valrubicin (Valstar)
Mitotic Inhibitors	
Cell Cycle Phase-Specific Agents	
Taxanes	
Antimicrotubule agents that interfere with mitosis. Act during the late G_2 phase and mitosis to stabilize microtubules, thus inhibiting cell division.	albumin-bound paclitaxel (Abraxane), docetaxel (Taxotere), paclitaxel (Taxol)
Vinca Alkaloids	
Act in M phase to inhibit mitosis.	vinblastine (Velban), vincristine (Oncovin), vinorelbine (Navelbine)
Others	
Microtubular inhibitors.	estramustine (Emcyt), ixabepilone (Ixempra), eribulin (Halaven)
Topoisomerase Inhibitors	
Cell Cycle Phase–Specific Agents	
Inhibit topoisomerases (normal enzymes) that function to make reversible breaks and repairs in DNA that allow for flexibility of DNA in replication.	etoposide (VePesid), irinotecan (Camptosar), teniposide (Vumon), topotecan (Hycamtin)
Corticosteroids	
Cell Cycle Phase–Nonspecific Agents	
Disrupt the cell membrane and inhibit synthesis of protein. Decrease circulating lymphocytes, inhibit mitosis, depress immune system, increase sense of well-being.	cortisone (Cortone), dexamethasone (Decadron), hydrocortisone (Cortef), methylprednisolone (Medrol), prednisone
Hormone Therapy	
Cell Cycle Phase–Nonspecific Agents	
Antiestrogens	
Selectively attach to estrogen receptors, causing down-regulation of them and inhibiting tumor growth. Also known as selective estrogen receptor modulators (SERMs).	fulvestrant (Faslodex), raloxifene (Evista), tamoxifen (Nolvadex), toremifene (Fareston)
Estrogens	
Interfere with hormone receptors and proteins.	estradiol (Estrace), estramustine (Emcyt), estrogen (Menest)
Aromatase Inhibitors	
Inhibit aromatase, an enzyme that converts adrenal androgen to estrogen.	anastrozole (Arimidex), exemestane (Aromasin), letrozole (Femara)
Miscellaneous	
Enzyme derived from the yeast Erwinia used to deplete the supply of asparagine (amino acid) for leukemic cells that are dependent on an exogenous source of this amino acid. Inhibits protein synthesis.	Erwinia asparaginase, L-asparaginase (Elspar)
Causes changes in DNA in leukemia cells and leads to cell death.	arsenic trioxide (Trisenox)
Suppresses mitosis. Appears to alter DNA, RNA, and protein.	procarbazine (Matulane, Natulan)

Preparation of Chemotherapy

It is important to know the specific guidelines for administration of chemotherapy drugs. In addition, it is important to understand that drugs may pose an occupational hazard to health care professionals who do not follow safe handling guidelines. A person preparing, transporting, or administering chemotherapy may absorb the drug through inhalation of particles when reconstituting a powder and through skin contact from exposure to droplets or powder from oral agents. There may also be some risk in handling the body fluids and excretions of people receiving chemotherapy immediately after administration for 48 hours. Only those personnel specifically trained in chemotherapy handling techniques should be involved with the preparation and administration of antineoplastic agents.

Guidelines for the safe handling of chemotherapy agents have been developed by the National Institute for Occupational Safety and Health (available at *www.cdc.gov/niosh/docs/2004-165*) and the Occupational Safety and Health Administration (OSHA) and the Oncology Nursing Society (ONS).[6]

Methods of Administration

Chemotherapy can be administered by multiple routes (Table 16-8). With advances in drug formulation techniques, more oral chemotherapy agents are available.

TABLE 16-8 DRUG THERAPY

Methods of Chemotherapy Administration

Method	Examples
Oral	cyclophosphamide (Cytoxan), capecitabine (Xeloda), temozolomide (Temodar)
Intramuscular	bleomycin (Blenoxane)
Intravenous	doxorubicin (Adriamycin), vincristine (Oncovin), cisplatin (Platinol), 5-fluorouracil (5-FU), paclitaxel (Taxol)
Intracavitary (pleural, peritoneal)	Radioisotopes, alkylating agents, methotrexate
Intrathecal	methotrexate (preservative free), cytarabine
Intraarterial	dacarbazine, 5-FU, methotrexate
Perfusion	Alkylating agents
Continuous infusion	5-FU, methotrexate, cytarabine
Subcutaneous	cytarabine
Topical	5-FU cream

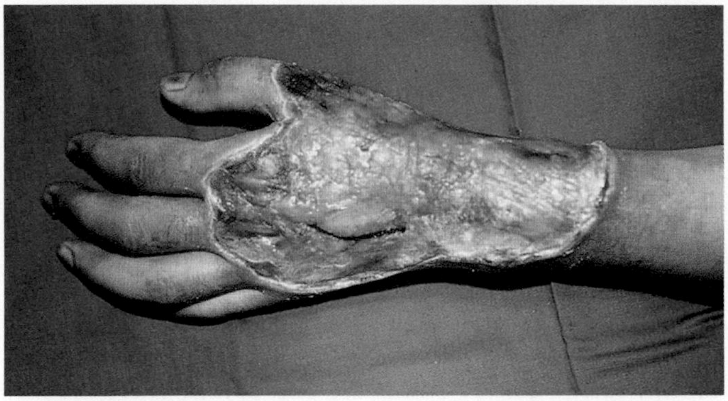

FIG. 16-11 Extravasation injury from infiltration of chemotherapy drug.

The IV route is most common. Major concerns associated with the IV administration of antineoplastic drugs include venous access difficulties, device- or catheter-related infection, and *extravasation* (infiltration of drugs into tissues surrounding the infusion site) causing local tissue damage (Fig. 16-11).

Many chemotherapy drugs are either irritants or vesicants. *Irritants* will damage the intima of the vein, causing phlebitis and sclerosis and limiting future peripheral venous access, but will not cause tissue damage if infiltrated. However, **vesicants,** if inadvertently infiltrated into the skin, may cause severe local tissue breakdown and necrosis. It is extremely important to monitor for and promptly recognize symptoms associated with extravasation of a vesicant and to take immediate action if it occurs. Immediately turn off the infusion and follow protocols for drug-specific extravasation procedures to minimize further tissue damage.

Although pain is the cardinal symptom of extravasation, it can occur without causing pain. Other signs of extravasation are swelling, redness, and vesicles on the skin. After a few days the tissue may begin to ulcerate and necrose. Complications of extravasation include sepsis, scarring, contractures, joint pain, and nerve loss.[6] Vesicants may cause partial- or full-thickness loss of skin. Patients may need surgical intervention varying from debridement to skin grafting.

To minimize the associated physical discomforts, emotional distress, and risks of infection and infiltration, IV chemotherapy can be administered by a *central venous access device* (CVAD). CVADs are placed in large blood vessels and permit frequent, continuous, or intermittent administration of chemotherapy, biologic and targeted therapy, and other products, thus avoiding multiple venipunctures for vascular access. (CVADs are discussed in Chapter 17 on p. 309.)

Regional Chemotherapy Administration

Regional treatment with chemotherapy involves delivery of the drug directly to the tumor site. The advantage of this method is that higher concentrations of the drug can be delivered to the tumor with reduced systemic toxicity. Several regional delivery methods have been developed, including intraarterial, intraperitoneal, intrathecal or intraventricular, and intravesical bladder chemotherapy.

Intraarterial Chemotherapy. Intraarterial chemotherapy delivers the drug to the tumor via the arteries supplying the tumor. This method has been used for the treatment of osteogenic sarcoma; cancers of the head and neck, bladder, brain, and cervix; melanoma; primary liver cancer; and metastatic liver disease. One method of intraarterial drug delivery involves the surgical placement of a catheter that is subsequently connected to an external infusion pump or an implanted infusion pump for infusion of the chemotherapy agent.

Intraperitoneal Chemotherapy. Intraperitoneal chemotherapy involves the delivery of chemotherapy to the peritoneal cavity for treatment of peritoneal metastases from primary colorectal and ovarian cancers and malignant ascites. Temporary Silastic catheters (Tenckhoff, Hickman, and Groshong) are percutaneously or surgically placed into the peritoneal cavity for short-term administration of chemotherapy. Alternatively, an implanted port can be used to administer chemotherapy intraperitoneally. Chemotherapy is generally infused into the peritoneum in 1 to 2 L of fluid and allowed to *dwell* in the peritoneum for 1 to 4 hours. After the *dwell time,* the fluid is drained from the peritoneum.

Intrathecal or Intraventricular Chemotherapy. Cancers that metastasize to the central nervous system (CNS) are difficult to treat because the blood-brain barrier often prevents distribution of chemotherapy to this area. One method used to treat metastasis to the CNS is intrathecal chemotherapy. This method involves a lumbar puncture and injection of chemotherapy into the subarachnoid space. However, this method has resulted in incomplete distribution of the drug in the CNS.

To ensure more uniform distribution of chemotherapy, an Ommaya reservoir is often inserted. An Ommaya reservoir is a Silastic, dome-shaped disk with an extension catheter that is surgically implanted through the cranium into a lateral ventricle. In addition to more consistent drug distribution, the Ommaya reservoir precludes the need for repeated, painful lumbar punctures.

Intravesical Bladder Chemotherapy. *Intravesical bladder chemotherapy* involves instillation of chemotherapy into the bladder. The chemotherapy agent is instilled into the bladder via a urinary catheter and retained for 1 to 3 hours.

Effects of Chemotherapy on Normal Tissues

Chemotherapy agents cannot selectively distinguish between normal cells and cancer cells. Chemotherapy-induced side effects are the result of the destruction of normal cells, especially those that are rapidly proliferating such as those in the bone marrow, the lining of the GI system, and the integumentary system (skin, hair, and nails)[7] (Table 16-9). The general and

TABLE 16-9 CELLS WITH RAPID RATE OF PROLIFERATION

Cells and Generation Time	Effect of Cell Destruction
Bone marrow stem cell, 6-24 hr	Myelosuppression (infection, bleeding, anemia)
Neutrophils, 12 hr	Leukopenia, infection
Epithelial cells lining the gastrointestinal tract, 12-24 hr	Anorexia, mucositis (including stomatitis, esophagitis), nausea and vomiting, diarrhea
Cells of the hair follicle, 24 hr	Alopecia
Ova or testes, 24-36 hr	Reproductive dysfunction

drug-specific adverse effects of these drugs are classified as acute, delayed, or chronic.

Acute toxicity occurs during and immediately after drug administration and includes anaphylactic and hypersensitivity reactions, extravasation or a flare reaction, anticipatory nausea and vomiting, and cardiac dysrhythmias.

Delayed effects are numerous and include delayed nausea and vomiting, mucositis, alopecia, skin rashes, bone marrow suppression, altered bowel function (diarrhea or constipation), and a variety of cumulative neurotoxicities.

Chronic toxicities involve damage to organs such as the heart, liver, kidneys, and lungs. Chronic toxicities can be either long-term effects that develop during or immediately after treatment and persist, or late effects that are absent during treatment and manifest later.

Some side effects fall into more than one category. For example, nausea and vomiting can be both acute and delayed.

Treatment Plan

Although single-drug chemotherapy is sometimes prescribed, combining agents in multidrug regimens has proven to be more effective in managing most cancers. The regimens with multiple agents involve drugs with different mechanisms of action and varying toxicity profiles. However, when chemotherapy agents are used in combination, patients can experience an increase in toxicities.

Drug regimens are selected based on evidence supporting their use in specific cancers. Sometimes they are customized to meet the needs of an individual patient. Chemotherapy is most effective when the tumor burden is low, therapy is not interrupted, and the patient receives the intended dose. The dose of each drug is based on the individual's body weight and height using the body surface area calculation.

Mutation of cancer cells within the tumor can result in cells that are resistant to chemotherapy. With the use of multiple drugs that work at different places in the cell cycle, cancer cells can be more effectively killed. Thus mutation and resistance of cancer cells can be prevented.

RADIATION THERAPY

Along with surgery, radiation therapy is one of the oldest methods of cancer treatment. It was first used by Emil Grubbe (a medical student) to treat an ulcerating breast cancer in 1896 (although the patient responded locally, she died later of metastatic disease). The observation that radiation exposure caused tissue damage led scientists to explore the use of radiation to treat tumors. The hypothesized association was that if radiation exposure resulted in the destruction of highly mitotic skin cells, it could be used in a controlled way to prevent the continued growth of cancer cells.

It was not until the 1960s that sophisticated equipment and treatment planning facilitated the delivery of adequate radiation doses to tumors and tolerable doses to normal tissues. Currently, about half of all cancer patients receive radiation therapy at some point in their treatment.[8]

Effects of Radiation

Radiation is energy that is emitted from a source and travels through space or some material. Delivery of high-energy beams, when absorbed into tissue, produces ionization of atomic particles. The energy in ionizing radiation acts to break the chemical bonds in DNA. The DNA is damaged, resulting in cell death.

Different types of ionizing radiation are used to treat cancer, including *electromagnetic radiation* (i.e., x-rays, gamma rays) and *particulate radiation* (alpha particles, electrons, neutrons, protons). High-energy x-rays (photons) are generated by an electric machine, such as a linear accelerator (sometimes referred to as a *linac*).

Technologic advances have expanded and refined the sources and methods of delivering radiation therapy, thus offering more accurate and less invasive radiation treatment options. Most radiation centers in the United States currently use megavoltage linear accelerator technology. Larger radiation facilities may offer a combination of machines that permit expanded options for patients at one treatment site.

Principles of Radiobiology

As the radiation beam passes through the treatment field, energy is deposited. *Low-energy beams* (such as electrons) expend energy quickly on impact with matter. Therefore they penetrate only a short distance. (They are clinically useful in treating superficial skin lesions.) *High-energy beams* (such as photons) have greater depth of penetration, not attaining full intensity until they reach a certain depth. Therefore they are suitable for delivering optimal doses to internal targets while sparing the skin. The principles of radiation therapy are guided by cell response to radiation, known as the four *R*s of radiobiology (see eTable 16-4 on the website for this chapter).

Technically, all cancer cells could be killed with radiation given in high enough doses. However, to avoid serious toxicity and long-term complications of treatment, radiation to surrounding healthy tissue must be limited to the *maximal tolerated dose* for that specific tissue. Advances in planning and in delivery technology (such as *intensity-modulated radiation therapy [IMRT]* and *image-guided radiation therapy [IGRT]*) have greatly improved the ability to deliver maximal doses to the target volume while sparing critical structures (e.g., spinal cord, carotid arteries, optic chiasm) as much as possible.

Historically, the radiation dose was expressed in units called *rads* (radiation absorbed doses). Current nomenclature is *gray* (Gy) or centigray (cGy). A *centigray* is equivalent to 1 rad, and 100 centigray equals 1 gray.

Once the total dose to be delivered is determined, that dose is divided into daily *fractions*. Doses between 180 and 200 cGy/day are considered *standard fractionation*, typically delivered once a day Monday through Friday for a period of 2 to 8 weeks (depending on the desired total dose). Other treatment schedules may be prescribed based on principles of radiobiologic effect. High daily doses of radiation may be given with fewer

TABLE 16-10 TUMOR RADIOSENSITIVITY*

High Radiosensitivity	Mild Radiosensitivity
• Ovarian dysgerminoma	• Soft tissue sarcomas (e.g., chondrosarcoma)
• Testicular seminoma	• Gastric adenocarcinoma
• Hodgkin's lymphoma	• Renal adenocarcinoma
• Non-Hodgkin's lymphoma	• Colon adenocarcinoma
• Wilms' tumor	
• Neuroblastoma	
Moderate Radiosensitivity	**Poor Radiosensitivity**
• Oropharyngeal carcinoma	• Osteosarcoma
• Esophageal carcinoma	• Malignant melanoma
• Breast adenocarcinoma	• Malignant glioma
• Uterine and cervical carcinoma	• Testicular nonseminoma
• Prostate carcinoma	
• Bladder carcinoma	

*Radiosensitivity is the relative susceptibility of cells and tissues to the effects of radiation.

fractions *(hypofractionated),* lower doses may be given more than once daily *(hyperfractionated),* or standard doses may be delivered twice daily over a shortened treatment time *(accelerated fractionation).*

The amount of time required for the manifestations of radiation damage is determined by the mitotic rate of the tissue, with rapidly proliferating tissues being more sensitive. Rapidly dividing cells in the GI tract, oral mucosa, and bone marrow die quickly and exhibit early acute responses to radiation. Tissues with slowly proliferating cells, such as cartilage, bone, and kidneys, manifest later responses to radiation. This differential rate of cell death explains the timing of clinical manifestations related to radiation therapy.

Certain cancers are more susceptible to the effects of radiation than others (Table 16-10). In responsive tumors (such as lymphomas), even a large tumor burden is affected by radiation therapy. In less responsive tumors, a large tumor burden may result in a slower and perhaps incomplete response. Localized prostate cancer responds very slowly to radiation (several months after treatment is completed).

Simulation and Treatment Planning

Simulation is a process by which the radiation treatment fields are defined, filmed, and marked out on the skin. The radiation oncologist specifies the dose and volume of area to be treated. Treatment volumes include the (1) *gross target v*olume (GTV), which is the gross extent of the tumor identified by examination or imaging; (2) the *clinical target* volume (CTV), which is the GTV plus additional margin to encompass any potential microscopic or subclinical disease; and (3) the *planning target volume* (PTV), which is the GTV/CTV plus additional margin to allow for organ motion or variance in daily set-up position.[9]

During the simulation, goals of the radiation plan are met by determining the orientation and size of radiation beams, defining the location of field-shaping blocks, and outlining the field on the patient's skin. The patient is positioned on a simulator, which is a diagnostic x-ray machine that re-creates the actions of the linear accelerator. Immobilization devices (e.g., casts, bite blocks, thermoplastic face masks) are typically used to help the patient maintain a stable position (Fig. 16-12).

The target is defined using a variety of possible imaging techniques (e.g., x-rays; CT, MRI, PET scans), physical examination, and surgical reports. Under fluoroscopy or with

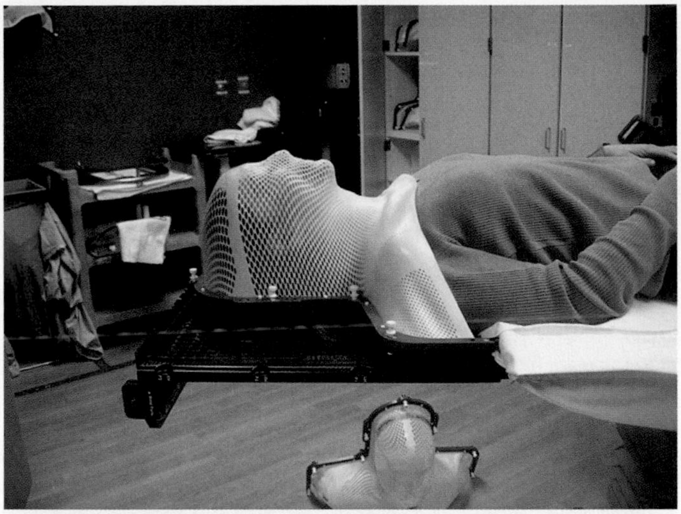

FIG. 16-12 Immobilization device. A head holder and an immobilization mask may be used to ensure accurate positioning for daily treatment of head and neck cancer.

CT-based treatment planning, the critical normal structures that will be included in the treatment field (or portal) are identified so they can be protected. A film is taken to verify the field, and marks are placed on the skin to delineate the "treatment port." Small tattoos may be placed to ensure the patient position is precisely reproduced on a daily basis.

Treatment

Radiation is used to treat a carefully defined area of the body. Since radiation only has an effect on tissues within the treatment field, it is not appropriate as the primary treatment for systemic disease. However, radiation may be used by itself, in combination with chemotherapy or surgery to treat primary tumors, or for palliation of metastatic lesions (see eTable 16-5 on the website for this chapter).

External Radiation. Radiation can be delivered externally (known as *teletherapy* or *external beam radiation therapy*) or internally *(brachytherapy).* **Teletherapy** *(external beam radiation)* is the most common form of radiation treatment delivery. With this technique, the patient is exposed to radiation from a megavoltage treatment machine. A linear accelerator, which generates ionizing radiation from electricity and can have multiple energies, is the most commonly used machine for delivering external beam radiation (Fig. 16-13). *Gamma knife technology* (used to deliver highly accurate stereotactic treatment to a localized treatment volume) uses a cobalt source. A cyclotron produces particulate energy, such as neutrons or protons. Proton therapy requires significant energy to generate, and only a small number of facilities in the United States are equipped to provide this treatment.

A linear accelerator may be used to deliver different types of treatment techniques (or plans). A *two-dimensional* plan is the simplest type of therapy, designed using x-rays, bony landmarks, and a simple beam arrangement. *Three-dimensional-conformal therapy* plans treatment based on three-dimensional anatomy using CT and/or other imaging, with the goal of improved dose distribution around the target volume. *Intensity-modulated radiation therapy* (IMRT) involves an inverse planning process, in which multiple beams of varying intensity deliver tailored treatment doses to a precise treatment field. It

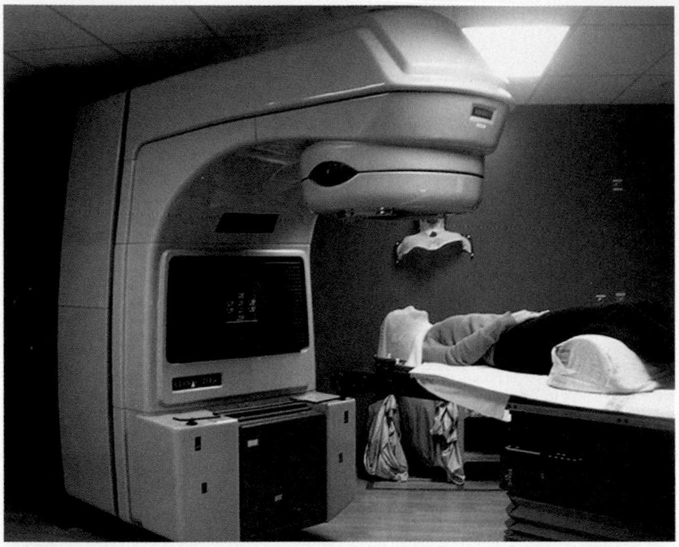

FIG. 16-13 Linear accelerator. Varian Clinac EX linear accelerator with multiple photon and electron energies available for use according to the treatment plan. Patient is positioned on radiation treatment table for treatment of head and neck cancer.

is more labor intensive to plan but has the advantage of tailoring beam intensity to optimize dose delivery to the target volume while minimizing dose to critical structures. It is particularly well suited to treating irregularly shaped fields and fields adjacent to sensitive structures (e.g., head and neck cancers).

Volumetric-modulated arc therapy (VMAT) and *tomotherapy* build on IMRT to further improve accuracy of dose delivery. With VMAT, the dose is delivered in one to three continuous arcs around the patient. An advantage of VMAT over standard IMRT is dramatically reduced treatment time, often delivering treatments in 3 to 5 minutes that previously would have taken 20 to 30 minutes.

Tomotherapy is a similar concept, but is done with a specialized linear accelerator built into a round gantry (similar to a CT scanner). The gantry rotates spirally around the patient advancing through the "doughnut," and treatment is thus delivered in "slice by slice" fashion. Dosimetry with tomotherapy appears to be comparable or superior to standard IMRT or VMAT, but is not as time efficient as VMAT.

Image-guided radiation therapy (IGRT) (sometimes referred to as *four-dimensional-conformal* therapy) further optimizes the delivery of conformal or IMRT treatment plans by addressing the element of physiologic movement over time. IGRT incorporates methods to control for physiologic movement during therapy, or anatomic changes (such as tumor shrinkage or weight loss), on a daily basis or over time during the treatment course. Imaging (usually CT, fluoroscopy, or ultrasound) may be performed in conjunction with the radiation treatment to detect any variations in tumor position or organ movement. Images are taken daily before treatment and compared with the original treatment plan so that "shifts" can be made if necessary to accommodate for any variations in target localization. Such tracking and visualization of tumor position during treatment may further improve the accuracy of dose delivery to the intended target volume. Although it is unclear how much these technologies will affect survival, IMRT treatment planning can reduce treatment toxicity, especially for prostate and head and neck cancers.

Internal Radiation. Radiation can also be delivered as **brachytherapy**, which means "close" or internal radiation treatment. It consists of the implantation or insertion of radioactive materials directly into the tumor (interstitial) or in close proximity to the tumor (intracavitary or intraluminal). This allows for direct delivery of radiation to the target with minimal exposure to surrounding healthy tissues. (In external radiation, the beam has to pass through external tissues to reach the internal target.) Brachytherapy is commonly used in combination with external radiation as a supplemental "boost" treatment, but may also be used as primary or adjuvant therapy.

Sources of radiation for brachytherapy include temporary sealed sources such as iridium-192 and cesium-137 and permanent sealed sources such as iodine-125, gold-198, and palladium-103. These are supplied in the form of seeds or ribbons. With a temporary implant, the source may be placed into a special catheter or metal tube that has been inserted into the tumor area. It is left in place until the prescribed dose of radiation has been reached in the calculated number of hours.

Brachytherapy may be delivered as high-dose-rate (HDR) treatment (i.e., several doses administered at varying intervals over a few minutes each time) or low-dose-rate (LDR) treatment (i.e., continuous treatment over several hours or days). A remote "afterloading" technique (i.e., the source is inserted after the applicator is in place) is designed to enhance physician and patient safety and is used for HDR brachytherapy with iridium-192. These methods are commonly used for head and neck, lung, breast, and gynecologic malignancies.

Permanent implants, such as for prostate brachytherapy, involve the insertion of radioactive seeds directly into the tumor tissue, where they remain permanently. As interstitial seeds used for treatment emit low energies with limited tissue penetration, patients are not considered radioactive. However, some initial radiation precautions may be recommended because of a small risk of seed dislodgement. Over time, the isotopes that are used decay and are no longer radioactive. The timeframe for side effects induced by treatment can be predicted based on the rate of decay for the specific isotope used.

Radiopharmaceutical therapy employs unsealed liquid radioactive sources that are administered orally as a drink, such as iodine-131 for thyroid cancer, or IV as with yttrium-90 given for refractory lymphomas or samarium-153 used to treat bone metastases.

Caring for the person undergoing brachytherapy or receiving radiopharmaceuticals requires that you be aware that the patient is emitting radioactivity. Patients with temporary implants are radioactive only while the source is in place. In patients with permanent implants, because the sources have fairly short half-lives and are weak emitters, the radioactive exposure to the outside and to others is low. These patients may be discharged with minimal precautions.

The principles of *ALARA (as low as reasonably achievable)* and *time, distance,* and *shielding* are vital to health care professional safety when caring for the person with a source of internal radiation. Organize care to limit the time spent in direct contact with the patient. To minimize anxiety and confusion, tell the patient the reason for time and distance limitations before the procedure.

The radiation safety officer will indicate how much time at a specific distance can be spent with the patient. This is determined by the dose delivered by the implant. Because the source is nonpenetrating, small differences in distance are critical.

Only care that must be delivered near the source, such as checking placement of the implant, is performed in close proximity. Use shielding, if available, and do not deliver care without wearing a film badge indicating cumulative radiation exposure. Do not share the film badge, do not wear it anywhere but at work, and return it according to the agency's protocol.

NURSING MANAGEMENT CHEMOTHERAPY AND RADIATION THERAPY

You have an important role in helping patients deal with the side effects of chemotherapy and radiation therapy. Before initiating teaching, assess the patient's ability to process information. Customize teaching to meet the patient's and the family's learning needs.

Common side effects of chemotherapy and radiation are presented in Table 16-11. Bone marrow suppression, fatigue, GI disturbances, integumentary and mucosal reactions, and pulmonary and reproductive effects are discussed in this section.

NURSING IMPLEMENTATION

BONE MARROW SUPPRESSION. Myelosuppression is one of the most common effects of chemotherapy and, to a lesser extent, it can also occur with radiation. Treatment-induced reductions in blood cell production can result in life-threatening and distressing effects, including infection, hemorrhage, and overwhelming fatigue. The major difference in manifestations between radiation therapy and chemotherapy is that with radiation (a local therapy), only bone marrow within the treatment field is affected, whereas chemotherapy (a systemic therapy) affects bone marrow function throughout the body. Therefore effects are more profound with chemotherapy and when the two therapies are combined.

In general, the onset of bone marrow suppression is related to the life span of the type of blood cell. WBCs (especially neutrophils) are affected most acutely (within 1 to 2 weeks), platelets in 2 to 3 weeks, and red blood cells (RBCs), with a longer life span of 120 days, at a later time. The severity of myelosuppression depends on the chemotherapy drugs used, dosages of drugs, and the specific radiation treatment field. Radiation to large marrow-containing regions of the body produces the most clinically significant myelosuppression. In the adult, most of the active marrow is in the pelvis or thoracic and lumbar vertebrae.

Monitor the complete blood count, particularly the neutrophil, platelet, and RBC counts, in patients receiving chemotherapy or radiation. Typically patients experience the lowest blood cell counts (called the **nadir**) between 7 and 10 days after initiation of therapy. However, the exact onset depends on the particular drug regimen.

Neutropenia is more common in patients receiving chemotherapy than radiation therapy. Neutropenia is a serious risk factor for life-threatening infection and sepsis. Significant neutropenia will prompt treatment delay or modification (i.e., lower dosages). Take every possible measure to prevent infections in these patients. Hand hygiene is the mainstay of patient protection. Patients and their contacts (including hospital staff) should follow hand-washing guidelines. Other precautions to minimize risks from neutropenia are presented in eTable 16-6, available on the website for this chapter.

Monitor temperature routinely. Any sign of infection should be treated promptly, since fever in the setting of neutropenia is a medical emergency. WBC growth factors (i.e., filgrastim [Neupogen], pegfilgrastim [Neulasta]) are routinely used to reduce the duration of chemotherapy-induced neutropenia. They are also used as a prophylactic measure to prevent neutropenia when highly myelosuppressive chemotherapy drugs are used.[10] (Neutropenia is discussed in Chapter 31; see also the patient teaching guide in Table 31-24 and eNursing Care Plan 31-2 on the website for that chapter.)

Thrombocytopenia can result in spontaneous bleeding or major hemorrhage. Avoid invasive procedures and advise patients to avoid activities that place them at risk for injury or bleeding (including excessive straining). Risk of serious bleeding is generally not apparent until the platelet count falls below 50,000/μL. Platelet transfusions may be necessary and are usually administered when platelet counts fall below 20,000/μL. (Thrombocytopenia is discussed in Chapter 31; see also the patient teaching guide in Table 31-16 and eNursing Care Plan 31-1 on the website for that chapter.)

Anemia is common in patients undergoing either radiation therapy or chemotherapy. It generally has a later onset (about 3 to 4 months after treatment initiation). For patients with low hemoglobin levels, RBC growth factors (i.e., darbepoetin [Aranesp], epoetin [Procrit]) may be given according to clinical guidelines for use. In extreme circumstances (i.e., symptomatic anemia), RBC transfusions may also be indicated. However, in general, RBC transfusions should be avoided. (Hematopoietic growth factors are discussed later in this chapter and presented in Table 16-14 on p. 274.)

FATIGUE. *Fatigue* is the persistent subjective sense of tiredness associated with cancer and its treatment that interferes with usual day-to-day functioning. Fatigue is a nearly universal symptom affecting most patients with cancer. It is commonly reported by patients as the most distressful of treatment-related side effects. Furthermore, it may persist long after treatment has ended.

Anemia is one cause of fatigue. Other causes may be related to (1) the accumulation of toxic substances that are left in the body after cells are killed by cancer treatment, (2) the need for extra energy to repair and heal body tissue damaged by treatment, and (3) lack of sleep caused by some chemotherapy drugs. Assess for reversible causes of fatigue, such as anemia, hypothyroidism, depression, anxiety, insomnia, dehydration, or infection.[11]

Help patients recognize that fatigue is a common side effect of therapy, and encourage energy conservation strategies. Help individuals identify days or times during the day when they typically feel better, and encourage them to remain more active during that time period. Resting before activity and having others assist with work or home management may be necessary. Ignoring the fatigue or overstressing the body when fatigue is tolerable may lead to an increase in symptoms. However, maintaining exercise and activity within tolerable limits is often helpful in managing fatigue. Walking programs are a way for most patients to keep active without overtaxing themselves. Remaining active helps to improve mood and avoid the debilitating cycle of fatigue-depression-fatigue that can occur in patients with cancer.

Published guidelines for the evaluation and management of cancer-related fatigue have been developed by the NCCN[11] and are available at *www.nccn.org*.

GASTROINTESTINAL EFFECTS. The cells of the mucosal lining of the GI tract are highly proliferative, with epithelial cells being replaced every 2 to 6 days. The intestinal mucosa is one of the

TABLE 16-11 NURSING MANAGEMENT OF PROBLEMS CAUSED BY CHEMOTHERAPY AND RADIATION THERAPY

Etiology	Nursing Management
Gastrointestinal System	
Stomatitis, Mucositis, Esophagitis	
• Epithelial cells are destroyed by chemotherapy or radiation treatment when located in field (e.g., head and neck, stomach, esophagus). • Inflammation and ulceration occur due to rapid cell destruction.	• Assess oral mucosa daily and teach patient to do this. • Encourage nutritional supplements (e.g., Ensure, Carnation Instant Breakfast) if intake decreasing. • Be aware that eating, swallowing, and talking may be difficult (may require analgesics). • Instruct in diet modification as necessary (avoidance of irritating spicy or acidic foods; selection of moist, bland, and softer foods). • Encourage patient to keep oral cavity clean and moist by performing frequent oral rinses with saline or salt and soda solution. • Encourage patient to use artificial saliva to manage dryness (radiation). • Discourage use of irritants such as tobacco and alcohol. • Apply topical anesthetics (e.g., viscous lidocaine, oxethazaine).
Nausea and Vomiting	
• Release of intracell breakdown products stimulates vomiting center in brain. • Drugs also stimulate vomiting center in brain (see Fig. 42-1). • GI lining destroyed with radiation and chemotherapy.	• Encourage patient to eat and drink when not nauseated. • Administer antiemetics prophylactically before chemotherapy and also on as-needed basis. • Instruct patient to take antiemetics on a scheduled basis for 2-3 days after highly emetogenic chemotherapy. • Use diversional activities (if appropriate).
Anorexia	
• Release of TNF and IL-1 from macrophages has appetite-suppressant effect. • Therapy-induced GI effects (mucositis, nausea and vomiting, bowel disturbances) and anxiety reduce appetite.	• Monitor weight. • Encourage patient to eat small, frequent meals of high-protein, high-calorie foods. • Gently encourage patient to eat, but avoid nagging. • Recommend keeping a food diary to track daily calories and fluids. • Serve food in pleasant environment.
Diarrhea	
• From denuding of epithelial lining of intestines. • Side effect of chemotherapy. • Follows radiation to abdomen, pelvis, lumbosacral areas.	• Give antidiarrheal drugs as needed. • Encourage low-fiber, low-residue diet. • Encourage fluid intake of at least 3 L/day.
Constipation	
• Decreased intestinal motility is related to autonomic nervous system dysfunction. • Caused by neurotoxic effects of plant alkaloids (vincristine, vinblastine).	• Instruct patient to take stool softeners as needed, eat high-fiber foods, and increase fluid intake. • Instruct patient to increase activity (e.g., walking) if tolerated.
Hepatotoxicity	
• Toxic effects from chemotherapy drugs (usually transient and resolve when drug is stopped).	• Monitor liver function tests.
Hematologic System	
Anemia	
• Bone marrow depressed secondary to therapy. • Malignant infiltration of bone marrow by cancer.	• Monitor hemoglobin and hematocrit levels. • Administer iron supplements and erythropoietin. • Encourage intake of foods that promote RBC production (see Table 31-5).
Leukopenia	
• Depression of bone marrow secondary to chemotherapy or radiation therapy. • Infection most frequent cause of morbidity and death in cancer patients. • Respiratory and genitourinary system usual sites of infection.	• Monitor WBC count, especially neutrophils. • Tell patient to report temperature elevation and any other manifestations of infection. • Teach patient to avoid large crowds and people with infections. • Administer WBC growth factors (see Table 16-14). • For patient teaching, see Table 31-24.
Thrombocytopenia	
• Bone marrow depressed secondary to chemotherapy. • Malignant infiltration of bone marrow crowds out normal marrow. • Spontaneous bleeding can occur with platelet counts $\leq 20,000/\mu L$.	• Observe for signs of bleeding (e.g., petechiae, ecchymosis). • Monitor platelet counts. • For patient teaching, see Table 31-16.
Integumentary System	
Alopecia	
• Destruction of hair follicles by chemotherapy or radiation to scalp. • Hair loss usually is temporary with chemotherapy, but usually permanent in response to radiation.	• Suggest ways to cope with hair loss (e.g., hair pieces, scarves, wigs). • Cut long hair before therapy. • Avoid excessive shampooing, brushing, and combing of hair. • Avoid use of electric hair dryers, curlers, and curling rods. • Discuss impact of hair loss on self-image.

TABLE 16-11 NURSING MANAGEMENT OF PROBLEMS CAUSED BY CHEMOTHERAPY AND RADIATION THERAPY—cont'd

Etiology	Nursing Management
Radiation Skin Changes (dry to moist desquamation)	
• Radiation damages skin.	• See Table 16-12 for patient management details.
Chemotherapy-Induced Skin Changes	
• Hyperpigmentation • Telangiectasia • Photosensitivity • Acneiform eruptions • Acral erythema	• Alert patient to potential skin changes. • Encourage patient to avoid sun exposure. • Implement symptomatic management as needed depending on specific skin effect (e.g., application of lotions, benzoyl peroxide for acne, corticosteroid creams).
Genitourinary Tract	
Hemorrhagic Cystitis	
• Cells lining bladder are destroyed by chemotherapy (e.g., cyclophosphamide, ifosfamide). • Side effect of radiation when located in treatment field.	• Encourage increased fluid intake 24-72 hr after treatment as tolerated. • Monitor manifestations such as urgency, frequency, and hematuria. • Administer cytoprotectant agent (mesna [Mesnex]) and hydration. • Administer supportive care agents to manage symptoms (e.g., flavoxate [Urispas]).
Reproductive Dysfunction	
• Cells of testes or ova are damaged by therapy.	• Discuss possibility with patients before treatment initiation. • Offer opportunity for sperm and ova banking before treatment for patients of childbearing age.
Nephrotoxicity	
• Direct renal cell damage from exposure to nephrotoxic agents (cisplatin and high-dose methotrexate). • Precipitation of metabolites of cell breakdown (tumor lysis syndrome [TLS]).	• Monitor BUN and serum creatinine levels. • Avoid potentiating drugs. • Alkalinize the urine with sodium bicarbonate and administer allopurinol (Zyloprim) or rasburicase for TLS prevention.
Nervous System	
Increased Intracranial Pressure	
• May result from radiation edema in central nervous system.	• Monitor neurologic status. • May be controlled with corticosteroids.
Peripheral Neuropathy	
• Paresthesias, areflexia, skeletal muscle weakness, and smooth muscle dysfunction can occur as a side effect of plant alkaloids, taxanes, and cisplatin.	• Monitor for these manifestations in patients on these drugs. • Consider temporary chemotherapy dose interruption or reduction until symptoms improve. • Antiseizure drugs (e.g., gabapentin [Neurontin]) may be considered.
Cognitive Changes ("chemo brain")	

• Occur during and after treatment (especially with chemotherapy).
• Difficulties in concentration, memory lapses, trouble remembering details, taking longer to finish tasks.
• May happen quickly and last a short time. Sometimes people have mild long-term effects.
	• Teach patients to do the following:
	  • Use detailed daily planner.
	  • Get enough sleep and rest.
	  • Exercise brain (learn something new, do word puzzles).
	  • Focus on one thing (no multitasking).

Respiratory System	
Pneumonitis	
• Radiation pneumonitis develops 2-3 mo after start of treatment. • After 6-12 mo, fibrosis occurs and is evident on x-ray. • Side effect of some chemotherapy drugs.	• Monitor for dry, hacking cough; fever; and exertional dyspnea.
Cardiovascular System	
Pericarditis and Myocarditis	
• Inflammation secondary to radiation injury. • Complication when chest wall is irradiated. May occur up to 1 yr after treatment. • Side effect of some chemotherapy drugs.	• Monitor for clinical manifestations of these disorders (e.g., dyspnea).
Cardiotoxicity	
• Some chemotherapy drugs (e.g., anthracyclines, taxanes) can cause ECG changes and rapidly progressive heart failure.	• Monitor heart with ECG and cardiac ejection fractions. • Drug therapy may need to be modified for symptoms or deteriorating cardiac function studies.
Biochemical	
Hyperuricemia	
• Increased uric acid levels due to chemotherapy-induced cell destruction. • Can cause secondary gout and obstructive uropathy.	• Monitor uric acid levels. • Allopurinol may be given as a prophylactic measure. • Encourage increased fluid intake.
Psychoemotional	
Fatigue	
• Anabolic processes result in accumulation of metabolites from cell breakdown.	• Assess for reversible causes of fatigue, and address them as indicated. • Reassure patient that fatigue is a common side effect of therapy. • Encourage patient to rest when fatigued, to maintain usual lifestyle patterns as much as possible, and to pace activities in accordance with energy level. • Encourage moderate exercise as tolerated.

BUN, Blood urea nitrogen; *IL-1,* interleukin-1; *TNF,* tumor necrosis factor.

most sensitive tissues to radiation and chemotherapy. The etiology of GI reactions is related to a variety of mechanisms, including (1) the release of serotonin from the GI tract, which then stimulates the chemoreceptor trigger zone (CTZ) and the vomiting center in the brain; and (2) cell death and resulting damage to GI mucosa. Additionally, radiation to treatment fields that contain GI structures (i.e., abdominopelvic, lumbosacral, and lower thoracic areas) and selected chemotherapy agents produce direct injury to GI epithelial cells. These injuries result in a variety of GI effects, including nausea and vomiting, diarrhea, mucositis, and anorexia. These problems can significantly affect the patient's hydration and nutritional status and sense of well-being.

Nausea and Vomiting. Nausea and vomiting are common sequelae of chemotherapy and, in some instances, radiation therapy. Vomiting may occur within 1 hour of chemotherapy administration or a few hours after radiation therapy to the chest or abdomen and may persist for 24 hours or more. Several antiemetic drugs are available (see Table 42-1). Metoclopramide (Reglan), prochlorperazine (Compazine), serotonin (5-HT$_3$) receptor antagonists (ondansetron [Zofran], granisetron [Kytril], dolasetron [Anzemet], and palonosetron [Aloxi]), and dexamethasone (Decadron) have been used to decrease nausea and vomiting caused by chemotherapy. Aprepitant (Emend), a neurokinin-1 receptor antagonist, is effective in preventing nausea and vomiting on the day of chemotherapy, as well as for delayed symptoms.[12,13]

Patients may also develop *anticipatory nausea and vomiting* if they experience poorly controlled nausea and vomiting after chemotherapy administration. In this phenomenon, encountering the cues even without receiving treatment may precipitate nausea and vomiting. Aggressive emesis control, including the prophylactic administration of antiemetic and antianxiety medication 1 hour before treatment, is recommended. The patient may find that eating a light meal of nonirritating food before treatment is also helpful.

Delayed nausea and vomiting can develop 24 hours to a week after treatment. Assess patients experiencing nausea and vomiting for signs and symptoms of dehydration and metabolic alkalosis. Nausea and vomiting can be successfully managed with antiemetic regimens, dietary modification, and other nondrug interventions (e.g., relaxation breathing).

Diarrhea. Diarrhea is a reaction of the bowel mucosa to radiation and to certain chemotherapy drugs. It is characterized by an increase in frequency and liquidity of stool. The small bowel is extremely sensitive and does not tolerate significant radiation doses. With pelvic radiation, patients may be treated with a full bladder to move the small bowel out of the treatment field. Both radiation- and chemotherapy-induced diarrhea are best managed with diet modification, antidiarrheals, antimotility agents, and antispasmodics (see Table 43-2).

Recommend a diet low in fiber and residue before treatment with chemotherapy known to cause diarrhea. This includes limiting foods that are high in roughage (e.g., fresh fruits, vegetables, seeds, nuts) (see Table 43-6). To prevent diarrhea, other foods to avoid include fried, fatty, or highly seasoned foods and other foods that are gas producing. Bowel mucosal injury from radiation may also result in temporary lactose intolerance. Therefore avoiding milk products is helpful for some patients during and immediately after treatment.

Depending on the severity of the diarrhea, hydration and electrolyte supplementation are also recommended. Lukewarm sitz baths may alleviate discomfort and cleanse the rectal area if significant rectal irritation has developed. The rectal area must be kept clean and dry to maintain skin integrity. You should visually inspect the perianal area for evidence of skin breakdown. Systemic analgesia may be warranted for the painful skin irritations that may develop. Note the number, volume, consistency, and character of stools per day. Teach patients to maintain a diary or log to record episodes and aggravating and alleviating factors.[14]

Mucositis. Mucositis (irritation, inflammation, and/or ulceration of the mucosa) is a common complication in almost all patients receiving radiation to the head and neck and in many patients receiving certain antineoplastic agents, especially 5-fluorouracil (5-FU). Similar to the bowel mucosa, the mucosal linings of the oral cavity, oropharynx, and esophagus are extremely sensitive to the effects of radiation and chemotherapy.

Certain factors can compound the problem. For example, patients undergoing head and neck radiation may face the additional challenge of radiation-induced parotid gland dysfunction. This may result in decreased salivary flow, causing acute or chronic *xerostomia* (dry mouth). Dryness or thick saliva compromises the protective salivary functions of assisting with cleansing teeth, moistening food, and swallowing. Meticulous oral care during and for a long time after treatment reduces the risk of cavities related to the radiation, which may develop as a result of diminished saliva. Advise patients to continue regular dental follow-up every 6 months and to use fluoride supplements as recommended by their dentist. Saliva substitutes may be offered to patients with xerostomia, although many patients find that drinking small amounts of water frequently has a similar effect.

Amifostine (a cytoprotectant) may be used during radiation treatment if a significant radiation dose to the parotid glands is expected. It may help to reduce radiation-related mucositis.

Dysgeusia (taste loss) may develop during therapy, and by the end of treatment patients often report that all food has lost its flavor. Ultimately, nutritional status may be compromised. *Dysphagia* (difficulty swallowing), which characterizes pharyngeal and/or esophageal involvement, further impedes eating. Patients may report feeling that they have a "lump" as they swallow and that "foods get stuck." *Odynophagia* (painful swallowing) caused by oropharyngeal or esophageal irritation and ulceration may require the use of analgesics before meals.

Oral assessment and meticulous intervention to keep the oral cavity moist, clean, and free of debris are essential to prevent infection and to facilitate nutritional intake. Implementing standard oral care protocols that address prevention and management of mucositis facilitates routine assessment, patient and family education, and intervention.

Routinely assess the oral cavity, mucous membranes, characteristics of saliva, and ability to swallow. Having a dentist perform all necessary dental work before the initiation of treatment is also recommended. Teach patients to self-examine the oral cavity and also how to perform oral care (proper tooth brushing with a soft-bristle toothbrush, flossing, and use of fluoride trays to prevent caries). Oral care should be performed at least before and after each meal, at bedtime, and as needed through the day. A saline solution of 1 tsp of salt in 1 L of water is an effective cleansing agent. One tsp of sodium bicarbonate may be added to the oral care solution to decrease odor, alleviate pain, and dissolve mucin.

Mucositis or pain in the throat can be alleviated by systemic and/or topical analgesics and antibiotics if infection is present. Monitor and get prompt treatment for oral candidiasis (which often occurs with mucositis). Frequent cleansing with saline and water and topical application of anesthetic gels directly to the lesions are standard care.

Palifermin (Kepivance), a synthetic version of keratinocyte growth factor, is available to prevent or shorten the duration of mucositis. It is given IV and stimulates growth of cells on the surface layer of the mouth. This leads to faster replacement of these cells when killed by cancer treatment. It may also speed up the healing process of mouth ulcers. Palifermin is currently recommended for mucositis prevention in patients with hematologic malignancies undergoing treatment. The safety and efficacy of palifermin have not been established in patients with nonhematologic malignancies.

Anorexia. Anorexia (loss of appetite) is a common occurrence in patients with cancer. It is a side effect of the cancer itself as well as of cancer treatment. Anorexia may be related to an inflamed mouth or esophagus, which creates difficulty chewing or swallowing, or to emotions such as anxiety or depression.

Patients experiencing nausea and vomiting, bowel disturbances, mucositis, and taste alterations typically have little desire to eat. Although it is highly individual, anorexia seems to peak at about 4 weeks of treatment and to resolve more quickly than fatigue when treatment ends.

Monitor the patient with anorexia during and after treatment to ensure that weight loss does not become excessive. Also observe for dehydration. Small, frequent meals of high-protein, high-calorie foods are better tolerated than large meals. Nutritional supplements can be helpful as well. Enteral or parenteral nutrition may be indicated if the patient is severely malnourished, if symptoms are expected to interfere with nutrition for a time, or if the bowel is being rested. Monitor for and manage other symptoms that may interfere with appetite (e.g., nausea, vomiting, pain, depression).[15]

SKIN REACTIONS

Radiation Skin Changes. With radiation, skin effects are local, occurring only in the treatment field. Radiation-induced skin changes can be acute or chronic depending on the area irradiated, dosage, and technique. The skin-sparing ability of modern radiation equipment limits the severity of these reactions. Erythema may develop 1 to 24 hours after a single treatment, but generally occurs progressively as the treatment dose accumulates. Erythema is an acute response followed by dry desquamation (Fig. 16-14). If the rate of cell sloughing is faster than the ability of the new epidermal cells to replace dead cells, a wet desquamation occurs with exposure of the dermis and weeping of serous fluid (Fig. 16-15). Skin reactions are particularly evident in areas of skinfolds or where skin is subjected to pressure, such as behind the ear; in gluteal folds; or on the perineum, breast, collar line, and bony prominences.

Although skin care protocols vary among institutions, basic skin care principles apply. The goal is to prevent infection and facilitate wound healing. Protect radiated skin from temperature extremes. Do not use heating pads, ice packs, and hot water bottles in the treatment field. Avoid constricting garments, rubbing, harsh chemicals, and deodorants, since they may traumatize the skin. Dry reactions are uncomfortable and result in pruritus. Lubricate dry skin with a nonirritating lotion emollient that contains no metal, alcohol, perfume, or additives, since these can be irritating. Calendula ointment and topical hyaluronic acid cream are effective for the management of radiation dermatitis. Aloe vera gel is also used, especially for prevention of skin problems.[16]

Wet desquamation of tissues generally produces pain, drainage, and increased risk of infection. Skin care to manage most desquamation includes keeping tissues clean with normal saline compresses or modified Burow's solution soaks and protected from further damage with moisture vapor–permeable dressings or Vaseline petrolatum gauze. Because protocols vary widely, the guidelines presented in Table 16-12 should be verified with your institution's radiation oncology department before using.

Chemotherapy Skin Changes. Chemotherapy produces a wide range of skin toxicities. These can range from mild erythema and hyperpigmentation to more distressing effects such as acral erythema and *erythrodysesthesia syndrome* (also called palmar-plantar erythrodysesthesia or hand-foot syndrome). Erythrodysesthesia syndrome can cause mild symptoms of redness and tingling of the palms of the hands and soles of the feet. It may also cause severe symptoms of painful moist desquamation, ulceration, blistering, and pain.

Alopecia is an easily recognizable effect of cancer therapy. It is frequently associated with varying degrees of emotional distress. Hair loss associated with radiation is local, whereas chemotherapy affects hair throughout the body. The degree and duration of hair loss experienced by patients depend on the type and dose of the chemotherapy agent.

Alopecia caused by the administration of chemotherapy agents is usually reversible. Sometimes the hair grows back while the patient is still receiving chemotherapy agents, but generally the hair does not grow back until 3 to 4 weeks after

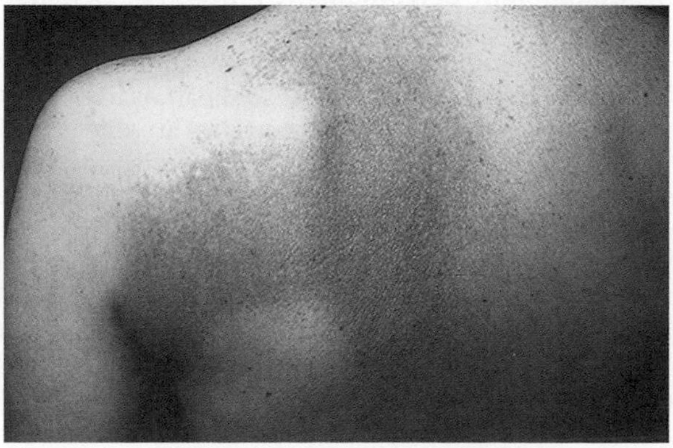

FIG. 16-14 Dry desquamation.

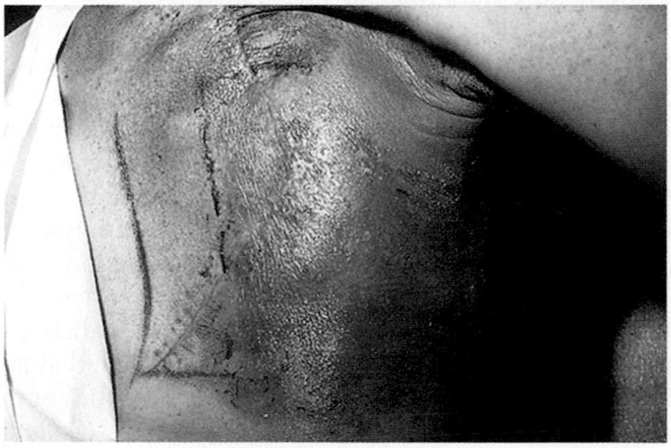

FIG. 16-15 Wet desquamation.

TABLE 16-12 PATIENT & CAREGIVER TEACHING GUIDE

Radiation Skin Reactions

Include the following instructions when teaching the patient and the caregiver to clean and protect the skin in a radiation treatment area.

1. Gently cleanse the skin in the treatment field using a mild soap (Ivory, Dove), tepid water, a soft cloth, and a gentle patting motion. Rinse thoroughly and pat dry.
2. Apply nonmedicated, nonperfumed, moisturizing lotion or cream, such as calendula ointment, aloe gel, Aquaphor, or Biafine cream, to alleviate dry skin. Some substances must be gently cleansed from the treatment field before each treatment and reapplied. Over-the-counter hydrocortisone cream 1% may reduce itching.
3. Rinse the area with saline solution. Expose the area to air as often as possible. If copious drainage is present, use astringent compresses (such as Domeboro solution) and nonadhesive absorbent dressings (they must be changed as soon as they become wet). Observe the area daily for signs of infection.
4. Avoid wearing tight-fitting clothing such as brassieres and belts over the treatment field.
5. Avoid wearing harsh fabrics, such as wool and corduroy. A lightweight cotton garment is best. If possible, expose the treatment field to air.
6. Use gentle detergents such as Dreft and Ivory Snow to wash clothing that will come in contact with the treatment field.
7. Avoid direct exposure to the sun. If the treatment field is in an area that is exposed to the sun, wear protective clothing such as a wide-brimmed hat when out in the sun and apply sunscreen lotion.
8. Avoid all sources of excessive heat (hot water bottles, heating pads, sunlamps) on the treatment field.
9. Avoid exposing the treatment field to cold temperatures (ice bags or cold weather).
10. Avoid swimming in saltwater or in chlorinated pools during the time of treatment.
11. Avoid the use of potential irritants (e.g., perfumes, powders, or cosmetics) on the skin in the treatment field; review use of other topical medications or lotions with your health care provider during treatment. Also avoid tape, dressings, and adhesive bandages unless permitted by the radiation therapist. Avoid shaving the hair in the treatment field.
12. Continue to protect sensitive skin after the treatment is completed. Do the following:
    - Avoid direct exposure to the sun. A sunscreen agent and protective clothing must be worn if the potential of exposure to the sun is present.
    - Use an electric razor if shaving is necessary in the treatment field.

the drugs are discontinued. Often the new hair has a different color and texture than the hair that was lost.

Patients experience a range of emotions at the prospect of losing their hair and when hair loss actually occurs. These may include anger, grief, embarrassment, or fear. Hair loss is a visible reminder of their cancer and the challenges of treatment. For some people, the loss of hair is one of the most stressful events experienced during the course of treatment. The American Cancer Society's "Look Good, Feel Better" program is an excellent support and resource for people experiencing not just hair loss but body image changes in general.

PULMONARY EFFECTS. Both chemotherapy and radiation have the potential to produce pulmonary tissue damage that is irreversible and progressive. Distinguishing between the complications of treatment and those related to disease is challenging. The effects of radiation on the lung include both acute and late reactions. Immediate pulmonary effects of radiation can be alarming to patients because they may mimic symptoms (e.g., cough, dyspnea) that precipitated the cancer diagnosis.

Pneumonitis is a delayed acute inflammatory reaction that may occur within 1 to 3 months after completion of thoracic radiation. This reaction is often asymptomatic, although an increase in cough, fever, and night sweats may occur. Some patients may develop pulmonary fibrosis (with or without prior pneumonitis), which is a late effect of therapy.

The most common pulmonary toxicities associated with chemotherapy include pulmonary edema (noncardiogenic) related to capillary leak syndrome or fluid retention, hypersensitivity pneumonitis, interstitial fibrosis, and pneumonitis produced by an inflammatory reaction or destruction of alveolar-capillary endothelium.

CARDIOVASCULAR EFFECTS. Radiation to the thorax can damage the pericardium, myocardium, valves, and coronary blood vessels. The pericardium is most commonly involved, with pericardial effusion or pericarditis the key problems. Patients with preexisting coronary artery disease are especially vulnerable.

Anthracyclines (e.g., doxorubicin [Adriamycin], daunorubicin) cause cardiotoxicity. Acute cardiotoxicities may cause electrocardiographic (ECG) abnormalities. Late effects of anthracyclines are left ventricular dysfunction and heart failure.

5-FU can cause cardiac ischemic syndrome. Trastuzumab (Herceptin), which is used in the treatment of breast cancer, is cardiotoxic and may result in ventricular dysfunction and heart failure. Baseline and periodic echocardiograms to monitor left ventricular function during treatment are usually done.

REPRODUCTIVE EFFECTS. Reproductive dysfunction secondary to radiation and chemotherapy varies according to the radiation treatment field and dosage, the particular chemotherapy agent and dose, and host factors (e.g., age). Treatment can cause temporary or permanent gonadal failure. Reproductive effects occur most often when reproductive organs are included in the radiation treatment field and when alkylating agents are used.

The testes are highly sensitive to radiation, and they should be protected with a testicular shield whenever possible. Pretreatment status may be a significant factor because a low sperm count and loss of motility are seen in individuals with testicular cancer and Hodgkin's lymphoma before any therapy is begun. Combined modality treatment or prior chemotherapy with alkylating agents enhances and prolongs the effects of radiation on the testes. When radiation is used alone with conventional doses and appropriate shielding, testicular recovery often occurs. Compromise of reproductive function in men may also result from erectile dysfunction after pelvic radiation.

The radiation dose that induces ovarian failure changes with age. Unlike the testes, there is no way to repair ovarian function. When radiation therapy is given, the ovaries are shielded whenever possible. Other factors that influence reproductive or sexual functioning in women include reactions in the cervix and endometrium. These tissues withstand a high radiation dose with minimal sequelae, accounting for the ability to treat endometrial and cervical cancer with high external and brachytherapy doses. Acute reactions such as tenderness, irritation, and loss of lubrication compromise sexual activity. Late effects of combined internal and external radiation therapy include vaginal shortening related to fibrosis and loss of elasticity and lubrication.

The patient and her or his partner require information about the expected effects of treatment relative to reproductive and sexual issues. Potential infertility can be a significant consequence for the individual, and counseling may be indicated. However, in no case should the patient think that conception is not possible during treatment. Pretreatment harvesting of sperm, ova, or ovarian tissue may be considered. Specific suggestions to manage side effects that have an impact on sexual functioning include using a water-soluble vaginal lubricant and routinely using a vaginal dilator after pelvic irradiation. Encourage discussion of issues related to sexuality, offer specific suggestions, and make referrals for ongoing counseling when indicated.

COPING WITH THERAPY. You have a key role in assisting patients in coping with the psychoemotional issues associated with cancer treatment. Anxiety is common—anxieties about various aspects of treatment administration (e.g., repeated venipuncture), dependency on others, ability to pay, potential side effects, and poor outcomes. Repetitive office visits or hospitalizations, continuing medications, and frequent laboratory testing force the individual to confront the cancer on a daily basis. Treatment-related uncertainties and fears are often most evident at the beginning of therapy, but anxiety may surface again when therapy is completed (e.g., fear of recurrence, less available support).

Telling patients that they will be followed and that support is ongoing can be reassuring. Providing information and support can help minimize the negative impact of cancer therapy on a person's quality of life. Patient teaching, symptom management, and interventions to help patients self-manage their illness (e.g., adjusting treatment schedules to permit patients to work when possible, making referrals to support groups) facilitate coping. Arranging for patients to meet with individuals who have successfully completed therapy can increase their hopefulness and confidence. In addition, make regular supportive telephone contacts between office visits and assist with planning for transportation, nutrition, and emotional support with available resources such as the American Cancer Society, Cancer Lifeline, churches, and other community resources.

LATE EFFECTS OF RADIATION AND CHEMOTHERAPY

Cancer survivors are achieving long-term remission and survival with advancements in treatment modalities. However, these forms of therapy (especially radiation therapy and chemotherapy) may produce long-term sequelae termed *late effects* that occur months to years after cessation of therapy. Every body system can be affected to some extent by chemotherapy or radiation therapy.

Acute radiation effects generally manifest as transient inflammatory changes in highly proliferative cells (e.g., epithelial tissues). In contrast, late radiation effects occur most commonly in post-mitotic cells (e.g., liver, kidney, lung, heart, muscle, bone, and connective tissues). Once they occur, the late effects may be progressive and generally are permanent. Examples range from skin telangiectasias to strictures, fistulas, or radiation necrosis. Alteration of the lymphatic channels (e.g., axillary lymph node dissection) may contribute to lymphedema. Secondary malignancies (particularly skin cancers) are other late radiation effects.

Long-term effects of chemotherapy include cataracts, arthralgias, endocrine alterations, renal insufficiency, hepatitis, osteoporosis, neurocognitive dysfunction, or other effects depending on the agents. The additive effects of multiagent chemotherapy before, during, or after a course of radiation therapy can significantly increase the resulting late effects.

The cancer survivor may also be at risk for secondary malignancies, including leukemia, angiosarcoma, and skin cancer. Approximately 8% of cancer survivors (most commonly breast and colon cancer survivors) face a secondary malignancy. Alkylating agents and high-dose radiation are the most frequent causes of secondary malignancies.

In general, the overall risk of developing neoplastic complications is low, and the latency period may be long. The potential risk for developing a secondary malignancy does not contraindicate the use of cancer treatment. Smoking may significantly increase the risk of secondary malignancies following some cancer treatment. Therefore counsel all patients about smoking cessation.

BIOLOGIC AND TARGETED THERAPY

Biologic and targeted therapy is the fourth cancer treatment modality. Biologic and targeted therapy can be effective alone or in combination with surgery, radiation therapy, and chemotherapy. **Biologic therapy**, or *biologic response modifier* therapy, consists of agents that modify the relationship between the host and the tumor by altering the biologic response of the host to the tumor cells. Biologic agents may affect host-tumor response in three ways: (1) they have direct antitumor effects; (2) they restore, augment, or modulate host immune system mechanisms; and (3) they have other biologic effects, such as interfering with the cancer cells' ability to metastasize or differentiate.

Targeted therapy interferes with cancer growth by targeting specific cell receptors and pathways that are important in tumor growth. Targeted therapies work at sites that are on the cell surface, at the intracellular level, or in the extracellular domain (Fig. 16-16 and Table 16-13). The targeted therapies are more selective for specific molecular targets than cytotoxic anticancer drugs. Thus they are able to kill cancer cells with less damage to normal cells compared with chemotherapy.

Targeted therapies include epidermal growth factor receptor (EGFR)–tyrosine kinase inhibitors, BCR-ABL tyrosine kinase inhibitors, CD20 monoclonal antibodies (MoAb), angiogenesis inhibitors, and proteasome inhibitors. As more oncogene targets are identified, such as BRAF (B-type Raf kinase) or ALK

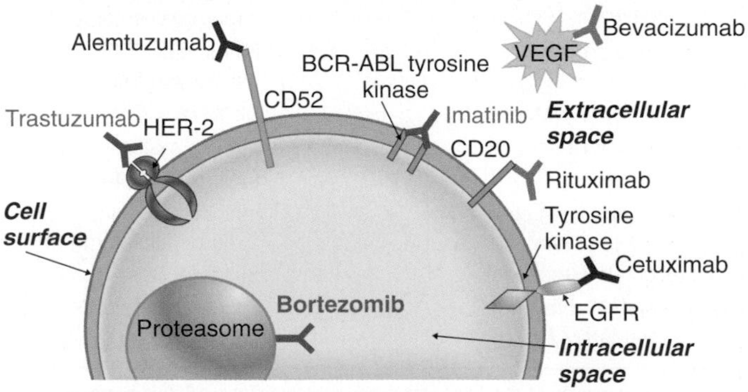

FIG. 16-16 Sites of action of targeted therapy. *EGFR,* Epidermal growth factor receptor; *HER-2,* human epidermal growth factor receptor 2; *VEGF,* vascular endothelial growth factor.

TABLE 16-13 DRUG THERAPY

Biologic and Targeted Therapy*

Drug	Mechanism of Action	Indications
α-interferon (Roferon-A, Intron A)	Inhibits DNA and protein synthesis Suppresses cell proliferation Increases cytotoxic effects of natural killer (NK) cells	Hairy cell leukemia, chronic myelogenous leukemia, malignant melanoma, renal cell carcinoma, ovarian cancer, multiple myeloma, Kaposi sarcoma
interleukin-2 (aldesleukin [Proleukin])	Stimulates proliferation of T and B cells Activates NK cells	Metastatic renal cell cancer, metastatic melanoma
BCG vaccine (TheraCys)	Induces an immune response that prevents angiogenesis of tumor	In situ bladder cancer
Epidermal Growth Factor Receptor (EGFR)–Tyrosine Kinase (TK) Inhibitors		
cetuximab (Erbitux)	Inhibits EGFR	Colorectal cancer, head and neck cancer
erlotinib (Tarceva)	Inhibits EGFR-TK	Non–small cell lung cancer, advanced pancreatic cancer
lapatinib (Tykerb)	Inhibits EGFR-TK and binds HER-2	Advanced breast cancer that is HER-2 positive
panitumumab (Vectibix)	Inhibits EGFR	Colorectal cancer
BCR-ABL Tyrosine Kinase Inhibitors		
dasatinib (Sprycel)	Inhibits BCR-ABL TK	Chronic myeloid leukemia
imatinib (Gleevec)	Inhibits BCR-ABL TK	Chronic myeloid leukemia, GI stromal tumors (GIST)
nilotinib (Tasigna)	Inhibits BCR-ABL TK	Chronic myeloid leukemia
CD20 Monoclonal Antibodies		
ibritumomab tiuxetan/yttrium-90 (Zevalin)	Binds CD20 antigen, causing cytotoxicity and radiation injury	Non-Hodgkin's lymphoma (B cell)
ofatumumab (Arzerra)	Binds CD20 antigen, causing cytotoxicity	Chronic lymphocytic leukemia
rituximab (Rituxan)	Binds CD20 antigen, causing cytotoxicity	Non-Hodgkin's lymphoma (B cell)
tositumomab/^{131}I tositumomab (Bexxar)	Binds CD20 antigen, causing immune attack and radiation injury	Non-Hodgkin's lymphoma (B cell)
Angiogenesis Inhibitors		
bevacizumab (Avastin)	Binds vascular endothelial growth factor (VEGF), thereby inhibiting angiogenesis	Colorectal cancer, non–small cell lung cancer, renal cell carcinoma
pazopanib (Votrient)	Binds VEGF, thereby inhibiting angiogenesis	Advanced renal cell carcinoma
Proteasome Inhibitors		
bortezomib (Velcade)	Inhibits proteasome activity, which functions to regulate cell growth	Multiple myeloma
carfilzomib (Kyprolis)	Inhibits proteasome activity, which functions to regulate cell growth	Multiple myeloma
Other Targeted Therapies		
alemtuzumab (Campath)	Binds CD52 antigen (found on T and B cells, monocytes, NK cells, neutrophils)	Chronic lymphocytic leukemia (B cell), GIST
axitinib (Inlyta)	Inhibits multiple TKs	Advanced renal cell carcinoma
crizotinib (Xalkori)	Inhibits anaplastic lymphoma kinase (ALK)	Locally advanced or metastatic non–small cell lung cancer that is ALK positive
everolimus (Afinitor)	Inhibits a specific protein known as the mammalian target of rapamycin (mTOR)	Advanced renal cell carcinoma, advanced breast cancer
ipilimumab (Yervoy)	Binds with CTLA-4 causing an antitumor-mediated immune response	Metastatic melanoma or unresectable melanoma
pertuzumab (Perjeta)	Binds HER-2	Breast cancer (HER-2 positive)
sorafenib (Nexavar)	Inhibits multiple TKs	Advanced renal cell carcinoma
sunitinib (Sutent)	Inhibits multiple TKs	Advanced renal cell carcinoma, GIST
temsirolimus (Torisel)	Inhibits a specific protein known as the mammalian target of rapamycin (mTOR)	Advanced renal cell carcinoma
trastuzumab (Herceptin)	Binds HER-2	Breast cancer (HER-2 positive)
vandetanib (Caprelsa)	Inhibits multiple TKs	Medullary thyroid cancer
vemurafenib (Zelboraf)	Inhibits BRAF serine threonine kinase	BRAF V600E mutated metastatic melanoma

*An enhanced version of this table listing side effects (eTable 16-7) is available on the website for this chapter.
BRAF, B-type Raf; *CTLA-4,* cytotoxic T lymphocyte antigen 4; *HER-2,* human epidermal growth factor receptor 2.

(anaplastic lymphoma kinase), agents are being developed that target specific oncogenes. Targeted therapies provide for use of personalized therapy based on the biology of an individual's tumor.[17]

EGFR is a transmembrane molecule that works through activation of intracellular tyrosine kinase (TK). Overexpression of EGFR is associated with unregulated cell growth and poor prognosis. Drugs that inhibit EGFR suppress cell proliferation and promote *apoptosis* (programmed cell death).

EGFRs belong to the same receptor family as human epidermal growth factor receptor 2 (HER-2), the target for trastuzumab (Herceptin). HER-2 is overexpressed in certain cancers (especially breast cancers) and is associated with more aggressive disease and decreased survival. Trastuzumab is a MoAb that binds to HER-2 and is given IV to inhibit the growth of breast cancer cells that overexpress the HER-2 protein. Lapatinib (Tykerb) is an oral agent used for breast cancer that overexpresses HER-2.

Chronic myeloid leukemia (CML) cells make an abnormal active enzyme called *BCR-ABL tyrosine kinase*. Drugs (e.g., imatinib [Gleevec]) that inhibit this enzyme suppress proliferation of CML cells and promote apoptosis.

Angiogenesis inhibitors work by preventing the mechanisms and pathways necessary for vascularization of tumors. Bevacizumab (Avastin), a recombinant human MoAb, binds with vascular endothelial growth factor (VEGF), a compound that stimulates blood vessel growth. When bevacizumab binds with VEGF, it prevents VEGF from binding with its receptors on vascular endothelial cells and promoting new vessel formation. As a result, further tumor growth is inhibited.

Proteasomes are intracellular multienzyme complexes that degrade proteins. In cancer cells, proteasome inhibitors (e.g., bortezomib [Velcade]) promote accumulation of proteins that lead to cell death.

Side Effects of Biologic and Targeted Therapy

The administration of one biologic agent usually induces the endogenous release of other biologic agents. The release and action of these biologic agents result in systemic immune and inflammatory responses. The toxicities and side effects of biologic agents are related to dose and schedule. (eTable 16-7 summarizes the potential side effects associated with specific biologic and targeted therapies.)

Common side effects include constitutional flu-like symptoms, including headache, fever, chills, myalgias, fatigue, malaise, weakness, photosensitivity, anorexia, and nausea. With interferon therapy, these flu-like symptoms almost invariably appear, but their severity generally decreases over time. Acetaminophen administered every 4 hours, as prescribed, often reduces the severity of the flu-like syndrome. The patient is commonly premedicated with acetaminophen in an attempt to prevent or decrease the intensity of these symptoms. In addition, large amounts of fluids help decrease the symptoms.

Tachycardia and orthostatic hypotension are also commonly reported. IL-2 and MoAbs can cause *capillary leak syndrome,* which can result in pulmonary edema. Other toxic and side effects may involve the CNS, renal and hepatic systems, and cardiovascular system. These effects are found particularly with interferons and IL-2.

A wide range of neurologic deficits has been observed with interferon and IL-2 therapy. The nature and extent of these problems are not yet completely understood. However, these problems are understandably frightening to the patient and the family, who must be taught to observe for neurologic problems (e.g., confusion, memory loss, difficulty making decisions, insomnia), report their occurrence, and institute appropriate safety and support measures.

MoAbs are administered by infusion. Patients may experience infusion-related symptoms, which can include fever, chills, urticaria, mucosal congestion, nausea, diarrhea, and myalgias. There is also a risk, although rare, of anaphylaxis associated with the administration of MoAbs. This potential exists because most MoAbs are produced by mouse lymphocytes and thus represent a foreign protein to the human body. The risk is significantly decreased with human MoAbs. Onset of anaphylaxis can occur within 5 minutes of administration and can be a life-threatening event. If this occurs, stop administration of the MoAb immediately, obtain emergency assistance, and implement resuscitation measures. (See Chapter 14 for a discussion of nursing management of anaphylaxis.)

Skin rashes are common in patients receiving EGFR inhibitors and manifest generally as erythema and acneiform-like rash that can cover up to 50% of the upper body. Angiogenesis inhibitors can cause problems of arterial thrombi, hemorrhage, hypertension, impaired wound healing, and proteinuria. Other toxicities of MoAbs include hepatotoxicity, bone marrow depression, and CNS effects. Individuals who receive rituximab may have a reactivation of hepatitis. Patients who receive trastuzumab may also experience cardiac dysfunction, especially when it is administered in higher doses or in combination with anthracycline antibiotics such as doxorubicin.

NURSING MANAGEMENT
BIOLOGIC AND TARGETED THERAPY

Some problems experienced by the patient receiving biologic and targeted therapy are different from those observed with more traditional forms of cancer therapy. These effects occur more acutely and are dose limited (i.e., effects resolve when the agent is discontinued). Capillary leak syndrome and pulmonary edema are problems that require critical care nursing. Bone marrow depression occurring with biologic therapy administration is generally more transient and less severe than that observed with chemotherapy. Fatigue associated with biologic therapy can be so severe that it constitutes a dose-limiting toxicity. As these agents are increasingly combined with cytotoxic therapies, the spectrum of therapy-related effects expands.

Nursing interventions for flu-like syndrome include the administration of acetaminophen before treatment and every 4 hours after treatment. IV meperidine (Demerol) has been used to control the severe chills or rigors associated with some biologic agents. Other nursing measures include monitoring vital signs and temperature, planning for periods of rest for the patient, assisting with activities of daily living (ADLs), and monitoring for adequate oral intake.

Many new targeted therapies are being developed and used more frequently. You need to become familiar with side effects associated with each agent.

HEMATOPOIETIC GROWTH FACTORS

Hematopoietic growth factors are used to support cancer patients through the treatment of the disease (Table 16-14). Colony-stimulating factors (CSFs) are a family of glycoproteins

TABLE 16-14 **DRUG THERAPY**

Hematopoietic Growth Factors Used in Cancer Treatment

Growth Factor	Drug Name	Indications	Side Effects
Granulocyte-macrophage colony-stimulating factor (GM-CSF)	sargramostim (Leukine)	Myeloid cell recovery after bone marrow transplantation	Nausea, vomiting, diarrhea, fever, chills, myalgia, headache, fatigue
Granulocyte colony-stimulating factor (G-CSF)	filgrastim (Neupogen), pegfilgrastim (Neulasta), tbo-filgrastim	Chemotherapy-induced neutropenia	Bone pain, nausea, vomiting
Erythropoietin	epoetin α (Epogen, Procrit)	Anemia of chronic cancer	Hypertension, thrombosis, headache
	darbepoetin α (Aranesp)	Anemia related to chemotherapy	Hypertension, thrombosis, headache
Interleukin-11 (platelet growth factor)	oprelvekin (Neumega)	Thrombocytopenia related to chemotherapy	Fluid retention, peripheral edema, dyspnea, tachycardia, nausea, mouth sores

produced by various cells. CSFs stimulate production, maturation, regulation, and activation of cells of the hematologic system. The name of the CSF is based on the specific cell line it affects (see Table 16-14).

Erythropoiesis-stimulating agents (ESAs) should be used only when treating anemia specifically caused by chemotherapy. ESA use is avoided in patients receiving chemotherapy with the intent to cure the disease. Use of these agents has raised safety concerns because they can cause thromboembolic events and increase the risk for death and for serious cardiovascular events when administered to achieve a target hemoglobin of greater than 12 g/dL. Therefore the lowest dose should be used that will gradually increase hemoglobin to the lowest level sufficient to avoid the need for blood transfusion. Monitor the hemoglobin level regularly.

HEMATOPOIETIC STEM CELL TRANSPLANTATION

Bone marrow transplantation (BMT) and **peripheral stem cell transplantation (PSCT)** are effective, lifesaving procedures for the treatment of a number of malignant and nonmalignant diseases (Table 16-15). BMT and PSCT allow for the safe use of very high doses of chemotherapy agents and/or radiation therapy in patients whose tumors have developed resistance or failed to respond to standard doses of chemotherapy and radiation. Although these procedures are lifesaving, patients may have long-term or delayed complications that can affect their quality of life.[18,19]

This therapeutic approach was typically referred to as BMT because the bone marrow was the original source of stem cells when the procedure was first developed. However, advances in harvesting and cryopreservation technologies have opened new pathways to the collection of stem cells from the peripheral blood. Consequently, the terminology has changed, and the procedure is now referred to as **hematopoietic stem cell transplantation (HSCT)**. Whether the diagnosis is a malignant or nonmalignant disease, the goal of HSCT is cure. Overall cure rates are still low but are steadily increasing. Even when cure is not achieved, transplantation can result in a period of remission.

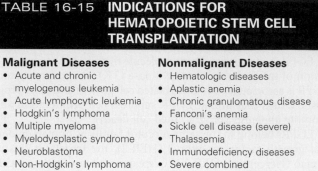

TABLE 16-15 **INDICATIONS FOR HEMATOPOIETIC STEM CELL TRANSPLANTATION**

Malignant Diseases	Nonmalignant Diseases
• Acute and chronic myelogenous leukemia	• Hematologic diseases
• Acute lymphocytic leukemia	• Aplastic anemia
• Hodgkin's lymphoma	• Chronic granulomatous disease
• Multiple myeloma	• Fanconi's anemia
• Myelodysplastic syndrome	• Sickle cell disease (severe)
• Neuroblastoma	• Thalassemia
• Non-Hodgkin's lymphoma	• Immunodeficiency diseases
• Ovarian cancer	• Severe combined immunodeficiency disease (SCID)
• Sarcoma	• Wiskott-Aldrich syndrome
• Testicular cancer	

The approach in HSCT is to eradicate diseased tumor cells and/or clear the marrow of its components to make way for engraftment of the transplanted, healthy stem cells. This is accomplished by administering higher than usual dosages of chemotherapy with or without radiation therapy, which can produce life-threatening consequences associated with pancytopenia and other adverse effects. After chemotherapy and radiation therapy are completed, healthy stem cells are infused. These healthy stem cells "rescue" the damaged bone marrow through subsequent proliferation and differentiation of the donated stem cells in the recipient.

HSCT is an intensive procedure with many risks. Some patients die from treatment-related complications or from recurrence of the original disease. Because it is a highly toxic therapy, the patient must weigh the significant risks of treatment-related death or treatment failure (relapse) against the hope of cure.

Types of Hematopoietic Stem Cell Transplants

HSCTs are categorized as allogeneic, syngeneic, or autologous. The sources of stem cells include the bone marrow, peripheral circulating blood, and umbilical cord blood. In *allogeneic transplantation,* stem cells are acquired from a donor who, through human leukocyte antigen (HLA) tissue typing, has been determined to be HLA matched to the recipient. HLA typing involves testing WBCs to identify genetically inherited antigens common to both donor and recipient that are important in compatibility of transplanted tissue. (HLA tissue typing is discussed in Chapter 14.) The donor is often a family member but may be an unrelated donor found through a national or international bone marrow registry (e.g., National Marrow Donor Program). Although more risks and toxicities may be associated with an unrelated allogeneic transplant, a benefit of this type of transplant is that it not only eradicates tumor cells with high-dose therapy, but also may stimulate the graft-versus-tumor effect in which donor WBCs identify and attack malignant cells in the

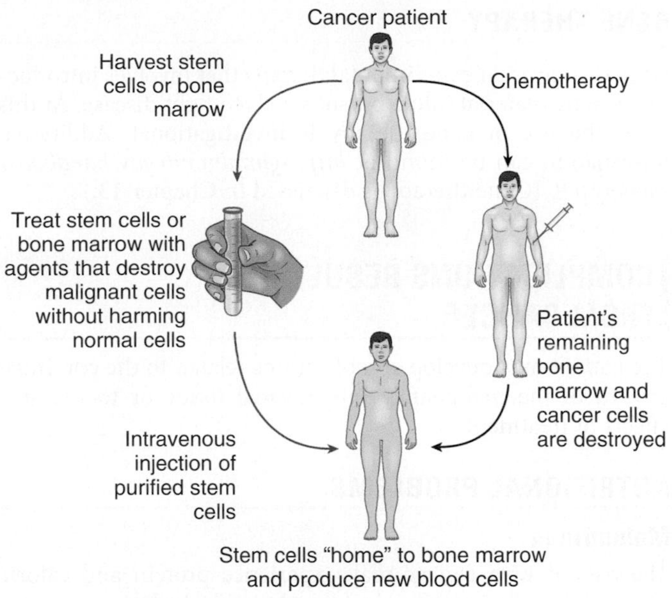

Cancer patient
Harvest stem cells or bone marrow
Chemotherapy
Treat stem cells or bone marrow with agents that destroy malignant cells without harming normal cells
Patient's remaining bone marrow and cancer cells are destroyed
Intravenous injection of purified stem cells
Stem cells "home" to bone marrow and produce new blood cells

FIG. 16-17 Autologous stem cell transplant.

recipient. Common indications for allogeneic transplant are certain leukemias, multiple myeloma, and lymphoma.

Syngeneic transplantation is a type of allogeneic transplant that involves obtaining stem cells from one identical twin and infusing them into the other. Identical twins have identical HLA types and are a perfect match. Therefore neither the graft-versus-host nor the graft-versus-tumor effect occurs.

In *autologous transplantation*, patients receive their own stem cells back after *myeloablative* (destroying bone marrow) chemotherapy (Fig. 16-17). The aim of this approach is purely "rescue." It enables patients to receive intensive chemotherapy and/or radiation by supporting them with their previously harvested stem cells until their marrow generates blood cells again on its own. Restoration usually takes about 4 to 6 weeks. Autologous transplants are typically used to treat hematologic malignancies if there is no suitable donor or the patient cannot undergo allogeneic transplantation.

The newer, nonmyeloablative or reduced intensity transplant uses lower doses of radiation or chemotherapy that result in less toxicity and myelosuppression. HSCT continues to be investigated in the management of some solid tumors refractory to treatment.

Procedures

Harvest Procedures. Hematopoietic stem cells are *harvested* from a donor (for allogeneic transplantation) or from the recipient (for autologous transplantation) via two different methods. In one type of procedure, used for harvesting stem cells residing in bone marrow (as the process was originally developed), the procedure is performed in the operating room using general or spinal anesthesia. Multiple bone marrow aspirations (usually from the iliac crest, but sometimes from the sternum) are carried out to obtain stem cells. The entire bone marrow harvest procedure takes about 1 to 2 hours, and the patient can be discharged after recovery. Post-harvest, the donor may experience pain at the collection site that lasts up to 7 days and can be treated with mild analgesics. The donor's body will replenish the removed bone marrow in a few weeks.

In the other type of procedure, peripheral stem cell transplants are obtained from the peripheral blood in an outpatient procedure. It is done using cell separator equipment that automatically separates the stem cells from the blood circulating through the machine and returns the remaining blood components to the donor. The process averages about 2 to 4 hours but can sometimes take longer depending on donor factors and the quality of the venous access. Often it takes more than one procedure to obtain enough stem cells. Because the blood has fewer stem cells than the bone marrow, "mobilization" of stem cells from the bone marrow into the peripheral blood can be accomplished using chemotherapy and/or hematopoietic growth factors.

Common growth factors that are used are granulocyte-macrophage colony-stimulating factor (GM-CSF) and granulocyte colony-stimulating factor (G-CSF) (see Table 16-14), but chemotherapy agents, typically cyclophosphamide, can also be used if there is a need to reduce tumor burden. When patients are given growth factors for mobilization, stem cells are harvested after 4 or 5 days of growth factor injections.

Plerixafor (Mozobil) is a drug given subcutaneously that, when used in combination with G-CSF, boosts the number of stem cells released from the bone marrow into the bloodstream. Plerixafor is intended to be used in combination with G-CSF for treatment of multiple myeloma or non-Hodgkin's lymphomas; it is not to be used for leukemia.

Harvested marrow is processed to strain out bone fragments (this is not necessary with peripheral collections). The marrow or peripherally collected stem cells are then bagged with preservative for cryopreservation and storage until they are needed, or they are used immediately. Since it is coming from the patient, autologous stem cells are sometimes treated (purged) to remove undetected cancer cells. Many different pharmacologic, immunologic, physical, and chemical agents have been used for this purpose.

Umbilical cord blood is also rich in hematopoietic stem cells, and successful allogeneic transplants have been performed using this source. Cord blood can be HLA-typed and cryopreserved. A disadvantage of cord blood is the possibility of insufficient numbers of stem cells to permit transplant to adults. Considerable research is currently ongoing to define the optimal application of this technology.

Preparative Regimens and Stem Cell Infusions. In malignant diseases, patients receive myeloablative dosages of chemotherapy with or without adjunctive radiation to treat underlying disease. Total-body irradiation (TBI) can be used for immunosuppression or to treat the disease. These preparative therapies are known as the *conditioning regimen*.

The timing of stem cell harvest and reinfusion is critical, particularly with autologous transplantation. To ensure the collection of optimally functioning stem cells in adequate numbers, conditioning is begun only after stem cells have already been harvested. They are thawed and reinfused only after chemotherapy has been eliminated from the body (i.e., usually about 24 to 48 hours) to avoid damage to newly infused cells.

Stem cell infusions are administered IV, and can be injected via the slow bolus method or infused much like a blood transfusion. The infused stem cells reconstitute the bone marrow elements, "rescuing" the recipient's hematopoietic system. Usually 2 to 4 weeks are required for the transplanted marrow to start producing hematopoietic blood cells. During this period, when the patient has pancytopenia, it is critical to protect the patient from exposure to infectious agents and support the patient with electrolyte supplements, nutrition, and blood component transfusions (as needed) to maintain adequate levels of circulating RBCs and platelets.

Complications. Bacterial, viral, and fungal infections are common after HSCT. Prophylactic antibiotic therapy may reduce their incidence. A potentially serious complication of allogeneic transplant is graft-versus-host disease. This occurs when the T lymphocytes from the donated marrow (graft) recognize the recipient (host) as foreign and begin to attack certain organs such as the skin, liver, and GI tract. (Graft-versus-host disease is discussed in Chapter 14.) The occurrence and severity of posttransplant complications also depend on the drugs used in the patient's particular conditioning regimen (some are more toxic than others) and the stem cell source. Because stem cells in the peripheral blood are more mature than those harvested from the marrow, the hematologic recovery period in PSCT is shorter, and fewer, less severe complications are seen.

TABLE 16-16 NUTRITIONAL THERAPY

Protein Foods With High Biologic Value

Milk

Whole milk (1 cup) = 9 g protein

Double-strength milk: 1 quart of whole milk plus 1 cup of dried skim milk blended and chilled: 1 cup = 14 g protein

Milk shake: 1 cup of ice cream plus 1 cup of milk = 15 g protein, 416 calories

Use evaporated milk, double-strength milk, or half-and-half to make casseroles, hot cereals, sauces, gravies, puddings, milk shakes, and soups.

Yogurt (regular and frozen): check labels and purchase brand with highest protein content: 1 cup = 10 g protein

Eggs

Egg = 6 g protein

Eggnog (1 cup) = 15.5 g protein

Add eggs to salads, casseroles, and sauces. Deviled eggs are especially well tolerated.

Desserts that contain eggs include angel food cake, sponge cake, custard, and cheesecake.

Cheese

Cottage	½ cup	15 g protein
American	1 slice	3 g protein
Cheddar	1 slice	6 g protein
Cream	1 tbs	1 g protein

Use cheese in a sandwich or as a snack.

Add cheese to salads, casseroles, sauces, and baked potatoes.

Cheese spread with crackers is a wholesome snack that can be made and stored in the refrigerator for easy accessibility.

Advise patient that cheese can be constipating.

Meat, Poultry, Fish

Pork	3 oz	approx. 19 g protein
Chicken	½ breast	approx. 26 g protein
Fish	3 oz	approx. 30 g protein
Tuna fish	6½ oz	approx. 44.5 g protein

Add meat, poultry, and fish to salads, casseroles, and sandwiches.

Add strained and junior baby meats to soups and casseroles.

Cocktail wieners and deviled ham on crackers are wholesome snacks. These snacks can be made and stored in the refrigerator for easy accessibility.

GENE THERAPY

Gene therapy is an experimental therapy that involves introducing genetic material into a person's cells to fight disease. At this time, the use of gene therapy is investigational. Additional information can be found at *http://ghr.nlm.nih.gov/handbook/therapy.pdf.* (Gene therapy is discussed in Chapter 13.)

COMPLICATIONS RESULTING FROM CANCER

The patient may develop complications related to the continual growth of the malignancy into normal tissue or to the side effects of treatment.

NUTRITIONAL PROBLEMS

Malnutrition

The patient with cancer may experience protein and calorie malnutrition characterized by fat and muscle depletion. (Assessment of malnutrition is discussed in Chapter 40.)

Soft, nonirritating high-protein and high-calorie foods should be eaten throughout the day. Foods suggested for increasing the protein intake are presented in Table 16-16. High-calorie foods that provide energy and minimize weight loss are presented in Table 16-17. (A sample high-calorie, high-protein diet is presented in Table 40-10.)

Teach the patient to avoid extremes of temperature, tobacco, alcohol, spicy or rough foods, and other irritants. Encourage nutritional supplements (e.g., Ensure) as an adjunct to meals and fluid intake. Weigh the patient at least twice each week to monitor for weight loss.

Suggest a referral for individualized nutritional counseling to the patient or the health care provider as soon as a 5% weight loss is noted or if the patient has the potential for protein and calorie malnutrition. Monitor albumin and prealbumin levels. Once a 10-lb (4.5-kg) weight loss occurs, it is difficult to maintain the nutritional status.

Teach the patient to use nutritional supplements in place of milk when cooking or baking. Foods to which nutritional supplements can be easily added include scrambled eggs, pudding, custard, mashed potatoes, cereal, and cream sauces. Packages of Instant Breakfast can be used as indicated or sprinkled on cereals, desserts, and casseroles.

Families are an integral part of the health care team. As symptom severity increases, the family's role in helping the patient eat becomes increasingly critical.

TABLE 16-17 NUTRITIONAL THERAPY

High-Calorie Foods

Mayonnaise	1 tbs	=	101 cal
Butter or margarine	1 tsp	=	35 cal
Sour cream	1 tbs	=	72 cal
Peanut butter	1 tbs	=	94 cal
Whipped cream	1 tbs	=	53 cal
Corn oil	1 tbs	=	119 cal
Jelly	1 tbs	=	49 cal
Ice cream	1 cup	=	256 cal
Honey	1 tbs	=	64 cal

If the malnutrition cannot be treated with dietary intake, it may be necessary to use enteral or parenteral nutrition. (Enteral and parenteral nutrition are discussed in Chapter 40.)

Altered Taste Sensation (Dysgeusia)

Cancer cells may release substances that stimulate the bitter taste buds. The patient may also experience an alteration in the sweet, sour, and salty taste sensations. Meat may taste bitter or bland. At this time, the physiologic basis of these varied taste alterations is unknown.

Teach the patient with an altered taste problem to avoid foods that are disliked. Frequently the patient may feel compelled to eat certain foods that are believed to be beneficial. Tell the patient to experiment with spices and other seasoning agents in an attempt to mask the taste alterations. Lemon juice, onion, mint, basil, and fruit juice marinades may improve the taste of certain meats and fish. Bacon bits, onion, and ham may enhance the taste of vegetables. Increasing the amount of spice or seasoning agent is usually not an effective way to enhance the taste.

INFECTION

Infection is a primary cause of death in the patient with cancer. The usual sites of infection include the lungs, GU system, mouth, rectum, peritoneal cavity, and blood (septicemia). Infection occurs as a result of the ulceration and necrosis caused by the tumor, compression of vital organs by the tumor, and neutropenia caused by the disease process or the treatment of cancer.

Instruct patients with a risk for neutropenia to call their health care provider if they have a temperature of 100.4° F (38° C) or greater. Assessment most often includes signs and symptoms of fever, determination of possible etiology (e.g., sinuses, mucous membranes, respiratory, GI, urinary, sites of any tubes or lines), and complete blood count.

Many patients are neutropenic when an infection develops. In these individuals, infection may cause significant morbidity and may be rapidly fatal if not treated promptly. The classic manifestations of infection are often subtle or absent in a patient with neutropenia and a depressed immune system. (Neutropenia is discussed in Chapter 31.)

ONCOLOGIC EMERGENCIES

Oncologic emergencies are life-threatening emergencies that can occur as a result of cancer or cancer treatment. These emergencies can be obstructive, metabolic, or infiltrative.

Obstructive Emergencies

Obstructive emergencies are primarily caused by tumor obstruction of an organ or blood vessel. Obstructive emergencies include superior vena cava syndrome, spinal cord compression syndrome, third space syndrome, and intestinal obstruction. (Chapter 43 presents a discussion of intestinal obstruction.)

Superior Vena Cava Syndrome. *Superior vena cava syndrome* (SVCS) results from obstruction of the superior vena cava by a tumor or thrombosis. The clinical manifestations include facial edema; periorbital edema; distention of veins of the head, neck, and chest (Fig. 16-18); headache; and seizures. A mediastinal mass is often visible on chest x-ray. The most common causes are lung cancer, non-Hodgkin's lymphoma, and metastatic breast cancer. The presence of a central venous catheter and previous radiation therapy to the mediastinum increase the risk for development of SVCS.

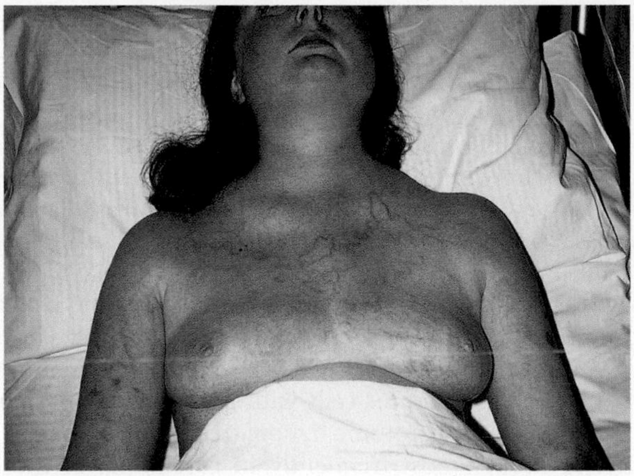

FIG. 16-18 Superior vena caval obstruction in bronchial carcinoma. Note the swelling of the face and neck and the development of collateral circulation in the veins.

SVCS is considered a serious medical problem. Management usually involves radiation therapy to the site of obstruction. However, chemotherapy may be administered for tumors more sensitive to this form of therapy.

Spinal Cord Compression. *Spinal cord compression* (SCC) is a neurologic emergency caused by a malignant tumor in the epidural space of the spinal cord. The most common cancers that cause this problem are breast, lung, prostate, GI, and renal tumors and melanomas. Lymphomas also pose a risk if diseased lymph tissue invades the epidural space.

Symptoms of SCC are back pain that is intense, localized, and persistent, accompanied by vertebral tenderness and aggravated by the Valsalva maneuver; motor weakness and dysfunction; sensory paresthesia and loss; and autonomic dysfunction. One of the clinical symptoms that reflects autonomic dysfunction is a reported change in bowel or bladder function.

The use of radiation therapy in conjunction with corticosteroids is generally associated with some initial improvement. Surgical decompressive laminectomy is used for those with tumors that are not responsive to radiation or when the tumor is in a previously irradiated area. Activity limitations and pain management are important nursing interventions.

Third Space Syndrome. *Third space syndrome* involves a shifting of fluid from the vascular space to the interstitial space that generally occurs secondary to extensive surgical procedures, biologic therapy, or septic shock. Initially patients exhibit signs of hypovolemia, including hypotension, tachycardia, low central venous pressure, and decreased urine output. Treatment includes fluid, electrolyte, and plasma protein replacement. During recovery hypervolemia can occur, resulting in hypertension, elevated central venous pressure, weight gain, and shortness of breath. Treatment generally involves reduction in fluid administration and fluid balance monitoring.

Metabolic Emergencies

Metabolic emergencies are caused by the production of ectopic hormones directly from the tumor or are secondary to metabolic alterations caused by the tumor or by cancer treatment.

Ectopic hormones arise from tissues that do not normally produce these hormones. Cancer cells return to a more embryonic form, thus allowing the cells' stored potential to become evident.

Metabolic emergencies include syndrome of inappropriate antidiuretic hormone secretion, hypercalcemia, tumor lysis syndrome, septic shock, and disseminated intravascular coagulation. (Septic shock is discussed in Chapter 67, and disseminated intravascular coagulation is discussed in Chapter 31.)

Syndrome of Inappropriate Antidiuretic Hormone Secretion. Syndrome of inappropriate antidiuretic hormone (SIADH) results from abnormal or sustained production of antidiuretic hormone (ADH) by tumor cells with resultant water retention and hyponatremia (hypotonic hyponatremia) (see Chapter 50).

SIADH occurs most frequently in carcinoma of the lung (especially small cell lung cancer), but can also occur in cancer of the pancreas, duodenum, brain, esophagus, colon, ovary, prostate, bronchus, and nasopharynx; leukemia; and Hodgkin's lymphoma. Cancer cells in these tumors are actually able to manufacture, store, and release ADH. Many chemotherapy agents may also contribute to ectopic ADH production, or potentiate ADH effects, including vincristine, cyclophosphamide, vinblastine, and cisplatin.[20]

Symptoms of SIADH include weight gain without edema, weakness, anorexia, nausea, vomiting, personality changes, seizures, oliguria, decrease in reflexes, and coma. Treatment of SIADH includes treating the underlying malignancy and measures to correct the sodium-water imbalance, including fluid restriction, oral salt tablets or isotonic (0.9%) saline administration, and, in severe cases, IV administration of 3% sodium chloride solution. Furosemide (Lasix) may also be a helpful treatment in the initial phases of SIADH. Demeclocycline (Declomycin) may be needed on an ongoing basis for moderate SIADH. Monitor the sodium level because correcting SIADH rapidly may result in seizures or death.

Hypercalcemia. Hypercalcemia can occur in metastatic disease of the bone or multiple myeloma, or when a parathyroid hormone–like substance is secreted by cancer cells. It occurs in approximately 10% to 20% of patients with advanced cancer.[21] Hypercalcemia resulting from malignancies that have metastasized occurs most frequently in patients with lung, breast, kidney, colon, ovarian, or thyroid cancer. Hypercalcemia resulting from secretion of parathyroid hormone–like substance occurs most frequently in squamous cell carcinoma of the lung; head and neck, cervical, and esophageal cancer; lymphomas; and leukemia. Immobility and dehydration can contribute to or exacerbate hypercalcemia.

The primary manifestations of hypercalcemia include apathy, depression, fatigue, muscle weakness, ECG changes, polyuria and nocturia, anorexia, nausea, and vomiting. Serum levels of calcium in excess of 12 mg/dL (3 mmol/L) often produce symptoms, and significant calcium elevations can be life threatening.

Serum calcium levels are affected by a low albumin level. A low albumin level will give a false-normal calcium level. Therefore the calcium level must be corrected for serum albumin values, or an ionized calcium level should be obtained.

Chronic hypercalcemia can result in nephrocalcinosis and irreversible renal failure. The long-term treatment of hypercalcemia is aimed at the primary disease. Acute hypercalcemia is treated by hydration (3 L/day) and bisphosphonate therapy. When hydration therapy is used in the frail or older adult, diuretics (particularly loop diuretics) may be used to avoid heart failure or edema. Bisphosphonates (the mainstay of treatment) are drugs that inhibit the action of osteoclasts and therefore reduce serum calcium levels. Infusion of the bisphosphonate zoledronate (Zometa) or pamidronate (Aredia) is the treatment of choice. Bisphosphonates are also used to prevent bone complications in patients with bone metastasis.

Tumor Lysis Syndrome. Acute *tumor lysis syndrome* (TLS) is a metabolic complication characterized by rapid release of intracellular components in response to chemotherapy. It occurs less commonly with radiation therapy. TLS is often associated with large tumors that have high growth rates and are sensitive to the effects of chemotherapy.[22] Massive cell destruction, associated with aggressive chemotherapy for rapidly growing tumors, releases a host of intracellular components into the bloodstream, including potassium, phosphate, and DNA and RNA components (which are metabolized to uric acid by the liver).

A rise in serum phosphate drives serum calcium levels down, with resultant hypocalcemia. Metabolic abnormalities and concentrated uric acid (which crystallizes in the distal tubules of the kidneys) lead quickly to acute renal failure if not identified and treated early.

The four hallmark signs of TLS are hyperuricemia, hyperphosphatemia, hyperkalemia, and hypocalcemia. Early symptoms include weakness, muscle cramps, diarrhea, nausea, and vomiting. TLS usually occurs within the first 24 to 48 hours after the initiation of chemotherapy and may persist for approximately 5 to 7 days.

The primary goal of TLS management is preventing renal failure and severe electrolyte imbalances. Patients at risk for TLS should be identified early, and preventive measures implemented concurrently with chemotherapy. The primary treatment includes increasing urine production using hydration therapy and decreasing uric acid concentrations using allopurinol.

Infiltrative Emergencies

Infiltrative emergencies occur when malignant tumors infiltrate major organs or secondary to cancer therapy. The most common infiltrative emergencies are cardiac tamponade and carotid artery rupture.

Cardiac Tamponade. *Cardiac tamponade* results from fluid accumulation in the pericardial sac, constriction of the pericardium by tumor, or pericarditis secondary to radiation therapy to the chest. Manifestations include a heavy feeling over the chest, shortness of breath, tachycardia, cough, dysphagia, hiccups, hoarseness, nausea, vomiting, excessive perspiration, decreased level of consciousness, distant or muted heart sounds, and extreme anxiety. Emergency management is aimed at reduction of fluid around the heart and includes surgical establishment of a pericardial window or an indwelling pericardial catheter. Supportive therapy includes administration of oxygen therapy, IV hydration, and vasopressor therapy.

Carotid Artery Rupture. Rupture of the carotid artery occurs most frequently in patients with cancer of the head and neck secondary to invasion of the arterial wall by tumor or to erosion following surgery or radiation therapy. Bleeding can manifest as minor oozing to spurting of blood in the case of a "blowout" of the artery. In the presence of a blowout, apply pressure to the site with a finger. IV fluids and blood products are administered in an attempt to stabilize the patient for surgery. Surgical management involves ligation of the carotid artery above and below the rupture site and reduction of local tumor.

CANCER PAIN

Moderate to severe pain occurs in approximately 50% of patients who are receiving active treatment for their cancer and in 80% to 90% of patients with advanced cancer. What is concerning is that these statistics have not changed in the past 30 years. Undertreatment of cancer pain is common and causes needless suffering, decreases quality of life, and increases the burden on family caregivers.[23]

Pain Assessment

Inadequate pain assessment is the single greatest barrier to effective pain management. Data such as vital signs and patient behaviors are not reliable indicators of pain, especially long-standing, chronic pain. It is important to distinguish between persistent and episodic, positional, or breakthrough pain. Therefore it is essential that a comprehensive pain assessment include a detailed history to elicit the following characteristics of pain: quality, location, intensity, duration, and precipitating and alleviating factors. Differentiating between types of pain (e.g., visceral, bone, neuropathic) is important in developing an effective pain management plan.

Assess pain on an ongoing basis to determine the effectiveness of the treatment plan. Obtain data and document at regular intervals the location and intensity of the pain, what it feels like, and how it is relieved. Assess change in pain (e.g., a significant change in the intensity, character, or location of pain) to determine the cause (e.g., progression of disease).

Always believe the patient report and accept it as the primary source of assessment data. Table 16-18 presents assessment questions that may facilitate data collection.

Pain Management

Pain management for the cancer patient needs to address both persistent and breakthrough components of pain if they are present. Adjuvant therapies need to be developed specific to the type or nature of the pain. In addition, teach patients how to keep a pain management diary.

Drug therapy, including nonsteroidal antiinflammatory drugs, opioids, and adjuvant pain medications, should be used and selected based on the character and/or cause of the pain. Opioids normally are prescribed for the treatment of moderate to severe cancer pain. Analgesic medications (e.g., morphine, fentanyl) should be given on a regular schedule (around the clock) with additional doses available as needed for breakthrough pain. In general, oral administration of the medication is preferred, but other routes (e.g., transdermal, transmucosal) are also available.

It is critical for you to pay attention to common side effects of pain medications (e.g., constipation) to ensure the patient's well-being and adherence with the pain management program. Nonsteroidal antiinflammatories (ibuprofen) often serve as helpful adjuncts to opioid therapy, particularly for bone pain. Other adjuvant therapies, such as antidepressant and antiseizure drugs, may beneficial in neuropathic pain, which is often resistant to opioids.

Radiopharmaceuticals (e.g., samarium-153) may benefit patients with diffuse bone pain (particularly if no further chemotherapy is planned). Patients may experience an initial pain *flare* after administration. Nerve blocks or epidural or intrathecal analgesia may also be used to treat patients with unrelieved pain or to minimize the requirements for opioids.

Remember that with opioid drugs (e.g., morphine) the appropriate dosage is whatever is necessary to control the pain with the fewest side effects. Fear of addiction is not warranted. However, it must be addressed as part of patient teaching, since it is a significant barrier for both patients and nurses in appropriate pain management. Discuss the goals of analgesic therapy with patients, especially those requiring large or chronic doses of opioids. Treatment plans should be developed that balance analgesia and side effects to maintain optimal functional status.

Patient teaching should clarify myths and misconceptions and reassure patients and family caregivers that cancer pain can be effectively relieved. Furthermore, addiction and tolerance are not problems associated with effective cancer pain management. Nondrug interventions, including relaxation therapy and imagery, can be effectively used to manage pain (see Chapter 7). Additional strategies to relieve pain are discussed in Chapter 9.

TABLE 16-18 PAIN ASSESSMENT IN CANCER PATIENTS

Characteristic	Questions to Ask
Location	• Where is the pain? • Is the pain in more than one place? Is the pain in a new location? • Does location of pain correlate with known diagnosis?
Intensity	• How bad is the pain? • Rate the pain on a scale of 0-10. (See Chapter 9 for rating scales.)
Quality	• What does the pain feel like—sharp, dull, burning, shooting, aching, or other? (See Chapter 9 for descriptors.)
Pattern	• Has the pain changed? • Is the pain getting better, worse, or unchanged? • What makes the pain better or worse?
Relief measures	• What do you do to control your pain? • Do you use medications? • Do the relief measures help much? How much?

PSYCHOLOGIC SUPPORT

Psychologic support of a patient with cancer is an important aspect of cancer care. The patient may experience a variety of psychosocial concerns, including fears of dependency, loss of control, family and relationship stress, financial burden, and fear of death. Distress may be experienced at many points throughout the cancer continuum, including at diagnosis, during or after treatment, and in association with long-term follow-up visits.

Adaptation and coping with a cancer diagnosis may be influenced by a variety of patient factors, including demographics, prior coping skills and strategies, social support, and religious and spiritual beliefs (Table 16-19). You are in a key position to assess the patient's and family's responses and support positive coping strategies.

To facilitate the development of effective coping and to support the patient and the family during the various stages of cancer, you should do the following.

TABLE 16-19 FACTORS AFFECTING HOW PATIENTS COPE WITH CANCER

Factor	Description
Ability to cope with stressful events in the past	How patients coped with previous stressful events (e.g., loss of job, major disappointment, significant traumatic event) affects how they cope with diagnosis of cancer.
Availability of significant others	Patients who have effective support systems cope more effectively than those who do not.
Ability to express feelings and concerns	Patients who express feelings and needs and ask for help cope more effectively than those who internalize feelings and needs.
Age at the time of diagnosis	Age determines coping strategies to a great degree. For example, a young mother with cancer may have concerns that differ from those of a 70-year-old woman with cancer.
Extent of disease	Cure or control of the disease process is usually easier to cope with than the reality of terminal illness.
Disruption of body image	Disruption of the body image (e.g., radical neck dissection, alopecia, mastectomy) may intensify the psychologic impact of cancer.
Presence of symptoms	Symptoms such as fatigue, nausea, diarrhea, and pain may intensify the psychologic impact of cancer.
Past experience with cancer	Negative experiences with cancer (personal or in others) influence perceptions about the current situation.
Attitude associated with the cancer	Patients who feel in control and have a positive attitude about cancer and cancer treatment cope better with the diagnosis and treatment of cancer than those who feel hopeless, helpless, and out of control.

- Be available and continue to be available, especially during difficult times.
- Exhibit a caring attitude.
- Listen actively to fears and concerns.
- Help provide relief from distressing symptoms.
- Provide essential information regarding cancer and cancer care that is accurate and establishes realistic expectations about what the patient will experience.
- Maintain a relationship based on trust and confidence. Be open, honest, and caring in the approach.
- Use touch to exhibit caring. A squeeze of the hand or a hug may at times be more effective than words.
- Assist the patient in setting realistic, reachable short-term and long-term goals.
- Assist the patient in maintaining usual lifestyle patterns.
- Maintain hope, which is the key to effective cancer care. Hope varies, depending on the patient's status—hope that the symptoms are not serious, hope that the treatment is curative, hope for independence, hope for relief of pain, hope for a longer life, hope to achieve meaningful goals, or hope for a peaceful death. Hope provides control over what is occurring and is the basis of a positive attitude toward cancer and cancer care.

Many patients with cancer benefit from a variety of psychosocial interventions, such as supportive listening, stress management techniques, individual or group counseling, and cognitive-behavioral therapy. Assess the psychosocial concerns and emotional responses of patients and their families so you can connect patients with appropriate supportive care resources. Organizations are listed in the Resources section at the end of this chapter. In many cities, local units of the American Cancer Society provide a wide variety of services.

ETHICAL/LEGAL DILEMMAS

Medical Futility

Situation

D.M., a 65-year-old Jewish woman, has breast cancer with metastasis to the liver and bone. The family asks you why their mother is not receiving chemotherapy. In addition, they want to make sure that she will be resuscitated should her heart stop. They are aware of her diagnosis and that she may have only a few months to live. In morning rounds you were told that D.M. does not want any treatment that would prolong her life.

Ethical/Legal Points for Consideration

- Although court decisions have varied, legally there is substantial consensus concerning right to privacy (a constitutional right), right to informed consent and refusal of treatment, and rights pertaining to end-of-life decision making.
- A patient who is an adult and is competent (defined as capable of understanding and interpreting information and making choices) solely retains the right to make personal health care decisions.
- The Patient Self-Determination Act requires that the patient be asked on admission whether he or she has an advance directive. It is placed in the medical record if available. If the patient does not have an advance directive, it must be documented.
- Often families have difficulty accepting the finality of a terminal diagnosis.
- Sometimes family members have conflicting interests (e.g., finances, property, inheritance rights) that influence their decision-making abilities.

Discussion Questions

1. How can you help D.M. communicate her wishes to her family?
2. How can you and the health care team assist the family in planning end-of-life care that incorporates the wishes of their mother?
3. What are the cultural issues in D.M.'s case?

GERONTOLOGIC CONSIDERATIONS

CANCER

Cancer is usually a disease of aging, with most cancers occurring in people over age 65. The cancer mortality rate is exceedingly high in older adults, with 70% of all deaths due to malignancies occurring in those over age 65. This is especially important since the normal life span is lengthening and the proportion of the population who are older than 65 years is increasing.[24,25]

Clinical manifestations of cancer in older adults may be mistakenly attributed to age-related changes and ignored by the person.[25] Older adults are particularly vulnerable to the complications of both cancer and cancer therapy. This is due to their decline in physiologic functioning, social and emotional resources, and cognitive function.

The older adult's functional status should be taken into consideration when developing a treatment plan. Age alone is not a good predictor of tolerance or response to treatment. Advances in the treatment of cancer are making cancer therapies beneficial to an increasing number of older adults, including patients with suboptimal health.

Conduct a Comprehensive Geriatric Assessment (CGA) at the time of diagnosis to identify important issues that might affect decisions about treatment options. Issues to assess include projected life expectancy, estimate of morbidity from cancer, co-morbidities that would affect treatment, and patient decision-making capacity and wishes.[24] The CGA also includes assessment of functional status, socioeconomic issues, psychosocial distress, cognitive function, nutrition, and medication-polypharmacy review.

Some important questions to consider when an older person is diagnosed with cancer include the following: Will the treatment provide more benefits than harm? Will he or she be able to tolerate the treatment safely? Is there need to optimize other co-morbidities or nutritional or functional status before starting treatment? What are the patient's preferences and wishes?

CANCER SURVIVORSHIP

It is estimated that there are currently more than 13.7 million cancer survivors in the United States, with breast cancer patients making up the largest portion of this group. Some of these individuals are cancer free, whereas others still have evidence of cancer and may be undergoing treatment.[1]

Over the past 20 years, the number of cancer survivors has increased threefold. With progressive advances in early detection and treatment, further increases in the number of cancer survivors are expected.[26]

The rapid increase in cancer survivors has been accompanied by a greater awareness of the long-term health and quality-of-life issues that a cancer diagnosis imposes. Cancer survivors experience a variety of long-term and late sequelae following treatment (discussed earlier in this chapter on pp. 265-271). The impact of cancer and its treatment confers greater risk of non-cancer-related death and co-morbidities (e.g., heart disease, diabetes, metabolic syndrome, endocrine dysfunction, osteoporosis) among cancer survivors. Furthermore, cancer survivors may continue to experience symptoms or functional impairment related to treatment for years after treatment.

The impact of a cancer diagnosis can affect many aspects of a patient's life, with cancer survivors commonly reporting financial, vocational, marital, and emotional concerns even long after treatment is over. These psychosocial effects can play a profound role in a patient's life after cancer, with issues related to living in uncertainty being frequently encountered.

To better assist cancer survivors, try to understand the meaning of the cancer experience from the individual's perspective.[27] Some patients may wish to return to their normal lives as soon as possible, and they might fail to attend scheduled follow-up appointments. Other survivors may become cancer advocates or active members of a cancer support group. Still others may allow their lives to revolve around the cancer and may even resist giving up the illness role. Some resources for survivors are listed in Table 16-20. Connecting diverse cancer survivors to culturally appropriate, evidence-based online support and resources is a strategy to enhance health outcomes.[28]

An important question that cancer survivors may ask is whether they should have children or whether their children will have genetic abnormalities. Recent and ongoing research suggests that children of cancer survivors are not at increased risk for genetic or congenital abnormalities. It is unknown whether humans have the ability to repair damage to germ cell DNA or whether processes such as infertility or miscarriages filter out any problems.[29]

TABLE 16-20 RESOURCES FOR CANCER SURVIVORS

Resource	Website
National Coalition for Cancer Survivorship (NCCS)	*www.canceradvocacy.org*
Office of Cancer Survivorship (OCS)	*http://cancercontrol.cancer.gov/ocs/office-survivorship.html*
Livestrong Survivor Care	*www.livestrong.org*
Cancer Survivors Network of the American Cancer Society	*http://csn.cancer.org*
Resources for Cancer Survivors	*www.cancerinformation.com/survivorship/resources.aspx*

You can help cancer survivors by doing the following:

- Provide all cancer patients with a treatment summary and care plan outlining treatment exposures, risk of late effects, preventive care recommendations, and follow-up surveillance plan after completion of treatment. Care plans should clearly identify all members of the care team and their responsibilities for follow-up care. Also include referrals to appropriate supportive care and community resources that would benefit the patient in recovery or ongoing care.
- Coordinate care among the oncology team, primary health care provider, and other specialists. Teach health care providers about the needs of cancer survivors, including long-term effects of cancer and cancer treatments.
- Teach cancer survivors to look for and report any ongoing symptoms resulting from treatment, including late effects of radiation therapy and chemotherapy.
- Promote healthy behaviors:
  - *Prevention:* good nutrition, exercise, smoking avoidance, maintenance of proper weight, cardiac risk reduction, bone health
  - *Early detection:* routine health screenings (e.g., breast, colon), cholesterol, diabetes, osteoporosis screening as recommended
- Encourage cancer survivors to have regular follow-up examinations with an identified primary health care provider.
- Assess for psychoemotional, financial, health insurance, or vocational problems related to cancer. Assist patients in getting appropriate help if necessary.

CULTURALLY COMPETENT CARE

CANCER

Both cancer incidence and death rates are disproportionately higher in African Americans than in whites and other minority groups (see Cultural and Ethnic Health Disparities box). Although overall racial disparities in cancer death rates have been declining, death rates continue to be 33% higher among African American men and 16% higher among African American women than whites. In addition, African Americans are more likely to have later stage disease at the time of diagnosis than whites.[30,31]

Differences in survival rates from cancer are attributed primarily to a combination of factors, including poverty, difficult access to and poorer quality of health care, more co-morbid conditions, and differences in tumor biology. Disparities in cancer care exist throughout the continuum from cancer pre-

CULTURAL & ETHNIC HEALTH DISPARITIES

Cancer

- Cancer incidence and death rates for men are highest among African Americans, followed by whites, Hispanics, and Asians/Pacific Islanders.
- Cancer incidence rates for women are highest among whites, followed by African Americans, Hispanics, and Asians/Pacific Islanders.
- However, cancer death rates for women are highest among African Americans, followed by whites, Hispanics, and Asians/Pacific Islanders.

vention and screening to end-of-life care and survivorship. The disparity in prevention and screening results in cancer being in advanced stages at the time of diagnosis.[32]

Culturally competent care in oncology is needed to meet the needs of diverse groups. Culturally competent care involves awareness of personal background, how culture affects care delivery, and how to adapt to meet cultural needs. Nurses need to actively seek to understand cultural differences to meet the individualized needs. (Culturally competent care related to specific cancers is presented in the chapters where the cancer is discussed.)

BRIDGE TO NCLEX EXAMINATION

The number of the question corresponds to the same-numbered outcome at the beginning of the chapter.

1. Trends in the incidence and death rates of cancer include the fact that
   a. lung cancer is the most common type of cancer in men.
   b. a higher percentage of women than men have lung cancer.
   c. breast cancer is the leading cause of cancer deaths in women.
   d. African Americans have a higher death rate from cancer than whites.
2. What features of cancer cells distinguish them from normal cells *(select all that apply)*?
   a. Cells lack contact inhibition.
   b. Cells return to a previous undifferentiated state.
   c. Oncogenes maintain normal cell expression.
   d. Proliferation occurs when there is a need for more cells.
   e. New proteins characteristic of embryonic stage emerge on cell membrane.
3. A characteristic of the stage of progression in the development of cancer is
   a. oncogenic viral transformation of target cells.
   b. a reversible steady growth facilitated by carcinogens.
   c. a period of latency before clinical detection of cancer.
   d. proliferation of cancer cells in spite of host control mechanisms.
4. The primary protective role of the immune system related to malignant cells is
   a. surveillance for cells with tumor-associated antigens.
   b. binding with free antigen released by malignant cells.
   c. production of blocking factors that immobilize cancer cells.
   d. responding to a new set of antigenic determinants on cancer cells.
5. The primary difference between benign and malignant neoplasms is the
   a. rate of cell proliferation.
   b. site of malignant tumor.
   c. requirements for cell nutrients.
   d. characteristic of tissue invasiveness.
6. The nurse is caring for a 59-year-old woman who had surgery 1 day ago for removal of a suspected malignant abdominal mass. The patient is awaiting the pathology report. She is tearful and says that she is scared to die. The most effective nursing intervention at this point is to use this opportunity to
   a. motivate change in an unhealthy lifestyle.
   b. teach her about the seven warning signs of cancer.
   c. instruct her about healthy stress relief and coping practices.
   d. allow her to communicate about the meaning of this experience.
7. The goals of cancer treatment are based on the principle that
   a. surgery is the single most effective treatment for cancer.
   b. initial treatment is always directed toward cure of the cancer.
   c. a combination of treatment modalities is effective for controlling many cancers.
   d. although cancer cure is rare, quality of life can be increased with treatment modalities.
8. The most effective method of administering a chemotherapy agent that is a vesicant is to
   a. give it orally.
   b. give it intraarterially.
   c. use an Ommaya reservoir.
   d. use a central venous access device.
9. The nurse explains to a patient undergoing brachytherapy of the cervix that she
   a. must undergo simulation to locate the treatment area.
   b. requires the use of radioactive precautions during nursing care.
   c. may experience desquamation of the skin on the abdomen and upper legs.
   d. requires shielding of the ovaries during treatment to prevent ovarian damage.
10. A patient on chemotherapy and radiation for head and neck cancer has a WBC count of $1.9 \times 10^3/\mu L$, hemoglobin of 10.8 g/dL, and a platelet count of $99 \times 10^3/\mu L$. Based on the CBC results, what is the most serious clinical finding?
    a. Cough, rhinitis, and sore throat
    b. Fatigue, nausea, and skin redness at site of radiation
    c. Temperature of 101.9° F, fatigue, and shortness of breath
    d. Skin redness at site of radiation, headache, and constipation
11. To prevent fever and shivering during an infusion of rituximab (Rituxan), the nurse should premedicate the patient with
    a. aspirin.
    b. acetaminophen.
    c. sodium bicarbonate.
    d. meperidine (Demerol).
12. The nurse counsels the patient receiving radiation therapy or chemotherapy that
    a. effective birth control methods should be used for the rest of the patient's life.
    b. if nausea and vomiting occur during treatment, the treatment plan will be modified.
    c. after successful treatment, a return to the person's previous functional level can be expected.
    d. the cycle of fatigue-depression-fatigue that may occur during treatment can be reduced by restricting activity.

13. A patient on chemotherapy for 10 weeks started at a weight of 121 lb. She now weighs 118 lb and has no sense of taste. Which nursing intervention would be a priority?
    a. Advise the patient to eat foods that are fatty, fried, or high in calories.
    b. Discuss with the physician the need for parenteral or enteral feedings.
    c. Advise the patient to drink a nutritional supplement beverage at least three times a day.
    d. Advise the patient to experiment with spices and seasonings to enhance the flavor of food.
14. A 70-year-old male patient has multiple myeloma. His wife calls to report that he sleeps most of the day, is confused when awake, and complains of nausea and constipation. Which complication of cancer is this most likely caused by?
    a. Hypercalcemia
    b. Tumor lysis syndrome
    c. Spinal cord compression
    d. Superior vena cava syndrome
15. A patient has recently been diagnosed with early stages of breast cancer. What is most appropriate for the nurse to focus on?
    a. Maintaining the patient's hope
    b. Preparing a will and advance directives
    c. Discussing replacement child care for the patient's children
    d. Discussing the patient's past experiences with her grandmother's cancer

1. d, 2. a, b, e, 3. d, 4. a, 5. d, 6. d, 7. c, 8. d, 9. b, 10. c, 11. b, 12. c, 13. d, 14. a, 15. a

evolve

For rationales to these answers and even more NCLEX review questions, visit *http://evolve.elsevier.com/Lewis/medsurg.*

REFERENCES

1. American Cancer Society: *Cancer facts and figures* 2012. Retrieved from *www.cancer.org/research/cancerfactsfigures/cancerfactsfigures/cancer-facts-figures-2013.*
2. Casey G: The biology of cancer, *Nurs N Z* 18(1):20, 2012.
3. Wu X, Watson M, Wilson R, et al: Human papillomavirus–associated cancers—United States, 2004-2008, *MMWR* 61(15):258, 2012.
4. Prenzel KL, Bollschweiler E, Schröder W, et al: Prognostic relevance of skip metastases in esophageal cancer, *Ann Thorac Surg* 90:1662, 2010.
*5. Zauber AG, Winawer SJ, O'Brien MJ, et al: Colonoscopic polypectomy and long-term prevention of colorectal-cancer deaths, *N Engl J Med* 366:687, 2012.
*6. Polovitch M, Whitford J, Olsen M: *Chemotherapy and biotherapy guidelines and recommendations for practice*, ed 3, Pittsburgh, 2009, Oncology Nursing Society. Retrieved from *www.ons.org.*
7. Held-Warmkessel J: Taming the three high-risk chemotherapy complications, *Nursing* 41:30, 2011.
8. National Cancer Institute: Radiation therapy for cancer Q&A. Retrieved from *www.cancer.gov/cancertopics/coping/radiation-therapy-and-you/page2.*
*9. Ma CM: The practice of radiation oncology. In Iwamoto RR, Haas ML, Gosselin TK, editors: *Manual for radiation oncology nursing practice and education*, ed 4, Pittsburgh, 2011, Oncology Nursing Society.
*10. National Comprehensive Cancer Network: NCCN clinical practice guidelines—myeloid growth factors. Retrieved from *www.nccn.org/professionals/physician_gls/pdf/myeloid_growth.pdf.*
*11. National Comprehensive Cancer Network: NCCN clinical practice guidelines—cancer related fatigue v1. 2012. Retrieved from *www.nccn.org.*
*12. Ettinger DS, Armstrong DK, Barbour S, et al: NCCN clinical practice guidelines in oncology: antiemesis, *J Natl Compr Cancer Network* 7:572, 2009.
*13. Feyer P, Maranzano E, Molassiotis A, et al: Radiotherapy-induced nausea and vomiting (RINV): MASCC/ESMO guideline for antiemetics in radiotherapy: update 2009, *Support Care Cancer* 19(Suppl 1):S5, 2011.
*14. Muehlbauer PM, Thrope D, Davis A: Putting evidence into practice: evidence-based interventions to prevent, manage, and treat chemotherapy- and radiotherapy-induced diarrhea, *Clin J Oncol Nurs* 13:336, 2009.
15. Cady J: Gastrointestinal/abdomen. In Iwamoto RR, Haas ML, Gosselin TK, editors: *Manual for radiation oncology nursing practice and education*, ed 4, Pittsburgh, 2012, Oncology Nursing Society.
16. Feight D, Baney T, Bruce S, et al: Putting evidence into practice: evidence-based interventions for radiation dermatitis, *Clin J Oncol Nurs* 15(5):481, 2011.
17. Camidge D, Doebele R: Treating Alk-positive lung cancer: early successes and future challenges, *Nature Rev Clin Oncol* 9:268, 2012.
18. National Cancer Institute: Bone marrow transplantation and peripheral blood stem cell transplantation, 2010. Retrieved from *http://cancer.gov.cancertopics/factsheet/Therapy/bone-marrow-transplant.*
19. Antin JH, Yolin DS: *Manual of cell and bone marrow transplantation*, Cambridge, Mass, 2009, Cambridge University Press.
20. Esposito P, Piotti G, Bianzina S, et al: The syndrome of inappropriate antidiuresis: pathophysiology, clinical management and new therapeutic options, *Nephron Clin Pract* 119:c62, 2011.
21. LeGrand S: Modern management of malignant hypercalcemia, *Am J Hospice Palliative Care* 28:515, 2011.
22. Held-Warmkessel J: How to prevent and manage tumor lysis syndrome, *Nursing* 40:27, 2010.
23. National Cancer Institute: Pain (PDQ). Retrieved from *www.cancer.gov/cancertopics/pdq/supportivecare/pain/HealthProfessional.*
24. National Comprehensive Cancer Network: NCCN clinical practice guidelines—senior adult oncology v2. 2012. Retrieved from *www.nccn.org.*
25. Hurria A, Cohen HJ: *Practical geriatric oncology*, Cambridge, Mass, 2009, Cambridge University Press.

*Evidence-based information for clinical practice.

26. Vachani C, Hampshire MK, Hill-Kayser CE, et al: Preparing patients for life after cancer treatment, *Am J Nurs* 111:51, 2011.
27. Stanton AL: What happens now? Psychosocial care for cancer survivors after medical treatment completion, *J Clin Oncol* 30:1215, 2012.
*28. Hong Y, Peña-Purcell NC, Ory MG: Outcomes of online support and resources for cancer survivors: a systematic literature review, *Patient Educ Couns* 86(3):288, 2012.
29. Signorella LB: Congenital anomalies in the children of cancer survivors: a report from the childhood cancer survivor study, *J Clin Oncol* 30:239, 2012.
30. National Cancer Institute: *Cancer trends progress report update, 2009/2010*, Bethesda, Md, 2010, National Institutes of Health. Retrieved from *http://progressreport.cancer.gov*.
31. American Cancer Society: *Cancer facts and figures for African Americans, 2011-2012*, Atlanta, 2012, The Society. Retrieved from *www.cancer.org/acs/groupscontent/@epidemiology surveilance/documents/document/acspc-027765.pdf*.
32. Pluth Yeo T, Phillips J, Delengowski A, et al: Oncology nursing: educating advanced practice nurses to provide culturally competent care, *J Professional Nurs* 27(4):245, 2011.

RESOURCES

American Association for Cancer Education (AACE)
www.aaceonline.com
American Cancer Society
www.cancer.org
American Society of Clinical Oncology (ASCO)
www.asco.org
Association of Community Cancer Centers (ACCC)
www.accc-cancer.org
Cancer Care, Inc.
www.cancercare.org
Cancer Guide
http://cancerguide.org
Cancer Hotlines
800-525-3777
800-638-6070 (Alaska)
800-636-5700 (District of Columbia)
800-524-1234 (Hawaii; call collect)
Cancer Information Service (CIS), a Program of the National Cancer Institute (NCI)
www.cancer.gov/aboutnci/cis
International Society of Nurses in Cancer Care (ISNCC)
www.isncc.org
National Cancer Institute (NCI)
www.cancer.gov
National Coalition for Cancer Survivorship (NCCS)
www.canceradvocacy.org
OncoLink (cancer information site)
www.oncolink.org
Oncology Nursing Society (ONS)
www.ons.org

CHAPTER 17

We never know the worth of water
till the well is dry.
Thomas Fuller

Fluid, Electrolyte, and Acid-Base Imbalances

Mariann M. Harding

evolve WEBSITE

http://evolve.elsevier.com/Lewis/medsurg

- NCLEX Review Questions
- Key Points
- Pre-Test
- Answer Guidelines for Case Study on p. 313
- Rationales for Bridge to NCLEX Examination Questions
- Case Studies
  - Patient With Hyponatremia/Fluid Volume Imbalance
- Concept Map Creator
- Glossary
- Fluids and Electrolytes Tutorial
- Content Updates

LEARNING OUTCOMES

1. Describe the composition of the major body fluid compartments.
2. Define processes involved in the regulation of movement of water and electrolytes between the body fluid compartments.
3. Describe the etiology, laboratory diagnostic findings, clinical manifestations, and nursing and collaborative management of the following disorders:
   a. Extracellular fluid volume imbalances: fluid volume deficit and fluid volume excess
   b. Sodium imbalances: hypernatremia and hyponatremia
   c. Potassium imbalances: hyperkalemia and hypokalemia
   d. Magnesium imbalances: hypermagnesemia and hypomagnesemia
   e. Calcium imbalances: hypercalcemia and hypocalcemia
   f. Phosphate imbalances: hyperphosphatemia and hypophosphatemia
4. Identify the processes to maintain acid-base balance.
5. Discuss the etiology, laboratory diagnostic findings, clinical manifestations, and nursing and collaborative management of the following acid-base imbalances: metabolic acidosis, metabolic alkalosis, respiratory acidosis, and respiratory alkalosis.
6. Describe the composition and indications of common IV fluid solutions.
7. Discuss the types and nursing management of commonly used central venous access devices.

KEY TERMS

acidosis, p. 302
active transport, p. 287
alkalosis, p. 302
anions, p. 286
buffers, p. 303
cations, p. 286
central venous access devices (CVADs), p. 309
electrolytes, p. 286
fluid spacing, p. 289
hydrostatic pressure, p. 288
hypertonic, p. 288
hypotonic, p. 288
isotonic, p. 288
oncotic pressure, p. 288
osmolality, p. 288
osmosis, p. 287
osmotic pressure, p. 287

HOMEOSTASIS

Body fluids and electrolytes play an important role in maintaining *homeostasis,* the stable internal environment of the body.[1] Body fluids are in constant motion transporting nutrients, electrolytes, and oxygen to cells and carrying waste products away from cells. The body uses a number of adaptive responses associated with these activities to keep the composition and volume of body fluids and electrolytes within the narrow limits of normal to maintain homeostasis and promote health.

Many diseases and their treatments can affect fluid and electrolyte balance. For example, a patient with metastatic breast or lung cancer may develop hypercalcemia because of bone destruction from tumor invasion. Chemotherapy prescribed to treat the cancer may result in nausea and vomiting and, subsequently, dehydration and acid-base imbalances. When correcting dehydration with IV fluids, the patient requires close monitoring to prevent fluid overload.

It is important for you to anticipate the potential for alterations in fluid and electrolyte balance associated with certain disorders and medical therapies, recognize the signs and symptoms of imbalances, and intervene with the appropriate action. This chapter describes the (1) normal control of fluids, electrolytes, and acid-base balance; (2) conditions that disrupt homeostasis and resultant manifestations; and (3) actions that

Reviewed by Dorothy (Dottie) M. Mathers, RN, DNP, CNE, Professor, School of Health Sciences, Pennsylvania College of Technology, Williamsport, Pennsylvania; and Jason Mott, RN, MSN, Instructor of Nursing, Bellin College: School of Nursing, Green Bay, Wisconsin.

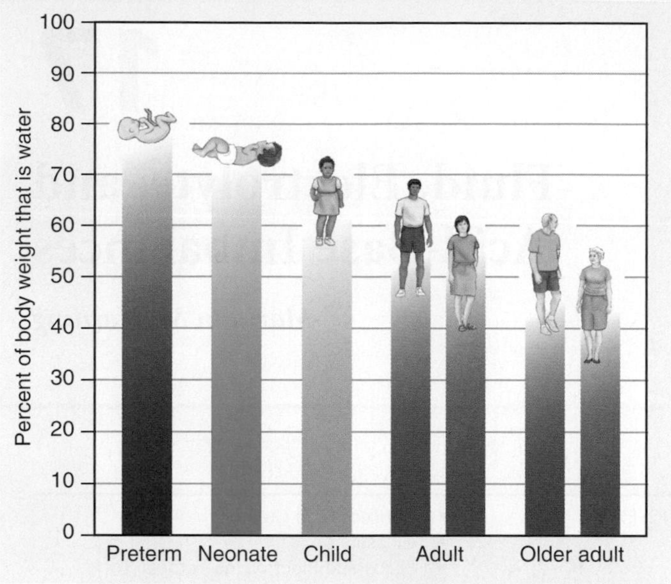

FIG. 17-1 Body water over the life span.

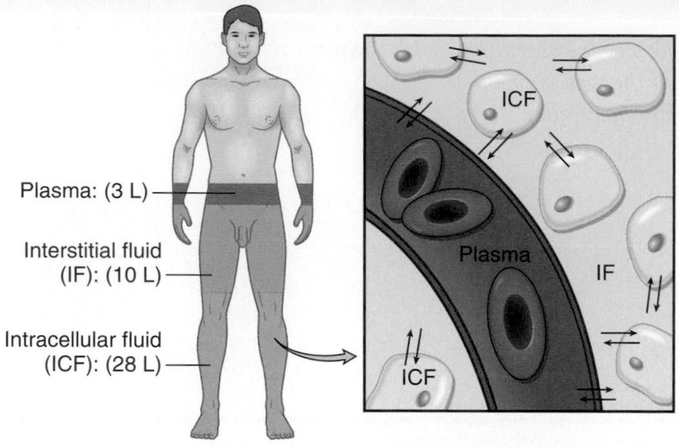

FIG. 17-2 Relative volumes of three body fluids. Values represent fluid distribution in a young male adult.

the health care provider and you can take to prevent fluid, electrolyte, and acid-base imbalances and restore homeostasis.

WATER CONTENT OF THE BODY

Water is the primary component of the body, accounting for approximately 50% to 60% of body weight in the adult. The water content varies with gender, body mass, and age (Fig. 17-1). The percentage of body weight that is composed of water is generally greater in men than in women because men tend to have more lean body mass. The more fat present in the body, the less the total water content. Therefore obese individuals have a lower percentage of body water than slender people do. Older adults, with less muscle mass and more fat content, have less body water for this same reason. In the older adult, body water content averages 45% to 55% of body weight, leaving them at a higher risk for fluid-related problems than young adults.

Body Fluid Compartments

The two fluid compartments in the body are the *intracellular space* (inside the cells) and the *extracellular space* (outside the cells) (Fig. 17-2). Approximately two thirds of the body water is located within cells and is termed *intracellular fluid* (ICF); ICF constitutes approximately 40% of body weight of an adult. The body of a 70-kg young man would contain approximately 42 L of water, of which 28 L would be located within cells.

The extracellular fluid (ECF) consists of *interstitial fluid* (the fluid in the spaces between cells), *plasma* (the liquid part of blood), and *transcellular fluid* (a very small amount of fluid contained within specialized cavities of the body). Transcellular fluids include cerebrospinal fluid; fluid in the gastrointestinal (GI) tract; and pleural, synovial, peritoneal, intraocular, and pericardial fluid. ECF consists of one third of the body water; this would amount to about 14 L in a 70-kg man. About 20% of ECF is in the intravascular space as plasma (3 L in a 70-kg man), and 70% is in the interstitial space (10 L in a 70-kg man). The fluid in the transcellular spaces totals about 1 L at any given time. However, because 3 to 6 L of fluid is secreted into and reabsorbed from the GI tract every day, loss of this fluid from vomiting or diarrhea can produce serious fluid and electrolyte imbalances.

Calculation of Fluid Gain or Loss

One liter of water weighs 2.2 lb (1 kg). Body weight change, especially sudden change, is an excellent indicator of overall fluid volume loss or gain. For example, if a patient drinks 240 mL (8 oz) of fluid, weight gain will be 0.5 lb (0.23 kg). A patient receiving diuretic therapy who loses 4.4 lb (2 kg) in 24 hours has experienced a fluid loss of approximately 2 L. An adult patient who is fasting might lose approximately 1 to 2 lb/day. A weight loss exceeding this is likely due to loss of body fluid.

ELECTROLYTES

Electrolytes are substances whose molecules dissociate, or split into ions, when placed in water. *Ions* are electrically charged particles. **Cations** are positively charged ions. Examples include sodium (Na^+), potassium (K^+), calcium (Ca^{2+}), and magnesium (Mg^{2+}) ions. **Anions** are negatively charged ions. Examples include bicarbonate (HCO_3^-), chloride (Cl^-), and phosphate (PO_4^{3-}) ions. Most proteins bear a negative charge and are thus anions.

Measurement of Electrolytes

The milliequivalent (mEq) is the commonly used unit of measure for electrolytes. Electrolytes in body fluids are active chemicals that unite in varying combinations, so it is more practical to express their concentration as a measure of chemical activity (or milliequivalents) rather than as a measure of weight. Ions combine milliequivalent for milliequivalent. For example, 1 mEq (1 mmol) of sodium combines with 1 mEq (1 mmol) of chloride.

Electrolyte Composition of Fluid Compartments

Electrolyte composition varies between ECF and ICF. The overall concentration of electrolytes is approximately the same in the two compartments. However, concentrations of specific ions differ greatly (Fig. 17-3). In ECF the main cation is sodium, with small amounts of potassium, calcium, and magnesium. The primary ECF anion is chloride, with small amounts of bicarbonate, sulfate, and phosphate anions. In ICF the most

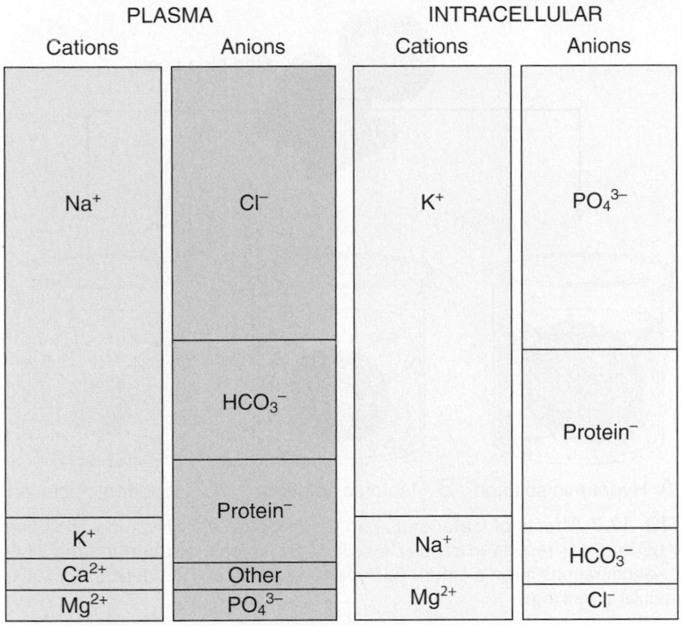

FIG. 17-3 The relative concentrations of the major cations and anions in the intracellular space and the plasma.

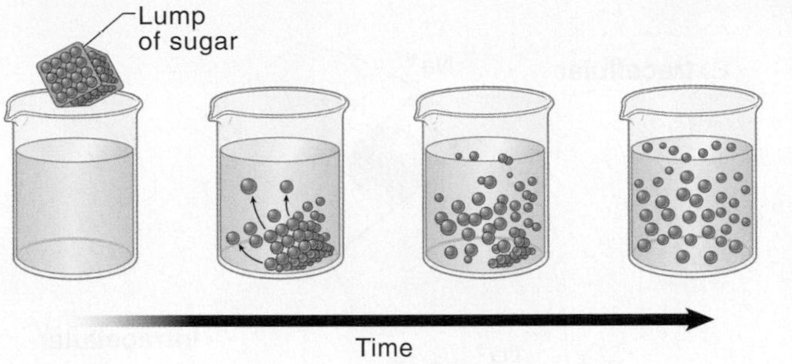

FIG. 17-4 Diffusion is the movement of molecules from an area of high concentration to an area of low concentration. Eventually the sugar molecules are evenly distributed.

TABLE 17-1 NORMAL SERUM ELECTROLYTE VALUES

Electrolyte	Reference Interval
Anions	
Bicarbonate (HCO_3^-)	22-26 mEq/L (22-26 mmol/L)
Chloride (Cl^-)	96-106 mEq/L (96-106 mmol/L)
Phosphate (PO_4^{3-})*	2.4-4.4 mg/dL (0.78-1.42 mmol/L)
Cations	
Potassium (K^+)	3.5-5.0 mEq/L (3.5-5.0 mmol/L)
Magnesium (Mg^{2+})	1.5-2.5 mEq/L (0.75-1.25 mmol/L)
Sodium (Na^+)	135-145 mEq/L (135-145 mmol/L)
Calcium (Ca^{2+}) (total)	8.6-10.2 mg/dL (2.15-2.55 mmol/L)
Calcium (ionized)	4.6-5.3 mg/dL (1.16-1.32 mmol/L)

*The majority of the phosphorus (P) in the body is found as phosphate (PO_4^{3-}). The terms are used interchangeably in this text.

prevalent cation is potassium, with small amounts of magnesium and sodium. The prevalent ICF anion is phosphate, with some protein and a small amount of bicarbonate. (Normal serum electrolyte values are presented in Table 17-1.)

MECHANISMS CONTROLLING FLUID AND ELECTROLYTE MOVEMENT

The movement of electrolytes and water between ICF and ECF involves many different processes, including simple diffusion, facilitated diffusion, and active transport. Water moves as driven by two forces: hydrostatic pressure and osmotic pressure.

Diffusion

Diffusion is the movement of molecules from an area of high concentration to one of low concentration (Fig. 17-4). It occurs in liquids, gases, and solids. Net movement of molecules across a membrane stops when the concentrations are equal in both areas. The membrane separating the two areas must be permeable to the diffusing substance for the process to occur. Simple diffusion requires no external energy.

Facilitated Diffusion

Facilitated diffusion involves the use of a protein carrier in the cell membrane. The protein carrier combines with a molecule, especially one too large to pass easily through the cell membrane, and assists in moving the molecule across the membrane from an area of high concentration to one of low concentration. Like simple diffusion, facilitated diffusion is passive and requires no energy. Glucose transport into the cell is an example of facilitated diffusion. The large glucose molecule must combine with a carrier molecule to be able to cross the cell membrane and enter most cells.

Active Transport

Active transport is a process in which molecules move against the concentration gradient. External energy is required for this process. An example is the sodium-potassium pump. The concentrations of sodium and potassium differ greatly intracellularly and extracellularly (see Fig. 17-3). To maintain this concentration difference, the cell uses active transport to move sodium out of the cell and potassium into the cell (Fig. 17-5). The energy source for this mechanism is adenosine triphosphate (ATP), produced in the cell's mitochondria.

Osmosis

Osmosis is the movement of water "down" a concentration gradient, that is, from a region of low solute concentration to one of high solute concentration, across a semipermeable membrane.[2] Imagine a chamber with two compartments separated by a semipermeable membrane, one that allows only the movement of water (Fig. 17-6). Water will move from the less concentrated side (has more water) to the more concentrated side of the chamber water (has less water). Osmosis requires no outside energy sources and stops when the concentration differences disappear or when hydrostatic pressure builds and is sufficient to oppose any further movement of water.

Whenever dissolved substances are contained in a space with a semipermeable membrane, they can pull water into the space by osmosis. The concentration of the solution determines the strength of the osmotic pull. The higher the concentration, the greater the solution's pulling, or **osmotic pressure.** Osmotic pressure is measured in milliosmoles (mOsm) and may be expressed as either fluid osmolarity or fluid osmolality. Although the terms *osmolarity* and *osmolality* are often used interchangeably, they are different measurements. *Osmolarity* measures the

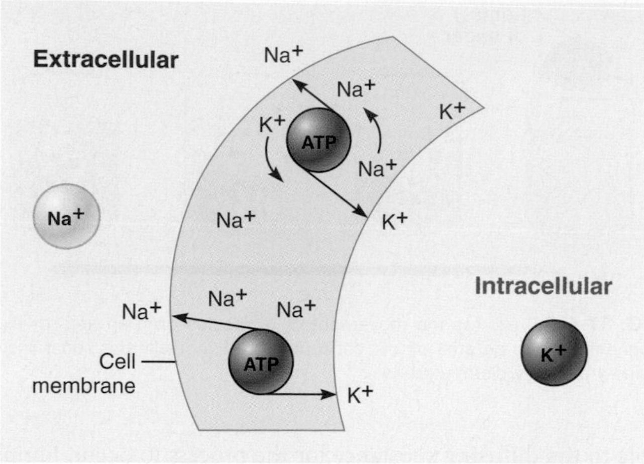

FIG. 17-5 Sodium-potassium pump. As sodium *(Na⁺)* diffuses into the cell and potassium *(K⁺)* diffuses out of the cell, an active transport system supplied with energy delivers Na^+ back to the extracellular compartment and K^+ to the intracellular compartment. *ATP*, Adenosine triphosphate.

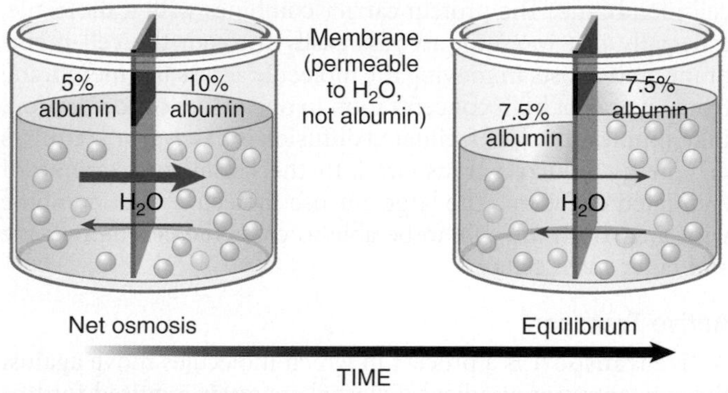

FIG. 17-6 Osmosis is the process of water movement through a semipermeable membrane from an area of low solute concentration to an area of high solute concentration.

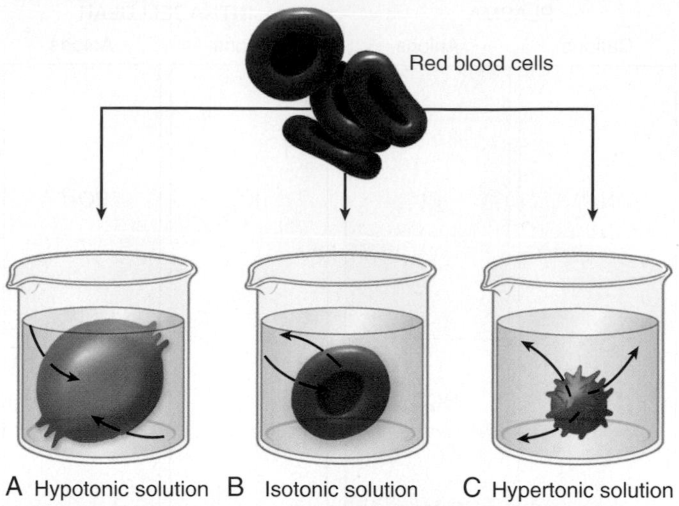

FIG. 17-7 Effects of water status on red blood cells. **A,** Hypotonic solution (H_2O excess) results in cellular swelling. **B,** Isotonic solution (normal H_2O balance) results in no change. **C,** Hypertonic solution (H_2O deficit) results in cellular shrinking.

total milliosmoles per liter of solution, or the concentration of molecules per volume of solution (mOsm/L). **Osmolality** measures the number of milliosmoles per kilogram of water, or the concentration of molecules per weight of water. Osmolality is the test typically performed to evaluate the concentration of plasma and urine.[2]

Measurement of Osmolality. Osmolality is approximately the same in the various body fluid spaces. Determining osmolality is important because it indicates the body's water balance. To assess the state of the body's water balance, one can measure or estimate plasma osmolality. Normal plasma osmolality is between 275 and 295 mOsm/kg. A value greater than 295 mOsm/kg indicates that the concentration of particles is too great or that the water content is too little. This condition is termed *water deficit.* A value less than 275 mOsm/kg indicates too little solute for the amount of water or too much water for the amount of solute. This condition is termed *water excess.* Both conditions are clinically significant. Because the major determinants of plasma osmolality are sodium and glucose, one can calculate the effective plasma osmolality based on the concentrations of those substances.

Osmolality of urine can range from 100 to 1300 mOsm/kg, depending on fluid intake and the amount of antidiuretic hormone (ADH) in circulation and the renal response to it.

Osmotic Movement of Fluids. The osmolality or tonicity of the fluid surrounding the cells affects them. Fluids with the same osmolality as the cell interior are termed **isotonic.** Normally, ECF and ICF are isotonic to one another, so no net movement of water occurs.

Changes in the osmolality of ECF alter the volume of cells. Solutions in which the solutes are less concentrated than in the cells are termed **hypotonic** (hypoosmolar). If a cell is surrounded by hypotonic fluid, water moves into the cell, causing it to swell and possibly to burst. Fluids with solutes more concentrated than in cells, or an increased osmolality, are termed **hypertonic** (hyperosmolar). If hypertonic fluid surrounds a cell, water leaves the cell to dilute ECF; the cell shrinks and may eventually die (Fig. 17-7).

Hydrostatic Pressure

Hydrostatic pressure is the force within a fluid compartment. In the blood vessels, hydrostatic pressure is the blood pressure generated by the contraction of the heart. Hydrostatic pressure in the vascular system gradually decreases as the blood moves through the arteries until it is about 30 mm Hg in the capillary bed. At the capillary level, hydrostatic pressure is the major force that pushes water out of the vascular system and into the interstitial space.

Oncotic Pressure

Oncotic pressure (colloidal osmotic pressure) is the osmotic pressure caused by plasma colloids in solution. The major colloid in the vascular system contributing to the total osmotic pressure is protein. Plasma has substantial amounts of protein, whereas the interstitial space has very little. The plasma protein molecules attract water, pulling fluid from the tissue space to the vascular space. Under normal conditions, plasma oncotic pressure is approximately 25 mm Hg. The small amount of protein found in the interstitial space exerts an oncotic pressure of approximately 1 mm Hg.

FLUID MOVEMENT IN CAPILLARIES

As plasma flows through the capillary bed, four factors determine if fluid moves out of the capillary and into the interstitial

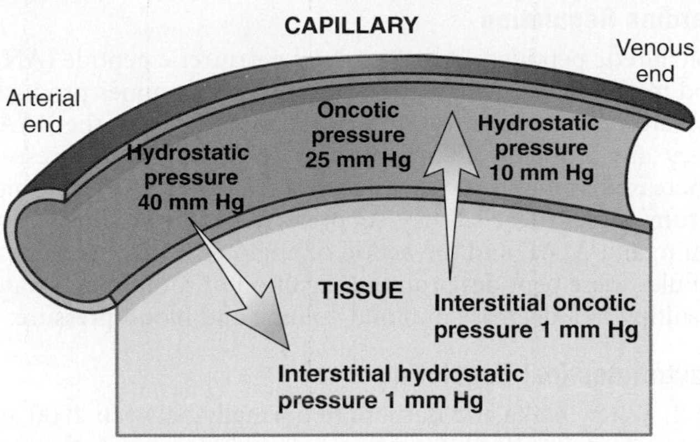

FIG. 17-8 Dynamics of fluid exchange between a capillary and tissue. An equilibrium exists between forces filtering fluid out of the capillary and forces absorbing fluid back into the capillary. Note that the hydrostatic pressure is greater at the arterial end of the capillary than at the venous end. The net effect of pressures at the arterial end of the capillary causes a movement of fluid into the tissue. At the venous end of the capillary, there is net movement of fluid back into the capillary.

space or if fluid moves back into the capillary from the interstitial space. The amount and direction of movement are determined by the interaction of (1) capillary hydrostatic pressure, (2) plasma oncotic pressure, (3) interstitial hydrostatic pressure, and (4) interstitial oncotic pressure.

Capillary hydrostatic pressure and interstitial oncotic pressure move water out of the capillaries. Plasma oncotic pressure and interstitial hydrostatic pressure move fluid into the capillaries. At the arterial end of the capillary, capillary hydrostatic pressure exceeds plasma oncotic pressure, and fluid moves into the interstitial space. At the venous end of the capillary, the capillary hydrostatic pressure is lower than plasma oncotic pressure, drawing fluid back into the capillary by the oncotic pressure created by plasma proteins (Fig. 17-8).

Fluid Shifts

If capillary or interstitial pressures change, fluid may abnormally shift from one compartment to another, resulting in edema or dehydration.

Shifts of Plasma to Interstitial Fluid. *Edema,* an accumulation of fluid in the interstitial space, occurs if venous hydrostatic pressure rises, plasma oncotic pressure decreases, or interstitial oncotic pressure rises. Edema may also develop if an obstruction of lymphatic outflow causes decreased removal of interstitial fluid.

Elevation of Venous Hydrostatic Pressure. Increasing the pressure at the venous end of the capillary inhibits fluid movement back into the capillary, which results in edema. Causes of increased venous pressure include fluid overload, heart failure, liver failure, obstruction of venous return to the heart (e.g., tourniquets, restrictive clothing, venous thrombosis), and venous insufficiency (e.g., varicose veins).

Decrease in Plasma Oncotic Pressure. Fluid remains in the interstitial space if the plasma oncotic pressure is too low to draw fluid back into the capillary. Low plasma protein content decreases oncotic pressure. This can result from excessive protein loss (renal disorders), deficient protein synthesis (liver disease), and deficient protein intake (malnutrition).

Elevation of Interstitial Oncotic Pressure. Trauma, burns, and inflammation can damage capillary walls and allow plasma proteins to accumulate in the interstitial space. This increases interstitial oncotic pressure, draws fluid into the interstitial space, and holds it there.

Shifts of Interstitial Fluid to Plasma. An increase in the plasma osmotic or oncotic pressure draws fluid into the plasma from the interstitial space. This could happen with administration of colloids, dextran, mannitol, or hypertonic solutions. Increasing the tissue hydrostatic pressure is another way of causing a shift of fluid into plasma. Wearing elastic compression gradient stockings or hose to decrease peripheral edema is a therapeutic application of this effect.

FLUID SPACING

Fluid spacing is a term used to describe the distribution of body water. *First spacing* describes the normal distribution of fluid in ICF and ECF compartments. *Second spacing* refers to an abnormal accumulation of interstitial fluid (i.e., edema). *Third spacing* occurs when fluid accumulates in a portion of the body from which it is not easily exchanged with the rest of the ECF. Third-spaced fluid is trapped and unavailable for functional use. Examples of third spacing are ascites; sequestration of fluid in the abdominal cavity with peritonitis; and edema associated with burns, trauma, or sepsis.[3]

REGULATION OF WATER BALANCE

Hypothalamic-Pituitary Regulation

Water balance is maintained via the finely tuned balance of water intake and excretion. Water ingestion will equal water loss in the individual who has free access to water, a normal thirst and ADH mechanism, and normally functioning kidneys.

An intact thirst mechanism is critical because it is the primary protection against the development of hyperosmolality. Osmoreceptors in the hypothalamus sense a body fluid deficit or increase in plasma osmolality, which in turn stimulates thirst and ADH release. Thirst causes the patient to drink water. The distal tubules and collecting ducts in the kidneys respond to ADH by becoming more permeable to water. The result is increased water reabsorption from the tubular filtrate into the blood and decreased excretion in the urine. Together these factors result in increased free water in the body and decreased plasma osmolality.

The patient who cannot recognize or act on the sensation of thirst is at risk for fluid deficit and hyperosmolality. Other factors that stimulate ADH release include stress, nausea, nicotine, and morphine. A decreased plasma osmolality or water excess suppresses secretion of ADH, resulting in urinary excretion of water. It is common for the postoperative patient to have a lower plasma osmolality, possibly because of the stress of surgery and opioid analgesia. Social and psychologic factors not related to fluid balance also affect the desire to consume fluids. A dry mouth will cause the patient to drink, even when there is no measurable body water deficit.

Renal Regulation

The kidneys are the primary organs for regulating fluid and electrolyte balance (see Chapter 45). The kidneys regulate water balance by adjusting urine volume and the urinary excretion of most electrolytes to maintain a balance between overall intake and output. The kidneys filter the total plasma volume many times each day. In the average adult the kidneys reabsorb 99% of this filtrate, producing approximately 1.5 L of urine per day.

As the filtrate moves through the renal tubules, selective reabsorption of water and electrolytes and secretion of electrolytes result in the production of urine that is greatly different in composition and concentration from plasma. This process helps maintain normal plasma osmolality, electrolyte balance, blood volume, and acid-base balance. The renal tubules are the site for the actions of ADH and aldosterone.

With severely impaired renal function, the kidneys cannot maintain fluid and electrolyte balance. This condition results in edema, potassium and phosphorus retention, acidosis, and other electrolyte imbalances (see Chapter 47).

Adrenal Cortical Regulation

Glucocorticoids and mineralocorticoids secreted by the adrenal cortex help regulate both water and electrolytes. The glucocorticoids (e.g., cortisol) primarily have an antiinflammatory effect and increase serum glucose levels, whereas the mineralocorticoids (e.g., aldosterone) enhance sodium retention and potassium excretion (Fig. 17-9). When sodium is reabsorbed, water follows because of osmotic changes.

Cortisol is the most abundant glucocorticoid. In large doses, cortisol has both glucocorticoid (glucose elevating and antiinflammatory) and mineralocorticoid (sodium-retention) effects. Normally cortisol secretion is in a diurnal or circadian pattern. Increased cortisol secretion occurs in response to physical and psychologic stress, affecting many body functions, including fluid and electrolyte balance (Fig. 17-10).

Aldosterone is a mineralocorticoid with potent sodium-retaining and potassium-excreting capabilities. Decreased renal perfusion or decreased sodium delivery to the distal portion of the renal tubule activates the renin-angiotensin-aldosterone system (RAAS), which results in aldosterone secretion (see Fig. 45-4). In addition to the RAAS, increased plasma potassium, decreased plasma sodium, and adrenocorticotropic hormone (ACTH) from the anterior pituitary act directly on the adrenal cortex to stimulate the secretion of aldosterone (see Fig. 17-9).

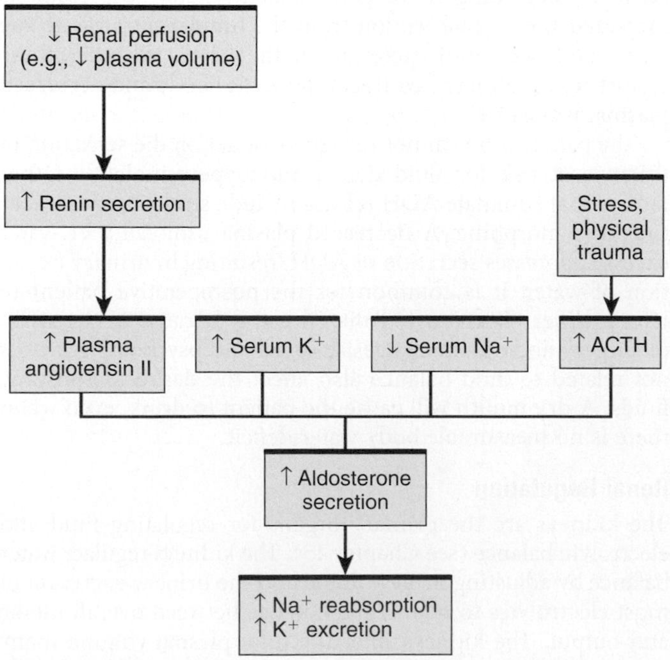

FIG. 17-9 Factors affecting aldosterone secretion. *ACTH,* Adrenocorticotropic hormone.

Cardiac Regulation

Natriuretic peptides, including atrial natriuretic peptide (ANP) and b-type natriuretic peptide (BNP), are hormones produced by cardiomyocytes. They are natural antagonists to the RAAS. They are produced in response to increased atrial pressure (increased volume, such as occurs in heart failure) and high serum sodium levels. They suppress secretion of aldosterone, renin, and ADH, and the action of angiotensin II. In the renal tubules these peptides promote excretion of sodium and water, resulting in a decrease in blood volume and blood pressure.

Gastrointestinal Regulation

Daily water intake and output are normally between 2000 and 3000 mL (Table 17-2). Oral intake of fluids accounts for most

TABLE 17-2 NORMAL FLUID BALANCE IN THE ADULT

Intake	
Fluids	1200 mL
Solid food	1000 mL
Water from oxidation	300 mL
Total	2500 mL
Output	
Insensible loss (skin and lungs)	900 mL
In feces	100 mL
Urine	1500 mL
Total	2500 mL

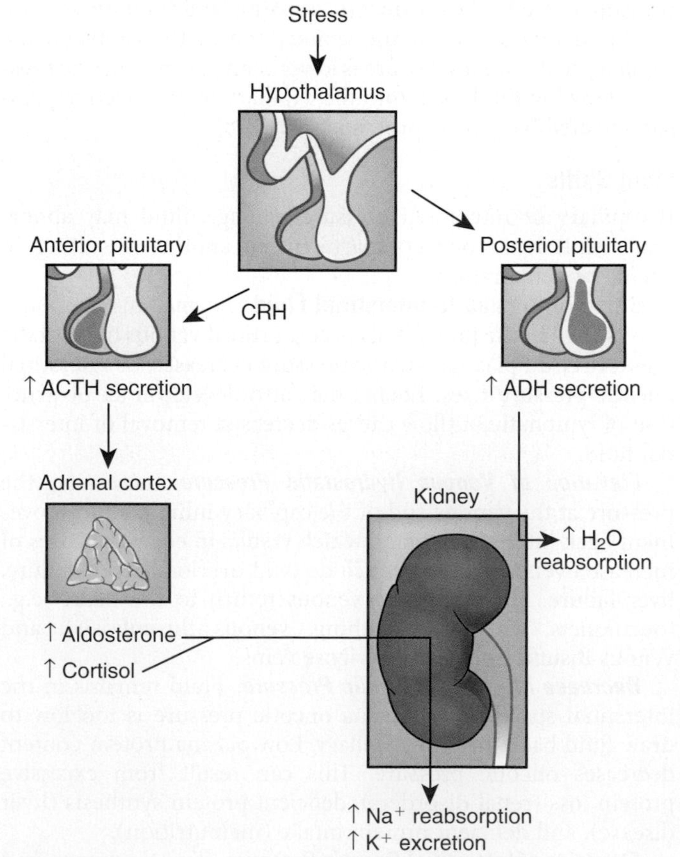

FIG. 17-10 Effects of stress on fluid and electrolyte balance. *ACTH,* Adrenocorticotropic hormone; *ADH,* antidiuretic hormone; *CRH,* corticotropin-releasing hormone.

of the water intake. Water intake also includes water from food metabolism and water present in solid foods. Lean meat is approximately 70% water, whereas the water content of many fruits and vegetables approaches 100%.

In addition to oral intake, the GI tract normally secretes approximately 8000 mL of digestive fluids each day. Most of this fluid is reabsorbed in the GI tract; only a small amount is normally eliminated in feces. Diarrhea and vomiting, which prevent GI reabsorption of this secreted fluid, can lead to significant fluid and electrolyte loss.

Insensible Water Loss

Insensible water loss, which is invisible vaporization from the lungs and skin, assists in regulating body temperature. Normally, about 600 to 900 mL/day is lost. Accelerated body metabolism, which occurs with increased body temperature and exercise, increases the amount of water loss.

Do not confuse water loss through the skin with the vaporization of water excreted by sweat glands. Insensible perspiration causes only water loss. Excessive sweating *(sensible perspiration)* caused by exercise, fever, or high environmental temperatures may lead to large losses of water and electrolytes.

GERONTOLOGIC CONSIDERATIONS

FLUID AND ELECTROLYTES

The older adult experiences normal physiologic changes with aging that increase susceptibility to fluid and electrolyte imbalances. Structural changes to the kidneys and a decrease in the renal blood flow lead to decreased glomerular filtration rate, decreased creatinine clearance, and loss of the ability to concentrate urine and conserve water. Hormonal changes include a decrease in renin and aldosterone and an increase in ADH and ANP.[4] Loss of subcutaneous tissue and thinning of the dermis lead to increased loss of moisture through the skin and an inability to respond to heat or cold quickly.

Older adults experience a decrease in the thirst mechanism, resulting in decreased fluid intake despite increases in osmolality and serum sodium level. Older adults, especially if they are ill, are at increased risk of free-water loss and subsequent development of hypernatremia secondary to impairment of the thirst mechanism and barriers to obtaining fluids to drink.[5]

Healthy older adults usually consume adequate fluids to remain well hydrated. However, functional changes may occur that affect the ability to independently obtain fluids. For example, musculoskeletal changes, such as stiffness of the hands and fingers, can lead to a decreased ability to hold a glass or cup. Mental status changes, such as confusion or disorientation, or changes in ambulation status may lead to a decreased ability to obtain fluids. To reduce incontinent episodes, the older adult may intentionally restrict fluid intake.

You should not automatically attribute older patients' fluid and electrolyte problems to the natural processes of aging. Adapt your assessment and nursing interventions to account for these physiologic and functional changes. Suggestions for alterations in nursing care for the older adult are presented throughout this chapter.

FLUID AND ELECTROLYTE IMBALANCES

Fluid and electrolyte imbalances occur to some degree in most patients with a major illness or injury because illness disrupts the normal homeostatic mechanism. Some fluid and electrolyte imbalances are directly caused by illness or disease (e.g., burns, heart failure). At other times, therapeutic measures (e.g., IV fluid replacement, diuretics) cause or contribute to fluid and electrolyte imbalances. Perioperative patients are at risk for the development of fluid and electrolyte imbalances because of fluid restrictions, blood or fluid loss, and the stress of surgery.[6]

Imbalances are commonly classified as *deficits* or *excesses.* Although each imbalance is discussed separately in this chapter, it is common for more than one imbalance to occur in the same patient. For example, a patient with prolonged nasogastric suction will lose sodium, potassium, hydrogen, and chloride ions. These imbalances may result in a deficiency of both sodium and potassium, a fluid volume deficit, and metabolic alkalosis caused by loss of hydrochloric acid.

EXTRACELLULAR FLUID VOLUME IMBALANCES

ECF volume deficit *(hypovolemia)* and ECF volume excess *(hypervolemia)* are common clinical conditions. ECF volume imbalances are typically accompanied by one or more electrolyte imbalances, particularly changes in the serum sodium level.

Fluid Volume Deficit

Fluid volume deficit can occur with abnormal loss of body fluids (e.g., diarrhea, fistula drainage, hemorrhage, polyuria), inadequate intake, or a shift of fluid from plasma into interstitial fluid. The term *fluid volume deficit* is not interchangeable with the term *dehydration. Dehydration* refers to loss of pure water alone without a corresponding loss of sodium. Causes and clinical manifestations of fluid volume deficit are listed in Table 17-3.

Collaborative Care

The goal of treatment for fluid volume deficit is to correct the underlying cause and to replace both water and any needed electrolytes. Balanced IV solutions, such as lactated Ringer's solution, are usually given. Isotonic (0.9%) sodium chloride is used when rapid volume replacement is indicated. Blood is administered when volume loss is due to blood loss.

Fluid Volume Excess

Fluid volume excess may result from excessive intake of fluids, abnormal retention of fluids (e.g., heart failure, renal failure), or a shift of fluid from interstitial fluid into plasma fluid. Although fluid shifts between the interstitial space and plasma do not alter the overall volume of ECF, these shifts result in changes in the intravascular volume. Causes and clinical manifestations of fluid volume excess are listed in Table 17-3.

Collaborative Care

The goal of treatment for fluid volume excess is removing fluid without producing abnormal changes in the electrolyte composition or osmolality of ECF. The primary cause must be identified and treated. Diuretics and fluid restriction are the primary forms of therapy. Restriction of sodium intake may also be indicated. If the fluid excess leads to ascites or pleural

TABLE 17-3 EXTRACELLULAR FLUID IMBALANCES: CAUSES AND CLINICAL MANIFESTATIONS

ECF Volume Deficit	ECF Volume Excess
Causes	
• ↑ Insensible water loss or perspiration (high fever, heatstroke) • Diabetes insipidus • Osmotic diuresis • Hemorrhage • GI losses: vomiting, NG suction, diarrhea, fistula drainage • Overuse of diuretics • Inadequate fluid intake • Third-space fluid shifts: burns, intestinal obstruction	• Excessive isotonic or hypotonic IV fluids • Heart failure • Renal failure • Primary polydipsia • SIADH • Cushing syndrome • Long-term use of corticosteroids
Clinical Manifestations	
• Restlessness, drowsiness, lethargy, confusion • Thirst, dry mucous membranes • Decreased skin turgor, ↓ capillary refill • Postural hypotension, ↑ pulse, ↓ CVP • ↓ Urine output, concentrated urine • ↑ Respiratory rate • Weakness, dizziness • Weight loss • Seizures, coma	• Headache, confusion, lethargy • Peripheral edema • Jugular venous distention • Bounding pulse, ↑ BP, ↑ CVP • Polyuria (with normal renal function) • Dyspnea, crackles, pulmonary edema • Muscle spasms • Weight gain • Seizures, coma

CVP, Central venous pressure; *ECF*, extracellular fluid; *SIADH*, syndrome of inappropriate antidiuretic hormone.

effusion, an abdominal paracentesis or thoracentesis may be necessary.

NURSING MANAGEMENT EXTRACELLULAR FLUID VOLUME IMBALANCES

NURSING DIAGNOSES

Nursing diagnoses and collaborative problems for the patient with fluid imbalances include, but are not limited to, the following:

ECF volume deficit:

- Deficient fluid volume *related to* excessive ECF losses or decreased fluid intake
- Decreased cardiac output *related to* excessive ECF losses or decreased fluid intake
- Risk for deficient fluid volume *related to* excessive ECF losses or decreased fluid intake
- Potential complication: hypovolemic shock

ECF volume excess:

- Excess fluid volume *related to* increased water and/or sodium retention
- Impaired gas exchange *related to* water retention leading to pulmonary edema
- Risk for impaired skin integrity *related to* edema
- Activity intolerance *related to* increased water retention, fatigue, and weakness
- Disturbed body image *related to* altered body appearance secondary to edema
- Potential complications: pulmonary edema, ascites

NURSING IMPLEMENTATION

INTAKE AND OUTPUT. The use of 24-hour intake and output records gives valuable information regarding fluid and electrolyte problems. An accurately recorded intake-and-output flow sheet can identify sources of excessive intake or fluid losses. Intake should include oral, IV, and tube feedings and retained irrigants. Output includes urine, excess perspiration, wound or tube drainage, vomitus, and diarrhea. Estimate fluid loss from wounds and perspiration. Measure the urine specific gravity according to agency policy. Readings of greater than 1.025 indicate concentrated urine, whereas those of less than 1.010 indicate dilute urine.

CARDIOVASCULAR CHANGES. Monitoring the patient for cardiovascular changes is necessary to prevent or detect complications from fluid and electrolyte imbalances. Signs and symptoms of ECF volume excess and deficit are reflected in changes in blood pressure, pulse force, and jugular venous distention. In fluid volume excess the pulse is full, bounding, and not easily obliterated. Increased volume causes distended neck veins (jugular venous distention) and increased blood pressure.

In mild to moderate fluid volume deficit, compensatory mechanisms include sympathetic nervous system stimulation of the heart and peripheral vasoconstriction. Stimulation of the heart increases the heart rate and, combined with vasoconstriction, maintains the blood pressure within normal limits. A change in position from lying to sitting or standing may elicit a further increase in the heart rate or a decrease in the blood pressure (orthostatic hypotension). If vasoconstriction and tachycardia provide inadequate compensation, hypotension occurs when the patient is recumbent. Severe fluid volume deficit can cause flattened neck veins and a weak, thready pulse that is easily obliterated. Severe, untreated fluid deficit will result in shock.

RESPIRATORY CHANGES. Both fluid excess and fluid deficit affect respiratory status. ECF excess can result in pulmonary congestion and pulmonary edema as increased hydrostatic pressure in the pulmonary vessels forces fluid into the alveoli. The patient will experience shortness of breath and moist crackles on auscultation. The patient with ECF deficit will demonstrate an increased respiratory rate because of decreased tissue perfusion and resultant hypoxia.

NEUROLOGIC CHANGES. Changes in neurologic function may occur with fluid volume excesses or deficits. ECF excess may result in cerebral edema from increased hydrostatic pressure in cerebral vessels. Alternatively, profound volume depletion may cause an alteration in sensorium secondary to reduced cerebral tissue perfusion.

Assessment of neurologic function includes evaluation of (1) the level of consciousness, which includes responses to verbal and painful stimuli and determination of a person's orientation to time, place, and person; (2) pupillary response to light and equality of pupil size; and (3) voluntary movement of the extremities, degree of muscle strength, and reflexes. Nursing care focuses on maintaining patient safety.

DAILY WEIGHTS. Accurate daily weights provide the easiest measurement of volume status. An increase of 1 kg (2.2 lb) is equal to 1000 mL (1 L) of fluid retention (provided the person has maintained usual dietary intake or has not been on nothing-by-mouth [NPO] status). Obtain the weight under standardized conditions, that is, weigh the patient at the same time every day, wearing the same garments, and on the same carefully calibrated scale. Remove excess bedding and empty all drainage

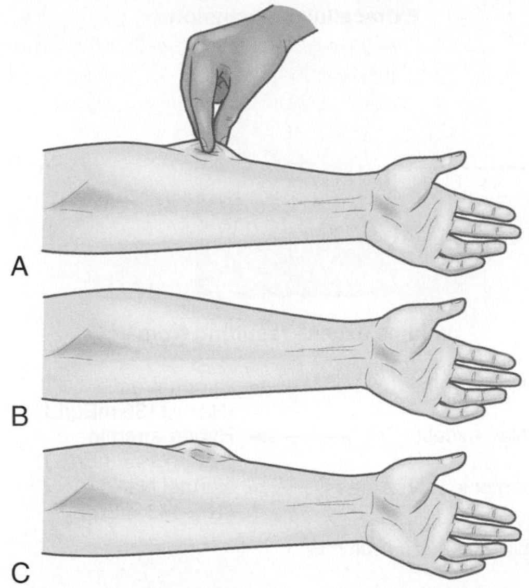

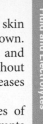

FIG. 17-11 Assessment of skin turgor. **A** and **B,** When normal skin is pinched, it resumes shape in seconds. **C,** If the skin remains wrinkled for 20 to 30 seconds, the patient has poor skin turgor.

bags before the weighing. If the patient has items present that are not there every day, such as bulky dressings or tubes, note this along with the weight.

SKIN ASSESSMENT AND CARE. Detect clues to ECF volume deficit and excess by inspecting the skin. Examine the skin for turgor and mobility. Normally a fold of skin, when pinched, will readily move and, on release, rapidly return to its former position. Skin areas over the sternum, abdomen, and anterior forearm are the usual sites for evaluation of tissue turgor (Fig. 17-11). In older people, decreased skin turgor is less predictive of fluid deficit because of the loss of tissue elasticity.[4] In ECF volume deficit, skin turgor is diminished, and there is a lag in the pinched skinfold's return to its original state (referred to as *tenting*).

The skin may be cool and moist if there is vasoconstriction to compensate for the decreased fluid volume. Mild hypovolemia usually does not stimulate this compensatory response. Consequently, the skin will be warm and dry. Volume deficit may also cause the skin to appear dry and wrinkled. These signs may be difficult to evaluate in the older adult because the patient's skin may be normally dry, wrinkled, and nonelastic. Oral mucous membranes will be dry, the tongue may be furrowed, and the individual often complains of thirst. Routine oral care is critical for the comfort of a patient who is dehydrated or fluid restricted for management of fluid volume excess.

Edematous skin may feel cool because of fluid accumulation and a decrease in blood flow secondary to the pressure of the fluid. The fluid can also stretch the skin, causing it to feel taut and hard. Assess edema by pressing with a thumb or forefinger over the edematous area. A grading scale is used to standardize the description if an indentation (ranging from 1+ [slight edema; 2-mm indentation] to 4+ [pitting edema; 8-mm indentation]) remains when pressure is released. Evaluate for edema in areas where soft tissues overlie a bone, with preferred sites being the tibia, fibula, and sacrum.

Good skin care for the person with ECF volume excess or deficit is important. Protect edematous tissues from extremes of heat and cold, prolonged pressure, and trauma. Frequent skin care and changes in position will prevent skin breakdown. Elevate edematous extremities to promote venous return and fluid reabsorption. Dehydrated skin needs frequent care without the use of soap. Applying moisturizing creams or oils increases moisture retention and stimulates circulation.

OTHER NURSING MEASURES. Carefully monitor the rates of infusion of IV fluid solutions. Be cautious about any attempts to "catch up," particularly when large volumes of fluid or certain electrolytes are involved. This is especially true in patients with cardiac, renal, or neurologic problems. Patients receiving tube feedings need supplementary water added to their enteral formula. The amount of additional water depends on the osmolarity of the feeding and the patient's condition.

Do not allow the patient with nasogastric suction to drink water because it will increase the loss of electrolytes. Occasionally the patient may be given small amounts of ice chips to suck. Irrigate nasogastric tubes with isotonic saline solution, not with water. Water causes diffusion of electrolytes into the gastric lumen from mucosal cells. The suction then removes the electrolytes, increasing the risk of electrolyte imbalances.

Nurses in hospitals and long-term care facilities should encourage and help the older or debilitated patient to maintain adequate oral intake. Assess the patient's ability to obtain adequate fluids independently, express thirst, and swallow effectively.[4] Fluids should be easily accessible. Assist older adults with physical limitations, such as arthritis, to open and hold containers. A variety of types of fluids should be available, and assess for individual preferences. Serve fluids at the temperature preferred by the patient. Seventy percent to 80% of the daily intake of fluids should be with meals, with fluid supplements between meals. Older adults may choose to decrease or eliminate fluids 2 hours before bedtime to decrease nocturia or incontinence. The unconscious or cognitively impaired patient is at increased risk because of an inability to express thirst and act on it. In these patients, accurately document fluid intake and losses and carefully evaluate the adequacy of intake and output.[4]

SODIUM IMBALANCES

Sodium, the main cation of ECF, plays a major role in maintaining the concentration and volume of ECF and influencing water distribution between ECF and ICF. Sodium plays an important role in the generation and transmission of nerve impulses, muscle contractility, and the regulation of acid-base balance.

Because sodium is the primary determinant of ECF osmolality, sodium imbalances are typically associated with parallel changes in osmolality. Serum sodium is measured in milliequivalents per liter (mEq/L) or millimoles per liter (mmol/L). The serum sodium level reflects the ratio of sodium to water, not necessarily the loss or gain of sodium. Changes in the serum sodium level may reflect a primary water imbalance, a primary sodium imbalance, or a combination of the two. Sodium imbalances are typically associated with imbalances in ECF volume (Figs. 17-12 and 17-13).

The GI tract absorbs sodium from foods. Typically, daily intake of sodium far exceeds the body's daily requirements. Sodium leaves the body through urine, sweat, and feces. The kidneys are the primary regulator of sodium balance. The kidneys regulate the ECF concentration of sodium by excreting or retaining water under the influence of ADH. Aldosterone

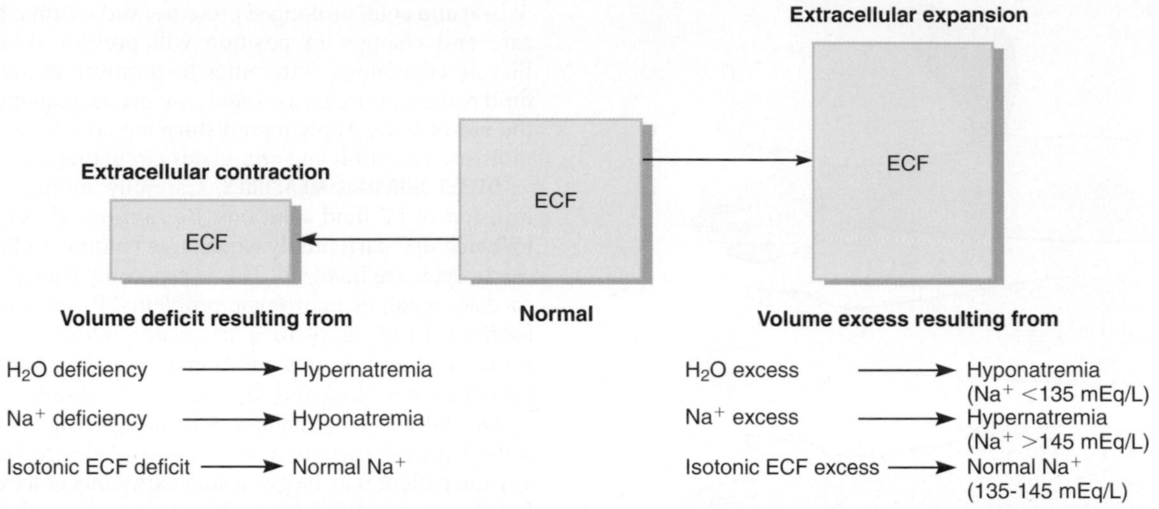

FIG. 17-12 Differential assessment of extracellular fluid *(ECF)* volume.

also plays a role in sodium regulation by promoting sodium reabsorption from the renal tubules.

Hypernatremia

Hypernatremia, an elevated serum sodium, may occur with water loss or sodium gain. Because sodium is the major determinant of the ECF osmolality, hypernatremia causes hyperosmolality. In turn, ECF hyperosmolality causes a shift of water out of the cells, which leads to cellular dehydration. As discussed earlier, the primary protection against the development of hyperosmolality is thirst. Hypernatremia is not a problem in an alert person who has access to water, can sense thirst, and is able to swallow. Hypernatremia secondary to water deficiency is often the result of an impaired level of consciousness or an inability to obtain fluids.

Several clinical states can produce hypernatremia from water loss (Table 17-4). A deficiency in the synthesis or release of ADH from the posterior pituitary gland (central diabetes insipidus) or a decrease in kidney responsiveness to ADH (nephrogenic diabetes insipidus) can result in profound diuresis, thus producing a water deficit and hypernatremia. Hyperosmolality with osmotic diuresis can result from administration of concentrated hyperosmolar tube feedings and hyperglycemia associated with uncontrolled diabetes mellitus. Other causes of hypernatremia include excessive sweating and increased sensible losses from high fever.

Excessive sodium intake with inadequate water intake can also lead to hypernatremia. Examples of sodium gain include IV administration of hypertonic saline or sodium bicarbonate, use of sodium-containing drugs, excessive oral intake of sodium (e.g., ingestion of seawater), and *primary aldosteronism* (hypersecretion of aldosterone) caused by a tumor of the adrenal glands.

Clinical Manifestations. The manifestations of hypernatremia are primarily the result of water shifting out of cells into ECF with resultant dehydration and shrinkage of cells (see Table 17-4). Dehydration of brain cells results in neurologic manifestations such as intense thirst, agitation, and decreased alertness, ranging from sleepiness to coma.[7] If there is any accompanying

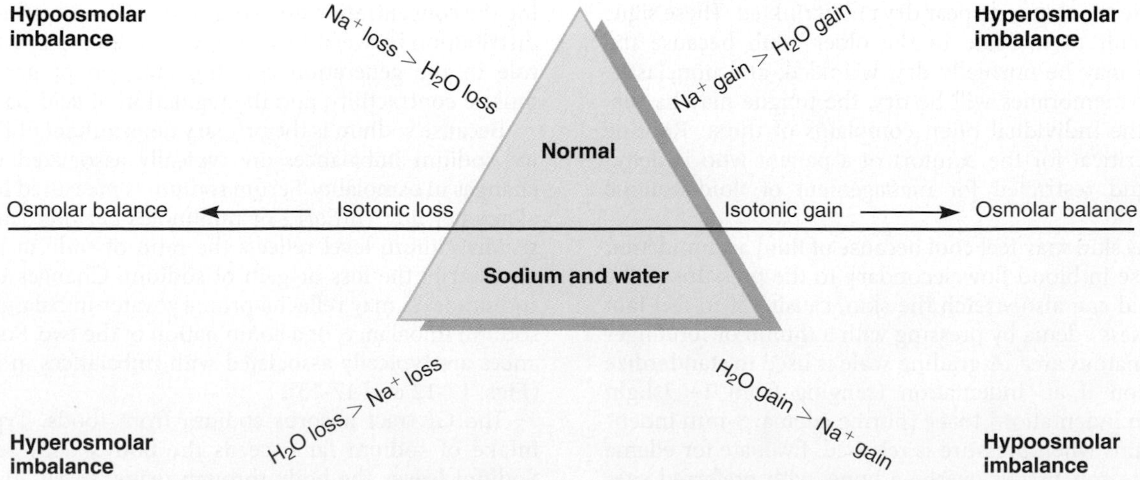

FIG. 17-13 Isotonic gains and losses affect mainly the extracellular fluid (ECF) compartment with little or no water movement into the cells. Hypertonic imbalances cause water to move from inside the cell into ECF to dilute the concentrated sodium, causing cell shrinkage. Hypotonic imbalances cause water to move into the cell, causing cell swelling.

TABLE 17-4 SODIUM IMBALANCES: CAUSES AND CLINICAL MANIFESTATIONS

Hypernatremia (Na^+ >145 mEq/L [mmol/L])	Hyponatremia (Na^+ <135 mEq/L [mmol/L])
Causes	
Excessive Sodium Intake	***Excessive Sodium Loss***
• IV fluids: hypertonic NaCl, excessive isotonic NaCl, IV sodium bicarbonate • Hypertonic tube feedings without water supplements • Near-drowning in salt water	• *GI losses:* diarrhea, vomiting, fistulas, NG suction • *Renal losses:* diuretics, adrenal insufficiency, Na^+ wasting renal disease • *Skin losses:* burns, wound drainage
Inadequate Water Intake	***Inadequate Sodium Intake***
• Unconscious or cognitively impaired individuals	• Fasting diets
Excessive Water Loss (↑ sodium concentration)	***Excessive Water Gain (↓ sodium concentration)***
• ↑ Insensible water loss (high fever, heatstroke, prolonged hyperventilation) • Osmotic diuretic therapy • Diarrhea	• Excessive hypotonic IV fluids • Primary polydipsia
Disease States	***Disease States***
• Diabetes insipidus • Primary hyperaldosteronism • Cushing syndrome • Uncontrolled diabetes mellitus	• SIADH • Heart failure • Primary hypoaldosteronism
Clinical Manifestations	
Hypernatremia With Decreased ECF Volume	***Hyponatremia With Decreased ECF Volume***
• Restlessness, agitation, twitching, seizures, coma • Intense thirst. Dry, swollen tongue. Sticky mucous membranes • Postural hypotension, ↓ CVP, weight loss, ↑ pulse • Weakness, lethargy	• Irritability, apprehension, confusion, dizziness, personality changes, tremors, seizures, coma • Dry mucous membranes • Postural hypotension, ↓ CVP, ↓ jugular venous filling, ↑ pulse, thready pulse • Cold and clammy skin
Hypernatremia With Normal or Increased ECF Volume	***Hyponatremia With Normal or Increased ECF Volume***
• Restlessness, agitation, twitching, seizures, coma • Intense thirst, flushed skin • Weight gain, peripheral and pulmonary edema, ↑ BP, ↑ CVP	• Headache, apathy, confusion, muscle spasms, seizures, coma • Nausea, vomiting, diarrhea, abdominal cramps • Weight gain, ↑ BP, ↑ CVP

CVP, Central venous pressure; *ECF,* extracellular fluid; *SIADH,* syndrome of inappropriate antidiuretic hormone.

ECF volume deficit, manifestations such as postural hypotension, weakness, and decreased skin turgor occur.

NURSING AND COLLABORATIVE MANAGEMENT HYPERNATREMIA

NURSING DIAGNOSES

Nursing diagnoses and collaborative problems for the patient with hypernatremia include, but are not limited to, the following:

- Risk for injury *related to* altered sensorium and seizures
- Risk for fluid volume deficit *related to* excessive intake of sodium and/or loss of water
- Risk for electrolyte imbalance *related to* excessive intake of sodium and/or loss of water
- Potential complication: seizures and coma leading to irreversible brain damage

NURSING IMPLEMENTATION

The primary goal of treatment of hypernatremia is to treat the underlying cause. In primary water deficit, fluid replacement is provided either orally or IV with isotonic or hypotonic fluids such as 5% dextrose in water or 0.45% sodium chloride saline solution.[8] The goal of treatment for sodium excess is to dilute the sodium concentration with sodium-free IV fluids, such as 5% dextrose in water, and to promote excretion of the excess sodium by administering diuretics. (See Chapter 50 for specific treatment of diabetes insipidus.)

Monitor serum sodium levels and the patient's response to therapy. Quickly reducing serum sodium levels can cause a rapid shift of water back into the cells, resulting in cerebral edema and neurologic complications. This risk is greatest in the patient who has developed hypernatremia over several days or longer. Dietary sodium intake is often restricted.

Hyponatremia

Hyponatremia (low serum sodium) may result from a loss of sodium-containing fluids, water excess in relation to the amount of sodium (dilutional hyponatremia), or a combination of both (see Table 17-4). Common causes of hyponatremia from loss of sodium-rich body fluids include profuse diaphoresis, draining wounds, excessive diarrhea or vomiting, and trauma with significant blood loss. Hyponatremia causes hypoosmolality with a shift of water into the cells.

A common cause of hyponatremia from water excess is inappropriate use of sodium-free or hypotonic IV fluids. This may occur in patients after surgery or major trauma or during administration of fluids in patients with renal failure. Patients with psychiatric disorders may have an excessive water intake. Syndrome of inappropriate antidiuretic hormone secretion (SIADH) will result in dilutional hyponatremia caused by abnormal retention of water. (See Chapter 50 for a discussion of the causes of SIADH.)

Clinical Manifestations. Manifestations of hyponatremia are due to cellular swelling and first manifested in the central nervous system (CNS) (see Table 17-4). The excess water lowers plasma osmolality, shifting fluid into brain cells, causing irritability, headache, confusion, seizures, and even coma. Severe acute hyponatremia, if untreated, can cause irreversible neurologic damage or death.[7]

NURSING AND COLLABORATIVE MANAGEMENT HYPONATREMIA

NURSING DIAGNOSES

Nursing diagnoses and collaborative problems for the patient with hyponatremia include, but are not limited to, the following:

- Risk for acute confusion *related to* electrolyte imbalance
- Risk for injury *related to* altered sensorium and decreased level of consciousness

- Risk for electrolyte imbalance *related to* excessive loss of sodium and/or excessive intake or retention of water
- Potential complication: severe neurologic changes

NURSING IMPLEMENTATION

In hyponatremia caused by water excess, fluid restriction is often the only treatment. If severe symptoms (seizures) develop, small amounts of IV hypertonic saline solution (3% sodium chloride) can restore the serum sodium level while the body is returning to a normal water balance. Treatment of hyponatremia associated with abnormal fluid loss includes fluid replacement with sodium-containing solutions.

The drugs conivaptan (Vaprisol) and tolvaptan (Samsca) are given to block the activity of ADH. Conivaptan results in increased urine output without loss of electrolytes such as sodium and potassium. It should not be used in patients with hyponatremia from excess water loss. Tolvaptan is used to treat hyponatremia associated with heart failure, liver cirrhosis, and SIADH.[9] Treatment with these drugs is started in a hospital setting so the patient's clinical status and serum sodium levels can be carefully monitored.

POTASSIUM IMBALANCES

Potassium is the major ICF cation, with 98% of the body potassium being intracellular. For example, potassium concentration within muscle cells is approximately 140 mEq/L; potassium concentration in ECF is 3.5 to 5.0 mEq/L. The sodium-potassium pump in cell membranes maintains this concentration difference by pumping potassium into the cell and sodium out. Because the ratio of ECF potassium to ICF potassium is the major factor in the resting membrane potential of nerve and muscle cells, neuromuscular and cardiac function are commonly affected by potassium imbalances.

Disruptions in the dynamic equilibrium between ICF and ECF potassium often cause clinical problems. Potassium regulates intracellular osmolality and promotes cellular growth. Potassium is required for glycogen to be deposited in muscle and liver cells. Potassium also plays a role in acid-base balance (discussed in the section on acid-base regulation later in this chapter).

Diet is the source of potassium. The typical Western diet contains approximately 50 to 100 mEq of potassium daily, mainly from fruits, dried fruits, and vegetables. Many salt substitutes used in low-sodium diets contain substantial potassium. Patients may receive potassium from parenteral sources, including IV fluids; transfusions of stored, hemolyzed blood; and medications (e.g., potassium penicillin).

The kidneys are the primary route for potassium loss, eliminating about 90% of the daily potassium intake. The remainder is lost in the stool and sweat. There is an inverse relationship between sodium and potassium reabsorption in the kidneys. Factors that cause sodium retention (e.g., low blood volume, increased aldosterone level) cause potassium loss in the urine. Large urine volumes can be associated with excess loss of potassium in the urine. If kidney function is significantly impaired, retained potassium can lead to toxic levels.

TABLE 17-5 POTASSIUM IMBALANCES: CAUSES AND CLINICAL MANIFESTATIONS

Hyperkalemia (K^+ >5.0 mEq/L [mmol/L])	Hypokalemia (K^+ <3.5 mEq/L [mmol/L])
Causes	
Excess Potassium Intake • Excessive or rapid parenteral administration • Potassium-containing drugs (e.g., potassium penicillin) • Potassium-containing salt substitute	***Potassium Loss*** • *GI losses:* diarrhea, vomiting, fistulas, NG suction • *Renal losses:* diuretics, hyperaldosteronism, magnesium depletion • *Skin losses:* diaphoresis • Dialysis
Shift of Potassium Out of Cells • Acidosis • Tissue catabolism (e.g., fever, sepsis, burns) • Crush injury • Tumor lysis syndrome	***Shift of Potassium Into Cells*** • Increased insulin (e.g., IV dextrose load) • Alkalosis • Tissue repair • ↑ Epinephrine (e.g., stress)
Failure to Eliminate Potassium • Renal disease • Potassium-sparing diuretics (e.g., amiloride [Midamor]) • Adrenal insufficiency • ACE inhibitors • NSAIDs	***Lack of Potassium Intake*** • Starvation • Diet low in potassium • Failure to include potassium in parenteral fluids if NPO
Clinical Manifestations	
• Irritability • Anxiety • Abdominal cramping, diarrhea • Weakness of lower extremities • Paresthesias • Irregular pulse • Cardiac arrest if hyperkalemia sudden or severe	• Fatigue • Muscle weakness, leg cramps • Nausea, vomiting, paralytic ileus • Soft, flabby muscles • Paresthesias, decreased reflexes • Weak, irregular pulse • Polyuria • Hyperglycemia
Electrocardiogram Changes • Tall, peaked T wave • Prolonged PR interval • ST segment depression • Loss of P wave • Widening QRS • Ventricular fibrillation • Ventricular standstill	***Electrocardiogram Changes*** • ST segment depression • Flattened T wave • Presence of U wave • Prolonged QRS • Ventricular dysrhythmias (e.g., PVCs) • Bradycardia

ACE, Angiotensin-converting enzyme; *PVCs,* premature ventricular contractions.

Hyperkalemia

Hyperkalemia (high serum potassium) may result from impaired renal excretion, a shift of potassium from ICF to ECF, a massive intake of potassium, or a combination of these factors (Table 17-5). The most common cause of hyperkalemia is renal failure. Adrenal insufficiency with a subsequent aldosterone deficiency leads to retention of potassium ions. Factors that cause potassium to move from ICF to ECF include acidosis, massive cell destruction (as in burn or crush injury, tumor lysis, severe infections), and exercise. In metabolic acidosis, potassium ions shift from ICF to ECF in exchange for hydrogen ions moving into the cell.

Both digoxin-like drugs and β-adrenergic blockers (beta blockers) (e.g., propranolol [Inderal]) can impair entry of potassium into cells, resulting in a higher ECF potassium concentration.[10] Certain drugs, such as potassium-sparing diuretics (e.g., amiloride [Midamor]), aldosterone receptor blockers (e.g., spi-

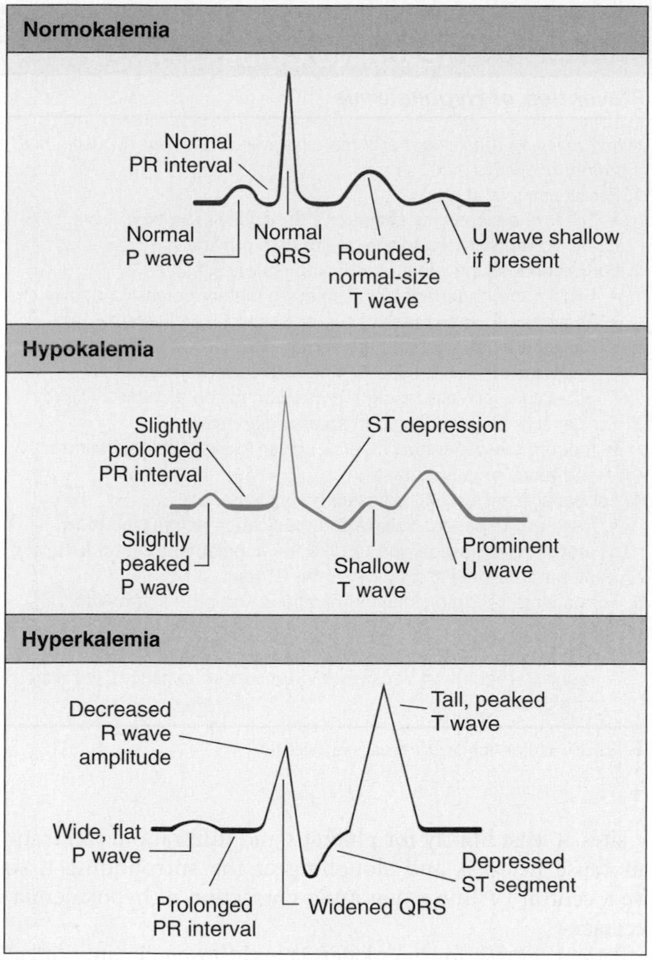

FIG. 17-14 Electrocardiographic changes associated with alterations in potassium status.

ronolactone [Aldactone]), and angiotensin-converting enzyme (ACE) inhibitors (e.g., enalapril [Vasotec], lisinopril [Prinivil]), may contribute to the development of hyperkalemia by reducing the kidney's ability to excrete potassium.

Clinical Manifestations. Hyperkalemia increases the concentration of potassium outside of the cell, altering the normal ECF and ICF ratio and resulting in increased cellular excitability (see Table 17-5). Initially, as the levels of potassium increase, the patient may experience cramping leg pain and weakness, followed by weakness or paralysis of other skeletal muscles, including the respiratory muscles. Abdominal cramping and diarrhea occur from hyperactivity of smooth muscles.

The most clinically significant manifestations of hyperkalemia are the disturbances in cardiac conduction[8] (Fig. 17-14). Cardiac depolarization is decreased, leading to flattening of the P wave and widening of the QRS complex. Repolarization occurs more rapidly, resulting in shortening of the QT interval and a T wave that is narrower and more peaked. Ventricular fibrillation or cardiac standstill may occur.

NURSING AND COLLABORATIVE MANAGEMENT HYPERKALEMIA

NURSING DIAGNOSES

Nursing diagnoses and collaborative problems for the patient with hyperkalemia include, but are not limited to, the following:

- Risk for activity intolerance *related to* lower extremity muscle weakness
- Risk for electrolyte imbalance *related to* excessive retention or cellular release of potassium
- Risk for injury *related to* lower extremity muscle weakness and seizures
- Potential complication: dysrhythmias

NURSING IMPLEMENTATION

Treatment of hyperkalemia consists of the following:

1. Eliminate oral and parenteral potassium intake (see Table 47-11).
2. Increase elimination of potassium. This is accomplished with diuretics, dialysis, and ion-exchange resins such as sodium polystyrene sulfonate (Kayexalate). Kayexalate, administered orally or rectally, binds potassium in exchange for sodium, and the resin is excreted in feces (see Chapter 47).
3. Force potassium from ECF to ICF. This is accomplished by IV administration of regular insulin (along with glucose so the patient does not become hypoglycemic) or IV sodium bicarbonate for the correction of acidosis. Occasionally, a β-adrenergic agonist (e.g., nebulized albuterol) is administered. This therapy is not indicated for patients with tachycardia or coronary artery disease.
4. Reverse the membrane potential effects of the elevated ECF potassium by administering IV calcium gluconate. Calcium ions can immediately reverse the membrane excitability.

In cases in which the elevation of potassium is mild and the kidneys are functioning, it may be sufficient to (1) withhold potassium from the diet and IV sources and (2) increase renal potassium elimination by administering fluids and loop or thiazide diuretics. Patients with moderate hyperkalemia should additionally receive one of the treatments to force potassium into cells, usually IV insulin and glucose. Monitor the electrocardiograms (ECGs) of all patients with clinically significant hyperkalemia to detect dysrhythmias and to monitor the effects of therapy. The patient experiencing dangerous cardiac dysrhythmias should receive IV calcium gluconate immediately. Monitor blood pressure because rapid administration of calcium can cause hypotension. Hemodialysis is an effective means of removing potassium from the body in the patient with renal failure.

Hypokalemia

Hypokalemia (low serum potassium) can result from increased loss of potassium, from an increased shift of potassium from ECF to ICF, or rarely from deficient dietary potassium intake. The most common causes of hypokalemia are abnormal losses from either the kidneys or the GI tract. GI tract losses of potassium are associated with diarrhea, laxative abuse, vomiting, and ileostomy drainage. Renal losses occur when the patient has a low magnesium level or is diuresing, particularly in the patient with an elevated aldosterone level. Aldosterone is released when the circulating blood volume is low, thus causing sodium retention in the kidneys with a loss of potassium in the urine. Low plasma magnesium stimulates renin release and subsequent increased aldosterone levels, which results in potassium excretion.

Among the factors causing potassium to move from ECF to ICF are insulin therapy (especially in conjunction with diabetic ketoacidosis) and β-adrenergic stimulation (catecholamine release in stress, coronary ischemia, delirium tremens, administration of β-adrenergic agonist drugs). Alkalosis can cause a shift of potassium into cells in exchange for hydrogen, thus lowering the potassium in ECF and causing symptomatic hypokalemia.

Clinical Manifestations. Hypokalemia alters the resting membrane potential, resulting in hyperpolarization (an increased negative charge within the cell) and impaired muscle contraction. Therefore the manifestations of hypokalemia involve changes in cardiac and muscle function (see Table 17-5).

The most serious clinical problems are cardiac changes, including impaired repolarization, resulting in a flattening of the T wave and eventually in emergence of a U wave. The P waves peak, and the QRS complex is prolonged (see Fig. 17-14). There is an increased incidence of potentially lethal ventricular dysrhythmias.

Skeletal muscle weakness and paralysis may occur with hypokalemia. As with hyperkalemia, hypokalemia initially affects leg muscles. Severe hypokalemia can cause weakness or paralysis of respiratory muscles, leading to shallow respirations and respiratory arrest. Alterations in smooth muscle function may lead to decreased GI motility (e.g., paralytic ileus), decreased airway responsiveness, and impaired regulation of arteriolar blood flow, possibly contributing to smooth muscle cell breakdown. Finally, hypokalemia can impair function in nonmuscle tissue by impairing insulin secretion, leading to hyperglycemia.

NURSING AND COLLABORATIVE MANAGEMENT HYPOKALEMIA

NURSING DIAGNOSES

Nursing diagnoses and collaborative problems for the patient with hypokalemia include, but are not limited to, the following:

- Risk for activity intolerance *related to* lower extremity muscle weakness
- Risk for electrolyte imbalance *related to* excessive loss of potassium
- Risk for injury *related to* muscle weakness and hyporeflexia
- Potential complication: dysrhythmias

NURSING IMPLEMENTATION

Treatment of hypokalemia consists of oral or IV potassium chloride (KCl) supplements and increased dietary intake of potassium. Except in severe deficiencies, KCl is not given unless there is urine output of at least 0.5 mL/kg of body weight per hour.

SAFETY ALERT

- IV KCl must always be diluted and never given in concentrated amounts.
- Never give KCl via IV push or as a bolus.
- Invert IV bags containing KCl several times to ensure even distribution in the bag.
- Never add KCl to a hanging IV bag to prevent giving a bolus dose.

The preferred maximum concentration is 40 mEq/L. However, stronger concentrations (up to 80 mEq/L) may be given for severe hypokalemia, with continuous cardiac monitoring.[11] The rate of IV administration of KCl should not exceed 10 mEq/hr and must be given by infusion pump to ensure correct administration rate. Because KCl is irritating to the vein, assess IV sites at least hourly for phlebitis and infiltration. Infiltration can cause necrosis and sloughing of the surrounding tissue. Use a central IV line when rapid correction of hypokalemia is necessary.

Patients at risk for hypokalemia and those who are critically ill should have cardiac monitoring to detect cardiac changes related to potassium imbalances. Monitor serum potassium levels and urine output as appropriate. Because patients on digoxin therapy have an increased risk of toxicity if their serum potassium level is low, monitor the patient for digitalis toxicity.

Teach patients methods to prevent hypokalemia (Table 17-6). Foods high in potassium are identified in Table 47-11. Patients at risk for hypokalemia should have regular serum potassium levels monitored.

TABLE 17-6 PATIENT & CAREGIVER TEACHING GUIDE

Prevention of Hypokalemia

When teaching the patient and the caregiver to prevent hypokalemia, do the following.

1. For all patients at risk:
   - Teach the signs and symptoms of hypokalemia (see Table 17-5) and to report them to the health care provider.
2. For patients taking potassium-losing diuretics:*
   - Explain the importance of increasing dietary potassium intake.
   - Teach which foods are high in potassium (see Table 47-11).
   - Explain that salt substitutes contain approximately 50 to 60 mEq of potassium per teaspoon, and help patients raise their potassium levels if taking a potassium-losing diuretic.
3. For patients taking potassium-sparing diuretics:*
   - Instruct the patient and the caregiver to avoid salt substitutes and foods high in potassium.
4. For patients taking oral potassium supplements:
   - Instruct the patient to take the medication as prescribed to prevent overdosage and to take the supplement with a full glass of water to help it dissolve in the GI tract.
5. For patients taking digitalis preparations and others at risk for hypokalemia:
   - Explain the importance of having serum potassium levels regularly monitored because low potassium enhances the action of digitalis.

*For specific information on diuretics, see Table 33-7.

CALCIUM IMBALANCES

Calcium is necessary for many metabolic processes. It is the major cation in the structure of bones and teeth. Other functions of calcium include blood clotting, transmission of nerve impulses, myocardial contractions, and muscle contractions. The source of calcium is dietary intake. Calcium absorption requires the active form of vitamin D. Vitamin D is either ingested in the diet or formed in the skin in the presence of sunlight.

The total body content of calcium is about 1200 g. More than 99% of the body's calcium is found in bones; the remainder is in plasma and body cells. Of the calcium in plasma, 50% is bound to plasma proteins (primarily albumin); 40% is in the free or ionized form; and the remainder is bound with phosphate, citrate, or carbonate. Ionized calcium is the biologically active form.

Calcium is measured in milligrams per deciliter (mg/dL) and milliequivalents per liter (mEq/L). Serum calcium levels usually

TABLE 17-7 CALCIUM IMBALANCES: CAUSES AND CLINICAL MANIFESTATIONS

Hypercalcemia (Ca^{2+} >10.2 mg/dL [2.55 mmol/L])	Hypocalcemia (Ca^{2+} <8.6 mg/dL [2.15 mmol/L])
Causes	
Increased Total Calcium	***Decreased Total Calcium***
• Multiple myeloma	• Chronic kidney disease
• Malignancies with bone metastasis	• Elevated phosphorus
• Prolonged immobilization	• Primary hypoparathyroidism
• Hyperparathyroidism	• Vitamin D deficiency
• Vitamin D overdose	• Magnesium deficiency
• Thiazide diuretics	• Acute pancreatitis
• Milk-alkali syndrome	• Loop diuretics (e.g., furosemide [Lasix])
	• Chronic alcoholism
	• Diarrhea
	• ↓ Serum albumin (patient is usually asymptomatic due to normal ionized calcium level)
Increased Ionized Calcium	***Decreased Ionized Calcium***
• Acidosis	• Alkalosis
	• Excess administration of citrated blood
Clinical Manifestations	
• Lethargy, weakness	• Easy fatigability
• Depressed reflexes	• Depression, anxiety, confusion
• Decreased memory	• Numbness and tingling in extremities and region around mouth
• Confusion, personality changes, psychosis	• Hyperreflexia, muscle cramps
• Anorexia, nausea, vomiting	• Chvostek's sign
• Bone pain, fractures	• Trousseau's sign
• Polyuria, dehydration	• Laryngeal spasm
• Nephrolithiasis	• Tetany, seizures
• Stupor, coma	
Electrocardiogram Changes	***Electrocardiogram Changes***
• Shortened ST segment	• Elongation of ST segment
• Shortened QT interval	• Prolonged QT interval
• Ventricular dysrhythmias	• Ventricular tachycardia
• Increased digitalis effect	

reflect the total calcium level (all three forms). Ionized calcium levels are analyzed and reported separately. The levels listed in Table 17-7 reflect total calcium levels. Changes in serum pH alter the level of ionized calcium without altering the total calcium level. A decreased plasma pH (acidosis) decreases calcium binding to albumin, leading to more ionized calcium. An increased plasma pH (alkalosis) increases calcium binding, leading to decreased ionized calcium. Alterations in serum albumin levels affect the interpretation of total calcium levels. Low albumin levels result in a drop in the total calcium level, although the level of ionized calcium is not affected.

Calcium balance is controlled by parathyroid hormone (PTH) and calcitonin. Since the bones serve as a readily available store of calcium, the body is usually able to maintain normal serum calcium levels by regulating the movement of calcium into or out of the bone. PTH is produced by the parathyroid gland. Its production and release are stimulated by low serum calcium levels. PTH increases bone resorption (movement of calcium out of bones), increases GI absorption of calcium, and increases renal tubule reabsorption of calcium. Calcitonin is produced by the thyroid gland and is stimulated by high serum calcium levels. It opposes the action of PTH and lowers the serum calcium level by decreasing GI absorption, increasing calcium deposition into bone, and promoting renal excretion.

Hypercalcemia

Hypercalcemia (high serum calcium) is caused by hyperparathyroidism in about two thirds of the cases. Malignancy, especially from myeloma and breast, lung, and kidney cancers, causes the remaining third.[12] Malignancies lead to hypercalcemia through bone destruction from tumor invasion or through tumor secretion of a parathyroid-related protein, which stimulates calcium release from bones. Hypercalcemia is also associated with prolonged immobilization, which results in bone mineral loss and increased plasma calcium concentration. Rare causes include vitamin D overdose or increased calcium intake (e.g., ingestion of antacids containing calcium, excessive administration during cardiac arrest).

Excess calcium leads to reduced excitability of both muscles and nerves. Table 17-7 outlines the causes and clinical manifestations of hypercalcemia.

NURSING AND COLLABORATIVE MANAGEMENT HYPERCALCEMIA

NURSING DIAGNOSES

Nursing diagnoses and collaborative problems for the patient with hypercalcemia include, but are not limited to, the following:

- Risk for activity intolerance *related to* generalized muscle weakness
- Risk for electrolyte imbalance *related to* excessive bone destruction
- Risk for injury *related to* neuromuscular and sensorium changes
- Potential complication: dysrhythmias

NURSING IMPLEMENTATION

The basic treatment for hypercalcemia is promoting urinary excretion of calcium by administering a loop diuretic (e.g., furosemide [Lasix]) and hydrating the patient with isotonic saline infusions. The patient must drink 3000 to 4000 mL of fluid daily to promote the renal excretion of calcium and decrease the possibility of kidney stone formation. Other supportive measures include a diet low in calcium and an increase in weight-bearing activity to enhance bone mineralization.

Bisphosphonates (e.g., pamidronate [Aredia], zoledronic acid [Zometa]) are the most effective agents in treating hypercalcemia caused by a malignancy.[12] They inhibit the activity of osteoclasts (cells that break down bone and result in calcium release). Synthetic calcitonin given intramuscularly (IM) or subcutaneously lowers serum calcium levels; the intranasal form is not effective.

Hypocalcemia

Hypocalcemia (low serum calcium) can be caused by any condition that decreases the production of PTH. This may occur with surgical removal of a portion of or injury to the parathyroid glands during thyroid or neck surgery. Acute pancreatitis is

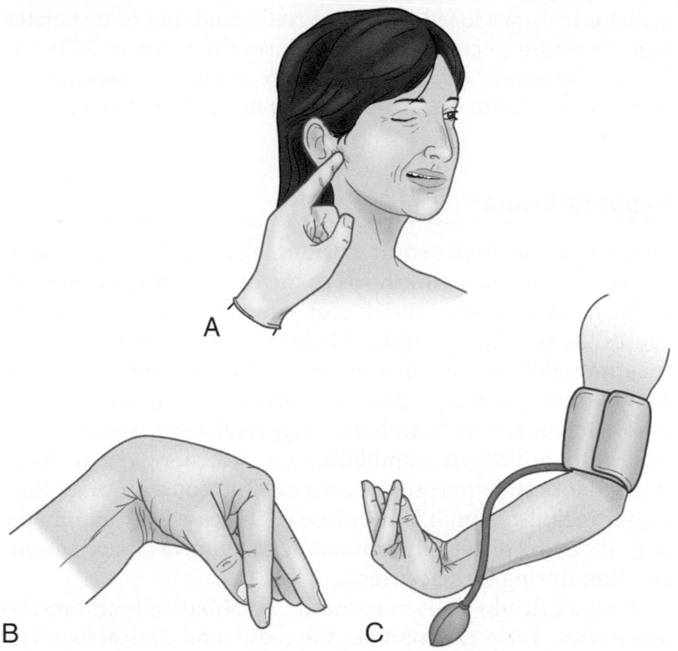

FIG. 17-15 Tests for hypocalcemia. **A,** Chvostek's sign is contraction of facial muscles in response to a light tap over the facial nerve in front of the ear. **B,** Trousseau's sign is a carpal spasm induced by, **C,** inflating a blood pressure cuff above the systolic pressure for a few minutes.

another potential cause of hypocalcemia. Lipolysis, a consequence of pancreatitis, produces fatty acids that combine with calcium ions, decreasing serum calcium levels. The patient who receives multiple blood transfusions can become hypocalcemic because the citrate used to anticoagulate the blood binds with the calcium. Sudden alkalosis may result in symptomatic hypocalcemia despite a normal total serum calcium level. The high pH increases calcium binding to protein, decreasing the amount of ionized calcium. Hypocalcemia can occur if there is increased loss of calcium due to laxative abuse and malabsorption syndromes. (See Table 17-7 for the causes of hypocalcemia.)

Low calcium levels allow sodium to move into excitable cells, decreasing the threshold of action potentials with subsequent depolarization of the cells. This results in increased nerve excitability and sustained muscle contraction, or *tetany.* Clinical signs of tetany include Chvostek's sign and Trousseau's sign. *Chvostek's sign* is contraction of facial muscles in response to a tap over the facial nerve in front of the ear (Fig. 17-15, *A*). *Trousseau's sign* refers to carpal spasms induced by inflating a blood pressure cuff on the arm (Fig. 17-15, *B* and *C*). After the cuff is inflated above the systolic pressure, carpal spasms occur within 3 minutes if hypocalcemia is present. Other manifestations of tetany are laryngeal stridor, dysphagia, and numbness and tingling around the mouth or in the extremities.

Cardiac effects of hypocalcemia include decreased cardiac contractility and ECG changes. A prolonged QT interval may develop into ventricular tachycardia. Table 17-7 outlines the clinical manifestations of hypocalcemia.

NURSING AND COLLABORATIVE MANAGEMENT HYPOCALCEMIA

NURSING DIAGNOSES

Nursing diagnoses and collaborative problems for the patient with hypocalcemia include, but are not limited to, the following:

- Acute pain *related to* sustained muscle contractions
- Ineffective breathing pattern *related to* laryngospasm
- Risk for electrolyte imbalance *related to* decreased production of PTH
- Risk for injury *related to* tetany and seizures
- Potential complications: fracture, respiratory arrest

NURSING IMPLEMENTATION

The primary goal of treatment of hypocalcemia is to treat the underlying cause. When severe manifestations of hypocalcemia occur, IV preparations of calcium (e.g., calcium gluconate, calcium chloride) are given. Treatment of mild hypocalcemia involves a diet high in calcium-rich foods along with vitamin D supplementation. Oral calcium supplements, such as calcium carbonate, can be used when patients are unable to consume enough dietary calcium, such as those who cannot tolerate dairy products. Measures to promote CO_2 retention, such as breathing into a paper bag or sedating the patient, can control muscle spasm and other symptoms of tetany until the calcium level is corrected. Adequately treat pain and anxiety because hyperventilation-induced respiratory alkalosis can precipitate hypocalcemic symptoms. Closely observe any patient who has had thyroid or neck surgery in the immediate postoperative period for manifestations of hypocalcemia because of the proximity of the surgery to the parathyroid glands.

PHOSPHATE IMBALANCES

Phosphorus is the primary anion in ICF and the second most abundant element in the body, second to calcium. Most phosphorus is in the bones and teeth as calcium phosphate. The remaining phosphorus is metabolically active and essential to the function of muscle, red blood cells (RBCs), and the nervous system. It is also involved in the acid-base buffering system; the mitochondrial formation of ATP; cellular uptake and use of glucose; and the metabolism of carbohydrates, proteins, and fats.

PTH maintains serum phosphorus levels and balance. Regulation of phosphate balance requires adequate renal functioning because the kidneys are the major route of phosphate excretion. When the phosphate level in the glomerular filtrate falls below the normal level or PTH levels are low, the kidneys reabsorb additional phosphorus. A reciprocal relationship exists between phosphorus and calcium in that a high serum phosphate level tends to cause a low calcium concentration in the serum. Low serum calcium levels stimulate the release of PTH, which decreases reabsorption of phosphorus.

Hyperphosphatemia

Hyperphosphatemia (high serum phosphate) is commonly caused by acute kidney injury or chronic kidney disease, which results in an altered ability of the kidneys to excrete phosphate. Other causes include chemotherapy for leukemia or lymphoma, excessive ingestion of milk or phosphate-containing laxatives, and large intakes of vitamin D that increase GI absorption of phosphorus. Table 17-8 summarizes causes and clinical manifestations of hyperphosphatemia.

Mild hyperphosphatemia is often asymptomatic. The clinical manifestations of more severe hyperphosphatemia primarily relate to the low serum calcium levels often associated with high serum phosphate levels. These include tetany, muscle cramps, paresthesias, and seizures. Increased levels of phosphate readily

TABLE 17-8 PHOSPHATE IMBALANCES: CAUSES AND CLINICAL MANIFESTATIONS

Hyperphosphatemia (PO_4^{3-} >4.4 mg/dL [1.42 mmol/L])	Hypophosphatemia (PO_4^{3-} <2.4 mg/dL [0.78 mmol/L])
Causes	
• Renal failure • Chemotherapy drugs • Enemas containing phosphorus (e.g., Fleet Enema) • Excessive ingestion (e.g., milk, phosphate-containing laxatives) • Hypoparathyroidism • Sickle cell anemia	• Malabsorption syndromes • Recovery from malnutrition or refeeding • Glucose or insulin therapy • Total parenteral nutrition • Alcohol withdrawal • Phosphate-binding antacids • Recovery from diabetic ketoacidosis • Respiratory alkalosis
Clinical Manifestations	
• Hypocalcemia • Numbness and tingling in extremities and region around mouth • Hyperreflexia, muscle cramps • Tetany, seizures • Deposition of calcium-phosphate precipitates in skin, soft tissue, cornea, viscera, blood vessels	• CNS depression (confusion, coma) • Muscle weakness, including respiratory muscle weakness and difficulty weaning from ventilator • Polyneuropathy, seizures • Cardiac problems (dysrhythmias, decreased stroke volume) • Osteomalacia • Rhabdomyolysis

precipitate with calcium, and calcified deposits occur outside of the bones. These metastatic calcium precipitates can be found in soft tissues such as joints, arteries, skin, kidneys, and corneas and produce organ dysfunction, notably renal failure (see Chapter 47).

The primary management of hyperphosphatemia is identifying and treating the underlying cause. Ingestion of foods and fluids high in phosphorus (e.g., dairy products) should be restricted. Phosphate-binding agents or gels (e.g., calcium carbonate) limit intestinal phosphate absorption and increase phosphate secretion into the intestine. With severe hyperphosphatemia, hemodialysis or an insulin and glucose infusion can rapidly decrease levels. If hypocalcemia is present, providing adequate hydration and instituting measures to correct calcium levels assist with returning phosphorus levels to normal.

Hypophosphatemia

Hypophosphatemia (low serum phosphate) is rare, but may occur in the patient who is malnourished or has a malabsorption syndrome. Other causes include alcohol withdrawal and use of phosphate-binding antacids. Hypophosphatemia may also occur during parenteral nutrition with inadequate phosphorus replacement. Table 17-8 summarizes causes and clinical manifestations of hypophosphatemia.

Most clinical manifestations of hypophosphatemia result from impaired cellular energy and O_2 delivery due to low levels of cellular ATP and 2,3-diphosphoglycerate (2,3-DPG), an enzyme in RBCs that facilitates O_2 delivery to the tissues. Mild to moderate hypophosphatemia is often asymptomatic. Severe hypophosphatemia may be fatal because of decreased cellular function. Acute manifestations include CNS depression, confusion, and other mental changes. Other manifestations include muscle weakness and pain, dysrhythmias, and cardiomyopathy.

Management of a mild phosphorus deficiency may involve oral supplementation (e.g., Neutra-Phos) and ingestion of foods high in phosphorus (e.g., dairy products). Symptomatic hypophosphatemia can be fatal and often requires IV administration of sodium phosphate or potassium phosphate.[13] Frequent monitoring of serum phosphate and calcium levels is necessary to guide IV therapy. Sudden symptomatic hypocalcemia, secondary to increased calcium phosphorus binding, is a potential complication of IV phosphorus administration.

MAGNESIUM IMBALANCES

Magnesium is the second most abundant intracellular cation. Magnesium plays an important role in many essential cellular processes. The most notable is the activation of a wide variety of enzyme systems. Magnesium is a coenzyme in the metabolism of carbohydrates and protein and is required for the synthesis of nucleic acids and proteins. Magnesium plays a role in maintaining normal calcium and potassium balance. Adequate intracellular magnesium is necessary for normal function of the sodium-potassium pump. Because magnesium acts directly on the myoneural junction, alterations in serum magnesium levels profoundly affect neuromuscular excitability and contractility.

Approximately 50% to 60% of the body's magnesium is contained in bone. Only a small amount (2%) is in ECF, with the remainder inside the cell. Magnesium is regulated by GI absorption and renal excretion. The kidneys are able to conserve magnesium in times of need and excrete excesses. Factors that regulate calcium balance (e.g., PTH) similarly influence magnesium balance. Manifestations of magnesium imbalance are often mistaken for calcium imbalances. Because magnesium, calcium, and potassium balance are closely related, assess all three cations together.[14]

Hypermagnesemia

Hypermagnesemia (high serum magnesium level) usually occurs only with an increase in magnesium intake accompanied by renal insufficiency or failure. (Table 17-9 lists the causes of hypermagnesemia.) A patient with chronic kidney disease who ingests products containing magnesium (e.g., Maalox, milk of magnesia) will have a problem with excess magnesium. Magnesium excess could develop in the pregnant woman who receives magnesium sulfate for the management of eclampsia.

Hypermagnesemia depresses neuromuscular and CNS functions. Initial clinical manifestations of a mildly elevated serum magnesium concentration include lethargy, nausea, and vomiting. As the levels of serum magnesium increase, deep tendon reflexes are lost, followed by somnolence, and then respiratory and, ultimately, cardiac arrest can occur (see Table 17-9).

Management of hypermagnesemia should focus on prevention. People with chronic kidney disease should not take magnesium-containing drugs and should limit ingestion of magnesium containing foods (e.g., green vegetables, nuts, bananas, oranges, peanut butter, chocolate).

The emergency treatment of hypermagnesemia is IV administration of calcium chloride or calcium gluconate to oppose the effects of the magnesium on cardiac muscle. If renal function is adequate, promoting urinary excretion with oral and parenteral fluids and IV furosemide decreases magnesium levels. The

TABLE 17-9 MAGNESIUM IMBALANCES: CAUSES AND CLINICAL MANIFESTATIONS

Hypermagnesemia (Mg^+ >2.5 mEq/L [1.25 mmol/L])	Hypomagnesemia (Mg^+ <1.5 mEq/L [0.75 mmol/L])
Causes	
• Renal failure • Adrenal insufficiency • Excessive administration of magnesium, especially for treatment of eclampsia • Tumor lysis syndrome • Diabetic ketoacidosis	• Diarrhea • Vomiting • Chronic alcoholism • Malabsorption syndromes • Prolonged malnutrition • ↑ Urine output • NG suction • Poorly controlled diabetes mellitus • Hyperaldosteronism
Clinical Manifestations	
• Lethargy, drowsiness • Nausea, vomiting • Diminished deep tendon reflexes • Flushed, warm skin • ↓ Pulse, ↓ BP • Muscle weakness • Dysphagia	• Confusion • Tremors, seizures • Hyperactive deep tendon reflexes • Insomnia • ↑ Pulse, ↑ BP • Muscle cramps

patient with impaired renal function requires dialysis because the kidneys are the major route of excretion for magnesium.

Hypomagnesemia

Hypomagnesemia (low serum magnesium level) occurs in patients with limited magnesium intake or increased renal losses. Major causes of hypomagnesemia from insufficient food intake include prolonged fasting or starvation and chronic alcoholism. Fluid loss from the GI tract interferes with magnesium absorption. Another potential cause of hypomagnesemia is prolonged parenteral nutrition without magnesium supplementation. Many diuretics increase the risk of magnesium loss through renal excretion.[14] In addition, osmotic diuresis caused by high glucose levels in uncontrolled diabetes mellitus increases renal excretion of magnesium.

Hypomagnesemia produces neuromuscular and CNS hyperirritability. Clinical manifestations include confusion, hyperactive deep tendon reflexes, muscle cramps, tremors, and seizures. Magnesium deficiency predisposes to cardiac dysrhythmias, such as premature ventricular contractions and ventricular fibrillation. Clinically, hypomagnesemia resembles hypocalcemia and may contribute to the development of hypocalcemia resulting from the decreased action of PTH. Hypomagnesemia may also be associated with hypokalemia that does not respond well to potassium replacement. This occurs because intracellular magnesium is critical to normal function of the sodium-potassium pump.

The primary goal of treatment of hypomagnesemia is to treat the underlying cause. Management of mild magnesium deficiencies involves oral supplements and increased dietary intake of foods high in magnesium. If hypomagnesemia is severe or if hypocalcemia is present, IV magnesium (e.g., magnesium sulfate) is given. Monitor vital signs and use an infusion pump, since too rapid administration of magnesium can lead to cardiac or respiratory arrest.

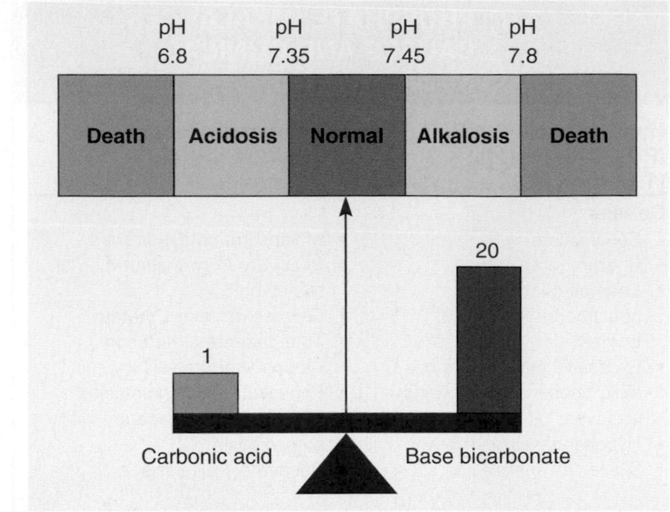

FIG. 17-16 The normal range of plasma pH is 7.35 to 7.45. A normal pH is maintained by a ratio of 1 part carbonic acid to 20 parts bicarbonate.

ACID-BASE IMBALANCES

The body normally maintains a steady balance between the acids produced during normal metabolism and the bases that neutralize and promote the excretion of the acids. Because these acids alter the body's internal environment, their regulation is necessary to maintain homeostasis and acid-base balance. Many health problems may lead to acid-base imbalances. Patients with diabetes mellitus, chronic obstructive pulmonary disease, and kidney disease frequently develop acid-base imbalances. Remember that an acid-base imbalance is not a disease but a symptom of an underlying health problem. Always consider the possibility of acid-base imbalance in patients with serious illnesses.

pH and Hydrogen Ion Concentration

The acidity or alkalinity of a solution depends on its hydrogen ion (H^+) concentration. An increase in H^+ concentration leads to acidity; a decrease leads to alkalinity. Despite the fact that acids are produced by the body daily, the H^+ concentration of body fluids is small (0.0004 mEq/L) and maintained within a narrow range to ensure optimal cellular function.

H^+ concentration is usually expressed as a negative logarithm (symbolized as *pH*) rather than in milliequivalents. The use of the negative logarithm means that the lower the pH, the higher the H^+ concentration. In contrast to a pH of 7, a pH of 8 represents a 10-fold decrease in H^+ concentration.

The pH of a chemical solution may range from 1 to 14. A solution with a pH of 7 is considered neutral. An acid solution has a pH less than 7, and an alkaline solution has a pH greater than 7. Blood is slightly alkaline (pH 7.35 to 7.45). Yet if it drops below 7.35, the person has **acidosis**, even though the blood may never become truly acidic. If the blood pH is greater than 7.45, the person has **alkalosis** (Fig. 17-16).

Acid-Base Regulation

Normally the body has three mechanisms by which it regulates the acid-base balance to maintain the arterial pH between 7.35 and 7.45. These mechanisms are the buffer systems, the respiratory system, and the renal system. The regulatory mechanisms react at different speeds. Buffers react immediately. The respiratory system responds in minutes and reaches maximum effectiveness in hours. The renal response takes 2 or 3 days to respond maximally, but the kidneys can maintain balance indefinitely in patients with chronic imbalances.

Buffer System. The buffer system is the fastest-acting system and the primary regulator of acid-base balance. **Buffers** act chemically to change strong acids into weaker acids or to bind acids to neutralize their effect. This minimizes the effect of acids on blood pH until their excretion from the body. The body buffers an acid load better than it neutralizes base excess. Buffers cannot maintain pH without the adequate functioning of the respiratory and renal systems.

A buffer consists of a weakly ionized acid or a base and its salt. The buffers in the body include carbonic acid–bicarbonate, monohydrogen–dihydrogen phosphate, intracellular and plasma protein, and hemoglobin buffers. The cell can also act as a buffer by shifting hydrogen in and out of the cell. With an accumulation of H^+ in ECF, the cells can accept H^+ in exchange for another cation (e.g., potassium ion).

The carbonic acid–bicarbonate (H_2CO_3/HCO_3^-) buffer system neutralizes hydrochloric acid (HCl) in the following manner:

$$\underset{\text{Strong acid}}{HCl} + \underset{\text{Strong base}}{NaH_2CO_3} \rightarrow \underset{\text{Salt}}{NaCl} + \underset{\text{Weak acid}}{H_2CO_3}$$

In this way, combining a strong acid with a strong base prevents the acid from making a large change in the blood's pH. The carbonic acid is broken down to H_2O and CO_2. The lungs excrete CO_2, either combined with insensible H_2O as carbonic acid, or alone as CO_2. In this process, the buffer system maintains a 20:1 ratio between bicarbonate and carbonic acid and the normal pH.

The phosphate buffer system is composed of sodium and other cations in combination with monohydrogen phosphate (HPO_4^{2-}) or dihydrogen phosphate ($H_2PO_4^-$). This intracellular buffer system acts in the same manner as the bicarbonate system. Bases neutralize strong acids, forming sodium chloride (NaCl) and sodium biphosphate (NaH_2PO_4), a weaker acid. Conversely, if a strong base, such as sodium hydroxide (NaOH), is present, sodium dihydrogen phosphate (NaH_2PO_4) neutralizes it to a weaker base (Na_2HPO_4) and H_2O.

The intracellular and extracellular protein buffering system acts like the bicarbonate system. Some of the amino acids of proteins contain free acid radicals (–COOH), which can dissociate into CO_2 and H^+. Other amino acids have basic radicals (NH_3OH [ammonium hydroxide]), which can dissociate into NH_3^+ (ammonia) and OH^- (hydroxide). The OH^- can combine with an H^+ to form H_2O. Hemoglobin is a protein and assists in regulation of pH by shifting chloride in and out of RBCs in exchange for bicarbonate.

Respiratory System. The lungs help maintain a normal pH by excreting CO_2 and water, which are by-products of cellular metabolism. When released into the circulation, CO_2 enters RBCs and combines with H_2O to form H_2CO_3. This carbonic acid dissociates into H^+ and HCO_3^-. Hemoglobin buffers the free H^+, and the HCO_3^- diffuses into the plasma. This process is reversed in the pulmonary capillaries, forming CO_2 that is then excreted by the lungs. The overall reversible reaction is expressed in the following manner:

$$CO_2 + H_2O \rightarrow H_2CO_3 \rightarrow H^+ + HCO_3^-$$

The amount of CO_2 in the blood directly relates to carbonic acid concentration and subsequently to H^+ concentration. With increased respirations, more CO_2 is expelled and less remains in the blood. This leads to less carbonic acid and less H^+. With decreased respirations, more CO_2 remains in the blood. This leads to increased carbonic acid and more H^+.

The respiratory center in the medulla in the brainstem controls the rate of excretion of CO_2. If increased amounts of CO_2 or H^+ are present, the respiratory center stimulates an increased rate and depth of breathing. If the center senses low H^+ or CO_2 levels, respirations are inhibited.

As a compensatory mechanism, the respiratory system acts on the $CO_2 + H_2O$ side of the reaction by altering the rate and depth of breathing to "blow off" (through hyperventilation) or "retain" (through hypoventilation) CO_2. If a respiratory problem (e.g., respiratory failure) is the cause of an acid-base imbalance, the respiratory system loses its ability to correct a pH alteration. The older adult has impaired compensatory ability because of decreased respiratory function.

Renal System. Under normal conditions, the body depends on the kidneys to reabsorb and conserve all of the HCO_3^- they filter and excrete a portion of the acid produced by cellular metabolism. The three mechanisms of acid elimination are (1) secretion of small amounts of free hydrogen into the renal tubule, (2) combination of H^+ with ammonia (NH_3) to form ammonium (NH_4^+), and (3) excretion of weak acids.

The kidneys normally excrete acidic urine (average pH is 6). As a compensatory mechanism, the pH of the urine can decrease to 4 or increase to 8. To compensate for acidosis, the kidneys can reabsorb additional HCO_3^- and eliminate excess H^+. Thus the pH of the blood increases and the pH of the urine decreases. If the renal system is the cause of an acid-base imbalance (e.g., renal failure), it loses its ability to correct a pH alteration. In the older adult the kidneys are less able to compensate for an acid load.

Alterations in Acid-Base Balance

An acid-base imbalance results when there is an alteration in the ratio of 20:1 between base and acid content. This occurs when a primary disease or process alters one side of the ratio (e.g., CO_2 retention in pulmonary disease) and the compensatory processes that maintain the other side of the ratio (e.g., increased renal HCO_3^- reabsorption) either fail or are inadequate. The compensatory process may be inadequate because either the pathophysiologic process is overwhelming or there is insufficient time for the compensatory process to function.

Acid-base imbalances are classified as respiratory or metabolic. *Respiratory imbalances* result from the retention or an excess of CO_2 altering carbonic acid concentrations; *metabolic imbalances* affect the base HCO_3^-. Therefore acidosis is caused by an increase in carbonic acid (respiratory acidosis) or a decrease in HCO_3^- (metabolic acidosis). Alkalosis is caused by a decrease in carbonic acid (respiratory alkalosis) or an increase in HCO_3^- (metabolic alkalosis). Imbalances may be further classified as acute or chronic. Chronic imbalances allow greater time for compensatory changes.

Respiratory Acidosis. *Respiratory acidosis* (carbonic acid excess) occurs whenever the person hypoventilates (Table 17-10). Hypoventilation leads to a buildup of CO_2, resulting in an accumulation of carbonic acid in the blood. Carbonic acid dissociates, liberating H^+, and there is a decrease in pH. If CO_2

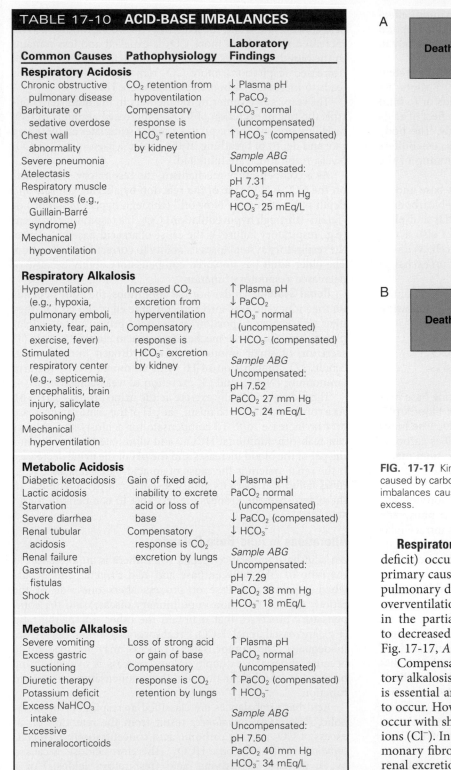

TABLE 17-10 ACID-BASE IMBALANCES

Common Causes	Pathophysiology	Laboratory Findings
Respiratory Acidosis		
Chronic obstructive pulmonary disease Barbiturate or sedative overdose Chest wall abnormality Severe pneumonia Atelectasis Respiratory muscle weakness (e.g., Guillain-Barré syndrome) Mechanical hypoventilation	CO_2 retention from hypoventilation Compensatory response is HCO_3^- retention by kidney	↓ Plasma pH ↑ $PaCO_2$ HCO_3^- normal (uncompensated) ↑ HCO_3^- (compensated) *Sample ABG* Uncompensated: pH 7.31 $PaCO_2$ 54 mm Hg HCO_3^- 25 mEq/L
Respiratory Alkalosis		
Hyperventilation (e.g., hypoxia, pulmonary emboli, anxiety, fear, pain, exercise, fever) Stimulated respiratory center (e.g., septicemia, encephalitis, brain injury, salicylate poisoning) Mechanical hyperventilation	Increased CO_2 excretion from hyperventilation Compensatory response is HCO_3^- excretion by kidney	↑ Plasma pH ↓ $PaCO_2$ HCO_3^- normal (uncompensated) ↓ HCO_3^- (compensated) *Sample ABG* Uncompensated: pH 7.52 $PaCO_2$ 27 mm Hg HCO_3^- 24 mEq/L
Metabolic Acidosis		
Diabetic ketoacidosis Lactic acidosis Starvation Severe diarrhea Renal tubular acidosis Renal failure Gastrointestinal fistulas Shock	Gain of fixed acid, inability to excrete acid or loss of base Compensatory response is CO_2 excretion by lungs	↓ Plasma pH $PaCO_2$ normal (uncompensated) ↓ $PaCO_2$ (compensated) ↓ HCO_3^- *Sample ABG* Uncompensated: pH 7.29 $PaCO_2$ 38 mm Hg HCO_3^- 18 mEq/L
Metabolic Alkalosis		
Severe vomiting Excess gastric suctioning Diuretic therapy Potassium deficit Excess $NaHCO_3$ intake Excessive mineralocorticoids	Loss of strong acid or gain of base Compensatory response is CO_2 retention by lungs	↑ Plasma pH $PaCO_2$ normal (uncompensated) ↑ $PaCO_2$ (compensated) ↑ HCO_3^- *Sample ABG* Uncompensated: pH 7.50 $PaCO_2$ 40 mm Hg HCO_3^- 34 mEq/L

ABG, Arterial blood gas.

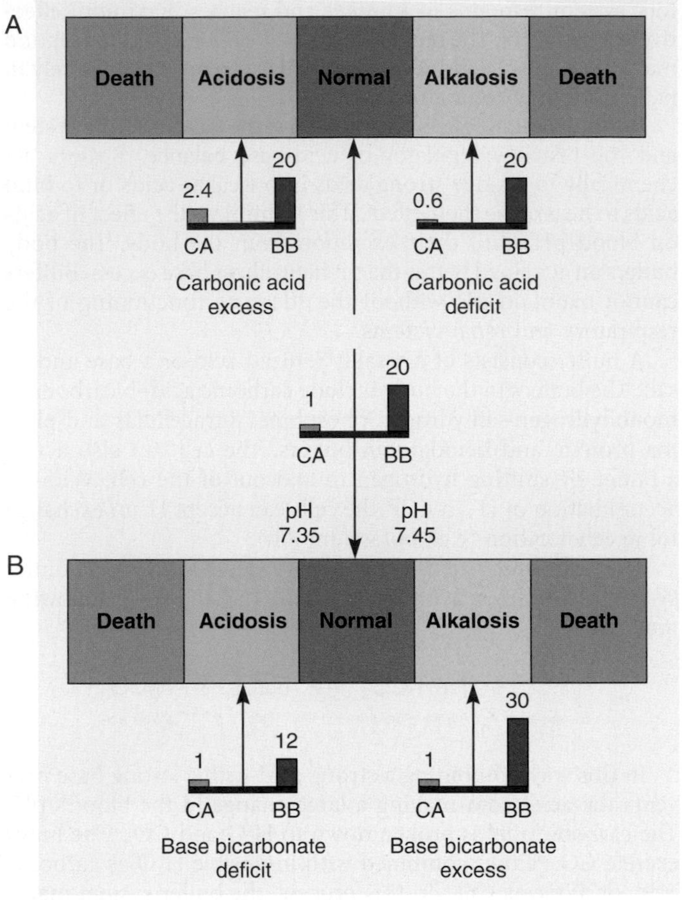

FIG. 17-17 Kinds of acid-base imbalances. **A,** Respiratory imbalances caused by carbonic acid *(CA)* excess and carbonic acid deficit. **B,** Metabolic imbalances caused by base bicarbonate *(BB)* deficit and base bicarbonate excess.

is not eliminated from the blood, acidosis results from the accumulation of carbonic acid (Fig. 17-17, *A*).

To compensate, the kidneys conserve HCO_3^- and secrete increased concentrations of H^+ into the urine. During acute respiratory acidosis, the renal compensatory mechanisms begin to operate within 24 hours. Until the renal mechanisms have an effect, the serum HCO_3^- level will usually be normal.

Respiratory Alkalosis. *Respiratory alkalosis* (carbonic acid deficit) occurs with hyperventilation (see Table 17-10). The primary cause of respiratory alkalosis is hypoxemia from acute pulmonary disorders. Anxiety, CNS disorders, and mechanical overventilation also increase the ventilation rate. The decrease in the partial pressure of arterial CO_2 ($PaCO_2$) level leads to decreased carbonic acid concentration and alkalosis (see Fig. 17-17, *A*).

Compensated respiratory alkalosis is rare. In acute respiratory alkalosis, aggressive treatment of the causes of hypoxemia is essential and usually does not allow time for compensation to occur. However, buffering of acute respiratory alkalosis may occur with shifting of HCO_3^- into cells in exchange for chloride ions (Cl^-). In chronic respiratory alkalosis that occurs with pulmonary fibrosis or CNS disorders, compensation may include renal excretion of HCO_3^-.

Metabolic Acidosis. *Metabolic acidosis* (base bicarbonate deficit) occurs when an acid other than carbonic acid accumulates in the body or when bicarbonate is lost from body fluids (see Table 17-10 and Fig. 17-17, *B*). Ketoacid accumulation in diabetic ketoacidosis and lactic acid accumulation with shock are examples of accumulation of acids. Severe diarrhea results in loss of HCO_3^-. In renal disease the kidneys lose their ability to reabsorb HCO_3^- and secrete H^+.

The compensatory response to metabolic acidosis is to increase CO_2 excretion by the lungs. The patient often develops

Kussmaul respiration (deep, rapid breathing). In addition, the kidneys attempt to excrete additional acid.

If metabolic acidosis is present, calculating the anion gap can help determine the source of the acidosis. The *anion gap* is the difference between the cations and the anions in ECF that are routinely measured. You calculate an anion gap by summing the chloride and bicarbonate levels and subtracting this number from the plasma sodium concentration. Ordinarily, the sum of the measured cations is greater than the sum of the measured anions. The anion gap is normally 10 to 14 mmol/L. The anion gap is increased in metabolic acidosis associated with acid gain (e.g., lactic acidosis, diabetic ketoacidosis) but remains normal in metabolic acidosis caused by bicarbonate loss (e.g., diarrhea).

Metabolic Alkalosis. *Metabolic alkalosis* (base bicarbonate excess) occurs when a loss of acid (e.g., from prolonged vomiting or gastric suction) or a gain in bicarbonate (e.g., from ingestion of baking soda) occurs (see Table 17-10 and Fig. 17-17, *B*). Renal excretion of bicarbonate occurs in response to metabolic alkalosis. The compensatory response to metabolic alkalosis is limited. There is a decreased respiratory rate to increase plasma CO_2. However, once plasma CO_2 reaches a certain level, stimulation of chemoreceptors results in ventilation.

Mixed Acid-Base Disorders. A mixed acid-base disorder occurs when two or more disorders are present at the same time. The pH depends on the type, severity, and acuity of each of the disorders involved and any compensatory mechanisms at work. Respiratory acidosis combined with metabolic alkalosis (e.g., a patient with chronic obstructive pulmonary disease also treated with a thiazide diuretic) may result in a near-normal pH, whereas respiratory acidosis combined with metabolic acidosis will cause a greater decrease in pH than either disorder alone. An example of a mixed acidosis is a patient in cardiopulmonary arrest. An example of a mixed alkalosis is a patient who is hyperventilating because of postoperative pain and losing acid secondary to nasogastric suctioning.

Clinical Manifestations

Clinical manifestations of acidosis and alkalosis are summarized in Tables 17-11 and 17-12. In both respiratory and metabolic acidosis, the CNS is depressed. Headache, lethargy, weakness, and confusion develop, leading eventually to coma and death. In both types of alkalosis, irritability of the CNS causes tingling and numbness of the fingers, restlessness, and tetany. If the severity of alkalosis increases, convulsions and coma may occur.[7]

The compensatory mechanisms also produce specific clinical manifestations. For example, the deep, rapid respirations of a patient with metabolic acidosis are an example of respiratory compensation. In alkalosis, hypocalcemia occurs due to increased calcium binding with albumin, lowering the amount of ionized, biologically active calcium. The hypocalcemia accounts for many of the clinical manifestations of alkalosis.

Blood Gas Values. Arterial blood gas (ABG) values provide objective information about a patient's acid-base status, the underlying cause of an imbalance, the body's ability to regulate pH, and the patient's overall O_2 status. Knowledge of the patient's clinical situation and the physiologic extent of renal and respiratory compensation enables you to identify acid-base disorders, as well as the patient's ability to compensate. Blood gas analysis also shows the partial pressure of arterial O_2 (PaO_2) and O_2 saturation. These values are used to identify hypoxemia.

TABLE 17-11 CLINICAL MANIFESTATIONS OF ACIDOSIS

Respiratory (↑ $PaCO_2$)	Metabolic (↓ HCO_3^-)
Neurologic	
Drowsiness	Drowsiness
Confusion	Confusion
Dizziness	Dizziness
Headache	Headache
Coma	Coma
Cardiovascular	
↓ BP	↓ BP
Ventricular fibrillation (related to hyperkalemia from compensation)	Dysrhythmias (related to hyperkalemia from compensation)
Warm, flushed skin (related to peripheral vasodilation)	Warm, flushed skin (related to peripheral vasodilation)
Gastrointestinal	
No significant findings	Nausea, vomiting, diarrhea, abdominal pain
Neuromuscular	
Seizures	No significant findings
Respiratory	
Hypoventilation with hypoxia (lungs are unable to compensate when there is a respiratory problem)	Deep, rapid respirations (compensatory action by the lungs)

TABLE 17-12 CLINICAL MANIFESTATIONS OF ALKALOSIS

Respiratory (↓ $PaCO_2$)	Metabolic (↑ HCO_3^-)
Neurologic	
Dizziness	Dizziness
Light-headedness	Light-headedness
Confusion	Confusion
Headache	Headache
Cardiovascular	
Tachycardia	Tachycardia
Dysrhythmias (related to hypokalemia from compensation)	Dysrhythmias (related to hypokalemia from compensation)
Gastrointestinal	
Nausea	Nausea
Vomiting	Vomiting
Epigastric pain	Anorexia
Neuromuscular	
Tetany	Tetany
Numbness	Tremors
Tingling of extremities	Tingling of fingers and toes
Hyperreflexia	Muscle cramps, hypertonic muscles
Seizures	Seizures
Respiratory	
Hyperventilation (lungs are unable to compensate when there is a respiratory problem)	Hypoventilation (compensatory action by the lungs)

To interpret the results of an ABG, perform the following six steps:

1. Determine whether the pH is acidotic or alkalotic. Label values less than 7.35 as acidotic and values greater than 7.45 as alkalotic.
2. Analyze the $PaCO_2$ to determine if the patient has respiratory acidosis or alkalosis. Since the lungs control $PaCO_2$, it is the respiratory component of the ABG. Because CO_2 forms carbonic acid when dissolved in blood, high $PaCO_2$ levels indicate acidosis, and low $PaCO_2$ levels indicate alkalosis.
3. Analyze the HCO_3^- level to determine if the patient has metabolic acidosis or alkalosis. Since the kidneys primarily control HCO_3^-, it is the metabolic component of the ABG. Because HCO_3^- is a base, high levels of HCO_3^- result in alkalosis and low levels result in acidosis.
4. At this point, if the pH is between 7.35 and 7.45, and the CO_2 and the HCO_3^- are within normal limits, the ABGs are normal.
5. Determine if the CO_2 or the HCO_3^- matches the acid or base alteration of the pH. For example, if the pH is acidotic (less than 7.35) and the CO_2 is high (respiratory acidosis) but the HCO_3^- is high (metabolic alkalosis), the CO_2 is the parameter that matches the pH alteration of acidosis. The patient's acid-base imbalance is diagnosed as respiratory acidosis.
6. Determine if the body is attempting to compensate for the pH change. If the parameter that does not match the pH is moving in the opposite direction, the body is attempting to compensate. In the example in step 5, the HCO_3^- level is alkalotic; this is in the opposite direction of respiratory acidosis and considered compensation. If compensatory mechanisms are functioning, the pH will return toward 7.40. When the pH is within normal limits, the patient has *full compensation*.

Table 17-13 lists normal blood gas values, and Table 17-14 explains how to analyze ABG results. The laboratory findings section of Table 17-10 provides ABG findings of the four major acid-base disturbances. Table 17-15 shows ROME, a quick memory device (mnemonic) for understanding acid-base imbalances. See Chapter 26 for further discussion of blood gases.

ASSESSMENT OF FLUID, ELECTROLYTE, AND ACID-BASE IMBALANCES

Assessing patients for fluid, electrolyte, and acid-base imbalances is an important part of your nursing practice. Clinical manifestations for specific imbalances are presented earlier in this chapter. In addition to assessing for those clinical manifestations, obtain subjective and objective data from any patient with suspected fluid, electrolyte, or acid-base imbalances as outlined below.

Subjective Data

Important Health Information

Past Health History. Question the patient about any past history of problems involving the kidneys, heart, GI system, or lungs that could affect the present fluid, electrolyte, and acid-base balance. Obtain information about specific diseases such as diabetes mellitus, diabetes insipidus, chronic obstructive pulmonary disease, renal failure, ulcerative colitis, and Crohn's disease. Ask the patient about any prior fluid, electrolyte, or acid-base disorders.

Medications. Assess the patient's current and past use of medications. The ingredients in many drugs, especially over-the-counter drugs, are often missed as sources of sodium, potassium, calcium, magnesium, and other electrolytes. Many prescription drugs, including diuretics, corticosteroids, and electrolyte supplements, can cause fluid and electrolyte imbalances.

Surgery or Other Treatments. Ask the patient about past or present renal dialysis, kidney surgery, or bowel surgery resulting

TABLE 17-13 NORMAL ARTERIAL BLOOD GAS VALUES*

Parameter	Reference Interval
pH	7.35-7.45
$PaCO_2$	35-45 mm Hg
Bicarbonate (HCO_3^-)	22-26 mEq/L (mmol/L)
PaO_2†	80-100 mm Hg
SaO_2	>95%
Base excess	±2.0 mEq/L

*Venous blood gas reference intervals are listed in Table 26-1.
†Decreases above sea level and with increasing age.
$PaCO_2$, Partial pressure of CO_2 in arterial blood; *PaO_2*, partial pressure of O_2 in arterial blood; *SaO_2*, arterial O_2 saturation.

TABLE 17-14 ARTERIAL BLOOD GAS (ABG) ANALYSIS

ABG Values	Analysis
pH 7.30 $PaCO_2$ 25 mm Hg HCO_3^- 16 mEq/L	1. pH <7.35 indicates acidosis. 2. $PaCO_2$ is low, indicating respiratory alkalosis. 3. HCO_3^- is low, indicating metabolic acidosis. 4. Metabolic acidosis matches the pH. 5. The CO_2 does not match, but is moving in the opposite direction, which indicates the lungs are attempting to compensate for the metabolic acidosis.

Interpretation
This ABG is interpreted as metabolic acidosis with partial compensation. If the pH returns to the normal range, the patient is said to have full compensation.

TABLE 17-15 ROME: MEMORY DEVICE FOR ACID-BASE IMBALANCES

For acid-base imbalances a quick memory device (mnemonic) can be used.

In ***Respiratory*** conditions, the pH and the $PaCO_2$ go in ***Opposite*** directions.

- In respiratory alkalosis, the pH is ↑ and the $PaCO_2$ is ↓.
- In respiratory acidosis the pH is ↓ and the $PaCO_2$ is ↑.

In ***Metabolic*** conditions, the pH and the HCO_3^- go in the same direction (equal or ***Equivalent***). The $PaCO_2$ may also go in the same direction.

- In metabolic alkalosis, pH and HCO_3^- are ↑ and the $PaCO_2$ is ↑ or normal.
- In metabolic acidosis, pH and HCO_3^- are ↓ and the $PaCO_2$ is ↓ or normal.

		pH	$PaCO_2$
Respiratory			
Opposite	Acidosis	↓	↑
	Alkalosis	↑	↓
Metabolic		**pH**	**HCO_3^-**
Equivalent	Acidosis	↓	↓
	Alkalosis	↑	↑

in a temporary or permanent external collecting system such as a colostomy.

Functional Health Patterns

Health Perception–Health Management Pattern. If the patient is currently experiencing a problem related to fluid, electrolyte, and acid-base balance, obtain a careful description of the illness, including onset, course, and treatment. Question the patient about any recent changes in body weight.

Nutritional-Metabolic Pattern. Ask the patient about diet and any special dietary practices. Weight reduction diets, fad diets, or any eating disorders, such as anorexia or bulimia, can lead to fluid and electrolyte problems. If the patient is on a special diet, such as low sodium or high potassium, assess the ability to adhere to the dietary prescription.

Elimination Pattern. Make note of the patient's usual bowel and bladder habits. Carefully document any deviations from the expected elimination pattern, such as diarrhea, oliguria, nocturia, polyuria, or incontinence.

Activity-Exercise Pattern. Inquire about the patient's exercise pattern and any complaints of excessive perspiration. Determine if the patient is exposed to extremely high temperatures as a result of leisure or work activity. Ask the patient what he or she does to replace fluid and electrolytes lost through excessive perspiration. Assess the patient's activity level to determine any functional problems that could lead to lack of ability to obtain food or fluids.

Cognitive-Perceptual Pattern. Ask about any changes in sensations, such as numbness, tingling, *fasciculations* (uncoordinated twitching of a single muscle group), or muscle weakness, that could indicate a fluid and electrolyte problem. Additionally, ask both the patient and the caregiver if there have been any changes in mentation or alertness, such as confusion, memory impairment, or lethargy.

Objective Data

Physical Examination. A complete physical examination is needed because fluid, electrolyte, and acid-base balance affects all body systems. As you assess each system, check for manifestations that you would expect with an imbalance. Common abnormal assessment findings of major body systems offer clues to possible imbalances (Table 17-16).

Laboratory Values. Assessment of serum electrolyte values is a good starting point for identifying fluid and electrolyte imbalance (see Table 17-1). However, serum electrolyte values often provide only limited information. They reflect the concentration of that electrolyte in ECF but not necessarily in ICF. For example, most of the potassium in the body is found intracellularly. Changes in serum potassium values may be the result of a true deficit or excess of potassium or may reflect the movement of potassium into or out of the cell during acid-base imbalances. An abnormal serum sodium level may reflect a sodium problem or, more likely, a water problem.

In addition to arterial and venous blood gases, serum electrolytes can provide important information about a patient's acid-base balance. Changes in the serum HCO_3^- (often reported as total CO_2 or CO_2 content on an electrolyte panel) indicate metabolic acidosis (low HCO_3^- level) or alkalosis (high HCO_3^- level).

Other laboratory tests helpful in evaluating the presence of or risk for fluid, electrolyte, and acid-base imbalances include serum and urine osmolality, serum glucose, blood urea nitrogen, serum creatinine, venous blood gas sampling, urine specific gravity, and urine electrolytes.

TABLE 17-16 ASSESSMENT ABNORMALITIES

Fluid and Electrolyte Imbalances

Finding	Possible Etiology
Skin	
Poor skin turgor	Fluid volume deficit
Cold, clammy skin	Na^+ deficit, shift of plasma to interstitial fluid
Pitting edema	Fluid volume excess
Flushed, dry skin	Na^+ excess
Pulse	
Bounding pulse	Fluid volume excess, shift of interstitial fluid to plasma
Rapid, weak, thready pulse	Shift of plasma to interstitial fluid, Na^+ deficit, fluid volume deficit
Weak, irregular, rapid pulse	Severe K^+ deficit
Weak, irregular, slow pulse	Severe K^+ excess
Blood Pressure	
Hypotension	Fluid volume deficit, shift of plasma to interstitial fluid, Na^+ deficit
Hypertension	Fluid volume excess, shift of interstitial fluid to plasma
Respirations	
Deep, rapid breathing	Compensation for metabolic acidosis
Shallow, slow, irregular breathing	Compensation for metabolic alkalosis
Shortness of breath	Fluid volume excess
Moist crackles	Fluid volume excess, shift of interstitial fluid to plasma
Restricted airway	Ca^{2+} deficit
Skeletal Muscles	
Cramping of exercised muscle	Ca^{2+} deficit, Mg^{2+} deficit, alkalosis
Carpal spasm (Trousseau's sign)	Ca^{2+} deficit, Mg^{2+} deficit, alkalosis
Flabby muscles	K^+ deficit
Positive Chvostek's sign	Ca^{2+} deficit, Mg^{2+} deficit, alkalosis
Behavior or Mental State	
Picking at bedclothes	K^+ deficit, Mg^{2+} deficit
Indifference	Fluid volume deficit, Na^+ deficit
Apprehension	Shift of plasma to interstitial fluid
Extreme restlessness	K^+ excess, Na^+ excess, fluid volume deficit
Confusion and irritability	K^+ deficit, fluid volume excess, Ca^{2+} excess, Mg^{2+} excess, H_2O excess, Na^+ deficit
Decreased level of consciousness	Na^+ deficit, H_2O excess

ORAL FLUID AND ELECTROLYTE REPLACEMENT

In all cases of fluid, electrolyte, and acid-base imbalances, the primary treatment involves correction of the underlying cause. Oral rehydration solutions containing water, potassium, sodium, and glucose may be used to correct mild fluid and electrolyte deficits. Glucose not only provides calories but also promotes sodium and water absorption in the small intestine. Commercial oral rehydration solutions are now available for home use.

Cola drinks are avoided because they do not contain adequate electrolyte replacement and the sugar content may lead to osmotic diuresis.

INTRAVENOUS FLUID AND ELECTROLYTE REPLACEMENT

IV fluid and electrolyte therapy is necessary to treat many different fluid and electrolyte imbalances. Many patients need maintenance IV fluid therapy while they cannot take oral fluids (e.g., during and after surgery). Other patients need corrective or replacement therapy for losses that have already occurred. The amount and type of solution are determined by the normal daily maintenance requirements and by imbalances identified by laboratory results. IV replacement solutions are classified by their concentration or tonicity (Table 17-17). Tonicity is an important factor in determining the appropriate solution to correct water and solute imbalances.

Solutions

Hypotonic. A hypotonic solution provides more water than electrolytes, diluting the ECF. Osmosis then produces a movement of water from ECF to ICF. After achieving osmotic equilibrium, ICF and ECF have the same osmolality and both compartments are expanded. Table 17-17 gives examples of commonly used hypotonic fluids. Maintenance fluids are usually hypotonic solutions (e.g., 0.45% NaCl) because normal daily losses are hypotonic. Additional electrolytes (e.g., KCl) may be added to maintain normal levels. Because hypotonic solutions have the potential to cause cellular swelling, monitor patients for changes in mentation that may indicate cerebral edema.[15]

Although 5% dextrose in water is considered an isotonic solution, the dextrose is quickly metabolized, and the net result is the administration of free water (hypotonic) with proportionately equal expansion of ECF and ICF. One liter of a 5% dextrose solution provides 50 g of dextrose, or 170 calories. Although this amount of dextrose is not enough to meet caloric requirements, it helps prevent ketosis associated with starvation.

Isotonic. Administration of an isotonic solution expands only ECF. There is no net loss or gain from ICF. An isotonic solution is the ideal fluid replacement for a patient with an ECF volume deficit. Examples of isotonic solutions include lactated Ringer's solution and 0.9% NaCl. Lactated Ringer's solution

TABLE 17-17 COMMONLY USED CRYSTALLOID SOLUTIONS

Solution	Tonicity	mOsm/kg	Glucose (g/L)	Indications and Considerations
Dextrose in Water				
5%	Isotonic, but physiologically hypotonic	278	50	• Provides free water necessary for renal excretion of solutes • Used to replace water losses and treat hypernatremia • Provides 170 cal/L • Does not provide any electrolytes
10%	Hypertonic	556	100	• Provides free water only, no electrolytes • Provides 340 cal/L
Saline				
0.45%	Hypotonic	154	0	• Provides free water in addition to Na^+ and Cl^- • Used to replace hypotonic fluid losses • Used as maintenance solution, although it does not replace daily losses of other electrolytes • Provides no calories
0.9%	Isotonic	308	0	• Used to expand intravascular volume and replace extracellular fluid losses • Only solution that may be administered with blood products • Contains Na^+ and Cl^- in excess of plasma levels • Does not provide free water, calories, other electrolytes • May cause intravascular overload or hyperchloremic acidosis
3.0%	Hypertonic	1026	0	• Used to treat symptomatic hyponatremia • Must be administered slowly and with extreme caution because it may cause dangerous intravascular volume overload and pulmonary edema
Dextrose in Saline				
5% in 0.225%	Isotonic	355	50	• Provides Na^+, Cl^-, and free water • Used to replace hypotonic losses and treat hypernatremia • Provides 170 cal/L
5% in 0.45%	Hypertonic	432	50	• Same as 0.45% NaCl except provides 170 cal/L
5% in 0.9%	Hypertonic	586	50	• Same as 0.9% NaCl except provides 170 cal/L
Multiple Electrolyte Solutions				
Ringer's solution	Isotonic	309	0	• Similar in composition to plasma except that it has excess Cl^-, no Mg^{2+}, and no HCO_3^- • Does not provide free water or calories • Used to expand the intravascular volume and replace extracellular fluid losses
Lactated Ringer's (Hartmann's) solution	Isotonic	274	0	• Similar in composition to normal plasma except does not contain Mg^{2+} • Used to treat losses from burns and lower GI • May be used to treat mild metabolic acidosis but should not be used to treat lactic acidosis • Does not provide free water or calories

contains sodium, potassium, chloride, calcium, and lactate (the precursor of bicarbonate) in about the same concentrations as those of ECF. It is contraindicated in patients with hyperkalemia and lactic acidosis because they have a decreased ability to convert lactate to bicarbonate.

Isotonic saline (0.9% NaCl) has a sodium concentration (154 mEq/L) somewhat higher than that of plasma (135 to 145 mEq/L) and a chloride concentration (154 mEq/L) significantly higher than the plasma chloride level (96 to 106 mEq/L). Thus excessive administration of isotonic saline can result in elevated sodium and chloride levels. Isotonic saline may be used when a patient has experienced both fluid and sodium losses or as vascular fluid replacement in hypovolemic shock.

Hypertonic. A hypertonic solution initially raises the osmolality of ECF and expands it. In addition, the higher osmotic pressure draws water out of the cells into ECF. It is useful in the treatment of hypovolemia and hyponatremia. Table 17-17 lists commonly used hypertonic solutions. Hypertonic solutions require frequent monitoring of blood pressure, lung sounds, and serum sodium levels because of the risk for intravascular fluid volume excess.[15]

Although concentrated dextrose and water solutions (10% dextrose or greater) are hypertonic solutions, once the dextrose is metabolized, the net result is the administration of water. The free water provided by these solutions ultimately expands both ECF and ICF. The primary use of these solutions is the provision of calories as part of parenteral nutrition. Parenteral nutrition is composed of concentrated dextrose solutions with amino acids, electrolytes, vitamins, and trace elements (see Chapter 40). You may administer solutions containing 10% dextrose or less through a peripheral line. However, you must use a central line to administer solutions with concentrations greater than 10% dextrose. (Central lines are discussed at right.)

Intravenous Additives. In addition to the basic solutions that provide water, electrolytes, and a minimum amount of calories, there are additives to replace specific losses. KCl, CaCl, $MgSO_4$, and HCO_3^- are common additives to the basic IV solutions. The use of these additives is mentioned previously in the discussion of the specific electrolyte deficiencies.

Plasma Expanders. Plasma expanders stay in the vascular space and increase the osmotic pressure. Plasma expanders include colloids, dextran, and hetastarch (Hespan). Colloids are protein solutions such as plasma, albumin, and commercial plasmas (e.g., Plasmanate). Albumin is available in 5% and 25% solutions. The 5% solution has an albumin concentration similar to that of plasma and results in plasma volume expansion equal to the volume infused. This makes the 5% concentration useful in treating hypovolemic patients. In contrast, 25% albumin solution is hypertonic and draws additional fluid from the interstitial space. The main use of the 25% concentration is as a volume expander following a paracentesis for ascites.[16] Dextran is a complex synthetic sugar. Because dextran metabolizes slowly, it remains in the vascular system for a prolonged period (but not as long as the colloids). It pulls additional fluid into the intravascular space. Hetastarch is a synthetic colloid that works similarly to dextran to expand plasma volume. (See Chapter 67 for a discussion of plasma volume expanders.)

If the patient has lost blood, whole blood or packed RBCs are necessary. Packed RBCs have the advantage of giving the patient primarily RBCs. Thus the blood bank can use the plasma for blood components. Although packed RBCs have a decreased plasma volume, they increase the oncotic pressure and pull fluid into the intravascular space. The use of whole blood, with its additional fluid volume, may cause circulatory overload, particularly in patients who are susceptible to complications from excess circulating volume (e.g., heart failure). To prevent manifestations of fluid volume excess, loop diuretics may be administered with blood. (See Chapter 31 for more information on the administration of blood and blood products.)

DELEGATION DECISIONS

Intravenous Therapy

Although many states permit licensed practical nurses (LPNs) to administer IV fluids and medications, administration of IV fluids or medications to unstable or critically ill patients should be done by the registered nurse (RN).

Role of Registered Nurse (RN)

- Assess patient for clinical manifestations of fluid and electrolyte disturbances.
- Determine whether ordered IV therapies are still appropriate based on monitoring of patient hydration and electrolyte levels.
- Choose and insert appropriate IV catheters and infusion devices.
- Administer IV fluids and medications to unstable and critically ill patients.
- Evaluate patient for clinical manifestations of fluid overload or hypovolemia and initiate appropriate changes in IV fluids.
- Evaluate whether patient fluid and electrolyte needs are being addressed with IV therapies.

Role of Licensed Practical/Vocational Nurse (LPN/LVN)

- Administer IV fluids and medications to stable patients (consider state nurse practice act and agency policy).
- Adjust IV flow rate for stable patients according to health care provider orders (consider state nurse practice act and agency policy).
- Insert IV catheters (consider state nurse practice act and agency policy).
- Monitor for clinical manifestations of adverse reactions to IV fluids or medications.

Role of Unlicensed Assistive Personnel (UAP)

- Measure and record oral intake and output.
- Report swelling or redness at IV site or patient complaints of discomfort at IV site to RN.

CENTRAL VENOUS ACCESS DEVICES

Central venous access devices (CVADs) are catheters placed in large blood vessels (e.g., subclavian vein, jugular vein) of people who require frequent or special access to the vascular system. There are three main types of CVADs: centrally inserted catheters, peripherally inserted central catheters (PICCs), and implanted ports. A physician may place any of these devices; a nurse with specialized training can insert PICCs.

Advantages of CVADs include immediate access to the central venous system, a reduced need for multiple venipunctures, and decreased risk of extravasation injury. CVADs permit frequent, continuous, rapid, or intermittent administration of fluids and medications. They allow for the administration of drugs that are potential vesicants, blood and blood products, and parenteral nutrition. CVADs can provide a means to perform hemodynamic monitoring and obtain venous blood samples. They are useful with patients who have limited peripheral vascular access or who have a projected need for long-term vascular access. Table 17-18 provides examples of conditions where CVADs are used.

TABLE 17-18 **INDICATIONS FOR CENTRAL VENOUS ACCESS DEVICE (CVAD)***

Medical Condition	Indications for Use
Medication administration	
• Cancer	• Chemotherapy, infusion of irritating or vesicant medications
• Infection	• Long-term administration of antibiotics
• Pain	• Long-term administration of pain medication
• Drugs at risk for causing phlebitis	• epoprostenol (Flolan) • calcium chloride • potassium chloride • amiodarone (Cordarone)
Nutritional replacement	• Infusion of parenteral nutrition • Able to infuse higher dextrose solutions through CVAD than peripheral line
Blood samples	• Multiple blood draws for diagnostic tests over time
Blood transfusions	• Infusion of blood or blood products
Renal failure	• Perform hemodialysis (especially on an acute basis) or continuous renal replacement therapy
Shock, burns	• Infusion of high volumes of fluid and electrolyte replacement
Hemodynamic monitoring	• Used to measure central venous pressure to assess fluid balance
Heart failure	• Perform ultrafiltration
Autoimmune disorders	• Perform plasmapheresis

*This list is not all-inclusive, and these are examples only.

Specifically indicated CVADs are safe for injections of radiopaque contrast media at high pressures and controlled rates. For patients who already have poor peripheral venous access, using the port to inject contrast media decreases discomfort from venipuncture and helps lower the risk for extravasation of vesicant contrast media.[17]

The major disadvantages of CVADs are an increased risk of systemic infection and the invasiveness of the procedure. Extravasation can still occur if there is displacement of or damage to the device.

Centrally Inserted Catheters

Centrally inserted catheters (also called central venous catheters [CVCs]) are inserted into a vein in the neck or chest (subclavian or jugular) or groin (femoral) with the tip resting in the distal end of the superior vena cava (Fig. 17-18). The other end of the catheter is either nontunneled or tunneled through subcutaneous tissue and exits through a separate incision on the chest or abdominal wall. A Dacron cuff serves to stabilize the catheter and may decrease the incidence of infection by impeding bacteria migration along the catheter beyond the cuff. Do not use a newly place CVAD until the tip position is verified with a chest x-ray.

These catheters are single-, double-, triple-, or quad-lumen catheters. Multi-lumen catheters are useful in the critically ill patient because all of the lumens can provide a different therapy simultaneously. For example, incompatible drugs infuse in separate lumens without mixing while a third lumen provides access for blood sampling. Specific types of long-term central

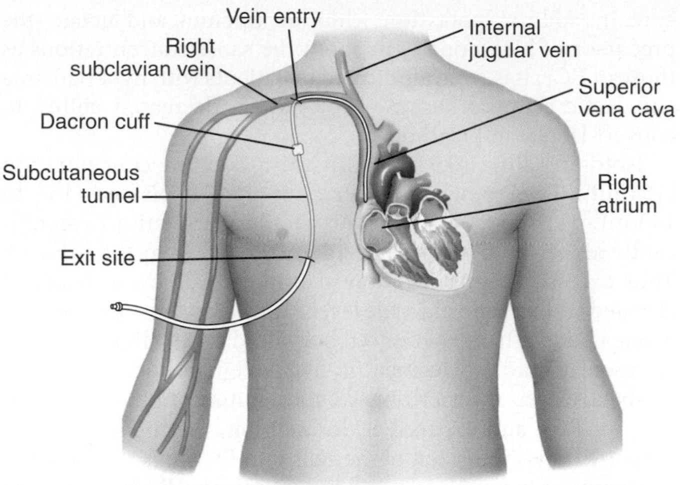

FIG. 17-18 Tunneled central venous catheter. Note tip of the catheter in the superior vena cava.

catheters are Hickman catheters, which require clamps to make sure the valve is closed, and Groshong catheters, which have a valve that opens as fluid is withdrawn or infused and remains closed when not in use.

Peripherally Inserted Central Catheters

PICCs are central venous catheters inserted into a vein in the arm rather than a vein in the neck or chest. They are inserted at or just above the antecubital fossa (usually cephalic or basilic vein) and advanced to a position with the tip ending in the distal one third of the superior vena cava. PICCs are single- or multiple-lumen, are nontunneled, and are up to 60 cm in length with gauges ranging from 24 to 16 (Fig. 17-19). They are used with patients who need vascular access for 1 week to 6 months but can be in place for longer periods.

Advantages of the PICC over a central venous catheter are lower infection rate, fewer insertion-related complications, decreased cost, and insertion at the bedside or outpatient area. Complications of PICCs include catheter occlusion and phlebitis (Table 17-19). If phlebitis occurs, it usually appears within 7 to 10 days after insertion. Do not use the arm with the PICC to obtain a blood pressure reading or draw blood.

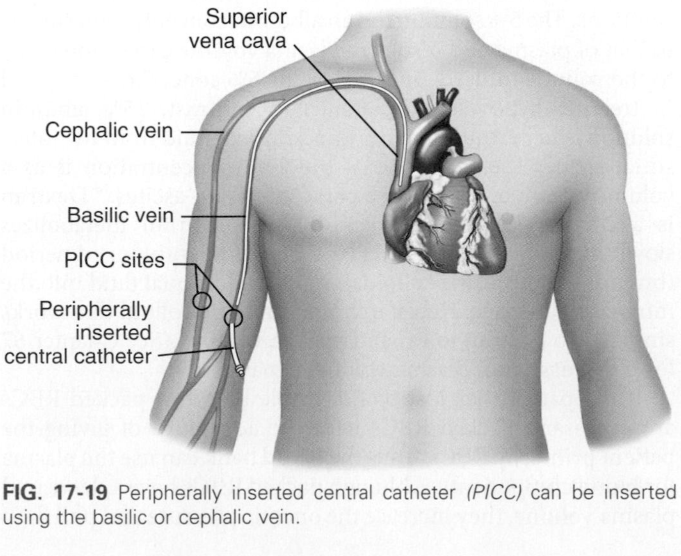

FIG. 17-19 Peripherally inserted central catheter *(PICC)* can be inserted using the basilic or cephalic vein.

TABLE 17-19 COMPLICATIONS OF CENTRAL VENOUS ACCESS DEVICES (CVADs)

Possible Cause	Clinical Manifestations	Management
Catheter Occlusion		
• Clamped or kinked catheter • Tip against wall of vessel • Thrombosis • Precipitate buildup in lumen	• Sluggish infusion or aspiration • Inability to infuse and/or aspirate	• Instruct patient to change position, raise arm, and cough. • Assess for and alleviate clamping or kinking. • Flush with normal saline using a 10-mL syringe. Do not force flush. • Perform fluoroscopy to determine cause and site. • Administer anticoagulant or thrombolytic agents.
Embolism		
• Catheter breaking • Dislodgment of thrombus • Entry of air into circulation	• Chest pain • Respiratory distress (dyspnea, tachypnea, hypoxia, cyanosis) • Hypotension • Tachycardia	• Administer O_2. • Clamp catheter. • Place patient on left side with head down (air emboli). • Notify physician.
Catheter-Related Infection (local or systemic)		
• Contamination during insertion or use • Migration of organisms along catheter • Immunosuppressed patient	• *Local:* redness, tenderness, purulent drainage, warmth, edema • *Systemic:* fever, chills, malaise	***Local*** • Culture drainage from site. • Apply warm, moist compresses. • Remove catheter if indicated. ***Systemic*** • Take blood cultures. • Give antibiotic therapy. • Give antipyretic therapy. • Remove catheter if indicated.
Pneumothorax		
• Perforation of visceral pleura during insertion	• Decreased or absent breath sounds • Respiratory distress (cyanosis, dyspnea, tachypnea) • Chest pain • Distended unilateral chest	• Administer O_2. • Position in semi-Fowler's position. • Prepare for chest tube insertion.
Catheter Migration		
• Improper suturing • Insertion site trauma • Changes in intrathoracic pressure • Forceful catheter flushing • Spontaneous	• Sluggish infusion or aspiration • Edema of chest or neck during infusion • Patient complaint of gurgling sound in ear • Dysrhythmias • Increased external catheter length	• Perform fluoroscopy to verify position. • Assist with removal and new CVAD placement.

Implanted Infusion Ports

Implanted infusion ports consist of a central venous catheter connected to an implanted, single or double subcutaneous injection port (Fig. 17-20, *A*). The catheter tip lies in the desired vein, and the other end is connected to a port that is surgically implanted in a subcutaneous pocket on the chest wall. The port consists of a metal sheath with a self-sealing silicone septum. To access these devices, a special Huber-point needle with a deflected tip is used to prevent damage to the rubber septum that could make the port useless (Fig. 17-20, *B*). Huber-point needles are also available with the tip at a 90-degree angle for longer infusions.

Drugs are placed in the port's reservoir either by a direct injection or through injection into an established IV line. After being filled, the reservoir slowly releases the medicine into the bloodstream. Implanted ports are good for long-term therapy and have a low risk of infection. The hidden port offers the patient cosmetic advantages and overall has less maintenance than other types of CVADs. Regular flushing is required to avoid the formation of "sludge" (clotted blood and drug precipitate) within the port septum.

Complications

CVADs always have a potential for complications. Astute monitoring and assessment may assist in early identification of potential complications. Table 17-19 lists common possible complications, potential causes, clinical manifestations, and interventions.

NURSING MANAGEMENT CENTRAL VENOUS ACCESS DEVICES

Nursing management of CVADs includes assessment, dressing changes and cleansing, injection cap changes, and maintenance of catheter patency. The exact frequency and procedures for these requirements vary by type of CVAD and institution, so it is important to follow your specific institution's policies and procedures. The following section discusses some general guidelines.

Catheter and insertion site assessment includes inspection of the site for redness, edema, warmth, drainage, and tenderness or pain. Observation of the catheter for misplacement or slippage is important. Perform a comprehensive pain assessment,

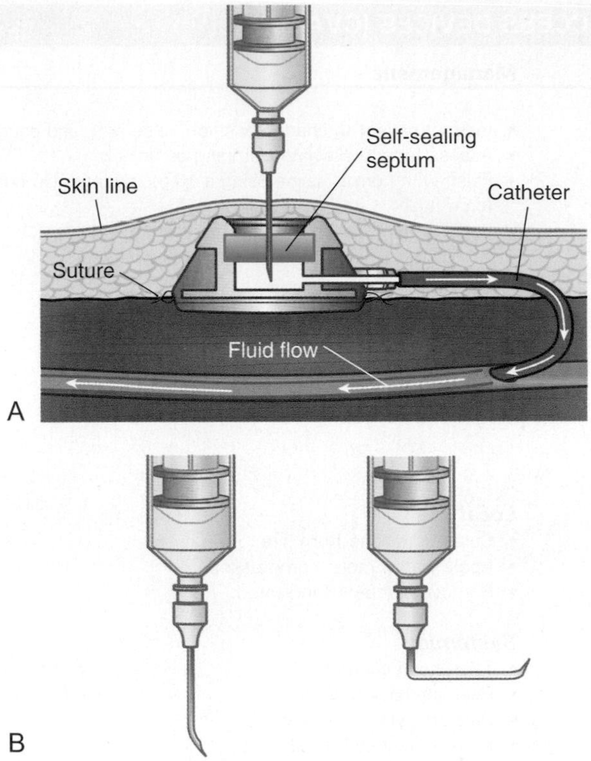

FIG. 17-20 A, Cross section of implantable port displaying access of the port with the Huber-point needle. Note the deflected point of the Huber-point needle, which prevents coring of the port's septum. **B,** Two Huber-point needles used to enter the implanted port. The 90-degree needle is used for top-entry ports for continuous infusion.

particularly noting any complaints of chest or neck discomfort, arm pain, or pain at the insertion site.[17] Before manipulating a catheter for any reason, perform hand hygiene.

Perform dressing changes and cleanse the catheter insertion site using strict sterile technique. Typical dressings include transparent semipermeable dressings or gauze and tape. If the site is bleeding, a gauze dressing may be preferable. Otherwise, transparent dressings are preferred. They allow observation of the site without having to remove the dressing. Transparent dressings may be left in place for up to 1 week if clean, dry, and intact. Change any dressing immediately if it becomes damp, loose, or visibly soiled.

Cleanse the skin around the catheter insertion site according to institution policy. A chlorhexidine-based preparation is the cleansing agent of choice. Its effects last longer than either povidone-iodine or isopropyl alcohol, offering improved killing of bacteria. When using chlorhexidine, cleansing the skin with friction is critical to infection prevention. When applying a new dressing, allow the area to air dry completely before application for chlorhexidine to be effective.[18] Secure the lumen ports to the skin above the dressing site. Document the date and time of the dressing change and initial the dressing.

Change injection caps at regular intervals according to institution policy or if they are damaged from excessive punctures. Use strict sterile technique. Teach the patient to turn the head to the opposite side of the CVAD insertion site during cap change. If the catheter cannot be clamped, instruct the patient to lie flat in bed and perform the Valsalva maneuver whenever the catheter is open to air to prevent an air embolism.

Flushing is one of the most effective ways to maintain lumen patency and to prevent occlusion of the CVAD.[19] It also keeps incompatible drugs or fluids from mixing. Use a normal saline solution in a syringe that has a barrel capacity of 10 mL or more to avoid excess pressure on the catheter. If you feel resistance, do not apply force. This could result in a ruptured catheter or create an embolism if a thrombus is present. Because of the risk of contamination and infection, prefilled syringes or single-dose vials are preferred over multiple-dose vials. If you are not using a positive-pressure valve cap, clamp any unused lines after flushing.

Use the push-pause technique when flushing all catheters. Push-pause creates turbulence within the catheter lumen, promoting the removal of debris that adheres to the catheter lumen and decreasing the chance of occlusion. This technique involves injecting saline with a rapid alternating push-pause motion, instilling 1 to 2 mL with each push on the syringe plunger. If you are using a negative-pressure cap or neutral pressure cap, clamp the catheter while maintaining positive pressure while instilling the last 1mL of saline in order to prevent reflux of blood back into the catheter. If a positive-pressure valve cap is present, it works to prevent the reflux of blood and resultant catheter lumen occlusion. Remove the syringe before clamping the catheter to allow the positive pressure valve to work correctly. Clamping the catheter during flushing with this cap may actually promote blood reflux.[19]

REMOVAL OF CVADs

Removal of CVADs is done according to institution policy and the nurse's scope of practice. In many agencies, nurses with demonstrated competency can remove PICCs and nontunneled central venous catheters. The procedure involves removing any sutures and then gently withdrawing the catheter. Instruct the patient to perform the Valsalva maneuver as the last 5 to 10 cm of the catheter is withdrawn. Immediately apply pressure to the site with sterile gauze to prevent air from entering and to control bleeding. Inspect the catheter tip to determine that it is intact. After bleeding has stopped, apply an antiseptic ointment and sterile dressing to the site.

CASE STUDY

Fluid and Electrolyte Imbalance

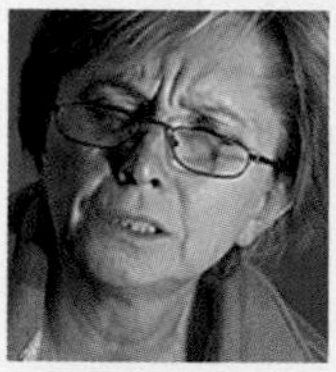

iStockphoto/Thinkstock

Patient Profile

S.S., a 63-year-old white woman with lung cancer, has been receiving chemotherapy on an outpatient basis. She completed her third treatment 5 days ago and has been experiencing nausea and vomiting for 2 days even though she has been using ondansetron (Zofran). S.S.'s daughter brings her to the hospital, where she is admitted to the medical unit. As the admitting nurse, you perform a thorough assessment.

Subjective Data

- Complains of lethargy, weakness, dizziness, and dry mouth
- States she has been too nauseated to eat or drink anything for 2 days

Objective Data

- Heart rate 110 beats/min, pulse thready
- BP 100/65
- Weight loss of 5 lb since she received her chemotherapy treatment 5 days ago
- Dry oral mucous membranes

Discussion Questions

1. Based on her clinical manifestations, what fluid imbalance does S.S. have?
2. What additional assessment data should you obtain?
3. What are her risk factors for fluid and electrolyte imbalances?
4. You draw blood for a serum chemistry evaluation. What electrolyte imbalances are likely and why?
5. S.S. is at risk for which acid-base imbalance? Describe the changes that would occur in S.S.'s ABGs with this acid-base imbalance. How would the body compensate?
6. The physician orders dextrose 5% in 0.45% saline to infuse at 100 mL/hr. What type of solution is this, and how will it help S.S.'s fluid imbalance?
7. ***Priority Decision:*** What are the priority nursing interventions for S.S.?
8. ***Evidence-Based Practice:*** S.S. has a double-lumen PICC in her left arm. One lumen is connected to the IV infusion; the other is unused. What is the recommended practice for maintaining the patency of the unused lumen?

evolve Answers available at *http://evolve.elsevier.com/Lewis/medsurg.*

BRIDGE TO NCLEX EXAMINATION

The number of the question corresponds to the same-numbered outcome at the beginning of the chapter.

1. During the postoperative care of a 76-year-old patient, the nurse monitors the patient's intake and output carefully, knowing that the patient is at risk for fluid and electrolyte imbalances primarily because
   a. older adults have an impaired thirst mechanism and need reminding to drink fluids.
   b. water accounts for a greater percentage of body weight in the older adult than in younger adults.
   c. older adults are more likely than younger adults to lose extracellular fluid during surgical procedures.
   d. small losses of fluid are more significant because body fluids account for only about 50% of body weight in older adults.
2. During administration of a hypertonic IV solution, the mechanism involved in equalizing the fluid concentration between ECF and the cells is
   a. osmosis.
   b. diffusion.
   c. active transport.
   d. facilitated diffusion.

3a. An older woman was admitted to the medical unit with dehydration. Clinical indications of this problem are *(select all that apply)*
   a. weight loss.
   b. dry oral mucosa.
   c. full bounding pulse.
   d. engorged neck veins.
   e. decreased central venous pressure.

3b. The nursing care for a patient with hyponatremia includes
   a. fluid restriction.
   b. administration of hypotonic IV fluids.
   c. administration of a cation-exchange resin.
   d. increased water intake for patients on nasogastric suction.

3c. The nurse should be alert for which manifestations in a patient receiving a loop diuretic?
   a. Restlessness and agitation
   b. Paresthesias and irritability
   c. Weak, irregular pulse and poor muscle tone
   d. Increased blood pressure and muscle spasms

3d. Which patient would be at greatest risk for the potential development of hypermagnesemia?
   a. 83-year-old man with lung cancer and hypertension
   b. 65-year-old woman with hypertension taking β-adrenergic blockers
   c. 42-year-old woman with systemic lupus erythematosus and renal failure
   d. 50-year-old man with benign prostatic hyperplasia and a urinary tract infection

3e. It is especially important for the nurse to assess for which clinical manifestation(s) in a patient who has just undergone a total thyroidectomy *(select all that apply)?*
   a. Confusion
   b. Weight gain
   c. Depressed reflexes
   d. Circumoral numbness
   e. Positive Chvostek's sign

3f. The nurse anticipates that treatment of the patient with hyperphosphatemia secondary to renal failure will include
   a. fluid restriction.
   b. calcium supplements.
   c. loop diuretic therapy.
   d. magnesium supplements.

4. The lungs act as an acid-base buffer by
   a. increasing respiratory rate and depth when CO_2 levels in the blood are high, reducing acid load.
   b. increasing respiratory rate and depth when CO_2 levels in the blood are low, reducing base load.
   c. decreasing respiratory rate and depth when CO_2 levels in the blood are high, reducing acid load.
   d. decreasing respiratory rate and depth when CO_2 levels in the blood are low, increasing acid load.
5. A patient has the following arterial blood gas results: pH 7.52; $PaCO_2$ 30 mm Hg; HCO_3^- 24 mEq/L. The nurse determines that these results indicate
   a. metabolic acidosis.
   b. metabolic alkalosis.
   c. respiratory acidosis.
   d. respiratory alkalosis.
6. The typical fluid replacement for the patient with a fluid volume deficit is
   a. dextran.
   b. 0.45% saline.
   c. lactated Ringer's.
   d. 5% dextrose in 0.45% saline.
7. The nurse is unable to flush a central venous access device and suspects occlusion. The best nursing intervention would be to
   a. apply warm moist compresses to the insertion site.
   b. attempt to force 10 mL of normal saline into the device.
   c. place the patient on the left side with head-down position.
   d. instruct the patient to change positions, raise arm, and cough.

1. d, 2. a, 3a. a, b, e, 3b. a, 3c. c, 3d. c, 3e. a, d, e, 3f. b, 4. a, 5. d, 6. c, 7. d

evolve

For rationales to these answers and even more NCLEX review questions, visit *http://evolve.elsevier.com/Lewis/medsurg.*

REFERENCES

1. Huether SE, McCance KL: *Understanding pathophysiology*, ed 5, St Louis, 2012, Mosby.
2. McCance K, Huether SE: *Pathophysiology: the biologic basis for disease in adults and children*, ed 6, St Louis, 2010, Mosby.
3. Herlihy B: *The human body in health and illness*, ed 5, St Louis, 2011, Saunders.
4. Touhy TA, Jett KF: *Gerontologic nursing and healthy aging*, ed 3, St Louis, 2010, Mosby.
5. Fillit H, Rockwood K, Woodhouse K, et al: *Brocklehurst's textbook of geriatric medicine and gerontology*, ed 7, St Louis, 2010, Mosby.
6. Rothrock J: *Alexander's care of the patient in surgery*, ed 14, St Louis, 2011, Mosby.
*7. Yee AH, Rabinstein AA: Neurologic presentations of acid-base imbalance, electrolyte abnormalities and endocrine emergencies, *Neurol Clin* 28:1, 2010.
8. Crawford A, Harris H: Balancing act: sodium and potassium, *Nursing* 41:44, 2011.
*9. Cyr PL, Slawsky KA, Olchanski N, et al: Effect of serum sodium concentration and tolvatapan treatment on length of hospitalization in patients with heart failure, *Am J Health System Pharm* 68:328, 2011.
10. Lehnhardt A, Kemper MJ: Pathogenesis, diagnosis and management of hyperkalemia, *Pediatr Nephrol* 26:377, 2011.
11. Gahart BL, Nazareno AR: *Intravenous medications*, ed 27, St Louis, 2011, Mosby.
12. Lewis MA, Hendrickson AW, Moynihan TJ: Oncologic emergencies, *CA-Cancer J Clin* 61:287, 2011.
*13. Geerse DA, Bindels AJ, Kuiper MA, et al: Treatment of hypophosphatemia in the intensive care unit: a review, *Crit Care* 14:147, 2010.
14. Crawford A, Harris H: Balancing act: hypermagnesemia and hypomagnesemia, *Nursing* 41:52, 2011.
15. Bope ET, Kellerman RD: *Conn's current therapy 2012*, St Louis, 2012, Saunders.
*16. Nieme TT, Miyashita R, Yamakage M: Colloid solutions: a clinical update, *J Anesth* 24:913, 2010.
*17. Earhart A, McMahon P: Vascular access and media, *J Infusion Nurs* 34:97, 2011.
18. Eisenberg S: Accessing implanted ports, *Clin J Oncol Nurs* 15:324, 2011.
19. Mathers D: Evidence-based practice: improving outcomes for patients with a central venous access device, *JAVA* 16:64, 2011.

*Evidence-based information for clinical practice.

RESOURCE

Infusion Nurses Society
www.ins1.org

CASE STUDY

Managing Multiple Patients

You are assigned to care for the following three patients in the intensive care unit (ICU). There are two other RNs and two unlicensed assistive personnel (UAP) on duty to care for a total of 12 patients currently in the unit.

Patients

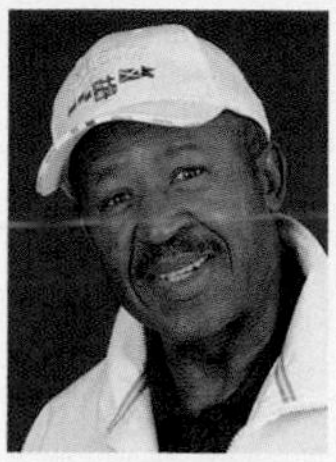

iStockphoto/Thinkstock

G.N., a 58-year-old African American man, was admitted to the ICU after falling out of a tree onto a lit gas grill. He has partial-thickness burns on his face, neck, and upper trunk. He has undergone surgical repair of right tibia and left hip fractures as well as debridement of a severely lacerated right leg. His voice is slightly hoarse and he is coughing up sooty sputum. He is receiving O_2 at 4 L/min via nasal cannula and his O_2 saturation is 93%. His WBC count is 26,400/μL (26.4×10^9/L) with 80% neutrophils (10% bands).

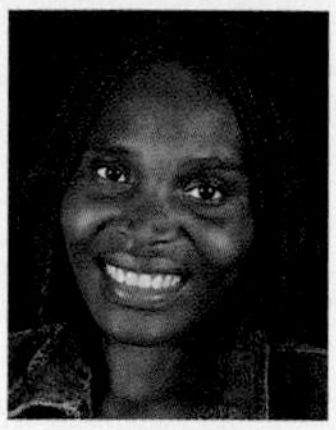

iStockphoto/Thinkstock

J.N., a 35-year-old African American woman, was transferred to the ICU from the clinical unit last evening with acute respiratory failure. She was diagnosed 2 days ago with AIDS and *Pneumocystis jiroveci* pneumonia (PCP). Prior to this hospital admission she had consistently refused antiretroviral therapy (ART) because she could not afford it. She was started on oral trimethoprim/sulfamethoxazole (Bactrim) and combination antiretroviral therapy. However, her respiratory distress worsened and she was transferred to the ICU for intubation and mechanical ventilation. She is started on IV Bactrim and corticosteroid therapy.

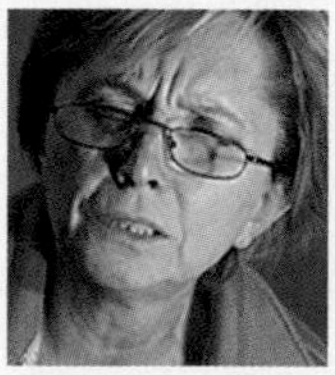

iStockphoto/Thinkstock

S.S., a 63-year-old white woman with lung cancer, has been receiving chemotherapy on an outpatient basis. She completed her third treatment 5 days ago and has been experiencing nausea and vomiting for 2 days even though she has been using ondansetron (Zofran). She was initially admitted to the medical unit but was transferred to the ICU for closer monitoring after becoming severely hypotensive overnight. Her most recent blood pressure was 98/50.

Management Discussion Questions

1. ***Priority Decision:*** After receiving report, which patient should you see first? Provide rationale.
2. ***Delegation Decision:*** Which of the following morning tasks should you delegate to the UAP *(select all that apply)?*
   a. Take blood pressure readings on S.S.
   b. Perform neurovascular checks on G.N.
   c. Document strict intake and output on S.S.
   d. Provide oral care around the endotracheal tube for J.N.
   e. Titrate S.S.'s IV infusion rate based on her blood pressure reading.
3. ***Priority and Delegation Decision:*** When you enter J.N.'s room, the ventilator alarms are going off. The UAP had just finished providing oral care and she tells you that J.N. has become increasingly agitated within the last 5 minutes. Which initial action would be most appropriate?
   a. Suction J.N.'s endotracheal tube.
   b. Have the UAP stay with J.N. while you obtain IV sedation for her.
   c. Ask the UAP to describe exactly what she did when she was performing oral care.
   d. Assess the ventilator to identify what alarm is going off and to make sure all connections are secure.

Case Study Progression

J.N.'s ventilator tubing had become disconnected. You quickly reconnect her tubing and she settles down as her oxygenation improves. You ask the UAP to obtain vital signs on all your patients while you begin a more thorough assessment of J.N.

4. During your assessment of J.N., you note grey-white patches on the inside of her mouth. You recognize these as most likely caused by
   a. *Candida albicans.*
   b. poor oral hygiene.
   c. *Coccidioides immitis.*
   d. irritation from recent mouth care.
5. G.N.'s family asks you why surgery was performed on his leg wound. Your response is based on the knowledge that debridement *(select all that apply)*
   a. is used to remove infected tissue.
   b. is used to remove nonviable tissue.
   c. prepares the wound bed for healing.
   d. can only be accomplished with surgery.
6. S.S.'s morning laboratory results reveal a serum potassium level of 2.8 mEq/L. You notify the health care provider and obtain an order for IV potassium. During infusion of the potassium aliquots, you prioritize assessment of S.S.'s
   a. bowel function.
   b. cardiac rhythm.
   c. muscle strength.
   d. level of consciousness.
7. ***Management Decision:*** While sitting at the computer charting your patients' morning assessments, you overhear the UAP telling a nursing student that J.N. deserves what she got because HIV is God's way of punishing those who sin. Your most appropriate response would be to
   a. report the UAP's actions to your supervisor.
   b. ask the UAP to keep her opinions to herself.
   c. ignore the conversation as it does not impact patient care.
   d. talk to the UAP and student about keeping personal feelings separate from patient care.

evolve Answers available at *http://evolve.elsevier.com/Lewis/medsurg.*

SECTION 3

Perioperative Care

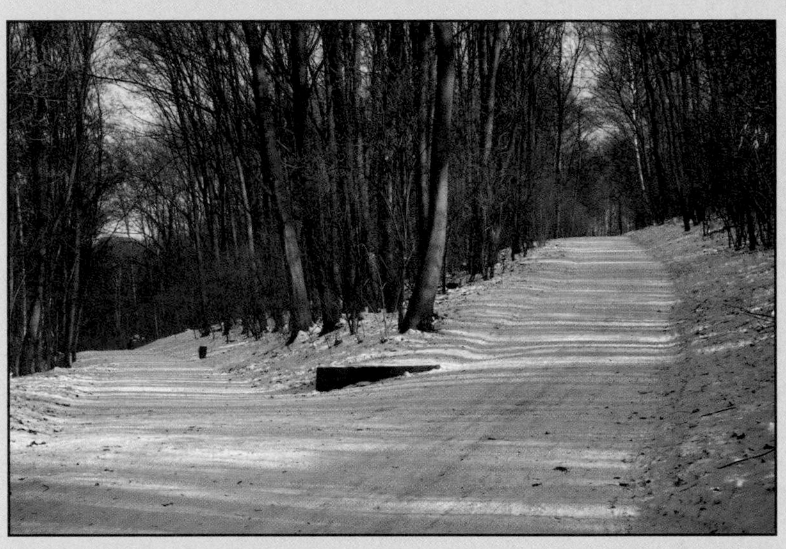

iStockphoto/Thinkstock

Two roads diverged in a wood, and I—I took the one less traveled by, and that has made all the difference.
Robert Frost

CHAPTER 18

The very first requirement in a hospital is that it should do the sick no harm.
Florence Nightingale

Nursing Management
Preoperative Care

Janice Neil

evolve WEBSITE

http://evolve.elsevier.com/Lewis/medsurg

- NCLEX Review Questions
- Key Points
- Pre-Test
- Answer Guidelines for Case Study on p. 330
- Rationales for Bridge to NCLEX Examination Questions
- Concept Map Creator
- Glossary
- Content Updates

LEARNING OUTCOMES

1. Differentiate the common purposes and settings of surgery.
2. Apply knowledge of the purpose and components of a preoperative nursing assessment.
3. Interpret the significance of data related to the preoperative patient's health status and operative risk.
4. Analyze the components and purpose of informed consent for surgery.
5. Examine the nursing role in the physical, psychologic, and educational preparation of the surgical patient.
6. Prioritize the nursing responsibilities related to day-of-surgery preparation for the surgical patient.
7. Differentiate the purposes and types of common preoperative medications.
8. Apply knowledge of the special considerations of preoperative preparation for the older adult surgical patient.

KEY TERMS

ambulatory surgery, p. 318
elective surgery, p. 318
emergency surgery, p. 318
informed consent, p. 325
same-day admission, p. 318
surgery, p. 317

Preparation of patients for surgery is an important nursing role. This chapter includes a discussion of preoperative care that is applicable to all surgical patients regardless of where the surgery is performed. Preparation measures for specific surgical procedures (e.g., abdominal, thoracic, or orthopedic surgery) are discussed in appropriate chapters of this text.

Surgery is the art and science of treating diseases, injuries, and deformities by operation and instrumentation. The surgical experience involves a multidisciplinary interaction among the patient, surgeon, anesthesia care provider (ACP), nurse, and other health care team members as needed. Surgery may be performed for any of the following purposes:

- *Diagnosis:* Determination of the presence and extent of a pathologic condition (e.g., lymph node biopsy, bronchoscopy).
- *Cure:* Elimination or repair of a pathologic condition (e.g., removal of ruptured appendix or benign ovarian cyst).
- *Palliation:* Alleviation of symptoms without cure (e.g., cutting a nerve root [rhizotomy] to remove symptoms of pain, creating a colostomy to bypass an inoperable bowel obstruction).
- *Prevention* (e.g., removal of a mole before it becomes malignant, removal of the colon in a patient with familial polyposis to prevent cancer).
- *Cosmetic improvement* (e.g., repairing a burn scar, breast reconstruction after a mastectomy).
- *Exploration:* Surgical examination to determine the nature or extent of a disease (e.g., laparotomy). With the advent of advanced diagnostic tests, exploration is less common because problems can be identified earlier and easier.

Reviewed by Lisa Kiper, RN, MSN, Assistant Professor of Nursing, Morehead State University, Morehead, Kentucky; Margaret Ochab-Ohryn, RN, MS, MBA, CRNA, Associate Professor, Oakland Community College, Farmington Hills, Michigan; and Cynthia Schoonover, RN, MS, CCRN, Associate Nursing Professor, Sinclair Community College, Dayton, Ohio and PACU Staff Nurse, Kettering Medical Center, Kettering, Ohio.

TABLE 18-1 SUFFIXES DESCRIBING SURGICAL PROCEDURES

Suffix	Meaning	Example
-ectomy	Excision or removal of	Appendectomy
-lysis	Destruction of	Electrolysis
-orrhaphy	Repair or suture of	Herniorrhaphy
-oscopy	Looking into	Endoscopy
-ostomy	Creation of opening into	Colostomy
-otomy	Cutting into or incision of	Tracheotomy
-plasty	Repair or reconstruction of	Mammoplasty

Specific suffixes are commonly used in combination with a body part or organ in naming surgical procedures (Table 18-1).

SURGICAL SETTINGS

Surgery may be a carefully planned event (**elective surgery**) or may arise with unexpected urgency (**emergency surgery**). Both elective and emergency surgery may be performed in a variety of settings. The setting in which a surgical procedure may be safely and effectively performed is influenced by the type of surgery, potential complications, and the patient's general health status.

For inpatient surgery, patients who are going to be admitted to the hospital are usually admitted on the day of surgery (**same-day admission**). Patients who are in the hospital before surgery are usually there because of acute or chronic medical conditions.

The majority of surgical procedures are performed as **ambulatory surgery** (also called *same-day* or *outpatient surgery*). Many of these surgeries use minimally invasive techniques (e.g., laparoscopic techniques). (The surgeries are described in chapters throughout the text in discussions of interventions for specific problems.) Ambulatory surgery may be conducted in endoscopy clinics, physicians' offices, freestanding surgical clinics, and outpatient surgery units in hospitals. These procedures can be performed using general, regional, or local anesthetic; have an operating time of less than 2 hours; and require less than a 24-hour stay postoperatively. Many patients go home with a caregiver within hours of surgery.

Ambulatory surgery is often preferred by patients and physicians. Generally, it involves minimal laboratory tests, requires fewer preoperative and postoperative medications, and reduces the patient's risk for health care–associated infections. Patients like the convenience of recovering at home, physicians prefer the flexibility in scheduling, and the cost is usually less for both the patient and the insurer.

Regardless of where the surgery is performed, you play an essential role in preparing the patient for surgery, caring for the patient during surgery, and facilitating the patient's recovery after surgery. To perform these functions effectively, first know the nature of the disorder requiring surgery and any coexisting medical problems. Second, identify the individual patient's response to the stress of surgery. Third, know the results of appropriate preoperative diagnostic tests. Finally, identify potential risks and complications associated with the surgical procedure and any coexisting medical problems that should be included in the plan of care. The nurse caring for the patient preoperatively is likely to be different from the nurse in the operating room (OR), postanesthesia care unit (PACU), surgical intensive care unit (SICU), or surgical unit. Thus communication and documentation of important preoperative assessment findings are essential for the continuity of care.

PATIENT INTERVIEW

One of the most important nursing actions is the preoperative interview. The nurse who works in the physician's office, the ambulatory surgery center, or the hospital preoperative area may do the interview. The site of the interview and the time before surgery dictate the depth and completeness of the interview. Important findings must be documented and communicated to others to maintain continuity of care.

The preoperative interview can occur in advance or on the day of surgery. The primary purposes of the patient interview are to (1) obtain the patient's health information; (2) provide and clarify information about the planned surgery, including anesthesia; and (3) assess the patient's emotional state and readiness for surgery, including his or her expectations about the surgical outcomes. Ensure that the patient's consent form for surgery has been signed and witnessed and that the appropriate laboratory and diagnostic tests have been ordered or completed.

The interview also provides the patient and the caregiver an opportunity to ask questions about surgery, anesthesia, and postoperative care. Often patients ask about taking their routine medications, such as insulin, anticoagulants, or cardiac medications, and if they will experience pain. By being aware of the patient's and caregiver's needs, you can provide the information and support needed during the perioperative period.

NURSING ASSESSMENT OF PREOPERATIVE PATIENT

The overall goal of the preoperative assessment is to identify risk factors and plan care to ensure patient safety throughout the surgical experience. Goals of the assessment are to

- Determine the patient's psychologic status in order to reinforce the use of coping strategies during the surgical experience.
- Determine physiologic factors directly or indirectly related to the surgical procedure that may contribute to operative risk factors.
- Establish baseline data for comparison in the intraoperative and postoperative period.
- Participate in the identification and documentation of the surgical site and/or side (of body) on which the surgical procedure will be performed.
- Identify prescription drugs, over-the-counter medications, and herbal supplements taken by the patient that may result in drug interactions affecting the surgical outcome.
- Document the results of all preoperative laboratory and diagnostic tests in the patient's record, and communicate this information to appropriate health care providers.
- Identify cultural and ethnic factors that may affect the surgical experience.
- Determine if the patient has received adequate information from the surgeon to make an informed decision to have surgery and that the consent form is signed and witnessed.

Subjective Data

Psychosocial Assessment. Surgery is a stressful event, even when the procedure is considered minor. The psychologic and physiologic reactions to surgery and anesthesia may elicit the stress response (e.g., elevated blood pressure [BP] and heart rate). The stress response enables the body to prepare to meet the demands in the perioperative period. If stressors or the responses to the stressors are excessive, the stress response can be magnified and may affect recovery. Many factors influence the patient's susceptibility to stress, including age, past experiences with illness and pain, current health, and socioeconomic status. Identifying a patient's perceived or actual stressors allows you to provide support during the preoperative period so that stress does not become distress.

The use of common language and avoidance of medical jargon are essential. Use words and language that are familiar to the patient to increase the patient's understanding of surgical consent and the surgery. Familiar language also helps reduce preoperative anxiety.

Your role in psychologically preparing the patient for surgery is to assess the patient for potential stressors that could negatively affect surgery (Table 18-2). Communicate all concerns to the appropriate surgical team member, especially if the concern requires intervention later in the surgical experience. Because many patients are admitted directly into the preoperative area from their homes, you must be skilled in assessing important psychologic factors in a short time. The most common psychologic factors are anxiety, fear, and hope.

Anxiety. Most people are anxious when facing surgery because of the unknown. This is normal and is an inborn survival mechanism. However, if the anxiety level is high, cognition, decision making, and coping abilities are reduced.

Anxiety can arise from lack of knowledge, which may range from not knowing what to expect during surgery to uncertainty about the outcome. This may be a result of past experiences or stories heard through friends or the media. You can decrease some anxiety for the patient by providing information about what to expect. This is often done through classes, or web-based or audiovisual educational materials before surgery. Inform the surgeon if the patient requires any additional information or if anxiety is excessive.

The patient may experience anxiety when surgery is in conflict with his or her religious and cultural beliefs. In particular, identify, document, and communicate the patient's religious and cultural beliefs about the possibility of blood transfusions. For example, Jehovah's Witnesses may choose to refuse blood or blood products.[1]

Common Fears. Patients fear surgery for a number of reasons. The most common fear is the risk of death or permanent disability resulting from surgery. Sometimes the fear arises after hearing or reading about the risks during the informed consent process. Other fears are related to pain, change in body image, or results of diagnostic procedures.

Fear of death can be extremely harmful. Notify the physician if the patient has a strong fear of death. A patient's strong fear of impending death may prompt the physician to delay the surgery until the situation improves because the emotional state influences the stress response, and thus the surgical outcome.

Fear of pain and discomfort during and after surgery is common. If the fear is extreme, notify the ACP or the surgeon. Reassure the patient that drugs are available for both anesthesia and analgesia during surgery. For pain after surgery, tell patients to ask for pain medication before pain becomes severe. Instruct the patient on the use of a pain intensity scale (e.g., 0 to 10, FACES [see eFig. 9-3, available on the website for Chapter 9]). (Pain scales are explained in Chapter 9.)

Drugs may also be given that provide an amnesic effect so the patient will not remember what occurs during surgery. Tell the patient that this effect assists in decreasing anxiety after surgery.

Fear of mutilation or alteration in body image can occur whether the surgery is radical, such as amputation, or minor, such as a bunion repair. Even a small scar on the body can be upsetting to some, and others fear keloid development (overgrowth of a scar). Listen to and assess the patient's concern about this fear with an accepting attitude.

Fear of anesthesia may arise from the unknown, personal experience, or tales of others' bad experiences. These concerns can also result from information about the risks (e.g., brain damage, paralysis) of anesthesia. Many patients fear losing control while under anesthesia. If these fears are identified, inform the ACP immediately so that he or she can talk further with the patient. Reassure the patient that a nurse and the ACP will be present at all times during surgery.

Fear of disruption of life functioning may be present in varying degrees. It can range from fear of permanent disability to concern about not being able to engage in activities of daily

TABLE 18-2 PSYCHOSOCIAL ASSESSMENT OF PREOPERATIVE PATIENT

Situational Changes
- Identify support systems, including family, other caregivers, group and institutional structures, and religious and spiritual groups.
- Define current degree of personal control, decision making, and independence.
- Consider the impact of surgery and hospitalization and the possible effects on lifestyle.
- Determine the presence of hope and anticipation of positive results.

Concerns With the Unknown
- Identify specific areas and degree of anxiety and fears related to the surgery (e.g., pain).
- Identify expectations of surgery, changes in current health status, effects on daily living, and sexual activity (if appropriate).

Concerns With Body Image
- Identify current roles or relationships and view of self.
- Determine perceived or potential changes in roles or relationships and their impact on body image.

Past Experiences
- Review previous surgical experiences, hospitalizations, and treatments.
- Determine responses to those experiences (positive and negative).
- Identify current perceptions of surgical procedure in relation to the above and information from others (e.g., a friend's view of a personal surgical experience).

Knowledge Deficit
- Identify the amount and type of preoperative information the patient wants.
- Assess understanding of the surgical procedure, including preparation, care, interventions, preoperative activities, restrictions, and expected outcomes.
- Identify the accuracy of information the patient has received from others, including health care team, family, friends, and the media.

living for a few weeks. Concerns about loss of role function, separation from family, and how the family will manage may be revealed. Financial concerns may be related to an anticipated loss of income or the costs of surgery.

If you identify any of these fears, a consult with the patient's caregiver, a social worker, a spiritual or cultural advisor, or a psychologist may be appropriate. Financial advisors at the hospital may be able to provide information about financial support.

Hope. Although many psychologic factors related to surgery seem to be negative, hope is a positive attribute.[2] Hope may be the patient's strongest method of coping. To deny or minimize hope may negate the positive mental attitude necessary for a quick and full recovery. Some surgeries are hopefully anticipated. These can be the surgeries that repair (e.g., plastic surgery for burn scars), rebuild (e.g., total joint replacement to reduce pain and improve function), or save and extend life (e.g., repair of aneurysm, organ transplant). Assess and support the presence of hope and the patient's anticipation of positive results.

Past Health History. Ask the patient about any previous medical problems and surgeries. Determine if the patient understands the need for surgery. For example, the patient scheduled for a total knee replacement may indicate that increasing pain and immobility are the reasons for the surgery.

Document the reason for any past hospitalizations, including previous surgeries and the dates. Also identify any problems with previous surgeries. For example, the patient may have experienced a wound infection or a reaction to a medication.

Ask women about their menstrual and obstetric history. This includes the date of their last menstrual period, the number of pregnancies, and any history of cesarean section.

When obtaining a family health history, ask both patient and caregiver about any inherited traits, since they may contribute to the surgical outcome. Record any family history of cardiac and endocrine diseases. For example, if a patient reports a parent with hypertension, sudden cardiac death, or myocardial infarction, this should alert you to the possibility that the patient may have a similar predisposition or condition. Also obtain information about the patient's family history of adverse reactions to or problems with anesthesia. For example, malignant hyperthermia has a genetic predisposition. Measures to decrease complications associated with this condition can be taken. (For further information on malignant hyperthermia, see Chapter 19.)

Medications. Document all current routine and intermittent medication use, including over-the-counter drugs and herbal supplements. In many ambulatory surgery centers, patients are asked to bring their medications with them when reporting for surgery. This helps to accurately assess and document both the name and the dosage of medications.

The interaction of the patient's current medications and anesthetics can increase or decrease the desired physiologic effect of anesthetics. Consider the effects of opioids and prescribed medications for chronic health conditions (e.g., heart disease, hypertension, depression, epilepsy, diabetes mellitus). For example, certain antidepressants can potentiate the effect of opioids, agents that can be used for anesthesia. Antihypertensive drugs may predispose the patient to shock from the combined effect of the drug and the vasodilator effect of some anesthetic agents. Insulin or oral hypoglycemic agents may require dose or agent adjustments during the perioperative period because of increased body metabolism, decreased oral intake, stress, and anesthesia. Antiplatelet drugs (e.g., aspirin, clopidogrel [Plavix]) and nonsteroidal antiinflammatory drugs (NSAIDs) inhibit platelet aggregation and may contribute to postoperative bleeding. Surgeons may instruct patients to withhold these medications before surgery. Specific timeframes for withholding drugs depend on the drug and the patient. Patients on long-term anticoagulation therapy (e.g., warfarin [Coumadin]) present a unique challenge. The options for these patients include (1) continuing therapy, (2) withholding therapy for a time before and after surgery, or (3) withholding the therapy and starting subcutaneous or IV heparin therapy during the perioperative period. The management strategy selected is determined by patient characteristics and the nature of the surgery.[3]

Ask about the use of herbs and dietary supplements because their use is so common. Many patients do not think to include supplements in their list of medications. They believe that herbal and dietary supplements are "natural" and do not pose a surgical risk.[4] (See the Complementary & Alternative Therapies box in Chapter 3 on p. 39 on how to assess for the use of herbal supplements.) Excessive use of vitamins and herbs can cause harmful effects in patients undergoing surgery. In patients taking anticoagulants or antiplatelets, herbal supplements can produce excessive postoperative bleeding that may require a return to the OR.[5] The effects of specific herbs that are of concern during the perioperative period are listed below in the Complementary & Alternative Therapies box.

Also ask the patient about possible recreational drug use, abuse, and addiction. The substances most likely to be abused include tobacco, alcohol, opioids, marijuana, cocaine, and amphetamines. Ask questions about the use of these substances in a frank manner. Stress that recreational drug use may affect the type and amount of anesthesia that will be needed. When patients become aware of the potential interactions of these substances with anesthetics, most patients respond honestly about using them. Chronic alcohol use can place the patient at risk because of lung, gastrointestinal, or liver damage. When liver function is decreased, metabolism of anesthetic agents is prolonged, nutritional status is altered, and the potential for postoperative complications is increased. Alcohol withdrawal can also occur during lengthy surgery or in the postoperative period. Although this can be a life-threatening event, it can be

COMPLEMENTARY & ALTERNATIVE THERAPIES

Herbal Products and Surgery

The following can be used as a guide for patient teaching:

- Notify your health care provider of all vitamins, herbal products, and dietary supplements that you are or have been taking.
- Avoid astragalus and ginseng, since they can increase blood pressure before and during surgery.
- Avoid garlic, vitamin E, ginkgo, and fish oils because they can increase bleeding.
- Avoid kava and valerian because they can cause excess sedation.
- In general, discontinue all herbal supplements 2 to 3 weeks before any surgical procedure. Consult your health care provider for specific instructions.

Helpful Herbs and Vitamins

- Ginger can be useful for preventing nausea associated with anesthesia. Consider ginger ale, crystallized ginger, or ginger tea.
- Arnica is a homeopathic remedy useful in soft tissue healing.
- Multivitamins can be taken until the day before surgery. Taking them on the day of surgery, on an empty stomach, may contribute to nausea and vomiting after surgery.

avoided with appropriate planning and management (see Chapter 11).

Document and communicate all findings of the medication history to the perioperative health care team. The ACP will determine the appropriate schedule and dose of the patient's routine medications before and after surgery. Ensure that all of the patient's medications are identified, implement any changes in the medication plan, and monitor the patient for potential interactions and complications.

Allergies. Question the patient about drug intolerances and drug allergies. Drug intolerance usually results in side effects that are uncomfortable or unpleasant for the patient but are not life threatening. These effects can include nausea, constipation, diarrhea, or *idiosyncratic* (opposite than expected) reactions. A true drug allergy produces hives and/or an anaphylactic reaction, causing cardiopulmonary compromise (e.g., hypotension, tachycardia, bronchospasm). Being aware of drug intolerances and drug allergies aids the health care team to maintain patient comfort and safety. For example, some anesthetic agents contain sulfur, so notify the ACP if a history of allergy to sulfur is reported. Document all drug intolerances and drug allergies and, if appropriate, place an allergy identification band on the patient on the day of surgery.

Also inquire about nondrug allergies, specifically food and environmental (e.g., latex, pollen, animals) allergies. The patient with a history of any allergic reactions has a greater potential for hypersensitivity reactions to drugs given during anesthesia. Patients need to be screened specifically for latex allergies by gathering data in the following areas:

- Risk factors
- Contact dermatitis
- Contact urticaria (e.g., hives)
- Aerosol reactions
- History of reactions that suggest an allergy to latex

Risk factors for latex allergy include long-term, multiple exposures to latex products, such as those experienced by health care and rubber industry workers. Additional risk factors include a history of hay fever, asthma, and allergies to certain foods (e.g., eggs, avocados, bananas, chestnuts, potatoes, peaches).[6] (Latex allergies are discussed in Chapter 14.)

Review of Systems. The last component of the patient history is the body systems review. Ask specific questions to confirm the presence or absence of any diseases. Current medical problems can alert you to areas that should be more closely examined in the preoperative physical examination. The combined review of systems and the patient history provide essential data to determine the specific preoperative tests that need to be ordered.

Cardiovascular System. Evaluate cardiovascular (CV) function to determine preexisting disease or problems (e.g., coronary artery disease, prosthetic heart valve). In reviewing the CV system, you may find a history of hypertension, angina, dysrhythmias, heart failure, or myocardial infarction. Inquire about the patient's current treatment for any CV condition (e.g., medications) and the level of functioning. A cardiology consult is often required before surgery if the patient has a significant CV history (e.g., recent myocardial infarction, valvular heart disease, implantable cardioverter-defibrillator).

If indicated, a 12-lead electrocardiogram (ECG) and coagulation studies should be ordered, and the results should be on the chart before surgery. The CV assessment provides data on what other measures need to be done. For example, the patient who is on diuretic therapy will need to have a serum potassium level drawn preoperatively. If the patient has a history of hypertension, the ACP may administer vasoactive drugs to maintain adequate BP during surgery. If the patient has a history of valvular heart disease, antibiotic prophylaxis often is given before surgery to decrease the risk of bacterial endocarditis (see Chapter 37).

Postoperative venous thromboembolism (VTE), a condition that includes deep vein thrombosis and pulmonary embolism, is a concern for any surgical patient. Patients at high risk for VTE include those with a history of previous thrombosis, blood-clotting disorders, cancer, varicosities, obesity, smoking, heart failure, or chronic obstructive pulmonary disease (COPD).[7] People are also at risk for developing a VTE because of immobility and positioning during the operative procedure. Antiembolism stockings or sequential compression devices may be applied to the legs in the preoperative holding area.

Respiratory System. Ask the patient about any recent or chronic respiratory disease or infections. Elective surgery may need to be postponed if the person has an upper respiratory tract infection. Upper airway infections increase the risk of bronchospasm, laryngospasm, decreased O_2 saturation, and problems with respiratory secretions. Also report a patient's history of dyspnea at rest or with exertion, coughing (dry or productive), or hemoptysis (coughing blood) to the ACP and the surgeon.

If a patient has a history of asthma, inquire about the use of inhaled or oral corticosteroids and bronchodilators, as well as the frequency and triggers of asthma attacks. The patient with a history of COPD is at high risk for postoperative pulmonary complications, including hypoxemia and atelectasis.

Encourage the patient who smokes to stop at least 6 weeks preoperatively to decrease the risk of intraoperative and postoperative respiratory complications. The greater the patient's pack-years of smoking (packs smoked per day times years), the greater the risk for pulmonary complications during or after surgery. Report conditions likely to affect respiratory function such as sleep apnea; obesity; and spinal, chest, and airway deformities. For example, patients may be asked to bring their sleep apnea devices with them to the hospital or surgical center. Depending on the patient's history and physical examination, baseline pulmonary function tests and arterial blood gases may be ordered preoperatively.

Neurologic System. Preoperative evaluation of neurologic functioning includes assessing the patient's ability to respond to questions, follow commands, and maintain orderly thought patterns. Alterations in the patient's hearing and vision may affect responses and the ability to follow directions throughout the perioperative assessment and evaluation. Document the patient's ability to pay attention, concentrate, and respond appropriately to establish a preoperative baseline for postoperative comparison.

If you note deficits in cognitive function, determine the extent of the problems and whether they can be corrected before surgery. If the problems cannot be corrected, it is important to involve a legal guardian or person with durable power of attorney for health care to assist the patient and provide informed consent for surgery.

Preoperative assessment of the older person's baseline cognitive function is especially crucial for intraoperative and postoperative evaluation.[8] The older adult may have intact mental abilities preoperatively, but is more prone to adverse outcomes during and after surgery than the younger adult. This is due to the additional stressors of the surgical procedure, dehydration, hypothermia, and anesthesia and adjunctive medications. These factors may contribute to the development of emergence delirium ("waking up wild"), a condition that may be falsely labeled as senility or dementia. Thus preoperative findings are critical for postoperative comparison.

In the review of the neurologic system, inquire about any history of strokes, transient ischemic attacks, or spinal cord injury. Also ask about neurologic diseases, such as myasthenia gravis, Parkinson's disease, and multiple sclerosis, and any treatments used.

Genitourinary System. Assess the preoperative patient for a history of renal or urinary tract diseases, such as glomerulonephritis, chronic kidney disease, or repeated urinary tract infections. Document the present disease state and treatment used to control the disease. Renal dysfunction is associated with a number of alterations, including fluid and electrolyte imbalances, coagulopathies, increased risk for infection, and impaired wound healing. Because many drugs are metabolized and excreted by the kidneys, a decrease in renal function can lead to an altered response to drugs and unpredictable drug elimination. Renal function tests, such as serum creatinine and blood urea nitrogen (BUN), are commonly ordered preoperatively.

Document and report to the perioperative team if the patient has problems voiding (e.g., incontinence, hesitancy). Male patients may have physical conditions, such as an enlarged prostate, that can interfere with the insertion of a urinary catheter during surgery or impair voiding in the postoperative period.

For women of childbearing age, determine if they are pregnant or think they could be pregnant. Most institutions require a pregnancy test for all women of childbearing age before surgery.[9] Immediately inform the surgeon if the patient states that she might be pregnant, since maternal and subsequent fetal exposure to anesthetics during the first trimester should be avoided.

Hepatic System. The liver is involved in glucose homeostasis, fat metabolism, protein synthesis, drug and hormone metabolism, and bilirubin formation and excretion. The liver detoxifies many anesthetics and adjunctive drugs. The patient with hepatic dysfunction may have an increased perioperative risk for clotting abnormalities and adverse responses to medications. Consider the presence of liver disease if there is a history of jaundice, hepatitis, alcohol abuse, or obesity.

Integumentary System. Inquire about a history of skin problems. Assess the current condition of the skin, especially at the incision site, for rashes, breakdown, or other dermatologic conditions. A patient with a history of pressure ulcers may require extra padding during surgery. Skin problems can affect postoperative healing.

Body art such as tattoos and piercings are increasingly common. When possible, select pigment-free areas for injections, IV sites, and laboratory draws.

Musculoskeletal System. Note any musculoskeletal and mobility problems, especially in the older adult. If the patient has arthritis, identify all affected joints. Mobility restrictions may influence intraoperative and postoperative positioning and ambulation. Spinal anesthesia may be difficult if the patient cannot flex his or her lumbar spine adequately to allow easy needle insertion. If the neck is affected, intubation and airway management may be difficult. Any mobility aids (e.g., cane, walker) should be brought with the patient on the day of surgery.

Endocrine System. The patient with diabetes is especially at risk for adverse effects of anesthesia and surgery. Hypoglycemia, hyperglycemia, delayed wound healing, and infection are common complications of diabetes during the perioperative period. Clarify with the patient's surgeon or ACP whether the patient should take the usual dose of insulin or oral hypoglycemic agents on the day of surgery. ACPs may vary the usual insulin dose based on the patient's current status and history of glucose control. Regardless of the preoperative insulin orders, determine serum or capillary glucose levels the morning of surgery to establish baseline levels. Assess the patient's glucose levels periodically and manage, if necessary, with short-acting or rapid-acting insulin.

Determine if the patient has a history of thyroid dysfunction. Hyperthyroidism or hypothyroidism can place the patient at surgical risk because of alterations in metabolic rate. If the patient takes a thyroid replacement drug, check with the ACP about administration of the drug on the day of surgery. If the patient has a history of thyroid dysfunction, laboratory tests may be ordered to determine current levels of thyroid function.

The patient with Addison's disease also requires special consideration during surgery. Addisonian crisis or shock can occur if a patient abruptly stops taking replacement corticosteroids, and the stress of surgery may require additional IV corticosteroid therapy[10] (see Chapter 50).

Immune System. If the patient has a history of a compromised immune system or takes immunosuppressive drugs, document it. Corticosteroids used in immunosuppressive doses may be tapered before surgery. Impairment of the immune system can lead to delayed wound healing and increased risk for postoperative infections.[11] If the patient has an acute infection (e.g., upper respiratory tract infection, sinusitis, influenza), elective surgery is often canceled. Patients with active chronic infections such as hepatitis B or C, acquired immunodeficiency syndrome, or tuberculosis may have surgery if indicated. However, when preparing the patient for surgery, remember to take infection control precautions for the protection of the patient and staff.[12] (Infection control guidelines are discussed in Chapter 15 and eTable 15-1, available on the website for Chapter 15.)

Fluid and Electrolyte Status. Ask the patient about any recent conditions that increase the risk for fluid and electrolyte imbalances, such as vomiting, diarrhea, or preoperative bowel preps. For example, surgery may be planned for a patient with cholecystitis who has been vomiting for several days. Also identify drugs that alter fluid and electrolyte status, such as diuretics. Serum electrolyte levels are often assessed before surgery. Many patients may have restricted fluids for some time before surgery. If the surgery is delayed, they could develop dehydration. A patient with or at risk for dehydration may require additional fluids and electrolytes before or during surgery.

Although a preoperative fluid balance history should be completed for all patients, it is especially critical for older adults. Their reduced adaptive capacity leaves a narrow margin of safety between overhydration and underhydration.

Nutritional Status. Nutritional deficits include overnutrition and undernutrition, both of which require considerable time to correct. However, knowing that a patient has a nutritional deficit can help the perioperative team provide more individualized care. For example, if the patient is thin, provide more padding than usual (pressure points on all patients are protected routinely) on the OR table. Notify the team if a patient is morbidly obese (body mass index [BMI] greater than 40 kg/m^2) to allow time to obtain special equipment needed for the patient's care (e.g., longer instruments for abdominal surgery).

Obesity stresses both the cardiac and pulmonary systems and makes access to the surgical site and anesthesia administration more difficult.[13] It predisposes the patient to wound dehiscence, wound infection, and incisional herniation postoperatively. Adipose tissue is less vascular than other types of tissue. In addition, the patient may be slower to recover from anesthesia because inhalation agents are absorbed and stored by adipose tissue, thus leaving the body more slowly. (See Chapter 41 for special needs of obese patients undergoing surgery.)

Nutritional deficiencies impair the ability to recover from surgery. Remember that the obese patient and the very thin patient can also be protein and vitamin deficient. If the nutritional problem is severe, surgery may be postponed. Protein and vitamins A, C, and B complex deficiencies are particularly significant because these substances are essential for wound healing.[14] Supplemental nutrition may be administered during the perioperative period to patients who are malnourished. The older adult is often at risk for malnutrition and fluid volume deficits.[8]

Identify patients who consume large quantities of coffee or soft drinks containing caffeine. In many cases, withholding caffeinated beverages preoperatively or for some time postoperatively can lead to severe withdrawal headaches.[15] Caffeine withdrawal headaches can be confused with spinal headaches if the preoperative data are not documented. Giving caffeinated beverages postoperatively, when possible, may prevent these headaches.

Objective Data

Physical Examination. The Joint Commission requires that all patients admitted to the OR have a documented history and physical examination (H&P) in their chart.[16] This may be done in advance of surgery or on the day of surgery. It may be performed by any qualified person, including advanced practice nurses, physicians, physician assistants, or ACPs. Findings from the patient's H&P will enable the ACP to assign the patient a physical status rating for anesthesia administration (Table 18-3). This rating is an indicator of the patient's perioperative risk and may influence perioperative decisions.

TABLE 18-3 AMERICAN SOCIETY OF ANESTHESIOLOGISTS' PHYSICAL CLASSIFICATION SYSTEM

Rating	Definition
P1	Normal healthy person
P2	Patient with mild systemic disease
P3	Patient with severe systemic disease
P4	Patient with severe systemic disease that is a constant threat to life
P5	Moribund patient who is not expected to survive without surgery
P6	Declared brain-dead patient whose organs are being removed for donor purposes

Source: American Society of Anesthesiologists: ASA physical status classification system, 2012. Retrieved from *www.asahq.org/clinical/physicalstatus.htm.*

NOTE: Patients selected for surgery in ambulatory or outpatient settings generally have ratings of P1, P2, or P3.

In addition to the health assessment, also complete a physical examination of the patient before surgery (Table 18-4). Review the documentation already present in the patient's chart, including the H&P, to better proceed with your examination. Document all findings and communicate any relevant findings immediately to the surgeon or the ACP.

Laboratory and Diagnostic Testing. Obtain and assess the results of laboratory and diagnostic tests ordered preoperatively (Table 18-5). For example, if the patient is taking an antiplatelet medication (e.g., aspirin), a coagulation profile will be ordered; if the patient is on diuretic therapy, a potassium level is assessed; if the patient is of childbearing age, a pregnancy test should be ordered; or if the patient is taking medications for dysrhythmias, a preoperative ECG is obtained. Blood glucose monitoring is done for patients with diabetes. In some settings, tests for methicillin-resistant *Staphylococcus aureus* are done preoperatively. Patients with positive results are prescribed antibiotics for several days before surgery.[17]

Ideally, preoperative tests are ordered based on the patient's H&P. However, many facilities and insurers have a written protocol for preoperative tests, which may not include all the identified areas. In addition, the preoperative tests may be done days before surgery. Ensure that all laboratory and diagnostic reports are in the patient's chart. Missing reports may result in a delay or cancellation of the surgery.

NURSING MANAGEMENT PREOPERATIVE PATIENT

Preoperative nursing interventions are derived from the nursing assessment and must reflect each patient's specific needs. Physical preparations are determined by the pending surgery and the routines of the surgery setting. Preoperative teaching may be minimal or extensive. The Association of periOperative Registered Nurses (AORN) provides standards and recommended practices to guide nursing interventions in all perioperative settings.[7]

PREOPERATIVE TEACHING

The patient has a right to know what to expect and how to participate effectively during the surgical experience. Preoperative teaching increases patient satisfaction and may reduce postoperative fear, anxiety, and stress.[18] Teaching may also decrease the development of complications, the length of hospitalization, and the recovery time after discharge.

In most surgical settings, patients often arrive only a short time before surgery is scheduled. Preoperative teaching for these patients is generally done in the surgeon's office or a preadmission surgical clinic and reinforced on the day of surgery. After ambulatory surgery the patient usually goes home several hours after recovery, depending on the patient's progress and procedure-specific needs. Teaching must include information that focuses on the patient's safety. Provide written materials for patients and caregivers to use for review and reinforcement at home. Discharge teaching is required for all patients[19,20] and is discussed in Chapter 20.

When doing preoperative teaching for a patient, provide a balance between explaining so much that the patient is overwhelmed and telling so little that the patient is unprepared. If you observe carefully and listen sensitively to the patient, you can usually determine how much information is enough. Remember that anxiety and fear may decrease learning ability.

TABLE 18-4 HEALTH ASSESSMENT AND PHYSICAL EXAMINATION OF PREOPERATIVE PATIENT*

Cardiovascular System
- Identify acute or chronic problems. Note presence of angina, hypertension, heart failure, recent myocardial infarction, renal disease, diabetes.
- Identify any drugs (e.g., aspirin) or herbal supplements (e.g., ginkgo) that may affect coagulation.
- Identify patients with prosthetic heart valves, pacemakers, or implantable cardioverter-defibrillators.
- Assess for edema (including dependent areas), noting location and severity.
- Inspect neck veins for distention.
- Obtain bilateral baseline blood pressures.
- Assess pulses (bilaterally when appropriate) for rate, rhythm, and quality: apical, radial, and pedal.

Respiratory System
- Identify acute or chronic problems. Note the presence of infection, chronic obstructive pulmonary disease, or asthma. Note use of CPAP machine.
- Assess history of smoking, including the time since the last cigarette and the number of pack-years.
- Determine baseline respiratory rate and rhythm and regularity of pattern.
- Observe for cough, dyspnea, and use of accessory muscles of respiration.
- Auscultate lungs for normal and adventitious breath sounds.

Neurologic System
- Determine orientation to person, place, and time.
- Assess baseline mental status. Note presence of confusion, disorderly thinking, or inability to follow commands.
- Identify past history of strokes, transient ischemic attacks, or neurologic diseases (e.g., Parkinson's disease, multiple sclerosis).

Genitourinary System
- Identify any infection or preexisting disease.
- Determine ability to void.
- Note color, amount, and characteristics of urine (if appropriate).
- Determine pregnancy status (if appropriate).

Hepatic System
- Review past history of substance abuse, especially alcohol and IV drug use.
- Inspect skin color and sclera of eyes for any signs of jaundice.

Integumentary System
- Identify any current or previous skin disorders (e.g., pressure ulcers, eczema).
- Determine skin status. Note drying, bruising, or breaks in surface.
- Inspect skin for rashes, boils, or infection, especially around the planned surgical site.
- Inspect the mucous membranes and skin turgor for signs of dehydration.
- Assess skin moisture and temperature.

Musculoskeletal System
- Examine skin around bone pressure points.
- Assess for limitations in joint range of motion and muscle strength.
- Assess for joint or muscle pain.
- Assess mobility, gait, and balance.

Gastrointestinal System
- Determine patterns of food and fluid intake and any recent changes in weight.
- Determine usual pattern of bowel movements, including date of last bowel movement.
- Assess for the presence of dentures and bridges (loose dentures or teeth may be dislodged during intubation).
- Weigh patient.
- Auscultate abdomen for presence of bowel sounds.

Immune System
- Identify any immunodeficiency or autoimmune disorders.
- Assess for use of corticosteroids or other immunosuppressant drugs.

Laboratory and Diagnostic Tests
- Review results of all laboratory and diagnostic tests completed preoperatively (see Table 18-5).

*See specific body system chapters for more detailed assessments and related laboratory studies.
CPAP, Continuous positive airway pressure.

Also assess what the patient wants to know and give priority to those concerns.

Generally, preoperative teaching includes three types of information: sensory, process, and procedural. Different patients, with varying cultures, backgrounds, and experience, may want different types of information.

With *sensory information,* patients find out what they will see, hear, smell, and feel during the surgery. For example, you may tell them that the OR will be cold, but they can ask for a warm blanket; the lights in the OR are bright; or many unfamiliar sounds and specific smells will be present.

Patients wanting *process information* may not want specific details but just the general flow of what is going to happen. This information would include the patient's transfer to the holding area, visits by the nurse and the ACP before transfer to the OR, and waking up in the PACU.

With *procedural information,* patients desire details that are more specific. For example, this information would include that an IV line will be started while the patient is in the holding area and the surgeon will mark the operative area with an indelible marker to verify site and side.[7]

Share the preoperative teaching provided to the patient with the nurses providing postoperative care to evaluate learning and avoid duplication of teaching. Because the time for teaching is limited, the team approach is often used. For example, teaching may be started in the outpatient setting. Your responsibility is to assess the patient's understanding of this teaching and fill in the gaps. The discharge nurse provides written instructions and additional information for reinforcement. Home care nurses may be involved if patients have complex learning needs that must be addressed after discharge.

Document all teaching in the patient's chart. A Patient & Caregiver Teaching Guide for preoperative preparation is presented in Table 18-6. Additional information related to patient and caregiver teaching is found in Chapter 4.

GENERAL SURGERY INFORMATION. Unless contraindicated (e.g., after craniotomy, tonsillectomy), all patients should receive instruction about deep breathing, coughing, and early ambulation (moving) postoperatively. This is essential because patients may not want to do these activities postoperatively unless they are taught the reason for them and practice them preoperatively. Tell patients and caregivers if tubes, drains, monitoring devices, or special equipment will be used after surgery. Explain that these devices help you to safely care for the patient. Examples of individualized teaching may include how to use incentive spirometers or postoperative patient-controlled analgesia

TABLE 18-5 COMMON PREOPERATIVE LABORATORY AND DIAGNOSTIC TESTS

Test	Assessment
ABGs, pulse oximetry	Respiratory and metabolic function, oxygenation status
Blood glucose	Metabolic status, diabetes mellitus
Blood urea nitrogen, creatinine	Renal function
Chest x-ray	Pulmonary disorders, cardiac enlargement, heart failure
Complete blood count: RBCs, Hgb, Hct, WBCs, WBC differential	Anemia, immune status, infection
Electrocardiogram	Cardiac disease, dysrhythmias
Electrolytes	Metabolic status, renal function, diuretic side effects
hCG	Pregnancy status
Liver function tests	Liver status
PT, PTT, INR, platelet count	Coagulation status
Pulmonary function studies	Pulmonary status
Serum albumin	Nutritional status
Type and crossmatch	Blood available for replacement (elective surgery patients may have own blood available)
Urinalysis	Renal status, hydration, urinary tract infection

hCG, Human chorionic gonadotropin; *Hct,* hematocrit; *Hgb,* hemoglobin; *INR,* international normalized ratio; *PT,* prothrombin time; *PTT,* partial thromboplastin time.

pumps. Patients should have a clear understanding of how to rate their pain intensity and how their pain will be managed.[21] (See Chapter 9 for additional information on pain.)

The patient should also receive accurate surgery-specific information. For example, a patient having a total joint replacement may have an immobilizer after surgery, or a patient with extensive neurosurgery should be told about waking up in the intensive care unit.

AMBULATORY SURGERY INFORMATION. The ambulatory surgery patient or the patient admitted to the hospital the day of surgery needs to receive information before admission. Some ambulatory surgical centers telephone the patients the evening before surgery to answer last-minute questions and to reinforce teaching. Each center has policies and procedures that direct this communication in a timely manner.

In addition to specifics on the procedure, patients need information on day-of-surgery events such as arrival time, registration, parking, what to wear, what to bring, and the need to have a responsible adult present for transportation home after surgery.

Traditionally, patients having elective surgery are instructed to have nothing by mouth (NPO) starting at midnight on the night before surgery. Current guidelines published by the American Society of Anesthesiologists are less strict[22] (Table 18-7). Restriction of fluids and food is designed to reduce the risk of pulmonary aspiration and postoperative nausea and vomiting. Protocols may vary for patients having local anesthesia or surgery scheduled late in the day. Follow the NPO protocol of each surgical facility. The patient who has not followed the NPO instructions may have surgery delayed or canceled. It is critical that the patient understands the reason for and follows all restrictions.

TABLE 18-6 PATIENT & CAREGIVER TEACHING GUIDE

Preoperative Preparation

Include the following information in the preoperative teaching plan for patient and caregiver.

Sensory Information

- Preoperative holding area may be noisy.
- Drugs and cleaning solutions may be cold and odorous.
- Operating room (OR) can be cold. Warm blankets are available and can be requested.
- Talking may be heard in the OR but may be distorted because of masks. Ask questions if something is not understood.
- OR bed will be narrow. A safety strap will be applied over the thighs.
- Lights in the OR may be bright.
- Monitoring machines may be heard (e.g., ticking and beeping noises) when awake.

Procedural Information

- What to bring and what type of clothing to wear to the surgery center.
- Any changes in time of surgery.
- Fluid and food restrictions.
- Physical preparation required (e.g., bowel or skin preparation).
- Purpose of frequent vital signs assessment.
- Pain control and other comfort measures.
- Why turning, coughing, and deep breathing postoperatively are important. Practice sessions need to be done preoperatively.
- Insertion of IV lines.
- Procedure for anesthesia administration.
- Expect surgical site and/or side to be marked with indelible ink or marker.

Process Information

Information About General Flow of Surgery

- Admission area.
- Preoperative holding area, OR, and recovery area.
- Caregivers can usually stay in preoperative holding area until surgery.
- Caregivers will be able to see the patient after discharge from the recovery area or possibly in the recovery area once the patient is awake.
- Identification of any technology that may be present on awakening, such as monitors and central lines.

Where Caregivers Can Wait During Surgery

- Encourage caregivers to ask questions and express any concerns.
- OR staff will update caregivers during surgery and when surgery is completed.
- Surgeon will usually talk with caregivers after surgery.

LEGAL PREPARATION FOR SURGERY

Legal preparation for surgery consists of checking that all required forms have been correctly signed and are present in the patient's chart, and that the patient and the caregiver clearly understand what is going to happen. Standard consent forms include those for the surgical procedure and blood transfusions. Other forms may include advance directives and durable power of attorney for health care (see Chapter 10).

CONSENT FOR SURGERY. Before nonemergency surgery can be legally performed, the patient must voluntarily sign an informed consent form in the presence of a witness. **Informed consent** is an active, shared decision-making process between the health care provider and the recipient of care.[23] Three conditions must be met for consent to be valid. First, there must be *adequate*

TABLE 18-7 PREOPERATIVE FASTING RECOMMENDATIONS*

Liquid and Food Intake	Minimum Fasting Period (Hr)
Clear liquids (e.g., water, clear tea, black coffee, carbonated beverages, fruit juice without pulp)	2
Breast milk	4
Nonhuman milk, including infant formula	6
Light meal (e.g., toast and clear liquids)	6
Regular meal (may include fried or fatty food, meat)	8 or more

Source: Practice guidelines for preoperative fasting and the use of pharmacologic agents to reduce the risk of pulmonary aspiration: application to healthy patients undergoing elective procedures: an updated report by the American Society of Anesthesiologists Task Force on Preoperative Fasting. Retrieved from *http://journals.lww.com/anesthesiology/Fulltext/2011/03000/Practice_Guidelines_for_Preoperative_Fasting_and.13.aspx?WT.mc_id=HPxADx20100319xMP.*

*For healthy patients of all ages undergoing elective surgery (excluding women in labor).

EVIDENCE-BASED PRACTICE

Applying the Evidence

G.L. is a 57-year-old woman scheduled for a knee replacement. She has been NPO since midnight and was scheduled to be the third surgical case of the day. Unfortunately, several emergency surgeries have resulted in delays, and she is not expected to leave for surgery for another 4 hours. She tells you that she has a "headache" from missing her "morning coffee." She says she is hungry and thirsty and, since surgery has been delayed, she would like a cup of coffee.

Best Available Evidence	Clinician Expertise	Patient Preferences and Values
For healthy adults, the minimum fasting period for clear liquids before surgery is 2 hr.	Nothing by mouth (NPO) restrictions are meant to prevent aspiration and vomiting during surgery. Patients who are NPO from midnight frequently complain of hunger and thirst while waiting for surgery. Patients who regularly drink caffeine in the morning often experience a "caffeine withdrawal" headache when fasting. You know that clear liquids consist of water, fruit juices without pulp, carbonated beverages, clear tea, and black coffee.	Patient is requesting something to drink given the extended period of fast due to the delay in surgery.

Your Decision and Action

You know that the current protocol of keeping all patients NPO after midnight for surgery does not reflect the best available evidence. You also know that there is a multidisciplinary task force working to review and revise the protocol. You decide to call the anesthesia care provider to discuss G.L.'s situation and request that clear liquids be ordered for her.

References for Evidence

American Society of Anesthesiologists Committee on Standards and Practice Parameters: Practice guidelines for preoperative fasting and the use of pharmacologic agents to reduce the risk of pulmonary aspiration: application to healthy patients undergoing elective procedures: an updated report by the ASA Committee on Standards and Practice Parameters, *Anesthesiology* 114(3):495, 2011.

Crenshaw JT: Preoperative fasting: will the evidence ever be put into practice? *Am J Nurs* 111:38, 2011.

disclosure of the diagnosis; the nature and purpose of the proposed treatment; the risks and consequences of the proposed treatment; the probability of a successful outcome; the availability, benefits, and risks of alternative treatments; and the prognosis if treatment is not instituted. Second, the patient must demonstrate clear *understanding* of the information being provided before receiving sedating preoperative medications. Third, the recipient of care must *give consent voluntarily.* The patient must not be persuaded or coerced in any way by anyone to undergo the procedure.[24]

The physician is ultimately responsible for obtaining the patient's consent for surgical treatment. You may be responsible for witnessing the patient's signature on the consent form. At this time, you can be a patient advocate, verifying that the patient (or caregiver) understands the information presented in the consent form and the implications of consent, and that consent for surgery is truly voluntary. If the patient is unclear about the surgical plans, contact the surgeon about the patient's need for additional information. The patient should also be aware that consent, even when signed, can be withdrawn at any time.

If the patient is a minor, unconscious, or mentally incompetent to sign the permit, a legally appointed representative or responsible family member may give written permission. An *emancipated minor* is one who is younger than the legal age of consent but is recognized as having the legal capacity to provide consent.[25] Procedures for obtaining consent vary among states and agencies. Follow specifics required by your state's nurse practice act and agency policies that apply to an individual situation.

ETHICAL/LEGAL DILEMMAS

Informed Consent

Situation

J.S., a 72-year-old woman, is waiting in the preoperative holding area. You are discussing her impending surgery when you realize that this competent adult does not fully understand her surgery and was not informed of the alternatives to this surgery. Although she has previously signed a consent form, your assessment is that she was not fully informed about her treatment options or does not recall them.

Ethical/Legal Points for Consideration

- Informed consent requires that patients have complete information about the proposed treatment, as well as alternative treatments, risks and benefits of each treatment option, and possible consequences of the surgical procedure. The person (usually the surgeon) performing the procedure usually has this responsibility.
- An opportunity to have questions answered about the various treatment options and their possible outcomes is also an important element of informed consent.
- A patient can revoke the consent at any time, even at the very last minute. It is essential that you report any circumstance that suggests that the patient does not understand the information or is revoking the informed consent to the person who obtained the consent.
- In most states, the registered nurse's legal role is to witness the signing of the document. This means that as a nurse, you attest to the fact that the patient's signature was valid.

Discussion Questions

1. What do you think you should do next?
2. What is your role as a patient advocate in the informed consent process?
3. What should you do if the patient states that she does not want to know about the surgical procedure or alternatives to surgery?

A true medical emergency may override the need to obtain consent. When immediate medical treatment is needed to preserve life or to prevent serious impairment to life or limb and the patient is incapable of giving consent, the next of kin may give consent. If reaching the next of kin is not possible, the physician may begin treatment without written consent. A note is written in the chart documenting the medical necessity of the procedure. In the case of an emergency where consent cannot be obtained, the perioperative nurse usually needs to complete an event report because it is an occurrence that is inconsistent with routine facility practices.[26]

DAY-OF-SURGERY PREPARATION

NURSING ROLE. Day-of-surgery preparation varies a great deal depending on whether the patient is an inpatient or an ambulatory surgical patient. Your responsibilities immediately before surgery include final preoperative teaching, assessment, and communication of pertinent findings. In addition, ensure that all preoperative orders are done and that the chart is complete and accompanies the patient to the OR. It is especially important to verify the presence of a signed informed consent, laboratory and diagnostic data, an H&P, a record of any consultations, baseline vital signs, and completed nursing notes. In addition, the site and side of the anticipated surgery are identified and marked with an indelible marker by the surgeon and documented to indicate the patient agrees.[9]

Hospitals often require that a patient wear a hospital gown with no underclothes. Surgical centers may allow the patient to wear underwear, depending on the procedure to be performed. The patient should remove any cosmetics, since observation of skin color is important. Nail polish and artificial nails should be removed so that capillary refill and pulse oximetry can be assessed. Place an identification band on the patient and, if applicable, an allergy band (Fig. 18-1). Return all patient valuables to a caregiver or secure according to institutional protocol. All prostheses, including dentures, contact lenses, and glasses, are generally removed to prevent loss or damage. If electrocautery devices will be used during surgery, jewelry in piercings needs to be removed as a safety measure. Hearing aids should be left in place to allow the patient to better follow instructions. Return glasses to the patient as soon as possible after surgery. Encourage the patient to void before preoperative medications are given and before transfer to the OR. Many preoperative medications interfere with balance and increase the risk for a fall during ambulation. An empty bladder prevents involuntary elimination under anesthesia and reduces the possibility of urinary retention during the early postoperative recovery.

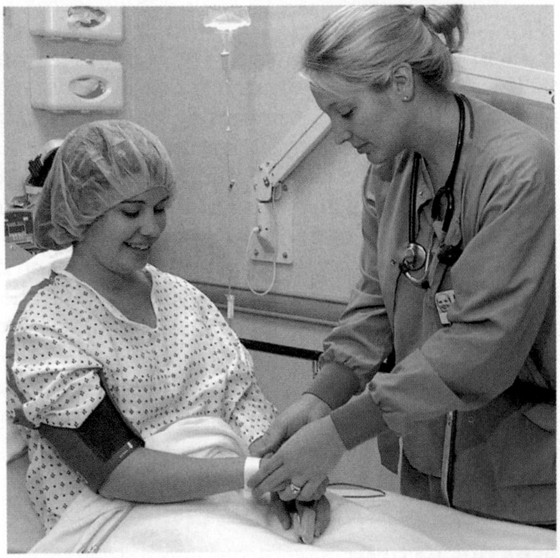

FIG. 18-1 The nurse performs a safety check by verifying that the patient has an identification band (wristband) as part of the preoperative preparations before she goes to surgery.

SAFETY ALERT

Use a preoperative checklist (Table 18-8) to ensure that all preoperative preparations have been completed before the patient is given any sedating medications.

PREOPERATIVE MEDICATIONS. Preoperative medications are used for a variety of reasons (Table 18-9). A patient may receive a single drug or a combination of drugs. Benzodiazepines are used for their sedative and amnesic properties. Anticholinergics are sometimes given to reduce secretions. Opioids may be given to decrease pain and intraoperative anesthetic requirements. Antiemetics may be given to decrease nausea and vomiting.

Other medications that may be administered preoperatively include antibiotics, eyedrops, and routine prescription drugs. Antibiotics may be administered throughout the perioperative period for patients with a history of congenital or valvular heart disease to prevent infective endocarditis and for patients with previous joint replacement. Antibiotics may also be ordered for the patient undergoing surgery where wound contamination is a potential risk (e.g., gastrointestinal surgery) or where wound infection could have serious postoperative consequences (e.g., cardiac and joint replacement surgery). Antibiotics are most commonly administered IV and are usually started preoperatively (e.g., 30 to 60 minutes before the surgical incision).

β-Adrenergic blockers (β-blockers) are sometimes used in people with known hypertension or coronary artery disease to control BP or reduce the chances of myocardial infarction and cardiac arrest.[27] People with diabetes are also carefully monitored and may receive insulin in the preoperative period.[28] Eyedrops are often ordered and given preoperatively for the patient undergoing cataract and other eye surgery. Many times the patient will require multiple sets of eyedrops given at 5-minute intervals. It is important to give these drugs as ordered and on time to adequately prepare the eye for surgery.

Medications that patients routinely take may or may not be used on the day of surgery. To facilitate patient teaching and eliminate confusion about which medications should be taken, carefully check written preoperative orders and clarify the orders with the surgeon and/or ACP if there is any question.

Preoperative medications may be ordered by mouth (PO), IV, or subcutaneously. Provide PO medications with a small sip

INFORMATICS IN PRACTICE

Computer-Based Timing for Antibiotic Administration

- A patient who receives the appropriate preoperative antibiotic has a decreased risk of a health care–associated infection.
- Using a computer to time the administration of preoperative antibiotics can decrease the incidence of wound infections.
- Computer-based timing systems assist with quality of care by tracking patient outcomes.
- You can look at the time patients received antibiotics and compare the rate of wound infections for those who did and did not receive timely treatment.

TABLE 18-8 PREOPERATIVE CHECKLIST

Preoperative Requirements	Initials
Height ____ Weight ____	
Isolation Y or N Type ____	
Allergies noted on chart Y or N	
Vital signs (baseline) T ____ P ____ R ____ BP ____ Pulse Ox ____	
Chart Review	
H&P on chart	
H&P within 30 days? Y or N	
Signed and witnessed informed consent form on chart Y or N	
Signed consent for blood administration Y or NA	
Blood type and crossmatch Y or NA	
Name plate on chart Y or N	
Diagnostic Results	
Hgb/Hct ____ / ____ NA	
PT/INR/PTT ____ / ____ / ____ NA	
CXR ____ NA	
ECG ____ NA	
hCG ____ Negative ____ Positive ____ NA	
Other labs	
Final Chart Review	
Additional forms attached	

Day of Surgery	Initials
Surgical site marked Y or NA	
ID band on patient Y or N	
Allergy band on patient Y or NA	
Vital signs Time ____ T ____ P ____ R ____ BP ____ Pulse Ox ____	
Procedures	
NPO since ____	
Capillary blood glucose Result: ____ NA	
Voided/catheter Time ____	
Preoperative medications given Time ____ NA	
Preoperative antibiotics given Time ____ NA	
Preoperative skin prep Y or NA Shower____ Scrub____ Clip____	
Makeup, nail polish, false fingernails, and false eyelashes removed Y or NA	
Hospital gown applied Y or NA	
Valuables	
Dentures Y or N	
Wig or hairpiece Y or N	
Eyeglasses Y or N	
Contact lenses Y or N	
Hearing aid Y or N	
Prosthesis Y or N	
Jewelry Y or N Piercings with jewelry Y or N	
Clothing Y or N	
Disposition of valuables: Hearing aid in place Y or NA	

Time to OR ____________ Date ____________
Transported to OR by ____________
Final check by ____________ RN ____________

of water 60 to 90 minutes before the patient goes to the OR unless otherwise ordered. Subcutaneous injections (e.g., insulin) and IV medications are usually given to the patient after arrival in the preoperative holding area or OR. Inform the patient about the expected effects of the medications (e.g., drowsiness).

TRANSPORTATION TO THE OPERATING ROOM

For inpatients, transport staff move the patient by stretcher to the OR. Assist the patient in moving from the hospital bed to the stretcher, raise the side rails, and ensure that the completed chart and any ordered preoperative equipment (e.g., sequential compression devices) goes with the patient. In many institutions the caregiver may accompany the patient to the holding area.

In an ambulatory surgical center the patient may be transported to the OR by stretcher or wheelchair. If no sedatives have been given, the patient may even walk accompanied to the OR. In all cases it is important to ensure patient safety during transport. Document the method of transportation and the person who transports the patient to the OR. You are also responsible for the hand-off communication to the nurse receiving the patient. This provides an opportunity for each of you to ensure that all pertinent information regarding the patient has been shared.[29] To avoid adverse events related to miscommunication, AORN recommends the use of the Situation-Background-Assessment-Recommendation (SBAR) model for the hand-off process in this setting[30,31] (see Table 1-7).

Show the caregiver where to wait for the patient during surgery. Many hospitals have a surgical waiting room where OR personnel communicate the patient's status to the caregiver(s) and notify them when the surgery is complete. The surgeon also can locate the caregiver in this room after surgery to discuss the outcome. Some hospitals provide pagers to caregivers so that they may eat or do errands during the surgery.

CULTURALLY COMPETENT CARE

PREOPERATIVE PATIENT

Include cultural considerations when assessing and implementing care for the patient's preoperative needs. For example,

TABLE 18-9 **DRUG THERAPY**

Commonly Used Preoperative Medications

Class	Drug	Purpose
Antibiotics	cefazolin (Ancef)	Prevent postoperative infection
Anticholinergics	atropine (Isopto Atropine) glycopyrrolate (Robinul)	↓ Oral and respiratory secretions
	scopolamine (Transderm-Scōp)	Prevent nausea and vomiting Provide sedation
Antidiabetics	insulin (Humulin R)	Stabilize blood glucose
Antiemetics	metoclopramide (Reglan)	↑ Gastric emptying
	ondansetron (Zofran)	Prevent nausea and vomiting
Benzodiazepines	midazolam (Versed) diazepam (Valium) lorazepam (Ativan)	↓ Anxiety, induce sedation, amnesic effects
β-Blockers	labetalol (Normodyne)	Manage hypertension
Histamine (H_2)-receptor antagonists	famotidine (Pepcid) ranitidine (Zantac)	↓ HCl acid secretion, ↑ pH, ↓ gastric volume
Opioids	morphine (Duramorph) fentanyl (Sublimaze)	Relieve pain during preoperative procedures

culture often determines one's expression of pain, family expectations, and ability to verbally express needs. One's culture may require that the family be included in any decision making. For example, many older Hispanic women may defer to their family for the decision to have or not to have surgery. Respect these decisions. If the patient or caregiver does not speak English, it is mandated that a qualified translator or translator communication system be used.[32] (Culturally competent care is discussed in Chapter 2.)

GERONTOLOGIC CONSIDERATIONS

PREOPERATIVE PATIENT

Many surgical procedures are performed on patients older than 65 years of age. Surgery on older adults requires careful evaluation.[33] Frequently performed procedures in older adults include cataract extraction, coronary and vascular procedures, prostate surgery, herniorrhaphy, cholecystectomy, and joint repair or replacement.

Be particularly alert when assessing and caring for the older adult surgical patient. An event that has little effect on a younger adult may be overwhelming to the older patient. Emotional reactions to impending surgery and hospitalization often intensify in the older adult. Hospitalization may represent a physical decline and loss of health, mobility, and independence. The older adult may view the hospital as a place to die or as a stepping-stone to nursing home placement. Help to decrease anxieties and fears, as well as maintaining and restoring the self-esteem of the older adult during the surgical experience.

The risks associated with anesthesia and surgery increase in the older patient.[33] In general, the older the patient, the greater the risk of complications after surgery. In planning care, consider the patient's physiologic status, not simply the chronologic age. The surgical risk in the older adult relates to normal physiologic aging and changes that compromise organ function, reduce reserve capacity, and limit the body's ability to adapt to stress. This decreased ability to cope with stress, often compounded by the burden of one or more chronic illnesses, and the surgery itself increase the risk of complications.

When preparing the older adult for surgery, obtain a detailed H&P. Preoperative laboratory tests, an ECG, and a chest x-ray are important in planning the choice and type of anesthesia. The patient's primary physician is usually not the surgeon, and frequently several physicians are involved in the patient's care. Help to coordinate the care for the older adult patient.

Many older adults have sensory deficits. Vision and hearing may be reduced, and bright lights may bother those with eye problems. Thought processes and cognitive abilities may be slowed or impaired. Assess and document baseline sensory and cognitive function. Physical reactions are often slowed as a result of mobility and balance problems. All these changes may require more time for the older adult to complete preoperative testing and understand preoperative instructions. These changes also require attention to promote patient safety and prevent injury. (See Chapter 5 for more discussion about older adults.)

When older adults live in some type of long-term care facility, you may need to coordinate transportation from these agencies so that timely arrival allows for surgery preparation. A legal representative of the patient must be present to provide consent for surgery if the patient cannot sign for himself or herself.

Finally, determine the presence of or need for caregiver support for the older adult undergoing surgery. With the increase in outpatient surgical procedures and shorter postoperative length of stays, caregiver support is often critical in the continuity of care for this population.

CASE STUDY

Preoperative Patient

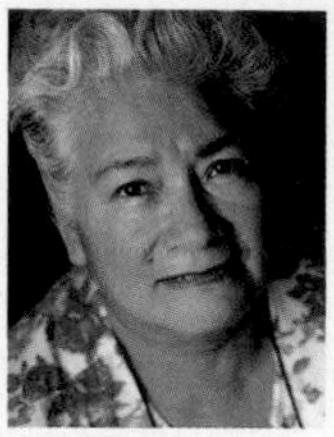

Ryan McVay/Photodisc/ Thinkstock

Patient Profile

F.D., a 72-year-old Hispanic retired librarian, is admitted to the hospital with compromised circulation of the right lower leg and a necrotic right foot. She has diabetes and takes insulin to maintain appropriate blood glucose levels. In addition, she has hypertension and kidney and peripheral vascular disease. She has been NPO since midnight. It is now 10 AM on the morning of the surgery.

Subjective Data

- History of type 2 diabetes mellitus for 30 years; states "my blood sugar is hard to control" and "I just started taking insulin"
- History of hypertension
- History of stage 2 chronic kidney disease
- History of peripheral vascular disease
- History of macular degeneration in right eye; reports poor vision
- Surgical history: cesarean section at age 30, cholecystectomy at age 65; reports poor wound healing after last surgery
- Social Security checks barely cover the cost of living
- States she often runs out of medications and cannot always afford to refill them right away
- Reports chronic burning pain in both legs and has trouble sleeping at night
- Lives alone but has family who want her to move in with them after surgery
- Uses herbs to control blood glucose levels and frequently skips her insulin

Objective Data

Physical Examination

- Alert, cognitively intact, anxious, older woman with complaints of numbness and lack of feeling in right leg
- Weight 190 lb, height 5 ft 3 in
- BP 180/94, pulse 84 and slightly irregular
- Wears glasses for close work and reading
- Has macular degeneration in right eye

Diagnostic Studies

- Admission serum blood glucose level 272 mg/dL (15.2 mmol/L); glycosylated hemoglobin (Hb A1C) 14%
- Morning capillary blood glucose level 198 mg/dL (11 mmol/L)
- Doppler pulses for right lower leg weak, absent in right foot
- Doppler pulses in left lower leg present, weak in left foot
- Serum creatinine 2.0 mg/dL (176 mmol/L)

Collaborative Care

- Scheduled for a below-the-knee amputation of the right leg at 1 PM today

Discussion Questions

1. What factors may influence F.D.'s response to hospitalization and surgery?
2. ***Priority Decision:*** Given F.D.'s history, what priority preoperative nursing assessments would you want to complete and why?
3. What potential perioperative complications might you expect for F.D.?
4. ***Priority Decision:*** What priority topics would you include in F.D.'s preoperative teaching plan?
5. ***Priority Decision:*** Based on the assessment data presented, identify the priority nursing diagnoses and related interventions. Are there any collaborative problems?
6. ***Delegation Decision:*** Identify appropriate preoperative interventions that need to be completed and could be delegated to unlicensed assistive personnel (UAP).
7. ***Evidence-Based Practice:*** F.D. asks you why she received insulin this morning when she has not eaten anything since midnight. How would you respond to her?

evolve Answers available at *http://evolve.elsevier.com/Lewis/medsurg.*

BRIDGE TO NCLEX EXAMINATION

The number of the question corresponds to the same-numbered outcome at the beginning of the chapter.

1. An overweight patient (BMI 28.1 kg/m^2) is scheduled for a laparoscopic cholecystectomy at an outpatient surgery setting. The nurse knows that
   a. surgery will involve multiple small incisions.
   b. this setting is not appropriate for this procedure.
   c. surgery will involve removing a portion of the liver.
   d. the patient will need special preparation because of obesity.
2. The patient tells the nurse in the preoperative setting that she has noticed she has a reaction when wearing rubber gloves. What is the most appropriate intervention?
   a. Notify the surgeon so the case can be cancelled.
   b. Ask additional questions to assess for a possible latex allergy.
   c. Notify the OR staff immediately so that latex-free supplies can be used.
   d. No intervention is needed because the patient's rubber sensitivity has no bearing on surgery.
3. A 59-year-old man is scheduled for a herniorrhaphy in 2 days. During the preoperative evaluation he reports that he takes ginkgo daily. What is the priority intervention?
   a. Inform the surgeon, since the procedure may need to be rescheduled.
   b. Notify the anesthesia care provider, since this herb interferes with anesthetics.
   c. Ask the patient if he has noticed any side effects from taking this herbal supplement.
   d. Tell the patient to continue to take the herbal supplement up to the day before surgery.

4. A 17-year-old patient with a leg fracture is scheduled for surgery. She reports that she is living with a friend and is an emancipated minor. She has a statement from the court for verification. Which intervention is most appropriate?
   a. Witness the permit after consent is obtained by the surgeon.
   b. Call a parent or legal guardian to sign the permit, since the patient is under 18.
   c. Obtain verbal consent, since written consent is not necessary for emancipated minors.
   d. Investigate your state's nurse practice act related to emancipated minors and informed consent.
5. A priority nursing intervention to assist a preoperative patient in coping with fear of postoperative pain would be to
   a. inform the patient that pain medication will be available.
   b. teach the patient to use guided imagery to help manage pain.
   c. describe the type of pain expected with the patient's particular surgery.
   d. explain the pain management plan, including the use of a pain rating scale.
6. A patient is scheduled for surgery requiring general anesthesia at an ambulatory surgical center. The nurse asks him when he ate last. He replies that he had a light breakfast a couple of hours before coming to the surgery center. What should the nurse do first?
   a. Tell the patient to come back tomorrow, since he ate a meal.
   b. Proceed with the preoperative checklist, including site identification.
   c. Notify the anesthesia care provider of when and what the patient last ate.
   d. Have the patient void before administering any preoperative medications.
7. A patient who normally takes 40 units of glargine insulin (long acting) at bedtime asks the nurse what to do about her dose the night before surgery. The best response would be to have her
   a. skip her insulin altogether the night before surgery.
   b. take her usual dose at bedtime and eat a light breakfast in the morning.
   c. eat a moderate meal before bedtime and then take half her usual insulin dose.
   d. get instructions from her surgeon or health care provider on any insulin adjustments.
8. Preoperative considerations for older adults include *(select all that apply)*
   a. only using large-print educational materials.
   b. speaking louder for patients with hearing aids.
   c. recognizing that sensory deficits may be present.
   d. providing warm blankets to prevent hypothermia.
   e. teaching important information early in the morning.

1. a, 2. b, 3. a, 4. a, 5. d, 6. c, 7. d, 8. c, d

evolve

For rationales to these answers and even more NCLEX review questions, visit *http://evolve.elsevier.com/Lewis/medsurg.*

REFERENCES

1. Jehovah's Witness Official Website: You have the right to choose. Retrieved from *www.watchtower.org/e/hb/article_04.htm.*

*2. Sanatani M, Schreier G, Stitt L: Level and direction of hope in cancer patients: an exploratory longitudinal study, *Support Care Cancer* 16:493, 2008.

3. Levy J, Key N, Azran M: Novel oral anticoagulants: implications in the perioperative setting. Retrieved from *http://journals.lww.com/anesthesiology/Fulltext/2010/09000/Novel_Oral_Anticoagulants__Implications_in_the.38.aspx.*

4. American Society of Anesthesiologists: Common questions by patients preparing for anesthesia. Retrieved from *www.asahq.org/sitecore/content/Lifeline/Anesthesia-Topics/Michigan/Common-Questions-for-Patients-Preparing-for-Anesthesia.aspx.*

5. American Society of Anesthesiologists: What you should know about your patients' use of herbal medicines and other dietary supplements. Retrieved from *https://ecommerce.asahq.org/p-131-considerations-for-anesthesiologists-what-you-should-know-about-your-patients-use-of-herbal-medicines.aspx.*

6. American Academy of Allergy, Asthma, and Immunology: Tips to remember: latex allergy, 2007. Retrieved from *www.aaaai.org/patients/publicedmat/tips/latexallergy.stm.*

7. Association of periOperative Registered Nurses: *Perioperative standards and recommended practices*, Denver, 2010, The Association.

*Evidence-based information for clinical practice.

*8. Slor C, de Jonghe J, Vreeswijk R, et al: Anesthesia and postoperative delirium in older adults undergoing hip surgery, *J Am Geriatr Society* 59:7, 2011.

*9. Hepner DL: The role of testing in the preoperative evaluation, *Cleve Clin J Med.* Retrieved from *www.ccjm.org/content/76/Suppl_4/S22.full.*

10. Yalamarthi S: Perioperative steroids in surgical patients. Retrieved from *www.hmjanaesthesia.4t.com/periopsteroid.htm.*

11. Neil JA: Perioperative care of the immunocompromised patient, *AORN J* 85:544, 2007.

12. Neil JA: Perioperative care of the patient with tuberculosis, *AORN J* 88:942, 2008.

13. Ide P, Farber E, Lautz D: Perioperative nursing care of the bariatric surgical patient, *AORN J* 88:30, 2008.

14. Posthauer M, Dorner B, Collins, N, et al: A critical component of wound healing, *Adv Skin Wound Care* 23:12, 2010.

15. Health News Feed, John Hopkins Medical Information: Caffeine withdrawal. Retrieved from *www.hopkinsmedicine.org/hnf/hnf_915.htm.*

16. Code of Federal Regulations for Hospitals: *Surgical services*, §482.45 42 CFR Ch. IV (10-1-04 Edition). Retrieved from *http://edocket.access.gpo.gov/cfr_2004/octqtr/pdf/42cfr482.51.pdf.*

17. Durai R, Ng P, Hogue H: Methicillin-resistant *Staphylococcus aureus*: an update, *AORN J* 91:5, 2010.

*18. Kruzik N: Benefits of preoperative education for adult elective surgery patients, *AORN J* 90:3, 2009.

19. Appendix L—Guidance for surveyors: ambulatory surgical. In *State operations manual*, Survey procedures §416.52(c)(1), US Department of Health and Human Services, Centers for

Medicare and Medicaid Services. Retrieved from *www.cms.gov/manuals/Downloads/som107ap_l_ambulatory.pdf*.
20. American Hospital Association: The patient care partnership: understanding expectations, rights and responsibilities. Retrieved from *www.aha.org/aha/content/2003/pdf/pcp_english_030730.pdf*.
*21. Odom-Forren J: Postoperative patient care and pain management. In JC Rothrock, editor: *Alexander's care of the patient in surgery*, ed 14, St Louis, 2011, Mosby.
*22. Practice guidelines for preoperative fasting and the use of pharmacologic agents to reduce the risk of pulmonary aspiration: application to healthy patients undergoing elective procedures: an updated report by the American Society of Anesthesiologists Committee on Standards and Practice Parameters, *Anesthesiology* 114:3, 2011.
23. American College of Surgeons: Public information from the American College of Surgeons: principle of informed consent. Retrieved from *www.facs.org/public_info/operation/consent.html*.
24. Phillips NF, Berry EC, Kohn ML: *Berry and Kohn's operating room technique*, ed 12, St Louis, 2013, Mosby.
25. DiFusco LA: Pediatric surgery. In Rothrock JC, editor: *Alexander's care of the patient in surgery*, ed 14, St Louis, 2011, Mosby.
26. Rothrock JC: *Alexander's care of the patient in surgery*, ed 14, St Louis, 2011, Mosby.
*27. Wolf A, McGoldrick K: Cardiovascular pharmacotherapeutic considerations in patients undergoing anesthesia, *Cardiol Rev* 19:1, 2011.
28. DeLamar LM: Anesthesia. In Rothrock JC, editor: *Alexander's care of the patient in surgery*, ed 14, St Louis, 2011, Mosby.
*29. American Society of PeriAnesthesia Nurses: *2010-2012 Perianesthesia nursing and practice recommendations*, Cherry Hill, NJ, 2010, The Society.
30. Association of periOperative Registered Nurses: Perioperative patient hand-off tool kit: AORN practice resources. Retrieved from *www.aorn.org/PracticeResources/ToolKits/PatientHandOffToolKit*.
31. Murphy EK: Patient safety and risk management. In Rothrock JC, editor: *Alexander's care of the patient in surgery*, ed 14, St Louis, 2011, Mosby.
32. Wilson-Stronks A, Lee KK, Cordero CL, et al: *One size does not fit all: meeting the health care needs of diverse populations*, Washington, DC, 2008, The Joint Commission. Retrieved from *www.jointcommission.org/assets/1/6/HLCOneSizeFinal.pdf*.
33. Chow WB, Ko CY, Rosenthal RA, et al: American College of Surgeons NSQIP®/AGS best practice guidelines: optimal preoperative assessment of the geriatric surgical patient. Retrieved from *www.jhartfound.org/blog/wp-content/upLoads/2012/10/ACS-NSQIP-AGS-Geriatric-2012-Guidelines6.pdf*.

RESOURCES

Resources for this chapter are listed in Chapter 20 on p. 366.

CHAPTER 19

The ultimate measure of a man is not where he stands in moments of comfort and convenience, but where he stands at times of challenge and controversy.
Martin Luther King, Jr.

Nursing Management
Intraoperative Care

Anita Jo Shoup and David M. Horner*

evolve WEBSITE

http://evolve.elsevier.com/Lewis/medsurg

- NCLEX Review Questions
- Key Points
- Pre-Test
- Rationales for Bridge to NCLEX Examination Questions
- Concept Map Creator
- Glossary
- Content Updates

eFigures
- eFig. 19-1: Surgical safety checklist
- eFig. 19-2: Emergency therapy for malignant hyperthermia

eTable
- eTable 19-1: Fire Risk Assessment Tool

LEARNING OUTCOMES

1. Differentiate the purposes of the various areas of the perioperative/surgery department and the proper attire for each area.
2. Differentiate the roles and responsibilities of the interdisciplinary surgical team members.
3. Prioritize needs of patients undergoing surgery.
4. Analyze the role of the perioperative nurse in the management of the patient undergoing surgery.
5. Apply basic principles of aseptic technique used in the operating room.
6. Evaluate the importance of safety in the operating room relative to patients, equipment, and anesthesia.
7. Differentiate the common types of and delivery systems for anesthesia.

KEY TERMS

anesthesia care provider (ACP), p. 336
anesthesiology, p. 336
epidural block, p. 345
general anesthesia, p. 341
local anesthesia, p. 342
malignant hyperthermia (MH), p. 346
nurse anesthetist, p. 336
regional anesthesia, p. 342
spinal anesthesia, p. 345

Historically, surgery took place in the traditional environment of the hospital operating room (OR). However, now the majority of surgical procedures are performed as ambulatory surgery (outpatient surgery). This chapter includes a discussion of the intraoperative care that is applicable to all surgical patients regardless of where the surgery if performed.

PHYSICAL ENVIRONMENT OF OPERATING ROOM

Department Layout

The *surgical suite* is a controlled environment designed to minimize the spread of pathogens and allow a smooth flow of patients, staff, and equipment needed to provide safe patient care. The suite is divided into three distinct areas: unrestricted, semirestricted, and restricted areas. The *unrestricted area* is where people in street clothes can interact with those in surgical attire. These areas typically include the points of entry for patients (e.g., holding area), staff (e.g., locker rooms), and information (e.g., nursing station or control desk). The *semirestricted area* includes the surrounding support areas and corridors. Only authorized staff are allowed access to the semirestricted areas. All staff in the semirestricted area must wear surgical attire and cover all head and facial hair. In the *restricted area* masks are required to supplement surgical attire.[1] The restricted area can include the OR, scrub sink area, and clean core.

In addition, the physical layout is designed to reduce cross-contamination. The flow of clean and sterile supplies and equipment should be separated from contaminated supplies,

*Contributed section on anesthesia content.
Reviewed by Ronald R. Castaldo, CRNA, MBA, MS, CCRN, Staff Nurse Anesthetist, Anesthesia Services, New Castle, Delaware; Lisa Kiper, RN, MSN, Assistant Professor of Nursing, Morehead State University, Morehead, Kentucky; Angela M. Martinelli, RN, PhD, CNOR, Science Officer, Congressionally Directed Medical Research Programs, Fort Detrick, Maryland; and Cynthia Schoonover, RN, MS, CCRN, Associate Nursing Professor, Sinclair Community College, Dayton, Ohio and PACU Staff Nurse, Kettering Medical Center, Kettering, Ohio.

equipment, and waste by space, time, and traffic patterns. Staff move supplies from clean areas, such as the clean core, through the OR for surgery, and on to the surrounding areas, such as the instrument decontamination area.[2]

Holding Area

The *holding area,* frequently called the *preoperative holding area,* is a special waiting area inside of or adjacent to the surgical suite. The size can range from a centralized area to accommodate numerous patients to a small designated area immediately outside the actual room scheduled for the surgical procedure. The holding area is where you identify and assess the patient before transferring him or her to the OR.

The *Surgical Care Improvement Project* (SCIP) is a national quality partnership of organizations focused on improving surgical care by significantly reducing the number of complications from surgery[3] (refer to *www.jointcommission.org/assets/1/6/Surgical%20Care%20Improvement%20Project.pdf*). Several SCIP measures may be implemented in the holding area, such as drug administration, patient warming, and application of sequential compression devices (SCDs). Many minor procedures (e.g., inserting IV catheters and arterial lines) can also be performed here.

The National Patient Safety Goals (NPSGs) require a preprocedure process, including the verification of relevant documentation (e.g., history and physical examination, signed consent form, nursing and preanesthesia assessment). In addition, any required blood products, implants, devices, and special equipment need to be available. Further, any diagnostic and radiology test results (e.g., x-rays, biopsy reports) need to be properly labeled and displayed.[4]

In addition, the NPSGs require that the surgeon mark the procedure site. If possible, the marking should be done with the patient's involvement.[4]

In some settings, another area for holding is identified as the *admission, observation, and discharge* (AOD) area. This area is designed to allow early-morning admission for outpatient surgery, same-day admission, and inpatient holding before surgery. In this area you can assess preoperative information, observe the patient both before and after surgery, and allow sufficient recovery time before the patient is discharged to either the home or an inpatient room. The AOD area is important in the patient's stay throughout outpatient surgery and prevents unnecessary overnight stays in the inpatient setting.

Separation from caregivers just before surgery can produce anxiety for the patient. This anxiety can be reduced when the caregiver is permitted to wait with the patient in the holding area until the patient is transferred to the OR.

Operating Room

The traditional surgical environment, or OR, is a unique setting removed from other hospital clinical units. It is controlled geographically, environmentally, and bacteriologically, and it is restricted in terms of the inflow and outflow of staff (Fig. 19-1). It is preferable to have the OR located next to the postanesthesia care unit (PACU) and the surgical intensive care unit. This allows for quick transport of the postoperative patient and close proximity to anesthesia staff if complications arise.

Several methods are used to prevent the transmission of infection. Filters and controlled airflow in the ventilating systems provide dust control. Positive air pressure in the rooms prevents air from entering the OR from the halls and corridors.

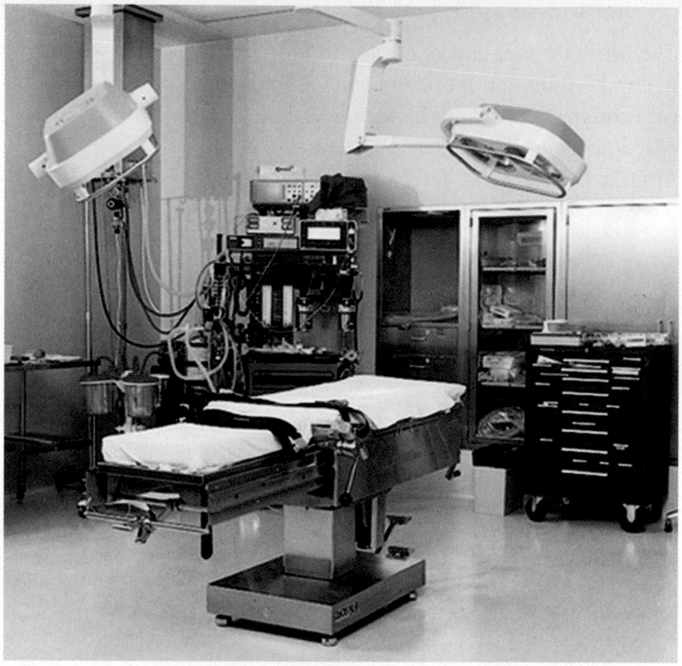

FIG. 19-1 Typical operating room.

Ultraviolet (UV) lighting may be used because UV radiation reduces the number of microorganisms in the air. Dust-collecting surfaces such as open shelves and tables are omitted. Materials that are resistant to the corroding effects of strong disinfectants are used.

Overall safety and comfort are aided by the use of OR furniture that is adjustable, easy to clean, and easy to move. All equipment is checked frequently to ensure proper functioning and electrical safety. The lighting is designed to provide a low- to high-intensity range for a precise view of the surgical site (see Fig. 19-2). A communication system provides a means for the delivery of routine and emergency messages.[5,6]

SURGICAL TEAM

Registered Nurse

The *perioperative nurse* is a registered nurse (RN) who implements patient care during the perioperative period. Through close collaboration with the other members of the surgical team, you prepare the OR for patients before they arrive. You are usually the first member of the surgical team who meets the patient. You are the patient's advocate throughout the intraoperative experience. This includes maintaining the patient's safety, privacy, dignity, and confidentiality; communicating with the patient; and providing physical care. Assess the patient to determine any additional needs or tasks to complete before surgery. Provide physical and emotional comfort and patient and caregiver teaching regarding the upcoming surgery. In addition, work with the patient's caregivers, keeping them informed and answering questions. This is particularly important in day-surgery areas where caregivers must assume greater responsibility for preoperative and postoperative care.

In the perioperative role, you assume functions that involve either sterile or unsterile activities (Table 19-1). When you serve in the role of *scrub nurse,* you follow the designated scrub procedure, are gowned and gloved in sterile attire, and remain in the sterile field (Fig. 19-2). When you serve in the role of *circu-*

TABLE 19-1 INTRAOPERATIVE ACTIVITIES OF PERIOPERATIVE NURSE

Circulating, Nonsterile Activities
- Reviews anatomy, physiology, and surgical procedure
- Assists in preparing room, ensuring that supplies and equipment are available, in working order, and sterile (if required)
- Maintains aseptic technique in all required activities
- Monitors practices of aseptic technique in self and others
- Checks mechanical and electrical equipment and environmental factors
- Conducts a preprocedure verification process
- Assesses patient's physical and emotional status
- Verifies and implements ordered SCIP measures
- Plans and coordinates intraoperative nursing care
- Checks chart and relates pertinent data to team members
- Participates in the application of monitoring devices and insertion of invasive lines and other devices
- Assists with and ensures patient safety in transferring and positioning patient
- Assists with induction of anesthesia
- Monitors draping procedure
- Participates in surgical time-out
- Documents intraoperative care
- Prepares, records, labels, and sends blood, pathology, and any anatomic specimens to proper locations
- Measures blood, urine output, and other fluid loss
- Verifies, dispenses, and records medications used, including local anesthetics
- Coordinates all intraoperative activities with team members and other health-related staff and departments
- Maintains accurate count of sponges, needles, instruments, and medical devices that could be retained in the patient
- Accompanies patient to PACU
- Provides hand-off report to PACU nurse with information relevant to care of patient

Scrubbed, Sterile Activities
- Reviews anatomy, physiology, and surgical procedure
- Assists in preparing the operating room
- Completes surgical hand and arm scrub, and gowns and gloves self and other members of surgical team
- Prepares instrument table and organizes sterile equipment for functional use
- Assists with draping procedure
- Participates in surgical time-out procedure
- Passes instruments to surgeon and assistants by anticipating their needs
- Maintains accurate count of sponges, needles, instruments, and medical devices that could be retained in the patient
- Monitors practices of aseptic technique in self and others
- Keeps track of irrigation solutions used for calculation of blood loss
- Accepts, verifies, and reports medications used by surgeon and/or ACP, including local anesthetics

ACP, Anesthesia care provider; *PACU,* postanesthesia care unit; *SCIP,* Surgical Care Improvement Project.

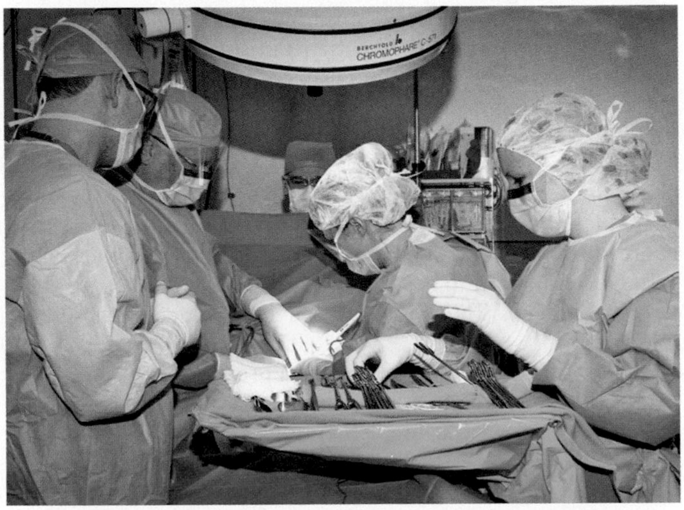

FIG. 19-2 The complexity of surgery requires maintaining asepsis.

lating nurse, you remain in the unsterile field and so you are not gowned and gloved in sterile attire.

Ongoing assessment of the patient is essential because the patient's condition may change quickly. You respond to these changes and revise the plan of care as needed. Examples of nursing activities that characterize each phase surrounding the surgical experience are presented in Table 19-2.

As patients move through the surgical experience, they are cared for by many team members. Opportunities for error are created whenever clinical information is shared among these members.[7] The Joint Commission requires that all health care providers implement a standardized approach to hand-off communication. The perioperative RN ensures that a complete and accurate hand-off using a consistent format, such as SBAR (see Table 1-7), occurs every time the responsibility for patient care is transferred to another professional. Examples of such transfers include change of shift, surgeon to nurse, and OR nurse to postanesthesia nurse.

You also have the opportunity to become a certified operating room nurse (CNOR). Certification reflects expertise in surgical nursing. The credential is a personal commitment to higher standards that inspires credibility and confidence with patients and peers in the workplace.[8]

Licensed Practical/Vocational Nurse and Surgical Technologist

Depending on your state nurse practice act, the role of the circulating or scrub nurse may be filled by a licensed practical/vocational nurse or a surgical technologist. Surgical technologists may attend an associate degree program, a vocational training program, or a hospital or military training program. The Association of Surgical Technologists is an organization that sets standards for education, provides continuing education opportunities, and offers certification for surgical technologists.[9]

If the circulating nurse is not an RN, the licensed practical/vocational nurse or surgical technologist must have access to an RN at all times. You are responsible for supervising the licensed practical/vocational nurse or surgical technologist in the performance of all delegated nursing tasks.[10]

Surgeon and Assistant

The *surgeon* is the physician who performs the surgical procedure. The surgeon is primarily responsible for the following:

- Preoperative medical history and physical assessment, including need for surgical intervention, choice of surgical procedure, management of preoperative testing, and discussion of the risks of and alternatives to surgical intervention

TABLE 19-2 NURSING ACTIVITIES DURING SURGICAL EXPERIENCE*

Before	During	After
Assessment and Planning	**Implementation**	**Evaluation**
Home, Clinic, Holding Area Initiates preoperative assessment Plans teaching appropriate to patient's needs Involves caregiver	**Safety Maintenance** Ensures integrity of sterile field Ensures that sponge, needle, instrument, and medical device counts are correct Positions patient to ensure correct alignment, exposure of surgical site, and prevention of injury Prevents chemical injury from prepping solutions, pharmaceuticals, etc. Ensures safe use of electrical equipment Safely administers medications	**Postanesthesia, Discharge Area** Determines patient's response to surgical intervention Monitors ABCs, vital signs, level of consciousness Safely administers medications
Surgical Unit Completes preoperative assessment Coordinates patient teaching with staff Develops a plan of care that reflects patient's level of function and ability	**Monitoring Physical Status** Monitors and reports changes in patient's vital signs Monitors blood loss and urine output	**Clinical Unit** Evaluates effectiveness of nursing care in OR using patient outcome criteria Determines patient's level of satisfaction with care given during perioperative period Determines patient's psychologic status Assists with discharge planning
Surgical Suite Conducts preprocedure verification Assesses patient's level of consciousness, skin integrity, mobility, emotional status, and functional limitations Reviews chart Ensures all supplies and equipment needed are available, functioning, and sterile, if appropriate	**Monitoring Psychologic Status** Provides emotional support to patient Stands near or touches patient during procedures Ensures patient's right to privacy is maintained Communicates patient's emotional status to health care team	**Home, Clinic** Seeks patient's perception of surgery in terms of effects of anesthetic agents, impact on body image, immobilization Determines caregiver's perceptions of surgery

*List of activities is not all-inclusive.
ABCs, Airway, breathing, circulation.

- Patient safety and management in the OR
- Postoperative management of the patient

The surgeon's assistant can be a physician who functions in an assisting role during the surgical procedure. The assistant usually holds retractors to expose surgical areas and assists with hemostasis and suturing. In some instances, especially in educational settings, the assistant may perform some portions of the surgery under the surgeon's direct supervision. In many institutions the surgeon's assistant is a registered nurse first assistant or a physician's assistant (PA) who functions under the physician's direct supervision.

Registered Nurse First Assistant

The *registered nurse first assistant* (RNFA) works in collaboration with the surgeon to produce an optimal surgical outcome for the patient. The Association of periOperative Registered Nurses (AORN) position statement on RNFAs states that the perioperative nurse must have formal education for this role and works collaboratively with the surgeon, patient, and surgical team by handling tissue, using instruments, providing exposure to the surgical site, assisting with hemostasis, and suturing.[6,11] RNFA education programs are designed to provide RNs with the education necessary to assume this expanded role.[12] The RNFA can also obtain certification.

Anesthesia Care Provider

The **anesthesia care provider (ACP)** is a person who administers anesthesia and can be an anesthesiologist, nurse anesthetist, or anesthesiologist assistant (AA). **Anesthesiology** is a discipline within the practice of medicine that specializes in the following:

- Medically managing patients who are unconscious or insensible to pain and emotional stress during surgical and other medical procedures
- Protecting functions and vital organs under the stress of anesthetic, surgical, or other medical procedures
- Managing pain
- Managing cardiopulmonary resuscitation
- Managing problems in pulmonary care
- Managing critically ill patients in special care units

ACPs who are anesthesiologists are responsible for administering anesthetic agents to relieve pain and manage vital life functions (e.g., breathing, blood pressure [BP]) during surgery. After surgery they provide care during recovery.[13]

A **nurse anesthetist** is an RN who has graduated from an accredited nurse anesthesia program (minimally a master's degree program) and successfully completed a national certification examination to become a certified registered nurse anesthetist (CRNA). The CRNA scope of practice includes the following:[14]

- Performing and documenting a preanesthetic assessment and evaluation
- Developing and implementing a plan for delivering anesthesia
- Selecting and initiating the planned anesthetic technique
- Selecting, obtaining, and administering the anesthesia, adjuvant drugs, and fluids
- Selecting, applying, and inserting appropriate noninvasive and invasive monitoring devices
- Managing a patient's airway and pulmonary status
- Managing emergence and recovery from anesthesia
- Releasing or discharging patients from a PACU
- Ordering, initiating, or modifying pain relief therapy
- Responding to emergency situations by providing airway management, and administering emergency fluids and drugs
- Assuming additional responsibilities within the expertise of the individual

An *anesthesiologist assistant* (AA) is a specialty PA who functions under the direction of an anesthesiologist in many states. The AA has graduated from an accredited program (minimally a master's degree program) and successfully completed a national certification examination. AAs participate in the provision of all types of anesthesia, including administering drugs, obtaining vascular access, applying and interpreting monitors, establishing and maintaining airways, and assisting with preoperative assessments.

NURSING MANAGEMENT PATIENT BEFORE SURGERY

The preoperative assessment of the surgical patient establishes baseline data for intraoperative and postoperative care. Preoperative care of the patient is discussed in Chapter 18. Some additional information is discussed in this chapter.

PSYCHOSOCIAL ASSESSMENT

Knowing about the activities that occur when a patient is moved into the surgical suite allows you to provide explanations and reassurances, especially to the anxious patient. You can usually answer general questions regarding surgery or anesthesia, such as "When will I go to sleep?" "Who will be in the room?" "When will my surgeon arrive?" "How much of my body will be exposed?" "Will I be cold?" "When will I wake up?" Specific questions relating to details of the surgical procedure and anesthesia may be referred to the surgeon or the ACP.

Performing a cultural and spiritual assessment can help you understand the patient's response to the surgical experience (see Tables 2-7 and Table 10-5 for additional information). For example, members of the Jehovah's Witness community may refuse blood transfusions.[15] For Muslims, the left hand is considered unclean, so you should use the right hand to give forms, drugs, and treatments.[16] Some Native American patients may request that surgically removed body tissue be preserved so that it may be buried. Some tattoos and body piercings may also have cultural meaning.[17] Some patients may have a prayer cloth or other traditional or sacred item with them. Consider spiritual needs and beliefs in the individualized plan of care. For patients who do not speak English, a qualified interpreter must be used (see Table 2-10).

PHYSICAL ASSESSMENT

Perform a thorough physical assessment during the preoperative preparation of the patient (see Chapter 18).

CHART REVIEW

Required chart data vary with agency policy, patient condition, and specific surgical procedures. Because ambulatory surgery facilities tend to have a healthier population, fewer tests may be required. Examples of data that are obtained during the preoperative assessment can be found in Tables 18-2 and 18-4. This information contributes to an understanding of past and present history, cardiopulmonary status, and potential for infection and other complications.

ADMITTING THE PATIENT

Hospital policy designates the protocol to be followed when admitting the patient to the holding area and OR. A general routine includes initial greeting, extension of human contact and warmth, and proper identification. A preprocedure verification process is conducted before the start of surgery. In some institutions this takes place in the holding area; in others it takes place in the OR itself.

COMPLEMENTARY & ALTERNATIVE THERAPIES

Music Therapy

Music is an ancient healing tool recognized in the writings of Plato.

Scientific Evidence

Strong scientific evidence for use in reducing stress and anxiety and enhancing mood.*

Nursing Implications

- To be effective, the music selected needs to be appropriate for the situation. Music can have many different physiologic effects.
  - Listening to calming music can result in slower, deeper breathing and a decrease in heart rate and blood pressure. Both of these indicate relaxation.
  - Music with a faster pace can energize a person and promote mental alertness.
- Music therapy is safe in combination with other treatment approaches.

*Based on a systematic review of scientific literature. Retrieved from *www.naturalstandard.com*.

Complementary and alternative therapies such as therapeutic touch, aromatherapy, music therapy, guided imagery, and even movies may be used for surgical patients. (See the Complementary & Alternative Therapies box above on music and Chapter 6.) These therapies may decrease anxiety, promote relaxation, reduce pain, and accelerate the healing process.[6,18] In some facilities these therapies are initiated before the patient's admission to the OR. In others, such as ambulatory settings, they may be started after the patient's arrival in the holding area.

The admitting procedure is continued with reassessment of the patient and with time allowed for last-minute questions. Complete the chart review for the previously mentioned data and note any abnormalities or changes. Question the patient concerning valuables, prostheses, and last intake of food and fluid. Validate that the correct preoperative medications were given (if ordered). Provide a pillow or position adjustment if the patient is uncomfortable. Most hospitals require the patient's hair to be covered just before transfer to the OR suite to reduce potential shedding. Specific SCIP measures may include a prophylactic antibiotic started within 30 to 60 minutes before the surgical incision, and application of a warming blanket and SCDs.

NURSING MANAGEMENT PATIENT DURING SURGERY

ROOM PREPARATION

Before transferring the patient into the OR, prepare the room to ensure privacy, prevention of infection, and safety. Individualization of this preparation is essential to achieve the expected patient outcomes. For example, when an obese patient is admitted to the OR, there are several special considerations (see Chapter 41). Ask such questions as, What equipment is needed to safely transfer the patient to and from the OR table? Will extra staff be required for safe transfer and positioning? Is special equipment needed (e.g., extra-long instrumentation)? What special precautions, if any, must be taken to ensure maintenance of the patient's airway? The unique needs of each patient must be addressed for a safe surgical experience.

Surgical attire (pants and shirts, masks, protective eyewear, and caps or hoods) is worn by all people entering the OR (Fig. 19-3). All electrical and mechanical equipment is checked

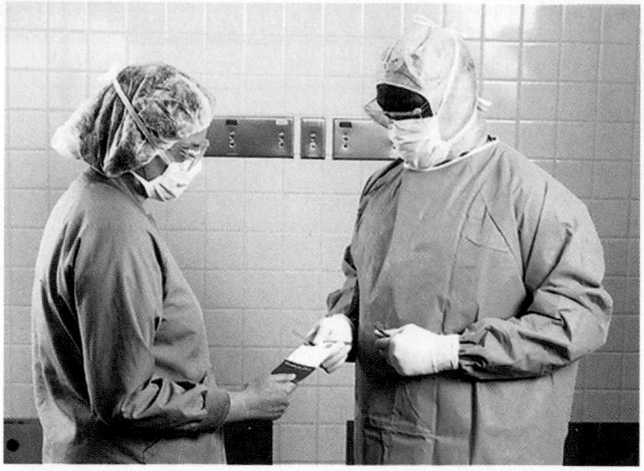

FIG. 19-3 Surgical attire is worn by all people entering the operating room.

for proper functioning. Aseptic technique is practiced as each surgical item is opened and placed on the instrument table.[19] Sponges, needles, instruments, and small medical devices (e.g., surgical clip cartridges, universal adapters) are counted according to strict processes to ensure accurate retrieval at the end of the procedure. Any retained surgical supplies, devices, or instruments are sentinel events that can result in negative outcomes for the patient.[20,21]

During room preparation and the surgical procedure, the scrub person performs surgical hand antisepsis, dons sterile gown and gloves, and touches only those items in the sterile field. The circulating nurse remains in the unsterile field and performs those activities that permit touching all unsterile items and the patient. This coordinated effort allows for smooth functioning throughout the procedure.

TRANSFERRING PATIENT

Once the patient's identity has been verified and the OR has been prepared, the patient is transported into the room for the surgery. Each time a patient is transferred from one bed to another, the wheels of the stretcher must be locked, and a sufficient number of personnel should be available to lift, guide, and prevent accidental falling or injury to self, other staff, or the patient. Once the patient is on the OR bed, place safety straps snugly across the patient's thighs. At this time the monitor leads (e.g., electrocardiogram [ECG] leads), BP cuff, and pulse oximeter are usually applied and an IV catheter is inserted if it was not done in the holding area.

SCRUBBING, GOWNING, AND GLOVING

Surgical hand antisepsis is required of all sterile members of the surgical team (scrub nurse, surgeon, and assistant). When the procedure of scrubbing is the chosen method for surgical hand antisepsis (often for the first case of the day), your fingers and hands should be scrubbed first with progression to the forearms and elbows. The hands should be held away from surgical attire and higher than the elbows at all times to prevent contamination from clothing or detergent suds and water from draining from the unclean area above the elbows to the clean and previously scrubbed areas of the hands and fingers.[6,22]

Waterless, alcohol-based agents are replacing traditional soap and water in many facilities. When using an alcohol-based surgical hand-scrub product, prewash hands and forearms with soap and dry completely before applying the alcohol-based product. After application of the alcohol-based product, allow hands and forearms to dry thoroughly before donning sterile gloves.[22,23]

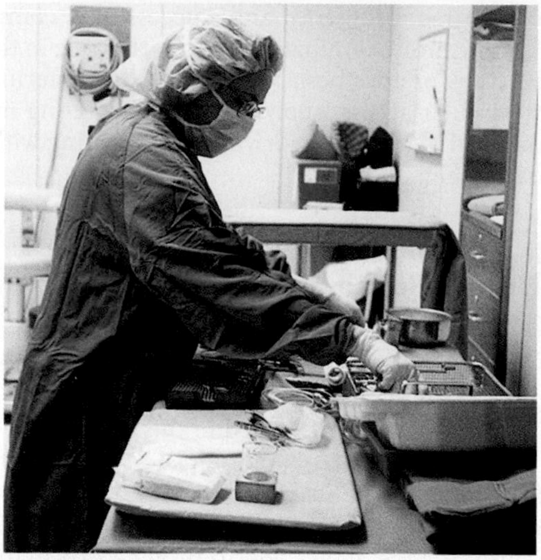

FIG. 19-4 A sterile field is created before surgery.

Once surgical hand antisepsis is completed, the team members enter the OR to put on surgical gowns and two pairs of gloves to protect patients and themselves from the transmission of microorganisms.[24,25] Because the gowns and gloves are sterile, those who have scrubbed can manipulate and organize all sterile items for use during the procedure.

BASIC ASEPTIC TECHNIQUE

Aseptic technique is practiced in the OR to prevent infection. This is implemented through the creation and maintenance of a sterile field (Fig. 19-4). The center of the sterile field is the site of the surgical incision. Inanimate items used in the sterile field, including surgical items and equipment, have been sterilized by appropriate sterilization methods.

Team members must understand specific principles to practice aseptic technique (Table 19-3). Unless these principles are followed, the patient's safety is compromised and the potential for postoperative infection is increased.[5,6,19]

In addition to following the principles of aseptic technique, the surgical team is responsible for following the guidelines established by the U.S. Occupational Safety and Health Administration (OSHA) and AORN to protect the patient and the team from exposure to blood-borne pathogens.[26] These guidelines emphasize standard and transmission-based precautions (see eTable 15-1, available on the website for Chapter 15); engineering and work practice controls; and the use of personal protective equipment such as gloves, gowns, caps, face shields, masks, and protective eyewear. This is especially important in the OR because of the high potential for exposure to blood-borne pathogens.

ASSISTING ANESTHESIA CARE PROVIDER

While you check the OR to complete the final preparations, the ACP prepares the patient for the administration of the anesthetic. You need to understand the effects of the anesthetic agents and know the location of all emergency drugs and equipment.

If you are the circulating nurse, you may be involved in placing monitoring devices to be used during the surgical pro-

TABLE 19-3 PRINCIPLES OF ASEPTIC TECHNIQUE IN OPERATING ROOM

- All materials that enter the sterile field must be sterile.
- If a sterile item comes in contact with an unsterile item, it is contaminated.
- Contaminated items are removed immediately from the sterile field. If the unsterile item is small (e.g., unopened suture), once it is removed, the area is marked off (i.e., covered with a sterile drape). If the entire field is contaminated, it should be set up again with all new materials.
- The surgical team working in the operative field must wear sterile gowns and gloves. Once dressed for procedure, they must recognize that the only parts of the gown considered sterile are front from chest to table level and sleeves to 2 inches above elbow.
- A wide margin of safety must be maintained between sterile and unsterile fields.
- Tables are considered sterile only at tabletop level. Items extending beneath this level are considered contaminated.
- The edges of a sterile package are considered contaminated once the package has been opened. If a sterile package (e.g., package of sutures) is placed on the sterile field, that entire package remains sterile even when opened.
- Microorganisms travel on airborne particles and will enter the sterile field with excessive air movements and currents.
- Microorganisms travel by capillary action through moist fabrics, resulting in contamination.
- Microorganisms harbor on the patient's and team members' hair, skin, and respiratory tracts and must be confined by appropriate attire.

cedure (e.g., ECG leads). If the patient is to have a general anesthetic, remain at the patient's side to ensure safety and to assist the ACP. These responsibilities may include measuring BP and assisting in the maintenance of the patient's airway. During the surgical procedure, you also provide a vital communication link for the ACP to other departments such as the laboratory or the blood bank.

SAFETY CONSIDERATIONS

All surgical procedures, regardless of where they take place, can put the patient at risk for injury. These injuries can be infections, physical trauma from positioning or equipment used, or physiologic effects of surgery itself. Be alert to all safety issues, since the patient in the OR is often compromised from the effects of anesthesia.

Fire in the OR can have devastating consequences for the patient. Fortunately, surgical fires can be prevented with awareness of the hazards and emphasis on safe practices.[27] Care must be taken to correctly place the grounding pad and all electrosurgical equipment to prevent injury from burns or fire[28] (Fig. 19-5).

Smoke particles produced during laser procedures may contain trace hydrocarbons (e.g., acetone, isopropanol, formaldehyde, cyanide). These airborne contaminants can cause respiratory irritation and have mutagenic and carcinogenic potential. Smoke evacuators may be used to minimize this exposure.[29]

The *Universal Protocol*, one of the NPSGs, is followed to prevent wrong site, wrong procedure, and wrong surgery.[30] A patient safety checklist for ORs is the cornerstone of a major focus to make surgery safer around the world (see eFig. 19-1 available on the website for this chapter). The use of the World Health Organization (WHO) Surgical Safety Checklist has

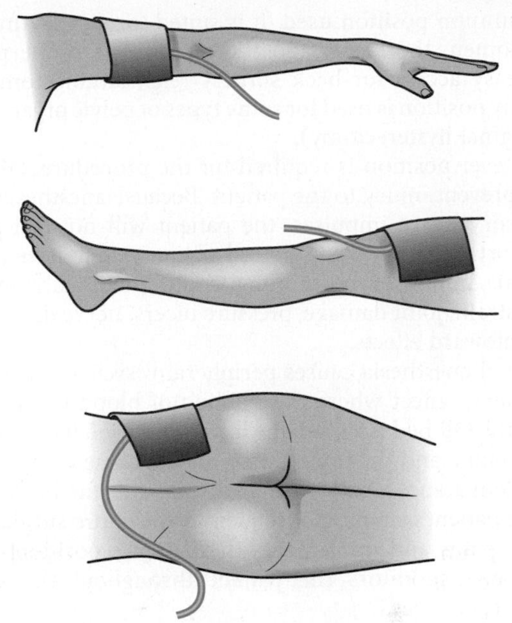

FIG. 19-5 When an electrosurgical unit is used, the patient must be properly grounded to prevent unintended injury. A well-vascularized muscle mass is an optimal site. Safety can be compromised by excessive hair, adipose tissue, bony prominences, fluid (edema), adhesive failure, and scar tissue.

improved compliance with standards and decreased complications from surgery.[31]

Similarly, AORN has developed a position statement regarding correct site surgery and guidelines for implementing the Universal Protocol.[32] All members of the surgical team stop what they are doing during a *surgical time-out* just before the procedure starts to verify patient identification, surgical procedure, and surgical site. In addition, it is becoming more common for OR personnel to complete a fire risk assessment protocol (see eTable 19-1 available on the website for this chapter) to identify and reduce the potential for an OR fire.

SAFETY ALERT: Take a Surgical Time-Out

- Before the induction of anesthesia, ask the patient to confirm name, birth date, operative procedure and site, and consent.
- Compare the hospital ID number with the patient's own ID band and chart.

POSITIONING PATIENT

Positioning the patient is a critical part of every procedure and usually follows administration of the anesthetic. The ACP indicates when to begin the positioning. The patient's position should allow for accessibility to the operative site, administration and monitoring of anesthetic agents, and maintenance of the patient's airway. When positioning for the surgical procedure, take care to (1) provide correct musculoskeletal alignment; (2) prevent undue pressure on nerves, skin over bony prominences, earlobes, and eyes; (3) provide for adequate thoracic excursion; (4) prevent occlusion of arteries and veins; (5) provide modesty in exposure; and (6) recognize and respect individual needs such as previously assessed aches, pains, or deformities. It is your responsibility to secure the extremities, provide adequate padding and support, and obtain sufficient physical or mechanical help to avoid unnecessary straining of self or patient.[33]

The patient may be placed in various positions, including supine, prone, lateral, lithotomy, or sitting. The supine is the most common position used. It is suited for surgery involving the abdomen, the heart, and the breast. The prone position allows easy access for back surgery (e.g., laminectomy). The lithotomy position is used for some types of pelvic organ surgery (e.g., vaginal hysterectomy).

Whatever position is required for the procedure, take great care to prevent injury to the patient. Because anesthesia blocks the sensory nerve impulses, the patient will not feel pain or discomfort or stress being placed on nerves, muscles, bones, and skin. Improper positioning could potentially result in muscle strain, joint damage, pressure ulcers, nerve damage, and other untoward effects.

General anesthesia causes peripheral vessels to dilate. Position changes affect where the pooling of blood occurs. If the head of the OR bed is raised, the lower torso will have increased blood volume and the upper torso may become compromised. Hypovolemia and cardiovascular disease can further compromise the patient's status. Consequently, the entire surgical team carefully plans and implements the patient's positioning, and then closely monitors the patient throughout the surgical procedure.

PREVENTING HYPOTHERMIA

Research has shown a correlation between unintended hypothermia and impaired wound healing, adverse cardiac events, altered drug metabolism, and coagulopathies. One study showed that the rate of culture-positive surgical site infections among those with mild perioperative hypothermia was three times higher than among normothermic patients.[34]

To prevent hypothermia, members of the surgical team need to closely monitor the patient's temperature and may apply a thermal warming blanket to the patient to maintain body temperature.[35,36]

PREPARING SURGICAL SITE

The purpose of skin preparation, or "prepping," is to reduce the number of microorganisms available to migrate to the surgical wound. The task of prepping is completed intraoperatively by the circulating nurse, surgeon, or surgical assistant.

The skin is prepared by mechanically scrubbing or cleansing around the surgical site with an antimicrobial agent identified as one that reduces microorganisms on intact skin, contains a nonirritating antimicrobial agent, has broad-spectrum activity, is fast acting and persistent, and is nonallergenic to the patient. A liberal area is scrubbed in a circular motion. The principle of scrubbing from the clean area (site of the incision) to the dirty area (distal to the incision) is observed at all times.[37,38]

Antiseptic agents used for skin preparation may contain alcohol and be flammable. Skin injury can occur if these agents are allowed to pool under the patient. Care must be taken to ensure that these agents are properly confined and allowed to fully dry. After the skin is prepped and the fumes are allowed to dispel, the sterile members of the surgical team drape the area. Only the site to be incised is left exposed.

PATIENT AFTER SURGERY

Through constant observation of the surgical process, the ACP anticipates the end of the surgical procedure. Appropriate types and doses of anesthetic agents are used so that their effects will be minimal at the end of the surgical procedure. This also allows greater physiologic control of the patient during the transfer to the PACU.

The patient's response to your care is evaluated based on outcome criteria established during the development of the patient's plan of care. These outcome criteria are published as the *Perioperative Nursing Data Set (PNDS)* by AORN. The PNDS reflects standards and recommended practices related to the delivery of nursing care in any perioperative setting.[6,39]

The ACP and you or another member of the surgical team accompany the patient to the PACU. A hand-off of the patient that includes his or her status and the procedure performed is communicated to the nurse receiving the patient in the PACU to promote safe, ongoing care.

ANESTHESIA

The art and science of anesthesia have dramatically changed over time. For example, the Bispectral Index monitor allows ACPs to track the level of patient awareness (i.e., *awareness monitoring*) during surgery and adjust sedation as needed. The use of regional anesthetics facilitates the smooth and rapid transition from patient recovery to early discharge.

The anesthetic technique and agents are selected by the ACP in collaboration with the surgeon and the patient. The ACP has ultimate responsibility for the choice of anesthetic. Factors contributing to the decision include the patient's current physical and mental status, allergy and pain history, expertise of the ACP, and factors relating to the operative procedure (e.g., length, site, discharge plans). An absolute contraindication to any anesthetic technique or agent is patient refusal.

The ACP obtains anesthesia consent, writes orders for preoperative and postoperative medications, and assigns the patient an anesthesia classification. The American Society of Anesthesiologists (ASA) physical status classification system is based on the patient's physiologic status with no regard to the surgical procedure to be performed. A scale of P1 to P6 is used, with a rating of P6 reserved for a brain-dead patient undergoing organ harvest (see Table 18-3). An intraoperative complication is more likely to develop with a higher classification number. Other designations can be added to the ASA status (e.g., "E" to designate an "emergent" procedure). ASA physical status is dynamic and represents the patient's status immediately before surgery. For example, a healthy 26-year-old adult who is severely injured in an automobile collision may be classified as ASA P5E because life-threatening injuries require emergent surgery.

CLASSIFICATION OF ANESTHESIA

The ASA classifies anesthesia according to the effect that it has on the patient's sensorium and pain perception. These classifications include general anesthesia, regional anesthesia, local anesthesia, monitored anesthesia care (MAC), and moderate sedation[40,41] (Table 19-4).

Monitored anesthesia care (MAC) is used for diagnostic or therapeutic procedures performed in or outside of the OR (e.g., eye clinic). It includes varying levels of sedation, analgesia, and anxiolysis. A critical component of MAC is the assessment and management of any physiologic problems that may develop. The provider of MAC must be an ACP, since it may be necessary to convert to general anesthesia during the procedure.

Moderate sedation is used for procedures performed outside of the OR (e.g., reduction of dislocated joints in the emergency department) and does not require the presence of an ACP. RNs

TABLE 19-4 CLASSIFICATION OF ANESTHESIA AND PATIENT EFFECTS

Classification	Anticipated Patient Effects
General anesthesia	• Loss of sensation with loss of consciousness • Combination of hypnosis, analgesia, and amnesia • Usually involves use of inhalation agents • Skeletal muscle relaxation • Elimination of coughing, gagging, vomiting, and sympathetic nervous system responsiveness • Requires advanced airway management
Regional anesthesia	• Loss of sensation to a region of body without loss of consciousness • Involves blocking a specific nerve or group of nerves with administration of a local anesthetic • Includes spinal, caudal, and epidural anesthesia and IV and peripheral nerve blocks (e.g., interscalene, axillary, infraclavicular or supraclavicular, popliteal, femoral, sciatic)
Local anesthesia	• Loss of sensation without loss of consciousness • Induced topically or via infiltration, intracutaneously, or subcutaneously • Topical applications may be aerosolized or nebulized
Monitored anesthesia care (MAC)	• Similar to general anesthesia • Sedative, anxiolytic, and/or analgesic medications used • Does not usually involve inhalation agents • Patients less responsive and may require airway management • Provides maximum flexibility to match sedation level to patient needs and procedural requirements • Often used in conjunction with regional or local anesthesia • Often used for minor therapeutic and diagnostic procedures (e.g., eye surgery, colonoscopy)
Moderate sedation (formerly called conscious sedation)	• Sedative, anxiolytic, and/or analgesic medications used • Does not include use of inhalation agents • Patients responsive and breathe without assistance • Not expected to induce levels of sedation that would impair patients' ability to protect their airway • Most often used for minor therapeutic procedures (e.g., realignment of a fracture in the emergency department)

Sources: American Society of Anesthesiologists: Frequently asked questions. Retrieved from *www.lifelinetomodernmedicine.com/FAQs.aspx*; and American Society of Anesthesiologists: Distinguishing monitored anesthesia care ("MAC") from moderate sedation/analgesia (conscious sedation). Retrieved from *www.asahq.org/~/media/For%20Members/Standards%20and%20Guidelines/DISTINGUISHING%20MONITORED%20ANESTHESIA%20CARE.ashx.*

who receive education in moderate sedation and are permitted by institutional protocols and state nurse practice acts can provide this type of anesthesia.[42] It is administered by the nurse under the direct supervision of a physician.

General Anesthesia

The present goals of anesthesiology include the (1) control of excessive biologic responses induced by a variety of stressors and (2) protection of patients from stress-induced complications. To this end, *total intravenous anesthesia (TIVA)* and newer inhalation agents have a fast onset, fast elimination, and fewer undesirable side effects than previous agents. These factors facilitate early discharge from the PACU and ambulatory surgery centers.

General anesthesia is the technique of choice for patients who are having surgical procedures that are of significant duration, require skeletal muscle relaxation, require uncomfortable operative positions because of the location of the incision site, or require control of ventilation. Additional reasons for general anesthesia include refusal of local or regional techniques, contraindications to other techniques, and uncooperative patients. Patients may be uncooperative due to intoxication, emotional lability, head injury, impaired cognition, or inability to remain immobile for any length of time. Phases of general anesthesia are presented in Table 19-5.

General anesthesia may be induced IV or by inhalation, and maintained by either one or a combination of the two (Table 19-6, p. 343). A *balanced technique,* using adjunctive drugs to complement the induction, is the most common approach used for general anesthesia.

Intravenous Agents. Virtually all routine general anesthetics begin with an IV induction agent, whether it is a hypnotic, an anxiolytic, or a dissociative agent. When used during the initial period of anesthesia, these agents induce a pleasant sleep with a rapid onset of action that patients find desirable. A single dose lasts only a few minutes, which is long enough for a laryngeal mask airway (LMA) or an endotracheal (ET) tube to be placed. Once this is done, the ACP uses the selected inhalation and IV agent(s).

Recent advances in IV hypnotics and opioids have led to the more frequent use of TIVA. However, the patient may still require advanced airway management (e.g., LMA, ET tube) and will receive oxygen/air mixtures via this route.

Inhalation Agents. Inhalation agents are the cornerstone of general anesthesia. These agents may be volatile liquids or gases. Volatile liquids are administered through a specially designed vaporizer after being mixed with oxygen as a carrier gas. This gas mixture is then delivered to the patient via the anesthesia circuit. Waste gases are removed using negative evacuation pressure venting to the outside of the institution.

Inhalation agents enter the body through the alveoli in the lungs. Ease of administration and rapid excretion by ventilation make them desirable agents. One undesirable trait is the irritating effect some inhalation agents (e.g., desflurane [Suprane]) have on the respiratory tract. Possible complications include coughing, laryngospasm (muscular constriction of the larynx), and increased secretions.[43]

Once the patient has been induced with an IV agent, the choice for delivering inhalation agents is usually through an ET tube or LMA. The ET tube permits control of ventilation and protects the airway from aspiration. LMAs are currently an important option for patients with difficult airways, but they do not provide access to the trachea with the same certainty as ETs. Complications of ET tube or LMA include those primarily associated with insertion and removal. These include failure to intubate, damage to teeth and lips, laryngospasm, laryngeal edema, postoperative sore throat, and hoarseness caused by injury or irritation of the vocal cords or surrounding tissues.

Adjuncts to General Anesthesia. The administration of general anesthesia is rarely limited to one agent. Drugs added to an inhalation anesthetic (other than an IV induction agent) are termed *adjuncts.* These agents are added to the anesthetic

TABLE 19-5 PHASES OF GENERAL ANESTHESIA

Preinduction	Induction	Maintenance	Emergence
Description			
• Period starting with preoperative medication, initiation of IV or arterial access, application of monitors (e.g., ECG).	• Initiation of medications that make patient unconscious. • Airway secured with airway assist devices.	• Period during which surgical procedure is performed. • Patient remains in an unconscious state with measures to ensure airway safety.	• Period when surgical procedure is completed. • Patient is prepared for return to consciousness and removal of airway assist devices.
Role of Anesthesia Care Provider			
• Determine final anesthetic care plan. • Insert and monitor IV or arterial access. • Confirm antibiotic prophylaxis. • Administer drugs for anxiety, aspiration prophylaxis.	• Administer appropriate drugs. • Secure airway. • Position patient appropriately for surgical procedure.	• Monitor patient's physiologic status. • Administer medications and titrate fluids as appropriate.	• Reverse residual neuromuscular blocking agents. • Assess for return of all protective reflexes. • Remove airway assist devices. • Assess pain.
Role of Perioperative Nurse			
• Complete preoperative assessment. • Check and confirm signed informed consent. • Complete surgical time-out.	• Assist with application of monitors (noninvasive and invasive). • Assist with airway management.	• Adjust patient position as necessary. • Monitor patient safety.	• Assist in placement of dressing. • Protect patient during return of reflexes. • Prepare patient to move to postanesthesia care unit.
Classes of Drugs Used (see Tables 18-9, 19-6, and 19-7)			

• Benzodiazepines
• Opioids
• Antibiotics
• Aspiration prophylaxis:
  • H_2-receptor blockers (e.g., ranitidine [Zantac])
  • Gastric motility agents (e.g., metoclopramide [Reglan])
  • Anticholinergics (e.g., scopolamine [Transderm-Scōp])
	• Benzodiazepines
	• Opioids
	• Barbiturates
	• Hypnotics
	• Volatile gases
		• Benzodiazepines
		• Opioids
		• Barbiturates
		• Hypnotics
		• Volatile gases
		• Neuromuscular blocking agents
			• Reversal agents:
			  • Anticholinesterases (e.g., neostigmine [Prostigmin])
			  • Opioid antagonists (PRN) (e.g., naloxone [Narcan])
			  • Benzodiazepine antagonists (PRN) (e.g., flumazenil [Romazicon])
			• Supplemental opioids (PRN)
			• Antiemetics (PRN)

regimen specifically to achieve unconsciousness, analgesia, amnesia, muscle relaxation, or autonomic nervous system control. Adjuncts include opioids, benzodiazepines, neuromuscular blocking agents (muscle relaxants), and antiemetics (Table 19-7, p. 344). It is important to know that these drugs are often given in combination and may have synergistic or antagonistic effects. You may observe deeper levels of sedation or more drug-related side effects beyond those seen with inhalation anesthetics alone. If needed, drugs are available to reverse the effects of some of these adjuncts.

Dissociative Anesthesia. Dissociative anesthesia interrupts associative brain pathways while blocking sensory pathways. The patient may appear catatonic, is amnesic, and experiences profound analgesia that lasts into the postoperative period. Ketamine (Ketalar) is a commonly administered dissociative anesthetic. Ketamine (administered IV or intramuscularly) is a potent analgesic and amnesic. It is used in asthmatic patients undergoing surgery because it promotes bronchodilation and in trauma patients requiring surgery because it increases heart rate and helps maintain cardiac output. Because ketamine is a phenylcyclohexylpiperidine (PCP) derivative, the drug may cause hallucinations and nightmares, greatly limiting its usefulness. Concurrent use of midazolam (Versed) can reduce or eliminate hallucinations associated with ketamine. Provide a quiet, unhurried environment in the PACU for all patients receiving dissociative anesthesia.[44]

Local and Regional Anesthesia

Local anesthesia interrupts the generation of nerve impulses by altering the flow of sodium into nerve cells through cell membranes. Volume and concentration of the local anesthetic agent will, in accelerating fashion, first block autonomic, then somatic sensory, and, last, somatic motor impulses. The result is autonomic nervous system blockade, anesthesia, and skeletal muscle flaccidity or paralysis. Local anesthetics are topical, ophthalmic, nebulized, or injectable.

A local anesthetic, such as lidocaine (Xylocaine), is applied to a specific area of the body by the surgeon or ACP and does not require sedation or loss of consciousness. **Regional anesthesia** (or block) using a local anesthetic is always injected and involves a central nerve (e.g., spinal) or group of nerves (e.g., plexus) that innervate a site remote to the point of injection.

Administration of a local or regional anesthetic may involve concurrent use of MAC or moderate sedation (see Table 19-4), either preinjection or intraoperatively. Regional blocks are used as preoperative analgesia, intraoperatively to manage surgical pain, and postoperatively to control pain. Indwelling catheters that deliver local anesthetic via a pump to the surgical site may be implanted before the patient emerges from anesthesia to provide continuous pain relief up to 72 hours postoperatively.

Certain advantages of local and regional anesthesia include rapid recovery and discharge with continued postoperative analgesia and without any accompanying cognitive dysfunc-

TABLE 19-6 DRUG THERAPY

General Anesthesia

Drugs	Advantages	Disadvantages	Nursing Interventions
Intravenous Agents			
Barbiturates			
thiopental (Pentothal) methohexital (Brevital)	Rapid induction, duration of action <5 min.	Adverse cardiac effects (e.g., myocardial depression), hypotension, respiratory depression. *thiopental:* histamine release. *methohexital:* excitation, involuntary movement.	Usually have minimal postoperative effects because of short duration of action. Increased incidence of postoperative nausea in patients with barbiturate sensitivity, histamine-triggered nausea, vomiting.
Nonbarbiturate Hypnotics			
etomidate (Amidate)	Produces little change in cardiovascular dynamics. Useful for hemodynamically unstable patients. Only minor respiratory depression. No histamine release.	Associated with adverse effects of myoclonia, nausea and vomiting, hiccups, and adrenocortical inhibition.	Observe for transient skeletal muscle movements (myoclonia), nausea and vomiting, hiccups, hypotension, hypoglycemia.
propofol (Diprivan)	Ideal for short outpatient procedures because of rapid onset of action, metabolic clearance. May be used for induction and maintenance of anesthesia.	May cause bradycardia and other dysrhythmias, hypotension, apnea, transient phlebitis, nausea and vomiting, hiccups. May cause hypertriglyceridemia.	Monitor for postoperative hypotension, bradycardia. Monitor serum triglycerides q24hr for sedation >24 hr.
Inhalation Agents			
Volatile Liquids			
isoflurane (Forane) desflurane (Suprane) sevoflurane (Ultane) halothane (Fluothane)	All cause skeletal muscle relaxation. *isoflurane*: No increase in ventricular irritability. Does not cause liver or renal toxicity. Resistant to metabolic breakdown. *desflurane*: Fastest onset and emergence, widely used in ambulatory settings. Least postoperative cognitive dysfunction. Potential airway irritant. *sevoflurane*: Predictable effects on cardiovascular and respiratory systems, rapid acting. Preferred for inhalation induction as nonirritating to respiratory tract. *halothane*: Bronchodilation, nonirritating to respiratory tract.	All cause respiratory depression, hypotension, myocardial depression. *isoflurane and desflurane*: May be unsuitable for patients with coronary artery disease. *sevoflurane*: May be associated with emergence delirium (see Chapter 20). Atypical seizure-like activity has been reported. *halothane*: Ventricular excitability, hepatotoxicity.	Assess and treat pain during early anesthesia recovery. Assess for adverse reactions such as cardiopulmonary depression with hypotension and prolonged respiratory depression. Monitor for nausea and vomiting.
Gaseous Agents			
nitrous oxide	Potentiates volatile agents, thus speeding induction and reducing total dosage and side effects. Good analgesic potency. Produces little or no toxicity at therapeutic concentrations.	Weak anesthetic, rarely used alone. Must be administered with O_2 to prevent hypoxemia. Avoid in patients with strong history of nausea and vomiting.	Avoid in patients with bone marrow depression.
Dissociative Anesthetic			
ketamine (Ketalar)	Can be administered IV or IM. Potent analgesic and amnesic.	May cause hallucinations and nightmares, increased intracranial and intraocular pressure, ↑ heart rate, ↑ blood pressure.	Anticipate administration of a benzodiazepine if agitation and hallucinations occur. Calm, quiet environment is essential in postoperative care.

tion.[45] Patients with co-morbidities that would preclude general anesthesia are now offered surgical solutions with increased safety. Some disadvantages to local and regional anesthesia include the potential for technical difficulties; discomfort at the injection site; and the risk of inadvertent vascular injection leading to refractory hypotension, dysrhythmias, and possible seizures. Finally, the inability to precisely match the agent's duration of action to the duration of the surgical procedure is a limiting factor.

In ambulatory or outpatient procedures, you may assist a physician in the administration of a peripheral or regional block. Consequently, you must be familiar with the drugs, the methods of administration, and adverse and toxic effects of the drugs. Initial assessment of the patient should include detailed questioning of the patient's history with local anesthetics and any adverse events associated with their use by the patient or blood relatives.

Many patients report "allergies" to local anesthetics. Although true allergies to local anesthetics occur, they are rare. Allergies are likely to be a result of additives or preservatives in the preparation. Moreover, many local anesthetics are combined with epinephrine solutions. They may be absorbed in the tissues or inadvertently injected IV. Once the agent enters the general circulation, the patient may experience tachycardia, hyperten-

TABLE 19-7 DRUG THERAPY

Adjuncts to General Anesthesia

Agents	Uses During Anesthesia	Adverse Effects	Nursing Interventions
Opioids fentanyl (Sublimaze) sufentanil (Sufenta) morphine sulfate hydromorphone (Dilaudid) alfentanil (Alfenta) remifentanil (Ultiva) methadone (Dolophine)	Induce and maintain anesthesia, reduce stimuli from sensory nerve endings, provide analgesia during surgery and recovery in PACU.	Respiratory depression, stimulation of vomiting center, possible bradycardia and peripheral vasodilation (when combined with anesthetics). High incidence of pruritus in both regional and IV administration.	Assess respiratory rate and rhythm, monitor pulse oximetry, protect airway in anticipation of vomiting. Use standing orders for antipruritics and antiemetics. Reverse opioid-induced respiratory depression with naloxone (Narcan). If used, reversal of analgesic effects also occurs.
Benzodiazepines midazolam (Versed) diazepam (Valium) lorazepam (Ativan)	Reduce anxiety preoperatively and postoperatively, induce and maintain anesthesia, induce amnesia, treat emergence delirium. Supplement sedation in local and regional anesthesia and MAC.	Synergistic effect with opioids, increasing potential for respiratory depression. Hypotension and tachycardia. Prolonged sedation or confusion.	Monitor level of consciousness. Assess for respiratory depression, hypotension, and tachycardia. Reverse severe benzodiazepine-induced respiratory depression with flumazenil (Romazicon).
Neuromuscular Blocking Agents *Depolarizing agent:* succinylcholine (Anectine) *Nondepolarizing agents:* vecuronium (Norcuron) pancuronium (Pavulon) pipecuronium (Arduan) doxacurium (Nuromax) rocuronium (Zemuron)	Facilitate endotracheal intubation, promote skeletal muscle relaxation (paralysis) to enhance access to surgical sites. Effects of nondepolarizing agents are usually reversed toward end of surgery by administration of anticholinesterase agents (e.g., neostigmine, pyridostigmine).	Apnea related to paralysis of respiratory muscles. Duration of action of nondepolarizing agents may be longer than surgery. Reversal agents may not completely eliminate effects. Confusion and nausea. Recurrence of muscle weakness with correction of hypothermia.	If intubated, monitor return of muscle strength, level of consciousness, and ventilation. Maintain patent airway. Monitor respiratory rate and rhythm until patient able to cough and return to previous levels of muscle strength. Ensure availability of nondepolarizing reversal agents (e.g., neostigmine [Prostigmin]) and emergency respiratory support equipment. Monitor temperature and levels of muscle strength with temperature changes.
Antiemetics ondansetron (Zofran) dolasetron (Anzemet) granisetron (Kytril) metoclopramide (Reglan) prochlorperazine (Compazine) promethazine (Phenergan) scopolamine (Transderm-Scōp) diphenhydramine (Benadryl)	Counteract emetic effects of inhalation agents and opioids. Prophylactic prevention of nausea and vomiting related to histamine release, vagal stimulation, vestibular disturbance, surgical procedure (e.g., abdominal and laparoscopic procedures).	Headache, dizziness, IV irritation, dysrhythmias, dysphoria, dystonia, dry mouth, central nervous system sedation.	Monitor heart rhythm, cardiopulmonary status, level of central nervous system excitation or sedation, ability to move limbs, presence of nausea or vomiting.
Miscellaneous dexamethasone (Decadron)	Counteract emetic effects of inhalation agents and opioids (off-label use).*	Insomnia, nervousness, abdominal distention.	Monitor for possible side effects.

*For an explanation of off-label drug use, see *www.cancer.org/docroot/ETO/content/ETO_1_2x_Off-Label_Drug_Use.asp.*
MAC, Monitored anesthesia care; *PACU,* postanesthesia care unit.

sion, and a general perception of panic. There are two classes of local anesthetics: esters and amides. It is highly unlikely that an individual is allergic to both. Therefore it is important to carefully question the patient concerning the agent and the symptoms experienced so that an agent in the proper class can be selected for the procedure.

Methods of Administration. Local anesthetics are injected at the surgical site, nebulized, or applied topically. Topical applications, with or without compression, of creams, ointments, aerosols, and liquids are all standard methods of administration. The agent is applied directly to the skin, mucous membranes, or open surface. Eutectic mixture of local anesthetics (EMLA cream, a combination of prilocaine and lidocaine) is an example of a cream applied to the site 30 to 60 minutes before the procedure for analgesia. The success of injected local anesthetics may be limited by prolonged duration of procedure or infection at the injection site, thus interfering with drug absorption.

Whenever a patient is prepared for regional anesthesia, airway equipment, emergency drugs, and a cardiac monitor/defibrillator should be immediately available to provide advanced airway and cardiopulmonary support if necessary. Inadvertent IV injection of the agent or excessive absorption of bupivacaine (Sensorcaine), in particular, may lead to cardiac depression, severe dysrhythmias, or cardiac arrest.[46]

Examples of common regional nerve blocks include brachial plexus block; IV regional anesthesia (IVRA) or Bier block anesthesia; and femoral, axillary, cervical, sciatic, ankle, and retrobulbar blocks. For IVRA or Bier block, the patient has a

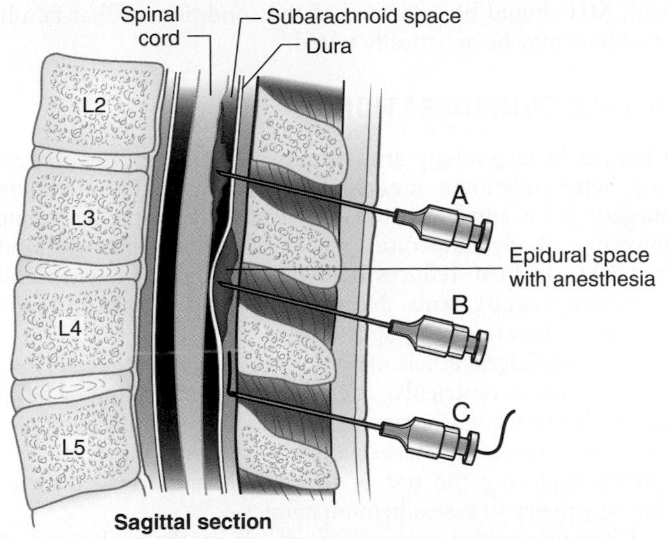

FIG. 19-6 Location of needle point and injected anesthetic relative to dura and spinal cord. **A,** Spinal anesthesia. **B,** Single-injection epidural. **C,** Epidural catheter. (Interspaces most commonly used are L2-3, L4-5, L3-4.)

double-cuff tourniquet applied as a safety measure. You can facilitate the success of regional anesthesia by assisting in patient positioning, monitoring vital signs during block delivery, administering oxygen therapy, and using supporting devices (at the direction of the ACP) that contribute to the anesthesia (e.g., ultrasound imaging, nerve stimulator, tourniquets).

Spinal and Epidural Anesthesia. Spinal anesthesia and epidural anesthesia are also types of regional anesthesia. **Spinal anesthesia** involves the injection of a local anesthetic into the cerebrospinal fluid found in the subarachnoid space, usually below the level of L2 (Fig. 19-6, *A*). The local anesthetic mixes with cerebrospinal fluid. Depending on the extent of its spread, various levels of anesthesia are achieved. Because the local anesthetic is administered directly into the cerebrospinal fluid, a spinal anesthetic produces an autonomic, sensory, and motor blockade. Patients experience vasodilation and may become hypotensive as a result of the autonomic block. They feel no pain as a result of the sensory block. They cannot move as a result of the motor block. The duration of action of the spinal anesthetic depends on the agent selected and the dose administered. A spinal anesthetic may be used for procedures involving the extremities (e.g., joint replacements) and lower gastrointestinal, prostate, and gynecologic surgeries.[47]

An **epidural block** involves injection of a local anesthetic into the epidural space via a thoracic or lumbar approach (see Fig. 19-6, *B*). The anesthetic agent does not enter the cerebrospinal fluid but binds to nerve roots as they enter and exit the spinal cord. With use of a low concentration of local anesthetic, sensory pathways are blocked but motor fibers remain intact. In higher doses, both sensory and motor fibers are blocked. Epidural anesthesia may be used as the sole anesthetic for a surgical procedure. In addition, a catheter may be placed to allow for intraoperative use and continued analgesia in the postoperative period (see Fig. 19-6, *C*). For postoperative analgesia, lower doses of epidurally administered local anesthetic, usually in combination with an opioid, are used.[47] Epidural anesthesia is commonly used for analgesia, or in combination with MAC or general anesthesia, in obstetrics, vascular procedures involving the lower extremities, lung resections, and renal and midabdominal surgeries. The desirable effects of vasodilation and analgesia contribute to better surgical outcomes.[48]

When spinal or epidural anesthesia is used, the patient can remain fully conscious, receive MAC, or choose general anesthesia. The onset of spinal anesthesia is more rapid than that of epidural anesthesia. Both spinal and epidural anesthesia may be extended in duration using indwelling catheters, thus allowing administration of additional doses of anesthetic. Closely observe the patient for signs of autonomic nervous system blockade. These include hypotension, bradycardia, nausea, and vomiting. There is less autonomic nervous system blockade with epidural anesthesia than with spinal anesthesia. Should "too high" a block be achieved, the patient may experience tingling in the arms and hands or inadequate breathing and apnea.[47] Other complications of spinal or epidural anesthesia include post-dural puncture headache, back pain, isolated nerve injury, and meningitis.

GERONTOLOGIC CONSIDERATIONS

PATIENT DURING SURGERY

Although anesthetic agents have become safer and more predictable, the aging process affects the pharmacokinetics of drugs, specifically the absorption, distribution, and metabolism of medications. This results in alterations in the onset, peak, and duration of medications independent of the route of administration. Because of this, anesthetic drugs should be carefully titrated when given to older adults. Physiologic changes in aging may alter the patient's response not only to the anesthetic but also to blood and fluid loss and replacement, hypothermia, pain, and tolerance of the surgical procedure and positioning. Carefully monitor the older adult's response to all anesthetic agents. Assess the postoperative recovery from these agents before the patient is transferred out of the PACU.

Some older adults may have difficulty communicating and following directions as a result of alterations in hearing or vision. These factors increase the need for clear and concise communication in the OR, especially when preoperative sedation is combined with already existing sensory deficits. Because of decreased ability to perceive discomfort or pressure on vulnerable areas and a loss of skin elasticity, the older adult's skin is at risk for injury from tape, electrodes, warming and cooling blankets, and certain types of dressings. In addition, pooling of solutions used to prepare the skin in dependent areas can quickly create skin burns or abrasions.

The care and vigilance of the entire surgical team are needed in preparing and positioning the older patient. The older adult often has osteoporosis and osteoarthritis. Misalignment, pressure, or other insults to arthritic joints that may be desensitized from administration of an anesthetic may create long-term injury and disability. Older adults are also at a greater risk of perioperative hypothermia. Consider the use of a variety of warming devices and carefully monitor them if used.

CATASTROPHIC EVENTS IN OPERATING ROOM

Unanticipated intraoperative events occasionally occur. Although some might be anticipated (e.g., cardiac arrest in an unstable patient, massive blood loss during trauma surgery), others may occur without warning, demanding immediate intervention by all members of the OR team. Two such events are anaphylactic reactions and malignant hyperthermia.

Anaphylactic Reactions

Anaphylaxis is the most severe form of an allergic reaction, manifesting with life-threatening pulmonary and circulatory complications. The initial clinical manifestations of anaphylaxis may be masked by anesthesia. ACPs administer an array of drugs to patients, such as anesthetics, antibiotics, blood products, and plasma expanders. Because any parenterally administered material can stimulate an allergic response, vigilance and rapid intervention are essential. An anaphylactic reaction causes hypotension, tachycardia, bronchospasm, and possibly pulmonary edema. Antibiotics and latex are responsible for many perioperative allergic reactions. (Anaphylaxis is discussed in Chapter 14.)

Latex allergy has become a particular concern in the perioperative setting, given the use of gloves, catheters, and many other devices containing natural rubber latex. Reactions to natural rubber latex range from urticaria to anaphylaxis with symptoms appearing immediately or at some time during the surgical procedure. Latex allergy protocols should be set up in each institution to provide a latex-safe environment for susceptible individuals.[49] (Latex allergies are discussed in Chapter 14.)

Malignant Hyperthermia

Malignant hyperthermia (MH) is a rare disorder characterized by hyperthermia with rigidity of skeletal muscles that can result in death. It occurs in susceptible people when they are exposed to certain anesthetic agents. Succinylcholine (Anectine), especially when given with volatile inhalation agents, appears to be the primary trigger of the disorder. Other factors, such as stress, trauma, and heat, also have been implicated. When MH does occur, it is usually during general anesthesia, but it may manifest in the recovery period as well.

MH is an autosomal dominant trait but is variable in its genetic manifestation, so predictions based on family history are important but not reliable. (Autosomal dominant disorders are discussed in Chapter 13.) The fundamental defect is hypermetabolism of skeletal muscle resulting from altered control of intracellular calcium. This leads to muscle contracture, hyperthermia, hypoxemia, lactic acidosis, and hemodynamic and cardiac alterations.

Tachycardia, tachypnea, hypercarbia, and ventricular dysrhythmias are generally seen but are nonspecific to MH. MH is generally diagnosed after all other causes of the hypermetabolism are ruled out. The rise in body temperature is not an early sign of MH. Unless promptly detected and treated, MH can result in cardiac arrest and death. The definitive treatment of MH is prompt administration of dantrolene (Dantrium). Dantrolene slows metabolism, reduces muscle contraction, and mediates the catabolic processes associated with MH.[44] A treatment protocol, available from the Malignant Hyperthermia Association of the United States, is often displayed in the OR[50] (see eFig. 19-2 available on the website for this chapter).

To prevent MH, obtain a careful family history and be alert to the development of MH perioperatively. The patient known or suspected to be at risk for this disorder can be anesthetized with minimal risks if appropriate precautions are taken. Patients with MH should be informed of the condition so that family members may be genetically tested.

FUTURE CONSIDERATIONS

Changes in technology and surgical techniques provide new and better treatment modalities for the patient undergoing surgery. For example, the use of *hypothermia,* or the deliberate lowering of body temperature, decreases metabolism and blood loss. This, in turn, reduces both the demand for oxygen and anesthetic requirements. Neurosurgery and selected trauma surgery benefit from this approach.

Transesophageal echocardiography (TEE) is used intraoperatively to assess ventricular function and competency of heart valves and to recognize venous air embolism. TEE is less invasive, inexpensive, and associated with few complications. It is quickly replacing the use of the pulmonary artery catheter during surgery to assess hemodynamics.

Ultrasonic-guided regional anesthesia is the technique of visualizing a nerve or plexus of nerves using ultrasound to place a regional block with more accuracy. This approach results in fewer side effects and increased patient satisfaction.

Minimally invasive surgery (MIS) is rapidly increasing as more procedures are performed using endoscopes. Incisions are smaller, blood loss is reduced, postoperative pain is decreased, and recovery time is shortened with MIS. Similarly, "bloodless surgery" is becoming more of a reality. Techniques to minimize blood loss during and after surgery include drug therapy and techniques for managing low hematocrit, hemostatic agents to enhance clotting and control bleeding, surgical devices and techniques to locate and stop internal bleeding, and surgical and anesthetic techniques to limit blood loss. The goal is to manage blood loss without the need for a blood transfusion.

Hydroxyethyl starch (Voluven, Hespan) is an IV synthetic starch solution approved for use as a blood volume expander during and after surgery. Blood volume expanders are administered to quickly restore some of the volume lost during surgery so that remaining red blood cells can continue to deliver oxygen to the body's tissues. There are also new alternatives to blood transfusions such as the perioperative use of erythropoietin (epoetin α [Epogen, Procrit]) to increase red blood cell count. Research on the development of a synthetic blood substitute (e.g., PolyHeme) is ongoing.

The number of procedures that can be performed using *robotic-assisted surgery* is rapidly growing. For example, laparoscopic procedures using robotics include prostatectomy, cholecystectomy, common bile duct injury repair, small bowel surgery, tubal reanastomosis, internal mammary artery harvesting, and video-assisted thoracoscopic surgery.

More recent technologic advancements have made *telesurgery,* or remote surgery, a reality. In telesurgery, a surgeon at a site separate from the patient performs the surgery using a robotic system located at the patient's site. Telesurgery allows surgeons to perform procedures in areas where their expertise is not readily available. In addition, they can perform procedures on patients in remote or hazardous locations (e.g., war zones).

BRIDGE TO NCLEX EXAMINATION

The number of the question corresponds to the same-numbered outcome at the beginning of the chapter.

1. Proper attire for the semirestricted area of the surgery department is
   a. street clothing.
   b. surgical attire and head cover.
   c. surgical attire, head cover, and mask.
   d. street clothing with the addition of shoe covers.
2. Activities that the nurse might perform in the role of a scrub nurse during surgery include *(select all that apply)*
   a. checking electrical equipment.
   b. preparing the instrument table.
   c. passing instruments to the surgeon and assistants.
   d. coordinating activities occurring in the operating room.
   e. maintaining accurate counts of sponges, needles, and instruments.
3. The nurse is caring for a patient undergoing surgery for a knee replacement. What is critical to the patient's safety during the procedure *(select all that apply)*?
   a. Universal protocol is followed.
   b. The ACP is an anesthesiologist.
   c. The patient has adequate health insurance.
   d. The circulating nurse is a registered nurse.
   e. The patient's allergies are conveyed to the surgical team.
4. The nurse's primary responsibility for the care of the patient undergoing surgery is
   a. developing an individualized plan of nursing care for the patient.
   b. carrying out specific tasks related to surgical policies and procedures.
   c. ensuring that the patient has been assessed for safe administration of anesthesia.
   d. performing a preoperative history and physical assessment to identify patient needs.
5. When scrubbing at the scrub sink, the nurse should
   a. scrub from elbows to hands.
   b. scrub without mechanical friction.
   c. scrub for a minimum of 10 minutes.
   d. hold the hands higher than the elbows.
6. When positioning a patient in preparation for surgery, the nurse understands that injury to the patient is most likely to occur as a result of
   a. incorrect musculoskeletal alignment.
   b. loss of perception of pain or pressure.
   c. pooling of blood in peripheral vessels.
   d. disregarding the patient's need for modesty.
7. Intravenous induction for general anesthesia is the method of choice for most patients because
   a. the patient is not intubated.
   b. the agents are nonexplosive.
   c. induction is rapid and pleasant.
   d. emergence is longer but with fewer complications.

1. b, 2. b, c, e, 3. a, e, 4. a, 5. d, 6. a, 7. c

evolve

For rationales to these answers and even more NCLEX review questions, visit *http://evolve.elsevier.com/Lewis/medsurg.*

REFERENCES

*1. Association of periOperative Registered Nurses: Recommended practices for surgical attire. In *Perioperative standards and recommended practices*, Denver, 2012, The Association.

*2. Association of periOperative Registered Nurses: Recommended practice for traffic patterns in the perioperative practice setting. In *Perioperative standards and recommended practices*, Denver, 2012, The Association.

3. The Joint Commission: Surgical care improvement project, 2011. Retrieved from *www.jointcommission.org/surgical_care_improvement_project.*

4. The Joint Commission: National patient safety goals. Retrieved from *www.jointcommission.org/assets/1/6/NPSG_Chapter_Jan2012_HAP.pdf.*

5. Phillips N: *Berry and Kohn's operating room technique*, ed 12, St Louis, 2013, Mosby.

6. Rothrock JC: *Alexander's care of the patient in surgery*, ed 14, St Louis, 2011, Mosby.

7. Agency for Healthcare Research and Quality: Patient safety network. Retrieved from *http://psnet.ahrq.gov/primer.aspx?primerID=9.*

8. Competency and Credentialing Institute: CNOR certification, 2012. Retrieved from *www.cc-institute.org/cnor.*

9. Association of Surgical Technologists: About the profession, 2011. Retrieved from *www.ast.org/professionals/about_prof.aspx.*

10. Association of periOperative Registered Nurses: AORN position statement on allied health care providers and support personnel in the perioperative practice setting, 2012. Retrieved from *www.aorn.org/Clinical_Practice/Position_Statements/Position_Statements.aspx.*

11. Association of periOperative Registered Nurses: AORN position statement on RN first assistants, 2011. Retrieved from *www.aorn.org/Clinical_Practice/Position_Statements/Position_Statements.aspx.*

*12. Association of periOperative Registered Nurses: AORN standards for RN first assistant education programs. In *Perioperative standards and recommended practices*, Denver, 2012, The Association.

13. American Society of Anesthesiologists: About ASA, 2011. Retrieved from *www.asahq.org/aboutASA.htm.*

14. American Association of Nurse Anesthetists: Nurse anesthetists at a glance. Retrieved from *www.aana.com/ceandeducation/becomeacrna/Pages/Nurse-Anesthetists-at-a-Glance.aspx.*

15. Jehovah's Witnesses: Teachings on blood transfusions and related procedures, 2008. Retrieved from *www.religioustolerance.org/witness5.htm.*

*Evidence-based information for clinical practice.

16. 30-Days Prayer Network: Customs and behavior: tips on how to behave in Muslim countries, 2011. Retrieved from *www.30-days.net/reveal/customs*.
17. About.com: The meanings behind common tattoo symbols and designs, 2009. Retrieved from *http://tattoo.about.com/cs/tatfaq/a/symbols_ancient.htm*.
*18. Shabanloei R, Golchin M, Esfahani A, et al: Effects of music therapy on pain and anxiety in patients undergoing bone marrow biopsy and aspiration, *AORN J* 91:746, 2010.
*19. Association of periOperative Registered Nurses: Recommended practice for sterile field-maintaining. In *Perioperative standards and recommended practices*, Denver, 2012, The Association.
*20. Association of periOperative Registered Nurses: Recommended practice for counts—sponge, sharp and instrument. In *Perioperative standards and recommended practices*, Denver, 2012, The Association.
*21. Steelman VM: Designing a safer process to prevent retained surgical sponges: a healthcare failure mode and effect analysis, *AORN J* 94:132, 2011.
*22. Association of periOperative Registered Nurses: Recommended practice for hand antisepsis—surgical. In *Perioperative standards and recommended practices*, Denver, 2012, The Association.
23. World Health Organization: WHO guidelines on hand hygiene in health care, 2009. Retrieved from *http://whqlibdoc.who.int/publications/2009/9789241597906_eng.pdf*.
*24. Centers for Disease Control and Prevention: Guideline for hand hygiene in health-care settings, 2002. Retrieved from *www.cdc.gov/mmwr/PDF/rr/rr5116.pdf*. (Classic)
*25. Association of periOperative Registered Nurses: Recommended practice for prevention of transmissible infections in the perioperative practice setting. In *Perioperative standards and recommended practices*, Denver, 2012, The Association.
*26. Cicconi L, Claypool M, Stevens W: Prevention of transmissible infections in the perioperative setting, *AORN J* 92:519, 2010.
27. ECRI Institute: Surgical fire safety update: best practices for prevention. Retrieved from *www.ecri.org/Conferences/Pages/Surgical_Fires.aspx*.
*28. Association of periOperative Registered Nurses: Recommended practice for electrosurgery. In *Perioperative standards and recommended practices*, Denver, 2012, The Association.
*29. Association of periOperative Registered Nurses: AORN position statement on surgical smoke and bio-aerosols, 2012. Retrieved from *www.aorn.org/Clinical_Practice/Position_Statements/Position_Statements.aspx*.
30. The Joint Commission: Universal protocol, 2012. Retrieved from *www.jointcommission.org/assets/1/6/NPSG_Chapter_Jan2012_HAP.pdf*.
*31. World Health Organization: Safe surgery saves lives. Retrieved from *www.who.int/patientsafety/safesurgery/en*.
32. Association of periOperative Registered Nurses: Preventing wrong-patient, wrong-site, wrong-procedure events. Retrieved from *www.aorn.org/Clinical_Practice/Position_Statements/Position_Statements.aspx*.
*33. Association of periOperative Registered Nurses: Recommended practice for positioning the patient in the perioperative practice setting. In *Perioperative standards and recommended practices*, Denver, 2012, The Association.
*34. American Society of PeriAnesthesia Nurses: ASPAN's evidence-based clinical practice guideline for the promotion of perioperative normothermia. Retrieved from *www.aspan.org/ClinicalPractice/ClinicalGuidelines/Normothermia/tabid/5599/Default.aspx*.
*35. Lynch S, Dixon J, Leary D: Reducing the risk of unplanned perioperative hypothermia, *AORN J* 92:553, 2010.
*36. Jardeleza A, Fleig D, Davis N, et al: The effectiveness and cost of passive warming in adult ambulatory surgery patients, *AORN J* 94:363, 2011.
*37. Association of periOperative Registered Nurses: Recommended practice for skin preparation of patients. In *Perioperative standards and recommended practices*, Denver, 2012, The Association.
*38. Centers for Disease Control and Prevention: Guideline for prevention of surgical site infection, 1999. Retrieved from *www.cdc.gov/hicpac/pdf/guidelines/SSI_1999.pdf*. (Classic)
*39. Association of periOperative Registered Nurses: *Perioperative nursing data set: the perioperative nursing vocabulary*, ed 3, Denver, 2011, The Association.
40. American Society of Anesthesiologists: Frequently asked questions. Retrieved from *www.lifelinetomodernmedicine.com/FAQs.aspx*.
41. American Society of Anesthesiologists: Distinguishing monitored anesthesia care ("MAC") from moderate sedation/analgesia (conscious sedation). Retrieved from *www.asahq.org/.../Distinguishing%20Monitored%20Anesthesia%20Care%20From.ashx*.
42. American Association of Nurse Anesthetists: Considerations for policy development number 4.2 registered nurses engaged in the administration of sedation and analgesia, 2010. Retrieved from *www.aana.com/resources2/professionalpractice/Documents/PPM%20Consid%204.2%20RNs%20Engaged%20in%20Sedation%20Analgesia.pdf*.
43. Kossick MA: Inhalation anesthetics. In Naglehout JJ, Plaus KL, editors: *Nurse anesthesia*, ed 4, St Louis, 2010, Saunders.
44. Hodgson BB, Kizior RJ: *Saunders nursing drug handbook 2012*. St Louis, 2012, Saunders.
45. Silverstein JH, Steinmetz J, Reichenberg A, et al: Postoperative cognitive dysfunction in patients with preoperative cognitive impairment: which domains are most vulnerable? *Anesthesiology* 106:431, 2007.
46. Morrell RC: Intralipid might save lives as a rescue from bupivacaine toxicity, 2007. Retrieved from *www.apsf.org/newsletters/html/2007/summer/03_intralipid.htm*.
47. Olson RL, Pellegrini JE, Movinsky BA: Regional anesthesia. In Naglehout JJ, Plaus KL, editors: *Nurse anesthesia*, ed 4, St Louis, 2010, Saunders.
48. Ballantyne JC: Does epidural analgesia improve surgical outcome? *Br J Anesthesia* 92:4, 2004. (Classic)
49. Shoup AJ: Latex allergy. In Watson DS, editor: *Perioperative safety*, St Louis, 2011, Mosby.
*50. Malignant Hyperthermia Association of the United States: Emergency therapy for malignant hyperthermia, 2008. Retrieved from *http://medical.mhaus.org/PubData/PDFs/treatmentposter.pdf*.

RESOURCES

Resources for this chapter are listed in Chapter 20 on p. 366.

CHAPTER

20

Life moves pretty fast. If you don't stop and look around once in a while, you could miss it.
Ferris Bueller

Nursing Management

Postoperative Care

Christine Hoch

evolve WEBSITE

http://evolve.elsevier.com/Lewis/medsurg

- NCLEX Review Questions
- Key Points
- Pre-Test
- Answer Guidelines for Case Study on p. 364
- Rationales for Bridge to NCLEX Examination Questions
- Case Study
  - Patient Undergoing Surgery
- Nursing Care Plan (Customizable)
  - eNCP 20-1: Postoperative Patient
- Concept Map Creator
- Glossary
- Content Updates

eTable

- eTable 20-1: Modified Aldrete Scoring System

LEARNING OUTCOMES

1. Prioritize nursing responsibilities in admitting patients to the postanesthesia care unit (PACU).
2. Prioritize nursing responsibilities in the prevention of postoperative complications of patients in the PACU.
3. Apply data from the initial nursing assessment to the management of the patient after transfer from the PACU to the general care unit.
4. Select appropriate nursing interventions to manage potential problems during the postoperative period.
5. Differentiate discharge criteria from Phase I and Phase II postanesthesia care.

KEY TERMS

airway obstruction, p. 351
atelectasis, p. 351
delayed emergence, p. 357
emergence delirium, p. 357
fast-tracking, p. 349
patient-controlled analgesia (PCA), p. 358
postoperative ileus, p. 359
rapid postanesthesia care unit progression (RPP), p. 349

The postoperative period begins immediately after surgery and continues until the patient is discharged from medical care. This chapter focuses on the common features of postoperative nursing care of the surgical patient. Specific surgical procedures are discussed in the appropriate chapters of this text.

POSTOPERATIVE CARE OF THE SURGICAL PATIENT

The patient's immediate recovery period is managed in a *postanesthesia care unit (PACU),* which is located adjacent to the operating room (OR). This location minimizes transportation of the patient immediately after surgery and provides ready access to anesthesia and OR personnel. During the three phases of postanesthesia care, different levels of care are provided depending on the patient's needs[1] (Table 20-1).

Postanesthesia Care Unit Admission

The patient's initial admission to the PACU is a joint effort among the anesthesia care provider (ACP), the OR nurse, and the PACU nurse. This collaborative effort fosters a smooth transfer of care to the PACU and helps determine the phase to which the patient is assigned.

PACU Progression. How patients move through the phases of care in the PACU is determined by their condition. If a patient assigned to Phase I care on admission to the PACU is stable and recovering well, the patient may rapidly progress through Phase I to discharge to either Phase II care or an inpatient unit. This accelerated progress is called **rapid postanesthesia care unit progression (RPP).** Another accelerated system of care is **fast-tracking,** which involves admitting ambulatory surgery patients directly to Phase II care.[1] Although both RPP and fast-tracking can potentially result in time and cost savings, the patient's safety is the primary

Reviewed by Lisa Kiper, RN, MSN, Assistant Professor of Nursing, Morehead State University, Morehead, Kentucky; Heidi E. Monroe, RN, MSN, CPAN, CAPA, Assistant Professor of Nursing, Bellin College, Green Bay, Wisconsin; and Cynthia Schoonover, RN, MS, CCRN, Associate Nursing Professor, Sinclair Community College, Dayton, Ohio and PACU Staff Nurse, Kettering Medical Center, Kettering, Ohio.

TABLE 20-1 PHASES OF POSTANESTHESIA CARE

Phase I
- Care during the immediate postanesthesia period
- ECG and more intense monitoring (e.g., arterial BP monitoring, mechanical ventilation)
- *Goal:* Prepare patient for transfer to Phase II or inpatient unit

Phase II
- Ambulatory surgery patients
- *Goal:* Prepare patient for transfer to extended observation, home, or extended care facility

Extended Observation
- Extended care or observation unit
- *Goal:* Prepare patient for self-care

Source: American Society of PeriAnesthesia Nurses: *Perianesthesia nursing standards and practice recommendations 2010-2012,* Cherry Hill, NJ, 2010, The Society.

determining factor of where and at what level postoperative care is provided.[2,3]

Phase I Initial Assessment. On admission of the patient to the PACU, the ACP gives you a complete postanesthesia admission report (Table 20-2). The goal of PACU care is to identify actual and potential patient problems that may occur as a result of anesthesia and surgery and to intervene appropriately. Potential problems in the postoperative period are identified in Fig. 20-1. Table 20-3 identifies key components of a PACU assessment.

Begin the assessment with an evaluation of the patient's airway, breathing, and circulation (ABC) status. During the initial assessment, identify signs of inadequate oxygenation and ventilation (Table 20-4). Any evidence of respiratory compromise requires prompt intervention.

Pulse oximetry monitoring provides a noninvasive means of assessing oxygenation and can provide an early warning of hypoxemia.[4] *Transcutaneous carbon dioxide* ($PTCCO_2$) and *end-tidal* CO_2 ($PETCO_2$) *(capnography) monitoring* are used to detect respiratory depression.[5-6] (Pulse oximetry, $PTCCO_2$, and $PETCO_2$ are discussed in Chapter 26.)

Note and evaluate deviations in electrocardiographic (ECG) results from preoperative findings. Measure the blood pressure (BP) and compare it with baseline readings. Invasive monitoring (e.g., arterial BP) is initiated if needed. Also assess body temperature, capillary refill, and skin condition (e.g., color, moisture). Any evidence of inadequate circulatory status requires prompt intervention.

The initial neurologic assessment focuses on level of consciousness; orientation; sensory and motor status; and size, equality, and reactivity of the pupils. The patient may be awake, drowsy but arousable, or asleep. Because hearing is the first sense to return in the unconscious patient, explain all activities to the patient from the moment of admission to the PACU. If the patient received a regional anesthetic (e.g., spinal, epidural), sensory and motor blockade may still be present and a

TABLE 20-2 PACU ADMISSION REPORT

General Information
- Patient name
- Age
- Anesthesia care provider
- Surgeon
- Surgical procedure
- Type of anesthesia (e.g., general, regional, monitored anesthesia care [MAC])

Patient History
- Indication for surgery
- Medical history, medications, allergies
- Preoperative or baseline vital signs, level of consciousness, orientation

Intraoperative Management
- Anesthetic medications
- Other medications received preoperatively or intraoperatively
- Last dose of opioid administration
- Total fluid replacements, including blood transfusions
- Total fluid losses (e.g., blood, nasogastric drainage)
- Urine output

Intraoperative Course
- Unexpected anesthetic events or reactions
- Unexpected surgical events
- Most recent vital signs and monitoring trends
- Results of intraoperative laboratory tests

PACU, Postanesthesia care unit.

TABLE 20-3 INITIAL PACU ASSESSMENT

Airway
- Patency
- Oral or nasal airway
- Laryngeal mask airway
- Endotracheal tube

Breathing
- Respiratory rate and quality
- Auscultated breath sounds
- Pulse oximetry
- Supplemental O_2

Circulation
- ECG monitoring—rate and rhythm
- Blood pressure
- Temperature
- Capillary refill
- Color and temperature of skin
- Peripheral pulses

Neurologic
- Level of consciousness
- Orientation
- Sensory and motor status
- Pupil size and reaction

Gastrointestinal
- Nausea, vomiting
- Intake (fluids, irrigations)

Genitourinary
- Output (urine, drains)

Surgical Site
- Dressings and drainage

Pain
- Incision
- Other

TABLE 20-4 MANIFESTATIONS OF INADEQUATE OXYGENATION

Central Nervous System
- Restlessness
- Agitation
- Confusion
- Muscle twitching
- Seizures
- Coma

Cardiovascular System
- Hypertension
- Hypotension
- Tachycardia
- Bradycardia
- Dysrhythmias
- Delayed capillary refill
- Decreased O_2 saturation

Integumentary System
- Flushed and moist skin
- Cyanosis

Respiratory System
- Increased to absent respiratory effort
- Use of accessory muscles
- Abnormal breath sounds
- Abnormal arterial blood gases

Renal System
- Urine output <0.5 mL/kg/hr

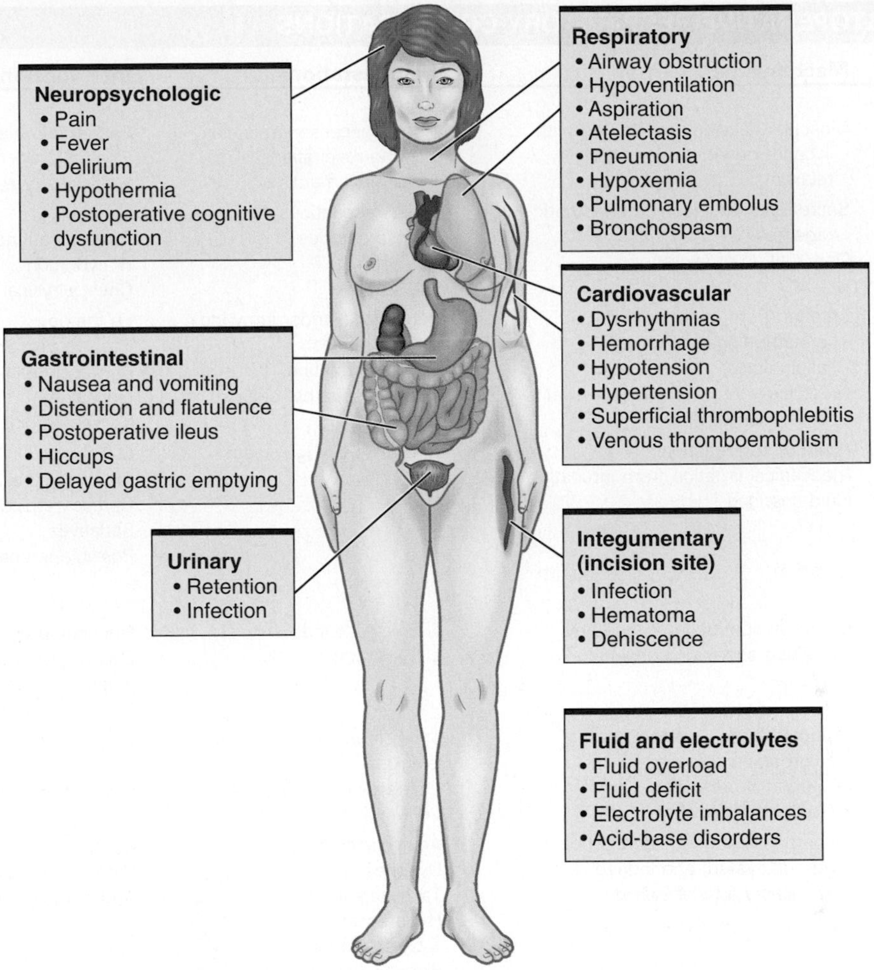

FIG. 20-1 Potential problems in the postoperative period.

dermatome level should be checked (see eFig. 9-1). (A dermatome is an area of the skin that is supplied by a single spinal nerve.) During recovery from regional anesthesia, sensory and motor function returns from the extremities to the site where the anesthetic was administered. Therefore the areas near the site of injections are the last to recover.

Assessment of the urinary system focuses on intake, output, and fluid balance. Intraoperative fluid totals are part of the anesthesia report. Note the presence of all IV lines; all irrigation solutions and infusions; and all output devices, including catheters and wound drains. Assess the surgical site, noting the condition of any dressings and the type and amount of any drainage. Implement postoperative orders related to incision care.

Nursing management of these problems is discussed in the following pages and can be applied to patients in both the PACU and the clinical unit.

RESPIRATORY PROBLEMS

Etiology

PACU. In the immediate postanesthesia period the most common causes of airway compromise include obstruction, hypoxemia, and hypoventilation (Table 20-5). Patients at high risk include those who have had general anesthesia; are older; have a smoking history; have obstructive sleep apnea or lung disease; are obese; or have undergone airway, thoracic, or abdominal surgery. However, respiratory problems may occur with any patient who has been anesthetized.

Airway obstruction is commonly caused by blockage of the airway by the patient's tongue (Fig. 20-2). The base of the tongue falls backward against the soft palate and occludes the pharynx. It is most pronounced in the supine position and in the patient who is extremely sleepy after surgery.

Hypoxemia, a partial pressure of arterial oxygen (PaO_2) less than 60 mm Hg, is characterized by a variety of nonspecific clinical signs and symptoms, ranging from agitation to somnolence, hypertension to hypotension, and tachycardia to bradycardia. Pulse oximetry will indicate low O_2 saturation (less than 90% to 92%).

The most common cause of postoperative hypoxemia is atelectasis. **Atelectasis** (alveolar collapse) may be the result of bronchial obstruction caused by retained secretions or decreased respiratory excursion. Atelectasis may also result from general anesthesia. Atelectasis occurs when mucus blocks bronchioles or when the amount of alveolar surfactant (the substance that holds the alveoli open) is reduced (Fig. 20-3). As air becomes trapped beyond the plug and is eventually absorbed, the alveoli collapse. Atelectasis may affect a portion of or an entire lobe of the lungs.

Other causes of hypoxemia include pulmonary edema, pulmonary embolism (PE), aspiration, and bronchospasm.

TABLE 20-5 **POSTOPERATIVE RESPIRATORY COMPLICATIONS**

Complications	Mechanisms	Manifestations	Interventions
Airway Obstruction			
Tongue falling back	Muscular flaccidity associated with ↓ consciousness and muscle relaxants	Use of accessory muscles Snoring respirations ↓ Air movement	Patient stimulation Head tilt, jaw thrust (see Fig. 20-2) Artificial airway
Retained thick secretions	Secretion stimulation by anesthetic agents Dehydration of secretions	Noisy respirations Coarse crackles	Suctioning Deep breathing and coughing IV hydration Chest physical therapy
Laryngospasm	Irritation from endotracheal tube, anesthetic gases, or gastric aspiration Most likely to occur after removal of endotracheal tube	Inspiratory stridor (crowing respirations) Sternal retraction Acute respiratory distress	O_2 therapy Positive pressure ventilation IV muscle relaxant Lidocaine Corticosteroids
Laryngeal edema	Allergic drug reaction Mechanical irritation from intubation Fluid overload	Similar to laryngospasm	O_2 therapy Antihistamines Corticosteroids Sedatives Possible intubation
Hypoxemia			
Atelectasis	Bronchial obstruction caused by retained secretions or ↓ lung volumes	↓ Breath sounds ↓ O_2 saturation	Humidified O_2 therapy Deep breathing Incentive spirometry Early mobilization
Pulmonary edema	Fluid overload ↑ Hydrostatic pressure ↓ Interstitial pressure ↑ Capillary permeability	↓ O_2 saturation Crackles Infiltrates on chest x-ray	O_2 therapy Diuretics Fluid restriction
Pulmonary embolism	Thrombus dislodged from peripheral venous system and lodged in pulmonary arterial system	Acute tachypnea Dyspnea Tachycardia Hypotension ↓ O_2 saturation Bronchospasm	O_2 therapy Cardiopulmonary support Anticoagulant therapy
Aspiration	Inhalation of gastric contents into lungs	Unexplained tachypnea Bronchospasm ↓ O_2 saturation Atelectasis Interstitial edema Alveolar hemorrhage Respiratory failure	O_2 therapy Cardiac support Antibiotics
Bronchospasm	↑ Smooth muscle tone with closure of small airways	Wheezing Dyspnea Tachypnea ↓ O_2 saturation	O_2 therapy Bronchodilators
Hypoventilation			
Depression of central respiratory drive	Medullary depression from anesthetics, opioids, sedatives	Shallow respirations ↓ Respiratory rate, apnea ↓ PaO_2 ↑ $PaCO_2$	Stimulation Reversal of opioids or benzodiazepines Mechanical ventilation
Poor respiratory muscle tone	Neuromuscular blockade Neuromuscular disease	As above	Reversal of paralysis Mechanical ventilation
Mechanical restriction	Tight casts, dressings, abdominal binders. Positioning and obesity preventing lung expansion	As above	Elevate head of bed Repositioning Loosen dressings
Pain	Shallow breathing to prevent incisional pain	↑ Respiratory rate Hypotension Hypertension ↓ $PaCO_2$ ↓ PaO_2 Complaints of pain Guarding behavior	Opioid analgesic drug therapy Nonsteroidal antiinflammatory drug therapy Adjunctive complementary and alternative therapies (e.g., music therapy, guided imagery)

$PaCO_2$, Partial pressure of arterial carbon dioxide; *PaO_2*, partial pressure of arterial oxygen.

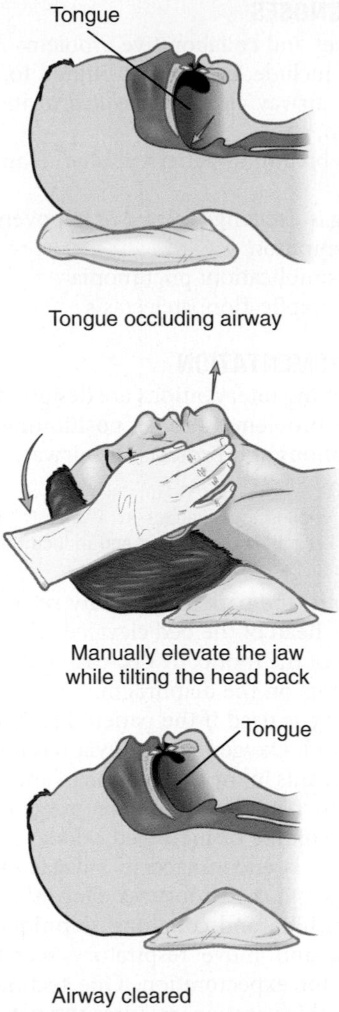

FIG. 20-2 Etiology and relief of airway obstruction.

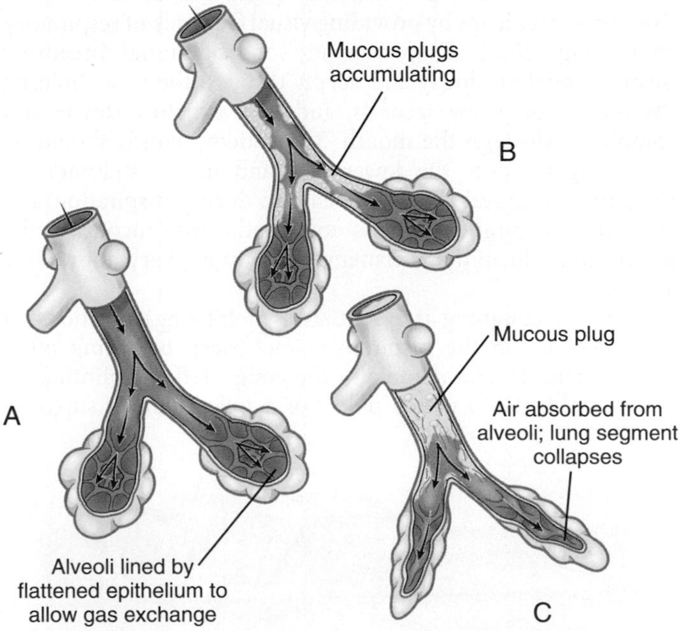

FIG. 20-3 Postoperative atelectasis. **A,** Normal bronchiole and alveoli. **B,** Mucous plug in bronchiole. **C,** Collapse of alveoli resulting from atelectasis after absorption of air.

Pulmonary edema is caused by an accumulation of fluid in the alveoli. It may be the result of fluid overload, left ventricular failure, prolonged airway obstruction, sepsis, or aspiration.

Aspiration of gastric contents into the lungs is a potentially serious emergency. Gastric aspiration may also cause laryngospasm, infection, and pulmonary edema. Because of the serious consequences of aspiration of gastric fluids, prevention is the goal.

Bronchospasm is the result of an increase in bronchial smooth muscle tone with resultant closure of small airways. Airway edema develops, causing secretions to build up in the airway. The patient will have wheezing, dyspnea, use of accessory muscles, hypoxemia, and tachypnea. Bronchospasm may be due to aspiration, endotracheal intubation, suctioning, or an allergic response. (Allergic responses are discussed in Chapter 14.) Bronchospasm may occur in any patient but is seen more frequently in patients with asthma and chronic obstructive pulmonary disease (COPD).

Hypoventilation, a common complication in the PACU, is characterized by a decreased respiratory rate or effort, hypoxemia, and an increasing partial pressure of arterial carbon dioxide ($PaCO_2$) *(hypercapnia)*. Hypoventilation may result from depression of the central respiratory drive (secondary to anesthesia or pain medication), poor respiratory muscle tone (secondary to neuromuscular blockade or disease), or a combination of both.

Clinical Unit. Common causes of respiratory problems for postoperative patients in the clinical unit are atelectasis and pneumonia, especially after abdominal and thoracic surgery. The postoperative development of mucous plugs and decreased surfactant production is directly related to hypoventilation, immobility and bed rest, ineffective coughing, and history of smoking. Increased bronchial secretions occur when the respiratory passages have been irritated by heavy smoking; acute or chronic pulmonary infection or disease; and the drying of mucous membranes that occurs with intubation, inhalation anesthesia, and dehydration. Without intervention, atelectasis can progress to pneumonia.

NURSING MANAGEMENT RESPIRATORY PROBLEMS

NURSING ASSESSMENT

For an adequate respiratory assessment, evaluate airway patency; chest symmetry; and the depth, rate, and character of respirations. Observe the chest wall for symmetry of movement. Impaired ventilation may initially be seen as slowed breathing or reduced chest and abdominal movement during breathing. Also assess for the use of abdominal or accessory muscles, which may indicate respiratory distress. Auscultate breath sounds, since decreased or absent breath sounds are found when airflow is diminished or obstructed.

Regular monitoring of vital signs, including pulse oximetry, and a thorough respiratory assessment permit you to recognize early signs of respiratory problems. Manifestations of hypoxemia include tachypnea, gasping, anxiety, restlessness, confusion, and a rapid or thready pulse.

Note and record the characteristics of sputum or mucus. Mucus from the trachea and throat is normally colorless and thin in consistency. Sputum from the lungs and bronchi is normally thick with a pale yellow tinge. Changes in sputum (e.g., color) may indicate a respiratory infection.

DELEGATION DECISIONS

Postoperative Patient

In the PACU, patients require frequent assessment and intervention by RNs. On the clinical units, the RN is responsible for assessment, development of an individualized plan of care, evaluation of the patient, and discharge teaching. Much of the care can be delegated to LPN/LVNs and UAP.

PACU	Clinical Unit
Registered Nurse (RN)	
• Assess patient's initial airway, breathing, and circulation status. • Evaluate for the return to consciousness, ability to maintain airway and breathing. • Provide ongoing assessments for postoperative problems (e.g., airway obstruction, hypoventilation, hypotension or hypertension, dysrhythmias, emergence delirium). • Evaluate patient's readiness to transfer to the clinical unit or be discharged from ambulatory surgery. • Provide oral and written report about patient status when transferring patient to RN on the clinical unit. • Provide discharge teaching for patient and caregiver after ambulatory surgery.	• Assess patient on initial admission to the clinical unit. • Assess for postoperative complications (e.g., atelectasis, hemodynamic instability, cognitive dysfunction, pain, fluid and electrolyte disturbance, fever or hypothermia, nausea and vomiting, urinary retention, wound infection). • Develop an individualized plan of care based on identification of patient risk factors and potential complications. • Develop and implement individualized patient and caregiver education, including discharge teaching.
Licensed Practical/Vocational Nurse (LPN/LVN)	
• Administer and titrate O_2 based on agency protocols. • Administer analgesics and IV fluids (consider state nurse practice act and agency policy).	• Titrate O_2 administration according to prescribed parameters. • Monitor pain level and administer prescribed analgesics. • Administer medications (consider state nurse practice act and agency policy for medications). • Provide wound care, including dressing changes. • Use bladder ultrasound to check for urinary retention. • Insert catheter as prescribed for urinary retention.
Unlicensed Assistive Personnel (UAP)	
• Assist with positioning of patients in the "recovery" position. • Obtain vital signs and pulse oximetry; report abnormal levels to RN. • Assist patient with elimination needs. • Assist in transfer of patient to clinical unit.	• Monitor vital signs, pulse oximetry, and intake and output. Report abnormal levels to RN. • Assist patient with deep breathing and coughing exercises. • Report complaints of pain to RN or LPN/LVN. • Reposition and ambulate patients. • Provide hygiene, including oral care. • Assist with nutrition and elimination needs.

NURSING DIAGNOSES

Nursing diagnoses and collaborative problems related to respiratory problems include, but are not limited to, the following:

- Ineffective airway clearance *related to* ineffective cough, obstruction, pain
- Ineffective breathing pattern *related to* anesthetic agents, pain
- Impaired gas exchange *related to* hypoventilation
- Risk for aspiration
- Potential complication: pneumonia
- Potential complication: atelectasis

NURSING IMPLEMENTATION

In the PACU, nursing interventions are designed to prevent and treat respiratory problems. Proper positioning of the patient facilitates respirations and protects the airway.

SAFETY ALERT

- Position the unconscious patient in a lateral "recovery" position (Fig. 20-4) to keep the airway open and reduce the risk of aspiration if vomiting occurs.

Once conscious, the patient is usually returned to a supine position with the head of the bed elevated. This position maximizes expansion of the thorax by decreasing the pressure of the abdominal contents on the diaphragm.

Oxygen therapy is used if the patient has had general anesthesia or if ordered. Oxygen is given via nasal cannula or face mask. The oxygen aids in the elimination of anesthetic gases and helps meet the increased demand for oxygen resulting from decreased blood volume or increased cellular metabolism.

Deep breathing is encouraged to aid gas exchange and to promote the return to consciousness. Once the patient is more awake, deep-breathing and coughing techniques help prevent alveolar collapse and move respiratory secretions to larger airway passages for expectoration. One technique, known as *sustained maximal inspiration,* requires the patient to inhale as deeply as possible and, at the peak of inspiration, hold the breath for a few seconds, and then exhale. This should be followed by a second deep breath and cough. The use of an incentive spirometer helps by providing visual feedback of respiratory effort (Fig. 20-5). Diaphragmatic or abdominal breathing involves inhaling slowly and deeply through the nose, holding the breath for a few seconds, and then exhaling slowly and completely through the mouth. The patient's hands should be placed lightly over the lower ribs and upper abdomen so the patient can feel the abdomen rise during inspiration and fall during expiration. Unless contraindicated, encourage the patient to perform these maneuvers 10 times every hour while awake.

Effective coughing is essential in mobilizing secretions. If secretions are in the respiratory tract, deep breathing often moves them up and stimulates the cough reflex. Splinting an abdominal incision with a pillow or a rolled blanket supports

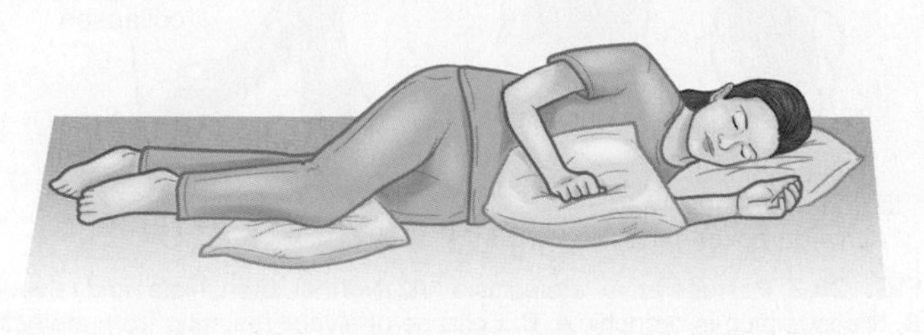

FIG. 20-4 Position of patient during recovery from general anesthesia.

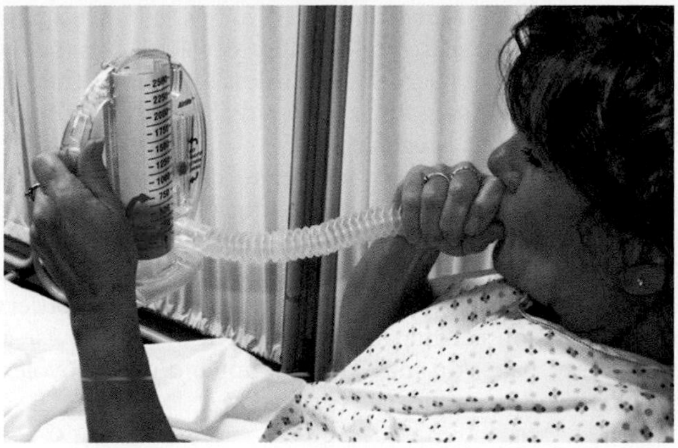

FIG. 20-5 Proper use of an incentive spirometer.

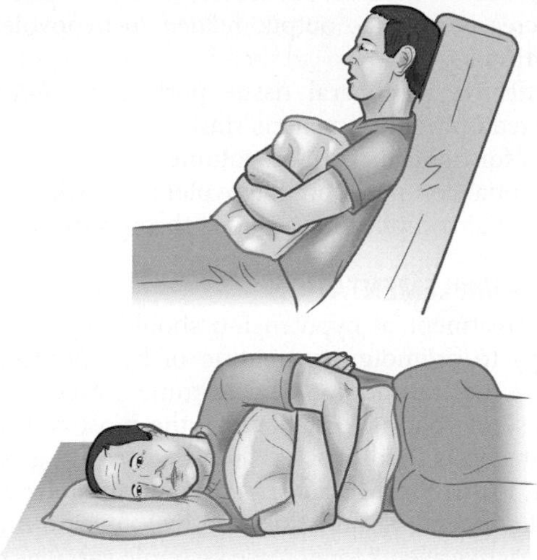

FIG. 20-6 Techniques for splinting incision when coughing.

the incision and aids in coughing and expectorating secretions (Fig. 20-6).

Change the patient's position every 1 to 2 hours to allow full chest expansion and to increase perfusion of both lungs. Sitting in a chair and ambulating should be carried out as soon as physician approval is given. Provide adequate and regular analgesic medication because incisional pain often is the greatest barrier to patient participation in effective breathing exercises and ambulation. Also reassure the patient that these activities will not cause the incision to open. Adequate hydration, either parenteral or oral, is essential to maintain the integrity of mucous membranes and to keep secretions thin and loose for easy expectoration.

Other nursing interventions appropriate for specific respiratory problems are detailed in Table 20-5. A nursing care plan for the postoperative patient (eNursing Care Plan 20-1) is available on the website for this chapter.

CARDIOVASCULAR PROBLEMS

Etiology

PACU. In the immediate postanesthesia period the most common cardiovascular problems include hypotension, hypertension, and dysrhythmias. Patients at greatest risk for alterations in cardiovascular function include those with alterations in respiratory function, those with a history of cardiovascular disease, older adults, the debilitated, and the critically ill.

Hypotension is evidenced by signs of hypoperfusion to the vital organs, especially the brain, heart, and kidneys. Clinical signs of disorientation, loss of consciousness, chest pain, and oliguria reflect hypoperfusion, hypoxemia, and the loss of physiologic compensation. Intervention must be timely to prevent the devastating complications of cardiac ischemia or infarction, cerebral ischemia, renal ischemia, and bowel infarction.

The most common cause of hypotension in the PACU is unreplaced fluid and blood loss, which may lead to hypovolemic shock. Hemorrhage is always a risk of surgery. Marked blood loss is possible when cauterization or sutures fail. Hemorrhage most often occurs internally, requiring assessment for changes in level of consciousness and vital signs. If changes are detected, treatment is directed toward restoring circulating volume. If there is no response to fluid administration, cardiac dysfunction should be considered the cause of hypotension.

Primary cardiac dysfunction, as may occur in myocardial infarction, cardiac tamponade, or PE, results in an acute fall in cardiac output. Secondary myocardial dysfunction occurs as a result of the negative *chronotropic* (rate of cardiac contraction) and negative *inotropic* (force of cardiac contraction) effects of drugs, such as β-adrenergic blockers, digoxin, or opioids. Other causes of hypotension include decreased systemic vascular resistance, dysrhythmias, and measurement errors (e.g., taking BP with an incorrectly sized cuff).

Hypertension, a common finding in the PACU, is most frequently the result of sympathetic nervous system stimulation that may be the result of pain, anxiety, bladder distention, or respiratory compromise. Hypertension may also be the result of hypothermia and preexisting hypertension.

In the PACU, *dysrhythmias* are caused by hypoxemia, hypercapnia, alterations in electrolyte and acid-base status, circulatory instability, and preexisting heart disease. Hypothermia, pain, surgical stress, and many anesthetic agents can also cause dysrhythmias.

Clinical Unit. In the clinical unit, postoperative fluid and electrolyte imbalances are contributing factors to cardiovascular problems. Such imbalances may result from a combination of the body's normal response to the stress of surgery, excessive fluid losses, and improper IV fluid replacement. The body's fluid status directly affects cardiac output.

Fluid retention during postoperative days 1 to 3 can result from the stress response, which serves to maintain both blood volume and BP. Fluid retention is caused by the secretion and release of two hormones by the pituitary—antidiuretic hormone (ADH) and adrenocorticotropic hormone (ACTH)—and activation of the renin-angiotensin-aldosterone system (RAAS). ADH release leads to increased water reabsorption and decreased urine output, increasing blood volume. ACTH stimulates the adrenal cortex to secrete cortisol and, to a lesser degree, aldosterone. Fluid losses resulting from surgery decrease kidney perfusion, stimulating the RAAS and causing marked release of aldosterone (see Chapter 17). Both mechanisms that increase aldosterone lead to significant sodium and fluid retention, thus increasing blood volume.

Fluid overload may occur during this period of fluid retention when IV fluids are administered too rapidly, when chronic (e.g., cardiac, renal) disease exists, or when the patient is an older adult. Fluid deficits from untreated preoperative dehydration, intraoperative blood losses, or slow or inadequate fluid replacement can lead to decreases in cardiac output and tissue perfusion. Postoperative losses from vomiting, bleeding, wound drainage, or suctioning can also contribute to fluid deficits.

Hypokalemia can be a consequence of urinary and gastrointestinal (GI) tract losses. Low serum potassium levels directly affect the contractility of the heart and may contribute to decreases in cardiac output and tissue perfusion. Potassium replacement, usually 40 mEq/day, should not be given until renal function is assessed. A urine output of at least 0.5 mL/kg/hr is generally considered indicative of adequate renal function.

Cardiovascular status is also affected by the state of tissue perfusion or blood flow. The stress response contributes to an increase in clotting tendencies by increasing platelet production. In addition, general anesthesia causes peripheral vasodilation, which may contribute to damage of the vascular lining.

A *venous thromboembolism* (VTE) may form in leg veins as a result of inactivity, body position, and pressure, all of which lead to venous stasis and decreased perfusion. VTE is especially common in older adults, obese individuals, immobilized patients, and patients with a history of PE. It is a potentially life-threatening complication because it may lead to PE and infarction. Suspect PE in any patient with tachypnea, dyspnea, and tachycardia, particularly when the patient is already receiving O_2 therapy. Other manifestations may include agitation, chest pain, hypotension, hemoptysis, dysrhythmias, and heart failure. Superficial thrombophlebitis is an uncomfortable but less serious complication that may develop in a leg vein as a result of venous stasis or in the arm veins as a result of irritation from IV catheters or solutions. (PE and VTE are discussed in Chapters 28 and 38, respectively.)

Syncope (fainting) may indicate decreased cardiac output, fluid deficits, or defects in cerebral perfusion. Syncope frequently occurs as a result of postural hypotension when the patient ambulates. It is more common in the older adult or in the patient who has been immobile for long periods. Normally when the patient stands up quickly, the arterial baroreceptors respond to the accompanying fall in BP with sympathetic nervous system stimulation. This produces vasoconstriction and thereby maintains BP. These sympathetic and vasomotor functions may be diminished in the older adult and the immobile or postanesthesia patient.

NURSING MANAGEMENT CARDIOVASCULAR PROBLEMS

NURSING ASSESSMENT

The most important aspect of the cardiovascular assessment is frequent monitoring of vital signs. They are usually monitored every 15 minutes in Phase I, or more often until stabilized, and then at less frequent intervals in Phase II. Compare postoperative vital signs with preoperative and intraoperative readings to determine when the signs are returning to baseline. Notify the ACP or the surgeon if any of the following occurs:

- Systolic BP less than 90 mm Hg or greater than 160 mm Hg
- Pulse rate less than 60 beats/minute or greater than 120 beats/minute
- Pulse pressure (difference between systolic and diastolic pressures) narrows
- BP trends gradually decrease over several consecutive readings
- Change in cardiac rhythm

ECG monitoring is recommended for patients who have a history of cardiac disease and for all older adult patients who have undergone major surgery, regardless of whether they have cardiac problems. Assess the apical-radial pulse carefully, and report any deficits or irregularities.

Assessment of skin color, temperature, and moisture provides valuable information in detecting cardiovascular problems. Hypotension accompanied by a normal pulse and warm, dry, pink skin usually represents the residual vasodilating effects of anesthesia and suggests only a need for continued observation. Hypotension accompanied by a rapid or weak pulse and cold, clammy, pale skin may indicate impending hypovolemic shock and requires immediate treatment.

NURSING DIAGNOSES

Nursing diagnoses and collaborative problems related to cardiovascular problems include, but are not limited to, the following:

- Decreased cardiac output *related to* hypovolemia, dysrhythmias
- Ineffective peripheral tissue perfusion *related to* prolonged immobility, venous stasis
- Risk for imbalanced fluid volume
- Potential complication: hypovolemic shock
- Potential complication: venous thromboembolism

NURSING IMPLEMENTATION

PACU. Treatment of hypotension should always begin with O_2 therapy to promote oxygenation of hypoperfused organs. Inspect the surgical incision to determine if excessive bleeding is the cause of volume loss. Because the most common cause of hypotension is fluid loss, IV fluid boluses are given to normalize BP. Primary cardiac dysfunction may require drug intervention. Peripheral vasodilation and hypotension may require vasoconstrictive agents to increase systemic vascular resistance.

Treatment of hypertension centers on eliminating the cause of sympathetic nervous system stimulation. Treatment may include the use of analgesics, assistance in voiding, and correction of respiratory problems. Rewarming corrects hypothermia-induced hypertension. If the patient has preexisting hypertension or has undergone cardiac or vascular surgery, drug therapy to reduce BP is usually required.

Because the majority of dysrhythmias seen in the PACU have identifiable causes, treatment is directed toward removing the cause. Correction of these physiologic alterations usually corrects the dysrhythmias. In the event of life-threatening dysrhythmias (e.g., ventricular tachycardia), protocols for advanced cardiac life support are followed.

CLINICAL UNIT. Maintaining an accurate intake and output record, monitoring laboratory findings (e.g., electrolytes, hematocrit), and managing IV therapy are key nursing responsibilities during the postoperative period. Ongoing assessment of the potential complications associated with IV potassium, such as cardiac dysrhythmias and pain at the infusion site, is essential.

Early ambulation is the most significant general nursing measure to prevent postoperative complications. The exercise associated with walking (1) increases muscle tone; (2) stimulates circulation, which prevents venous stasis and VTE, and speeds wound healing; and (3) increases vital capacity and maintains normal respiratory function.

Recommendations for the prevention of VTE for patients who undergo a major surgical procedure or who have multiple risk factors for VTE (e.g., nonambulatory, older, history of VTE) include prophylaxis with low-molecular-weight heparin (LMWH) (e.g., dalteparin [Fragmin], enoxaparin [Lovenox]) or low-dose unfractionated heparin. In addition, sequential compression devices (SCDs) are often used in combination with drug prophylaxis.[7] (SCDs are discussed in Chapter 38.)

You can prevent syncope by slowly making changes in the patient's position. Progression to ambulation can be achieved by first raising the head of the patient's bed for 1 to 2 minutes and then assisting the patient to sit, with legs dangling, while monitoring the pulse rate. If no changes or complaints are noted, start ambulation with ongoing monitoring of the pulse. If changes in the pulse are noted or dizziness occurs, sit the patient in a nearby chair. The patient should remain in this location until the BP and pulse are stable. Then help the patient back to the bed. If dizziness occurs, it is often frightening for the patient and you. Injury can result from a fall, so take measures to ensure patient safety.

NEUROLOGIC AND PSYCHOLOGIC PROBLEMS

Etiology

PACU. Postoperatively, **emergence delirium**, or *waking up wild,* is the neurologic alteration that causes the most concern. It is manifested by behaviors such as restlessness, agitation, disorientation, thrashing, and shouting. This condition may be caused by hypoxia, anesthetic agents, bladder distention, pain, residual neuromuscular blockade, or the presence of an endotracheal tube.[8] If delirium occurs, first suspect hypoxia.

Delayed emergence may also be a problem postoperatively. Fortunately, the most common cause of delayed emergence is prolonged drug action, particularly of opioids, sedatives, and inhalation anesthetics, as opposed to neurologic injury. Normal awakening can be predicted by the ACP based on the drugs used in surgery.

Clinical Unit. Two types of postoperative cognitive impairments seen in surgical patients are *postoperative cognitive dysfunction* (POCD) and *delirium.* POCD is a decline in the patient's cognitive function (e.g., memory, ability to concentrate) for weeks or months after surgery. POCD is primarily seen in the older surgical patient. Preexisting cognitive impairment, age, duration of anesthesia, intraoperative complications, and postoperative infections are related to the development of POCD.[9]

Postoperative delirium is more common in the older patient, but it can occur in patients of any age. Delirium may be the result of severe postoperative pain, fluid and electrolyte imbalances, hypoxemia, drug effects, sleep deprivation, and sensory deprivation or overload. It is characterized by cognitive dysfunction, varying levels of consciousness, altered psychomotor activity, and a disturbed sleep/wake cycle. (Delirium is discussed in Chapter 60.)

Anxiety and depression may also occur in postoperative patients. Any patient may experience these responses as part of grieving for lost body parts or functions or for decreased independence during the recovery and rehabilitation process.

Alcohol withdrawal delirium occurs as a result of alcohol withdrawal in a postoperative patient. It is characterized by restlessness, insomnia and nightmares, irritability, and auditory or visual hallucinations. Identification and management of alcohol withdrawal delirium are discussed in Chapter 11.

NURSING MANAGEMENT NEUROLOGIC AND PSYCHOLOGIC PROBLEMS

NURSING ASSESSMENT

Assess the patient's level of consciousness, orientation, memory, and ability to follow commands. Determine the size, reactivity, and equality of the pupils. Also assess the patient's sleep/wake cycle and sensory and motor status. If the neurologic status is altered, try to determine possible causes. If the patient was mentally alert before surgery and becomes cognitively impaired postoperatively, you should suspect delirium or POCD.

NURSING DIAGNOSES

Nursing diagnoses related to neurologic or psychologic problems include, but are not limited to, the following:

- Acute confusion *related to* hypoxia, postoperative cognitive dysfunction, delirium
- Anxiety *related to* change in health status, hospital environment
- Disturbed body image *related to* loss of body part(s), function
- Disturbed sleep pattern *related to* pain, hospital environment

NURSING IMPLEMENTATION

PACU. The most common cause of postoperative agitation in the PACU is hypoxemia. As a result, focus your attention on evaluating respiratory function. Once you have ruled out hypoxemia or other known causes of postoperative delirium, sedation may be beneficial in controlling the agitation. Because the most common cause of delayed emergence is prolonged drug action, delays in awakening usually spontaneously resolve with time. If necessary, benzodiazepines and opioids may be reversed with drug antagonists.

Until the patient is awake and able to communicate effectively, be a patient advocate and maintain patient safety at all times. This includes having the side rails up, securing equipment (e.g., IV lines, artificial airways), monitoring physiologic status, and verifying the presence of identification and allergy bands.

Clinical Unit. To prevent or manage postoperative delirium or POCD, address factors that are known to contribute to the condition. Maintenance of normal physiologic function is important and includes fluid and electrolyte balance, adequate nutrition and sleep, pain management, proper bowel and bladder function, and early mobilization. To help orient the patient, use specific aids, such as clocks, calendars, and photos.

To prevent or limit psychologic problems, provide adequate support for the patient. This includes listening to and talking with the patient, offering explanations and reassurance, and encouraging the presence and assistance of the patient's caregiver(s). Evaluate the patient's behavior to distinguish a normal reaction to a stressful situation from one that is becoming abnormal or excessive. The recognition of alcohol withdrawal delirium presents a particular challenge. Document and report any unusual or disturbed behavior so that a diagnosis and treatment may be made.

PAIN AND DISCOMFORT

Etiology

Despite the availability of pain-relieving drugs and techniques, pain remains a common problem and a significant fear for patients. Postoperative pain is caused by the interaction of a number of physiologic and psychologic factors. The skin and underlying tissues have been traumatized by the incision and retraction during surgery. In addition, there may be reflex muscle spasms around the incision. Anxiety and fear, sometimes related to the anticipation of pain, create tension and further increase muscle tone and spasm. Positioning during surgery or the use of internal devices such as an endotracheal tube or catheters may also result in pain. The effort and movement associated with deep breathing, coughing, and ambulating may aggravate pain by creating tension on the incision area.

When the internal viscera are cut, no pain is felt. However, pressure in the internal viscera elicits pain. Therefore deep visceral pain may signal a complication such as intestinal distention, bleeding, or abscess formation. Pain also increases the risk of atelectasis and impaired respiratory function.[10]

NURSING MANAGEMENT PAIN

NURSING ASSESSMENT

The patient's self-report is the single most reliable indicator of pain. Since this is not always possible in the PACU, observe the patient for other indications of pain (e.g., restlessness, changes in vital signs, diaphoresis). Identifying the location of the pain is important. Incisional pain is to be expected, but other causes of pain, such as a full bladder, may also be present.

The American Society for Pain Management Nursing and American Society of PeriAnesthesia Nurses have developed evidence-based guidelines for the nursing management of pain throughout the perioperative experience.[11,12] In addition, The Joint Commission requires that effective pain management strategies be implemented for all patients experiencing pain.[13] (Pain is discussed in Chapter 9.)

NURSING DIAGNOSES

A nursing diagnoses for the patient experiencing pain includes, but is not limited to, the following:

- Acute pain *related to* inflammation or injury in surgical area

NURSING IMPLEMENTATION

The most effective interventions for postoperative pain management include using a variety of analgesics. IV opioids provide the most rapid relief.[14] More sustained relief may be obtained using epidural catheters, patient-controlled analgesia (PCA), or regional anesthetic blockade.

Orders for analgesic medication and other comfort measures are often written on an as-needed (PRN) basis. During the first 48 hours or longer, opioid analgesics (e.g., morphine) are required to relieve moderate to severe pain. A combination of two analgesics (e.g., an opioid and a nonsteroidal antiinflammatory drug [NSAID]) may be used to provide the lowest dose of medication and decrease side effects.[15] Nonopioid analgesics, such as NSAIDs, may be sufficient as pain decreases.

Time the administration of analgesics to ensure that they are in effect during activities that may be painful, such as walking. Although opioid analgesics are often essential for the postoperative patient's comfort, there are undesirable side effects. The most common include constipation, nausea and vomiting, respiratory and cough depression, and hypotension. Before administering any analgesic, first assess the patient's pain, including location, quality, and intensity; respiratory rate; and level of consciousness. If it is incisional pain, analgesic administration is appropriate. If it is chest or leg pain, medication may simply mask a complication (e.g., VTE). If it is gas pain, opioids can aggravate it. If the analgesic either fails to relieve the pain or makes the patient excessively lethargic or somnolent, notify the physician and request a change in the order.

Patient-controlled analgesia (PCA) and epidural analgesia are two alternative approaches for pain control. The goals of PCA are to provide immediate analgesia and to maintain a constant, steady blood level of the analgesic agent. PCA involves self-administration of predetermined doses of analgesia by the patient. The route of delivery may be IV, oral, epidural, or transdermal. The transdermal route is designed for short-term pain management and may offer advantages over the IV route (e.g., needleless, low infection risk, decreased medication errors associated with inaccurate pump function or programming).[14] Some advantages of PCA are early ambulation, better pain management than with PRN analgesia, and greater patient satisfaction. (PCA is discussed in Chapter 9.)

Epidural analgesia is the infusion of opioid analgesics through a catheter placed into the epidural space surrounding the spinal cord (see Fig. 19-6). The goal of epidural analgesia is delivery of medication directly to opiate receptors in the spinal cord. Administration methods include intermittent bolus dosing, continuous infusion, and patient-controlled epidural analgesia. This technique results in a constant circulating level and a reduced total dose of medication. The use of epidural analgesia for postoperative pain is increasing. Superior pain relief and improved functional outcomes after major surgery have been found in patients who receive epidural analgesia compared with those who receive IV opioids.[16,17]

Postoperative pain can also be managed by the infiltration of a nonopioid medication into the surgical site. A single dose of bupivacaine liposome injectable suspension (Exparel) provides pain relief with reduced opioid requirements for up to 72 hours.

The acute pain of surgery almost always requires the use of analgesics. However, nondrug approaches such as repositioning, massage, distraction, and deep breathing can enhance pain management. Complementary and alternative therapies such as music therapy, guided imagery, relaxation exercises, and aromatherapy have also been shown to be effective adjuncts in pain management.[18,19]

ALTERATIONS IN TEMPERATURE

Etiology

The patient's temperature in the postoperative period provides valuable information (Table 20-6).

Hypothermia. *Hypothermia,* a core temperature less than 96.8° F (36° C), occurs when heat loss exceeds heat production. Heat loss may occur due to skin exposure by the surgical procedure and the use of cold irrigants and unwarmed inhaled gases.[20] Although all patients are at risk for hypothermia, patients with a systolic BP less than 140 mm Hg, older patients, and female patients are at a higher risk of developing hypothermia postoperatively.[21] Long surgical procedures and prolonged anesthetic administration lead to redistribution of body heat from the core to the periphery. This places the patient at an increased risk for hypothermia.

Hypothermia can affect the patient's perception of the perioperative experience. The complications associated with hypo-

TABLE 20-6 POSTOPERATIVE TEMPERATURE CHANGES

Time After Surgery	Temperature	Possible Causes
Up to 12 hr	Hypothermia: ≤96.8° F (36° C)	Effects of anesthesia, body heat loss during surgical procedure
First 48 hr (postop days 1 and 2)	Mild elevation: ≤100.4° F (38° C)	Inflammatory response to surgical stress
	Moderate elevation: >100.4° F (38° C)	Lung congestion, dehydration
After first 48 hr (postop day 3 and later)	Elevation >100° F (37.8° C)	Infection (e.g., wound, urinary, respiratory)

thermia can include compromised immune function, bleeding, untoward cardiac events, impaired wound healing, altered drug metabolism, and postoperative pain and shivering.[22] Shivering can increase oxygen consumption, carbon dioxide production, and cardiac output, as well as significantly affect the patient's comfort level.

Fever. Fever may occur at any time during the postoperative period (see Table 20-6). Wound infection, particularly from aerobic organisms, is often accompanied by a fever that spikes in the afternoon or evening and returns to near-normal levels in the morning. The respiratory tract may be infected secondary to stasis of secretions in areas of atelectasis. The urinary tract may be infected secondary to catheterization. Superficial thrombophlebitis may occur at the IV site. VTE in the leg veins may produce a temperature elevation.

Surgical patients who receive antibiotics for a period of time are at risk for *Clostridium difficile* infections. Manifestations of *C. difficile* may include fever, diarrhea, and abdominal pain.

Intermittent high fever accompanied by shaking chills and diaphoresis suggests septicemia. This may occur at any time during the postoperative period because microorganisms may have been introduced into the bloodstream during surgery, especially in GI or genitourinary (GU) procedures. Septicemia may also occur later from a wound or urinary tract infection.

NURSING MANAGEMENT ALTERED TEMPERATURE

NURSING ASSESSMENT

Frequent assessment of the patient's temperature is important to detect patterns of hypothermia or fever. Temperature may be taken orally, temporally, or via the tympanic membrane. The same route of temperature measurement should be used while the patient is in the PACU.[21] Also assess the color and temperature of the skin. Observe the patient for early signs of inflammation and infection that may precede a fever so that any complications can be treated in a timely manner.

NURSING DIAGNOSES

Nursing diagnoses related to an altered temperature include, but are not limited to, the following:

- Hypothermia *related to* long surgical procedures, prolonged use of anesthetics
- Risk for imbalanced body temperature

NURSING IMPLEMENTATION

Passive warming measures include the use of warmed cotton blankets, socks, and reflective blankets and limiting skin exposure. *Active warming measures* involve the application of external warming devices, including forced air warmers; heated water mattresses; radiant warmers; heated, humidified oxygen; and warmed IV fluids. When using any external warming device, assess body temperature and the patient's comfort level at 15-minute intervals.[21] In addition, take care to prevent skin injuries. Oxygen therapy via nasal prongs or mask is used to treat the increased demand for oxygen caused by shivering. Shivering can be treated with opioids (e.g., meperidine [Demerol]).

Measure the patient's temperature every 4 hours for the first 24 hours postoperatively and then less frequently if no problem develops. Meticulous asepsis is required with wound and IV site care. Airway clearance is encouraged with deep breathing, coughing, and the use of the incentive spirometer. If fever develops, chest x-rays may be taken and antipyretic drugs given. Depending on the suspected cause of the fever, cultures of the wound, sputum, urine, or blood are obtained. If a bacterial infection is the source of the fever, antibiotics are started as soon as cultures have been obtained. If the fever rises above 103° F (39.4° C), body-cooling measures may be used.

GASTROINTESTINAL PROBLEMS

Etiology

Nausea and vomiting remain the most common postoperative complications. Risk factors include gender (female), history of motion sickness or previous postoperative nausea and vomiting, action of anesthetics or opioids, and duration and type of surgery.[1,21] Delayed gastric emptying and slowed peristalsis that result from handling of the bowel during abdominal surgery also contribute to nausea and vomiting, as does the resumption of oral intake too soon after surgery.

Postoperative ileus, or the temporary impairment of gastric and bowel motility after surgery, is another common problem and is an expected result of major abdominal surgery.[23] It results from the handling or reconstruction of the intestine during surgery and limited dietary intake before and after surgery. After abdominal surgery, motility in the large intestine may be reduced for 3 to 5 days, although motility in the small intestine resumes within 24 hours. Use of opioid analgesia prolongs the duration of postoperative ileus.[23] Abdominal distention and gas pains can occur as a result of decreased bowel motility, swallowed air, and the accumulation of GI secretions.

Hiccups (singultus) are intermittent spasms of the diaphragm caused by irritation of the phrenic nerve, which innervates the diaphragm. The phrenic nerve may be irritated postoperatively by gastric distention, intestinal obstruction, intraabdominal bleeding, and a subphrenic abscess. Indirect irritation of the phrenic nerve may be produced by acid-base and electrolyte imbalances. Reflex irritation may come from drinking hot or cold liquids or from the presence of a nasogastric (NG) tube. Hiccups usually last a short time and subside spontaneously.

NURSING MANAGEMENT GASTROINTESTINAL PROBLEMS

NURSING ASSESSMENT

Ask the patient about feelings of nausea. If vomiting occurs, determine the quantity, characteristics, and color of the vomitus.

Assess the abdomen for distention and the presence of bowel sounds. Because bowel sounds are frequently absent or diminished in the immediate postoperative period, auscultate all four quadrants to determine the presence, frequency, and characteristics of the sounds. The return of normal bowel motility is usually accompanied by the passage of gas or stool and the patient's ability to tolerate oral intake without complaints of nausea or vomiting.[24]

NURSING DIAGNOSES

Nursing diagnoses and collaborative problems related to GI problems include, but are not limited to, the following:

- Nausea *related to* anesthetic agents, manipulation of abdominal contents
- Imbalanced nutrition: less than body requirements *related to* vomiting, decreased appetite, decreased peristalsis
- Risk for imbalanced fluid volume
- Risk for electrolyte imbalance
- Potential complication: hiccups

NURSING IMPLEMENTATION

Postoperative nausea and vomiting are treated with antiemetic or prokinetic drugs (see Chapter 42, Table 42-1). In the PACU, oral fluids should be given only as ordered and tolerated. IV fluids will provide hydration until the patient is able to tolerate oral fluids. Be alert to prevent aspiration if the patient vomits while still sleepy from anesthesia. Position the patient in the lateral recovery position and have suction equipment readily available at the bedside. Complementary and alternative therapy interventions for nausea and vomiting include guided imagery, music therapy, aromatherapy, distraction, and acupressure.[25]

Depending on the type of the surgery, the patient may begin oral intake as soon as the gag reflex returns. The patient who has abdominal surgery is usually allowed nothing by mouth (NPO) until the return of peristalsis. Chewing gum has been found to aid in the return of bowel motility.[26,27] When the patient is NPO, IV infusions are given to maintain fluid and electrolyte balance. An NG tube may be used to decompress the stomach to prevent nausea, vomiting, and abdominal distention. Regular oral care is essential for comfort and stimulation of salivary glands when the patient is NPO or has an NG tube. When oral intake is allowed, clear liquids are offered first and the IV infusion is continued, usually at a reduced rate. If oral intake is well tolerated, the IV infusion is discontinued, and the diet is advanced until a regular diet is tolerated.

Despite limited evidence to support early ambulation for abdominal distention, it is a standard postoperative intervention.[28] Assess the patient regularly to detect the return of peristalsis as evidenced by the passage of gas or stool. The NG tube must be clamped or the suction turned off when the abdomen is auscultated. Resumption of a normal diet after bowel sounds have returned also enhances the return of normal peristalsis.

Encourage the patient to expel gas. Gas pains, which tend to become pronounced on the second or third postoperative day, may be relieved by ambulation and frequent repositioning. Positioning the patient on the right side permits gas to rise along the transverse colon and aids its release. Bisacodyl (Dulcolax) suppositories may be ordered to stimulate colonic peristalsis and expulsion of gas and stool.

URINARY PROBLEMS

Etiology

Low urine output (800 to 1500 mL) in the first 24 hours after surgery may be expected, regardless of fluid intake. This low output is caused by increased aldosterone and ADH secretion resulting from the stress of surgery; fluid restriction before surgery; and fluid loss through surgery, drainage, and diaphoresis. By the second or third day, after fluid has been mobilized and the immediate stress reaction subsides, the patient will begin to have increasing urine output.

Acute urinary retention can occur in the postoperative period for a variety of reasons. Anesthesia depresses the nervous system, including the micturition reflex arc and the higher centers that influence it. This allows the bladder to fill more completely than normal before the urge to void is felt. Anesthesia also impedes voluntary micturition. Anticholinergic and opioid drugs may also interfere with the ability to initiate voiding or to empty the bladder completely.

Urinary retention is more likely to occur after lower abdominal or pelvic surgery because spasms or guarding of the abdominal and pelvic muscles interferes with their normal function in micturition. Pain may alter perception and interfere with the patient's awareness of bladder filling. Voiding ability is probably impaired to the greatest extent by immobility and bed rest. The supine position reduces the ability to relax the perineal muscles and external sphincter.

Oliguria (the diminished output of urine) can be a manifestation of renal failure and is a less common, although more serious, problem after surgery. It may result from renal ischemia caused by inadequate renal perfusion.

NURSING MANAGEMENT URINARY PROBLEMS

NURSING ASSESSMENT

Examine the urine for both quantity and quality. Note the color, amount, and odor of the urine. Assess indwelling catheters for patency. Urine output should be at least 0.5 mL/kg/hr. To decrease the risk of catheter-associated urinary tract infection (CAUTI), remove the catheter as soon as possible or within 24 hours, unless there is a reason to continue its use.[29] Most patients urinate within 6 to 8 hours after surgery. If no voiding occurs, scan or percuss the suprapubic area for signs of bladder fullness or distention.

NURSING DIAGNOSES

Nursing diagnoses and collaborative problems related to urinary problems include, but are not limited to, the following:

- Urinary retention *related to* anesthetic agents, pain
- Potential complication: acute kidney injury

NURSING IMPLEMENTATION

You can aid voiding by normal positioning of the patient—sitting for women and standing for men. Reassure the patient regarding the ability to void. Helpful techniques include providing privacy, running water, offering water for the patient to drink, or pouring warm water over the perineum. Walking, preferably to the bathroom, and the use of a bedside commode are additional helpful measures to assist in voiding.

The surgeon often leaves an order to catheterize the patient in 6 to 8 hours if voiding has not occurred. Because of the possibility of CAUTI, first try to validate that the bladder is actually full. Consider fluid intake during and after surgery and determine bladder fullness (e.g., discomfort when the bladder is palpated). Scan the bladder with a portable ultrasound to assess volume of urine in the bladder and avoid unnecessary catheterization. If catheterization is required, a straight catheterization (as compared to an indwelling catheter) is preferred to limit the possibility of CAUTI.

INTEGUMENTARY PROBLEMS

Etiology

Surgery generally involves an incision through the skin and underlying tissues, disrupting the protective skin barrier. Therefore wound healing is one of the major concerns during the postoperative period.

Wound infection may result from contamination of the wound from three major sources: (1) exogenous flora present in the environment and on the skin, (2) oral flora, and (3) intestinal flora. The incidence of wound sepsis is higher in patients who are malnourished, immunosuppressed, or older, or who have had a long hospital stay or a lengthy surgical procedure (more than 3 hours). Patients needing bowel surgery, particularly after a traumatic injury, are at high risk. Infection may involve the entire incision and may extend downward through deeper tissues. An abscess may form locally, or it may spread throughout entire body cavities, as in peritonitis.

Evidence of wound infection usually does not become apparent before the third to fifth postoperative day. Local manifestations include redness, swelling, and increasing pain and tenderness at the site. Systemic manifestations are fever and leukocytosis.

An accumulation of fluid in a wound may create pressure, impair circulation and wound healing, and predispose the patient to infection. To allow for drainage, the surgeon may place a drain in the incision or make a stab wound adjacent to the incision. These drains may be made of soft rubber and drain into a dressing, or they may be firm catheters attached to a Hemovac or other source of gentle suction.

An adequate nutritional state is essential for wound healing. Obesity affects abdominal wound healing. Wound healing is also a concern for the older adult. The patient who was well nourished preoperatively can tolerate the postoperative delay in nutritional intake for several days. However, the patient with preexisting nutritional deficits that occur with chronic diseases (e.g., diabetes, ulcerative colitis, alcoholism) is more prone to problems of wound healing. The patient who is unable to meet nutritional needs postoperatively may be provided with enteral or parenteral nutrition to promote healing.

NURSING MANAGEMENT SURGICAL WOUNDS

NURSING ASSESSMENT

Nursing assessment of the wound and dressing requires knowledge of the type of wound, the drains inserted, and expected drainage related to the specific type of surgery. A small amount of serous drainage is common from any type of wound. If a drain is in place, a moderate to large amount of drainage may be expected. For example, an abdominal incision with an accompanying drain is expected to have a moderate amount of serosanguineous drainage in the first 24 hours. In contrast, an inguinal herniorrhaphy should have only minimal serous drainage during the postoperative period.

In general, drainage is expected to change from sanguineous (red) to serosanguineous (pink) to serous (clear yellow). The drainage should decrease over hours or days, depending on the type of surgery. Wound infection may be accompanied by purulent drainage. *Wound dehiscence* (separation and disruption of previously joined wound edges) may be preceded by a sudden discharge of brown, pink, or clear drainage. (Wound dehiscence is discussed in Chapter 12.)

NURSING DIAGNOSES

Nursing diagnoses related to surgical wounds include, but are not limited to, the following:

- Impaired skin integrity *related to* surgical incision
- Risk for infection

NURSING IMPLEMENTATION

When drainage appears on the dressing, document the type, amount, color, and odor of drainage. Expected drainage from tubes is outlined in Table 20-7. Also assess the effect of position changes on drainage. Notify the surgeon of any excessive or abnormal drainage or significant changes in vital signs.

TABLE 20-7 DRAINAGE FROM TUBES AND CATHETERS

Substance	Daily Amount	Color	Odor	Consistency
Indwelling Catheter				
Urine	800-1500 mL for first 24 hr Minimum expected output: 0.5 mL/kg/hr	Clear, yellow	Ammonia	Watery
Nasogastric Tube or Gastrostomy Tube				
Gastric contents	<1500 mL/day	Pale, yellow-green Bloody after GI surgery	Sour	Watery
Hemovac				
Wound drainage	Varies with procedure May decrease over hours or days	Varies with procedure Initially, may be sanguineous or serosanguineous, changing to serous	Same as wound dressing	Variable
T Tube				
Bile	500 mL	Bright yellow to dark green	Acid	Thick

The incision may be covered with a dressing immediately after surgery. If there is no drainage after 24 to 48 hours, the dressing may be removed and the incision left open to the air. If the initial operative dressing is saturated, agency policy determines whether you may change the dressing or simply reinforce it.

When a dressing is changed, note the number and type of drains present, and avoid dislodging the drains. Inspect the incision site carefully. The area around the sutures may be slightly reddened and swollen, which is an expected inflammatory response. However, the skin around the incision should be of normal color and temperature. If the wound is healing by primary intention, has little or no drainage, or has no drains in place, a single-layer dressing or no dressing is sufficient. A multilayer dressing is used when drains are in place, when moderate to heavy drainage is occurring, or when healing occurs other than by primary intention. (Wound healing and care are discussed in Chapter 12.)

DISCHARGE FROM THE PACU

The choice of discharge site is based on patient acuity, access to follow-up care, and the potential for postoperative complications. The decision to discharge the patient from the PACU is based on written discharge criteria (Table 20-8). A standardized scoring system, such as the *Modified Aldrete Scoring System,* is often used to determine the patient's general condition and readiness for discharge from the PACU. (The Modified Aldrete Scoring System is presented in eTable 20-1 on the website for this chapter.)

Discharge to the Clinical Unit

Before discharging the patient from the PACU to the clinical unit, provide a verbal report about the patient to the receiving nurse. The report summarizes the operative and postanesthesia period. It should also include information as to where the patient's caregivers are waiting. Nurse-to-nurse communication must be accurate and allow for questions. The use of a standardized communication tool, such as SBAR *(Situation-Background-Assessment-Recommendation),* provides a complete report and enhances a safe transfer of the patient from PACU to the clinical unit (Table 20-9). (Handoff communication is discussed in Chapter 1, and SBAR is presented in Table 1-7.)

If you are the nurse who receives the patient on the clinical unit, assist the PACU transport staff to move the patient from the stretcher to the bed. Take care to protect IV lines, drains, and traction devices. Use a draw sheet, transfer board or sling, and sufficient staff to facilitate the safe transfer of the patient. Obtain vital signs and compare the patient status with the report provided by the PACU nurse. After this, perform a more in-depth assessment and initiate postoperative orders and nursing care as appropriate (Table 20-10).

AMBULATORY SURGERY

Phase II and Extended Observation

Advances in minimally invasive and noninvasive procedures, anesthesia, and analgesia have resulted in an increase in ambulatory surgical procedures.[30] Ambulatory surgery patients include those patients receiving Phase II and extended observation postoperative care (see Table 20-1). Postoperative nausea and vomiting and pain are significant problems after ambulatory surgery. These can lead to delirium, prolonged PACU stay, delayed discharge, readmission, delayed resumption of usual activities, and decreased patient satisfaction.[31,32]

Ambulatory Surgery Discharge

The patient leaving an ambulatory surgery setting must be mobile and alert to provide a degree of self-care when discharged to home (see Table 20-8). Postoperative pain, nausea,

TABLE 20-8 SURGERY DISCHARGE CRITERIA

PACU Discharge Criteria (Phase I)

- Patient awake (or baseline)
- Vital signs at baseline or stable
- No excess bleeding or drainage
- No respiratory depression
- O_2 saturation >90%
- Pain controlled or acceptable
- Minimal nausea and vomiting
- Report given

Ambulatory Surgery Discharge Criteria (Phase II or Extended Observation)

- All PACU discharge criteria (Phase I) met
- No IV opioid drugs for last 30 min
- Voided if appropriate to surgical procedure or orders
- Able to ambulate if not contraindicated
- Responsible adult present to accompany and drive patient home
- Written discharge instructions given and patient and caregiver understanding confirmed

TABLE 20-9 POSTOPERATIVE SBAR HANDOFF COMMUNICATION

Situation

Patient transferring to Room # ________ Date ________
Surgeon ________ Anesthesia ________
Procedure ________
Surgical site(s) ________

Background

Allergies ________
Medications received in PACU ________
IV site/fluids ________
Dressings and/or drains ________
Operative comments ________

Assessment

PACU vital signs T ____ P ____ RR ____ BP ____ O_2 Sat ____
Oxygen source ________ FIO_2 ________
Pain rating at discharge ________
Method of pain management ________
Last dose of pain medication ________
Nausea/vomiting at discharge ________
Intake ________ Output ________
Recovery comments ________

Recommendations

Equipment needed ________
Physician orders to be completed ________
Other notes ________
Transferring RN ________ Phone # for questions ________
Receiving RN ________

Modified from Sandlin D: Improving patient safety by implementing a standardized and consistent approach to hand-off communication, *J Perianesth Nurs* 22:290, 2007.

TABLE 20-10 NURSING ASSESSMENT

Care of Patient on Admission to Clinical Unit

1. Record time of patient's return to unit and assess airway, breathing, and circulation.
2. Obtain baseline vital signs, including O_2 saturation.
3. Assess neurologic status, including level of consciousness and movement of extremities.
4. Assess level of pain:
   - Last dose and type of pain control
   - Current pain rating
5. Assess wound, dressing, and drainage tubes:
   - Type and amount of drainage
   - Tubing connected to gravity or suction drainage (per orders)
6. Assess color, temperature, and appearance of skin.
7. Assess urinary status:
   - Time of voiding
   - Presence of catheter, patency, and total output
   - Bladder distention or urge to void
8. Position for airway maintenance, comfort, and safety (bed in low position, side rails up).
9. Check IV infusion:
   - Type of solution
   - Amount of fluid remaining
   - Patency and flow rate
   - Condition of insertion site and size of catheter
10. Position call light within reach, and orient patient to use of call light.
11. Assess for any nausea or vomiting.
    - Availability of emesis basin and tissues
12. Determine emotional state and provide support as needed.
13. Check for presence of caregiver.
    - Patient and caregiver oriented to immediate environment
14. Check and carry out postoperative orders.

and vomiting must be controlled. Overall, the patient must be stable and near the level of preoperative functioning for discharge from the unit. At discharge, provide teaching for the patient and the caregiver specific to the type of anesthesia and surgery, and reinforce with written instructions. The patient may not drive and must be accompanied by a responsible adult at the time of discharge. A follow-up evaluation of the patient's status is made by telephone, and any specific questions and concerns are addressed.

Carefully assess the patient's readiness for discharge and home care needs. Determine availability of caregivers (e.g., family, friends) and access to a (1) pharmacy for prescriptions, (2) phone in the event of an emergency, and (3) follow-up care.

Discuss the patient's expectations regarding activity and assistance needed after discharge. The patient and caregiver must be included in discharge planning and provided with the information and support to make informed decisions about continuing care.

Planning for Discharge and Follow-up Care

Preparation for the patient's discharge is an ongoing process that begins during the preoperative period. The informed patient is prepared as events unfold and gradually assumes more responsibility for self-care during the postoperative period. As discharge approaches, be certain that the patient and any caregivers have the following information:

- Symptoms to be reported (e.g., fever, increased incisional drainage, unrelieved incisional pain, discomfort in other parts of the body)
- When and how to take drugs, and possible side effects

INFORMATICS IN PRACTICE

Discharge Teaching

- If you are discharging a patient who requires a complex dressing change and think that written instructions are not adequate, consider using a video. This may be available on the hospital's television system or the Internet (e.g.,YouTube). You could also take a series of pictures that show how to perform the procedure.
- If using a video from the Internet, check it to ensure that the procedure is properly done.
- The patient and caregiver can view the video or pictures at home as a reference when performing the procedure.

- Care of incision and any dressings, including bathing recommendations
- Activities allowed and prohibited. When various activities can be resumed safely (e.g., driving a car, returning to work, sexual intercourse, leisure activities)
- Dietary restrictions or modifications
- Where and when to return for follow-up care
- Answers to any individual questions or concerns

Common reasons patients seek help after discharge include unrelieved pain, need for advice about medications, and wound issues (e.g., drainage). Attention to complete discharge instructions may prevent needless distress for the patient and the caregiver. Standardized, preprinted discharge instructions that are surgery specific and easy to read ensure that information is complete.[33,34]

Document the discharge instructions in the medical record. For the patient, the postoperative phase of care continues and extends into the recuperative period. Assessment and evaluation of the patient after discharge may be accomplished by a follow-up call or by a visit from a nurse (e.g., home health nurse).

Increasingly, patients are being discharged from the hospital with many care needs. They may be transferred to transitional care facilities, to long-term care facilities, or directly to their homes. When discharged directly to home, the patient is expected to continue self-care, with assistance from family, friends, or home health care personnel. The care may include dressing changes, wound care, catheter or drain care, home antibiotics, or continued physical therapy. Working with the discharge planner or case manager, facilitate the patient's safe transition from hospital-based care to community- or home-based care.

GERONTOLOGIC CONSIDERATIONS

POSTOPERATIVE PATIENT

The older postoperative patient deserves special consideration. The older adult has decreased respiratory function, including decreased ability to cough and decreased thoracic compliance. These alterations lead to an increase in the work of breathing and a decreased ability to eliminate drugs. Carefully monitor reactions to anesthetic drugs. Pneumonia is a common postoperative complication in older adults.

Vascular function in the older adult is altered due to atherosclerosis and decreased elasticity in the blood vessels. Cardiac function is often compromised, and compensatory responses to changes in BP and volume are limited. Circulating blood volume is decreased, and hypertension is common. Cardiovascular parameters must be closely monitored throughout surgery and the postoperative period.

Drug toxicity is a potential problem in the older adult. Renal perfusion in the older adult normally decreases, with a reduction in the ability to eliminate drugs that are excreted by the kidneys. Decreased liver function also leads to decreased drug metabolism and increased drug activity. Carefully assess renal and liver function in the postoperative phase to prevent drug overdose and toxicity.[35]

Observing for changes in mental status is an important part of postoperative care in older adults. Factors such as age, history of alcohol abuse, poor baseline cognition, hypoxia, severe metabolic derangement, hypotension, and polypharmacy can contribute to postoperative delirium. Anesthetics, especially anticholinergic drugs and benzodiazepines, also increase the risk for delirium. Despite knowledge of risk factors, postoperative delirium in older adults is poorly understood.[36] Research suggests that recovery from postoperative delirium is delayed in older patients with high pain levels. This may affect the length of hospital stay and the patient's condition at the time of discharge.[37]

Pain control in the older patient is challenging because of possible preexisting cognitive deficits, impaired communication, and physiologic changes that affect how drugs are metabolized. Older patients may hesitate to request pain medication because they believe that pain is an inevitable result of surgery that should be tolerated. Some older patients may be nervous about using PCA machines.

Thoroughly assess pain in a surgical patient who does not report any pain. Encourage the use of analgesics, and explain to the patient and caregiver that untreated pain has a negative effect on recovery.[35]

CASE STUDY

Postoperative Patient

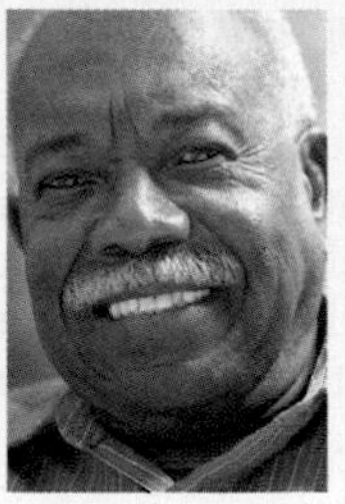

Stockbyte/Thinkstock

Patient Profile

E.G., a 74-year-old African American retired college professor, has just undergone surgery for a fractured hip. He fell off a ladder while painting his house. The surgery, performed while the patient was under general anesthesia, lasted 3 hours.

Subjective Data

- Was in good health before his fall
- Played tennis three times each week
- Smokes 1 pack of cigarettes per day × 58 years
- Always had problems sleeping
- Difficulty hearing, wears hearing aid
- Upset with injury and its impact on activity
- Is a widower and has no relatives nearby or friends to assist with care
- Reports pain is 8 on a 0-10 scale on arrival to PACU

Objective Data

- Admitted to PACU with abduction pillow between his legs, one peripheral IV catheter, a self-suction drain from the hip dressing, an indwelling urinary catheter
- O_2 saturation 91% on 40% O_2 face mask

Collaborative Care

Postoperative Orders

- Vital signs per PACU routine
- Dextrose 5% in 0.45 normal saline at 100 mL/hr
- Morphine via patient-controlled analgesia 1 mg q10min (20 mg max in 4 hr) for pain
- Advance diet as tolerated
- Incentive spirometry q1hr × 10 while awake
- O_2 therapy to keep O_2 saturation >90%
- Neurovascular checks q1hr × 4 hr
- Empty and measure self-suction drain every shift
- Strict intake and output

Discussion Questions

1. What are the potential postanesthesia problems that you might expect with E.G.?
2. ***Priority Decision:*** What priority nursing interventions would be appropriate to prevent these complications from occurring?
3. ***Delegation Decision:*** Which of these interventions could you delegate to unlicensed assistive personnel (UAP)?
4. What factors may predispose E.G. to the following problems: atelectasis, infection, pulmonary embolism, nausea and vomiting?
5. How can you determine when E.G. is sufficiently recovered from general anesthesia to be discharged to the clinical unit?
6. What potential postoperative problems on the clinical unit might you expect?
7. What are risk factors for this patient developing postoperative delirium? What are the signs and symptoms of delirium?
8. Why is drug toxicity a potential problem for E.G.?
9. ***Priority Decision:*** Based on the assessment data presented, identify two priority nursing diagnoses. Are there any collaborative problems?
10. ***Evidence-Based Practice:*** E.G. asks you why he has to use the incentive spirometer. How would you respond to this question?

evolve Answers available at *http://evolve.elsevier.com/Lewis/medsurg.*

BRIDGE TO NCLEX EXAMINATION

The number of the question corresponds to the same-numbered outcome at the beginning of the chapter.

1. When a patient is admitted to the PACU, what are the priority interventions the nurse performs?
   - **a.** Assess the surgical site, noting presence and character of drainage.
   - **b.** Assess the amount of urine output and the presence of bladder distention.
   - **c.** Assess for airway patency and quality of respirations, and obtain vital signs.
   - **d.** Review results of intraoperative laboratory values and medications received.
2. A patient is admitted to the PACU after major abdominal surgery. During the initial assessment the patient tells the nurse he thinks he is going to "throw up." A priority nursing intervention would be to
   - **a.** increase the rate of the IV fluids.
   - **b.** obtain vital signs, including O_2 saturation.
   - **c.** position patient in lateral recovery position.
   - **d.** administer antiemetic medication as ordered.
3. After admission of the postoperative patient to the clinical unit, which assessment data require the most immediate attention?
   - **a.** Oxygen saturation of 85%
   - **b.** Respiratory rate of 13/min
   - **c.** Temperature of 100.4° F (38° C)
   - **d.** Blood pressure of 90/60 mm Hg

4. A 70-kg postoperative patient has an average urine output of 25 mL/hr during the first 8 hours. The priority nursing intervention(s) given this assessment would be to
   a. perform a straight catheterization to measure the amount of urine in the bladder.
   b. notify the physician and anticipate obtaining blood work to evaluate renal function.
   c. continue to monitor the patient because this is a normal finding during this time period.
   d. evaluate the patient's fluid volume status since surgery and obtain a bladder ultrasound.

5. Discharge criteria for the Phase II patient include *(select all that apply)*
   a. no nausea or vomiting.
   b. ability to drive self home.
   c. no respiratory depression.
   d. written discharge instructions understood.
   e. opioid pain medication given 45 minutes ago.

1. c, 2. c, 3. a, 4. d, 5. c, d, e

evolve

For rationales to these answers and even more NCLEX review questions, visit *http://evolve.elsevier.com/Lewis/medsurg.*

REFERENCES

*1. American Society of PeriAnesthesia Nurses: *Perianesthesia nursing standards and practice recommendations 2010-2012*, Cherry Hill, NJ, 2012, The Society.
2. Varadhan KK, Lobo DN, Ljungqvist O: Enhanced recovery after surgery: the future of improving surgical care, *Crit Care Clin* 26(3):527, 2010.
*3. Larsson G, Holgers K: Fast-track care for patients with suspected hip fracture, *Injury* 42:1257, 2011.
*4. Pedersen T, Hovhannisyan K, Moller AM: Pulse oximetry for perioperative monitoring, *Cochrane Database Syst Rev* 4:CD002013, 2009. doi:10.1002/14651858.CD002013.pub2.
*5. Xue Q, Wu X, Jin J, et al: Transcutaneous carbon dioxide monitoring accurately predicts arterial carbon dioxide partial pressure in patients undergoing prolonged laparoscopic surgery, *Anesth Analg* 111:417, 2010.
6. Godden B: Where does capnography fit into the PACU? *J Perianesth Nurs* 26(6):408, 2011.
*7. Geerts WH, Bergqvist D, Pineo GF, et al: Prevention of venous thromboembolism: American College of Chest Physicians evidence-based clinical practice guidelines, ed 8, *Chest* 133(Suppl 6):381S, 2008.
8. Hudek K: Emergence delirium: a nursing perspective, *JAORN* 89:509, 2009.
9. Rudolph JL, Marcantonio ER: Postoperative delirium: acute change with long-term implications, *Anesth Analg* 112:1202, 2011.
10. Shander A, Fleisher LA, Barie PS, et al: Clinical and economic burden of postoperative pulmonary complications: patient safety summit on definition, risk-reducing interventions, and preventive strategies, *Crit Care Med* 39:2163, 2011.
*11. Czarnecki ML, Turner HN, Collins PM, et al: Procedural pain management: a position statement with clinical practice recommendations, *Pain Manag Nurs* 12:95, 2011.
*12. American Society of PeriAnesthesia Nurses: Pain and comfort clinical guidelines, 2003. Retrieved from *www.aspan.org/Portals/6/docs/ClinicalPractice/Guidelines/ASPAN_Clinical Guideline_PainComfort.pdf.*
13. The Joint Commission: Provision of care, treatment, and services: standard PC 01.02.07. In comprehensive accreditation manual for hospitals E-dition, 2009. Retrieved from *www.educode.com/Images/aacn-pharm04-16.pdf.*
14. Comerford D: Techniques of opioid administration, *Anes Intens Care Med* 12:16, 2011.
15. Buvanendran A, Kroin JS: Multimodal analgesia for controlling acute postoperative pain, *Curr Opin Anaesthesiol* 22:588, 2009.
16. Manion SC, Brennan TJ: Thoracic epidural analgesia and acute pain management, *Anesthesiology* 115:181, 2011.
*17. van Lier F, van der Geest PJ, Hoeks SE, et al: Epidural analgesia is associated with improved health outcomes of surgical patients with chronic obstructive pulmonary disease, *Anesthesiology* 115:315, 2011.
*18. Easter B, DeBoer L, Settlemyre G, et al: The impact of music on the PACU patient's perception of discomfort, *J Perianesth Nurs* 25:70, 2010.
*19. Topcu SY, Findik UY: Effect of relaxation exercises on controlling postoperative pain, *Pain Manag Nurs* 13:11, 2012.
20. Burns SM, Piotrowski K, Caraffa G, et al: Incidence of postoperative hypothermia and the relationship to clinical variables, *J Perianesth Nurs* 25:286, 2010.
*21. Hooper VD, Chard R, Clifford T, et al: ASPAN's evidence-based clinical practice guideline for the promotion of perioperative normothermia: ed 2, *J Perianesth Nurs* 25:346, 2010.
*22. Pikus E, Hooper VD: Postoperative rewarming: are there alternatives to warm hospital blankets? *J Perianesth Nurs* 25:11, 2010.
23. Miaskowski C: A review of the incidence, causes, consequences, and management of gastrointestinal effects associated with postoperative opioid administration, *J Perianesth Nurs* 24:222, 2009.
24. Artinyan A, Nunoo-Mensah JW, Balasubramaniam S, et al: Prolonged postoperative ileus: definition, risk factors, and predictors after surgery, *World J Surg* 32:1495, 2008.
25. Makic MB: Management of nausea, vomiting, and diarrhea during critical illness, *AACN Adv Crit Care* 22:265, 2011.
*26. Hocevar BJ, Robinson B, Gray M: Does chewing gum shorten the duration of postoperative ileus in patients undergoing abdominal surgery and creation of a stoma? *J Wound Ostomy Continence Nurs* 37:140, 2010.
*27. Crainic C, Erickson K, Gardner J, et al: Comparison of methods to facilitate postoperative bowel function, *Medsurg Nurs* 18:235, 2009.
*28. McNicol ED, Boyce D, Schumann R, et al: Mu-opioid antagonists for opioid-induced bowel dysfunction, *Cochrane Database Syst Rev* 2:CD006332, 2008. doi:10.1002/14651858.CD006332.pub2.
*29. Gould CV, Umscheid CA, Agarwal RK, et al: *Health care infection control practices advisory committee: guideline for prevention of catheter-associated urinary tract infections*, 2009, Centers for Disease Control and Prevention. Retrieved from *www.cdc.gov/hicpac/pdf/CAUTI/CAUTIguideline2009final.pdf.*
30. Cullen KA, Hall MJ, Golosinskiy A: Ambulatory surgery in the United States, *Natl Health Stat Report* 11:1, 2009.

*Evidence-based information for clinical practice.

31. Le TP, Gan TJ: Update on the management of postoperative nausea and vomiting and postdischarge nausea and vomiting in ambulatory surgery, *Anesthesiol Clin* 28:225, 2010.
32. Elvir-Lazo OL, White PF: Postoperative pain management after ambulatory surgery: role of multimodal analgesia, *Anesthesiol Clin* 28:217, 2010.
33. Ortoleva C: An approach to consistent patient education, *JAORN* 92:437, 2010.
*34. Shuilain L, Stuenkel DI, Rodriguez L: The impact of diagnosis-specific discharge instructions on patient satisfaction, *J Perianesth Nurs* 24:156, 2009.
35. Coldrey JC, Upton RN, Macintyre PE: Advances in analgesia in the older patient, *Best Pract Res Clin Anaesthesiol* 25:367, 2011.
36. Krenk L, Rasmussen LS: Postoperative delirium and postoperative cognitive dysfunction in the elderly—what are the differences? *Minerva Anestesiol* 77:742, 2011.
37. DeCrane SK, Sands L, Ashland M, et al: Factors associated with recovery from early postoperative delirium, *J Perianesth Nurs* 26:231, 2011.

RESOURCES

American Association of Nurse Anesthetists (AANA)
www.aana.com

American Latex Allergy Association
www.latexallergyresources.org

American Society of Anesthesiologists
www.asahq.org

American Society of PeriAnesthesia Nurses (ASPAN)
www.aspan.org

Association of periOperative Registered Nurses (AORN)
www.aorn.org

CASE STUDY

Managing Multiple Patients

You have been called into work at 10 AM to cover patients for a nurse who had a family emergency. You take over care for the following three patients on an orthopedic surgical unit. You have one UAP available who is assigned to help you and two other RNs.

Patients

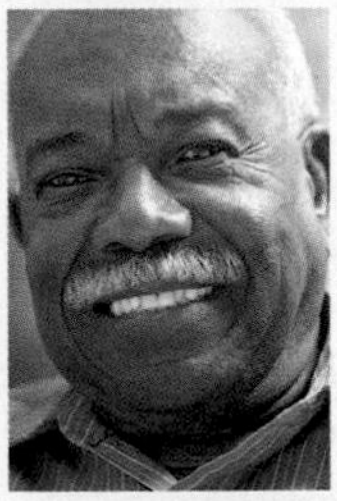

Stockbyte/Thinkstock

E.G., a 74-year-old man, underwent surgery for a fractured hip yesterday. He is currently receiving dextrose 5% in 0.45 normal saline at 100 mL/hr, morphine via patient-controlled analgesia at 1 mg q10min (20 mg max in 4 hr) for pain, and O_2 to keep O_2 saturation >93%. He has a self-suction drain in place at the surgical site. He has good respiratory effort when using his incentive spirometer.

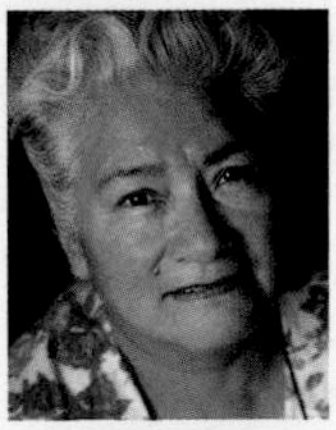

Ryan McVay/Photodisc/Thinkstock

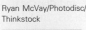

F.D., a 72-year-old woman, was admitted to the hospital with compromised circulation of the right lower leg and a necrotic right foot as a complication of her diabetes. She is scheduled for a below-the-knee amputation of the right leg at 1 PM today. She has been NPO since midnight. Her morning capillary blood glucose level was 198 mg/dL. She received 4 units of regular insulin at 8 AM. She has an IV of NSS infusing at 125 mL/hr.

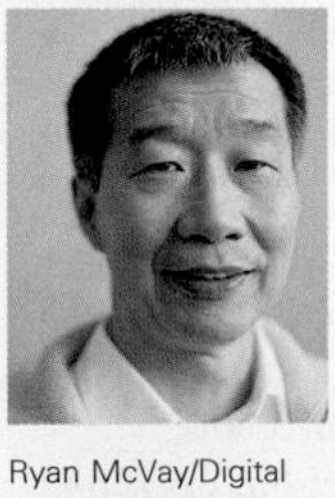

Ryan McVay/Digital Vision/Thinkstock

A.T., a 56-year-old man, is 2 days post lumbar laminectomy. He has been ambulating in the hallway without difficulty and his pain is controlled with the prescribed analgesic medication, last administered at 4 AM. His discharge orders have been written but teaching has yet to be completed.

Management Discussion Questions

1. ***Priority Decision:*** After receiving report, which patient should you see first? Provide a rationale for your decision.
2. ***Delegation Decision:*** Which tasks should you delegate to the UAP? *(select all that apply)*
   a. Explain discharge instructions to A.T.
   b. Obtain noon vital signs on E.G. and F.D.
   c. Obtain capillary blood glucose level on F.D.
   d. Remind E.G. and A.T. to use their incentive spirometers every hour.
   e. Confirm E.G.'s understanding of how to use the PCA pump.
3. ***Priority and Delegation Decision:*** When you enter F.D.'s room, you find her somewhat withdrawn and lethargic. Her face is cool and slightly clammy. What initial action would be most appropriate?
   a. Give 1 ampule of D_{50} IV stat
   b. Increase F.D.'s IV rate to 150 mL/hour.
   c. Ask the UAP to give F.D. a glass of orange juice.
   d. Have the UAP obtain a stat capillary blood glucose level.

Case Study Progression

F.D.'s capillary blood glucose reading was 64 mg/dL. You notify her health care provider and administer IV dextrose as ordered. You also change her IV infusion to D5 ½NS and monitor her capillary blood glucose levels on an hourly basis.

4. A preoperative checklist for F.D. is used to ensure completion of *(select all that apply)*
   a. removal of nail polish and jewelry.
   b. signed and witnessed informed consent.
   c. patient understanding of sensory information.
   d. identification of surgical site with indelible marker.
   e. notifying family of where to wait for surgeon postoperatively.
5. F.D. tells you that she is afraid they might amputate the wrong leg. She tells you she has read stories of that happening at other hospitals. Your best response to F.D. would be to
   a. ask her if she would like a sedative to calm her fears.
   b. reassure her that it has never happened in this hospital.
   c. explain the "time-out" procedure for preventing such errors.
   d. offer to go to the operating room with her to ensure the correct leg is amputated.
6. The UAP reports that E.G.'s blood pressure is 92/54 mm Hg, his heart rate is 110 bpm, his respirations are 30 breaths/min, and his O_2 saturation is 90%. On entering E.G.'s room, you find him clutching his chest, complaining of shortness of breath and chest pain. His lungs are clear to auscultation but you note unilateral swelling of his left leg. You suspect that E.G. is likely experiencing
   a. anxiety.
   b. atelectasis.
   c. pulmonary edema.
   d. pulmonary emboli.
7. ***Management Decision:*** When providing discharge instructions to A.T., he tells you that the UAP told him that he could do whatever activity he was comfortable doing—to let pain guide his progress. Your initial reaction to this statement should be to
   a. ask the UAP to clarify what was said to A.T.
   b. report the UAP's actions to the nurse manager.
   c. teach A.T. about the reason for activity restrictions.
   d. clarify the discharge instructions with the health care provider.

evolve Answers available at *http://evolve.elsevier.com/Lewis/medsurg.*

SECTION 4

Problems Related to Altered Sensory Input

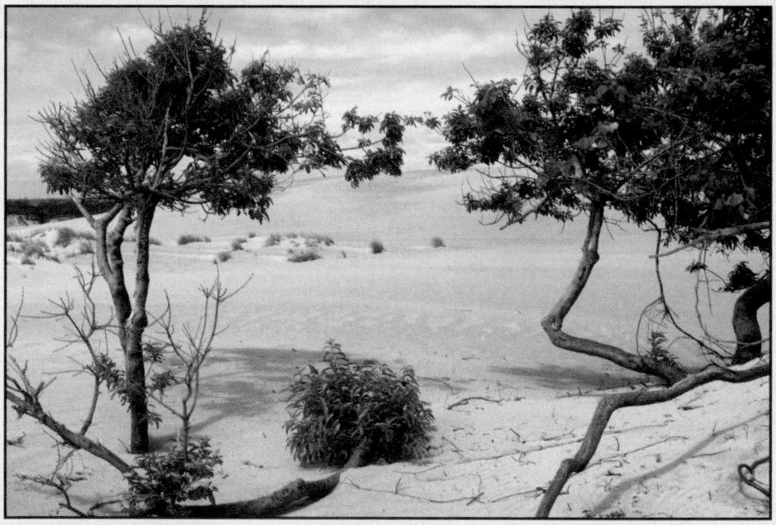

Courtesy Peter Bonner

It's fun to be a little bit different in the world,
to make a few new trails of your own.
Dennis Weaver

CHAPTER

21

The health of the eye seems to demand a horizon. We are never tired, so long as we can see far enough.
Ralph Waldo Emerson

Nursing Assessment

Visual and Auditory Systems

Mary Ann Kolis

evolve WEBSITE

http://evolve.elsevier.com/Lewis/medsurg

- NCLEX Review Questions
- Key Points
- Pre-Test
- Answer Guidelines for Case Study in this chapter
- Rationales for Bridge to NCLEX Examination Questions
- Concept Map Creator
- Glossary
- Animation
  - Weber Test
- Videos
  - Evaluation: Central Vision and Visual Acuity
  - Evaluation: Pupil Responses, Direct and Consensual
  - Inspection and Palpation: External Ear
  - Inspection and Palpation: External Eye
  - Inspection: Ear Canal
  - Physical Examination: Ears
  - Physical Examination: Eyes
- Content Updates

eFigures

- eFig. 21-1: Six cardinal positions of gaze
- eFig. 21-2: Tono-pen tonometry
- eFig. 21-3: Pneumatic otoscopic examination of the adult ear

eTable

- eTable 21-1: Diagnostic Tuning Fork Tests: Auditory System

LEARNING OUTCOMES

1. Describe the structures and functions of the visual and auditory systems.
2. Explain the physiologic processes involved in normal vision and hearing.
3. Evaluate the significant subjective and objective assessment data related to the visual and auditory systems that should be obtained from a patient.
4. Select the appropriate techniques to use in the physical assessment of the visual and auditory systems.
5. Differentiate normal from common abnormal findings of a physical assessment of the visual and auditory systems.
6. Link the age-related changes in the visual and auditory systems to differences in assessment findings.
7. Describe the purpose, significance of results, and nursing responsibilities related to diagnostic studies of the visual and auditory systems.

KEY TERMS

astigmatism, p. 369
conjunctiva, p. 370
hyperopia, p. 369
lens, p. 370
myopia, p. 369
nystagmus, p. 379
presbycusis, p. 379
presbyopia, p. 369
refraction, p. 369
retina, p. 371
sclera, p. 370
tinnitus, p. 379
vertigo, p. 379

VISUAL SYSTEM

STRUCTURES AND FUNCTIONS OF VISUAL SYSTEM

The visual system consists of the external tissues and structures surrounding the eye, the external and internal structures of the eye, the refractive media, and the visual pathway. The external structures are the eyebrows, eyelids, eyelashes, lacrimal system, conjunctiva, cornea, sclera, and extraocular muscles. The internal structures are the iris, lens, ciliary body, choroid, and retina. The entire visual system is important for visual function. Light reflected from an object in the field of vision passes through the transparent structures of the eye and, in doing so, is *refracted* (bent) so that a clear image can fall on the retina. From the retina, the visual stimuli travel through the visual pathway to the occipital cortex, where they are perceived as an image.

Reviewed by Sarah Smith, RN, MA, CRNO, COT, Nurse Manager, Department of Ophthalmology, University of Iowa Health Care, Oxford, Iowa; and Helen Stegall, RN, BSN, CORLN, Nurse Manager of Department of Ophthalmology, University of Iowa Hospitals and Clinics, Iowa City, Iowa.

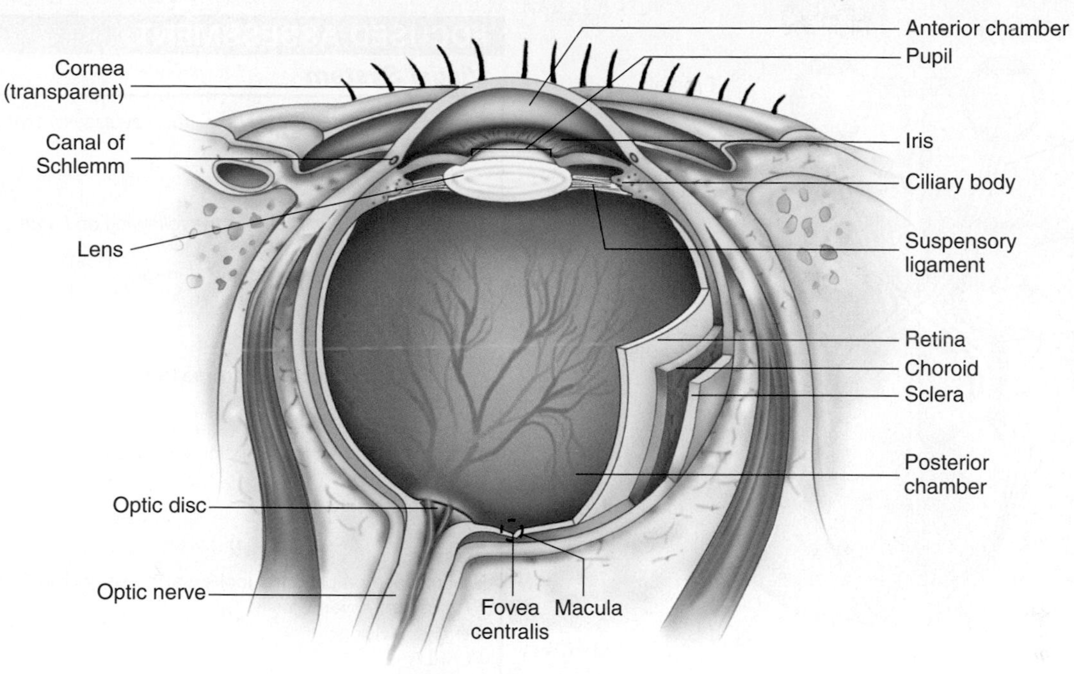

FIG. 21-1 The human eye.

Structures and Functions of Vision

Eyeball. The eyeball, or globe, is composed of three layers (Fig. 21-1). The tough outer layer is composed of the sclera and the transparent cornea. The middle layer consists of the uveal tract (iris, choroid, and ciliary body), and the innermost layer is the retina. The *anterior cavity* is divided into the anterior and posterior chambers. The anterior chamber lies between the iris and the posterior surface of the cornea, and the posterior chamber lies between the anterior surface of the lens and the posterior surface of the iris. The *posterior cavity* lies in the large space behind the lens and in front of the retina.

Refractive Media. For light to reach the retina, it must pass through a number of structures: the cornea, aqueous humor, lens, and vitreous. All these structures must remain clear for light to reach the retina and stimulate the photoreceptor cells. The transparent cornea is the first structure through which light passes. It is responsible for the majority of light refraction necessary for clear vision.

Aqueous humor, a clear watery fluid, fills the anterior and posterior chambers of the anterior cavity of the eye. Aqueous humor is produced from capillary blood in the ciliary body. It is drained away by the scleral veins *(canal of Schlemm),* which enter the circulation of the body. The aqueous humor bathes and nourishes the lens and the endothelium of the cornea. Excess production or decreased outflow can elevate intraocular pressure above the normal 10 to 21 mm Hg, a condition termed *glaucoma.*

The lens is a biconvex structure located behind the iris and supported in place by small fibers collectively called *zonule.* The zonule is a "scaffolding," a series of microscopic wire-like threads that connect the lens to the ciliary body. The primary function of the lens is to bend light rays, allowing the rays to fall onto the retina. The lens shape is modified by action of the ciliary body as part of *accommodation,* a process that allows a person to focus on near objects, such as when reading. Anything altering the clarity of the lens affects light transmission.

Vitreous humor is a transparent gel-like substance that fills the posterior chamber (see Fig. 21-1). Light passing through the vitreous may be blocked by any nontransparent substance within the vitreous. The effect on vision varies, depending on the amount, type, and location of the substance blocking the light.

Refractive Errors. **Refraction** is the eye's ability to bend light rays so that they fall on the retina. In the normal eye, parallel light rays are focused through the lens into a sharp image on the retina. When the light does not focus properly, it is called a *refractive error.*

The individual with **myopia** (nearsightedness) can see near objects clearly, but objects in the distance are blurred. The individual with **hyperopia** (farsightedness) can see distant objects clearly, but close objects are blurred. **Astigmatism** is caused by unevenness in the cornea, which results in visual distortion. **Presbyopia** is a loss of accommodation, causing an inability to focus on near objects. It occurs as a normal process of aging, usually around age 40.

Visual Pathways. Once the image travels through the refractive media, it is focused on the retina (Fig. 21-2). From the retina, the impulses travel through the optic nerve to the optic chiasm where the nasal fibers of each eye cross over to the other side. Fibers from the left field of both eyes form the left optic tract and travel to the left occipital cortex. The fibers from the right field of both eyes form the right optic tract and travel to the right occipital cortex. This arrangement of the nerve fibers in the visual pathways allows determination of the anatomic location of abnormalities.

External Structures and Functions

The eyebrows, eyelids, and eyelashes serve an important role in protecting the eye. They provide a physical barrier to dust and foreign particles (Fig. 21-3). The eye is further protected by the surrounding bony orbit and by fat pads located below and behind the *globe,* or eyeball.

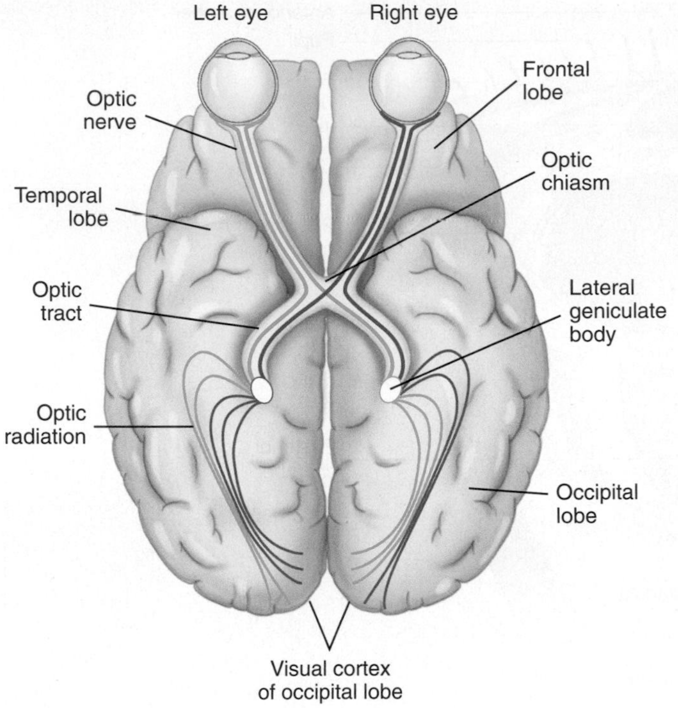

FIG. 21-2 The visual pathway. Fibers from the nasal portion of each retina cross over to the opposite side of the optic chiasma, terminating in the lateral geniculate body of the opposite side. Location of a lesion in the visual pathway determines the resulting visual defect.

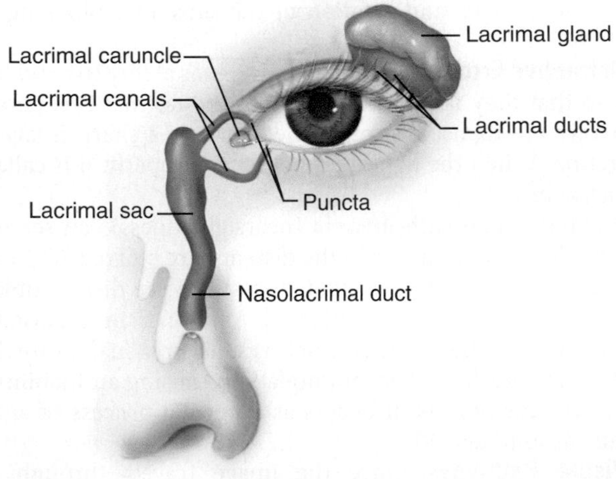

FIG. 21-3 External eye and lacrimal apparatus. Tears produced in the lacrimal gland pass over the surface of the eye and enter the lacrimal canal. From there the tears are carried through the nasolacrimal duct to the nasal cavity.

The upper and lower eyelids join at the medial and lateral canthi. Blinking of the upper eyelid distributes tears over the anterior surface of the eyeball and helps control the amount of light entering the visual pathway. The eyelids open and close through the action of muscles innervated by cranial nerve (CN) VII, the facial nerve.

The **conjunctiva** is a transparent mucous membrane that covers the inner surfaces of the eyelids and also extends over the sclera, forming a "pocket" under each eyelid. Glands in the conjunctiva secrete mucus and tears. The **sclera** is composed of collagen fibers meshed together to form an opaque structure commonly referred to as the "white" of the eye. The sclera forms a tough shell that helps protect the intraocular structures.

The transparent and avascular cornea allows light to enter the eye (see Fig. 21-1). The curved cornea refracts (bends) incoming light rays to help focus them on the retina. The cornea consists of six layers: the epithelium, Bowman's layer, the stroma, Descemet's membrane, Dua's layer, and the endothelium. The lacrimal system consists of the lacrimal gland and ducts, lacrimal canals and puncta, lacrimal sac, and nasolacrimal duct (see Fig. 21-3). In addition to the lacrimal gland, other glands provide secretions to make up the mucous, aqueous, and lipid layers of the tear film. The tear film moistens the eye and provides oxygen to the cornea.

Each eye is moved by three pairs of extraocular muscles: (1) superior and inferior rectus muscles, (2) medial and lateral rectus muscles, and (3) superior and inferior oblique muscles. Neuromuscular coordination produces simultaneous movement of the eyes in the same direction.

FOCUSED ASSESSMENT
Visual System

Use this checklist to make sure the key assessment steps have been done.

Subjective

Ask the patient about any of the following and note responses.

Changes in vision (e.g., acuity, blurred)	Y	N
Eye redness, itching, discomfort	Y	N
Drainage from eyes	Y	N

Objective: Physical Examination

Inspect

Eyes for any discoloration or drainage	✓
Conjunctiva and sclera for color and vascularity	✓
Lens for clarity	✓
Eyelid for ptosis	✓

Assess

Vision based on patient's looking at nurse or Snellen chart	✓
Extraocular movements	✓
Peripheral vision	✓
PERRLA	✓

PERRLA, Pupils equal, round, reactive to light and accommodation.

Internal Structures and Functions

The iris provides the color of the eye. The iris has a small round opening in its center, the *pupil,* which allows light to enter the eye. The pupil constricts via action of the iris sphincter muscle (innervated by CN III [oculomotor nerve]) and dilates via action of the iris dilator muscle (innervated by CN V [trigeminal nerve]) to control the amount of light that enters the eye.

The **lens** is a biconvex, avascular, transparent structure located behind the iris. The primary function of the lens is to bend light rays so that they focus onto the retina. Accommodation occurs when the eye focuses on a near object and is facilitated by contraction of the ciliary body, which changes the shape of the lens. The ciliary body consists of the ciliary muscles, which surround the lens and lie parallel to the sclera. The ciliary processes lie behind the peripheral part of the iris and secrete aqueous humor. The *choroid* is a highly vascular structure that nourishes the ciliary body, the iris, and the outer portion of the retina. It lies inside and parallel to the sclera (see Fig. 21-1).

TABLE 21-1 GERONTOLOGIC ASSESSMENT DIFFERENCES

Visual System

Changes	Differences in Assessment Findings
Eyebrows and Eyelashes	
Loss of pigment in hair	Graying of eyebrows, eyelashes
Eyelids	
Loss of orbital fat, decreased muscle tone	Entropion, ectropion, mild ptosis
Tissue atrophy, prolapse of fat into eyelid tissue	Blepharodermachalasis (excessive upper lid skin)
Conjunctiva	
Tissue damage related to chronic exposure to ultraviolet light or to other chronic environmental exposure	Pinguecula (small yellowish spot usually on medial aspect of conjunctiva)
Sclera	
Lipid deposition	Scleral color yellowish as opposed to bluish
Cornea	
Cholesterol deposits in peripheral cornea	Arcus senilis (milky white-gray ring encircling periphery of cornea) (Fig. 21-4)
Tissue damage related to chronic exposure	Pterygium (thickened, triangular bit of pale tissue that extends from inner canthus of eye to nasal border of cornea)
Decrease in water content, atrophy of nerve fibers	Decreased corneal sensitivity and corneal reflex
Epithelial changes	Loss of corneal luster
Accumulation of lipid deposits	Blurring of vision
Lacrimal Apparatus	
Decreased tear secretion	Dryness
Malposition of eyelid resulting in tears overflowing lid margins instead of draining through puncta	Tearing, irritated eyes
Iris	
Increased rigidity of iris	Decreased pupil size
Dilator muscle atrophy or weakness	Slower recovery of pupil size after light stimulation
Loss of pigment	Change of iris color
Ciliary muscle becoming smaller, stiffer	Decrease in near vision and accommodation
Lens	
Biochemical changes in lens proteins, oxidative damage, chronic exposure to ultraviolet light	Cataracts
Increased rigidity of lens	Presbyopia
Opacities in lens (may also be related to opacities in cornea and vitreous)	Complaints of glare, night vision impaired
Accumulation of yellow substances	Yellow color of lens
Retina	
Retinal vascular changes related to atherosclerosis and hypertension	Narrowed, pale, straighter arterioles. Acute branching
Decrease in cones	Changes in color perception, especially blue and violet
Loss of photoreceptor cells, retinal pigment, epithelial cells, and melanin	Decreased visual acuity
Age-related macular degeneration as a result of vascular changes	Loss of central vision
Vitreous	
Liquefaction and detachment of vitreous	Increased complaints of "floaters"

The **retina** is the innermost layer of the eye that extends and forms the optic nerve. Neurons make up the major portion of the retina. Therefore retinal cells are unable to regenerate if destroyed. The retina lines the inside of the eyeball, extending from the area of the optic nerve to the ciliary body (see Fig. 21-1). It is responsible for converting images into a form that the brain can understand and process as vision. The retina is composed of two types of photoreceptor cells: rods and cones. Rods are stimulated in dim or darkened environments, and cones are receptive to colors in bright environments. The center of the retina is the *fovea centralis,* a pinpoint depression composed only of densely packed cones.[1] This area of the retina provides the sharpest visual acuity. Surrounding the fovea is the *macula,* an area less than 1 mm^2, which has a high concentration of cones and is relatively free of blood vessels.

GERONTOLOGIC CONSIDERATIONS

EFFECTS OF AGING ON VISUAL SYSTEM

Every structure of the visual system is subject to changes as the individual ages. Whereas many of these changes are relatively benign, others may result in severely compromised visual acuity in the older adult. The psychosocial impact of poor vision or blindness can be highly significant. Age-related changes in the visual system and differences in assessment findings are presented in Table 21-1.

ASSESSMENT OF VISUAL SYSTEM

Assessment of the visual system may be as simple as determining a patient's visual acuity or as complex as collecting complete subjective and objective data pertinent to the visual system. To do an appropriate visual evaluation, determine which parts of the data collection are important for each individual patient.

Subjective Data

Important Health Information

Past Health History. Obtain information about the patient's past health history, including both the ocular and nonocular history. Question the patient specifically about systemic diseases, such as diabetes, hypertension, cancer, rheumatoid arthritis, syphilis and other sexually transmitted infections

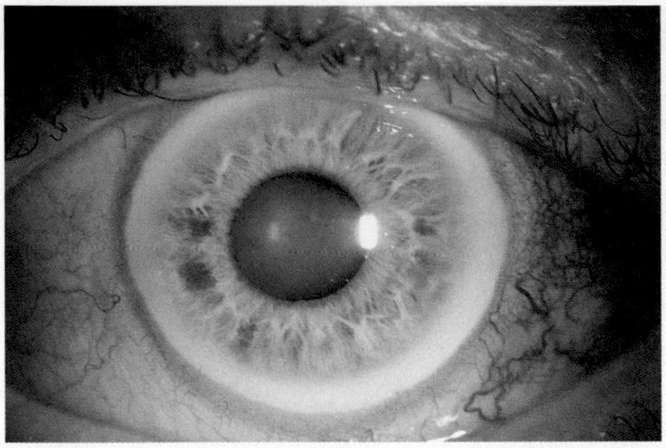

FIG. 21-4 Arcus senilis, or age-related degeneration of the cornea.

CASE STUDY

Patient Introduction

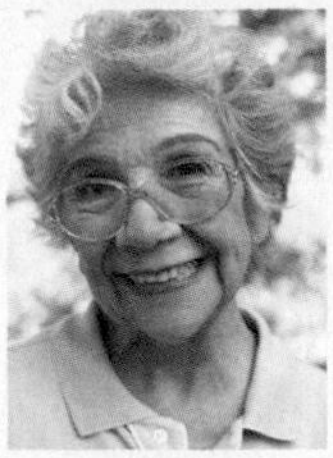

Jack Hollingsworth/ Photodisc/Thinkstock

F.M. is an 81-year-old Hispanic woman who comes to the emergency department with complaints of visual disturbances. F.M. states that her vision "looks like everything is covered with a spider web." She also reports seeing periodic light flashes and small white spots "floating" in the air.

Critical Thinking

As you read through this assessment chapter, think about F.M. with the following questions in mind:

1. What are the possible causes of F.M.'s visual disturbances?
2. What type of assessment would be most appropriate for F.M.: comprehensive, focused, or emergency?
3. What questions would you ask?
4. What should be included in the physical assessment? What would you be looking for?
5. What diagnostic studies might you expect to be ordered?

evolve Answers available at *http://evolve.elsevier.com/Lewis/medsurg.*

(STIs), acquired immunodeficiency syndrome (AIDS), muscular dystrophy, myasthenia gravis, multiple sclerosis, inflammatory bowel disease, and hypothyroidism or hyperthyroidism; many of these diseases have ocular manifestations. It is particularly important to determine whether the patient has any history of cardiac or pulmonary disease because β-adrenergic blockers are often used to treat glaucoma. These medications can slow heart rate, decrease blood pressure, and exacerbate asthma or chronic obstructive pulmonary disease (COPD).[2]

Obtain a history of tests for visual acuity, including the date of the last examination and change in glasses or contact lenses. Ask the patient about a history of strabismus, amblyopia, cataracts, retinal detachment, refractive surgery, or glaucoma. Note any trauma to the eye, its treatment, and sequelae.

The patient's nonocular history can be significant in assessing or treating the ophthalmic condition. Ask the patient about previous surgeries, treatments, or trauma related to the head.

Medications. If the patient takes medication, obtain a complete list, including dosage and frequency of over-the-counter (OTC) medicines, eyedrops, and herbal therapies or dietary supplements. Many patients do not think of these as "real" drugs and may not mention their use unless specifically questioned. However, many of these drugs have ocular effects. For example, many cold preparations contain a form of epinephrine (e.g., pseudoephedrine) that can dilate the pupil. Note the use of any antihistamine or decongestant, since these drugs can cause ocular dryness. In addition, specifically ask whether the patient uses any prescription drugs such as corticosteroids, thyroid medications, or agents such as oral hypoglycemics and insulin to lower blood glucose levels. Long-term use of corticosteroid preparations can contribute to the development of glaucoma or cataracts. Also note whether the patient is taking any β-adrenergic blockers, since these can be potentiated by the β-adrenergic blockers used to treat glaucoma.

Surgery or Other Treatments. Note any surgical procedures related to the eye or brain. Brain surgery and the subsequent swelling can cause pressure on the optic nerve or tract, resulting in visual alterations. Also document any laser procedures to the eye. The effect of any eye surgery or laser treatment on visual acuity is important information to obtain.

Functional Health Patterns. Ocular problems do not always affect the patient's visual acuity. For example, patients with blepharitis or diabetic retinopathy may not have noticeable visual deficits. The focus of the functional health pattern assessment depends on the presence or absence of vision loss and whether the loss is permanent or temporary. Table 21-2 lists suggested health history questions related to the functional health patterns.

Health Perception–Health Management Pattern. Patient characteristics such as gender, ethnicity, and age are important in assessing ophthalmic conditions. Men are more likely than women to have color blindness. The leading cause of blindness among African Americans is glaucoma.[3] Older individuals are also at greater risk for glaucoma.

The ophthalmic patient in a clinic or office setting is often seeking routine eye care or a change in the prescription of eyewear. However, the patient may have some underlying concerns that he or she does not mention or even recognize. Ask the patient, "Why are you here today?"

The patient's visual health can affect activities at home or at work. It is important to know how the patient perceives the current health problem. As outlined in Table 21-2, guide the patient in describing the current problem. Assess the patient's ability to accomplish necessary self-care, especially any eye care related to the patient's ophthalmic problem.

The patient may not recognize the importance of eye-safety practices such as wearing protective eyewear during potentially hazardous activities or avoiding noxious fumes and other eye irritants. Obtain information about the use of sunglasses in bright light. Prolonged exposure to ultraviolet (UV) light can affect the retina. Ask about night driving habits and any problems encountered. Today, millions of people wear contact lenses, but many do not care for them properly. The type of contact lenses used and the patient's wearing and care habits may provide information for teaching.

Obtain information about allergies. Allergies often cause eye symptoms such as itching, burning, watering, drainage, and blurred vision.

Hereditary systemic diseases (e.g., sickle cell anemia) can significantly affect ocular health. In addition, many refractive errors and other eye problems are hereditary. Specifically, ask whether the patient has a family history of diseases such as atherosclerosis, diabetes, thyroid disease, hypertension, arthritis, or cancer. In addition, determine whether the patient has a family history of ocular problems such as cataracts, tumors,

TABLE 21-2 HEALTH HISTORY

Visual System

Health Perception–Health Management
- Describe the change in your vision. Describe how this affects your daily life.
- Do you wear protective eyewear (sunglasses, safety goggles, hats)?*
- Do you wear contact lenses? If so, how do you take care of them?
- If you use eyedrops, how do you instill them?
- Do you have any allergies that cause eye symptoms?*
- Do you have a family history of cataracts, glaucoma, or macular degeneration?*

Nutritional-Metabolic
- Do you take any nutritional supplements?*
- Does your visual problem affect your ability to obtain and prepare food?*

Elimination
- Do you have to strain to void or defecate?*

Activity-Exercise
- Are your activities limited in any way by your eye problem?*
- Do you participate in any leisure activities that have the potential for eye injury?*

Sleep-Rest
- Is your vision affected by the amount of sleep you get?*
- Does your eye problem affect your sleeping patterns?*

Cognitive-Perceptual
- Does your eye problem affect your ability to read?*
- Do you have any eye pain?* Do you have any eye itching, burning, or foreign body sensation?*

Self-Perception–Self-Concept
- How does your eye problem make you feel about yourself?

Role-Relationship
- Do you have any problems at work or home because of your eyes?*
- Have you made any changes in your social activities because of your eyes?*

Sexuality-Reproductive
- Has your eye problem caused a change in your sex life?*
- For women: Are you pregnant? Do you use birth control pills?*
- For men: Do you use any erectile dysfunction drugs? Any vision problems with their use?*

Coping–Stress Tolerance
- Do you feel able to cope with your eye problem?*
- Are you able to acknowledge the effects of your eye problem on your life?*

Value-Belief
- Do you have any conflicts about the treatment of your eye problem?*

*If yes, describe.

glaucoma, refractive errors (especially myopia and hyperopia), or retinal degenerative conditions (e.g., macular degeneration, retinal detachment).

GENETIC RISK ALERT

Glaucoma
- Certain types of glaucoma have a strong genetic link. Many different glaucoma genes have been discovered.
- People with a family history of glaucoma have a much greater risk of developing it.

Age-Related Macular Degeneration (AMD)
- Some cases of AMD have a genetic link. Multiple genes may be associated with AMD.

Nutritional-Metabolic Pattern. High doses of vitamins containing antioxidants (vitamins C and E and beta-carotene) may be important to ocular health. Some patients with AMD may benefit from supplements of these vitamins.

Elimination Pattern. Straining to defecate (Valsalva maneuver) can raise the intraocular pressure. After eye surgery, many surgeons do not want the patient to strain. Assess the patient's usual pattern of elimination and determine whether there is the potential for constipation in the patient who has had ophthalmic surgical procedures.

Activity-Exercise Pattern. The patient's usual level of activity or exercise may be affected by reduced vision, symptoms accompanying an ocular problem, or activity restrictions after a surgical procedure. Inquire about leisure activities during which the patient may incur an ocular injury. For example, gardening, woodworking, and other craft activities can result in corneal or conjunctival foreign bodies or even penetrating injuries of the globe. Sports activities such as racquetball, baseball, and tennis carry risks for blunt trauma to the eyes. Protection goggles should be worn for these sports.

Sleep-Rest Pattern. In the otherwise healthy person, lack of sleep may cause ocular irritation, especially if the patient wears contact lenses. Normal sleep patterns may be disrupted in the patient with painful eye problems such as corneal abrasions.

Cognitive-Perceptual Pattern. The entire assessment of the ophthalmic patient focuses on the sense of sight, but do not overlook other cognitive or perceptual problems. For example, the functional ability of a patient with a visual deficit will be further compromised if the patient also has hearing problems. The patient who cannot see to read has increased difficulty following postoperative instructions if he or she also has trouble hearing or remembering verbal instructions. Eye pain is always an important symptom to assess. If eye pain is present, question the patient about treatment and response.

Self-Perception–Self-Concept Pattern. The loss of independence that can follow a partial or complete loss of vision, even if the condition is temporary, can have devastating effects on the patient's self-concept. Carefully evaluate the potential effect of vision loss on the patient's self-image. For instance, disabling glare from a cataract may prevent nighttime driving. In today's highly mobile society, the loss of ability to drive can represent a significant loss of independence and self-esteem.

Role-Relationship Pattern. Ocular problems can negatively affect the patient's ability to maintain the necessary or desired roles and responsibilities in the home, work, and social environments. For example, AMD may decrease visual acuity so that the patient can no longer adequately function at work. Many occupations place workers in conditions in which eye injury may occur. For example, factory workers may be at risk from flying metal debris. Eye-safety practices, such as the use of goggles or safety glasses, are now a legal requirement in the workplace. The patient with diabetes may not be able to see well enough to self-administer insulin. This patient may resent dependence on a family member who takes over this function.

CASE STUDY

Subjective Data

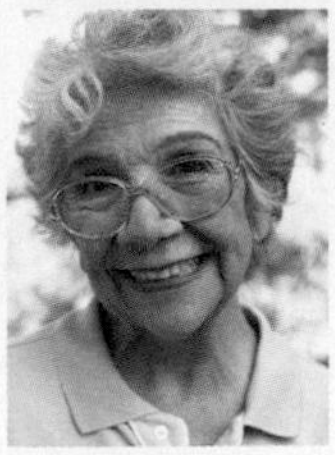

Jack Hollingsworth/ Photodisc/Thinkstock

A focused subjective assessment of F.M. revealed the following information:

- ***PMH:*** Extraocular extraction of cataract on R eye with implantation of intraocular lens 2 mo ago. Type 2 diabetes mellitus, hypothyroidism, and hypertension.
- ***Medications:*** Glyburide (DiaBeta) 5 mg/day, levothyroxine (Synthroid) 100 mcg/day, metoprolol (Lopressor) 50 mg PO daily.
- ***Health Perception–Health Management:*** States she was compliant with postoperative antibiotic and corticosteroid eyedrops and with office follow-up with eye surgeon. Recovery from surgery was uneventful, and eyedrops were discontinued 2 wk ago. Does not have allergies. Had excellent eyesight until today. Is afraid she might be having a stroke.
- ***Elimination:*** Has had difficulty moving bowels with increased straining. Trying prune juice to help.
- ***Activity-Exercise:*** Walks in the mall at least ½ mile three times a week. No resistance or isotonic exercises.
- ***Cognitive-Perceptual:*** Denies eye pain, itching, or tearing. Having difficulty reading.
- ***Coping–Stress Tolerance:*** Afraid she is having a stroke.

Sensitively inquire if the ocular problem has affected the patient's preferred roles and responsibilities.

Sexuality-Reproductive Pattern. The patient with severe vision loss may develop such a poor self-image that the ability to be sexually intimate is lost. Assure the patient that low vision or blindness does not affect a person's ability to be sexually expressive. Often touch is more important than vision.

Coping–Stress Tolerance Pattern. The patient with temporary or permanent visual problems may experience emotional stress. Assess the patient's coping level, coping mechanisms, and availability of social and personal support systems.

Value-Belief Pattern. Be sensitive to each patient's individual values and spiritual beliefs, since these may guide the patient's decisions regarding ophthalmic care. It can be difficult to understand why a patient refuses treatment that has potential benefit or wants treatment that may have limited potential benefit.

Objective Data

Physical Examination. Physical examination of the visual system includes inspecting the ocular structures and determining the status of their respective functions. Physiologic functional assessment includes determining the patient's visual acuity, ability to judge closeness and distance, and extraocular muscle (EOM) function; evaluating visual fields; observing pupil function; and measuring the intraocular pressure.[4] Assessment of ocular structures should include examining the ocular adnexa, the external eye, and internal structures. Some structures, such as the retina and blood vessels, must be visualized with the ophthalmoscope.

Assessment of the visual system may include all of the components discussed in the following sections, or it may be as brief as measuring the patient's visual acuity. Assess what is appropriate and necessary for the specific patient. Many of the following assessments are within your scope of practice, but some require special training.

TABLE 21-3 NORMAL PHYSICAL ASSESSMENT OF VISUAL SYSTEM

- Visual acuity 20/20 OU. No diplopia.
- External eye structures symmetric and without lesions or deformities.
- Lacrimal apparatus nontender and without drainage.
- Conjunctiva clear. Sclera white.
- PERRLA.
- Lens clear.
- EOMI.
- Optic nerve margins sharp.
- Retinal vessels normal, with no hemorrhages or spots.

EOMI, Extraocular movements intact; *OU,* both eyes; *PERRLA,* pupils equal, round, reactive to light and accommodation.

Normal physical assessment of the visual system is outlined in Table 21-3. Age-related visual changes and differences in assessment findings are listed in Table 21-1. Assessment techniques related to vision are summarized in Table 21-4, and assessment abnormalities are listed in Table 21-5 on p. 376.

A *focused assessment* is used to evaluate the status of previously identified visual problems and to monitor for signs of new problems (see Table 3-6). A focused assessment of the visual system is presented in the box on p. 370.

Initial Observation. Your initial observation of the patient can provide information that will help focus the assessment. When first encountering the patient, you may observe that the patient is dressed in clothing with unusual color combinations. This may indicate a color-vision deficit. Also note an unusual head position. The patient with diplopia may hold the head in a skewed position in an attempt to see a single image. The patient with a corneal abrasion or photophobia will cover the eyes with the hands to try to block out room light. Make a crude estimate of depth perception by extending a hand for the patient to shake.

During the initial observation, observe the patient's overall facial and ophthalmic appearance. The eyes should be symmetric and normally placed on the face. The globes should not have a bulging or sunken appearance.

Assessing Functional Status

Visual Acuity. Always record the patient's visual acuity for medical and legal reasons. Document the patient's visual acuity before the patient receives any ophthalmic care. Position the person on a mark exactly 20 ft (6 m) from the Snellen eye chart. If the person wears glasses or contacts, leave them on. Cover one eye at a time during the test. Ask the person to read down the lines of the chart to the smallest line of letters possible. Record the result using the numeric fraction at the end of the last successful line read. Indicate whether any letters were missed and if corrective lenses were worn (e.g., "Left eye, 20/30-2, with contacts"). Next ask the patient to cover the other eye, and repeat the process. Normal visual acuity is 20/20. The first number indicates the distance the person is standing or sitting from the chart; the second number gives the distance at which a normal eye can read the particular line. *Legal blindness* is defined as the best-corrected vision in the better eye of 20/200 or less.

If the patient reports near vision difficulty or is 40 years of age or older, you would also use a hand-held vision screener with varying print sizes (e.g., a Jaeger chart). Hold the card at

TABLE 21-4 NURSING ASSESSMENT

Assessment Techniques: Visual System

Description	Purpose
Visual Acuity Testing	
Patient reads from Snellen chart at 20 ft (distance vision test) or Jaeger chart at 14 in (near vision test). Examiner notes smallest print patient can read on each chart.	Determines distance and near visual acuity
Confrontation Visual Field Test	
Patient faces examiner, covers one eye, fixates on examiner's face, and counts number of fingers that examiner brings into patient's field of vision.	Determines if patient has a full field of vision, without obvious scotomas
Pupil Function Testing	
Examiner shines light into patient's pupil and observes pupillary response. Each pupil is examined independently. Examiner also checks for consensual and accommodative response.	Determines if patient has normal pupillary response
Intraocular Pressure Testing: Tono-pen	
Covered end of probe is gently touched several times to anesthetized corneal surface. Examiner records several readings to obtain a mean intraocular pressure (see eFig. 21-2).	Measures intraocular pressure (normal pressure is 10-21 mm Hg)
Ophthalmoscopy	
Examiner holds ophthalmoscope close to patient's eye, shining light into back of eye and looking through aperture on ophthalmoscope. Examiner adjusts dial to select one of lenses in ophthalmoscope that produces desired amount of magnification to inspect retina.	Provides magnified view of retina and optic nerve head (see Fig. 21-5)
Color Vision Testing	
In the Ishihara test, a patient identifies numbers or paths formed by pattern of dots in series of color plates.	Determines ability to distinguish colors
Keratometry	
Examiner aligns projection and notes readings of corneal curvature.	Measures corneal curvature. Often done before fitting contact lenses, before refractive surgery, or after corneal transplantation

14 in (35 cm) from the eye in good light to assess near vision. Examine each eye separately with glasses on. A normal result is "14/14" in each eye, read without hesitancy and without the patient moving the card.

Hand motion or light perception may be used for distance vision assessment if a specific vision chart for distance assessment is not available. If you must assess near visual acuity without access to a Jaeger eye chart, an accurate assessment is still possible using newsprint or the label on a container. Record the acuity as "reads newspaper headline at *X* inches."

Extraocular Muscle Functions. Observe the corneal light reflex to evaluate for weakness or imbalance of the extraocular muscles (EOM). In a darkened room, ask the patient to look straight ahead while shining a penlight directly on the cornea. The light reflection should be located in the center of both corneas as the patient faces the light source.

To assess eye movement, hold a finger or an object within 10 to 12 in of the patient's nose. Ask the patient to follow with eyes only the movement of the object or finger in the six cardinal positions of gaze. (This is demonstrated in eFig. 21-1 available on the website for this chapter.) This test can indicate weakness or paralysis in the EOM and cranial nerves (oculomotor nerve [CN III], trochlear nerve [CN IV], and abducens nerve [CN VI]).

Pupil Function and Intraocular Pressure. Pupil function is determined by inspecting the pupils and their reactions to light. The normal finding is commonly abbreviated as PERRL (pupils are equal [in size], round, and reactive to light). To test for accommodation, ask the person to focus on a distant object. This process dilates the eyes. Then have the person shift the focus to a near object (e.g., your finger held about 3 inches from the person's nose). A normal response is constriction of the eyes and convergence (inward movement of both eyes toward each other). When accommodation is assessed in addition to the pupillary light reflex, a normal response is *PERRLA* (pupils are equal, round, and reactive to light and accommodation).

In a small percentage of the population the pupils are unequal in size *(anisocoria)*. The pupils should react to light directly (the pupil constricts when a light shines into the eye) and consensually (the pupil constricts when a light shines into the opposite eye).

Intraocular pressure (see Table 21-4) can be measured by a variety of methods, including the Tono-pen[5] (shown in eFig. 21-2 available on the website for this chapter). Normal intraocular pressure ranges from 10 to 21 mm Hg.

Assessing Structures. The visual system structures are assessed primarily by inspection. The visual system is unique because not only the external structures but also many of the internal structures can be directly inspected. The iris, lens, vitreous, retina, and optic nerve can all be visualized directly through the clear cornea and pupil opening.

This direct inspection requires special observation equipment such as the slit lamp microscope and the ophthalmoscope. This equipment permits examination of the conjunctiva, sclera, cornea, anterior chamber, iris, lens, vitreous, and retina under magnification. The *ophthalmoscope* is a hand-held instrument with a light source and magnifying lenses that is held close to the patient's eye to visualize the posterior part of the eye. Little pain or discomfort is associated with these examinations.

Eyebrows, Eyelashes, and Eyelids. All structures should be present and symmetric, without deformities, redness, or swelling. Eyelashes extend outward from the lid margins. In normal closing the upper and lower eyelid margins just touch. The lacrimal puncta should be open and positioned properly against the globe.

Conjunctiva and Sclera. The conjunctiva and sclera can easily be examined at the same time. Evaluate the color, smoothness, and presence of lesions or foreign bodies. The conjunctiva covering the sclera is normally clear, with fine blood vessels visible. These blood vessels are more common in the periphery.

The sclera is normally white, but it may take on a yellowish hue in the older individual because of lipid deposition. A pale blue cast caused by scleral thinning can also be normal in older adults and in infants (who have naturally thinner sclerae). A

TABLE 21-5 ASSESSMENT ABNORMALITIES

Visual System

Finding	Description	Possible Etiology and Significance
Subjective Data		
Pain	Foreign body sensation	Superficial corneal erosion or abrasion. Can result from contact lens wear or trauma. Conjunctival or corneal foreign body
	Severe, deep, throbbing	Anterior uveitis, acute glaucoma, infection. Acute glaucoma also associated with nausea, vomiting
Photophobia	Persistent abnormal intolerance to light	Inflammation or infection of cornea or anterior uveal tract (iris and ciliary body)
Blurred vision	Gradual or sudden inability to see clearly	Refractive errors, corneal opacities, cataracts, migraine aura, retinal changes (detachment, macular degeneration)
Spots, floaters	Patient describes seeing spots, "spiderwebs," "curtain," or floaters within the field of vision	Most common cause is vitreous liquefaction (benign phenomenon). Other possible causes include hemorrhage into the vitreous humor, retinal holes or tears
Dryness	Discomfort, sandy, gritty, irritation, or burning	Decreased tear formation or changes in tear composition because of aging or various systemic diseases
Diplopia	Double vision	Abnormalities of extraocular muscle action related to muscle or cranial nerve pathologic condition
Objective Data		
Eyelids		
Allergic reactions	Redness, excessive tearing, and itching of lid margins	Many possible allergens. Associated eye trauma can occur from rubbing itchy eyelids
Hordeolum (sty)	Small, superficial white nodule along lid margin	Infection of sebaceous gland of eyelid. Causative organism is usually bacterial (most commonly *Staphylococcus aureus*)
Blepharitis	Redness, swelling, and crusting along lid margins	Bacterial invasion of lid margins. Often chronic
Ptosis	Drooping of upper lid margin, unilateral or bilateral	Mechanical causes as a result of eyelid tumors or excess skin. Myasthenia gravis
Entropion	Inward turning of upper or lower lid margin, unilateral or bilateral	Congenital causes resulting in development abnormalities
Ectropion	Outward turning of lower lid margin	Mechanical causes as a result of eyelid tumors, herniated orbital fat, or extravasation of fluid
Conjunctiva		
Conjunctivitis	Redness, swelling of conjunctiva. May be itchy	Bacterial or viral infection. May be allergic response or inflammatory response to chemical exposure
Subconjunctival hemorrhage	Appearance of blood spot on sclera. May be small or can affect entire sclera	Conjunctival blood vessels rupture, leaking blood into the subconjunctival space
Cornea		
Corneal abrasion	Localized painful disruption of the epithelial layer of cornea. Can be visualized with fluorescein dye	Trauma. Overwear or improper fit of contact lenses
Globe		
Exophthalmos	Protrusion of globe beyond its normal position within bony orbit. Sclera often visible above iris when eyelids are open	Intraocular or periorbital tumors. Hyperthyroidism
Pupil		
Anisocoria	Pupils unequal (constricted)	Central nervous system disorders. Slight difference in pupil size is normal in some people
Abnormal response to light or accommodation	Pupils respond asymmetrically or abnormally to light stimulus or accommodation	Central nervous system disorders, general anesthesia
Extraocular Muscles		
Strabismus	Deviation of eye position in one or more directions	Overaction or underaction of one or more extraocular muscles
Lens		
Cataract	Opacification of lens. Pupil can appear cloudy or white when opacity is visible behind pupil opening	Aging, trauma, diabetes, long-term systemic corticosteroid therapy
Visual Field Defect		
Peripheral	Partial or complete loss of peripheral vision	Glaucoma. Interruption of visual pathway (e.g., tumor). Migraine headache
Central	Loss of central vision	Macular disease

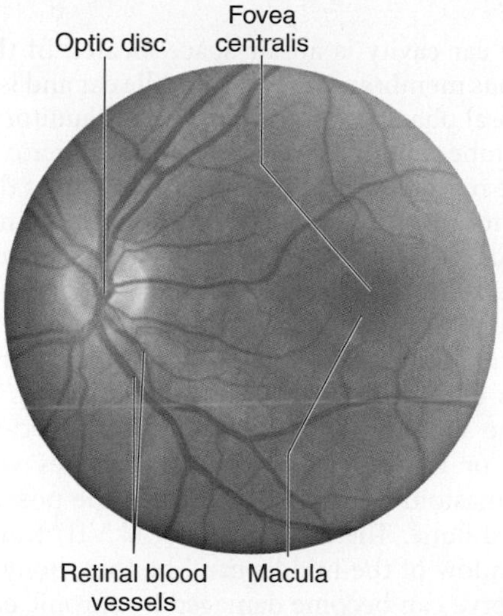

FIG. 21-5 Magnified view of retina through the ophthalmoscope.

slight yellow cast may also be found in some dark-skinned people, such as African Americans and Native Americans.

Cornea. The cornea should be clear, transparent, and shiny. The iris should appear flat and not bulge toward the cornea. The area between the cornea and the iris should be clear, with no blood or purulent material visible in the anterior chamber.

Iris. Both irides should be of similar color and shape. However, a color difference between the irides occurs normally in a small portion of the population.

Retina and Optic Nerve. An ophthalmoscope is used to magnify the retina and optic nerves and bring them into crisp focus (Fig. 21-5). Examine the optic nerve or disc for size, color, and abnormalities. The optic disc is creamy yellow with distinct margins. A central depression in the disc, called the *physiologic cup,* may be seen. This area is the exit site for the optic nerve. The cup should be less than one half the diameter of the disc. Normally, no hemorrhages or exudates are present in the fundus (retinal background). Careful inspection of the fundus can reveal retinal holes, tears, detachments, or lesions. Small hemorrhages can be associated with diabetes or hypertension and can appear in various shapes, such as dots or flames. Finally, examine the macula for shape and appearance. This area of high reflectivity is devoid of any blood vessels.

Important information about the vascular system and the central nervous system (CNS) can be obtained through direct visualization with an ophthalmoscope. Skilled use of this instrument requires practice.

Special Assessment Techniques

Color Vision. Testing the patient's ability to distinguish colors can be an important part of the overall assessment because some occupations may require accurate color discrimination. The Ishihara color test determines the patient's ability to distinguish a pattern of color in a series of color plates.[6]

Stereopsis. *Stereoscopic vision* allows a patient to see objects in three dimensions. Any event that causes a patient to have monocular vision (e.g., enucleation, patching) results in the loss of stereoscopic vision. Without stereopsis, the individual's ability to judge distances or the height of a step is impaired. This disability can have serious consequences if the patient trips over a step when walking or follows too closely behind another vehicle when driving.

CASE STUDY

Objective Data

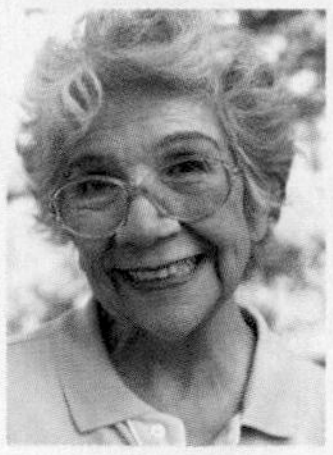

Jack Hollingsworth/
Photodisc/Thinkstock

Physical Examination

Physical examination findings of F.M. were as follows:

- PERRL. No abnormalities noted on visual examination of external eye structures. EOM intact and symmetric.

As you continue to read this chapter, consider diagnostic studies you would anticipate being performed for F.M.

Diagnostic Studies

The health care provider performs an ophthalmoscopic examination on F.M. and identifies a partial retinal detachment. This diagnosis is confirmed via ultrasonography.

DIAGNOSTIC STUDIES OF VISUAL SYSTEM

Diagnostic studies provide important information in monitoring the patient's condition and planning appropriate interventions. These studies are considered objective data. Table 21-6 presents the most common diagnostic studies of the visual system.

AUDITORY SYSTEM

STRUCTURES AND FUNCTIONS OF AUDITORY SYSTEM

The auditory system is composed of the peripheral auditory system and the central auditory system. The peripheral system includes the structures of the ear itself: the external, middle, and inner ear (Fig. 21-6). This system is concerned with the reception and perception of sound. The inner ear functions in hearing and balance. The central system integrates and assigns meaning to what is heard. This system includes the vestibulocochlear nerve (CN VIII) and the auditory cortex of the brain. The brain and its pathways transmit and process sound and sensations that maintain a person's equilibrium.

The role of the external and middle portion of the ear is to conduct and amplify sound waves from the environment. This portion of sound conduction is termed *air conduction.* Problems in these two parts of the ear may cause *conductive hearing loss,* resulting in a decrease in sound intensity and/or a distortion in sound.

Disturbances in equilibrium can impair coordination, balance, and orientation. Damage to or an abnormality of the inner ear or along the nerve pathways results in *sensorineural hearing loss.* In addition to causing distortion or faintness of sound, sensorineural hearing loss may affect the ability to understand speech or cause complete hearing loss. Impairment within the auditory pathways of the brain causes *central hearing loss.* This type of hearing loss causes difficulty in understanding the meaning of words that are heard. (Types of hearing loss are discussed in Chapter 22 on pp. 406-407.)

External Ear

The external ear consists of the *auricle* (pinna), external auditory canal, and tympanic membrane (TM). The auricle is composed of cartilage and connective tissue covered with epithelium,

TABLE 21-6 DIAGNOSTIC STUDIES

Visual System

Description and Purpose	Nursing Responsibility*
Refractometry	
Subjective measure of refractive error. Multiple lenses are mounted on rotating wheels. Patient sits looking through apertures at Snellen acuity chart, and lenses are changed. Patient chooses lenses that make acuity sharpest. Comprehensive examination requires dilation of eyes to visualize retina and optic nerves.	Procedure is painless. Patient may need help to hold head still. Pupil dilation makes it difficult to focus on near objects. Dilation may last 3-4 hr.
Ultrasonography	
A-scan probe is applanated against patient's anesthetized cornea. Used primarily for axial length measurement for calculating power of intraocular lens implanted after cataract extraction. *B-scan* probe is applied to patient's closed lid. Used more often than A-scan for diagnosis of ocular pathologic conditions such as intraocular foreign bodies or tumors, vitreous opacities, retinal detachments.	Procedure is painless (cornea is anesthetized).
Fluorescein Angiography	
Fluorescein (a nonradioactive, non-iodine dye) injected IV into antecubital or other peripheral vein, followed by serial photographs (over 10-min period) of the retina through dilated pupils. Provides diagnostic information about flow of blood through pigment epithelial and retinal vessels. Often used in diabetic patients to accurately locate areas of diabetic retinopathy before laser destruction of neovascularization.	If extravasation occurs, fluorescein is toxic to tissue. Although systemic allergic reactions are rare, be familiar with emergency equipment and procedures. Tell patient that dye can sometimes cause transient nausea or vomiting. Transient yellow-orange discoloration of urine and skin is normal.
Amsler Grid Test	
Test is self-administered using a hand-held card printed with a grid of lines (similar to graph paper). Patient fixates on center dot and records any abnormalities of the grid lines, such as wavy, missing, or distorted areas. Used to monitor macular problems.	Regular testing is necessary to identify any changes in macular function.

*Patient teaching regarding the purpose and method of testing is a nursing responsibility for all diagnostic procedures.

which also lines the external auditory canal (see Fig. 21-6). The external auditory canal is a slightly S-shaped tube about 1 in (2.5 cm) in length in the adult. The lining of the canal contains fine hairs (cilia), sebaceous (oil) glands, and ceruminous (wax) glands. The oil and wax lubricate the ear canal, keep it free from debris, and kill bacteria.

The function of the external ear and canal is to collect and transmit sound waves to the *tympanic membrane* (eardrum). This shiny, translucent, pearl-gray membrane is composed of epithelial cells, connective tissue, and mucous membrane. It serves as a partition and an instrument of sound transmission between the external auditory canal and the middle ear.

Middle Ear

The middle ear cavity is an air space located in the temporal bone. Mucous membrane lines the middle ear and is continuous from the nasal pharynx via the eustachian (auditory) tube. The eustachian tube functions to equalize atmospheric air pressure between the middle ear and the throat and allows the tympanic membrane to move freely. It opens during yawning and swallowing. Blockage of this tube can occur with allergies, nasopharyngeal infections, or enlarged adenoids.

The middle ear contains the three smallest bones in the body: *malleus, incus,* and *stapes* (ossicles). Vibrations of the TM cause the ossicles to move and transmit sound waves to the oval window. The superior part of the middle ear is called the *epitympanum,* or the attic. It also communicates with air cells within the mastoid bone. The mastoid is the posterior part of the temporal bone. The facial nerve (CN VII) traverses above the oval window of the middle ear. The thin, bony covering of the facial nerve can become damaged by chronic ear infection, skull fracture, or trauma during ear surgery. Problems may occur related to voluntary facial movements, eyelid closure, and taste discrimination. Permanent damage to the facial nerve can also result.

Inner Ear

The inner ear is composed of a bony labyrinth (maze) surrounding a membrane. Perilymphatic fluid lies between the bone and the membrane. The fluid inside the membrane is called *endolymph.* The inner ear contains the functional organs for hearing and balance. The receptor organ for hearing is the *cochlea,* which is a coiled structure. It contains the *organ of Corti,* whose tiny hair cells respond to stimulation of selected portions of the basilar membrane according to pitch. This stimulus is converted into an electrochemical impulse and then transmitted by the acoustic portion of the vestibulocochlear nerve (CN VIII) to the temporal lobe of the brain to process and interpret the sound.

Three semicircular canals and the vestibule make up the organ of balance. These structures comprise the membranous labyrinth, which is housed within the bony labyrinth. The membranous labyrinth is filled with endolymphatic fluid, and the bony labyrinth is filled with perilymphatic fluid. Nervous stimuli are communicated by the vestibular portion of CN VIII. Debris such as loose crystals of calcium or excessive pressure within the lymphatic fluid can produce disorders such as benign paroxysmal positional vertigo (BPPV).

Transmission of Sound. Sound waves are conducted by air (air conduction) and picked up by the auricles and auditory canal. The TM is struck by the sound waves, causing it to vibrate. The central area of the TM is connected to the malleus, which also starts to vibrate. The malleus transmits the vibration to the incus and then the stapes. As the stapes moves back and forth, it pushes the membrane of the oval window in and out. Movement of the oval window produces waves in the perilymph.

Once sound has been transmitted to the liquid medium of the inner ear, the vibration is picked up by the tiny sensory hair cells of the cochlea, which initiate nerve impulses. These impulses are carried by nerve fibers to the main branch of the acoustic portion of CN VIII and then to the brain.

The bones of the skull can also transmit sound directly to the inner ear (bone conduction). This can be demonstrated by placing the stem of a vibrating tuning fork on the skull.

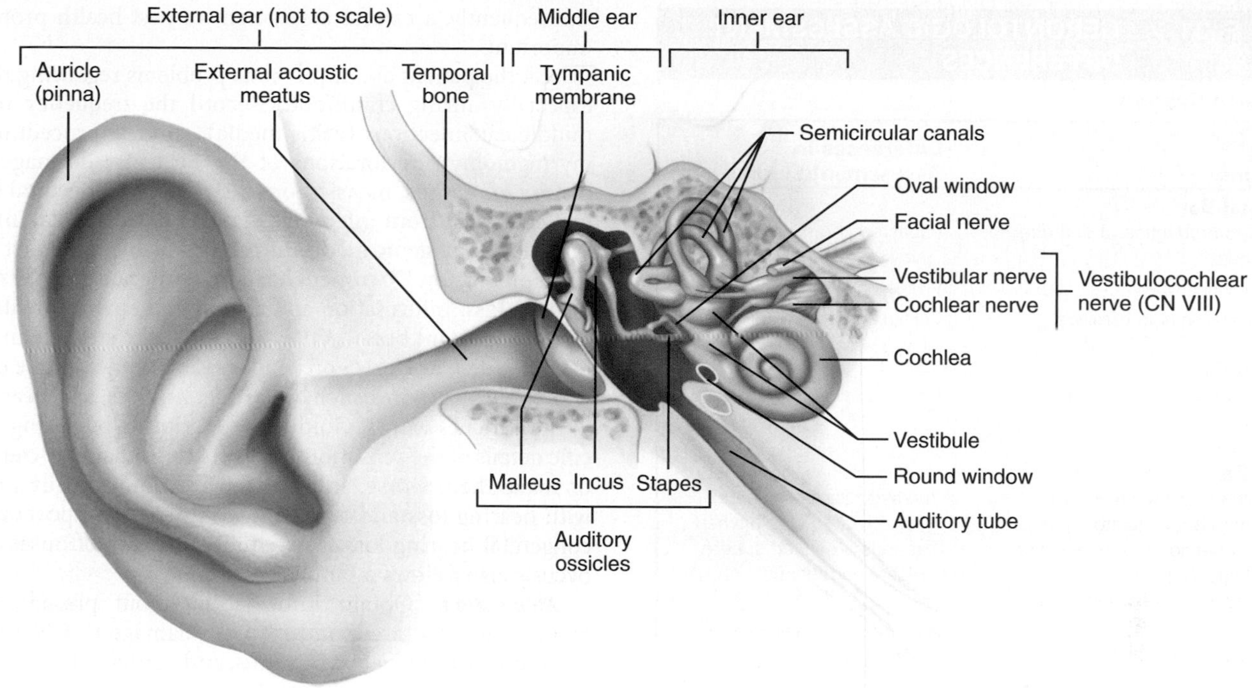

FIG. 21-6 External, middle, and inner ear.

GERONTOLOGIC CONSIDERATIONS

EFFECTS OF AGING ON AUDITORY SYSTEM

Approximately 36 million American adults report some degree of hearing loss, with aging being the primary cause.[7] **Presbycusis,** or hearing loss due to aging, can result from a variety of sources. Noise exposure, systemic diseases, poor nutrition, ototoxic drugs, and pollution exposure over the life span can damage the delicate hair cells of the organ of Corti or atrophy lymph-producing cells. Sound transmission is also diminished by calcification of the ossicles. The loss associated with presbycusis is usually greater for high-pitched sounds. Accumulation of dry cerumen (earwax) in the external canal can also interfere with the transmission of sound.[8] **Tinnitus,** or ringing in the ears, may accompany the hearing loss that results from the aging process. As the average life span increases, the number of people with hearing loss will also increase. Prevention and early identification of problems will ensure a more active and healthy aging population.

Age-related changes in the auditory system and differences in assessment findings are presented in Table 21-7.

FOCUSED ASSESSMENT

Auditory System

Use this checklist to make sure the key assessment steps have been done.

Subjective

Ask the patient about any of the following and note responses.

Changes in hearing	Y	N
Ear pain	Y	N
Ear drainage	Y	N

Objective: Physical Examination

Inspect

Alignment and position of ears on head	✓
Size, shape, symmetry, color, and skin intactness	✓
External auditory meatus for discharge or lesions	✓

Assess

Hearing based on ability to respond to conversation, respond to a whisper, or hear a ticking watch	✓

ASSESSMENT OF AUDITORY SYSTEM

Assessment of the auditory system should include assessment of hearing and equilibrium because the auditory and *vestibular* (balance) systems are closely related. It is often difficult to separate symptoms related to these two systems. Help the patient describe symptoms and problems to differentiate the source of the problems. Health history questions to ask a patient with an auditory problem are listed in Table 21-8.

Problems with balance may manifest as vertigo or nystagmus. **Vertigo** is a sense that the person or objects around the person are moving or spinning and is usually stimulated by movement of the head. *Dizziness* is a sensation of being off-balance that occurs when standing or walking. **Nystagmus** is an abnormal eye movement that may be observed as a twitching of the eyeball or described by the patient as a blurring of vision with head or eye movement.

Initially try to categorize symptoms related to balance and separate them from symptoms related to hearing loss or tinnitus. The symptoms can be combined later in the assessment to help make the diagnosis and plan for the patient.

Subjective Data

Important Health Information

Past Health History. Many problems related to the ear may result from childhood illnesses or problems of adjacent organs.

TABLE 21-7 GERONTOLOGIC ASSESSMENT DIFFERENCES

Auditory System

Changes	Differences in Assessment Findings
External Ear	
Increased production of and drier cerumen	Impacted cerumen, potential hearing loss
Increased hair growth	Visible hair, especially in men
Loss of elasticity in cartilage	Collapsed ear canal
Middle Ear	
Atrophic changes of tympanic membrane	Conductive hearing loss
Inner Ear	
Hair cell degeneration, neuron degeneration in auditory nerve and central pathways, reduced blood supply to cochlea, calcification of ossicles	Presbycusis, diminished sensitivity to high-pitched sounds, impaired speech reception, tinnitus
Less effective vestibular apparatus in semicircular canals	Alterations in balance and body orientation
Brain	
Decline in ability to filter out unwanted and unnecessary sound	Difficulty hearing in a noisy environment, heightened sensitivity to loud sounds

Consequently, a careful assessment of past health problems is important.

Ask the patient about previous problems regarding the ears, especially during childhood. Record the frequency of acute middle ear infections (otitis media); surgical procedures (e.g., myringotomy); perforations of the eardrum; drainage; and a history of mumps, measles, or scarlet fever. Congenital hearing loss can result from infectious diseases (e.g., rubella, influenza, syphilis), teratogenic medications, or hypoxia in the first trimester of pregnancy. Document head injury because it may result in hearing loss. Information about food and environmental allergies is important because they can cause the eustachian tube to become edematous and prevent aeration of the middle ear.

Record symptoms such as vertigo, tinnitus, and hearing loss in the patient's words. Guide the description by asking for specific details of the sensations and situations that may cause them or make them worse. Information regarding family members with hearing loss and type of hearing loss is important. Some congenital hearing loss is hereditary. The age of onset of presbycusis also follows a familial pattern.

Medications. Obtain information about present or past medications that are *ototoxic* (cause damage to CN VIII) and can produce hearing loss, tinnitus, and vertigo. The amount and frequency of aspirin use are important because tinnitus can result from high aspirin intake. Aminoglycosides, any other antibiotics, salicylates, antimalarial agents, chemotherapeutic drugs, diuretics, and nonsteroidal antiinflammatory drugs

TABLE 21-8 HEALTH HISTORY

Auditory System

Health Perception–Health Management

Hearing

- Have you had a change in your hearing?* If yes, how does this change affect your daily life?
- Do you use any devices to improve your hearing (e.g., hearing aid, special volume control, headphones for television or stereo)?*
- How do you protect your hearing?
- Do you have any allergies that result in ear problems?*

Equilibrium

- When did the dizziness or spinning sensation first occur?
- Does this sensation occur when you first stand up, when you are lying down, or both?
- Have you ever fallen because of the dizziness?*
- Can you drive or walk alone? If no, elaborate.
- Are there any times of the day when your symptoms are worse?*

Tinnitus

- How long have you experienced ringing in your ears? Has it changed?* Describe the ringing (e.g., buzzing, ringing, roaring). Do you also have a feeling of fullness or pressure?*
- When does it bother you the most?
- What things have you tried that help or have not helped?
- What medications are you taking?

Nutritional-Metabolic

- Do you notice any differences in symptoms with changes in diet?*
- Does your ear problem cause nausea that interferes with your food intake?*
- Does chewing or swallowing cause you any ear discomfort?*

Elimination

- Does straining during a bowel movement cause ear pain?*

Activity-Exercise

- Do you need help with certain activities (e.g., lifting, bending, climbing stairs, driving, speaking) because of symptoms?*

Sleep-Rest

- Is your sleep disturbed by noises or ringing in the ears or by a sensation of spinning?*

Cognitive-Perceptual

- Do you experience ear pain?* What relieves the pain? What makes it worse? Does the pain affect your hearing or balance?
- Have you noticed any problem with communicating or understanding what people are saying?*

Self-Perception–Self-Concept

- Have changes in your hearing affected how you feel about yourself or your feeling of independence?*

Role-Relationship

- What effect has your ear problem had on your work, family, or social life?
- Are you able to recognize the effects of your ear problems on your life?*

Sexuality-Reproductive

- Has your ear problem caused a change in your sex life?*

Coping–Stress Tolerance

- Do you consider your ear problem a source of stress?*
- How do you cope when you are experiencing symptoms?

Value-Belief

- Do you have a conflict between what your health care provider would like you to do and what you believe you should do?

*If yes, describe.

(NSAIDs) are groups of drugs that are potentially ototoxic. Monitor for hearing and balance problems in patients receiving these drugs. Many drugs produce hearing loss that may be reversible if treatment is stopped.

Surgery or Other Treatments. Document previous hospitalizations for ear surgery, including *myringotomy* (ventilation holes placed in the TM with or without tubes), *tympanoplasty* (surgical repair of TM), tonsillectomy, and adenoidectomy (removal of tonsils and adenoids). Record the use of and satisfaction with a hearing aid. Also note any problems with impacted cerumen.

Functional Health Patterns. Hearing and balance problems can affect all aspects of a person's life. To assess the impact of hearing loss, ask health history questions based on a functional health patterns approach (see Table 21-8).

Health Perception–Health Management Pattern. Note the onset of hearing loss, whether sudden or gradual, and who noted the onset (e.g., patient, family, significant others). Gradual hearing losses are most often noted by those who communicate with the patient. Sudden losses and those exacerbated by some other condition are most often reported by the patient.

Assess the patient for personal measures used to preserve hearing. The use of protective ear covers or earplugs is good practice for people in high-noise environments. Document if the patient is a swimmer and the frequency and duration of swimming and use of ear protection. Note the type of water (pool, lake, or ocean) in which the swimming takes place to help identify contact with contaminated water. Assess for the placement of any item in the ear, including hearing aids, which can cause trauma to the canal and TM.

Nutritional-Metabolic Pattern. Alcohol, sodium, and dietary supplements affect the amount of endolymph in the inner ear system. Patients with Ménière's disease may notice some improvement in their symptoms with alcohol restriction and a low-sodium diet.[9] Note changes in symptoms with food intake. Question the patient about any ear pain (otalgia) or discomfort associated with chewing or swallowing that might decrease nutritional intake. This situation is often associated with a problem in the middle ear.

Assessment of clenching or grinding of the teeth helps differentiate problems of the ear from referred pain of the temporomandibular joint (TMJ). Ask about dental problems and dentures.

Elimination Pattern. Elimination patterns are mainly of interest in the patient with perilymph fistula and after surgical procedures. Frequent constipation or straining with bowel or bladder elimination may interfere with healing or repair of a perilymph fistula. After middle ear surgery (stapedectomy) the patient needs to prevent increased intracranial (and consequent inner ear) pressure associated with straining during bowel movements. Stool softeners may be ordered postoperatively for the patient who reports chronic problems with constipation.

Activity-Exercise Pattern. A review of the patient's activity-exercise pattern is essential when assessing for equilibrium problems. Question the patient specifically about the onset, duration, and frequency of symptoms. Identify activities that relieve or worsen symptoms and how they relate to the time of the day. For example, patients with Ménière's disease are less able to compensate for environmental input as the day progresses.

Sleep-Rest Pattern. Ask the patient with chronic tinnitus about sleep problems. Find out if the patient has tried any techniques to drown out the tinnitus (e.g., having fan on, using white noise devices). Also assess for snoring because it can be caused by swelling or hypertrophy of tissue in the nasopharynx. This excessive tissue can impair the functioning of the eustachian tube and cause the sensation of ear fullness or pain.

Cognitive-Perceptual Pattern. Pain is associated with some ear problems, particularly those involving the middle ear and auditory canal. If pain is present, ask the patient to describe the pain, presence of drainage (otorrhea), history of teeth grinding, and the treatments used for relief. Note the effect on the pain level when the auricle is moved or the tragus is palpated.

Note the patient's ability to pay attention and follow directions. Problems with these tasks may be an early indicator of hearing loss. The patient may not recognize a gradual hearing loss. Ask significant others if they have noted any change in the patient's hearing.

Self-Perception–Self-Concept Pattern. Ask the patient to describe how the ear problem has affected his or her personal life and feelings about himself or herself. Hearing loss and chronic vertigo are particularly distressing for the patient. Hearing loss can result in embarrassing social situations that affect the patient's self-concept. Sensitively question the patient about such situations.

At times the patient with chronic vertigo may be accused of acting intoxicated. Clarify the symptom history with the patient and consider an evaluation with a hearing specialist.

Role-Relationship Pattern. Question the patient about the effect that the ear problem has had on family life, work responsibilities, and social relationships. Hearing loss can result in strained family relations and misunderstandings.

Also ask about employment or contact with environments that have excessive noise levels, such as work with jet engines and machinery and electronically amplified music. Document the use of preventive devices worn in noisy environments. Many jobs rely on the ability to hear accurately and respond appropriately. If a hearing loss is present, gather detailed information on the effect this has on the patient's job.

The unpredictability of vertigo attacks can have devastating effects on all aspects of a patient's life. Ordinary activities such as driving or cooking and work that requires balance all have an element of danger. Assess the effect of the vertigo on the patient's many roles and responsibilities.

Sexuality-Reproductive Pattern. Determine whether hearing loss or vertigo has interfered with the establishment of a satisfactory sex life. Although intimacy does not depend on the ability to hear, a hearing loss could interfere with establishing or maintaining a relationship.

Coping–Stress Tolerance Pattern. Ask the patient about his or her usual coping style, stress-reducing techniques, and available support. If the patient seems unable to manage the situation, outside intervention may be required. Denial is a common response to a hearing problem and should be assessed.

Value-Belief Pattern. Question the patient about any conflicts produced by the problem or treatment related to values or beliefs. Every effort should be made to resolve the problem so the patient does not experience additional stress. Ask about the use of home remedies such as hot oil in the ear.

Objective Data

Physical Examination. During the health-history interview, collect objective data regarding the patient's ability to hear. Note clues such as posturing of the head and appropriateness of

TABLE 21-9 NORMAL PHYSICAL ASSESSMENT OF AUDITORY SYSTEM

- Ears symmetric in location and shape.
- Auricles and tragus nontender, without lesions.
- Canal clear, tympanic membrane intact, landmarks and light reflex intact.
- Able to hear low whisper at 30 cm. Weber test results, no lateralization. Rinne test results AC > BC.

AC, Air conduction; *BC,* bone conduction.

responses. Does the patient ask to have certain words repeated? Does the patient intently watch the examiner but miss comments when *not* looking at the examiner? Is the patient lip reading? Record these significant observations. This is also important because the patient is often unaware of hearing loss or does not admit to changes in hearing until moderate losses have occurred.

A normal assessment of the auditory system is listed in Table 21-9. Age-related changes of the auditory system and differences in assessment findings are listed in Table 21-7.

A *focused assessment* is used to evaluate the status of previously identified auditory problems and to monitor for signs of new problems (see Table 3-6). A focused assessment of the auditory system is presented in the box on p. 379.

External Ear. Inspect and palpate the external ear before examining the external canal and tympanum.[4] Observe the auricle, preauricular area, and mastoid area for symmetry, color of skin, swelling, redness, and lesions. Then palpate the auricle and mastoid areas for tenderness and nodules. Grasping the auricle or pressing on the tragus may elicit pain, especially if the external ear or canal is inflamed.

External Auditory Canal and Tympanum. Before inserting an otoscope, inspect the canal opening for patency, palpate the tragus, and gently move the auricle to check for discomfort. Select a speculum slightly smaller than the size of the ear canal. Tip the patient's head to the opposite shoulder. Grasp the top of the auricle and gently pull up and backward to straighten the canal. Hold the otoscope while stabilizing it with your fingers on the patient's cheek, and then insert it slowly. A pneumatic otoscope creates negative pressure to pull at the TM and is helpful in confirming TM retraction or fluid behind the membrane (see eFig. 21-3 available on the website for this chapter). A tight seal of the speculum is essential during this step of the examination. Observe the canal for size and shape and the color, amount, and type of cerumen. Be careful when clearing the canal of cerumen. Damage can occur to the middle ear if the TM is perforated.

Inspect the TM for color, fluid behind the membrane, landmarks, contour, and intactness (Fig. 21-7). The TM is normally pearl gray, white, or pink; shiny; and translucent. The handle *(manubrium)* of the malleus and its short process *(umbo)* should be visible through the membrane. The position and dome (concave) shape of the TM causes the light from the otoscope to reflect back in a cone shape with crisp edges. If the TM is bulging or retracted, the edges of the light reflex will be fuzzy (diffuse) and may spread over the TM. The middle and inner ear cannot be examined with the otoscope because of the TM.

Table 21-10 summarizes assessment abnormalities of the auditory system.

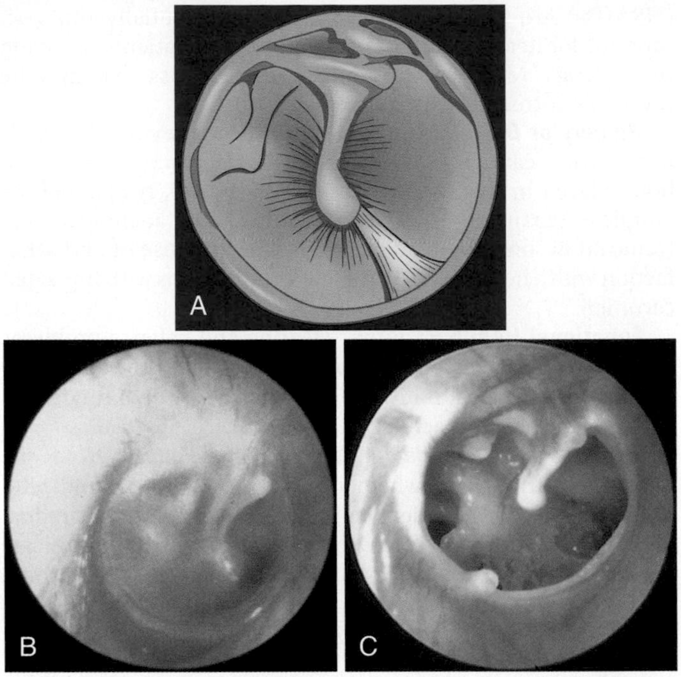

FIG. 21-7 The tympanic membrane. **A,** Landmarks of right tympanic membrane. **B,** Normal-appearing tympanic membrane. **C,** Perforated tympanic membrane.

DIAGNOSTIC STUDIES OF AUDITORY SYSTEM

Table 21-11 describes diagnostic studies commonly used to assess the auditory system.

Tests for Hearing Acuity

Tests involving the whispered and spoken voice can provide general screening information about the patient's ability to hear. Audiometric testing provides more detailed information that can be used for diagnosis and treatment.

In the *whisper test,* stand 12 to 24 in (30.5 to 61 cm) to the side of the patient and, after exhaling, speak in a low whisper. Ask the patient to repeat numbers or words or answer questions. Use a louder whisper if the patient does not respond correctly. Test each ear separately. The ear not being tested is covered by the patient.

Tuning Fork Tests. Tuning fork tests aid in differentiating between conductive and sensorineural hearing loss. Tuning forks of 512 Hz are generally used for this examination. Both skill and experience are required to ensure accurate results. If a problem is suspected, further evaluation by pure-tone audiometry is needed. The most common tuning fork tests are the *Weber test* and the *Rinne test*[10] (described in eTable 21-1 available on the website for this chapter). These tests measure hearing by bone conduction or by air conduction. Results of tuning fork tests are subjective. The patient with inconsistent or questionable test results should be referred for more objective audiometric evaluation.

Audiometry. *Audiometry* is beneficial as a screening test for hearing acuity and as a diagnostic test for determining the degree and type of hearing loss. The audiometer produces pure tones at varying intensities to which the patient can respond. Sound is characterized by the number of vibrations or cycles that occur each second. *Hertz* (Hz) is the unit of measurement used to classify the frequency of a tone; the higher the fre-

TABLE 21-10 ASSESSMENT ABNORMALITIES

Auditory System

Finding	Description	Possible Etiology and Significance
External Ear and Canal		
Sebaceous cyst behind ear	Usually within skin, possible presence of black dot (opening to sebaceous gland)	Removal or incision and drainage if painful
Tophi	Hard nodules in the helix or antihelix consisting of uric acid crystals	Associated with gout, metabolic disorder. Further diagnosis needed
Impacted cerumen	Wax that has not normally been excreted from the ear. No visualization of eardrum	Decreased hearing possible, pain, sensation of fullness in auditory canal, removal necessary before otoscopic examination
Discharge in canal	Infection of external ear, usually painful	Swimmer's ear, infection of external ear. Possibly caused by ruptured eardrum and otitis media
Swelling of pinna, pain	Infection of glands of skin, hematoma caused by trauma	Aspiration (for hematoma)
Scaling or lesions	Change in usual appearance of skin	Seborrheic dermatitis, actinic keratosis, basal or squamous cell carcinoma
Exostosis	Bony growth extending into canal causing narrowing of canal	Possible interference with visualization of tympanum. Usually asymptomatic
Tympanum		
Retracted eardrum	Appearance of shorter, more horizontal malleus. Absent or bent cone of light	Vacuum in middle ear, blockage of eustachian tube, negative pressure in middle ear
Hairline fluid level, yellow-amber bubbles above fluid level	Caused by transudate of blood and serum, meniscus of fluid producing hairline appearance	Serous otitis media
Bulging red or blue eardrum, lack of landmarks	Fluid-filled middle ear, pus, blood	Acute otitis media, perforation possible
Perforation of eardrum (see Fig. 21-7)	Previous perforations of the eardrum that have failed to heal. Thin, transparent layer of epithelium surrounding eardrum	Chronic otitis media, mastoiditis, drainage
Recruitment	Disproportionate loudness of sound from malfunction of inner ear	Hearing aid difficult to use

TABLE 21-11 DIAGNOSTIC STUDIES

Auditory System

Study	Description and Purpose	Nursing Responsibility
Auditory		
Pure-tone audiometry	Sounds are presented through earphones in soundproof room. Patient responds nonverbally when sound is heard. Response is recorded on an audiogram. Purpose is to determine patient's hearing range in terms of decibels (dB) and Hertz (Hz) for diagnosing conductive and sensorineural hearing loss. Tinnitus can cause inconsistent results.	Nurse does not usually participate in examination.
One- and two-syllable word lists	Words are presented and recorded at comfortable level of hearing to determine percentage correct and word understanding.	Nurse may perform test.
Auditory evoked potential (AEP)	Procedure is similar to electroencephalogram (see Chapter 56 and Table 56-8). Electrodes are attached to patient in a darkened room. Electrodes are placed typically at vertex, mastoid process, or earlobes and forehead. A computer is used to isolate auditory from other electrical activity of brain.	Explain procedure to patient. Do not leave patient alone in darkened room.
Electrocochleography	Test is useful for uncooperative patient or patient who cannot volunteer useful information. Test records electrical activity in cochlea and auditory nerve.	Nurse does not usually participate in examination.
Auditory brainstem response (ABR)	Study measures electrical peaks along auditory pathway of inner ear to brain and provides diagnostic information related to acoustic neuromas, brainstem problems, and stroke.	Nurse does not usually participate in examination.
Tympanometry (impedance audiometry)	Useful in diagnosis of middle ear effusions. A probe is placed snugly in external ear canal, and positive and negative pressures are then applied. Compliance of middle ear is then noted in response to pressures.	Nurse does not usually participate in examination.

Continued

TABLE 21-11 DIAGNOSTIC STUDIES—cont'd

Auditory System

Study	Description and Purpose	Nursing Responsibility
Vestibular		
Caloric test stimulus	Endolymph of semicircular canals is stimulated by irrigation of cold (68° F [20° C]) or warm (97° F [36° C]) solution into ear. Patient is seated or in supine position. Observation of type of nystagmus, nausea and vomiting, falling, or vertigo is helpful in diagnosing disease of labyrinth. Decreased function is indicated by decreased response and indicates disease of vestibular system. Other ear is tested similarly and results are compared.	Instruct patient to eat light meal before test to avoid nausea. Observe patient for vomiting. Assist if necessary. Ensure patient safety.
Electronystagmography (ENG)	Electrodes are placed near patient's eyes, and movement of eyes (nystagmus) is recorded on graph during specific eye movements and when ear is irrigated. Used to diagnose diseases of vestibular system.	Instruct patient to eat light meal before test to avoid nausea. Observe patient for vomiting. Assist if necessary. Ensure patient safety.
Posturography	Balance test that can isolate one semicircular canal from others to determine site of lesion. Test is done in a boxlike device in which floor moves in response to a correction in balance by patient.	Inform patient that test is time consuming and uncomfortable. Test can be discontinued at any time at patient's request.
Rotary chair testing	Evaluates peripheral vestibular system. Patient is seated in a chair driven by a motor under computer control. Test is usually done in the dark.	Instruct patient to eat light meal before test to avoid nausea. Observe patient for vomiting. Assist if necessary. Ensure patient safety.

quency, the higher the pitch. Hearing loss can affect certain sound frequencies. The specific pattern produced on the audiogram by these losses can assist in the diagnosis of the type of hearing loss. The intensity or strength of a sound wave is expressed in terms of decibels (dB), ranging from 0 to 110 dB. The intensity of a sound required to make any frequency barely audible to the average normal ear is 0 dB. *Threshold* refers to the signal level at which pure tones are detected (pure-tone thresholds) or the signal level at which the patient correctly hears 50% of the signals (speech detection thresholds).

Normal speech is approximately 40 to 65 dB; a soft whisper is 20 dB. Normally, a child and a young adult can hear frequencies from about 16 to 20,000 Hz, but hearing is most sensitive between 500 and 4000 Hz. This is similar to the frequencies of normal speech. A 40- to 45-dB loss in these frequencies causes moderate difficulty in hearing normal speech. A hearing aid may be helpful because it makes sound information louder but not clearer. A hearing aid may not be helpful to the patient who has problems with discrimination of sounds or sound information because the consonants are still not heard enough to make speech understandable.

Screening Audiometry. Screening audiometry is the testing of large numbers of people with a fast, simple test to detect possible hearing problems. A pass-fail criterion is used to screen people who will or will not be given additional diagnostic testing. People who fail the screening should be referred to an audiologist for pure-tone (threshold) audiometry.

Specialized Tests

The more specialized tests of the auditory system are frequently performed in an outpatient setting by an audiologist. An audiologist can perform many additional tests with the use of audiometers and computers that record electrical activity from the middle ear, inner ear, and brain (see Table 21-11). The most common test performed by the audiologist is pure-tone audiometry. A pure-tone audiometer produces pure tones at varied frequencies (pitch) and intensity (volume). Testing determines the patient's hearing range in decibels and Hertz.

More sophisticated tests are available to determine the origin of certain hearing losses. These include evoked potential studies (also called auditory brainstem response) and electrocochleography. Computed tomography (CT) and magnetic resonance imaging (MRI) scans are used to diagnose the site of a lesion, such as a tumor of the auditory nerve.

Test for Vestibular Function

Table 21-11 describes diagnostic studies commonly used to assess vestibular function.

BRIDGE TO NCLEX EXAMINATION

The number of the question corresponds to the same-numbered outcome at the beginning of the chapter.

1. In a patient who has a hemorrhage in the posterior cavity of the eye, the nurse knows that blood is accumulating
   a. in the aqueous humor.
   b. between the lens and the retina.
   c. between the cornea and the lens.
   d. in the space between the iris and the lens.
2. Increased intraocular pressure may occur as a result of
   a. edema of the corneal stroma.
   b. dilation of the retinal arterioles.
   c. blockage of the lacrimal canals and ducts.
   d. increased production of aqueous humor by the ciliary process.

3. Question patients using eyedrops to treat their glaucoma about
   a. use of corrective lenses.
   b. their usual sleep pattern.
   c. a history of heart or lung disease.
   d. sensitivity to opioids or depressants.
4. Always assess the patient with an ophthalmic problem for
   a. visual acuity.
   b. pupillary reactions.
   c. intraocular pressure.
   d. confrontation visual fields.
5. During an assessment of hearing, the nurse would expect to find normal finding of
   a. absent cone of light.
   b. bluish purple tympanic membrane.
   c. midline tone heard equally in both ears.
   d. fluid level at hairline in the tympanum.
6. Age-related changes in the auditory system commonly include *(select all that apply)*
   a. drier cerumen.
   b. tinnitus in both ears.
   c. auditory nerve degeneration.
   d. atrophy of the tympanic membrane.
   e. greater ability to hear high-pitched sounds.
7. Before injecting fluorescein for angiography, it is important for the nurse to *(select all that apply)*
   a. obtain an emesis basin.
   b. ask if the patient is fatigued.
   c. administer a topical anesthetic.
   d. inform patient that skin may turn yellow.
   e. assess for allergies to iodine-based contrast media.

1. b, 2. d, 3. c, 4. a, 5. c, 6. a, c, d, 7. a, d

evolve

For rationales to these answers and even more NCLEX review questions, visit *http://evolve.elsevier.com/Lewis/medsurg.*

REFERENCES

1. Thibodeau G, Patton K: *Structure and function of the body,* ed 14, St Louis, 2012, Mosby.
2. *Saunders nursing drug handbook 2012,* St Louis, 2012, Saunders.
3. American Foundation for the Blind: AFB senior site. Retrieved from *www.afb.org/seniorsite.asp?SectionID=63&TopicID=286&DocumentID=3198.*
4. Goldman L, Schafer A, editors: *Goldman's Cecil medicine,* ed 24, St Louis, 2011, Saunders.
5. Rakel R, Rakel D, editors: *Textbook of family medicine,* ed 8, St Louis, 2011, Saunders.

*6. Almog Y, Nemet A: The correlation between visual acuity and color vision as an indicator of the cause of visual loss, *Am J Ophthalmol* 149:1000, 2010.

7. National Institute on Deafness and Other Communication Disorders: Quick statistics. Retrieved from *www.nided.nih.gov/health/statistics.*
8. Ko J: Presbycusis and its management, *Br J Nurs* 19:160, 2010.
9. Bope E, Kellerman R, editors: *Conn's current therapy 2012,* St Louis, 2011, Saunders.
10. Isaacson B: Hearing loss, *Med Clin North Am* 94:973, 2010.

*Evidence-based information for clinical practice.

RESOURCES

Resources for this chapter are listed after Chapter 22 on p. 413.

CHAPTER

22

The most important thing in communication is to hear what isn't being said.
Peter Drucker

Nursing Management
Visual and Auditory Problems

Mary Ann Kolis

evolve WEBSITE

http://evolve.elsevier.com/Lewis/medsurg

- NCLEX Review Questions
- Key Points
- Pre-Test
- Answer Guidelines for Case Study on p. 411
- Rationales for Bridge to NCLEX Examination Questions
- Case Study
  - Patient Undergoing Cataract Surgery
- Nursing Care Plan (Customizable)
  - eNCP 22-1: Patient After Eye Surgery
- Concept Map Creator
- Glossary
- Content Updates

eFigures

- eFig. 22-1: Refractive errors
- eFig. 22-2: Strabismus with right exotropia and fixation of the left eye

eTables

- eTable 22-1: Ocular Manifestations of Systemic Diseases
- eTable 22-2: Patient & Caregiver Teaching Guide: After Ear Surgery

LEARNING OUTCOMES

1. Compare and contrast the types of refractive errors and appropriate corrections.
2. Describe the etiology and collaborative care of extraocular disorders.
3. Explain the pathophysiology, clinical manifestations, and nursing management and collaborative care of the patient with selected intraocular disorders.
4. Discuss the nursing measures that promote the health of the eyes and ears.
5. Elaborate on the general preoperative and postoperative care of patients undergoing surgery of the eye or ear.
6. Summarize the action and uses of drug therapy for treating problems of the eyes and ears.
7. Explain the pathophysiology, clinical manifestations, and nursing and collaborative management of common ear problems.
8. Compare the causes, management, and rehabilitative potential of conductive and sensorineural hearing loss.
9. Explain the use, care, and patient teaching related to assistive devices for eye and ear problems.
10. Describe the common causes and assistive measures for uncorrectable visual impairment and deafness.
11. Describe the measures used to assist the patient in adapting psychologically to decreased vision and hearing.

KEY TERMS

acoustic neuroma, p. 406
age-related macular degeneration (AMD), p. 397
astigmatism, p. 387
benign paroxysmal positional vertigo (BPPV), p. 406
cataract, p. 393
conjunctivitis, p. 390
enucleation, p. 402
external otitis, p. 403
glaucoma, p. 398
hordeolum, p. 389
hyperopia, p. 387
keratitis, p. 391
Ménière's disease, p. 405
myopia, p. 387
otosclerosis, p. 405
presbycusis, p. 410
presbyopia, p. 387
refractive error, p. 387
retinal detachment, p. 396
retinopathy, p. 395
strabismus, p. 392

Reviewed by Sarah Smith, RN, MA, CRNO, COT, Nurse Manager, Department of Ophthalmology, University of Iowa Health Care, Oxford, Iowa; and Helen Stegall, RN, BSN, CORLN, Nurse Manager of Department of Ophthalmology, University of Iowa Hospitals and Clinics, Iowa City, Iowa.

The chapter describes visual and auditory problems, with an emphasis on their pathophysiology, clinical manifestations, collaborative care, and nursing management. Discussion of assistive devices for visual and hearing impairment is also included.

VISUAL PROBLEMS

CORRECTABLE REFRACTIVE ERRORS

The most common visual problem is refractive error. This defect prevents light rays from converging into a single focus on the retina. Defects are a result of irregularities of the corneal curvature, the focusing power of the lens, or the length of the eye. The major symptom is blurred vision. In some cases the patient may also complain of ocular discomfort, eyestrain, or headaches. The principal refractive errors of the eye can be corrected by the use of lenses in the form of eyeglasses or contact lenses, refractive surgery, or surgical implantation of an artificial lens. Contrary to popular belief, failure to correct refractive errors does not worsen the error, nor does it cause any further pathologic conditions after age 6.

Myopia (nearsightedness) is an inability to accommodate for objects at a distance. It causes light rays to be focused in front of the retina. Myopia may occur because of excessive light refraction by the cornea or lens or because of an abnormally long eye. (Refractive errors are depicted in eFig. 22-1 available on the website for this chapter.) Myopia is the most common refractive error, with approximately 25% of Americans having this disorder.

Hyperopia (farsightedness) is an inability to accommodate for near objects. It causes the light rays to focus behind the retina and requires the patient to use accommodation to focus the light rays on the retina for near objects. This type of refractive error occurs when the cornea or lens does not have adequate focusing power or when the eyeball is too short.

Presbyopia is the loss of accommodation associated with age. This condition generally appears at about age 40. As the eye ages, the lens becomes larger, firmer, and less elastic. These changes, which progress with aging, result in an inability to focus on near objects.[1]

Astigmatism is caused by an irregular corneal curvature. This irregularity causes the incoming light rays to be bent unequally. Consequently, the light rays do not come to a single point of focus on the retina. Astigmatism can occur in conjunction with any of the other refractive errors.

Aphakia is the absence of the lens. Rarely, the lens may be absent congenitally, or it may be removed during cataract surgery. A lens that is traumatically injured is removed and replaced with an intraocular lens (IOL) implant. The lens accounts for approximately 30% of ocular refractive power. The absence of the lens results in a significant refractive error. Without the focusing ability of the lens, images are projected behind the retina.

Nonsurgical Corrections

Corrective Glasses. Myopia, hyperopia, presbyopia, and astigmatism can be modified by using the appropriate corrective lenses. Glasses for presbyopia are often called "reading glasses" because they are usually worn for close work only. The presbyopic correction may also be combined with a correction for another refractive error, such as myopia or astigmatism. In these combined glasses the presbyopic correction is in the lower portion of the spectacle lens. A traditional bifocal or trifocal has visible lines. However, most lenses today that correct vision at various distances do not have visible lines. The prescription varies throughout the lens, allowing distance focusing in the top two thirds and near focus in the bottom one third of the lens.

Contact Lenses. Contact lenses are another way to correct refractive errors. Contact lenses are made from various plastic and silicone substances that are highly permeable to oxygen and have a high water content. These features allow for increased wearing time with greater comfort. If the oxygen supply to the cornea is decreased, it becomes swollen, visual acuity decreases, and the patient experiences severe discomfort.

Altered or decreased tear formation can make wearing contact lenses difficult. Tear production can be decreased by medications such as antihistamines, decongestants, diuretics, and birth control pills, as well as the hormones produced during pregnancy. Environmental factors such as wind, fans, and dust may also decrease the tear film. Allergic conjunctivitis with itching, tearing, and redness can also affect contact lens wear.

In general, you need to know whether the patient wears contact lenses, the pattern of wear (daily versus extended), and care practices. Shining a light obliquely on the eyeball can help visualize a contact lens. Contact lenses are associated with microbial keratitis, a severe sight-threatening complication. Risk factors for keratitis include poor hand cleaning, poor lens case hygiene, and inadequate lens cleaning.[2] Teach the patient the importance of following recommended cleaning practices and reporting redness, sensitivity, vision problems, and pain to the eye care professional. Instruct the patient to remove contact lenses immediately if any of these problems occur.

Surgical Therapy

Surgical procedures are designed to eliminate or reduce the need for eyeglasses or contact lenses and correct refractive errors by changing the focus of the eye. Surgical management for refractive errors includes laser surgery and IOL implantation.

Laser. *Laser-assisted in situ keratomileusis* (LASIK) may be considered for patients with low to moderately high amounts of myopia or hyperopia, with or without astigmatism. The procedure first involves using a laser or surgical blade to create a flap in the cornea. The flap is folded back on the middle section, or stroma, of the cornea.[3] Pulses from a computer-controlled laser vaporize a part of the stroma. The flap is then repositioned, adhering on its own without sutures in a few minutes.

Photorefractive keratectomy (PRK) is indicated for low to moderate amounts of myopia or hyperopia, with or without astigmatism and is a good option for a patient with insufficient corneal thickness for a LASIK flap. In PRK only the epithelium is removed, and the laser sculpts the cornea to correct the refractive error. *Laser-assisted subepithelial keratomileusis* (LASEK) is similar to PRK except that the epithelium is replaced after surgery.

Implant. *Refractive intraocular lens* (refractive IOL) implantation is an option for patients with a high degree of myopia or hyperopia. Like cataract surgery, it involves removal of the patient's natural lens and implantation of an IOL, which is a small plastic lens to correct a patient's refractive error. Since this requires entering the eye, the risk of complications is higher. New accommodating IOLs correct both myopia and presbyopia.

CULTURAL & ETHNIC HEALTH DISPARITIES
Visual and Auditory Problems

- Whites have a higher incidence of hearing impairment than African Americans or Asian Americans.
- Glaucoma has an increased incidence and severity among African Americans compared with whites.
- Hispanic Americans have an increased incidence of diabetic retinopathy.
- Native Americans have an increased incidence of otitis media when compared with whites.
- Whites have a higher incidence of macular degeneration than Hispanics, African Americans, and Asian Americans.

Phakic intraocular lenses (phakic IOLs) are sometimes referred to as implantable contact lenses. They are implanted into the eye without removing the eye's natural lens. They are used for patients with high degrees of myopia or hyperopia. Unlike refractive IOLs, the phakic IOL is placed in front of the eye's natural lens. Leaving the natural lens in the eye preserves the eye's ability to focus for reading vision. Artisan is one type of phakic IOL used for moderate to severe myopia.

UNCORRECTABLE VISUAL IMPAIRMENT

In the United States, 6.5 million people over age 65 have *severe visual impairment,* which is defined as the inability to read newsprint even with glasses.[4] Of those individuals, 9% have no useful vision, and the remaining 91% are considered partially sighted. The *partially sighted* individual may still have significant visual abilities.

A patient with visual impairment may be categorized by the level of visual loss. *Total blindness* is defined as no light perception and no usable vision. *Functional blindness* is present when the patient has some light perception but no usable vision.

The patient with either total or functional blindness is considered legally blind. *Legal blindness* refers to central visual acuity of 20/200 or less in the better eye with correction, or a peripheral visual field of 20 degrees or less. It is estimated that about 1.3 million people in the United States are legally blind. Almost all blindness in the United States is the result of common eye diseases, including cataracts, glaucoma, age-related macular degeneration, and diabetic retinopathy. Less than 4% of blindness is the result of injuries.[4]

NURSING MANAGEMENT VISUAL IMPAIRMENT

NURSING ASSESSMENT

It is important to assess how long the patient has had a visual impairment, since recent loss of vision has different implications for nursing care. Determine how the patient's visual impairment affects normal functioning. Question the patient about the level of difficulty involved in doing certain tasks. For example, ask how much difficulty the patient has when reading a newspaper, writing a check, moving from one room to the next, or viewing television. Other questions can help determine the personal meaning that the patient attaches to the visual impairment. Ask how the vision loss has affected specific aspects of the patient's life, whether the patient has lost a job, or what activities the patient does not engage in because of the visual impairment. The patient may attach many negative meanings to the impairment because of societal views of blindness. For example, the patient may view the impairment as punishment or view himself or herself as useless and burdensome. Determine the patient's primary coping strategies, the patient's emotional reactions, and the availability and strength of the patient's support systems.

PLANNING

The overall goals are that the patient with recently impaired vision or the patient with poor adjustment to long-standing visual impairment will (1) make a successful adjustment to the impairment, (2) verbalize feelings related to the loss, (3) identify personal strengths and external support systems, and (4) use appropriate coping strategies. If the patient has been functioning at an appropriate or acceptable level, the goal is to maintain the current level of function.

NURSING IMPLEMENTATION

HEALTH PROMOTION. Encourage the partially sighted patient with preventable causes of further visual impairment to seek appropriate health care. For example, the patient with vision loss from glaucoma may prevent further visual impairment by complying with prescribed therapies and suggested ophthalmic evaluations.

ACUTE INTERVENTION. Provide emotional support and direct care to the patient with recent visual impairment. Allow the patient to express anger and grief, and help the patient identify fears and successful coping strategies. The family is intimately involved in the experiences that follow vision loss. With the patient's knowledge and permission, include family members in discussions and encourage them to express their concerns.

Many people are uncomfortable around a blind or partially sighted individual because they are not sure what behaviors are appropriate. Being sensitive to the patient's feelings without being overly worried or smothering the patient's independence is vital in creating a therapeutic nursing presence. Always communicate in a normal conversational tone and manner with the patient, and address the patient, not the caregiver. Common courtesy dictates introducing oneself and any other people who approach the blind or partially sighted patient and saying goodbye on leaving. Making eye contact with the partially sighted patient accomplishes several objectives. It ensures that you are speaking while facing the patient so the patient has no difficulty hearing. Your head position validates that you are attentive to the patient. In addition, establishing eye contact ensures that you can observe the patient's facial expressions and reactions.

Assist the patient using a *sighted-guide technique*. Stand slightly in front and to one side of the patient, and offer an elbow for the patient to hold. Serve as the sighted guide, walking slightly ahead of the patient with the patient holding the back of your arm. As you walk, describe the environment to help orient the patient. For example, "We're going through an open doorway and approaching two steps down." Help the patient sit by placing one of his or her hands on the seat of the chair.

AMBULATORY AND HOME CARE. In working with the visually impaired patient, remember that a person classified as legally blind may have some useful vision. Rehabilitation after partial or total loss of vision can foster independence, self-esteem, and productivity. Know what services and devices are available for the partially sighted or blind patient, and make appropriate referrals. For the legally blind patient the primary resource for services is the state agency for rehabilitation of the blind. Legally blind individuals are eligible for federal and state assistance and income tax benefits. A list of agencies that serve the partially sighted or blind patient is available from the American Foundation for the Blind *(www.afb.org)*. Many of these agencies are listed in the resources section at the end of the chapter.

Braille or audio books for reading and a cane or guide dog for ambulation are examples of vision substitution techniques. These are usually most appropriate for the patient with no functional vision. For most patients who have some remaining vision, vision enhancement techniques can provide help in learning to ambulate, read printed material, and accomplish activities of daily living (ADLs).

Optical Devices for Vision Enhancement. A wide range of newer technologies are available to assist people with low vision.[5] These devices include desktop video magnification/closed circuit units, electronic hand-held magnifiers, text-to-speech scanners (material read aloud to you), E-readers, and computer tablets (material read aloud, magnification, image zooming, brighter screen, voice recognition). Many of these devices require some training by an assistive technology professional. Encourage patients to practice with the technologic device to ensure they can use it successfully.

Nonoptical Methods for Vision Enhancement. *Approach magnification* is a simple way to enhance the patient's residual vision. Recommend that the patient sit closer to the television or hold books closer to the eyes. Contrast enhancement techniques include watching television in black and white, using a black felt-tip marker, and using contrasting colors (e.g., a red stripe at the edge of steps or curbs). Increased lighting can be provided by halogen lamps, direct sunlight, or gooseneck lamps that can be aimed directly at the reading material or other near objects.[6] Large type is often helpful, especially in conjunction with other optical or nonoptical vision enhancements.

EVALUATION

The overall expected outcomes are that the patient with severe visual impairment will

- Have no further loss of vision
- Be able to use adaptive coping strategies
- Not experience a decrease in self-esteem or social interactions
- Function safely within her or his own environment

GERONTOLOGIC CONSIDERATIONS

VISUAL IMPAIRMENT

The older adult is at an increased risk for vision loss caused by eye disease. This older person may have other deficits, such as cognitive impairment or limited mobility, that further affect the ability to function in usual ways. Societal devaluation of the elderly may compound the self-esteem or isolation issues associated with the older patient's visual impairment. Financial resources may meet normal needs but can be inadequate to meet the increased demands of vision services or assistive devices.

The older patient may become confused or disoriented when visually compromised. The combination of decreased vision and confusion increases the risk of falls, which have potentially serious consequences for the older adult. Decreased vision may compromise the older patient's ability to function, resulting in concerns about maintaining independence and a diminished self-image. Decreased manual dexterity may make the instillation of prescribed eyedrops difficult for some older adults.

HEALTHY PEOPLE

Health Impact of Responsible Eye Care

- Regular hand washing prevents the spread of disease from one eye to the other.
- Seeking appropriate health care can lead to early detection of disease and prevent further loss of vision in patients with certain types of partial vision loss.
- Wearing sunglasses and practicing proper nutrition may help prevent cataract development and age-related macular degeneration.
- Wearing eye protection during potentially hazardous work, hobby, and sport activities reduces the risk of eye injuries.

EYE TRAUMA

Although the eyes are well protected by the bony orbit and fat pads, everyday activities can result in ocular trauma. In the United States an estimated 2.5 million eye injuries occur each year. Of those injured, more than 10% will lose useful vision in the affected eye. Table 22-1 outlines emergency management of the patient with an eye injury. The most common ocular injuries in the United States occur in the home due to gardening, power tool use, and home repair work.[7] Sport and work-related injuries are additional causes of eye trauma.

Trauma is often a preventable cause of visual impairment. Many eye injuries could be prevented by wearing protective eyewear. Your role in individual and community education is extremely important in reducing the incidence of ocular trauma.

EXTRAOCULAR DISORDERS

INFLAMMATION AND INFECTION

One of the most common conditions encountered by the ophthalmologist is inflammation or infection of the external eye. Many external irritants or microorganisms can affect the eye, conjunctiva, and avascular cornea. It is your responsibility to teach the patient appropriate interventions related to the specific disorder.

An external **hordeolum** (commonly called a *sty*) is an infection of the sebaceous glands in the lid margin (Fig. 22-1). The most common bacterial infective agent is *Staphylococcus aureus*. A red, swollen, circumscribed, and acutely tender area develops rapidly. Instruct the patient to apply warm, moist compresses at least four times a day until it improves. This may be the only treatment necessary. If it tends to recur, teach the patient to perform lid scrubs daily. In addition, appropriate antibiotic ointments or drops may be indicated.

A *chalazion* is a chronic inflammatory granuloma of the meibomian (sebaceous) glands in the lid. It may evolve from a hordeolum or occur in response to the material released into the lid when a blocked gland ruptures. The chalazion usually appears on the upper lid as a swollen, tender, reddened area that may be painful. Initial treatment is similar to that for a hordeolum. If warm, moist compresses are ineffective in promoting spontaneous drainage, the ophthalmologist may surgically remove the lesion (this is normally an office procedure) or inject the lesion with corticosteroids.

Blepharitis is a common chronic bilateral inflammation of the lid margins.[8] The lids are red rimmed with many scales or

TABLE 22-1 EMERGENCY MANAGEMENT

Eye Injury

Etiology	Assessment Findings	Interventions
Trauma • Blunt (e.g., fist) • Penetrating (e.g., glass, metal, or wood fragments. Knife, stick, or other object) **Chemical Burn** • Alkaline • Acid **Thermal Burn** • Direct burn from hot surface • Indirect burn from UV light (e.g., welding torch, looking directly at sun) **Foreign Bodies** • Glass • Metal • Wood • Plastic • Ceramics	• Pain • Photophobia • Redness—diffuse or localized • Swelling • Ecchymosis • Tearing • Blood in the anterior chamber • Absent eye movements • Fluid drainage from eye (e.g., blood, CSF, aqueous humor) • Abnormal or decreased vision • Visible foreign body • Prolapsed globe • Abnormal intraocular pressure • Visual field defect	**Initial** • Determine mechanism of injury. • Ensure airway, breathing, circulation. • Assess for other injuries. • Assess for chemical exposure. • Begin ocular irrigation *immediately* in case of chemical exposure. Do not stop until emergency personnel arrive to continue irrigation. Use sterile saline or water if saline is unavailable. • Assess visual acuity. • Do not put pressure on the eye. • Instruct patient not to blow nose. • Do not attempt to treat the injury (except as noted above for chemical exposure). • Stabilize foreign objects. • Cover the eye(s) with dry, sterile patches and a protective shield. • Do not give the patient food or fluids. • Elevate head of bed 45 degrees. • Do not put medication or solutions in the eye unless ordered by physician. • Administer analgesia as appropriate. **Ongoing Monitoring** • Reassure the patient. • Monitor pain. • Anticipate surgical repair for penetrating injury, globe rupture, or globe avulsion.

CSF, Cerebrospinal fluid; *UV*, ultraviolet.

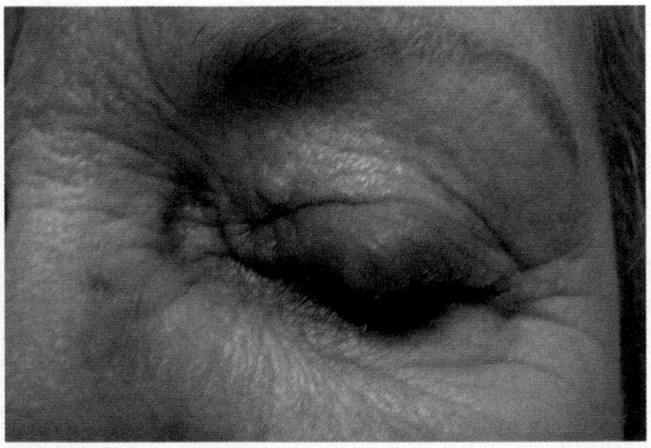

FIG. 22-1 Hordeolum (sty) on the upper eyelid caused by staphylococcal infection.

crusts on the lid margins and lashes. The patient may primarily complain of itching but may also experience burning, irritation, and photophobia. Conjunctivitis may occur simultaneously.

If the blepharitis is caused by a staphylococcal infection, collaborative care includes the use of an appropriate ophthalmic antibiotic ointment. Often blepharitis is caused by both staphylococcal and seborrheal microorganisms, and the treatment must be more vigorous to avoid hordeolum, *keratitis* (inflammation of the cornea), and other eye infections. Emphasize thorough cleaning practices of the skin and scalp. Gentle cleansing of the lid margins with baby shampoo can effectively soften and remove crusting.

Conjunctivitis

Conjunctivitis is an infection or inflammation of the conjunctiva. These infections may be caused by bacteria or viruses. Conjunctival inflammation may result from exposure to allergens or chemical irritants. The tarsal conjunctiva (lining the interior surface of the lids) may become inflamed as a result of a chronic foreign body in the eye, such as a contact lens. Careful hand washing and use of individual or disposable towels help prevent spreading the condition.

Bacterial Infections. Acute bacterial conjunctivitis *(pinkeye)* is a common infection. Although it occurs in every age-group, epidemics are common among children because of their poor hygienic habits. *S. aureus* is the most common cause. The patient with bacterial conjunctivitis may complain of discomfort, pruritus, redness, and a mucopurulent drainage.[9] Although this typically occurs initially in one eye, it generally spreads to the unaffected eye. It is usually self-limiting, but treatment with antibiotic drops (e.g., besifloxacin [Besivance]) shortens the course of the disorder.

Viral Infections. Conjunctival infections may be caused by many different viruses. The patient with viral conjunctivitis may complain of tearing, foreign body sensation, redness, and mild photophobia. This condition is usually mild and self-limiting. However, it can be severe, with increased discomfort and subconjunctival hemorrhaging. Adenovirus conjunctivitis may be contracted in contaminated swimming pools and through direct contact with an infected patient. Treatment is usually palliative. If the patient is severely symptomatic, topical corticosteroids can provide temporary relief but have no effect on the final outcome. Antiviral drops are ineffective and therefore not indicated.

Chlamydial Infections. Trachoma is a chronic conjunctivitis caused by *Chlamydia trachomatis* (serotypes A through C). It is a major cause of blindness worldwide. An estimated 84 million people have active disease in need of treatment if blindness is to be prevented, with 8 million people already living with irreversible vision loss.[10]

This preventable eye disease is transmitted mainly by the hands and by flies. Adult inclusion conjunctivitis (AIC) is caused by *C. trachomatis* (serotypes D through K). AIC is becoming more prevalent in the United States because of the increase in sexually transmitted chlamydial infection.

Manifestations of both trachoma and AIC are mucopurulent ocular discharge, irritation, redness, and lid swelling. For unknown reasons, AIC does not carry the long-term consequences of trachoma. AIC also differs from trachoma in that it is common in economically developed countries, whereas trachoma is most commonly seen in underdeveloped countries. Antibiotic therapy is usually effective for trachoma and AIC.

Although antibiotic treatment may be successful, patients with AIC have a high risk of concurrent chlamydial genital infection, as well as other sexually transmitted infections. In your teaching plan for these patients, include the sexual implications of AIC.

Allergic Conjunctivitis. Conjunctivitis caused by exposure to an allergen can be mild and transitory, or it can be severe enough to cause significant swelling, sometimes ballooning the conjunctiva beyond the eyelids. The defining symptom of allergic conjunctivitis is itching. The patient may also complain of burning, redness, and tearing. In addition to pollens, the patient may develop allergic conjunctivitis in response to animal dander, ocular solutions, and medications. Instruct the patient to avoid the allergen if it is known. Artificial tears can be effective in diluting the allergen and washing it from the eye. Effective topical medications include antihistamines and corticosteroids.

Keratitis

Keratitis is an inflammation or infection of the cornea that can be caused by a variety of microorganisms or by other factors. The condition may involve the conjunctiva and/or the cornea. When it involves both, the disorder is termed *keratoconjunctivitis.*

Bacterial Infections. The cornea can become infected by a variety of bacteria. Topical antibiotics are generally effective, but eradicating the infection may require subconjunctival antibiotic injection or, in severe cases, IV antibiotics. Risk factors include mechanical or chemical corneal epithelial damage, contact lens wear, nutritional deficiencies, immunosuppressed states, and contaminated products (e.g., lens care solutions and cases, topical medications, cosmetics).

Viral Infections. Herpes simplex virus (HSV) keratitis is the most frequently occurring infectious cause of corneal blindness in the Western hemisphere. It is a growing problem, especially with immunosuppressed patients. The corneal ulcer has a characteristic dendritic (tree-branching) appearance. Pain and photophobia are common. Up to 40% of patients with herpetic keratitis heal spontaneously.

Antiviral treatments include trifluridine drops (Viroptic), oral acyclovir (Zovirax), and topical vidarabine (Vira-A) ointment.[11] Therapy may also involve corneal debridement. Topical corticosteroids are usually contraindicated because they contribute to a longer course and possible deeper ulceration of the cornea.

The varicella-zoster virus (VZV) causes both chickenpox and herpes zoster ophthalmicus (HZO). HZO may occur by reactivation of an endogenous infection that has persisted in a latent form after an earlier attack of varicella or by contact with a patient with chickenpox or herpes zoster. It occurs most frequently in the older adult and in the immunosuppressed patient. Collaborative care of the patient with acute HZO may include analgesics for the pain, topical corticosteroids to reduce inflammation, antiviral agents such as acyclovir to reduce viral replication, mydriatic agents to dilate the pupil and relieve pain, and topical antibiotics to combat secondary infection. The patient may apply warm compresses and povidone-iodine gel to the affected skin (gel should not be applied near the eye).

Epidemic keratoconjunctivitis (EKC) is the most serious ocular adenoviral disease. EKC is spread by direct contact, including sexual activity. In the medical setting, contaminated hands and instruments can be the source of spread. The patient may complain of tearing, redness, photophobia, and foreign body sensation. In most patients the disease involves only one eye. Treatment is primarily palliative and includes ice packs and dark glasses. In severe cases therapy can include mild topical corticosteroids to temporarily relieve symptoms and topical antibiotic ointment. Teach the patient and the caregiver the importance of good hygiene practices to avoid spreading the disease.

Other Causes of Keratitis. Keratitis may also be caused by fungi (most commonly *Aspergillus, Candida,* and *Fusarium* species), especially in the case of ocular trauma in an outdoor setting where fungi are prevalent in the soil and moist organic matter.

Acanthamoeba keratitis is caused by a parasite that is associated with contact lens wear, probably as a result of contaminated lens care solutions or cases. Homemade saline solution is particularly susceptible to *Acanthamoeba* contamination. Instruct the patient who wears contact lenses about good lens care practices. Medical treatment of *Acanthamoeba* keratitis is difficult, since the organism is resistant to most drugs. Only one antifungal eyedrop (natamycin [Natacyn]) is approved by the U.S. Food and Drug Administration (FDA). If antimicrobial therapy fails, the patient may require a corneal transplant.

Exposure keratitis occurs when the patient cannot adequately close the eyelids. The patient with *exophthalmos* (protruding eyeball) from thyroid eye disease or masses posterior to the globe is susceptible to exposure keratitis.

Corneal Ulcer. Tissue loss caused by infection of the cornea produces a *corneal ulcer* (infectious keratitis) (Fig. 22-2). The infection can be due to bacteria, viruses, or fungi. Corneal ulcers are often painful, and patients may feel as if there is a foreign body in their eye. Other symptoms can include tearing, purulent or watery discharge, redness, and photophobia. Treatment is generally aggressive to avoid permanent loss of vision.

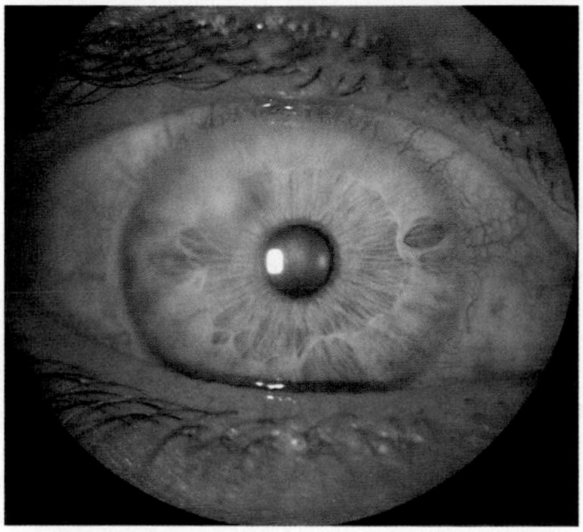

FIG. 22-2 Corneal ulcer. Infection associated with poor contact lens care.

Antibiotic, antiviral, or antifungal eyedrops may be prescribed as frequently as every hour night and day for the first 24 hours. An untreated corneal ulcer can result in corneal scarring and perforation (hole in the cornea). A corneal transplant may be indicated.

NURSING MANAGEMENT INFLAMMATION AND INFECTION

Assess ocular changes, such as edema, redness, decreased visual acuity, feelings that a foreign body is present, or discomfort. Document the findings in the patient's record. Also consider the psychosocial aspects of the patient's condition, especially when vision is impaired.

Careful asepsis and frequent, thorough hand washing are essential to prevent spreading organisms from one eye to the other, to other patients, to family members, and to health care professionals. Teach the patient and the family about avoiding sources of ocular irritation or infection and responding appropriately if an ocular problem occurs. Inform the patient about appropriate use and care of lenses and lens care products. The patient with infective disorders that may have a sexual mode of transmission needs specific information about those disorders.

Apply warm or cool compresses if indicated for the patient's condition. Darkening the room and providing an appropriate analgesic are other comfort measures. If the patient's visual acuity is decreased, modify the patient's environment or activities for safety.

The patient may require eyedrops as frequently as every hour. If the patient receives two or more different drops, stagger the eyedrops to promote maximum absorption. For example, if two different eyedrops are ordered hourly, administer one drop on the hour and one drop on the half hour (unless otherwise prescribed). The patient who needs frequent eyedrop administration may experience sleep deprivation.

The patient's primary need in the home environment is for information about required care and how to accomplish that care. Also instruct the patient and the caregiver about the proper techniques for medication administration. If the patient's vision is compromised, suggest alternative ways to accomplish necessary daily activities and self-care. Inform the patient who wears contact lenses and develops infections to discard all opened or used lens care products and cosmetics to decrease the risk of reinfection from contaminated products (a common problem and a probable source of infection for many patients).

DRY EYE DISORDERS

Keratoconjunctivitis sicca (dry eyes) is a common complaint, particularly of older adults and individuals with certain systemic diseases such as scleroderma and systemic lupus erythematosus. Patients with dry eyes complain of irritation or "sand in my eye" and that the sensation typically worsens through the day. This condition is caused by a decrease in the quality or quantity of the tear film, and treatment is directed at the underlying cause. With decreased tear secretion, the patient may use artificial tears or ointments. In severe cases, closure of the lacrimal puncta may be necessary. Patients with dry eyes associated with dry mouth may have Sjögren's syndrome (see Chapter 65).

STRABISMUS

Strabismus is a condition in which the patient cannot consistently focus two eyes simultaneously on the same object. One eye may deviate in *(esotropia)*, out *(exotropia)*, up *(hypertropia)*, or down *(hypotropia)* (see eFig. 22-2 available on the website for this chapter). Strabismus in the adult may be caused by thyroid disease, neuromuscular problems of the eye muscles, retinal detachment repair, or cerebral lesions. In the adult the primary complaint with strabismus is double vision.

CORNEAL DISORDERS

Corneal Scars and Opacities

The cornea is an optically transparent tissue that allows light rays to enter the eye and focus on the retina, thus producing a visual image. Any wound causes the cornea to become abnormally hydrated and decreases the normal transparency. The treatment for corneal scars or opacities is *penetrating keratoplasty* (corneal transplant). The ophthalmic surgeon removes the full thickness of the patient's cornea and replaces it with a donor cornea that is sutured into place (Fig. 22-3). Vision may not be restored for up to 12 months. Newer procedures in which only the damaged cornea epithelial layer is replaced are Descemet's stripping endothelial keratoplasty (DSEK) and Descemet's membrane endothelial keratoplasty (DMEK).[12] Patients report faster visual recovery with less astigmatism and changes in their glass lens prescription with these surgeries.

Approximately 40,000 corneal transplants are performed in the United States each year. The surgery is one of the fastest and safest of all tissue or organ transplant surgeries. The time between the donor's death and the removal of the tissue should be as short as possible. The eye banks test donors for human immunodeficiency virus (HIV) and hepatitis B and C. The tissue is preserved in a special nutritive solution. Improved methods of tissue procurement and preservation, postoperative topical corticosteroids, and careful follow-up have decreased graft rejection. Matching the blood type of the donor and the recipient may also improve the success rate.

Keratoconus

Keratoconus is a noninflammatory, usually bilateral disease that has a familial tendency. Keratoconus usually appears during adolescence and slowly progresses between ages 20 and 60

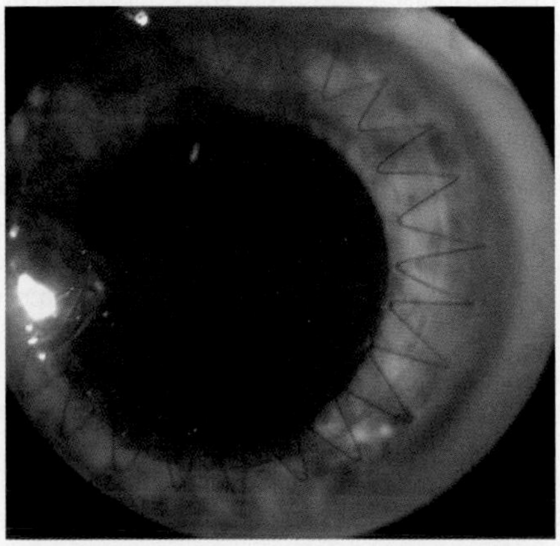

FIG. 22-3 Sutures on a donated cornea after penetrating keratoplasty (corneal transplant).

years. The anterior cornea thins and protrudes forward, taking on a cone shape. The only symptom is blurred vision. The astigmatism may be corrected with glasses or rigid contact lenses.

Intacs inserts are two clear plastic lenses surgically inserted on the cornea perimeter to reduce astigmatism and myopia. Intacs are generally used to delay the need for a corneal transplant when contact lenses or glasses no longer help a patient achieve adequate vision.

The cornea can perforate as central corneal thinning progresses. In advanced cases a penetrating keratoplasty is indicated before perforation.

INTRAOCULAR DISORDERS

CATARACT

A **cataract** is an opacity within the lens. The patient may have a cataract in one or both eyes. If cataracts are present in both eyes, one may affect the patient's vision more than the other. Almost 22 million Americans ages 40 years and older have cataracts, and by age 80 more than 50% have cataracts. Direct medical costs for cataract treatment are estimated at $6.8 billion annually. Cataract removal is the most common surgical procedure in the United States.[13]

Etiology and Pathophysiology

Although most cataracts are age related *(senile cataracts),* they can be associated with other factors. These include blunt or penetrating trauma, congenital factors such as maternal rubella, radiation or ultraviolet (UV) light exposure, certain drugs such as systemic corticosteroids or long-term topical corticosteroids, and ocular inflammation. The patient with diabetes mellitus tends to develop cataracts at a younger age.

Cataract development is mediated by a number of factors. In senile cataract formation it appears that altered metabolic processes within the lens cause an accumulation of water and alterations in the lens fiber structure. These changes affect lens transparency, causing vision changes.

Clinical Manifestations and Diagnostic Studies

The patient with cataracts may complain of a decrease in vision, abnormal color perception, and glare. Glare is due to light scatter caused by the lens opacities, and it may be significantly worse at night when the pupil dilates. The visual decline is gradual, but the rate of cataract development varies from patient to patient. Diagnosis is based on decreased visual acuity or other complaints of visual dysfunction. The opacity is directly observable by ophthalmoscopic or slit lamp microscopic examination. As noted earlier, a totally opaque lens creates the appearance of a white pupil. Table 22-2 lists other diagnostic studies that may be helpful in evaluation of a cataract.

Collaborative Care

The presence of a cataract does not necessarily indicate a need for surgery. For many patients the diagnosis is made long before they actually decide to have surgery. Nonsurgical therapy may postpone the need for surgery. Collaborative care for cataracts is presented in Table 22-2.

TABLE 22-2 COLLABORATIVE CARE

Cataract

Diagnostic / Collaborative Therapy	Acute Care: Surgical Therapy

Diagnostic
• History and physical examination
• Visual acuity measurement
• Ophthalmoscopy (direct and indirect)
• Slit lamp microscopy
• Glare testing, potential acuity testing in selected patients
• Keratometry and A-scan ultrasound (if surgery is planned)
• Other tests (e.g., visual field perimetry) to determine cause of visual loss
	Preoperative
	• Mydriatic, cycloplegic agents
	• Nonsteroidal antiinflammatory drugs
	• Topical antibiotics
	• Antianxiety medications
	Surgery
	• Removal of lens
	  • Phacoemulsification
	  • Extracapsular extraction
	• Correction of surgical aphakia
	• Intraocular lens implantation (most frequent type of correction)
	• Contact lens

Collaborative Therapy ***Nonsurgical*** • Change in glasses prescription • Strong reading glasses or magnifiers • Increased lighting • Lifestyle adjustment	***Postoperative*** • Topical antibiotic • Topical corticosteroid or other antiinflammatory agent • Mild analgesia if necessary • Eye shield and activity as preferred by patient's surgeon

Nonsurgical Therapy. Currently, no treatment is available to "cure" cataracts other than surgical removal. Often changing the patient's eyewear prescription can improve visual acuity, at least temporarily. Other visual aids, such as strong reading glasses or magnifiers of some type, may help the patient with close vision. Increasing the amount of light to read or accomplish other near-vision tasks is another useful measure. The patient may be willing to adjust his or her lifestyle to adjust to visual decline. For example, if glare makes it difficult to drive at night, a patient may elect to drive only during daylight hours or to have a family member drive at night. Sometimes informing and reassuring the patient about the disease process makes the patient comfortable about choosing nonsurgical measures, at least temporarily.

Surgical Therapy. When palliative measures no longer provide an acceptable level of visual function, the patient is an appropriate candidate for surgery. The patient's occupational needs and lifestyle changes are also factors affecting the decision to have surgery. In some instances, factors other than the patient's visual needs may influence the need for surgery. Lens-induced problems such as increased intraocular pressure (IOP) may require lens removal. Opacities may prevent the ophthalmologist from obtaining a clear view of the retina in the patient with diabetic retinopathy or other sight-threatening pathologic conditions. In those cases the cataract may be removed to allow visualization of the retina and adequate management of the problem.

Preoperative Phase. The patient's preoperative preparation should include an appropriate history and physical examination. Because almost all patients have local anesthesia, many physicians and surgical facilities do not require an extensive preoperative physical assessment. However, most patients with cataracts are older adults who may have several medical problems that should be evaluated and controlled before surgery. Almost all patients with cataracts are admitted to a surgical facility on an outpatient basis. The patient is normally admitted several hours before surgery to allow time for preoperative procedures.

The patient receives dilating drops and a nonsteroidal anti-inflammatory eyedrop to reduce inflammation. One type of drug used for dilation is a *mydriatic,* an α-adrenergic agonist that produces pupillary dilation by contraction of the iris dilator muscle. Another type of drug is a *cycloplegic,* an anticholinergic agent that produces paralysis of accommodation (cycloplegia) by blocking the effect of acetylcholine on the ciliary body muscles. Cycloplegics (tropicamide [Mydriacyl, Tropicacyl]) produce pupillary dilation (mydriasis) by blocking the effect of acetylcholine on the iris sphincter muscle. The patient often receives preoperative antianxiety medication before the local anesthesia injection.

DRUG ALERT: Cycloplegics and Mydriatics

- Instruct patient to wear dark glasses to minimize photophobia.
- Monitor for signs of systemic toxicity (e.g., tachycardia, central nervous system [CNS] effects).

Intraoperative Phase. Cataract extraction is an intraocular procedure. The anterior capsule is opened and the lens nucleus and cortex are removed, leaving the remaining capsular bag intact. In extracapsular extraction the surgeon removes the lens nucleus by *phacoemulsification,* in which the nucleus is fragmented by ultrasonic vibration and aspirated from inside the capsular bag.[14] The remaining cortex is aspirated with an irrigation and aspiration instrument. Larger incisions require closure with sutures, whereas smaller incisions are self-sealing and may require no closing suture.

Almost all patients now have an IOL implanted at the time of cataract extraction surgery (Fig. 22-4). The lens of choice is a posterior chamber lens that is implanted in the capsular bag behind the iris. At the end of the procedure, additional medications such as antibiotics and corticosteroids may be administered. Depending on the type of anesthesia, the patient's eye may be covered with a patch or protective shield, which is usually worn overnight and removed during the first postoperative visit.

Postoperative Phase. Unless complications occur, the patient is usually ready to go home as soon as the effects of sedative agents have worn off. Postoperative medications usually include antibiotic drops to prevent infection and corticosteroid drops to decrease the postoperative inflammatory response. Although postoperative activity restrictions and nighttime eye shielding are probably unnecessary, many ophthalmologists still prefer that the patient avoid activities that increase the IOP, such as bending or stooping, coughing, or lifting.

During each postoperative examination the surgeon measures the patient's visual acuity, checks anterior chamber depth, assesses corneal clarity, and measures IOP. Even on the operative day the patient's uncorrected visual acuity in the operative eye may be good. However, it is not unusual or indicative of any problem if the patient's visual acuity is reduced immediately after surgery.

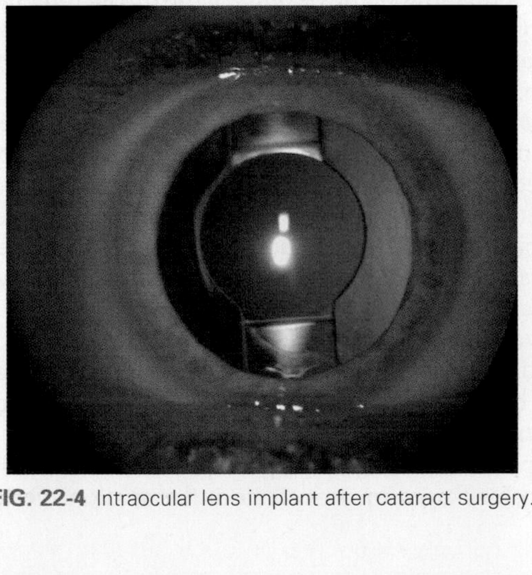

FIG. 22-4 Intraocular lens implant after cataract surgery.

The postoperative eyedrops are gradually reduced in frequency and finally discontinued when the eye has healed. When the eye is fully recovered, the patient receives a final prescription for glasses. The newest innovation is a multifocal IOL that corrects for both near and far vision. Regardless of the type of IOL used, patients may still need glasses to achieve their best visual acuity.

NURSING MANAGEMENT CATARACTS

NURSING ASSESSMENT

Assess the patient's distance and near visual acuity. If the patient is going to have surgery, especially note the visual acuity in the patient's unoperated eye. Use this information to determine how visually compromised the patient may be while the operative eye is healing. In addition, assess the psychosocial impact of the patient's visual disability and the level of knowledge regarding the disease process and therapeutic options. Postoperatively, assess the patient's level of comfort and ability to follow the postoperative regimen.

NURSING DIAGNOSES

Nursing diagnoses for the patient with a cataract include, but are not limited to, the following:

- Self-care deficits *related to* visual deficit
- Anxiety *related to* lack of knowledge about the surgical and postoperative experience

PLANNING

Preoperatively, the overall goals are that the patient with a cataract will (1) make informed decisions regarding therapeutic options and (2) experience minimal anxiety. Postoperatively, the overall goals are that the patient with a cataract will (1) understand and comply with postoperative therapy, (2) maintain an acceptable level of physical and emotional comfort, and (3) remain free of infection and other complications.

NURSING IMPLEMENTATION

HEALTH PROMOTION. There are no proven measures to prevent cataract development. However, it is probably wise (and certainly does no harm) to suggest that the patient wear sunglasses, avoid extraneous or unnecessary radiation, and maintain appropriate intake of antioxidant vitamins (e.g., vitamins C and E) and good nutrition. Also provide information about vision enhancement techniques for the patient who chooses not to have surgery.

ACUTE INTERVENTION. Preoperatively, the patient with cataracts needs accurate information about the disease process and the treatment options, especially because cataract surgery is considered an elective procedure. Be available to give the patient and the family information to help them make an informed decision about appropriate treatment. For the patient who elects to have surgery, provide information, support, and reassurance about the surgical and postoperative experience to reduce or alleviate anxiety.

TABLE 22-3 PATIENT & CAREGIVER TEACHING GUIDE

After Eye Surgery

Include the following information in the teaching plan for the patient and the caregiver after eye surgery.

- Proper hygiene and eye care techniques to ensure that medications, dressings, and/or surgical wound is not contaminated during eye care
- Signs and symptoms of infection and when and how to report these to allow for early recognition and treatment of possible infection
- Importance of complying with postoperative restrictions on head positioning, bending, coughing, and Valsalva maneuver to optimize visual outcomes and prevent increased intraocular pressure
- How to instill eye medications using aseptic techniques and adherence with prescribed eye medication routine to prevent infection
- How to monitor pain, take pain medication, and report pain not relieved by medication
- Importance of continued follow-up as recommended to maximize potential visual outcomes

Source: Lamb P, Simms-Eaton S: *Core curriculum for ophthalmic nursing*, ed 3, Dubuque, 2008, Kendall-Hunt.

Photophobia is common when administering pupil dilation medications. Therefore decreasing the room lighting is helpful. These medications produce transient stinging and burning. Table 22-3 outlines patient and caregiver teaching after eye surgery. Inform patients with a patch that they will not have depth perception until the patch is removed. This necessitates special considerations to avoid falls or other injuries. The patient with significant visual impairment in the unoperated eye requires more assistance while the operative eye is patched. Some patients may require 1 or 2 weeks for the visual acuity in the operated eye to reach an adequate level for most visual needs. These patients also need some special assistance until the vision improves.

After cataract surgery the patient usually experiences little or no pain but may have some scratchiness in the operative eye. Mild analgesics are usually sufficient to relieve any pain. If the pain is intense, the patient should notify the surgeon because this may indicate hemorrhage, infection, or increased IOP. Also instruct the patient to notify the surgeon if there is increased or purulent drainage, increased redness, or any decrease in visual acuity. A nursing care plan for the patient after eye surgery (eNursing Care Plan 22-1) is available on the website for this chapter.

AMBULATORY AND HOME CARE. Patients with cataracts who have surgery remain in the surgical facility for only a few hours. The patient and caregiver are responsible for almost all postoperative care. Give them written and verbal instructions before discharge, including information about postoperative eye care, activity restrictions, medications, follow-up visit schedule, and signs and symptoms of possible complications. Include the patient's caregiver in the instruction because some patients may have difficulty with self-care activities, especially if the vision in the unoperated eye is poor. Provide an opportunity for the patient and the caregiver to perform return demonstrations of any self-care activities.

Most patients experience little visual impairment after surgery.[15] IOL implants provide immediate visual rehabilitation, and many patients achieve a usable level of visual acuity within a few days after surgery.

A few patients may have significant visual impairment postoperatively. These include patients who do not have an IOL implanted at the time of surgery, those who require several weeks to achieve a usable level of visual acuity following surgery, or those with poor vision in their unoperated eye. For those patients the time between surgery and receiving glasses or contacts can be a period of significant visual disability. Suggest ways the patient and caregiver can modify activities and the environment to maintain an adequate level of safe functioning. Suggestions may include getting assistance with steps, removing area rugs and other potential obstacles, preparing meals for freezing before surgery, or obtaining audio books for diversion until visual acuity improves.

EVALUATION

The overall expected outcomes are that the patient following cataract surgery will

- Have improved vision
- Be better able to take care of self
- Have minimal to no pain
- Be optimistic about expected outcomes

GERONTOLOGIC CONSIDERATIONS

CATARACTS

Most patients with cataracts are older. When the older patient is visually impaired, even temporarily, the patient may experience a loss of independence, lack of control over her or his life, and a significant change in self-perception. Societal devaluation of the older individual complicates these experiences. The older patient often needs emotional support and encouragement, as well as specific suggestions to allow a maximum level of independent function. Assure the older patient that cataract surgery can be accomplished safely and comfortably with minimal sedation.

RETINOPATHY

Retinopathy is a process of microvascular damage to the retina. It can develop slowly or rapidly and lead to blurred vision and progressive vision loss. Retinopathy occurs most often in adults with diabetes mellitus or hypertension.

Diabetic retinopathy is a common complication of diabetes mellitus, especially in patients with long-standing uncontrolled diabetes. It is estimated that 40% of patients with diabetes over the age of 40 years have some evidence of retinopathy. (Diabetes is discussed in Chapter 49.) *Nonproliferative retinopathy* is the most common form of diabetic retinopathy and is characterized by capillary microaneurysms, retinal swelling, and hard exudates. Macular edema represents a worsening of the retinopathy as plasma leaks from macular blood vessels. As capillary walls weaken, they can rupture, leading to intraretinal "dot or blot" hemorrhaging (Fig. 22-5). A severe loss in central vision can result. As the disease advances, *proliferative retinopathy* may occur. New blood vessels grow, but they are abnormal, fragile, and predisposed to leak, thus causing severe vision loss. Fluorescein angiography is used to detect retinopathy, which may be treated with laser photocoagulation.[16]

Hypertensive retinopathy is caused by high blood pressure creating blockages in retinal blood vessels. (Hypertension is

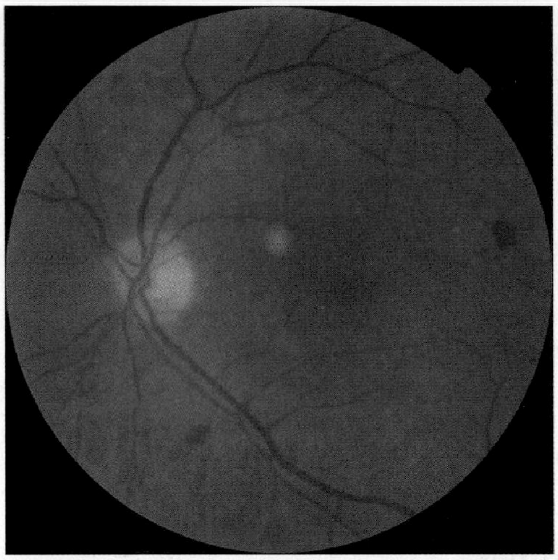

FIG. 22-5 Diabetic retinopathy. Intraretinal dot or blot hemorrhages.

discussed in Chapter 33.) These changes may not initially affect a person's vision. On a routine eye examination, retinal hemorrhages, anoxic cotton-wool spots, and macular swelling can be noted. Sustained, severe hypertension can cause sudden visual loss from swelling of the optic disc and nerve *(papilledema)*. Treatment, which may be an emergency, focuses on lowering the blood pressure. Normal vision is restored in most patients with treatment of the underlying cause of the hypertension.

RETINAL DETACHMENT

A **retinal detachment** is a separation of the sensory retina and the underlying pigment epithelium, with fluid accumulation between the two layers. The incidence of retinal detachment is approximately 1 out of every 15,000 individuals each year. In the patient with no other risk factors who has had a retinal detachment in one eye, the risk of detachment in the second eye is 2% to 25%. Almost all patients with an untreated, symptomatic retinal detachment become blind in the involved eye.

Etiology and Pathophysiology

Retinal detachment has many causes, the most common of which is a retinal break. *Retinal breaks* are an interruption in the full thickness of the retinal tissue, and they can be classified as tears or holes. *Retinal holes* are atrophic retinal breaks that occur spontaneously. *Retinal tears* can occur as the vitreous humor shrinks during aging and pulls on the retina. The retina tears when the traction force exceeds the strength of the retina. Once the retina has a break, liquid vitreous can enter the subretinal space between the sensory layer and the retinal pigment epithelium layer, causing a *rhegmatogenous* retinal detachment. Risk factors for retinal detachment are listed in Table 22-4.

Clinical Manifestations and Diagnostic Studies

Patients with a detaching retina describe symptoms that include *photopsia* (light flashes); floaters; and a "cobweb," "hairnet," or ring in the field of vision. Once the retina has detached, the patient describes a painless loss of peripheral or central vision, "like a curtain" coming across the field of vision. The area of visual loss corresponds to the area of detachment. If the detachment is small or develops slowly, the patient may not be aware of a visual problem. Visual acuity measurements should be the first diagnostic procedure with any complaint of vision loss

TABLE 22-4 RISK FACTORS FOR RETINAL DETACHMENT

- Increasing age
- Severe myopia
- Eye trauma
- Cataract surgery
- Family or personal history of retinal detachment

Source: National Eye Institute, National Institutes of Health: Retinal detachment. Retrieved from *www.nei.nih.gov/health/retinaldetach*.

TABLE 22-5 COLLABORATIVE CARE

Retinal Detachment

Diagnostic
- History and physical examination
- Visual acuity measurement
- Ophthalmoscopy (direct and indirect)
- Slit lamp microscopy
- Ultrasound if cornea, lens, or vitreous is hazy or opaque

Collaborative Therapy
Preoperative
- Mydriatic, cycloplegic agents
- Photocoagulation of retinal break that has not progressed to detachment

Surgery
- Laser photocoagulation
- Cryotherapy (cryopexy)
- Scleral buckling procedure
- Vitrectomy
- Intravitreal bubble

Postoperative
- Topical antibiotic
- Topical corticosteroid
- Analgesia
- Mydriatics
- Positioning and activity as preferred by patient's surgeon

(Table 22-5). The retinal detachment can be directly visualized using direct and indirect ophthalmoscopy or slit lamp microscopy in conjunction with a special lens to view the far periphery of the retina. Ultrasound may be useful in identifying a retinal detachment if the retina cannot be directly visualized (e.g., when the cornea, lens, or vitreous is hazy or opaque).

Collaborative Care

Some retinal breaks are not likely to progress to detachment. In these situations the ophthalmologist simply monitors the patient, giving precise information about the warning signs and symptoms of impending detachment and instructing the patient to seek immediate evaluation if any of those signs or symptoms is recognized. The ophthalmologist usually refers the patient with a detachment to a retinal specialist. Treatment objectives are to seal any retinal breaks and to relieve inward traction on the retina. Several techniques are used to accomplish these objectives.[17]

Surgical Therapy

Laser Photocoagulation and Cryopexy. These techniques seal retinal breaks by creating an inflammatory reaction that causes a chorioretinal adhesion or scar. *Laser photocoagulation* involves using an intense, precisely focused light beam to create an inflammatory reaction. The light is directed at the area of the retinal break. For retinal breaks accompanied by significant detachment, the retinal specialist may use photocoagulation intraoperatively in conjunction with scleral buckling. Tears or holes without accompanying retinal detachment may be treated prophylactically with laser photocoagulation if there is a high risk of progression to a retinal detachment. When used alone, laser therapy is an outpatient procedure that usually requires only topical anesthesia. The patient may experience minimal adverse symptoms during or after the procedure.

Another method used to seal retinal breaks is cryotherapy (also called *cryopexy*). This procedure involves using extreme cold to create the inflammatory reaction that produces the sealing scar. The ophthalmologist applies the cryoprobe instrument to the external globe in the area over the tear. This is usually done on an outpatient basis and using local anesthesia. As with photocoagulation, cryotherapy may be used alone or during scleral buckling surgery. The patient may experience significant discomfort and eye pain after cryotherapy. Encourage the patient to take the prescribed pain medication.

Scleral Buckling. *Scleral buckling* is an extraocular surgical procedure that involves indenting the globe so that the pigment epithelium, the choroid, and the sclera move toward the detached retina. The retinal surgeon sutures a silicone implant against the sclera, causing the sclera to buckle inward. The surgeon may place an encircling band over the implant if there are multiple retinal breaks, if suspected breaks cannot be located, or if there is widespread inward traction on the retina (Fig. 22-6). If present, subretinal fluid may be drained by inserting a small-gauge needle to facilitate contact between the retina and the buckled sclera. Scleral buckling is usually done with the patient under local anesthesia as an outpatient procedure.

Intraocular Procedures. In addition to the extraocular procedures described, retinal surgeons may also use one or more intraocular procedures in treating some retinal detachments. *Pneumatic retinopexy* is the intravitreal injection of a gas to form a temporary bubble in the vitreous that closes retinal breaks and provides apposition of the separated retinal layers.

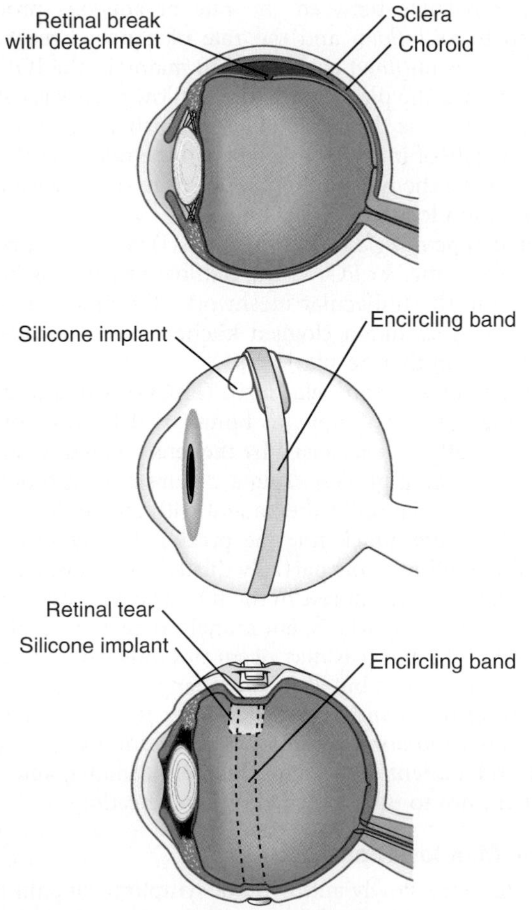

FIG. 22-6 Retinal break with detachment and surgical repair by scleral buckling technique.

Because the intravitreal bubble is temporary, this technique is combined with laser photocoagulation or cryotherapy (also called cryopexy). The patient with an intravitreal bubble must position the head so that the bubble is in contact with the retinal break. The patient may need to maintain this position as much as possible for up to several weeks.

Vitrectomy (surgical removal of the vitreous) may be used to relieve traction on the retina, especially when the traction results from proliferative diabetic retinopathy. Vitrectomy may be combined with scleral buckling to provide a dual effect in relieving traction.

Postoperative Considerations. Reattachment is successful in 90% of retinal detachments.[17] Visual prognosis varies, depending on the extent, length, and area of detachment. Postoperatively, the patient may be on bed rest and may require special positioning to maintain proper position of an intravitreal bubble. The patient may need multiple topical medications, including antibiotics, antiinflammatory agents, or dilating agents. The level of activity restriction after retinal detachment surgery varies greatly. Verify the prescribed level of activity with each patient's surgeon, and help the patient plan for any necessary assistance related to activity restrictions.

In most cases, retinal detachment is an urgent situation, and the patient is confronted suddenly with the need for surgery. The patient needs emotional support, especially during the immediate preoperative period when preparations for surgery can lead to additional anxiety. When the patient experiences postoperative pain, administer prescribed pain medications and teach the patient to take the medication as necessary after discharge. The patient may go home within a few hours of surgery or may remain in the hospital for several days, depending on the surgeon and the type of repair.

Discharge planning and teaching are important and should begin as early as possible because the patient does not remain hospitalized long. Patient and caregiver teaching after eye surgery is discussed in Table 22-5. The patient is at risk for retinal detachment in the other eye. Therefore teach the patient the signs and symptoms of retinal detachment. Also promote the use of proper protective eyewear to help avoid retinal detachments related to trauma.

AGE-RELATED MACULAR DEGENERATION

Age-related macular degeneration (AMD) is the most common cause of irreversible central vision loss in people over age 60 in the United States. AMD is divided into two forms: dry (nonexudative) and wet (exudative). People with *dry AMD,* which is the more common form (90% of all cases), often notice that close vision tasks are becoming more difficult. In this form the macular cells start to atrophy, leading to a slowly progressive and painless vision loss.

Wet AMD is the more severe form. Wet AMD accounts for 90% of the cases of AMD-related blindness. Wet AMD has a more rapid onset and is characterized by the development of abnormal blood vessels in or near the macula. Patients with wet AMD had dry AMD first.[18]

Etiology and Pathophysiology

AMD is related to retinal aging. Genetic factors also play a major role, and family history is a major risk factor for AMD. A gene responsible for some cases of AMD has been recently identified.

Long-term exposure to UV light, hyperopia, cigarette smoking, and light-colored eyes may be additional risk factors. Nutritional factors may play a role in the progression of AMD. A dietary supplement of vitamin C, vitamin E, beta-carotene, and zinc decreases the progression of advanced AMD but has no effect on people with minimal AMD or those with no evidence of AMD.[19] Eating lots of dark green, leafy vegetables containing lutein (e.g., kale and spinach) may help reduce the risk of AMD *(www.nei.nih.gov/health/maculardegen/armd_facts.asp)*.

The dry form of AMD starts with the abnormal accumulation of yellowish extracellular deposits called *drusen* in the retinal pigment epithelium. The atrophy and degeneration of macular cells then result. Wet AMD is characterized by the growth of new blood vessels from their normal location in the choroids to an abnormal location in the retinal epithelium. As the new blood vessels leak, scar tissue gradually forms. Acute vision loss may occur in some cases with bleeding from subretinal neovascular membranes.

Clinical Manifestations and Diagnostic Studies

The patient may complain of blurred and darkened vision, *scotomas* (blind spots in the visual field), and *metamorphopsia* (distortion of vision). If patients have only one eye affected, they may not notice early changes in their vision. In addition to visual acuity measurement, the primary diagnostic procedure is ophthalmoscopy. The examiner looks for drusen and other fundus changes associated with AMD. The Amsler grid test may help define the involved area, and it provides a baseline for future comparison. Fundus photography and IV angiography with fluorescein and/or indocyanine green dyes may help to further determine the extent and type of AMD.

Collaborative Care

Vision does not improve for most people with AMD. Limited treatment options for patients with wet AMD include several medications that are injected directly into the vitreous cavity. Ranibizumab (Lucentis), bevacizumab (Avastin), aflibercept (Eylea), and pegaptanib (Macugen) are selective inhibitors of endothelial growth factor, thus helping to slow vision loss in wet AMD. Side effects can include blurred vision, eye irritation, eye pain, and photosensitivity. The injections are given at 4- to 6-week intervals, depending on which drug is used. Retinal stability is determined by ocular coherence tomography (OCT). OCT allows the physician to identify fluid in the central retina that determines the need for continued intravitreal injections.

Photodynamic therapy (PDT) uses verteporfin (Visudyne) IV and a "cold" laser to excite the dye. This procedure is used in wet AMD and destroys the abnormal blood vessels without permanent damage to the retinal pigment epithelium and photoreceptor cells. Verteporfin is a photosensitizing drug that becomes active when exposed to the low-level laser light wave. Until the drug is completely excreted by the body, it can be activated by exposure to sunlight or other high-intensity light such as halogen. Therefore caution patients to avoid direct exposure to sunlight and other intense forms of light for 5 days after treatment. After receiving therapy, patients must be completely covered because any exposure of the skin to sunlight could activate the drug in that area, resulting in a thermal burn.

People at risk for developing advanced AMD should consider supplements of vitamins and minerals (in consultation with their health care provider). The cessation of smoking may also help in halting the progression of dry AMD to a more advanced stage.

Many patients with low-vision assistive devices can continue reading and retain a license to drive during the daytime and at lowered speeds. The permanent loss of central vision has significant psychosocial implications for nursing care. Management of the patient with uncorrectable visual impairment is discussed on p. 388 and is appropriate for the patient with AMD. Avoid giving the impression that "nothing can be done" about the problem when caring for the patient with AMD. Although therapy will not recover lost vision, much can be done to augment the remaining vision.

GLAUCOMA

Glaucoma is a group of disorders characterized by increased IOP and the consequences of elevated pressure, optic nerve atrophy, and peripheral visual field loss. Glaucoma is the second leading cause of permanent blindness in the United States and the leading cause of blindness among African Americans. At least 2 million people have glaucoma, and, of these, more than 50% are unaware of their condition. Another 10 million people have elevated IOP, placing them at increased risk of developing the disease. The incidence of glaucoma increases with age. Blindness from glaucoma is largely preventable with early detection and appropriate treatment. Genetic factors have been identified in some types of glaucoma.[20]

Etiology and Pathophysiology

A proper balance between the rate of aqueous production (referred to as *inflow*) and the rate of aqueous reabsorption (referred to as *outflow*) is essential to maintain the IOP within normal limits. The place where the outflow occurs is called the *angle* because it is the angle where the iris meets the cornea. When the rate of inflow is greater than the rate of outflow, IOP can rise above the normal limits. If IOP remains elevated, permanent vision loss may occur.

Primary open-angle glaucoma (POAG) is the most common type of glaucoma. In POAG the outflow of aqueous humor is decreased in the trabecular meshwork. The drainage channels become clogged, like a clogged kitchen sink. Damage to the optic nerve can then result.

Primary angle-closure glaucoma (PACG) is due to a reduction in the outflow of aqueous humor that results from angle closure. Usually this is caused by the lens bulging forward as a result of the aging process. Angle closure may also occur as a result of pupil dilation in the patient with anatomically narrow angles. An acute attack may be precipitated by situations in which the pupil remains partially dilated long enough to cause an acute and significant rise in the IOP. This may occur because of drug-induced mydriasis, emotional excitement, or darkness. Drug-induced mydriasis may occur not only from topical ophthalmic preparations but also from many systemic medications (both prescription and over-the-counter [OTC] drugs). Check drug records and documentation before administering medications to the patient with angle-closure glaucoma, and instruct the patient not to take any mydriatic medications.

Clinical Manifestations

POAG develops slowly and without symptoms of pain or pressure. The patient usually does not notice the gradual visual field loss until peripheral vision has been severely compromised.

Eventually the patient with untreated glaucoma has "tunnel vision" in which only a small center field can be seen, and all peripheral vision is absent.

Acute angle-closure glaucoma causes definite symptoms, including sudden, excruciating pain in or around the eye. This is often accompanied by nausea and vomiting. Visual symptoms include seeing colored halos around lights, blurred vision, and ocular redness.

Manifestations of subacute or chronic angle-closure glaucoma appear more gradually. The patient who has had a previous, unrecognized episode of subacute angle-closure glaucoma may report a history of blurred vision, seeing colored halos around lights, ocular redness, or eye or brow pain.

Diagnostic Studies

IOP is usually elevated in glaucoma (normal is 10 to 21 mm Hg). In the patient with elevated pressures, the ophthalmologist usually repeats the measurements over time to verify the elevation. In open-angle glaucoma, IOP is usually between 22 and 32 mm Hg. In acute angle-closure glaucoma, IOP may be over 50 mm Hg.

In open-angle glaucoma, slit lamp microscopy reveals a normal angle. In angle-closure glaucoma the examiner may note a markedly narrow or flat anterior chamber angle, an edematous cornea, a fixed and moderately dilated pupil, and ciliary injection (hyperemia of the ciliary blood vessels produces a red color).

Measures of peripheral and central vision provide other diagnostic information. Whereas central acuity may remain 20/20 even in the presence of severe peripheral visual field loss, visual field perimetry may reveal subtle changes in the peripheral retina early in the disease process, long before actual scotomas develop. In acute angle-closure glaucoma, central visual acuity is reduced if the patient has corneal edema, and the visual fields may be markedly decreased. As glaucoma progresses, *optic disc cupping* may be one of the first signs of chronic open-angle glaucoma. The optic disc becomes wider, deeper, and paler (light gray or white), which is visible with direct or indirect ophthalmoscopy (Fig. 22-7).

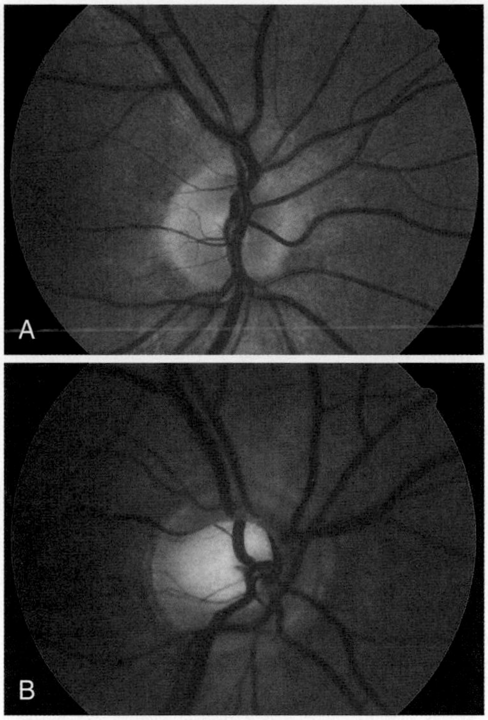

FIG. 22-7 **A,** In the normal eye the optic cup is pink with little cupping. **B,** In glaucoma the optic cup is bleached and optic cupping is present. (Note the appearance of the retinal vessels, which travel over the edge of the optic cup and appear to dip into it.)

Collaborative Care

The primary focus of glaucoma therapy is to keep the IOP low enough to prevent the patient from developing optic nerve damage. Therapy varies with the type of glaucoma. The diagnostic and collaborative care of glaucoma is summarized in Table 22-6.

TABLE 22-6 COLLABORATIVE CARE
Glaucoma

Diagnostic
- History and physical examination
- Visual acuity measurement
- Tonometry
- Ophthalmoscopy (direct and indirect)
- Slit lamp microscopy
- Gonioscopy
- Visual field perimetry

Collaborative Therapy
Chronic Open-Angle Glaucoma
Drug Therapy (see Table 22-7)
- β-Adrenergic blockers
- α-Adrenergic agonists
- Cholinergic agents (miotics)
- Carbonic anhydrase inhibitors

Surgical Therapy
- Argon laser trabeculoplasty (ALT)
- Trabeculectomy with or without filtering implant

Acute Angle-Closure Glaucoma
- Topical cholinergic agent
- Hyperosmotic agent
- Laser peripheral iridotomy
- Surgical iridectomy

Chronic Open-Angle Glaucoma

Initial treatment in chronic open-angle glaucoma is with drugs (Table 22-7). The patient must understand that continued treatment and supervision are necessary because the drugs control, but do not cure, glaucoma.

Argon laser trabeculoplasty (ALT) is a noninvasive option to lower IOP when medications are not successful or when the patient either cannot or will not use the drug therapy as recommended. ALT is an outpatient procedure that requires only topical anesthetic. The laser stimulates scarring and contraction of the trabecular meshwork, which opens the outflow channels. ALT reduces IOP approximately 75% of the time. The patient uses topical corticosteroids for 3 to 5 days after the procedure. The most common postoperative complication is an acute rise in IOP. The ophthalmologist examines the patient 1 week and again at 4 to 6 weeks after surgery.

Filtration surgery, also called a *trabeculectomy,* may be indicated if medical management and laser therapy are not successful. The success rate of this surgery is 75% to 85%.

Acute Angle-Closure Glaucoma. Acute angle-closure glaucoma is an ocular emergency that requires immediate intervention. Miotics (see Table 22-7) and oral or IV hyperosmotic agents, including glycerin liquid (Ophthalgan), isosorbide solution (Ismotic), and mannitol solution (Osmitrol), are usually successful in immediately lowering the IOP. A laser peripheral iridotomy or surgical iridectomy is necessary for long-term treatment and prevention of subsequent episodes. These procedures allow the aqueous humor to flow through a newly created opening in the iris and into normal outflow channels. One of these procedures may also be performed on the other eye as a

TABLE 22-7 DRUG THERAPY

Acute and Chronic Glaucoma

Drug	Action	Side Effects	Nursing Considerations
β-Adrenergic Blockers			
betaxolol (Betoptic)	β_1 Cardioselective blocker. ↓ IOP, ↓ aqueous humor production	Transient discomfort. Systemic reactions rarely reported but include bradycardia, heart block, pulmonary distress, headache, depression	Topical drugs. Minimal effect on pulmonary and cardiovascular parameters. Contraindicated in patient with bradycardia, cardiogenic shock, or overt cardiac failure. Systemic absorption can have additive effect with systemic β_1-blocking agents.
carteolol (Ocupress) levobunolol (Betagan) metipranolol (OptiPranolol) timolol maleate (Timoptic, Istalol)	β_1 and β_2 noncardioselective blockers. ↓ IOP, ↓ aqueous humor production	Transient ocular discomfort, blurred vision, photophobia, bradycardia, decreased BP, bronchospasm, headache, depression	Topical drops. Same as betaxolol. These noncardioselective β_2-blockers are also contraindicated in patients with asthma or COPD.
α-Adrenergic Agonists			
dipivefrin (Propine)	α- and β-adrenergic agonist. Converted to epinephrine inside the eye. ↓ aqueous humor production, enhances outflow facility	Ocular discomfort and redness, tachycardia, hypertension	Topical drops. Contraindicated in patient with narrow-angle glaucoma. Teach punctal occlusion if patient at risk of systemic reactions.
epinephrine (Epifrin, Eppy, Glaucon, Epitrate, Epinal, Eppy/N)	Same as dipivefrin	Same as dipivefrin, but can be more pronounced	Topical drops. Same as dipivefrin.
apraclonidine (Iopidine) brimonidine (Alphagan)	α-Adrenergic agonists. ↓ aqueous humor production	Ocular redness. Irregular heart rate	Topical drops. Used to control or prevent acute postlaser IOP rise (used before and immediately after ALT and iridotomy, Nd:YAG laser capsulotomy). Teach patient at risk of systemic reactions to occlude puncta.
latanoprost (Xalatan) travoprost (Travatan) bimatoprost (Lumigan)	Prostaglandin F analogs	Increased brown iris pigmentation, ocular discomfort and redness, dryness, itching, and foreign body sensation	Topical drops. Teach patient to not exceed 1 drop per evening. Have patient remove contact lens 15 min before instilling.
Cholinergic Agents (Miotics)			
carbachol (Isopto Carbachol)	Parasympathomimetic. Stimulates iris sphincter contraction, causing miosis and opening of trabecular meshwork, facilitating aqueous outflow. Also partially inhibits cholinesterase	Transient ocular discomfort, headache, blurred vision, decreased adaptation to the dark, syncope, salivation, dysrhythmias, vomiting, diarrhea, hypotension	Topical drops. Caution patient about ↓ visual acuity caused by miosis, particularly in dim light.
pilocarpine (Akarpine, Isopto Carpine, Pilocar, Pilopine-HS, Piloptic, Pilostat)	Parasympathomimetic. Stimulates iris sphincter contraction, causing miosis and opening of trabecular meshwork, facilitating aqueous humor outflow	Same as carbachol	Topical drops. Same as carbachol.
Carbonic Anhydrase Inhibitors			
Systemic			
acetazolamide (Diamox) dichlorphenamide (Daranide) methazolamide (Neptazane)	↓ Aqueous humor production	Paresthesias, especially "tingling" in extremities. Hearing dysfunction or tinnitus. Loss of appetite, taste alteration, GI disturbances. Drowsiness, confusion	Oral nonbacteriostatic sulfonamides. Anaphylaxis and other sulfa-type allergic reactions may occur in patient allergic to sulfa. Diuretic effect can ↓ electrolyte levels. Should not be given to patient on high-dose aspirin therapy.
Topical			
brinzolamide (Azopt) dorzolamide (Trusopt)	—	Transient stinging, blurred vision, redness	Same as above.

ALT, Argon laser trabeculoplasty; *IOP*, intraocular pressure.

precaution because many patients often experience an acute attack in the other eye.

DRUG ALERT: Miotics

- Warn patients about decreased visual acuity, especially in dim light.

NURSING MANAGEMENT GLAUCOMA

NURSING ASSESSMENT

Because glaucoma is a chronic condition requiring long-term management, assess the patient's ability to understand and adhere to the rationale and regimen of the prescribed therapy. In addition, assess the patient's psychologic reaction to the diagnosis of a potentially sight-threatening chronic disorder. Include the patient's caregiver in the assessment process because the chronic nature of this disorder affects the family in many ways. Some families may become the primary providers of necessary care, such as eyedrop administration, if the patient is unwilling or unable to accomplish these self-care activities.

NURSING DIAGNOSES

Nursing diagnoses for the patient with glaucoma include, but are not limited to, the following:

- Risk for injury *related to* visual acuity deficits
- Self-care deficits *related to* visual acuity deficits
- Acute pain *related to* pathophysiologic process and surgical correction
- Noncompliance *related to* the inconvenience and side effects of glaucoma medications

PLANNING

The overall goals are that the patient with glaucoma will (1) have no progression of visual impairment, (2) understand the disease process and rationale for therapy, (3) comply with all aspects of therapy (including medication administration and follow-up care), and (4) have no postoperative complications.

NURSING IMPLEMENTATION

HEALTH PROMOTION. Loss of vision as a result of glaucoma is a preventable problem. Teach the patient and the caregiver about the risk of glaucoma and that it increases with age. Stress the importance of early detection and treatment in preventing visual impairment. A comprehensive ophthalmic examination is important in identifying people with glaucoma or those at risk of developing glaucoma. The current recommendation is for an ophthalmologic examination every 2 to 4 years for people between ages 40 and 64 years, and every 1 to 2 years for people age 65 years or older. African Americans in every age category should have examinations more often because of the increased incidence and more aggressive course of glaucoma in these individuals.[21]

ACUTE INTERVENTION. Acute nursing interventions are directed primarily toward the patient with acute angle-closure glaucoma and the surgical patient. The patient with acute angle-closure glaucoma requires immediate medication to lower the IOP. It must be administered in a timely and appropriate manner according to the ophthalmologist's prescription. Most surgical procedures for glaucoma are outpatient procedures. Acutely, the patient needs postoperative instructions and may require nursing measures to relieve discomfort related to the procedure. Patient and caregiver teaching after eye surgery is discussed in Table 22-3.

AMBULATORY AND HOME CARE. Because of the chronic nature of glaucoma, remind the patient to follow the therapeutic regimen and follow-up recommendations prescribed by the ophthalmologist. Provide accurate information about the disease process and treatment options, including the rationale underlying each option. In addition, the patient needs information about the purpose, frequency, and technique for administration of antiglaucoma drugs. Encourage adherence by helping the patient identify the most convenient and appropriate times for medication administration or advocating a change in therapy if the patient reports unacceptable side effects.

EVALUATION

The overall expected outcomes are that the patient with glaucoma will

- Have no further loss of vision
- Adhere to the recommended therapy
- Safely function within own environment
- Obtain relief from pain associated with the disease and surgery

GERONTOLOGIC CONSIDERATIONS

GLAUCOMA

Many older patients with glaucoma have systemic illnesses or take systemic medications that may affect their therapy. In particular, the patient using a β-adrenergic blocking glaucoma agent may experience an additive effect if a systemic β-adrenergic blocking drug is also being taken. All β-adrenergic blocking glaucoma agents are contraindicated in the patient with bradycardia, heart block greater than first-degree heart block, cardiogenic shock, and overt cardiac failure. The noncardioselective β-adrenergic blocking glaucoma agents are also contraindicated in the patient with chronic obstructive pulmonary disease (COPD) or asthma. The hyperosmolar agents may precipitate heart failure or pulmonary edema in the susceptible patient. The older patient on high-dose aspirin therapy for rheumatoid arthritis should not take carbonic anhydrase inhibitors. The α-adrenergic agonists can cause tachycardia or hypertension, which may have serious consequences in the older patient. Teach the older patient to occlude the puncta to limit the systemic absorption of glaucoma medications.

INTRAOCULAR INFLAMMATION AND INFECTION

The term *uveitis* is used to describe inflammation of the uveal tract, retina, vitreous body, or optic nerve. This inflammation may be caused by bacteria, viruses, fungi, or parasites. *Cytomegalovirus retinitis* (CMV retinitis) is an opportunistic infection that occurs in patients with acquired immunodeficiency syndrome (AIDS) and in other immunosuppressed patients. The etiology of sterile intraocular inflammation includes autoimmune disorders, AIDS, malignancies, or those disorders associated with systemic diseases such as inflammatory bowel disease. Pain and photophobia are common symptoms.

Endophthalmitis is an extensive intraocular inflammation of the vitreous cavity. Bacteria, viruses, fungi, or parasites can all induce this serious inflammatory response. The mechanism of infection may be endogenous, in which the infecting agent arrives at the eye through the bloodstream, or exogenous, in which the infecting agent is introduced through a surgical wound or a penetrating injury. Although rare, endophthalmitis is a devastating complication of intraocular surgery or penetrating ocular injury. It can lead to irreversible blindness within hours or days. Manifestations include ocular pain, photophobia, decreased visual acuity, headaches, reddened and swollen conjunctiva, and corneal edema.

Treatment of intraocular inflammation depends on the underlying cause. Intraocular infections require antimicrobial agents, which may be delivered topically, subconjunctivally, intravitreally, systemically, or in some combination. Sterile inflammatory responses require antiinflammatory medications such as corticosteroids. The patient with intraocular inflammation is usually uncomfortable and may be noticeably anxious and frightened. Provide accurate information and emotional support to the patient and family. In severe cases, enucleation may be necessary. When the patient has lost visual function or even the entire eye, the patient will grieve the loss. Your role includes helping the patient through the grieving process.

OCULAR TUMORS

Benign and malignant tumors can occur in many areas of the eye, including the conjunctiva, retina, and orbit. Malignancies of the eyelid include basal cell and squamous cell carcinomas (see Chapter 24).

Uveal melanoma is a cancerous neoplasm of the iris, choroid, or ciliary body. It is the most common primary intraocular malignancy in adults with an incidence of 2610 new cases diagnosed annually in the United States.[22] It is more frequently found in light-skinned people over age 60 with chronic UV exposure. Genetic factors such as a mutated gene may also increase a person's risk. Uveal melanoma can arise from preexisting nevi in the eye. Tumors may be asymptomatic or associated with vision loss depending on their size and location and presence of hemorrhage and retinal detachment. As with other cancers, cancer stage and cell type are important variables in the patient's prognosis. Diagnostic testing may include ultrasonography, magnetic resonance imaging (MRI), and fine-needle aspiration biopsy. Uveal melanoma commonly appears as a dome-shaped, well-circumscribed, solid brown to golden colored pigment in the iris, choroid, or ciliary body (Fig. 22-8). Many patients do not lose their eye, and some may experience good vision after treatment in the affected eye.

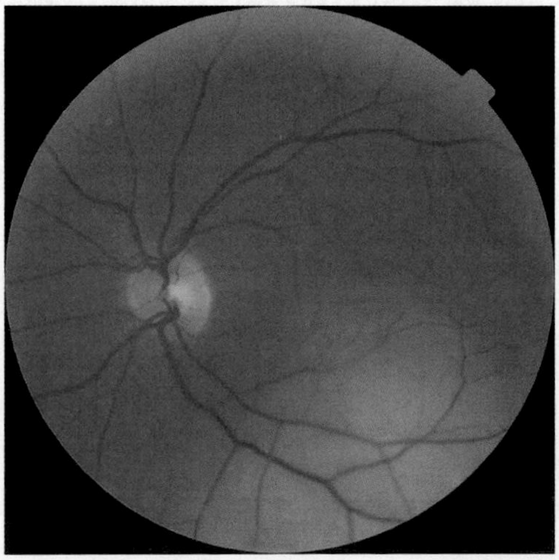

FIG. 22-8 Uveal melanoma. A large tumor in the choroid, the most common location in the eye for melanoma.

Depending on the status of the involved eye, treatment options can include enucleation, plaque radiation therapy (brachytherapy), external beam radiation, transpupillary photocoagulation, eye wall resection, and exenteration. Within 15 years, about 50% of all patients with uveal melanoma will develop metastases, with the liver the most common site.

ENUCLEATION

Enucleation is the removal of the eye. The primary indication for enucleation is a blind, painful eye. This may result from glaucoma, infection, or trauma. Enucleation may also be indicated in ocular malignancies. The surgical procedure includes severing the extraocular muscles close to their insertion on the globe, inserting an implant to maintain the intraorbital anatomy, and suturing the ends of the extraocular muscles over the implant. The conjunctiva covers the joined muscles, and a clear conformer is placed over the conjunctiva until the permanent prosthesis is fitted. A pressure dressing helps prevent postoperative bleeding.

Postoperatively, observe the patient for signs of complications, including excessive bleeding or swelling, increased pain, displacement of the implant, or temperature elevation. Patient teaching should include the instillation of topical ointments or drops and wound cleansing. Instruct the patient in the method of inserting the conformer into the socket in case it falls out. The patient is often devastated by the loss of an eye, even when enucleation occurs after a lengthy period of painful blindness. Recognize and validate the patient's emotional response and provide support to the patient and the family.

Approximately 6 weeks after surgery the wound is sufficiently healed for the permanent prosthesis. The prosthesis is fitted by an ocularist and designed to match the remaining eye. Teach the patient how to remove, cleanse, and insert the prosthesis. Special polishing is required periodically to remove dried protein secretions.

OCULAR MANIFESTATIONS OF SYSTEMIC DISEASES

Many systemic diseases have significant ocular manifestations. Ocular signs and symptoms may be the first finding or complaint in the patient with a systemic disease. One example is the patient with undiagnosed diabetes who seeks ophthalmic care for blurred vision. A careful history and examination of the patient can reveal that the underlying cause of the blurred vision is lens swelling caused by hyperglycemia. Another example is the patient who seeks care for a conjunctival lesion. The ophthalmologist may be the first health care professional to make the diagnosis of AIDS based on the presence of a conjunctival Kaposi sarcoma (KS). eTable 22-1 (available on the website for this chapter) lists some systemic diseases and disorders and the associated ophthalmic manifestations.

AUDITORY PROBLEMS

EXTERNAL EAR AND CANAL

TRAUMA

Trauma to the external ear can cause injury to the subcutaneous tissue that may result in a hematoma. If the hematoma is not aspirated, inflammation of the membranes of the ear cartilage (perichondritis) can result. Blows to the ear can also cause conductive hearing loss if the ossicles in the middle ear are damaged or the tympanic membrane (TM) is perforated. Head trauma that injures the temporal lobe of the cerebral cortex can impair the ability to understand the meaning of sounds.

EXTERNAL OTITIS

The skin of the external ear and canal is subject to the same problems as skin anywhere on the body. **External otitis** involves inflammation or infection of the epithelium of the auricle and ear canal. Swimming may alter the flora of the external canal because of chemicals and contaminated water. This can result in an infection often referred to as "swimmer's ear." Trauma from picking the ear or using sharp objects (e.g., hairpins) frequently causes the initial break in the skin. Piercing of cartilage in the upper part of the auricle also places the patient at higher risk for infection.

Infections and skin conditions may cause external otitis. Bacteria or fungi may be the cause. *Pseudomonas aeruginosa* is the most common bacterial cause. Fungi, including *Candida albicans* and *Aspergillus,* especially thrive in warm, moist climates. The warm, dark environment of the ear canal provides a good growth medium for microorganisms.

Malignant external otitis is a serious infection caused by *P. aeruginosa.* It occurs mainly in older patients with diabetes. The infection, which can spread from the external ear to the parotid gland and temporal bone (osteomyelitis), is usually treated with antibiotics.

Ear pain *(otalgia)* is one of the first signs of external otitis. Even in mild cases, the patient may experience significant discomfort with chewing, moving the auricle, or pressing on the tragus. Swelling of the ear canal can muffle hearing. There may be serosanguineous (blood-tinged fluid) or purulent (white to green thick fluid) drainage. Fever occurs when the infection spreads to surrounding tissue.

NURSING AND COLLABORATIVE MANAGEMENT EXTERNAL OTITIS

Diagnosis of external otitis is made by otoscopic examination of the ear canal. Care must be taken to avoid pain when pulling on the pinna to straighten out the canal or when inserting the otoscope speculum. The eardrum may be difficult to see due to swelling in the canal. Culture and sensitivity studies of the drainage may be done. Moist heat, mild analgesics, and topical anesthetic drops usually control the pain. Topical treatments may include antibiotics for infection and corticosteroids for inflammation. If the surrounding tissue is involved, systemic antibiotics are prescribed.[23] Improvement should occur in 48 hours, but the patient needs to adhere to the prescribed therapy for 7 to 14 days for complete resolution.

Hands should be washed before and after administration of otic drops (eardrops). The drops should be administered at room temperature. Cold drops can cause vertigo due to stimulation of the semicircular canals, and heated drops can burn the tympanum. The tip of the dropper should not touch the ear during administration to prevent contamination of the entire bottle of drops. The ear is positioned so that the drops can run into the canal. The patient should maintain this position for 2 minutes to allow the drops to spread. Sometimes the drops are placed onto a wick of cotton that is placed in the canal. Instruct the patient not to push the cotton farther into the ear. Careful handling and disposal of material saturated with drainage are important. Instruct the patient on methods to reduce the risk of external otitis (Table 22-8).

TABLE 22-8 PATIENT & CAREGIVER TEACHING GUIDE

Prevention of External Otitis

Include the following instructions when teaching the patient and caregiver.

1. Do not put anything in your ear canal unless requested by your health care provider.
2. Report itching if it becomes a problem.
3. Earwax is normal.
   - It lubricates and protects the canal.
   - Report chronic excessive cerumen if it impairs your hearing.
4. Keep your ears as dry as possible.
   - Use earplugs if you are prone to swimmer's ear.
   - Turn your head to each side for 30 seconds at a time to help water run out of the ears.
   - Do not dry with cotton-tipped applicators.
   - A hair dryer set to low and held at least 6 in from the ear can speed water evaporation.

CERUMEN AND FOREIGN BODIES IN EXTERNAL EAR CANAL

Impacted cerumen (earwax) can cause discomfort and decreased hearing. In the older person the cerumen becomes dense and drier. The hair in the ear becomes thicker and coarser, entrapping the hard, dry cerumen in the canal. Symptoms of cerumen impaction include hearing loss, otalgia, tinnitus, and vertigo.

Management involves irrigation of the canal with body-temperature solutions to soften the cerumen. Special syringes can be used and vary from a simple bulb syringe to special irrigating equipment. Place the patient in a sitting position with an emesis basin under the ear. Pull the auricle up and back, and direct the flow of solution above or below the impaction. It is important that the ear canal not be completely occluded with the syringe tip. If irrigation does not remove the wax, mild lubricant drops may be used to soften the earwax. Severe impactions may need to be removed by the health care provider.

Attempts to remove a foreign object from the ear may result in pushing it farther into the canal. Vegetable matter in the ear tends to swell and may create a secondary inflammation, making removal more difficult. Mineral oil or lidocaine drops can be used to kill an insect before removal with microscope guidance. Removal of impacted objects should be performed by the health care provider.

Ears should be cleaned with a washcloth and finger. Cotton-tipped applicators should be avoided. Penetration of the middle ear by a cotton-tipped applicator can cause serious injury to the TM and ossicles. The use of cotton-tipped applicators can also cause cerumen to become impacted against the TM and impair hearing.

MALIGNANCY OF EXTERNAL EAR

Skin cancers are the only common malignancies of the ear. Rough sandpaper-like changes to the upper border of the auricle are premalignant lesions (actinic keratoses) associated with chronic sun exposure. They are often removed with liquid nitrogen. Malignancies in the external ear canal include basal cell carcinoma in the pinna and squamous cell carcinoma in the ear canal. If left untreated, they can invade underlying tissue. Teach the patient about the dangers of sun exposure and the importance of using hats and sunscreen when outdoors.

MIDDLE EAR AND MASTOID

OTITIS MEDIA

Acute Otitis Media

Acute otitis media is an infection of the tympanum, ossicles, and space of the middle ear. Swelling of the auditory tube from colds or allergies can trap bacteria, causing a middle ear infection. Pressure from the inflammation pushes on the TM, causing it to become red, bulging, and painful. Acute otitis media is usually a childhood disease because, in children, the auditory tube that normally drains fluid and mucus from the middle ear is shorter and narrower and its position is flatter than in adults. Infection can be due to viruses or bacteria. Pain, fever, malaise, and reduced hearing are signs and symptoms of infection. Referred pain from the temporomandibular joint, teeth, gums, sinuses, or throat may also cause ear pain.

Collaborative care involves the use of antibiotics if an infection is present.[24] Surgical intervention is generally reserved for the patient who does not respond to medical treatment. A *myringotomy* involves an incision in the tympanum to release the increased pressure and exudate from the middle ear. A tympanostomy tube may be placed for short- or long-term use. Prompt treatment of an episode of acute otitis media generally prevents spontaneous perforation of the TM. If allergies are a causative factor, antihistamines may also be prescribed.

Otitis Media With Effusion

Otitis media with effusion is an inflammation of the middle ear with a collection of fluid in the middle ear space. The fluid may be thin, mucoid, or purulent. If the auditory tube does not open and allow equalization of atmospheric pressure, negative pressure within the middle ear pulls fluid from surrounding tissues. This problem commonly follows upper respiratory tract or chronic sinus infections, barotrauma (caused by pressure change), or otitis media.

Complaints include a feeling of fullness of the ear, a "plugged" feeling or popping, and decreased hearing. The patient does not experience pain, fever, or discharge from the ear. It is common to have otitis media with effusion for weeks to months after an episode of acute otitis media. It usually resolves without treatment but may recur.

Chronic Otitis Media and Mastoiditis

Repeated attacks of otitis media may lead to chronic otitis media, especially in adults who have a history of recurrent otitis in childhood. Because the mucous membrane of the middle ear is continuous with the air cells of the mastoid bone, both can be involved in the chronic infectious process.

Chronic otitis media is characterized by a purulent exudate and inflammation that can involve the ossicles, the auditory tube, and the mastoid bone. It is often painless. Hearing loss, nausea, and episodes of dizziness can occur. Hearing loss is a complication from inflammatory destruction of the ossicles, a TM perforation, or accumulation of fluid in the middle ear space. A mass of epithelial cells and cholesterol in the middle ear *(cholesteatoma)* may also develop. The cholesteatoma enlarges and can destroy the adjacent bones. Unless removed surgically, it can cause extensive damage to the ossicles and impair hearing.

Otoscopic examination of the TM may reveal changes in color and mobility or a perforation (Fig. 22-9). Culture and sensitivity tests of the drainage are necessary to identify the organisms involved so that appropriate antibiotic therapy can be prescribed. The audiogram may demonstrate a hearing loss as great as 50 to 60 dB if the ossicles have been damaged or separated. Sinus x-rays, MRI, or a computed tomography (CT) scan of the temporal bone is done to assess for bone destruction and the presence of a mass.

NURSING AND COLLABORATIVE MANAGEMENT CHRONIC OTITIS MEDIA

The aims of treatment are to clear the middle ear of infection, repair any perforations, and preserve hearing (Table 22-9). Otic and systemic (oral and IV) antibiotic therapy is started based on the culture and sensitivity results. In many cases of chronic otitis media, antibiotic resistance is present. The patient may need to undergo frequent evacuation of drainage and debris in an outpatient setting.

Often chronic TM perforations do not heal with conservative treatment, and surgery is necessary. *Tympanoplasty (myringoplasty)* involves reconstruction of the TM and/or the ossicles. A *mastoidectomy* is often performed with a tympanoplasty to

TABLE 22-9 COLLABORATIVE CARE

Chronic Otitis Media

Diagnostic	Collaborative Therapy

• History and physical examination
• Otoscopic examination
• Culture and sensitivity of middle ear drainage
• Mastoid x-ray
	• Ear irrigations
	• Otic, oral, or parenteral antibiotics
	• Analgesics
	• Antiemetics
	• Surgery
	  • Tympanoplasty (see eTable 22-2)
	  • Mastoidectomy

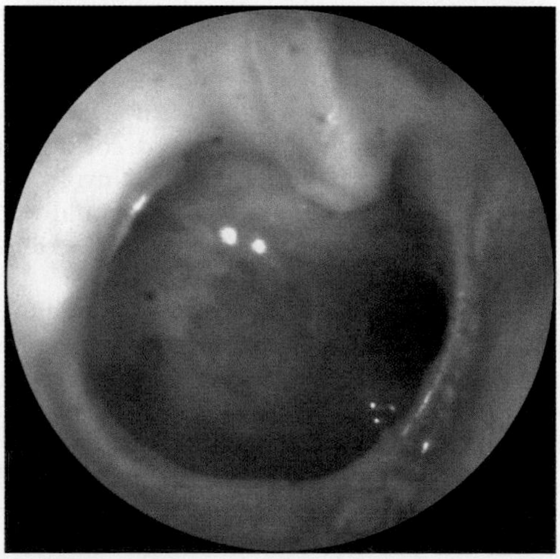

FIG. 22-9 Perforation of the tympanic membrane (TM).

remove infected portions of the mastoid bone. Removal of tissue stops at the middle ear structures that appear capable of conducting sound. Sudden pressure changes in the ear and postoperative infections can disrupt the surgical repair during the healing phase or cause facial nerve paralysis.

Impaired hearing is expected during the postoperative period if there is packing in the ear. A cotton ball dressing is used for the incision made through the external auditory canal (endaural). Instruct the patient to change the cotton packing as needed. If a postauricle (behind the ear) incision is used and a drain is in place, place a dressing over the mastoid area. A small gauze pad is cut to fit behind the ear, and soft dressing material is applied over the ear to prevent the outer circular head dressing from placing pressure on the auricle. Monitor the tightness of the dressing to prevent tissue necrosis and assess the amount and type of drainage. Keep the suture line dry. Postoperative teaching is presented in eTable 22-2, available on the website for this chapter.

OTOSCLEROSIS

Otosclerosis is a hereditary autosomal dominant disease. It is the most common cause of hearing loss in young adults.[25] Spongy bone develops from the bony labyrinth, preventing movement of the footplate of the stapes in the oval window. This reduces the transmission of vibrations to the inner ear fluids and results in conductive hearing loss. Although otosclerosis is typically bilateral, one ear may show faster progression of hearing loss. The patient is often unaware of the problem until the loss becomes so severe that communication is difficult.

Otoscopic examination may reveal a reddish blush of the tympanum (Schwartz's sign) caused by the vascular and bony changes within the middle ear. Tuning fork tests and an audiogram demonstrate good hearing by bone conduction but poor hearing by air conduction (air-bone gap). Usually a difference of at least 20 to 25 dB between air and bone conduction levels of hearing is seen in otosclerosis.

The hearing loss associated with otosclerosis may be stabilized by the oral administration of sodium fluoride with vitamin D and calcium carbonate. These medications retard bone resorption and encourage the calcification of bony lesions. Amplification of sound by a hearing aid can be effective because the inner ear function is normal.

Collaborative care of otosclerosis is shown in Table 22-10. Microdrill or laser surgical treatment involves opening the footplate (stapedotomy) or replacing the stapes with a metal or Teflon substitute (prosthesis). These procedures are usually performed with the patient under conscious sedation. The ear with poorer hearing is repaired first, and the other ear may be operated on within a year. Immediately after surgery the patient often reports a significant improvement in hearing in the operative ear. Because of the accumulation of blood and fluid in the middle ear during the postoperative period, the hearing level decreases initially, but it improves gradually with healing.

Nursing management of the patient undergoing surgery to correct otosclerosis is similar to that for the patient having a tympanoplasty. Use Gelfoam on the incision flap to limit bleeding. Place a cotton ball in the ear canal, and cover the ear with a small dressing. The patient may experience dizziness, nausea, and vomiting as a result of stimulation of the labyrinth during surgery. Some patients demonstrate nystagmus because of disturbance of the perilymph fluid. The patient should take care to avoid sudden movements that may bring on or exacerbate vertigo. Actions that increase inner ear pressure, such as coughing, sneezing, lifting, bending, and straining during bowel movements, should be avoided.

TABLE 22-10 COLLABORATIVE CARE

Otosclerosis

Diagnostic	Collaborative Therapy

• History and physical examination
• Otoscopic examination
• Rinne test
• Weber test
• Audiometry
• Tympanometry
	• Hearing aid
	• Surgery (stapedectomy or stapes prosthesis)
	• Drug therapy
	  • Sodium fluoride with vitamin D
	  • Calcium carbonate

INNER EAR PROBLEMS

Three symptoms that indicate disease of the inner ear are vertigo, sensorineural hearing loss, and tinnitus. Symptoms of vertigo arise from the vestibular labyrinth, whereas hearing loss and tinnitus arise from the auditory labyrinth. There is an overlap between manifestations of inner ear problems and CNS disorders.

MÉNIÈRE'S DISEASE

Ménière's disease (endolymphatic hydrops) is characterized by symptoms caused by inner ear disease, including episodic vertigo, tinnitus, fluctuating sensorineural hearing loss, and aural fullness. The patient experiences significant disability because of sudden, severe attacks of vertigo with nausea, vomiting, sweating, and pallor. Symptoms usually begin between 30 and 60 years of age.

The cause of the disease is unknown, but it results in an excessive accumulation of endolymph in the membranous labyrinth. The volume of endolymph increases until the membranous labyrinth ruptures. Attacks may be preceded by a sense of fullness in the ear, increasing tinnitus, and muffled hearing. The patient may experience the feeling of being pulled to the ground ("drop attacks"). Some patients report that they feel like they are whirling in space. Attacks may last hours or days and may occur several times a year. The clinical course of the disease is highly variable.

NURSING AND COLLABORATIVE MANAGEMENT MÉNIÈRE'S DISEASE

Collaborative care of Ménière's disease (Table 22-11) includes diagnostic tests to rule out other causes of the symptoms, including CNS disease. Results that suggest Ménière's disease include a mild, low-frequency sensorineural hearing loss on audiogram and abnormalities with vestibular tests. A glycerol test may aid in diagnosis. An oral dose of glycerol is given, followed by serial audiograms over 3 hours. Improvement in hearing or speech discrimination supports a diagnosis of Ménière's disease. The improvement is attributed to the osmotic effect of glycerol that pulls fluid from the inner ear.

During the acute attack, antihistamines (e.g., diphenhydramine [Benadryl]), anticholinergics (e.g., atropine), and benzodiazepines (e.g., lorazepam [Ativan]) can be used to decrease

TABLE 22-11 COLLABORATIVE CARE
Ménière's Disease

Diagnostic
- History and physical examination
- Audiometric studies (including speech discrimination, tone decay)
- Vestibular tests (including caloric test, positional test)
- Electronystagmography
- Neurologic examination
- Glycerol test

Collaborative Therapy
Acute Care
Drug Therapy (one or more)
- Sedatives
- Benzodiazepines
- Anticholinergics
- Antihistamines
- Antiemetics

Surgical Therapy
- Endolymphatic sac decompression
- Endolymphatic shunt
- Vestibular nerve section
- Labyrinthectomy

Ambulatory or Home Care
- Diuretics
- Antihistamines
- Calcium channel blockers
- Sedatives
- Hydrops diet: restriction of sodium, caffeine, nicotine, alcohol, and foods with monosodium glutamate (MSG)

the abnormal sensation and lessen nausea and vomiting. Acute vertigo is treated symptomatically with bed rest, sedation, and antiemetics (e.g., prochlorperazine [Compazine]) or antivertigo drugs (e.g., meclizine [Antivert]) for motion sickness. The patient requires reassurance and counseling that the condition is not life threatening. Management between attacks may include diuretics, antihistamines, calcium channel blockers, and a low-sodium diet. Diazepam (Valium), meclizine, and fentanyl with droperidol (Innovar) may be used to reduce the vertigo. Over time, most patients respond to the prescribed medications but must learn to live with the unpredictability of the attacks and the loss of hearing.

Frequent and incapacitating attacks are indications for surgical intervention. Decompression of the endolymphatic sac and shunting are performed to reduce the pressure on the cochlear hair cells and to prevent further damage and hearing loss. If relief is not achieved, vestibular nerve section (cutting the nerve) may be performed. When involvement is unilateral, surgical ablation of the labyrinth, resulting in loss of the vestibular and hearing cochlear function, is performed. Some patients with severe attacks of vertigo have shown improvement with the injection of gentamicin through the TM.[26] This results in inner ear damage and a reduction in endolymph production.

Plan nursing interventions to minimize vertigo and provide for patient safety. During an acute attack keep the patient in a quiet, darkened room in a comfortable position. Teach the patient to avoid sudden head movements or position changes. Fluorescent or flickering lights or a television may exacerbate symptoms and should be avoided. Make an emesis basin available because vomiting is common. To minimize the risk of falling, keep the side rails up and the bed in a low position when the patient is in bed. Instruct the patient to call for assistance when getting out of bed. Medications and fluids are administered parenterally, and intake and output are monitored. When the attack subsides, assist the patient with ambulation because unsteadiness may remain.

BENIGN PAROXYSMAL POSITIONAL VERTIGO

Benign paroxysmal positional vertigo (BPPV) is a common cause of vertigo. Approximately 50% of the cases of vertigo may be due to BPPV. In BBPV, free-floating debris in the semicircular canal causes vertigo with specific head movements, such as getting out of bed, rolling over in bed, and sitting up from lying down. The debris ("ear rocks") is composed of small crystals of calcium carbonate that derive from the utricle in the inner ear. The utricle may be injured by head trauma, infection, or degeneration from the aging process. However, for many patients a cause cannot be found.

Symptoms include nystagmus, vertigo, light-headedness, loss of balance, and nausea. There is no hearing loss, and symptoms tend to be intermittent. The symptoms of BPPV may be confused with those of Ménière's disease. Diagnosis is based on the results of auditory and vestibular tests.

Although BPPV is bothersome, it is rarely serious unless a person falls. The Epley maneuver, or canalith repositioning procedure, is effective in providing symptom relief for many patients.[27] In this maneuver the ear debris is moved from areas in the inner ear that cause symptoms and repositioned into less sensitive areas where they do not cause these problems. The Epley maneuver does not address the actual presence of debris but rather changes their location. A trained health care provider can instruct the patient in how to perform the maneuver.

ACOUSTIC NEUROMA

An **acoustic neuroma** is a unilateral benign tumor that occurs where the vestibulocochlear nerve (cranial nerve [CN] VIII) enters the internal auditory canal. Early diagnosis is important because the tumor can compress the trigeminal and facial nerves and arteries within the internal auditory canal. Symptoms usually begin between 40 and 60 years of age.

Early symptoms are associated with CN VIII compression and destruction. They include unilateral, progressive, sensorineural hearing loss; reduced touch sensation in the posterior ear canal; unilateral tinnitus; and mild, intermittent vertigo. Diagnostic tests include neurologic, audiometric, and vestibular tests; CT scans; and MRI.

Surgery to remove small tumors generally preserves hearing and vestibular function. Large tumors (larger than 3 cm) and the surgery required to remove them can leave the patient with permanent hearing loss and facial paralysis. Stereotactic radiosurgery may slow tumor growth and preserve the facial nerve. Instruct the patient to report any clear, colorless discharge from the nose. This may be cerebrospinal fluid (CSF), which increases the risk of infection. Teach the importance of follow-up care after surgery to monitor hearing and for recurrence of the tumor.

HEARING LOSS AND DEAFNESS

Hearing disorders are a common cause of disability in the United States. Nearly half of the people who need assistance with hearing disorders are 65 years of age or older. With the aging of the population, the incidence of hearing loss is increasing. Causes of hearing loss are shown in Fig. 22-10.

Types of Hearing Loss

Conductive Hearing Loss. *Conductive hearing loss* occurs when conditions in the outer or middle ear impair the transmission of sound through air to the inner ear. A common cause is otitis media with effusion. Other causes are impacted cerumen,

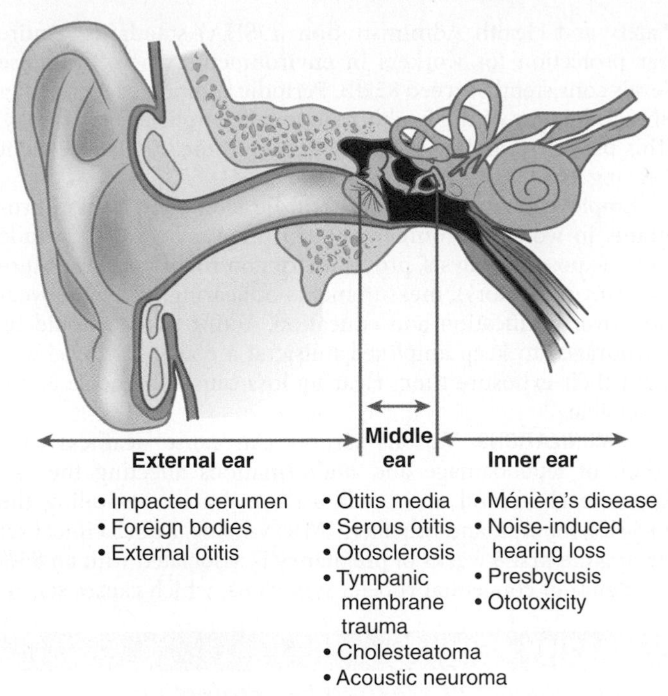

FIG. 22-10 Causes of hearing loss.

perforation of the TM, otosclerosis, and narrowing of the external auditory canal.[28]

The audiogram demonstrates better hearing through bone than through air (air-bone gap).The patient often speaks softly because hearing his or her own voice (which is conducted by bone) seems loud. This patient hears better in a noisy environment. The first step is to identify and treat the cause if possible. If correction of the cause is not possible, a hearing aid may help if the loss is greater than 40 to 50 dB.

Sensorineural Hearing Loss. *Sensorineural hearing loss* is caused by impairment of function of the inner ear or the vestibulocochlear nerve (CN VIII). Congenital and hereditary factors, noise trauma over time, aging (presbycusis), Ménière's disease, and ototoxicity can cause sensorineural hearing loss. Ototoxic drugs include aspirin, nonsteroidal antiinflammatory drugs, antibiotics (aminoglycosides, erythromycin, vancomycin), loop diuretics, and chemotherapy drugs (e.g., vincristine [Oncovin], cisplatin [Platinol]).

Systemic infections, such as Paget's disease of the bone, immune diseases, diabetes mellitus, bacterial meningitis, and trauma, are associated with this type of hearing loss. The main problems are the ability to hear sound but not to understand speech, and the lack of understanding of the problem by others. The ability to hear high-pitched sounds, including consonants, diminishes. Sounds become muffled and difficult to understand. An audiogram demonstrates a loss in decibel levels of the 4000-Hz range and eventually the 2000-Hz range. A hearing aid may help some patients, but it only makes sounds and speech louder, not clearer.

Mixed Hearing Loss. Mixed hearing loss occurs due to a combination of conductive and sensorineural causes. Careful evaluation is needed if corrective surgery for conductive loss is planned because the sensorineural component of the hearing loss will still remain.

Central and Functional Hearing Loss. Central hearing loss involves an inability to interpret sound, including speech, because of a problem in the brain (CNS). A careful history is helpful because there are usually cases of deafness in the family. Refer the patient to a qualified hearing and speech service if indicated.

Functional hearing loss may be caused by an emotional or a psychologic factor. The patient does not seem to hear or respond to pure-tone subjective hearing tests, but no physical reason for hearing loss can be identified. Psychologic counseling may help.

Classification of Hearing Loss. Hearing loss can also be classified by the decibel (dB) level or loss as recorded on the audiogram. Normal hearing is in the 0- to 15-dB range. Table 22-12 describes the levels of hearing loss.

TABLE 22-12 CLASSIFICATION OF HEARING LOSS

Decibel (dB) Loss	Meaning
0-15	Normal hearing
16-25	Slight hearing loss
26-40	Mild impairment
41-55	Moderate impairment
56-70	Moderately severe impairment
71-90	Severe impairment
>90	Profound deafness*

*Most people in this category have been deaf since birth (congenitally deaf).

Clinical Manifestations

Common early signs of hearing loss are answering questions inappropriately, not responding when not looking at the speaker, asking others to speak up, and showing irritability with others who do not speak up. Other behaviors that suggest hearing loss include straining to hear, cupping the hand around the ear, reading lips, and an increased sensitivity to slight increases in noise level. Often the patient is unaware of minimal hearing loss. Family and friends who get tired of repeating or talking loudly are often the first to notice hearing loss. Pressure exerted by significant others is a significant factor in whether the patient seeks help for hearing impairment.

Deafness is often called the "unseen handicap" because the difficulty in communication with a deaf person is not realized until you initiate a conversation with that person. You need to thoroughly validate the deaf person's understanding of health teaching. Descriptive visual aids can be helpful. If the significantly hearing-impaired individual uses sign language to communicate, the Americans with Disabilities Act[29] requires providing an interpreter when significant information is presented such as for patient consent or discharge teaching.

Interference in communication and interaction with others can be the source of many problems for the patient and caregiver. Often the patient refuses to admit or may be unaware of impaired hearing. Irritability is common because the patient must concentrate so hard to understand speech. The loss of clarity of speech in the patient with sensorineural hearing loss is most frustrating. The patient may hear what is said but not understand it. Withdrawal, suspicion, loss of self-esteem, and insecurity are commonly associated with advancing hearing loss.

Tinnitus and Hearing Loss. *Tinnitus* is the perception of *sound* in the ears where no external source is present. It is "ringing in the ears" or "head noise" (see *www.ata.org*). Tinnitus is sometimes the first symptom of hearing loss, especially in older people. It may be soft or loud, high pitched or low pitched.

Tinnitus and hearing loss are directly related. Both are caused by inner ear nerve damage. The main difference between tinnitus and hearing loss is the extent of the damage (since tinnitus can still be heard).

Although the most common cause of tinnitus is noise, it can also be a side effect of medications (see discussion on drugs causing sensorineural hearing loss on p. 407). More than 200 drugs are known to cause tinnitus.

NURSING AND COLLABORATIVE MANAGEMENT HEARING LOSS AND DEAFNESS

HEALTH PROMOTION

ENVIRONMENTAL NOISE CONTROL. Noise is the most preventable cause of hearing loss. (Fig. 22-11 lists the levels of environmental noise generated by common indoor and outdoor sounds.) Sudden severe loud noise (acoustic trauma) and chronic exposure to loud noise (noise-induced hearing loss) can damage hearing. Acoustic trauma causes hearing loss by destroying the hair cells of the organ of Corti. Sensorineural hearing loss as a result of increased and prolonged environmental noise, such as amplified sound, is occurring in young adults at an increasing rate. Amplified music (e.g., on iPods or MP3 players) should not exceed 50% of maximum volume. Ear protection should be worn when firing a gun and during other recreational pursuits with high noise levels. Health teaching regarding avoidance of continued exposure to noise levels greater than 70 dB is essential.

In work environments known to have high noise levels (more than 85 dB), ear protection should be worn. Occupational Safety and Health Administration (OSHA) standards require ear protection for workers in environments where the noise levels consistently exceed 85 dB. Periodic audiometric screening should be part of the health maintenance policies of industry. This provides baseline data on hearing to measure subsequent hearing loss.

Employees should participate in hearing conservation programs in work environments. Such programs should include noise exposure analysis, provision for control of noise exposure (hearing protectors), measurements of hearing, and employee-employer notification and education. Young adults should be encouraged to keep amplified music at a reasonable level and limit their exposure time. Hearing loss caused by noise is not reversible.

IMMUNIZATIONS. Various viruses can cause deafness as a result of fetal damage and malformations affecting the ear. Promote childhood and adult immunizations, including the measles, mumps, and rubella (MMR) vaccine. Rubella infection during the first 8 weeks of pregnancy is associated with an 85% incidence of congenital rubella syndrome, which causes senso-

HEALTHY PEOPLE

Health Impact of Wearing Ear Protection

- Ear protection should be worn during all recreational and work activities involving high noise levels.
- Ear protection can greatly reduce the damage to the ear from loud noise.
- Periodic audiometric screening is important to detect loss before it progresses.

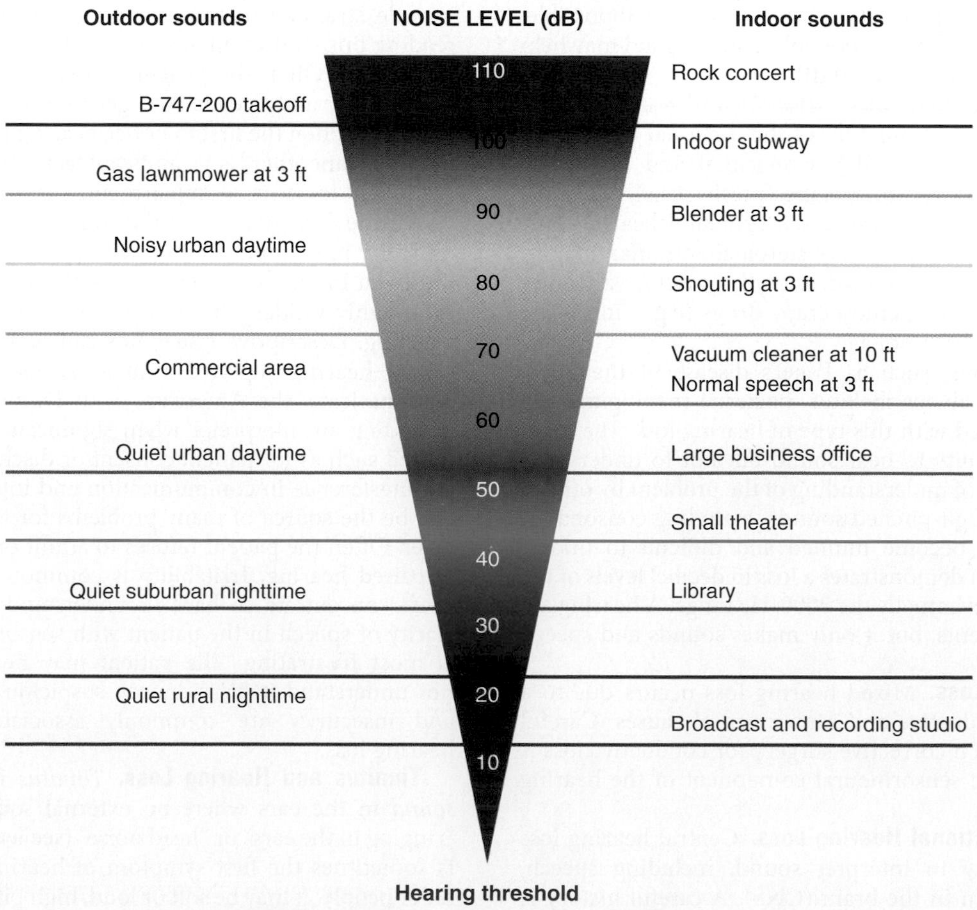

FIG. 22-11 Range of common environmental sounds.

rineural deafness. Women of childbearing age should be tested for antibodies to these viral diseases. Women should avoid pregnancy for at least 3 months after being immunized. Immunization must be delayed if the woman is pregnant. Women who are susceptible to rubella can be vaccinated safely during the postpartum period.

OTOTOXIC SUBSTANCES. Drugs commonly associated with ototoxicity include salicylates, loop diuretics, cancer chemotherapy drugs, and antibiotics.[30] Chemicals used in industry (e.g., toluene, carbon disulfide, mercury) may damage the inner ear. The patient who is receiving ototoxic drugs or is exposed to ototoxic chemicals should be monitored for signs and symptoms associated with ototoxicity, including tinnitus, diminished hearing, and changes in equilibrium. If these symptoms develop, immediate withdrawal of the drug may prevent further damage and may cause the symptoms to disappear.

ASSISTIVE DEVICES AND TECHNIQUES

HEARING AIDS. The patient with a suspected hearing loss should have a hearing assessment by a qualified audiologist. If a hearing aid is indicated, it should be fitted by an audiologist or a speech and hearing specialist. Many types of hearing aids are available, each with advantages and disadvantages (Table 22-13). The conventional hearing aid serves as a simple amplifier. For the patient with bilateral hearing impairment, binaural hearing aids provide the best sound lateralization and speech discrimination.

The goal of hearing aid therapy is improved hearing with consistent use. Patients who are motivated and optimistic about using a hearing aid are more successful users. Determine the patient's readiness for hearing aid therapy, including acknowledgment of a hearing problem, the patient's feelings about wearing a hearing aid, the degree to which the hearing loss affects life, and any difficulties the patient has manipulating small objects such as putting a battery in a hearing aid.

Initially, use of the hearing aid should be restricted to quiet situations in the home. The patient must first adjust to voices (including the patient's own voice) and household sounds. The patient should also experiment by increasing and decreasing the volume as situations require. As the patient adjusts to the increase in sounds and background noise, he or she can progress to situations where several people will be talking simultaneously. Next, the environment can be expanded to the outdoors and then the shopping mall or grocery store. Adjustment to

TABLE 22-13 TYPES OF HEARING AIDS

Type	Advantages	Disadvantages
Completely in the canal (mild to moderate hearing loss) 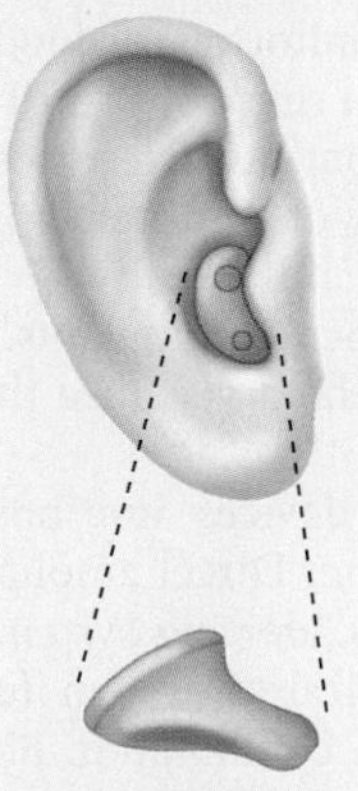	Smallest and least visible aid. Protected from sounds such as wind noise.	Costly. No space for add-ons such as directional microphones or volume controls. Small, short-lived batteries.
In the canal (mild to severe hearing loss) 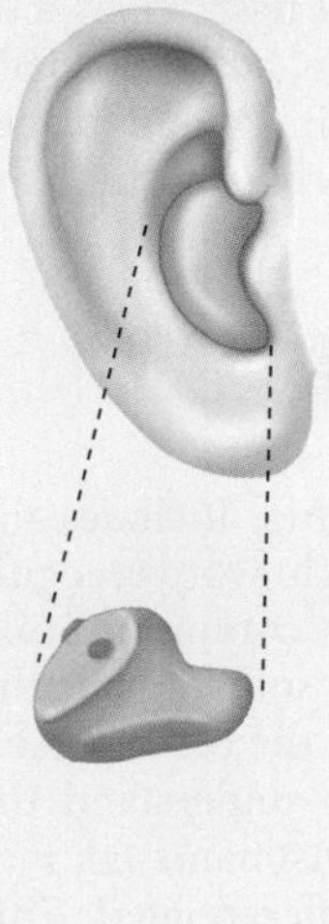	More powerful than aids completely in the canal. Has adjustable features such as noise reduction.	Small size of aid with its additional features may be difficult to operate for patients with visual loss or arthritis.
In the ear (mild to severe hearing loss) 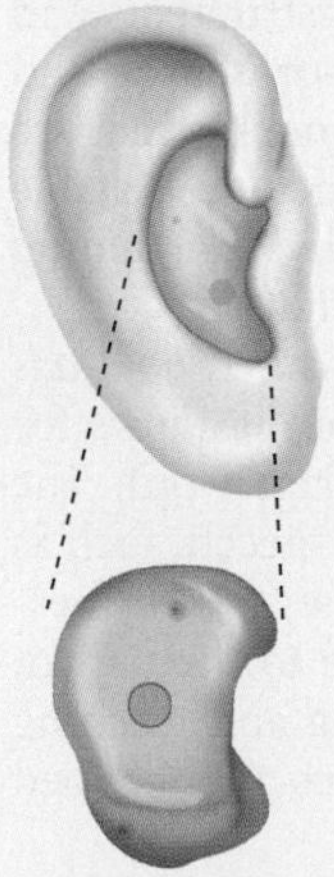	Powerful amplification. Inserts and adjusts easily. Longer-lasting batteries.	Visible. May pick up wind noise readily.
Behind the ear (all types of hearing loss) 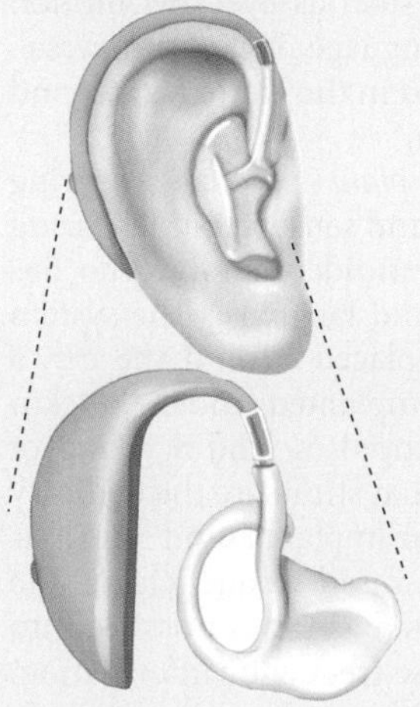	Most powerful aid. Adjusts easily. Longest battery life.	Largest, most visible aid. Newer models may be smaller and less obvious.

TABLE 22-14 COMMUNICATION WITH HEARING-IMPAIRED PATIENT

Nonverbal Aids	Verbal Aids
• Draw attention with hand movements. • Have speaker's face in good light. • Avoid covering mouth or face with hands. • Avoid chewing, eating, smoking while talking. • Maintain eye contact. • Avoid distracting environments. • Avoid careless expression that the patient may misinterpret. • Use touch. • Move close to better ear. • Avoid light behind speaker.	• Speak normally and slowly. • Do not overexaggerate facial expressions. • Do not overenunciate. • Use simple sentences. • Rephrase sentence. Use different words. • Write name or difficult words. • Do not shout. • Speak in normal voice directly into better ear.

different environments occurs gradually, depending on the individual patient.

When the hearing aid is not being worn, it should be placed in a dry, cool area where it will not be inadvertently damaged or lost. The battery should be disconnected or removed when not in use. Battery life averages 1 week, and patients should be advised to purchase only a month's supply at a time. Ear molds should be cleaned weekly or as needed. Toothpicks or pipe cleaners may be used to clear a clogged ear tip.

An implanted hearing system (i.e., Esteem) is available to treat moderate to severe sensorineural hearing loss. The system consists of external testing and programming instruments and three implantable components: a sound processor, sensor, and driver. The device does not have external components that are visible. Criteria for placement of the device include a stable bilateral sensorineural hearing loss, a normally functioning eustachian tube, and normal middle ear anatomy.

SPEECH READING. *Speech reading,* commonly called *lip reading,* can be helpful in increasing communication. It allows for approximately 40% understanding of the spoken word. The patient is able to use visual cues associated with speech, such as gestures and facial expression, to help clarify the spoken message. In speech reading, many words look alike to the patient (e.g., rabbit, woman). Help the patient by using and teaching verbal and nonverbal communication techniques as described in Table 22-14.

SIGN LANGUAGE. *Sign language* is used as a form of communication for people with profound hearing impairment. It involves gestures and facial features such as eyebrow motion and lip-mouth movements. Sign language is not universal. American Sign Language (ASL) is used in the United States and the English-speaking parts of Canada.

COCHLEAR IMPLANT. The *cochlear implant* is used as a hearing device for people with severe to profound sensorineural hearing loss in one or both ears. The ideal candidate is one who has become deaf after acquiring speech and language. The system consists of an external microphone placed behind the ear, a speech processor and a transmitter implanted under the skin that change sounds into electrical impulses, and a group of electrodes placed within the cochlea that stimulate the auditory nerves in the ear (Fig. 22-12). Cochlear implants send information that covers the entire range of sound frequencies.[31] The cochlear implant electrodes are inserted as far as possible into the cochlea to send both high- and low-frequency information.

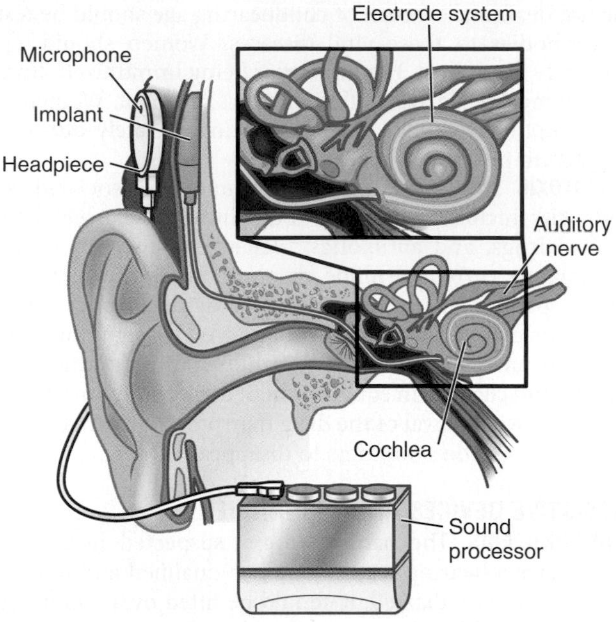

FIG. 22-12 Cochlear implant.

For patients with conductive and mixed hearing loss, the cochlear Baha system may be surgically implanted. The system works through direct bone conduction and integrates with the skull bone over time.

Extensive training and rehabilitation are essential to receive maximum benefit from these implants. The positive aspects of a cochlear implant include providing sound to the person who heard none, improving lip-reading ability, monitoring the loudness of the person's own speech, improving the sense of security, and decreasing feelings of isolation. With continued research, the cochlear implant may offer the possibility of aural rehabilitation for a wider range of hearing-impaired individuals.

The FDA has an information website on cochlear implants.[32] The website includes an animated movie to help visualize the implants and how they work.

ASSISTED LISTENING DEVICES. Numerous devices are now available to assist the hearing-impaired person. Direct amplification devices, amplified telephone receivers, alerting systems that flash when activated by sound, an infrared system for amplifying the sound of the television, and a combination FM receiver and hearing aid are all devices that you can explore based on patient needs. People with profound deafness may be assisted by text-telephone alerting systems that flash when activated by sound, closed captioning on television, and a specially trained dog. The dogs are trained to alert their owners to specific sounds within the environment, thus increasing the person's safety and independence.

GERONTOLOGIC CONSIDERATIONS

HEARING LOSS

Presbycusis, hearing loss associated with aging, includes the loss of peripheral auditory sensitivity, a decline in word recognition ability, and associated psychologic and communication issues. Because consonants (high-frequency sounds) are the letters by which spoken words are recognized, the older person with presbycusis has a diminished ability to understand the spoken word. Vowels are heard, but some consonants fall into the high-frequency range and cannot be differentiated. This may lead to confusion and embarrassment because of the difference in what was said and what was heard.

The cause of presbycusis is related to degenerative changes in the inner ear. Noise exposure is thought to be a common factor. Table 22-15 describes the classification of specific causes and associated hearing changes of presbycusis. Often a person may have more than one type of presbycusis. The prognosis for hearing depends on the cause of the loss. Sound amplification with the appropriate device is often helpful in improving the understanding of speech. In other situations an audiologic rehabilitation program can be valuable.

The older adult is often reluctant to use a hearing aid for sound amplification.[30] Reasons cited most often include cost, appearance, insufficient knowledge about hearing aids, amplification of competing noise, and unrealistic expectations. Most hearing aids and batteries are small, and neuromuscular changes such as stiff fingers, enlarged joints, and decreased sensory perception often make the care and handling of a hearing aid difficult and frustrating for an older person. Some older adults may also tend to accept their losses as part of getting older and believe there is no need for improvement.

TABLE 22-15 CLASSIFICATION OF PRESBYCUSIS

Type	Hearing Change and Prognosis
Sensory	
Atrophy of auditory nerve. Loss of sensory hair cells	Loss of high-pitched sounds. Little effect on speech understanding. Good response to sound amplification.
Neural	
Degenerative changes in cochlea and spinal ganglion	Loss of speech discrimination. Amplification alone not sufficient.
Metabolic	
Atrophy of blood vessels in wall of cochlea with interruption of essential nutrient supply	Uniform loss for all frequencies accompanied by recruitment.* Good response to hearing aid.
Cochlear	
Stiffening of basilar membrane, which interferes with sound transmission in the cochlea	Hearing loss increases from low to high frequencies. Speech discrimination affected with higher-frequency losses. Helped by appropriate forms of amplification.

*Abnormally rapid increase in loudness as sound intensity increases.

DELEGATION DECISIONS

Corrective Lenses and Hearing Aids

Role of Registered Nurse (RN)
- Assess patient vision and hearing with and without corrective devices.
- Teach patient about the use of and care for corrective lenses and hearing aids.
- Evaluate whether corrective lenses or hearing aids are effective in maintaining or improving vision or hearing.
- Evaluate for problems that may occur with contact lenses (e.g., conjunctivitis) or with hearing aids (e.g., external ear irritation).

Role of Licensed Practical/Vocational Nurse (LPN/LVN)
- Perform Snellen and/or Jaeger testing as delegated by the RN (consider state nurse practice act and agency policy).
- Monitor for adverse effects of contact lenses (e.g., redness, complaints of irritation) and report these to the RN.

Role of Unlicensed Assistive Personnel (UAP)
- Clean corrective lenses with ordered solutions.
- Help patients with hearing aid placement.
- Clean and replace batteries in hearing aids.

CASE STUDY

Glaucoma and Diabetic Retinopathy

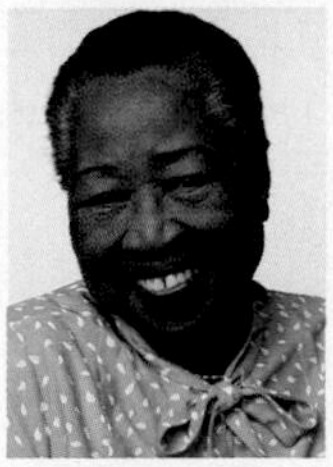
Kevin Peterson/
Stockbyte/Thinkstock

Patient Profile

J.K. is a 68-year-old African American woman who has been diagnosed with osteoarthritis and type 2 diabetes mellitus for the past 15 years. She now has diabetic retinopathy. She returns to the eye clinic with her daughter for continued care of primary open-angle glaucoma (POAG) and reexamination for changes in diabetic retinopathy. Her current medical regimen for POAG includes topical timolol maleate 0.5% extended (Timoptic-XE) once daily OU and latanoprost (Xalatan) 0.005% OU hs. At her last examination it was noted that she had microaneurysms and hard exudates of the retina.

Subjective Data
- She can no longer read the newspaper and reports that medication labels are difficult to read.
- States she is not always successful in getting the eyedrops instilled because her hands are gnarled and painful from osteoarthritis.

Objective Data
- Distant and near visual acuity are stable at 20/60 (OD) and 20/50 (OS). This is a reduction from 20/40 (OU) at her last visit.
- Intraocular pressures are stable at 20 mm Hg (OU). There is a new scotoma on visual field testing in the OS.
- Fluorescein angiography reveals diabetic macular edema OU.

Collaborative Care
- Brimonidine (Alphagan) 0.15% (OS) 15 min before and immediately after argon laser trabeculoplasty (ALT)
- Argon laser (OU) to seal leaking microaneurysms from macular edema
- Check intraocular pressure (IOP) 1 hr after ALT
- Continue previous glaucoma drop regimen
- Follow-up examination for glaucoma in 2 wk for possible ALT (OD)
- Follow-up examination for diabetic macular edema in 8 wk

Discussion Questions
1. Explain the etiology of the new scotoma.
2. Why might ALT be an appropriate therapy for J.K.?
3. What is the purpose of the eyedrops before and immediately after ALT?
4. ***Priority Decision:*** What are the priority topics that should be discussed in discharge teaching with J.K.?
5. What is the etiology of the vision loss from diabetic retinopathy?
6. ***Priority Decision:*** What are the priority nursing interventions for J.K.?
7. ***Priority Decision:*** Based on the assessment data, what are the priority nursing diagnoses? Are there any collaborative problems?
8. ***Evidence-Based Practice:*** J.K. wants to know if her glaucoma is related to her diabetes. How would you respond to her question?

evolve Answers available at *http://evolve.elsevier.com/Lewis/medsurg.*

BRIDGE TO NCLEX EXAMINATION

The number of the question corresponds to the same-numbered outcome at the beginning of the chapter.

1. Presbyopia occurs in older individuals because
   a. the eyeball elongates.
   b. the lens becomes inflexible.
   c. the corneal curvature becomes irregular.
   d. light rays are focusing in front of the retina.
2. The most important intervention for the patient with epidemic keratoconjunctivitis is
   a. cleansing the affected area with baby shampoo.
   b. monitoring spread of infection to the opposing eye.
   c. regular instillation of artificial tears to the affected eye.
   d. teaching the patient and family members good hygiene techniques.
3. Inflammation and infection of the eye
   a. are caused by irritants and microorganisms.
   b. have a higher incidence in sexually active patients.
   c. are chronic problems that result in a loss of vision.
   d. are frequently treated with cold compresses and antibiotics.
4. Which patient behaviors would the nurse promote for healthy eyes and ears *(select all that apply)*?
   a. Wearing protective sunglasses when bicycling
   b. Supplemental intake of B vitamins and magnesium
   c. Playing amplified music at 75% of maximum volume
   d. Patient notifying the health care provider of tinnitus while on antibiotics
   e. A woman avoiding pregnancy for 4 weeks after receiving measles, mumps, rubella (MMR) immunization
5. What should be included in the postoperative teaching of the patient who has undergone cataract surgery *(select all that apply)*?
   a. Eye discomfort is often relieved with mild analgesics.
   b. A decline in visual acuity is common for the first week.
   c. Stay on bed rest and limit activity for the first few days.
   d. Notify surgeon if an increase in redness or drainage occurs.
   e. Nighttime eye shielding and activity restrictions are essential to prevent eyestrain.
6. What should be included in the nursing plan for a patient who needs to administer antibiotic eardrops?
   a. Cool the drops so that they decrease swelling in the canal.
   b. Avoid placing a cotton wick to assist in administering the drops.
   c. Be careful to avoid touching the tip of the dropper bottle to the ear.
   d. Keep the head tilted 5 to 7 minutes after administration of the drops.
7. What is important for the nurse to include in the postoperative care of the patient following tympanoplasty?
   a. Check the gag reflex.
   b. Encourage independence.
   c. Avoid changing the cotton padding.
   d. Instruct patient to refrain from forceful nose blowing.
8. The patient who has a conductive hearing loss
   a. hears better in a noisy environment.
   b. hears sound but does not understand speech.
   c. often speaks loudly because his or her own voice seems low.
   d. experiences clearer sound with a hearing aid if the loss is less than 30 dB.
9. Instruct the patient who is newly fitted with bilateral hearing aids to *(select all that apply)*
   a. replace the batteries monthly.
   b. clean the ear molds weekly or as needed.
   c. clean ears with cotton-tipped applicators daily.
   d. disconnect or remove the batteries when not in use.
   e. initially restrict usage to quiet listening in the home.
10. Which strategies would best assist the nurse in communicating with a patient who has a hearing loss *(select all that apply)*?
    a. Overenunciate speech.
    b. Speak normally and slowly.
    c. Exaggerate facial expressions.
    d. Raise the voice to a higher pitch.
    e. Write out names or difficult words.
11. Patients with permanent visual impairment
    a. feel most comfortable with other visually impaired people.
    b. may feel threatened when others make eye contact during a conversation.
    c. usually need others to speak louder so they can communicate appropriately.
    d. may experience the same grieving process that is associated with other losses.

1. b, 2. d, 3. a, 4. a, d, 5. a, d, 6. c, 7. d, 8. a, 9. b, d, e, 10. b, e, 11. d

evolve

For rationales to these answers and even more NCLEX review questions, visit *http://evolve.elsevier.com/Lewis/medsurg.*

REFERENCES

1. Shagam JY: Diagnosis and treatment of ocular disorders, *Radiol Technol* 81:565, 2010.

*2. Wu Y, Carnt N, Stapleton F: Contact lens user profile, attitudes and level of compliance to lens care, *Contact Lens Anterior Eye* 33:183, 2010.

3. US Food and Drug Administration: LASIK. Retrieved from *www.fda.gov/MedicalDevices/ProductsandMedicalProcedures/SurgeryandLifeSupport/LASIK/default.htm.*

4. American Foundation for the Blind: Aging and vision fact sheet. Retrieved from *www.afb.org/seniorsite.*

5. Johns Hopkins University: New technologies brighten up low vision, *Johns Hopkins Med Lett Health After 50* 28:3, 2011.

6. American Foundation for the Blind: Maximize your lighting. Retrieved from *www.afb.org/seniorsite.asp?SectionID=66&TopicID=321&SubTopicID=206&DocumentID=4813.*

7. Boyle E: Preparedness critical to minimizing ocular trauma in emergencies, *Ocular Surgery News* 28:1, 2010.

8. Bernardes T, Bonfioli A: Blepharitis, *Semin Ophthalmol* 25:79, 2010.

9. Selby M: The red and painful eye, *Practice Nurse* 41:34, 2011.

*Evidence-based information for clinical practice.

10. World Health Organization: Trachoma and world-wide blindness. Retrieved from *www.who.int/blindness/causes/trachoma.*

*11. Wilhelmus K: Antiviral treatment and other therapeutic interventions for herpes simplex virus epithelial keratitis, *Cochrane Database Syst Rev* vol. 1, CD002898, 2010.

12. John T: Descemet's membrane endothelial keratoplasty: a useful technique for selective tissue corneal transplantation, *Ocular Surgery News* 28:4, 2010.

13. Chan E, Mahroo O, Spalton D: Complications of cataract surgery, *Clin Experiment Optometry* 93:379, 2010.

14. Mayo Clinic: Cataract surgery. Retrieved from *www.mayoclinic.com/health/cataract-surgery/MY00164/DSECTION=what-you-can-expect.*

15. National Eye Institute, National Institutes of Health: Facts about cataracts. Retrieved from *www.nei.nih.gov/health/cataract/cataract_facts.asp#5a.*

16. Bressler N, Beck R, Ferris F: Panretinal photocoagulation for proliferative diabetic retinopathy, *N Engl J Med* 365:1520, 2011.

17. Schaal S, Sherman M, Barr C, et al: Primary retinal detachment repair: comparison of 1-year outcomes of four surgical techniques, *Retina* 31:1500, 2011.

18. National Eye Institute, National Institutes of Health: Age-related macular degeneration. Retrieved from *www.nei.nih.gov/health/maculardegen/armd.*

19. Age-Related Eye Disease Study Research Group: A randomized, placebo-controlled, clinical trial of high-dose supplementation with vitamins C and E, beta-carotene, and zinc for age-related macular degeneration and vision loss, *Arch Ophthalmol* 119:1417, 2001. (Classic)

20. Khan A: Genetics of primary glaucoma, *Curr Opin Ophthalmol* 22:347, 2011.

*21. Wise L, Rosenberg L, Radin R, et al: A prospective study of diabetes, lifestyle factors, and glaucoma among African-American women, *Ann Epidemiol* 21:430, 2011.

22. American Cancer Society: Eye cancer (melanoma and lymphoma). Retrieved from *www.cancer.org/acs/groups/cid/documents/webcontent/003100-pdf.pdf.*

23. Centers for Disease Control and Prevention: Estimated burden of acute otitis externa—United States 2003-2007, *MMWR* 60:605, 2011.

*24. Ebell M: Short course of antibiotics for acute otitis media treatment, *Am Fam Physician Cochrane Briefs* 83:37, 2011.

25. Ferri F: *Ferri's clinical advisor 2012*, St Louis, 2011, Mosby.

26. Vibert D, Caversaccio M, Hausler R: Ménière's disease in the elderly, *Otolaryngol Clin North Am* 43:1041, 2010.

27. Balatsouras D: Subjective benign paroxysmal positional vertigo, *Otolaryngol Head Neck Surg* 146:98, 2012.

28. Harkin H, Kelleher C: Caring for older adults with hearing loss, *Nursing Older People* 23:9, 2011.

29. American Disabilities Act. Retrieved from *www.ada.gov/pubs/ada.htm.*

30. Laubach G: Speaking up for older patients with hearing loss, *Nursing* 40:60, 2010.

31. National Institute on Deafness and Other Communication Disorders: Cochlear implants. Retrieved from *www.nidcd.nih.gov/health/hearing/coch.asp.*

32. Cochlear implants. Retrieved from *www.fda.gov/MedicalDevices/ProductsandMedicalProcedures/ImplantsandProsthetics/CochlearImplants/default.htm.*

RESOURCES

Alexander Graham Bell Association for the Deaf and Hard of Hearing
www.agbell.org

American Academy of Audiology
www.audiology.org

American Academy of Ophthalmology
www.aao.org

American Foundation for the Blind
www.afb.org

American Society of Cataract and Refractive Surgery
www.ascrs.org

American Society of Ophthalmic Registered Nurses
www.asorn.org

Association for Education and Rehabilitation of the Blind and Visually Impaired
www.aerbvi.org

Guide Dogs for the Blind
www.guidedogs.com

Hearing Loss Association of America
www.hearingloss.org

International Hearing Dog, Inc.
www.ihdi.org

International Hearing Society
www.ihsinfo.org

Lighthouse International
http://lighthouse.org

National Association of the Deaf
www.nad.org

National Braille Association
www.nationalbraille.org

National Institute on Deafness and Other Communication Disorders, National Institutes of Health
www.nidcd.nih.gov

TDI (telecommunications for the deaf and hard of hearing)
www.tdi-online.org

CHAPTER

23

Nursing Assessment

Integumentary System

Shannon Ruff Dirksen

Nobody grows old merely by living a number of years. We grow old by deserting our ideals. Years may wrinkle the skin, but to give up enthusiasm wrinkles the soul.
Samuel Ullman

evolve WEBSITE

http://evolve.elsevier.com/Lewis/medsurg

- NCLEX Review Questions
- Key Points
- Pre-Test
- Answer Guidelines for Case Study in this chapter
- Rationales for Bridge to NCLEX Examination Questions
- Concept Map Creator
- Glossary
- Content Updates
- Videos
  - Physical Examination: Back and Posterior Chest
  - Physical Examination: Feet, Legs, and Hips
  - Physical Examination: Head and Face

LEARNING OUTCOMES

1. Describe the structures and functions of the integumentary system.
2. Link the age-related changes in the integumentary system to differences in assessment findings.
3. Select the significant subjective and objective data related to the integumentary system that should be obtained from a patient.
4. Describe specific assessments to be made during the physical examination of the skin and the appendages.
5. Compare and contrast the critical components for describing primary and secondary lesions.
6. Select appropriate techniques to use in the physical assessment of the integumentary system.
7. Specify the structural and assessment differences in light- and dark-skinned individuals.
8. Differentiate normal from common abnormal findings of a physical assessment of the integumentary system.
9. Describe the purpose, significance of results, and nursing responsibilities related to diagnostic studies of the integumentary system.

KEY TERMS

alopecia, Table 23-8, p. 422
dermis, p. 415
epidermis, p. 414
erythema, Table 23-8, p. 422
hirsutism, Table 23-8, p. 422
intertriginous, p. 419
keloid, p. 423
keratinocytes, p. 415
melanocytes, p. 414
mole (nevus), Table 23-8, p. 422
pruritus, p. 419
sebaceous glands, p. 416

The integumentary system is the largest body organ and is composed of the skin, hair, nails, and glands. The skin is further divided into two layers: the epidermis and the dermis. The subcutaneous tissue is immediately under the dermis (Fig. 23-1).

STRUCTURES AND FUNCTIONS OF SKIN AND APPENDAGES

Structures

The epidermis is the outermost layer of the skin. The dermis, the second skin layer, contains collagen bundles and supports the nerve and vascular network. The subcutaneous layer is composed primarily of fat and loose connective tissue.

Epidermis. The **epidermis,** the thin avascular superficial layer of the skin, is made up of an outer dead cornified portion that serves as a protective barrier and a deeper, living portion that folds into the dermis. Together these layers measure 0.05 to 0.1 mm in thickness. The epidermis is nourished by blood vessels in the dermis. The epidermis regenerates with new cells every 28 days. The two major types of epidermal cells are melanocytes (5%) and keratinocytes (90%).

Melanocytes are contained in the deep, basal layer (stratum germinativum) of the epidermis. They contain melanin, a pigment that gives color to the skin and hair and protects the body from damaging ultraviolet (UV) sunlight. Sunlight and hormones stimulate the melanosome (within the melanocyte) to increase the production of melanin.[1] The wide range of skin

Reviewed by Brenda C. Morris, RN, EdD, CNE, Senior Director, Baccalaureate Nursing and Clinical Associate Professor, College of Nursing and Health Innovation, Arizona State University, Phoenix, Arizona; and Rosalynde D. Peterson, RN, DNP, Nursing Instructor, Shelton State Community College, Tuscaloosa, Alabama.

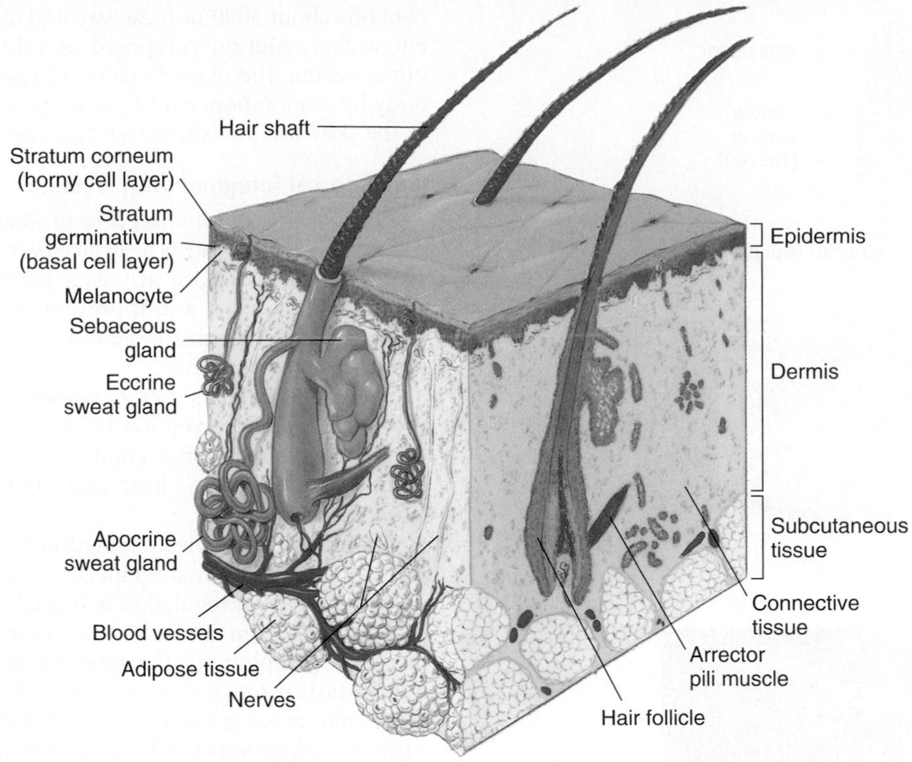

FIG. 23-1 Microscopic view of the skin in longitudinal section. From Jarvis C: *Physical examination and health assessment,* ed 6, St Louis, 2012, Saunders.

color is caused by the amount of melanin produced; more melanin results in darker skin color.[2]

Keratinocytes are synthesized from epidermal cells in the basal layer. Initially these cells are undifferentiated. As they mature (keratinize), they move to the surface, where they flatten and die to form the outer skin layer (stratum corneum). Keratinocytes produce a fibrous protein, keratin, which is vital to the skin's protective barrier function. The upward movement of keratinocytes from the basement membrane to the stratum corneum takes approximately 4 weeks. If dead cells slough off too rapidly, the skin will appear thin and eroded. If new cells form faster than old cells are shed, the skin becomes scaly and thickened. Changes in this cell cycle are reflected in many skin problems, such as psoriasis.

Dermis. The dermis is the connective tissue below the epidermis. Dermal thickness varies from 1 to 4 mm. The dermis is very vascular.

The dermis is divided into two layers, an upper thin papillary layer and a deeper, thicker reticular layer. The papillary layer is folded into ridges, or papillae, which extend into the upper epidermal layer. These exposed surface ridges form congenital patterns called fingerprints and footprints. The reticular layer contains collagen and elastic and reticular fibers.

Collagen forms the greatest part of the dermis and is responsible for the skin's mechanical strength. The primary cell type in the dermis is the *fibroblast.* Fibroblasts produce collagen and elastin fibers and are important in wound healing. Nerves, lymphatic vessels, hair follicles, and sebaceous glands are also found in the dermis.

Subcutaneous Tissue. The subcutaneous tissue lies below the dermis and is not part of the skin. The subcutaneous tissue is often discussed with the skin because it attaches the skin to underlying tissues such as muscle and bone. The subcutaneous tissue contains loose connective tissue and fat cells that provide insulation. The anatomic distribution of subcutaneous tissue varies according to gender, heredity, age, and nutritional status. This layer also stores lipids, regulates temperature, and provides shock absorption.

Skin Appendages. Appendages of the skin include the hair, nails, and glands (sebaceous, apocrine, and eccrine). These structures develop from the epidermal layer and receive nutrients, electrolytes, and fluids from the dermis. Hair and nails form from specialized keratin that becomes hardened.

Hair grows on most of the body except for the lips, the palms of the hands, and the soles of the feet.[3] The color of the hair is a result of heredity and is determined by the type and amount of melanin in the hair shaft. Hair grows approximately 1 cm per month. On average 100 hairs are lost each day. The rate of growth is not affected by cutting.[2] When lost hair is not replaced, baldness results. The absence of hair may be related to disease, treatment, or heredity.

Nails grow from the matrix. The nail matrix is located at the proximal area of the nail plate. The matrix is commonly called the *lunula,* which is the white crescent-shaped area visible through the nail plate (Fig. 23-2). The nail bed that is under the nail matrix and nail plate is normally pink and contains blood vessels. The nail plate adheres to and is supported by the nail bed. The cuticle is part of the skin that extends a small distance on the nail plate before being shed (like the stratum corneum). The nail root is bordered by the cuticle and hidden by a fold of skin. Fingernails grow at a rate of 0.7 to 0.84 mm per week, with toenail growth 30% to 50% slower. Nails can be injured by direct trauma. A lost fingernail usually regenerates in 3 to 6 months, whereas a lost toenail may require 12 months or longer for

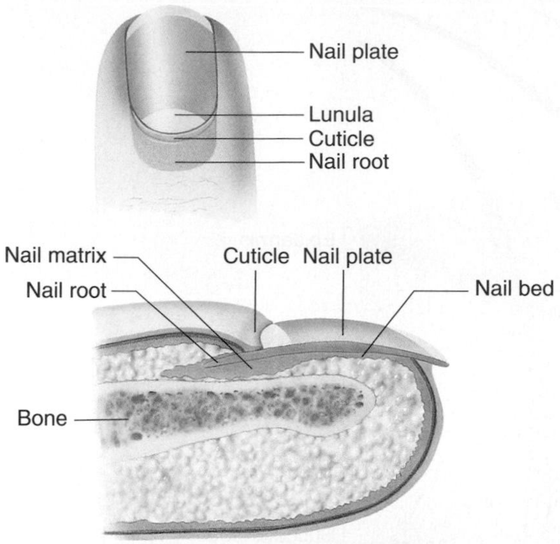

FIG. 23-2 Structure of a nail.

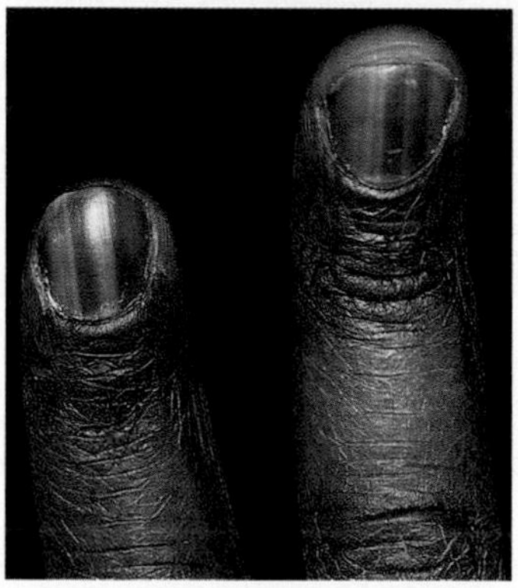

FIG. 23-3 Pigmented nail bed normally seen with dark skin color.

regeneration. Nail growth may vary according to the person's age and health. Nail color ranges from pink to yellow or brown depending on skin color. Pigmented longitudinal bands (melanonychia striata) may commonly occur in the nail bed in approximately 90% or more of all people with dark skin (Fig. 23-3).

Two major types of glands are associated with the skin: sebaceous and sweat (apocrine and eccrine) glands. The **sebaceous glands** secrete *sebum,* which is emptied into the hair follicles. Sebum prevents the skin and hair from becoming dry. Sebum is somewhat bacteriostatic and fungistatic and consists mainly of lipids. These glands depend on sex hormones, particularly testosterone, to regulate sebum secretion and production. Sebum secretion varies across the life span according to sex hormone levels. Sebaceous glands are present on all areas of the skin except the palms and the soles. These glands are most abundant on the face, scalp, upper chest, and back.

The *apocrine sweat glands* are located in the axillae, breast areolae, umbilical and anogenital areas, external auditory canals, and eyelids. They secrete a thick milky substance of unknown composition that becomes odoriferous when altered by skin surface bacteria. These glands enlarge and become active at puberty because of reproductive hormones.

The *eccrine sweat glands* are widely distributed over the body, except in a few areas, such as the lips. One square inch of skin contains about 3000 of these sweat glands. Sweat is a transparent watery solution composed of salts, ammonia, urea, and other wastes. The main function of these glands is to cool the body by evaporation, excrete waste products through the pores of the skin, and moisturize surface cells.

Functions of Integumentary System

The skin's primary function is to protect the underlying tissues of the body by serving as a surface barrier to the external environment. The skin also acts as a barrier against invasion by bacteria and viruses, and it prevents excessive water loss. The fat of the subcutaneous layer insulates the body and provides protection from trauma.

The skin with its nerve endings and special receptors provides sensory perception for environmental stimuli. These highly specialized nerve endings supply information to the brain related to pain, heat and cold, touch, pressure, and vibration.

The skin controls heat regulation by responding to changes in internal and external temperature with vasoconstriction or vasodilation. Heat regulation is related to the skin's function of excretion. Between 600 and 900 mL of water is lost daily through insensible perspiration. This function of the skin helps maintain homeostasis through fluid and electrolyte balance. In addition, sebum and sweat are secreted by the skin and lubricate the skin surface. Endogenous synthesis of vitamin D, which is critical to calcium and phosphorus balance, occurs in the epidermis. Vitamin D is synthesized by the action of UV light on vitamin D precursors in epidermal cells.

The esthetic functions of the skin include the expression of various emotions, such as anger or embarrassment, and the person's individual appearance. The skin is also used as a system for the delivery of drugs. An increasing number of systemic drugs are effectively delivered via patches or creams applied directly to the skin.

GERONTOLOGIC CONSIDERATIONS

EFFECTS OF AGING ON INTEGUMENTARY SYSTEM

Many skin changes are associated with aging. Although many changes are not serious except for their cosmetic value, others are more serious and need careful evaluation. Age-related changes of the integumentary system and differences in assessment findings are listed in Table 23-1.

The rate of age-related skin changes is influenced by heredity, a personal history of sun exposure, hygiene practices, nutrition, and general state of health. Skin changes that are related to aging include decreased turgor, thinning, dryness, wrinkling, vascular lesions, increased skin fragility, and benign neoplasms.

The junction between the dermis and the epidermis becomes flattened and the epidermis contains fewer melanocytes, which decreases the production of melanin, resulting in gray or white hair. In addition, the dermis loses volume and has fewer blood vessels. Scalp, pubic, and axillary hair becomes depigmented and thinner. The nail plate thins, and nails become brittle and more prone to splitting and yellowing. Nails, especially the toenails, may also thicken with age.

Chronic UV exposure is the major contributor to the photoaging and wrinkling of skin.[4] Sun damage to the skin is cumulative (Fig. 23-4). The wrinkling of sun-exposed areas such as the face and hands is more marked than that of a sun-shielded area such as the buttocks. Poor nutrition, with decreased intake

TABLE 23-1 GERONTOLOGIC ASSESSMENT DIFFERENCES

Integumentary System

Changes	Differences in Assessment Findings
Skin	
Decreased subcutaneous fat, muscle laxity, degeneration of elastic fibers, collagen stiffening	Increased wrinkling, sagging breasts and abdomen, redundant flesh around eyes, slowness of skin to flatten when pinched (tenting).
Decreased extracellular water, surface lipids, and sebaceous gland activity	Dry, flaking skin with possible signs of excoriation caused by scratching.
Decreased activity of apocrine and sebaceous glands	Dry skin with minimal to no perspiration, skin color uneven.
Increased capillary fragility and permeability	Bruising.
Increased focal melanocytes in basal layer with pigment accumulation	Solar lentigines on face and back of hands.
Diminished blood supply	Decrease in rosy appearance of skin and mucous membranes. Skin cool to touch. Diminished awareness of pain, touch, temperature, peripheral vibration.
Decreased proliferative capacity	Diminished rate of wound healing.
Decreased immunocompetence	Increase in neoplasms.
Hair	
Decreased melanin and melanocytes	Gray or white hair.
Decreased oil	Dry, coarse hair. Scaly scalp.
Decreased density of hair	Thinning and loss of hair. Loss of hair in outer half or outer third of eyebrow and back of legs.
Cumulative androgen effect; decreasing estrogen levels	Facial hirsutism, baldness.
Nails	
Decreased peripheral blood supply	Thick, brittle nails with diminished growth.
Increased keratin	Longitudinal ridging.
Decreased circulation	Prolonged return of blood to nails on blanching.

of protein, calories, and vitamins, also contributes to aging of the skin. With aging, collagen fibers stiffen, elastic fibers degenerate, and the amount of subcutaneous tissue decreases. These changes, with the added effects of gravity, lead to wrinkling.

Benign neoplasms related to the aging process can occur on the skin. These growths include seborrheic keratoses, vascular lesions such as cherry angiomas, and skin tags. *Actinic keratoses* appear on areas of chronic sun exposure, especially in the person who has a fair complexion and light eyes (blue, green, or hazel). These premalignant cutaneous lesions place an individual at increased risk for squamous cell and basal cell carcinomas. The photoaged person is more susceptible to skin cancers because UV exposure decreases the capacity to repair cellular damage (especially deoxyribonucleic acid [DNA]). Chronic UV exposure from tanning beds causes the same damage as UV from the sun.

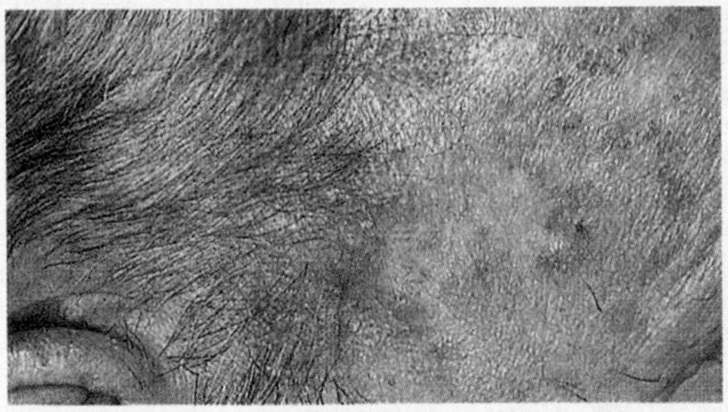

FIG. 23-4 Photoaging. Irregular pigmentation and keratoses occur on sun-damaged skin on forehead.

TABLE 23-2 NORMAL PHYSICAL ASSESSMENT OF INTEGUMENTARY SYSTEM

Skin	• Evenly pigmented; no petechiae, purpura, lesions, or excoriations. • Warm, good turgor.
Nails	• Pink, oval, adhere to nail bed with 160-degree angle.
Hair	• Shiny and full; amount and distribution appropriate for age and gender. • No flaking of scalp, forehead, or pinna.

In older adults decreased subcutaneous fat leads to an increased risk of traumatic injury, hypothermia, and skin shearing, which may lead to pressure ulcers. With aging, the apocrine and eccrine sweat glands atrophy, causing dry skin and decreased body odor. The growth rate of the hair and nails decreases as a result of atrophy of the involved structures. Hormonal and vitamin deficiencies can cause dry, thin hair and alopecia (partial or complete lack of hair).

The visible effects of aging on the skin and hair may have a profound psychologic effect. A youthful look may be tied to a person's self-image. Although fine wrinkling of the skin, thinning hair, and brittle nails are normal changes with aging, they may result in an altered self-image.[5]

ASSESSMENT OF INTEGUMENTARY SYSTEM

A general assessment of the skin begins at the initial contact with the patient and continues throughout the examination. Specific areas of the skin are assessed during the examination of other body systems unless the chief complaint is a dermatologic problem. Record a general statement about the skin's physical condition (Table 23-2). In addition, ask the health history questions presented in Table 23-3 when a skin problem is noted.

Subjective Data

Individuals with skin problems may have complaints that are not readily observed. A thorough health history yields information about possible causes and the effect of the problem on the individual's life.

Important Health Information

Past Health History. Past health history indicates previous trauma, surgery, or disease that involves the skin. Determine if the patient has noticed any dermatologic manifestations of systemic problems such as jaundice (liver disease), delayed wound

CASE STUDY

Patient Introduction

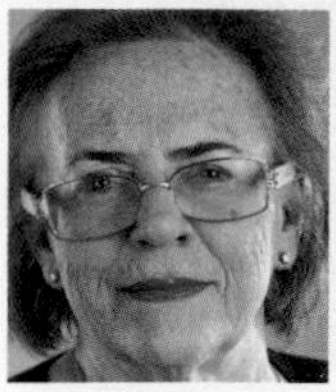

iStockphoto/Thinkstock

D.A. is a 74-year-old woman who comes to the medical clinic with concerns related to various "spots" on her face. She says they have been there for a while and she thought they were just "age spots" but got concerned after her friend was diagnosed with a malignant melanoma.

Critical Thinking

As you read through this assessment chapter, think about D.A. with the following questions in mind:

1. What are the possible causes of D.A.'s facial lesions?
2. What questions would you ask D.A. to determine the possible causes?
3. What should be included in the physical assessment? What specific characteristics of the skin lesions would you be looking for?
4. What diagnostic studies might you expect to be ordered?

evolve Answers available at *http://evolve.elsevier.com/Lewis/medsurg.*

healing (diabetes mellitus), cyanosis (respiratory disorder), or pallor (anemia). eTable 24-1 lists diseases with dermatologic manifestations. Obtain specific information related to food sensitivities, pet or drug allergies, and skin reactions to insect bites and stings. Note any history of chronic or unprotected exposure to UV light, including tanning bed use and radiation treatments.

Medications. Ask the patient about skin-related problems that occurred as a result of taking prescription or over-the-counter (OTC) medications. A thorough medication history is important, especially in relation to vitamins, hormones, antibiotics, corticosteroids, and antimetabolites because these may cause side effects that are manifested in the skin.

Document the use of prescription or OTC medications used specifically to treat a primary skin problem such as acne or a secondary skin problem such as itching. If a medication is used, record the name, length of use, method of application, and effectiveness.

Surgery or Other Treatments. Determine if any surgical procedures, including cosmetic surgery, were performed on the skin. If a biopsy was done, record the result. Note any treatments specific for a skin problem (e.g., phototherapy) or for a health problem (e.g., radiation therapy). In addition, document any treatments undergone primarily for cosmetic purposes, such as tanning booth use, laser resurfacing, or cosmetic "peels."

Functional Health Patterns

Health Perception–Health Management Pattern. Question the patient about health practices related to the integumentary system, such as self-care habits related to daily hygiene. Document the frequency of use and sun protection factor (SPF) of sunscreen products. Assess the use of personal care products (e.g., shampoos, moisturizing agents, cosmetics), including brand name, quantity, and frequency. Record a description of any current skin problem, including onset, symptoms, course, and treatment. Note any medications used for treating hair loss.

GENETIC RISK ALERT

- The primary risk factor leading to skin cancer and melanoma is environmental exposure to UV radiation. UV radiation damages DNA, causing an error in the genetic code and resulting in abnormal skin cells.
- Inherited genetic factors can also increase the risk for skin cancer. A person has an increased risk for developing melanoma if he or she has a first-degree relative (e.g., parent, full sibling) who had a melanoma.
- The risk for skin cancer is increased for people who have a fair complexion (light-colored skin that easily freckles, red or blond hair, and blue or light-colored eyes).

Obtain information about the family history of any skin diseases, including congenital and familial diseases (e.g., alopecia, psoriasis) and systemic diseases with dermatologic

TABLE 23-3 HEALTH HISTORY

Integumentary System

Health Perception–Health Management
- Describe your daily hygiene practices.
- What skin products are you currently using?
- Describe any current skin condition, including onset, course, and treatment (if any).

Nutritional-Metabolic
- Describe any changes in the condition of your skin, hair, nails, and mucous membranes.
- Have you noticed any recent changes in the way sores or wounds heal?*
- Have you had any weight loss or dietary changes, including supplemental vitamins and minerals?*

Elimination
- Have you noticed recent changes in your skin related to excessive sweating, dryness, or swelling?*

Activity-Exercise
- Do your leisure or work activities involve the use of any chemicals that are irritating to your skin?*
- Do you do anything to protect yourself from the sun?*

Sleep-Rest
- Does your skin condition keep you awake or awaken you after you have fallen asleep?*

Cognitive-Perceptual
- Do you have any unusual sensations of heat, cold, or touch?*
- Do you have any pain associated with your skin condition?*
- Do you have any joint pain?*

Self-Perception–Self-Concept
- How does your skin condition make you feel about yourself?

Role-Relationship
- Has your skin condition changed your relationships with others?*
- Have you changed your lifestyle because of your skin condition?*

Sexuality-Reproductive
- Has your skin condition changed your intimate relationships with others?*
- Has your birth control method (if used) caused a skin problem?*

Coping–Stress Tolerance
- Are you aware of any situation or stressor that changes your skin condition?*
- Do you think that stress plays a role in your skin condition?*
- How do you handle stress?

Value-Belief
- Are there any cultural beliefs that influence your thinking or feelings about your skin condition?*
- Are there any treatment options that you would be opposed to using?

*If yes, describe.

manifestations (e.g., diabetes, thyroid disease, cardiovascular diseases, immune disorders). In addition, note any family and personal history of skin cancer, particularly melanoma.

Nutritional-Metabolic Pattern. Question the patient about any changes in the condition of skin, hair, nails, and mucous membranes and whether they are related to dietary changes. A diet history reveals the adequacy of nutrients essential to healthy skin such as vitamins A, D, E, and C; dietary fat; and protein. Note any food allergies that cause a skin reaction. Ask obese patients if they have areas of chafing or a rash in **intertriginous** areas, where skin surfaces overlap and rub on each other (e.g., below the breasts, axillae, and groin). Note any excessive or absent sweating. Question the patient about poor or delayed wound healing.

Elimination Pattern. Ask the patient about conditions of the skin such as dehydration, edema, and **pruritus** (itching), which can indicate alterations in fluid balance. If urinary or fecal incontinence is a problem, determine the condition of the skin in the anal and perineal areas.

Activity-Exercise Pattern. Obtain information about environmental hazards in relation to hobbies and recreational activities, including exposure to known carcinogens, chemical irritants, and allergens. Ask the patient if any changes occur in the skin during exercise or other activities.

Sleep-Rest Pattern. Question the patient about disturbances in sleep patterns caused by a skin condition. For example, pruritus can be distressing and cause major alterations in normal sleep patterns. Also, poor sleep and resulting tiredness are often reflected in a patient's face by dark circles under the eyes and a decreased firmness in the facial skin.

Cognitive-Perceptual Pattern. Determine the patient's perception of the sensations of heat, cold, pain, and touch. Note any discomfort associated with a skin condition, especially when observed in intact skin. Assess and record any joint pain. Assess the mobility of the joints, since the patient's skin condition may cause alterations in mobility.

Self-Perception–Self-Concept Pattern. Assess any feelings related to the patient's skin condition such as sadness, anxiety, despair, or altered body image. These feelings can occur with visible skin problems such as acne, rosacea, and psoriasis, which alter a person's physical appearance.

Role-Relationship Pattern. Determine how the patient's skin condition affects relationships with family members, peers, and work associates. In addition, question the patient regarding the effect of environmental factors on the skin such as occupational exposure to irritants, sun, and unusually cold or unhygienic conditions. Contact dermatitis caused by allergies and irritants is a common skin problem associated with occupation.

Sexuality-Reproductive Pattern. Tactfully question and assess the effect of the patient's skin condition on sexual activity. In particular, note the reproductive status of the female patient relative to possible therapeutic interventions. For example, isotretinoin (Accutane), used to treat acne, and topical fluorouracil (Efudex, Fluoroplex), used to treat actinic keratoses, are teratogenic drugs that may cause abnormal fetal development. These medications should not be used by pregnant women or women who could become pregnant.

Coping–Stress Tolerance Pattern. Assess and question the patient about the role that stress may play in creating or exacerbating the skin condition. Ask the patient what coping strategies are used to manage the skin condition.

CASE STUDY—cont'd

Subjective Data

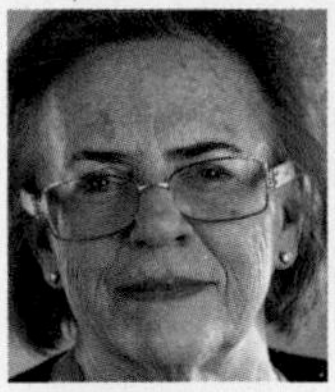

iStockphoto/Thinkstock

A focused subjective assessment of D.A. reveals the following:

- ***PMH:*** Negative except for an appendectomy at age 16.
- ***Medications:*** None at present. NKA.
- ***Health Perception–Health Management:*** Currently washes her face with a skin cleanser in the morning and nighttime. After cleansing, she applies a moisturizer with SPF 15. She has used these facial products for the past 3 years since she first started noticing small age spots appearing. Before that she just used soap and water.
- ***Nutritional:*** D.A. reports that her skin seems to be drier as she ages but otherwise no changes besides the "age spots" or "whatever they are." Denies any changes in the way cuts or sores heal. No weight loss. Does not take any supplemental vitamins or minerals.
- ***Elimination:*** Although skin is a little dry, D.A. does not perceive it to be excessively dry. Denies excessive sweating or any swelling.
- ***Activity-Exercise:*** Loves to garden and go for walks outdoors. Reports a history of frequent, sometimes severe, sunburns as a child. No use of sunscreen growing up but does remember her mother making her wear T-shirts over her bathing suits to help prevent sunburn. Has used sunscreen for the past 20 years when outdoors. Reapplies as needed.
- ***Cognitive-Perceptual:*** Denies any pain or discomfort associated with skin lesions.
- ***Coping–Stress Tolerance:*** Fearful that she might have skin cancer.

Value-Belief Pattern. Ask about cultural or religious beliefs that could influence the patient's self-image as related to the skin condition. Also, assess values and beliefs that might influence or limit the choice of treatment options.

Objective Data

Physical Examination. Primary skin lesions develop on previously unaltered skin. The common characteristics of primary skin lesions are shown in Table 23-4. Secondary skin lesions are lesions that change with time or occur because of factors such as scratching or infection. Secondary skin lesions are shown in Table 23-5. General principles when assessing the skin are as follows:

- Have a private examination room of moderate temperature with good lighting; a room with exposure to daylight is preferred.
- Ensure that the patient is comfortable and in a dressing gown that allows easy access to all skin areas.
- Be systematic and proceed from head to toe.
- Compare symmetric parts.
- Perform a general inspection and then a lesion-specific examination.
- Use the metric system when taking measurements.
- Use appropriate terminology and nomenclature when reporting or documenting.

Photographs are useful when accurate findings are needed. Follow clinical agency protocol regarding obtaining a patient's consent to photograph skin lesions for inclusion in the medical record.

Inspection. Inspect the skin for general color and pigmentation, vascularity, bruising, and lesions or discolorations. The critical factor in assessment of skin color is change. A skin color

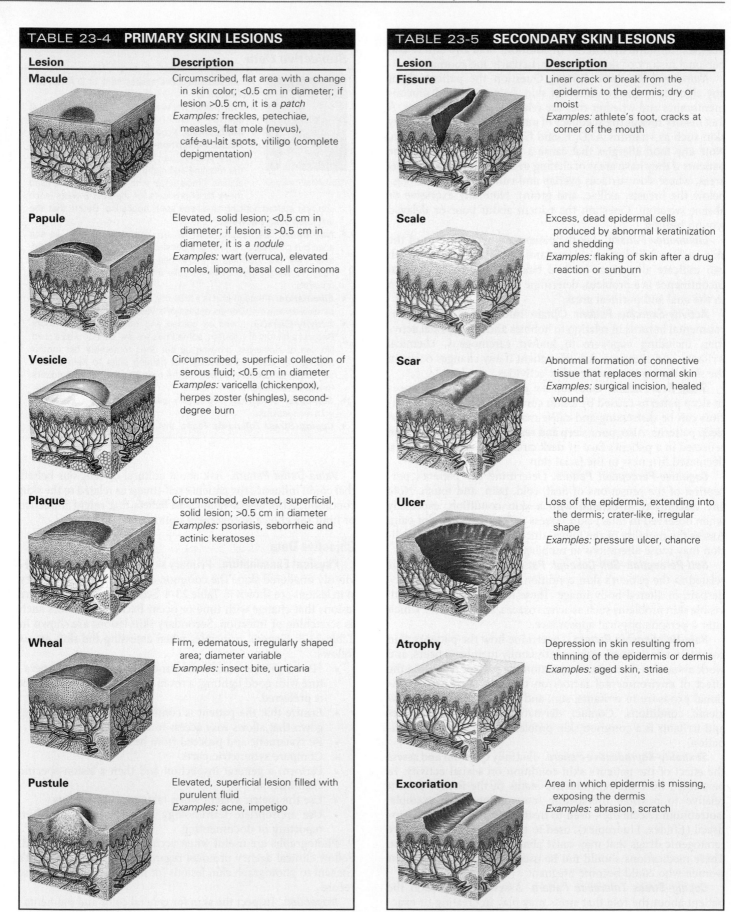

TABLE 23-4 PRIMARY SKIN LESIONS

Lesion	Description
Macule 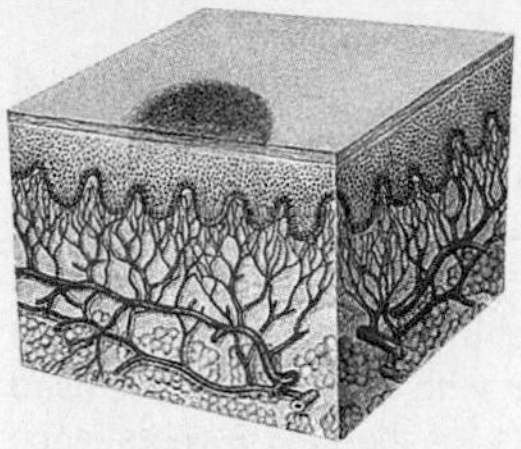	Circumscribed, flat area with a change in skin color; <0.5 cm in diameter; if lesion >0.5 cm, it is a *patch* *Examples:* freckles, petechiae, measles, flat mole (nevus), café-au-lait spots, vitiligo (complete depigmentation)
Papule 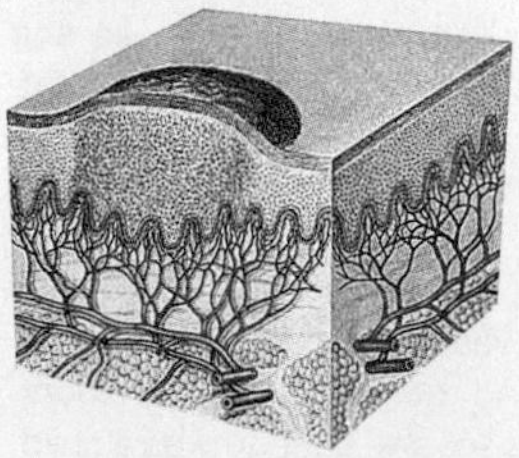	Elevated, solid lesion; <0.5 cm in diameter; if lesion is >0.5 cm in diameter, it is a *nodule* *Examples:* wart (verruca), elevated moles, lipoma, basal cell carcinoma
Vesicle 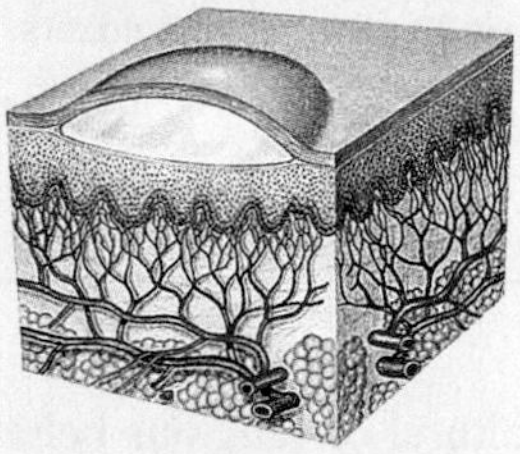	Circumscribed, superficial collection of serous fluid; <0.5 cm in diameter *Examples:* varicella (chickenpox), herpes zoster (shingles), second-degree burn
Plaque 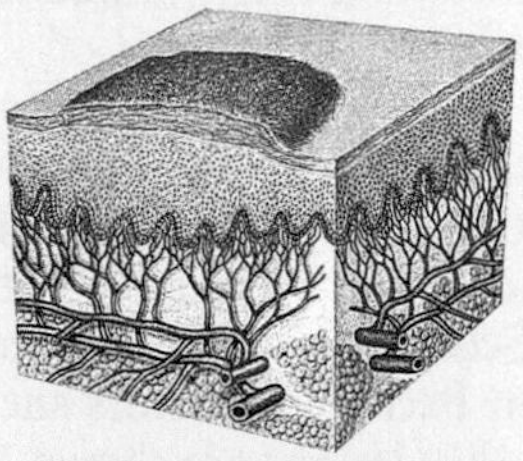	Circumscribed, elevated, superficial, solid lesion; >0.5 cm in diameter *Examples:* psoriasis, seborrheic and actinic keratoses
Wheal 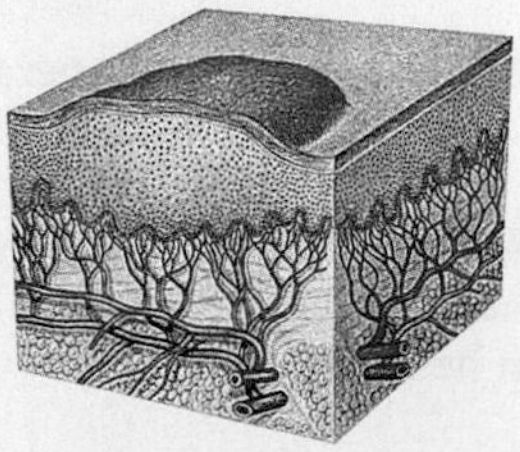	Firm, edematous, irregularly shaped area; diameter variable *Examples:* insect bite, urticaria
Pustule 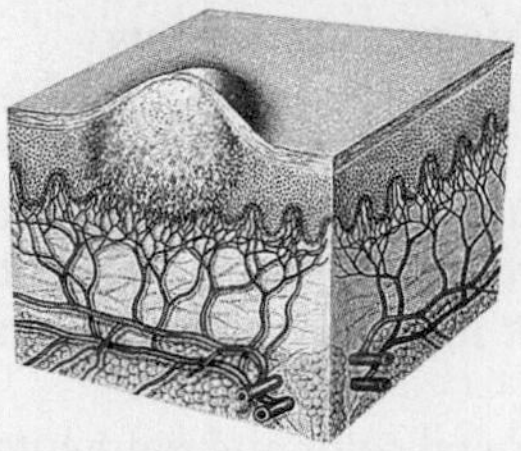	Elevated, superficial lesion filled with purulent fluid *Examples:* acne, impetigo

TABLE 23-5 SECONDARY SKIN LESIONS

Lesion	Description
Fissure 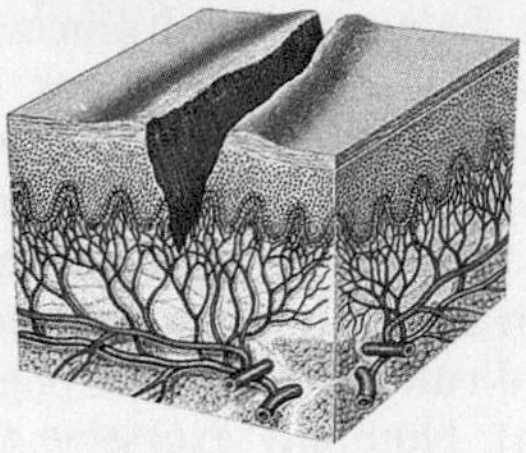	Linear crack or break from the epidermis to the dermis; dry or moist *Examples:* athlete's foot, cracks at corner of the mouth
Scale 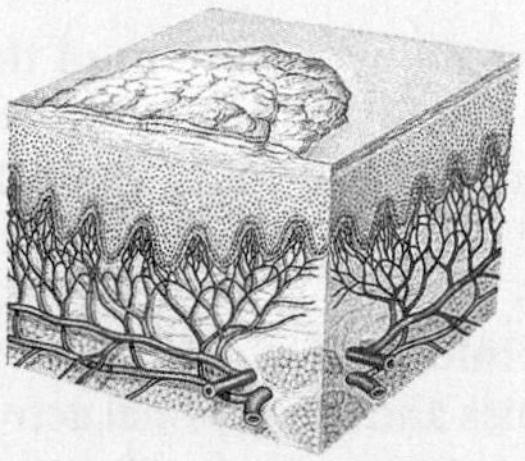	Excess, dead epidermal cells produced by abnormal keratinization and shedding *Examples:* flaking of skin after a drug reaction or sunburn
Scar 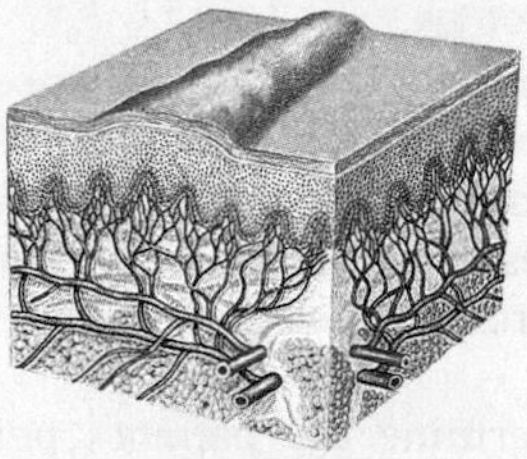	Abnormal formation of connective tissue that replaces normal skin *Examples:* surgical incision, healed wound
Ulcer 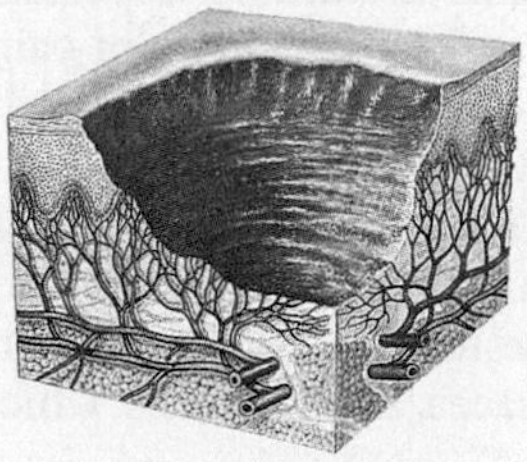	Loss of the epidermis, extending into the dermis; crater-like, irregular shape *Examples:* pressure ulcer, chancre
Atrophy 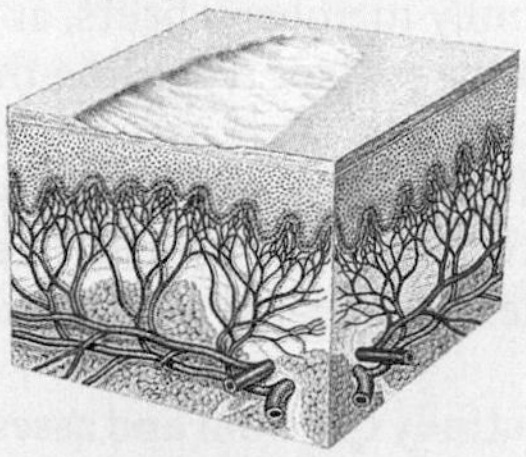	Depression in skin resulting from thinning of the epidermis or dermis *Examples:* aged skin, striae
Excoriation 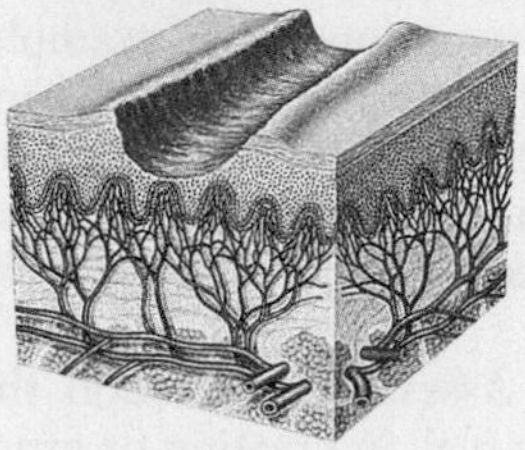	Area in which epidermis is missing, exposing the dermis *Examples:* abrasion, scratch

that is normal for a particular patient can be a sign of a pathologic condition in another patient. The skin color depends on the amount of melanin (brown), carotene (yellow), oxyhemoglobin (red), and reduced hemoglobin (bluish red) present at a particular time. The most reliable areas to assess erythema, cyanosis, pallor, and jaundice are the areas of least pigmentation, such as the sclerae, conjunctivae, nail beds, lips, and buccal mucosa. The true skin color is best observed in photo-protected areas such as the buttocks. Activity, sun (UV) exposure, emotions, cigarette smoking, and edema, as well as respiratory, renal, cardiovascular, and hepatic disorders, can all directly affect skin color. Table 23-6 describes assessment variations in light- and dark-skinned individuals.

TABLE 23-6 NURSING ASSESSMENT

Assessment Variations in Light- and Dark-Skinned Individuals

Light Skin	Dark Skin
Cyanosis	
Grayish blue tone, especially in nail beds, earlobes, lips, mucous membranes, palms, and soles	Ashen or gray color most easily seen in the conjunctiva of the eye, mucous membranes, and nail beds
Ecchymosis	
Dark red, purple, yellow, or green color, depending on age of bruise	Purple to brownish black. Difficult to see unless occurring in an area of light pigmentation
Erythema	
Reddish tone, possibly accompanied by increased skin temperature secondary to localized inflammation	Deeper brown or purple skin tone with evidence of increased skin temperature secondary to inflammation
Jaundice	
Yellowish color of skin, sclera, fingernails, palms, and oral mucosa	Yellowish green color most obviously seen in sclera of eye (do not confuse with yellow eye pigmentation, which may be evident in dark-skinned patients), palms, and soles
Pallor	
Pale skin color that may appear white or ashen; also evident on lips, nail beds, and mucous membranes	Lack of underlying red tone in brown or black skin. In light-skinned African Americans, yellowish brown skin. In dark-skinned African Americans, ashen or gray skin
Petechiae	
Lesions appearing as small, reddish purple pinpoints, best observed on abdomen and buttocks	Difficult to see. May be evident in the buccal mucosa of the mouth or conjunctiva of the eye
Rash	
May be visualized and felt with light palpation	Not easily visualized, but may be felt with light palpation
Scar	
Generally heals, showing narrow scar line	Higher incidence of keloid development, resulting in a thickened, raised scar (see Table 23-5)

In your general inspection, note the presence of body art such as piercings and tattoos. The nose, ears, eyebrows, lips, navel, and nipples are common sites of piercing. Tattoo pigments deposited in the skin may cause itching, pain, and sensitivity for several weeks after the tattoo is placed.

Examine the skin for possible problems related to vascularity, including bruising and vascular and purpuric lesions such as *angioma* (benign tumor of blood or lymph vessels), *petechiae* (tiny purple spots on skin), or *purpura* (bleeding disorder caused by ecchymosis or petechiae). Note the reaction to direct pressure. If a lesion blanches on direct pressure and then refills, the redness is due to dilated blood vessels. If the discoloration remains, it is the result of subcutaneous or intradermal bleeding or a nonvascular lesion. Note any pattern of bruising such as discoloration in the shape of the hand or fingers or bruises at different stages of resolution. These may indicate other health problems or abuse and should be further investigated.

If lesions are found on the skin, record their color, size, distribution, location, and shape. Skin lesions are usually described in terms related to the lesions' configuration (solitary or pattern in relation to other lesions) and distribution (arrangement of lesions over an area of skin) (Table 23-7).

During systematic inspection, note any unusual odors. Skin sites with lesions, such as rashes, may be colonized with yeast or bacteria, which can be associated with distinctive odors in intertriginous areas (Fig. 23-5). Examine tattoos and needle-track marks and note the location and characteristics of the surrounding skin area.

TABLE 23-7 LESION DISTRIBUTION TERMINOLOGY

Term	Description
Asymmetric	Unilateral distribution
Confluent	Merging together
Diffuse	Wide distribution
Discrete	Separate from other lesions
Generalized	Diffuse distribution
Grouped	Cluster of lesions
Localized	Limited areas of involvement that are clearly defined
Solitary	A single lesion
Symmetric	Bilateral distribution
Zosteriform	Bandlike distribution along a dermatome area

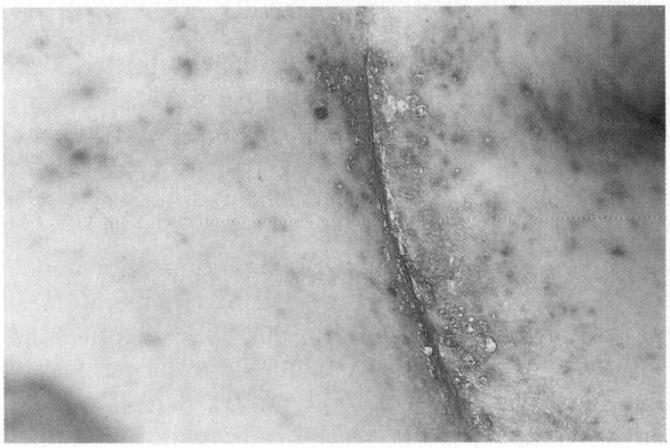

FIG. 23-5 Intertrigo. Rash in body folds with *Candida* infection.

TABLE 23-8 ASSESSMENT ABNORMALITIES

Integumentary System

Finding	Description	Possible Etiology and Significance
Alopecia	Loss of hair (localized or general)	Heredity, friction, rubbing, traction, trauma, stress, infection, inflammation, chemotherapy, pregnancy, emotional shock, tinea capitis, immunologic factors
Angioma	Tumor consisting of blood or lymph vessels	Normal increase in incidence with aging, liver disease, pregnancy, varicose veins
Carotenemia (carotenosis)	Yellow discoloration of skin, no yellowing of sclerae, most noticeable on palms and soles	Vegetables containing carotene (e.g., carrots, squash), hypothyroidism
Comedo (acne lesion)	Enlarged hair follicle plugged with sebum, bacteria, and skin cells; can be open (blackhead) or closed (whitehead)	Heredity, certain drugs, hormonal changes with puberty and pregnancy
Cyanosis	Slightly bluish gray or dark purple discoloration of the skin and mucous membranes caused by excessive amounts of reduced hemoglobin in capillaries	Cardiorespiratory problems, vasoconstriction, asphyxiation, anemia, leukemia, and malignancies
Cyst	Sac containing fluid or semisolid material	Obstruction of a duct or gland, parasitic infection
Ecchymosis	Large, bruise-like lesion caused by collection of extravascular blood in dermis and subcutaneous tissue	Trauma, bleeding disorders
Erythema	Redness occurring in patches of variable size and shape	Heat, certain drugs, alcohol, ultraviolet rays, any problem that causes dilation of blood vessels to the skin
Hematoma	Extravasation of blood of sufficient size to cause visible swelling	Trauma, bleeding disorders
Hirsutism	Male distribution of hair in women	Abnormality of ovaries or adrenal glands, decrease in estrogen level, familial trait
Hypopigmentation	Loss of pigmentation resulting in lighter patches than the normal skin	Chemical agents, nutritional factors, burns, inflammation, infection
Intertrigo	Dermatitis of overlying surfaces of the skin	Moisture, irritation, obesity; may be complicated by *Candida* infection (see Fig. 23-5)
Jaundice	Yellow (in white patients) or yellowish brown (in African Americans) discoloration of the skin, best observed in the sclera, secondary to increased bilirubin in the blood	Liver disease, red blood cell hemolysis, pancreatic cancer, common bile duct obstruction
Keloid	Hypertrophied scar beyond wound margins (see Fig. 23-6)	Predisposition more common in African Americans
Lichenification	Thickening of the skin with accentuated normal skin markings	Repeated scratching, rubbing, and irritation usually as a result of pruritus or neurosis
Mole (nevus)	Benign overgrowth of melanocytes	Defects of development; excessive numbers and large, irregular moles; often familial
Petechiae	Pinpoint, discrete deposits of blood <1-2 mm in the extravascular tissues and visible through the skin or mucous membrane	Inflammation, marked vasodilation, blood vessel trauma, blood dyscrasia that results in bleeding tendencies (e.g., thrombocytopenia)
Telangiectasia	Visibly dilated, superficial, cutaneous small blood vessels, commonly found on face and thighs	Aging, acne, sun exposure, alcohol, liver failure, corticosteroids, radiation, certain systemic diseases, skin tumors
Tenting	Failure of skin to return immediately to normal position after gentle pinching	Aging, dehydration, cachexia
Varicosity	Increased prominence of superficial veins	Interruption of venous return (e.g., from tumor, incompetent valves, inflammation), commonly found on lower legs with aging
Vitiligo	Complete absence of melanin (pigment) resulting in chalky white patch (see Fig. 23-7)	Autoimmune, familial, thyroid disease

Inspection of the hair should include an examination of all body hair. Note the distribution, texture, and quantity of hair. Changes in the normal distribution of body hair and growth may indicate an endocrine or vascular disorder. Carefully inspect the nails, including nail shape, thickness, curvature, and surface. Note any grooves, pitting, ridges, or detachment from nail bed. Changes in nail smoothness or thickness can occur with anemia, psoriasis, thyroid problems, decreased vascular circulation, and some infections.

Palpation. Palpate the skin to obtain information about temperature, turgor, moisture, and texture. Temperature of the patient's skin is best assessed using the back of your hand. The skin should be warm without being hot. The temperature of the skin increases when blood flow to the dermis is increased. A localized temperature increase occurs with burns and local inflammation. A generalized increase in skin temperature occurs when a person has a fever. A decreased body temperature may occur when shock or other circulatory problems, chilling, or infection is present.

Turgor refers to the elasticity of the skin. Assess turgor by gently pinching an area of skin under the clavicle or on the back of the hand. Skin with good turgor should move easily when lifted and should immediately return to its original position when released. In patients with dehydration and aging, a loss of turgor occurs and can cause tenting of the skin (Table 23-8).

Moisture of the skin (the dampness or dryness of the skin) increases in intertriginous areas and with high humidity. Skin moisture varies with environmental temperature, muscular activity, body weight, and body temperature. The skin should be intact with no flaking, scaling, or cracking. Skin generally becomes drier with increasing age.

FOCUSED ASSESSMENT

Integumentary System

Use this checklist to make sure the key assessment steps have been done.

Subjective

Ask the patient about any of the following and note responses.

Hair loss (unusual or rapid)	Y	N
Changes in skin (e.g., lesions, bruising)	Y	N
Nail discoloration	Y	N

Objective: Diagnostic

Check the following for results and critical values.

Biopsy results	✓
Albumin	✓

Objective: Physical Examination

Inspect

Skin for color, integrity, scars, lesions, signs of breakdown	✓
Facial and body hair for distribution, color, quantity, hygiene	✓
Nails for shape, contour, color, thickness, cleanliness	✓
Dressings if present	✓

Palpate

Skin for temperature, texture, moisture, thickness, turgor, mobility	✓

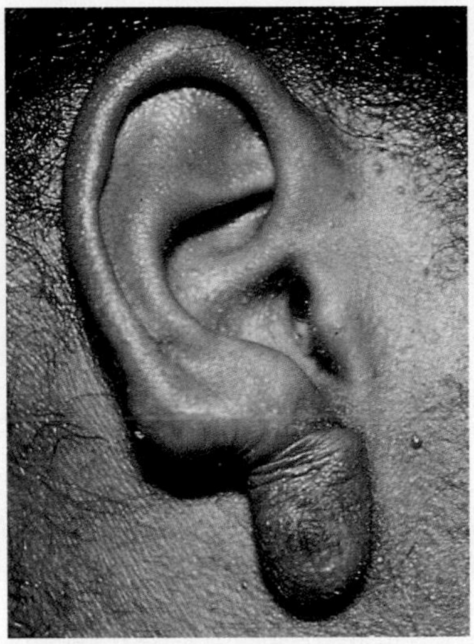

FIG. 23-6 Keloid. Hypertrophic scarring after skin injury, which is more common in dark-skinned individuals.

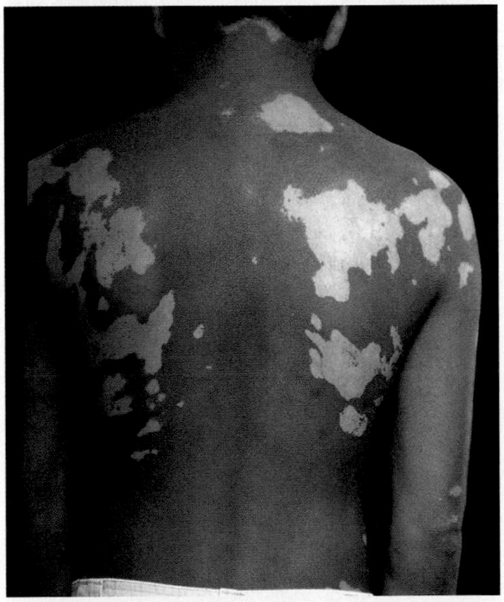

FIG. 23-7 Vitiligo. Total loss of pigment in the affected area.

Texture refers to the fineness or coarseness of the skin. The skin should feel smooth and firm with the surface evenly thin in most areas. Thickened callus areas are normal on the soles and palms and relate to weight bearing. Increased thickness is often work related and the result of excessive pressure.

A *focused assessment* is used to evaluate the status of previously identified integumentary problems and to monitor for signs of new problems (see Table 3-6). A focused assessment of the integumentary system is presented in the box on this page. Assessment abnormalities of the skin are described in Table 23-8.

Assessment of Dark Skin

A normal range of differences occurs in the physical examination of skin, hair, and nails. Genetic factors determine a person's skin color, which can vary from white to dark brown with overtones of yellow, olive, and red. The darker skin tones result from the reflection of light as it strikes the underlying skin pigment. An increased amount of melanin pigment produced by the melanocytes causes the darker skin color. This increased melanin forms a natural sun shield for dark skin and results in a decreased incidence of skin cancer in these individuals.

The structures of dark skin are no different from those of lighter skin, but they are often more difficult to assess (see Table 23-6). Color is more easily assessed in areas where the epidermis is thin and pigmentation is not influenced by sun exposure such as the lips, mucous membranes, nail beds, and protected areas (e.g., buttocks). Palmar and plantar surfaces are lighter than other skin areas in darker-skinned individuals. Rashes are often more difficult to observe and may need to be palpated.[6] Wrinkling is more apparent in light-skinned individuals than in dark-skinned individuals.

Individuals with dark skin are predisposed to certain skin and hair conditions. **Keloid** is an overgrowth of collagenous tissue at the site of a skin injury (e.g., ear piercing) (Fig. 23-6). *Vitiligo* is total loss of pigment in the affected area (Fig. 23-7). In *dermatosis papulosa nigra,* small, pigmented wartlike papules are commonly found on the face. *Nevus of Ota* is a slate-gray or blue-gray birthmark located on the forehead and face around the eye area; it may also involve the sclera (Fig. 23-8). *Traction alopecia* may be noted due to trauma from hair rollers or from tight braiding of the hair (Fig. 23-9). The hair loss may be temporary or permanent. *Pseudofolliculitis* is an inflammatory response to ingrown hairs that occurs after shaving too closely in the beard area. It is characterized by pustules and papules.

Because of the darkness of the skin of some individuals, color often cannot be used as an indicator of systemic conditions (e.g., flushed skin with fever). Cyanosis may be difficult to determine because a normal bluish hue occurs in dark-skinned people.

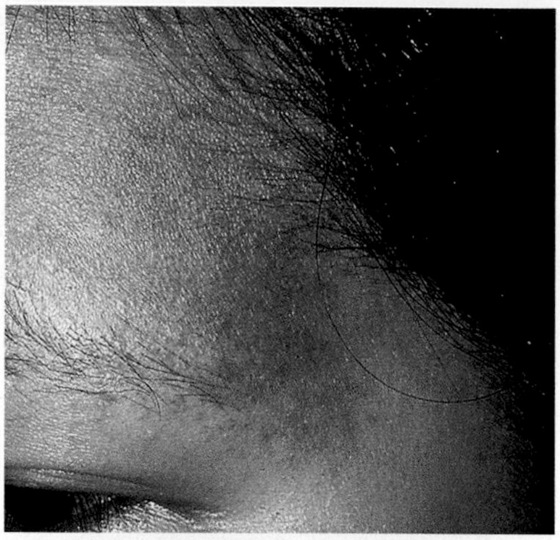

FIG. 23-8 Nevus of Ota. Flat gray to blue pigmentation in the upper trigeminal area, which is more common in dark-skinned individuals.

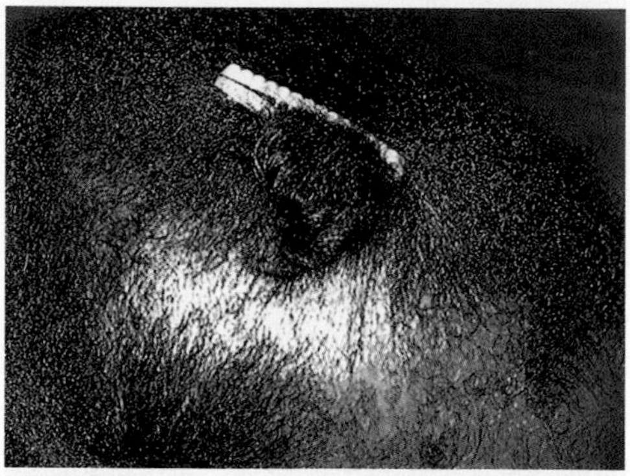

FIG. 23-9 Traction alopecia. Hair loss in scalp because of prolonged tension from hair rollers, braiding, or straightening combs.

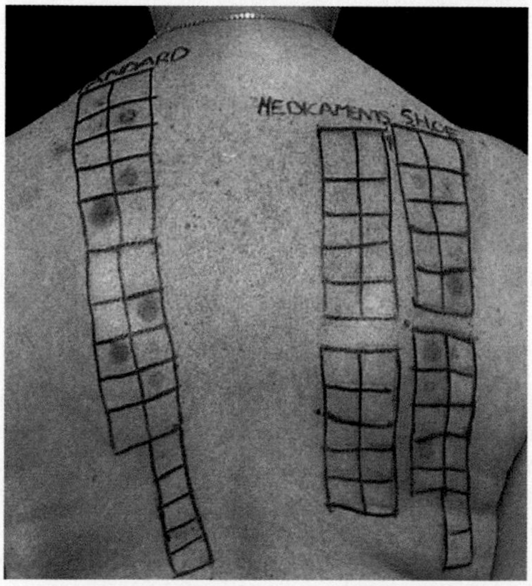

FIG. 23-10 Patch test. Results from an application of possible allergens to the skin shows positive reactions in the sites labeled "standard" and "shoe."

CASE STUDY—cont'd

Objective Data

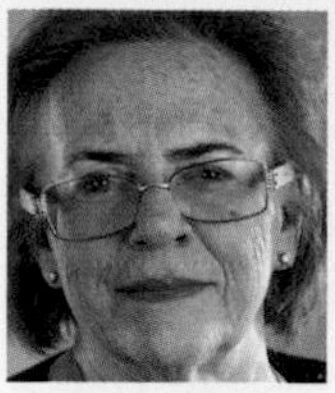

iStockphoto/Thinkstock

Physical Examination

Physical examination findings of D.A.'s skin are as follows:

- Complexion fair. Wrinkles around eyes, above upper lip, and on sides of cheeks bilaterally. Normal skin temperature and turgor.
- Lesion on upper right forehead measuring 2 × 3 mm; on left forehead near hairline measuring 1 × 2 mm; and on left lower cheek measuring 2 × 2.5 mm.
- All lesions are slightly erythematous but do not blanch when direct pressure is applied. Borders distinct. Minimal elevation noted on palpation.
- No other skin lesions noted on rest of body.

As you continue to read this chapter, consider diagnostic studies you would anticipate being performed for D.A. Also identify patient problems and appropriate nursing interventions for D.A. while she is a patient in the clinic.

Diagnostic Studies

The health care provider examines the lesion via dermatoscopy and also uses a Wood's lamp to rule out a fungal infection. The provider suspects basal cell carcinoma, which is confirmed by a shave biopsy.

DIAGNOSTIC STUDIES OF INTEGUMENTARY SYSTEM

Diagnostic studies provide important information in monitoring the patient's condition and planning interventions. These studies are considered to be objective data. Table 23-9 contains diagnostic studies commonly used for the integumentary system.

The main diagnostic techniques related to skin problems are inspection of an individual lesion and a careful history related to the problem. If a definitive diagnosis cannot be made by these techniques, additional tests may be indicated, such as *dermatoscopy* (examination of the skin through a lighted instrument with optical magnification).[6]

Biopsy is one of the most common diagnostic tests used to evaluate a skin lesion. A biopsy is indicated in all conditions in which a malignancy is suspected or a specific diagnosis is questionable. Techniques include punch, incisional, excisional, and shave biopsies. The method used is related to factors such as the site of the biopsy, the cosmetic result desired, and the type of tissue to be obtained.

Other diagnostic procedures include stains and cultures for fungal, bacterial, and viral infections. Direct immunofluorescence is a special diagnostic technique used on biopsy specimens and may be indicated in certain conditions such as bullous diseases and systemic lupus erythematosus. Indirect immunofluorescence is performed on a sample of blood. Patch testing (Fig. 23-10) and photopatch testing may be used to evaluate allergic dermatitis and photoallergic reactions.[2]

TABLE 23-9 DIAGNOSTIC STUDIES

Integumentary System

Study	Description and Purpose	Nursing Responsibility
Biopsy		
Punch	Special punch biopsy instrument of appropriate size used. Instrument rotated to appropriate level to include dermis and some fat. Suturing may or may not be done. Provides full-thickness skin for diagnostic purposes.	Verify that consent form is signed (if needed). Assist with preparation of site, anesthesia, procedure, and hemostasis. Apply dressing, give postprocedure instructions to patient. Properly identify specimen.
Excisional	Used when good cosmetic results and/or entire lesion removal desired. Skin closed with subcutaneous and skin sutures.	Same as above.
Incisional	Wedge-shaped incision made in lesion too large for excisional biopsy. Useful when larger specimen than shave or punch biopsy is needed.	Same as above.
Shave	Single-edged razor blade used to shave off superficial lesions or small sample of a large lesion. Provides thin specimen for diagnostic purposes.	Same as above.
Microscopic Tests		
Potassium hydroxide (KOH)	Hair, scales, or nails examined for superficial fungal infection. Specimen put on glass slide and 10%-20% concentration of KOH added.	Instruct patient regarding purpose of test. Prepare slide.
Tzanck test (Wright's and Giemsa's stain)	Fluid and cells from vesicles examined. Used to diagnose herpes infections. Specimen put on slide, stained, and examined microscopically.	Inform patient of purpose of test. Use sterile technique for collection of fluid.
Culture	Test identifies fungal, bacterial, and viral organisms. For *fungi,* scraping or swab of skin performed. For *bacteria,* material obtained from intact pustules, bullae, or abscesses. For *viruses,* vesicle or bulla and exudate taken from base of lesion.	Instruct patient regarding purpose and procedure. Properly identify specimen. Follow instructions for storage of specimen if not immediately sent to laboratory.
Mineral oil slides	To check for infestations, scrapings are placed on slide with mineral oil and viewed microscopically.	Instruct patient about purpose of test. Prepare slide.
Immunofluorescent studies	Some skin diseases have specific, abnormal antibody proteins that can be identified by fluorescent studies. Both skin tissue and serum can be examined.	Inform patient about purpose of test. Assist in obtaining specimen. For punch biopsy of tissue, place specimen in special fixative (e.g., Michel's) and not formalin.
Miscellaneous		
Wood's lamp (black light)	Examination of skin with long-wave ultraviolet light causes specific substances to fluoresce (e.g., *Pseudomonas* organisms, fungal infections, vitiligo).	Explain purpose of examination. Inform patient it is not painful. Room is darkened for examination.
Patch test	Used to determine whether patient is allergic to specific testing material. Small amount of potentially allergenic material applied, usually to skin on back.	Explain purpose and procedure to patient. Instruct patient to return in 48-72 hr for removal of allergens and at 96 hr for preliminary evaluation (see Fig. 23-10).

BRIDGE TO NCLEX EXAMINATION

The number of the question corresponds to the same-numbered outcome at the beginning of the chapter.

1. The primary function of the skin is
   a. insulation.
   b. protection.
   c. sensation.
   d. absorption.
2. Age-related changes in the hair and nails include *(select all that apply)*
   a. oily scalp.
   b. scaly scalp.
   c. thinner nails.
   d. thicker, brittle nails.
   e. longitudinal nail ridging.
3. When assessing the nutritional-metabolic pattern in relation to the skin, the nurse questions the patient regarding
   a. joint pain.
   b. the use of moisturizing shampoo.
   c. recent changes in wound healing.
   d. self-care habits related to daily hygiene.
4. During the physical examination of a patient's skin, the nurse would
   a. use a flashlight in a poorly lit room.
   b. note cool, moist skin as a normal finding.
   c. pinch up a fold of skin to assess for turgor.
   d. perform a lesion-specific examination first and then a general inspection.
5. The nurse assessed the patient's skin lesions as firm, edematous, irregularly shaped with a variable diameter. They would be called
   a. wheals.
   b. papules.
   c. pustules.
   d. plaques.
6. To assess the skin for temperature and moisture, the most appropriate technique for the nurse to use is
   a. palpation.
   b. inspection.
   c. percussion.
   d. auscultation.

7. Individuals with dark skin are more likely to develop
   a. keloids.
   b. wrinkles.
   c. skin rashes.
   d. skin cancer.
8. On inspection of a patient's dark skin, the nurse notes a blue-gray birthmark on the forehead and eye area. This assessment finding is called
   a. vitiligo.
   b. intertrigo.
   c. telangiectasia.
   d. Nevus of Ota.
9. Diagnostic testing is recommended for skin lesions when
   a. a health history cannot be obtained.
   b. a more definitive diagnosis is needed.
   c. percussion reveals an abnormal finding.
   d. treatment with prescribed medication has failed.

1. b, 2. b, d, e, 3. c, 4. c, 5. a, 6. a, 7. a, 8. d, 9. b

evolve

For rationales to these answers and even more NCLEX review questions, visit *http://evolve.elsevier.com/Lewis/medsurg.*

REFERENCES

1. Patton KT, Thibodeau GA, Douglas M: *Essentials of anatomy and physiology*, St Louis, 2012, Mosby.
2. Goldsmith L, Katz S, Gilcrest B, et al: *Fitzpatrick's dermatology in general medicine*, ed 8, New York, 2012, McGraw-Hill.
3. Thibodeau GA, Patton KT: *Structure and function of the body*, ed 14, St Louis, 2011, Mosby.
4. Burnett C, Ozog D: Aging gracefully, *Dermatol Nurs* 22:11, 2010.
5. Jarvis C: *Physical examination and health assessment*, ed 6, Philadelphia, 2012, Saunders.
6. Micali MD, Lacarrubba F, Massimino D, et al: Dermatoscopy: alternative daily uses in clinical practice, *J Am Acad Dermatol* 64:1135, 2011.

RESOURCES

Resources for this chapter are listed after Chapter 24 on p. 449.

Though we travel the world over to find the beautiful, we must carry it with us or we will not find it.
Ralph Waldo Emerson

CHAPTER 24

Nursing Management Integumentary Problems

Shannon Ruff Dirksen

evolve WEBSITE

http://evolve.elsevier.com/Lewis/medsurg

- NCLEX Review Questions
- Key Points
- Pre-Test
- Answer Guidelines for Case Study on p. 447
- Rationales for Bridge to NCLEX Examination Questions
- Nursing Care Plans (Customizable)
  - eNCP 24-1: Patient With Chronic Skin Lesions
- Concept Map Creator
- Glossary
- Content Updates

eFigures

- eFig. 24-1: Squamous cell carcinoma of the finger
- eFig. 24-2: Candidiasis in interdigital cleft
- eFig. 24-3: Scabies infestation on hand
- eFig. 24-4: Seborrheic keratosis
- eFig. 24-5: PUVA unit for phototherapy
- eFig. 24-6: Curettage

eTable

- eTable 24-1: Diseases With Dermatologic Manifestations

LEARNING OUTCOMES

1. Specify health promotion practices related to the integumentary system.
2. Explain the etiology, clinical manifestations, and nursing and collaborative management of common acute dermatologic problems.
3. Summarize the psychologic and physiologic effects of chronic dermatologic conditions.
4. Explain the etiology, clinical manifestations, and nursing and collaborative management of malignant dermatologic disorders.
5. Explain the etiology, clinical manifestations, and nursing and collaborative management of bacterial, viral, and fungal infections of the integument.
6. Describe the etiology, clinical manifestations, and nursing and collaborative management of infestations and insect bites.
7. Explain the etiology, clinical manifestations, and nursing and collaborative management of allergic dermatologic disorders.
8. Explain the etiology, clinical manifestations, and nursing and collaborative management related to benign dermatologic disorders.
9. Distinguish the dermatologic manifestations of common systemic diseases.
10. Explain the indications and nursing management related to common cosmetic procedures and skin grafts.

KEY TERMS

acne vulgaris, Table 24-9, p. 439
actinic keratosis, p. 431
basal cell carcinoma (BCC), p. 431
cellulitis, Table 24-4, p. 434
cryosurgery, p. 442
curettage, p. 442
dysplastic nevi (DN), p. 434
herpes zoster, Table 24-5, p. 436
impetigo, Table 24-4, p. 434
lichenification, p. 444
malignant melanoma, p. 432
psoriasis, p. 437
squamous cell carcinoma (SCC), p. 431
sun protection factor (SPF), p. 428
urticaria, Table 24-8, p. 438

In this chapter health promotion of the skin, common dermatologic conditions, and malignant skin neoplasms are discussed. Nursing management of patients with dermatologic conditions is emphasized.

HEALTH PROMOTION

Health promotion practices related to the skin often parallel practices for general good health. The skin reflects both physical and psychologic well-being. Specific health promotion activities appropriate to good skin health include avoidance of environmental hazards, adequate hygiene and nutrition, and skin self-examination.

Environmental Hazards

Sun Exposure. Years of exposure to the sun are cumulative and damaging. The ultraviolet (UV) rays of the sun cause degenerative changes in the dermis, resulting in premature

Reviewed by Lakshi M. Aldredge, RN, MSN, ANP-BC, Nurse Practitioner, Dermatology Service, Portland VA Medical Center, Portland, Oregon; and Brenda C. Morris, RN, EdD, CNE, Senior Director, Baccalaureate Nursing and Clinical Associate Professor, College of Nursing and Health Innovation, Arizona State University, Phoenix, Arizona.

aging (e.g., loss of elasticity, thinning, wrinkling, drying of the skin). Prolonged and repeated sun exposure is a major factor in precancerous and cancerous lesions. Actinic keratosis, basal cell carcinoma, squamous cell carcinoma, and malignant melanoma are dermatologic problems that are associated with direct or indirect sun exposure.

Safe sun practices are important for you to emphasize to the patient. Specific wavelengths of the sun (Table 24-1) have different effects on the skin. Sunlight is composed of visible light and UV light. There are two types of UV light: UVA and UVB. UVA light is responsible for tanning and UVB for sunburn. Both types can damage the skin and increase the risk of skin cancer. Both UVA and UVB can cause collagen damage and accelerate the aging of skin. Tanning is the skin's response to injury and is caused by the increased production of melanin. When sun exposure is excessive, the turnover time of the skin becomes shortened, which can result in peeling. Fair-skinned persons should be especially cautious about excessive sun exposure because they have less melanin and thus less natural protection.

TABLE 24-1 WAVELENGTHS OF SUN AND EFFECTS ON SKIN

Wavelength	Effect
Long (ultraviolet A [UVA])	Can produce elastic tissue damage and actinic skin damage. Contributes to formation of skin cancer.
Middle (ultraviolet B [UVB])	Causes sunburn and cumulative effect of sun damage. Major factor in development of skin cancer.
Short (ultraviolet C [UVC])	Does not reach earth, since it is blocked by atmosphere.

EVIDENCE-BASED PRACTICE

Applying the Evidence

You are a nurse helping in a skin cancer screening clinic. W.S., a 24-year-old woman with a fair skin type (blond hair and blue eyes), is completing her health history before her screening examination. She indicates that she visits an indoor tanning salon every other week. She tells you that being tan makes her feel "more attractive." You spend time explaining the increased risk of skin cancer associated with the use of tanning booths.

Best Available Evidence	Clinician Expertise	Patient Preferences and Values
American Academy of Dermatology reports a strong link between exposure to indoor tanning devices and development of skin cancer and melanoma.	You note that W.S. has the following skin cancer risk factors: fair skin, blond hair, blue eyes, frequent use of tanning booths.	After listening, the patient tells you that she will consider reducing the frequency of her visits—going only when she has an important event to attend.

Your Decision and Action

As her nurse, you accept her decision, tell her that this is a step in the right direction, and encourage her to consider completely stopping her usage of the tanning booth.

Reference for Evidence

American Academy of Dermatology: The dangers of indoor tanning. Retrieved from *www.aad.org/skin-care-and-safety/skin-cancer-prevention/indoor-tanning*.

Patients should recognize that sun safety guidelines include sun avoidance (especially during the midday hours), protective clothing, and sunscreen. Advise the patient on ways to avoid the damaging effects of the sun, such as wearing a large-brimmed hat, sunglasses, and a long-sleeved shirt of a lightly woven fabric or carrying an umbrella. Patients need to know that the rays of the sun are most dangerous between 10:00 AM and 2:00 PM standard time or 11:00 AM and 3:00 PM daylight saving time, regardless of the latitude. Even on overcast days, serious sunburn can occur because up to 80% of the sun's UV rays can penetrate the clouds.

Other factors that increase the possibility of sunburn include being at high altitude, being in snow (reflects 80% of the sun's rays), or being in or near water. Warn people of the dangers of tanning booths and sun lamps, which are UVA. Tanning booths increase the risk of sunburn and contribute to the development of skin cancer.[1]

Sunscreens can filter both UVA and UVB wavelengths. The two types of topical sunscreens are chemical and physical. Chemical sunscreens are light creams or lotions designed to absorb or filter UV light, resulting in diminished UV light penetration. Physical sunscreens are thick, opaque, heavy creams that reflect UV radiation.

The U.S. Food and Drug Administration (FDA) rates sunscreen products on their **sun protection factor (SPF).** The SPF

EVIDENCE-BASED PRACTICE

Translating Research Into Practice

Is Sun-Protective Counseling Effective?

Clinical Question

In adults (P) does sun-protective counseling (I) improve safe sun behaviors (O)?

Best Available Evidence

Systematic review of randomized controlled trials (RCTs)

Critical Appraisal and Synthesis of Evidence

- Five RCTs (n = 6949) of middle-aged white men and women and three RCTS (n = 897) of young adults examined the effect of counseling on sun-protective behaviors. Trials ranged from one to several sessions of in-person counseling, phone counseling, or tailored risk written feedback.
- Counseling with tailored feedback influenced sun-protective behaviors in older adults.
- Appearance-focused counseling reduced indoor tanning use among young adult women.

Conclusion

- Relevant counseling by primary health care providers can increase sun-protective behaviors and decrease indoor tanning.

Implications for Nursing Practice

- Promote safe sun behaviors for patients to decrease ultraviolet exposure, including sunscreen use, sun avoidance hours, and protective clothing.
- Emphasize the dangers of tanning booth use among college students.
- Tailor sun safety interventions to the target population.

Reference for Evidence

Lin J, Eder M, Weinmann S: Behavioral counseling to prevent skin cancer: a systematic review for the U.S. Preventive Services Task Force, *Ann Intern Med* 154:190, 2011.

P, Patient population of interest; *I*, intervention or area of interest; *O*, outcomes of interest (see p. 12).

measures the effectiveness of a sunscreen in filtering and absorbing UV radiation. All sunscreen labels in the United States must state which rays they protect against. Products labeled with "broad protection" block both UVA and UVB.[2] Sunscreen broad protection labeling is allowed only if the product has an SPF of at least 15. Sunscreen should no longer be labeled as "waterproof" and "sweat proof." The product should only state if it is "water resistant."

Consumers need to select the sunscreen most appropriate for their needs. Para-aminobenzoic acid (PABA) and PABA esters, cinnamates, salicylates, and methyl anthranilate block UVB rays. PABA has been removed from many sunscreen products because it stains clothing and can cause allergic reactions, including contact dermatitis. Avobenzone (Parsol) blocks UVA rays and has been added to some sunscreens. The benzophenones block both UVA and UVB rays.

The general recommendation is that everyone should use a sunscreen with a minimum SPF of 15 daily. Teach patients to look for the term *broad spectrum* on sunscreen packaging. Sunscreens with an SPF of 15 or more filter 92% of the UVB rays that are responsible for erythema, and make sunburn unlikely when applied appropriately. Patients who have a history of skin cancer or problems with sun sensitivity should use a product with an SPF of at least 30. Sunscreens should be applied 20 to 30 minutes before going outdoors, even in cloudy weather. The SPF value of all sunscreens decreases with time after application, and therefore sunscreen should be reapplied every 2 hours in a sufficient amount. One ounce per total body application is recommended. The ears, toes, and lips also need sunscreen. Sunscreens are not "waterproof" and should be reapplied immediately after swimming. Regular sunscreen use decreases the rate of developing melanoma.[3]

Certain topical and systemic medications potentiate the effect of the sun, even with brief exposure. Categories of drug therapy that may contain common photosensitizing medications are listed in Table 24-2. Be aware that many drugs are included in these categories. Examine the photosensitivity of each individual drug. The chemicals in these medications absorb light when exposed to natural sunlight and release energy that harms cells and tissues. The clinical manifestations of drug-induced photosensitivity (Fig. 24-1) are similar to those of exaggerated sunburn. These include swelling; erythema; vesicles; and papular, plaquelike lesions. Skin that is at risk for photosensitivity reactions can be protected by the use of sunscreen products. Teach patients who are taking these drugs about their photosensitizing effect.

CULTURAL & ETHNIC HEALTH DISPARITIES

Integumentary Problems

- African Americans and Native Americans have a lower incidence of skin cancer than whites.
- Melanoma can occur in dark-skinned individuals, but often goes unrecognized until the advanced stages.
- Skin assessment may be difficult in individuals with darker skin. The oral mucous membranes and conjunctiva are areas where pallor, cyanosis, and jaundice are more readily detected. The palms of the hands and soles of the feet can also be used for assessment of the skin of darker individuals.
- When darker skin heals after injury or inflammation, it tends to be hypopigmented or hyperpigmented.

Irritants and Allergens. Patients can seek treatment for irritant or allergic dermatitis, which are two types of contact dermatitis. *Irritant contact dermatitis* is produced by direct chemical injury to the skin. *Allergic contact dermatitis* is an antigen-specific, type IV delayed hypersensitivity response. This response requires sensitization and occurs only in individuals who are predisposed to react to a particular antigen (see Chapter 14).

Counsel patients to avoid known irritants (e.g., ammonia, harsh detergents). Skin patch testing (application of allergens) can sometimes help determine the most likely sensitizing agent. Sometimes the health care provider is the first to detect a contact

TABLE 24-2 DRUG THERAPY

Drugs That May Cause Photosensitivity

Categories	Examples
Anticancer drugs	methotrexate, vinorelbine (Navelbine)
Antidepressants	amitriptyline (Elavil), clomipramine (Anafranil), doxepin (Sinequan)
Antidysrhythmics	quinidine, amiodarone (Cordarone)
Antihistamines	diphenhydramine (Benadryl), chlorpheniramine, clemastine (Tavist)
Antimicrobials	tetracycline, sulfamethoxazole, azithromycin (Zithromax), ciprofloxacin (Cipro)
Antifungals	griseofulvin, ketoconazole (Nizoral)
Antipsychotics	chlorpromazine (Thorazine), haloperidol (Haldol)
Diuretics	furosemide (Lasix), hydrochlorothiazide (HydroDIURIL)
Hypoglycemics	tolbutamide (Orinase), glipizide (Glucotrol), chlorpropamide (Diabinese)
Nonsteroidal antiinflammatory drugs	diclofenac (Voltaren), piroxicam (Feldene), sulindac (Clinoril)

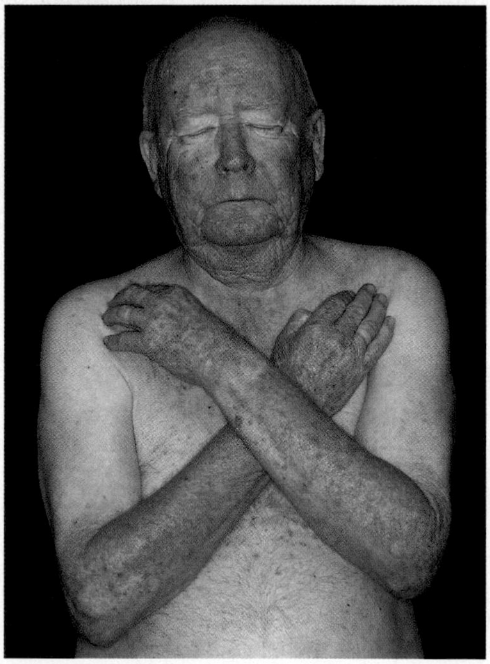

FIG. 24-1 Intense eruption in areas exposed to sunlight after patient started on hydrochlorothiazide.

allergy to various metals, gloves (latex), and adhesives. Prescribed and over-the-counter (OTC) topical and systemic medications used to treat a variety of conditions may contain fragrances and preservatives that can cause dermatologic reactions.

Radiation. Although most radiology departments are extremely cautious in protecting both themselves and their patients from the effects of excessive radiation, it is important for you to help the patient make decisions about radiologic procedures. X-rays are valuable in both diagnosis and therapy but can cause serious side effects to the skin, including erythema, dry and moist desquamation, edema, and hypopigmentation or hyperpigmentation. In the past (30 years ago), acne and hirsutism were treated with radiation. This information is important for you to obtain because of an increased incidence of carcinoma for these patients.

Rest and Sleep

Sleep is restorative to the skin, as well as to the rest of the body. Pruritic skin diseases often interfere with sleep. Therefore helping patients obtain high-quality sleep is an important health-promotion consideration. Adequate rest increases the patient's ability to tolerate itching, thereby decreasing skin damage from the resultant scratching.

Exercise

Exercise increases circulation and dilates the blood vessels. In addition to the healthy glow produced by exercise, the psychologic effects can also improve one's appearance and mental outlook. However, caution must be used to prevent overexposure to heat, cold, and sun during outdoor exercise.

Hygiene

Hygienic practices are influenced by the patient's skin type, lifestyle, culture, age, and gender. The normal acidity of the skin and perspiration protect against bacterial overgrowth. Most soaps are alkaline and neutralize the skin surface, leading to a loss of protection. The use of mild, moisturizing soaps (e.g., Ivory) and lipid-free cleansers, plus avoidance of hot water and vigorous scrubbing, can noticeably decrease local skin irritation and inflammation. Skin piercings where jewelry has been inserted can be cared for with antibacterial soaps that do not contain sulfites.

In general, the skin and hair should be washed often enough to remove excess oil and excretions and to prevent odor. Older persons should avoid harsh soaps and shampoos and frequent bathing because of the dryness of their skin and scalp. Moisturizers should be used immediately after a bath or shower while the skin is still damp to seal in this moisture.

Nutrition

A well-balanced diet adequate in all food groups can produce healthy skin, hair, and nails. Important elements of skin nutrition include the following:

- *Vitamin A:* Essential for maintenance of normal cell structure, specifically epithelial cells. It is necessary for normal wound healing. The absence of vitamin A causes dryness of the conjunctiva and poor wound healing.
- *Vitamin B complex:* Essential for complex metabolic functions. Deficiencies of niacin and pyridoxine (B_6) manifest as dermatologic symptoms such as erythema, bullae, and seborrhea-like lesions.
- *Vitamin C (ascorbic acid):* Essential for connective tissue formation and normal wound healing. Absence of vitamin C causes symptoms of scurvy, including petechiae, bleeding gums, and purpura.
- *Vitamin D_3 (cholecalciferol):* Essential for bone health. It is produced naturally by cutaneous photosynthesis after UVB exposure. A deficiency manifests as bone and muscle weakness and pain.
- *Vitamin K:* Essential for synthesizing blood clotting factors. A deficiency interferes with normal prothrombin synthesis in the liver and can lead to bruising.
- *Protein:* Necessary in amounts adequate for cell growth and maintenance. It is also necessary for normal wound healing.
- *Unsaturated fatty acids:* Necessary to maintain the function and integrity of cellular and subcellular membranes in tissue metabolism. Linoleic and arachidonic acids are particularly important.

A deficiency of biotin, a water-soluble B-complex vitamin, may result in rashes and alopecia. The effectiveness of biotin supplements has not been proven. Foods high in biotin include liver, cauliflower, salmon, carrots, bananas, soy flour, cereals, and yeast.

Obesity has adverse effects on the skin. The increase in subcutaneous fat can lead to stretching and overheating (see Chapter 41). Overheating secondary to the greater insulation provided by fat causes increased sweating, which inflames and dries the skin. Obesity is also a risk factor for poor wound healing. Obesity can be associated with the development of type 2 diabetes mellitus, which may cause skin symptoms such as velvety dark skin of neck and body folds *(acanthosis nigricans)*, rash in intertriginous sites *(intertrigo)*, skin tags *(acrochordons)*, and impaired arterial and venous flow (see Chapter 49).

Self-Treatment

Determine if the patient is aware of the dangers of self-diagnosis and treatment. The increasing variety of OTC skin preparations can be confusing.

In your general instructions to the patient, stress the duration of the treatment and the need to closely follow package directions. Skin problems may be slow to produce symptoms and slow to resolve. If the package insert of an OTC drug says its use should not exceed 7 days, patients should heed this warning. Tell the patient to always follow package directions for use of OTC drugs. If any systemic signs of inflammation or extensions of the skin problem (e.g., an increased number of lesions or increased erythema or swelling) develop, the patient should stop self-care and seek the help of a health care provider.

MALIGNANT SKIN NEOPLASMS

Skin cancer is the most commonly diagnosed cancer.[4] Skin cancers are either nonmelanoma or melanoma. A persistent skin lesion that does not heal is highly suspicious for malignancy and should be examined by a health care provider. Early detection and treatment can often lead to a highly favorable prognosis. The fact that skin lesions are so visible increases the likelihood of early detection and diagnosis.

Teach patients to self-examine their skin at least on a monthly basis. The cornerstone of skin self-examination is the ABCDE rule,[5] which is easy to teach and remember. Examine skin lesions for ***A****symmetry,* ***B****order* irregularity, ***C****olor* change and

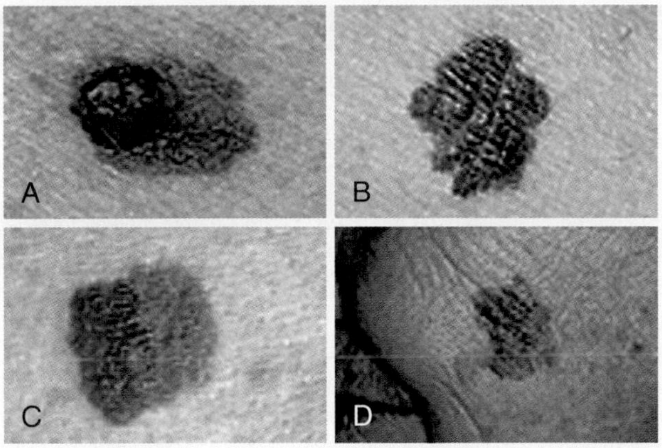

FIG. 24-2 The ABCDEs of melanoma. **A,** Asymmetry: one half unlike the other half. **B,** Border irregularity: edges are ragged, notched, or blurred. **C,** Color: varied pigmentation; shades of tan, brown, and black. **D,** Diameter: greater than 6 mm (diameter of a pencil eraser). **E,** (not pictured) Evolving; changing appearance (change in shape, size, color, or other characteristic is noted over time).

variation, ***Diameter*** of 6 mm or more, and ***Evolving*** in appearance (Fig. 24-2). Emphasize that lesions once flat and now raised, or once small and recently growing or changing in appearance, are warning signs and should be examined by a health care provider.

Risk Factors

Risk factors for skin malignancies include having a fair skin type (blond or red hair and blue or green eyes), history of chronic sun exposure, family history of skin cancer, and exposure to tar and systemic arsenicals.[6] Environmental factors that increase the risk of skin malignancies include living near the equator, outdoor occupations, and frequent outdoor recreational activities. Behavioral factors such as using indoor tanning booths and outdoor sunbathing are controllable risk factors for skin malignancies. Patients treated with oral methoxsalen (psoralen) and psoralen plus ultraviolet A radiation (PUVA) may be at greater risk for melanoma.

Dark-skinned persons are less susceptible to skin cancer because of the naturally occurring increased melanin, which is a sunscreen. However, although dark skin lowers the risk of melanoma, people with dark skin can develop melanoma, most often on the palms, soles, and mucous membranes.

The Fitzpatrick classification of skin type can assist you in determining how a patient will respond or react to facial treatments, and how likely they are to get skin cancer. This system classifies skin into six different skin types, skin color, and reaction to sun exposure.

- Type I (very white or freckled): Always burn
- Type II (white): Usually burn
- Type III (white to olive): Sometimes burn
- Type IV (brown): Rarely burn
- Type V (dark brown): Very rarely burn
- Type VI (black): Never burn

NONMELANOMA SKIN CANCERS

Nonmelanoma skin cancers, either basal cell or squamous cell carcinoma, are the most common forms of skin cancer.[7] More than 2.2 million new cases are diagnosed every year. Nonmelanoma skin cancers develop in the epidermis. They do not develop from melanocytes, the skin cells that make melanin, as melanoma skin cancers do. The most common sites for the development of nonmelanoma skin cancer are in sun-exposed areas, such as the face, head, neck, back of the hands, and arms.

Although relatively few deaths are attributable to nonmelanoma skin cancer, the tumors have an inherent potential for severe local destruction, permanent disfigurement, and disability. The most common etiologic factor is sun exposure. Avoidance of exposure to the midday sun and the use of protective clothing and sunscreens beginning early in life can prevent the formation of skin malignancies later in life.

Actinic Keratosis

Actinic keratosis, also known as solar keratosis, consists of hyperkeratotic papules and plaques on sun-exposed areas. Actinic keratoses are premalignant skin lesions that affect nearly all of the older white population. These are the most common of all precancerous skin lesions. The clinical appearance of actinic keratoses can be highly varied. The typical lesion is an irregularly shaped, flat, slightly erythematous papule with indistinct borders and an overlying hard keratotic scale or horn (Table 24-3).

Many forms of treatment are used, including cryosurgery, fluorouracil (5-FU), surgical removal, tretinoin (Retin-A), imiquimod (Aldara), diclofenac (Solaraze), chemical peeling agents, dermabrasion, laser resurfacing, and photodynamic therapy (PDT, with 5-aminolevulinic acid [5-ALA] or methyl aminolevulinate [MAL] followed by light irradiation). (These treatments are discussed later in this chapter.) Any lesion that persists should be evaluated for a possible biopsy.

Basal Cell Carcinoma

Basal cell carcinoma (BCC) is a locally invasive malignancy arising from epidermal basal cells. It is the most common type of skin cancer and also the least deadly. BCC usually occurs in middle-aged to older adults. Clinical manifestations are described in Table 24-3. The cancerous cells of BCC almost never spread beyond the skin (Fig. 24-4). However, if BCC is left untreated, massive tissue destruction may result. Some BCCs are pigmented with curled borders and an opaque appearance and may be misinterpreted as a melanoma. A tissue biopsy is needed to confirm the diagnosis.[8]

Multiple treatment modalities are used depending on the tumor location and histologic type, history of recurrence, and patient characteristics. Treatment modalities include surgical excision, electrodesiccation and curettage, cryosurgery, radiation therapy, topical or systemic chemotherapy, and photodynamic therapy. (These treatments are discussed later in this chapter.) Electrodesiccation and curettage, cryosurgery, and surgical excision all have a cure rate of greater than 90% when used correctly on primary lesions. Location and size are important factors in determining the best treatment.

Squamous Cell Carcinoma

Squamous cell carcinoma (SCC) is a malignant neoplasm of keratinizing epidermal cells (see eFig. 24-1 available on the website for this chapter). It frequently occurs on sun-exposed skin at the base of an actinic keratosis or another lesion. SCC is less common than BCC. SCC can be highly aggressive, has the potential to metastasize, and may lead to death if not treated early and correctly. Pipe, cigar, and cigarette smoking contribute

TABLE 24-3 **PREMALIGNANT AND MALIGNANT CONDITIONS OF THE SKIN**

Etiology and Pathophysiology	Clinical Manifestations	Treatment and Prognosis
Actinic Keratosis		
Actinic (sun) damage. Premalignant skin lesions. Common in older whites.	Flat or elevated, dry, hyperkeratotic scaly papule. Possibly flat, rough, or verrucous (wartlike). Adherent scale, which returns when removed. Often multiple. Rough scale on red base. Often on erythematous sun-exposed area. Increase in number with age.	Cryosurgery, chemical peels, laser resurfacing, topical application of 5-FU over entire area for 14-28 days or topical application of imiquimod (Aldara) for 16 wk, photodynamic therapy followed by light irradiation. Recurrence possible even with adequate treatment.
Atypical or Dysplastic Nevi		
Morphologically between common acquired nevi and melanoma. May be precursor of malignant melanoma.	Often >5 mm. Irregular border, possibly notched. Variegated color of tan, brown, black, red, or pink within single mole. Presence of at least one flat portion, often at edge of mole. Frequently multiple. Most common site on back, but possible in uncommon mole sites such as scalp or buttocks (Fig. 24-3).	Increased risk for melanoma. Careful monitoring of persons suspected of familial tendency to melanoma or dysplastic nevi. Excisional biopsy for suspicious lesions.
Basal Cell Carcinoma		
Change in basal cells. No maturation or normal keratinization. Continuing division of basal cells and formation of enlarging mass. Related to excessive sun exposure, genetic skin type, x-ray radiation, scars, and some types of nevi.	*Nodular and ulcerative:* Small, slowly enlarging papule. Borders semitranslucent or "pearly," with overlying telangiectasia. Erosion, ulceration, and depression of center. Normal skin markings lost (see Fig. 24-2). *Superficial:* Erythematous, pearly, sharply defined, barely elevated plaques.	Surgical excision, chemosurgery, electrosurgery, chemotherapy, cryosurgery. 90% cure rate. Slow-growing tumor that invades local tissue. Metastasis rare. 5-FU and imiquimod for superficial lesions, photodynamic therapy for small lesions, vismodegib (Erivedge) for metastatic or recurrent locally invasive lesions.
Squamous Cell Carcinoma		
Frequent occurrence on previously damaged skin (e.g., from sun, radiation, scar). Malignant tumor of squamous cell of epidermis. Invasion of dermis, surrounding skin.	*Superficial:* Thin, scaly erythematous plaque without invasion into the dermis. *Early:* Firm nodules with indistinct borders, scaling and ulceration (see eFig. 24-1). *Late:* Covering of lesion with scale or horn from keratinization, ulceration. Most common on sun-exposed areas such as face and hands.	Surgical excision, cryosurgery, radiation therapy, chemotherapy, electrodesiccation and curettage. Untreated lesion may metastasize to regional lymph nodes and distant organs. High cure rate with early detection and treatment.
Malignant Melanoma		
Neoplastic growth of melanocytes anywhere on skin, eyes, or mucous membranes. Classification according to major histologic mode of spread. Potential invasion and widespread metastases.	Irregular color, surface, and border. Variegated color, including red, white, blue, black, gray, brown. Flat or elevated. Eroded or ulcerated. Often <1 cm in size. Most common sites in males are back, then chest. In females are legs, then back (see Fig. 24-2).	Surgical excision and possible sentinel lymph node evaluation depending on the depth. Correlation of survival rate with depth of invasion. Poor prognosis unless diagnosed and treated early. Spreading by local extension, regional lymphatic vessels, and bloodstream. Possible use of adjuvant therapy after surgery if lesion >1.5 mm in depth.
Cutaneous T-Cell Lymphoma		
Origination in skin. Localized chronic, slowly progressing disease. Possibly related to environmental toxins and chemical exposure. Mycosis fungoides (MF) is most common form. Sézary syndrome is an advanced form of MF. Prevalence twice as high in men as in women in United States.	Classic presentation involves three stages—patch (early), plaque, and tumor (advanced). History of persistent macular eruption followed by gradual appearance of indurated erythematous plaques on the trunk that appear similar to psoriasis. Pruritus, lymphadenopathy.	Treatment usually controls symptoms, not curative. UVB, PUVA, corticosteroids, topical nitrogen mustard, radiation therapy in patch and plaque stage disease. Interferon, systemic chemotherapy, extracorporeal photopheresis, romidepsin (Istodax) for progressive disease. Bexarotene (Targretin), denileukin diftitox (Ontak), and vorinostat (Zolinza) for advanced disease. Disease course is unpredictable, 10% will have progressive disease.

5-FU, Fluorouracil; *PUVA,* psoralen ultraviolet A; *UVB,* ultraviolet B.

to the formation of SCC on the mouth and lips. The clinical manifestations of SCC are described in Table 24-3. A biopsy should always be performed when a lesion is suspected to be SCC.

MALIGNANT MELANOMA

Malignant melanoma is a tumor arising in melanocytes, which are the cells producing melanin. Melanoma causes the majority of skin cancer deaths. More than 132,000 new cases are diagnosed every year worldwide. Melanoma has the ability to metastasize to any organ, including the brain and the heart. The death rate of melanoma is 10 times higher in white persons than in African Americans.[4]

Although the exact cause of melanoma is unknown, a combination of environmental and genetic factors is involved. The use of immunosuppressive drugs and a history of dysplastic nevi also increase a person's risk. UV radiation from the sun is

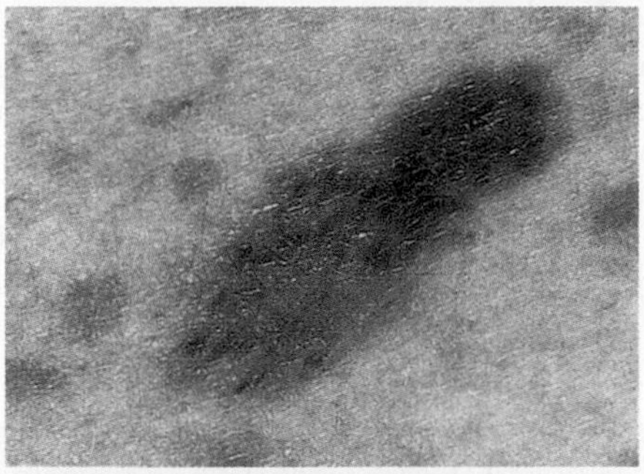

FIG. 24-3 Dysplastic nevus. Irregular border and color.

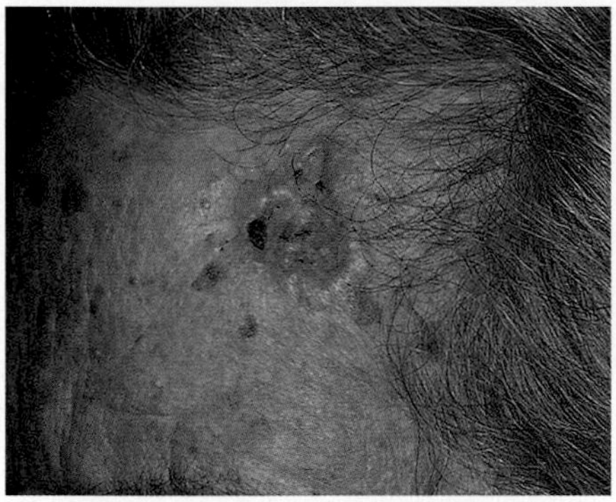

FIG. 24-4 Basal cell carcinoma. Rolled, well-defined border and central erosion.

the main cause of melanomas and other skin cancer, but artificial sources of UV radiation, such as sunlamps and tanning booths, also play a role. UV radiation damages the deoxyribonucleic acid (DNA) in skin cells, creating "misspellings" in their genetic code. As a result, these cells are altered.

Although anyone can develop melanoma, the risk is greatest for people who have red or blond hair, blue or light-colored eyes, and light-colored skin that freckles easily. These people have less melanin and thus less protection from UV radiation.

A person may have a genetic predisposition toward getting melanoma. Between 5% and 10% of people who develop melanoma have a first-degree relative (e.g., parent, full sibling) who developed melanoma. This risk increases significantly if multiple relatives have a history of melanoma. Mutated genes have been identified in some families who have a high familial incidence of melanoma.

Clinical Manifestations

About one fourth of melanomas occur in existing nevi or moles; about 20% occur in dysplastic nevi (see Table 24-3). Melanoma frequently occurs on the lower legs and backs in women and on the trunk, head, and neck in men. Because most melanoma cells continue to produce melanin, melanoma tumors are often dark brown or black. Individuals should consult their health care provider immediately if their moles or lesions show any of the clinical signs (ABCDEs) of melanoma (see Fig. 24-2). Any sudden or progressive change or increase in the size, color, or shape of a mole should be evaluated.

When melanoma begins in the skin, it is called *cutaneous melanoma.* Melanoma can also occur in the eye (see Fig. 22-8), meninges, lymph nodes, digestive tract, and anywhere else in the body where melanocytes are found.

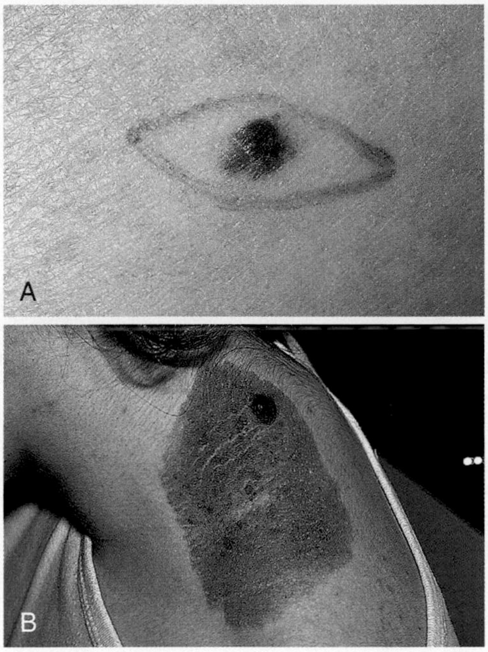

FIG. 24-5 Breslow measurement of tumor thickness. **A,** Thin (0.08 mm) superficial spreading melanoma, good prognosis. **B,** Thick nodular melanoma with lymph node involvement, poor prognosis.

Collaborative Care

Pigmented lesions suspicious for melanoma should not be shave-biopsied, shave-excised, or electrocauterized. Handheld screening devices (e.g., MelaFind) can assist the health care provider in determining if a lesion without the obvious ABCDE signs should be biopsied. All suspicious lesions should be biopsied using an excisional biopsy technique.

The most important prognostic factor is tumor thickness at the time of diagnosis. Two methods to determine thickness are currently being used. The *Breslow measurement* indicates the depth of the tumor in millimeters (Fig. 24-5), and the *Clark level* indicates the depth of invasion of the tumor; the higher the number, the deeper the melanoma.

Treatment depends on the site of the original tumor, the stage of the cancer, and the patient's age and general health. The staging of melanoma (stages 0 to IV) is based on tumor size (thickness), nodal involvement, and metastasis. In stage 0 the melanoma is confined to one place (in situ) in the epidermis. Melanoma is nearly 100% curable by excision if diagnosed at stage 0. The 5-year survival rate depends on sentinel node biopsy results, which indicate if metastasis has occurred. If metastasis to other organs is found (stage IV), treatment then becomes palliative.

Initial treatment of malignant melanoma is surgical excision, which may require a skin graft to close (discussed later in the chapter). Melanoma that has spread to the lymph nodes or nearby sites usually requires additional (adjuvant) therapy such as chemotherapy, biologic therapy (e.g., α-interferon, interleukin-2), and/or radiation therapy. Examples of chemotherapy agents used are dacarbazine (DTIC), temozolomide (Temodar), procarbazine (Matulane), carmustine (BCNU), and lomustine (CCNU).

Newer treatment options for patients with metastatic melanoma are ipilimumab (Yervoy), vemurafenib (Zelboraf), dabrafenib (Tafinlar), and trametinib (Mekinist). Ipilimumab, a type of immunotherapy, is a monoclonal antibody that locks onto CTLA-4, a protein that normally helps keep T cells in check. By blocking the action of CTLA-4, ipilimumab boosts the immune response against melanoma cells.[9] Vemurafenib, dabrafenib, and trametinib are used for patients whose melanoma tumors express a gene mutation called *BRAF V600*.

Atypical or Dysplastic Nevus

An abnormal nevus pattern called *dysplastic nevus syndrome* identifies an individual at increased risk of melanoma. Approximately 2% to 8% of the white population has moles classified as atypical or dysplastic nevi. **Dysplastic nevi (DN),** or atypical moles, are nevi that are larger than usual (greater than 5 mm across) with irregular borders and various shades of color (see

TABLE 24-4 COMMON BACTERIAL INFECTIONS OF THE SKIN

Etiology and Pathophysiology	Clinical Manifestations	Treatment and Prognosis
Impetigo		
Group A β-hemolytic streptococci, staphylococci, or combination of both. Associated with poor hygiene. Primary or secondary infection. Contagious.	Vesiculopustular lesions that develop thick, honey-colored crust surrounded by erythema. Pruritic. Most common on face as primary infection.	*Systemic antibiotics:* Oral penicillin, benzathine penicillin, erythromycin. *Local treatment:* Warm saline or aluminum acetate soaks followed by soap-and-water removal of crusts. Topical antibiotic cream or ointment (mupirocin [Bactroban], retapamulin [Altabax]). With no treatment, glomerulonephritis possible when streptococcal strain nephritogenic. Meticulous hygiene essential.
Folliculitis		
Usually staphylococci. Present in areas subjected to friction, moisture, rubbing, or oil. Increased incidence in patients with diabetes mellitus.	Small pustule at hair follicle opening with minimal erythema. Development of crusting. Most common on scalp, beard, extremities in men. Tender to touch.	Antistaphylococcal soap (e.g., Hibiclens, Lever 2000, Dial) and water cleansing. Topical antibiotics (e.g., mupirocin). Warm compresses of water or aluminum acetate solution. Healing usually without scarring. If lesions extensive and deep, possible scarring, loss of involved hair follicles, and treatment with systemic antibiotics.
Furuncle		
Deep infection with staphylococci around hair follicle, often associated with severe acne or seborrheic dermatitis.	Tender erythematous area around hair follicle. Draining pus and core of necrotic debris on rupture. Most common on face, back of neck, axillae, breasts, buttocks, perineum, thighs. Painful.	Incision and drainage, possibly with packing, antibiotics, meticulous care of involved skin, frequent application of warm, moist compresses.
Furunculosis		
Increased incidence in patients who are obese, diabetic, chronically ill, or regularly exposed to moisture, pressure.	Lesions as above. Malaise, regional adenopathy, elevated body temperature.	Incision and drainage of painful nodules. Warm, moist compresses to erythematous plaques. Systemic antibiotic after culture and sensitivity study of drainage (usually semisynthetic, penicillinase-resistant, oral penicillin such as cloxacillin and oxacillin). Measures to reduce surface staphylococci include antimicrobial cream to nares, armpits, and groin and antiseptic to entire skin. Often recurrent with scarring. Prevention or correction of predisposing factors. Meticulous personal hygiene.
Carbuncle		
Multiple, interconnecting furuncles.	Many pustules appearing in erythematous area, most common at nape of neck.	Treatment same as for furuncles. Often recurrent despite production of antibodies. Healing slow with scar formation.
Cellulitis		
Inflammation of subcutaneous tissues. Possibly secondary complication or primary infection. Often following break in skin. *Staphylococcus aureus* and streptococci usual causative agents. Deep inflammation of subcutaneous tissue from enzymes produced by bacteria.	Hot, tender, erythematous, and edematous area with diffuse borders. Chills, malaise, and fever (Fig. 24-6).	Moist heat, immobilization and elevation, systemic antibiotic therapy, hospitalization if severe. Progression to gangrene possible if untreated.
Erysipelas		
Superficial cellulitis primarily involving the dermis. Group A β-hemolytic streptococci.	Red, hot, sharply demarcated plaque that is indurated and painful. Bacteremia possible. Most common on face and extremities. Toxic signs, such as fever, ↑ white blood cell count, headache, malaise.	Systemic antibiotics, usually penicillin. Hospitalization often required.

Fig. 24-3). These nevi may have the same ABCDE characteristics as melanoma, but they are less pronounced. The earliest clinically detectable abnormality associated with DN is an increase in the number of morphologically normal-looking nevi that occur in children between 2 and 6 years of age. Another proliferation occurs around adolescence, and new nevi continue to appear throughout the person's life. The average number of normal nevi in adults is about 40. Individuals with DN may have more than 100 normal-appearing nevi. Obtain a detailed family history related to melanoma and DN. The risk of developing melanoma doubles with the presence of one DN, and having multiple DN increases the risk up to 12-fold.

SKIN INFECTIONS AND INFESTATIONS

Bacterial Infections

The skin provides an ideal environment for bacterial growth with an abundant supply of nutrients, water, and warm temperature. Bacterial infection occurs when the balance between the host and the microorganisms is altered. This can occur as a primary infection after a break in the skin. It can also occur as a secondary infection to already damaged skin or as a sign of a systemic disease (Table 24-4). *Staphylococcus aureus* and group A β-hemolytic streptococci are the major types of bacteria responsible for primary and secondary skin infections.

Healthy persons can develop bacterial skin infections. Predisposing factors such as moisture, obesity, atopic dermatitis, systemic corticosteroids and antibiotics, and chronic disease such as diabetes mellitus all increase the likelihood of infection. Good hygiene practices and general good health inhibit bacterial infections. If an infection is present, the resulting drainage is infectious. Good skin hygiene and infection control practices are necessary to prevent the spread of the infection.

Viral Infections

Viral infections of the skin are as difficult to treat as viral infections anywhere in the body. When a virus infects a cell, a skin lesion may develop. Lesions can also result from an inflammatory response to viral infections. Herpes simplex, herpes zoster (Fig. 24-7), and warts (Fig. 24-8) are the most common viral infections affecting the skin (Table 24-5).

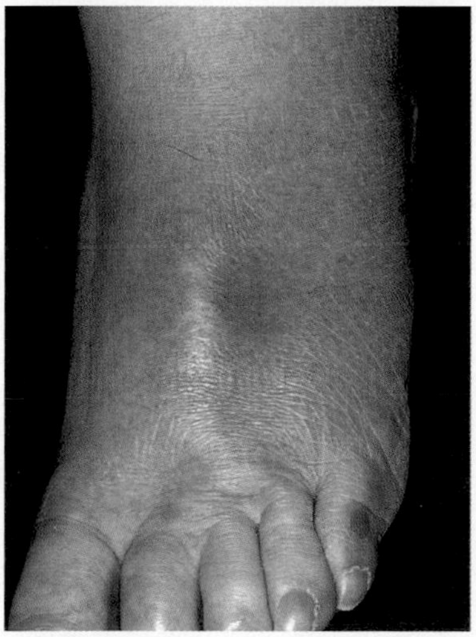

FIG. 24-6 Cellulitis with characteristic erythema, tenderness, and edema.

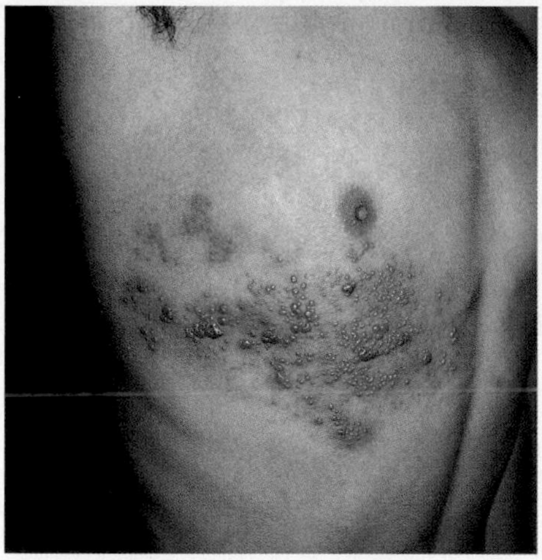

FIG. 24-7 Herpes zoster (shingles) on the anterior chest, classic dermatomal distribution.

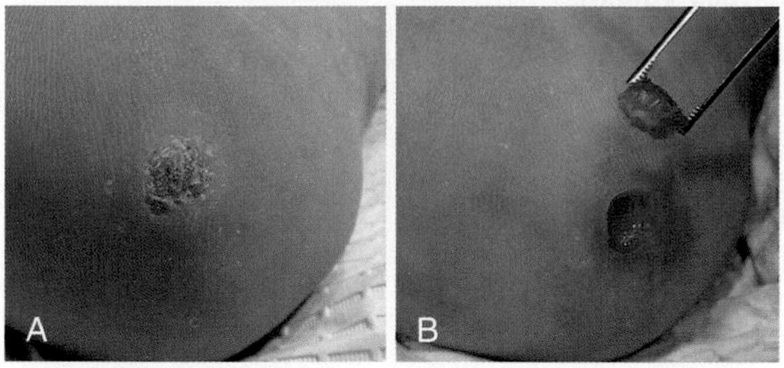

FIG. 24-8 Plantar wart. **A,** Keratotic lesion. **B,** After excision.

Fungal Infections

Because of the large number of fungi that are present everywhere, exposure to some pathologic varieties may occur. Skin, hair, and nails may all become infected with fungi, including candidiasis (see eFig. 24-2 available on the website for this chapter) and tinea unguium (Fig. 24-9). Common fungal infections of the skin are presented in Table 24-6. Most infections are relatively harmless in healthy adults, but they can be embarrassing and distressing to the patient.[10]

The microscopic examination of the scraping of suspicious scaly skin lesions in 10% to 20% potassium hydroxide (KOH) is an inexpensive diagnostic measure to determine the presence of a fungus. The appearance of microscopic hyphae (threadlike structures) is indicative of a fungal infection.

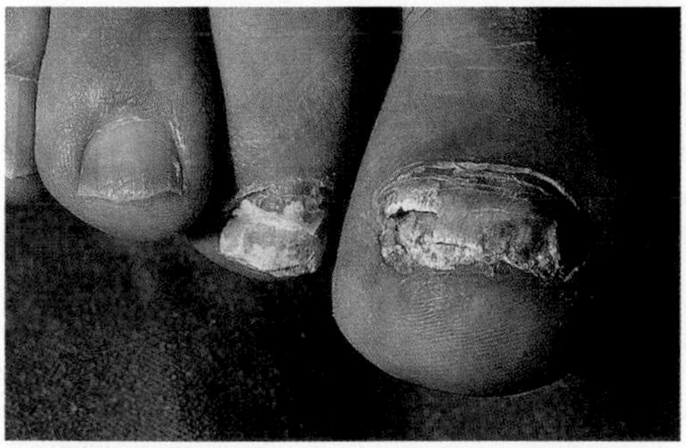

FIG. 24-9 Tinea unguium (onychomycosis). Fungal infection of toenails. Crumbly, discolored, and thickened nails.

TABLE 24-5 COMMON VIRAL INFECTIONS OF THE SKIN

Etiology and Pathophysiology	Clinical Manifestations	Treatment and Prognosis
Herpes Simplex Virus (HSV) Types 1 and 2		
Oral or genital HSV infections can be serotyped as either HSV-1 or HSV-2. Both are recurrent lifelong viral infections. Exacerbated by sunlight, trauma, menses, stress, and systemic infection. Contagious to those not previously infected. Transmission by respiratory droplets or virus-containing fluid (e.g., saliva, cervical secretions). Infection in one area is readily transmitted to another site by contact.	*First episode:* Symptoms occurring 3-7 days or more after contact, Painful local reaction. Single or grouped vesicles on erythematous base. Systemic symptoms (e.g., fever, malaise) possible or no symptoms possible. *Recurrent:* Small. Recurrence in similar spot. Characteristic grouped vesicles on erythematous base.	Symptomatic medication. Soothing, moist compresses. White petrolatum to lesions. Scarring not usual result. Antiviral agents such as acyclovir (Zovirax), famciclovir (Famvir), and valacyclovir (Valtrex). Vaccine not currently available for HSV-1 or HSV-2.
Herpes Zoster (Shingles)		
Activation of the varicella-zoster virus. Incidence increases with age. Potentially contagious to anyone who has not had varicella or who is immunosuppressed. >1 million cases annually in the United States.	Linear distribution along a dermatome of grouped vesicles and pustules on erythematous base resembling chickenpox. Usually unilateral on trunk, face, and lumbosacral areas. Burning, pain, and neuralgia preceding outbreak. Mild to severe pain during outbreak (see Fig. 24-7).	Symptomatic. Antiviral agents such as acyclovir, famciclovir, and valacyclovir within 72 hr to prevent postherpetic neuralgia. Wet compresses, silver sulfadiazine (Silvadene) to ruptured vesicles. Analgesia. Mild sedation at bedtime. Gabapentin (Neurontin) to treat postherpetic neuralgia. Usually heals without complications, but scarring and postherpetic neuralgia possible. Vaccine (Zostavax) to prevent shingles is available for adults ≥50 yr.
Verruca Vulgaris		
Caused by human papillomavirus (HPV). Spontaneous disappearance in 1-2 yr possible. Mildly contagious by autoinoculation. Specific response dependent on body part affected. Prevalence greater in youth and immunosuppressed.	Circumscribed, hypertrophic, flesh-colored papule limited to epidermis. Painful on lateral compression.	Multiple treatments, including surgery using blunt dissection with scissors or curette. Liquid nitrogen therapy. Blistering agent (cantharidin). Keratolytic agent (salicylic acid). CO_2 laser destruction.
Plantar Warts		
Caused by HPV.	Wart on bottom surface of foot, growing inward because of pressure of walking or standing. Painful when pressure applied. Interrupted skin markings. Cone shaped with black dots (thrombosed vessels) when wart removed (see Fig. 24-8).	Topical immunotherapy (imiquimod), cryosurgery, salicylic acid, duct tape.

TABLE 24-6 COMMON FUNGAL INFECTIONS OF THE SKIN

Etiology and Pathophysiology	Clinical Manifestations	Treatment and Prognosis
Candidiasis		
Caused by *Candida albicans*. Also known as moniliasis. 50% of adults symptom-free carriers. Appears in warm, moist areas such as groin area, oral mucosa, and submammary folds. HIV infection, chemotherapy, radiation, and organ transplantation related to depression of cell-mediated immunity that allows yeast to become pathogenic.	*Mouth:* White, cheesy plaque, resembles milk curds. *Vagina:* Vaginitis with red, edematous, painful vaginal wall, white patches. Vaginal discharge. Pruritus. Pain on urination and intercourse. *Skin:* Diffuse papular erythematous rash with pinpoint satellite lesions around edges of affected area (see eFig. 24-2).	Microscopic examination and culture. Azole antifungals (e.g., fluconazole, ketoconazole) or other specific medication such as vaginal suppository or oral lozenge. Sexual abstinence or use of condom. Skin hygiene to keep area clean and dry. Powder is effective on nonmucosal surfaces of skin to prevent recurrence.
Tinea Corporis		
Various dermatophytes, commonly referred to as ringworm.	Typical annular (ringlike) scaly appearance, well-defined margins. Erythematous.	Cool compresses. Topical antifungals for isolated patches. Creams or solutions of miconazole, ketoconazole, clotrimazole, butenafine.
Tinea Cruris		
Various dermatophytes, commonly referred to as jock itch.	Well-defined scaly plaque in groin area. Does not affect mucous membranes.	Topical antifungal cream or solution.
Tinea Pedis		
Various dermatophytes, commonly referred to as athlete's foot.	Interdigital scaling and maceration. Scaly plantar surfaces sometimes with erythema and blistering. May be pruritic. Possibly painful.	Topical antifungal cream, gel, solution, spray, or powder.
Tinea Unguium (Onychomycosis)		
Various dermatophytes. Incidence increases with age.	Only few nails on one hand may be affected. Toenails more commonly affected. Scaliness under distal nail plate. Brittle, thickened, broken, or crumbling nails with yellowish discoloration (see Fig. 24-9).	Oral antifungal (terbinafine [Lamisil], itraconazole [Sporanox]). Topical antifungal cream or solution (minimal effectiveness) if unable to tolerate systemic treatment. Thinning of toenails if needed. Nail avulsion (removal) is an option.

TABLE 24-7 COMMON INFESTATIONS AND INSECT BITES

Etiology and Pathophysiology	Clinical Manifestations	Treatment and Prognosis
Bees and Wasps		
Hymenoptera species.	Intense, burning, local pain. Swelling and itching. Severe hypersensitivity possibly leading to anaphylaxis.	Cool compresses. Local application of antipruritic lotion. Antihistamines if indicated. Usually uneventful recovery.
Bedbugs		
Cimicidae species. Feeding periodic, usually at night. Present in furniture, walls during day.	Wheal surrounded by vivid flare. Firm urticaria transforming into persistent lesion. Severe pruritus. Often grouped in threes appearing on uncovered parts of body.	Bedbug controlled by chlorocyclohexane. Lesions usually requiring no treatment. Severe itching possibly requiring use of antihistamines or topical corticosteroids.
Pediculosis (Head Lice, Body Lice, Pubic Lice)		
Pediculus humanus var. *capitis, Pediculus humanus* var. *corporis, Phthirus pubis.* Obligate parasites that suck blood, leave excrement and eggs on skin and hair, live in seams of clothing (if body lice) and in hair as nits. Transmission of pubic lice often by sexual contact.	Minute, red, noninflammatory. Points flush with skin. Progression to papular wheal-like lesions. Pruritus. Secondary excoriation, especially parallel linear excoriations in intrascapular region. Firmly attached to hair shaft in head and body lice.	γ-Benzene hexachloride or pyrethrins to treat various parts of body. Application as directed. Spinosad (Natroba) topical suspension 0.9% to treat scalp and hair. Close contacts (e.g., bed partners and playmates) should be screened and treated. Do not share head gear.
Scabies		
Sarcoptes scabiei. Mite penetrates stratum corneum, deposits eggs. Allergic reaction to eggs, feces, mite parts. Transmission by direct physical contact, only occasionally by shared personal items. Rarely seen in dark-skinned people.	Severe itching, especially at night, usually not on face. Presence of burrows, especially in interdigital webs, flexor surface of wrists, genitalia, and anterior axillary folds. Erythematous papules (may be crusted), possible vesiculation, interdigital web crusting (see eFig. 24-3).	5% permethrin topical lotion, one overnight application with second application 1 wk later, may yield 95% eradication. Treat all family members, treat environment with plastic covering for 5 days, launder all clothes and linen with bleach. Treat sexual partner. Antibiotics if secondary infections present. Possible residual pruritus up to 4 wk after treatment. Recurrence possible if inadequately treated.
Ticks		
Borrelia burgdorferi (spirochete transmitted by ticks in certain areas) causes Lyme disease. Endemic areas include Northeast, Mid-Atlantic states, parts of Midwest and West (see Chapter 65).	Spreading, ringlike rash 3-4 wk after bite (see Fig. 65-7). Rash commonly in groin, buttocks, axillae, trunk, and upper arms and legs. Warm, itchy, or painful rash. Flu-like symptoms. Cardiac, arthritic, and neurologic manifestations possible. Unreliable laboratory test. No acquired immunity.	Oral antibiotics, such as doxycycline, tetracycline. IV antibiotics for arthritic, neurologic, and cardiac symptoms. Rest and healthy diet. Most patients recover.

Infestations and Insect Bites

The possibilities for exposure to *infestations* (harboring insects or worms) and insect bites are numerous. In many instances an allergy to the venom plays a major role in the reaction. In other cases the clinical manifestations are a reaction to the eggs, feces, or body parts of the invading organism. Some individuals react with a severe hypersensitivity (anaphylaxis), which can be life threatening. (Anaphylaxis is discussed in Chapter 14.)

Prevention of insect bites by avoidance or by the use of repellents is somewhat effective. Meticulous hygiene related to personal articles, clothing, bedding, and examination and care of pets, as well as careful selection of sexual partners, can reduce the incidence of infestations. Routine skin inspection is necessary in geographic areas where there is a risk of tick bites (Table 24-7). (Lyme disease, which is caused by a tick, is discussed in Chapter 65.)

ALLERGIC DERMATOLOGIC PROBLEMS

Dermatologic problems associated with allergies and hypersensitivity reactions may present a challenge to the clinician (Table 24-8). The pathophysiology related to allergic and contact dermatitis is discussed in Chapter 14. A careful family history and discussion of exposure to possible offending agents can provide valuable data. Patch testing involves the application of allergens to the patient's skin (usually on the back) for 48 hours with reevaluation at 96 hours. Test sites are examined for erythema, papules, vesicles, or all of these. Patch testing is used to aid in determining possible causative agents (see Fig. 23-10). The best treatment of allergic dermatitis is avoidance of the causative agent. The extreme pruritus of contact dermatitis and its potential for chronicity make it a frustrating problem for you and the patient, especially if the offending agent cannot be identified.

BENIGN DERMATOLOGIC PROBLEMS

Although the list of benign dermatoses is extensive, some of the most commonly seen and distressing problems include acne vulgaris (Fig. 24-10), psoriasis (Fig. 24-11), and seborrheic keratoses (see eFig. 24-4 available on the website for this chapter). Benign problems are summarized in Table 24-9.

Psoriasis is a common benign disorder that currently affects 125 million people worldwide.[11] The disease usually develops in individuals between 15 and 35 years old. One third of people

TABLE 24-8 COMMON ALLERGIC CONDITIONS OF THE SKIN

Etiology and Pathophysiology	Clinical Manifestations	Treatment and Prognosis
Allergic Contact Dermatitis		
Manifestation of delayed hypersensitivity, absorbed agent acting as antigen, sensitization after one or more exposures, appearance of lesions 2-7 days after contact with allergen.	Red papules and plaques. Sharply circumscribed with occasional vesicles. Usually pruritic. Area of dermatitis frequently takes shape of causative agent (e.g., metal allergy and bandlike dermatitis on ring finger) (see Fig. 14-9).	Topical or oral corticosteroids, antihistamines. Skin lubrication. Elimination of contact allergen. Avoidance of irritating affected area. Systemic corticosteroids if sensitivity severe.
Urticaria		
Usually allergic phenomenon. Erythema and edema in upper dermis resulting from a local increase in permeability of capillaries (usually from histamine release).	Spontaneously occurring, raised or irregularly shaped wheals, varying size, usually multiple. A single lesion usually resolves in 24 hr. Can occur anywhere on the body.	Removal of triggering agent, if known. Oral antihistamine therapy. Possibly systemic corticosteroids.
Drug Reaction		
May be caused by any drug that acts as antigen and causes hypersensitivity reaction. Certain drugs (e.g., penicillin) more likely to cause reactions. Not all reactions are allergic, some are intolerance (e.g., gastric upset).	Rash of any morphology. Often red, macular and papular, semiconfluent, generalized rash with abrupt onset. Appearance as late as 14 days after cessation of drug. Possibly pruritic. Some reactions may be life threatening requiring immediate and intensive care.	Withdrawal of drug if possible. Antihistamines, topical or systemic corticosteroids may be necessary depending on severity of symptoms.
Atopic Dermatitis		
Genetically influenced, chronic, relapsing disease associated with immunologic irregularity involving inflammatory mediators, exaggerated by a cutaneous response to environmental allergens. Associated with allergic rhinitis and asthma.	Multiple presentations, including acute, subacute, and chronic stages. All are pruritic. *Acute stage* with bright erythema, oozing vesicles, with extreme pruritus. *Subacute stage* with scaly, light red to red-brown plaques. *Chronic stage* with thickened skin with accentuation of skin markings (lichenification), possible hypopigmentation or hyperpigmentation. Dry skin. Common in antecubital and popliteal space.	Lubrication of dry (xerotic) skin, restoration of skin barrier function. Topical immunomodulators (pimecrolimus [Elidel], tacrolimus [Protopic]). Corticosteroids, phototherapy for severe inflammation and pruritus. Reduction of stress reduces flares. Antibiotics for secondary infection as needed.

with psoriasis have at least one relative with the disease. Diagnosis is often based on the appearance of the skin (see Fig. 24-11). Most people have mild disease that affects at least 3% of the body. Severe disease is when psoriasis affects more than 10% of the body. Patients with severe disease often have a weakened immune system and are at risk for cardiovascular disease. Monitor the laboratory values (e.g., cholesterol, triglycerides) of patients with severe psoriasis to assist in early detection and intervention strategies for cardiovascular disease.

The chronicity of psoriasis can be severe and disabling as people withdraw from social contacts because of visible lesions. Quality of life is also negatively affected. Psoriatic arthritis affects 10% to 30% of all persons with psoriasis. (Psoriatic arthritis is discussed in Chapter 65.)

DRUG ALERT: Isotretinoin (Accutane)

- Can cause serious damage to fetus
- Blood donation prohibited for those taking the drug and for 1 month after treatment ends
- Contraindicated in women who are pregnant or who are intending to become pregnant while on the drug
- Linked to liver function test abnormalities

DISEASES WITH DERMATOLOGIC MANIFESTATIONS

Dermatologic manifestations of various diseases are listed in eTable 24-1 (available on the website for this chapter). Always consider the possibility that a particular skin manifestation is a clue to an internal, less obvious disease or disorder.

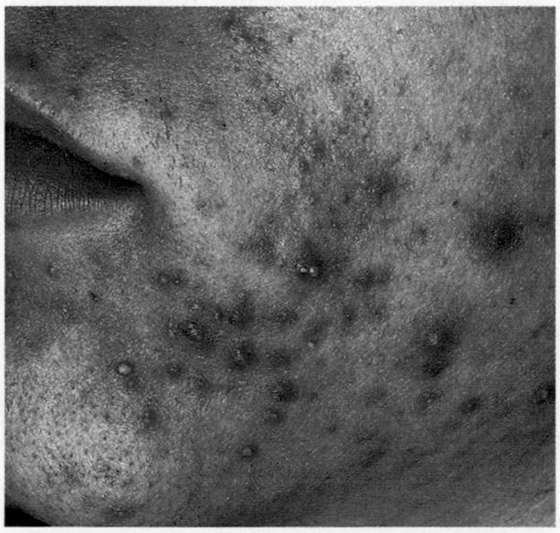

FIG. 24-10 Acne vulgaris. Papules and pustules.

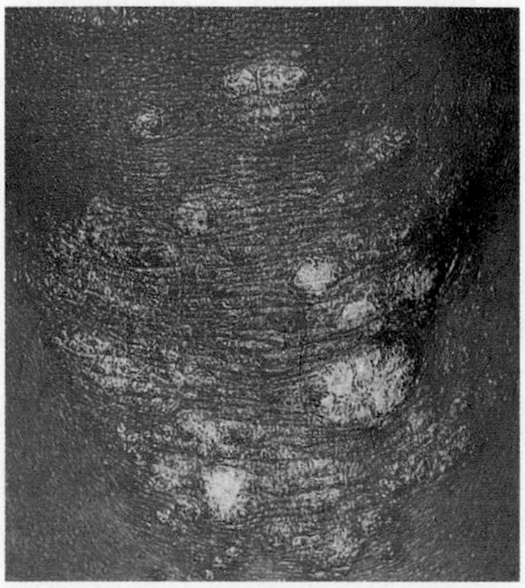

FIG. 24-11 Psoriasis. Characteristic inflammation and scaling.

TABLE 24-9 COMMON BENIGN CONDITIONS OF THE SKIN

Etiology and Pathophysiology	Clinical Manifestations	Treatment and Prognosis
Acne Vulgaris		
Inflammatory disorder of sebaceous glands. More common in teenagers but possible development and persistence in adulthood. Flare can occur with use of corticosteroids and androgen-dominant birth control pills and before menses.	Noninflammatory lesions, including open comedones (blackheads) and closed comedones (whiteheads). Inflammatory lesions, including papules and pustules. Most common on face, neck, and upper back (see Fig. 24-10).	Mechanical removal of multiple lesions with comedo extractor. Topical benzoyl peroxide or other antimicrobials. Veltin gel (clindamycin and tretinoin). Topical retinoids, systemic antibiotics. Aim of treatment to suppress new lesions and minimize scarring. Spontaneous remission possible. Often improvement with exposure to sun. May last many years. Use of isotretinoin (Accutane) for severe nodulocystic acne to possibly provide lasting remission (see Drug Alert on p. 438 for contraindications). Pregnancy tests, monitoring of liver function, cholesterol, triglycerides, and for depression essential.
Nevi (Moles)		
Grouping of normal cells derived from melanocyte-like precursor cells.	Hyperpigmented areas that vary in form and color. Flat, slightly elevated, verrucoid, polypoid, dome-shaped, sessile, or papillomatous. Preservation of normal skin markings. Hair growth possible.	No treatment necessary except for cosmetic reasons. Skin biopsy for suspicious nevi.
Psoriasis		
Autoimmune chronic dermatitis that involves excessively rapid turnover of epidermal cells. Family predisposition. Usually develops before age 40.	Sharply demarcated silvery scaling plaques on reddish colored skin commonly on the scalp, elbows, knees, palms, soles, and fingernails. Itching, burning, pain. Localized or general, intermittent or continuous. Symptoms vary in intensity from mild to severe (see Fig. 24-11).	Goal to reduce inflammation and suppress rapid turnover of epidermal cells. No cure, but control is possible. *Topical treatments:* corticosteroids, tar, calcipotriene, anthralin. Intralesional injection of corticosteroids for chronic plaques. *Systemic treatments:* natural or artificial UVB. PUVA (UVA with topical or systemic photosensitizer (psoralen). Antimetabolite (methotrexate), retinoid (acitretin), immunosuppressant (cyclosporine), biologic therapy (adalimumab [Humira], alefacept [Amevive], etanercept [Enbrel], infliximab [Remicade], ustekinumab [Stelara]) for moderate to severe plaque disease.
Seborrheic Keratoses		
Benign, familial, exact etiology unknown. Usually occur after age 40, increase in number with age.	Irregularly round or oval, often verrucous papules or plaques. Well-defined shape, appearance of being stuck on. Increase in pigmentation with time. Usually multiple and possibly itchy (see eFig. 24-4).	Removal by curettage or cryosurgery for cosmetic reasons or to eliminate source of irritation. Biopsy if unable to distinguish from melanoma.
Acrochordons (Skin Tags)		
Common after midlife. Appearance on neck, axillae, and upper trunk secondary to mechanical friction or redundant skin (associated with obesity).	Small, skin-colored, soft, pedunculated papules. May become irritated.	No treatment medically necessary. Surgical removal when needed. Usually just snipping without anesthesia.
Lipoma		
Benign tumor of adipose tissue, often encapsulated, most common in 40- to 60-yr-old age-group.	Rubbery, compressible, round mass of adipose tissue. Single or multiple. Variable in size, possibly extremely large. Most common on trunk, back of neck, and forearms.	Usually no treatment, biopsy to differentiate from liposarcoma, excision usual treatment (when indicated).
Lentigo		
Increased number of normal melanocytes in basal layer of epidermis related to sun exposure and aging. Also called "liver spots" or "age spots."	Hyperpigmented, brown to black macule or patch (flat lesion) on sun-exposed areas.	Evaluate carefully for progression. Treatment only for cosmetic purposes: liquid nitrogen, laser resurfacing. May recur. Biopsy when suspicious of melanoma.

PUVA, Psoralen ultraviolet A; *UBA*, ultraviolet A; *UVB*, ultraviolet B.

COLLABORATIVE CARE DERMATOLOGIC PROBLEMS

Diagnostic Studies

A careful history is of prime importance in the diagnosis of skin problems. The clinician must be skilled at detecting any evidence that could lead to the cause of many different skin diseases and conditions. After a careful history and physical examination, inspect individual lesions. Based on the history, physical examination, and appropriate diagnostic tests, either medical, surgical, or combination therapy is planned.

Collaborative Therapy

Many different treatment methods are used in dermatology. Advances in this field have brought relief to many previously chronic, untreatable conditions. Many of the specific therapeutic treatments require specialized equipment and are usually reserved for use by the dermatologist. Many clinicians prescribe drug therapy. The effectiveness of topical therapy can often be related to the base (or vehicle) in which the medication is prepared. Table 24-10 summarizes the common agents used as bases for topical preparations and their therapeutic considerations.

Phototherapy. Ultraviolet light (UVL) of different wavelengths may be used to treat many dermatologic conditions, including psoriasis, cutaneous T-cell lymphoma, atopic dermatitis, vitiligo, and pruritus. Light sources available to treat skin problems include broadband UVB, narrowband UVB, and long-wave UV (UVA1). One form of phototherapy involves the use of psoralen plus UVA light (PUVA). The photosensitizing drug psoralen is given to patients for a prescribed amount of time before exposure to UVA (see eFig. 24-5 available on the website for this chapter).

Treatments are generally given two to four times a week. Side effects of oral psoralen include nausea and vomiting, sunburn, and persistent pruritus. Perform frequent skin assessments on all patients receiving phototherapy, since erythema is a side effect of treatment. Topical corticosteroids may be given for painful erythema. Psoralen should be used with extreme caution in patients with liver or renal disease because slower metabolism and excretion can lead to prolonged photosensitivity.

Caution patients about the potential hazards of using photosensitizing chemicals and further exposure to UV rays from sunlight or artificial UVL during the course of phototherapy. Protective eyewear that blocks 100% of UVL is prescribed for patients receiving PUVA because psoralen is absorbed by the lens of the eye. The eyewear is used to prevent cataract formation. Instruct patients to use the eyewear for 24 hours after taking the medication when outdoors or near a bright window because UVA penetrates glass. Ongoing monitoring of these patients is essential because of the immunosuppressive effects of PUVA, including an increased risk of squamous and basal cell carcinomas and melanoma.

Photodynamic therapy is a special type of phototherapy that may be used in the treatment of actinic keratosis and malignant skin tumors.[12] This therapy uses a photosensitizing agent in a different way than some phototherapy treatments to selectively cause tumor necrosis.

Radiation Therapy. The use of radiation for the treatment of basal and squamous cell carcinomas and malignant melanoma varies greatly according to local practice and availability.[13] Even if radiation therapy is planned, a biopsy must first be performed to obtain a pathologic diagnosis.

Radiation to malignant cutaneous lesions may be given to reduce tumor size or in palliative treatment. One advantage of this therapy is minimal damage to surrounding tissue, which is of prime consideration in locations such as the nose, eyelids, and canthal areas. Careful shielding is necessary to prevent ocular lens damage if the irradiated area is around the eyes. Radiation therapy is particularly effective for the older adult or debilitated patient who cannot tolerate even a minor surgical procedure.

Radiation therapy usually requires multiple visits to a radiology department. It can produce permanent hair loss *(alopecia)* of the irradiated areas. Other adverse effects, depending on anatomic location and dose of radiation delivered, include telangiectasia, atrophy, hyperpigmentation, depigmentation, ulceration, hearing loss, ocular damage, atrophy, and mucositis. (Radiation therapy is discussed in Chapter 16.)

Total-body skin irradiation (body is bombarded with high-energy electrons) is one treatment for cutaneous T-cell lymphoma. Treatment follows a lengthy course and causes premature aging of the skin. Patients experience varying degrees of permanent alopecia and radiation dermatitis with a transient loss of sweat gland function.

Laser Technology. Laser treatment is expanding rapidly as an efficient surgical tool for many types of dermatologic problems (Table 24-11). Lasers are able to produce measurable, repeatable, consistent zones of tissue damage. They can cut, coagulate, and vaporize tissue to some degree. The wavelength determines the type of delivery system used and the intensity of the energy delivered.

The surgical use of laser energy requires a focusing device to produce a small, high-density spot of energy. Written policies and procedures should cover laser safety and be reviewed by all personnel working with laser equipment. Laser light does not

TABLE 24-10 DRUG THERAPY

Common Bases for Topical Medications

Agent	Therapeutic Considerations
Powder	Promotion of dryness. Lubricates skinfold areas to prevent irritation. Base for antifungal preparations. Protect patient from inhaling
Lotion	Oil and water emulsions. Cooling and drying. Some leave residual powder film after evaporation of water. Useful in subacute pruritic eruptions
Cream	Emulsions of oil and water. Most common base for topical medications. Lubrication and protection
Ointment	Oil with differing amounts of water added in suspension. Lubrication and prevention of dehydration. Petrolatum most common
Paste	Mixture of powder and ointment, used when drying effect necessary because moisture is absorbed
Gel	Nongreasy combination of propylene glycol and water. May contain alcohol

TABLE 24-11 SKIN CONDITIONS TREATED BY LASER

- Acne scars
- Skin lesions
- Hemangiomas
- Leg veins
- Rosacea
- Pigmented nevi
- Hair removal
- Port wine stain
- Vascular lesions
- Tattoo removal
- Resurfacing of skin
- Psoriasis
- Wrinkles
- Pigment discoloration in epidermis

accumulate in body cells and cannot cause cumulative cellular changes or damage.

Several types of lasers are available in most offices and hospitals. The CO_2 laser, the most common, has numerous applications as a vaporizing and cutting tool for most tissues. The argon laser emits light that is primarily absorbed by hemoglobin and helps in the treatment of vascular and other pigmented lesions. Other, less common lasers include the use of copper and gold vapors and neodymium:yttrium-aluminum-garnet (Nd:YAG).

Drug Therapy

Antibiotics. Antibiotics are used both topically and systemically to treat dermatologic problems, and are often used in combination. When using topical antibiotics, apply a thin film lightly to clean skin. Common OTC topical antibiotics include bacitracin-neomycin-polymyxin (Neosporin), bacitracin, and polymyxin B. Many health care providers do not recommend Neosporin because it often causes allergic contact dermatitis. Prescription topical antibiotics include mupirocin (for superficial *Staphylococcus* infections such as impetigo), gentamicin (used for *Staphylococcus* and most gram-negative organisms), and erythromycin (used for gram-positive cocci [staphylococci and streptococci] and gram-negative cocci and bacilli). Topical erythromycin and clindamycin (Cleocin solutions or gels) are used in the treatment of acne vulgaris. Topical metronidazole is used to treat rosacea and bacterial vaginosis. Many of the more popular systemic antibiotics are not used topically because of the danger of allergic contact dermatitis.

If there are manifestations of systemic infection, a systemic antibiotic should be used. Systemic antibiotics are useful in the treatment of bacterial infections and acne vulgaris. The most frequently used are synthetic sulfur, penicillin, minocycline, erythromycin, and tetracycline (or doxycycline). These drugs are particularly useful for erysipelas, cellulitis, carbuncles, and severe infected eczema. Culture and sensitivity of the lesion can guide the choice of antibiotic. Patients require drug-specific instructions on the proper technique of taking or applying antibiotics. For instance, oral tetracycline must be taken on an empty stomach. It should never be taken within 1 hour before consuming a dairy product or 2 hours after, since this would interfere with its absorption.

Corticosteroids. Corticosteroids are particularly effective in treating a wide variety of dermatologic conditions and can be used topically, intralesionally, or systemically. Topical corticosteroids are used for their local antiinflammatory and antipruritic effects. Attempts to diagnose a skin problem should be made *before* a corticosteroid preparation is applied, since corticosteroids may alter the clinical manifestations. Once a sufficient amount of medication is dispensed, limits should be set on the duration and frequency of application.

The potency of a particular preparation is related to the concentration of active drug. With prolonged use, more potent corticosteroid formulations can cause adrenal suppression, especially if a large surface area is covered and occlusive dressings are used. Over time, high-potency corticosteroids may produce side effects, including atrophy of the skin resulting from impaired cell mitosis, capillary fragility, and susceptibility to bruising. In general, dermal and epidermal atrophy does not occur until a corticosteroid has been used for 2 to 3 weeks. If drug use is discontinued at the first sign of atrophy, recovery usually occurs in several weeks. Rosacea eruptions and severe exacerbations of acne vulgaris may also occur. Rebound dermatitis is not uncommon when therapy is stopped. This can be reduced by tapering the use of high-potency topical corticosteroids when improvement is noted.

Low-potency corticosteroids such as hydrocortisone act more slowly but can be used for a longer time without producing serious side effects. Low-potency corticosteroids are safe to use on the face and intertriginous areas, such as the axillae and groin.

The most potent delivery system for a topical corticosteroid is an ointment form. Creams and ointments should be applied in thin layers and slowly massaged into the site one to three times a day as prescribed. Accurate and adequate topical therapy is often the key to a successful outcome.

Intralesional corticosteroids are injected directly into or just beneath the lesion. This method provides a reservoir of medication with an effect lasting several weeks to months. Intralesional injection is commonly used in the treatment of psoriasis, alopecia areata (patchy hair loss), cystic acne, hypertrophic scars, and keloids. Triamcinolone acetonide (Kenalog) is the most common drug used for intralesional injection.

Systemic corticosteroids can have remarkable results in the treatment of dermatologic conditions. However, they often have undesirable systemic effects (see Chapter 50). Corticosteroids can be administered as short-term therapy for acute conditions such as contact dermatitis caused by poison ivy. Long-term corticosteroid therapy for dermatologic conditions is reserved for severe disease such as bullous (blistering) disorders.

Antihistamines. Oral antihistamines are used to treat conditions that exhibit urticaria, angioedema, and pruritus.[14] Dermatologic problems such as atopic dermatitis, allergic dermatitis, and other allergic cutaneous reactions can be reduced with the use of histamine blockers. Antihistamines compete with histamine for the receptor site, thus preventing its effect. Antihistamines may have anticholinergic and/or sedative effects. Several different antihistamines may have to be tried before the satisfactory therapeutic effect is achieved. Sedating antihistamines, such as hydroxyzine (Atarax) and diphenhydramine (Benadryl), are often preferred for pruritic conditions because the tranquilizing and sedative effects offer symptomatic relief. Warn the patient about sedative effects, a particular problem when driving or operating heavy machinery. Antihistamines such as loratadine (Claritin), fexofenadine (Allegra), and cetirizine (Zyrtec) bind to peripheral histamine receptors, providing antihistamine action without sedation. These nonsedating antihistamines are not effective for controlling pruritus. Antihistamines should be used with particular caution in older adults because of their long half-life and their anticholinergic effects.

Topical Fluorouracil. Fluorouracil (5-FU) is a topical cytotoxic agent with selective toxicity for sun-damaged cells. 5-FU is available in four strengths (0.5%, 1%, 2%, and 5%) and is used for the treatment of premalignant (especially actinic keratosis) and some malignant skin diseases. Because systemic absorption of the drug is minimal, systemic side effects are virtually nonexistent. Patient compliance is a consideration in the use of 5-FU. The medication produces erythema and pruritus within 3 to 5 days and painful, eroded areas over the damaged skin within 1 to 3 weeks, depending on skin thickness at the site. Low-potency topical corticosteroids are often prescribed to be applied 20 minutes after 5-FU to reduce erythema and pruritus and increase patient adherence with therapy. Treatment must continue with applications one (only in the 0.5% strength) or two times a day for 2 to 6 weeks. Healing may take up to 4 weeks after medication is stopped.

Because 5-FU is a photosensitizing drug, instruct the patient to avoid sunlight during treatment. Teach patients about the effect of the medication and that they will look worse before they look better. Adherence depends on thoroughness of your instruction, which should include a written handout. After effective treatment, treated skin is smooth and free of actinic keratosis. Actinic keratosis may recur in treated areas, and multiple courses of chemotherapy may be necessary over the years for individuals with severely sun-damaged skin.

Immunomodulators. Topical immunomodulators, such as pimecrolimus (Elidel) and tacrolimus (Protopic), are used to treat atopic dermatitis. They work by suppressing an overreactive immune system. The side effects are minimal and may include a transient burning or feeling of heat at the application site. An increased risk of skin cancer and precancerous lesions may be associated with these drugs.

Another topical immunomodulator, imiquimod, acts to stimulate the production of α-interferon and other cytokines to enhance cell-mediated immunity. It boosts the immune response only where applied and is safe for transplant patients. This medication is used for external genital warts, actinic keratoses, and superficial BCC. Most patients using this cream experience skin reactions, including redness, swelling, blistering, excoriations, peeling, itching, and burning.

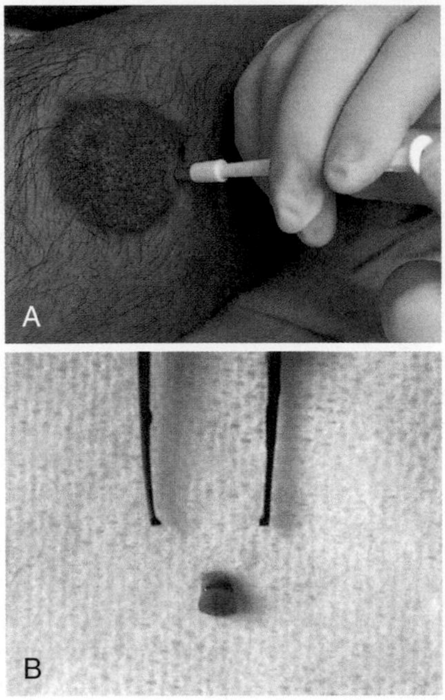

FIG. 24-12 Punch biopsy. **A,** Removal of skin for diagnostic purposes. **B,** Specimen obtained.

Diagnostic and Surgical Therapy

Skin Scraping. Scraping is done with a scalpel blade to obtain a sample of surface cells (stratum corneum) for microscopic inspection and diagnosis. The most common tests of skin scrapings are potassium hydroxide (KOH) for fungus and mineral oil examination for scabies.

Electrodesiccation and Electrocoagulation. Electrical energy can be converted to heat with the tip of an electrode. This results in tissue being destroyed by burning. The major uses of this type of therapy are coagulation of bleeding vessels to obtain hemostasis and destruction of small *telangiectasias* (dilation of groups of superficial capillaries and venules). *Electrodesiccation* usually involves more superficial destruction, and a monopolar electrode is used. *Electrocoagulation* has a deeper effect, with better hemostasis and an increased possibility of scarring. A dipolar electrode is used for electrocoagulation.

Curettage. Curettage is the removal and scooping away of tissue using an instrument with a circular cutting edge attached to a handle (see eFig. 24-6 available on the website). Although the curette is not usually strong enough to cut normal skin, it is useful for removing many types of small, soft skin tumors and superficial lesions, such as warts, actinic keratoses, and small basal and squamous cell carcinomas. The area to be curetted is anesthetized before the procedure. Hemostasis is obtained by one of several methods: electrodesiccation, ferric subsulfate (Monsel solution), gelatin foam, aluminum chloride (Drysol), or a gauze pressure dressing. A small scar and hypopigmentation can result. The curetted tissue should be sent for biopsy.

Punch Biopsy. Punch biopsy is a common dermatologic procedure used to obtain a tissue sample for histologic study or to remove small lesions (Fig. 24-12). It is generally reserved for lesions smaller than 0.5 cm.[15] Before local anesthesia is used, the biopsy area is outlined so that landmarks will not be obscured by the anesthetizing agent. The punch biopsy instrument is twirled between the fingers, and its sharp edge cores out a small cylinder of skin. The core of skin is snipped from the subcutaneous fat and appropriately preserved for examination in a fixative solution. Hemostasis is achieved by using methods similar to those used with curettage, but sites of 4 mm or larger are usually closed with sutures. Other types of biopsies are discussed in Table 23-9 and Chapter 23.

Cryosurgery. Cryosurgery is the use of subfreezing temperatures to destroy epidermal lesions. Cryosurgery is a useful treatment for common benign, precancerous conditions, including common and genital warts, cutaneous tags, thin seborrheic keratoses, lentigines, actinic keratoses, and nonmelanoma skin cancers. Topical liquid nitrogen (−196° F) is the agent most commonly used for cryosurgery.[15] The mechanism of injury involves direct cellular freezing and vascular stasis (stoppage or slowdown in the flow of blood), which develops after thawing. Intracellular ice formation causes the cell to rupture during thaw, leading to cell death and necrosis of the treated tissue.

Liquid nitrogen can be applied topically (directly onto the lesion) with a direct spray or a cotton-tipped applicator. Patients are informed that they will feel a stinging cold sensation. The lesion first becomes swollen and red, and it may blister. A scab forms and falls off in 1 to 3 weeks. The skin lesion is sloughed along with the scab. Growth of new skin follows.

Because of the temperature of the liquid nitrogen, melanocytes can easily be destroyed, leaving an area of hypopigmentation resembling a scar. The size of an affected area to be treated may limit the use of cryotherapy. The disadvantages of this treatment are (1) the lack of a tissue specimen for histologic confirmation of cell type before destruction and (2) the potential for destruction of adjacent healthy tissue.

Excision. Excision should be considered if the lesion to be removed involves the dermis. Complete closure of the excised area usually results in a good cosmetic result.

A specific type of excision is *Mohs' surgery,* which is a microscopically controlled removal of a cutaneous malignancy. This procedure sections the surgical specimen horizontally, so that

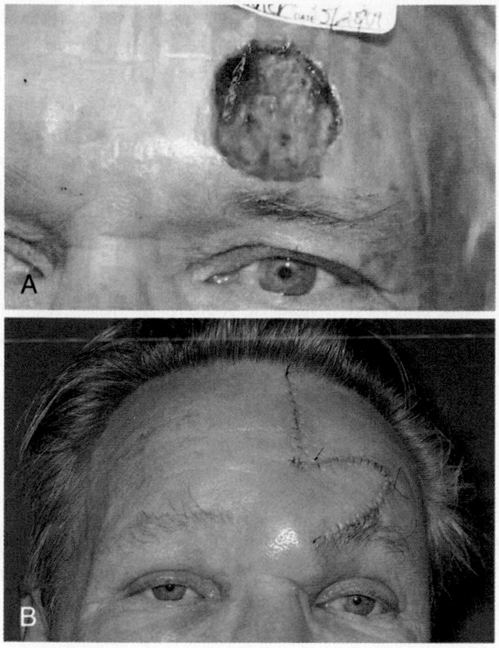

FIG. 24-13 **A,** Removal of melanoma by Mohs' surgery. **B,** After plastic surgery using a skin flap to repair defect.

100% of the surgical margin can be examined. Tissue is removed in thin layers, and all margins of the specimen are mapped to determine whether any malignant cells remain (Fig. 24-13). Any residual tumor not removed by the first surgical excision can be removed in serial excisions performed the same day. The benefits of this treatment are preserving normal tissue, producing the smallest possible wound, and completely removing the cancer before surgical closure. Although this can become a lengthy procedure, it is performed in an outpatient setting with the patient under local anesthesia.

NURSING MANAGEMENT DERMATOLOGIC PROBLEMS

AMBULATORY AND HOME CARE

Dermatologic conditions are not usually the primary reason for hospitalization. Nevertheless, many hospitalized patients exhibit concurrent skin problems that warrant nursing intervention and patient education.

If the patient is in an acute care setting, you both administer and teach the appropriate treatments. In an outpatient setting the focus is on patient teaching, with opportunities provided for demonstration and repeated demonstration. Subsequent visits allow you to evaluate patient understanding and treatment effectiveness.

Nursing interventions related to dermatologic conditions fall into broad categories. They are applicable to many skin problems in both inpatient and outpatient settings. (A nursing care plan for the patient with chronic skin lesions [eNursing Care Plan 24-1] is available on the website for this chapter.)

WET DRESSINGS. Wet dressings are commonly used when there is oozing from the skin. Oozing usually indicates an infection and/or inflammation. Salt water or a prescribed solution (e.g., Domeboro powder) is used on the skin by soaking (a foot or hand) or applying compresses to a larger area. Wet dressings are also used to relieve itching, suppress inflammation, and debride a wound. In addition, wet dressings increase penetration of topical medications; promote sleep by relieving discomfort; and enhance removal of scales, crusts, and exudate. Materials such as thin sheeting, gauze sponges, thermal underwear, or tube socks can be used for dressings. Ingenuity is sometimes required when odd-shaped body parts must be covered.

Place the prescribed dressing material into fresh solution, and squeeze until it is no longer dripping. Then apply it to the affected area, avoiding normal skin tissue. If the desired effect is drying, soaks or compresses are left in place for 20 minutes, three times daily for 2 or 3 days. Take care to avoid overdrying, since new problems such as fissuring may result. Wet dressings for uses other than drying should be left in place 10 to 30 minutes, two to four times a day as ordered. If the skin appears *macerated* (softens and turns white), discontinue the dressings for 2 to 3 hours. Protect the patient from discomfort and chilling by using linens and bedclothes with pads or plastic.

Wet dressings do not need to be sterile. Tap water at room temperature is the most common solution where water quality is adequate. Filtered or sterile water may be indicated in some locations. Wet dressings should be cool when an antiinflammatory effect is desired and tepid when the purpose is to debride an infected, crusted lesion. These treatments are excellent ways to remove the scabs left by the collection of debris at a wound site.

BATHS. Baths are appropriate when large body areas need to be treated. They also have sedative and antipruritic effects. Some agents, such as oilated oatmeal (Aveeno) and sodium bicarbonate, can be added directly to bath water. Fill the tub to cover the affected areas. Both the bath water and the prescribed solution should be at a lukewarm (tepid) temperature. Have the patient soak for 15 to 20 minutes three or four times a day, depending on the severity of the dermatitis and the patient's discomfort. Stress to the patient that the skin must not be rubbed dry with a towel but gently patted to prevent increased irritation and inflammation. The addition of oils makes the bathtub extremely slippery and should be avoided. If oils are used in the tub, use caution in transferring patients to prevent accidents. To sustain the hydrating effect, apply cream or ointment emollients (moisturizers) or other prescribed topical agents after the bath. This helps retain the moisture in the hydrated cells and increases the absorption of a prescribed topical medication.

TOPICAL MEDICATIONS. A thin layer of ointment, cream, lotion or solution, or gel should be applied to clean skin and spread evenly in a downward motion. Thickly applied topical medications waste medication and leave the skin greasy. An alternative method is for you to apply the medication directly onto a dressing. Pastes are designed to protect the affected area. Apply pastes thickly with a tongue blade or a gloved hand. Draining lesions and lesions with oily medication can be covered with a light dressing to avoid soiling clothes. Provide specific directions to patients on the proper application technique of prescribed topical medications.

CONTROL OF PRURITUS. *Pruritus* (itching) can be caused by dry skin, almost any physical or chemical stimulus to the skin (such as drugs or insects), and any scaling skin disorder. The itch sensation is carried by the same nonmyelinated nerve fibers as pain. If the epidermis is damaged or absent, the sensation will be felt as pain rather than an itch.

The itch/scratch cycle must be broken to prevent excoriation and lichenification. Control of pruritus is also important because it is difficult to diagnose a lesion that is excoriated and inflamed. Certain circumstances make itching worse. Anything that causes vasodilation, such as heat or rubbing, should be avoided. Dryness of the skin lowers the itch threshold and increases the itch sensation.

Inform the patient of the various methods that may be helpful in breaking the itch/scratch cycle. A cool environment may cause vasoconstriction and decrease itching. Topically applied menthol, camphor, or phenol can be used to numb the itch receptors.[16] Systemic antihistamines may provide relief while the underlying cause of the patient's pruritus is diagnosed and treated. The principal side effect of most antihistamines is sedation. This may be desirable because pruritus is often worse at night and can interfere with sleep.

Wet dressings may also relieve pruritus. Thin cotton sheets or thermal underwear should be placed in cool water, wrung out, and placed over the pruritic area. After 10 to 15 minutes remove the dressing, pat the skin dry, and then apply a lubricant or medication. This procedure can be repeated as necessary for comfort.

Lichenification is a thickening of skin as a result of the proliferation of keratinocytes with accentuation of the normal markings of the skin. Lichenification is caused by chronic scratching or rubbing of the skin and is often associated with atopic dermatoses and pruritic conditions. Although any area of the body may be affected, the hands, forearms, shins, and nape of the neck are common sites. Excoriations may be evident in the lichenified skin as a result of persistent pruritus and scratching. Treatment of the cause of the itching is the key to prevention of lichenification.

PREVENTION OF SPREAD. Although most skin problems are not contagious, infection control precautions indicate the need for gloves with open or bleeding wounds or any lesion with purulent drainage. Explain procedures to the patient to avoid provoking undue anxiety. Careful hand washing and the safe disposal of soiled dressings are the best means of preventing the spread of skin problems. The most common contagious lesions include impetigo, staphylococcal infections, pyoderma, fungal infections, primary chancre, scabies, and pediculosis.

PREVENTION OF SECONDARY INFECTIONS. Open lesions on the skin are susceptible to invasion by other viral, bacterial, or fungal organisms. Meticulous hygiene, hand washing, and dressing changes are important to minimize the potential for secondary infections. Warn the patient about scratching the lesions, which can cause excoriations and create a portal of entry for pathogens. Trim the patient's nails short to minimize trauma from scratching.

SPECIFIC SKIN CARE. You are often in a position to advise patients regarding care of the skin after simple dermatologic surgical procedures, such as skin biopsy, excision, and cryosurgery. Patient follow-up should be individualized. In general, your instructions should include dressing changes, use of topical antibiotics, and the signs and symptoms of infection. After a dermatologic procedure, any oozing wound should be cleansed with a saline solution twice daily or as ordered by the provider. A wound that is not oozing may be washed with soap and plain water. An antibiotic ointment or plain petrolatum ointment may then be applied with a dressing that is both absorbent and nonadherent.

Wounds that are kept moist and covered heal more rapidly and with less scarring. The initial crust that forms should be left undisturbed as a protective coating for the damaged skin beneath it. Healing crusts that have been moisturized and protected will separate naturally from healed epidermis.

A wound that required sutures can be covered with a variety of different dressings. Sutures are generally removed in 4 to 14 days, depending on the placement site. Sometimes alternating sutures are removed after the third day. Incision lines may require daily cleansing, usually with plain tap water. If necessary, a topical antibiotic is applied and the wound is either covered with a dry sterile dressing or left open to air. The patient may experience some swelling and discomfort in the first 24 hours, during the first phase of wound healing. Ice packs may be applied over the surgical dressing to reduce edema. Mild analgesics such as acetaminophen or a nonsteroidal antiinflammatory medication should control the discomfort. Teach the patient the manifestations of inflammation, such as redness, fever, or increased pain or swelling, and signs of infection, such as purulent drainage. If these manifestations occur, they should be reported to the health care provider.

PSYCHOLOGIC EFFECTS OF CHRONIC DERMATOLOGIC PROBLEMS. Emotional stress can occur for persons who suffer from chronic skin problems such as psoriasis, atopic dermatitis, or acne. The sequelae of chronic skin problems could result in social and employment problems with subsequent financial implications, a poor self-image, problems with sexuality, and increasing and progressive frustration. The usual lack of systemic overt illness coupled with the visibility of the skin lesions often presents a real problem to the patient.

Help the patient comply with the prescribed regimen. The patient must be allowed to verbalize the "Why me?" question, even though there is no ready answer. Dermatology patient support groups are listed on the American Academy of Dermatology website *(www.aad.org)*. These groups are extremely helpful for patient support and accurate education materials.

Many lesions can be camouflaged with the skillful use of cosmetics. Individual sensitivity to product ingredients must always be considered in the selection of a cosmetic product. Oil-free, hypoallergenic cosmetics are available and may be beneficial to the allergic patient. Rehabilitative cosmetics are available to help camouflage and deemphasize such lesions as *vitiligo* (loss of pigmentation), *melasma* (tan to brown patches on the face), or healed postoperative wound sites. These commercially available products are opaque, smudge resistant, and water resistant.

In addition to specific skin conditions that tend to be chronic, other factors affecting the outcome of long-term dermatologic problems include skin type, history of previous exacerbations, family history, complications, intolerance to therapy, environmental factors, lack of adherence to the prescribed regimen, endocrine factors, and psychologic factors.

PHYSIOLOGIC EFFECTS OF CHRONIC DERMATOLOGIC PROBLEMS. Scarring and lichenification are the results of chronic dermatologic problems. Scars occur when ulceration takes place. Scars are pink and vascular at first. With time, they become avascular and white (scars on individuals with darker skin may be hyperpigmented) with increasing strength. Different regions of the body scar differently. For example, the face and neck heal fairly rapidly because they are well vascularized. Regions of the lower body with less vascularization tend to scar more easily and heal more slowly. Scar formation is described in Chapter 12.

The location of the scar is the determining factor with respect to its cosmetic implications. Facial scars are the most damaging

TABLE 24-12 COMMON COSMETIC TOPICAL PROCEDURES

Tretinoin (Retin-A, Renova)	Chemical Peels	Microdermabrasion	α-Hydroxy Acids (e.g., Glycolic Acid, Lactic Acid)
Indications			
Improves appearance of photodamaged skin, especially fine wrinkling. Reduces actinic keratoses.	Improves appearance of photodamaged skin, acne scarring, actinic and seborrheic keratoses.	Smoothes appearance of photodamaged and wrinkled skin, acne scarring.	Similar indications as microdermabrasion. Also called a "light chemical peel."
Description			
Applied initially qod, nightly applications as tolerated, since preparation is inactivated by light. Treatment stopped if severe inflammation occurs. Maximum response in 8-12 mo.	Solution applied (e.g., trichloroacetic acid, phenol) in varying amounts to the skin, causing a controlled burn with a loss of melanin.	Epidermis and top dermal layer removed by applying aluminum oxide or baking soda crystals. Re-epithelialization of abraded surface then occurs.	Low concentrations (<10%) in many skin care products consumers can apply to the skin. Higher concentrations (50%-70%) given only by a health care provider.
Side Effects			
Erythema, swelling, flaking, pigmentation changes. Teratogenic. Increases phototoxicity if also taking other photosensitive drugs (see Table 24-2).	Moderate swelling and crusting for 1 wk. Redness for 6-8 wk. Pink tone possible for several mo. Photosensitivity.	Light pink tone that resolves within 24 hr. Photosensitivity.	Photosensitivity, slight irritation at lower concentrations, severe redness, oozing, and flaking skin possible with higher concentrations.
Patient Teaching			
Apply emollients, use sunscreen (SPF 15 or higher), use sun avoidance measures, avoid use of abrasive or drying facial cleansers for severe sensitivity (e.g., excess irritation).	Use sunscreen, avoid sun for 6 mo to prevent hyperpigmentation.	Generous application of emollients and sunscreen.	Use sunscreen.

qod, Every other day; *SPF,* sun protection factor.

psychologically, because they are so visible. Creative use of cosmetics can do much to mask the scarring of chronic skin conditions. The best treatment is the prevention of scarring by controlling the problem in the acute phase.

COSMETIC PROCEDURES

A vast array of cosmetic procedures is available, including chemical peels, toxin injections, fillers, laser surgery, breast enlargement and reduction (see Chapter 52), face-lift, eyelid-lift, and liposuction. Common cosmetic topical procedures are presented in Table 24-12. Other types of cosmetic procedures include the injection of botulinum toxin (Botox), calcium hydroxylapatite (Radiesse), collagen (Zyplast), and hyaluronic acid fillers (Restylane, Perlane). Transitory side effects may occur such as mild redness, pain, swelling, and bruising. Uncommon side effects from cosmetic procedures include allergic reaction, infection, or lumps at the injection sites; undercorrection or overcorrection of wrinkles; and reactivation of human papillomavirus (HPV). Instruct the patient that he or she will need to repeat the procedure at prescribed intervals to maintain the appearance desired.

The reasons for undergoing these procedures are as varied as the techniques. The most common reason that people suffer the discomfort and financial expense (most are not covered by health insurance) of a cosmetic procedure is to improve their body image. If they feel better about themselves after having cosmetic procedures, they often act more confident and self-assured. Often social position and economic considerations are part of the decision. Increased longevity provides a larger population to whom cosmetic procedures are especially appealing.

Regardless of the patient's reasons for seeking cosmetic procedures, maintain a supportive, nonjudgmental attitude about these procedures. If the patient wishes to change or enhance a body feature perceived as unattractive and has realistic expectations about the outcome, you should support this decision.

Elective Surgery

Laser Surgery. When a laser beam enters the skin, the light can affect skin structures by scattering, absorbing, or passing through different layers. The spectrum of clinical application for each laser depends on the depth of the wavelength emitted and the operator technique. Alterations in technique, such as pulse duration and the number of passes over the skin, vary the result. New handpiece technology with multiple spot size and cooling device additions has also generated new flexibility in laser surgery.

Lasers can reduce scarring and fine wrinkles around the lips or eyes and remove facial lesions[17] (see Table 24-11). Swelling, redness, and bruising are common after treatment. The treated areas usually are kept moist with ointment or occlusive dressings (surgical bandages) for the first few days. The treated skin must be protected from the sun.

Face-Lift. A face-lift *(rhytidectomy)* is the lifting and repositioning of the lower two thirds of the face and neck to improve appearance (Fig. 24-14). Indications for this procedure include the following:

- Redundant soft tissue or scarring resulting from disease (e.g., acne scarring)
- Asymmetric redundancy of soft tissues (e.g., facial palsy)
- Redundant soft tissue resulting from trauma
- Preauricular lesions

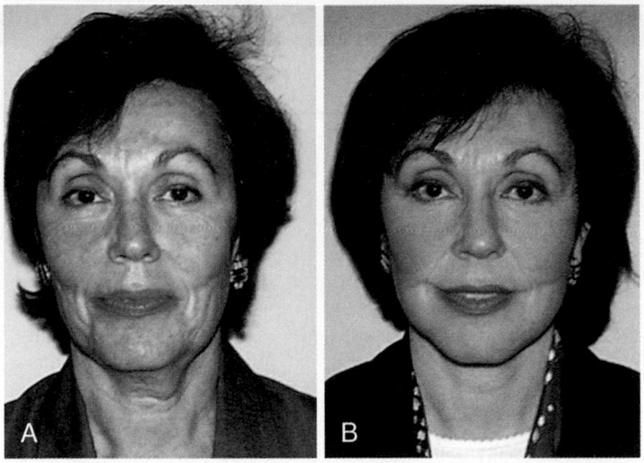

FIG. 24-14 Face-lift. **A,** Preoperative. **B,** Postoperative.

- Redundant soft tissues resulting from *solar elastosis* (sagging of the skin as a result of sun damage), changes in body weight, and the effects of gravity
- Restoration of body image

The surgical approach and lines of incisions vary according to the desired correction and the position of the hairline. Eyelid-lifts *(blepharoplasty)* with similar indications are performed to remove redundant tissue and possibly improve the field of vision. Prevention of hematoma formation is the most important postoperative consideration. Ice packs are usually applied for the first 24 to 48 hours to reduce swelling and decrease the possibility of hematoma formation. Complications can occur if the person smokes or is involved in vigorous exercise. Usually the pain is minimal. Antibiotics are used at the surgeon's discretion.

Liposuction. Liposuction is a technique for removing subcutaneous fat to improve facial and body contours. Although not a substitute for diet and exercise, it can be successful in removing areas of fat from virtually any body area that is resistant to other techniques.

Liposuction is relatively free of complications, but possible contraindications include use of anticoagulants, uncontrolled hypertension, diabetes mellitus, and poor cardiovascular status. Persons under 40 years of age with good skin elasticity are the best candidates. However, patients ranging in age from 16 to 70 years can be treated successfully.

The procedure is usually performed on an outpatient basis with the aid of local anesthesia. One or more sessions may be necessary, depending on the size of the area to be treated. A blunt-tipped cannula is inserted through a 0.5-in incision and pushed into the fat to break it loose from the fibrous stroma. Multiple repeated thrusts disrupt the fat and create tunnels. The loosened fat is removed with a powerful suction. The incision sites are taped because firm, absorbent bandaging reduces the amount of postoperative bleeding and fluid accumulation.[18] Bandaging also helps to contour the skin. It may take several months for the final results to be evident.

NURSING MANAGEMENT COSMETIC SURGERY

Many cosmetic surgical procedures are performed in well-equipped day-surgery units or in dermatology surgeons' or plastic surgeons' office surgery suites.

DELEGATION DECISIONS

Skin Care

Role of Registered Nurse (RN)

- Assess patient's skin for acute and chronic integumentary problems.
- Assess patient's risk factors for integumentary problems.
- Document skin condition and risk factor assessment, and develop a plan of care.
- Determine whether patient is taking drugs that increase photosensitivity.
- Teach about risks associated with sun exposure and methods for decreasing exposure to the sun.
- Teach about therapies that are used for integumentary disorders, including dressings, baths, and oral or topical medications used on an outpatient basis.
- Evaluate treatment for effectiveness and any adverse effects.

Role of Licensed Practical/Vocational Nurse (LPN/LVN)

- Administer prescribed therapies such as dressings and oral or topical medications.
- Monitor the skin for changes in appearance or texture that may indicate worsening of integumentary problem or adverse reactions to treatment.
- Reinforce teaching done by the RN.

Role of Unlicensed Assistive Personnel (UAP)

- Assist patient with bathing.
- Apply wet dressings to skin or add medications (such as oilated oatmeal) to patient baths (consider state nurse practice act and agency policy).
- Report changes in skin appearance or patient complaints of discomfort to the RN.

PREOPERATIVE MANAGEMENT

A major preoperative management consideration relates to informed consent and realistic expectations of what cosmetic surgery can accomplish. Although the surgeon should provide this information, reinforce it and answer questions and concerns. For instance, a face-lift has little or no effect on deep wrinkling of the forehead and temples, deep nasolabial grooves, or vertical lip wrinkles. Before-and-after treatment photographs of similar cases are often useful in helping the patient to set realistic expectations.

Your teaching plan should include patient understanding of the timeframe for healing. Because wound healing may not be complete for 1 year, immediate, complete results should not be anticipated. Explain the oozing, crusting stage of the abrasive procedure so the patient can plan time off from work if necessary. The final results of the cosmetic procedure are affected by the patient's age, general state of health, and skin type and the extent (severity) of the condition being treated. If a health problem is present, efforts should be made to correct or control the problem before the procedure is performed.

POSTOPERATIVE MANAGEMENT

Most cosmetic procedures are not extremely painful. Usually mild analgesics are sufficient to keep the patient comfortable.

Although infection is not a common problem after cosmetic surgery, assess the surgical sites for signs of infection. Inform the patient of the signs and symptoms of infection with instructions to report them immediately so that appropriate antibiotic intervention can be started.

If the surgery involved an alteration in the circulation to the skin, as in a face-lift, carefully monitor for adequate circulation.

Warm, pink skin that blanches on pressure indicates that adequate circulation is present in the surgical area. Supportive, compressive dressings and ice packs may be necessary early in the postoperative period.

SKIN GRAFTS

Uses

Skin grafts may be necessary to protect underlying structures or to reconstruct areas for cosmetic or functional purposes. Ideally, wounds heal by primary intention. However, large wounds, surgically created wounds, trauma, and chronic wounds can cause extensive tissue destruction, making primary intention healing impossible. In these cases, skin grafting may be necessary to close the defect. Improved surgical techniques make it possible to graft skin, bone, cartilage, fat, fascia, muscles, and nerves. For cosmetically pleasing results, the color, thickness, texture, and hair-growing nature of skin used for grafting must be chosen to match the recipient site. (Skin grafting is also discussed in Chapter 25.)

Types

The two types of skin grafts are free grafts and skin flaps. Free grafts are further classified according to the method of providing a blood supply to the grafted skin. One method is to transfer the graft (epidermis and part or all of the dermis) to the recipient site from the donor site. If the graft is an *autograft* (from the patient's own body) or an *isograft* (from an identical twin), it will revascularize and become fixed to the new site. Chapter 25 discusses full- and split-thickness skin grafts. Another method of free skin grafting is by *reconstructive microsurgery.* With the use of an operating microscope, circulation is immediately established in the free flap by anastomosis of the blood vessels from the skin flap to the vessels in the recipient site.

Skin flaps involve moving a section of skin and subcutaneous tissue from one part of the body to another without terminating the vascular attachment.[19] The vascular attachment is called a *pedicle.* Skin flaps are used to cover wounds with a poor vascular bed, to provide padding when needed, and to cover wounds over cartilage and bone. The patient may need intermediate flap placement if the recipient site is far removed from the donor site. For instance, a skin flap from the thigh to the head would require an intermediate graft. The flap is advanced to the recipient site when circulation is well established at the intermediate site. The type of flap and the route of transfer are determined according to the patient's needs and the defect being repaired.

Soft tissue expansion is a technique for providing skin for resurfacing of a defect, such as a burn scar; for removal of a disfiguring mark (e.g., a tattoo); or as a preliminary step in breast reconstruction. A subcutaneous tissue expander of an appropriate size and shape is placed under the skin, usually as an outpatient procedure. Weekly expansion with saline solution can be done in a health care setting or by the patient at home. This expansion procedure is repeated until the skin reaches the size needed for the repair. This may take from several weeks to 3 to 4 months. Once sufficient skin is available, the old incision is opened, the expander is removed, and the soft tissue is ready to be used as an advancement flap. The tissue expander next to a defect retains the primary tissue characteristics such as color and texture.

CASE STUDY

Malignant Melanoma and Dysplastic Nevi

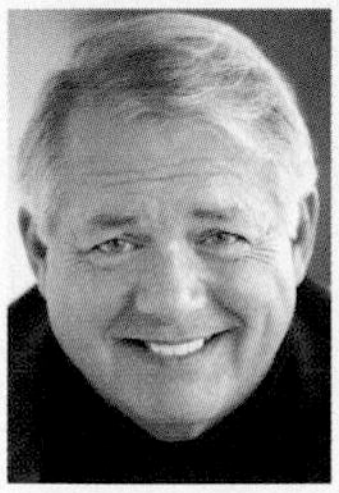

Hemera/Thinkstock

Patient Profile

G.L. is a 59-year-old white fair-skinned man who is a long-distance truck driver. In his leisure time, he enjoys swimming. He comes to the clinic for evaluation of a changing lesion on his left arm.

Subjective Data

- History of a basal cell carcinoma (BCC) on his left ear in the last 4 years
- Father treated for metastatic malignant melanoma in the last 2 years
- First noted the lesion 5 months ago when it started changing size
- Anxious the lesion might have spread and require extensive, disfiguring surgery

Objective Data

Physical Examination

- Has a 4-mm lesion, dark brown, scalloped with vaguely defined borders
- Four dysplastic nevi found on back

Diagnostic Studies

- Excisional biopsy confirmed malignant melanoma.
- Sentinel node biopsy results were negative.
- Diagnostic tests indicate melanoma stage I.

Discussion Questions

1. What risk factors for malignant melanoma does he have?
2. What are the usual clinical manifestations associated with malignant melanoma?
3. What is the prognosis for a patient with this stage of malignant melanoma?
4. What treatment options are available for him?
5. How would you help G.L. deal with his anxiety over the treatment outcomes?
6. ***Priority Decision:*** What is the priority of care for G.L.?
7. What would you include in his patient teaching plan to address future sun exposure?
8. ***Delegation Decision:*** Which of the following nursing personnel should be responsible for teaching G.L.: RN, LPN/LVN, or UAP?
9. ***Priority Decision:*** Based on the assessment data presented, what are the priority nursing diagnoses? Are there any collaborative problems?
10. ***Evidence-Based Practice:*** G.L. wants to know whether regularly applying sunscreen will reduce his risk for developing a second melanoma. How would you reply?

evolve Answers available at *http://evolve.elsevier.com/Lewis/medsurg.*

BRIDGE TO NCLEX EXAMINATION

The number of the question corresponds to the same-numbered outcome at the beginning of the chapter.

1. Which safe sun practices would the nurse include in the teaching care plan for a patient who has photosensitivity *(select all that apply)*?
   a. Wear protective clothing.
   b. Apply sunscreen liberally and often.
   c. Emphasize the short-term use of a tanning booth.
   d. Avoid exposure to the sun, especially during midday.
   e. Wear any sunscreen as long as it is purchased at a drugstore.
2. In teaching a patient who is using topical corticosteroids to treat acute dermatitis, the nurse should tell the patient that *(select all that apply)*
   a. the cream form is the most efficient system of delivery.
   b. short-term use of topical corticosteroids usually does not cause systemic side effects.
   c. creams and ointments should be applied with a glove in small amounts to prevent further infection.
   d. abruptly discontinuing the use of topical corticosteroids may cause a reappearance of the dermatitis.
   e. systemic side effects may be experienced from topical corticosteroids if the person is malnourished.
3. A patient with acne vulgaris tells the nurse that she has quit her job as a receptionist because she believes her facial appearance is unattractive to customers. The nursing diagnosis that best describes this patient response is
   a. ineffective coping related to lack of social support.
   b. impaired skin integrity related to presence of lesions.
   c. anxiety related to lack of knowledge of the disease process.
   d. social isolation related to decreased activities secondary to fear of rejection.
4. In teaching a patient with malignant melanoma about this disorder, the nurse recognizes that the patient's prognosis is most dependent on
   a. the thickness of the lesion.
   b. the degree of asymmetry in the lesion.
   c. the amount of ulceration in the lesion.
   d. how much the lesion has spread superficially.
5. The nurse determines that a patient with a diagnosis of which disorder is most at risk for spreading the disease?
   a. Tinea pedis
   b. Impetigo on the face
   c. Candidiasis of the nails
   d. Psoriasis on the palms and soles
6. A mother and her two children have been diagnosed with pediculosis corporis at a health care center. An appropriate measure in treating this condition is
   a. applying pyrethrins to the body.
   b. topical application of griseofulvin.
   c. moist compresses applied frequently.
   d. administration of systemic antibiotics.
7. A common site for the lesions associated with atopic dermatitis is the
   a. buttocks.
   b. temporal area.
   c. antecubital space.
   d. plantar surface of the feet.
8. During the assessment of a patient, you note an area of red, sharply defined plaques covered with silvery scales that are mildly itchy on the patient's knees and elbows. You recognize this finding as
   a. lentigo.
   b. psoriasis.
   c. actinic keratosis.
   d. seborrheic keratosis.
9. Dermatologic manifestation(s) of Addison's disease can include *(select all that apply)*
   a. urticaria.
   b. loss of body hair.
   c. increased sweating.
   d. generalized hyperpigmentation.
   e. hypopigmentation in the legs and trunk.
10. Important patient teaching after a chemical peel includes
    a. avoidance of sun exposure.
    b. application of firm bandages.
    c. limitation of vigorous exercise.
    d. use of moist heat to relieve discomfort.

1. a, b, d, 2. b, d, 3. d, 4. a, 5. b, 6. a, 7. c, 8. b, 9. b, d, 10. a

evolve

For rationales to these answers and even more NCLEX review questions, visit *http://evolve.elsevier.com/Lewis/medsurg.*

REFERENCES

1. Lim HW, James WD, Rigel D, et al: Adverse effects of ultraviolet radiation from the use of indoor tanning equipment: time to ban the tan, *J Am Acad Dermatol* 64:e51, 2011.
2. US Food and Drug Administration: FDA announces changes to better inform consumers about sunscreen. Retrieved from *www.fda.gov/NewsEvents/Newsroom/PressAnnouncements/ucm258940.htm.*

*3. Green A, Williams G, Logan V, et al: Reduced melanoma after regular sunscreen use: randomized trial follow-up, *J Clin Oncol* 29:257, 2010.

4. American Cancer Society: *Cancer facts and figures* 2011, Atlanta, American Cancer Society. Retrieved from *www.cancer.org.*
5. Rigel D, Russak J, Friedman R: The evolution of melanoma diagnosis: 25 years beyond the ABCDs, *CA-Cancer J Clin* 60:301, 2010.
6. Madan V, Lear J, Szeimies R: Non-melanoma skin cancer, *Lancet* 375:673, 2010.
7. Miller SJ, Alam M, Andersen J, et al: Basal cell and squamous cell skin cancers, *J Natl Compr Cancer Network* 8:836, 2010.
8. Pfenninger J: Approach to various lesions. In Pfenninger J, Fowler G, editors: *Pfenninger and Fowler's procedures for primary care*, ed 3, St Louis, 2010, Saunders.
9. US Food and Drug Administration: FDA approves new treatment for a type of late-stage skin cancer. Retrieved from

*Evidence-based information for clinical practice.

www.fda.gov/newsevents/newsroom/pressannouncements/ucm1193237.htm.
10. Gould D: Diagnosis, prevention and treatment of fungal infections, *Nurs Stand* 33:38, 2011.
11. National Psoriasis Foundation: About psoriasis. Retrieved from *www.psoriasis/org/about.*
12. Agostinis O, Berg K, Cengel K, et al: Photodynamic therapy of cancer, *CA-Cancer J Clin* 61:250, 2011.
13. Hulyalkar R, Rakkhit T, Garcia-Zuazaga J: The role of radiation therapy in the management of skin cancers, *Dermatol Clin* 29:287, 2011.
14. Saunders nursing drug handbook 2012, St Louis, 2012, Mosby.
15. Pfenninger J: Skin biopsy. In Pfenninger J, Fowler G, editors: *Pfenninger and Fowler's procedures for primary care*, ed 3, St Louis, 2010, Saunders.
16. Karim K: Diagnosis, treatment and management of pruritus, *Br J Nurs* 20:356, 2011.
17. Goel A, Krupashankar D, Aurangabadkar S, et al: Fractional lasers in dermatology: current status and recommendations, *Indian J Dermatol Venereol Leprol* 77:369, 2011.
18. Pelosi M, Pelosi M: Liposuction, *Obstet Gynecol Clin* 37:507, 2010.
19. Zhang A, Meine J: Flaps and grafts reconstruction, *Dermatol Clin* 29:217, 2011.

RESOURCES

AcneNet
www.skincarephysicians.com/acnenet
American Academy of Cosmetic Surgery
www.cosmeticsurgery.org
American Academy of Dermatology
www.aad.org
American Academy of Facial Plastic and Reconstructive Surgery
www.aafprs.org
American Society of Plastic Surgical Nurses
https://aspsn.org
Dermatology Foundation
www.dermfnd.org
Dermatology Nurses' Association
www.dnanurse.org
National Institute of Arthritis and Musculoskeletal and Skin Diseases, National Institutes of Health
www.niams.nih.gov
National Psoriasis Foundation
www.psoriasis.org
Skin Cancer Foundation
www.skincancer.org

CHAPTER 25

Holding onto anger is like grasping onto a hot coal with the intent of throwing it at someone else. You are the one who gets burned.
Gautama Buddha

Nursing Management
Burns

Judy Knighton

evolve WEBSITE

http://evolve.elsevier.com/Lewis/medsurg

- NCLEX Review Questions
- Key Points
- Pre-Test
- Answer Guidelines for Case Study on p. 470
- Rationales for Bridge to NCLEX Examination Questions
- Case Study
  - Patient With Burns
- Nursing Care Plan (Customizable)
  - eNCP 25-1: Patient With a Thermal Burn Injury
- Concept Map Creator
- Glossary
- Content Updates

eFigure
- eFig. 25-1: Foot contractures

LEARNING OUTCOMES

1. Relate the causes of and prevention strategies for burn injuries.
2. Differentiate between partial-thickness and full-thickness burns.
3. Apply the tools used to determine the severity of burns.
4. Compare the pathophysiology, clinical manifestations, complications, and collaborative management throughout the three burn phases.
5. Compare the fluid and electrolyte shifts during the emergent and acute burn phases.
6. Differentiate the nutritional needs of the burn patient throughout the three burn phases.
7. Compare the various burn wound care techniques and surgical options for partial-thickness versus full-thickness burn wounds.
8. Prioritize nursing interventions in the management of the burn patient's physiologic and psychosocial needs.
9. Examine the various physiologic and psychosocial aspects of burn rehabilitation.
10. Design a plan of care to prepare the burn patient and caregiver for discharge.

KEY TERMS

burn, p. 450
carboxyhemoglobin, p. 452
chemical burns, p. 451
contracture, p. 468
cultured epithelial autograft (CEA), p. 466
debridement, p. 461
electrical burns, p. 452
escharotomy, p. 458
excision and grafting, p. 465
full-thickness burns, p. 453
partial-thickness burns, p. 453
smoke and inhalation injuries, p. 451
thermal burns, p. 451

The focus of this chapter is the care of patients who have experienced a burn. A **burn** is an injury to the tissues of the body caused by heat, chemicals, electric current, or radiation. The resulting effects are influenced by the temperature of the burning agent, duration of contact time, and type of tissue that is injured.

An estimated 450,000 Americans seek medical care each year for burns.[1,2] Approximately 45,000 people are hospitalized, one half of whom require care in specialized burn centers. About 3500 Americans die annually as a direct result of their injuries. The highest fatality rates occur in children ages 4 years and younger and adults over age 65. Around the world, nearly 11 million people need medical attention annually for burn injuries, and about 300,000 die.[3]

Although burn incidence has decreased over the past 20 years, burn injuries still occur too frequently and mainly to people at a lower socioeconomic level. Most burn incidents should be viewed as preventable. Today, the focus of burn prevention programs has shifted from blaming individuals and changing behaviors to making legislative changes and collecting global burn data to address the unique prevention needs of developing countries.[4]

Coordinated national programs in developed countries have focused on child-resistant lighters, nonflammable children's clothing, tap water anti-scald devices, fire-safe cigarettes, stricter building codes, hardwired smoke detectors and alarms, and fire sprinklers. As a nurse, you can advocate for burn risk reduction strategies in the home and at work, and

Reviewed by Cecilia M. Bidigare, RN, MSN, Associate Professor of Nursing, Sinclair Community College, Beavercreek, Ohio; and Patricia S. Regojo, RN, MSN, Nurse Manager, Burn Center, Temple University Hospital, Philadelphia, Pennsylvania.

TABLE 25-1 SOURCES OF BURN INJURY*

Home Hazards	Occupational Hazards
Kitchen and Bathroom • Microwaved food • Steam, hot grease or liquids from cooking • Hot water heaters set at 140° F (60° C) or higher	• Tar • Chemicals • Hot metals • Steam pipes • Combustible fuels • Fertilizers, pesticides • Electricity from power lines • Sparks from live electric sources
General Household • Fireplaces (e.g., gas, wood) • Open space heaters • Radiators (e.g., home, automobile) • Outdoor grills (e.g., propane, charcoal) • Frayed or defective wiring • Multiple extension cords per outlet • Flammables (e.g., starter fluid, gasoline, kerosene) • Carelessness with cigarettes, matches, candles	

*List is not all-inclusive.

TABLE 25-2 STRATEGIES TO REDUCE BURN INJURY

Flame or Contact
- Never leave candles unattended or near open windows or curtains.
- Use "child-resistant" lighters.
- Hold regular home fire exit drills.
- Never use gasoline or other flammable liquids to start a fire.
- Never leave hot oil unattended while cooking.
- Never smoke in bed.
- Consider a flame-retardant smoking apron for older or "at-risk" people.
- Exercise caution when microwaving food and beverages.

Scald
- Lower hot water temperature to the "lowest point" or 120° F (40° C).
- Use "anti-scald" devices with showerhead or faucet fixtures.
- Supervise bathing with small children, older adults, or anyone with impaired physical movement, physical sensation, or judgment.
- After running bath water, check temperature with back of hand or bath thermometer.

Inhalation
- Install smoke and carbon monoxide detectors.

Chemical
- Store chemicals safely in approved containers and label clearly.
- Ensure safety of workers and students handling chemicals (education, protective eyewear, gloves, masks, clothing).

Electrical
- Avoid or repair frayed wiring.
- Ensure electrical power source is shut off before beginning repairs.
- Wear protective eyewear and gloves when making electrical repairs.
- Avoid outdoor activities during electrical (i.e., lightning) storms.

you can teach workers to reduce burn injuries in both settings (Tables 25-1 and 25-2).

TYPES OF BURN INJURY

Thermal Burns

Thermal burns, caused by flame, flash, scald, or contact with hot objects, are the most common type of burn injury (Fig. 25-1). The severity of the injury depends on the temperature of the burning agent and the duration of contact time. Scald injuries can occur in the bathroom or while cooking. Flash, flame, or contact burns can occur while cooking, smoking, burning leaves in the backyard, or using gasoline or hot oil.

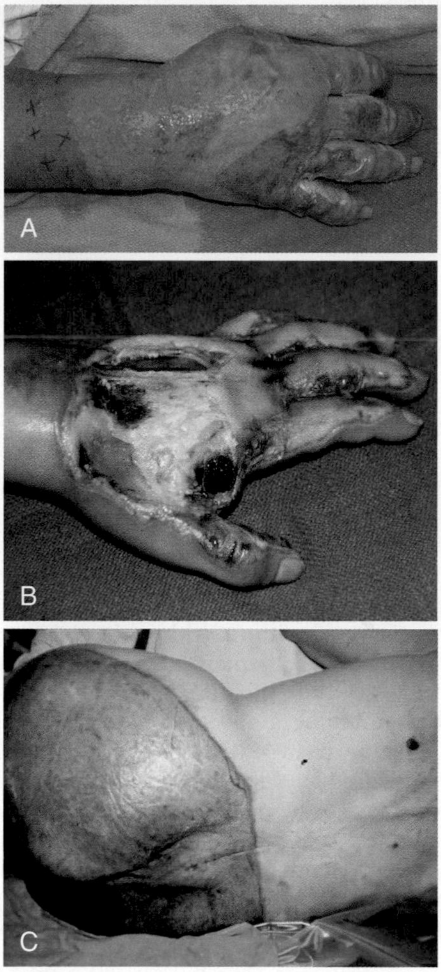

FIG. 25-1 Types of burn injury. **A,** Partial-thickness thermal hand burn. **B,** Full-thickness thermal hand burn. **C,** Full-thickness scald burn to the buttock and lower back secondary to immersion in hot water.

Chemical Burns

Chemical burns are the result of contact with acids, alkalis, and organic compounds. In addition to tissue damage, eyes can be injured if they are splashed with the chemical. Acids are found in the home and at work and include hydrochloric, oxalic, and hydrofluoric acid. Alkali burns can be more difficult to manage than acid burns, since alkalis adhere to tissue, causing protein hydrolysis and liquefaction. Alkalis are found in oven and drain cleaners, fertilizers, and heavy industrial cleansers. Organic compounds, including phenols (chemical disinfectants) and petroleum products (creosote and gasoline), produce contact burns and systemic toxicity.

Smoke and Inhalation Injury

Smoke and inhalation injuries from breathing hot air or noxious chemicals can cause damage to the respiratory tract. Three types of smoke and inhalation injuries can occur: metabolic asphyxiation, upper airway injury, and lower airway injury. Because smoke inhalation injuries are a major predictor of mortality in burn patients, rapid assessment is critical.[5]

TABLE 25-3 MANIFESTATIONS OF LUNG INJURY ASSOCIATED WITH BURNS

Upper Airway	Lower Airway
• Blisters, edema	• High degree of suspicion if patient was trapped in a fire in an enclosed space or clothing caught fire
• Hoarseness	• Presence of facial burns or singed nasal or facial hair
• Difficulty swallowing	• Dyspnea
• Copious secretions	• Carbonaceous sputum
• Stridor	• Wheezing
• Substernal and intercostal retractions	• Hoarseness
• Total airway obstruction	• Altered mental status

Metabolic Asphyxiation. The majority of deaths at a fire scene are the result of inhaling certain smoke elements, primarily carbon monoxide (CO) or hydrogen cyanide. Oxygen delivery to or consumption by tissues is impaired. The result is hypoxia and, ultimately, death when **carboxyhemoglobin** (i.e., hemoglobin combined with CO) blood levels are greater than 20%. CO and hydrogen cyanide poisoning may occur in the absence of burn injury to the skin.

Upper Airway Injury. Upper airway injury results from an inhalation injury to the mouth, oropharynx, and/or larynx. The injury may be caused by thermal burns or the inhalation of hot air, steam, or smoke. Mucosal burns of the oropharynx and the larynx are manifested by redness, blistering, and edema (Table 25-3). The swelling can be massive and the onset rapid. Flame burns to the neck and the chest may make breathing more difficult because of the burn eschar, which becomes tight and constricting from the underlying edema. Swelling from scald burns to the face and the neck can also be lethal, as can external pressure from edema pressing on the airway. Mechanical obstruction can occur quickly, presenting a true medical emergency.

Carefully assess the patient for facial burns, singed nasal hair, hoarseness, painful swallowing, darkened oral and nasal membranes, carbonaceous sputum, history of being burned in an enclosed space, and clothing burns around the chest and neck.

Lower Airway Injury. An inhalation injury to the trachea, bronchioles, and alveoli is usually caused by breathing in toxic chemicals or smoke. Tissue damage is related to the duration of exposure to toxic fumes or smoke. Clinical manifestations of lower airway lung injury are presented in Table 25-3. Pulmonary edema may not appear until 12 to 24 hours after the burn, and then it may manifest as acute respiratory distress syndrome (ARDS) (see Chapter 68).

Electrical Burns

Electrical burns result from intense heat generated from an electric current. Direct damage to nerves and vessels, causing tissue anoxia and death, can also occur. The severity of the electrical injury depends on the amount of voltage, tissue resistance, current pathways, surface area in contact with the current, and length of time that the current flow was sustained (Fig. 25-2). Tissue densities offer various amounts of resistance to electric current. For example, fat and bone offer the most resistance, whereas nerves and blood vessels offer the least resistance. Current that passes through vital organs (e.g., brain, heart, kidneys) produces more life-threatening sequelae than that which passes through other tissues. In addition, electric sparks may ignite the patient's clothing, causing a flash injury.

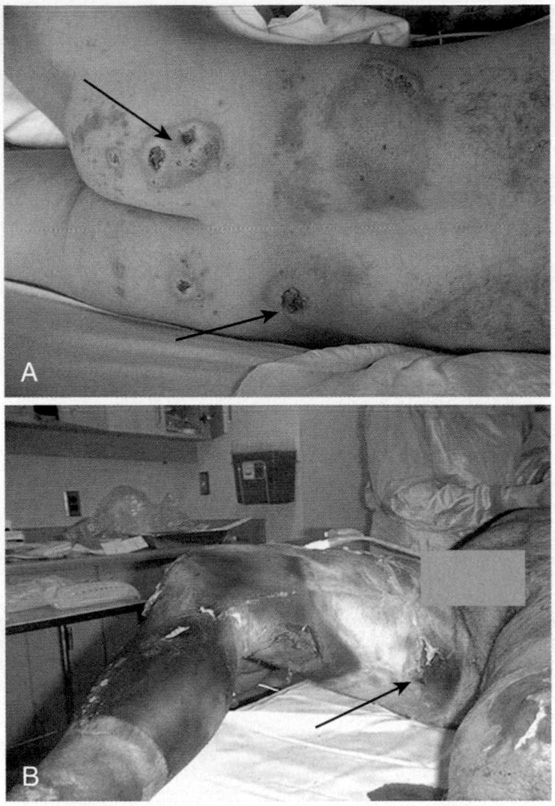

FIG. 25-2 Electrical injury produces heat coagulation of blood supply and contact area as electric current passes through the skin. **A,** Back and buttock (arrows). **B,** Leg (arrow).

As with inhalation injury, perform a rapid assessment of the patient with electrical injury. Transfer to a burn center is indicated. The severity of an electrical injury can be difficult to determine, since most of the damage is below the skin (known as the *iceberg effect*). Determination of electric current contact points and history of the injury may help determine the probable path of the current and potential areas of injury. Contact with electric current can cause muscle contractions strong enough to fracture the long bones and vertebrae. Another reason to suspect long bone or spinal fractures is a fall resulting from the electrical injury. For this reason, all patients with electrical burns should be considered at risk for a potential cervical spine injury. Cervical spine immobilization must be used during transport and subsequent diagnostic testing completed to rule out any injury.

Electrical injury puts the patient at risk for dysrhythmias or cardiac arrest, severe metabolic acidosis, and myoglobinuria. The electric shock event can cause immediate cardiac standstill or ventricular fibrillation. Delayed cardiac dysrhythmias or arrest may also occur without warning during the first 24 hours after injury. Myoglobin from injured muscle tissue and hemoglobin from damaged red blood cells (RBCs) are released into the circulation whenever massive muscle and blood vessel damage occurs. The released myoglobin pigments travel to the kidneys and can block the renal tubules, which can result in acute tubular necrosis (ATN) and acute kidney injury (see Chapter 47).

Cold Thermal Injury

Cold thermal injury, or frostbite, is discussed in Chapter 69.

TABLE 25-4 BURN CENTER REFERRAL CRITERIA

Burn injuries that should be referred to a burn center include the following:

1. Partial-thickness burns >10% of total body surface area (TBSA).
2. Burns that involve the face, hands, feet, genitalia, perineum, or major joints.
3. Third-degree burns in any age-group.
4. Electrical burns, including lightning injury.
5. Chemical burns.
6. Inhalation injury.
7. Burn injury in patients with preexisting medical disorders that could complicate management, prolong recovery, or affect mortality risk (e.g., heart or kidney disease).
8. Any patients with burns and concomitant trauma (e.g., fractures) in which the burn injury poses the greatest risk of morbidity or mortality. In such cases, if the trauma poses the greater immediate risk, the patient may be initially stabilized in a trauma center before being transferred to a burn center. The health care provider will need to use his or her judgment, in consultation with the regional medical control plan and triage protocols.
9. Burn injury in children in hospitals without qualified personnel or equipment needed to care for them.
10. Burn injury in patients who will require special social, emotional, or long-term rehabilitative intervention.

Source: Guidelines for the operation of burn centers. In American College of Surgeons, Committee on Trauma: Resources for optimal care of the injured patient, 2006. Retrieved from *www.ameriburn.org/Chapter14.pdf.*

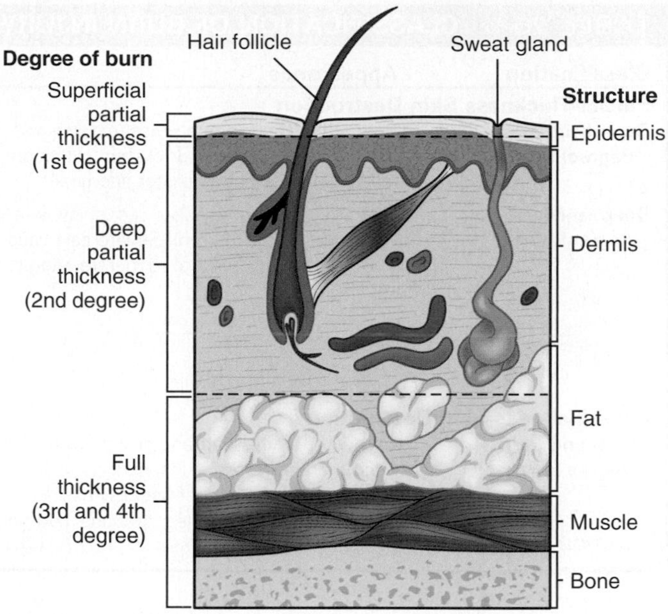

FIG. 25-3 Cross section of skin indicating the depth of burn and structures involved.

CLASSIFICATION OF BURN INJURY

The treatment of burns is related to the severity of the injury.[6] Severity is determined by (1) depth of burn, (2) extent of burn calculated in percent of total body surface area (TBSA), (3) location of burn, and (4) patient risk factors (e.g., age, past medical history). The American Burn Association (ABA) has established referral criteria to determine which burn injuries should be treated in burn centers with specialized facilities (Table 25-4). The majority of patients with minor burn injuries can be managed in community hospitals.[7]

Depth of Burn

Burn injury involves the destruction of the integumentary system. The skin is divided into three layers: epidermis, dermis, and subcutaneous tissue (Fig. 25-3). The *epidermis,* or nonvascular protective outer layer of the skin, is approximately as thick as a sheet of paper. (The structure and function of the skin are discussed in Chapter 23.)

The *dermis,* which lies below the epidermis, is approximately 30 to 45 times thicker than the epidermis. The dermis contains connective tissues with blood vessels, hair follicles, nerve endings, sweat glands, and sebaceous glands.

Under the dermis lies the *subcutaneous tissue,* which contains major vascular networks, fat, nerves, and lymphatics. The subcutaneous tissue acts as a heat insulator for underlying structures, including muscles, tendons, bones, and internal organs.

Burns continue to be defined by degrees: first, second, third, and fourth degree. The ABA recommends a more precise definition and classifies burns according to depth of skin destruction: **partial-thickness burns** and **full-thickness burns** (see Fig. 25-3). Skin-reproducing (re-epithelializing) cells are located along the shafts of the hair follicles, sweat glands, and oil glands. If significant damage occurs to the dermis (i.e., a full-thickness burn), not enough skin cells remain to regenerate new skin. A permanent, alternative source of skin needs to be found. Table 25-5 compares the various burn classifications according to the depth of injury.

Extent of Burn

Two commonly used guides for determining the TBSA affected or the extent of a burn wound are the *Lund-Browder chart* (Fig. 25-4, *A*) and the *Rule of Nines* (Fig. 25-4, *B*). (First-degree burns, equivalent to a sunburn, are not included when calculating TBSA.) The Lund-Browder chart is considered more accurate because it considers the patient's age in proportion to relative body-area size. The Rule of Nines is often used for initial assessment of a burn patient because it is easy to remember. For irregular- or odd-shaped burns, the patient's hand (including the fingers) is approximately 1% TBSA. The *Sage Burn Diagram* is a free, Internet-based tool for estimating TBSA burned *(www.sagediagram.com).*

Location of Burn

The severity of the burn injury is also determined by the location of the burn wound. Burns to the face and neck and circumferential burns to the chest or back may interfere with breathing as a result of mechanical obstruction from edema or leathery, devitalized burn tissue *(eschar).* These burns may also indicate possible inhalation injury and respiratory mucosal damage.

Burns to the hands, feet, joints, and eyes are of concern because they make self-care difficult and may jeopardize future function. Burns to the hands and feet are challenging to manage because of superficial vascular and nerve supply systems that need to be protected while the burn wounds are healing.

Burns to the ears and the nose are susceptible to infection because of poor blood supply to the cartilage. Burns to the buttocks or perineum are highly susceptible to infection from urine or feces contamination. Circumferential burns to the extremi-

TABLE 25-5 CLASSIFICATION OF BURN INJURY DEPTH

Classification	Appearance	Possible Cause	Structures Involved
Partial-Thickness Skin Destruction			
Superficial (first-degree) burn	Erythema, blanching on pressure, pain and mild swelling, no vesicles or blisters (although after 24 hr skin may blister and peel).	Superficial sunburn Quick heat flash	Superficial epidermal damage with hyperemia. Tactile and pain sensation intact.
Deep (second-degree) burn	Fluid-filled vesicles that are red, shiny, wet (if vesicles have ruptured). Severe pain caused by nerve injury. Mild to moderate edema.	Flame Flash Scald Contact burns Chemical Tar Electric current	Epidermis and dermis involved to varying depths. Skin elements, from which epithelial regeneration occurs, remain viable.
Full-Thickness Skin Destruction			
Third- and fourth-degree burns	Dry, waxy white, leathery, or hard skin; visible thrombosed vessels. Insensitivity to pain because of nerve destruction. Possible involvement of muscles, tendons, and bones.	Flame Scald Chemical Tar Electric current	All skin elements and local nerve endings destroyed. Coagulation necrosis present. Surgical intervention required for healing.

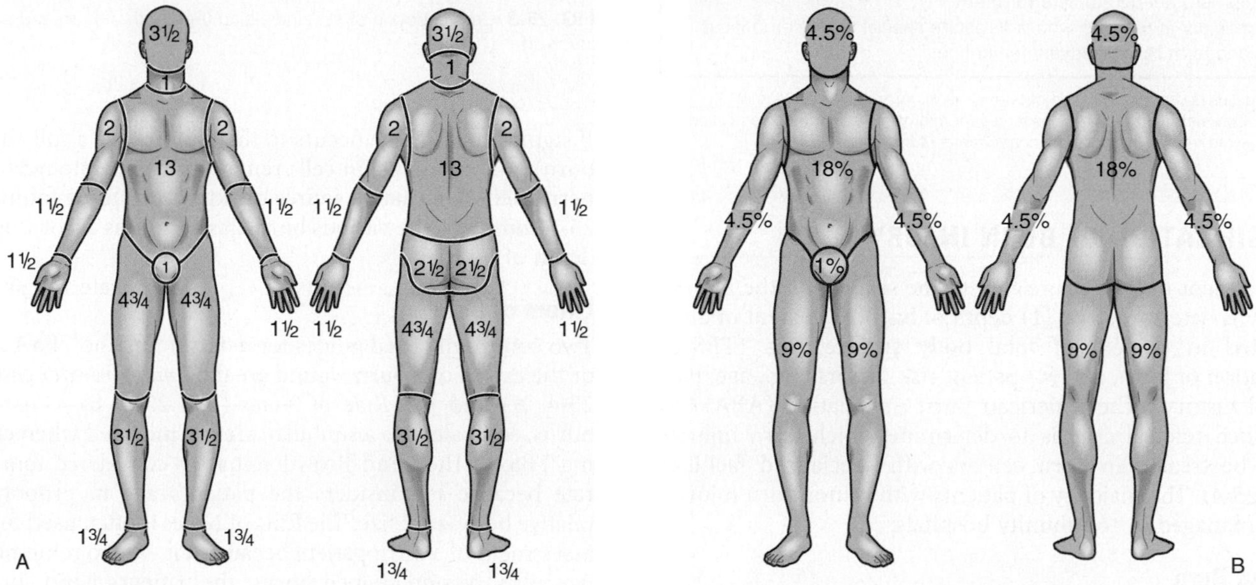

FIG. 25-4 A, Lund-Browder chart. By convention, areas of partial-thickness injury are colored in blue and areas of full-thickness injury in red. Superficial partial-thickness burns are not calculated. **B,** Rule of Nines chart.

ties can cause circulation problems distal to the burn, with possible nerve damage to the affected extremity. Patients may also develop compartment syndrome (see Chapter 63) from direct heat damage to the muscles, swelling, and/or preburn vascular problems.

Patient Risk Factors

Any patient with preexisting cardiovascular, respiratory, or renal disease has a poorer prognosis for recovery because of the tremendous demands placed on the body by a burn injury. The patient with diabetes mellitus or peripheral vascular disease is at high risk for poor healing, especially with foot and leg burns.[8] General physical debilitation from any chronic disease, including alcoholism, drug abuse, or malnutrition, makes it challenging for the patient to fully recover from a burn injury. In addition, the burn patient who has also sustained fractures, head injuries, or other trauma has a more difficult time recovering.

PHASES OF BURN MANAGEMENT

Burn management can be organized chronologically into three phases: emergent (resuscitative), acute (wound healing), and rehabilitative (restorative). Overlap in care does exist. For example, the emergent phase begins at the time of the burn injury, and care often begins in the prehospital phase, depending on the skill level of providers at the scene. Planning for rehabilitation begins on the day of the burn injury or admission to the burn center. Formal rehabilitation begins as soon as functional assessments can be performed. Wound care is the primary focus of the acute phase, but wound care also takes place in both the emergent and rehabilitation phases.

PREHOSPITAL CARE

At the scene of the injury, priority is given to removing the person from the source of the burn and stopping the burning

TABLE 25-6 EMERGENCY MANAGEMENT

Thermal Burns

Etiology	Assessment Findings	Interventions
• Hot liquids or solids • Flash flame • Open flame • Steam • Hot surface • Ultraviolet rays	***Partial-Thickness (superficial; first-degree) Burn*** • Redness • Pain • Moderate to severe tenderness • Minimal edema • Blanching with pressure ***Partial-Thickness (deep; second-degree) Burn*** • Moist blebs, blisters • Mottled white, pink to cherry-red • Hypersensitive to touch or air • Moderate to severe pain • Blanching with pressure ***Full-Thickness (third- and fourth-degree) Burns*** • Dry, leathery eschar • Waxy white, dark brown, or charred appearance • Strong burn odor • Impaired sensation when touched • Absence of pain with severe pain in surrounding tissues • Lack of blanching with pressure	**Initial** • Assess airway, breathing, and circulation. • Stabilize cervical spine. • Assess for inhalation injury. • Provide supplemental O_2 as needed. • Anticipate endotracheal intubation and mechanical ventilation with circumferential full-thickness burns to the neck and chest or large TBSA burn. • Monitor vital signs, level of consciousness, respiratory status, O_2 saturation, and heart rhythm. • Remove nonadherent clothing, shoes, watches, jewelry, glasses or contact lenses (if face was exposed). • Cover burned areas with dry dressings or clean sheet. • Establish IV access with two large-bore catheters if burn >15% TBSA. • Begin fluid replacement. • Insert indwelling urinary catheter if burn >15% TBSA. • Elevate burned limbs above heart to decrease edema. • Administer IV analgesia and assess effectiveness frequently. • Identify and treat other associated injuries (e.g., fractures, head injury). **Ongoing Monitoring** • Monitor airway. • Monitor vital signs, heart rhythm, level of consciousness, respiratory status, and O_2 saturation. • Monitor urine output.

TBSA, Total body surface area.

process. Rescuers must also protect themselves from being injured. In the case of electrical and chemical injuries, initial management involves removal of the patient from contact with the electrical or chemical source.

Small thermal burns (10% or less of TBSA) should be covered with a clean, cool, tap water–dampened towel for the patient's comfort and protection until medical care is available.[9] Cooling of the injured area (if small) within 1 minute helps minimize the depth of the injury. If the burn is large (greater than 10% TBSA) or an electrical or inhalation burn is suspected, first focus your attention on the ABCs:

- *Airway:* Check for patency, soot around nares and on the tongue, singed nasal hair, darkened oral or nasal membranes.
- *Breathing:* Check for adequacy of ventilation.
- *Circulation:* Check for presence and regularity of pulses, and elevate the burned limb(s) above the heart to decrease pain and swelling.

To prevent hypothermia, cool large burns for no more than 10 minutes. Do not immerse the burned body part in cool water because it may cause extensive heat loss. Never cover a burn with ice, since this can cause hypothermia and vasoconstriction of blood vessels, thus further reducing blood flow to the injury. Gently remove as much burned clothing as possible to prevent further tissue damage. Leave adherent clothing in place until the patient is transferred to a hospital. Wrap the patient in a dry, clean sheet or blanket to prevent further contamination of the wound and to provide warmth.

Chemical burns are best treated by quickly removing any chemical particles or powder from the skin. Remove all clothing containing the chemical because the burning process continues while the chemical is in contact with the skin. Flush the affected area with copious amounts of water to irrigate the skin anywhere from 20 minutes to 2 hours postexposure. Tap water is acceptable for flushing eyes exposed to chemicals. Tissue destruction may continue for up to 72 hours after contact with some chemicals.

Observe patients with inhalation injuries closely for signs of respiratory distress. These patients need to be treated quickly and efficiently if they are to survive. If CO poisoning is suspected, treat the patient with 100% humidified O_2. Patients who have both body burns and an inhalation injury must be transferred to the nearest burn center.

Always remember that the burn patient may also have sustained other injuries that could take priority over the burn itself. Individuals involved in the prehospital phase of burn care must adequately communicate the circumstances of the injury to hospital providers. This is especially important when the patient's injury involves being trapped in a closed space, exposure to hazardous chemicals or electricity, or a possible traumatic injury (e.g., fall).

Prehospital care and emergency management are presented in tables that describe thermal burns (Table 25-6), inhalation injury (Table 25-7), electrical burns (Table 25-8), and chemical burns (Table 25-9).

EMERGENT PHASE

The *emergent (resuscitative) phase* is the time required to resolve the immediate, life-threatening problems resulting from the burn injury. This phase usually lasts up to 72 hours from the time the burn occurred. The primary concerns are the onset of hypovolemic shock and edema formation. The emergent phase ends when fluid mobilization and diuresis begin.

TABLE 25-7 EMERGENCY MANAGEMENT

Inhalation Injury

Etiology	Assessment Findings	Interventions
• Exposure of respiratory tract to intense heat or flames • Inhalation of noxious chemicals, smoke, or CO	• History of being trapped in an enclosed space, being in an explosion, or having clothing catch fire • Rapid, shallow respirations • Increasing hoarseness • Coughing • Singed nasal or facial hair • Darkened oral or nasal membranes • Smoky breath • Carbonaceous sputum • Productive cough with black, gray, or bloody sputum • Irritation of upper airways or burning pain in throat or chest • Difficulty swallowing • Cherry-red skin color (CO levels >20%) • Restlessness, anxiety • Altered mental status, including confusion, coma • Decreased O_2 saturation • Dysrhythmias	**Initial** • Assess airway, breathing, and circulation. • Stabilize cervical spine. • Assess for thermal burn. • Provide 100% humidified O_2. • Anticipate endotracheal intubation and mechanical ventilation with significant inhalation injury. • Monitor vital signs, level of consciousness, O_2 saturation, and heart rhythm. • Remove nonadherent clothing, jewelry, glasses, or contact lenses (if face was exposed). • Establish IV access with two large-bore catheters if burn >15% TBSA. • Begin fluid replacement. • Insert indwelling urinary catheter if burn >15% TBSA. • Elevate burned limb(s) above heart to decrease edema. • Obtain arterial blood gas, carboxyhemoglobin levels, and chest x-ray. • Administer IV analgesia and assess effectiveness frequently. • Identify and treat other associated injuries (e.g., fractures, pneumothorax, head injury). • Cover burned areas with dry dressings or clean sheet. • Anticipate need for fiberoptic bronchoscopy or intubation. **Ongoing Monitoring** • Monitor airway. • Monitor vital signs, level of consciousness, respiratory status, O_2 saturation, and heart rhythm. • Monitor urine output.

CO, Carbon monoxide; *TBSA,* total body surface area.

TABLE 25-8 EMERGENCY MANAGEMENT

Electrical Burns

Etiology	Assessment Findings	Interventions
Alternating Current • Electric wires • Utility wires **Direct Current** • Lightning • Defibrillator	• Leathery, white, or charred skin • Burn odor • Loss of consciousness • Impaired touch sensation • Minimal or absent pain • Dysrhythmias • Cardiac arrest • Location of contact points • Diminished peripheral circulation in injured extremity • Thermal burns if clothing ignites • Fractures or dislocations from force of current • Head or neck injury if fall occurred • Depth and extent of wound difficult to visualize. Assume injury greater than what is seen	**Initial** • Remove patient from electrical source while protecting rescuer. • Assess airway, breathing, and circulation. • Stabilize cervical spine. • Provide supplemental O_2 as needed. • Monitor vital signs, heart rhythm, level of consciousness, respiratory status, and O_2 saturation. • Check pulses distal to burns. • Remove nonadherent clothing, shoes, watches, jewelry, glasses or contact lenses (if face was exposed). • Cover burned areas with dry dressings or clean sheet. • Establish IV access with two large-bore catheters if burn >15% TBSA. • Begin fluid replacement. • Obtain arterial blood gas to assess acid-base balance. • Insert indwelling urinary catheter if burn >15% TBSA. • Elevate burned limb(s) above heart to decrease edema. • Administer IV analgesia and assess effectiveness frequently. • Identify and treat other associated injuries (e.g., fractures, head injury, thermal burns). **Ongoing Monitoring** • Monitor airway. • Monitor vital signs, heart rhythm, level of consciousness, respiratory status, O_2 saturation, and neurovascular status of injured limbs. • Monitor urine output. • Monitor urine for development of myoglobinuria secondary to muscle breakdown and hemoglobinuria secondary to RBC breakdown. • Anticipate possible administration of $NaHCO_3$ to alkalinize the urine and maintain serum pH >6.0.

$NaHCO_3$, Sodium bicarbonate; *TBSA,* total body surface area.

TABLE 25-9 EMERGENCY MANAGEMENT

Chemical Burns

Etiology	Assessment Findings	Interventions
• Acids • Alkalis • Organic compounds	• Burning • Redness, swelling of injured tissue • Degeneration of exposed tissue • Discoloration of injured skin • Localized pain • Edema of surrounding tissue • Tissue destruction continuing for up to 72 hr • Respiratory distress if chemical inhaled • Decreased muscle coordination (if organophosphate) • Paralysis	**Initial** • Assess airway, breathing, and circulation before decontamination procedures. • Stabilize cervical spine. • Provide supplemental O_2 as needed. • Brush dry chemical from skin before irrigation. • Remove nonadherent clothing, shoes, watches, jewelry, glasses or contact lenses (if face was exposed). • Flush chemical from wound and surrounding area with copious amounts of saline solution or water. • For chemical burn of the eye(s), flush from inner to outer corner of eye with water or lactated Ringer's (if available). • Cover burned areas with dry dressings or clean sheet. • Establish IV access with two large-bore catheters if burn >15% TBSA. • Begin fluid replacement. • Insert indwelling urinary catheter if burn >15% TBSA. • Elevate burned limb(s) above heart to decrease edema. • Administer IV analgesia and assess effectiveness frequently. • Contact poison control center for assistance. **Ongoing Monitoring** • Monitor airway if exposed to chemicals. • Monitor urine output. • Consider possibility of systemic impact of identified chemical, and monitor and treat accordingly. • Monitor pH of eye if exposed to chemicals.

TBSA, Total body surface area.

Pathophysiology

Fluid and Electrolyte Shifts. The greatest initial threat to a patient with a major burn is hypovolemic shock (Fig. 25-5). It is caused by a massive shift of fluids out of the blood vessels as a result of increased capillary permeability and can begin as early as 20 minutes postburn. As the capillary walls become more permeable, water, sodium, and plasma proteins (especially albumin) move into the interstitial spaces and other surrounding tissue. The colloidal osmotic pressure decreases with progressive loss of protein from the vascular space. This results in more fluid shifting out of the vascular space into the interstitial spaces (Fig. 25-6). Fluid accumulation in the interstitium is termed *second spacing.*

Fluid also moves to areas that normally have minimal to no fluid, a phenomenon termed *third spacing.* Examples of third spacing in burn injury are exudate and blister formation, as well as edema in nonburned areas.

Other sources of fluid loss are insensible losses by evaporation from large, denuded body surfaces and the respiratory system. The normal insensible loss of 30 to 50 mL/hr is increased in the severely burned patient. The net result of the fluid shifts and losses is termed *intravascular volume depletion.* Clinical signs of hypovolemic shock are decreased blood pressure (BP) and increased heart rate. If hypovolemic shock is not corrected, irreversible shock and death may result. (Shock is discussed in Chapter 67.)

The circulatory system is also affected by the hemolysis of RBCs from circulating factors (e.g., oxygen free radicals) released at the time of the burn, as well as by the direct insult of the burn injury. Thrombosis in the capillaries of burned tissue causes an additional loss of circulating RBCs. An elevated hematocrit is commonly caused by hemoconcentration resulting from fluid loss. After fluid balance has been restored, dilution causes the hematocrit levels to drop.

PATHOPHYSIOLOGY MAP

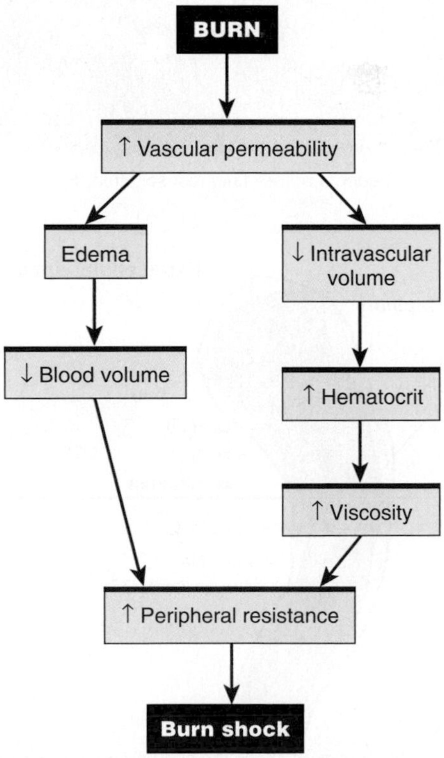

FIG. 25-5 At the time of major burn injury, there is increased capillary permeability. All fluid components of the blood begin to leak into the interstitium, causing edema and a decreased blood volume. Hematocrit increases, and the blood becomes more viscous. The combination of decreased blood volume and increased viscosity produces increased peripheral resistance. Burn shock, a type of hypovolemic shock, rapidly ensues and, if not corrected, can result in death.

Major electrolyte shifts of sodium and potassium also occur during this phase. Sodium rapidly moves to the interstitial spaces and remains there until edema formation ceases (Fig. 25-7). A potassium shift develops initially because injured cells and hemolyzed RBCs release potassium into the circulation.

Toward the end of the emergent phase, capillary membrane permeability is restored if fluid replacement is adequate. Fluid loss and edema formation end. Interstitial fluid gradually returns to the vascular space (see Fig. 25-7). Diuresis occurs, and the urine has a low specific gravity.

Inflammation and Healing. Burn injury to tissues and vessels causes coagulation necrosis. Neutrophils and monocytes accumulate at the site of injury. Fibroblasts and newly formed collagen fibrils appear and begin wound repair within the first 6 to 12 hours after injury. (The inflammatory response is discussed in Chapter 12.)

Immunologic Changes. The body's immune system is challenged when a burn injury occurs. The skin barrier to invading organisms is destroyed, bone marrow depression occurs, and circulating levels of immunoglobulins are decreased. Defects occur in the function of white blood cells (WBCs). The inflammatory cytokine cascade, triggered by tissue damage, impairs the function of lymphocytes, monocytes, and neutrophils. Thus the patient is at a greater risk for infection.

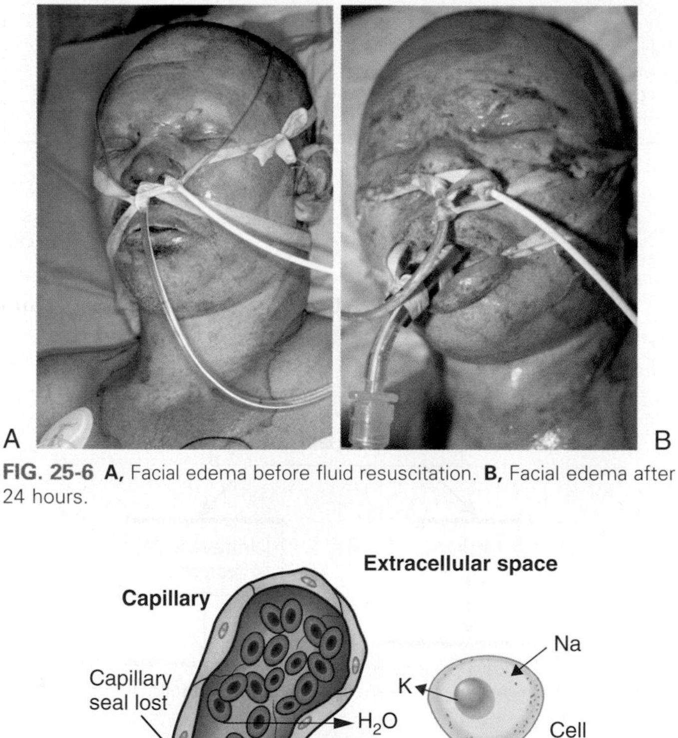

FIG. 25-6 **A,** Facial edema before fluid resuscitation. **B,** Facial edema after 24 hours.

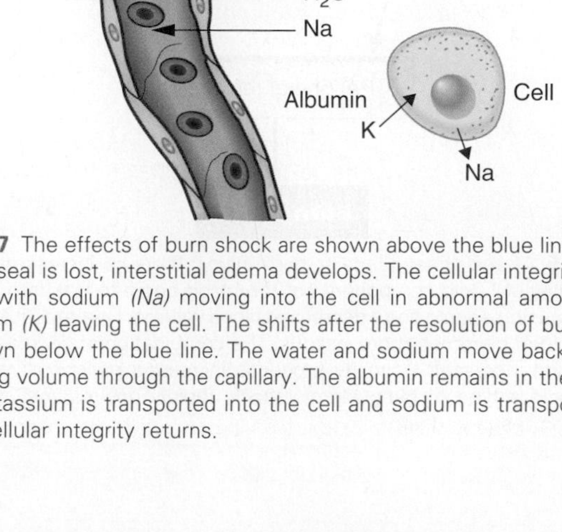

FIG. 25-7 The effects of burn shock are shown above the blue line. As the capillary seal is lost, interstitial edema develops. The cellular integrity is also altered, with sodium *(Na)* moving into the cell in abnormal amounts and potassium *(K)* leaving the cell. The shifts after the resolution of burn shock are shown below the blue line. The water and sodium move back into the circulating volume through the capillary. The albumin remains in the interstitium. Potassium is transported into the cell and sodium is transported out as the cellular integrity returns.

Clinical Manifestations

The patient with severe burns is likely to be in shock from hypovolemia. Frequently the areas of full-thickness and deep partial-thickness burns are initially anesthetic because the nerve endings have been destroyed. Superficial to moderate partial-thickness burns are very painful. Blisters, filled with fluid and protein, are common in partial-thickness burns. The patient with a larger burn area may develop a paralytic ileus, with absent or decreased bowel sounds. Shivering may occur as a result of chilling that is caused by heat loss, anxiety, or pain. The patient may be alert and able to answer questions shortly after admission or until he or she is intubated (if there is an inhalation injury). Patients are often frightened and benefit from your calm reassurances and simple explanations of what to expect as you provide care. Unconsciousness or altered mental status in a burn patient is usually not a result of the burn but of the hypoxia associated with smoke inhalation. Other possibilities include head trauma, substance abuse, or excessive amounts of sedation or pain medication.

Complications

The three major organ systems most susceptible to complications during the emergent phase of burn injury are the cardiovascular, respiratory, and urinary systems.

Cardiovascular System. Cardiovascular system complications include dysrhythmias and hypovolemic shock, which, if untreated, may progress to irreversible shock. Circulation to the extremities can be severely impaired by deep circumferential burns and subsequent edema formation, which act like a tourniquet. If untreated, ischemia, paresthesias, and necrosis can occur. An **escharotomy** (a scalpel or electrocautery incision through the full-thickness eschar) is frequently performed after transfer to a burn center to restore circulation to compromised extremities (Fig. 25-8). Initially, blood viscosity increases because of the fluid loss. Microcirculation is impaired because of the damage to skin structures that contain small capillary systems. These two events result in a phenomenon termed *sludging*. Sludging can be corrected by adequate fluid replacement.

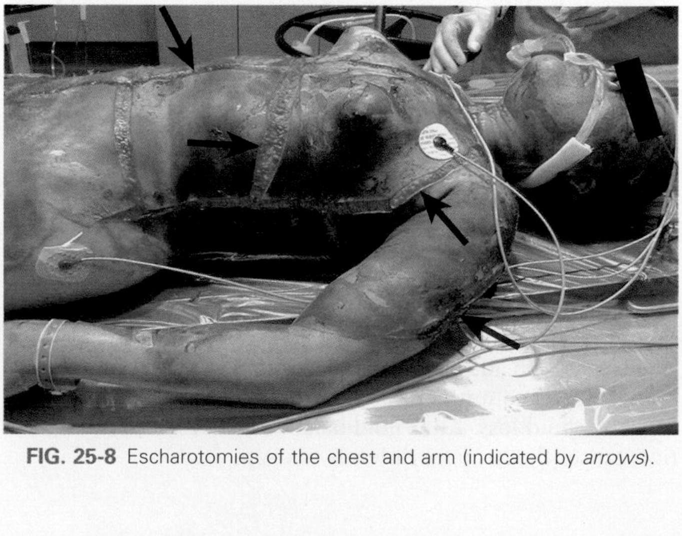

FIG. 25-8 Escharotomies of the chest and arm (indicated by *arrows*).

Respiratory System. The respiratory system is vulnerable to two types of injury: (1) upper airway burns and (2) lower airway injury (see Table 25-3). Upper airway distress may occur with or without smoke inhalation, and airway injury at either level may occur in the absence of burn injury to the skin. (Smoke and inhalation injuries are discussed earlier in this chapter on pp. 451-452.)

The patient may require a fiberoptic bronchoscopy and carboxyhemoglobin blood levels to confirm a suspected inhalation injury. Look in the prehospital notes to see if the patient was exposed to smoke or fumes. Examine any sputum for carbon. Watch for signs of impending respiratory distress, such as increased agitation, anxiety, restlessness, or a change in the rate or character of the patient's breathing, since symptoms may not be present immediately. In general, there is no correlation between the extent of TBSA burn and severity of inhalation injury. In a patient with inhalation injury, a chest x-ray may appear normal on admission, but changes usually occur over the next 24 to 48 hours. Arterial blood gas (ABG) values may also be within the normal range on admission and change over time.

Other Cardiopulmonary Problems. Patients with preexisting heart disease (e.g., myocardial infarction) or lung disease (e.g., chronic obstructive pulmonary disease) are at an increased risk for complications. If fluid replacement is too vigorous, watch for early signs of heart failure or pulmonary edema. Invasive measures (e.g., hemodynamic monitoring) may be necessary to monitor fluid resuscitation.

Patients with preexisting respiratory problems are more likely to develop a respiratory tract infection. Pneumonia, a common complication of major burns, is the leading cause of death in patients with an inhalation injury.

Burn patients are at an increased risk for venous thromboembolism (VTE) if one or more of the following conditions are present: advanced age, morbid obesity, extensive or lower-extremity burns, concomitant lower-extremity trauma, and prolonged immobility.[10] VTE prophylaxis should be started and should include medications such as enoxaparin (Lovenox) unless contraindicated.[11]

Urinary System. The most common complication of the urinary system in the emergent phase is acute tubular necrosis (ATN). If your patient becomes hypovolemic, blood flow to the kidneys is decreased, causing renal ischemia. If this continues, acute kidney injury may develop.

With full-thickness and major electrical burns, myoglobin (from muscle cell breakdown) and hemoglobin (from RBC breakdown) are released into the bloodstream and occlude renal tubules. Carefully monitor the adequacy of fluid replacement because this can counteract obstruction of the tubules.

NURSING AND COLLABORATIVE MANAGEMENT EMERGENT PHASE

In the emergent phase the patient's survival depends on rapid and thorough assessment and appropriate interventions. Usually the physician and you make an initial assessment of the depth and extent of the burn and coordinate the actions of others on the health care team. In a community hospital, determine whether the patient requires inpatient or outpatient care. In the case of inpatient care, decide whether the patient remains in the hospital or should be transferred to the closest burn center (see Table 25-4).

Nursing and collaborative management predominantly consists of airway management, fluid therapy, and wound care (Table 25-10). Patients often improve and worsen, unpredictably, on an almost daily basis.

Although physical and occupational therapy are important in both the acute and rehabilitation phases, proper positioning and splinting begin on the day of admission. Emotional support and teaching of patients and caregivers begin on admission. A nursing care plan for the patient with burn injury (eNursing Care Plan 25-1) is available on the website for this chapter.

AIRWAY MANAGEMENT

Airway management frequently involves early endotracheal (preferably orotracheal) intubation. Early intubation eliminates the need for emergency tracheostomy after respiratory problems have become apparent. In general, the patient with burns to the face and neck requires intubation within 1 to 2 hours after injury. (Intubation is discussed in Chapter 66.) After intubation the patient is placed on ventilatory support, with the delivered oxygen concentration based on ABG values. Extubation may be indicated when the edema resolves, usually 3 to 6 days after burn injury, unless severe inhalation injury is involved. Escharotomies of the chest wall may be needed to relieve respiratory distress secondary to circumferential, full-thickness burns of the neck and trunk (see Fig. 25-8).

Within 6 to 12 hours after injury in which smoke inhalation is suspected, a fiberoptic bronchoscopy should be performed to assess the lower airway. When intubation is not performed, treatment of inhalation injury includes administration of 100% humidified O_2 as needed. Place the patient in a high Fowler's position, unless contraindicated (e.g., spinal injury), and encourage deep breathing and coughing every hour. Reposition the patient every 1 to 2 hours and provide suctioning and chest physiotherapy (as ordered). If severe respiratory distress (e.g., hoarseness, shortness of breath) develops, intubation and mechanical ventilation are initiated. Positive end-expiratory pressure (PEEP) may be used to prevent collapse of the alveoli and progressive respiratory failure (see Chapters 66 and 68). Bronchodilators may be administered to treat severe bronchospasm. CO poisoning is treated by administering 100% O_2 until carboxyhemoglobin levels return to normal.

FLUID THERAPY

Establishing IV access is critical for fluid resuscitation and drug administration. At least two large-bore IV access sites must be in place for patients with burns that are 15% TBSA or more. It is critical to establish IV access that can handle large volumes of fluid. For patients with burns greater than 30% TBSA, consider a central line for fluid and drug administration and blood sampling (central lines are discussed in Chapter 17). An arterial line is often placed if frequent ABGs or invasive BP monitoring is needed.

Assess the extent of the burn wound using a standardized chart (see Fig. 25-4). Then use a standardized formula to estimate the patient's fluid resuscitation requirements. Fluid replacement is achieved with crystalloid solutions (usually lactated Ringer's), colloids (albumin), or a combination of the two.[12] Paramedics generally give IV saline until the patient's arrival at the hospital.

The Parkland (Baxter) formula for fluid replacement is the most common formula used (Table 25-11, or *www.mdcalc.com/parkland-formula-for-burns*). Remember that all formulas are

TABLE 25-10 COLLABORATIVE CARE

Burn Injury

Emergent Phase	Acute Phase	Rehabilitation Phase
Fluid Therapy (see Table 25-11) • Assess fluid needs. • Begin IV fluid replacement. • Insert indwelling urinary catheter. • Monitor urine output. **Wound Care** • Start daily shower and wound care. • Debride as necessary. • Assess extent and depth of burns. • Administer tetanus toxoid or tetanus antitoxin. **Pain and Anxiety** • Assess and manage pain and anxiety. **Physical and Occupational Therapy** • Place patient in position that prevents contracture formation and reduces edema. • Assess need for splints. **Nutritional Therapy** • Assess nutritional needs and begin feeding patient by most appropriate route as soon as possible. **Respiratory Therapy** • Assess oxygenation needs. • Provide supplemental O_2 as needed. • Intubate if necessary. • Monitor respiratory status. **Psychosocial Care** • Provide support to patient and caregiver during initial crisis phase.	**Fluid Therapy** • Continue to replace fluids, depending on patient's clinical response. **Wound Care** • Continue daily shower and wound care. • Continue debridement (if necessary). • Assess wound daily and adjust dressing protocols as necessary. • Observe for complications (e.g., infection). **Early Excision and Grafting** • Provide temporary allografts. • Provide permanent autografts. • Care for donor sites. **Pain and Anxiety** • Continue to assess for and treat pain and anxiety. **Physical and Occupational Therapy** • Begin daily therapy program for maintenance of range of motion. • Assess need for splints and anticontracture positioning. • Encourage and assist patient with self-care as possible. **Nutritional Therapy** • Continue to assess diet to support wound healing. **Respiratory Therapy** • Continue to assess oxygenation needs. • Continue to monitor respiratory status. • Monitor for signs of complications (e.g., pneumonia). **Psychosocial Care** • Provide ongoing support, counseling, and teaching to patient and caregiver about physical and emotional aspects of care and recovery. • Begin to anticipate discharge needs. **Drug Therapy** (see Table 25-13) • Assess need for medications (e.g., antibiotics). • Continue to monitor effectiveness and adjust dosage as needed.	• Continue to counsel and teach patient and caregiver. • Continue to encourage and assist patient in resuming self-care. • Continue to prevent or minimize contractures and assess likelihood for scarring (surgery, physical and occupational therapy, splinting, pressure garments). • Discuss possible reconstructive surgery. • Prepare for discharge home or transfer to rehabilitation hospital.

TABLE 25-11 FLUID RESUSCITATION

Parkland (Baxter) Formula*

4 mL lactated Ringer's solution per kilogram (kg) of body weight per percent of total body surface area (% TBSA) burned = Total fluid requirements for first 24 hr after burn

Application

½ of total in first 8 hr
¼ of total in second 8 hr
¼ of total in third 8 hr

Example

For a 70 kg patient with a 50% TBSA burn:
4 mL × 70 kg × 50 TBSA burned = 14,000 mL in 24 hr

½ of total in first 8 hr = 7000 mL (875 mL/hr)
¼ of total in second 8 hr = 3500 mL (437 mL/hr)
¼ of total in third 8 hr = 3500 mL (437 mL/hr)

*Formulas are guidelines. Fluid is administered at a rate to produce 0.5-1.0 mL/kg/hr of urine output. The American Burn Association Consensus Fluid Resuscitation Formula of 2-4 mL lactated Ringer's solution per kg of body weight per %TBSA burned = Total fluid requirements for first 24 hr after burn has been suggested as a strategy to avoid over-resuscitation, or "fluid creep."

estimates, and fluids must be titrated based on the patient's response (e.g., hourly urine output, vital signs). Patients with an electrical injury have greater than normal fluid requirements and generally require an osmotic diuretic (mannitol [Osmitrol]) to increase their urine output and overcome high levels of hemoglobin and myoglobin in the urine. Too much fluid and overestimation of TBSA contribute to the development of "fluid creep."[13] For the first 24 hours, the recommendation is 2 to 4 mL lactated Ringer's/kg/%TBSA burned.

Colloidal solutions (e.g., 5% albumin) may also be given. However, administration is recommended after the first 12 to 24 hours postburn when capillary permeability returns to normal or near normal. After this time, the plasma remains in the vascular space and expands the circulating volume. The replacement volume is calculated based on the patient's body weight and TBSA burned (e.g., 0.3 to 0.5 mL/kg/%TBSA burned).

Hourly assessments of the adequacy of fluid resuscitation are best made using clinical parameters. Urine output, the most commonly used parameter, and cardiac parameters are defined as follows.

- *Urine output:* 0.5 to 1 mL/kg/hr; 75 to 100 mL/hr for electrical burn patient with evidence of hemoglobinuria or myoglobinuria.
- *Cardiac parameters:* Mean arterial pressure (MAP) greater than 65 mm Hg, systolic BP greater than 90 mm Hg, heart rate less than 120 beats/minute. MAP and BP are best measured by an arterial line. Manual BP measurement is often invalid because of edema and vasoconstriction.

WOUND CARE

Once a patent airway, effective circulation, and adequate fluid replacement have been established, priority is given to care of the burn wound. Partial-thickness burn wounds appear pink to cherry-red and are wet and shiny with serous exudate. These wounds may or may not have intact blisters; are painful when touched; and have only minor, localized sensation because nerve endings have been destroyed in the burned dermis.

You and appropriate personnel can perform cleansing and gentle debridement, using scissors and forceps, on a cart shower (Fig. 25-9), regular shower, or patient bed or stretcher.[14] Extensive, surgical debridement is performed in the operating room (OR) (Fig. 25-10). During **debridement,** necrotic skin is removed. Releasing escharotomies and fasciotomies are carried out in the emergent phase, usually in burn centers by burn physicians.

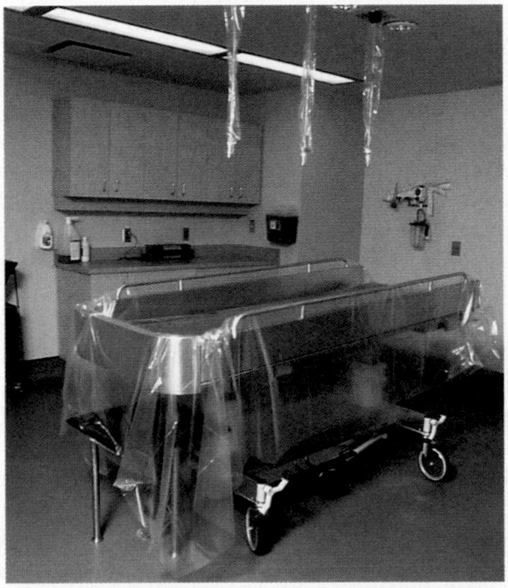

FIG. 25-9 Cart shower. Showering presents an opportunity for physical therapy and wound care.

Patients find the initial wound care to be both physically and psychologically demanding. Provide emotional support and begin to build trust during this activity. A once-daily shower and dressing change in the morning, with an evening dressing change in the patient's room, are part of the routine in many burn centers. Others opt to shower the patient on admission and then perform all other dressing changes in the patient's room. Some of the newer antimicrobial dressings can be left in place from 3 to 14 days, thereby decreasing the frequency of dressing changes.

Infection may cause further tissue injury and possible sepsis.[15] The source of infection in burn wounds is likely the patient's own flora, predominantly from the skin, respiratory tract, and gastrointestinal (GI) tract. The prevention of cross-contamination from one patient to another is a priority.

Two approaches to burn wound treatment are (1) the open method and (2) the use of multiple dressing changes (closed method). In the *open method* the patient's burn is covered with a topical antimicrobial and has no dressing over the wound. In the *multiple dressing change,* or *closed method,* sterile gauze dressings are impregnated with or laid over a topical antimicrobial (Fig. 25-11). These dressings are changed anywhere from every 12 to 24 hours to once every 14 days (depending on the product). Most burn centers support the concept of moist wound healing and use dressings to cover the burned areas, with the exception of facial burns.

When the patient's open burn wounds are exposed, always wear personal protective equipment (PPE) (e.g., disposable hats, masks, gowns, gloves). When removing contaminated dressings and washing the dirty wound, use nonsterile, disposable gloves. Use sterile gloves when applying ointments and sterile dressings. In addition, prevent shivering by keeping the room warm (approximately 85° F [29.4° C]). Before leaving one patient, remove your PPE. Don new equipment before you treat another patient. Perform thorough hand washing both before and after patient contact to prevent cross-contamination.

Permanent skin coverage is the primary goal for burn wound care. There is rarely enough unburned skin in the major (greater than 50% TBSA) burn patient for immediate skin grafting. This situation requires the use of temporary wound closure methods. *Allograft (homograft) skin* (from skin donor cadavers) is used, along with newer biosynthetic options. The treatment approaches vary among burn centers (Table 25-12).

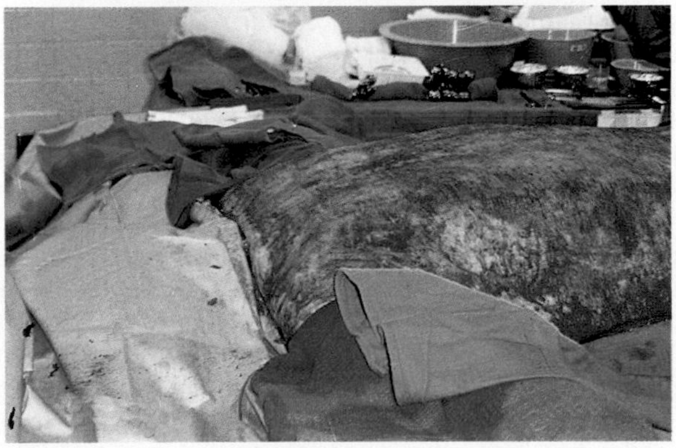

FIG. 25-10 Surgical debridement of full-thickness burns is necessary to prepare the wound for grafting.

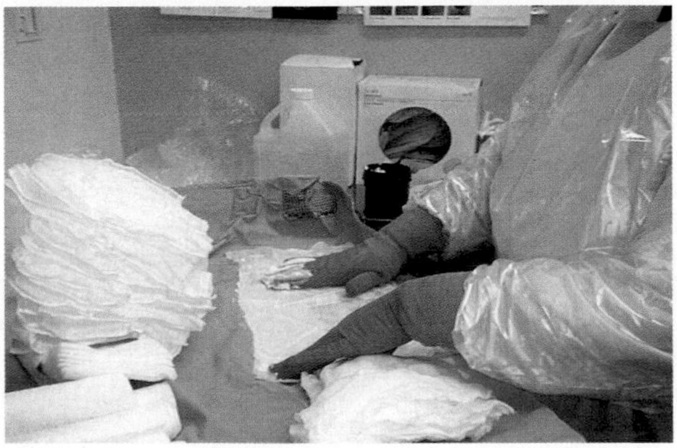

FIG. 25-11 Application of silver sulfadiazine cream to saline-moistened gauze.

TABLE 25-12 SOURCES OF GRAFTS

Source	Graft Name	Coverage
Porcine skin	Xenograft (or heterograft) (different species)	Temporary (3 days to 2 wk)
Cadaveric skin	Allograft (or homograft) (same species)	Temporary (3 days to 2 wk)
Patient's own skin	Autograft	Permanent
Patient's own skin and cell cultures	Cultured epithelial autograft (CEA)	Permanent
Porcine collagen bonded to silicone membrane	Biobrane	Temporary (10-21 days)
Bovine collagen and glycosaminoglycan bonded to silicone membrane	Integra	Permanent
Acellular dermal matrix derived from donated human skin	AlloDerm	Permanent

OTHER CARE MEASURES

Certain parts of the body (e.g., face, eyes, hands, arms, ears, perineum) require particularly vigilant nursing care. The face is highly vascular and can become very swollen. It is often covered with ointments and gauze but not wrapped to limit pressure on delicate facial structures. Eye care for corneal burns or edema includes antibiotic ointments. An ophthalmology examination should occur soon after admission for all patients with facial burns. Periorbital edema can prevent eye opening and is often frightening for the patient. Provide assurance that the swelling is not permanent. Instill methylcellulose drops or artificial tears into the eyes for moisture and additional comfort.

Ears should be kept free from pressure because of their poor vascularization and tendency to become infected. Do not use pillows for the patient with ear burns. The pressure on the cartilage may cause chondritis. Further, the ear may stick to the pillowcase, causing pain and bleeding. Elevate your patient's head using a rolled towel placed under the shoulders, being careful to avoid pressure necrosis. Follow the same strategy for the patient with neck burns to hyperextend the neck and prevent neck wound contracture.

Extend your patient's burned hands and arms and elevate them on pillows or plastic-covered foam wedges to minimize edema. Ask the occupational therapist and the physician if splints need to be applied to burned hands and feet to maintain them in positions of function. Remove the splints frequently and inspect the skin and bony prominences to avoid areas of pressure from inappropriate or prolonged application.

Keep your patient's perineum as clean and dry as possible after each voiding or bowel movement. In addition to monitoring hourly urine outputs, an indwelling catheter prevents urine contamination of the perineal area. Regular once- or twice-daily perineal and catheter care, in the presence or absence of a perineal burn wound, is essential. Assess the need for an indwelling urinary catheter on a daily basis and remove when no longer necessary to avoid development of a urinary tract infection. If your patient has frequent, loose stools, consider the temporary insertion of a fecal diversion device.

Perform necessary laboratory tests to monitor fluid and electrolyte balance. Draw ABGs, as necessary, to determine adequacy of ventilation and perfusion in patients with suspected or confirmed inhalation or electrical injury.

Work in collaboration with the physical therapist to perform range-of-motion (ROM) exercises during dressing changes and throughout the day. Movement facilitates mobilization of the leaked fluid back into the vascular bed. Active and passive exercise of body parts also maintains function, prevents contractures, and reassures the patient that movement is still possible.

DRUG THERAPY

ANALGESICS AND SEDATIVES. Promote the use of analgesics for the patient's comfort.[16] Early in the postburn period, IV pain medications should be given because (1) onset of action is fastest with this route; (2) oral medications have a slower onset of action and are not as effective when GI function is slowed or impaired because of shock or paralytic ileus; and (3) intramuscular (IM) injections will not be absorbed adequately in burned or edematous areas, causing pooling of medications in the tissues. Consequently, when fluid mobilization begins, the patient could be inadvertently overdosed from the interstitial accumulation of previous IM medications.

Common opioids used for pain control are listed in Table 25-13. Reevaluate analgesic requirements, since the patient's needs may change and tolerance to medications may develop over time. Initially, opioids are the drug of choice for pain control. When given appropriately, these drugs should provide adequate pain relief. Sedatives/hypnotics and antidepressants can also be given with analgesics to control the anxiety, insomnia, or depression that patients may experience (see Table 25-13). Analgesic requirements can vary widely from one patient to another, so consider a multimodal approach to pain management.[17] Remember that the patient's pain intensity may not directly correlate with the extent and depth of burn.

TETANUS IMMUNIZATION. Tetanus toxoid is given routinely to all burn patients because of the likelihood of anaerobic burn wound contamination. If the patient has not received an active immunization within 10 years before the burn injury, tetanus immunoglobulin should be considered. (Tetanus immunization is discussed in Table 69-6.)

ANTIMICROBIAL AGENTS. After the wound is cleansed, topical antimicrobial agents may be applied (see Fig. 25-11) and covered with a light dressing.[18] Systemic antibiotics are not routinely used to control burn wound flora because the burn eschar has little or no blood supply and consequently little antibiotic is delivered to the wound. In addition, the routine use of systemic antibiotics increases the chance of developing multidrug-resistant organisms. Some topical burn agents penetrate the eschar and inhibit bacterial invasion of the wound. Silver-impregnated dressings (e.g., Acticoat, Silverlon, Aquacel AG) can be left in place from 3 to 14 days, depending on the patient's clinical situation and the particular product. Silver sulfadiazine (Silvadene, Flamazine) and mafenide acetate (Sulfamylon) creams are also used.

SAFETY ALERT

- Check the patient for any allergies to sulfa, since many burn antimicrobial creams contain sulfa.

Sepsis remains a primary cause of death in the patient with major burns and may lead to multiple organ dysfunction syndrome (see Chapter 67). Systemic antibiotic therapy is initiated when the diagnosis of sepsis is made, or when some other source of infection is identified (e.g., pneumonia).[19]

TABLE 25-13 DRUG THERAPY

Burn Care

Drugs	Purpose
Analgesics	
morphine (Avinza)	Relieve pain
sustained-release morphine (MS Contin)	
hydromorphone (Dilaudid)	
sustained-release hydromorphone (Dilaudid CR)	
fentanyl (Sublimaze)	
oxycodone and acetaminophen (Percocet)	
methadone (Dolophine)	
Nonsteroidal antiinflammatory (e.g., ketorolac [Toradol])	
Adjuvant analgesics (e.g., gabapentin [Neurontin])	
Sedatives/Hypnotics	
lorazepam (Ativan)	Reduce anxiety
midazolam (Versed)	Provide short-acting amnesic effects
zolpidem (Ambien)	Promote sleep
Antidepressants	
sertraline (Zoloft)	Reduce depression, improve mood
citalopram (Celexa)	
Anticoagulants	
enoxaparin (Lovenox)	Prevent venous thromboembolism
heparin	
Nutritional Support	
Vitamins A, C, E, and multivitamins	Promote wound healing
Minerals: zinc, iron (ferrous sulfate)	Promote cell integrity and hemoglobin formation
oxandrolone (Oxandrin)	Promote weight gain and preservation of lean body mass
Gastrointestinal Support	
ranitidine (Zantac)	Decrease stomach acid and risk of Curling's ulcer
esomeprazole (Nexium)	
calcium carbonate and magnesium carbonate (Mylanta), aluminum hydroxide and magnesium hydroxide (Maalox)	Neutralize stomach acid
nystatin (Mycostatin)	Prevent overgrowth of *Candida albicans* in oral mucosa

Fungal infections may develop in the patient's mucous membranes (mouth and genitalia) as a result of systemic antibiotic therapy and low resistance. The offending organism is usually *Candida albicans.* Oral infection is treated with nystatin (Mycostatin) mouthwash. When a normal diet is resumed, yogurt or *Lactobacillus* (Lactinex) may be given by mouth to reintroduce the normal intestinal flora that was destroyed by antibiotic therapy.

VENOUS THROMBOEMBOLISM PROPHYLAXIS. Burn patients are at risk for VTE. If there are no contraindications, it is recommended that low-molecular-weight heparin (enoxaparin) or low-dose unfractionated heparin be started as soon as it is considered safe. For burn patients who have a high bleeding risk, VTE prophylaxis with sequential compression devices and/or graduated compression stockings are used until the bleeding risk decreases and heparin can be started (see Table 25-13). (VTE prophylaxis is discussed in Chapter 38.)

EVIDENCE-BASED PRACTICE

Translating Research Into Practice

Does the Type of Enteral Feeding Affect Outcomes in Burn Patients?

Clinical Question

In patients with burns (P), what is the effect of high-carbohydrate enteral feeding (I) versus high-fat enteral feeding (C) in reducing mortality, days on ventilator, and incidence of pneumonia (O)?

Best Available Evidence

Systematic review of randomized controlled trials (RCTs)

Critical Appraisal and Synthesis of Evidence

- Two RCTs (*n* = 93) of hospitalized patients in the immediate postburn period, with burns covering ≥10% of the total body surface area (TBSA).
- Two types of enteral feeding were compared: high-carbohydrate, high-protein, low-fat feeding (high-carbohydrate formula) and low-carbohydrate, high-protein, high-fat feeding (high-fat formula).
- High-carbohydrate enteral feeding resulted in a reduced incidence of pneumonia compared with high-fat enteral feeding.
- Inconclusive results on type of enteral feeding and patient outcomes of mortality and days on ventilator.

Conclusion

- High-carbohydrate enteral feedings may be of benefit in reducing the risk of pneumonia.

Implications for Nursing Practice

- Further research is needed to determine if enteral feeds are significantly different related to patient outcomes.

Reference for Evidence

Masters B, Aarabi S, Sidhwa F, et al: High-carbohydrate, high-protein, low-fat versus low-carbohydrate, high-protein, high-fat enteral feeds for burns, *Cochrane Database Syst Rev* (1):CD006122, 2012.

P, Patient population of interest; *I*, intervention or area of interest; *C*, comparison of interest or comparison group; *O*, outcomes of interest (see p. 12).

NUTRITIONAL THERAPY

Once fluid replacement needs have been addressed, nutrition takes priority in the initial emergent phase.[20] Early and aggressive nutritional support within several hours of the burn injury can decrease mortality risks and complications, optimize healing of the burn wound, and minimize the negative effects of hypermetabolism and catabolism.[21] Nonintubated patients with a burn of less than 20% TBSA will generally be able to eat enough to meet their nutritional needs.

Intubated patients and those with larger burns require additional support. Enteral feedings (gastric or intestinal) have almost entirely replaced parenteral feeding. Early enteral feeding, usually with smaller-bore tubes, preserves GI function, increases intestinal blood flow, and promotes optimal conditions for wound healing. In general, begin the feedings slowly at a rate of 20 to 40 mL/hr and increase to the goal rate within 24 to 48 hours. If a large nasogastric tube is inserted, gastric residuals should be checked to rule out delayed gastric emptying. Assess bowel sounds every 8 hours.

A *hypermetabolic state* proportional to the size of the wound occurs after a major burn injury.[21] Resting metabolic expenditure may be increased by 50% to 100% above normal in patients with major burns. Core temperature is elevated. Catecholamines, which stimulate catabolism and heat production, are increased. Massive catabolism can occur and is characterized by protein breakdown and increased gluconeogenesis. Failure to supply adequate calories and protein leads to malnutrition and delayed healing. Calorie-containing nutritional supplements and milkshakes are often given to meet the caloric needs. Protein powder can also be added to food and liquids. Supplemental vitamins may be started in the emergent phase, with iron supplements often given in the acute phase (see Table 25-13).

ACUTE PHASE

The *acute phase* of burn care begins with the mobilization of extracellular fluid and subsequent diuresis. It concludes when partial-thickness wounds are healed or full-thickness burns are covered by skin grafts. This may take weeks or months.

Pathophysiology

A healing burn injury causes many pathophysiologic changes in the body. Diuresis from fluid mobilization occurs, and the patient is less edematous. Bowel sounds return. The depth of the burn wounds may be more apparent as they "declare" themselves as partial or full thickness. The patient may now become more aware of the enormity of his or her situation and will benefit from psychosocial support and information.

Some healing begins as WBCs surround the burn wound and phagocytosis occurs. Necrotic tissue begins to slough. Fibroblasts lay down matrices of the collagen precursors that eventually form granulation tissue. A partial-thickness burn will heal, from both the wound edges and the dermal bed below, if kept free from infection and *desiccation* (dryness). However, full-thickness burn wounds, unless extremely small, must have the burn eschar surgically removed (excised) and skin grafts applied in order to heal. In some cases, healing time and length of hospitalization are decreased by early excision and grafting.

Clinical Manifestations

Partial-thickness wounds form eschar, which begins separating fairly soon after injury. Once the eschar is removed, reepithelialization begins at the wound margins and appears as red or pink scar tissue. Epithelial buds, from the hair follicles and glands in the dermal bed, eventually close the wound. Healing is spontaneous and usually occurs within 10 to 21 days.

Margins of full-thickness eschar take longer to separate. As a result, full-thickness burn wounds require surgical debridement and skin grafting to heal.

Laboratory Values

Because the body is attempting to reestablish fluid and electrolyte balance in the initial acute phase, it is important to follow serum electrolyte levels closely.

Sodium. *Hyponatremia* can develop from excessive GI suction, diarrhea, and water intake. Manifestations of hyponatremia include weakness, dizziness, muscle cramps, fatigue, headache, tachycardia, and confusion. The patient may also develop a dilutional hyponatremia called *water intoxication.* To avoid this condition, encourage the patient to drink fluids other than water, such as juice or nutritional supplements.

Hypernatremia may be seen after successful fluid resuscitation if copious amounts of hypertonic solutions were required. Hypernatremia may also be related to tube feeding therapy or inappropriate fluid administration. Manifestations of hypernatremia include thirst; dried, furry tongue; lethargy; confusion; and possibly seizures. Sodium restrictions may be applied to IV fluids and enteral or oral feedings until levels return to safe limits.

Potassium. *Hyperkalemia* may occur if the patient has renal failure, adrenocortical insufficiency, or massive deep muscle injury (e.g., electrical burn) with large amounts of potassium released from damaged cells. Cardiac dysrhythmias and arrest can occur with elevated potassium levels. Muscle weakness, cramping, and paralysis are found clinically (see Chapters 17 and 36).

Hypokalemia occurs with vomiting, diarrhea, prolonged GI suction, and IV therapy without potassium supplementation. Potassium is also lost through the patient's burn wounds. Signs and symptoms of hypokalemia include fatigue, muscle weakness, leg cramps, cardiac dysrhythmias (e.g., premature ventricular contractions), paresthesias, and decreased reflexes (see Chapter 17).

Complications

Infection. The body's first line of defense, the skin, is destroyed by a burn injury. The burn wound is now colonized with the person's own organisms that were on the skin before the burn. If the levels of bacteria between the eschar and the viable wound bed rise to greater than 10^5/g of tissue, the patient has a burn wound infection. Localized inflammation, induration, and sometimes suppuration can be seen at the burn wound margins. Partial-thickness burns can convert to full-thickness wounds when these organisms invade viable, adjacent, unburned tissue. Invasive wound infections may be treated with systemic antibiotics based on culture and sensitivity wound swab results.

Watch for signs and symptoms, including hypothermia or hyperthermia, increased heart and respiratory rate, decreased BP, and decreased urine output. The patient may have mild confusion, chills, malaise, and loss of appetite. The WBC count usually is between 10,000/μL (10×10^9/L) and 20,000/μL (20×10^9/L). The WBCs have functional defects and the patient remains immunosuppressed for many months after the burn injury.

The causative organisms of sepsis are usually gram-negative bacteria (e.g., *Pseudomonas, Proteus* organisms), putting the patient at further risk for septic shock. When sepsis is suspected, immediately obtain cultures from all possible sources, including the burn wound, blood, urine, sputum, oropharynx and perineal regions, and IV site. Treatment immediately begins with antibiotics appropriate for the usual residual flora of the particular burn center. When the culture and sensitivity results are known, the antibiotic in use may be continued or changed based on the results. At this stage the patient's condition is considered critical, requiring close monitoring of vital signs.

Cardiovascular and Respiratory Systems. The same cardiovascular and respiratory system complications present in the emergent phase may continue into the acute phase of care. In addition, new problems might arise, requiring timely intervention.

Neurologic System. Neurologically, the patient probably has no physical symptoms unless severe hypoxia from respiratory injuries or complications from electrical injuries occur. Probable causes of neurologic complications include electrolyte imbalance, stress, cerebral edema, sepsis, sleep disturbances, and the use of analgesics and antianxiety drugs. However, some patients may demonstrate certain behaviors that are not completely understood. The patient can become extremely disoriented, may withdraw or become combative, and may have hallucinations and frequent nightmare-like episodes. Delirium is more acute at night and occurs more often in the older patient. Use a screening tool to diagnose delirium (see Table 60-16) and initiate appropriate nursing interventions to prevent delirium, whenever possible. Focus on nursing strategies to orient and reassure your patient if he or she is confused or agitated. This state is usually transient, lasting from a day or two to several weeks, but complications and sequelae can last for years and be quite serious.

Musculoskeletal System. The musculoskeletal system is particularly prone to complications during the acute phase, and the involvement of both the physical and occupational therapist is vitally important.[22] As the burns begin to heal and scar tissue forms, the skin is less supple and pliant. ROM may be limited, and contractures can occur. Because of pain, the patient likely prefers a flexed position for comfort. Encourage the patient to stretch and move the burned body parts as much as possible. Consult with the occupational therapist about proper positioning and splinting to prevent or reduce contracture formation.

Gastrointestinal System. The GI system may also experience complications during this phase. Paralytic ileus can be caused by sepsis. Diarrhea may result from the use of enteral feedings or antibiotics. Constipation can occur as a side effect of opioid analgesics, decreased mobility, and a low-fiber diet. *Curling's ulcer* is a type of gastroduodenal ulcer characterized by diffuse superficial lesions (including mucosal erosion). It is caused by a generalized stress response to decreased blood flow to the GI tract. The patient has increased gastric acid secretion. Aim to prevent Curling's ulcer by feeding the patient as soon as possible after the burn injury. Antacids, H_2-histamine blockers (e.g., ranitidine [Zantac]), and proton pump inhibitors (e.g., esomeprazole [Nexium]) are used prophylactically to neutralize stomach acids and inhibit histamine and the secretion of hydrochloric acid (see Table 25-13). Patients with major burns may also have occult blood in their stools during the acute phase and require close monitoring for bleeding.

Endocrine System. Observe for transient increases in the patient's blood glucose levels as a result of stress-mediated cortisol and catecholamine release. There is an increased mobilization of glycogen stores and gluconeogenesis. Subsequently, glucose is produced, along with an increase in insulin production. However, insulin's effectiveness is decreased because of relative insulin insensitivity. This results in an elevated blood glucose level. Hyperglycemia may also be caused by the increased caloric intake necessary to meet some patients' metabolic requirements. When this occurs, the treatment is supplemental IV insulin, not decreased feeding. Check blood glucose levels frequently and give insulin as ordered. Point-of-care testing of glucose can be done, but serum glucose testing is more accurate. As the patient's metabolic demands are met and less stress is placed on the entire system, this stress-induced condition is reversed.

NURSING AND COLLABORATIVE MANAGEMENT ACUTE PHASE

The predominant therapeutic interventions in the acute phase are (1) wound care, (2) excision and grafting, (3) pain management, (4) physical and occupational therapy, and (5) nutritional therapy.

WOUND CARE

The goals of wound care are to (1) prevent infection by cleansing and debriding the area of necrotic tissue that would promote bacterial growth and (2) promote wound re-epithelialization and/or successful skin grafting.

Wound care consists of ongoing observation, assessment, cleansing, debridement, and dressing reapplication. Nonsurgical debridement, dressing changes, topical antimicrobial therapy, graft care, and donor site care are performed as often as necessary, depending on the topical cream or dressing ordered. Enzymatic debriders made of natural ingredients, such as collagen, may be used for *enzymatic debridement* of burn wounds, which speeds up the removal of dead tissue from the healthy wound bed.

Cleanse wounds with soap and water or normal saline-moistened gauze to gently remove the old antimicrobial agent and any loose necrotic tissue, scabs, or dried blood. During the debridement phase, cover the wound with topical antimicrobial creams (e.g., silver sulfadiazine) or silver-impregnated dressings. When the partial-thickness burn wounds have been fully debrided, a protective, coarse or fine-meshed, greasy-based (paraffin or petroleum) gauze dressing is applied to protect the re-epithelializing keratinocytes as they resurface and close the open wound bed.

If grafting is necessary, protect the skin graft (discussed below) with the same greasy gauze dressings next to the graft, followed by saline-moistened middle, and dry gauze outer dressings. With facial grafts the unmeshed sheet graft is left open, so it is possible for *blebs* (serosanguineous exudate) to form between the graft and the recipient bed. Blebs prevent the graft from permanently attaching to the wound bed. The evacuation of blebs is best performed by aspiration with a tuberculin syringe and only by those who have received instruction in this specialized skill. (Dressings are discussed in Table 12-10.)

EXCISION AND GRAFTING

Management of full-thickness burn wounds involves early removal (surgical excision) of the necrotic tissue followed by application of split-thickness autograft skin.[23] This aggressive and definitive approach has improved the management and survival rate of burn patients. In the past, patients with major burns had low rates of survival because healing and wound coverage took so long that the patient usually died of sepsis or malnutrition.

Many patients, especially those with major burns, are taken to the OR for wound excision on day 1 or 2 (emergent phase). The wounds are covered with a biologic dressing or allograft for temporary coverage until permanent grafting can occur (see Table 25-12).

During the procedure of **excision and grafting,** devitalized tissue (eschar) is excised down to the subcutaneous tissue or fascia, depending on the degree of injury. Surgical excision can result in massive blood loss.[24] To decrease surgical blood loss, topical application of epinephrine or thrombin, injection of saline and epinephrine, application of extremity tourniquets, or application of a new fibrin sealant (Artiss) is used. Once hemostasis has been achieved, a graft is then placed on clean, viable tissue to achieve good adherence. Whenever possible, the freshly excised wound is covered with *autograft* (the person's own) skin (see Table 25-12). Recently, fibrin sealant has been used to attach skin grafts to the wound bed. Grafts can also be stapled or sutured into place (Fig. 25-12, *A*). A temporary

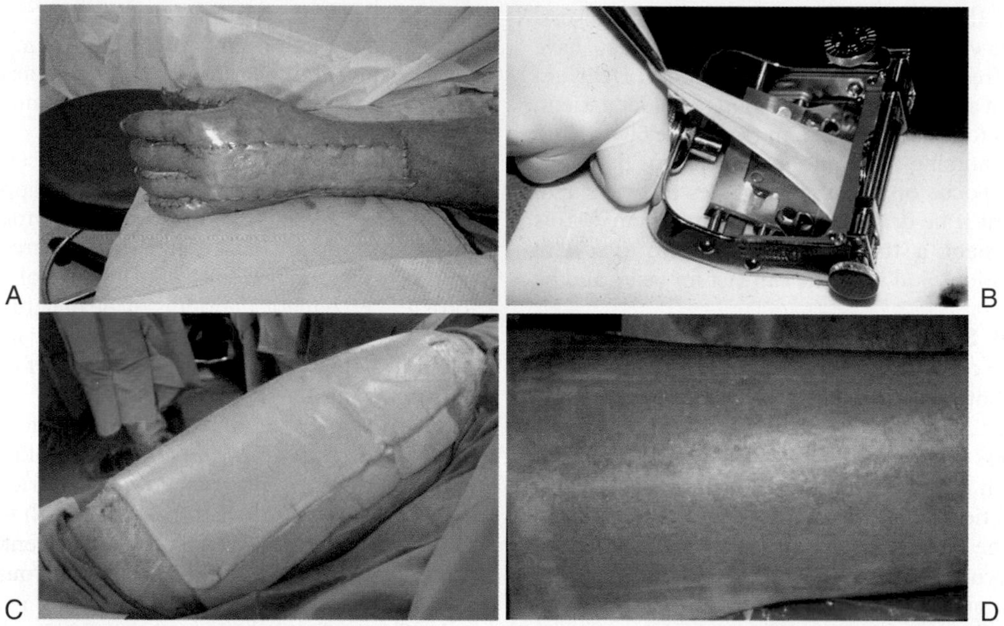

FIG. 25-12 **A,** Freshly applied split-thickness sheet skin graft to the hand. **B,** Split-thickness skin graft is harvested from a patient's thigh using a dermatome. **C,** Donor site is covered with a hydrophilic foam dressing after harvesting. **D,** Healed donor site.

allograft can be used to test the suitability of the recipient site to accept a graft.[25] The allograft is then removed several days later in the OR and an autograft applied.

With early excision, function is restored and scar tissue formation is minimized. Clots between the graft and the wound keep the graft from adhering to the wound. Outer occlusive dressings apply just enough pressure to promote adherence of the graft to the wound bed and help control bleeding. Protect the grafted area from shearing, friction, and pressure. Facial, neck, and hand burns require skillful nursing care to identify and manage clots quickly for the best functional and esthetic outcomes.

Donor skin is taken from the patient for grafting by means of a *dermatome,* which removes a thin (14/1000 to 16/1000 inch) split-thickness layer of skin from an unburned site (Fig. 25-12, *B*). The donor skin can be meshed (usually ratio of 1.5:1) to allow for greater wound coverage, or it may be applied as an unmeshed sheet for a better cosmetic result when grafting the face, neck, and hands. The donor site now becomes a new open wound.

The goals of donor site care are to promote rapid, moist wound healing; decrease pain at the site; and prevent infection. The choices of dressings for donor sites vary among burn centers and include transparent dressings (e.g., Opsite), xenograft, silver sulfadiazine, silver-impregnated dressings, calcium alginate, and hydrophilic foam dressings (Fig. 25-12, *C*). Nursing care of the donor site is specific to the dressing selected.[26] Several of the newer dressing materials offer decreased healing time, which facilitates earlier reharvesting of skin at the same site. The average healing time for a donor site is 10 to 14 days (Fig. 25-12, *D*).

CULTURED EPITHELIAL AUTOGRAFTS. In the patient with large body burns, only a limited amount of unburned skin may be available as donor sites for grafting, and some of that skin may be unsuitable for harvesting. **Cultured epithelial autograft (CEA)** is a method of obtaining permanent skin from a person with limited skin available for harvesting. CEA is grown from biopsy specimens obtained from the patient's own unburned skin.[27] This procedure is performed in suitable patients in some burn centers as soon as possible. The specimens are sent to a commercial laboratory, where the biopsied keratinocytes are grown in a culture medium containing epidermal growth factor. After approximately 18 to 25 days, the keratinocytes have expanded up to 10,000 times and form sheets that can be used as skin grafts. The cultured skin is returned to the burn center, where it is placed on the patient's excised burn wounds (Fig. 25-13, *A*). CEA grafts generally form a seamless, smooth replacement skin tissue (Fig. 25-13, *B*). Problems related to CEA include a poor graft take because of thin epidermal skin, graft loss during healing, infection, and contracture development.

ARTIFICIAL SKIN. Artificial skin must replace all functions of the skin and consist of both dermal and epidermal elements.[27] The Integra artificial skin dermal regeneration template is an example of a skin replacement system. As with CEA, it is indicated for use in the treatment of life-threatening, full-thickness or deep partial-thickness burn wounds when conventional autograft is not available or advisable, as in older or high anesthetic-risk patients. It has also been successfully used in reconstructive burn surgery procedures. It needs to be applied within a few days postburn for greatest success.

Integra artificial skin has a bilayer membrane composed of acellular dermis and silicone. The wound is excised, the bilayer membrane is placed dermal layer down, and the wound is wrapped with dressings in the OR. The dermal layer functions as a biodegradable template that induces organized regeneration of new dermis by the body. The silicone layer remains intact for 3 weeks as the dermal layer degrades and epidermal autografts become available. At this point, the silicone is removed during a second surgical procedure and replaced by the patient's own epidermal autografts. Some burn centers use CEA as the source of the epidermis.

Another dermal replacement is AlloDerm, a cryopreserved allogenic dermis. Human allograft dermis, harvested from

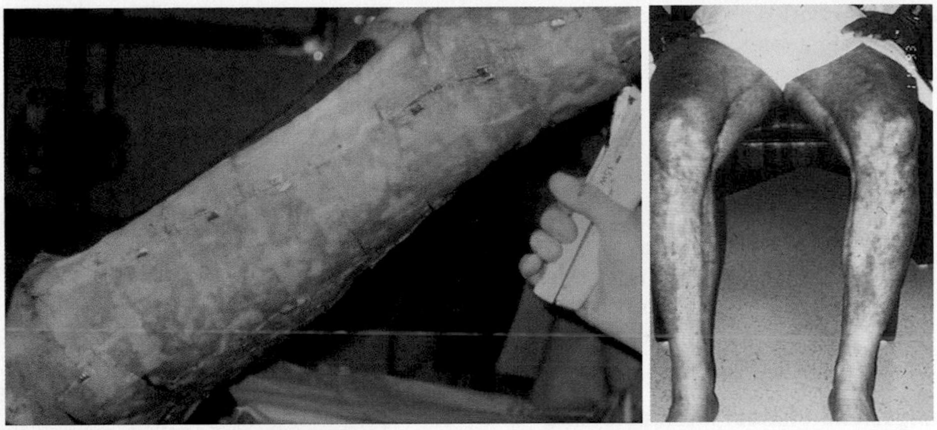

A B

FIG. 25-13 Patient with cultured epithelial autograft (CEA). **A,** Intraoperative application of CEA. **B,** Appearance of healed CEA.

cadavers, is decellularized to render it immunogenic and then freeze-dried. Once thawed, AlloDerm is rehydrated with ultra-thin epidermal autografts immediately before placement on a freshly excised wound.

PAIN MANAGEMENT

Many aspects of burn care cause pain. However, patients experience moments of relative comfort if they receive adequate analgesia. To provide effective pain management, you must understand both the physiologic and psychologic aspects of pain. (Pain management is discussed in Chapter 9.)

Burn patients experience two kinds of pain: (1) *continuous, background pain* that might be present throughout the day and night; and (2) *treatment-induced pain* associated with dressing changes, ambulation, and rehabilitation activities. The first line of treatment is drugs (see Table 25-13). With background pain, a continuous IV infusion of an opioid (e.g., hydromorphone [Dilaudid]) allows for a steady, therapeutic level of medication. If an IV infusion is not present, slow-release, twice-a-day opioid medications (e.g., morphine [MS Contin]) are indicated. Around-the-clock oral analgesics can also be used. Breakthrough doses of pain medication need to be available regardless of the regimen selected. Anxiolytics, which can potentiate analgesics, are also indicated and include lorazepam (Ativan) and midazolam (Versed). Adjuvant analgesics, such as gabapentin (Neurontin) and pregabalin (Lyrica), also potentiate opioids. The use of these drugs can help reduce the opioid dosage and undesirable side effects.

For treatment-induced pain, premedicate with an analgesic and an anxiolytic via the IV or oral route. For patients with an IV infusion, a potent, short-acting analgesic, such as fentanyl (Sublimaze), is often effective. During treatment and activity, small doses should be given to keep the patient as comfortable as possible. Elimination of all the pain is difficult, and most patients indicate acceptance of "tolerable" levels of discomfort.

Pain management is complex and ever-changing throughout the patient's hospital stay and after discharge.[28] Some pain can be managed using nondrug strategies. Mind-body interventions, such as relaxation breathing, guided imagery, hypnosis, biofeedback, and music therapy, can be effective in helping patients cope with pain (see Chapters 6 and 7).

Remember, the more control the patient has in managing pain, the more successful the chosen strategies will be. Active participation in requesting time-outs and scheduling treatments and rest periods can help the patient manage feelings of anticipatory pain. Patient-controlled analgesia (PCA) is used in selected circumstances in some burn centers, with varying degrees of success. (PCA is discussed in Chapter 9.)

PHYSICAL AND OCCUPATIONAL THERAPY

Continuous physical therapy, throughout burn recovery, is imperative if the patient is to regain and maintain muscle strength and optimal joint function. A good time for exercise is during and after wound cleansing, when the skin is softer and bulky dressings are removed. Passive and active ROM should be performed on all joints. Ensure that the patient with neck burns continues to sleep without pillows or with the head hanging slightly over the top of the mattress to encourage hyperextension. Maintain the occupational therapy schedule for wearing custom-fitted splints, which are designed to keep joints in functional position. Examine the splints frequently to ensure an optimal fit, with no undue pressure that might lead to skin breakdown or nerve damage.

NUTRITIONAL THERAPY

The goal of nutritional therapy during the acute burn phase is to provide adequate calories and protein to promote healing. When the wounds are still open, the burn patient is in a hypermetabolic and highly catabolic state.

The patient may benefit from an antioxidant protocol, which includes selenium, acetylcysteine, ascorbic acid, vitamin E, zinc, and a multivitamin. Meeting daily caloric requirements is crucial and should begin within the first 1 to 2 days postburn. The daily estimated caloric needs must be regularly calculated by a dietitian and readjusted as the patient's condition changes (e.g., wound healing improves, sepsis develops). Monitor laboratory values (e.g., albumin, prealbumin, total protein, transferrin) on a regular basis.

If the patient is on a mechanical ventilator or unable to consume adequate calories by mouth, a small-bore feeding tube is placed and enteral feedings are initiated. When the patient is extubated, contact the speech pathologist to perform a swallowing assessment before an oral diet is started.[29] Encourage the patient to eat high-protein, high-carbohydrate foods to meet caloric needs. Ask caregivers to bring in favorite foods from home. Appetite is usually diminished, and you will need to reinforce whatever steps are necessary to achieve adequate intake. Ideally, weight loss should not be more than 10% of preburn weight. Record the patient's daily caloric intake using calorie count sheets, which are monitored by the dietitian. Weigh your patient weekly to evaluate progress.

REHABILITATION PHASE

The formal *rehabilitation phase* begins when the patient's wounds have healed and he or she is engaging in some level of self-care. This may happen as early as 2 weeks or as long as 7 to 8 months after the burn injury. Goals for the patient now are to (1) work toward resuming a functional role in society and (2) rehabilitate from any functional and cosmetic postburn reconstructive surgery that may be necessary.[30]

Pathophysiologic Changes and Clinical Manifestations

Burn wounds heal either by spontaneous re-epithelialization or by skin grafting. Layers of keratinocytes begin rebuilding the tissue structure destroyed by the burn injury. Collagen fibers, present in the new scar tissue, assist with healing and add strength to weakened areas. The new skin appears flat and pink. In approximately 4 to 6 weeks, the area becomes raised and hyperemic. If adequate ROM is not instituted, the new tissue will shorten, causing a contracture. Mature healing is reached in about 12 months when suppleness has returned, and the pink or red color has faded to a slightly lighter hue than the surrounding unburned tissue.

Counsel patients who have more heavily pigmented skin that it will take longer for it to regain its dark color because many of the melanocytes have been destroyed. Frequently, the skin does not regain its original color. Provide teaching and psychosocial support to assist the patient with grieving about these changes to his or her body image. In particular, teenagers and female patients may need more support, but explore potential body image concerns with everyone.[31] Cosmetic camouflage, the implantation of pigment within the skin, can help even out unequal skin tones and improve the patient's overall appearance and self-image.

Scarring has two characteristics: discoloration and contour. The discoloration of scars fades somewhat with time. However, scar tissue tends to develop altered contours; that is, it is no longer flat or slightly raised but becomes elevated and enlarged above the original burned area. Some burn care providers believe that pressure can eventually help keep a scar flat.[32] Gentle pressure is maintained on the healed burn with custom-fitted pressure garments and clear, thermoplastic face masks. Pressure garments and masks should never be worn over unhealed wounds and, once a wearing schedule has been established, are removed only for short periods while bathing. Pressure garments are worn up to 24 hours a day for as long as 12 to 18 months.

The patient typically experiences discomfort from itching where healing is occurring. Teach your patient about the application of water-based moisturizers and selective, short-term use of oral antihistamines (e.g., hydroxyzine [Atarax]) to help reduce the itching. Massage oil, silicone gel sheeting (e.g., Biodermis), gabapentin, and injectable corticosteroids also may be helpful.[33]

As "old" epithelium is replaced by new cells, flaking occurs. The newly formed skin is extremely sensitive to trauma. Blisters and skin tears are likely to develop from slight pressure or friction. Additionally, these newly healed areas can be hypersensitive or hyposensitive to cold, heat, and touch. Grafted areas are more likely to be hyposensitive until peripheral nerve regeneration occurs. Teach your patients to protect healed burn areas from direct sunlight for about 3 months to prevent hyperpigmentation and sunburn injury. They should always wear sunscreen when they are outside.[34]

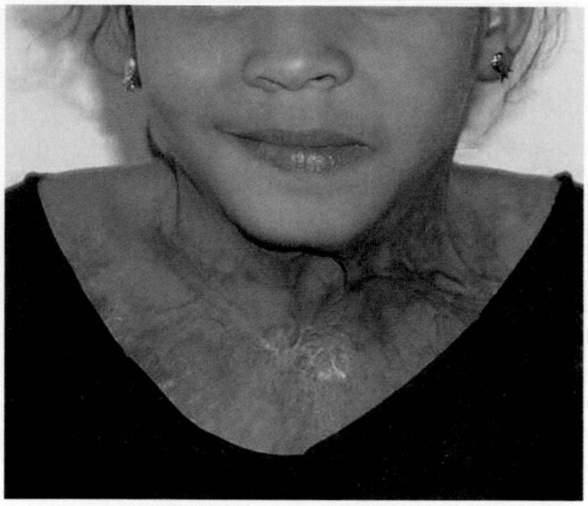

FIG. 25-14 Neck contractures.

Complications

The most common complications during the rehabilitation phase are skin and joint contractures and hypertrophic scarring (Fig. 25-14) and eFig. 25-1 (available on the website for this chapter). A **contracture** (an abnormal condition of a joint characterized by flexion and fixation) develops as a result of the shortening of scar tissue in the flexor tissues of a joint. Areas that are most susceptible to contracture formation include the anterior and lateral neck areas, axillae, antecubital fossae, fingers, groin areas, popliteal fossae, knees, and ankles. Some areas encompass major joints. Not only does the skin over these areas develop contractures, but the underlying tissues, such as the ligaments and tendons, also have a tendency to shorten during the healing process.

Carefully observe the patient for these potential problems. Encourage proper positioning, splinting, and exercise to minimize this complication. Tell the patient to continue with these strategies until the skin matures at around 1 year posthealing. Rehabilitative therapy is aimed at the extension of body parts because the flexors are stronger than the extensors. Burned legs may first be wrapped with elastic (e.g., tensor, Ace) bandages to assist with circulation to leg-graft and donor sites before ambulation. Burned arms can be wrapped with a layer of tubular elastic gauze (e.g., Tubigrip). This interim pressure prevents blister formation, promotes venous return, and decreases pain and itchiness. Once the skin is completely healed and less fragile, custom-fitted pressure garments replace the elastic bandages and tubular gauze.

NURSING AND COLLABORATIVE MANAGEMENT REHABILITATION PHASE

During the rehabilitation phase, encourage both the patient and the caregiver to participate in care. Since the patient may go home with small, unhealed wounds, teach your patient and caregiver the skills for dressing changes and wound care.[34] Pain management and nutritional needs continue to be based on individual patient status. If needed, arrange home care nursing services to assist with care after discharge. Water-based creams that penetrate into the dermis (e.g., Vaseline Intensive Rescue, Sween, Complex 15) should be used routinely on healed areas to keep the skin supple and well moisturized, which will decrease itching and flaking. Occasionally low-dose antihistamines may be used at bedtime if itching persists.

Postburn reconstructive surgery is frequently required after a major burn. The need for further surgery is reviewed at the outpatient burn clinic appointments after discharge.

Continue to encourage the patient to perform the physical and occupational therapy routines. Constant encouragement and reassurance are necessary to maintain a patient's morale, particularly once the patient realizes that recovery can be slow. Rehabilitation may need to be a primary focus for at least the next 6 to 12 months.

GERONTOLOGIC CONSIDERATIONS

BURNS

The older patient presents many challenges for the burn team. The normal aging process puts the patient at risk for injury because of unsteady gait, limited eyesight, and diminished hearing. As people age, skin becomes drier and more wrinkled. Older adults have thinning of the dermal layer, a loss of elastic fibers, a reduction in subcutaneous adipose tissue, and a decrease in vascularity. As a result, the thinner dermis, with reduced blood flow, sustains deeper burns with poorer rates of healing.[35]

Once injured, the older adult has more complications in the emergent and acute phases of burn resuscitation because of preexisting medical conditions. For example, older patients with diabetes, heart failure, or chronic obstructive pulmonary disease have morbidity and mortality rates exceeding those of healthy, younger patients. In older patients, pneumonia is a frequent complication, burn wounds and donor sites take longer to heal, and surgical procedures are less well tolerated. Weaning from a ventilator can be a challenge. Although usually self-limiting, delirium, if it develops, may be distressing. It usually takes longer for these patients to rehabilitate to the point where they can safely return home.[36] For some, a return home to independent living may not be possible. As the population ages, developing strategies to prevent burn injuries in older adults is a priority.

EMOTIONAL/PSYCHOLOGIC NEEDS OF PATIENTS AND CAREGIVERS

Patients and caregivers have many emotional/psychologic needs during the often lengthy, unpredictable, and complex course of care.[37,38] You have an important supportive and counseling role as patients struggle to get their lives back on track.

To manage the enormous range of emotional responses that the burn patient may exhibit, assess the circumstances of the burn (e.g., cause, people involved), family relationships, and previous coping experiences with stressful stimuli. At any time the patient may experience a variety of emotions such as fear, anxiety, anger, guilt, and depression (Table 25-14).

Burn survivors frequently experience thoughts and feelings that are frightening and disturbing, such as guilt about the burn incident, reliving of the frightening burn experience, fear of dying, concern about future therapy and surgery, frustrations with ongoing discomfort and treatment, and hopelessness about the future. During recovery, as more independence is expected from the patient, new fears may occur: "Can I really do this?" "Am I a desirable person?" "How can I go outside looking like this?" These challenges confront patients throughout their recovery and perhaps for years to come.

TABLE 25-14 EMOTIONAL RESPONSES OF BURN PATIENTS*

Emotion	Possible Verbal Expression
Fear	Will I die? What will happen next? Will I be disfigured? Will my family and friends still love me?
Anxiety	I feel out of control. What's going to happen to me? When will I look normal again?
Anger	Why did this happen to me? The nurses enjoy hurting me. I hope the person who did this to me dies.
Guilt	If only I'd been more careful. I'm being punished because I did something wrong.
Depression	It's no use going on like this. I don't care what happens to me. I wish people would leave me alone.

*List is not all-inclusive.

A person's self-esteem may be adversely affected by a burn injury. Some individuals may fear the loss of relationships because of perceived or actual physical disfigurement. In a society that values physical beauty, alterations in body image can result in psychologic distress.

Open and frequent communication among the patient, caregivers, close friends, and burn team members is essential. Because of the tremendous psychologic impact of a burn injury, be particularly sensitive to the patient's emotions and concerns. Encourage the patient to discuss fears regarding loss of life as he or she once knew it, loss of function, temporary or permanent deformity and disfigurement, return to work and home life, and financial burdens resulting from a long and costly hospitalization and rehabilitation.[39]

Encourage appropriate independence and an eventual return to preburn activities, such as school or work.[40] Peer counseling and informal interactions with other burn survivors may bring comfort and help to restore confidence. Reassure patients that their feelings, during this period of adjustment, are a normal reaction to an extraordinary life event. Their frustration and impatience are to be expected as they work to establish a new life. Assist patients in adapting to a realistic, yet positive appraisal of their particular situation, emphasizing what they *can* do instead of what they *cannot* do.

Caregivers may share some or all of these challenges and feelings. At times, they may feel helpless or too exhausted to assist their loved one. Continued support from trusted and familiar burn team members is essential. Helping caregivers assist with aspects of the patient's care helps them to reconnect with their loved one and eases the transition home. Many burn survivors and their caregivers remark on the powerful learning experience of the burn and a renewed appreciation of life, despite the ongoing challenges of a prolonged recovery. You need to acknowledge that their feelings are real and common. Most burn survivors speak of a real satisfaction with their postburn life and are more empowered as time goes on.

It is important to address individual spiritual and cultural needs because both have a role in treatment decisions and recovery. Pastoral care may be a helpful resource for the patient and the caregiver. The need for support, information, and family involvement may vary among cultures. Identify what is important to your patient and caregiver, and communicate that information in the patient's plan of care. Encourage the burn care team to remain culturally aware of and sensitive to the individual patient's and caregiver's cultural needs.

The difficult issue of sexuality must be met with honesty.[41] Physical appearance is altered in the patient who has sustained a major burn. Acceptance of any changes is difficult at first for the patient and significant other. The nature of skin injury in itself can cause modifications in processing sexual stimuli. Touch is an important part of sexuality, and immature scar tissue may make the sensation of touch unpleasant or may dull it. This may only be transient, but the patient and partner need to know that it is normal and receive anticipatory guidance from the burn team to avoid undue emotional strain.

The stress of the burn injury occasionally precipitates a psychologic crisis. Many patients realize this experience is beyond their ability to cope. Assessment by a psychiatrist who can prescribe appropriate medication, if needed, and begin short-term counseling is frequently helpful. Early psychiatric intervention is essential if the patient has been previously treated for a psychiatric illness or if the injury was a suicide attempt. The diagnosis of posttraumatic stress disorder is made in a number of burn patients. Treatment typically begins in the hospital, but links to community resources must be made before discharge to ensure continuity of psychologic care. A referral to a psychiatrist, psychologist, mental health counselor, social worker, or psychiatric advanced practice nurse (APN) should be discussed if concerns are raised at burn clinic follow-up.

Caregiver and patient support groups may be beneficial in meeting the patient's and caregiver's emotional needs at any phase of the recovery process.[42] Speaking with others who have experienced burn trauma can be beneficial, both in terms of reaffirming that the patient's feelings are normal and in sharing helpful advice. The Phoenix Society *(www.phoenix-society.org)* is an international, highly respected burn survivors' support group. For many years the society has offered invaluable support and resources (e.g., annual World Burn Congress conference) to burn survivors, caregivers, and burn team personnel.

SPECIAL NEEDS OF NURSES

Warm, trusting, and mutually satisfying relationships frequently develop between burn patients and nursing staff, not only during hospitalization but also during the long-term rehabilitation period.[43] Sometimes the bond can be so strong that the patient has difficulty separating from the hospital and staff. The frequency and intensity of family contact can be rewarding as well as draining to you. You may find it difficult to cope with the deformities caused by the burn injury, the odors, the unpleasant sight of the wound, and the reality of the pain that accompanies the burn and its treatment. Do not hesitate to seek help from co-workers, a manager, or the employee assistance program should you feel the need.

In time, you will come to know that the specialized burn care you provide makes a critical difference in helping patients not only survive, but also cope with and triumph over an intense and multifaceted injury.

Ongoing support services or critical incident stress debriefings led by a psychiatrist, psychologist, psychiatric APN, or social worker may also be helpful. Peer support groups (e.g., ABA, International Society for Burn Injuries) can serve a similar purpose by helping you cope with difficult feelings experienced when caring for burn patients. Because burn nursing is physically, psychologically, and intellectually demanding, it has many challenges and inherent rewards. Attention to your own self-care is important to maintain a positive attitude and healthy work-life balance.[44] Time with family and friends and rest and relaxation at home are essential parts of self-care and a balanced life with purpose and meaning.

CASE STUDY

Burn Injury

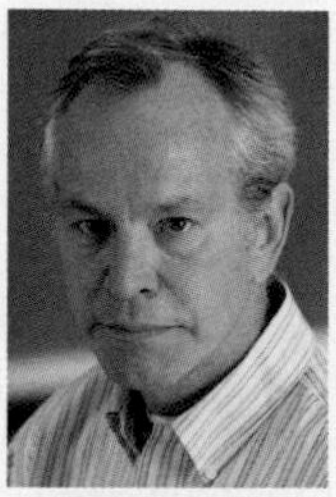

Comstock/Thinkstock

Patient Profile

G.M., a 52-year-old married white man, arrives at the emergency department with burns to his face, neck, chest, right arm and hand, and right foot. He was burning brush on his farm when the fire went out of control. He has an 18-gauge IV with NSS running at 100 mL/hr, and he is receiving 100% humidified O_2 by mask.

Subjective Data

- Complains of blurry vision and trouble swallowing
- States his burns are painful and that he is scared
- States he is a "diabetic" and has "high blood pressure"

Objective Data

Physical Examination

- Is awake, alert, and oriented, but in some distress
- Eyes are red, irritated
- Voice is hoarse; nasal hair is singed
- Face is reddened with blisters noted on the nose and forehead
- Right arm, right hand, chest, neck, and right foot have shiny, bright red, wet wounds
- Patient is shivering

Discussion Questions

1. ***Priority Decision:*** What are the priorities of care in the prehospital environment? How should his airway, breathing, and circulation be managed?
2. ***Priority Decision:*** What factors place G.M. at high risk for an inhalation injury? What priority interventions can be anticipated?
3. What pain medications might be considered to relieve his pain?
4. Which of the criteria for burn center referral does G.M. meet for admission to the hospital burn unit?
5. What metabolic disturbances would be expected soon after G.M.'s admission? Explain the physiologic basis for these changes.
6. How might G.M.'s co-morbidities affect his burn care and rehabilitation?
7. What measures should be taken to support G.M.'s caregivers?
8. ***Priority Decision:*** Based on the assessment data presented, develop three priority nursing diagnoses. Identify any collaborative problems.
9. ***Evidence-Based Practice:*** What are the most effective wound care strategies to manage G.M.'s burn wounds?

evolve Answers available at *http://evolve.elsevier.com/Lewis/medsurg.*

BRIDGE TO NCLEX EXAMINATION

The number of the question corresponds to the same-numbered outcome at the beginning of the chapter.

1. Knowing the most common causes of household fires, which prevention strategy would the nurse focus on when teaching about fire safety?
   a. Set hot water temperature at 140° F (60° C).
   b. Use only hardwired smoke detectors.
   c. Encourage regular home fire exit drills.
   d. Never permit older adults to cook unattended.
2. The injury that is least likely to result in a full-thickness burn is
   a. sunburn.
   b. scald injury.
   c. chemical burn.
   d. electrical injury.
3. When assessing a patient with a partial-thickness burn, the nurse would expect to find *(select all that apply)*
   a. blisters.
   b. exposed fascia.
   c. exposed muscles.
   d. intact nerve endings.
   e. red, shiny, wet appearance.
4. A patient is admitted to the burn center with burns of his head and neck, chest, and back after an explosion in his garage. On assessment, the nurse auscultates wheezes throughout the lung fields. On reassessment, the wheezes are gone and the breath sounds are greatly diminished. Which action is the most appropriate for the nurse to take next?
   a. Obtain vital signs and a STAT arterial blood gas.
   b. Encourage the patient to cough and auscultate the lungs again.
   c. Document the findings and continue to monitor the patient's breathing.
   d. Anticipate the need for endotracheal intubation and notify the physician.
5. Fluid and electrolyte shifts that occur during the early emergent phase of a burn injury include
   a. adherence of albumin to vascular walls.
   b. movement of potassium into the vascular space.
   c. sequestering of sodium and water in interstitial fluid.
   d. hemolysis of red blood cells from large volumes of rapidly administered fluid.
6. To maintain a positive nitrogen balance in a major burn, the patient must
   a. eat a high-protein, low-fat, high-carbohydrate diet.
   b. increase normal caloric intake by about three times.
   c. eat at least 1500 calories/day in small, frequent meals.
   d. eat rice and whole wheat for the chemical effect on nitrogen balance.
7. A patient has 25% TBSA burned from a car fire. His wounds have been debrided and covered with a silver-impregnated dressing. The nurse's priority intervention for wound care would be to
   a. reapply a new dressing without disturbing the wound bed.
   b. observe the wound for signs of infection during dressing changes.
   c. apply cool compresses for pain relief in between dressing changes.
   d. wash the wound aggressively with soap and water three times a day.
8. Pain management for the burn patient is most effective when *(select all that apply)*
   a. a pain rating tool is used to monitor the patient's level of pain.
   b. painful dressing changes are delayed until the patient's pain is completely relieved.
   c. the patient is informed about and has some control over the management of the pain.
   d. a multimodal approach is used (e.g., sustained-release and short-acting opioids, NSAIDs, adjuvant analgesics).
   e. nonpharmacologic therapies (e.g., music therapy, distraction) replace opioids in the rehabilitation phase of a burn injury.
9. A therapeutic measure used to prevent hypertrophic scarring during the rehabilitation phase of burn recovery is
   a. applying pressure garments.
   b. repositioning the patient every 2 hours.
   c. performing active ROM at least every 4 hours.
   d. massaging the new tissue with water-based moisturizers.
10. A patient is recovering from second- and third-degree burns over 30% of his body and is now ready for discharge. The first action the nurse should take when meeting with the patient would be to
    a. arrange a return-to-clinic appointment and prescription for pain medications.
    b. teach the patient and the caregiver proper wound care to be performed at home.
    c. review the patient's current health care status and readiness for discharge to home.
    d. give the patient written discharge information and websites for additional information for burn survivors.

1. c, 2. a, 3. a, d, e, 4. d, 5. c, 6. a, 7. b, 8. a, c, d, 9. a, 10. c

evolve

For rationales to these answers and even more NCLEX review questions, visit *http://evolve.elsevier.com/Lewis/medsurg.*

REFERENCES

1. American Burn Association: Burn incidence and treatment in the US: 2011 fact sheet. Retrieved from *www.ameriburn.org/resources_factsheet.php.*
2. Centers for Disease Control and Prevention: Fire deaths and injuries: fact sheet, Atlanta, 2011. Retrieved from *www.cdc.gov/HomeandRecreationalSafety/Fire-Prevention/fires-factsheet.html.*
*3. Peck M: Epidemiology of burns throughout the world—part I: distribution and risk factors, *Burns* 37:1087, 2011.
*4. Edwards D, Heard J, Latenser B, et al: Burn injuries in Eastern Zambia: impact of multidisciplinary teaching teams, *J Burn Care Res* 32:31, 2011.
5. Cancio L: Airway management and smoke inhalation injury in the burn patient, *Clin Plast Surg* 36:555, 2009.
6. Latenser B: Critical care of the burn patient: the first 48 hours, *Crit Care Med* 37:2819, 2009.
7. Moss L: Treatment of the burn patient in primary care, *Skin Wound Care* 23:517, 2010.
*8. Schwartz S, Rothrock M, Barron-Vaya Y, et al: Impact of diabetes on burn injury: preliminary results from prospective study, *J Burn Care Res* 32:435, 2011.

*Evidence-based information for clinical practice.

9. Arnstein P: What's the best way to cool my patient's burn pain, *Nursing* 40:61, 2010.
*10. Pannucci C, Osborne N, Wahl W: Venous thromboembolism in thermally-injured patients: analysis of the National Burn Repository, *J Burn Care Res* 32:6, 2011.
*11. Garcia DA, Baglin TP, Weitz JI, et al: Parenteral anticoagulants: antithrombotic therapy and prevention of thrombosis, ed 9: American College of Chest Physicians evidence-based clinical practice guidelines, *Chest* 141:e24S, 2012.
12. Dries DJ, Mohr WJ: *Yearbook of intensive care and emergency medicine*, Berlin, 2010, Springer-Verlag.
13. Cartotto R: Fluid resuscitation of the thermally-injured patient, *Clin Plast Surg* 36:569, 2009.
*14. Davison P, Loiselle F, Nickerson D: Survey on current hydrotherapy use among North American burn centers, *J Burn Care Res* 31:540, 2010.
*15. Rafla K, Tredget E: Infection control in the burn unit, *Burns* 37:5, 2011.
*16. Trupkovic T, Kinn M, Kleinschmidt S: Analgesia and sedation in the intensive care of burn patients: results of a European survey, *J Intens Care Med* 26:397, 2011.
*17. Wong L, Turner L: Treatment of post-burn neuropathic pain: evaluation of pregabalin, *Burns* 36:769, 2010.
18. Greenhalgh D: Topical antimicrobial agents for burn wounds, *Clin Plast Surg* 36:597, 2009.
*19. Posluszny J, Conrad P, Halerz M, et al: Surgical burn wound infections and their clinical implications, *J Burn Care Res* 32:324, 2011.
*20. Mosier M, Pham T, Klein M, et al: Early enteral nutrition in burns: compliance with guidelines and associated outcomes in a multicenter study, *J Burn Care Res* 32:104, 2011.
*21. Williams I, Herndon D, Jeschke M, et al: The hypermetabolic response to burn injury and interventions to modify this response, *Clin Plast Surg* 36:583, 2009.
*22. Holavanahalli R, Helm P, Parry I, et al: Select practices in management and rehabilitation of a survey report, *J Burn Care Res* 32:210, 2011.
23. Mosier M, Gibran N: Surgical excision of the burn wound, *Clin Plast Surg* 36:617, 2009.
*24. Curinga G, Jain A, Feldman M, et al: RBC transfusion following burns, *Burns* 37:742, 2011.
25. Saffle J: Closure of the excised burn wound: temporary skin substitutes, *Clin Plast Surg* 36:627, 2009.
*26. Demirtas Y, Yagmur C, Soylemez S, et al: Management of split-thickness skin graft donor sites: a prospective clinical trial for comparison of five different dressing materials, *Burns* 36:999, 2010.
27. Sheridan R: Closure of the excised burn wound: autograft, semipermanent skin substitutes and permanent skin substitutes, *Clin Plast Surg* 36:643, 2009.
*28. Tengvall O, Wickman M, Wengstrom Y: Memories of pain after burn injury—the patient's experience, *J Burn Care Res* 31:319, 2010.
*29. Rumbach A, Ward E, Cornwell P, et al: Incidence and predictive factors for dysphagia after thermal burn injury: a prospective cohort study, *J Burn Care Res* 32:608, 2011.
*30. Reeve J, James F, McNeill R, et al: Functional and psychological outcomes following burn injury: reduced income and hidden emotions are predictors of greater distress, *J Burn Care Res* 32:468, 2011.
*31. Sundara D: A review of issues and concerns of family members of adult burn survivors, *J Burn Care Res* 32:349, 2011.
*32. Engrav L, Heimbach D, Rivara F, et al: Twelve-year within-wound study of the effectiveness of custom pressure garment therapy, *Burns* 36:975, 2010.
*33. Gautos I: Burns pruritus—a study of current practices in the UK, *Burns* 36:42, 2010.
*34. Richards R: Burn rehabilitation and research: proceedings of a consensus summit, *J Burn Care Res* 30:543, 2009.
*35. Holavanahalli R, Helm P, Kowalske K, et al: Long-term outcomes in patients surviving large burns: the skin, *J Burn Care Res* 31:631, 2010.
*36. Brown-Guttovz H: Burn injury, *Nursing* 41:68, 2011.
*37. Elsherbiny O, Salem M, El-Sabbagh A, et al: Quality of life of adult burn patients with severe burns, *Burns* 37:776, 2011.
*38. Schneider J, Bassi S, Ryna C: Employment outcomes after burn injury: a comparison of those burned at work and those burned outside of work, *J Burn Care Res* 32:294, 2011.
*39. Klein M, Lezotte D, Heltshe S, et al: Functional and psychosocial outcomes of older adults after burn injury: results from a multicenter database of severe burn injury, *J Burn Care Res* 32:66, 2011.
*40. Solanki N, Greenwood J, Kavanagh S, et al: Social issues prolong elderly burn patient hospitalization, *J Burn Care Res* 32:387, 2011.
*41. Rimmer R, Rutter C, Lessard C, et al: Burn care professionals' attitudes and practices regarding discussions of sexuality and intimacy with adult burn survivors, *J Burn Care Res* 31:579, 2010.
*42. Orcutt T: Developing family support groups in the ICU, *Nurs Crit Care* 5:33, 2010.
43. Greenfield E: The pivotal role of nursing personnel in burn care, *Indian J Plast Surg* 43:594, 2010.
*44. Kornhaber R, Wilson A: Psychosocial needs of burns nurses: a descriptive, phenomenological inquiry, *J Burn Care Res* 32:286, 2011.

RESOURCES

American Burn Association
www.ameriburn.org

Burn Survivor.org
www.burnsurvivor.org

Changing Faces
www.changingfaces.org.uk

International Society for Burn Injuries
www.worldburn.org

Phoenix Society for Burn Survivors
www.phoenix-society.org

World Burn Foundation
www.burnfoundation.com

CASE STUDY

Managing Multiple Patients

Introduction

You are working the day shift on a medical-surgical unit and have been assigned to care for the following five patients. You have 1 UAP who is assigned to work with you. There are 15 other patients on the unit being cared for by an additional 3 RNs and 3 UAPs.

Patients

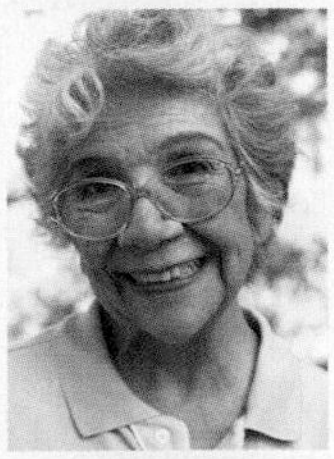

Jack Hollingsworth/Photodisc/Thinkstock

F.M., an 81-year-old Hispanic woman, had pneumatic retinopexy surgery yesterday to repair a partially detached retina. She has a history of diabetes, hypothyroidism, and hypertension. She is scheduled to be discharged today, but the night nurse is concerned because her blood pressure is elevated at 150/94 mm Hg.

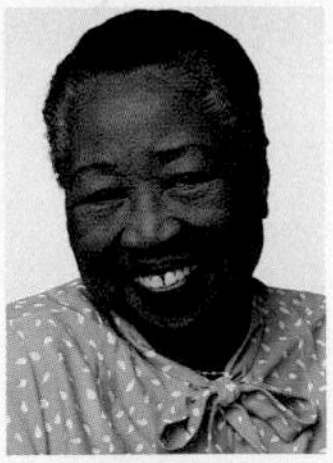

Kevin Peterson/Stockbyte/Thinkstock

J.K., a 68-year-old African American woman with osteoarthritis and type 2 diabetes mellitus for the past 15 years, now has diabetic retinopathy. She had argon laser therapy to her right eye yesterday to seal leaking microaneurysms from macular edema. She was admitted with uncontrolled postoperative hyperglycemia.

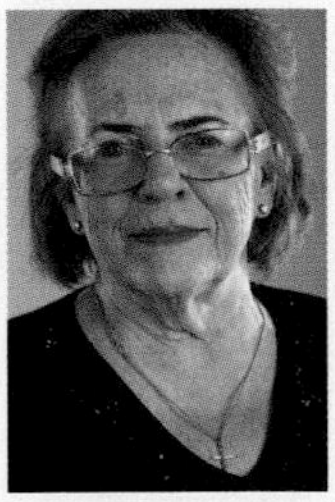

iStockphoto/Thinkstock

D.A., a 74-year-old woman, is admitted to the hospital with complaints of chest tightness and shortness of breath. Her past medical history is negative except for a recent diagnosis of basal cell carcinoma (BCC) on her face. She was scheduled to have the BCC surgically removed tomorrow. The health care provider suspects D.A.'s symptoms are caused by anxiety but first needs to rule out any coronary artery disease before surgery.

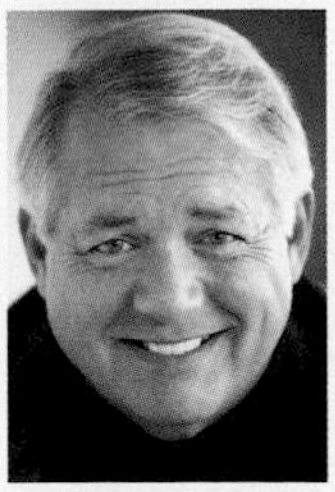

Hemera/Thinkstock

G.L., a 59-year-old white man, just arrived for admission. He is scheduled for surgical removal of malignant melanoma lesions on his face at 1200. He is worried that the surgery will be disfiguring.

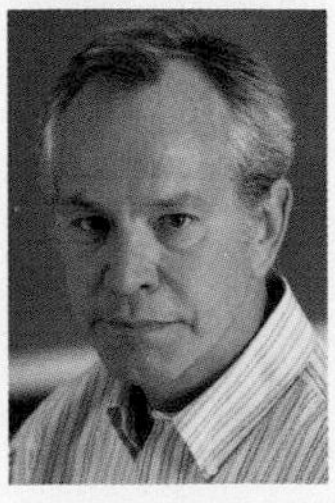

Comstock/Thinkstock

G.M., a 52-year-old white man, is transferred from the ICU following burns to his face, neck, chest, right arm and hand, and right foot. He has a tracheostomy and is receiving 35% O_2 via a humidified trach collar. He has a history of diabetes and hypertension. In the ICU he had been on a mechanical ventilator for respiratory failure caused by inhalation injury. His burns are shiny, bright red, and wet. There are a few blisters on his face.

Management Discussion Questions

1. ***Priority Decision:*** After receiving report, which patient should you see first? Provide rationale.
2. ***Delegation Decision:*** Which tasks could you delegate to the UAP *(select all that apply)?*
   a. Obtain vital signs on F.M.
   b. Take a blood pressure reading on G.M.
   c. Perform an admission assessment on G.L.
   d. Explain planned diagnostic testing to D.A.
   e. Obtain a capillary blood glucose reading on J.K.
3. ***Priority and Delegation Decision:*** When you enter G.M.'s room, he tells you he is not feeling well. He says he has a headache and his legs are "cramping up." He is also somewhat confused as he is unaware that he is in the hospital. What initial action would be most appropriate?
   a. Administer acetaminophen for headache relief.
   b. Have the UAP obtain a stat capillary blood glucose reading.
   c. Notify G.M.'s health care provider of his altered level of consciousness.
   d. Have the UAP obtain vital signs on G.M. while you look at his most recent laboratory test results.

Case Study Progression

G.M.'s vital signs are BP 154/88 mm Hg, his heart rate is 112 bpm, his respirations are 18 breaths/min, and his temperature is 98° F (36.8° C). His most recent lab work reveals a serum sodium level of 125 mEq/L (125 mmol/L). You notify his health care provider, who orders a normal saline IV to infuse at 100 mL/hr.

4. G.M. complains of thirst and asks for something to drink. Which fluid would be appropriate to give him *(select all that apply)?*
   a. Gatorade
   b. Tap water
   c. Cola soda
   d. Apple juice
   e. Orange juice
5. In addition to teaching F.M. how to administer postoperative eye drops, you will also explain
   a. position and activity restrictions.
   b. how to change the dressing on her eye.
   c. the necessity for restricting fluid intake.
   d. that protective eyewear will no longer be required.
6. When giving report to your UAP regarding your assigned patients, she asks if there is a significant difference between D.A. and G.L.'s skin cancers. You reply based on knowledge that
   a. basal cell carcinoma is the most deadly form of skin cancer.
   b. malignant melanoma typically appears as red, rough patches on the skin.
   c. basal cell carcinoma typically presents during the second and third decades of life.
   d. melanoma has the ability to metastasize to any organ, including the brain and heart.
7. ***Management Decision:*** Another RN offers to help you by providing wound care for G.M. Which observed action by the RN would require your immediate intervention?
   a. G.M.'s hands are elevated on pillows.
   b. G.M.'s burns are cleansed with soap and water.
   c. G.M. is promised analgesia as soon as wound care is complete.
   d. G.M.'s burns are covered with a very thin layer of prescribed ointment.

evolve Answers available at *http://evolve.elsevier.com/Lewis/medsurg.*

SECTION 5

Problems of Oxygenation: Ventilation

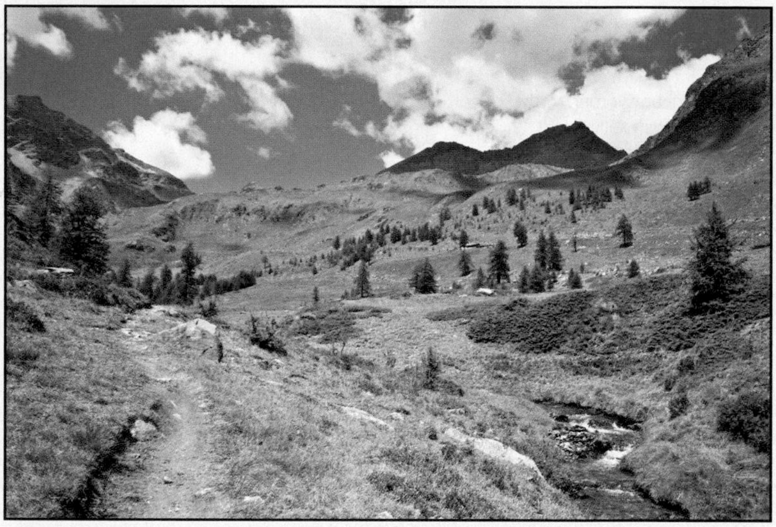

iStockphoto

May your trails be crooked, winding, lonesome, dangerous, leading to the most amazing view. May your mountains rise into and above the clouds.
Edward Abbey

CHAPTER

26

When you own your breath, nobody can steal your peace.
Author Unknown

Nursing Assessment
Respiratory System

Susan J. Eisel

evolve WEBSITE

http://evolve.elsevier.com/Lewis/medsurg

- NCLEX Review Questions
- Key Points
- Pre-Test
- Answer Guidelines for Case Study in this chapter
- Rationales for Bridge to NCLEX Examination Questions
- Concept Map Creator
- Glossary
- Animations
  - Patterns of Respiration
  - Percussion Tones Throughout Chest
  - Pulmonary Circulation
- Videos
  - Inspection and Palpation: Breathing and Respiratory Excursion, Anterior Chest
  - Inspection and Palpation: Respirations, Respiratory Excursion, and Tactile Fremitus, Posterior Chest
  - Inspection and Percussion: Diaphragmatic Excursion
  - Inspection: Nose
  - Palpation: Tactile Fremitus, Posterior Chest
  - Percussion: Anterior Thorax
  - Physical Examination: Anterior Chest, Lungs, Heart
  - Physical Examination: Lung
- Content Updates
- Audio
  - Bronchial Breath Sounds
  - Bronchovesicular Breath Sounds
  - High-Pitched Crackles
  - High-Pitched Wheeze
  - Low-Pitched Crackles
  - Low-Pitched Wheeze
  - Pleural Friction Rub
  - Stridor
  - Vesicular Breath Sounds

eFigures

- eFig 26-1: Oxygen-hemoglobin dissociation curve
- eFig. 26-2: Pulse oximeter
- eFig. 26-3: Finger clubbing
- eFig. 26-4: Relationship of lung volumes and capacities

eTable

- eTable 26-1: Oxygen-Hemoglobin Dissociation Curve

LEARNING OUTCOMES

1. Differentiate among the structures and functions of the upper respiratory tract, the lower respiratory tract, and the chest wall.
2. Describe the process that initiates and controls inspiration and expiration.
3. Describe the process of gas diffusion within the lungs.
4. Identify the respiratory defense mechanisms.
5. Describe the significance of arterial blood gas values in relation to respiratory function.
6. Relate the signs and symptoms of inadequate oxygenation to implications of these findings.
7. Link the age-related changes of the respiratory system to the differences in assessment findings.
8. Select the significant subjective and objective data related to the respiratory system that should be obtained from a patient.
9. Select appropriate techniques to use in the physical assessment of the respiratory system.
10. Differentiate normal from common abnormal findings in a physical assessment of the respiratory system.
11. Describe the purpose, significance of results, and nursing responsibilities related to diagnostic studies of the respiratory system.

KEY TERMS

adventitious sounds, p. 488
chemoreceptor, p. 480
compliance, p. 478
crackles, Table 26-8, p. 489
dyspnea, p. 478
elastic recoil, p. 478
fremitus, p. 486
mechanical receptors, p. 480
pleural friction rub, Table 26-8, p. 490
rhonchi, Table 26-8, p. 489
surfactant, p. 477
tidal volume (VT), p. 477
ventilation, p. 478
wheezes, Table 26-8, p. 489

STRUCTURES AND FUNCTIONS OF RESPIRATORY SYSTEM

The primary purpose of the respiratory system is gas exchange. This involves the transfer of oxygen (O_2) and carbon dioxide (CO_2) between the atmosphere and the blood. The respiratory system is divided into two parts: the upper respiratory tract and the lower respiratory tract (Fig. 26-1).

Upper Respiratory Tract

The *upper respiratory tract* includes the nose, mouth, pharynx, epiglottis, larynx, and trachea. Air enters into the respiratory tract through the nose. The nose is made of bone and cartilage and is divided into two nares by the nasal septum. The inside of the nose is shaped into three passages by projections called *turbinates.* The turbinates increase the surface area of the nasal

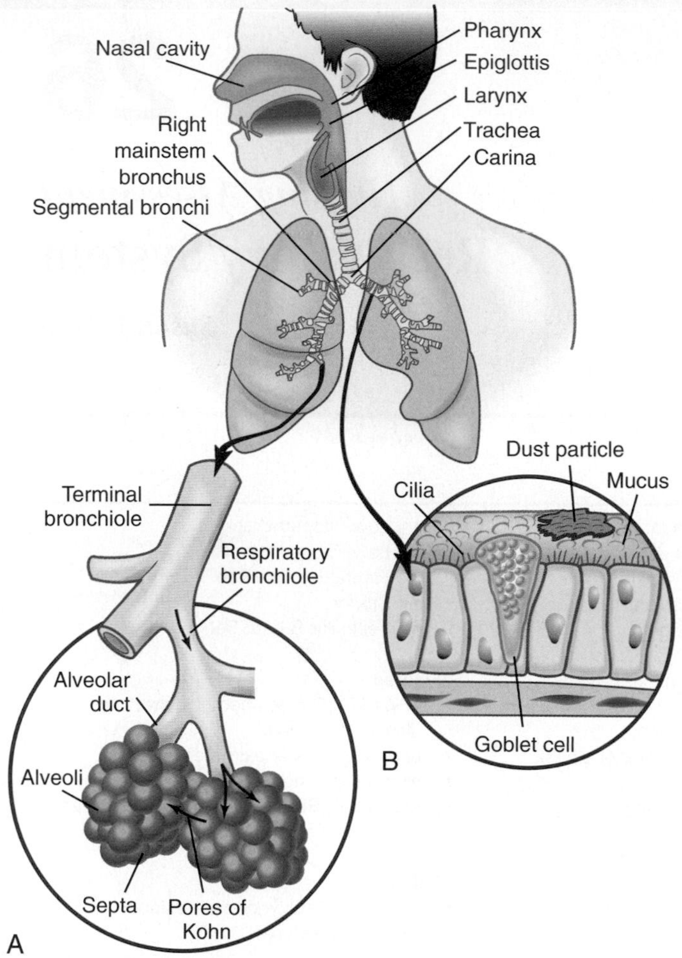

FIG. 26-1 Structures of the respiratory tract. **A,** Pulmonary functional unit. **B,** Ciliated mucous membrane.

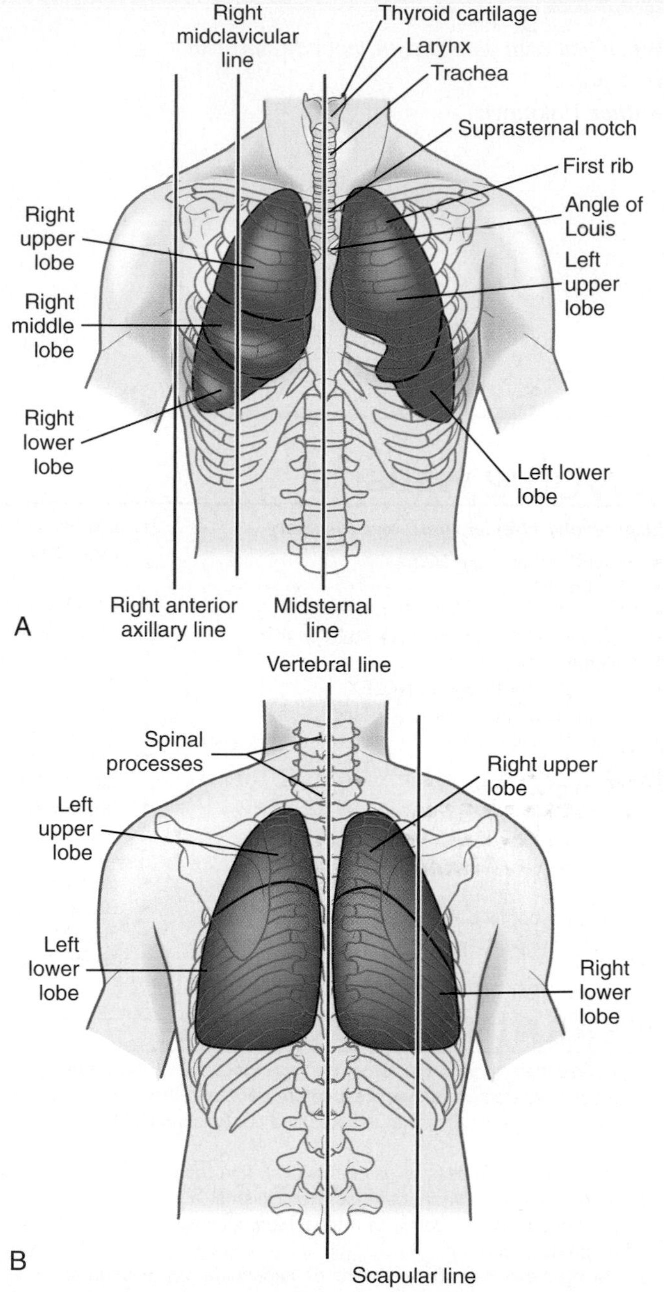

FIG. 26-2 Landmarks and structures of the chest wall. **A,** Anterior view. **B,** Posterior view.

mucosa, which warms and moistens the air as it enters the nose. The internal nose opens directly into the sinuses. The nasal cavity connects with the pharynx, a tubular passageway that is subdivided into three parts: the *nasopharynx, oropharynx,* and *laryngopharynx.*

The nose functions to protect the lower airway by warming and humidifying air and filtering small particles before air enters the lungs. Olfactory nerve endings, located in the roof of the nose, are responsible for the sense of smell.

Air moves through the oropharynx to the laryngopharynx. It then travels through the epiglottis to the larynx before moving into the trachea. The *epiglottis* is a small flap located behind the tongue that closes over the larynx during swallowing. This prevents solids and liquids from entering the lungs. The vocal cords are located in the larynx. Vibrational sounds are made during respiration leading to vocalization. Air passes through the glottis, the opening between the vocal cords, and into the trachea. The trachea is a cylindric tube about 5 in (10 to 12 cm) long and 1 in (1.5 to 2.5 cm) in diameter. U-shaped cartilages keep the trachea open but allow the adjacent esophagus to expand for swallowing. The trachea bifurcates into the right and left mainstem bronchi at a point called the *carina.* The carina is located at the level of the manubriosternal junction, also called the *angle of Louis.* The carina is highly sensitive, and touching it during suctioning causes vigorous coughing.[1]

Lower Respiratory Tract

The *lower respiratory tract* consists of the bronchi, bronchioles, alveolar ducts, and alveoli. With the exception of the right and left mainstem bronchi, all lower airway structures are located inside the lungs. The right lung is divided into three lobes (upper, middle, and lower) and the left lung into two lobes (upper and lower) (Fig. 26-2). The structures of the chest wall (ribs, pleura, muscles of respiration) are also important for respiration.

Once air passes the carina, it is in the lower respiratory tract. The mainstem bronchi, pulmonary vessels, and nerves enter the lungs through a slit called the *hilus.* The right mainstem bronchus is shorter, wider, and straighter than the left mainstem bronchus. For this reason, aspiration is more likely to occur in the right lung than in the left lung.

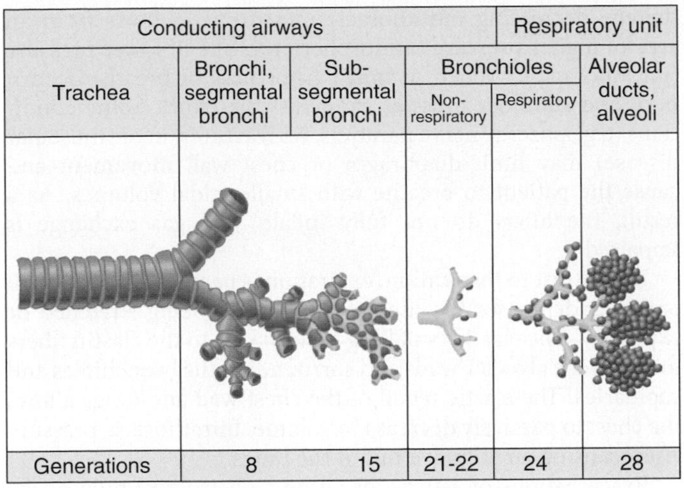

Conducting airways
Respiratory unit
Trachea
Bronchi, segmental bronchi
Sub-segmental bronchi
Bronchioles
Non-respiratory
Respiratory
Alveolar ducts, alveoli
Generations
8
15
21-22
24
28

FIG. 26-3 Structures of lower airways.

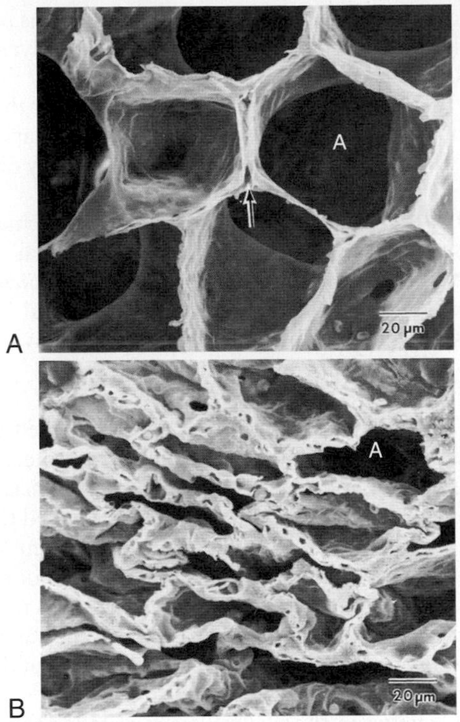

FIG. 26-4 Scanning electron micrograph of lung parenchyma. **A,** Alveoli *(A)* and alveolar-capillary membrane *(arrow)*. **B,** Effects of atelectasis. Alveoli *(A)* are partially or totally collapsed.

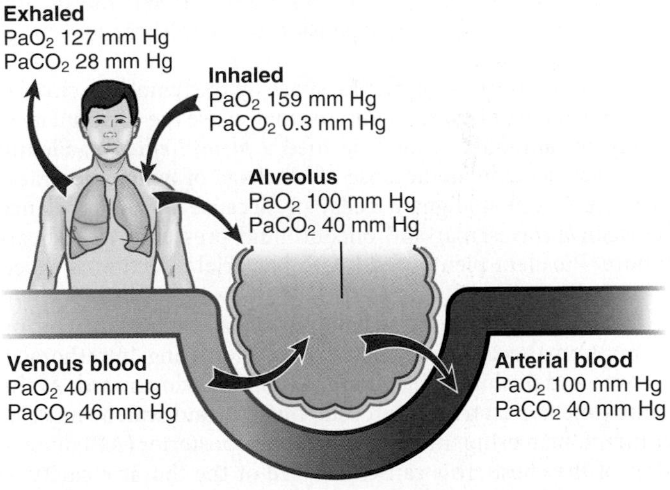

FIG. 26-5 Partial pressure of respiratory gases in normal respiration. The pressures are shown in inhaled and exhaled air from the lungs and at the level of the alveoli and pulmonary venous and arterial blood vessels.

The mainstem bronchi subdivide several times to form the lobar, segmental, and subsegmental bronchi. Further divisions form the bronchioles. The most distant bronchioles are called the respiratory bronchioles. Beyond these lie the alveolar ducts and alveolar sacs (Fig. 26-3). The bronchioles are encircled by smooth muscles that constrict and dilate in response to various stimuli. The terms *bronchoconstriction* and *bronchodilation* refer to a decrease or increase in the diameter of the airways caused by contraction or relaxation of these muscles.

Oxygen and carbon dioxide exchange takes place in the alveoli. The trachea and bronchi act as a pathway to conduct gases to the alveoli. The trachea plus the bronchi are called *anatomic dead space* (VD).The air filling this space with every breath is not available for gas exchange. In adults a normal **tidal volume (VT)**, or volume of air exchanged with each breath, is about 500 mL (in a 150 lb man). Of each 500 mL inhaled, about 150 mL is VD.

After moving through the VD, air reaches the respiratory bronchioles and alveoli (Fig. 26-4). *Alveoli* are small sacs that are the primary site of gas exchange in the lungs. The alveoli are interconnected by pores of Kohn, which allow movement of air from alveolus to alveolus (see Fig. 26-1). Deep breathing promotes air movement through these pores and assists in moving mucus out of the respiratory bronchioles. Bacteria can also move through these pores, spreading infection to previously uninfected areas. The adult lung has 300 million alveoli. Alveoli have a total volume of about 2500 mL and a surface area for gas exchange that is about the size of a tennis court.

Gases are exchanged at the alveolar-capillary membrane where the alveoli come in contact with pulmonary capillaries (Fig. 26-5). In conditions such as pulmonary edema, excess fluid fills the interstitial space and alveoli, markedly reducing gas exchange.

Surfactant. The lungs are a collection of 300 million alveoli, each 0.3 mm in diameter. Because alveoli are unstable, they have a natural tendency to collapse. Alveolar cells secrete surfactant. **Surfactant** is a lipoprotein that lowers the surface tension in the alveoli. It reduces the amount of pressure needed to inflate the alveoli and makes them less likely to collapse. Normally, each person takes a slightly larger breath, termed a *sigh*, after every five or six breaths. This sigh stretches the alveoli and promotes surfactant secretion.

When not enough surfactant is present, the alveoli collapse. The term *atelectasis* refers to collapsed, airless alveoli (see Fig. 26-4, *B*). The postoperative patient is at risk for atelectasis because of the effects of anesthesia and restricted breathing with pain (see Chapter 20). In acute respiratory distress syndrome (ARDS), lack of surfactant contributes to widespread atelectasis (see Chapter 68).

Blood Supply. The lungs have two different types of circulation: pulmonary and bronchial. The *pulmonary circulation* provides the lungs with blood that participates in gas exchange. The pulmonary artery receives deoxygenated blood from the right ventricle of the heart and delivers it to pulmonary capillaries that are directly connected with alveoli. Oxygen–carbon dioxide exchange occurs at this point. The pulmonary veins return oxygenated blood to the left atrium, which then delivers it to the left ventricle. This oxygenated blood is pumped by the left ventricle into the aorta, which supplies the arteries of the systemic circulation. Venous blood is collected from capillary networks of the body and returned to the right atrium by way of the venae cavae.

The *bronchial circulation* starts with the bronchial arteries, which arise from the thoracic aorta. The bronchial circulation provides oxygen to the bronchi and other pulmonary tissues. Deoxygenated blood returns from the bronchial circulation through the azygos vein into the superior vena cava.

Chest Wall

The chest wall is shaped, supported, and protected by 24 ribs (12 on each side). The ribs and the sternum protect the lungs and the heart from injury and are called the *thoracic cage.*

The chest cavity is lined with a membrane called the *parietal pleura,* and the lungs are lined with a membrane called the *visceral pleura.* The parietal and visceral pleurae join to form a closed, double-walled sac. The visceral pleura does not have any sensory pain fibers or nerve endings, whereas the parietal pleura does have sensory pain fibers. Therefore irritation of the parietal pleura causes pain with each breath.

The space between the pleural layers is called the *intrapleural space.* Normally this space contains 20 to 25 mL of fluid. This fluid serves two purposes: (1) it provides lubrication, allowing the pleural layers to slide over each other during breathing; and (2) it increases cohesion between the pleural layers, thereby facilitating expansion of the pleurae and lungs during inspiration.

Fluid drains from the pleural space by the lymphatic circulation. Several pathologic conditions may cause the accumulation of greater amounts of fluid, termed a *pleural effusion.* Pleural fluid may accumulate because of blockage of lymphatic drainage (e.g., from malignant cells) or because of an imbalance between intravascular and oncotic fluid pressures, as in heart failure. Purulent pleural fluid with bacterial infection is called *empyema.*

The *diaphragm* is the major muscle of respiration. During inspiration the diaphragm contracts, increasing intrathoracic volume and pushing the abdominal contents downward. At the same time the external intercostal muscles and scalene muscles contract, increasing the lateral and anteroposterior (AP) dimension of the chest. This causes the size of the thoracic cavity to increase and intrathoracic pressure to decrease, so air enters the lungs.

The diaphragm is made up of two hemidiaphragms, each innervated by the right and left phrenic nerves. The phrenic nerves arise from the spinal cord between C3 and C5, the third and fifth cervical vertebrae. Injury to the phrenic nerve results in hemidiaphragm paralysis on the side of the injury. Complete spinal cord injuries above the level of C3 result in total diaphragm paralysis and dependence on a mechanical ventilator.

Physiology of Respiration

Ventilation. **Ventilation** involves *inspiration,* or inhalation (movement of air into the lungs), and *expiration,* or exhalation (movement of air out of the lungs). Air moves in and out of the lungs because intrathoracic pressure changes in relation to pressure at the airway opening. Contraction of the diaphragm and intercostal and scalene muscles increases chest dimensions, thereby decreasing intrathoracic pressure. Gas flows from an area of higher pressure (atmospheric) to one of lower pressure (intrathoracic).[2] When **dyspnea** (shortness of breath) occurs, neck and shoulder muscles can assist the effort. Some conditions (e.g., phrenic nerve paralysis, rib fractures, neuromuscular disease) may limit diaphragm or chest wall movement and cause the patient to breathe with smaller tidal volumes. As a result, the lungs do not fully inflate, and gas exchange is impaired.

In contrast to inspiration, expiration is passive. **Elastic recoil** is the tendency for the lungs to relax after being stretched or expanded. The elasticity of lung tissue is due to the elastin fibers found in the alveolar walls and surrounding the bronchioles and capillaries. The elastic recoil of the chest wall and lungs allows the chest to passively decrease in volume. Intrathoracic pressure rises, causing air to move out of the lungs.

Exacerbations of asthma or chronic obstructive pulmonary disease (COPD) cause expiration to become an active, labored process (see Chapter 29). Abdominal, intercostal, and accessory muscles (e.g., scalene, trapezius) assist in expelling air during labored breathing.

Compliance. **Compliance** (distensibility) is a measure of the ease of expansion of the lungs. This is a product of the elasticity of the lungs and the elastic recoil of the chest wall. When compliance is decreased, the lungs are more difficult to inflate. Examples include conditions that increase fluid in the lungs (e.g., pulmonary edema, ARDS, pneumonia), conditions that make lung tissue less elastic or distensible (e.g., pulmonary fibrosis, sarcoidosis), and conditions that restrict lung movement (e.g., pleural effusion). Compliance is increased when there is destruction of alveolar walls and loss of tissue elasticity, as in COPD.

Diffusion. Oxygen and carbon dioxide move back and forth across the alveolar-capillary membrane by diffusion. The overall direction of movement is from the area of higher concentration to the area of lower concentration. Thus oxygen moves from alveolar gas (atmospheric air) into the arterial blood and carbon dioxide from the arterial blood into the alveolar gas. Diffusion continues until equilibrium is reached.

The lungs' ability to oxygenate arterial blood adequately is assessed by examination of the partial pressure of oxygen in arterial blood (PaO_2) and arterial oxygen saturation (SaO_2). Oxygen is carried in the blood in two forms: dissolved oxygen and hemoglobin-bound oxygen. The PaO_2 represents the amount of oxygen dissolved in the plasma and is expressed in millimeters of mercury (mm Hg). The SaO_2 is the amount of oxygen bound to hemoglobin in comparison with the amount of oxygen the hemoglobin can carry. The SaO_2 is expressed as a percentage. For example, if the SaO_2 is 90%, this means that 90% of the hemoglobin attachments for oxygen have oxygen bound to them.

Arterial Blood Gases. Two methods are used to assess the efficiency of gas transfer in the lung and tissue oxygenation: analysis of *arterial blood gases* (ABGs) and pulse oximetry. ABGs are measured to determine oxygenation status and acid-base balance. ABG analysis includes measurement of the PaO_2, $PaCO_2$, acidity (pH), and bicarbonate (HCO_3^-) in arterial blood. The SaO_2 is either calculated or measured during this analysis. Normal values for ABGs are given in Table 26-1.

Blood for ABG analysis can be obtained by arterial puncture or from an arterial catheter, usually in the radial or femoral artery. Both techniques allow only intermittent analysis. Con-

TABLE 26-1 NORMAL ARTERIAL AND VENOUS BLOOD GAS VALUES*

Arterial Blood Gases			Venous Blood Gases	
Laboratory Value	**Sea Level BP 760 mm Hg**	**1 Mile Above Sea Level BP 629 mm Hg**	**Mixed Venous Blood Gases**	
pH	7.35-7.45	7.35-7.45	pH	7.32-7.43
PaO_2†	80-100 mm Hg	65-75 mm Hg	PvO_2	38-42 mm Hg
SaO_2†	>95%‡	>95%‡	SvO_2	60%-80%‡
$PaCO_2$	35-45 mm Hg	35-45 mm Hg	$PvCO_2$	38-55 mm Hg
HCO_3^-	22-26 mEq/L (mmol/L)	22-26 mEq/L (mmol/L)	HCO_3^-	22-26 mEq/L (mmol/L)

*Assumes patient is ≤60 yr of age and breathing room air.
†Values decrease with age.
‡The same normal values apply when SpO_2 and SvO_2 are obtained by oximetry.
BP, Barometric pressure; *HCO_3^-*, bicarbonate; *$PaCO_2$*, partial pressure of arterial CO_2; *$PvCO_2$*, partial pressure of CO_2 in venous blood; *PaO_2*, partial pressure of O_2 in arterial blood; *PvO_2*, partial pressure of O_2 in venous blood; *SaO_2*, arterial O_2 saturation; *SvO_2*, venous O_2 saturation.

TABLE 26-2 MANIFESTATIONS OF INADEQUATE OXYGENATION

Manifestations	Onset: Early	Onset: Late	Manifestations	Onset: Early	Onset: Late
Central Nervous System			**Cardiovascular**		
Unexplained apprehension	X		Tachycardia	X	
Unexplained restlessness or irritability	X		Mild hypertension	X	
Unexplained confusion or lethargy	X	X	Dysrhythmias	X	X
Combativeness		X	Hypotension		X
Coma		X	Cyanosis		X
			Cool, clammy skin		X
Respiratory			**Other**		
Tachypnea	X		Diaphoresis	X	X
Dyspnea on exertion	X		Decreased urine output	X	X
Dyspnea at rest		X	Unexplained fatigue	X	X
Use of accessory muscles		X			
Retraction of interspaces on inspiration		X			
Pause for breath between sentences, words		X			

tinuous intraarterial blood gas monitoring is also possible via a fiberoptic sensor or an oxygen electrode inserted into an arterial catheter. An arterial catheter permits ABG sampling without repeated arterial punctures.

The normal PaO_2 decreases with advancing age. It also varies in relation to the distance above sea level. At higher altitudes the barometric pressure is lower, resulting in a lower inspired oxygen pressure and a lower PaO_2 (see Table 26-1).

Mixed Venous Blood Gases. For the patient with a normal or near-normal cardiac status, an assessment of PaO_2 or SaO_2 is usually sufficient to determine the level of oxygenation. The patient with impaired cardiac output or hemodynamic instability may have inadequate tissue oxygen delivery or abnormal oxygen consumption.[3]

The amount of oxygen delivered to the tissues or consumed can be calculated. A catheter positioned in the pulmonary artery, termed a *pulmonary artery (PA) catheter,* is used for mixed venous sampling (see Chapter 66). Blood drawn from a PA catheter is termed a *mixed venous blood gas* sample because it consists of venous blood that has returned to the heart and "mixes" in the right ventricle. Normal mixed venous values are given in Table 26-1. When tissue oxygen delivery is inadequate or when inadequate oxygen is transported to the tissues by the hemoglobin, the PvO_2 and SvO_2 fall.

Oximetry. Arterial oxygen saturation can be monitored noninvasively and continuously using a *pulse oximetry* probe on the finger, toe, ear, or bridge of the nose[4] (see eFig. 26-2 available on the website). The abbreviation SpO_2 is used to indicate the oxygen saturation of hemoglobin as measured by pulse oximetry. SpO_2 and heart rate are displayed on the monitor as digital readings (see eFig. 26-2).

Pulse oximetry is particularly valuable in intensive care and perioperative situations, in which sedation or decreased consciousness might mask hypoxia (Table 26-2). SpO_2 is assessed with each routine vital sign check in many inpatient areas. Changes in SpO_2 can be detected quickly and treated (Table 26-3). Oximetry is also used during exercise testing and when adjusting flow rates during long-term oxygen therapy.

Values obtained by pulse oximetry are less accurate if the SpO_2 is less than 70%. At this level the oximeter may display a value that is ±4% of the actual value. For example, if the SpO_2 reading is 70%, the actual value can range from 66% to 74%. Pulse oximetry is also inaccurate if hemoglobin variants (e.g., carboxyhemoglobin, methemoglobin) are present. Other factors that can alter the accuracy of pulse oximetry include motion, low perfusion, anemia, cold extremities, bright fluorescent lights, intravascular dyes, thick acrylic nails, and dark skin color. If there is doubt about the accuracy of the SpO_2 reading, obtain an ABG analysis to verify the results.

Oximetry can also be used to monitor SvO_2 via a PA catheter. A decrease in SvO_2 suggests that less oxygen is being delivered to the tissues or that more oxygen is being consumed. Changes in SvO_2 provide an early warning of a change in cardiac output or tissue oxygen delivery. Normal SvO_2 is 60% to 80%.

Carbon Dioxide Monitoring. Carbon dioxide can be monitored using transcutaneous CO_2 ($PTCCO_2$) and end-tidal CO_2

TABLE 26-3 CRITICAL VALUES FOR PaO_2 AND SpO_2*

PaO_2 (%)	SpO_2 (%)	Significance
≥70	≥94	Adequate unless patient is hemodynamically unstable or hemoglobin (Hgb) has difficulty releasing O_2 to the tissues.
60	90	Adequate in almost all patients. Provides adequate oxygenation but with less margin for error than above.
55	88	Adequate for patients with chronic hypoxemia if no cardiac problems occur. These values are also used as criteria for prescription of continuous O_2 therapy.
40	75	Inadequate but may be acceptable on a short-term basis if the patient also has CO_2 retention. In this situation, respirations may be stimulated by a low PaO_2. Thus the PaO_2 cannot be raised rapidly.
<40	<75	Inadequate. Tissue hypoxia and cardiac dysrhythmias can be expected.

*The same critical values apply for SpO_2 and SaO_2. Values pertain to rest or exertion.

($PETCO_2$) (capnography). Transcutaneous measurement of CO_2 is a noninvasive method of estimating arterial pressure of CO_2 ($PaCO_2$) using an electrode placed on the skin.

$PETCO_2$ is the noninvasive measurement of alveolar CO_2 at the end of exhalation when CO_2 concentration is at its peak. It is used to monitor and assess trends in the patient's ventilatory status. Expired gases are sampled from the patient's airway and are analyzed by a CO_2 sensor that uses infrared light to measure exhaled CO_2. The sensor may be attached to an adaptor on the endotracheal tube or the tracheostomy tube. A nasal cannula with a sidestream capnometer can be used in patients without an artificial airway. Capnography is usually presented as a graph of expiratory CO_2 plotted against time.

In the past, capnography was used mainly intraoperatively, postoperatively, and in critical care units. Today's monitors are portable and practical for use on inpatient units and emergency departments.

Measurement of oxygen saturation (oximetry) is primarily used to assess for hypoxia. CO_2 monitoring assesses for hypoventilation. The use of both measures together is important in determining patients' oxygenation and ventilatory status.

Control of Respiration

The respiratory center in the medulla (located in the brainstem) responds to chemical and mechanical signals. Impulses are sent from the medulla to the respiratory muscles through the spinal cord and the phrenic nerves.

Chemoreceptors. A chemoreceptor is a receptor that responds to a change in the chemical composition ($PaCO_2$ and pH) of the fluid around it. Central chemoreceptors are located in the medulla and respond to changes in the hydrogen ion (H^+) concentration. An increase in the H^+ concentration *(acidosis)* causes the medulla to increase the respiratory rate and tidal volume (VT). A decrease in H^+ concentration *(alkalosis)* has the opposite effect. Changes in $PaCO_2$ regulate ventilation primarily by their effect on the pH of the cerebrospinal fluid. When the $PaCO_2$ level is increased, more CO_2 is available to combine with H_2O and form carbonic acid (H_2CO_3). This lowers the cerebrospinal fluid pH and stimulates an increase in respiratory rate. The opposite process occurs with a decrease in $PaCO_2$ level.

Peripheral chemoreceptors are located in the carotid bodies at the bifurcation of the common carotid arteries and in the aortic bodies above and below the aortic arch. The peripheral chemoreceptors respond to decreases in PaO_2 and pH and to increases in $PaCO_2$. These changes also stimulate the respiratory center.

In a healthy person an increase in $PaCO_2$ or a decrease in pH causes an immediate increase in the respiratory rate. The $PaCO_2$ does not vary more than about 3 mm Hg if lung function is normal. Conditions such as COPD alter lung function and may result in chronically elevated $PaCO_2$ levels. In these instances the patient is relatively insensitive to further increases in $PaCO_2$ as a stimulus to breathe and may be maintaining ventilation largely because of a hypoxic drive from the peripheral chemoreceptors (see Chapter 29).

Mechanical Receptors. Mechanical receptors (juxtacapillary and irritant) are located in the lungs, upper airways, chest wall, and diaphragm. They are stimulated by a variety of physiologic factors, such as irritants, muscle stretching, and alveolar wall distortion. Signals from the stretch receptors aid in the control of respiration. As the lungs inflate, pulmonary stretch receptors activate the inspiratory center to inhibit further lung expansion. This is termed the *Hering-Breuer reflex,* and it prevents overdistention of the lungs. Impulses from the mechanical sensors are sent through the vagus nerve to the brain. Juxtacapillary (J) receptors are believed to cause the rapid respiration (tachypnea) seen in pulmonary edema. These receptors are stimulated by fluid entering the pulmonary interstitial space.

Respiratory Defense Mechanisms

Respiratory defense mechanisms are efficient in protecting the lungs from inhaled particles, microorganisms, and toxic gases. The defense mechanisms include filtration of air, the mucociliary clearance system, the cough reflex, reflex bronchoconstriction, and alveolar macrophages.

Filtration of Air. Nasal hairs filter inspired air. In addition, the abrupt changes in direction of airflow that occur as air moves through the nasopharynx and larynx increase air turbulence. This causes particles and bacteria to contact the mucosa lining these structures. Most large particles (greater than 5 μm) are less dangerous because they are removed in the nasopharynx or bronchi and do not reach the alveoli.

The velocity of airflow slows greatly after it passes the larynx, facilitating the deposition of smaller particles (1 to 5 μm). They settle out the way sand does in a river, a process termed *sedimentation.* Particles less than 1 μm in size are too small to settle in this manner and are deposited in the alveoli. An example of small particles that can build up is coal dust, which can lead to pneumoconiosis (see Chapter 28).

Mucociliary Clearance System. Below the larynx, the movement of mucus is accomplished by the mucociliary clearance system, commonly referred to as the *mucociliary escalator.* This term is used to indicate the relationship between the secretion of mucus and the ciliary activity. Mucus is continuously secreted at a rate of about 100 mL/day by goblet cells and submucosal glands. It forms a mucous blanket that contains the impacted particles and debris from distal lung areas (see Fig. 26-1). The small amount of mucus normally secreted is swallowed without being noticed. Secretory immunoglobulin A (IgA) in the mucus helps protect against bacteria and viruses.

Cilia cover the airways from the level of the trachea to the respiratory bronchioles (see Fig. 26-1). Each ciliated cell contains approximately 200 cilia, which beat rhythmically about 1000 times per minute in the large airways, moving mucus toward the mouth. The ciliary beat is slower further down the tracheobronchial tree. As a consequence, particles that penetrate more deeply into the airways are removed less rapidly. Ciliary action is impaired by dehydration; smoking; inhalation of high oxygen concentrations; infection; and ingestion of drugs such as atropine, anesthetics, alcohol, or cocaine. Patients with COPD and cystic fibrosis have repeated lower respiratory tract infections. Cilia are often destroyed during these infections, resulting in impaired secretion clearance; a chronic productive cough; and chronic colonization by bacteria, which leads to frequent respiratory tract infections.

Cough Reflex. The cough is a protective reflex action that clears the airway by a high-pressure, high-velocity flow of air. It is a backup for mucociliary clearance, especially when this clearance mechanism is overwhelmed or ineffective. Coughing is only effective in removing secretions above the subsegmental level (large or main airways). Secretions below this level must be moved upward by the mucociliary mechanism before they can be removed by coughing.

Reflex Bronchoconstriction. *Reflex bronchoconstriction* is another defense mechanism. In response to the inhalation of large amounts of irritating substances (e.g., dusts, aerosols), the bronchi constrict in an effort to prevent entry of the irritants. A person with hyperreactive airways, such as a person with asthma, may experience bronchoconstriction after inhalation of triggers such as cold air, perfume, or other strong odors.

Alveolar Macrophages. Because ciliated cells are not found below the level of the respiratory bronchioles, the primary defense mechanism at the alveolar level is alveolar macrophages. *Alveolar macrophages* rapidly phagocytize inhaled foreign particles such as bacteria. The debris is moved to the level of the bronchioles for removal by the cilia or removed from the lungs by the lymphatic system. Particles (e.g., coal dust, silica) that cannot be adequately phagocytized tend to remain in the lungs for indefinite periods and can stimulate inflammatory responses (see Chapter 28). Because alveolar macrophage activity is impaired by cigarette smoke, the smoker who is employed in an occupation with heavy dust exposure (e.g., mining, foundries) is at an especially high risk for lung disease.

GERONTOLOGIC CONSIDERATIONS

EFFECTS OF AGING ON RESPIRATORY SYSTEM

Age-related changes in the respiratory system can be divided into alterations in structure, defense mechanisms, and respiratory control (Table 26-4). Structural changes include calcification of the costal cartilages, which can interfere with chest expansion. The outward curvature of the spine is marked, especially with osteoporosis, and the lumbar curve flattens. Therefore the chest may appear barrel shaped, and the older person may need to use accessory muscles to breathe. Respiratory muscle strength progressively declines after age 50. Overall, the lungs in the older adult are harder to inflate.[5]

Many older adults lose subcutaneous fat, and bony prominences are pronounced. Within the lung, the number of functional alveoli decreases, and they become less elastic. Small airways in the lung bases close earlier in expiration. As a consequence, more inspired air is distributed to the lung apices and ventilation is less well matched to perfusion, lowering the PaO_2. Therefore older adults have less tolerance for exertion, and dyspnea can occur if their activity exceeds their normal exercise.[6]

TABLE 26-4 GERONTOLOGIC ASSESSMENT DIFFERENCES

Respiratory System

Changes	Differences in Assessment Findings
Structures	
Chest wall stiffening Costal cartilage calcification ↓ Elastic recoil ↓ Chest wall compliance ↑ Anteroposterior diameter ↓ Functioning alveoli ↓ Respiratory muscle strength	Barrel chest appearance, kyphotic posture, ↓ chest wall movement, ↓ deep breathing; mucus thickened ↓ Vital capacity, ↑ residual volume, ↑ functional residual capacity Diminished breath sounds, particularly at lung bases; ↓ PaO_2 and SaO_2, normal pH and $PaCO_2$
Defense Mechanisms	
↓ Cell-mediated immunity ↓ Specific antibodies ↓ Cilia function ↓ Cough force ↓ Alveolar macrophage function ↓ Sensation in pharynx	↓ Cough effectiveness, ↓ secretion clearance ↑ Risk of upper respiratory aspiration, infection, influenza, pneumonia Respiratory infections may be more severe and last longer
Respiratory Control	
↓ Response to hypoxemia ↓ Response to hypercapnia	Greater ↓ in PaO_2 and ↑ in $PaCO_2$ before respiratory rate changes ↓ Ability to maintain acid-base balance Significant hypoxemia or hypercapnia may develop from relatively small incidents Retained secretions, excessive sedation, or positioning that impairs chest expansion may substantially alter PaO_2 or SpO_2 values

Respiratory defense mechanisms are less effective because of a decline in both cell-mediated and humoral immunity (ability to produce antibodies). The alveolar macrophages are less effective at phagocytosis. An older patient has a less forceful cough and fewer and less functional cilia. Mucous membranes tend to be drier. Retained mucus predisposes the older adult to respiratory tract infections. Formation of secretory IgA, an important defense mechanism, is diminished. Swallowing is slower because of transit time in the pharyngeal area, and there is reduced sensation in the pharynx. If the older adult patient has a superimposed neurologic condition, aspiration is likely.

Respiratory control is altered, resulting in a more gradual response to changes in blood oxygen or carbon dioxide level. The PaO_2 drops to a lower level and the $PaCO_2$ rises to a higher level before the respiratory rate changes.

The extent of these changes in people of the same age varies greatly. The older adult who has a significant smoking history, is obese, and is diagnosed with a chronic illness is at greatest risk of adverse outcomes.

ASSESSMENT OF RESPIRATORY SYSTEM

Determining a patient's needs related to the respiratory system requires an accurate health history and a thorough physical examination. A respiratory assessment can be done as part of a comprehensive physical examination or as a focused respiratory

CASE STUDY

Patient Introduction

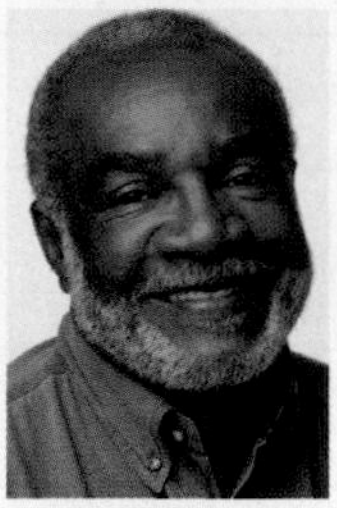

Kevin Peterson/
Photodisc/Thinkstock

F.T. is a 70-year-old African American man who comes to the emergency department complaining of increased shortness of breath. He states that he started using his albuterol inhaler every 4 hours a few days ago, but it does not seem to be helping. He has been having trouble sleeping or doing any activity because of the shortness of breath.

Critical Thinking

As you read through this assessment chapter, think about F.T. with the following questions in mind:

1. What are the possible causes of F.T.'s shortness of breath?
2. What type of assessment would be most appropriate for F.T.: comprehensive, focused, or emergency?
3. What questions would you ask?
4. What should be included in the physical assessment? What would you be looking for?
5. What diagnostic studies might you expect to be ordered?

evolve Answers available at *http://evolve.elsevier.com/Lewis/medsurg.*

examination. Use judgment in determining whether all or part of the history and physical examination will be completed based on the patient's problems and degree of respiratory distress. If respiratory distress is severe, only obtain pertinent information and defer a thorough assessment until the patient's condition stabilizes.

Subjective Data

Important Health Information

Past Health History. It is important to determine the frequency of upper respiratory problems (e.g., colds, sore throats, sinus problems, allergies) and whether seasonal changes have an effect on these problems. Question the patient with allergies about possible precipitating factors or triggers such as medications, pollen, smoke, mold, or pet exposure. Document characteristics and severity of the allergic reaction such as runny nose, wheezing, scratchy throat, or chest tightness. Inquire about a past history of lower respiratory problems, such as asthma, COPD, pneumonia, and tuberculosis (TB). Also determine the frequency of asthma exacerbations and triggers, if known. Because respiratory symptoms are often manifestations of problems that involve other body systems, it is important to ask about a history of additional health problems. For example, the patient with cardiac dysfunction may experience dyspnea (shortness of breath) as a consequence of heart failure. The patient with human immunodeficiency virus (HIV) infection may experience frequent respiratory tract infections because immune function is compromised.

Medications. Take a thorough medication history, including both prescription and over-the-counter medications. Ask about the reason for taking the medication, its name, the dose and frequency, length of time taken, its effect, and any side effects. Assess for overuse of short-term bronchodilators as a key indicator of symptom control, since this information will help guide management. Inquire about the use of an angiotensin-converting enzyme (ACE) inhibitor, since cough is a relatively common side effect of this class of drugs. Encourage the patient to bring her or his medication bottles to each visit with a health care provider.

If the patient is using oxygen to ease a breathing problem, document the fraction of inspired oxygen concentration (FIO_2), liter flow, method of administration, number of hours used per day, and effectiveness of the therapy. Assess safety practices, including the patient's mechanical and cognitive ability related to using oxygen.

Surgery or Other Treatments. Determine if the patient has been hospitalized for a respiratory problem. Note the dates, therapy (including surgery), and current status of the problem. Determine if the patient has ever been intubated because of a respiratory problem. Ask about the use and the response to respiratory treatments such as a nebulizer, humidifier, airway clearance modalities (see Chapter 29), high-frequency chest wall oscillation, postural drainage, and percussion.

Functional Health Patterns. Health history questions to ask a patient with a respiratory problem are presented in Table 26-5.

Health Perception–Health Management Pattern. Ask the patient if there has been a perceived change in health status within the last several days, months, or years. In COPD, lung function declines slowly over many years. The patient may not notice this decline because activity is altered to accommodate reduced exercise tolerance. If an upper respiratory tract infection is superimposed on a chronic problem, dyspnea and decreased exercise tolerance may occur very quickly. In asthma, symptoms may occur or worsen during exercise, if animals are present, or following a change in temperature.

Explore and document common signs of respiratory problems (e.g., cough, dyspnea). Also describe the course of the patient's illness, including when it began, the type of symptoms, and factors that alleviate or aggravate these symptoms. Because of the chronic nature of respiratory problems, the patient may relate a change in symptoms rather than the onset of new symptoms when describing the present illness. Carefully document any changes because they often suggest the cause of illness. For example, increased shortness of breath or increased purulence of sputum may suggest an acute exacerbation of COPD.

If a cough is present, evaluate its quality. For example, a loose-sounding cough indicates secretions; a dry, hacking cough indicates airway irritation or obstruction; a harsh, barky cough suggests upper airway obstruction from inhibited vocal cord movement related to subglottic edema. Assess whether the cough is strong enough to clear secretions, and note whether it is productive or nonproductive of secretions. Determine if a cough is acute or chronic (longer than 3 weeks in duration) or if it first began with an upper respiratory tract infection. The pattern and etiology of the cough are determined by asking questions such as the following: What has been the pattern of coughing? Has it been regular or paroxysmal (i.e., sudden, periodic onset), or related to a time of day, the weather, certain activities, talking, or deep breaths? Any change over time? Do you clear your throat a lot? What have you tried to alleviate the coughing? Did you try any prescription or over-the-counter drugs?

If the patient has a productive cough, evaluate the following characteristics of sputum: amount, color, consistency, and odor. Quantify the amount of sputum in teaspoons, tablespoons, or cups per day. Note any recent increases or decreases in the amount. The normal color is clear or slightly whitish. If a patient is a cigarette smoker, the sputum is usually clear to gray with occasional specks of brown. The patient with COPD may exhibit clear, whitish, or slightly yellow sputum, especially in the morning on rising. If the patient reports any change from base-

TABLE 26-5 HEALTH HISTORY

Respiratory System

Health Perception–Health Management
- Describe your daily activities. Have breathing problems changed activities that you could perform in the past several days?* Months?* Years?* Are your breathing problems better, worse, or about the same compared with 6 months ago?
- How do your breathing problems affect your self-care abilities?
- Have you ever smoked? Do you smoke now? If yes, how many cigarettes each day and for how long? Are you interested in stopping smoking? Are there aids we can tell you about that would assist your quitting? Would you be willing to come back for a visit so we can explore your quitting? If you stopped smoking, did you do so because of your health?* How did you stop?
- Have you ever smoked street drugs?*
- Have you had a Pneumovax vaccination? When was your last flu shot?
- What equipment helps you manage your respiratory problems? How often do you use it? Does it help? Cause problems?

Nutritional-Metabolic
- Have you recently lost weight because of difficulty eating secondary to a respiratory problem? How much? Voluntarily?
- Do any particular foods affect your sputum production or breathing?*

Elimination
- Does your respiratory problem make it difficult for you to get to the toilet?*
- Are you inactive because of dyspnea to the point that it causes constipation?*

Activity-Exercise
- Are you ever short of breath during exercise?* At rest?*
- Do you get too short of breath to do the things you want to do?*
- Is your home one story? Two stories? How many steps from the street to your door?
- Can you walk up a flight of steps without stopping?
- Are you able to maintain your typical activity pattern? If not, explain.
- What do you do when you get short of breath?

Sleep-Rest
- Do breathing problems cause you to awaken during the night?*
- Can you lie flat at night? If not, how many pillows do you use?
- Do you need to sleep upright in a chair?*
- Are you or your sleep partner aware of any snoring?
- Do you awaken in the morning feeling rested?
- Do you have a morning headache?*
- Do you fall asleep easily during the day?*

Cognitive-Perceptual
- Do you have any pain associated with breathing?* On a scale from 0 to 10, with 10 being the worst pain you can imagine, where would you rate your pain? Does it hurt more on inspiration?*
- Do you ever feel restless, irritable, or confused without a reason?*
- Do you have difficulty remembering things?*

Self-Perception–Self-Concept
- Describe how your respiratory problems have changed your life.
- If you use oxygen, do you ever go out without bringing it with you? When and why?

Role-Relationship
- Has your respiratory problem caused any difficulties in your work, family, or social relationships?*

Sexuality-Reproductive
- Has your respiratory problem caused a change in your sexual activity?*
- Do you want to discuss ways to decrease dyspnea during sexual activity?

Coping–Stress Tolerance
- How often do you leave your home?
- Would you want to join a support group? Pulmonary rehabilitation program?
- Does stress have an effect on your breathing?*
- What effect does your respiratory problem have on your emotions?

Value-Belief
- What do you believe causes your respiratory problems?
- Do you think the things you have been told to do for your respiratory problems really help? If not, why?

*If yes, describe.

line color, suspect pulmonary complications. Note any changes in consistency of sputum to thick, thin, or frothy and pink tinged. These changes may indicate dehydration, postnasal drip or sinus drainage, or possible pulmonary edema. Normally sputum should be odorless. A foul odor or exceptionally bad breath or taste in the mouth suggests an infectious process. Ask the patient if the sputum was produced along with a change in position (e.g., increased with lying down) or activity.

When assessing mucus, determine if the patient has a history of coughing up blood *(hemoptysis)*. Hemoptysis can range from a slight streaking of blood in the mucus to massive coughing up of blood, in which the patient loses 100 to 600 mL of blood in a 24-hour period. This situation is a medical emergency.

Frequently the patient cannot differentiate between hemoptysis and *hematemesis* (vomiting blood). Carefully question and then test the mucus for an acidic pH (which is present with hematemesis), since this will help differentiate the two. Hemoptysis can be found with a variety of conditions such as pneumonia, TB, lung cancer, and severe bronchiectasis.

Assess for a history of wheezing. *Wheezes* are musical sounds that can be audible. Wheezing indicates some degree of airway obstruction, such as asthma, foreign body aspiration, and emphysema. Assess for any history of family exposure to *Mycobacterium tuberculosis.*

GENETIC RISK ALERT
- Respiratory problems that have a strong genetic link include cystic fibrosis, COPD resulting from α_1-antitrypsin deficiency, and asthma.
- If people have a family history of these respiratory problems, they have a much greater risk of developing them.
- Although cigarette smoking is a major risk factor for COPD, only a minority of cigarette smokers develop symptomatic disease. The risk for COPD related to cigarette smoking is genetically related.
- Determine if there is a family history of any of these respiratory problems that may have genetic or familial tendencies.

Smoking is the most important risk factor for COPD and lung cancer. Discuss current and past smoking habits. Quantify smoking habits in *pack-years.* This is done by multiplying the number of packs smoked per day by the number of years smoked. For example, a person who smoked 1 pack per day for

15 years has a 15 pack-year history. In addition to asking about cigarette use, find out about the use of any tobacco products, including cigars, pipes, chewing tobacco, and smokeless tobacco products. Also find out about exposure to secondhand smoke. Determine if the patient has tried to quit using tobacco products, including using prescription, over-the-counter, and herbal remedies.

Assess if the patient received immunization for influenza (flu) and pneumococcal pneumonia (Pneumovax). Influenza vaccine should be administered yearly in the fall. Pneumovax is administered any time during the year. (The recommendations for use of Pneumovax are presented in Table 28-5.)

Ask where the patient has lived and traveled. Risk factors for TB include prior residence in Asia, Africa, the former Soviet Republic, Latin America, or any third-world country. Other TB risk factors include exposure to people with high rates of TB transmission such as the homeless, injection drug users, and people with HIV infection. Risk factors for fungal infections of the lung include living or traveling in the Southwest (coccidioidomycosis) and the Mississippi River Valley (histoplasmosis).

Ask the patient about the use of equipment to manage respiratory symptoms (e.g., home O_2 therapy equipment, inhalers, devices for sleep apnea). Question the patient about the type of equipment used, cleaning of the device, frequency of use, its effect, and any side effects. Have patients demonstrate the use of their inhalers. Many patients do not know how to use these devices correctly (see Chapter 29).

Nutritional-Metabolic Pattern. Weight loss is a symptom of many respiratory diseases. Determine if weight loss was intentional and, if not, if food intake is altered by anorexia (from medications), fatigue (from hypoxemia, increased work of breathing), or feeling full quickly (from lung hyperinflation). Anorexia, weight loss, and chronic malnutrition are common in patients with COPD, lung cancer, TB, and chronic severe infection (bronchiectasis). Also note fluid intake. Dehydration can cause mucus to thicken and obstruct the airway.

Excessive weight interferes with normal ventilation and may cause sleep apnea (see Chapter 8). Morbidly obese individuals may hypoventilate while awake or asleep, and weight loss can improve ABGs. Rapid weight gain from fluid retention may decrease pulmonary gas exchange.

Elimination Pattern. Healthy elimination habits depend on the ability to reach a toilet when necessary. Activity intolerance secondary to dyspnea could result in incontinence. Dyspnea can also be the cause of limited mobility, which can cause constipation. Question the patient with dyspnea about incontinence and constipation. People with a chronic cough, especially women, may be troubled with urinary incontinence during paroxysms of coughing.

Activity-Exercise Pattern. Determine if the patient's activity is limited by dyspnea at rest or during exercise. Also note whether the patient's residence (e.g., number of steps, levels) poses a problem that increases social isolation. Record and objectively measure the degree of the patient's dyspnea. For example, can the patient walk up one flight of stairs without stopping because of dyspnea? Is dyspnea that is associated with an activity better, worse, or about the same in the last few months? Determine if the patient has difficulty breathing in a certain position, or if relief of dyspnea can be obtained by assuming a different position (e.g., tripod position in COPD).

Discuss whether the patient is able to carry out activities of daily living without dyspnea or other respiratory symptoms. If unable, document the amount and type of care needed. Immobility and sedentary habits can be risk factors for hypoventilation leading to atelectasis or pneumonia.

Sleep-Rest Pattern. Determine if the patient wakes up because of pulmonary problems. The patient with asthma or COPD may awaken at night with chest tightness, wheezing, or coughing. This suggests a need for adjunct therapy or other medication changes. The patient with cardiovascular disease (e.g., heart failure) may sleep with the head elevated on several pillows to avoid respiratory problems brought on by lying flat *(orthopnea)*. Signs of sleep apnea include snoring, insomnia, abrupt awakenings, daytime drowsiness, and early morning headaches. Night sweats may be a manifestation of TB.

Cognitive-Perceptual Pattern. Because hypoxia can cause neurologic symptoms, ask the patient about apprehension, restlessness, irritability, and memory changes, which can indicate inadequate cerebral oxygenation (see Table 26-2). Hypoxemia interferes with the ability to learn and retain information. For this reason, teaching may be more effective if the caregiver is present during teaching sessions to provide reinforcement at a later date.

Assess the patient's cognitive ability to cooperate with treatment. Failure or inability to participate in needed therapy can result in exacerbation of respiratory problems.

Inquire about any discomfort or pain with breathing. Explore a complaint of chest pain carefully to rule out cardiac involvement. Problems such as pleurisy, fractured ribs, and costochondritis cause chest pain. Pleuritic pain is described as a sharp, localized, stabbing pain associated with movement or deep breathing. Fractured ribs cause localized sharp pain associated with breathing.

Self-Perception–Self-Concept Pattern. Dyspnea limits activity, impairs ability to fulfill normal roles, and often alters self-esteem. A patient may be reluctant to appear in public with a highly visible nasal cannula and O_2 equipment. Discuss with the patient his or her personal body image. A barrel chest, clubbed fingers, pursed-lip breathing, and frequent expectoration of sputum or throat clearing can be embarrassing and can lead to social isolation. Referral to a support group or pulmonary rehabilitation program may be beneficial in developing a support system and coping strategies.

Role-Relationship Pattern. Acute or chronic respiratory problems can seriously affect performance in work or other activities. Discuss the impact of medications, O_2 therapy, and special routines (e.g., pulmonary hygiene for cystic fibrosis) on the patient's family, job, and social life.

Document the nature of the patient's work and the frequency and intensity of exposure to fumes, toxins, asbestos, coal, fibers, or silica. Inquire whether symptoms are worse in specific situations (e.g., home versus work environments). Investigate any patient-specific allergens, such as dust or fumes, that could be present in the work environment. Hobbies such as woodworking (sawdust) or pottery (silica) and exposure to animals (allergies) may also cause respiratory problems. Because of hyperreactive airways, exposure to fumes, smoke, and other chemicals may trigger an attack in the patient with asthma.

Sexuality-Reproductive Pattern. Most patients can continue to have satisfactory sexual relationships despite marked physical limitations. In a tactful manner, determine whether breathing difficulties have caused alterations in sexual activity. If so, provide teaching about positions that decrease dyspnea during sexual activity and alternative strategies for sexual fulfillment.

CASE STUDY—cont'd

Subjective Data

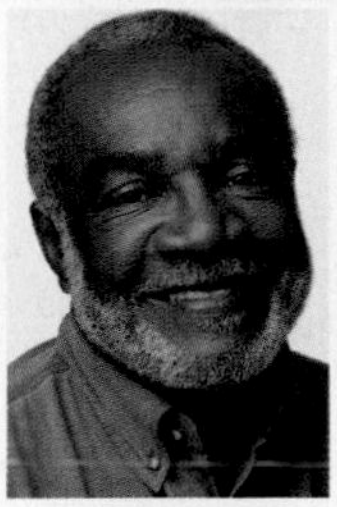

Kevin Peterson/ Photodisc/Thinkstock

A focused subjective assessment of F.T. revealed the following information:

PMH: COPD, hypertension, and benign prostatic hyperplasia. No history of environmental allergies. Denies history of coronary artery disease or heart failure.

Medications: Metoprolol (Lopressor) 50 mg/day PO, finasteride (Proscar) 5 mg/day PO, Advair inhaler (fluticasone and salmeterol) 2 puffs bid, and albuterol inhaler 2 puffs q4hr PRN. Does not use O_2 at home.

Health Perception–Health Management: F.T. states that he usually manages his COPD well with just the Advair inhaler and occasional use of the albuterol inhaler as needed. However, he caught a cold from his granddaughter last week and has had increasing difficulty breathing, even with the use of albuterol.

Has a history of 30 pack-years of smoking, quitting 5 years ago. Had a Pneumovax vaccination 5 years ago and receives the flu vaccine on an annual basis.

Activity-Exercise: States that he can typically walk at least 2 blocks and up and down stairs without getting short of breath. However, at this point, he can't walk 100 feet without feeling short of breath, nor can he walk up one flight of stairs without stopping to catch his breath.

Sleep-Rest: Has been having difficulty sleeping with this most recent episode of shortness of breath. Typically uses just one pillow to sleep with but needed three pillows this week, and last night he slept upright in his recliner.

Cognitive-Perceptual: Denies any pain or confusion associated with shortness of breath. Feels slightly irritable because of lack of sleep.

Coping–Stress Tolerance: Denies any stress or emotional disturbance that could be having an impact on his breathing.

Many patients need to perform good pulmonary hygiene (bronchodilators, coughing and deep breathing) before intimacy. This is similar to what they would do before strenuous physical activity. They may need to use O_2 therapy equipment during intercourse.

Coping–Stress Tolerance Pattern. Dyspnea causes anxiety, and anxiety exacerbates dyspnea. The result is a vicious cycle—the patient avoids activities that cause dyspnea, becoming more deconditioned and more dyspneic. The outcome is often physical and social isolation. Assess how often the patient leaves home and interacts with others. Referral to a support group or pulmonary rehabilitation program may be beneficial.

The chronic nature of many respiratory problems such as COPD and asthma can cause prolonged stress. Inquire about the patient's coping strategies to manage this stress.

Value-Belief Pattern. Determine the patient's adherence to the management regimen. Explore reasons for lack of adherence, including conflict with cultural beliefs, financial constraints (e.g., costs of prescriptions), or failure to understand benefit. Including the patient and the caregiver in the planning of care can improve adherence.

Objective Data

Physical Examination. Vital signs, including temperature, pulse, respirations, blood pressure, and SpO_2 (oxygen saturation obtained by pulse oximetry), are important data to collect before examination of the respiratory system.

Nose. Inspect the nose for patency, inflammation, deformities, symmetry, and discharge. Check each naris for air patency with respiration while the other naris is briefly occluded. Tilt the patient's head backward and push the tip of the nose upward gently. With a nasal speculum and a good light, inspect the interior of the nose. The mucous membrane should be pink and moist, with no evidence of edema (bogginess), exudate, or bleeding.[7] Inspect the nasal septum for deviation, perforations, and bleeding. Some nasal deviation is normal in an adult. Inspect the turbinates for polyps, which are abnormal, fingerlike projections of swollen nasal mucosa. Polyps may result from long-term irritation of the mucosa (e.g., from allergies). Assess any discharge for color and consistency. Purulent and malodorous discharge could indicate the presence of a foreign body. Watery discharge could be secondary to allergies or from cerebrospinal fluid. Bloody discharge could be from trauma or dryness. Thick mucosal discharge could indicate infection.

Mouth and Pharynx. Using a good light source, inspect the interior of the mouth for color, lesions, masses, gum retraction, bleeding, and poor dentition. Inspect the tongue for symmetry and lesions. Observe the pharynx by pressing a tongue blade against the middle of the back of the tongue. If the oropharynx is tight, have the patient yawn, since this usually allows more structures to be visible. The pharynx should be smooth and moist, with no evidence of exudate, ulcerations, swelling, or postnasal drip. Note the color, symmetry, and any enlargement of the tonsils. Stimulate the gag reflex by placing a tongue blade along the side of the pharynx behind the tonsil. A normal response (gagging) indicates that cranial nerves IX (glossopharyngeal) and X (vagus) are intact and that the airway is protected.

Neck. Inspect the neck for symmetry and tender or swollen areas. Palpate the lymph nodes while the patient is sitting erect with the neck slightly flexed. Progression of palpation is from the nodes around the ears, to the nodes at the base of the skull, and then to those located under the angles of the mandible to the midline. The patient may have small, mobile, nontender nodes *(shotty nodes),* which are not a sign of a pathologic condition. Tender, hard, or fixed nodes indicate disease. Describe the location and characteristics of any palpable nodes.

Thorax and Lungs. Picture imaginary lines on the chest to help identify abnormalities (see Fig. 26-2). Describe abnormalities in terms of their location relative to these lines (e.g., 2 cm from the right midclavicular line).[8]

Chest examination is best performed in a well-lighted, warm room with measures taken to ensure the patient's privacy. Perform all physical assessment maneuvers (inspection, palpation, percussion, auscultation) on either the anterior or the posterior chest rather than moving from anterior to posterior or vice versa with each maneuver. It is best to begin on the posterior chest, particularly with female patients, since more information can be obtained without interference from the breast tissue. In addition, if the patient tires or you are interrupted, baseline data with the most information will have been obtained from examining the posterior of the chest.

Inspection. When inspecting the *anterior chest,* have the patient sit upright or with the head of the bed upright. The patient may need to lean forward for support on the bedside table to facilitate breathing. First, observe the patient's appearance and note any evidence of respiratory distress, such as tachypnea or use of accessory muscles. Next, determine the shape and symmetry of the chest. Chest movement should be equal on both sides, and the AP diameter should be less than the side-to-side or transverse diameter by a ratio of 1:2. An increase in AP diameter (e.g., barrel chest) may be a normal aging change or result from lung hyperinflation. Observe for abnormalities in the sternum (e.g., *pectus carinatum* [a prominent protrusion of the sternum] and *pectus excavatum* [an indentation of the lower sternum above the xiphoid process]).

Next observe the respiratory rate, depth, and rhythm. The normal rate is 12 to 20 breaths/minute; in the older adult, it is 16 to 25 breaths/minute. Inspiration (I) should take half as long as expiration (E) (I:E ratio = 1:2). Observe for abnormal breathing patterns, such as Kussmaul (rapid, deep breathing), Cheyne-Stokes (abnormal respirations characterized by alternating periods of apnea and deep, rapid breathing), or Biot's (irregular breathing with apnea every four to five cycles) respirations.

Skin color provides clues to respiratory status. Cyanosis, a late sign of hypoxemia, is best observed in a dark-skinned patient in the conjunctivae, lips, and palms and under the tongue. Causes of cyanosis include hypoxemia or decreased cardiac output. Inspect the fingers for evidence of long-standing hypoxemia known as *clubbing* (an increase in the angle between the base of the nail and the fingernail to 180 degrees or more, usually accompanied by an increase in the depth, bulk, and sponginess of the end of the finger) (see eFig. 26-3 available on the website for this chapter).

When inspecting the *posterior chest,* ask the patient to lean forward with arms folded. This position moves the scapulae away from the spine, exposing more of the area to be examined. The same sequence of observations that was done on the anterior part of the chest is performed on the posterior part. In addition, any spinal curvature is noted. Spinal curvatures that affect breathing include kyphosis, scoliosis, and kyphoscoliosis.

Palpation. Determine tracheal position by gently placing the index fingers on either side of the trachea just above the suprasternal notch and gently pressing backward. Normal tracheal position is midline; deviation to the left or right is abnormal. Tracheal deviation occurs away from the side of a tension pneumothorax or a neck mass, but toward the side of a pneumonectomy or lobar atelectasis.

Symmetry of chest expansion and extent of movement are determined at the level of the diaphragm. Place your hands over the lower anterior chest wall along the costal margin and move them inward until the thumbs meet at midline. Ask the patient to breathe deeply. Observe the movement of the thumbs away from each other. Normal expansion is 1 in (2.5 cm). Hand placement on the posterior side of the chest is at the level of the tenth rib. Move the thumbs until they meet over the spine (Fig. 26-6). Check expansion anteriorly or posteriorly, but it is not necessary to check both.

Normal chest movement is equal. Unequal expansion occurs when air entry is limited by conditions involving the lung (e.g., atelectasis, pneumothorax) or the chest wall (e.g., incisional pain). Equal but diminished expansion occurs in conditions that produce a hyperinflated or barrel chest or in neuromuscular diseases (e.g., amyotrophic lateral sclerosis, spinal cord lesions). Movement may be absent or unequal over a pleural effusion, an atelectasis, or a pneumothorax.

Fremitus is the vibration of the chest wall produced by vocalization. Tactile fremitus can be felt by placing the palmar surface of the hands with hyperextended fingers against the patient's chest. Ask the patient to repeat a phrase such as "ninety-nine" in a deeper, louder than normal voice. Move your hands from side to side at the same time from top to bottom on the patient's chest (Fig. 26-7). When performing percussion, palpate all areas of the chest and compare vibrations from similar areas. Tactile fremitus is most intense adjacent to the sternum and between the scapulae because these areas are closest to the major bronchi. Fremitus is less intense farther away from these areas.

Note an increase, decrease, or absence of fremitus. Increased fremitus occurs when the lung becomes filled with fluid or is denser. As the patient's voice moves through a dense tissue or fluid, you can feel that the vibration is increased. This is found in pneumonia, in lung tumors, with thick bronchial secretions, and above a pleural effusion (the lung is compressed upward). Fremitus is decreased if the hand is farther from the lung (e.g., pleural effusion) or the lung is hyperinflated (e.g., barrel chest). Absent fremitus may be noted with pneumothorax or atelectasis. The anterior of the chest is more difficult to palpate for fremitus because of the large muscles and breast tissue.

Percussion. Percussion is performed to assess the density or aeration of the lungs. Percussion sounds are described in Table 26-6. (The technique for percussion is described in Chapter 3.)

The anterior chest is usually percussed with the patient in a semi-sitting or supine position. Starting above the clavicles, percuss downward, interspace by interspace (see Fig. 26-7). The area over lung tissue should be resonant, with the exception of the area of cardiac dullness (Fig. 26-8). For percussion of the posterior chest, have the patient sit leaning forward with arms

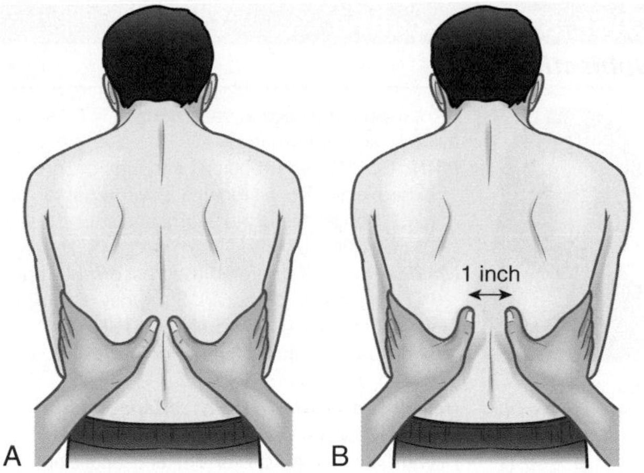

FIG. 26-6 Estimation of thoracic expansion. **A,** Exhalation. **B,** Maximal inhalation.

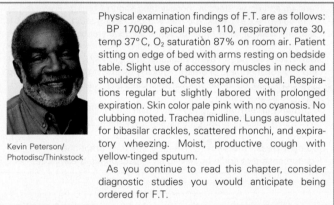

CASE STUDY—cont'd

Objective Data: Physical Examination

Kevin Peterson/
Photodisc/Thinkstock

Physical examination findings of F.T. are as follows:

BP 170/90, apical pulse 110, respiratory rate 30, temp 37° C, O_2 saturation 87% on room air. Patient sitting on edge of bed with arms resting on bedside table. Slight use of accessory muscles in neck and shoulders noted. Chest expansion equal. Respirations regular but slightly labored with prolonged expiration. Skin color pale pink with no cyanosis. No clubbing noted. Trachea midline. Lungs auscultated for bibasilar crackles, scattered rhonchi, and expiratory wheezing. Moist, productive cough with yellow-tinged sputum.

As you continue to read this chapter, consider diagnostic studies you would anticipate being ordered for F.T.

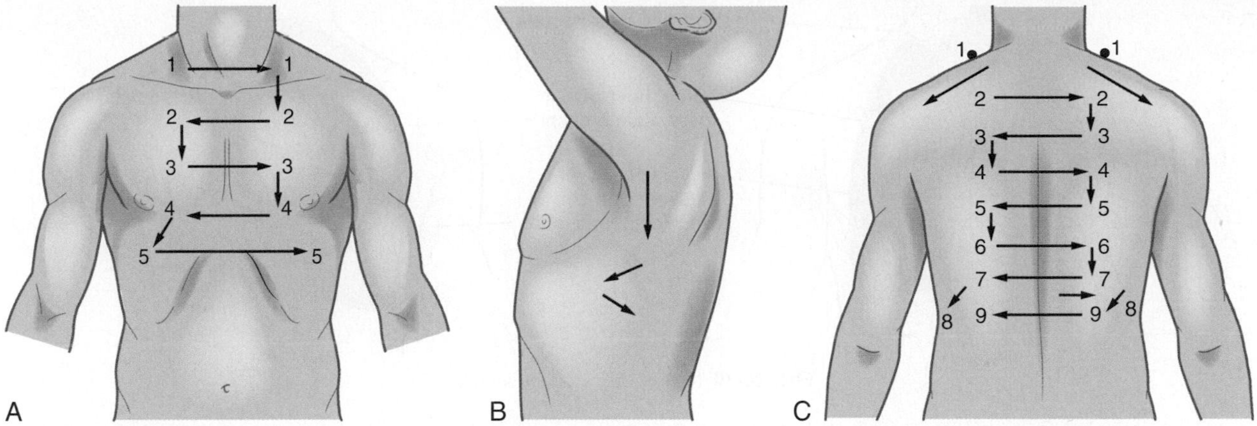

FIG. 26-7 Sequence for examination of the chest. **A,** Anterior sequence. **B,** Lateral sequence. **C,** Posterior sequence. For palpation, place the palms of the hands in the position designated as *"1"* on the right and left sides of the chest. Compare the intensity of vibrations. Continue for all positions in each sequence. For percussion, tap the chest at each designated position, moving downward from side to side. Compare percussion sounds at all positions. For auscultation, place the stethoscope at each position and listen to at least one complete inspiratory and expiratory cycle. Keep in mind that, with a female patient, the breast tissue will modify the completeness of the anterior examination.

TABLE 26-6 **PERCUSSION SOUNDS**

Sound	Description
Resonance	Low-pitched sound heard over normal lungs
Hyperresonance	Loud, lower-pitched sound than normal resonance heard over hyperinflated lungs, such as in chronic obstructive pulmonary disease and acute asthma
Tympany	Sound with drumlike, loud, empty quality heard over gas-filled stomach or intestine, or pneumothorax
Dull	Sound with medium-intensity pitch and duration heard over areas of "mixed" solid and lung tissue, such as over top area of liver, partially consolidated lung tissue (pneumonia), or fluid-filled pleural space
Flat	Soft, high-pitched sound of short duration heard over very dense tissue where air is not present, such as posterior chest below level of diaphragm

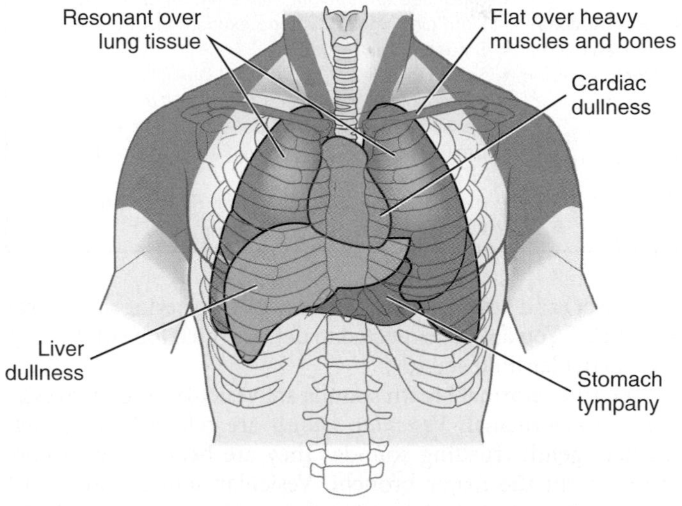

FIG. 26-8 Diagram of percussion areas and sounds in the anterior side of the chest.

folded. The posterior chest should be resonant over lung tissue to the level of the diaphragm (Fig. 26-9).

Auscultation. During chest auscultation, instruct the patient to breathe slowly and a little more deeply than normal through the mouth. Auscultation should proceed from the lung apices to the bases, comparing opposite areas of the chest, unless the patient is in respiratory distress or will tire easily; if so, start at the bases (see Fig. 26-7). Place the stethoscope over lung tissue, not over bony prominences. At each placement of the stethoscope, listen to at least one cycle of inspiration and expiration. Note the pitch (e.g., high, low), duration of sound, and presence of adventitious or abnormal sounds.[9] The location of normal auscultatory sounds is more easily understood by visualization of a lung model (Fig. 26-10).

The lung sounds are heard anteriorly from a line drawn perpendicular to the xiphoid process lateral to the midclavicular line. Palpate inferiorly (down) two ribs in the midaxillary line and around to the posterior chest. This gives you a fairly accurate and easy way to determine the lung fields to be auscultated. When documenting the location of the lung sounds, divide the anterior and posterior lung into thirds (upper, middle,

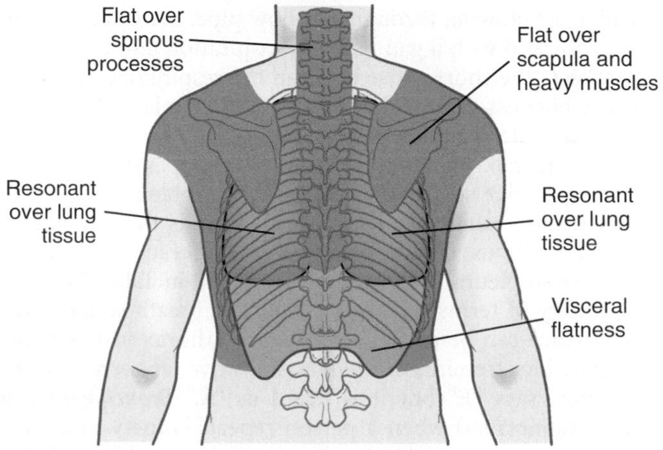

FIG. 26-9 Diagram of percussion areas and sounds in the posterior side of the chest. Percussion proceeds from the lung apices to the lung bases while comparing sounds in opposite areas of the chest.

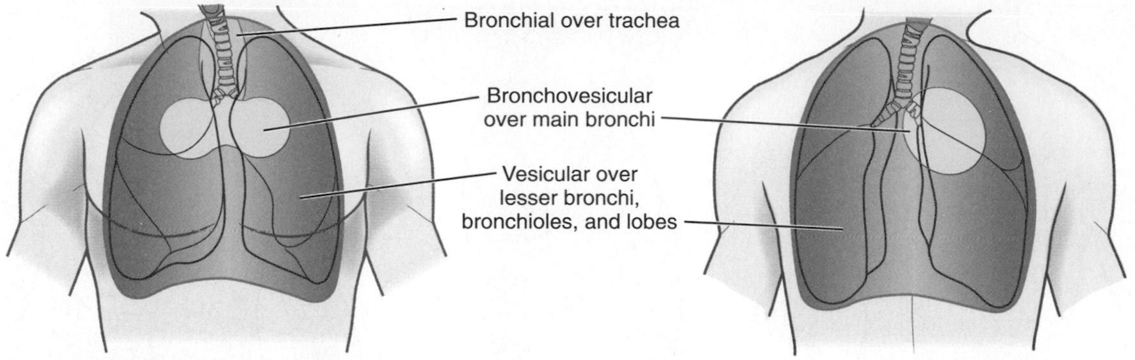

FIG. 26-10 Normal auscultatory sounds.

TABLE 26-7 NORMAL PHYSICAL ASSESSMENT OF THE RESPIRATORY SYSTEM

Nose	• Symmetric with no deformities • Nasal mucosa pink, moist with no edema, exudate, blood, or polyps • Nasal septum straight; nares patent bilaterally
Oral mucosa	• Light pink, moist, with no exudate or ulcerations
Pharynx	• Smooth, moist, and pink
Neck	• Trachea midline
Chest	• Anteroposterior to lateral diameter 1:2 • Respirations nonlabored at 14 breaths/min • Breath sounds vesicular without crackles, rhonchi, or wheezes • Excursion equal bilaterally with no increase in tactile fremitus

and lower) and note, for example, "crackles posterior right lower lung field." You are not expected to define which lobe of the lung has particular lung sounds.

The three normal breath sounds are vesicular, bronchovesicular, and bronchial. *Vesicular sounds* are relatively soft, low-pitched, gentle, rustling sounds. They are heard over all lung areas except the major bronchi. Vesicular sounds have a 3:1 ratio, with inspiration three times longer than expiration. *Bronchovesicular sounds* have a medium pitch and intensity and are heard anteriorly over the mainstem bronchi on either side of the sternum and posteriorly between the scapulae. Bronchovesicular sounds have a 1:1 ratio, with inspiration equal to expiration. *Bronchial sounds* are louder and higher pitched and resemble air blowing through a hollow pipe. Bronchial sounds have a 2:3 ratio with a gap between inspiration and expiration. This reflects the short pause between the respiratory cycles. To hear the likeness of bronchial breath sounds, place the stethoscope alongside the trachea in the neck.

The term *abnormal breath sounds* describes bronchial or bronchovesicular sounds heard in the peripheral lung fields. **Adventitious sounds** are extra breath sounds that are abnormal. Adventitious breath sounds include crackles, rhonchi, wheezes, and pleural friction rub (described in Table 26-7).

A variety of terms are used to describe breath sounds. The spoken voice can be auscultated over the thorax just as it can be palpated for fremitus. *Egophony* is positive (abnormal) when the person says "E" but it is heard as "A." *Bronchophony* is positive (abnormal) when a person repeats "ninety-nine" and the words are easily understood and are clear and loud. *Whispered pectoriloquy* is positive (abnormal) when the patient whispers "one-two-three" and the almost inaudible voice is transmitted clearly and distinctly. Conditions that increase lung density or a consolidated lung (e.g., pneumonia) have positive (abnormal) voice sounds.

A record of the normal physical assessment of the respiratory system is shown in Table 26-7. Assessment abnormalities of the thorax and lungs are presented in Table 26-8. Chest examination findings in common pulmonary problems are presented in Table 26-9. Age-related changes in the respiratory system and assessment findings are presented in Table 26-4.

A *focused assessment* is used to evaluate the status of previously identified respiratory problems and to monitor for signs of new problems (see Chapter 3, Table 3-6). A focused assessment of the respiratory system is presented in the box above.

FOCUSED ASSESSMENT

Respiratory System

Use this checklist to make sure the key assessment steps have been done.

Subjective

Ask the patient about any of the following and note responses.

Shortness of breath	Y	N
Wheezing	Y	N
Sputum production (color, quantity)	Y	N
Pain with breathing	Y	N
Cough	Y	N

Objective: Diagnostic

Check the following laboratory tests for critical values.

Arterial blood gases	✓
Chest x-ray	✓
Hct, Hgb	✓

Objective: Physical Examination

Observe

Respirations for rate, quality, and pattern	✓

Inspect

Skin and nails for integrity and color	✓
Neck for position of trachea	✓
Shape, symmetry, and movement of chest wall	✓

Palpate

Chest and back for masses	✓

Auscultate

Lung (breath) sounds	✓

Hct, Hematocrit; *Hgb,* hemoglobin.

TABLE 26-8 ASSESSMENT ABNORMALITIES

Respiratory System

Finding	Description	Possible Etiology and Significance*
Inspection		
Pursed-lip breathing	Exhalation through mouth with lips pursed together to slow exhalation.	COPD, asthma. Suggests ↑ breathlessness. Strategy taught to slow expiration, ↓ dyspnea.
Tripod position; inability to lie flat	Learning forward with arms and elbows supported on overbed table.	COPD, asthma in exacerbation, pulmonary edema. Indicates moderate to severe respiratory distress.
Accessory muscle use; intercostal retractions	Neck and shoulder muscles used to assist breathing; muscles between ribs pull in during inspiration.	COPD, asthma in exacerbation, secretion retention. Indicates severe respiratory distress, hypoxemia.
Splinting	Voluntary ↓ in tidal volume to ↓ pain on chest expansion.	Thoracic or abdominal incision, chest trauma, pleurisy.
↑ AP diameter	AP chest diameter equal to lateral; slope of ribs more horizontal (90 degrees) to spine.	COPD, asthma, cystic fibrosis, lung hyperinflation, advanced age.
Tachypnea	Rate >20 breaths/min; >25 breaths/min in older adults.	Fever, anxiety, hypoxemia, restrictive lung disease. Magnitude of ↑ above normal rate reflects increased work of breathing.
Kussmaul respirations	Regular, rapid, and deep respirations.	Metabolic acidosis. Increases CO_2 excretion.
Cyanosis	Bluish color of skin best seen in lips and on the palpebral conjunctiva (inside the lower eyelid).	Reflects 5-6 g of hemoglobin not bound with O_2. ↓ O_2 transfer in lungs, ↓ cardiac output. Nonspecific, unreliable indicator.
Finger clubbing	↑ Depth, bulk, sponginess of distal portion of finger (see eFig. 26-3 on the website for this chapter).	Chronic hypoxemia, cystic fibrosis, lung cancer, bronchiectasis.
Abdominal paradox	Inward (rather than normal outward) movement of abdomen during inspiration.	Inefficient and ineffective breathing pattern. Nonspecific indicator of severe respiratory distress.
Palpation		
Tracheal deviation	Leftward or rightward movement of trachea from normal midline position.	Nonspecific indicator of change in position of mediastinal structures. Medical emergency if caused by tension pneumothorax. Trachea deviates to the side opposite the collapsed lung.
Altered tactile fremitus	Increase or decrease in vibrations.	↑ In pneumonia, pulmonary edema. ↓ In pleural effusion, lung hyperinflation. Absent in pneumothorax, atelectasis.
Altered chest movement	Unequal or equal but diminished movement of two sides of chest with inspiration.	Unequal movement caused by atelectasis, pneumothorax, pleural effusion, splinting. Equal but diminished movement caused by barrel chest, restrictive disease, neuromuscular disease.
Percussion		
Hyperresonance	Loud, lower-pitched sound over areas that normally produce a resonant sound.	Lung hyperinflation (COPD), lung collapse (pneumothorax), air trapping (asthma).
Dullness	Medium-pitched sound over areas that normally produce a resonant sound.	↑ Density (pneumonia, large atelectasis), ↑ fluid in pleural space (pleural effusion).
Auscultation		
Fine crackles	Series of short-duration, discontinuous, high-pitched sounds heard just before the end of inspiration. Result of rapid equalization of gas pressure when collapsed alveoli or terminal bronchioles suddenly snap open. Similar sound to that made by rolling hair between fingers just behind ear.	Idiopathic pulmonary fibrosis, interstitial edema (early pulmonary edema), alveolar filling (pneumonia), loss of lung volume (atelectasis), early phase of heart failure.
Coarse crackles	Series of long-duration, discontinuous, low-pitched sounds caused by air passing through airway intermittently occluded by mucus, unstable bronchial wall, or fold of mucosa. Evident on inspiration and, at times, expiration. Similar sound to blowing through straw under water. Increase in bubbling quality with more fluid.	Heart failure, pulmonary edema, pneumonia with severe congestion, COPD.
Rhonchi	Continuous rumbling, snoring, or rattling sounds from obstruction of large airways with secretions. Most prominent on expiration. Change often evident after coughing or suctioning.	COPD, cystic fibrosis, pneumonia, bronchiectasis.
Wheezes	Continuous high-pitched squeaking or musical sound caused by rapid vibration of bronchial walls. First evident on expiration but possibly evident on inspiration as obstruction of airway increases. Possibly audible without stethoscope.	Bronchospasm (caused by asthma), airway obstruction (caused by foreign body, tumor), COPD.
Stridor	Continuous musical or crowing sound of constant pitch. Result of partial obstruction of larynx or trachea.	Croup, epiglottitis, vocal cord edema after extubation, foreign body.
Absent breath sounds	No sound evident over entire lung or area of lung.	Pleural effusion, mainstem bronchi obstruction, large atelectasis, pneumonectomy, lobectomy.

Continued

TABLE 26-8 ASSESSMENT ABNORMALITIES—cont'd

Respiratory System

Finding	Description	Possible Etiology and Significance*
Auscultation—cont'd		
Pleural friction rub	Creaking or grating sound from roughened, inflamed pleural surfaces rubbing together. Evident during inspiration, expiration, or both and no change with coughing. Usually uncomfortable, especially on deep inspiration.	Pleurisy, pneumonia, pulmonary infarct.
Bronchophony, whispered pectoriloquy	Spoken or whispered syllable more distinct than normal on auscultation.	Pneumonia.
Egophony	Spoken "E" similar to "A" on auscultation because of altered transmission of voice sounds.	Pneumonia, pleural effusion.

*Limited to common etiologic factors. (Further discussion of conditions listed may be found in Chapters 27 through 29.)

TABLE 26-9 CHEST EXAMINATION FINDINGS IN PULMONARY PROBLEMS

Problem	Inspection	Palpation	Percussion	Auscultation
Chronic obstructive pulmonary disease	Barrel chest, cyanosis, tripod position, use of accessory muscles	↓ Movement	Hyperresonant or dull if consolidation	Crackles, rhonchi, wheezes, distant breath sounds
Asthma				
In exacerbation	Prolonged expiration, tripod position, pursed lips	↓ Movement	Hyperresonance	Wheezes, ↓ breath sounds ominous sign (severely diminished air movement)
Not in exacerbation	Normal	Normal	Normal	Normal
Pneumonia	Tachypnea, use of accessory muscles, duskiness or cyanosis	↑ Fremitus over affected area	Dull over affected areas	*Early:* Bronchial sounds *Later:* Crackles, rhonchi, egophony, whispered pectoriloquy
Atelectasis	No change unless involves entire segment, lobe	If small, no change If large, ↓ movement, ↓ fremitus	Dull over affected area	Crackles (may disappear with deep breaths) Absent sounds if large
Pulmonary edema	Tachypnea, labored respirations, cyanosis	↓ Movement or normal movement	Dull or normal depending on amount of fluid	Fine or coarse crackles at bases moving upward as condition worsens
Pleural effusion	Tachypnea, use of accessory muscles	↑ Movement ↑ Fremitus above effusion Absent fremitus over effusion	Dull	Diminished or absent over effusion, egophony over effusion
Pulmonary fibrosis	Tachypnea	↓ Movement	Normal	Crackles or sounds like Velcro being pulled apart

DIAGNOSTIC STUDIES OF RESPIRATORY SYSTEM

Numerous diagnostic studies are available to assess the respiratory system. Table 26-10 identifies the most common studies, and select studies are described in more detail below.

Sputum Studies

Sputum samples can be obtained by expectoration, tracheal suction, or bronchoscopy (discussed below). When the patient is unable to expectorate spontaneously, sputum may also be collected by inhalation of an irritating aerosol, usually hypertonic saline. This is called sputum induction. The specimens may be examined for culture and sensitivity to identify an infecting organism (e.g., *Mycobacterium, Pneumocystis jiroveci*) or to confirm a diagnosis (e.g., malignant cells). Regardless of whether specimen tests are ordered, observe the sputum for color, blood, volume, and viscosity.

Skin Tests

Skin tests may be performed to test for allergic reactions (see Chapter 14) or exposure to TB bacilli or fungi. Skin tests involve the intradermal injection of an antigen. A positive result on a TB skin test indicates that the patient has been exposed to the antigen. It does not indicate that TB is currently present. A negative result indicates either no exposure or a depression of cell-mediated immunity such as occurs in HIV infection. Table 26-11 on p. 494 describes reactions that indicate a positive TB skin test.

Nursing responsibilities are similar for all skin tests. First, to prevent a false-negative reaction, be certain that the injection is intradermal and not subcutaneous. After the injection, circle the site(s) and instruct the patient not to remove the marks. When charting administration of the antigen, draw a diagram of the forearm and hand and label the injection sites. The diagram is especially helpful when more than one test is administered.

When reading test results, use a good light. If an induration is present, use a marking pen to indicate the periphery on all four sides of the induration. As the pen touches the raised area, make a mark. Then determine the diameter of the induration in millimeters. Reddened, flat areas are not measured.

Endoscopic Examinations

Bronchoscopy. *Bronchoscopy* is a procedure in which the bronchi are visualized through a fiberoptic tube (Fig. 26-11). Bronchoscopy may be used for diagnostic purposes to obtain

TABLE 26-10 DIAGNOSTIC STUDIES

Respiratory System

Study	Description and Purpose	Nursing Responsibility
Blood Studies		
Hemoglobin	Test reflects amount of hemoglobin available for combination with O_2. Venous blood is used. *Male:* 13.2-17.3 g/dL (132-173 g/L) *Female:* 11.7-16.0 g/dL (117-160 g/L)	Explain procedure and its purpose.
Hematocrit	Test reflects ratio of red blood cells to plasma. Increased hematocrit (polycythemia) found in chronic hypoxemia. Venous blood is used. *Male:* 39%-50% (0.39-0.50) *Female:* 35%-47% (0.35-0.47)	Explain procedure and its purpose.
Arterial blood gases (ABGs)	Arterial blood is obtained through puncture of radial or femoral artery or through arterial catheter. Performed to assess acid-base balance, ventilation status, need for O_2 therapy, change in O_2 therapy, or change in ventilator settings.* Continuous ABG monitoring is also possible via a sensor or electrode inserted into arterial catheter.	Indicate whether patient is using O_2 (percentage, L/min). Avoid change in O_2 therapy or interventions (e.g., suctioning, position change) for 20 min before obtaining sample. Assist with positioning (e.g., palm up, wrist slightly hyperextended if radial artery is used). Collect blood in heparinized syringe. To ensure accurate results, expel all air bubbles and place sample in ice, unless it will be analyzed in <1 min. Apply pressure to artery for at least 5 min after specimen is obtained to prevent hematoma at the arterial puncture site.
O_2 Monitoring		
Oximetry	Monitors arterial or venous O_2 saturation. Probe attaches to finger, toe, earlobe, bridge of the nose for SpO_2 monitoring (see eFig. 26-2) or is contained in a pulmonary artery catheter for SvO_2 monitoring. Oximetry is used for intermittent or continuous monitoring and exercise testing.	Apply probe. When interpreting SpO_2 and SvO_2 values, first assess patient status and presence of factors that can alter accuracy of pulse oximeter reading. For SpO_2 these include motion, low perfusion, cold extremities, bright lights, acrylic nails, dark skin color, carbon monoxide, and anemia. For SvO_2, these include change in O_2 delivery or O_2 consumption.
CO_2 Monitoring		
End-tidal CO_2 ($PETCO_2$) (capnography)	Assesses the level of CO_2 in exhaled air. Graphically displays partial pressure of CO_2. Expired gases are sampled from the patient's airway and are analyzed by a CO_2 sensor that uses infrared light to measure exhaled CO_2. The sensor may be attached to an adaptor on the endotracheal or tracheostomy tube. A nasal cannula with a sidestream capnometer can be used in patients without an artificial airway. Can be used as a diagnostic measure to detect lung disease and for monitoring patients. Normal difference between $PaCO_2$ and $PETCO_2$ is 2-5 mm Hg ($PaCO_2$: 35-45 mm Hg; $PETCO_2$: 37-50 mm Hg).	Teach patient and caregiver about the purpose of capnography monitoring, emphasizing the benefit of continuous monitoring. Make sure that sensor is properly attached. Record and document data per institution policy.
Sputum Studies		
Culture and sensitivity	Purpose is to diagnose bacterial infection, select antibiotic, and evaluate treatment. Sputum specimen is collected in a sterile container. Takes 48-72 hr for results.	Instruct patient on how to produce a good specimen (see Gram stain). If patient cannot produce specimen, bronchoscopy may be used (see Fig. 26-11).
Gram stain	Staining of sputum permits classification of bacteria into gram-negative and gram-positive types. Results guide therapy until culture and sensitivity results are obtained.	Instruct patient to expectorate sputum into container after coughing deeply. Obtain sputum (mucoidlike), not saliva. Obtain specimen in early morning after mouth care because secretions collect during night. If unsuccessful, try increasing oral fluid intake unless fluids are restricted. Collect sputum in sterile container (sputum trap) during suctioning or by aspirating secretions from the trachea. Send specimen to laboratory promptly.
Acid-fast smear and culture	Assesses sputum for acid-fast bacilli (e.g., *Mycobacterium tuberculosis*). A series of three early-morning specimens is used.	Instruct patient how to produce a good specimen (see Gram stain). Cover specimen and send to laboratory for analysis.
Cytology	Determines presence of abnormal cells that may indicate malignant condition. Single sputum specimen is collected in special container with fixative solution.	Instruct patient on how to produce a good specimen (see Gram stain). If patient cannot produce specimen, bronchoscopy may be used (see Fig. 26-11). Send specimen to laboratory promptly.

*For reference intervals, see Table 26-1.

Continued

TABLE 26-10 DIAGNOSTIC STUDIES—cont'd

Respiratory System

Study	Description and Purpose	Nursing Responsibility
Radiology		
Chest x-ray	Used to screen, diagnose, and evaluate changes in respiratory system. Most common views are anteroposterior (AP) and lateral.	Instruct patient to undress to waist, put on gown, and remove any metal between neck and waist.
Computed tomography (CT)	Performed for diagnosis of lesions difficult to assess (e.g., mediastinum, hilum, pleura) by conventional x-ray studies. Common types are helical or spiral CT (contrast medium is usually used) and high-resolution CT scan (contrast medium is not used). Spiral CT used to diagnose a pulmonary embolism.	Same as for chest x-ray. Contrast medium may be given IV. Evaluation of BUN and serum creatinine is done before contrast to assess renal function. Assess if patient is allergic to shellfish (iodine), since the contrast is iodine based. Be sure the patient is well hydrated before and after procedure (to excrete contrast). Warn patient that contrast injection may cause a feeling of being warm and flushed. Instruct the patient that he or she will need to lie still on a hard table and the scanner will revolve around the body with clicking noises.
Magnetic resonance imaging (MRI)	Used for diagnosis of lesions difficult to assess by CT scan (e.g., lung apex) and for distinguishing vascular from nonvascular structures.	Same as for chest x-ray and CT scan, except contrast medium is not iodine based. If closed MRI is used and patient has claustrophobia, provide with relaxation or other modes to cope. Patient must remove all metal (e.g., jewelry, watch) before test. Patients with pacemakers and implantable cardioverter-defibrillators may not be able to have MRI.
Ventilation-perfusion (V/Q) scan	Used to assess ventilation and perfusion of lungs. IV radioisotope given to assess perfusion. For the ventilation portion, the patient inhales a radioactive gas (xenon or krypton), which outlines the alveoli. Normal scans show homogeneous radioactivity. Diminished or absent radioactivity suggests lack of perfusion or airflow. Ventilation without perfusion suggests a pulmonary embolus.	Same as for chest x-ray. No precautions needed afterward because the gas and isotope transmit radioactivity for only a brief interval.
Pulmonary angiogram	Used to visualize pulmonary vasculature and locate obstruction or pathologic conditions (e.g., pulmonary embolus). Contrast medium is injected through a catheter threaded into pulmonary artery or right side of the heart. Series of x-rays are taken after contrast medium is injected into pulmonary artery. Chest CT is replacing angiography, since it is less invasive.	Same as for chest x-ray. (See CT scan for contrast media precautions.) Check pressure dressing site after procedure. Monitor blood pressure, pulse, and circulation distal to injection site. Report and record significant changes.
Positron emission tomography (PET) scan	Used to distinguish benign and malignant pulmonary nodules. Because malignant lung cells have an increased uptake of glucose, the PET scan, which uses an IV radioactive glucose preparation, can demonstrate increased uptake of glucose in malignant lung cells.	*Preprocedure:* Check the blood glucose levels as high levels may interfere with test. Food and fluids other than water may be restricted for 4-6 hr. *Postprocedure:* Encourage fluids to excrete radioactive substance.
Endoscopy		
Bronchoscopy (see Fig. 26-11)	Flexible fiberoptic scope is used for diagnosis, biopsy, specimen collection, or assessment of changes. It may also be done to suction mucous plugs, lavage the lungs, or remove foreign objects.	Instruct patient to be on NPO status for 6-12 hr before the test. Obtain signed permit. Give sedative if ordered. After procedure, keep patient NPO until gag reflex returns. Monitor for recovery from sedation. Blood-tinged mucus is not abnormal. If biopsy was done, monitor for hemorrhage and pneumothorax.

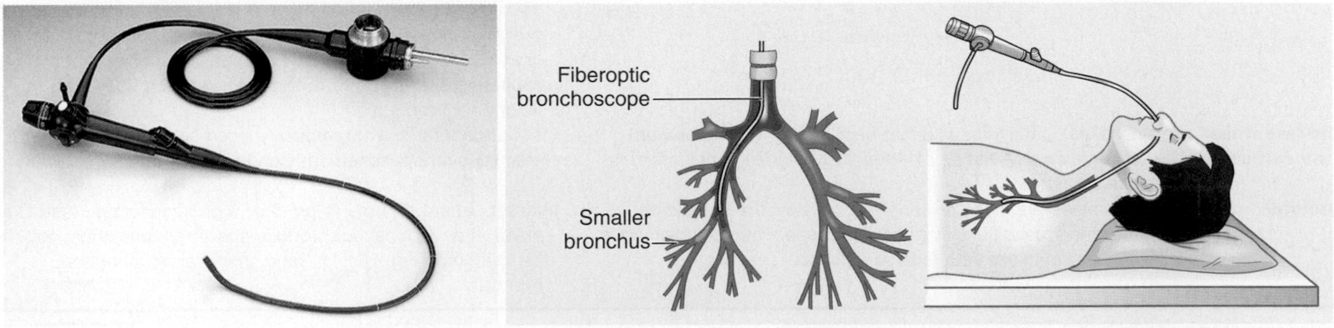

A B

FIG. 26-11 Fiberoptic bronchoscope. **A,** The transbronchoscopic balloon-tipped catheter and the flexible fiberoptic bronchoscope. **B,** The catheter is introduced into a small airway and the balloon inflated with 1.5 to 2 mL of air to occlude the airway. Bronchoalveolar lavage is performed by injecting and withdrawing 30-mL aliquots of sterile saline solution, gently aspirating after each instillation. Specimens are sent to the laboratory for analysis.

TABLE 26-10 DIAGNOSTIC STUDIES—cont'd

Respiratory System

Study	Description and Purpose	Nursing Responsibility
Mediastinoscopy	Scope is inserted through a small incision in the suprasternal notch and advanced into the mediastinum to inspect and biopsy lymph nodes. Used to diagnose lung cancer, non-Hodgkin's lymphoma, granulomatous infections, and sarcoidosis.	Prepare patient for surgical intervention. Obtain signed informed consent. Performed in the operating room (OR) using a general anesthetic. Afterward, monitor as for bronchoscopy.
Lung Biopsy	Specimens may be obtained by transbronchial or percutaneous biopsy or via transthoracic needle aspiration (TTNA), video-assisted thoracoscopic surgery (VATS), or open lung biopsy. Transbronchial biopsy and VATS can be performed in the bronchoscopy suite. TTNA is done under CT guidance in radiology department. Open lung is performed in the OR. VATS can also be done in the OR. These tests are used to obtain specimens for laboratory analysis.	Same as bronchoscopy if procedure done with bronchoscope, and same as thoracotomy if open lung biopsy done. With TTNA, check breath sounds q4hr for 24 hr and report any respiratory distress. Check incision site for bleeding. A chest x-ray should be done after TTNA or transbronchial biopsy to check for pneumothorax. With VATS a chest tube may be in postprocedure until lung has reexpanded. Monitor breath sounds to follow chest reexpansion. Encourage deep breathing for lung reinflation. Obtain signed informed consent for all procedures.
Thoracentesis	Used to obtain specimen of pleural fluid for diagnosis, to remove pleural fluid, or to instill medication. Chest x-ray is always obtained after procedure to check for pneumothorax.	Explain procedure to patient and obtain signed informed consent before procedure, which is usually performed in the patient's room. Position patient upright with elbows on an overbed table and feet supported. Instruct the patient not to talk or cough, and assist during procedure. Observe for signs of hypoxia and pneumothorax, and verify breath sounds in all fields after procedure. Encourage deep breaths to expand lungs. Send labeled specimens to laboratory.
Pulmonary Function Tests	Used to evaluate lung function. Involves use of spirometer to assess air movement as patient performs prescribed respiratory maneuvers.†	Avoid scheduling immediately after mealtime. Avoid administration of inhaled bronchodilator 6 hr before procedure. Explain procedure to patient. Assess for respiratory distress before procedure and report. Provide rest after the procedure.
Exercise Testing	Used in diagnosis and in determining exercise capacity. A *complete test* involves walking on a treadmill while expired O_2 and CO_2, respiratory rate, heart rate, and heart rhythm are monitored. In a *modified test* (desaturation test) only SpO_2 is monitored.	Instruct patient to wear comfortable shoes. Encourage patient to walk as quickly as possible.
6-Min walk test	Used to measure functional capacity and response to treatment in patients with heart or lung disease. Pulse oximetry is usually monitored during the walk. The distance walked is measured and used to monitor progression of disease or improvement after rehabilitation.	The patient is instructed by a trained practitioner to walk as far as possible during 6 min, stopping when short of breath and continuing when able.

†For reference intervals, see Tables 26-12 and 26-13.

biopsy specimens and assess results of treatment. Small amounts (30 mL) of sterile saline may be injected through the scope and withdrawn and examined for cells, a technique termed *bronchoalveolar lavage* (BAL). Bronchoscopy is also used for treatment, for example, to remove mucous plugs or foreign bodies. Laser therapy, electrocautery, cryotherapy, and stents may be placed through a bronchoscope to achieve patency of an airway that has been completely or partially obstructed by tumors.

Bronchoscopy can be performed in an outpatient procedure room, in a surgical suite, or at the bedside in the intensive care unit or on a medical-surgical unit, with the patient lying down or seated. After the nasopharynx and oropharynx are anesthetized with local anesthetic, the bronchoscope is coated with lidocaine (Xylocaine) and inserted, usually through the nose, and threaded down into the airways. Bronchoscopy can be done on mechanically ventilated patients through the endotracheal tube.

Lung Biopsy

Lung biopsy may be done (1) transbronchially, (2) percutaneously or via transthoracic needle aspiration (TTNA), (3) by video-assisted thoracic surgery (VATS), or (4) as an open lung biopsy. The purpose of a lung biopsy is to obtain tissue, cells, or secretions for evaluation. Transbronchial lung biopsy involves passing a forceps or needle through the bronchoscope for a specimen (Fig. 26-12). Specimens can be cultured or examined for malignant cells. A combination of transbronchial lung biopsy and BAL is used to differentiate infection and rejection in lung transplant recipients.

Percutaneous needle aspiration or TTNA involves inserting a needle through the chest wall, usually under computed tomography (CT) guidance. Because of the risk of a pneumothorax, a chest x-ray is ordered after TTNA.

In VATS a rigid scope with a lens is passed through a trocar placed into the pleura via one or two small incisions in the intercostal muscles. The physician views the lesions on a monitor

TABLE 26-11 INTERPRETING RESPONSES TO TUBERCULIN SKIN TESTING

Types of Responses	Consider Positive in the Following Groups
Positive Reactions	
≥5-mm induration	• HIV-infected people • People who had recent contact with a person with TB disease • People with fibrotic lesions on chest x-ray consistent with prior TB • Patients with organ transplants • People who are immunosuppressed (e.g., taking the equivalent of ≥15 mg/day of prednisone for ≥1 mo)
≥10-mm induration	• Recent immigrants (<5 yr) from high-prevalence countries • Injecting drug users • Residents and employees of high-risk congregate settings • Mycobacteriology laboratory personnel • People with clinical conditions (e.g., diabetes mellitus, end-stage kidney disease) that place them at high risk
≥15-mm induration	• All other people who are at low risk
False Reactions	**Possible Causes**
False-negative reactions (do not react even though infected)	• Anergy, immunosuppression • Recent TB infection (within 8-10 wk of exposure) • Overwhelming TB infection • Very old TB infection (many years) • Recent live virus vaccination (e.g., measles, chickenpox)
False-positive reactions (react even though not infected)	• Nontuberculous mycobacteria (e.g., *Mycobacterium avium-intracellulare* [MAI] or *Mycobacterium avium* complex [MAC]) • Previous BCG vaccine

Source: Centers for Disease Control and Prevention: Tuberculosis (TB) fact sheet: tuberculin skin testing. Retrieved from *www.cdc.gov/tb/publications/factsheets/testing/skintesting.htm.*

CASE STUDY—cont'd

Objective Data: Diagnostic Studies

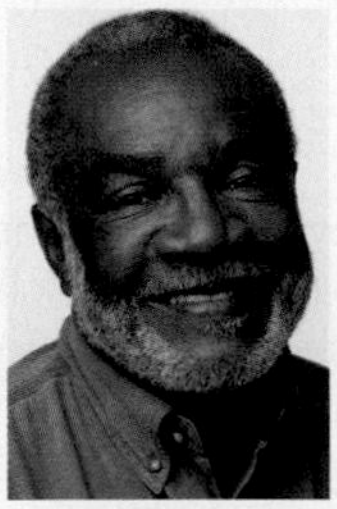

Kevin Peterson/ Photodisc/Thinkstock

The health care provider orders the following diagnostic studies for F.T.:

- CBC, basic metabolic panel (electrolytes, BUN, creatinine)
- ABGs
- Chest x-ray
- Sputum for culture and sensitivity

The ABGs demonstrate a compensated respiratory acidosis with hypoxemia. The WBC is 14,350/μL, and the chest x-ray shows lower lobe pneumonia. F.T. is admitted to the cardiopulmonary medical-surgical nursing unit.

directly via the lens, and biopsy specimens can be taken. A chest tube is kept in place until the lung expands. Lesions in the pleura or peripheral lung are biopsied via VATS. VATS is much less invasive than open lung biopsy and is the procedure of choice when appropriate.

Open lung biopsy is used when pulmonary disease cannot be diagnosed by other procedures. The patient is anesthetized, the chest is opened with a thoracotomy incision, and a biopsy

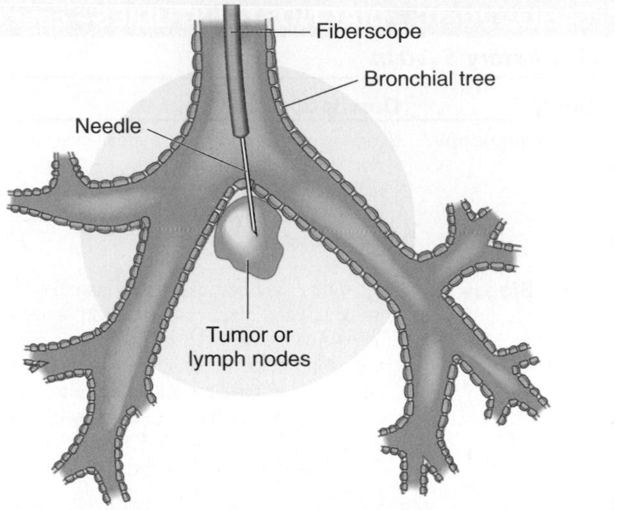

FIG. 26-12 Transbronchial biopsy needle penetrating the bronchial wall and entering a mass of subcarinal lymph nodes or tumor.

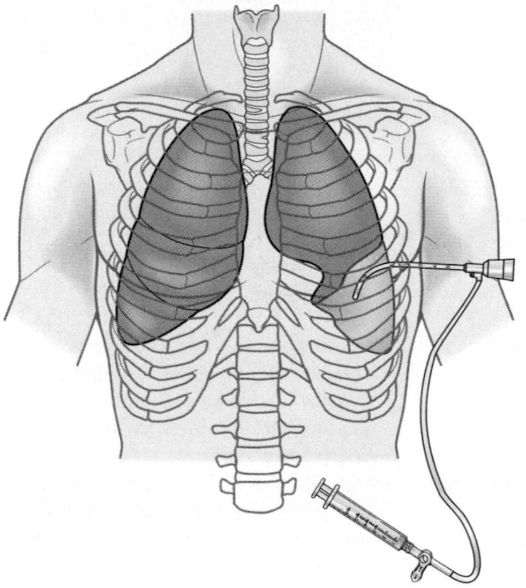

FIG. 26-13 Thoracentesis. A catheter is positioned in the pleural space to remove accumulated fluid.

specimen is obtained. Nursing care for the procedure is the same as after thoracotomy (see Chapter 28).

Thoracentesis

Thoracentesis is the insertion of a large-bore needle through the chest wall into the pleural space to obtain specimens for diagnostic evaluation, remove pleural fluid, or instill medication into the pleural space (Fig. 26-13). The patient is positioned sitting upright with elbows on an overbed table and feet supported. The skin is cleansed and a local anesthetic (lidocaine) is instilled subcutaneously. A chest tube may be inserted to permit further drainage of fluid.

Pulmonary Function Tests

Pulmonary function tests (PFTs) measure lung volumes and airflow. The results of PFTs are used to diagnose pulmonary disease, monitor disease progression, evaluate disability, and assess response to bronchodilators. Airflow measurement is administered by trained personnel using a spirometer. The patient inserts a mouthpiece, takes as deep a breath as possible,

TABLE 26-12 LUNG VOLUMES AND CAPACITIES

Parameter	Definitions	Normal Values*
Volumes		
Tidal volume (V_T)	Volume of air inhaled and exhaled with each breath. Only a small proportion of total capacity of lungs.	0.5 L
Expiratory reserve volume (ERV)	Additional air that can be forcefully exhaled after normal exhalation is complete.	1.0 L
Residual volume (RV)	Amount of air remaining in lungs after forced expiration. Air available in lungs for gas exchange between breaths.	1.5 L
Inspiratory reserve volume (IRV)	Maximum volume of air that can be inhaled forcefully after normal inhalation.	3.0 L
Capacities		
Total lung capacity (TLC)	Maximum volume of air that lungs can contain (TLC = IRV + V_T + ERV + RV).	6.0 L
Functional residual capacity (FRC)	Volume of air remaining in lungs at end of normal exhalation (FRC = ERV + RV). Increase or decrease possible with lung disease.	2.5 L
Vital capacity (VC)	Maximum volume of air that can be exhaled after maximum inspiration (VC = IRV + V_T + ERV); higher VC for men (generally).	4.5 L
Inspiratory capacity (IC)	Maximum volume of air that can be inhaled after normal expiration (IC = V_T + IRV).	3.5 L

*Normal values vary with patient's height, weight, age, race, and gender.

TABLE 26-13 COMMON MEASURES OF PULMONARY FUNCTION AIRFLOW

Measure	Description	Normal Value*
Forced vital capacity (FVC)	Amount of air that can be quickly and forcefully exhaled after maximum inspiration.	>80% of predicted
Forced expiratory volume in first second of expiration (FEV_1)	Amount of air exhaled in first second of FVC. Grades severity of airway obstruction.	>80% of predicted
FEV_1/FVC ratio	Dividing value for FEV_1 by value for FVC. Useful in differentiating obstructive and restrictive pulmonary dysfunction.	Age <50: ≥75% of predicted Age ≥50: ≥70% of predicted
Forced midexpiratory flow rate ($FEF_{25\%-75\%}$)	Measurement of airflow rate in middle half of forced expiration; early indicator of disease of small airways.	Age <50: ≥75% of predicted Age ≥50: ≥70% of predicted
Maximal voluntary ventilation (MVV)	Deep breathing as rapidly as possible for specified period. Fairly nonspecific test that gives information about exercise capacity. Used in conjunction with exercise stress test.	About 170 L/min
Peak expiratory flow rate (PEFR)	Maximum airflow rate during forced expiration. Aids in monitoring bronchoconstriction in asthma. Can be measured with peak flow meter.	Up to 600 L/min

*Normal values vary with patient's height, age, race, and gender.

and exhales as hard, fast, and long as possible. Verbal coaching is given to ensure that the patient continues blowing out until exhalation is complete.

The computer calculates the patient's percentage of predicted values, that is, how well the performance compares with an average based on age, gender, race, and height. Normal values are approximately 80% to 120% of the predicted value.[10] Normal values for PFTs are shown in Tables 26-12 and 26-13 and in eFig. 26-4, available on the website for this chapter.

Spirometry may be ordered before and after the administration of a bronchodilator to determine the patient's response. This may help document reversibility of airway obstruction (e.g., asthma). A positive response to the bronchodilator is greater than 200 mL increase or greater than 12% increase between preadministration and postadministration values.

Home spirometry may be used to monitor lung function in people with asthma, cystic fibrosis, or COPD, as well as before and after lung transplantation or other thoracic surgeries.[11] A peak flow meter is the instrument used at home. It is a handheld device through which one blows forcefully and quickly after taking a deep breath. Spirometry changes at home can warn of early lung transplant rejection or infection. Data from a peak flow meter provide important feedback to patients with asthma so they can learn to modify activities and medications in response to changes in peak expiratory flow rates (see Chapter 29).

Pulmonary function parameters can also be used to determine the need for mechanical ventilation or the readiness to be weaned from ventilatory support (see Table 66-13).

BRIDGE TO NCLEX EXAMINATION

The number of the question corresponds to the same-numbered outcome at the beginning of the chapter.

1. To promote the release of surfactant, the nurse encourages the patient to
   a. take deep breaths.
   b. cough five times per hour to prevent alveolar collapse.
   c. decrease fluid intake to reduce fluid accumulation in the alveoli.
   d. sit with head of bed elevated to promote air movement through the pores of Kohn.
2. A patient with a respiratory condition asks "How does air get into my lungs?" The nurse bases her answer on her knowledge that air moves into the lungs because of
   a. contraction of the accessory abdominal muscles.
   b. increased carbon dioxide and decreased oxygen in the blood.
   c. stimulation of the respiratory muscles by the chemoreceptors.
   d. decrease in intrathoracic pressure relative to pressure at the airway.

3. The nurse can best determine adequate arterial oxygenation of the blood by assessing
   a. heart rate.
   b. hemoglobin level.
   c. arterial oxygen tension.
   d. arterial carbon dioxide tension.
4. When teaching a patient about the most important respiratory defense mechanism distal to the respiratory bronchioles, which topic would the nurse discuss?
   a. Alveolar macrophages
   b. Impaction of particles
   c. Reflex bronchoconstriction
   d. Mucociliary clearance mechanism
5. A student nurse asks the RN what can be measured by arterial blood gases (ABGs). The RN tells the student that the ABGs can measure *(select all that apply)*
   a. acid-base balance.
   b. oxygenation status.
   c. acidity of the blood.
   d. glucose bound to hemoglobin.
   e. bicarbonate (HCO_3^-) in arterial blood.
6. To detect early signs or symptoms of inadequate oxygenation, the nurse would examine the patient for
   a. dyspnea and hypotension.
   b. apprehension and restlessness.
   c. cyanosis and cool, clammy skin.
   d. increased urine output and diaphoresis.
7. During the respiratory assessment of the older adult, the nurse would expect to find *(select all that apply)*
   a. a vigorous cough.
   b. increased chest expansion.
   c. increased residual volume.
   d. increased breath sounds in the lung apices.
   e. increased anteroposterior (AP) chest diameter.
8. When assessing activity-exercise patterns related to respiratory health, the nurse inquires about
   a. dyspnea during rest or exercise.
   b. recent weight loss or weight gain.
   c. ability to sleep through the entire night.
   d. willingness to wear oxygen equipment in public.
9. When auscultating the chest of an older patient in respiratory distress, it is best to
   a. begin listening at the apices.
   b. begin listening at the lung bases.
   c. begin listening on the anterior chest.
   d. ask the patient to breathe through the nose with the mouth closed.
10. Which assessment finding of the respiratory system does the nurse interpret as abnormal?
   a. Inspiratory chest expansion of 1 in
   b. Percussion resonance over the lung bases
   c. Symmetric chest expansion and contraction
   d. Bronchial breath sounds in the lower lung fields
11. The nurse is preparing the patient for a diagnostic procedure to remove pleural fluid for analysis. The nurse would prepare the patient for which test?
   a. Thoracentesis
   b. Bronchoscopy
   c. Pulmonary angiography
   d. Sputum culture and sensitivity

1. a, 2. d, 3. c, 4. a, 5. a, b, c, e, 6. b, 7. c, e, 8. a, 9. b, 10. d, 11. a

evolve

For rationales to these answers and even more NCLEX review questions, visit *http://evolve.elsevier.com/Lewis/medsurg*.

REFERENCES

1. Thibodeau GA, Patton KT: *Anthony's textbook of anatomy and physiology*, St Louis, 2013, Mosby.
2. Kaneko H, Horie J: Breathing movements of the chest and abdominal wall in healthy subjects, *Respir Care* 57(9):1442, 2012.
3. Kelly AM: Review article: can venous blood gas analysis replace arterial in emergency medical care, *Emerg Med Australas* 22(6):493, 2010.
4. Valdez-Lowe C, Ghareeb SA, Artinian NT: Pulse oximetry in adults, *Am J Nurs* 109(6):52, 2009.
5. Touhy TA: *Ebersole and Hess' toward healthy aging: human needs and nursing response*, ed 8, St Louis, 2012, Mosby.
6. Taylor BJ, Johnson BD: The pulmonary circulation and exercise responses in the elderly, *Semin Respir Crit Care Med* 31(5):528, 2010.
7. Pullen RL: Assessing the paranasal sinuses, *Nursing* 40(5):49, 2010.
8. Jarvis C: *Physical examination and health assessment*, ed 6, St Louis, 2012, Mosby.
9. Page B: Lung sound assessment: the lost art of using a stethoscope, *JEMS* 36(8):26, 2011.
10. Liang BM, Lam DC, Feng YL: Clinical applications of lung function tests: a revisit. *Respirology* 17(4):611, 2012.
11. Lam DC, Hui CK, Ip MS: Issues in pulmonary function testing for the screening and diagnosis of chronic obstructive pulmonary disease, *Curr Opin Pulm Med* 18(2):104, 2012.

RESOURCES

Resources for this chapter are listed after Chapter 29 on p. 610.

For breath is life, and if you breathe well you will live long on earth.
Sanskrit Proverb

CHAPTER

27

Nursing Management
Upper Respiratory Problems

Dorothy (Dottie) M. Mathers

evolve WEBSITE

http://evolve.elsevier.com/Lewis/medsurg

- NCLEX Review Questions
- Key Points
- Pre-Test
- Answer Guidelines for Case Study on p. 519
- Rationales for Bridge to NCLEX Examination Questions
- Case Study
  - Patient With Head and Neck Cancer/ Laryngectomy With Tracheostomy
- Nursing Care Plans (Customizable)
  - eNCP 27-1: Patient With a Tracheostomy
  - eNCP 27-2: Patient Having Total Laryngectomy and/or Radical Neck Surgery
- Concept Map Creator
- Glossary
- Animation
  - Anatomic Location of Sinuses
- Content Updates

eFigure

- eFig. 27-1: Placing posterior nasal pack in epistaxis

LEARNING OUTCOMES

1. Describe the clinical manifestations and nursing and collaborative management of problems of the nose.
2. Discuss the clinical manifestations and nursing and collaborative management of problems of the paranasal sinuses.
3. Describe the clinical manifestations and nursing and collaborative management of problems of the pharynx and larynx.
4. Discuss the nursing management of the patient who requires a tracheostomy.
5. Identify the steps involved in performing tracheostomy care and suctioning an airway.
6. Describe the risk factors and warning symptoms associated with head and neck cancer.
7. Discuss the nursing management of the patient with a laryngectomy.
8. Explain the methods used in voice restoration for the patient with temporary or permanent loss of speech.

KEY TERMS

allergic rhinitis, p. 499
deviated septum, p. 497
epistaxis, p. 498
esophageal speech, p. 516
nasal polyps, p. 506
rhinoplasty, p. 498
sinusitis, p. 504
tracheostomy, p. 507

Disorders of the nose, sinuses, pharynx, and larynx are presented in this chapter. Nursing management of patients with a tracheostomy or total laryngectomy is also discussed.

PROBLEMS OF NOSE AND PARANASAL SINUSES

DEVIATED SEPTUM

Deviated septum is a deflection of the normally straight nasal septum. Although up to 80% of the adult population may have septums that are slightly off center, the diagnosis of deviated septum is generally reserved for those that are severely shifted.[1] Trauma to the nose, either at birth or later in life, is the most common cause of deviated septum.[2] Deviation from midline can interfere with airflow and sinus drainage through the narrowed passageway. Symptoms vary depending on the degree of deviation. Minor septal deviations may be asymptomatic. Common manifestations of septal deviation include obstruction to nasal breathing, nasal congestion, frequent sinus infections and nosebleeds *(epistaxis),* and facial pain.

Medical management of deviated septum is focused on symptom control of nasal inflammation and congestion (see Table 27-2). For recurrent or severe symptoms, a nasal septoplasty is performed to reconstruct and properly align the deviated septum.

NASAL FRACTURE

Nasal fracture is the most common facial fracture and the third most common fracture of any bone. Fracture of the nose occurs as a result of blunt trauma, such as occurs with fights, automobile accidents, falls, and sports injuries. Many cases of facial trauma can be prevented by using protective sports

Reviewed by Sharon A. Willadsen, RN, PhD, Nursing Instructor, Lakeshore Technical College, Cleveland, Wisconsin.

equipment and protecting against falls. Complications associated with nasal fractures include airway obstruction, epistaxis, meningeal tears causing cerebrospinal fluid (CSF) leakage, septal hematoma, and cosmetic deformity.

Nasal fractures can be classified as simple or complex. *Simple fractures* may be unilateral or bilateral and typically produce little or no displacement.[3] Powerful frontal blows can cause *complex fractures,* which may also involve subsequent damage to adjacent facial structures such as the teeth, eyes, or other facial bones. Orbital fractures may be seen with midfacial trauma.

Diagnosis of a nasal fracture is based on the health history and physical examination. Clinical manifestations suggestive of a nasal fracture include localized pain, crepitus on palpation, swelling, ecchymosis, cosmetic deformity, epistaxis, and difficulty breathing out of the nostrils. Although facial deformity with a nasal fracture is common, often epistaxis may be the only initial sign.

On inspection, assess the patient's ability to breathe through each side of the nose and note the presence of edema, bleeding, or hematoma. Ecchymosis may be under one or both eyes. Ecchymosis involving both eyes is often termed *raccoon eyes* and may suggest an orbital or basilar skull fracture (see Chapter 57). Inspect the nose internally for evidence of septal deviation, hemorrhage, or clear drainage. Clear, pink-tinged, or persistent drainage after control of epistaxis suggests a CSF leak. Perform a quick test at the bedside or send a specimen to the laboratory to determine if glucose is present; the presence of glucose indicates that the fluid is CSF.

Injury of sufficient force to fracture nasal bones results in considerable swelling of soft tissues. With extensive swelling, it may be necessary to wait to repair the fracture until the edema subsides, which may be 5 to 10 days.

Goals of nursing management are to maintain the airway, reduce edema and pain, prevent complications, and provide emotional support. The best way to maintain the airway is to keep the patient in an upright position. Apply ice to the face and nose in 10- to 20-minute intervals to help reduce edema and bleeding. Administer analgesia as ordered to control pain. Acetaminophen is preferred over nonsteroidal antiinflammatory drugs (NSAIDs) or acetylsalicylic acid (ASA; aspirin) for the first 48 hours to avoid prolonging clotting time and increasing the risk for bleeding. Nasal stuffiness may be relieved with nasal decongestants, saline nasal sprays, and a humidifier. Tell the patient to avoid hot showers and alcohol for the first 48 hours to prevent an increase in swelling. Encourage the patient to quit or decrease smoking to maximize tissue healing.

When a fracture is confirmed, the goals are to realign the fracture using closed or open reduction (septoplasty, rhinoplasty) and to ensure that a septal hematoma does not develop, since this increases the patient's risk for infection. In addition to reestablishing cosmetic appearance, these surgical procedures provide an adequate airway and function of the nose.

RHINOPLASTY

Rhinoplasty, the surgical reconstruction of the nose, is performed for cosmetic reasons or to improve airway function when trauma or developmental deformities result in nasal obstruction. When caring for rhinoplasty patients before surgery, assess the patient's expectations of the surgery. Any actual or perceived alteration in body image (e.g., a deformed or enlarged nose) can affect self-esteem and interactions with others. Computerized photographs can be used to show the patient's appearance after the surgery. These images often help patients decide whether to undergo rhinoplasty. Explain expected results of surgery frankly and truthfully to avoid disappointment.

Rhinoplasty is performed as an outpatient procedure using regional or general anesthesia. Sometimes nasal tissue is added or removed, and the nose may be lengthened or shortened. Plastic implants are sometimes used to reshape the nose. Incisions are typically inside the nose and are thus hidden. Sonic rhinoplasty incorporates the use of an ultrasonic device to gently aspirate bone, enabling a refined cosmetic result.[4]

After surgery, nasal packing may be inserted to apply pressure and prevent bleeding or septal hematoma formation. An external plastic splint protects and supports the new shape of the nose during the healing process. Nasal packing is usually removed the day after surgery, and the splint is left in place for approximately 1 week.

NURSING MANAGEMENT NASAL SURGERY

Examples of nasal surgery include rhinoplasty, septoplasty, and nasal fracture reductions. Before surgery, instruct the patient not to take aspirin-containing drugs or NSAIDs for 2 weeks to reduce the risk of bleeding. Encourage preoperative smoking cessation to promote postoperative wound healing. Nursing interventions during the immediate postoperative period include maintenance of the airway; assessment of respiratory status; pain management; and observation of the surgical site for bleeding, infection, and edema. Teaching is important because the patient must be able to detect early and late complications at home. The patient typically experiences temporary edema and ecchymosis. Cold compresses and elevation of the head can help minimize swelling and discomfort. Teach activity restrictions aimed at preventing bleeding and injury (no nose blowing, swimming, heavy lifting, strenuous exercise).[5] Subtle swelling may be slow to resolve, delaying the achievement of a full cosmetic result for up to a year.

EPISTAXIS

Epistaxis (nosebleed) occurs in a bimodal distribution, with children 2 to 10 years of age and adults over age 50 most affected. Epistaxis can be caused by low humidity, allergies, upper respiratory tract infections, sinusitis, trauma, foreign bodies, hypertension, chemical irritants such as street drugs, overuse of decongestant nasal sprays, facial or nasal surgery, anatomic malformation, and tumors.[6] Any condition that prolongs bleeding time or alters platelet counts will predispose the patient to epistaxis. Bleeding time may also be prolonged if the patient takes aspirin, NSAIDs, warfarin, or other anticoagulant drugs.

Approximately 90% of nosebleeds occur in the anterior portion of the nasal cavity and are easily visualized. Posterior bleeding occurs more commonly with older adults secondary to other health problems. Anterior bleeding usually stops spontaneously or can be self-treated. Posterior bleeding may require medical treatment.

NURSING AND COLLABORATIVE MANAGEMENT EPISTAXIS

Use simple first aid measures to control epistaxis: (1) keep the patient quiet; (2) place the patient in a sitting position, leaning slightly forward with head tilted forward; and (3) apply direct pressure by pinching the entire soft lower portion of the nose against the nasal septum for 10 to 15 minutes. If bleeding does not stop within 15 to 20 minutes, seek medical assistance.

Medical management involves identifying the bleeding site and applying a vasoconstrictive agent, cauterization, or anterior packing. Pledgets (nasal tampon) impregnated with anesthetic solution (lidocaine) and/or vasoconstrictive agents such as cocaine or epinephrine are placed into the nasal cavity and left in place for 10 to 15 minutes. Silver nitrate may be used to chemically cauterize an identified bleeding point after epistaxis is controlled. Thermal cauterization is reserved for more severe bleeding and requires the use of local or general anesthesia.[7]

If bleeding does not stop, packing may be used. Packing with compressed sponges (e.g., Merocel) or epistaxis balloons (e.g., Rapid Rhino) is preferred over the use of traditional Vaseline ribbon gauze because of the ease of placement. Packing is inserted into the nares and advanced along the floor of the nasal cavity. The sponge expands with moisture to fill the nasal cavity and tamponade bleeding. The balloon is inflated with air to achieve the same pressure effect (Fig. 27-1). Alternatively, absorbable materials such as oxidized cellulose (surgical), gelatin foam (Gelfoam), or a gelatin-thrombin combination (Floseal) may be used as packing for anterior bleeds. In addition to providing pressure to stop bleeding, these materials increase clot formation and protect the nasal mucosa from further trauma.[7] A nasal sling (a folded 2 × 2-in gauze pad) may be taped under the nares to absorb drainage.

Nasal packing may impair respiratory status, especially in older adults. Closely monitor respiratory rate, heart rate and rhythm, oxygen saturation using pulse oximetry (SpO_2), and level of consciousness, and observe for signs of aspiration. Because of the risk of complications, all patients with posterior packing should be admitted to a monitored unit to permit closer observation.

Packing is painful because sufficient pressure must be applied to stop the bleeding. Nasal packing predisposes patients to infection from bacteria (e.g., *Staphylococcus aureus*) present in the nasal cavity. The patient should receive a mild opioid analgesic for pain (e.g., acetaminophen with codeine) and an antibiotic effective against staphylococci to protect against infection.

Nasal packing may be left in place for a few days. Before removal, medicate the patient for pain because this procedure is very uncomfortable. After removal, cleanse the nares gently and lubricate them with water-soluble jelly.

Teach the patient about home care before discharge. Instruct the patient to avoid vigorous nose blowing, engaging in strenuous activity, lifting, and straining for 4 to 6 weeks. Teach the patient to use saline nasal spray and/or a humidifier, to sneeze with the mouth open, and to avoid the use of aspirin-containing products or NSAIDs.

ALLERGIC RHINITIS

Allergic rhinitis is the reaction of the nasal mucosa to a specific allergen. Allergic rhinitis can be classified according to the causative allergen (seasonal or perennial) or the frequency of symptoms (episodic, intermittent, or persistent).[8] *Episodic* refers to symptoms related to sporadic exposure to allergens that are not typically encountered in the patient's normal environment, such as exposure to animal dander when visiting another person's home. *Intermittent* means that the symptoms are present less than 4 days a week or less than 4 weeks per year. *Persistent* means that the symptoms are present more than 4 days a week and for more than 4 weeks per year.

Seasonal rhinitis usually occurs in the spring and fall and is caused by allergy to pollens from trees, flowers, or grasses. The typical attack lasts for several weeks during times when pollen counts are high; then it disappears and recurs at the same time the following year. *Perennial rhinitis* occurs from exposure to environmental allergens, such as animal dander, dust mites, indoor molds, or cockroaches. Both seasonal and perennial rhinitis can be classified as episodic, intermittent, or persistent, depending on the duration and frequency of symptoms.

Sensitization to an allergen occurs with initial allergen exposure, which results in the production of antigen-specific immu-

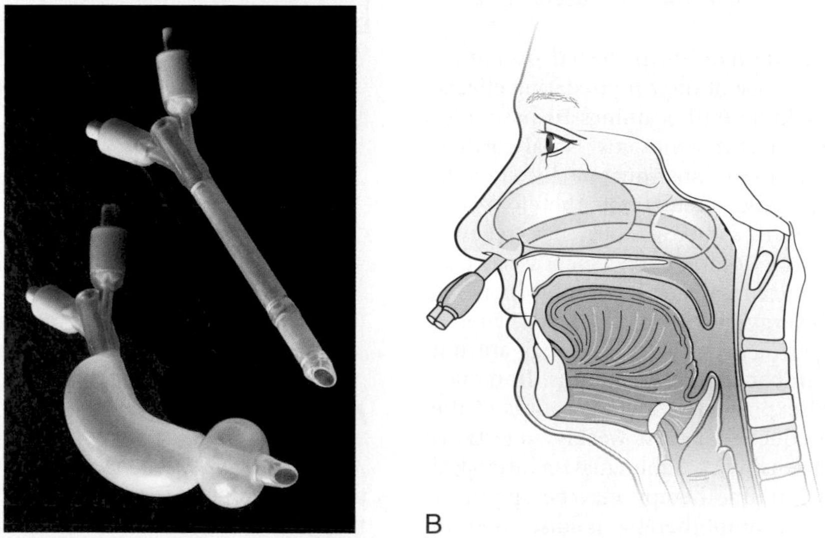

A B

FIG. 27-1 **A,** Epistaxis balloon. The balloon is inflated after insertion. **B,** Epistaxis balloon in proper position in nares.

noglobulin E (IgE) (see Fig. 14-6). After exposure, mast cells and basophils release histamine, cytokines, prostaglandins, and leukotrienes, which cause the early symptoms of sneezing, itching, rhinorrhea, and congestion. Four to 8 hours after exposure, inflammatory cells infiltrate the nasal tissues, causing and maintaining the inflammatory response. Because symptoms of rhinitis resemble those of the common cold, the patient may believe the condition is a continuous or repeated cold.

Clinical Manifestations

Manifestations of allergic rhinitis are initially sneezing; watery, itchy eyes and nose; altered sense of smell; and thin, watery nasal discharge that can lead to a more sustained mucus production and nasal congestion. The nasal turbinates appear pale, boggy, and swollen. The turbinates may fill the air space and press against the nasal septum. The posterior ends of the turbinates can become so enlarged that they obstruct sinus aeration or drainage and result in sinusitis. With chronic exposure to allergens, the patient's responses include headache, congestion, pressure, nasal polyps, and postnasal drip as the most common cause of cough. The patient may complain of cough, hoarseness, and the recurrent need to clear the throat. Congestion may cause snoring.

NURSING AND COLLABORATIVE MANAGEMENT ALLERGIC RHINITIS

The most important step in managing allergic rhinitis is identifying and avoiding triggers of allergic reactions (Table 27-1). Instruct the patient to keep a diary of times when the allergic reaction occurs and the activities that precipitate the reaction. Patients are often more aware of intermittent exposure to an allergen such as pets than they are of a more persistent exposure to allergens such as dust mites, cockroaches, or mold. Identifying such triggers is the first step toward avoiding them.

The goal of medications is to reduce inflammation associated with allergic rhinitis, reduce nasal symptoms, minimize associated complications, and maximize quality of life. Appropriate oral medication options include H_1-antihistamines, corticosteroids, decongestants, and leukotriene receptor antagonists (LTRAs). Intranasal medications include antihistamines, anticholinergics, corticosteroids, cromolyn, and decongestants[9] (Table 27-2).

Second-generation antihistamines are preferred over first-generation antihistamines because of their nonsedating effects. Remind patients who are taking antihistamines to have adequate fluid intake to reduce adverse symptoms. Nasal corticosteroid sprays are used to decrease inflammation locally with little absorption in the systemic circulation. Therefore systemic side effects are rare. If symptoms are not relieved with monotherapy, a two-drug combination (such as an oral H_1-antihistamine and an intranasal corticosteroid) may be helpful. Immunotherapy (allergy shots) may be used when a specific, unavoidable allergen is identified and drugs are not tolerated or are ineffective in controlling symptoms. Immunotherapy involves controlled exposure to small amounts of the known allergen through frequent (at least weekly) injections with the goal of decreasing sensitivity. Sublingual or intranasal administration of allergen immunotherapy may be appropriate for selected patients. (Immunotherapy is discussed in Chapter 14.)

TABLE 27-1 PATIENT & CAREGIVER TEACHING GUIDE

Avoiding Allergens in Allergic Rhinitis

Include the following instructions when teaching a patient or caregiver about allergic rhinitis.

What to Avoid	Specific Approaches
House dust	• Focus on the bedroom. Remove carpeting. Limit furniture. • Put the pillows, mattress, and springs in airtight vinyl bags or containers. • Limit clothing in the bedroom to items used frequently. Place clothing in airtight, zipper-sealed vinyl clothes bags. • Install an air filter. Close the air conditioning vent into the room. Use blinds rather than draperies.
House dust mites	• Wash bedding in hot water (130° F [54° C]) weekly. • Wear a mask when vacuuming. Install a filter on the outlet port of the vacuum cleaner. • Avoid sleeping or lying on upholstered furniture. • Keep house temperature and conditions cool and dry.
Pet allergens	• Remove pets from interior of home. • Clean the living area thoroughly. • Do not expect instant relief. Symptoms usually do not improve significantly for 2 mo after pet removal.
Mold spores	• The three *D*s that promote growth of mold spores are darkness, dampness, and drafts. • Ventilate closed rooms and open doors. Consider adding windows to dark rooms. Consider keeping a small light on in closets. • Basement light with a timer that provides light several hours a day may decrease mold growth. • Avoid places where humidity is high (e.g., basements, clothes hampers, greenhouses, barns). Dehumidifiers are rarely helpful.
Pollens	• Stay inside with closed doors and windows during high-pollen season. • Install an air conditioner with a good air filter. Wash filters weekly during high-pollen season. • Put the car air conditioner on "recirculate" when driving. • Avoid having plants, especially in the bedroom.
Smoke	• Presence of a smoker will sabotage the best of all possible symptom reduction programs.

DRUG ALERT: Antihistamines
- First-generation antihistamines (e.g., chlorpheniramine [Chlor-Trimeton]) can cause drowsiness and sedation.
- Warn patients that operating machinery and driving may be dangerous because of the sedative effect.

DRUG ALERT: Pseudoephedrine (Sudafed)
- Large doses may produce tachycardia and palpitations, especially in patients with cardiac disease.
- Overdosage in those over 60 years of age may result in central nervous system depression, seizures, and hallucinations.

ACUTE VIRAL RHINITIS

Acute viral rhinitis (common cold or acute coryza) is an infection of the upper respiratory tract that can be caused by more than 200 different viruses. The majority of colds, which are caused by rhinoviruses, are mild and self-limiting. Other

TABLE 27-2 **DRUG THERAPY**

Rhinitis and Sinusitis

Drug	Mechanism of Action	Side Effects	Nursing Actions
Corticosteroids			
Nasal Spray beclomethasone (Beconase) budesonide (Rhinocort) ciclesonide (Omnaris) flunisolide (Nasalide) fluticasone (Flonase) fluticasone furoate (Veramyst) mometasone (Nasonex) triamcinolone (Nasacort)	Inhibits inflammatory response of allergic rhinitis. At recommended dose, systemic side effects are unlikely because of low systemic absorption. Systemic effects may occur with higher than recommended doses.	Mild transient nasal burning and stinging, mucosal drying. In rare instances, localized fungal infection with *Candida albicans*.	• Instruct patient to use on regular basis and not PRN. • Instruct patient to clear nasal passages before use. • Reinforce that spray acts to decrease inflammation and it may take several days or weeks to achieve maximum effects. • Discontinue use if nasal infection develops.
Mast Cell Stabilizer			
Nasal Spray cromolyn spray (NasalCrom)	Suppresses release of histamine and other inflammatory mediators from mast cells.	Minimal side effects. Occasional burning or nasal irritation.	• Reinforce that spray prevents symptoms. • Begin 2 wk before pollen season starts and use throughout pollen season. • If isolated allergy, such as cat, use prophylactically (i.e., 10-15 min before exposure to allergen).
Leukotriene Receptor Antagonists (LTRAs) and Inhibitors			
Antagonists zafirlukast (Accolate) montelukast (Singulair) ***Inhibitors*** zileuton (Zyflo)	Suppress leukotriene activity, thereby inhibiting airway edema, bronchoconstriction, mucus production, and inflammation (see Fig. 12-2).	Generally well tolerated. May cause headaches, dizziness, rash, altered liver function tests, GI disturbances. *Zafirlukast and zileuton:* Monitor PT levels and theophylline levels if patient is taking warfarin or theophylline.	• Monitor liver function tests periodically while on therapy. Discontinue if elevated. • Administer on empty stomach. • Do not discontinue therapy without consulting health care professional. • Not to be used for acute attacks.
Anticholinergic			
Nasal Spray ipratropium bromide (Atrovent)	Blocks nasal cholinergic receptors, reducing nasal secretions in the common cold and nonallergic rhinitis.	Nasal dryness and irritation may occur. Does not cause systemic side effects.	• Need to prime pump with seven actuations before initial use • May reduce the need for other rhinitis medications.
Antihistamines			
First-Generation Agents (Oral) azatadine (Optimine) brompheniramine (Dimetane) chlorpheniramine (Chlor-Trimeton) clemastine (Tavist) dexchlorpheniramine (Polaramine) diphenhydramine (Benadryl) levocetirizine (Xyzal)	Bind with H_1 receptors on target cells, blocking histamine binding. Relieve acute symptoms of allergic response (itching, sneezing, rhinorrhea).	Cross blood-brain barrier, frequently causing sedation and somnolence. Can also cause paradoxical stimulation (restlessness, nervousness, insomnia). Anticholinergic side effects (e.g., palpitations, dry mouth, constipation, urinary hesitancy).	• Warn patient that operating machinery and driving may be dangerous because of sedative effect. • Teach patient to report palpitations, change in heart rate, change in bowel or bladder habits. • Instruct patient not to use alcohol with antihistamines because of additive depressant effect. • Rapid onset of action, no drug tolerance with prolonged use.
Second-Generation Agents (Oral) loratadine (Claritin) cetirizine (Zyrtec) fexofenadine (Allegra) desloratadine (Clarinex) levocetirizine (Xyzal)	Same as above.	Limited affinity for brain H_1 receptors. Cause minimal sedation, few effects on psychomotor activities or bladder function.	• Teach patient to expect few, if any, side effects. • More expensive than classic antihistamines. • Rapid onset of action, no drug tolerance with prolonged use.
Second-Generation Agents (Intranasal) azelastine (Astelin) olopatadine (Patanase)	Same as above.	Headache, bitter taste, somnolence, nasal irritation.	Longer use increases risk of rebound vasodilation, which can increase congestion.

Continued

TABLE 27-2 DRUG THERAPY—cont'd

Rhinitis and Sinusitis

Drug	Mechanism of Action	Side Effects	Nursing Actions
Decongestants			
Oral			
pseudoephedrine (Sudafed)	Stimulates adrenergic receptors on blood vessels, promotes vasoconstriction, reduces nasal congestion.	CNS stimulation, causing insomnia, excitation, headache, irritability, increased blood and ocular pressure, dysuria, palpitations, tachycardia.	• Advise patient of adverse reactions. • Advise that some preparations are contraindicated for patients with cardiovascular disease, hypertension, diabetes, glaucoma, benign prostatic hyperplasia, hepatic and renal disease.
Topical (Nasal Spray)			
oxymetazoline (Dristan 12-Hour) phenylephrine (Neo-Synephrine)	Same as above.	Same as above, plus rebound nasal congestion.	• Teach patient that these drugs should not be used for >3 days or >3-4 times/day.
Combination Cold Medications			
Zutripro oral solution (hydrocodone, chlorpheniramine, and pseudoephedrine) Rezira oral solution (hydrocodone and pseudoephedrine)	Hydrocodone suppresses cough. Mechanism of action of chlorpheniramine and pseudoephedrine discussed above.	See individual drugs above.	• Avoid in patients with head injury or increased intracranial pressure. • Use with caution in patients with acute abdominal conditions.

PT, Prothrombin time.

viruses, such as coxsackieviruses and adenoviruses, can cause a more severe illness. Acute viral rhinitis is the most prevalent infectious disease, with the average adult contracting one to three colds per year.

The virus is spread by airborne droplet sprays emitted by the infected person while breathing, talking, sneezing, or coughing. Because the virus can survive on inanimate objects for up to 3 days, transmission can also occur by direct hand contact. Frequency of the infection increases in the winter months when people stay indoors and overcrowding is more common. Other factors that increase susceptibility include fatigue, physical and emotional stress, allergies that affect the nose and throat, and compromised immune status. Exercise can significantly reduce the number of upper respiratory tract infections.[10]

Symptoms of acute viral rhinitis typically begin 2 or 3 days after infection and may include runny nose, watery eyes, nasal congestion, sneezing, cough, sore throat, fever, headache, and fatigue. Cold symptoms may last 2 to 14 days, with typical recovery in 7 to 10 days.

NURSING AND COLLABORATIVE MANAGEMENT ACUTE VIRAL RHINITIS

Interventions are directed toward relieving symptoms. Rest, fluids, proper diet, antipyretics, and analgesics are recommended. Warm salt water gargles, ice chips, throat lozenges, or throat sprays alleviate a sore throat. Petroleum jelly soothes a raw nose. Saline nasal spray reduces nasal congestion. Antihistamine and decongestant therapy reduces postnasal drip and significantly decreases severity of cough, nasal obstruction, and nasal discharge. Caution patients to use the intranasal decongestant sprays for no more than 3 days to prevent rebound congestion from occurring. Cough suppressants may be used.

COMPLEMENTARY & ALTERNATIVE THERAPIES

Echinacea

Scientific Evidence

- Echinacea may have some benefit in reducing the incidence and duration of the common cold.
- However, there is conflicting evidence on its use in prevention and treatment of upper respiratory tract infections.

Nursing Implications

- Echinacea is considered safe when used in recommended doses.
- Patients with asthma or allergies to plants in the daisy family (including ragweed, mums, marigolds, and daisies) are more likely to have allergic reactions.
- It may interfere with drugs that suppress the immune system and those that are metabolized by the liver.
- Caution is advised in patients with autoimmune disorders.

Complications of acute viral rhinitis include pharyngitis, sinusitis, otitis media, tonsillitis, and lung infections. Unless symptoms of complications are present, antibiotic therapy is not indicated. Antibiotics have no effect on viruses and, if taken injudiciously, may produce antibiotic-resistant bacteria. If symptoms remain for 10 to 14 days with no improvement, acute bacterial sinusitis may be present, and antibiotics will be prescribed.

Teach the patient to recognize the symptoms of secondary bacterial infection, such as a temperature higher than 100.4° F (38° C); tender, swollen glands; severe sinus or ear pain; or significantly worsening symptoms. Green, purulent nasal drainage during the later stages of a cold is not uncommon and is not considered indicative of bacterial infection. In the patient with pulmonary disease, signs of infection include a change in consistency, color, or volume of the sputum. Because infection

EVIDENCE-BASED PRACTICE

Translating Research Into Practice

Do Probiotics Prevent Upper Respiratory Tract Infections?

Clinical Question

In healthy patients (P) what is the effect of probiotics (I) versus placebo (C) in preventing acute upper respiratory tract infections (O)?

Best Available Evidence

Systematic review of randomized controlled trials (RCTs)

Critical Appraisal and Synthesis of Evidence

- Ten RCTs ($n = 3451$) including healthy children and adults up to age 40.
- Intervention was ingestion of any probiotic (single or mixture of strains, any dosage regimen or route of administration) for more than 7 days, compared with placebo or no treatment.
- Most common probiotics were lactic acid bacteria and bifidobacteria, often consumed in fermented foods (e.g., yogurt) or as dietary supplements.
- Probiotics were better than placebo in reducing the occurrence of acute URIs.
- The number of URIs requiring antibiotics was lower in patients using probiotics compared with those using placebo.

Conclusion

- Probiotics are effective in reducing the incidence of URIs.

Implications for Nursing Practice

- Encourage continued probiotic use to prevent acute URIs.
- Yogurt is an excellent food source for probiotics.
- Probiotics are also available as a dietary supplement.
- Advise patients with frequent URIs of potential benefit from probiotic ingestion.
- Probiotics are typically well tolerated, but can cause gastrointestinal (GI) side effects
- Counsel patients of minor probiotic side effects, including flatulence and increased GI irritability.

Reference for Evidence

Hao Q, Lu Z, Dong B, et al: Probiotics for preventing acute upper respiratory tract infections, *Cochrane Database Syst Rev* 9:CD006895, 2011.

P, Patient population of interest; *I*, intervention or area of interest; *C*, comparison of interest or comparison group; *O*, outcomes of interest (see p. 12).

can progress rapidly, teach the patient with chronic respiratory disease to immediately report sputum changes, increased shortness of breath, and chest tightness. During the cold season, advise patients with a chronic illness or a compromised immune system to avoid crowded situations and other persons who have obvious cold symptoms. Frequent hand washing and avoiding hand-to-face contact help prevent direct spread.

INFLUENZA

Influenza (flu) is a highly contagious respiratory illness that causes significant morbidity and mortality. Millions of Americans (about 5% to 20% of U.S. population) contract influenza each year. The flu season begins in September and continues through April of each year, peaking anywhere from November to March. More than 200,000 people are hospitalized each year for flu-related complications.[11] Death rates vary from season to season. On average, influenza is responsible for 20,000 deaths annually. Vaccination of high-risk groups can prevent many of these deaths.

Etiology and Pathophysiology

Influenza viruses are classified into three serotypes (A, B, and C), but only A and B cause significant illness in humans. Influenza A is subtyped based on the presence of two surface proteins: hemagglutinin (H) and neuraminidase (N). The H antigens enable the virus to enter the cell, and the N antigens facilitate cell-to-cell transmission. Influenza A viruses are thus named according to their H and N type (e.g., H3N2).

Influenza A can infect a variety of animals as well as humans. More than 100 types of influenza A are found in birds (avian flu), pigs (swine flu), horses, seals, and dogs. The virus mutates to allow it to infect different species. When a new viral strain reaches humans, people do not have immunity, and the virus can spread quickly around the globe, causing a *pandemic*. The type A H1N1 influenza (swine flu) emerged in 2009 having never been seen in humans before. A worldwide pandemic resulted. Pandemics can also be triggered by the reemergence of a viral strain that has not circulated for many years. *Epidemics* are more localized outbreaks, usually occurring yearly, caused by variants of already circulating strains. Influenza A is the most common flu virus and also the most virulent.

Influenza B and C viruses are not divided into subtypes and only infect humans. Outbreaks of influenza B can also cause regional epidemics, but the disease it produces is generally milder than that caused by influenza A. Influenza C causes mild illness and does not cause epidemics or pandemics.

Influenza viruses have a remarkable ability to change over time. This accounts for widespread disease and the need for annual vaccination against new strains. Fewer cases of influenza result when a minor change in the virus occurs because most persons have partial immunity.

Influenza is transmitted from animals to humans by direct contact with infected animals or through exposure to water and surfaces contaminated with animal feces. Influenza is communicable between humans through droplet contact and inhalation of aerosolized particles. The virus has an incubation period of 1 to 4 days, with peak transmission risk starting at approximately 1 day before onset of symptoms and continuing for 5 to 7 days.

Clinical Manifestations

The onset of flu is typically abrupt, with systemic symptoms of chills, fever, anorexia, malaise, and generalized myalgia often accompanied by a headache, cough, rhinorrhea, and sore throat. Physical findings are usually minimal, with normal assessment on chest auscultation. Dyspnea and diffuse crackles are signs of pulmonary complications. In uncomplicated cases, symptoms subside within 7 days. Some patients, particularly older adults, experience weakness or lassitude that persists for weeks. Hyperactive airways and a chronic cough often occur during recovery.

The most common complication of influenza is pneumonia, which can be either primary influenza (viral) pneumonia or secondary bacterial pneumonia. The patient who develops secondary bacterial pneumonia usually experiences gradual improvement of influenza symptoms, then worsening cough and purulent sputum. Treatment with antibiotics is usually effective if started early.

Diagnostic Studies

Important diagnostic factors in influenza include the patient's health history, clinical findings, and other cases of influenza in the community. Although a diagnosis of flu is frequently based on clinical findings, rapid flu tests can help in the diagnosis by detecting the virus in nasal secretions. Depending on the method, the test may be completed in the physician's office in less than 30 minutes or be sent to a laboratory, with results available the same day. The test can help differentiate influenza from other viral and bacterial infections with similar symptoms that may be serious and must be treated differently. Rapid flu tests are best used within the first 48 hours of the onset of symptoms to help diagnose influenza and determine whether antiviral drugs are a treatment option.[12] The main disadvantages of the rapid flu test are that it will miss some cases or occasionally be positive when a person does not actually have the flu.

Viral cultures are considered the "gold standard" for diagnosing influenza, but they can take up to 3 to 10 days for results. A viral culture has the advantage of identifying which virus (A, B, or another respiratory virus) and which strains of virus are present. These data are used in the formulation of the following season's flu vaccine.

NURSING AND COLLABORATIVE MANAGEMENT INFLUENZA

The most effective strategy for managing influenza is prevention. Two types of flu vaccines are available: inactivated and live attenuated (Table 27-3). The influenza vaccine may be changed on a yearly basis, depending on the virus strains identified by the Centers for Disease Control and Prevention as being most likely to cause illness in the upcoming flu season. The best time to receive the vaccine is in September (before flu exposure) because it takes 2 weeks for full protection to occur. Patients can receive it later if needed.

TABLE 27-3 TYPES OF INFLUENZA IMMUNIZATION

Trivalent Inactivated Influenza Vaccine (TIV)	Live Attenuated Influenza Vaccine (LSIV)
Given by injection	Given by nasal spray
Approved for use in people ≥6 mo of age	Approved for healthy people ages 2-49 yr
Can be used in people at increased risk: • People of any age with chronic medical conditions • Residents of nursing homes and long-term care facilities • People who are immunocompromised • Pregnant women	Should NOT be used in: • Children <2 yr or adults >50 yr • Pregnant women • People with known immunodeficiency • Children or adolescents receiving aspirin or other salicylates • People who have medical conditions that place them at increased risk for complications from influenza (chronic cardiovascular, pulmonary, or neurologic diseases; diabetes mellitus; renal or hepatic dysfunction; hemoglobinopathies) • Health care providers of high-risk patients because of risk of viral transmission from vaccine (should not care for high-risk patients for 7 days after vaccination)
Most common side effects are injection site reactions, such as pain, redness, and swelling	Most common side effects are runny nose and nasal congestion in all ages, fever in children ages 2-6 yr, and sore throat in adults

SAFETY ALERT

- Advocate for vaccination of all people older than 6 months of age but especially for those at high risk (e.g., health care workers, residents of long-term care facilities).
- Give high priority to groups, such as health care workers, that can transmit influenza to high-risk persons.

Vaccination of healthy people decreases the incidence and the risk of transmitting influenza to those who have less ability to cope with the effects of this illness. Despite obvious benefits, many persons are reluctant to be vaccinated. Current vaccines are highly purified, and reactions are extremely uncommon. Soreness at the injection site is usually the only side effect. Contraindications are history of Guillain-Barré syndrome within 6 weeks following a previous influenza vaccine and anaphylactic hypersensitivity to eggs.[13]

The primary nursing goals in influenza are relief of symptoms and prevention of secondary infection. Unless the patient with influenza is at high risk or complications develop, only supportive therapy is necessary. Rest, hydration, analgesics, and antipyretics can provide symptom relief. Older adults and those with a chronic illness may require hospitalization.

Two antiviral medications, zanamivir (Relenza) and oseltamivir (Tamiflu), are available to prevent and treat influenza A and B.[14] These drugs are neuraminidase inhibitors that prevent the virus from budding and spreading to other cells. These drugs shorten the duration of influenza symptoms and reduce the risk of complications. Treatment should be initiated as soon as possible in patients who are hospitalized with influenza, have severe or complicated illness, or are at high risk for complications. For maximum benefit in the treatment of influenza, therapy should begin within 2 days of the onset of symptoms, but it can be started later based on clinical judgment. Zanamivir is administered using an inhaler. Oseltamivir is available as an oral capsule.

SINUSITIS

Sinusitis affects one out of every seven adults in the United States. It develops when inflammation or hypertrophy (swelling) of the mucosa blocks the openings (ostia) in the sinuses through which mucus drains into the nose (Fig. 27-2). *Rhinosinusitis* is concurrent inflammation of the nasal mucosa. Obstruction of mucus drainage can also be caused by nasal polyps, foreign bodies, deviated septa, or tumors. The secretions

CULTURAL & ETHNIC HEALTH DISPARITIES

Immunizations in Hispanics

- Older Hispanics have lower influenza and pneumonia vaccination rates than non-Hispanic whites.
- Fifty-five percent of Hispanic older adults report receiving the "flu shot," compared with 67% of non-Hispanic older adults.
- Spanish-preferring Hispanic seniors are less likely to be immunized than English-preferring Hispanic seniors.
- Those living in newer immigration destinations are at greater risk for health disparities because of limited access to health care compared with persons in established Hispanic communities.
- Health care providers and policymakers need to target vulnerable subgroups of Hispanic seniors and identify areas of linguistic isolation to minimize these disparities.

Source: Haviland AM, Elliott MN, Hambarsoomian K, et al: Immunization disparities by Hispanic ethnicity and language preference, *Arch Intern Med* 171:158, 2011.

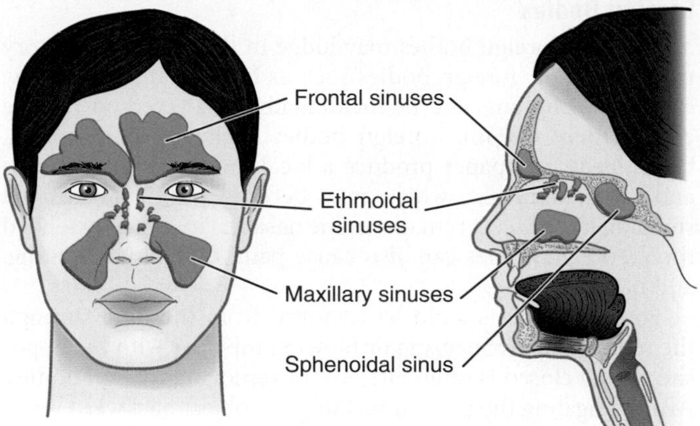

FIG. 27-2 Location of the sinuses.

that accumulate behind the blocked ostia provide a rich medium for growth of bacteria, viruses, and fungi, all of which may cause infection.

Viral sinusitis typically follows an upper respiratory tract infection in which the virus penetrates the mucous membrane and decreases ciliary function. Viral infections usually resolve without treatment in less than 14 days. If symptoms worsen after 3 to 5 days or persist for longer than 10 days, a secondary bacterial infection may be present. Only 5% to 10% of patients with viral sinusitis develop a bacterial infection requiring antibiotic therapy.[15] *Streptococcus pneumoniae, Haemophilus influenzae,* and *Moraxella catarrhalis* are the most common causes of bacterial sinusitis. Fungal sinusitis is uncommon, usually occurring in patients who are debilitated or immunocompromised.

Sinusitis can be classified as acute, subacute, or chronic. *Acute sinusitis* typically begins within 1 week of an upper respiratory tract infection and lasts less than 4 weeks. *Subacute sinusitis* is present when symptoms progress over 4 to 12 weeks. *Chronic sinusitis* (lasting longer than 12 weeks) is a persistent infection usually associated with allergies and nasal polyps. Chronic sinusitis generally results from repeated episodes of acute sinusitis that result in irreversible loss of the normal ciliated epithelium lining the sinus cavity.

COMPLEMENTARY & ALTERNATIVE THERAPIES

Zinc

Scientific Evidence

- When administered within 24 hr of onset of symptoms, zinc reduces the duration and severity of cold symptoms in healthy people.
- When zinc supplementation is taken for at least 5 mo, the incidence of colds is reduced.

Nursing Implications

- Zinc is regarded as relatively safe when taken at recommended doses.
- Zinc lozenges are more apt to cause adverse effects (bad taste, nausea) than syrup or tablets.
- Oral zinc should not be taken with foods that will reduce its absorption, such as caffeine and dairy products.

Source: Singh M, Das RR: Zinc for the common cold, *Cochrane Database Syst Rev* 16(2):CD001364, 2011.

Clinical Manifestations

Acute sinusitis causes significant pain over the affected sinus, purulent nasal drainage, nasal obstruction, congestion, fever, and malaise. The patient looks and feels sick. Assessment involves inspection of the nasal mucosa and palpation of the sinus points for pain. Findings that indicate acute sinusitis include hyperemic and edematous mucosa, discolored purulent nasal drainage, enlarged turbinates, and tenderness over the involved frontal and/or maxillary sinuses. Some patients have recurrent headaches that change in intensity with position changes or when secretions drain.

Chronic sinusitis is difficult to diagnose because symptoms are often nonspecific. The patient is rarely febrile. The patient may have facial or dental pain, nasal congestion, and increased drainage, but severe pain and purulent drainage are often absent. Some symptoms mimic those seen with allergies. X-rays or computed tomography (CT) scan of the sinuses may be done to confirm the diagnosis. CT scans may show the sinuses to be filled with fluid or a thickened mucous membrane. Nasal endoscopy with a flexible scope may be used to examine the sinuses, obtain drainage for culture, and restore normal drainage.

As many as 50% of patients with moderate to severe asthma have chronic sinusitis. The exact link between these diseases is unclear. Postnasal drip associated with sinusitis may trigger asthma by stimulating bronchoconstriction. Gastroesophageal reflux disease (GERD) and smoking may increase the risk of a person with asthma developing sinusitis. Appropriate treatment of sinusitis often causes a reduction in asthma symptoms.

NURSING AND COLLABORATIVE MANAGEMENT SINUSITIS

If allergies are the precipitating cause of sinusitis, instruct the patient about ways to reduce sinus inflammation and infection, including environmental control of allergens and appropriate drug therapy (see section on allergic rhinitis, earlier in this chapter).

Initial treatment for acute sinusitis focuses on symptom relief. Medications include oral or topical decongestants to promote drainage, nasal corticosteroids to decrease inflammation, analgesics to relieve pain, and saline nasal spray to relieve congestion. Instruct patients using topical decongestants to use the medication for no longer than 3 days to prevent rebound congestion caused by vasodilation. Saline irrigation of the nasal cavity can be used to rinse nasal passages, facilitate drainage, and decrease inflammation. Saline nasal spray is available over the counter as sterile physiologic saline solution in spray bottles. Alternatively, a saline solution can be prepared at home with ¼ tsp of salt dissolved in 8 oz of tap water. Patients may also add a pinch of baking soda to soften the effect of salt. Two to four puffs of nasal saline should be administered at least three times a day. The alternative, more aggressive method is lavage with a squeeze bottle, neti pot, or syringe while leaning over the sink with the mouth open.[16] Repeated full-syringe wash is recommended at least once a day to wash out the secretions if they cannot be effectively removed with saline spray alone. Alternatively, patients can use a Waterpik device on the lowest setting.

If symptoms worsen or persist for longer than 10 days, antibiotic therapy may be prescribed. Antibiotic therapy, consisting of amoxicillin as the first-line drug of choice, is continued for 10 to 14 days to prevent the formation of antibiotic-resistant

TABLE 27-4 PATIENT & CAREGIVER TEACHING GUIDE

Acute or Chronic Sinusitis

Include the following instructions when teaching the patient and caregiver about management of sinusitis.

1. Get plenty of rest to help body fight infection and promote recovery.
2. Keep well hydrated by drinking six to eight glasses of water to loosen secretions.
3. Take hot showers twice daily. Use a steam inhaler (15-min vaporization of boiled water), bedside humidifier, or nasal saline spray to promote secretion drainage.
4. Apply warm, damp towels around nose, cheeks, and eyes to ease facial pain.
5. Sleep with head elevated to help sinuses drain and reduce congestion.
6. Report a temperature of 100.4° F (38° C) or higher, which indicates infection.
7. Follow prescribed medication regimen:
   - Take analgesics to relieve pain.
   - Take decongestants/expectorants to relieve swelling.
   - Take antibiotics (as prescribed) for infection. Be sure to take entire prescription and report continued symptoms or a change in symptoms.
   - Administer nasal sprays correctly.
8. Perform large-volume nasal saline washes once or twice a day to wash sinuses.
9. Do not smoke, and avoid exposure to smoke. Smoke is an irritant and will worsen symptoms.
10. If allergies predispose to sinusitis, follow instructions regarding environmental control, drug therapy, and immunotherapy to reduce the inflammation and prevent sinus infection.

organisms. If symptoms do not resolve, the antibiotic should be changed to a broader spectrum cephalosporin antibiotic. With chronic sinusitis, mixed bacterial flora is often present and infections are difficult to eliminate. Broad-spectrum antibiotics may be used for 4 to 6 weeks. Patient and caregiver teaching for acute and chronic sinusitis is presented in Table 27-4.

Medical therapy may not relieve the symptoms of some patients with persistent or recurrent sinus complaints. They may require nasal endoscopic surgery to relieve blockage caused by hypertrophy or septal deviation. This is an outpatient procedure usually performed using local anesthesia. Propel, a self-expanding dissolvable implant, can be placed directly in the sinus during surgery to maintain postoperative patency and provide localized corticosteroid delivery directly to the sinus lining[17] (see Nursing Management: Nasal Surgery on p. 498).

OBSTRUCTION OF NOSE AND SINUSES

Nasal Polyps

Nasal polyps are soft, painless, benign growths that form slowly in response to repeated inflammation of the sinus or nasal mucosa. Polyps, which appear as gray-blue, semitransparent projections in the naris, can exceed the size of a grape. The patient may be anxious, fearing they are malignant. Small polyps are typically asymptomatic. Clinical manifestations of larger polyps include nasal obstruction, nasal discharge (usually clear mucus), and speech distortion. Topical and systemic corticosteroids are the primary medical therapy used to shrink nasal polyps. Endoscopic or laser surgery can remove nasal polyps, but recurrence is common.

Foreign Bodies

A variety of foreign bodies may lodge in the upper respiratory tract. Inorganic foreign bodies such as buttons and beads may cause no symptoms and be incidentally discovered on routine examination. Organic foreign bodies such as wood, cotton, beans, peas, and paper produce a local inflammatory reaction and nasal discharge, which may become purulent and foul smelling if the object remains in the nasal cavity for an extended time. Foreign bodies can also cause pain, difficulty breathing, and nasal bleeding.

Foreign bodies should be removed from the nose through the route of entry. Sneezing or blowing the nose with the opposite nostril closed is often effective in removing foreign bodies. Avoid irrigating the nose or pushing the object backward, since either could cause aspiration and airway obstruction. If sneezing or blowing the nose does not remove the object, the patient should see a health care provider.

PROBLEMS OF PHARYNX

ACUTE PHARYNGITIS

Acute pharyngitis is an acute inflammation of the pharyngeal walls. It may include the tonsils, palate, and uvula. It can be caused by a viral, bacterial, or fungal infection. Viral pharyngitis accounts for approximately 90% of cases in adults. Bacterial pharyngitis ("strep throat") usually results from β-hemolytic streptococci and accounts for 10% of cases in adults. Fungal pharyngitis, such as candidiasis, can develop with prolonged use of antibiotics or inhaled corticosteroids. It can also occur in immunosuppressed patients, especially those with human immunodeficiency virus (HIV) infection. Other causes of pharyngitis include dry air, smoking, GERD, allergy and postnasal drip, chemicals, neoplasia, and endotracheal intubation.[18]

Clinical Manifestations

Symptoms of acute pharyngitis range in severity from complaints of a "scratchy throat" to pain so severe that swallowing is difficult. Both viral and strep infections appear as a red and edematous pharynx, with or without patchy exudates. Fever, anterior cervical lymph node enlargement, tonsillar exudates, and the absence of cough are highly suggestive of bacterial pharyngitis. However, appearance is not always diagnostic. When two or three of the above criteria are present, a rapid strep antigen test and/or a culture is done to establish the cause and direct appropriate management. White, irregular patches on the oropharynx suggest fungal infection with *Candida albicans.*

NURSING AND COLLABORATIVE MANAGEMENT ACUTE PHARYNGITIS

The goals of nursing management are infection control, symptom relief, and prevention of secondary complications. Penicillin is the drug of choice for bacterial pharyngitis. This antibiotic needs to be taken several times a day for a full 10 days to prevent rheumatic fever, a sequela to the infection. Other antibiotics (amoxicillin, azithromycin [Zithromax], cephalosporins) may also be used. Most people with strep infections are contagious until they have been on antibiotics for 24 to 48 hours.

Candida infections are treated with nystatin (Mycostatin), an antifungal antibiotic. Tell patients to swish the preparation in their mouth as long as possible before swallowing it. Treatment should continue until symptoms are gone. Patients taking inhaled corticosteroids are at risk for infection with *Candida* organisms. Thoroughly rinsing the mouth out with water after using corticosteroids can prevent this infection.

Instruct patients to use ibuprofen or acetaminophen for pain relief. Encourage the patient with pharyngitis to increase fluid intake. To relieve the symptoms, instruct the patient to gargle with warm salt water (½ tsp of salt in 8 oz of water); drink warm or cold liquids; and suck on popsicles, hard candies, or throat lozenges. Cool, bland liquids and gelatin will not irritate the pharynx; citrus juices are often irritating. Encourage the patient to use a cool-mist vaporizer or humidifier.

PERITONSILLAR ABSCESS

Peritonsillar abscess is a complication of acute pharyngitis and is most often caused by β-hemolytic streptococci. The abscess causes pain, swelling, and (when severe) blockage of the throat, threatening airway patency. The patient also experiences a high fever, chills, leukocytosis, difficulty swallowing, and a muffled voice. IV antibiotic therapy is given along with needle aspiration or incision and drainage of the abscess. In some cases an emergency tonsillectomy is performed, or an elective tonsillectomy is scheduled after the infection has subsided.

PROBLEMS OF TRACHEA AND LARYNX

AIRWAY OBSTRUCTION

Acute airway obstruction is a medical emergency. Airway obstruction can be caused by aspiration of food or a foreign body, allergic reactions, edema and inflammation caused by infections or burns, peritonsillar or retropharyngeal abscesses, malignancy, laryngeal or tracheal stenosis, and trauma. Symptoms include choking, stridor, use of accessory muscles, suprasternal and intercostal retractions, flaring nostrils, wheezing, restlessness, tachycardia, cyanosis, and change in level of consciousness. Airway obstruction may be partial or complete. Prompt assessment and treatment are essential because partial obstruction may quickly progress to complete obstruction. Complete airway obstruction can result in permanent brain damage or death if not corrected within 3 to 5 minutes.

Interventions to reestablish a patent airway include the obstructed airway (Heimlich) maneuver (see Appendix A), cricothyroidotomy, endotracheal intubation, and tracheostomy. Unexplained or recurrent symptoms indicate the need for additional tests, such as a chest x-ray, laryngoscopy, and bronchoscopy.

TRACHEOSTOMY

A **tracheostomy** is a surgically created stoma (opening) in the trachea to establish an airway. It is used to (1) bypass an upper airway obstruction, (2) facilitate removal of secretions, or (3) permit long-term mechanical ventilation. Most patients who require mechanical ventilation are initially managed with an endotracheal tube, which can be quickly inserted in an emergency. (Care of the patient with an endotracheal tube is discussed in Chapter 66.)

Most *surgical tracheostomies* are performed in the operating room using general anesthesia. These are typically done electively on patients already intubated who require prolonged mechanical ventilation. When swelling, trauma, or upper airway obstruction prevents endotracheal intubation, an emergent surgical tracheostomy may be performed at the bedside.

A minimally invasive *percutaneous tracheostomy* can also be performed at the bedside using local anesthesia and sedation. A needle is placed into the trachea, followed by a guide wire. The opening is progressively dilated until it is large enough for insertion of a tracheostomy tube.

A tracheostomy provides a more secure airway, is less likely to be displaced, and allows more freedom of movement than an endotracheal tube. There is less risk of long-term damage to the vocal cords. Airway resistance and work of breathing are decreased, facilitating independent breathing.[19] Patient comfort may be increased because no tube is present in the mouth. The patient can eat with a tracheostomy because the tube enters lower in the airway (Fig. 27-3). Speaking is also permitted once the tracheostomy cuff can be deflated.

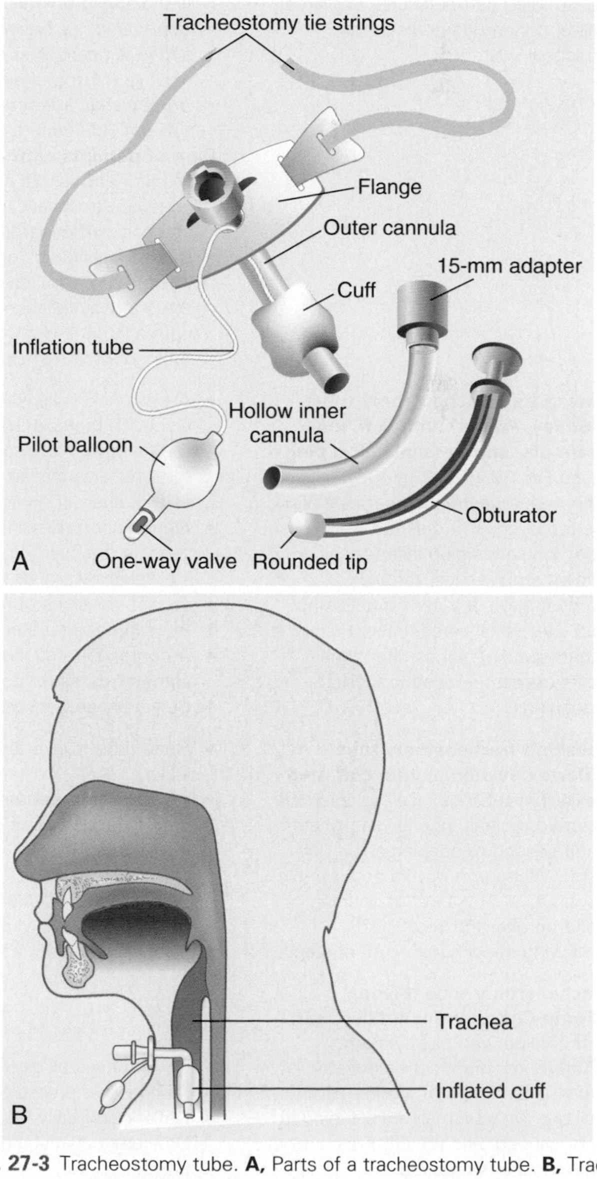

FIG. 27-3 Tracheostomy tube. **A,** Parts of a tracheostomy tube. **B,** Tracheostomy tube inserted in airway with inflated cuff. (See Table 27-5 and eNursing Care Plan 27-1 [on the website for this chapter] for related nursing management.)

NURSING MANAGEMENT TRACHEOSTOMY

PROVIDING TRACHEOSTOMY CARE

Before the tracheostomy procedure, explain to the patient and the caregiver the purpose of the procedure. Also inform them that the patient will not be able to speak while an inflated cuff is used.

A variety of tubes are available to meet individual patient needs (Table 27-5; see Fig. 27-3). All tracheostomy tubes contain a faceplate, or *flange,* which rests on the neck between the clavicles and outer cannula. In addition, all tubes have an *obturator,* which is used when inserting the tube (see Fig. 27-3, *A*). During insertion of the tube, place the obturator inside the outer cannula with its rounded tip protruding from the end of the tube to ease insertion. After insertion, immediately remove the obturator so air can flow through the tube. Keep the obturator in an easily accessible place at the bedside (e.g., taped to the wall) so that it can be used quickly in case of accidental decannulation.

TABLE 27-5 NURSING MANAGEMENT OF TRACHEOSTOMIES

Tube and Characteristics	Nursing Management
Tracheostomy tube with cuff and pilot balloon (see Fig. 27-3, *A* and *B*) When properly inflated, low-pressure, high-volume cuff distributes cuff pressure over large area, minimizing pressure on tracheal wall.	**Procedure for cuff inflation** • *Mechanically ventilated patient:* Inflate the cuff using *minimal occlusion volume (MOV) technique* by slowly injecting air into the cuff until no leak (sound) is heard at peak inspiratory pressure (end of ventilator inspiration) when a stethoscope is placed over the trachea. An alternative approach, termed *minimal leak technique* (MLT), involves inflating the cuff to minimal occlusion pressure and then withdrawing 0.1 mL of air. • *Spontaneously breathing patient:* Inflate cuff using MOV by slowly injecting air into the cuff until no sound is heard after deep breath or during inhalation with manual resuscitation bag. If using MLT, remove 0.1 mL of air while maintaining seal. MLT should not be used if there is risk of aspiration. • *Immediately after cuff inflation (both groups):* Verify pressure is within accepted range (≤20 mm Hg or ≤25 cm H_2O) with a manometer. Record cuff pressure and volume of air used for cuff inflation in chart. **Care of patients with an inflated cuff** • Monitor and record cuff pressure q8hr. Cuff pressure should be ≤20 mm Hg or ≤25 cm H_2O to allow adequate tracheal capillary perfusion. If needed, remove or add air to the pilot tubing using a syringe and stopcock. Afterward, verify cuff pressure is within accepted range with manometer. • Report inability to keep the cuff inflated or need to use progressively larger volumes of air to keep cuff inflated. Potential causes include tracheal dilation at the cuff site or a crack or slow leak in the housing of the one-way inflation valve. If the leak is due to tracheal dilation, the physician may intubate the patient with a larger tube. Cracks in the inflation valve may be temporarily managed by clamping the small-bore tubing with a hemostat. The tube should be changed within 24 hr.
Fenestrated tracheostomy tube (Shiley, Portex) with cuff, inner cannula, and decannulation plug (see Fig. 27-7, *A*) When nonfenestrated inner cannula is removed, cuff deflated, and decannulation plug inserted, air flows around tube, through fenestration in outer cannula, and up over vocal cords. Patient can then speak. A fenestrated inner cannula can be used to facilitate cleaning.	• Assess risk of aspiration before removing inner cannula. This is best accomplished by consulting with a speech therapist. An alternative but less reliable method is the use of colored liquid (e.g., Kool-Aid). Deflate cuff. Note coughing. Have patient swallow a small amount of colored liquid. Observe secretions for color after patient coughs or is suctioned. Severe coughing or cyanosis after drinking is also indicative of aspiration. If no aspiration is noted, a fenestrated tube may be used. • ***Never*** insert decannulation plug in tracheostomy tube until cuff is deflated and nonfenestrated inner cannula removed. Prior insertion will prevent patient from breathing (no air inflow). This may precipitate a respiratory arrest. • Assess for signs of respiratory distress when a fenestrated cannula is first used. If this occurs, remove the cap, insert a nonfenestrated inner cannula, and reinflate the cuff. • A nonfenestrated inner cannula must be used to suction patient to prevent tracheal damage from suction catheter passing through fenestrated openings. • Cuff management as described above.
Speaking tracheostomy tube (Portex, National) with cuff, two external tubings (see Fig. 27-7, *B*) Has two tubings, one leading to cuff and second to opening above the cuff. When port is connected to air source, air flows out of opening and up over the vocal cords, allowing speech with cuff inflated.	• Once tube is inserted, wait 2 days before use so that the stoma can close around the tube and prevent leaks. • When patient desires to speak, connect port to compressed air (or O_2). Be certain to identify correct tubing. If gas enters the cuff, it will overinflate and rupture, requiring an emergency tube change. Use lowest flow (typically 4-6 L/min) that results in speech. High flows dehydrate mucosa. • Cover port adapter. This will cause the air to flow upward. Instruct patient to speak in short sentences because voice becomes a whisper with long sentences. • Disconnect flow when patient does not want to speak to prevent mucosal dehydration. • Cuff management as described above.
Tracheostomy tube (Bivona Fome-Cuf) with foam-filled cuff Cuff is filled with plastic foam. Before insertion, cuff is deflated. After insertion, cuff is allowed to fill passively with air. Pilot tubing is not capped, and no cuff pressure monitoring is required.	• Before insertion, withdraw all air from the cuff using a 20-mL syringe. Cap pilot balloon tubing to prevent reentry of air. After tracheostomy is inserted, remove cap from pilot tubing, allowing cuff to passively reinflate. • Do not inject air into tubing or cap pilot balloon tubing while it is in patient. Air will flow in and out in response to pressure changes (head turning). Place tag on tubing to alert staff not to cap or inflate cuff. • Deflate cuff daily via pilot balloon to evaluate integrity of cuff. Also assess ability to easily deflate cuff. Difficulty deflating cuff indicates a need for tube change. If aspirate returns with air, cuff is no longer intact. • Tube can be used for up to 1 mo in patients on home mechanical ventilation. • Good choice for patients who require inflated cuff at home, since teaching about cuff pressure is simplified.

Some tracheostomy tubes also have an inner cannula, which can be removed for cleaning (see Fig. 27-3, *A*). The inner cannula can be disposable or nondisposable. If it is disposable, replace per manufacturer and institutional guidelines. If nondisposable, clean the inner cannula at least every 8 hours (Table 27-6). Cleaning removes mucus from the inside of the tube to prevent airway obstruction. If humidification is adequate, mucus may not accumulate and a tube without an inner cannula can be used. Suction the airway via the tracheostomy tube as needed (Fig. 27-4 and Table 27-6). Also, clean around the stoma at least every 8 hours and change the tracheostomy ties as needed (Fig. 27-5 and Table 27-7). A two-person technique, one to stabilize the tracheostomy and one to change the ties, is best to ensure that the tracheostomy does not become accidentally dislodged during the procedure. Place two fingers underneath the ties to ensure they are not too tight around the neck.[20]

Both cuffed and uncuffed tracheostomy tubes are available. A tracheostomy tube with an inflated cuff is used if the patient is at risk of aspiration or needs mechanical ventilation. Because an inflated cuff exerts pressure on the tracheal mucosa, it is important to inflate the cuff with the minimum volume of air required to obtain an airway seal. Cuff inflation pressure should not exceed 20 mm Hg or 25 cm H_2O because higher pressures may compress tracheal capillaries, limit blood flow, and predispose the patient to tracheal necrosis. The minimal leak technique (MLT) and the minimal occlusion volume (MOV) are two commonly used methods to inflate the tracheostomy cuff (see Table 27-5).

Routine cuff deflation is no longer recommended.[21] When the patient is not at risk for aspiration, the cuff may be deflated to allow the patient to talk and swallow more easily. Before deflation, have the patient cough up secretions, if possible, and suction the tracheostomy tube and then the mouth (see Table 27-6). This step is important to prevent secretions from being aspirated during deflation. The cuff is deflated during exhalation because the exhaled gas helps propel secretions into the mouth. Have the patient cough, and then suction the tube after cuff deflation. Assess the patient's ability to protect the airway from aspiration. Remain with the patient when the cuff is initially deflated. If needed, reinflate the cuff during inspiration.

Retention sutures may be placed in the tracheal cartilage when the tracheostomy is performed. Tape the free ends of the sutures to the skin in a place and manner that leaves them accessible in case the tube is dislodged. Take care not to dislodge the tracheostomy tube during the first 5 to 7 days when the stoma is not mature (healed). Because tube replacement is difficult, several precautions are required: (1) keep a replacement tube of equal or smaller size at the bedside, readily available for emergency reinsertion; (2) do not change tracheostomy tapes for at least 24 hours after the insertion procedure; and (3) a physician

TABLE 27-6 SUCTIONING A TRACHEOSTOMY TUBE

1. Assess the need for suctioning q2hr. Indications include coarse crackles or rhonchi over large airways, moist cough, increase in peak inspiratory pressure on mechanical ventilator, and restlessness or agitation if accompanied by decrease in SpO_2 or PaO_2. Do not suction routinely or if patient is able to clear secretions with cough.
2. If suctioning is indicated, explain procedure to patient.
3. Collect necessary sterile equipment: suction catheter (no larger than half the lumen of the tracheostomy tube), gloves, sterile water, cup, and drape. If a closed tracheal suction system is used, the catheter is enclosed in a plastic sleeve and reused (see Fig. 27-4). No additional equipment is needed.
4. Check suction source and regulator. Adjust suction pressure until the dial reads −120 to −150 mm Hg pressure with tubing occluded.
5. Assess SpO_2 and heart rate and rhythm to provide baseline for detecting change during suctioning.
6. Wash hands and put on goggles.
7. Use sterile technique to open package, fill cup with sterile water, put on sterile gloves, and connect catheter to suction tubing. Designate one hand as contaminated for (1) connecting and disconnecting the tubing at the suction catheter, (2) using the resuscitation bag, and (3) operating the suction control. Suction sterile water through the catheter to test the system.
8. Provide preoxygenation for a minimum of 30 seconds by (1) adjusting ventilator to deliver 100% O_2; (2) using a reservoir-equipped manual resuscitation bag (MRB) connected to 100% O_2; or (3) asking the patient to take 5-6 deep breaths while administering O_2. The method chosen depends on the patient's underlying disease and acuity of illness. The patient who has had a tracheostomy for an extended period and is not acutely ill may be able to tolerate suctioning without use of an MRB or the ventilator.
9. Gently insert catheter *without suction* to minimize the amount of O_2 removed from the lungs. Insert the catheter to the point where the patient coughs or resistance is met, or 0.5-1.0 cm beyond the length of the artificial airway. Withdraw the catheter 0.5-1.0 cm before applying suction to prevent trauma to the carina.
10. Apply suction intermittently, while withdrawing catheter in a rotating manner. If secretion volume is large, apply suction continuously. Suction should be applied for as short a time as possible to minimize decreases in arterial oxygenation levels.
11. *Limit suction time to 10 seconds.* Discontinue suctioning if heart rate decreases from baseline by 20 beats/min, increases from baseline by 40 beats/min, a dysrhythmia occurs, or SpO_2 decreases to less than 90%.
12. After each suction pass, oxygenate for at least 30 sec with 5-6 breaths by ventilator or MRB or deep breaths with O_2.
13. Rinse catheter with sterile water between suction passes.
14. Repeat procedure until airway is clear. Limit insertions of suction catheter to as few as needed. If airway is not clear after three suction passes, allow the patient to rest before additional suctioning.
15. Return O_2 concentration to prior setting.
16. Rinse catheter, and suction the oropharynx or use mouth suction.
17. Dispose of catheter by wrapping it around fingers of gloved hand and pulling glove over catheter. Discard equipment in proper waste container.
18. Auscultate to assess changes in lung sounds. Record time, amount, and character of secretions and response to suctioning.

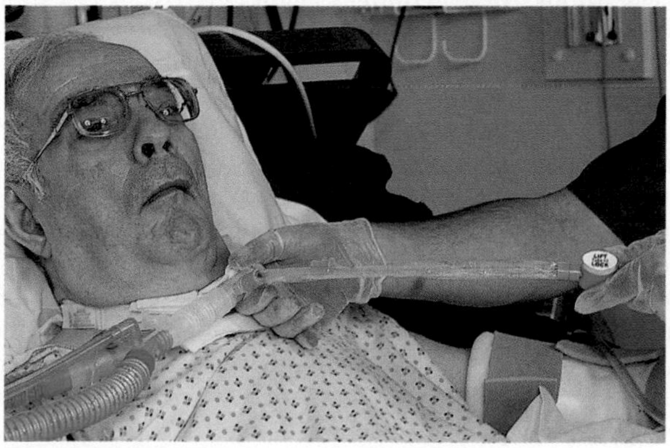

FIG. 27-4 Suctioning tracheostomy with closed system suction catheter.

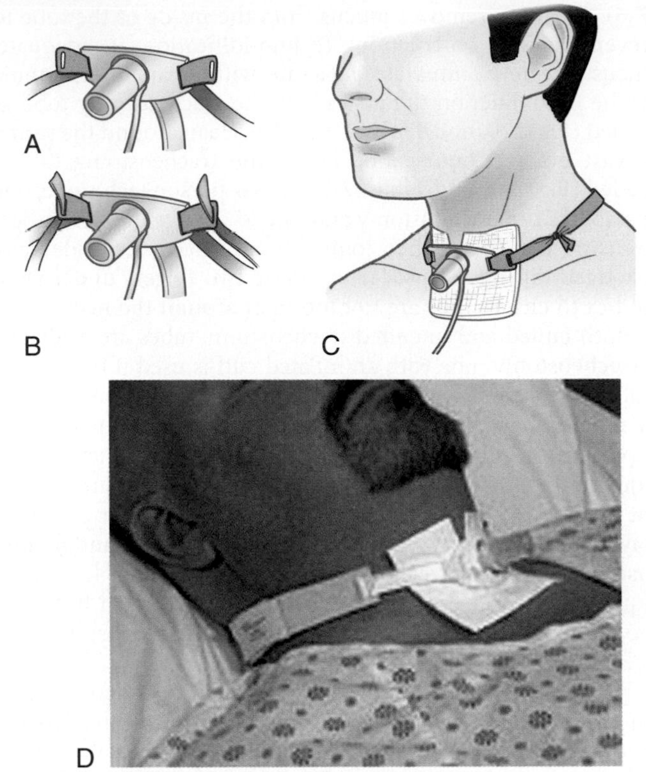

FIG. 27-5 Changing tracheostomy ties. **A,** A slit is cut about 1 in (2.5 cm) from the end. The slit end is put into the opening of the cannula. **B,** A loop is made with the other end of the tape. **C,** The tapes are tied together with a double knot on the side of the neck. **D,** A Velcro tracheostomy tube holder can be used instead of twill ties to make tracheostomy tube stabilization more secure.

performs the first tube change usually no sooner than 7 days after the tracheostomy.

If the tube is accidentally dislodged, immediately attempt to replace it. Grasp the retention sutures (if present) or use a hemostat to spread the opening to facilitate replacing the tube. Insert the obturator in the replacement tube, lubricated with saline poured over the tip, and insert the tube into the stoma at a 45-degree angle to the neck. Once the tube is inserted, remove the obturator immediately so that air can flow through the tube. Another method is to insert a suction catheter to allow passage of air and to serve as a guide for insertion. Thread the tracheostomy tube over the catheter and remove the suction catheter. If the tube cannot be replaced, assess the level of respiratory distress. Position the patient in the semi-Fowler's position to alleviate minor dyspnea until assistance arrives. Severe dyspnea may progress to respiratory arrest. If this situation occurs, cover the stoma with a sterile dressing, and ventilate the patient with bag-mask ventilation over the nose and mouth until help arrives. If a patient has had a total laryngectomy, there will be complete separation between the upper airway and the trachea. Ventilate this patient through the tracheostomy stoma.

Initially, tracheostomy patients should receive humidified air to compensate for the loss of the upper airway to warm and moisturize secretions. Humidification is essential to prevent retention of tenacious secretions and formation of mucous plugs. Change the tube approximately once a month after the first tube change. When a tracheostomy has been in place for several months, the healed tract will be well formed. Teach the patient to change the tube using a clean technique at home

TABLE 27-7 TRACHEOSTOMY CARE

1. Explain procedure to patient.
2. Use tracheostomy care kit or collect necessary sterile equipment (e.g., suction catheter, gloves, water basin, drape, tracheostomy ties, tube brush or pipe cleaners, 4 × 4 gauze pads, sterile water or normal saline, and tracheostomy dressing [optional]). NOTE: Clean rather than sterile technique is used at home.
3. Position patient in semi-Fowler's position.
4. Assemble needed materials on bedside table next to patient.
5. Wash hands. Put on goggles and clean gloves.
6. Auscultate chest sounds. If rhonchi or coarse crackles are present, suction the patient if unable to cough up secretions (see Table 27-6). Remove soiled dressing and clean gloves.
7. Open sterile equipment, pour sterile H_2O or normal saline into two compartments of sterile container or two basins, and put on sterile gloves. NOTE: Hydrogen peroxide (3%) is no longer recommended unless an infection is present. If it is used, rinse the inner cannula and skin with sterile H_2O or normal saline afterward to prevent trauma to tissue.
8. Unlock and remove inner cannula, if present. Many tracheostomy tubes do not have inner cannulas. Care for these tubes includes all steps except for inner cannula care.
9. If disposable inner cannula is used, replace with new cannula. If a nondisposable cannula is used:
   - Immerse inner cannula in sterile solution and clean inside and outside of cannula using tube brush or pipe cleaners.
   - Rinse cannula in sterile solution. Remove from solution and shake to dry.
   - Insert inner cannula into outer cannula with the curved part downward, and lock in place.
10. Remove dried secretions from stoma using 4 × 4 gauze pad soaked in sterile water or saline. Gently pat area around the stoma dry. Be sure to clean under the tracheostomy faceplate, using cotton swabs to reach this area.
11. Maintain position of tracheal retention sutures (if present) by taping above and below the stoma.
12. Change tracheostomy ties. Use two-person change technique or secure new ties to flanges before removing the old ones. Tie tracheostomy ties securely with room for two fingers between ties and skin (see Fig. 27-5). To prevent accidental tube removal, secure the tracheostomy tube by gently applying pressure to the flange of the tube during the tie changes. *Do not change tracheostomy ties for 24 hr after the tracheostomy procedure.*
13. As an alternative, some patients prefer tracheostomy ties made of Velcro, which are easier to adjust.
14. If drainage is excessive, place dressing around tube (see Fig. 27-5). A tracheostomy dressing or unlined gauze should be used. Do not cut the gauze because threads may be inhaled or wrap around the tracheostomy tube. Change the dressing frequently. Wet dressings promote infection and stoma irritation.
15. Repeat care three times/day and as needed.

(Fig. 27-6). Monitor the patient for potential complications[22] (Table 27-8).

SWALLOWING DYSFUNCTION

The patient with a tracheostomy who cannot protect the airway from aspiration requires an inflated cuff. However, an inflated cuff may result in swallowing dysfunction by interfering with the normal function of muscles used to swallow. It is important to evaluate the patient's swallowing ability and risk for aspiration with the cuff deflated. If the patient is able to swallow without aspiration when the cuff is deflated, the cuff may be left deflated or a cuffless tube substituted. Clinical assessment of the patient's ability to swallow is done by a speech therapist, videofluoroscopy, or fiberoptic endoscopic evaluations.[23]

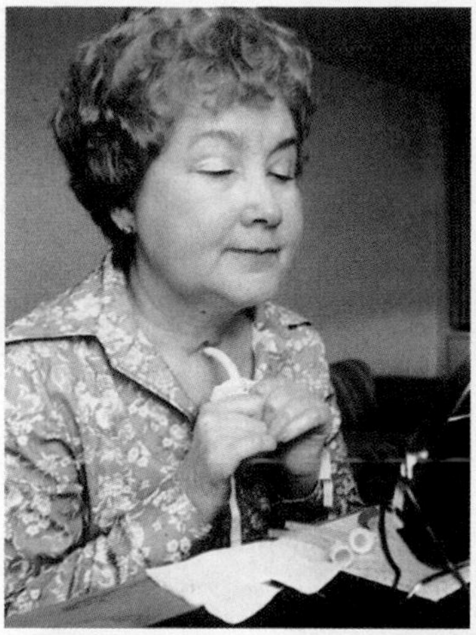

FIG. 27-6 Changing the tracheostomy tube at home. When a tracheostomy has been in place for several months, the tract will be well formed. The patient can be taught to change the tube using a clean technique at home.

TABLE 27-8 COMPLICATIONS OF TRACHEOSTOMY

Closely monitor patients with a tracheostomy for the following potential complications:

• Airway obstruction	• Impaired cough
• Air leak	• Infection—wound or respiratory tract
• Altered body image	• Subcutaneous emphysema
• Aspiration	• Tracheal stenosis
• Bleeding	• Tracheal necrosis
• Fistula formation	• Tube displacement

SPEECH WITH A TRACHEOSTOMY TUBE

A number of techniques promote speech in the patient with a tracheostomy. The spontaneously breathing patient may be able to talk by deflating the cuff, which allows exhaled air to flow upward over the vocal cords. This can be enhanced by the patient occluding the tube. However, this method is discouraged because bacteria from the fingers can lead to infection. Specialized tracheostomy tubes and speaking valves are available to facilitate speech. Advocating for the use of these devices will provide psychologic benefits and facilitate self-care for the patient with a tracheostomy.

A *fenestrated tube* has openings on the surface of the outer cannula that permit air from the lungs to flow over the vocal cords (see Fig. 27-7, *A*). A fenestrated tube allows the patient to breathe spontaneously through the larynx, speak, and cough up secretions while the tracheostomy tube remains in place. Air passes from the lungs through the openings in the tracheostomy into the upper airway and out the mouth and nose. Only patients who can swallow without risk of aspiration can use this tube. The inner cannula can be fenestrated or nonfenestrated. Use a nonfenestrated inner cannula when suctioning to decrease the risk of tracheal damage caused by the suction catheter going through the openings. The nonfenestrated inner cannula is also used whenever the patient needs to be mechanically ventilated.

Before using the fenestrated tube, determine the patient's ability to swallow without aspiration (see Table 27-5 and eNursing Care Plan 27-1, available on the website for this chapter). If there is no aspiration, (1) remove the inner cannula (if nonfenestrated), (2) deflate the cuff, and (3) place the decannulation cap in the tube (see Fig. 27-7, *A*). It is important to perform the

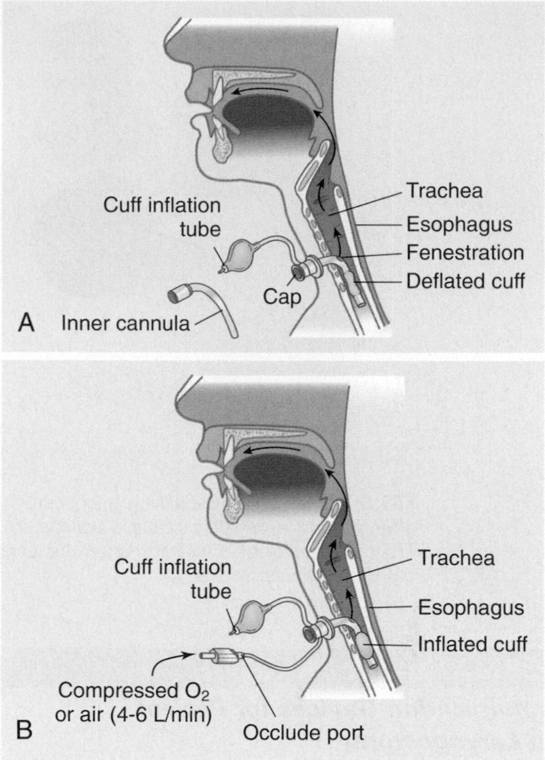

FIG. 27-7 Speaking tracheostomy tubes. **A,** Fenestrated tracheostomy tube with cuff deflated, inner cannula removed, and tracheostomy tube capped to allow air to pass over the vocal cords. **B,** Speaking tracheostomy tube. One tube is used for cuff inflation. The second tube is connected to a source of compressed air or O_2. When the port on the second tube is occluded, air flows up over the vocal cords, allowing speech with an inflated cuff. (See Table 27-5 and eNursing Care Plan 27-1 for related nursing management.)

steps in order because severe respiratory distress may result if the tube is capped before removing the inner cannula and deflating the cuff. When a fenestrated cannula is first used, frequently assess the patient for signs of respiratory distress. If the patient is not able to tolerate the procedure, remove the cap, insert a nonfenestrated inner cannula, and reinflate the cuff. A disadvantage of fenestrated tubes is the potential for development of tracheal polyps from tracheal tissue granulating into the fenestrated openings.

A speaking tracheostomy tube has two pigtail tubings. One tubing connects to the cuff and is for cuff inflation, and the second connects to an opening just above the cuff (see Fig. 27-7, *B*). When the second tubing is connected to a low-flow (4 to 6 L/minute) air source, sufficient air moves up over the vocal cords to permit speech. This device allows a patient at risk for aspiration to speak with the tracheostomy cuff inflated. However, speech quality is typically poor, with the patient barely speaking above a whisper.

A variety of speaking valves are available that can be attached to the tracheostomy tube (Fig. 27-8). These valves contain a thin plastic diaphragm that opens on inspiration and closes on expiration. During inspiration, air flows in through the valve. During expiration, the valve prevents exhalation and air flows upward over the vocal cords and into the mouth, allowing normal speech patterns. When a speaking tracheostomy valve is used, a cuffless tube must be in place or the cuff needs to be deflated to allow exhalation. Before attaching a speaking valve, evaluate the patient's ability to tolerate cuff deflation without

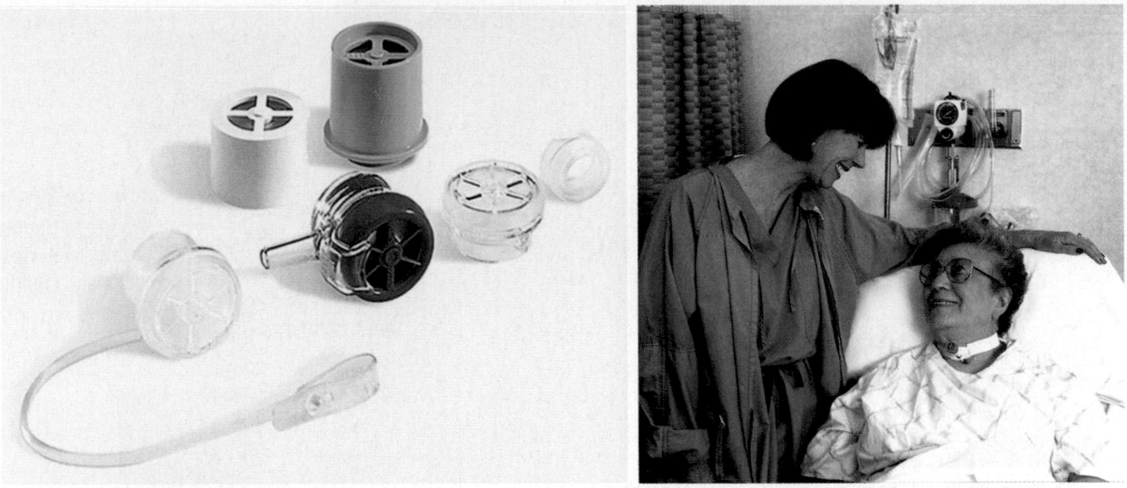

FIG. 27-8 Passy-Muir speaking tracheostomy valve. The valve is placed over the hub of the tracheostomy tube after the cuff is deflated. Multiple options are available and can be used for ventilated and nonventilated patients. The one-way valve allows air to enter the lungs during inspiration and redirects air upward over the vocal cords into the mouth during expiration.

INFORMATICS IN PRACTICE

Communication Devices for Patient With Laryngectomy

- Assisting with communication will improve a patient's quality of life after a laryngectomy.
- Use an iPad or iPhone and download a text-to-speech application. These applications allow the patient to type in text, and then a computer voice says the text aloud.
- You can also teach the patient how to use a keyboard-based communication program. The patient types on a traditional keyboard and generates speech that is transmitted through hand-held speakers.

aspiration or respiratory distress. Once the speaking valve is in place, carefully assess the patient's ability to breathe. The patient may initially be able to tolerate only short periods of use until he or she becomes acclimated to exhaling through the mouth. Remove the valve immediately if the patient demonstrates any signs of respiratory distress.

If speaking devices are not used, provide the patient with a paper and pencil or Magic Slate. A communication board with pictures of common needs and an alphabet for spelling words is useful for patients who are weak or have difficulty writing.

DECANNULATION

When the patient can adequately exchange air and expectorate secretions, the tracheostomy tube can be removed. Close the stoma with tape strips and cover it with an occlusive dressing. The dressing must be changed if it gets soiled or wet. Instruct the patient to splint the stoma with the fingers when coughing, swallowing, or speaking. Epithelial tissue begins to form in 24 to 48 hours, and the opening closes within 4 or 5 days. Surgical intervention to close the tracheostomy is not required.

LARYNGEAL POLYPS

Laryngeal polyps develop on the vocal cords from vocal abuse (e.g., excessive talking, singing) or irritation (e.g., intubation, cigarette smoking). The most common symptom is hoarseness. Polyps are treated conservatively with voice rest and adequate hydration. Surgical removal may be indicated for large polyps, which may cause dysphagia, dyspnea, and stridor. Polyps are usually benign but may be removed because they can become malignant.

HEAD AND NECK CANCER

Most head and neck cancers arise from squamous cells that line the mucosal surfaces of the head and neck region. The cancer is identified according to the area of origin (e.g., paranasal sinuses, oral cavity, nasopharynx, oropharynx, larynx). (Cancer of the oral cavity is discussed in Chapter 42.)

An estimated 52,600 new cases of head and neck cancer are diagnosed each year in the United States. Eighty-five percent are caused by tobacco use. Excessive alcohol consumption is also a major risk factor. Head and neck cancer occurs most frequently in patients 50 to 60 years of age. Cancers in patients younger than 50 have been associated with human papillomavirus (HPV) infection. Other risk factors include sun exposure (oral cavity), radiation therapy to the head and neck, exposure to asbestos and other industrial carcinogens, and poor oral hygiene.[24] Men are affected twice as often as women.[25]

Most people have locally advanced disease at the time of diagnosis. Disability from the disease and the treatment is great because of the potential loss of voice, disfigurement, and social consequences.

Clinical Manifestations

Early signs and symptoms of head and neck cancer vary with the tumor location. Cancer of the oral cavity may initially be seen as a white or red patch in the mouth, an ulcer that does not heal, or a change in the fit of dentures. Hoarseness that lasts more than 2 weeks may be a symptom of early laryngeal cancer. Some patients experience what feels like a lump in the throat or a change in voice quality. Other clinical manifestations include a sore throat that does not get better with treatment, unilateral sore throat or otalgia (ear pain), swelling or lumps in the neck, and coughing up blood. Difficulties chewing, swallowing, moving the tongue or jaw, and breathing are typically late symptoms. Unintentional weight loss and pain are also late symptoms of head and neck cancer.

Diagnostic Studies

Early detection is key to patient survival. Thoroughly examine the oral cavity, including the area under the tongue and dentures, with a flashlight. Bimanually palpate the floor of the mouth, tongue, and lymph nodes in the neck. There may be thickening of the normally soft and pliable oral mucosa. *Leukoplakia* (white patch) or *erythroplakia* (red patch) may be seen and should be noted for later biopsy. Both leukoplakia and carcinoma in situ (localized to a defined area) may precede invasive carcinoma by many years.

If lesions are suspected, the upper airways may be examined using indirect laryngoscopy, which involves using a laryngeal mirror or a flexible nasopharyngoscope to visualize the larynx. The larynx and vocal cords are visually inspected for lesions and tissue mobility. A CT scan or magnetic resonance imaging (MRI) may be performed to detect local and regional spread. Neoplastic tissue is identifiable because it has a greater density or because it distorts, displaces, or destroys normal anatomic structures. The use of positron emission tomography (PET) scanning along with CT has been successful in diagnosing recurrent cases of head and neck cancer. Typically, multiple biopsy specimens are obtained to determine the extent of the disease.

Collaborative Care

Head and neck cancer is staged based on tumor size (T), number and location of involved nodes (N), and extent of metastasis (M). TNM staging classifies disease as stage I to stage IV. Choice of treatment is based on exact location of tumor, disease stage, patient age and general health, cosmetic and functional considerations (e.g., ability to talk, swallow, and chew), urgency of treatment, and patient choice. Treatment modalities include surgery, radiation therapy, chemotherapy, and targeted therapy. Stage I and II cancers are potentially curable with single-modality radiation therapy or larynx-sparing surgery. Radiation therapy is often preferred for patients with early laryngeal cancer because it offers the patient good results with voice preservation. Surgery can then be reserved for recurrence or poor response to radiation. Patients with advanced disease (stages III and IV) are treated with various combinations of surgery, radiation, chemotherapy, and targeted therapy. Radiation therapy can be delivered by either external-beam therapy or internal implants (brachytherapy). Brachytherapy is a concentrated and localized method of delivering radiation that involves placing a radioactive source into or near the tumor. The goal is to deliver high doses of radiation to the target area while limiting exposure of surrounding tissues. Thin, hollow, plastic needles are inserted into the tumor area, and radioactive iridium seeds are placed in the needles. The seeds emit continuous radiation. (Radiation therapy and brachytherapy are discussed in Chapter 16.)

Surgical treatment varies depending on tumor location and stage. A *cordectomy* (partial removal of one vocal cord) is used for a superficial tumor involving one cord (Fig. 27-9). If the tumor is deeper but does not involve the entire larynx, one of several partial laryngectomy procedures are available that preserve speech and swallowing functions. A *hemilaryngectomy* involves removal of one side of the larynx. A *supraglottic laryngectomy* involves removing structures above the true cords—the false vocal cords and epiglottis. A *supracricoid laryngectomy* involves removal of the entire supraglottis; the false and true vocal cords; and the thyroid cartilage, including the paraglottic and preepiglottic spaces. The patient is at high risk of aspiration after these procedures and requires a temporary tracheostomy. Although speech is preserved, the quality and ease of speech vary. Voice quality is breathy, hoarse, and rough.

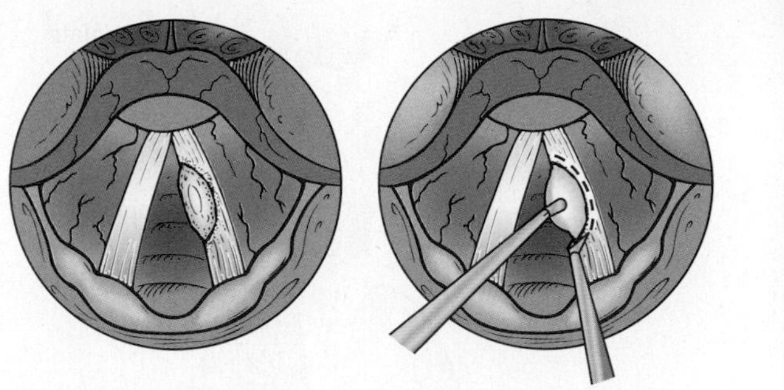

FIG. 27-9 Excision of laryngeal cancer. This cancer of the right vocal cord meets criteria for resection by transoral cordectomy. The cord is fully mobile, and the lesion can be fully exposed. It does not approach or cross the anterior commissure.

Advanced lesions are treated by a total laryngectomy, in which the entire larynx and preepiglottic region are removed and a permanent tracheostomy is performed. Airflow patterns before and after total laryngectomy are shown in Fig. 27-10. *Radical neck dissection* frequently accompanies total laryngectomy to decrease the risk of lymphatic spread. Depending on the extent of involvement, extensive dissection and reconstruction may be performed (Fig. 27-11). This procedure involves wide excision of the lymph nodes and their lymphatic channels. The following structures may also be removed or transected: sternocleidomastoid muscle and other closely associated muscles, internal jugular vein, mandible, submaxillary gland, part of the thyroid and parathyroid glands, and spinal accessory nerve.

A *modified neck dissection* is performed whenever possible as an alternative to a radical neck dissection. The dissection is modified by sparing as many structures as possible to limit disfigurement and functional loss. This usually involves dissection of the major cervical lymphatic vessels and lateral cervical space with preservation of nerves and vessels, including the sympathetic and vagus nerves, spinal accessory nerves, and internal jugular vein. Neck dissection with vocal cord cancer usually involves one side of the neck. However, if the lesion is midline, a bilateral neck dissection may be performed, with a modification on at least one side to minimize structural and functional deficits.

Some patients refuse surgical intervention for advanced lesions because of the extent of the procedure and the potential risk. In this situation, external radiation therapy is used as the sole treatment or in combination with chemotherapy. Your support and counseling are extremely important.

Chemotherapy is used in combination with radiation therapy for patients with stage III or IV cancers. A three-drug chemotherapeutic regimen using cisplatin (Platinol), docetaxel (Taxotere), and fluorouracil (5-FU) is used to treat locally advanced head and neck cancer.[26] Cetuximab (Erbitux), a targeted therapy, is also used in combination with radiation (first-line treatment) or as monotherapy for cancer that has metastasized after stan-

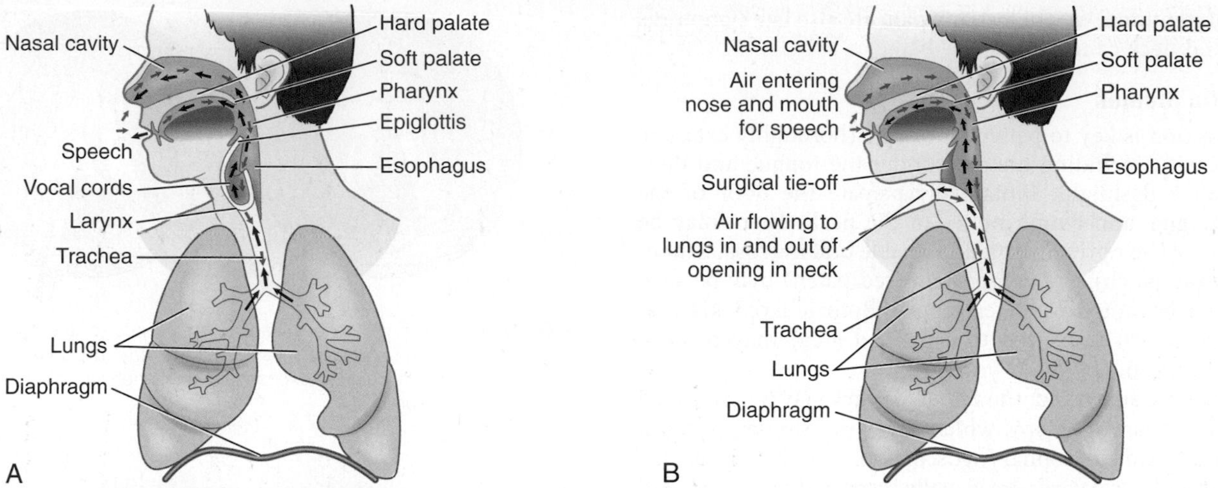

FIG. 27-10 **A,** Normal airflow in and out of the lungs. **B,** Airflow in and out of the lungs after total laryngectomy. Patients using esophageal speech trap air in the esophagus and release it to create sound.

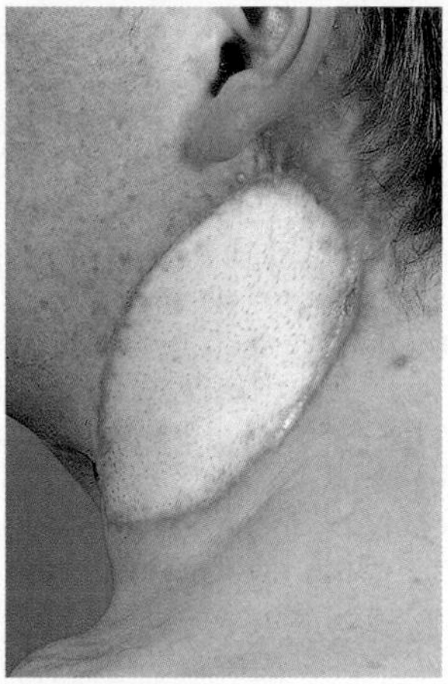

FIG. 27-11 Reconstructive surgery involving skin grafts may be needed after a radical neck dissection.

dard chemotherapy. (Targeted therapy is discussed in Chapter 16 and Table 16-13.)

Isotretinoin (13-*cis*-retinoic acid) is currently under clinical evaluation for use as a chemopreventive agent. This drug is given daily for 1 year to prevent recurrence of head and neck cancer.[27]

Nutritional Therapy. As many as 50% of patients with head and neck cancer are malnourished even before treatment begins.[28] Treatment modalities increase the risk of malnutrition. After radical neck surgery the patient may be unable to take in nutrients orally because of swelling, the location of sutures, or difficulty with swallowing. Side effects from chemotherapy and radiation therapy can impair the patient's ability to maintain adequate nutrition. Painful oral mucositis frequently leads to breaks in treatment if the patient is relying solely on oral intake for nutrition.

A thorough nutritional assessment and prophylactic placement of a gastrostomy tube in high-risk patients are vital to maintaining adequate nutrition. Enteral nutrition may be started before initiation of treatment to obtain and maintain optimal nutritional status needed for tissue repair. (Enteral nutrition is described in Chapter 40.) Observe for tolerance of the feedings and adjust the amount, time, and formula if nausea, vomiting, diarrhea, or distention occurs. Instruct the patient and caregiver about the tube feedings.

Patients who are not candidates for or who refuse enteral feedings need to be monitored closely for weight loss. Antiemetics or analgesics may be given before meals to reduce nausea and mouth pain. Bland foods are easier for patients to tolerate. Patients can increase caloric intake by adding dry milk to foods during preparation, selecting foods high in calories, and using oral supplements. It is helpful to add sauces and gravies to food, which adds calories and moistens food so it is more easily swallowed. Elevate the head of the bed while the patient is eating.

Anticipate swallowing problems when the patient resumes eating after surgery. The type and degree of difficulty vary, depending on the procedure. Videofluoroscopic swallowing studies may be used to evaluate the safety of patient swallowing. When the patient can swallow, give small amounts of thickened liquids or pureed foods with the patient in high Fowler's position. Closely observe for choking. Suctioning may be necessary to prevent aspiration.

Avoid thin, watery fluids because they are difficult to swallow and increase the risk of aspiration. A better choice is nonpourable pureed foods, which are thicker and allow more control during swallowing. Using a commercially available thickening agent (Thick-It) to thicken liquids will enhance swallowing.

When a supraglottic laryngectomy is performed, the upper portion of the larynx is excised, including the epiglottis and false vocal cords. The patient can speak because the true vocal cords remain intact. However, the patient must learn a new technique, the *supraglottic swallow,* to compensate for removal of the epiglottis and minimize the risk of aspiration (Table 27-9). When learning this technique, the patient should start with carbonated beverages because the effervescence helps determine the liquid's position.

NURSING MANAGEMENT HEAD AND NECK CANCER

NURSING ASSESSMENT

Table 27-10 presents subjective and objective data to obtain from a person with head and neck cancer.

TABLE 27-9 PATIENT TEACHING GUIDE

Supraglottic Swallow

Include the following instructions when teaching a patient to perform a supraglottic swallow.

1. Its purpose is to voluntarily control the closure of the vocal cords before and after swallowing. It protects the trachea from aspiration.
2. To do the technique, take a deep breath and hold it tightly.*
3. Take a bite of food or sip of fluid in your mouth.
4. Swallow while holding your breath. Some food will enter airway and remain on top of closed vocal cords.
4. Cough immediately after swallow to remove food from top of vocal cords.
5. Swallow again.
6. Breathe after cough-swallow sequence to prevent aspiration of food collected on top of vocal cords.

*If patient aspirates with this technique, the super-supraglottic swallow may be useful. This involves having the patient perform the Valsalva maneuver to close the vocal cords while holding breath and during swallow.

TABLE 27-10 NURSING ASSESSMENT

Head and Neck Cancer

Subjective Data

Important Health Information

Past health history: Positive family history; prolonged tobacco use (cigarettes, pipes, cigars, chewing tobacco, smokeless tobacco); prolonged, heavy alcohol use; poor intake of fruits and vegetables

Medications: Prolonged use of over-the-counter medication for sore throat, decongestants

Functional Health Patterns

Health perception–health management: Does not participate in preventive health measures, long history of alcohol and tobacco use

Nutritional-metabolic: Mouth ulcer that does not heal, change in fit of dentures, change in appetite, weight loss, swallowing difficulty (e.g., sensation of lump in throat, pain with swallowing, aspiration when swallowing)

Activity-exercise: Fatigue with minimal exertion

Cognitive-perceptual: Sore throat, pain on swallowing, referred ear pain

Objective Data

Respiratory

Hoarseness, change in voice quality, chronic laryngitis, nasal voice, palpable neck mass and lymph nodes (tender, hard, fixed), tracheal deviation; dyspnea, stridor (late sign)

Gastrointestinal

White (leukoplakia) or red (erythroplakia) patches inside mouth, ulceration of mucosa, asymmetric tongue, exudate in mouth or pharynx, mass or thickening of mucosa

Possible Diagnostic Findings

Mass on direct or indirect laryngoscopy; tumor on soft tissue x-ray, computed tomography (CT) scan, or magnetic resonance imaging (MRI); positive biopsy

NURSING DIAGNOSES

Nursing diagnoses for the patient with head and neck cancer include, but are not limited to, the following:

- Ineffective airway clearance *related to* presence of artificial airway and excessive mucus
- Risk for aspiration *related to* presence of tracheostomy tube and impaired swallowing
- Anxiety *related to* lack of knowledge regarding surgical procedure and pain management
- Acute pain *related to* tissue injury from surgery
- Impaired verbal communication *related to* removal of vocal cords

Additional information on nursing diagnoses for the patient with head and neck cancer is presented in eNursing Care Plan 27-2 on the website for this chapter.

PLANNING

The overall goals are that the patient will have (1) a patent airway, (2) no spread of cancer, (3) no complications related to therapy, (4) adequate nutritional intake, (5) minimal to no pain, (6) the ability to communicate, and (7) an acceptable body image.

NURSING IMPLEMENTATION

HEALTH PROMOTION. Development of head and neck cancer is closely related to personal habits, primarily tobacco use and excessive alcohol ingestion. Although tobacco use (including smokeless tobacco, also called "chewing tobacco" or "snuff") has been linked to most head and neck cancers, people who use both tobacco and alcohol are at greater risk than those who use just one.[24] Poor oral hygiene and HPV infection are also risk factors for head and neck cancer.

Include information about risk factors in health teaching. Encourage good oral hygiene. Teach patients about safe sex practices to prevent HPV infection (e.g., use condoms for every sex act, be in a monogamous relationship, and choose a partner who has had no or few previous partners). If cancer has been diagnosed, tobacco and alcohol cessation is still important. The likelihood of a cure, by any treatment modality, for a patient with head and neck cancer who continues to smoke and ingest alcoholic beverages is diminished. Additionally, risk of a second primary cancer is significantly increased. Give patients information about smoking cessation programs and techniques for success. If necessary, refer to an alcohol treatment program.

ACUTE INTERVENTION. Teach the patient and the caregiver about the type of therapy to be performed and care required. Help prepare them to deal with the psychologic impact of the diagnosis of cancer, alteration of physical appearance, possible need for enteral feedings, and potential for altered methods of communication because of the loss of a voice. The care plan should include assessment of the patient's support system. The patient may not have someone to provide assistance after discharge, may be unemployed, or may have a job that cannot be continued.

Radiation Therapy. Suggest interventions to reduce side effects of radiation therapy. Because the oral mucosa is frequently affected, patients should consult a dentist before starting radiation therapy. Dry mouth *(xerostomia),* the most frequent and annoying problem, typically begins within a few weeks of treatment. The patient's saliva decreases in volume and becomes thick. The change may be temporary or permanent. Pilocarpine hydrochloride (Salagen) is often effective in increasing saliva production and should be started before the initiation of radiation therapy. Amifostine (Ethyol) subcutaneous injection may also be ordered to decrease xerostomia. Patients can get symptom relief by increasing fluid intake, chewing sugarless gum or sugarless candy, using nonalcoholic mouth rinses (baking soda or glycerin solutions), and using artificial saliva. Over-the-counter mucous thinning agents (e.g., guaifenesin) two or three times daily and/or mucous solvents can be used to control thickening secretions. Instruct patients to always carry a water bottle with them. Fluoride gels or treatments can help prevent dental deterioration caused by xerostomia. Acupuncture has also been found to improve discomfort related to xerostomia.[27]

Oral mucositis can cause irritation, ulceration, and pain. Empty fluoride gel trays, along with bite blocks, athletic mouth guards, or gauze pads, can be worn during radiation treatments to prevent radiation scatter to the tongue and cheek from metal work in the mouth that contributes to development of mucositis.[28] Instruct the patient on oral care basics, including the use of a soft toothbrush and regular flossing. Warm bland rinses such as salt and baking soda should be done four to six times daily. Sucking on ice chips can also help with the pain. Encourage patients to eat soft, bland foods. Patients should avoid commercial mouthwashes and hot, spicy, or acidic foods because they are irritating. If the problem is severe, a mixture of equal parts antacid, diphenhydramine (Benadryl), and topical lidocaine can be used. Instruct the patient to rinse the mouth with the mixture without swallowing it.

Fatigue is a common side effect of radiation therapy and usually begins a few weeks into therapy. Encourage patients to walk 15 to 30 minutes each day, since regular exercise can give them more energy. Instruct patients to do activities that are most important to them and to rest during periods of low energy. Identify support systems and encourage patients to ask for help.

Skin over the irradiated area often becomes reddened and sensitive to touch. Instruct patients to use only prescribed lotions and skin products while undergoing radiation therapy, and to not use any lotions within 2 hours before treatment. (Skin care for patients having radiation therapy is discussed in Chapter 16.)

Surgical Therapy. Preoperatively assess the patient's physical and psychosocial needs. Physical preparation is the same as for any major surgery, with an emphasis on oral hygiene. Explanations and emotional support are of special significance and should include postoperative measures relating to communication and feeding. Assess knowledge and understanding of the planned surgical procedure, and clarify information as needed. Include the caregiver in preoperative teaching.

Tailor teaching to the planned surgical procedure. For surgeries that involve a laryngectomy, include information about expected changes in speech. Establish a means of communication for the immediate postoperative period. Magic Slates, alphabet boards, writing materials, pictorial guides, or hand signals are useful methods for communicating. Programmable speech-generating devices allow use of recorded messages that are matched with a graphic representing each message. Integration of this technology into patient care enhances the patient's ability to communicate basic needs postoperatively.[29]

Immediately after surgery, focus your nursing care on airway management, wound care, nutrition, communication, and psychosocial issues related to body-image changes. Maintenance of a patent airway is essential. The inflammation in the surgical area may compress the trachea. A tracheostomy tube will be in place. Keep the patient in semi-Fowler's position to decrease edema and limit tension on the suture lines. The patient with a laryngectomy requires frequent suctioning via the tracheostomy tube. Secretions typically change in amount and consistency over time. The patient may initially have copious blood-tinged secretions that diminish and thicken. Normal saline bolus via the tracheostomy tube is not recommended to assist with removal of thickened secretions, since this causes hypoxia and damage to the epithelial cells. Maintain adequate fluid intake (IV, enteral, and oral when allowed) and humidification of inspired gases to keep secretions liquid and mucous membranes moist. Encourage deep breathing and coughing. Provide tracheostomy care as needed (see Table 27-7).

Monitor vital signs frequently because of the risk of hemorrhage and respiratory compromise. Pressure dressings, packing, or drainage tubes may be used for wound management, depending on the type of surgical procedure. If skin flaps are employed, dressings are typically not used. This allows better visualization of the incision and avoids excessive pressure on tissue (see Fig. 27-11). When a radical neck dissection is performed, the wound is suctioned with a portable system, such as a Hemovac. The drainage should be serosanguineous and gradually decrease in volume over 24 hours. Monitor patency of drainage tubes every 4 hours to ensure proper functioning. In addition, monitor the amount and character of drainage. If the tubing becomes obstructed, fluid will accumulate under the skin flap and predispose the patient to formation of hematomas or seromas, impair wound healing, and increase the risk for infection. After drainage tubes are removed, closely monitor the area to detect any swelling. If fluid continues to accumulate, aspiration may be necessary. Closely monitor incision sites for signs of infection.

The patient may have a nasogastric tube inserted during surgery to remove gastric contents via intermittent suction for the first 24 to 48 hours until peristalsis returns. Because the nasogastric tube lies close to internal incision lines, do not manipulate or move the tube. When bowel sounds return, enteral feedings may be started slowly and advanced to meet nutritional needs. Monitor daily weights and blood chemistries to evaluate the patient's nutritional status.

After a neck dissection, teach the patient to use the upper extremities to assist with support and movement of the head. After the immediate postoperative period the patient should begin an exercise program to maintain strength and movement in the affected shoulder and neck. This is especially important when the spinal accessory nerve and sternocleidomastoid muscles are removed or damaged. Without exercise, the patient will be left with a "frozen" shoulder and limited range of neck motion. The patient should continue this exercise program after discharge to prevent future functional disabilities.

Voice Rehabilitation. Preoperatively a speech therapist should meet with the patient having a total laryngectomy to discuss voice restoration options. The International Association of Laryngectomees, an association of laryngectomy patients, focuses on helping patients reestablish speech. Local groups, called "Lost Chord" or "New Voice" Clubs, often provide volunteers to visit the patient, preferably preoperatively. Three options are available to restore speech: esophageal speech, electrolarynx, and transesophageal puncture.

Esophageal speech involves swallowing air, trapping it in the esophagus, and releasing it to create sound. The air causes vibration of the pharyngoesophageal segment and sound (which initially is similar to a belch). With practice, many patients develop some speech skills, but few develop fluent speech.

An *electrolarynx* is a hand-held, battery-powered device that creates speech with the use of sound waves. The two most common types of electrolarynx devices are classified as neck and intraoral. The *neck type* is placed against the neck, under the chin (Fig. 27-12, *A*), or on the cheek. The patient moves the lips to articulate sound that is conducted into the oropharynx

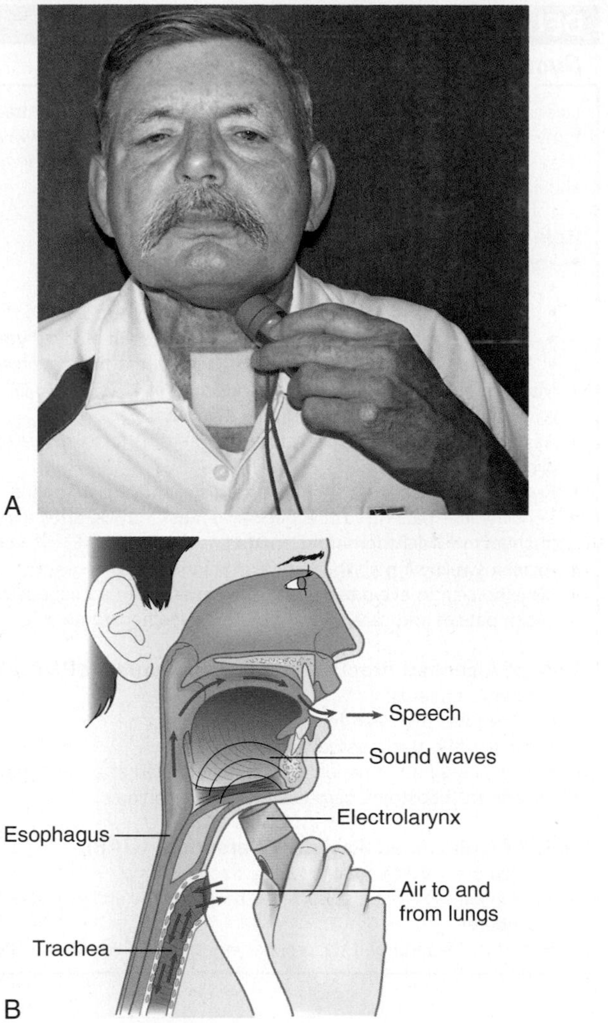

FIG. 27-12 Artificial larynx. **A,** Battery-powered electronic artificial larynx for patient who has had a total laryngectomy. **B,** The sound waves created by the electrolarynx allow the person to speak.

(Fig. 27-12, *B*). This option allows for speech immediately after surgery, is easy to learn, and requires little maintenance. Intraoral devices are used for patients who cannot achieve adequate sound conduction on the skin. The *intraoral electrolarynx* uses a plastic tube placed in the corner of the roof of the mouth to create vibrations. A hands-free device, using an electromyograph (EMG) transducer in the strap muscles of the neck, is also available.[30] With all devices, voice pitch is low and the sound is mechanical.

Transesophageal puncture, the most common voice rehabilitation method, offers the best speech quality with the highest patient satisfaction.[31] A transesophageal puncture creates a surgical fistula or tract between the esophagus and trachea. The puncture may be created at the same time as the total laryngectomy surgery or afterward if postoperative radiation is planned. A red rubber catheter is placed in the tracheoesophageal puncture as a stent. Several days later, the catheter is removed and a one-way valved prosthesis is placed in the tract. The valve prevents aspiration of food or saliva from the esophagus into the tracheostomy. To speak, the patient manually blocks the stoma with the finger. Air moves from the lungs, through the prosthesis, into the esophagus, and out the mouth. Speech is produced

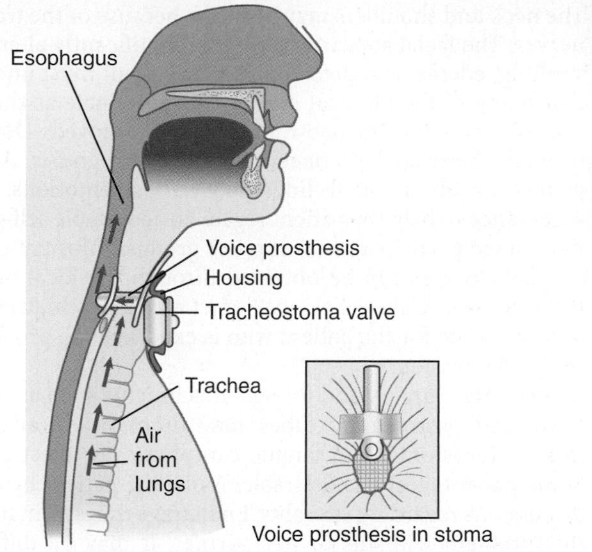

FIG. 27-13 Blom-Singer voice prosthesis and tracheostoma valve. With this prosthesis and valve, patients with a laryngectomy can speak normally. *Inset* shows laryngectomy stoma and voice prosthesis with tracheostoma valve removed.

by the air vibrating against the esophagus and is formed into words by moving the tongue and lips. The use of a hands-free external-airflow valve eliminates the need for finger occlusion of the stoma. The prosthesis must be cleaned regularly and replaced when it becomes blocked with mucus. The most commonly used voice prosthesis is the Blom-Singer prosthesis (Fig. 27-13).

Stoma Care. Before discharge, instruct the patient in the care of the laryngectomy stoma. The patient should wash the area around the stoma daily with a moist cloth. A nasal wash spray (e.g., Alkalol) can be used every 1 to 2 hours to keep the stoma moist and prevent crusting. Dried secretions can be removed with tweezers. If a laryngectomy tube is in place, the patient must remove the entire tube at least daily and clean it in the same manner as a tracheostomy tube. The inner cannula may need to be removed and cleaned more frequently. A scarf, a loose shirt, or a crocheted shield can be used to hide the stoma.

The patient should cover the stoma when coughing (because mucus may be expectorated) and during any activity (e.g., shaving, applying makeup) that might lead to inhalation of foreign materials. Because water can easily enter the stoma, the patient should wear a plastic collar when taking a shower. Swimming is contraindicated. Initially, humidification is administered via a tracheostomy mask. After discharge, the patient can use a bedside humidifier. The patient must also maintain a high oral fluid intake, especially in dry weather.

Inform the patient about the importance of wearing a Medic Alert bracelet or other identification that alerts emergency personnel of the neck breathing status. Because the patient no longer breathes through the nose, the ability to smell smoke and food is often lost. Advise the patient to install smoke and carbon monoxide detectors in the home. Encourage preparation of food that is colorful, attractive, and nutritious because taste may also be diminished secondary to the loss of smell and radiation therapy.

Depression. Depression is common in the patient who has had a radical neck dissection. The patient may not be able to speak because of the laryngectomy and cannot control saliva.

The neck and shoulders may be numb because of the transected nerves. The facial appearance may be significantly altered, with swelling, edema, and deformities. The patient must understand that many of the physical changes are reversible as the edema subsides and the tracheostomy tube is removed. Depression may also be related to concern about the prognosis. Allow the patient to talk about feelings and express emotions. Convey acceptance to help the patient regain an acceptable self-concept. Encourage participation in support groups. Information about available groups can be obtained through the local branch of the American Cancer Society. Sometimes a psychiatric referral is appropriate for the patient who is experiencing prolonged or severe depression.

Sexuality. Surgery and foreign attachments such as tracheostomy and gastrostomy tubes may dramatically affect body image. Xerostomia and fatigue can physically affect sexuality. Some patients feel less desirable. Assist the patient by allowing discussions regarding sexuality. Encourage the patient to discuss this problem with his or her partner. It may be difficult for the patient to talk about sexual problems because of the alteration in communication. Assist the patient in planning how to communicate with the sexual partner. Offer support and guidance to the sexual partner. Helping the patient see that sexuality involves much more than appearance may relieve some anxiety.

AMBULATORY AND HOME CARE. The patient is often discharged with a tracheostomy and a nasogastric or gastrostomy feeding tube. Some patients need home health care initially to evaluate the caregiver's or the patient's ability to perform self-care activities. The patient and the caregiver need to learn how to manage tubes and who to call if there are problems. Provide pictorial instructions for tracheostomy care, suctioning, stoma care, and enteral feeding as appropriate. The patient can resume exercise, recreation, and sexual activity when able. Most patients can return to work 1 to 2 months after surgery. However, many never return to full-time employment. The changes that follow a total laryngectomy can be upsetting. Loss of speech, loss of the ability to taste and smell, inability to produce audible sounds (including laughing and weeping), and the presence of a permanent tracheal stoma that produces undesirable mucus are often overwhelming to the patient. Although changes are discussed before surgery, the patient may not be prepared for the extent of these changes. If the patient has a significant other, this person's reaction to the patient's altered appearance is important. Acceptance by another person can promote an improved self-image. Encouraging the patient to participate in self-care is another important part of rehabilitation.

DELEGATION DECISIONS

Suctioning and Tracheostomy Care

Licensed practical nurses (LPNs) may do suctioning and give tracheostomy care to stable patients. In patients who have acute airway problems requiring an endotracheal or tracheostomy tube, these interventions should be done by the registered nurse (RN).

Role of Registered Nurse (RN)

- For unstable patients:
  - Assess for the need for suctioning.
  - Suction the endotracheal or tracheostomy tube.
  - Evaluate for adverse effects of suctioning such as dysrhythmias.
  - Evaluate whether patient status is improved after suctioning.
- Maintain appropriate cuff inflation pressure at 20-25 cm H_2O, or use minimal leak technique to maintain cuff pressure.
- Assess tracheostomy and any retention sutures for evidence of complications (e.g., infection).
- Replace the tracheostomy tube after accidental dislodgment.
- Ventilate the patient with a bag-valve-mask device after accidental tracheostomy dislodgment if needed.
- Assess swallowing ability and risk for aspiration.
- Develop plan to avoid aspiration in a patient with a tracheostomy.
- Teach patient and caregiver about home tracheostomy care.

Role of Licensed Practical/Vocational Nurse (LPN/LVN)

- For stable patients:
  - Determine the need for suctioning.
  - Suction the tracheostomy.
  - Evaluate whether patient status is improved after suctioning.
- Provide tracheostomy care using sterile technique.

Role of Unlicensed Assistive Personnel (UAP)

- Provide oral care to patient with a tracheostomy.
- Suction patient's oropharynx (after being trained and evaluated in this procedure).
- Report increased need for oropharyngeal suctioning to the RN.

EVALUATION

Expected outcomes for the patient with head and neck cancer who is treated surgically are that the patient will

- Demonstrate effective coughing and secretion clearance
- Demonstrate the ability to swallow oral foods without aspiration
- Report satisfaction with pain relief
- Use written and nonverbal techniques to effectively communicate with others

Other outcomes for the patient with head and neck cancer who is treated surgically are addressed in eNursing Care Plans 27-1 and 27-2 on the website for this chapter.

CASE STUDY

Laryngeal Cancer

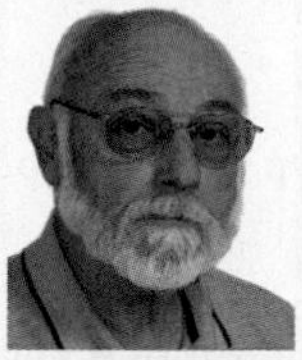

iStockphoto/Thinkstock

Patient Profile

M.R., a 60-year-old white man, was admitted for evaluation of mild pain on swallowing and a persistent sore throat over the past year. He has a history of type 2 diabetes mellitus.

Subjective Data

- States that his symptoms worsened in the past 2 mo
- Has used various cold remedies to relieve symptoms without relief
- Has lost weight because of decrease in appetite and difficulty swallowing
- Has smoked three packs of cigarettes a day for 40 yr
- Consumes 4-6 cans of beer a day

Objective Data

Laryngoscopy

- Subglottic mass

Physical Examination

- Enlarged cervical nodes

Computed Tomography Scan

- Subglottic lesion with lymph node involvement

Collaborative Care

- Percutaneous gastrostomy tube inserted preoperatively for enteral tube feeding
- Total laryngectomy with tracheostomy with inflated cuff
- Nasogastric tube postoperatively

Discussion Questions

1. What information in the assessment suggests that M.R. is at risk for cancer of the larynx?
2. ***Priority Decision:*** What are your priority teaching strategies for M.R. before and after laryngectomy?
3. Discuss methods used to restore speech after laryngectomy.
4. Is there anything in his history that may affect wound healing after surgery?
5. ***Priority Decision:*** While in the recovery room, M.R. develops shortness of breath. What are your priority nursing interventions?
6. What teaching is required to help this patient assume self-care after his surgery? What precautions should the patient take because of his stoma?
7. While on the medical-surgical unit, M.R. is tearful and is staring at the wall. What should you do?
8. ***Priority Decision:*** Based on the assessment data presented, what are your priority nursing diagnoses? Are there any collaborative problems?
9. ***Delegation Decision:*** What role can unlicensed assistive personnel (UAP) have in relation to the tracheostomy?
10. ***Evidence-Based Practice:*** How could you best meet M.R.'s communication needs during the first few postoperative days?

evolve Answers available at *http://evolve.elsevier.com/Lewis/medsurg.*

BRIDGE TO NCLEX EXAMINATION

The number of the question corresponds to the same-numbered outcome at the beginning of the chapter.

1. A patient was seen in the clinic for an episode of epistaxis, which was controlled by placement of anterior nasal packing. During discharge teaching, the nurse instructs the patient to
   a. use aspirin for pain relief.
   b. remove the packing later that day.
   c. skip the next dose of antihypertensive medication.
   d. avoid vigorous nose blowing and strenuous activity.
2. A patient with allergic rhinitis reports severe nasal congestion; sneezing; and watery, itchy eyes and nose at various times of the year. To teach the patient to control these symptoms, the nurse advises the patient to
   a. avoid all intranasal sprays and oral antihistamines.
   b. limit the usage of nasal decongestant spray to 10 days.
   c. use oral decongestants at bedtime to prevent symptoms during the night.
   d. keep a diary of when the allergic reaction occurs and what precipitates it.
3. A patient is seen at the clinic with fever, muscle aches, sore throat with yellowish exudate, and headache. The nurse anticipates that the collaborative management will include *(select all that apply)*
   a. antiviral agents to treat influenza.
   b. treatment with antibiotics starting ASAP.
   c. a throat culture or rapid strep antigen test.
   d. supportive care, including cool, bland liquids.
   e. comprehensive history to determine possible etiology.
4. The best method for determining the risk of aspiration in a patient with a tracheostomy is to
   a. consult a speech therapist for swallowing assessment.
   b. have the patient drink plain water and assess for coughing.
   c. assess for change of sputum color 48 hours after patient drinks small amount of blue dye.
   d. suction above the cuff after the patient eats or drinks to determine presence of food in trachea.
5. Which nursing action would be of highest priority when suctioning a patient with a tracheostomy?
   a. Auscultating lung sounds after suctioning is complete
   b. Providing a means of communication for the patient during the procedure
   c. Assessing the patient's oxygenation saturation before, during, and after suctioning
   d. Administering pain and/or antianxiety medication 30 minutes before suctioning
6. When planning health care teaching to prevent or detect early head and neck cancer, which people would be the priority to target *(select all that apply)?*
   a. 65-year-old man who has used chewing tobacco most of his life
   b. 45-year-old rancher who uses snuff to stay awake while driving his herds of cattle
   c. 78-year-old woman who has been drinking hard liquor since her husband died 15 years ago
   d. 21-year-old college student who drinks beer on weekends with his fraternity brothers
   e. 22-year-old woman who has been diagnosed with human papilloma virus (HPV) of the cervix

7. While in the recovery room, a patient with a total laryngectomy is suctioned and has bloody mucus with some clots. Which nursing interventions would apply?
   - **a.** Notify the physician immediately.
   - **b.** Place the patient in the prone position to facilitate drainage.
   - **c.** Instill 3 mL of normal saline into the tracheostomy tube to loosen secretions.
   - **d.** Continue your assessment of the patient, including O_2 saturation, respiratory rate, and breath sounds.

8. When using a prosthesis for transesophageal speech, the patient
   - **a.** places a vibrating device in the mouth.
   - **b.** blocks the stoma entrance with a finger.
   - **c.** swallows air using a Valsalva maneuver.
   - **d.** places a speaking valve next to the stoma.

1. d, 2. d, 3. c, d, e, 4. a, 5. c, 6. a, b, c, e, 7. d, 8. b

evolve

For rationales to these answers and even more NCLEX review questions, visit *http://evolve.elsevier.com/Lewis/medsurg.*

REFERENCES

1. American Academy of Otolaryngology–Head and Neck Surgery: Fact sheet: deviated septum. Retrieved from *www.entnet.org/HealthInformation/deviatedSeptum.cfm.*
2. Reitzen SD, Chung W, Shah AR: Nasal septal deviation in the pediatric and adult populations, *Ear Nose Throat J* 90:112, 2011.
*3. Eiff MP, Hatch RL: *Fracture management for primary care*, ed 3, St Louis, 2011, Saunders.
*4. Lewis R: Ultrasound device adds precision to rhinoplasty. Retrieved from *www.medscape.com/viewarticle/750055.*
5. American Academy of Facial, Plastic, and Reconstructive Surgery: Rhinoplasty. Retrieved from *www.aafprs.org/patient/procedures/rhinoplasty.html.*
6. US National Library of Medicine, NIH National Institutes of Health: MedlinePlus: nosebleed. Retrieved from *www.nlm.nih.gov/medlineplus/ency/article/003106.htm.*
7. Bamimore O, Dronen SC: Management of acute epistaxis. Retrieved from *http://emedicine.medscape.com/article/764719-overview.*
*8. Dykewicz MS: Management of rhinitis: guidelines, evidence basis, and systematic clinical approach for what we do, *Immunol Allergy Clin North Am* 31:619, 2011.
*9. Brozek JL, Bousquet J, Baena-Cagnani CE, et al: Allergic rhinitis and its impact on asthma (ARIA) guidelines: 2010 revision, *J Allergy Clin Immunol* 126:466, 2010.
10. National Institute of Allergy and Infectious Diseases: Common cold. Retrieved from *http://niaid.nih.gov/topics/commoncold/Pages/default.aspx.*
11. Centers for Disease Control and Prevention: Seasonal influenza. Retrieved from *www.cdc.gov/flu/about/qa/disease.htm.*
12. American Association for Clinical Chemistry: Influenza tests. Retrieved from *http://labtestsonline.org/understanding/analytes/flu/tab/test.*
13. Centers for Disease Control and Prevention: Key facts about influenza (flu) and flu vaccine. Retrieved from *www.cdc.gov/flu/keyfacts.htm.*
*14. Centers for Disease Control and Prevention: 2011-2012 influenza antiviral medications: a summary for clinicians. Retrieved from *www.cdc.gov/flu/pdf/professionals/antivirals/clinician-antivirals-2011.pdf.*
15. Brook I, Cunha BA, Cohen AJ, et al: Acute sinusitis. Retrieved from *http://emedicine.medscap.com/articl/232670-overview.*
16. WebMD: Nasal irrigation: natural relief for cold and allergy symptoms. Retrieved from *www.webmd.com/allergies/ss/slideshow-nasal-irrigation.*
17. Shantouf R: Intersect ENT's Propel sinus implant receives green light from FDA. Retrieved from *http://medgadget.com/2011/08/intersect-ent%e2%80%99s-propel-sinus-implant-receives-green-light-from-fda.html.*
18. Acerra JR, Dyne PL: Pharyngitis in emergency medicine. Retrieved from *http://emedicine.medscape.com/article/764304-clinical.*
19. Lindman JP, Morgan CE, Schweinfurth J, et al: Tracheostomy. Retrieved from *http://emedicine,medscape.com/article/865968.*
*20. Wiegand DJL, editor: *AACN procedure manual for critical care*, ed 6, St Louis, 2011, Saunders.
21. Frace MA: Tracheostomy care on the medical-surgical unit, *MEDSURG Nurs* 19:58, 2010.
*22. Freman S: Care of adult patients with a temporary tracheostomy, *Nurs Stand* 26:49, 2011.
*23. Regan K, Hunt K: Tracheostomy management: weaning and decannulation. Retrieved from *www.medscape.com/viewarticle/574271.*
24. National Cancer Institute: Head and neck cancer: questions and answers. Retrieved from *www.cancer.gov/cancertopics/factsheet/Sites-Types/head-and-neck.*
25. American Cancer Society: Cancer facts and figures 2011. Retrieved from *www.cancer.org/acs/groups/content/@epidemiologysurveilance/documents/document/acspc-029771.pdf.*
*26. Lowry F: Three-drug combo best for head and neck cancer. Retrieved from *http://medscape.com/viewarticle/735730.*
27. National Cancer Institute: Laryngeal cancer treatment. Retrieved from *www.cancer.gov/cancertopics/pdq/treatment/laryngeal/HealthProfessional/page1.*
28. Lambertz CK, Gruell J, Robenstein V, et al: NO SToPS: reducing treatment breaks during chemoradiation for head and neck cancer, *Clin J Oncol Nurs* 14:585. 2010.
*29. Rodriguez C, Rowe M: Use of a speech-generating device for hospitalized postoperative patients with head and neck cancer experiencing speechlessness, *Oncol Nurs Forum* 37:199, 2010.
30. Lombard LE: Laryngectomy rehabilitation. Retrieved from *http://emedicine.medscape.com/article/883689-overview.*
*31. Xi S, Li Z, Huang X: The effectiveness of voice rehabilitation on vocalization in post-laryngectomy patients: a systematic review, *J Adv Nurs* 66:962, 2010.

*Evidence-based information for clinical practice.

RESOURCES

International Association of Laryngectomees
www.theial.com

National Cancer Institute
www.cancer.gov

CHAPTER

28

Breath is the bridge which connects life to consciousness, which unites your body to your thoughts.
Thich Nhat Hanh

Nursing Management

Lower Respiratory Problems

Dorothy (Dottie) M. Mathers

evolve WEBSITE

http://evolve.elsevier.com/Lewis/medsurg

- NCLEX Review Questions
- Key Points
- Pre-Test
- Answer Guidelines for Case Study on p. 557
- Rationales for Bridge to NCLEX Examination Questions
- Case Studies
  - Patient With Lung Cancer
  - Patient With Pulmonary Embolism and Respiratory Failure
- Nursing Care Plans (Customizable)
  - eNCP 28-1: Patient With Pneumonia
  - eNCP 28-2: Patient After Thoracotomy
- Concept Map Creator
- Glossary
- Content Updates

eTables

- eTable 28-1: Environmental Lung Diseases
- eTable 28-2: Traumatic Chest Injuries and Mechanisms of Injury
- eTable 28-3: Causes of Restrictive Lung Disease

LEARNING OUTCOMES

1. Compare and contrast the clinical manifestations and collaborative and nursing management of patients with acute bronchitis and pertussis.
2. Differentiate among the types of pneumonia and their etiology, pathophysiology, clinical manifestations, and collaborative care.
3. Prioritize the nursing management of the patient with pneumonia.
4. Describe the pathogenesis, classification, clinical manifestations, complications, diagnostic abnormalities, and nursing and collaborative management of patients with tuberculosis.
5. Describe the causes, clinical manifestations, and collaborative management of patients with pulmonary fungal infections.
6. Explain the pathophysiology, clinical manifestations, and collaborative management of patients with lung abscesses.
7. Identify the causative factors, clinical manifestations, and nursing and collaborative management of patients with environmental lung diseases.
8. Describe the etiology, risk factors, pathophysiology, clinical manifestations, and nursing and collaborative management of lung cancer.
9. Compare and contrast the pathophysiology, clinical manifestations, and nursing and collaborative management of pneumothorax, fractured ribs, and flail chest.
10. Describe the purpose, function, and nursing responsibilities related to chest tubes and various drainage systems.
11. Explain the types of chest surgery and appropriate preoperative and postoperative care.
12. Describe the etiology, clinical manifestations, and nursing and collaborative management of patients with restrictive lung disorders such as pleural effusion, pleurisy, and atelectasis.
13. Describe the pathophysiology, clinical manifestations, and management of pulmonary embolism, pulmonary hypertension, and cor pulmonale.
14. Discuss the use of lung transplantation as a treatment for pulmonary disorders.

KEY TERMS

acute bronchitis, p. 522
community-acquired pneumonia (CAP), p. 523
cor pulmonale, p. 555
empyema, p. 549
flail chest, p. 543
hemothorax, p. 543
lung abscess, p. 534
medical care–associated pneumonia (MCAP), p. 523
pertussis, p. 522
pleural effusion, p. 549
pleurisy (pleuritis), p. 550
pneumoconiosis, p. 535
pneumonia, p. 522
pneumothorax, p. 542
pulmonary edema, p. 551
pulmonary embolism (PE), p. 551
pulmonary hypertension, p. 553
tension pneumothorax, p. 543
thoracentesis, p. 550
thoracotomy, p. 548
tuberculosis (TB), p. 528

Reviewed by Sharon A. Willadsen, RN, PhD, Nursing Instructor, Lakeshore Technical College, Cleveland, Wisconsin.

HEALTHY PEOPLE
Prevention of Respiratory Diseases

- Avoid cigarette smoking and exposure to environmental smoke.
- Wash hands frequently to prevent and avoid spreading infections.
- Avoid exposure to allergens, indoor pollutants, and ambient air pollutants.
- Get a pneumococcal vaccine and yearly flu vaccine as directed by health care provider.
- Wear proper protection when working in an occupation with prolonged exposure to dust, fumes, or gases.

A wide variety of problems affect the lower respiratory system. Lung diseases that are characterized primarily by an obstructive disorder, such as asthma, chronic obstructive pulmonary disease (COPD), and cystic fibrosis, are discussed in Chapter 29. This chapter discusses other lower respiratory tract diseases, including infectious, oncologic, traumatic, restrictive, and vascular disorders.

LOWER RESPIRATORY TRACT INFECTIONS

Lower respiratory tract infection is both a common and a serious occurrence. It is the third leading cause of death worldwide.[1] Pneumonia and influenza are the eighth leading cause of death in the United States, accounting for more than 56,000 deaths annually.[2]

ACUTE BRONCHITIS

Acute bronchitis is an inflammation of the bronchi in the lower respiratory tract. Up to 90% of acute bronchial infections are viral in origin. Cough, which is the most common symptom, lasts for up to 3 weeks. Clear, mucoid sputum is often present, although some patients produce purulent sputum. The presence of colored (e.g., green) sputum is not a reliable indicator of bacterial infection.[3] Associated symptoms include headache, fever, malaise, hoarseness, myalgias, dyspnea, and chest pain.

Assessment may reveal normal breath sounds or rhonchi, crackles, or wheezes, usually with expiration and exertion. Diagnosis is based on clinical assessment. Evidence of consolidation (e.g., fremitus, rales, egophony), which is suggestive of pneumonia, is absent with bronchitis. (*Consolidation* in the lungs occurs when fluid accumulates, causing the lung tissue to become stiff and unable to exchange gases.) Chest x-rays would be normal and are therefore not indicated unless pneumonia is suspected. (Chronic bronchitis is discussed in Chapter 29.)

Acute bronchitis is usually self-limiting, and treatment is supportive. Cough suppressants, β_2-agonist (bronchodilator) inhalers in patients with wheezing, and high-dose inhaled corticosteroids may be used.[3] Antibiotics generally are not prescribed unless the person has a prolonged infection associated with systemic symptoms. Explain to the patient that antibiotics are not effective in treating a viral infection and that they may cause side effects and antibiotic-resistant germs. Complementary and alternative therapies (e.g., echinacea, honey) may be useful for symptom relief. If the acute bronchitis is due to an influenza virus, treatment with antiviral drugs, either zanamivir (Relenza) or oseltamivir (Tamiflu), can be started. These drugs should be initiated within 48 hours of the onset of symptoms.

PERTUSSIS

Pertussis is a highly contagious infection of the respiratory tract caused by a gram-negative bacillus, *Bordetella pertussis*. Pertussis is characterized by uncontrollable, violent coughing. Despite improved childhood vaccination in the United States, the incidence of pertussis has been steadily increasing since the 1980s, with the largest increase noted in adults.[4] It is thought that immunity resulting from childhood vaccination with DPT (diphtheria, pertussis, tetanus) may wane over time, resulting in a milder infection that is still distressing and contagious. Therefore the Centers for Disease Control and Prevention (CDC) currently recommends that all adults age 18 years and older receive a one-time dose of Tdap (tetanus, diphtheria, and pertussis) vaccination.[4]

Clinical manifestations of pertussis occur in stages. The first (catarrhal) stage manifests as a mild upper respiratory tract infection (URI) with a low-grade or no fever, runny nose, watery eyes, and mild nonproductive cough. The second (paroxysmal) stage is characterized by paroxysms of cough. Inspiration after each cough produces the typical "whooping" sound as the patient tries to breathe in air against an obstructed glottis. Vomiting may also occur with the coughing. Like acute bronchitis, the coughing is more frequent at night. Unlike bronchitis, the cough with pertussis may last from 6 to 10 weeks.

Treatment is antibiotics, usually macrolides (erythromycin, azithromycin [Zithromax]), to minimize symptoms and prevent spread of the disease. Cough suppressants and antihistamines should not be used, since they are ineffective and may induce coughing episodes. Corticosteroids and bronchodilators are not useful in reducing symptoms.

PNEUMONIA

Pneumonia is an acute infection of the lung parenchyma. Until 1936, pneumonia was the leading cause of death in the United States. The discovery of sulfa drugs and penicillin was pivotal in the treatment of pneumonia. Since that time, remarkable progress has been made in the development of antibiotics to treat pneumonia. However, despite new antimicrobial agents, pneumonia is still associated with significant morbidity and mortality rates. Community-acquired pneumonia (CAP) is the sixth leading cause of death for people ages 65 years or older in the United States.[5]

Etiology

Normally, the airway distal to the larynx is protected from infection by various defense mechanisms. Mechanisms that create a mechanical barrier to microorganisms include air filtration, epiglottis closure over the trachea, cough reflex, mucociliary escalator mechanism, and reflex bronchoconstriction (see Chapter 26). Immune defense mechanisms include secretion of immunoglobulins A and G and alveolar macrophages.

Pneumonia is more likely to occur when the defense mechanisms become incompetent or are overwhelmed by the virulence or quantity of infectious agents. Decreased consciousness depresses the cough and epiglottal reflexes, which may allow aspiration of oropharyngeal contents into the lungs. Tracheal intubation interferes with the normal cough reflex and the mucociliary escalator mechanism. Air pollution, cigarette smoking, viral URIs, and normal changes that occur with aging can impair the mucociliary mechanism. Chronic diseases can

TABLE 28-1 RISK FACTORS FOR PNEUMONIA

- Abdominal or thoracic surgery
- Age >65 yr
- Air pollution
- Altered consciousness: alcoholism, head injury, seizures, anesthesia, drug overdose, stroke
- Bed rest and prolonged immobility
- Chronic diseases: chronic lung and liver disease, diabetes mellitus, heart disease, cancer, chronic kidney disease
- Debilitating illness
- Exposure to bats, birds, rabbits, farm animals
- Immunosuppressive disease and/or therapy (corticosteroids, cancer chemotherapy, human immunodeficiency virus [HIV] infection, immunosuppressive therapy after organ transplant)
- Inhalation or aspiration of noxious substances
- Intestinal and gastric feedings via nasogastric or nasointestinal tubes
- IV drug use
- Malnutrition
- Recent antibiotic therapy
- Resident of a long-term care facility
- Smoking
- Tracheal intubation (endotracheal intubation, tracheostomy)
- Upper respiratory tract infection

suppress the immune system's ability to inhibit bacterial growth. The risk factors for pneumonia are listed in Table 28-1.

Organisms that cause pneumonia reach the lung by three methods:

1. *Aspiration* of normal flora from the nasopharynx or oropharynx. Many of the organisms that cause pneumonia are normal inhabitants of the pharynx in healthy adults.
2. *Inhalation* of microbes present in the air. Examples include *Mycoplasma pneumoniae* and fungal pneumonias.
3. *Hematogenous spread* from a primary infection elsewhere in the body. An example is *Staphylococcus aureus.*

Types of Pneumonia

Bacteria, viruses, *Mycoplasma* organisms, fungi, parasites, and chemicals are all potential causes of pneumonia. Although pneumonia can be classified according to the causative organism, a clinically effective way is to classify it as *community-acquired* or *medical care–associated* pneumonia. Classifying pneumonia is important because of the differences in the likely causative organisms (Table 28-2) and the selection of appropriate antimicrobial therapy.

Community-Acquired Pneumonia. Community-acquired pneumonia (CAP) is an acute infection of the lung occurring in patients who have not been hospitalized or resided in a long-term care facility within 14 days of the onset of symptoms.[5] The decision to treat the patient at home or admit him or her to the hospital is based on several factors such as the patient's age, vital signs, mental status, and presence of co-morbid conditions. Clinicians can use tools such as the CURB-65 scale (Table 28-3) or the Pneumonia Patient Outcomes Research Team (PORT) Pneumonia Severity Index (PSI) to supplement clinical judgment. (The PSI calculator is available online at *http://pda.ahrq.gov/clinic/psi/psicalc.asp*). Empiric antibiotic therapy should be started as soon as possible. (*Empiric therapy* is the initiation of treatment before a definitive diagnosis. It is based on experience and knowledge of drugs known to be effective for the likely causative agent.)

TABLE 28-2 ORGANISMS CAUSING PNEUMONIA

Community-Acquired Pneumonia	Medical Care–Associated Pneumonia
*Streptococcus pneumoniae**	*Pseudomonas aeruginosa*†
Mycoplasma pneumoniae	*Escherichia coli*†
Haemophilus influenzae	*Klebsiella pneumoniae*†
Respiratory viruses	*Acinetobacter* species†
Chlamydophila pneumoniae	*Haemophilus influenzae*
Chlamydophila psittaci	*Staphylococcus aureus*
Coxiella burnetti	*Streptococcus pneumoniae*
Legionella pneumophila	*Proteus* species
Oral anaerobes	*Enterobacter* species
Moraxella catarrhalis	Oral anaerobes
Staphylococcus aureus	
Pseudomonas aeruginosa	
Enteric aerobic gram-negative bacteria (e.g., *Klebsiella* species)	
Fungi	
Mycobacterium tuberculosis	

*Most common cause of community-acquired pneumonia (CAP).
†Most common causes of medical care–associated pneumonia (MCAP).

TABLE 28-3 ASSESSING PNEUMONIA USING CURB-65

The CURB-65 scale may be used as a supplement to clinical judgment to determine the severity of pneumonia and if patients need to be hospitalized.

Identifying the Level of Risk

Patients receive 1 point for each of the following indicators:

- **C:** Confusion (compared to baseline)
- **U:** BUN >20 mg/dL
- **R:** Respiratory rate ≥30 breaths/min
- **B:** Systolic blood pressure <90 mm Hg or diastolic blood pressure ≤60 mm Hg
- **65:** ≥Age 65 yr

Scoring and Decision Making

Score	Decision
0	Treat at home
1-2	Consider hospital admission
3 or more	Hospital admission
4-5	Consider admission to intensive care unit

Source: Lim WS, van der Eerden MM, Laing R, et al: Defining community acquired pneumonia severity on presentation to hospital: an international derivation and validation study, *Thorax* 58(5):377, 2003.

Medical Care–Associated Pneumonia. Medical care–associated pneumonia (MCAP) encompasses three forms of pneumonia: hospital-associated pneumonia, ventilator-associated pneumonia, and health care–associated pneumonia.[6]

Hospital-associated pneumonia (HAP) is pneumonia that occurs 48 hours or longer after hospital admission and was not incubating at the time of hospitalization. *Ventilator-associated pneumonia* (VAP) refers to pneumonia that occurs more than 48 hours after endotracheal intubation. (VAP is discussed in Chapter 66.) *Health care–associated pneumonia* (HCAP) is a new-onset pneumonia in a patient who (1) was hospitalized in an acute care hospital for 2 days or longer within 90 days of the infection; (2) resided in a long-term care facility; (3) received IV antibiotic therapy, chemotherapy, or wound care within the past 30 days of the current infection; or (4) attended a hospital or hemodialysis clinic.[6]

These infections cause significant morbidity and increase the risk of death. HAP, VAP, and HCAP also increase health care costs with longer hospital stays and associated costs.

Once the diagnosis is made, empiric treatment of the pneumonia is initiated based on known risk factors, early versus late onset, and probable organism. Antibiotic therapy can be adjusted once the results of sputum cultures identify the exact pathogen.

A major problem in treating MCAP is multidrug-resistant (MDR) organisms. Antibiotic susceptibility tests can identify MDR organisms. The virulence of these organisms can severely limit the available and appropriate antimicrobial therapy. In addition, MDR organisms can increase the morbidity and mortality risks associated with pneumonia. (Chapter 15 discusses MDR organisms.)

Aspiration Pneumonia. *Aspiration pneumonia,* occurring as either CAP or MCAP, results from the abnormal entry of material from the mouth or stomach into the trachea and lungs. Conditions that increase the risk of aspiration include decreased level of consciousness (e.g., seizure, anesthesia, head injury, stroke, alcohol intake), difficulty swallowing, and nasogastric intubation with or without tube feeding. With loss of consciousness, the gag and cough reflexes are depressed, and aspiration is more likely to occur. Other high-risk groups are those who are seriously ill, have poor dentition, or are receiving acid-reducing medications.[7]

The aspirated material (food, water, vomitus, or oropharyngeal secretions) triggers an inflammatory response. The most common form of aspiration pneumonia is a primary bacterial infection. Typically, more than one organism is identified on sputum culture, including both aerobes and anaerobes, since they comprise the flora of the oropharynx. Until the cultures are completed, the choice of antibiotic therapy is based on an assessment of the severity of illness, where the infection was acquired (community versus medical care), and the probable causative organism. In contrast, aspiration of acidic gastric contents causes *chemical (noninfectious) pneumonitis,* which may not require antibiotic therapy. However, secondary bacterial infection can occur 48 to 72 hours later.

Opportunistic Pneumonia. Individuals at risk for opportunistic pneumonia include those with altered immune responses. This can include people with severe protein-calorie malnutrition or immunodeficiencies (e.g., human immunodeficiency virus [HIV] infection), and those receiving radiation therapy, chemotherapy, and any immunosuppressive therapy, including long-term corticosteroid therapy. In addition to the risk of bacterial and viral pneumonia, the immunocompromised person may develop an infection from microorganisms that do not normally cause disease, such as *Pneumocystis jiroveci* (formerly *carinii*) and cytomegalovirus (CMV).

P. jiroveci pneumonia (PCP) rarely occurs in the healthy individual but is the most common form of pneumonia in people with HIV disease. The onset is slow and subtle with symptoms of fever, tachypnea, tachycardia, dyspnea, nonproductive cough, and hypoxemia. The chest x-ray usually shows diffuse bilateral infiltrates. In widespread disease the lungs have massive consolidation. PCP can be life threatening, causing acute respiratory failure and death. Infection can also spread to other organs, including the liver, bone marrow, lymph nodes, spleen, and thyroid. Bacterial and viral pneumonias must first be ruled out because of the vague presentation of PCP. Treatment consists of a course of trimethoprim/sulfamethoxazole

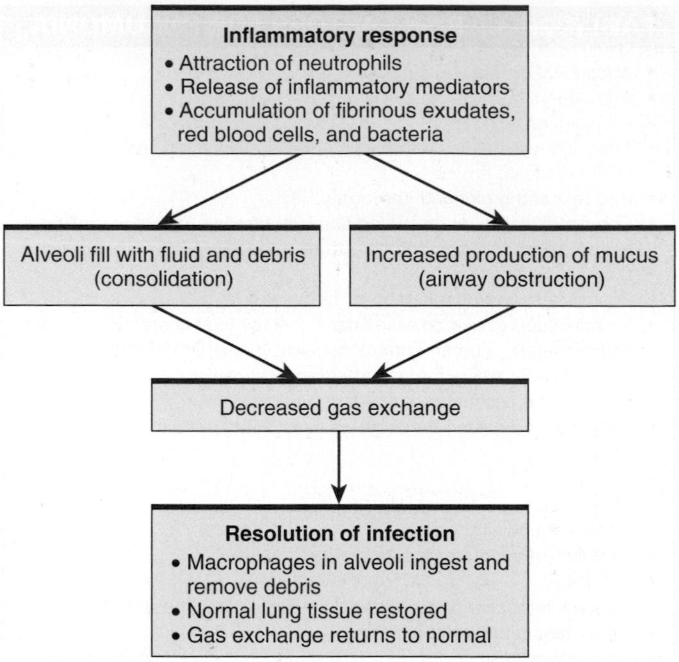

FIG. 28-1 Pathophysiologic course of pneumonia.

(Bactrim, Septra) either IV or orally depending on the severity of disease and the patient's response.

CMV, a herpes virus, can cause viral pneumonia. Most CMV infections are asymptomatic or mild, but severe disease can occur in people with an impaired immune response. CMV is the most common life-threatening infectious complication after hematopoietic stem cell transplantation.[8] Antiviral medications (e.g., ganciclovir [Cytovene], foscarnet [Foscavir], cidofovir [Vistide]) and high-dose immunoglobulin are used for treatment.

Pathophysiology

Specific pathophysiologic changes related to pneumonia vary according to the offending organism. Some viruses cause direct injury and cell death. The majority of organisms, however, trigger an inflammatory response in the lung (Fig. 28-1). A vascular reaction occurs, characterized by an increase in blood flow and vascular permeability. Neutrophils are activated to engulf and kill the offending organisms. The neutrophils, the offending organism, and fluid from surrounding blood vessels fill the alveoli and interrupt normal oxygen transportation, leading to clinical manifestations of hypoxia (e.g., tachypnea, dyspnea, tachycardia). Mucus production is also increased, which can obstruct airflow and further decrease gas exchange. Consolidation, a feature typical of bacterial pneumonia, occurs when the normally air-filled alveoli become filled with fluid and debris. Complete resolution and healing occur if there are no complications. Macrophages lyse and process the debris, normal lung tissue is restored, and gas exchange returns to normal.

Clinical Manifestations

The most common presenting symptoms of pneumonia are cough, fever, shaking chills, dyspnea, tachypnea, and pleuritic chest pain. The cough may or may not be productive. Sputum may appear green, yellow, or even rust colored (bloody). Viral pneumonia may initially be seen as influenza, with respiratory symptoms appearing and/or worsening 12 to 36 hours after onset.[9] The older or debilitated patient may not have classic symptoms of pneumonia. Confusion or stupor (possibly related to hypoxia) may be the only finding. Hypothermia, rather than fever, may also be noted with the older patient. Nonspecific clinical manifestations include diaphoresis, anorexia, fatigue, myalgias, headache, and abdominal pain.

On physical examination, rhonchi and crackles may be auscultated over the affected region. If consolidation is present, bronchial breath sounds, egophony, and increased fremitus (vibration of the chest wall produced by vocalization) may be noted. Patients with pleural effusion may exhibit dullness to percussion over the affected area.

Complications

Complications develop more frequently in older individuals and those with underlying chronic diseases. Potential complications include the following:

- *Pleurisy* (inflammation of the pleura) is relatively common.
- *Pleural effusion* (fluid in the pleural space) can occur. In most cases, the effusion is sterile and is reabsorbed in 1 to 2 weeks. Occasionally, effusions require aspiration by thoracentesis.
- *Atelectasis* (collapsed, airless alveoli) of one or part of one lobe may occur. These areas usually clear with effective coughing and deep breathing.
- *Bacteremia* (bacterial infection in the blood) is more likely to occur in infections with *Streptococcus pneumoniae* and *Haemophilus influenzae.*
- *Lung abscess* is not a common complication of pneumonia. However, it may occur with pneumonia caused by *S. aureus* and gram-negative organisms.
- *Empyema*, the accumulation of purulent exudate in the pleural cavity, occurs in less than 5% of cases and requires antibiotic therapy and drainage of the exudate by a chest tube or open surgical drainage.
- *Pericarditis* results from spread of the infecting organism from infected pleura or via a hematogenous route to the pericardium.
- *Meningitis* can be caused by *S. pneumoniae*. The patient with pneumonia who is disoriented, confused, or drowsy may have a lumbar puncture to evaluate the possibility of meningitis.
- *Sepsis* can occur when bacteria within alveoli enter the bloodstream. Severe sepsis can lead to shock and multisystem organ dysfunction syndrome (MODS) (see Chapter 67).
- *Acute respiratory failure* is one of the leading causes of death in patients with severe pneumonia. Failure occurs when pneumonia damages the lungs' ability to exchange oxygen for carbon dioxide.
- *Pneumothorax* can occur when air collects in the pleura space, causing the lungs to collapse.

Pleurisy, pleural effusion, atelectasis, lung abscess, and pneumothorax are discussed later in this chapter.

Diagnostic Studies

The common diagnostic measures for pneumonia are presented in Table 28-4. History, physical examination, and chest x-ray often provide enough information to make management decisions without costly laboratory tests. Chest x-ray often shows a typical pattern characteristic of the infecting organism and is important in the diagnosis of pneumonia. X-ray can also show pleural effusions. A thoracentesis and/or bronchoscopy with washings may be used to obtain fluid samples for patients not responding to initial therapy.

TABLE 28-4 COLLABORATIVE CARE

Pneumonia

Diagnostic	Collaborative Therapy
• History and physical examination • Chest x-ray • Gram stain of sputum • Sputum culture and sensitivity test • Pulse oximetry or ABGs (if indicated) • Complete blood count, WBC differential, and routine blood chemistries (if indicated) • Blood cultures (if indicated)	• Appropriate antibiotic therapy (see Table 28-6) • Increased fluid intake (at least 3 L/day) • Limited activity and rest • Antipyretics • Analgesics • O_2 therapy (if indicated)

Ideally, a sputum specimen for culture and Gram stain to identify the organism is obtained before beginning antibiotic therapy. However, antibiotic administration should not be delayed if a specimen cannot be readily obtained. Delays in antibiotic therapy can increase morbidity and mortality risks. Blood cultures are done for patients who are seriously ill. Arterial blood gases (ABGs) may be obtained to assess for hypoxemia (partial pressure of oxygen in arterial blood [PaO_2] less than 80 mm Hg), hypercapnia (partial pressure of carbon dioxide in arterial blood [$PaCO_2$] greater than 45 mm Hg), and acidosis. Leukocytosis occurs in the majority of patients with bacterial pneumonia; the white blood cell (WBC) count is usually greater than 15,000/μL (15×10^9/L) with the presence of bands (immature neutrophils).

The use of biologic markers of infection to guide clinical decisions for treatment of pneumonia is under investigation. Serum levels of C-reactive protein (CRP) and procalcitonin have shown promise in providing information to guide the duration of antibiotic therapy.[10]

Collaborative Care

Pneumococcal vaccine is used to prevent *S. pneumoniae* (pneumococcus) pneumonia. Vaccination is recommended for individuals 65 years of age or older and younger patients who are at high risk. A one-time repeat vaccination in 5 years is recommended for those who received their initial vaccination when less than 65 years of age (Table 28-5).

Prompt treatment with the appropriate antibiotic almost always cures bacterial and mycoplasmal pneumonia. In uncomplicated cases the patient responds to drug therapy within 48 to 72 hours. Indications of improvement include decreased temperature, improved breathing, and reduced chest pain. Abnormal physical findings can last more than 7 days. A repeat chest x-ray is obtained in 6 to 8 weeks to assess for resolution.

In addition to antibiotic therapy, supportive measures are individualized to the patient's needs. These may include O_2 therapy to treat hypoxemia, analgesics to relieve chest pain, and antipyretics such as aspirin or acetaminophen for significantly elevated temperature. Although cough suppressants, mucolytics, bronchodilators, and corticosteroids are often prescribed as adjunctive therapy, there is insufficient evidence to support their use.[11]

Individualize rest and activity to the patient's tolerance. Benefits of mobility include improved diaphragm movement and

TABLE 28-5 PNEUMOVAX VACCINATION

Groups for Which Initial Vaccination Is Recommended

- People age ≥65 yr
- People ages 2-64 yr with long-term health problem (e.g., chronic cardiovascular disease, chronic pulmonary disease, sickle cell disease, diabetes mellitus, alcoholism, cirrhosis, leaks of cerebrospinal fluid, or cochlear implant)
- People ages 19-64 yr who smoke cigarettes or have asthma
- People ages 2-64 yr who have a disease or condition that lowers the body's resistance to infection (e.g., Hodgkin's disease, leukemia, lymphoma, kidney failure, multiple myeloma, HIV infection, nephrotic syndrome; those receiving immunosuppressive chemotherapy, radiation therapy, or long-term corticosteroids; asplenia; and after organ or bone marrow transplantation)
- People living in long-term care facilities

Groups for Which Revaccination Is Recommended

People age ≥65 yr	Patients who received vaccine ≥5 yr previously and were <65 yr at the time of vaccination
People ages 2-64 yr who have a disease or condition that lowers the body's resistance to infection (same as above for initial vaccination)	If ≥5 yr have elapsed since receipt of first dose

Source: Centers for Disease Control and Prevention: Pneumococcal polysaccharide vaccine: what you need to know. Retrieved from *www.cdc.gov/vaccines/pubs/vis/downloads/vis-ppv.pdf.*

chest expansion, mobilization of secretions, and prevention of venous stasis.

Currently, no definitive treatment exists for the majority of viral pneumonias. Care is generally supportive. Antiviral therapy may be used to treat pneumonia caused by influenza (e.g., oseltamivir or zanamivir) and a few other select viruses (e.g., acyclovir [Zovirax] for herpes simplex virus).[12]

Drug Therapy. Once the pneumonia is classified, the health care provider bases empiric therapy on the likely infecting organism (see Table 28-2). Table 28-6 presents the drug therapy for bacterial CAP.

For HAP, VAP, and HCAP, empiric antibiotic therapy is based on whether the patient has risk factors for MDR organisms. The prevalence and resistance patterns of MDR pathogens vary among localities and institutions. Therefore the antibiotic regimen needs to be adapted to the local patterns of antibiotic resistance. Appropriate initial antibiotic therapy for HAP, VAP, and HCAP may also vary markedly. Multiple regimens exist, but all should include antibiotics that are effective against both resistant gram-negative and gram-positive organisms. Clinical improvement usually occurs in 3 to 5 days. Patients who deteriorate or fail to respond to therapy require aggressive evaluation to assess for noninfectious etiologies, complications, coexisting infectious processes, or pneumonia caused by a drug-resistant pathogen.

IV antibiotic therapy should be switched to oral therapy as soon as the patient is hemodynamically stable, is improving clinically, is able to ingest oral medication, and has a normally functioning gastrointestinal (GI) tract. Patients on oral therapy do not need to be observed in the hospital and can be discharged to home. Total treatment time for patients with CAP should be a minimum of 5 days, and the patient should be afebrile for 48 to 72 hours before stopping treatment. Longer treatment time may be needed if initial therapy was not active against the identified pathogen or complications occur.

TABLE 28-6 DRUG THERAPY

Bacterial Community-Acquired Pneumonia

Patient Variable	Treatment Options
Outpatient	
Previously Healthy	
No recent antibiotic therapy in past 3 mo and no risk for drug-resistant *Staphylococcus pneumoniae* (DRSP)	Macrolide OR doxycycline
Co-morbidities (e.g., COPD; diabetes; chronic heart, liver, lung, or renal disease; malignancy; use of antibiotics in past 3 mo)	Respiratory fluoroquinolone OR β-Lactam plus macrolide (doxycycline may be substituted for macrolide)
***Regions with ≥25% Macrolide-Resistant* S. pneumoniae**	Respiratory fluoroquinolone OR β-Lactam plus macrolide
Inpatient	
Medical Unit	Respiratory fluoroquinolone OR β-Lactam plus macrolide
ICU	β-Lactam plus either azithromycin or respiratory fluoroquinolone
Special Conditions	
• *Pseudomonas* infection	Antipneumococcal, antipseudomonal β-lactam plus either ciprofloxacin or levofloxacin OR Antipneumococcal, antipseudomonal β-lactam plus aminoglycoside and azithromycin OR Antipneumococcal, antipseudomonal β-lactam plus an aminoglycoside and an antipneumococcal fluoroquinolone
• *Pseudomonas* infection but patient has penicillin allergy	Substitute aztreonam for the above β-lactam
• Community-acquired methicillin-resistant *Staphylococcus aureus* (CA-MRSA)	Add vancomycin or linezolid (Zyvox)
Types of Antibiotics	
Macrolides	erythromycin, azithromycin (Zithromax), clarithromycin (Biaxin)
Fluoroquinolones	moxifloxacin (Avelox, Vigamox), levofloxacin (Levaquin), gemifloxacin (Factive)
β-Lactams	High-dose amoxicillin, amoxicillin/clavulanate (Augmentin), cefpodoxime (Vantin), ceftriaxone (Rocephin), cefuroxime (Ceftin)
Antipneumococcal, antipseudomonal β-lactams	imipenem/cilastatin (Primaxin), meropenem (Merrem), cefepime (Maxipime), piperacillin/tazobactam (Zosyn)

Source: Adapted from the Infectious Diseases Society of America Practice Guidelines for CAP. Retrieved from *http://www.idsociety.org/Organ_System/#CommunityAcquiredPneumoniaCAP.*

Nutritional Therapy. Hydration is important in the supportive treatment of pneumonia to prevent dehydration and loosen secretions. Individualize and carefully monitor fluid intake if the patient has heart failure. If the patient cannot maintain adequate oral intake, IV administration of fluids and electrolytes may be necessary.

Weight loss often occurs in patients with pneumonia because of increased metabolic needs and difficulty eating due to shortness of breath and pleuritic pain. Small, frequent meals are easier for dyspneic patients to tolerate. Offer foods high in calories and nutrients.

NURSING MANAGEMENT PNEUMONIA

NURSING ASSESSMENT

Table 28-7 presents subjective and objective data to obtain from a patient with pneumonia.

TABLE 28-7 NURSING ASSESSMENT

Pneumonia

Subjective Data

Important Health Information

Past health history: Lung cancer, COPD, diabetes mellitus, chronic debilitating disease, malnutrition, altered consciousness, immunosuppression, exposure to chemical toxins, dust, or allergens

Medications: Antibiotics; corticosteroids, chemotherapy, or any other immunosuppressants

Surgery or other treatments: Recent abdominal or thoracic surgery, splenectomy, endotracheal intubation, or any surgery with general anesthesia; tube feedings

Functional Health Patterns

Health perception–health management: Cigarette smoking, alcoholism; recent upper respiratory tract infection, malaise

Nutritional-metabolic: Anorexia, nausea, vomiting; chills

Activity-exercise: Prolonged bed rest or immobility; fatigue, weakness; dyspnea, cough (productive or nonproductive); nasal congestion

Cognitive-perceptual: Pain with breathing, chest pain, sore throat, headache, abdominal pain, muscle aches

Objective Data

General

Fever, restlessness or lethargy; splinting of affected area

Respiratory

Tachypnea; pharyngitis; asymmetric chest movements or retraction; decreased excursion; nasal flaring; use of accessory muscles (neck, abdomen); grunting; crackles, friction rub on auscultation; dullness on percussion over consolidated areas, increased tactile fremitus on palpation; pink, rusty, purulent, green, yellow, or white sputum (amount may be scant to copious)

Cardiovascular

Tachycardia

Neurologic

Changes in mental status, ranging from confusion to delirium

Possible Diagnostic Findings

Leukocytosis; abnormal ABGs with ↓ or normal PaO_2, ↓ $PaCO_2$, and ↑ pH initially, and later ↓ PaO_2, ↑ $PaCO_2$, and ↓ pH; positive sputum on Gram stain and culture; patchy or diffuse infiltrates, abscesses, pleural effusion, or pneumothorax on chest x-ray*

*In the older dehydrated patient, chest x-ray may not be indicative of pneumonia until patient is rehydrated.

NURSING DIAGNOSES

Nursing diagnoses for the patient with pneumonia may include, but are not limited to, the following:

- Impaired gas exchange *related to* fluid and exudate accumulation at the capillary-alveolar membrane
- Ineffective breathing pattern *related to* inflammation and pain
- Acute pain *related to* inflammation and ineffective pain management and/or comfort measures

Additional information on nursing diagnoses for the patient with pneumonia can be found in eNursing Care Plan 28-1 on the website for this chapter.

PLANNING

The overall goals are that the patient with pneumonia will have (1) clear breath sounds, (2) normal breathing patterns, (3) no signs of hypoxia, (4) normal chest x-ray, and (5) no complications related to pneumonia.

NURSING IMPLEMENTATION

HEALTH PROMOTION. To reduce the risk of pneumonia, teach individuals to practice good health habits, such as frequent hand washing, proper nutrition, adequate rest, regular exercise, and coughing or sneezing into the elbow rather than hands. Avoidance of cigarette smoke is one of the most important health-promoting behaviors. If possible, people should avoid exposure to people with URIs. If a URI occurs, it requires prompt attention with supportive measures (e.g., rest, fluids). If symptoms persist for longer than 7 days, the person should seek medical care. Encourage those at risk for pneumonia (e.g., the chronically ill, older adult) to obtain both influenza and pneumococcal vaccines (see Tables 27-3 and Table 28-5).

Identifying patients at risk (see Table 28-1) and taking measures to prevent pneumonia are priority interventions. Place the patient with altered consciousness in positions (e.g., side-lying, upright) that will prevent or minimize the risk of aspiration. Turn and reposition the patient at least every 2 hours to facilitate adequate lung expansion and to discourage pooling of secretions. Encourage and assist with ambulation and positioning in a chair. In the intensive care unit, strict adherence to all aspects of the ventilator bundle (see Table 68-8), a group of interventions aimed at reducing the risk of VAP, has been shown to significantly reduce VAP.[13]

Patients who have orogastric or nasogastric tubes are at risk for aspiration pneumonia (see Chapter 40). Although the feeding tube is small, an interruption in the integrity of the lower esophageal sphincter can allow reflux of gastric contents. To prevent aspiration, elevate the head of the bed 30 to 45 degrees and monitor gastric residual volumes (see Table 40-12).

Elevate the patient's head-of-bed to at least 30 degrees and have patient sit up for all meals. The patient who has difficulty swallowing needs assistance in eating, drinking, and taking medication to prevent aspiration. Assess for a gag reflex before giving food or fluids in patients who have received local anesthesia to the throat. Patients with impaired mobility from any cause need assistance with turning and moving, as well as encouragement to breathe deeply at frequent intervals. Early mobilization, the use of an incentive spirometer, and twice-daily oral hygiene with chlorhexidine swabs have been shown to significantly reduce the incidence of pneumonia in postoperative patients.[14] Treat pain to a comfort level that permits the patient to deep breathe, cough, and achieve optimum mobility.

Practice strict medical asepsis and adherence to infection control guidelines to reduce the incidence of health care–associated infections. Staff and visitors should wash their hands on entering and leaving the patient's room. Staff must wash or use sanitizing hand gel before and after providing care and on removing gloves. Respiratory devices, which can harbor microorganisms, have been associated with outbreaks of pneumonia. Use strict sterile aseptic technique when suctioning the patient's trachea, and use caution when handling ventilator circuits, tracheostomy tubing, and nebulizer circuits that can become contaminated from patient secretions. Avoid inappropriate use of antibiotics to prevent the development of drug-resistant organisms.

ACUTE INTERVENTION. Although many patients with pneumonia are treated on an outpatient basis, the nursing care plan for a patient with pneumonia (see eNursing Care Plan 28-1) applies to both these individuals and in-hospital patients. Essential nursing care for patients with pneumonia includes monitoring physical assessment parameters, providing treatment, and monitoring the patient's response to treatment. Along with physical assessment (including pulse oximetry monitoring), prompt collection of specimens and initiation of antibiotics are critical. Oxygen therapy, hydration, nutritional support, breathing exercises, early ambulation, and therapeutic positioning are part of nursing management. Collaboration with respiratory therapy for postural drainage and chest percussion is important.

AMBULATORY AND HOME CARE. Teach the patient about the importance of taking every dose of the prescribed antibiotic, any drug-drug and food-drug interactions for the prescribed antibiotic, and the need for adequate rest to continue recovery. Instruct the patient to drink plenty of liquids (at least 6 to 10 glasses/day, unless contraindicated) and to avoid alcohol and smoking. A cool mist humidifier or warm bath may help the patient breathe easier. Tell patients that it may be several weeks before their usual vigor and sense of well-being return. Explain that a follow-up chest x-ray will be done in 6 to 8 weeks to evaluate resolution of pneumonia. A prolonged period of convalescence may be necessary for the older adult or chronically ill patient.

Teaching should also include information about available influenza and pneumococcal vaccines. Patients can receive the pneumococcal vaccine and influenza vaccine at the same time in different arms.

EVALUATION

The expected outcomes are that the patient with pneumonia will

- Have effective respiratory rate, rhythm, and depth of respirations
- Lungs clear to auscultation

Additional outcomes for the patient with pneumonia are presented in eNursing Care Plan 28-1.

TUBERCULOSIS

Tuberculosis (TB) is an infectious disease caused by *Mycobacterium tuberculosis.* It usually involves the lungs, but any organ can be infected. TB is a primary cause of death worldwide from a potentially curable infectious disease. It is the leading cause of mortality in patients with HIV infection.[15] The incidence of TB worldwide declined until the mid-1980s when HIV disease emerged. The major factors contributing to the resurgence of TB were (1) high rates of TB among patients with HIV infection and (2) the emergence of MDR strains of *M. tuberculosis.* Worldwide, more than two billion people (one third of the population) are currently infected with TB. Although the prevalence of TB has increased in Europe, in the United States it has steadily declined since reaching a resurgence peak in 1992.[16,17]

CULTURAL & ETHNIC HEALTH DISPARITIES

Tuberculosis

- Of the reported tuberculosis (TB) cases in the United States, 82% occur in racial and ethnic minorities.
- Asians have the highest TB rate of any ethnic group in the United States. Native Hawaiian and other Pacific Islanders have the second-highest TB rate.
- African Americans have 40% of the TB cases in U.S.-born people.
- Of all the TB cases in the United States, 60% occur in foreign-born people. This rate is 11 times higher than in U.S.-born people.
- The percentage of foreign-born people with multidrug-resistant TB has increased from 25% in 1993 to 82% in 2010.
- Eleven U.S. states (California, Connecticut, Delaware, Iowa, Maine, Minnesota, Nebraska, New Hampshire, New York, North Dakota, and Utah) have ≥75% of their total cases of TB among foreign-born people.

Source: Centers for Disease Control and Prevention. Trends in tuberculosis—United States 2010, *Morbidity and Mortality Weekly Report* 60:11, 2011.

TB occurs disproportionately in the poor, the underserved, and minorities. In the United States, people at risk include the homeless, residents of inner-city neighborhoods, foreign-born people, those living or working in institutions (long-term care facilities, prisons, shelters, hospitals), IV injecting drug users, people at poverty level, and those with poor access to health care. Immunosuppression from any etiology (e.g., HIV infection, malignancy, long-term corticosteroid use) increases the risk of active TB infection. The prevalence of TB in the United States is highest in those of Asian descent (see Cultural & Ethnic Health Disparities box).

Once a strain of *M. tuberculosis* develops resistance to two of the most potent first-line antituberculous drugs (e.g., isoniazid [INH], rifampin [Rifadin]), it is defined as *multidrug-resistant tuberculosis* (MDR-TB). Extensively drug-resistant TB (XDR-TB) occurs when the organism is also resistant to any of the fluoroquinolones plus any injectable antibiotic agent. Resistance results from several problems, including incorrect prescribing, lack of public health case management, and patient nonadherence to the prescribed regimen.[18]

Etiology and Pathophysiology

M. tuberculosis is a gram-positive, acid-fast bacillus (AFB) that is usually spread from person to person via airborne droplets produced by breathing, talking, singing, sneezing, and coughing. A process of evaporation leaves small droplet nuclei, 1 to 5 μm in size, suspended in the air for minutes to hours. These droplet nuclei are then transmitted via inhalation to another person. TB is not highly infectious, and transmission usually requires close, frequent, or prolonged exposure. Brief exposure to a few tubercle bacilli rarely causes an infection. The disease cannot be spread by touching, sharing food utensils, kissing, or any other type of physical contact.

Factors that influence the likelihood of transmission include the (1) number of organisms expelled into the air, (2) concentration of organisms (small spaces with limited ventilation

TABLE 28-8 CLASSIFICATION OF TUBERCULOSIS (TB)

Class	Exposure or Infection	Description
0	No TB exposure	No TB exposure, not infected (no history of exposure, negative tuberculin skin test)
1	TB exposure, no infection	TB exposure, no evidence of infection (history of exposure, negative tuberculin skin test)
2	Latent TB infection, no disease	TB infection without disease (significant reaction to tuberculin skin test, negative bacteriologic studies, no x-ray findings compatible with TB, no clinical evidence of TB)
3	TB, clinically active	TB infection with clinically active disease (positive bacteriologic studies or both a significant reaction to tuberculin skin test and clinical or x-ray evidence of current disease)
4	TB, but not clinically active	No current disease (history of previous episode of TB or abnormal, stable x-ray findings in a person with a significant reaction to tuberculin skin test; negative bacteriologic studies if done; no clinical or x-ray evidence of current disease)
5	TB suspect	TB suspect (diagnosis pending); person should not be in this classification for >3 mo

Source: American Thoracic Society.

TABLE 28-9 LATENT TUBERCULOSIS (TB) INFECTION COMPARED WITH TB DISEASE

Latent TB Infection	TB Disease
Has no symptoms	Has symptoms that may include the following: • Bad cough that lasts ≥3 wk • Pain in the chest • Coughing up blood or sputum • Weakness or fatigue • Weight loss • No appetite • Chills • Fever • Sweating at night
Does not feel sick	Usually feels sick
Cannot spread TB bacteria to others	May spread TB bacteria to others
Usually has a skin test or blood test result indicating TB infection	Usually has a skin test or blood test result indicating TB infection
Has a normal chest x-ray and a negative sputum smear	May have an abnormal chest x-ray or positive sputum smear or culture
Needs treatment for latent TB infection to prevent active TB disease	Needs treatment for active TB disease

Source: Centers for Disease Control and Prevention: Tuberculosis (TB): basic TB facts. Retrieved from *www.cdc.gov/tb/topic/basics/default.htm.*

would mean higher concentration), (3) length of time of exposure, and (4) immune system of the exposed person. Once inhaled, these small particles lodge in the bronchiole and alveolus. A local inflammatory reaction occurs, and the focus of infection is established. This is called the *Ghon focus,* which develops into a *granuloma,* the hallmark of TB. The formation of a granuloma is a defense mechanism aimed at walling off the infection and preventing further spread. Replication of the bacillus is inhibited and the infection is stopped.

Seventy percent of immunocompetent adults infected with TB are able to completely kill the mycobacteria. The rest of them contain the mycobacteria in a nonreplicating dormant state. Of these individuals, 5% to 10% go on to develop active TB infection when the bacteria begin to multiply months or years later. *M. tuberculosis* is aerophilic (oxygen loving) and thus has an affinity for the lungs. However, the infection can spread via the lymphatic system and find favorable environments for growth in other organs, including the kidneys, epiphyses of the bone, cerebral cortex, and adrenal glands.

Classification

Several systems can be used to classify TB. The American Thoracic Society classifies TB based on development of the disease (Table 28-8). TB can also be classified according to its (1) presentation (primary, latent, or reactivated) and (2) whether it is pulmonary or extrapulmonary.

Primary infection occurs when the bacteria are inhaled and initiate an inflammatory reaction. The majority of people mount effective immune responses to encapsulate these organisms for the rest of their lives, preventing primary infection from progressing to disease.

Latent TB infection (LTBI) occurs in a person who does not have active TB disease (Table 28-9). These individuals are asymptomatic and cannot transmit the TB bacteria to others. An estimated 10 million to 15 million Americans have LTBI; of these, 5% to 10% will develop active TB disease at some point. Therefore treatment of LTBI is important (discussed later in this chapter).

If the initial immune response is not adequate, the body cannot contain the organisms, the bacteria replicate, and *active TB disease* results. When active disease develops within the first 2 years of infection, it is termed *primary TB.* Postprimary TB, or *reactivation TB,* is defined as TB disease occurring 2 or more years after the initial infection. Individuals co-infected with HIV are at greatest risk for developing active TB. Immunosuppression, diabetes mellitus, poor nutrition, aging, pregnancy, stress, and chronic disease can also precipitate the reactivation of LTBI.[18] If the site of TB is pulmonary or laryngeal, the individual is considered infectious and can transmit the disease to others.

Clinical Manifestations

People with LTBI have a positive skin test but are asymptomatic (see Table 28-9). Symptoms of pulmonary TB usually do not develop until 2 to 3 weeks after infection or reactivation. The characteristic pulmonary manifestation is an initial dry cough that frequently becomes productive with mucoid or mucopurulent sputum. Active TB disease may initially manifest with constitutional symptoms such as fatigue, malaise, anorexia, unexplained weight loss, low-grade fevers, and night sweats. Dyspnea is a late symptom that may signify considerable pulmonary disease or a pleural effusion. Hemoptysis, which occurs in less than 10% of patients with TB, is also a late symptom.

Sometimes TB has a more acute, sudden presentation. The patient may have a high fever, chills, generalized flu-like symptoms, pleuritic pain, and a productive cough. Auscultation of the lungs may be normal or reveal crackles, rhonchi, and/or bronchial breath sounds.

Immunosuppressed (e.g., HIV-infected) people and older adults are less likely to have fever and other signs of an infection. In patients with HIV, classic manifestations of TB such as fever, cough, and weight loss may be wrongly attributed to PCP or other HIV-associated opportunistic diseases. Clinical manifestations of respiratory problems in patients with HIV must be carefully investigated to determine the cause. A change in cognitive function may be the only initial presenting sign of TB in an older person.

The clinical manifestations of extrapulmonary TB depend on the organs infected. For example, renal TB can cause dysuria and hematuria. Bone and joint TB may cause severe pain. Headaches, vomiting, and lymphadenopathy may be present with TB meningitis.

Complications

Appropriately treated pulmonary TB typically heals without complications except for a scar and residual cavitation within the lung. Significant pulmonary damage, although rare, can occur in patients who are poorly treated or who do not respond to anti-TB treatment.

Miliary TB is the widespread dissemination of the mycobacterium. The bacteria are spread via the bloodstream to distant organs. The infection is characterized by a large amount of TB bacilli and may be fatal if left untreated. It can occur as a result of primary disease or reactivation of latent infection. Clinical manifestations of miliary TB slowly progress over a period of days, weeks, or even months. Symptoms vary depending on which organs are infected. Hepatomegaly, splenomegaly, and generalized lymphadenopathy may be present.

Pleural TB can result from either primary disease or reactivation of a latent infection. A pleural effusion is caused by bacteria in the pleural space, which trigger an inflammatory reaction and a pleural exudate of protein-rich fluid. Empyema is less common than effusion but may occur from large numbers of tubercular organisms in the pleural space.

Acute pneumonia may result when large amounts of tubercle bacilli are discharged from granulomas into the lung or lymph nodes. The clinical manifestations are similar to those of bacterial pneumonia.

Because TB can infect organs throughout the body, various acute and long-term complications can result. TB in the spine (Pott's disease) can lead to destruction of the intervertebral disc and adjacent vertebrae. Central nervous system TB can cause severe bacterial meningitis. Abdominal TB can lead to peritonitis, especially in HIV-positive patients. The kidneys, adrenal glands, lymph nodes, and urogenital tract may also be affected.

Diagnostic Studies

Tuberculin Skin Test. The tuberculin skin test (TST) (Mantoux test) using purified protein derivative (PPD) is the standard method to screen people for *M. tuberculosis.* The test is administered by injecting 0.1 mL of PPD intradermally on the ventral surface of the forearm. The test is read by inspection and palpation 48 to 72 hours later for the presence or absence of induration. Induration (not redness) at the injection site means the person has been exposed to TB and has developed antibodies. (Antibody formation would occur 2 to 12 weeks after the initial exposure to the organisms.) The indurated area (if present) is measured and recorded in millimeters. Based on the size of the induration and the risk factors, an interpretation is made according to diagnostic standards for determining a positive test reaction.[15] (The procedure for performing the TST is described in Chapter 26.) Because the immunocompromised patient may have a decreased response to TST, smaller induration reactions (5 mm or larger) are considered positive. (See Table 26-11 for guidelines in interpreting responses to the TST.)

Some people who were previously infected with TB may have a waning immune response to the TST, resulting in a false negative result. However, the repeated TST may stimulate (boost) the body's ability to react to tuberculin in future tests. A positive reaction to a subsequent test could then be misinterpreted as a new infection, rather than the result of the boosted reaction to an old infection. To prevent misinterpretation in future testing, a two-step testing process is recommended for initial testing for health care workers (who get repeated testing) and for individuals who have a decreased response to allergens. A negative two-step TST ensures that any future positive results can be accurately interpreted as being caused by a new infection.[19]

Interferon-γ Release Assays. Interferon-γ (INF-γ) release assays (IGRAs) provide another screening tool for TB. These whole blood assays detect INF-γ released from T lymphocytes in response to mycobacterial antigens. Examples of IGRAs include QuantiFERON-TB test and the T-SPOT.TB test. Test results are available in a few hours.

IGRAs offer several advantages over the TST in that they require only one patient visit, are not subject to reader bias, have no booster phenomenon, and are not affected by prior bacillus Calmette-Guérin (BCG) vaccination.[15] The cost of an IGRA is substantially higher than the TST. Current guidelines suggest that both tests are viable options and that selection should be based on context and reasons for testing. Neither IGRAs nor TST can distinguish between LTBI and active TB infection. LTBI can only be diagnosed by excluding active TB.

Chest X-Ray. Although the findings on chest x-ray examination are important, it is not possible to make a diagnosis of TB solely on chest x-ray findings, since other diseases can mimic the appearance of TB. The chest x-ray may also appear normal in a patient with TB. Findings suggestive of TB include upper lobe infiltrates, cavitary infiltrates, and lymph node involvement.

Bacteriologic Studies. The diagnosis of TB requires the demonstration of tubercle bacilli bacteriologically by sputum culture. The initial testing also involves a microscopic examination of stained sputum smears for AFB. Three consecutive sputum specimens collected on different days are obtained and sent for smear and culture. The culture, which can take up to 8 weeks, must grow the organisms for confirmatory diagnosis. Treatment is warranted pending results for patients in whom clinical suspicion of TB is high. Samples for other suspected TB sites can be collected from gastric washings, cerebrospinal fluid (CSF), or fluid from an effusion or abscess.

Collaborative Care

Most patients with TB are treated on an outpatient basis (Table 28-10). Many people can continue to work and maintain their lifestyles with few changes. Patients with sputum smear–positive TB are generally considered infectious for the first 2 weeks after starting treatment. Advise these patients to restrict visitors and avoid travel on public transportation and trips to public places. Hospitalization may be needed for the severely ill or debilitated.

TABLE 28-10 COLLABORATIVE CARE

Pulmonary Tuberculosis

Diagnostic	Collaborative Therapy
• History and physical examination • Tuberculin skin test (TST) • QuantiFERON-TB test • Chest x-ray • Bacteriologic studies • Sputum smear for acid-fast bacilli (AFB) • Sputum culture	• Long-term treatment with antimicrobial drugs (see Tables 28-11 and 28-12) • Follow-up bacteriologic studies and chest x-rays

TABLE 28-11 DRUG THERAPY

Tuberculosis (TB)

Drug	Side Effects*
isoniazid (INH)	Hepatitis, asymptomatic elevation of aminotransferases (ALT, AST) Monitor liver function tests monthly
rifampin (Rifadin)	Hepatitis, thrombocytopenia, orange discoloration of bodily fluids (sputum, urine, sweat, tears)
pyrazinamide (PZA)	Hepatitis, arthralgias, hyperuricemia
ethambutol (Myambutol)	Ocular toxicity (decreased red-green color discrimination) Monitor visual acuity and color discrimination regularly
rifabutin (Mycobutin)	Hepatitis, thrombocytopenia, neutropenia, orange discoloration of bodily fluids (sputum, urine, sweat, tears)
rifapentine (Priftin)	Similar to those of rifampin
streptomycin	Ototoxicity, neurotoxicity, nephrotoxicity
bedaquiline (Sirturo)	Dysrhythmias
aminoglycosides	Ototoxicity, nephrotoxicity
capreomycin (Capastat) kanamycin (Kantrex) amikacin (Amikin)	Used in selected cases for treatment of resistant strains
fluoroquinolones	GI disturbance, neurologic effects (dizziness, headache), rash
levofloxacin (Levaquin) moxifloxacin (Avelox, Vigamox)	Used in drug-resistant TB

*Only common side effects are listed.
ALT, Alanine transaminase; *AST,* aspartate aminotransferase.

The mainstay of TB treatment is drug therapy (Table 28-11). Promoting and monitoring adherence are critical for treatment to be successful.

Drug Therapy

Active TB Disease. Because of the growing prevalence of MDR-TB, it is important to manage the patient with active TB aggressively. Drug therapy is divided into two phases: initial and continuation (Table 28-12). In most circumstances the treatment regimen for patients with previously untreated TB consists of a 2-month initial phase with four-drug therapy (INH, rifampin, pyrazinamide [PZA], and ethambutol). If drug susceptibility test results indicate that the bacteria are susceptible to all drugs, ethambutol may be discontinued. If PZA cannot be included in the initial phase (because of liver disease, pregnancy, etc.), the remaining three drugs are used for the initial phase.

TABLE 28-12 DRUG THERAPY

Tuberculosis Disease Regimens

Initial Phase	Continuation Phase
Option 1 4-drug regimen consisting of INH, rifampin, pyrazinamide, ethambutol Given daily for 56 doses (8 wk) OR 5 days/wk DOT for 40 doses (8 wk)	INH, rifampin daily for 126 doses (18 wk) OR 5 days/wk DOT for 90 doses (18 wk)
Option 2 4-drug regimen consisting of INH, rifampin, pyrazinamide, ethambutol Given daily for 14 doses (2 wk), followed by twice weekly for 12 doses (6 wk) OR 5 days/wk DOT for 10 doses (2 wk), then twice weekly for 12 doses (6 wk)	INH, rifampin twice weekly for 36 doses (18 wk) OR once weekly for 18 doses (18 wk)
Option 3 4-drug regimen consisting of INH, rifampin, pyrazinamide, ethambutol Given 3 times weekly for 24 doses (8 wk)	INH, rifampin 3 times weekly for 54 doses (18 wk)
Option 4 3-drug regimen consisting of INH, rifampin, ethambutol Given daily for 56 doses (8 wk) OR 5 days/wk DOT for 40 doses (8 wk)	INH, rifampin daily for 217 doses (31 wk) OR 5 days/wk DOT for 155 doses (31 wk) OR twice weekly for 62 doses (31 wk)

Source: American Thoracic Society, Centers for Disease Control and Prevention, and Infectious Diseases Society of America: Treatment of tuberculosis. Retrieved from *www.cdc.gov/mmwr/PDF/rr/rr5211.pdf.*
DOT, Directly observed therapy; *INH,* isoniazid.

DRUG ALERT: Isoniazid (INH)
- Alcohol may increase hepatotoxicity of the drug. Instruct patient to avoid drinking alcohol during treatment.
- Monitor for signs of liver damage before and while taking drug.

Other drugs can be used if the patient develops a toxic reaction to the primary drugs. The newer rifamycins, rifabutin and rifapentine (Priftin), should be considered first line in special situations: rifabutin for patients receiving medications that have interactions with rifampin or who have an intolerance to rifampin, and rifapentine with INH in once-weekly dosing for selected patients. Treatment for drug-resistant TB is guided by sensitivity testing. MDR-TB therapy typically includes a fluoroquinolone and an injectable antibiotic (see Table 28-11). Bedaquiline (Sirturo), a relatively new drug, is used in combination with other drugs to treat MDR-TB. It works by inhibiting an enzyme needed for *M. tuberculosis* to replicate.

Directly observed therapy (DOT) involves providing the antituberculous drugs directly to patients and watching as they swallow the medications. It is the preferred strategy for all patients with TB to ensure adherence and is recommended for all patients at risk for nonadherence.[15] Nonadherence is a major factor in the emergence of multidrug resistance and treatment failures. Many individuals do not adhere to the treatment program in spite of understanding the disease process and the value of treatment. DOT is an expensive but essential public health measure. The risk for reactivation of TB and MDR-TB is increased in patients who do not complete the full course of therapy. In many areas the public health nurse administers DOT at a clinic site.

ETHICAL/LEGAL DILEMMAS

Patient Adherence

Situation

The health clinic for the homeless discovers that F.C., a 64-year-old African American man with tuberculosis (TB), has not been taking his prescribed medication. He tells you that it is hard for him to get to the clinic to obtain the medication, much less to keep on a schedule. You are concerned not only about this patient, but also about the risks for the other people at the shelter, in the park, and at the meal sites.

Ethical/Legal Points for Consideration

- Adherence is a complex issue involving a person's culture and values, perceived risk of disease, availability of resources, access to treatment, and perceived consequences of available choices.
- Advocacy for the patient and the community obliges you to involve other members of the health care team, such as social services, to assist in obtaining the necessary resources or support for the patient to complete a course of treatment.
- Legally the constitutionally granted right to control one's own body may be limited by the state and federal obligation to protect public health and safety. Most of these laws have provisions for the protection of constitutional rights such as right to counsel, the right to least restrictive alternative in terms of confinement setting, and the right to prompt judicial review.
- The federal government and many states have provisions for quarantine, detention, and treatment. With the threats of bioterrorism and the globalization of exposure to highly lethal infectious diseases, it seems unlikely that the government's power to detain will be removed.

Discussion Questions

1. What alternatives of care can be offered to F.C.?
2. Under what circumstances are health care providers justified in overriding a patient's autonomy or decision making?

When DOT is not used, fixed-dose combination drugs may enhance adherence. Combinations of INH and rifampin (Rifamate) and of INH, rifampin, and PZA (Rifater) are available to simplify therapy. The therapy for people with HIV follows the same therapy options outlined in Table 28-12. However, alternative regimens that include once-weekly INH plus rifapentine continuation dosing in any HIV-infected patient and twice-weekly INH plus rifampin or rifabutin should not be used if $CD4^+$ counts are less than 100/μL. Health care providers must also be alert for possible drug interactions between antiretrovirals (used to treat HIV) and rifamycins.

Teaching patients about the side effects of these drugs and when to seek prompt medical attention is critical. The major side effect of INH, rifampin, and PZA is nonviral hepatitis. Baseline liver function tests (LFTs) are done at the start of treatment. Monthly monitoring of LFTs is done if baseline tests are abnormal.

Latent Tuberculosis Infection. In people with LTBI, drug therapy helps prevent a TB infection from developing into active TB disease. Because a person with LTBI has fewer bacteria, treatment is much easier. Usually only one drug is needed. Drug therapy regimens for LTBI are presented in Table 28-13.

The standard treatment regimen for LTBI is 9 months of daily INH. It is an effective and inexpensive drug that the patient can take orally. The 9-month regimen is more effective, but adherence issues may make a 6-month regimen preferable. For HIV patients and those with fibrotic lesions on chest x-ray, INH

TABLE 28-13 DRUG THERAPY

Latent Tuberculosis Infection Regimens

Drugs	Duration	Interval	Minimum Doses
isoniazid	9 mo	Daily	270
		Twice weekly*	76
isoniazid	6 mo	Daily	180
		Twice weekly*	52
isoniazid and rifapentine	3 mo	Once weekly*	12
rifampin	4 mo	Daily	120

Source: Centers for Disease Control and Prevention: Tuberculosis (TB): treatment options for latent tuberculosis infection. Retrieved from *www.cdc.gov/tb/publications/factsheets/treatment/LTBItreatmentoptions.htm.*
* Use directly observed therapy (DOT).

is given for 9 months. An alternative 3-month regimen of INH and rifapentine may be used for otherwise healthy patients who are not presumed to be infected with drug-resistant bacilli. Four-month therapy with rifampin may be indicated if the patient is resistant to INH. Because of reports of severe liver injury and deaths, the CDC does not recommend the combination of rifampin and PZA for treatment of LTBI.

Vaccine. BCG vaccine is a live, attenuated strain of *Mycobacterium bovis.* The vaccine is given to infants in parts of the world with a high prevalence of TB. In the United States it is typically not recommended because of the low risk of infection, the vaccine's variable effectiveness against adult pulmonary TB, and potential interference with TB skin test reactivity. The BCG vaccination can result in a false-positive TST. IGRA results are not affected. The BCG vaccine should be considered only for select individuals who meet specific criteria (e.g., health care workers who are continually exposed to patients with MDR-TB and when infection control precautions are not successful).

NURSING MANAGEMENT TUBERCULOSIS

NURSING ASSESSMENT

Ask the patient about a previous history of TB, chronic illness, or any immunosuppressive medications. Obtain a social and occupational history to determine risk factors for transmission of TB. Assess the patient for productive cough, night sweats, afternoon temperature elevation, weight loss, pleuritic chest pain, and abnormal lung sounds. If the patient has a productive cough, early morning is the ideal time to collect sputum.

NURSING DIAGNOSES

Nursing diagnoses for the patient with TB may include, but are not limited to, the following:

- Ineffective breathing pattern *related to* decreased lung capacity
- Ineffective airway clearance *related to* increased secretions, fatigue, and decreased lung capacity
- Noncompliance *related to* lack of knowledge of disease process, lack of motivation, long-term nature of treatment, and lack of resources
- Ineffective self-health management *related to* lack of knowledge about the disease process and therapeutic regimen

PLANNING

The overall goals are that the patient with TB will (1) comply with the therapeutic regimen, (2) have no recurrence of disease, (3) have normal pulmonary function, and (4) take appropriate measures to prevent the spread of the disease.

NURSING IMPLEMENTATION

HEALTH PROMOTION. The ultimate goal is to eradicate TB worldwide. Screening programs in known risk groups are of value in detecting individuals with TB. Treatment of LTBI reduces the number of TB carriers in the community. The person with a positive TST should have a chest x-ray to assess for active TB disease. Individuals with a diagnosis of TB must be reported to the public health authorities for identification and assessment of contacts and risk to the community.

Programs to address the social determinants of TB are necessary to decrease transmission of TB.[20] Reducing HIV infection, poverty, overcrowded living conditions, malnutrition, smoking, and drug and alcohol abuse can help minimize TB infection rates. Improving access to health care and education is also important.

ACUTE INTERVENTION. Patients admitted to the emergency department or directly to the nursing unit with respiratory symptoms should be triaged for the possibility of TB. Those strongly suspected of having TB should (1) be placed on airborne isolation; (2) receive a medical workup, including chest x-ray, sputum smear, and culture; and (3) receive appropriate drug therapy. Airborne infection isolation is indicated for the patient with pulmonary or laryngeal TB until the patient is noninfectious. *Airborne infection isolation* refers to isolation of patients infected with organisms spread by the airborne route. It requires a single-occupancy room with negative pressure and airflow of 6 to 12 exchanges per hour.

High-efficiency particulate air (HEPA) masks are worn whenever entering the patient's room. These masks are highly effective at protecting from small particles 5 μm or less in diameter. Health care providers should be "fit tested" to ensure proper mask size. To be effective, the mask must be molded to fit tightly around the nose and mouth.

Teach patients to cover the nose and mouth with paper tissues every time they cough, sneeze, or produce sputum. The tissues should be thrown into a paper bag and disposed of with the trash, burned, or flushed down the toilet. Emphasize careful hand washing after handling sputum and soiled tissues. If patients need to be out of the negative-pressure room, they must wear a standard isolation mask to prevent exposure to others. Minimize prolonged visitation to other parts of the hospital.

Identify and screen close contacts of the person with TB. Anyone testing positive for TB infection will undergo further evaluation and needs to be treated for either LTBI or active TB disease.

AMBULATORY AND HOME CARE. Patients who respond clinically are discharged home (even with positive cultures) if their household contacts have already been exposed and the patient is not posing a risk to susceptible people. Negative cultures are needed to declare the patient not infectious. Monthly sputum cultures are obtained until two consecutive specimens are culture negative.[15]

Teach the patient how to minimize exposure to close contacts and household members. Homes should be well ventilated, especially the areas where the infected person spends a lot of time. While still infectious, the patient should sleep alone, spend as much time as possible outdoors, and minimize time in congregate settings or on public transportation.

Teach the patient and caregiver about adherence with the prescribed regimen. This is important, since most treatment failures occur because the patient neglects to take the drug, discontinues it prematurely, or takes it irregularly. Strategies to improve adherence to drug therapy include teaching and counseling, reminder systems, incentives or rewards, contracts, and DOT.

Notification of the public health department is required. The public health nurse is responsible for follow-up on household contacts and assessment of the patient for adherence. If adherence is an issue, the public health agency may be responsible for DOT. Most individuals can be considered adequately treated when the therapy regimen has been completed and there is evidence of negative cultures, clinical improvement, and improvement on chest x-ray.

Because about 5% of individuals experience relapses, teach the patient to recognize the symptoms that indicate recurrence of TB. If these symptoms occur, the patient should seek immediate medical attention. Instruct the patient about certain factors that could reactivate TB, such as immunosuppressive therapy, malignancy, and prolonged debilitating illness. If the patient experiences any of these events, the health care provider must be told so that reactivation of TB can be closely monitored. In some situations it is necessary to put the patient on anti-TB therapy. Because smoking is associated with poor outcomes in TB, patients should be encouraged to quit. Provide patients with teaching and resources to help them stop smoking.

EVALUATION

The expected outcomes are that the patient with TB will have

- Complete resolution of the disease
- Normal pulmonary function
- Absence of any complications
- No transmission of TB

ATYPICAL MYCOBACTERIA

There are more than 30 varieties of acid-fast mycobacteria that do not cause TB but can cause pulmonary disease, lymphadenitis, skin or soft tissue disease, or disseminated disease. Pulmonary disease is indistinguishable from TB clinically and radiologically but can be differentiated by bacteriologic culture. Atypical mycobacteria are not airborne and thus are not transmitted by droplets.

Mycobacterium avium complex (MAC), found in aerosols generated from baths, hot spas, and swimming pools, is the most common cause of atypical mycobacteria pulmonary infection. Only a small number of people exposed to the organism actually develop MAC lung disease. People who are immunosuppressed (e.g., HIV/AIDS) or have chronic pulmonary disease are most susceptible. Treatment is similar to that for TB.

PULMONARY FUNGAL INFECTIONS

Pulmonary fungal pneumonia is an infectious process in the lungs caused by endemic (native and common) or opportunis-

TABLE 28-14 FUNGAL INFECTIONS OF THE LUNG

Infection	Organism
Endemic Fungal Infections	
Histoplasmosis	*Histoplasma capsulatum*
Coccidioidomycosis	*Coccidioides immitis*
Blastomycosis	*Blastomyces dermatitidis*
Opportunistic Fungal Infections	
Candidiasis	*Candida albicans*
Aspergillosis	*Aspergillus niger* or *Aspergillus fumigatus*
Cryptococcosis	*Cryptococcus neoformans*

tic fungi (Table 28-14). *Endemic* fungal pathogens cause infection in healthy people and in immunocompromised people in certain geographic locations in the United States. For example, *Coccidioides*, which cause coccidioidomycosis, is a fungus found in the soil of dry, low rainfall areas. It is endemic in many areas of the southwestern United States. *Opportunistic* fungal infections occur in immunocompromised patients (e.g., those being treated with corticosteroids, chemotherapy, and immunosuppressive drugs) and in patients with HIV and cystic fibrosis. These infections can be very serious.

Fungal infections are acquired by inhalation of spores. These infections are not transmitted from person to person, and the patient does not have to be placed in isolation. The clinical manifestations are similar to those of bacterial pneumonia. Skin testing, serology, and biopsy methods assist in identifying the infecting organism.

Amphotericin B remains the standard therapy for treating serious systemic fungal infections. It must be given IV to achieve adequate blood and tissue levels because the GI tract does not absorb it well. Less serious infections can be treated with oral antifungals such as ketoconazole (Nizoral), fluconazole (Diflucan), voriconazole (Vfend), and itraconazole (Sporanox). Effectiveness of therapy can be monitored with fungal serology titers.[21]

LUNG ABSCESS

Etiology and Pathophysiology

A **lung abscess** is caused by necrosis of lung tissue typically resulting from bacteria aspirated from the GI tract or from the oral cavity in patients with periodontal disease. Because oral secretions can contain large amounts of bacteria, even small amounts *(microaspiration)* can cause infection. The abscess usually develops slowly, beginning with an enlarging area of infection that becomes necrotic and eventually forms a cavity filled with purulent material. Lung abscesses can also result from IV drug use, malignancy, pulmonary emboli, TB, and various parasitic and fungal diseases. Abscesses usually contain more than one type of microbe, most commonly reflecting the anaerobic flora of the mouth.

The area of the lung most often affected is the posterior segment of the right upper lobe. The abscess may erode into the bronchial system, causing the production of foul-smelling or sour-tasting sputum. It may grow toward the pleura and cause pleuritic pain. Multiple small abscesses, sometimes referred to as necrotizing pneumonia, can occur within the lung.

Clinical Manifestations and Complications

Clinical manifestations usually occur slowly over a period of weeks to months, especially if anaerobic organisms are the primary cause. Symptoms of abscess caused by aerobic bacteria develop more acutely and resemble bacterial pneumonia. The most common manifestation is cough-producing purulent sputum (often dark brown) that is foul smelling and foul tasting. Hemoptysis is common, especially when an abscess ruptures into a bronchus. Other common manifestations are fever, chills, prostration, night sweats, pleuritic pain, dyspnea, anorexia, and weight loss.

Physical examination of the lungs indicates dullness to percussion and decreased breath sounds on auscultation over the involved segment of lung. Bronchial breath sounds may be transmitted to the periphery if the communicating bronchus becomes patent and the segment begins to drain. Crackles may also be present in the later stages as the abscess drains.

Complications include chronic pulmonary abscess, bronchopleural fistula, bronchiectasis, and empyema from perforation of the abscess into the pleural cavity. The infection can also spread via the bloodstream, resulting in a brain abscess.

Diagnostic Studies

A chest x-ray is often the only test needed. The presence of a solitary cavitary lesion with an air-fluid level and local infiltrate can confirm the diagnosis. Computed tomography (CT) scanning may be helpful if the cavitation is not clear on chest x-ray. As long as there is drainage via the bronchus, sputum will contain the microorganisms that are present in the abscess. However, expectorated sputum samples are contaminated with oral flora, making it difficult to determine the offending organisms. Bronchoscopy may be used (1) to avoid oropharyngeal contamination, (2) to collect a specimen if drainage is delayed, or (3) to investigate if there is a possibility of an underlying malignancy. Pleural fluid and blood cultures may be useful to identify the offending organisms. Although nonspecific, an elevated neutrophil count from a complete blood count (CBC) indicates an infectious process.

NURSING AND COLLABORATIVE MANAGEMENT LUNG ABSCESS

Monitor the patient's vital signs, level of consciousness, and respiratory status for any signs of hypoxia. Note any cyanosis or clubbing of the fingers. Administer oxygen as needed. Broad-spectrum antibiotic coverage is necessary because of mixed bacteria in an abscess. IV antibiotic therapy should be started as soon as possible. Clindamycin is first-line therapy. Parenteral antibiotics are switched to oral antibiotics once the patient shows clinical and x-ray evidence of improvement.

Because of the need for prolonged antibiotic therapy, the patient must be aware of the importance of continuing the medication for the prescribed period. Sometimes the patient is asked to return periodically during the course of antibiotic therapy for repeat cultures and sensitivity tests to ensure that the infecting organism is not becoming resistant to the antibiotic. When antibiotic therapy is completed, the patient is reevaluated.

Teach the patient how to cough effectively (see Table 29-23). Chest physiotherapy and postural drainage are not recommended because they may cause spillage of infection into other bronchi, extending the infection. Rest, good nutrition, and adequate fluid intake are supportive measures to facilitate recovery. If dentition is poor and dental hygiene is not adequate, encourage the patient to obtain dental care. Consider collaboration with the social worker to evaluate available options for dental care if the patient has limited resources.

Percutaneous drainage of the abscess may be necessary if the patient does not adequately respond to antibiotic treatment. A CT- or ultrasound-guided catheter is placed to drain the abscess. Surgery is rarely indicated but occasionally necessary when reinfection of a large cavitary lesion occurs or to establish a diagnosis when there is evidence of an underlying problem such as a neoplasm. The usual procedure in such cases is a lobectomy. A pneumonectomy may be necessary for multiple abscesses.

ENVIRONMENTAL LUNG DISEASES

Environmental or occupational lung diseases result from inhaled dust or chemicals. The extent of lung damage is influenced by the toxicity of the inhaled substance, amount and duration of exposure, and individual susceptibility. Environmentally induced lung disease includes pneumoconiosis, chemical pneumonitis, hypersensitivity pneumonitis, and asthma. (Asthma is discussed in Chapter 29.)

Pneumoconiosis is a general term for a group of lung diseases caused by inhalation and retention of mineral or metal dust particles. The literal meaning of *pneumoconiosis* is "dust in the lungs." These diseases are classified according to the origin of the dust (e.g., silicosis, asbestosis, berylliosis). Black lung is caused by inhalation of large amounts of coal dust, an occupational hazard for underground coal miners. The inhaled substance is ingested by macrophages, which releases substances that cause cell injury and death. Fibrosis occurs as a result of tissue repair. Repeated exposure eventually results in diffuse *pulmonary fibrosis* (excess connective tissue). Fibrosis is the result of tissue repair after inflammation. Pneumoconiosis and other environmental lung diseases are presented in eTable 28-1 available on the website for this chapter.

Chemical pneumonitis results from exposures to toxic chemical fumes. Acutely, there is diffuse lung injury characterized as pulmonary edema. Chronically, the clinical picture is that of *bronchiolitis obliterans* (obstruction of the bronchioles due to inflammation and fibrosis), which is usually associated with a normal chest x-ray or one that shows hyperinflation. An example is silo filler's disease.

Hypersensitivity pneumonitis, or extrinsic allergic alveolitis, is a form of parenchymal lung disease seen when an individual inhales antigens to which he or she is allergic. Examples include bird fancier's lung and farmer's lung.

Lung cancer, either squamous cell carcinoma or adenocarcinoma, is the most frequent cancer associated with asbestos exposure. People with more exposure are at a greater risk of disease. There is a minimum lapse of 15 to 19 years between first exposure and development of lung cancer. Mesotheliomas, both pleural and peritoneal, are also associated with asbestos exposure.

Clinical Manifestations

Symptoms of many environmental lung diseases may not occur until at least 10 to 15 years after the initial exposure to the inhaled irritant. Clinical manifestations common to all pneumoconioses include dyspnea, cough, wheezing, and weight loss. Pulmonary function studies often show reduced vital capacity. A chest x-ray often reveals lung involvement specific to the primary problem. CT scans have been useful in detecting early lung involvement.

Cor pulmonale (described later in this chapter) is a late complication, especially in conditions characterized by diffuse pulmonary fibrosis. COPD is the most common complication of environmental lung disease. Other associated disorders include lung cancer, mesothelioma, and TB. Manifestations of these complications are often the reason the patient seeks health care.

Manifestations of acute hypersensitivity pneumonitis occur 4 to 6 hours after exposure and include chills, fever, cough, shortness of breath, and malaise. Symptoms of chronic hypersensitivity pneumonitis include cough, anorexia, and weight loss. Acute pulmonary edema may occur after exposure to chemical fumes.

Collaborative Care

The best approach to management of environmental lung diseases is to try to prevent or decrease environmental and occupational exposure. Teach the public about the risk and the appropriate protective equipment. Using well-designed, effective ventilation systems and wearing masks are appropriate for some occupations and household activities. Inhalation of smoke by nonsmoking workers has led to regulations requiring a smoke-free workplace. Periodic inspections and monitoring of workplaces by agencies such as the Occupational Safety and Health Administration (OSHA) and the National Institute for Occupational Safety and Health (NIOSH) reinforce the employers' obligations to provide a safe work environment. NIOSH is responsible for workplace safety and health regulations in the United States *(www.cdc.gov/niosh/homepage.html).*

Early diagnosis is essential to halting the disease process. Strategies are directed toward preventing disease progression and improving or controlling respiratory symptoms. Discontinuation of exposure to the offending inhalant and smoking cessation may or may not be effective in stopping disease progression. Strategies to improve respiratory status include O_2 therapy, inhaled bronchodilators, percussion therapy, and pulmonary rehabilitation. Patients should also be immunized against pneumococcal pneumonia and influenza.

LUNG CANCER

Lung cancer is the leading cause of cancer-related deaths in the United States. Lung cancer accounts for 28% of all cancer deaths, more than those caused by breast, prostate, and colon cancer combined. An estimated 225,000 new cases of lung cancer are diagnosed and 160,000 deaths occur each year in the United States. Although lung cancer is associated with a high mortality and low cure rate, advances in medical treatment are improving the response to treatment.[22]

Etiology

Smoking is responsible for 80% to 90% of all lung cancers. Tobacco smoke contains 60 carcinogens in addition to substances (carbon monoxide, nicotine) that interfere with normal cell development. Exposure to tobacco smoke causes changes in the bronchial epithelium, which usually returns to normal when smoking is discontinued. The risk of lung cancer gradually

CULTURAL & ETHNIC HEALTH DISPARITIES
Lung Cancer

African Americans
- Have the highest incidence of lung cancer
- Are more likely to die from lung cancer than any other ethnic group
- Have a higher rate of lung cancer among men than in other ethnic groups

Whites
- Have the second-highest death rate from lung cancer
- Have a higher rate of lung cancer among women than in other ethnic groups

Asian/Pacific Islanders and Hispanics
- Have the lowest rates of lung cancer in both men and women

Other
- Regional variations among ethnic groups may be due to smoking prevalence, exposure to cancer-causing substances, and other factors.
- Cigarette consumption has decreased dramatically in developed countries such as the United States and Canada.
- Cigarette smoking is increasing in developing countries (e.g., nations in Africa, Asia, Latin America).

Source: Centers for Disease Control and Prevention: Racial/ethnic disparities and geographic differences in lung cancer incidence—38 states and the District of Columbia, 1998-2006. Retrieved from *www.cdc.gov/mmwr/PDF/wk/mm5944.pdf.*

decreases with smoking cessation, reaching that of nonsmokers within 10 to 15 years of quitting.

Assessment of the risk of lung cancer is now divided into three categories: (1) smokers, people who are currently smoking; (2) nonsmokers, people who formerly smoked; and (3) never smokers. The Memorial Sloan-Kettering Cancer Center has developed a tool that calculates risk for developing lung cancer for smokers and former smokers who quit 20 years ago or less *(www.mskcc.org/cancer-care/adult/lung/prediction-tools).*

The risk of developing lung cancer is directly related to total exposure to tobacco smoke, measured by total number of cigarettes smoked in a lifetime, age of smoking onset, depth of inhalation, tar and nicotine content, and the use of unfiltered cigarettes. Sidestream smoke (smoke from burning cigarettes, cigars) contains the same carcinogens found in mainstream smoke (smoke inhaled and exhaled by the smoker). This exposure to secondhand smoke creates a health risk to nonsmoking adults and children.

Other common causes of lung cancer include high levels of pollution, radiation (especially radon exposure), and asbestos.[22] Heavy or prolonged exposure to industrial agents such as ionizing radiation, coal dust, nickel, uranium, chromium, formaldehyde, and arsenic can also increase the risk of lung cancer, especially in smokers.

Marked variations exist in a person's propensity to develop lung cancer. Although genetic factors are not yet well understood, mutations in the epidermal growth factor receptor gene *(EGFR)* may be linked to familial lung cancer.[22] It is also theorized that people have different genetic carcinogen-metabolizing pathways. This may explain why some smokers develop lung cancer and others do not.

Differences in lung cancer incidence, risk factors, and survival exist between men and women (see Gender Differences box above). Genetic, hormonal, and molecular influences may contribute to these differences. Female smokers have a higher relative risk of developing lung cancer than male smokers.

GENDER DIFFERENCES
Lung Cancer

Men	Women
• More men than women are diagnosed with lung cancer. • More men than women die from lung cancer. • Male smokers are 10 times more likely to develop lung cancer than nonsmokers. • Men with lung cancer have a worse prognosis than women. • Lung cancer incidence and deaths are decreasing in men.	• Lung cancer incidence and deaths are increasing in women. • Women develop lung cancer after fewer years of smoking than men do. • Women develop lung cancer at a younger age than men. • Women are more likely to develop small cell carcinoma than men. • Nonsmoking women are at greater risk of developing lung cancer than men. • Women with lung cancer live, on the average, 12 months longer than men.

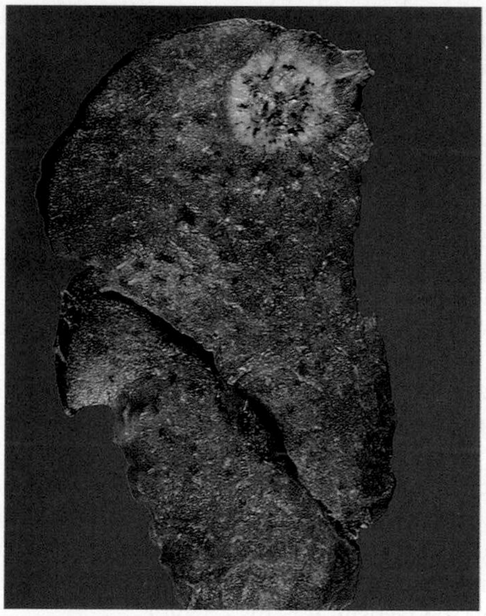

FIG. 28-2 Lung cancer (peripheral adenocarcinoma). The tumor shows prominent black pigmentation, suggestive of having evolved in an anthracotic scar.

Pathophysiology

Most primary lung tumors are believed to arise from mutated epithelial cells. The development of mutations, which are caused by carcinogens, are also influenced by various genetic factors.[23] Once started, continued tumor development is promoted by epidermal growth factor. These cells grow slowly, taking 8 to 10 years for a tumor to reach 1 cm in size, the smallest lesion detectable on an x-ray. Lung cancers occur primarily in the segmental bronchi or beyond and have a preference for the upper lobes of the lungs (Figs. 28-2 and 28-3).

Primary lung cancers are categorized into two broad subtypes (Table 28-15): non–small cell lung cancer (NSCLC) (80%) and small cell lung cancer (SCLC) (20%).[22] Lung cancers metastasize primarily by direct extension and via the blood and lymph system. The common sites for metastasis are the liver, brain, bones, lymph nodes, and adrenal glands.

Paraneoplastic Syndrome. *Paraneoplastic syndrome* is caused by humoral factors (hormones, cytokines) excreted by tumor cells or by an immune response against the tumor.

TABLE 28-15 **TYPES OF PRIMARY LUNG CANCER**

Type	Growth Rate	Characteristics	Response to Therapy
Non–Small Cell Lung Cancer (NSCLC)			
Squamous cell carcinoma	Slow	Accounts for 20%-30% of lung cancers. More common in men. Centrally located, producing early symptoms of nonproductive cough and hemoptysis. Does not have a strong tendency to metastasize.	Surgical resection may be attempted. Adjuvant chemotherapy and radiation. Depending on the staging, life expectancy is better than for small cell lung cancer.
Adenocarcinoma	Moderate	Accounts for 30%-40% of lung cancers. Most common lung cancer in people who have not smoked; more common in women. Peripherally located. Often has no clinical manifestations until widespread metastasis is present.	Surgical resection may be attempted depending on the staging. Does not respond well to chemotherapy.
Large cell (undifferentiated) carcinoma	Rapid	Accounts for 10% of lung cancers. Composed of large cells that are anaplastic and often arise in the bronchi. Is highly metastatic via lymphatics and blood.	Surgery is not usually attempted because of high rate of metastases. Tumor may be radiosensitive but often recurs.
Small Cell Lung Cancer (SCLC)			
Small cell carcinoma	Very rapid	Accounts for about 20% of lung cancers. Most malignant form of lung cancer. Spreads early via lymphatics and bloodstream; frequent metastasis to brain. Associated with endocrine disturbances.	Chemotherapy mainstay of treatment but overall poor prognosis. Radiation is used as adjuvant therapy and palliative measure.

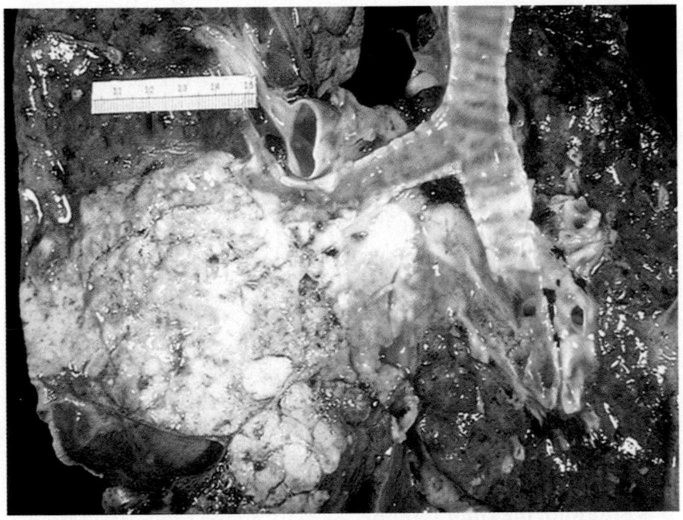

FIG. 28-3 Lung carcinoma. The gray-white tumor tissue is infiltrating the lung. Histologically this tumor is identified as a squamous cell carcinoma.

Sometimes the symptoms of paraneoplastic syndrome manifest even before the diagnosis of a malignancy.

Examples of paraneoplastic syndrome include hypercalcemia, syndrome of inappropriate antidiuretic hormone (SIADH), adrenal hypersecretion, hematologic disorders, and neurologic syndromes. SCLCs are most often associated with the paraneoplastic syndrome. These conditions may stabilize with treatment of the underlying neoplasm.[24] (These effects are discussed in the section on metabolic emergencies in Chapter 16 on pp. 277-278.)

Clinical Manifestations

The clinical manifestations of lung cancer are usually nonspecific and appear late in the disease process. Symptoms may be masked by a chronic cough attributed to smoking or smoking-related lung disease. Manifestations depend on the type of primary lung cancer, its location, and metastatic spread. Lung

EVIDENCE-BASED PRACTICE

Translating Research Into Practice

Which Interventions Improve Well-Being in Lung Cancer?

Clinical Question

In patients with lung cancer (P), what is the effectiveness of nonpharmacologic interventions (I) on symptoms, psychologic functioning, and quality of life (O)?

Best Available Evidence

Systematic review of randomized controlled trials (RCTs) and quasi-randomized clinical trials

Critical Appraisal and Synthesis of Evidence

- Fifteen trials ($n = 1440$) of patients diagnosed with lung cancer receiving various nonpharmacologic interventions, including exercise and nutrition, breathlessness and pain management, progressive muscle relaxation, foot reflexology, and counseling.
- Significant benefits resulted from nurse-led breathlessness programs.
- Counseling may assist patients in coping with emotional symptoms.
- Exercise and nutrition interventions did not improve quality of life in the long term.
- Reflexology may provide short-term help for pain and anxiety.

Conclusion

- Nonpharmacologic interventions can improve anxiety, depression, and symptoms such as breathlessness.

Implications for Nursing Practice

- Encourage patients to participate in programs that help reduce breathlessness and other distressful symptoms.
- Follow-up with patients who are self-managing their symptoms.
- Engage in educational programs to increase your ability to deliver high-quality supportive care.

Reference for Evidence

Rueda J, Solà I, Pascual A, et al: Non-invasive interventions for improving well-being and quality of life in patients with lung cancer, *Cochrane Database Syst Rev* 9:CD004282, 2011.

P, Patient population of interest; I, intervention or area of interest; *O*, outcomes of interest (see p. 12).

TABLE 28-16 COLLABORATIVE CARE

Lung Cancer

Diagnostic	Collaborative Therapy
• History and physical examination • Chest x-ray • Cytologic study of sputum, bronchial washings, or pleural space fluid • Bronchoscopy • Computed tomography (CT) scan • Magnetic resonance imaging (MRI) • Positron emission tomography (PET) • Mediastinoscopy • Video-assisted thoracoscopic surgery (VATS) • Transbronchial or percutaneous fine-needle aspiration	• Surgery • Radiation therapy • Chemotherapy • Biologic and targeted therapy • Prophylactic cranial radiation • Bronchoscopic laser therapy • Photodynamic therapy • Airway stenting • Cryotherapy

cancer frequently manifests as a lobar pneumonia that does not respond to treatment.

One of the most common symptoms of lung cancer, and often the one reported first, is a persistent cough. Blood-tinged sputum may be produced because of bleeding caused by the malignancy. The patient may complain of dyspnea or wheezing. Chest pain, if present, may be localized or unilateral, ranging from mild to severe.

Later manifestations include nonspecific systemic symptoms such as anorexia, fatigue, weight loss, and nausea and vomiting. Hoarseness may be present as a result of laryngeal nerve involvement. Unilateral paralysis of the diaphragm, dysphagia, and superior vena cava obstruction may occur because of intrathoracic spread of the malignancy. Sometimes there are palpable lymph nodes in the neck or axillae. Mediastinal involvement may lead to pericardial effusion, cardiac tamponade, and dysrhythmias.

Diagnostic Studies

A chest x-ray is the initial diagnostic test used for patients with suspected lung cancer. Approximately 5% of cases are found incidentally on a chest x-ray performed for unrelated conditions.[22] The x-ray may identify a lung mass or infiltrate. Evidence of metastasis to the ribs or vertebrae and a pleural effusion may also be seen on chest x-ray. CT scanning is used to further evaluate the lung mass. CT scans can identify the location and extent of masses in the chest, any mediastinal involvement, and lymph node enlargement.

Sputum cytologic studies can identify malignant cells, but results are positive in only 20% to 30% of specimens because the malignant cells are not always present in the sputum. Biopsy is necessary for a definitive diagnosis. Cells for biopsy can be obtained by CT-guided needle aspiration, bronchoscopy, mediastinoscopy, or video-assisted thoracoscopic surgery (VATS) (see Chapter 26). If a thoracentesis is performed to relieve a pleural effusion, the fluid is also analyzed for malignant cells.

Accurate assessment of lung cancer is critical for staging and determining appropriate treatment. Bone scans and CT scans of the brain, pelvis, and abdomen are used to determine if metastatic disease is present. A complete history and physical examination, CBC with differential, chemistry panel, LFTs, renal function tests, and pulmonary function tests are necessary. Magnetic resonance imaging (MRI) and/or positron emission tomography (PET) may also be used to evaluate and stage lung cancer. Table 28-16 summarizes the diagnostic management of lung cancer.

TABLE 28-17 STAGING OF NON–SMALL CELL LUNG CANCER

Stages		Characteristics
I		Tumor is small and localized to lung. No lymph node involvement.
	A	Tumor <3 cm.
	B	Tumor 3-5 cm and invading surrounding local areas.
II		Increased tumor size, some lymph node involvement.
	A	Tumor 3-5 cm with invasion of lymph nodes on same side of chest OR Tumor 5-7 cm without lymph node involvement.
	B	Tumor 5-7 cm involving the bronchus and lymph nodes on same side of chest and tissue of other local organs OR Tumor >7 cm without lymph node involvement.
III		Increased spread of tumor
	A	Tumor spread to the nearby structures (chest wall, pleura, pericardium) and regional lymph nodes.
	B	Extensive tumor involving heart, trachea, esophagus, mediastinum, malignant pleural effusion, contralateral lymph nodes, scalene or supraclavicular lymph nodes.
IV		Distant metastasis.

Staging. Staging of NSCLC is performed according to the TNM staging system (see Table 16-5). Under the TNM system, the tumor is grouped into four stages with A or B subtypes. A simplified version of staging of NSCLC is presented in Table 28-17. Patients with stages I, II, and IIIA disease may be surgical candidates. However, stage IIIB or IV disease is usually inoperable and has a poor prognosis.

Staging of SCLC by TNM has not been useful because this cancer is aggressive and is always considered systemic. The stages of SCLC are *limited* and *extensive*. Limited means that the tumor is confined to one side of the chest and regional lymph nodes. Extensive SCLC means that the cancer extends beyond the limited stage. Approximately 65% to 70% of patients with SCLC have extensive disease. On average, patients with extensive SCLC survive only 12 months with treatment and 6 weeks without.[25]

Screening for Lung Cancer. Screening for high-risk patients is supported by the recent National Lung Screening Trial (NLST). This study showed a 20% decrease in deaths from lung cancer in patients who underwent screening with low-dose spiral CT scanning, compared with those who had chest x-rays.[26] Only those patients who meet the following criteria should be considered for screening: 55 to 74 years old, current or former smokers with at least a 30 pack-year smoking history, former smokers who quit within the past 15 years, no history of lung cancer, not on home O_2 therapy.[27-29]

Collaborative Care

Surgical Therapy. Surgical resection is the treatment of choice in NSCLC stages I to IIIA without mediastinal involvement, since resection provides the best chance for a cure. The 5-year survival rate in stage I and II disease ranges from 30% to 50%. Factors that affect survival include the size of the primary tumor and co-morbidities. For other NSCLC stages, patients may require surgery in conjunction with radiation therapy and/or chemotherapy. Fifty percent of NSCLCs are not resectable at the time of diagnosis.

The surgical procedures that may be performed include pneumonectomy (removal of one entire lung), lobectomy (removal of one or more lobes of the lung), or segmental or wedge resection procedures. VATS may be used to treat lung cancers near the outside of the lung. Surgery is generally not indicated for SCLC because of its rapid growth and dissemination at the time of diagnosis.

When the tumor is considered operable, the patient's cardiopulmonary status must be evaluated to determine the ability to withstand surgery. Pulmonary function studies and ABGs are often used to assess the patient's cardiopulmonary status.

Radiation Therapy. Radiation therapy may be used as treatment for both NSCLC and SCLC. Radiation therapy may be given as curative therapy, palliative therapy (to relieve symptoms), or adjuvant therapy in combination with surgery or chemotherapy.

Radiation therapy may be used as primary therapy in the individual who is unable to tolerate surgical resection because of co-morbidities. Radiation therapy also relieves symptoms of dyspnea and hemoptysis resulting from bronchial obstructive tumors and treats superior vena cava syndrome. It can also be used to treat pain that is caused by metastatic bone lesions or cerebral metastasis. Sometimes radiation is used preoperatively to reduce the tumor mass before surgical resection. Complications of radiation therapy include esophagitis, skin irritation, nausea and vomiting, anorexia, and radiation pneumonitis (see Chapter 16).

Stereotactic Body Radiotherapy. Stereotactic body radiotherapy (SBRT), also called stereotactic surgery or radiosurgery, is a new lung cancer treatment. It is a type of radiation therapy that uses high doses of radiation delivered accurately to the tumor. SBRT provides an option for patients with early stage lung cancers who are not surgical candidates for other medical reasons. SBRT is an outpatient procedure that uses special positioning procedures and radiology techniques so that a higher dose of radiation can be delivered to the tumor, and only a small part of the healthy lung is exposed. Therapy is given over 1 to 3 days.

Chemotherapy. Chemotherapy is the primary treatment for SCLC. In NSCLC, chemotherapy may be used in the treatment of nonresectable tumors or as adjuvant therapy to surgery. A variety of chemotherapy drugs and multidrug regimens (i.e., protocols) have been used. Chemotherapy for lung cancer typically consists of combinations of two or more of the following drugs: etoposide (VePesid), carboplatin (Paraplatin), cisplatin (Platinol), paclitaxel (Taxol), vinorelbine (Navelbine), cyclophosphamide (Cytoxan), ifosfamide (Ifex), docetaxel (Taxotere), gemcitabine (Gemzar), and pemetrexed (Alimta).

Targeted Therapy. Targeted therapy uses drugs that block the growth of molecules involved in specific aspects of tumor growth (see Chapter 16). Because it inhibits growth rather than directly kills cancer cells, targeted therapy may be less toxic than chemotherapy. One type of targeted therapy for patients with NSCLC inhibits tyrosine kinase, an enzyme associated with epidermal growth factor receptor. These drugs (e.g., erlotinib [Tarceva]) block signals for growth in the cancer cells.

Another kinase inhibitor, crizotinib (Xalkori), is used to treat patients with NSCLC who have an abnormal anaplastic lymphoma kinase *(ALK)* gene. This drug directly inhibits the kinase protein produced by the *ALK* gene that is responsible for cancer development and growth.

Other drugs, such as bevacizumab (Avastin), inhibit the growth of new blood vessels (angiogenesis) by targeting vascular endothelial growth factor.

Other Therapies

Prophylactic Cranial Radiation. Patients with SCLC have early metastases, especially to the central nervous system. Most chemotherapy does not penetrate the blood-brain barrier. Therefore after successful systemic treatment, the patient is at risk for cerebral metastases. Prophylactic radiation has been shown to decrease the incidence of cerebral metastases and improve the survival rate in patients with limited SCLC.[22]

Bronchoscopic Laser Therapy. Bronchoscopic laser therapy makes it possible to remove obstructing bronchial lesions. The neodymium: yttrium-aluminum-garnet (Nd:YAG) laser is most commonly used for laser resection using either the flexible or the rigid bronchoscope. The laser's thermal energy is transmitted to the target tissue. It is a safe and effective treatment of endobronchial obstructions from tumors. Symptoms of airway obstruction are relieved as a result of thermal necrosis and shrinkage of the tumor. The procedure may be repeated as needed.[27]

Photodynamic Therapy. Photodynamic therapy can be used to treat very early stage lung cancers that are confined to the outer layers of the airways. It can also remove lesions obstructing the airway. Porfimer (Photofrin) is injected IV and selectively concentrates in tumor cells. After a set time (usually 48 hours), the tumor is exposed to laser light via bronchoscopy, activating the drug and causing cell death. Necrotic tissue is removed with bronchoscopy a few days later.[27] This process can also be repeated as needed.

Airway Stenting. Stents are used alone or in combination with other techniques for relief of dyspnea, cough, or respiratory insufficiency. The advantage of an airway stent is that it supports the airway wall against collapse or external compression and can delay extension of tumor into the airway lumen.

Radiofrequency Ablation. Radiofrequency ablation therapy is being used to treat small NSCLC lung tumors that are near the outer edge of the lungs. This therapy is an alternative to surgery in patients who cannot or elect not to have surgery. A thin, needle-like probe is inserted through the skin into the tumor. CT scans are used to guide placement. An electric current is then passed through the probe, which heats and destroys tumor cells. Local anesthesia is used for this outpatient procedure.[27]

NURSING MANAGEMENT LUNG CANCER

NURSING ASSESSMENT

It is important to determine the patient and caregiver's understanding of diagnostic tests (those completed as well as those planned), the diagnosis or potential diagnosis, the treatment options, and the prognosis. At the same time, assess the patient's level of anxiety and support provided by the patient's significant others. Subjective and objective data that should be obtained from a patient with lung cancer are presented in Table 28-18.

NURSING DIAGNOSES

Nursing diagnoses for the patient with lung cancer may include, but are not limited to, the following:

- Ineffective airway clearance *related to* increased tracheobronchial secretions and presence of tumor

TABLE 28-18 NURSING ASSESSMENT
Lung Cancer

Subjective Data

Important Health Information

Past health history: Exposure to secondhand smoke, airborne carcinogens (e.g., asbestos, radon, hydrocarbons), or other pollutants; urban living environment; chronic lung disease (e.g., TB, COPD, bronchiectasis)

Medications: Cough medicines or other respiratory medications

Functional Health Patterns

Health perception–health management: Smoking history, including amount per day and number of years; family history of lung cancer; frequent respiratory tract infections

Nutritional-metabolic: Anorexia, nausea, vomiting, dysphagia (late); weight loss; chills

Activity-exercise: Fatigue; persistent cough (productive or nonproductive); dyspnea at rest or with exertion, hemoptysis (late symptom)

Cognitive-perceptual: Chest pain or tightness, shoulder and arm pain, headache, bone pain (late symptom)

Objective Data

General

Fever, neck and axillary lymphadenopathy, paraneoplastic syndrome (e.g., syndrome of inappropriate ADH secretion)

Integumentary

Jaundice (liver metastasis); edema of neck and face (superior vena cava syndrome), digital clubbing

Respiratory

Wheezing, hoarseness, stridor, unilateral diaphragm paralysis, pleural effusions (late signs)

Cardiovascular

Pericardial effusion, cardiac tamponade, dysrhythmias (late signs)

Neurologic

Unsteady gait (brain metastasis)

Musculoskeletal

Pathologic fractures, muscle wasting (late)

Possible Diagnostic Findings

Observance of lesion on chest x-ray, CT scan, or PET scan; MRI findings of vertebral, spinal cord, or mediastinal invasion; positive sputum or bronchial washings for cytologic studies; positive fiberoptic bronchoscopy and biopsy findings

ADH, Antidiuretic hormone.

- Anxiety *related to* lack of knowledge of diagnosis or unknown prognosis and treatments
- Ineffective self-health management *related to* lack of knowledge about the disease process and therapeutic regimen
- Ineffective breathing pattern *related to* decreased lung capacity
- Impaired gas exchange *related to* tumor obstructing airflow

PLANNING

The overall goals are that the patient with lung cancer will have (1) effective breathing patterns, (2) adequate airway clearance, (3) adequate oxygenation of tissues, (4) minimal to no pain, and (5) a realistic attitude about treatment and prognosis.

NURSING IMPLEMENTATION

HEALTH PROMOTION. The best way to halt the epidemic of lung cancer is to prevent people from starting to smoke and help smokers stop smoking. Because most smokers start in the teenage years, prevention of teen smoking has the most significant role in reducing the incidence of lung cancer. A wealth of material is available to the smoker who is interested in smoking cessation. The CDC provides an index of tools *(www.cdc.gov/tobacco/quit_smoking/cessation/index.htm).* (Smoking cessation is discussed in Chapter 11.)

Modeling healthy behavior by not smoking, promoting smoking cessation programs, and actively supporting education and policy changes related to smoking are important nursing activities. Many changes have occurred as a result of the recognition that passive smoke is a health hazard. Laws prohibit smoking in most public places and limit public smoking to designated areas. Most hospital environments are now completely smoke-free, prohibiting smoking by employees and patients. A new trend is for hospitals to refuse employment to anyone testing positive for nicotine. This includes not only smokers but also nonsmokers who are routinely exposed to secondhand smoke.

ACUTE INTERVENTION. Care of the patient with lung cancer initially involves support and reassurance during the diagnostic evaluation. It is important to recognize the multiple stressors that occur when someone is diagnosed with lung cancer. The stress response is a normal and adaptive response, but can become detrimental when it is overwhelming and intense. Patients suffer the stress of their symptoms, including dyspnea and cough. Diagnostic and therapeutic procedures provide additional stress by placing patients in unfamiliar environments with unusual and perhaps painful results. Emotional stressors include the knowledge of the high mortality rate of lung cancer and the causal effect of cigarette smoking. Worries about role performance and ability to care for their family while undergoing cancer treatment provide further stress. Carefully assess each individual, since he or she will experience unique stressors. The insight gained will help the patient and caregiver cope with the stress of the illness and treatment.[30]

Care of the patient undergoing thoracic surgery is discussed later in this chapter on p. 548. Care of the patient undergoing radiation therapy and chemotherapy is discussed in Chapter 16. Individualized care depends on the plan for treatment. Assessment and intervention in symptom management are pivotal, as is teaching the patient to recognize signs and symptoms that may indicate progression or recurrence of disease. Provide patient comfort, teach methods to reduce pain, monitor for side effects of prescribed medications, foster appropriate coping strategies for the patient and caregiver, assess smoking cessation readiness, and help patients access resources to deal with the illness.

AMBULATORY AND HOME CARE. Teach signs and symptoms to report, such as hemoptysis, dysphagia, chest pain, and hoarseness. Counseling patients on smoking cessation and prevention is essential in decreasing morbidity and mortality risks associated with lung cancer. Encourage the patient and the family to provide a smoke-free environment. This may include smoking cessation for multiple family members. If the treatment plan includes home oxygen, the teaching plan must include the safe use of oxygen.

For many individuals who have lung cancer, little can be done to significantly prolong their lives. Radiation therapy and chemotherapy can provide palliative relief from distressing symptoms. Constant pain may become a major problem. (Measures used to relieve pain are discussed in Chapter 9. Care of the patient with cancer is discussed in Chapter 16.) The palliative care team should be involved as the patient and the family move toward the end of life (see Chapter 10). The team can provide information about disability, financial planning, and community resources for end-of-life care such as hospice.

EVALUATION

The expected outcomes are that the patient with lung cancer will have

- Adequate breathing patterns
- Adequate oxygenation
- Minimal to no pain
- Realistic attitude about prognosis

OTHER TYPES OF LUNG TUMORS

SCLC and NSCLC account for 95% of lung tumors. The other 5% include the following:

- *Hamartomas*, the most common benign tumor, is a slow-growing congenital tumor composed of fibrous tissue, fat, and blood vessels.
- *Mucous gland adenoma* is a benign tumor arising in the bronchi that consists of columnar cystic spaces.
- *Mesotheliomas* are either malignant or benign and originate from the visceral pleura. Malignant mesotheliomas are associated with exposure to asbestos. Benign mesotheliomas are localized lesions.
- Secondary metastases from other malignancies can occur. Malignant cells from another part of the body reach the lungs via the pulmonary capillaries or the lymphatic network. The primary malignancies that spread to the lungs often originate in the GI or genitourinary tract and in the breast. General symptoms of lung metastases are chest pain and nonproductive cough.

CHEST TRAUMA AND THORACIC INJURIES

Traumatic injuries to the chest contribute to 75% of all traumatic deaths.[31] Thoracic injuries range from simple rib fractures to complex life-threatening rupture of organs. The mechanisms of injuries causing chest trauma are separated into two categories: blunt trauma and penetrating trauma.

Blunt trauma occurs when the chest strikes or is struck by an object. The impact can cause deceleration, acceleration, shearing, and compression of thoracic structures. The external injury may appear minor, but internally the organs may have severe injuries. The injuries can occur on the same side as the impact and on the opposite side as the tissue moves back and forth. Rib and sternal fractures can lacerate lung tissue. In a high-velocity impact the shearing force may result in laceration or tearing of the aorta. Compression of the chest may result in contusion, crush injury, and organ rupture.

Penetrating trauma is an open injury in which a foreign body impales or passes through the body tissues, creating an open wound. Examples include knife wounds, gunshot wounds, and injuries with other sharp objects. eTable 28-2 (available on the website for this chapter) describes traumatic injuries as they relate to the categories of trauma and the mechanism of injury. Emergency care of the patient with a chest injury is presented in Table 28-19.

The most common thoracic emergencies and their management are described in Table 28-20.

TABLE 28-19 EMERGENCY MANAGEMENT

Chest Trauma

Etiology	Assessment Findings	Interventions
Blunt • Motor vehicle accident • Pedestrian accident • Fall • Assault with blunt object • Crush injury • Explosion **Penetrating** • Knife • Gunshot • Stick • Arrow • Other missiles	**Respiratory** • Dyspnea, respiratory distress • Cough with or without hemoptysis • Cyanosis of mouth, face, nail beds, mucous membranes • Tracheal deviation • Audible air escaping from chest wound • Decreased breath sounds on side of injury • Decreased O_2 saturation • Frothy secretions **Cardiovascular** • Rapid, thready pulse • Decreased BP • Narrowed pulse pressure • Asymmetric BP values in arms • Distended neck veins • Muffled heart sounds • Chest pain • Crunching sound synchronous with heart sounds • Dysrhythmias **Surface Findings** • Bruising • Abrasions • Open chest wound • Asymmetric chest movement • Subcutaneous emphysema	**Initial** • Ensure patent airway. • Administer O_2 to keep SpO_2 >90%. • Establish IV access with two large-bore catheters. Begin fluid resuscitation as appropriate. • Remove clothing to assess injury. • Cover sucking chest wound with nonporous dressing taped on three sides. • Stabilize impaled objects with bulky dressings. *Do not remove object.* • Assess for other significant injuries and treat appropriately. • Stabilize flail rib segment with hand followed by application of large pieces of tape horizontal across the flail segment. • Place patient in a semi-Fowler's position or position patient on the injured side if breathing is easier *after* cervical spine injury has been ruled out. • Prepare for emergency needle decompression if tension pneumothorax or cardiac tamponade present. **Ongoing Monitoring** • Monitor vital signs, level of consciousness, O_2 saturation, cardiac rhythm, respiratory status, and urine output. • Anticipate intubation for respiratory distress. • Release dressing if tension pneumothorax develops after sucking chest wound is covered.

TABLE 28-20 EMERGENCY MANAGEMENT

Thoracic Injuries

Injury	Definition	Manifestations	Interventionist
Pneumothorax	Air in pleural space (see Fig. 28-4).	Dyspnea, decreased movement of involved chest wall, diminished or absent breath sounds on the affected side, hyperresonance to percussion	Chest tube insertion with flutter valve or chest drainage system.
Hemothorax	Blood in the pleural space, may or may not occur in conjunction with pneumothorax.	Dyspnea, diminished or absent breath sounds, dullness to percussion, decreased Hgb, shock depending on blood volume lost	Chest tube insertion with chest drainage system. Autotransfusion of collected blood, treatment of hypovolemia as necessary.
Tension pneumothorax	Air in pleural space that does not escape. The increased air in the pleural space shifts organs and increases intrathoracic pressure (see Fig. 28-5).	Cyanosis, air hunger, violent agitation, tracheal deviation away from affected side, subcutaneous emphysema, neck vein distention, hyperresonance to percussion	Medical emergency: needle decompression followed by chest tube insertion with chest drainage system.
Flail chest	Fracture of two or more adjacent ribs in two or more places with loss of chest wall stability (see Fig. 28-6).	Paradoxic movement of chest wall, respiratory distress. May be associated hemothorax, pneumothorax, pulmonary contusion	O_2 as needed to maintain O_2 saturation, analgesia. Stabilize flail segment with positive pressure ventilation (CPAP, BiPAP) or intubation and mechanical ventilation. Treat associated injuries. Surgical fixation.
Cardiac tamponade	Blood rapidly collects in pericardial sac, compresses myocardium because the pericardium does not stretch, and prevents ventricles from filling.	Muffled, distant heart sounds, hypotension, neck vein distention, increased central venous pressure	Medical emergency: pericardiocentesis with surgical repair as appropriate.

BiPAP, Bilevel positive airway pressure; *CPAP,* continuous positive airway pressure.

PNEUMOTHORAX

A **pneumothorax** is caused by air entering the pleural cavity. Normally, negative pressure exists between the visceral pleura (surrounding the lung) and the parietal pleura (lining the thoracic cavity), allowing the lung to be filled by chest wall expansion. The pleural space contains only a few milliliters of lubricating fluid to reduce friction when the tissues move. When air enters this space, the change to positive pressure causes a partial or complete lung collapse. As the volume of air in the pleural space increases, the lung volume decreases. This condition should be suspected after any trauma to the chest wall. Pneumothorax can be classified as *open* (air entering through an opening in the chest wall) or *closed* (no external wound).

If a pneumothorax is small, mild tachycardia and dyspnea may be the only manifestations. If the pneumothorax occupies a large area, respiratory distress may be present, including shallow, rapid respirations; dyspnea; air hunger; and oxygen desaturation. Chest pain and a cough with or without hemoptysis may be present. On auscultation, no breath sounds are detected over the affected area. A chest x-ray shows air or fluid in the pleural space and reduction in lung volume.

Types of Pneumothorax

Spontaneous Pneumothorax. A spontaneous pneumothorax typically occurs due to the rupture of small blebs (air-filled blisters) located on the apex of the lung. These blebs can occur in healthy, young individuals *(primary spontaneous pneumothorax)* or as a result of lung disease such as COPD, asthma, cystic fibrosis, and pneumonia *(secondary spontaneous pneumothorax).* Smoking increases the risk for bleb formation. Other risk factors include being tall and thin, male gender, family history, and previous spontaneous pneumothorax.

Iatrogenic Pneumothorax. *Iatrogenic pneumothorax* can occur due to laceration or puncture of the lung during medical procedures. Transthoracic needle aspiration is the leading cause

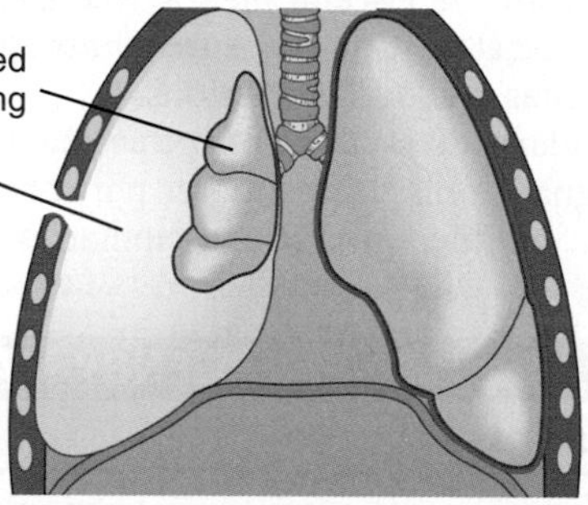

FIG. 28-4 Open pneumothorax resulting from collapse of lung due to disruption of chest wall and outside air entering.

of iatrogenic pneumothorax.[32] Other causes include subclavian catheter insertion, thoracentesis, pleural biopsy, and transbronchial lung biopsy. Barotrauma from excessive ventilatory pressure during manual or mechanical ventilation can rupture alveoli or bronchioles. Esophageal procedures may also be involved in the development of a pneumothorax. Tearing during insertion of a gastric tube can allow air from the esophagus to enter the mediastinum and the pleural space.

Traumatic Pneumothorax. *Traumatic pneumothorax* can occur from either penetrating (open) or nonpenetrating (closed) chest trauma. Penetrating trauma allows air to enter the pleural space through an opening in the chest wall (Fig. 28-4). Examples include stab or gunshot wounds and surgical thoracotomy. A penetrating chest wound may be referred to as a *sucking chest wound,* since air enters the pleural space through the chest wall during inspiration.

Emergency treatment consists of covering the wound with an occlusive dressing that is secured on three sides (vent dressing). During inspiration, as negative pressure is created in the chest, the dressing pulls against the wound, preventing air from entering the pleural space. During expiration, as the pressure rises in the pleural space, the dressing is pushed out and air escapes through the wound and from under the dressing. If the

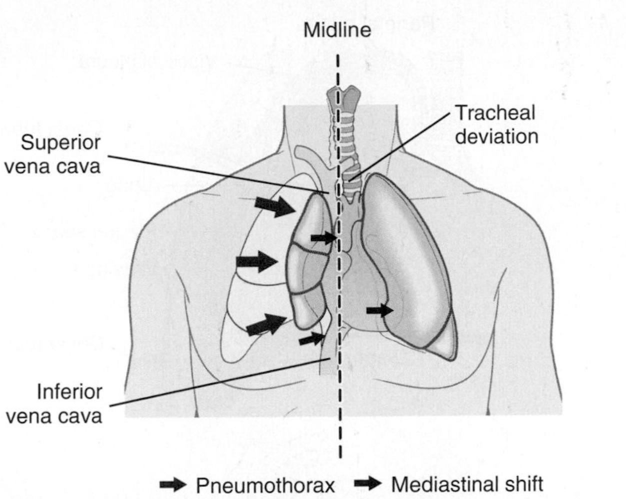

FIG. 28-5 Tension pneumothorax. As pleural pressure on the affected side increases, mediastinal displacement ensues with resultant respiratory and cardiovascular compromise. Tracheal deviation is an external manifestation of the mediastinal shift.

object that caused the open chest wound is still in place, do not remove it until a physician is present. Stabilize the impaled object with a bulky dressing.

Nonpenetrating chest trauma, such as rib fractures, can lacerate the lung and cause air to enter the pleural space. Blunt trauma can also cause alveolar rupture secondary to sudden chest compression.

Tension Pneumothorax. Tension pneumothorax occurs when air enters the pleural space but cannot escape. The continued accumulation of air in the pleural space causes increasingly elevated intrapleural pressures. This results in compression of the lung on the affected side and pressure on the heart and great vessels, pushing them away from the affected side (Fig. 28-5). The mediastinum shifts toward the unaffected side, compressing the "good" lung, which further compromises oxygenation. As the pressure increases, venous return is decreased and cardiac output falls. Tension pneumothorax may result from either an open or a closed pneumothorax. In an open chest wound, a flap may act as a one-way valve. Thus air can enter on inspiration but cannot escape. Tension pneumothorax can occur with mechanical ventilation and resuscitative efforts. It can also occur if chest tubes are clamped or become blocked in a patient with a pneumothorax. Unclamping the tube or relieving the obstruction will remedy this situation.

Tension pneumothorax is a medical emergency, with both the respiratory and cardiovascular systems affected. Manifestations include dyspnea, marked tachycardia, tracheal deviation, decreased or absent breath sounds on the affected side, neck vein distention, cyanosis, and profuse diaphoresis.[32] If the tension in the pleural space is not relieved, the patient is likely to die from inadequate cardiac output or severe hypoxemia.

Hemothorax. Hemothorax is an accumulation of blood in the pleural space resulting from injury to the chest wall, diaphragm, lung, blood vessels, or mediastinum.[32] When it occurs with pneumothorax, it is called a *hemopneumothorax*. The patient with a traumatic hemothorax requires immediate insertion of a chest tube for evacuation of the blood, which can be recovered and reinfused for a short time after the injury. (Autotransfusion is discussed in Chapter 31.)

Chylothorax. *Chylothorax* is the presence of lymphatic fluid in the pleural space. The thoracic duct is disrupted either traumatically or from a malignancy, and the lymphatic fluid fills the pleural space. This milky white fluid is high in lipids. Normal lymphatic flow through the thoracic duct is 1500 to 2500 mL/day. This amount can be increased up to tenfold after ingestion of fats. Fifty percent of cases heal with conservative treatment (chest drainage, bowel rest, and parenteral nutrition). Octreotide has been used with some success to reduce the flow of lymphatic fluid.[29] Surgery and pleurodesis are options if conservative therapy fails. *Pleurodesis* is the artificial production of adhesions between the parietal and visceral pleura, usually done with a chemical sclerosing agent, such as talc or doxycycline.

Collaborative Care

Treatment of a pneumothorax depends on its severity and the underlying disease. If the patient is stable and minimal air and fluid is accumulated in the intrapleural space, no treatment may be necessary, since the condition may resolve spontaneously. The pleural space can also be aspirated with a large-bore needle. This procedure is called a thoracentesis.

The most definitive and common treatment of pneumothorax and hemothorax is to insert a chest tube and connect it to water-seal drainage. Repeated spontaneous pneumothorax may need to be treated surgically by a partial pleurectomy, stapling, or pleurodesis to promote adherence of the pleurae to one another. Tension pneumothorax is a medical emergency, requiring urgent needle decompression followed by chest tube insertion to water-seal drainage.

FRACTURED RIBS

Rib fractures are the most common type of chest injury resulting from blunt trauma. Ribs 5 through 9 are most frequently fractured because they are the least protected by chest muscles. If the fractured rib is splintered or displaced, it may damage the pleura and lungs.

Clinical manifestations of fractured ribs include pain at the site of injury, especially during inspiration and coughing. The patient splints the affected area and takes shallow breaths to try to decrease the pain. Atelectasis and pneumonia may develop because of decreased ventilation and retained secretions.

The main goal in treatment is to decrease pain so that the patient can breathe adequately and clear secretions. Strapping the chest with tape or using a binder is not recommended, since it limits chest expansion and predisposes the individual to atelectasis. Nonsteroidal antiinflammatory drugs (NSAIDs), opioids, and nerve blocks can be used to reduce pain and aid with deep breathing and coughing. Patient teaching should emphasize deep breathing, coughing, incentive spirometry, and appropriate use of pain medications.

FLAIL CHEST

Flail chest results from the fracture of several consecutive ribs, in two or more separate places, causing an unstable segment (Fig. 28-6). It can also be caused by fracture of the sternum and several consecutive ribs. The resultant instability of the chest wall causes paradoxic movement during breathing. The affected (flail) area moves in the opposite direction with respect to the intact portion of the chest. During inspiration, the affected portion is sucked in, and during expiration, it bulges out. This paradoxic chest movement prevents adequate ventilation of the lung in the injured area and increases the work of breathing.

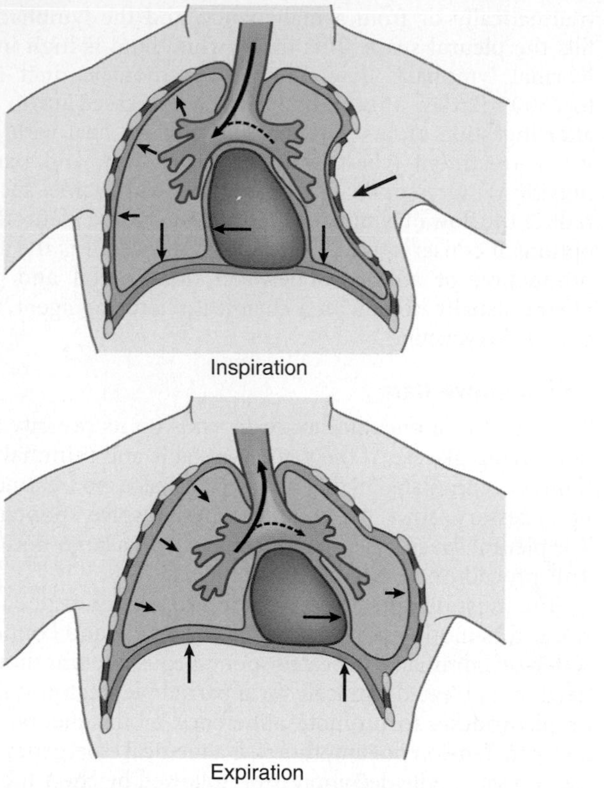

FIG. 28-6 Flail chest produces paradoxic respiration. On inspiration, the flail section sinks in with mediastinal shift to the uninjured side. On expiration, the flail section bulges outward with mediastinal shift to the injured side.

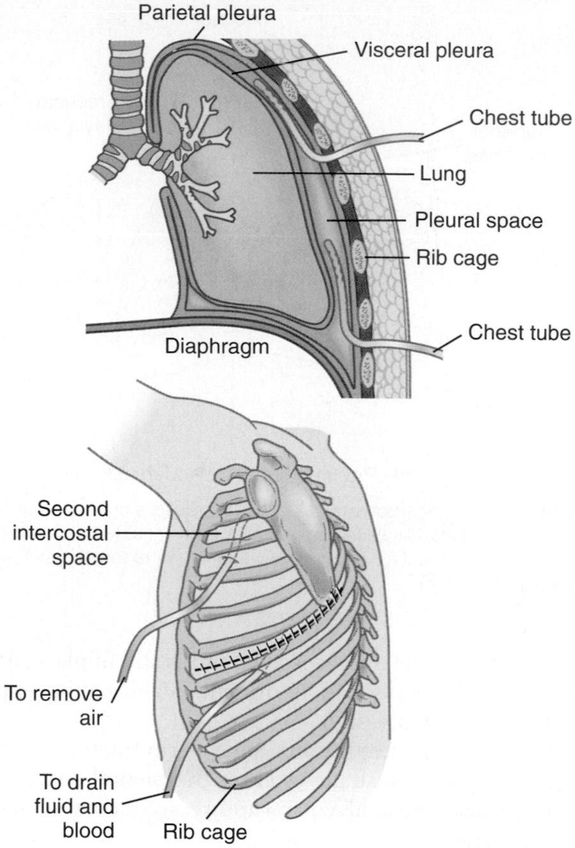

FIG. 28-7 Placement of chest tubes.

The underlying lung may have a pulmonary contusion aggravating hypoxemia.

In an unconscious patient a flail chest is usually apparent on visual examination. The patient manifests rapid, shallow respirations and tachycardia. In a conscious patient a flail chest may not be initially apparent as a result of splinting of the chest wall. The patient moves air poorly, and movement of the thorax is asymmetric and uncoordinated. Palpation of abnormal respiratory movements, evaluation for crepitus near the rib fractures, chest x-ray, and ABGs all assist in the diagnosis.

Initial therapy consists of airway management, adequate ventilation, supplemental oxygen therapy, careful administration of IV solutions, and pain control. The definitive therapy is to reexpand the lung and ensure adequate oxygenation. Although many patients can be managed without mechanical ventilation, intubation and ventilation may be necessary. Surgical fixation of the flail segment may be done.[33] The lung parenchyma and fractured ribs heal with time. Some patients continue to experience intercostal pain after the flail chest has resolved.

CHEST TUBES AND PLEURAL DRAINAGE

Whenever fluid or air accumulates in the pleural space, the pressure becomes positive instead of negative and the lungs collapse. Chest tubes are inserted to drain the pleural space and reestablish negative pressure, allowing for proper lung expansion. Tubes may also be inserted in the mediastinal space to drain air and fluid postoperatively.

Chest tubes are approximately 20 inches (51 cm) long and vary in size from 12F to 40F. The size inserted is determined by the patient's condition. Large (36F to 40F) tubes are used to drain blood, medium (24F to 36F) tubes are used to drain fluid, and small (12F to 24F) tubes are used to drain air.[34] Pigtail tubes are very small (10F to 14F) tubes with a curly end designed to keep them in place. They are a safe and effective alternative to larger-bore chest tubes for treatment of pneumothorax.[35]

Chest Tube Insertion

Insertion of a chest tube can take place in the emergency department, at the patient's bedside, or in the operating room. The patient is positioned with the arm raised above the head on the affected side to expose the midaxillary area, the standard site for insertion. Elevate the patient's head 30 to 60 degrees, when possible, to lower the diaphragm and reduce the risk of injury.

A chest x-ray is used to confirm the affected side. The area is cleansed with an antiseptic solution. The chest wall is prepared with a local anesthetic, and a small incision is made over a rib. The chest tube is advanced up and over the top of the rib to avoid the intercostal nerves and blood vessels that are behind the rib inferiorly (Fig. 28-7). Once inserted, the tube is connected to a pleural drainage system (Fig. 28-8). Two tubes may be connected to the same drainage unit with a Y-connector.

The incision is closed with sutures, and the chest tube is secured. The wound is covered with an occlusive dressing. Some clinicians prefer to seal the wound around the chest tube with petroleum gauze. Proper tube placement is confirmed by chest x-ray.

The insertion of a chest tube and its presence in the pleural space are painful. Monitor the patient's comfort at frequent intervals and use the appropriate pain-relieving interventions.

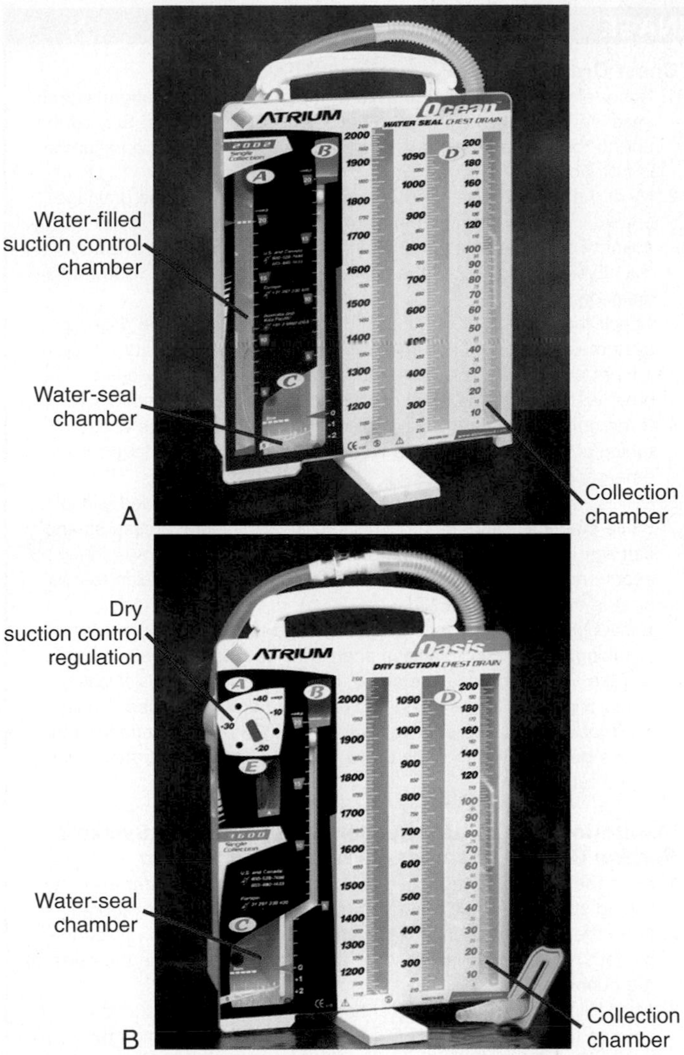

FIG. 28-8 Chest drainage unit. Both units have three chambers: (1) collection chamber; (2) water-seal chamber; and (3) suction control chamber. Suction control chamber requires a connection to a wall suction source that is dialed up higher than the prescribed suction for the suction to work. **A,** Water suction. This unit uses water in the suction control chamber to control the wall suction pressure. **B,** Dry suction. This unit controls wall suction by using a regulator control dial.

Flutter or Heimlich Valve

A flutter valve (also called the Heimlich valve after its inventor) is used to evacuate air from the pleural space (Fig. 28-9). This device consists of a one-way rubber valve within a rigid plastic tube. It is attached to the external end of the chest tube. The valve opens whenever the pressure in the chest is greater than atmospheric pressure, such as during expiration, and it closes when intrathoracic pressure is less than atmospheric pressure, such as during inspiration.

The flutter valve can be used for emergency transport and for a small- to moderate-sized pneumothorax. It also allows for patient mobility, since the smaller drainage bag can be hidden under the clothes while the patient ambulates. Drainage bags attached to the flutter valve must have a vent to the atmosphere to prevent a potential tension pneumothorax. This can be accomplished by simply cutting a small slit in the top of any drainage bag that does not have a built-in vent. Patients may go home with a flutter valve in place.

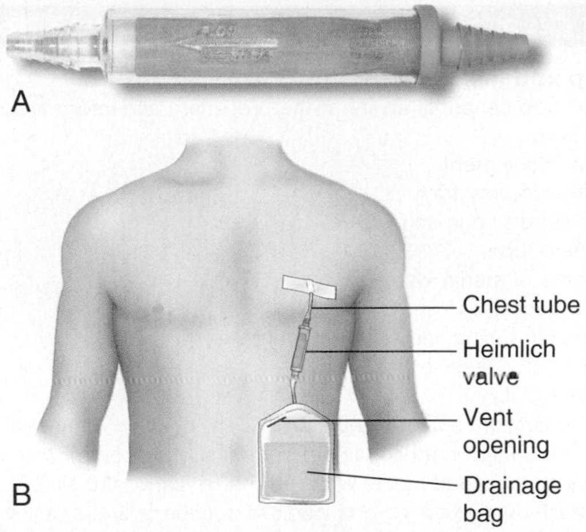

FIG. 28-9 A, Heimlich chest drain valve is a specially designed flutter valve that is used in place of a chest drainage unit for small uncomplicated pneumothorax with little or no drainage and no need for suction. The valve allows for escape of air but prevents the reentry of air into the pleural space. **B,** Placement of valve between chest tube and vented drainage bag, which can be worn under a person's clothes.

Pleural Drainage

The second type of chest drainage is larger and less portable, and it contains three basic compartments, each with a separate function (see Fig. 28-8). The *first compartment*, or collection chamber, receives fluid and air from the pleural or mediastinal space. The drained fluid stays in this chamber while the air vents to the second compartment.

The *second compartment,* called the water-seal chamber, contains 2 cm of water, which acts as a one-way valve. The incoming air enters from the collection chamber and bubbles up through the water. The water prevents backflow of air into the patient from the system. Initially, brisk bubbling of air occurs in this chamber when a pneumothorax is evacuated. Intermittent bubbling during exhalation, coughing, or sneezing (when the patient's intrathoracic pressure is increased) will continue as long as there is air in the pleural space. As the source of the air in the pleural space gets smaller, it will take more and more positive intrapleural pressure to force air out. Eventually, the air leak seals and the lung is fully expanded.

Normal fluctuation of the water within the water-seal chamber is called *tidaling.* This up and down movement of water in concert with respiration reflects the intrapleural pressure changes during inspiration and expiration. Investigate any sudden cessation of tidaling, since this may signify an occluded chest tube. Gradual reduction and eventual cessation of tidaling are expected as the lung reexpands. The parietal and visceral pleura will form a tight seal around the chest tube openings, obliterating the response to changes in intrapleural pressures with respiration.

The *third compartment,* the suction control chamber, applies suction to the chest drainage system. There are two types of suction control: water and dry. The water suction control chamber uses a column of water with the top end vented to the atmosphere to control the amount of suction from the wall regulator. The chamber is typically filled with 20 cm of water. When the negative pressure generated by the suction source exceeds the set 20 cm, air from the atmosphere enters the chamber through the vent on top and the air bubbles up through

TABLE 28-21 CHEST TUBES AND WATER-SEAL DRAINAGE

Set-Up and Insertion
1. Make sure patient is aware of the procedure and informed consent is obtained.
2. Gather equipment.
   - Thoracotomy tray
   - Chest drainage unit (CDU)
   - Chest tube
   - Bottle of sterile water
   - 1% lidocaine
   - Suction tubing and collection container
   - Occlusive dressing
3. Prepare CDU.
   - Wet suction: add sterile water to 2-cm mark in water-seal chamber and to 20-cm mark (or as ordered) in suction control chamber.
   - Dry suction: add sterile water to the fill line of the air leak meter. Attach suction tubing and increase suction until the bellows-like float moves across the display window.
4. Position and support the patient to minimize movement during procedure.

Drainage System
1. Keep all tubing loosely coiled below chest level. Tubing should drop straight from bed or chair to drainage unit. Do not let it be compressed.
2. Keep all connections between chest tubes, drainage tubing, and the drainage collector tight, and tape at connections.
3. Observe for air fluctuations (tidaling) and bubbling in the water-seal chamber.
   - If tidaling (rising with inspiration and falling with expiration in the spontaneously breathing patient) is not observed, the drainage system is blocked, the lungs are reexpanded, or the system is attached to suction.
   - If bubbling increases, there may be an air leak in the drainage system or a leak from the patient (bronchopleural leak).
4. If the chest tube is connected to suction, disconnect from wall suction to check for tidaling.
5. Suspect a system leak when bubbling is continuous.
   - Retape tubing connections.
   - Ensure that dressing is air-occlusive.
   - If leak persists, briefly clamp the chest tube at the patient's chest. If the leak stops, then the air is coming from the patient.
   - If the air leak persists, briefly and methodically move the clamps down the tubing away from the patient until the air leak stops. The leak will then be present between the last two clamp points. If the air leak persists all the way to the drainage unit, replace the unit.
6. High fluid levels in the water seal indicate residual negative pressure.
   - The chest system may need to be vented by using the high-negativity release valve available on the drainage system to release residual pressure from the system.
   - Do not lower water-seal column when wall suction is not operating or when patient is on gravity drainage.

Patient's Clinical Status
1. Monitor the patient's clinical status. Assess vital signs, lung sounds, and pain.
2. Assess for manifestations of reaccumulation of air and fluid in the chest (↓ or absent breath sounds), significant bleeding (>100 mL/hr), chest drainage site infection (drainage, erythema, fever, ↑ WBC), or poor wound healing. Notify physician for management plan.
3. Evaluate for subcutaneous emphysema at chest tube site.
4. Encourage the patient to breathe deeply periodically to facilitate lung expansion and encourage range-of-motion exercises to the shoulder on the affected side. Encourage use of incentive spirometry every hour while awake to prevent atelectasis or pneumonia.

Chest Drainage
1. Never elevate the drainage system to the level of the patient's chest because this will cause fluid to drain back into the lungs. Secure the unit to the drainage stand. Change the unit if the collection chamber is full. Do not try to empty it.
2. Mark the time of measurement and the fluid level on the drainage unit according to the unit standards. Report any change in the quantity or characteristics of drainage (e.g., clear yellow to bloody) to the physician and record the change. Notify physician if >100 mL/hr drainage.
3. Check the position of the chest drainage container. If the drainage system is overturned and the water seal is disrupted, return it to an upright position and encourage the patient to take a few deep breaths, followed by forced exhalations and cough maneuvers.
4. If the drainage system breaks, place the distal end of the chest tubing connection in a sterile water container at a 2-cm level as an emergency water seal.
5. Milking or stripping chest tubes is no longer recommended, since these practices can dangerously increase intrapleural pressures and damage lung tissues. Position tubing so that drainage flows freely to negate need for milking or stripping. If ordered by physician to milk or strip tubes, do so GENTLY.
   - *Milking:* Alternately fold or squeeze and then release drainage tubing. Milk only if drainage and evidence of clots or obstruction. Take 15-cm strips of the chest tube and squeeze and release starting close to the chest and repeating down the tube distally.
   - *Stripping:* Squeeze drainage tube with thumb and forefinger and use gentle pulling motion down tube with other hand, then release the tubing.

Monitoring Wet vs. Dry Suction Chest Drainage Systems
Suction Control Chamber in Wet Suction System
1. Keep the suction control chamber at the appropriate water level by adding sterile water as needed to replace water lost to evaporation.
2. Keep the muffler covering the suction control chamber in place to prevent more rapid evaporation of water and to decrease the noise of the bubbling.
3. After filling the suction control chamber to the ordered suction amount (generally 20 cm H_2O suction), connect the suction tubing to the wall suction.
4. Dial the wall suction regulator until continuous gentle bubbling is seen in the suction control chamber (generally 80-120 mm Hg). Vigorous bubbling is not necessary and will increase the rate of evaporation.
5. If no bubbling is seen in the suction control chamber, (1) there is no suction, (2) suction is not high enough, or (3) the pleural air leak is so large that suction is not high enough to evacuate it.

Suction Control Chamber in Dry Suction System (see manufacturer's directions)
1. After connecting patient to system, turn the dial on the chest drainage system to amount ordered (generally –20 cm pressure), connect suction tubing to wall suction source, and increase the suction until the correct amount of negative pressure is indicated.
2. If ordered to decrease suction, turn the dial down, depress the high-negativity vent, and assess for a rise in the water level of the water-seal chamber.

Chest Tube Dressings
1. Change dressing according to unit protocol and physician preference.
2. Remove old dressing carefully to avoid removing unsecured chest tube. Assess the site and culture site as indicated.
3. Cleanse the site according to protocol, maintaining asepsis.
4. Redress with occlusive dressing (e.g., Opsite or gauze with occlusive tape). Some physicians prefer the use of petroleum gauze dressing around the tube to prevent air leak. Date the dressing and document dressing change.

INFORMATICS IN PRACTICE

Chest Drainage System

- You find yourself in a situation where you need to set up a chest drainage system. You have not done this since simulation lab in nursing school.
- On the Internet, find a procedure manual or watch a video or podcast on the procedure.

the water, causing a suction-breaker effect. As a result, excess pressure is relieved.

The amount of suction applied is regulated by the amount of water in this chamber and not by the amount of suction applied to the system. An increase in suction does not result in an increase in negative pressure to the system because any excess suction merely draws in air through the vent on the top of the third chamber. The suction pressure is usually ordered to be −20 cm H_2O, although higher pressures (−40 cm H_2O) are sometimes necessary to evacuate the pleural space; lower pressure (−10 cm H_2O) may be used for frail patients at risk for tissue damage with higher pressures.

To initiate suction, turn up the vacuum source until gentle bubbling is present in the chamber. Excessive bubbling does not increase the amount of applied suction, but does increase the rate of evaporation of the column of water and the amount of noise made by the device.

The dry suction control chamber system contains no water. It has a visual alert that indicates if the suction is working. It uses either a restrictive device or a regulator to dial the desired negative pressure; this is internal in the chest drainage system. To increase the suction pressures, turn the dial on the drainage system. Increasing the vacuum source does not increase the pressure. When decreasing suction, depress the manual vent to reduce excess vacuum to the lower prescribed level.

The addition of wall suction (active suction) to the chest drainage unit may actually promote the development of air leaks and thus prolong the number of days the chest tube needs to remain in place.[36] Patients with just water-seal drainage (passive suction) have a shorter duration of air leaks. Although the majority of clinicians continue to use active suction, the use of water-seal drainage alone is gaining popularity.

A variety of commercial disposable plastic chest drainage systems are available. Manufacturers include directions for set-up and use with each unit. Atrium Medical Corporation offers online educational videos of the principles of chest drainage and products at *www.atriummed.com/Products/Chest_Drains/education.asp*.

NURSING MANAGEMENT CHEST DRAINAGE

General guidelines for nursing care of the patient with chest tubes and water-seal drainage systems are presented in Table 28-21.

Clamping of chest tubes during transport or when the tube is accidentally disconnected is no longer advocated. The danger of rapid accumulation of air in the pleural space, causing tension pneumothorax, is far greater than that of a small amount of atmospheric air entering the pleural space. If a chest tube becomes disconnected, immediately reestablish the water-seal system and attach a new drainage system as soon as possible. In some hospitals, when disconnection occurs, the chest tube is immersed in sterile water (about 2 cm) until the system can be reestablished. It is important to know the unit protocol, individual clinical situation (whether an air leak exists), and physician preference before resorting to prolonged chest tube clamping.

Chest tubes may be momentarily clamped to change the drainage apparatus or to check for air leaks. Appearance of a new air leak warrants assessment of the drainage system to identify whether the air leak is coming from the patient or the system. Although it is controversial, some clinicians clamp the chest tube for a few hours before removal. This is done to assess how the patient will tolerate chest tube removal. Generally this occurs 4 to 6 hours before the tube is removed, and the patient is monitored closely for any signs of respiratory distress.

Closely monitor the patient for complications associated with chest tube placement and drainage. If volumes from 1 to 1.5 L of pleural fluid are removed rapidly, reexpansion pulmonary edema or a vasovagal response with symptomatic hypotension can occur. Subcutaneous emphysema can occur from air leaking into the tissue surrounding the chest tube insertion site. A "crackling" sensation will be felt when palpating the skin. A small amount of subcutaneous air is harmless and will be reabsorbed. However, severe subcutaneous emphysema can cause drastic swelling of the head and the neck with potential airway compromise.[37]

Meticulous sterile technique during dressing changes can reduce the incidence of infected sites. Nursing care and patient teaching can minimize the risk of atelectasis and shoulder stiffness. Encourage coughing, deep breathing, incentive spirometer use, and range-of-motion exercises.

CHEST TUBE REMOVAL

The chest tubes are removed when the lungs are reexpanded and fluid drainage has ceased or is minimal. Generally suction is discontinued and the chest drain is on gravity drainage for 24 hours before the tube is removed. Give the patient pain medication about 30 to 60 minutes before tube removal. Gather dressing supplies and petroleum jelly dressing. Explain the procedure to the patient. The tube is removed by the physician or an advanced practice nurse in most settings. The suture is cut, and a sterile airtight petroleum jelly gauze dressing is prepared. With the patient holding his or her breath or bearing down (Valsalva maneuver), the tube is removed. The site is immediately covered with the airtight dressing to prevent air from entering the pleural space. The pleura will seal off, and the wound usually heals in several days. A chest x-ray is done to evaluate for pneumothorax or reaccumulation of fluid. Observe the wound for drainage, and reinforce the dressing if necessary. Assess the patient for respiratory distress, which may signify a recurrence of the original problem.

CHEST SURGERY

Chest surgery is performed for various reasons, including lung, heart, vascular, and esophageal disorders. The most common types of chest surgery are described in Table 28-22.

Preoperative Care

The patient's cardiopulmonary status is assessed to determine his or her ability to tolerate the surgery and to provide a baseline reference for postoperative care. Diagnostic studies include pulmonary function studies, chest x-ray, electrocardiogram (ECG),

TABLE 28-22 **CHEST SURGERIES**

Type	Indications	Description
Lobectomy Removal of one lobe of lung	Lung cancer, bronchiectasis, TB, emphysematous bullae, benign lung tumors, fungal infections	Most common lung surgery. Need chest tubes postoperatively. Lung tissue expands to fill up space left by resected lobe.
Pneumonectomy Removal of entire lung	Lung cancer (most common)	Done only when lobectomy or segmental resection will not remove all diseased lung. May have clamped chest tube postoperatively. Fluid will gradually fill space where lung has been removed. Position patient on operative side to facilitate expansion of remaining lung.
Segmental resection Removal of one or more lung segments	Lung cancer, bronchiectasis	Done to remove bronchovascular lung segment. Need chest tubes postoperatively. Remaining lung tissue expands to fill space. Indicated for a patient unable to handle more extensive surgery.
Wedge resection Removal of small, localized lesion that occupies only part of a segment	Lung biopsy, excision of small nodules	Most conservative approach. Need chest tubes postoperatively. Done to remove small peripheral nodules or for patients unable to handle more extensive surgery.
Decortication Removal or stripping of thick, fibrous membrane from visceral pleura	Empyema or other inflammatory process unresponsive to conservative management	Need chest tubes postoperatively.
Exploratory thoracotomy Incision into thorax to look for injured or bleeding tissues	Chest trauma	Need chest tubes postoperatively.
Thoracotomy (not involving lungs) Incision into thorax for surgery on other organs	Hiatal hernia repair, open heart surgery, esophageal surgery, tracheal resection, thoracic aorta repair	Postoperative care related to thoracotomy and to primary reason for surgical procedure; need chest tubes postoperatively.
Video-assisted thoracoscopic surgery (VATS)	VATS done under general anesthesia in operating room. Procedures performed using VATS include lung biopsy, lobectomy, resection of nodules, repair of fistulas	Video-assisted technique with a rigid scope with a distal lens inserted into the pleura and image shown on a monitor screen. Allows surgeon to manipulate instruments passed into the pleural space through separate small intercostal incisions. Need one chest tube postoperatively.
Lung volume reduction surgery (LVRS)	Advanced bullous emphysema, α_1-antitrypsin emphysema	Involves reducing lung volume by multiple wedge excisions or VATS.

ABGs, blood urea nitrogen (BUN), serum creatinine, blood glucose, serum electrolytes, prothrombin time/international normalized ratio (PT/INR), activated partial thromboplastin time (aPTT), and CBC. Additional cardiac function studies are often done for the patient who is to undergo a pneumonectomy. An anesthesia consult is also completed.

The patient should be in optimal health and stop smoking, if applicable, before elective surgery. Anxiety associated with anticipated surgery makes smoking cessation more difficult. Provide encouragement, support, and teaching regarding various methods to help stop smoking (see Chapter 11).

Teach the patient what to expect postoperatively, including the use of oxygen, possible intubation, administration of blood and fluids, and the purpose and function of chest tubes. Reassure the patient that adequate medication will be used to reduce pain. Explain how to use patient-controlled analgesia (PCA), if planned. Preoperative teaching also includes exercises for effective deep breathing and use of incentive spirometry. If the patient practices these techniques before surgery, they will be easier to perform postoperatively. Show the patient how to splint the incision with a pillow to facilitate deep breathing. Teach and have the patient provide a return demonstration of range-of-motion exercises on the surgical side (similar to those for the mastectomy patient [see Fig. 52-9]).

The thought of losing part of a vital organ is frequently frightening. Reassure the patient that the lungs have a large degree of functional reserve. Even after the removal of one lung, enough lung tissue is left to maintain adequate oxygenation. Be available to answer the patient and caregiver's questions. Answer questions honestly. Try to facilitate the expression of concerns, feelings, and questions. (General preoperative care and teaching are discussed in Chapter 18.)

Surgical Procedures

Thoracotomy. A **thoracotomy** is a surgical incision into the chest to gain access to the heart, lungs, esophagus, thoracic aorta, or anterior spine. The two most common approaches to a thoracotomy are the medial sternotomy and the lateral thoracotomy. The medial sternotomy involves splitting the sternum and is primarily used for surgery involving the heart. The lateral thoracotomy incision can be done using a posterolateral or anterolateral incision. The *posterolateral incision* is used for most surgeries involving the lung. The incision is made from front to back at the level of the fourth, fifth, or sixth intercostal space. Strong mechanical retractors are used to separate the ribs and gain access to the lung. The *anterolateral incision* is made in the fourth or fifth intercostal space from the sternal border to the midaxillary line. This procedure is commonly used for surgery or trauma victims, mediastinal operations, and wedge resections of the upper and middle lobes of the lung.

Video-Assisted Thoracic Surgery. *Video-assisted thoracoscopic surgery* (VATS) is a widely used, minimally invasive surgical approach. It provides a real-time two-dimensional video image of the inside of the chest cavity. It is used for diagnosis and treatment of diseases of the pleura, pulmonary masses and nodules, mediastinal masses, and interstitial lung disease. Through incisions just large enough to insert the instruments, the surgeon can inspect the chest cavity, biopsy suspicious areas, obtain samples of fluids for analysis, and remove tissue. VATS is increasingly being used for patients with thoracic trauma. The surgeon can inspect, diagnose, and manage intrathoracic injuries in both blunt and penetrating trauma, including injuries to the diaphragm. A chest tube is placed in the pleural space through one or more of the incisions at the end of the procedure, secured with sutures, and connected to a drainage unit in the usual manner.

The advantages of minimally invasive surgery include less discomfort, faster return to normal activity level, reduced length of hospital stay, lower postoperative morbidity risk, and fewer complications.[38] Patients who have marginal respiratory reserve or are too debilitated to tolerate an open thoracotomy approach may benefit from the VATS procedure.

Postoperative Care

Postoperative pain after a thoracotomy is typically intense because respiratory muscles are cut during surgery. Adequate pain management is a priority to prevent respiratory compromise. The use of PCA and intercostal nerve blocks enables the patient to breathe deeply, cough, and move the arm and shoulder on the operative side.

For most chest surgeries, chest tubes are placed in the pleural space to allow for lung reexpansion. In a pneumonectomy, chest tubes may or may not be placed in the space from which the lung was removed. If a chest tube is used, it is clamped and only released by the surgeon to adjust the volume of serosanguineous fluid that will fill the space vacated by the lung. If the cavity overfills, it could compress the remaining lung and compromise the cardiovascular and pulmonary function. Daily chest x-rays assess the volume and space.

Nursing care priorities in the postoperative period include assessment of respiratory function, including observation of respiratory rate and effort, sputum volume and color, breath sounds, and chest tube function and drainage. Assessment of pain, monitoring of temperature, and observation of the surgical site are similar to care provided for other postoperative patients (see Chapter 20). Care after thoracotomy is presented in eNursing Care Plan 28-2 (available on the website for this chapter).

RESTRICTIVE RESPIRATORY DISORDERS

Disorders that impair the ability of the chest wall and diaphragm to move with respiration are called *restrictive respiratory disorders*. There are two categories: *extrapulmonary conditions,* in which the lung tissue is normal, and *intrapulmonary conditions,* in which the cause is the lung or the pleura. Examples of extrapulmonary conditions that alter respirations are listed in Table 28-23. These disorders are further described in their respective chapters.

Examples of intrapulmonary causes are listed in Table 28-24. Lung damage can be caused by inflammation and scarring of lung tissue (interstitial lung disease), air spaces (pneumonitis), or pleura (empyema).

Pulmonary function tests are the best means of differentiating between restrictive and obstructive respiratory disorders. Restrictive lung disorders are characterized by reduced vital capacity (VC) and total lung capacity (TLC).[39] Mixed obstructive and restrictive disorders sometimes occur together. For example, a patient may have both chronic bronchitis (an obstructive problem) and pulmonary fibrosis (a restrictive problem).

TABLE 28-23 EXTRAPULMONARY CAUSES OF RESTRICTIVE LUNG DISEASE*

Central Nervous System (CNS)	Chest Wall
• Head injury, CNS lesion (e.g., tumor, stroke) • Opioid and barbiturate use **Neuromuscular System** • Spinal cord injury • Guillain-Barré syndrome • Amyotrophic lateral sclerosis • Myasthenia gravis • Muscular dystrophy	• Chest wall trauma (e.g., flail chest, fractured rib) • Obesity-hypoventilation syndrome (Pickwickian syndrome) • Kyphoscoliosis

*See eTable 28-3 for more detailed descriptions on extrapulmonary causes of restrictive lung disease.

TABLE 28-24 INTRAPULMONARY CAUSES OF RESTRICTIVE LUNG DISEASE*

Pleural Disorders	Parenchymal Disorders
• Pleural effusion • Pleurisy (pleuritis) • Pneumothorax	• Atelectasis • Pneumonia • Interstitial lung diseases • Acute respiratory distress syndrome (ARDS)

*See eTable 28-3 for more detailed descriptions on intrapulmonary causes of restrictive lung disease.

PLEURAL EFFUSION

Types

The pleural space normally contains 5 to 15 mL of fluid that acts as a lubricant between the chest wall (parietal pleura) and the lung (visceral pleura). **Pleural effusion** is an abnormal collection of fluid in this space. It is not a disease but rather an indication of disease. A balance between hydrostatic pressure, oncotic pressure, and membrane permeability governs movement of fluid in and out of the pleural space. Fluid accumulation can be a result of increased pulmonary capillary pressure, decreased oncotic pressure, increased pleural membrane permeability, or obstruction of lymphatic flow.[40]

Pleural effusion is classified as transudative or exudative according to the protein content. A *transudate* occurs primarily in noninflammatory conditions and is an accumulation of protein-poor, cell-poor fluid. Transudative pleural effusions are clear, pale yellow, and caused by (1) increased hydrostatic pressure found in heart failure or (2) decreased oncotic pressure (from hypoalbuminemia) found in chronic liver or renal disease. An *exudative effusion* results from increased capillary permeability characteristic of the inflammatory reaction. It is most commonly associated with infections and malignancies.

An **empyema** is the collection of purulent fluid in the pleural space. It is caused by conditions such as pneumonia, TB, lung

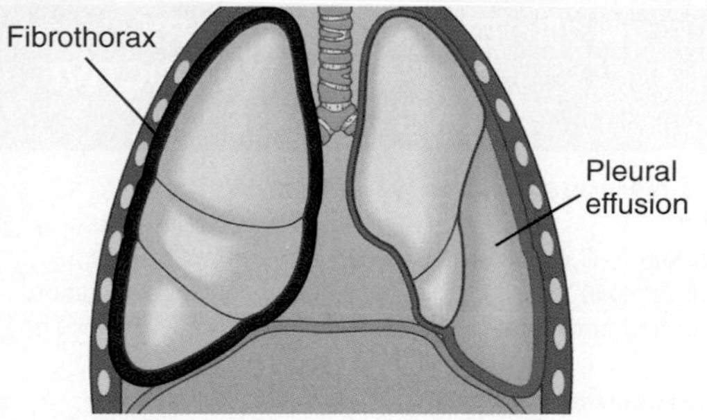

FIG. 28-10 Fibrothorax resulting from an organization of inflammatory exudate and pleural effusion.

abscess, and infection of surgical wounds of the chest. A complication of empyema is *fibrothorax,* in which there is fibrous fusion of the visceral and parietal pleurae (Fig. 28-10).

Clinical Manifestations

Common clinical manifestations of pleural effusion are dyspnea; cough; and occasional sharp, nonradiating chest pain that is worse on inhalation. Physical examination of the chest may indicate decreased movement of the chest on the affected side, dullness to percussion, and diminished breath sounds over the affected area. A chest x-ray and CT reveal the volume and location of the effusion. Manifestations of empyema include the manifestations of pleural effusion, as well as fever, night sweats, cough, and weight loss.

Thoracentesis

Thoracentesis is aspiration of intrapleural fluid for diagnostic and therapeutic purposes. For a thoracentesis, the patient sits on the edge of a bed and leans forward over a bedside table. Chest x-ray results, ultrasound images, and percussion of chest for maximal dullness are used to determine the optimal puncture site. The skin is cleansed with an antiseptic solution and injected with a local anesthetic. The thoracentesis needle is inserted into the intercostal space. Fluid is aspirated with a syringe, or tubing is connected to the needle to allow fluid to drain into a sterile container. After the fluid is removed, the needle is withdrawn, and a bandage is applied over the insertion site.

Usually only 1000 to 1200 mL of pleural fluid is removed at one time. Rapid removal of a large volume can result in hypotension, hypoxemia, or pulmonary edema. A chest x-ray may be done after the procedure to assess for possible complications such as pneumothorax or pulmonary edema. During and after the procedure, monitor vital signs and pulse oximetry, and observe the patient for any manifestations of respiratory distress.

Collaborative Care

The management of pleural effusions is to treat the underlying cause. For example, adequate treatment of heart failure with diuretics and sodium restriction will result in decreased incidence of pleural effusion. The treatment of pleural effusions secondary to malignant disease represents a more difficult problem. These types of pleural effusions are frequently recurrent and accumulate quickly after thoracentesis.

Chemical pleurodesis is performed to obliterate the pleural space and prevent reaccumulation of effusion fluid in both malignant and nonmalignant pleural effusions. This procedure first requires chest tube drainage of the effusion. Once the fluid is drained, a chemical slurry is instilled into the pleural space. Talc is the most effective agent for pleurodesis.[41] Other agents such as doxycycline and bleomycin can also be used. The chest tube is clamped for 8 hours while the patient is turned in different positions to allow the chemical to contact the entire pleural space. After 8 hours the chest tube is unclamped and attached to a drainage unit. Fever and chest pain are the most common side effects associated with pleurodesis. Chest tubes are left in place until fluid drainage is less than 150 mL/day and no air leaks are noted.

Treatment of empyema is generally with chest tube drainage. Appropriate antibiotic therapy is also necessary to eradicate the causative organism. Intrapleural fibrinolytic therapy (instilled via the chest tube) may be considered for some patients to dissolve fibrous adhesions. If this therapy is unsuccessful, a *decortication* surgical procedure may be needed to remove the pleural peel.

PLEURISY

Pleurisy (pleuritis) is an inflammation of the pleura. Inflammation can be caused by infectious diseases, neoplasms, autoimmune disorders, chest trauma, GI disease, and certain medications. The inflammation usually subsides with adequate treatment of the primary disease. The pain of pleurisy is typically abrupt and sharp in onset and is aggravated by inspiration. The patient's breathing is shallow and rapid to avoid unnecessary movement of the pleura and chest wall. A pleural friction rub may occur, which is the sound over areas where inflamed visceral pleura and parietal pleura rub over one another during inspiration. This sound, like a squeaking door, is usually loudest at peak inspiration but may be heard during exhalation as well.

Treatment of pleurisy is aimed at treating the underlying disease and providing pain relief. Taking NSAIDs or analgesics and lying on or splinting the affected side may provide some relief. Teach the patient to splint the rib cage when coughing. Intercostal nerve blocks may be done if the pain is severe.

ATELECTASIS

Atelectasis is a lung condition characterized by collapsed, airless alveoli. There may be diminished or absent breath sounds and dullness to percussion over the affected area. The most common cause of atelectasis is obstruction of the small airways with secretions. This is common in bedridden patients and in postoperative abdominal and thoracic surgery patients. Normally the pores of Kohn (see Fig. 26-1) provide collateral passage of air from one alveolus to another. Deep inspiration is necessary to open the pores effectively. For this reason, deep-breathing exercises and coughing are important to prevent atelectasis and treat the patient at risk. (The prevention and treatment of atelectasis are discussed in Chapter 20.)

INTERSTITIAL LUNG DISEASES

Interstitial lung disease (ILD), also called *diffuse parenchymal lung disease,* refers to more than 200 lung disorders in which the tissue between the air sacs of the lungs (the interstitium) is affected by inflammation or scarring (fibrosis). ILDs can be caused by inhalation of occupational and environmental toxins, certain medications, radiation therapy, connective tissue disorders, malignancy, and infection. Treatment is aimed at reducing exposure to the causative agent and/or treating the underlying disease process. Although scarring is irreversible, treatment with corticosteroids and immunosuppressant drugs can minimize progression. A lung transplant may be an option for some patients.

Many times the cause of ILD is unknown. The most common ILDs of unknown etiology are idiopathic pulmonary fibrosis and sarcoidosis.

IDIOPATHIC PULMONARY FIBROSIS

Idiopathic pulmonary fibrosis (IPF) is a chronic, progressive disorder characterized by chronic inflammation and formation of scar tissue in the connective tissue. A history of cigarette smoking is a risk factor for IPF. It affects more men than women and typically first appears between the ages of 50 and 70 years.

Clinical manifestations of IPF include exertional dyspnea, nonproductive cough, clubbing of the fingers, and inspiratory crackles. Fatigue, weakness, anorexia, and weight loss may occur as the disease progresses. Chest x-ray shows changes characteristic of IPF. High-resolution CT scan provides detailed images. Pulmonary function tests are abnormal with evidence of restriction (reduced vital capacity) and impaired gas exchange. Open lung biopsy using VATS often helps to confirm the pathology and is considered the "gold standard" for diagnosis.

The clinical course of IPF is variable and the prognosis is poor, with a 5-year survival rate of 30% to 50% after diagnosis. Many people diagnosed with IPF are initially treated with a corticosteroid (prednisone), sometimes in combination with other drugs that suppress the immune system (e.g., methotrexate, cyclosporine). None of these combinations has proved very effective.[42] O_2 therapy should be prescribed for all patients. Lung transplantation is an option for those who meet the criteria. (Lung transplantation is discussed later in this chapter on p. 556.)

SARCOIDOSIS

Sarcoidosis is a chronic, multisystem granulomatous disease of unknown cause that primarily affects the lungs. The disease may also involve the skin, eyes, liver, kidney, heart, and lymph nodes. African Americans and those with a family history are at higher risk for developing sarcoidosis. Signs and symptoms vary depending on what organs are affected. Pulmonary symptoms include dyspnea, cough, and chest pain. Many patients do not have symptoms.

The disease is staged and treatment decisions are based on pulmonary function and progression of the disease. Some patients have a spontaneous remission. Treatment is aimed at suppression of the inflammatory response. Patients are followed every 3 to 6 months with pulmonary function tests, chest x-ray, and CT scan to monitor disease progression.

VASCULAR LUNG DISORDERS

PULMONARY EDEMA

Pulmonary edema is an abnormal accumulation of fluid in the alveoli and interstitial spaces of the lungs. It is a complication of various heart and lung diseases (Table 28-25). Pulmonary edema is considered a life-threatening medical emergency.

TABLE 28-25 CAUSES OF PULMONARY EDEMA

- Heart failure
- Overhydration with IV fluids
- Hypoalbuminemia: nephrotic syndrome, hepatic disease, nutritional disorders
- Altered capillary permeability of lungs: inhaled toxins, inflammation (e.g., pneumonia), severe hypoxia, near-drowning
- Malignancies of the lymph system (e.g., non-Hodgkin's lymphoma)
- Respiratory distress syndrome (e.g., O_2 toxicity)
- Unknown causes: neurogenic condition, opioid overdose, reexpansion pulmonary edema, high altitude

The most common cause of pulmonary edema is left-sided heart failure. (Pathophysiology, clinical manifestations, and management of pulmonary edema are described in Chapter 35.)

PULMONARY EMBOLISM

Etiology and Pathophysiology

Pulmonary embolism (PE) is the blockage of pulmonary arteries by a thrombus, fat or air embolus, or tumor tissue. The word *embolus* derives from a Greek word meaning "plug" or "stopper." *Emboli* are mobile clots that generally do not stop moving until they lodge at a narrowed part of the circulatory system. A pulmonary embolus consists of material that gains access to the venous system and then to the pulmonary circulation. The embolus travels with the blood flow through ever-smaller blood vessels until it lodges and obstructs perfusion of the alveoli (Fig. 28-11). Because of higher blood flow, the lower lobes of the lung are commonly affected. Approximately 10% of patients with PE die within the first hour. An additional 30% die from recurrent embolism. Treatment with anticoagulants reduces the mortality rate to less than 5%.[43]

More than 90% of pulmonary emboli arise from deep vein thrombosis (DVT) in the deep veins of the legs.[7] *Venous thromboembolism* (VTE) is the preferred term to describe the spectrum of pathologic conditions from DVT to PE (see Table 38-7). Lethal pulmonary emboli most commonly originate in the femoral or iliac veins. Generally, DVTs that are below the knee are not considered a risk factor for PE, since they rarely migrate to the pulmonary circulation without first extending above the knee. The highest rate of DVT is in spinal cord injury patients (60% to 80%).[43]

Other sites of origin of PE include the right side of the heart (especially with atrial fibrillation), the upper extremities (rare),

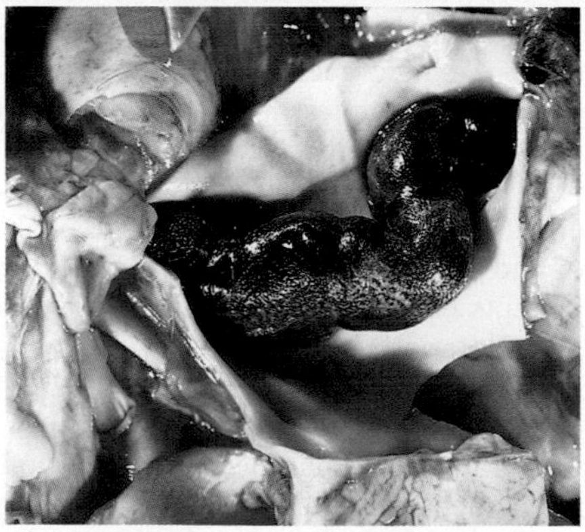

FIG. 28-11 Large embolus from the femoral vein lying in the main left and right pulmonary arteries.

and the pelvic veins (especially after surgery or childbirth). Upper extremity DVT occasionally occurs in the presence of central venous catheters or cardiac pacing wires. These cases may resolve with the removal of the catheter.

In addition to dislodged thrombi, less common causes of PE include fat emboli (from fractured long bones), air emboli (from improperly administered IV therapy), bacterial vegetations, amniotic fluid, and tumors. Risk factors for PE include immobility or reduced mobility, surgery within the last 3 months (especially pelvic and lower extremity surgery), history of DVT, malignancy, obesity, oral contraceptives and hormone therapy, heavy cigarette smoking, prolonged air travel, heart failure, pregnancy, and clotting disorders.

Clinical Manifestations

The signs and symptoms in PE are varied and nonspecific, making diagnosis difficult. Symptoms may begin slowly or suddenly. Dyspnea is the most common presenting symptom, occurring in 85% of patients with PE.[7] A mild to moderate hypoxemia with a low $PaCO_2$ is a common finding. Other manifestations are tachypnea, cough, chest pain, hemoptysis, crackles, wheezing, fever, accentuation of the pulmonic heart sound, tachycardia, syncope, and sudden change in mental status as a result of hypoxemia.

Clinical manifestations depend on the size and extent of emboli. Massive emboli may produce abrupt hypotension and shock. The mortality rate for massive PE is 30% to 60%, with most deaths occurring within 1 to 2 hours of onset.[43]

Conversely, small emboli may go undetected or produce vague, transient symptoms. The exception to this is the patient with underlying cardiopulmonary disease. In these patients, even small or medium-sized emboli may result in severe cardiopulmonary compromise. Repeated pulmonary emboli gradually cause a reduction in the capillary bed and eventual pulmonary hypertension. Right ventricular hypertrophy can develop secondary to pulmonary hypertension.

Complications

Pulmonary infarction (death of lung tissue) is most likely when the following factors are present: (1) occlusion of a large or medium-sized pulmonary vessel (more than 2 mm in diameter), (2) insufficient collateral blood flow from the bronchial circulation, or (3) preexisting lung disease. Infarction results in alveolar necrosis and hemorrhage. Occasionally the necrotic tissue becomes infected, and an abscess may develop. Concomitant pleural effusion is frequent.

Pulmonary hypertension results from hypoxemia or from involvement of more than 50% of the area of the normal pulmonary bed. As a single event, an embolus does not cause pulmonary hypertension unless it is massive. Recurrent emboli may result in chronic pulmonary hypertension. Pulmonary hypertension eventually results in dilation and hypertrophy of the right ventricle. Depending on the degree of pulmonary hypertension and its rate of development, outcomes can vary, with some patients dying within months of the diagnosis and others living for decades.

Diagnostic Studies

D-dimer is a laboratory test that measures the amount of cross-linked fibrin fragments. These fragments are the result of clot degradation and are rarely found in healthy individuals. The disadvantage of D-dimer is that it is neither specific (other conditions cause elevation) nor sensitive, because up to 50% of patients with small pulmonary emboli have normal results. Patients with suspected PE and an elevated D-dimer level but normal venous ultrasound may need a spiral CT or lung scan.

TABLE 28-26 COLLABORATIVE CARE

Acute Pulmonary Embolism

Diagnostic	Collaborative Therapy
• History and physical examination • Chest x-ray • Continuous ECG monitoring • ABGs • Venous ultrasound • CBC count with WBC differential • Spiral (helical) CT scan • Ventilation-perfusion (V/Q) lung scan • D-dimer level • Troponin level, BNP level • Pulmonary angiography	• Supplemental O_2, intubation if necessary • Fibrinolytic agent • Unfractionated heparin IV • Low-molecular-weight heparin (e.g., enoxaparin [Lovenox]) • Warfarin (Coumadin) for long-term therapy • Monitoring of aPTT and INR levels • Limited activity • Opioids for pain relief • Inferior vena cava filter • Pulmonary embolectomy in life-threatening situation

ABGs, Arterial blood gases; *aPTT,* activated partial thromboplastin time; *BNP,* b-type natriuretic peptide; *INR,* international normalized ratio.

A *spiral (helical) CT scan* (also known as CT angiography or CTA) is the most frequently used test to diagnose PE (Table 28-26). An IV injection of contrast media is required to view the blood vessels. The scanner continuously rotates while obtaining slices and does not start and stop between each slice. This allows visualization of all anatomic regions of the lungs. The computer reconstructs the data to provide a three-dimensional picture and assist in emboli visualization.

If a patient cannot have contrast media, a ventilation-perfusion (V/Q) scan is done. The V/Q scan has two components and is most accurate when both are performed:

1. *Perfusion scanning* involves IV injection of a radioisotope. A scanning device images the pulmonary circulation.
2. *Ventilation scanning* involves inhalation of a radioactive gas such as xenon. Scanning reflects the distribution of gas through the lung. The ventilation component requires the patient's cooperation and may be impossible to perform in the critically ill patient, particularly if the patient is intubated.

Pulmonary angiography is the most sensitive and specific test for PE. However, it is an expensive and invasive procedure that involves insertion of a catheter through the antecubital or femoral vein, advancement to the pulmonary artery, and injection of contrast medium. The reliability of the spiral CT has greatly diminished the need for pulmonary angiography.

ABG analysis is important, but not diagnostic. The PaO_2 is low because of inadequate oxygenation secondary to an occluded pulmonary vasculature preventing matching of perfusion to ventilation. The pH remains normal unless respiratory alkalosis develops as a result of prolonged hyperventilation or to compensate for lactic acidosis caused by shock. Abnormal findings are usually reported on the chest x-ray (atelectasis, pleural effusion) and the ECG (ST segment and T wave changes), but they are not diagnostic for PE. Serum troponin levels and b-type natriuretic peptide (BNP) levels are frequently elevated. Although not diagnostic, elevated levels of these markers are associated with increased mortality in patients with PE.[44]

Collaborative Care

Prevention of PE begins with prevention of DVT. DVT prophylaxis includes the use of sequential compression devices, early ambulation, and anticoagulant medications.

To reduce mortality risk, treatment is begun as soon as PE is suspected (see Table 28-26). The objectives are to (1) prevent further growth or multiplication of thrombi in the lower extremities, (2) prevent embolization from the upper or lower extremities to the pulmonary vascular system, and (3) provide cardiopulmonary support if indicated.

Supportive therapy for the patient's cardiopulmonary status varies according to the severity of the PE. O_2 can be given via mask or cannula, and the concentration is determined by ABG analysis. In some situations, endotracheal intubation and mechanical ventilation are necessary to maintain adequate oxygenation. Respiratory measures such as turning, coughing, deep breathing, and using incentive spirometry are important to help prevent or treat atelectasis. If manifestations of shock are present, IV fluids are administered followed by vasopressor agents as needed to support perfusion (see Chapter 67). If heart failure is present, diuretics are used (see Chapter 35). Pain resulting from pleural irritation or reduced coronary blood flow is treated with opioids (usually morphine).

Drug Therapy. Immediate anticoagulation is required for patients with PE. Subcutaneous administration of low-molecular-weight heparin (LMWH) (e.g., enoxaparin [Lovenox]) has been found to be safer and more effective than use of unfractionated heparin. It is the recommended choice of treatment for patients with nonmassive PE. Unfractionated IV heparin can be as effective but is more difficult to titrate to therapeutic levels. Monitoring the aPTT is not necessary or useful when using LMWH.

Warfarin (Coumadin) should be initiated within the first 3 days of heparinization and is typically administered for 3 to 6 months. Some health care providers use direct thrombin inhibitors (see Table 38-10) in the treatment of PE. Anticoagulant therapy may be contraindicated if the patient has complicating factors such as blood dyscrasias, hepatic dysfunction causing alteration in the clotting mechanism, injury to the intestine, overt bleeding, a history of hemorrhagic stroke, or neurologic conditions.

Fibrinolytic agents, such as tissue plasminogen activator (tPA) or alteplase (Activase), dissolve the pulmonary embolus and the source of the thrombus in the pelvis or deep leg veins, thereby decreasing the likelihood of recurrent emboli. Indications for thrombolytic therapy in PE include hemodynamic instability and right ventricular dysfunction. (Fibrinolytic therapy is discussed in Chapter 34.)

Surgical Therapy. Hemodynamically unstable patients with massive PE with contraindications for fibrinolytic therapy are candidates for immediate pulmonary embolectomy. This can be achieved via a vascular (catheter) or surgical approach. Pulmonary embolectomy has a high mortality rate and is thus not recommended for patients who can be successfully treated otherwise.

To prevent further emboli, an inferior vena cava (IVC) filter may be the treatment of choice in patients who remain at high risk and patients for whom anticoagulation is contraindicated. This device is percutaneously placed at the level of the diaphragm in the inferior vena cava via the femoral vein. It prevents migration of large clots into the pulmonary system. The complications associated with this device are rare and include misplacement, migration, and perforation.

NURSING MANAGEMENT PULMONARY EMBOLISM

NURSING IMPLEMENTATION

Nursing measures aimed at prevention of PE are similar to those for prophylaxis of DVT (see Chapter 38, pp. 849-850).

The prognosis of a patient with PE is good if therapy is promptly instituted. Keep the patient on bed rest in a semi-Fowler's position to facilitate breathing. Maintain an IV line for medications and fluid therapy. Administer oxygen therapy as ordered. Assess the patient's cardiopulmonary status with careful monitoring of vital signs, cardiac rhythm, pulse oximetry, ABGs, and lung sounds. Monitor laboratory results to ensure therapeutic ranges of INR (for warfarin) and aPTT (for IV heparin). Monitor the patient for complications of anticoagulant and fibrinolytic therapy (e.g., bleeding, hematomas, bruising). Provide appropriate interventions related to immobility and fall precautions.

The patient is usually anxious because of pain, a sense of doom, inability to breathe, and fear of death. Carefully explain the situation and provide emotional support and reassurance to help relieve the patient's anxiety.

Patient teaching regarding long-term anticoagulant therapy is critical. Anticoagulant therapy continues for at least 3 to 6 months. Patients with recurrent emboli are treated indefinitely. INR levels are drawn at intervals and warfarin dosage is adjusted. Some patients are monitored by nurses in an anticoagulation clinic.

Long-term management is similar to that for the patient with DVT (see discussion of DVT in Chapter 38 on pp. 847-856). Discharge planning is aimed at limiting progression of the condition and preventing complications and recurrence. Reinforce the need for the patient to return to the health care provider for regular follow-up examinations.

EVALUATION

The expected outcomes are that the patient who has a PE will have

- Adequate tissue perfusion and respiratory function
- Adequate cardiac output
- Increased level of comfort
- No recurrence of PE

PULMONARY HYPERTENSION

Pulmonary hypertension is characterized by elevated pulmonary artery pressure, resulting from an increase in resistance to blood flow through the pulmonary circulation. Normally the pulmonary circulation is characterized by low resistance and low pressure. In pulmonary hypertension the pulmonary pressures are elevated with the mean pulmonary artery pressure greater than 25 mm Hg at rest (normal is 12 to 16 mm Hg) or greater than 30 mm Hg with exercise.

The disease commonly manifests with shortness of breath and fatigue. Pulmonary hypertension can occur as a primary disease *(idiopathic pulmonary arterial hypertension)* or as a secondary complication of a respiratory, cardiac, autoimmune, hepatic, or connective tissue disorder *(secondary pulmonary arterial hypertension)*.

IDIOPATHIC PULMONARY ARTERIAL HYPERTENSION

Idiopathic pulmonary arterial hypertension (IPAH) is pulmonary hypertension that occurs without an apparent cause. (It was previously known as *primary pulmonary hypertension* [PPH].) If untreated, this disorder can be rapidly progressive, causing right-sided heart failure and death within a few years. Although new drug therapy has greatly improved survival, the disease remains incurable.

Etiology and Pathophysiology

The etiology of IPAH is unknown. It affects females more than males. The pathophysiology of IPAH is poorly understood. Some type of insult (e.g., hormonal, mechanical) to the pulmonary endothelium may occur, causing a cascade of events leading to vascular scarring, endothelial dysfunction, and smooth muscle proliferation[44] (Fig. 28-12).

Clinical Manifestations and Diagnostic Studies

Classic symptoms of pulmonary hypertension are dyspnea on exertion and fatigue. Exertional chest pain, dizziness, and exertional syncope are other symptoms. These symptoms are related to the inability of cardiac output to increase in response to increased oxygen demand. Eventually, as the disease progresses, dyspnea occurs at rest. Pulmonary hypertension increases the workload of the right ventricle and causes right ventricular hypertrophy (a condition called *cor pulmonale*) and eventually heart failure.

Right-sided cardiac catheterization is the definitive test to diagnose any type of pulmonary hypertension. In addition to providing an accurate measurement of pulmonary artery pressures, it also determines cardiac output and pulmonary vascular resistance. Confirmation of IPAH requires a thorough workup to exclude conditions that may cause secondary pulmonary hypertension. Diagnostic evaluation includes ECG, chest x-ray, pulmonary function tests, echocardiogram, and CT scans.

The mean time between onset of symptoms and the diagnosis is about 2 years. By the time patients become symptomatic, the disease is already in the advanced stages and the pulmonary artery pressure is two to three times normal.

PATHOPHYSIOLOGY MAP

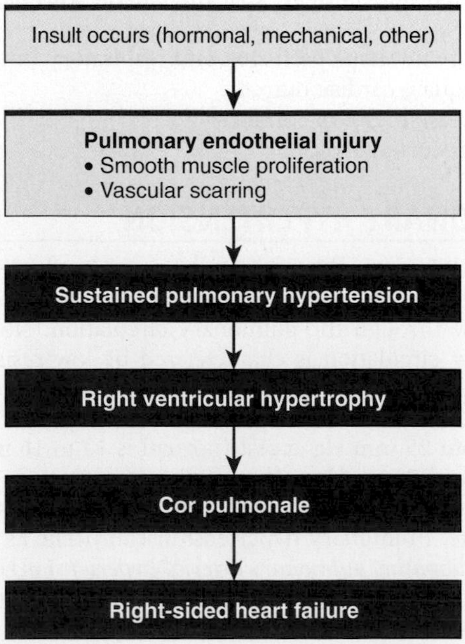

FIG. 28-12 Pathogenesis of pulmonary hypertension and cor pulmonale.

NURSING AND COLLABORATIVE MANAGEMENT PULMONARY HYPERTENSION

Early recognition of pulmonary hypertension is essential to interrupt the vicious cycle responsible for progression of the disease (see Fig. 28-12). Patients are classified using the New York Heart Association functional classification (see Chapter 35, Table 35-5).

Although IPAH has no cure, treatment can relieve symptoms, improve quality of life, and prolong life. Drug therapy consists of several drug classifications that promote vasodilation of the pulmonary blood vessels, reduce right ventricular overload, and reverse remodeling (Table 28-27). Diuretics are used to manage peripheral edema. The use of anticoagulants is also beneficial in pulmonary complications related to thrombus formation. Because hypoxia is a potent pulmonary vasoconstrictor, low-flow O_2 provides symptomatic relief. The goal is to keep O_2 saturation at 90% or greater.

Surgical interventions for pulmonary hypertension include atrial septostomy (AS) and lung transplantation. AS is a palliative procedure that involves the creation of an intraatrial right-to-left shunt to decompress the right ventricle. It is used for a select group of patients awaiting lung transplantation.

Lung transplantation is indicated for those patients who do not respond to drug therapy and progress to severe right-sided heart failure. Recurrence of the disease has not been reported in individuals who have undergone transplantation. A patient teaching and support website for pulmonary hypertension is located at *www.phassociation.org*.

SECONDARY PULMONARY ARTERIAL HYPERTENSION

Secondary pulmonary arterial hypertension (SPAH) occurs when a primary disease causes a chronic increase in pulmonary artery pressures. SPAH can develop as a result of parenchymal lung disease, left ventricular dysfunction, intracardiac shunts, chronic pulmonary thromboembolism, or systemic connective tissue disease. The specific primary disease pathology can result in anatomic or vascular changes causing the pulmonary hypertension.

The symptoms can reflect the underlying disease, but some are directly attributable to SPAH, including dyspnea, fatigue, lethargy, and chest pain. The initial physical findings can include right ventricular hypertrophy and signs of right ventricular failure (increased pulmonic heart sound, right-sided fourth heart sound, peripheral edema, and hepatomegaly).

Diagnosis of SPAH is similar to that of IPAH. Treatment of SPAH consists mainly of treating the underlying primary disorder. When irreversible pulmonary vascular damage has occurred, therapies used for IPAH are initiated. A pulmonary thromboendarterectomy (PTE) may offer a cure for patients with chronic pulmonary hypertension caused by thromboembolism. It is a technically demanding procedure and is performed only at selected centers.

TABLE 28-27 DRUG THERAPY

Pulmonary Hypertension

Drug	Mechanism of Action	Considerations
Calcium Channel Blockers		
nifedipine (Adalat CC, Nifedical XL, Procardia) diltiazem (Cardizem, Cardizem LA, Cartia XT, Tiazac)	• Act on vascular smooth muscle, causing dilation • Lower pulmonary artery pressure	• Can only be used in patients who do not have right-sided heart failure. • Used at high doses in comparison to other uses of calcium channel blockers.
Phosphodiesterase (Type 5) Enzyme Inhibitors		
sildenafil (Revatio) tadalafil (Adcirca)	• Promote selective smooth muscle relaxation in lung vasculature	• Given orally. • Contraindicated in patients taking nitroglycerin, since may cause refractory hypotension.
Vasodilators (Parenteral)		
epoprostenol (Flolan, Veletri) treprostinil (Remodulin) adenosine (Adenocard)	• Prostacyclin analog • Promote pulmonary vasodilation and reduce pulmonary vascular resistance	• Given IV to patients who do not respond to calcium channel blockers or have New York Heart Association (NYHA) class III or IV right-sided heart failure. • Given by continuous IV (central line) or continuous subcutaneous route (see Fig. 28-13). Half life of epoprostenol is short. Potential clinical deterioration from abrupt withdrawal if infusion disrupted.
Vasodilators (Inhaled)		
iloprost (Ventavis) treprostinil (inhaled) (Tyvaso)	• Synthetic analogs of prostacyclin (PGI_2) • Dilate systemic and pulmonary arterial vasculature	• Indicated for patients with NYHA class III or IV heart failure. • Administered 6-9 times a day using a disk inserted into a nebulizer. • Can cause orthostatic hypotension. Do not give to patients with systolic BP <85 mm Hg.
Endothelin Receptor Antagonists		
bosentan (Tracleer) ambrisentan (Letairis)	• Bind to endothelin-1 receptors, causing a reduction in pulmonary artery pressure, pulmonary vascular resistance, and mean atrial pressure • Significantly increase cardiac index	• Given orally. • Indicated for patients with NYHA class II to IV symptoms. • Hepatotoxic. • Monitor liver function tests monthly.

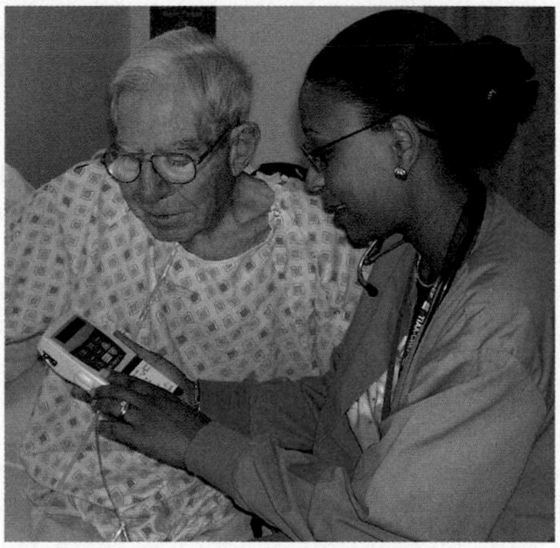

FIG. 28-13 A patient with pulmonary hypertension who is on continuous epoprostenol infusion is being taught how to use the portable infusion pump.

COR PULMONALE

Cor pulmonale is enlargement of the right ventricle caused by a primary disorder of the respiratory system. Pulmonary hypertension is usually a preexisting condition in cor pulmonale. Cor pulmonale may be present with or without overt cardiac failure. The most common cause of cor pulmonale is COPD. Almost any disorder that affects the respiratory system can cause cor pulmonale. Fig. 28-12 outlines the etiology and pathogenesis of pulmonary hypertension and cor pulmonale.

Clinical Manifestations and Diagnostic Studies

Clinical manifestations are subtle and often masked by the symptoms of the pulmonary condition. Common symptoms include exertional dyspnea, tachypnea, cough, and fatigue. Physical signs include evidence of right ventricular hypertrophy on ECG and an increase in intensity of the second heart sound. Chronic hypoxemia leads to polycythemia and increased total blood volume and viscosity of the blood. (Polycythemia is often present in cor pulmonale secondary to COPD.)

If heart failure accompanies cor pulmonale, additional manifestations such as peripheral edema; weight gain; distended neck veins; full, bounding pulse; and enlarged liver will also be found. (Heart failure is discussed in Chapter 35.) Various laboratory tests and imaging studies are used to confirm the diagnosis of cor pulmonale (Table 28-28).

Collaborative Care

The primary management of cor pulmonale is directed at treating the underlying pulmonary problem (see Table 28-28). Long-term O_2 therapy to correct the hypoxemia reduces vasoconstriction and pulmonary hypertension. If fluid, electrolyte, and acid-base imbalances are present, they must be corrected. Diuretics and a low-sodium diet help decrease the plasma volume and reduce the workload on the heart. Bronchodilator therapy is indicated if the underlying respiratory problem is due to an obstructive disorder. Other treatments include those for pulmonary hypertension, such as vasodilator therapy, calcium channel blockers, and anticoagulants. Theophylline may help

TABLE 28-28 COLLABORATIVE CARE

Cor Pulmonale

Diagnostic	Collaborative Therapy
• History and physical examination	• O_2 therapy
• ABGs, SpO_2	• Bronchodilators
• Serum and urine electrolytes	• Diuretics
• b-Type natriuretic peptide (BNP)	• Low-sodium diet
• ECG	• Vasodilators (if indicated)
• Chest x-ray	• Calcium channel blockers (if indicated)
• Echocardiography	• Inotropic agents
• CT scans	
• MRI	
• Cardiac catheterization	

due to its weak inotropic effect on the heart. Digitalis may also be used to increase cardiac contractility. Phlebotomy is indicated in patients with chronic cor pulmonale and chronic hypoxia causing severe polycythemia (hematocrit 65% or greater). Chronic management of cor pulmonale resulting from COPD is similar to that described for COPD (see Chapter 29).

LUNG TRANSPLANTATION

Lung transplantation has become an important mode of therapy for patients with end-stage lung disease. The limiting factor for this therapy is the availability of donors. A variety of pulmonary disorders are potentially treatable with lung transplantation (Table 28-29). Improved patient selection criteria, technical advances, and better methods of immunosuppression have resulted in improved survival rates.

Preoperative Care

Patients being considered for lung transplantation need to undergo extensive evaluation. Absolute contraindications for lung transplant include malignancy within past 2 years (except for skin cancer), chronic active hepatitis B or C, HIV, untreatable advanced dysfunction of another major organ system (e.g., liver or renal failure), current smoker, poor nutritional status, poor rehabilitation potential, and significant psychosocial problems. The patient and the family must be able to cope with a complex postoperative regimen (e.g., strict adherence to immunosuppressive therapy, continuous monitoring for early signs of infection, prompt reporting of manifestations of infection). Many transplant centers require preoperative outpatient pulmonary rehabilitation to maximize physical conditioning.

The United Network for Organ Sharing (UNOS) designates recipients of donor lungs based on a lung allocation score (LAS). The LAS prioritizes waiting list recipients based on the urgency of need and posttransplant survival expectations.

TABLE 28-29 INDICATIONS FOR LUNG TRANSPLANTATION*

- Chronic obstructive pulmonary disease
- Idiopathic pulmonary fibrosis
- Cystic fibrosis
- Idiopathic pulmonary arterial hypertension
- α_1-Antitrypsin deficiency

* These are the most common indications.

Patients who are accepted as good potential transplant candidates must carry a pager with them at all times in case a donor organ becomes available. These patients must be prepared to move to their chosen transplant center at a moment's notice. Such patients may be encouraged to limit their travel within a certain geographic region to facilitate rapid transportation to a transplant center.

Surgical Procedure

Four types of transplant procedures are available: single-lung transplantation, bilateral lung transplantation, heart-lung transplantation, and transplantation of lobes from a living-related donor. *Single-lung transplantation* involves an incision on the side of the chest. The opposite lung is ventilated while the diseased lung is excised. The lung is removed and the donor lung implanted. Three anastomoses are done: the bronchus, the pulmonary artery, and the pulmonary veins. In *bilateral lung transplantation* the incision is made across the sternum, and the donor lungs are implanted separately. A median sternotomy incision is used for a *heart-lung transplant* procedure. *Lobar transplantation* from living donors is reserved for candidates who urgently need transplantation and are unlikely to survive until a donor becomes available. The majority of these transplant recipients are patients with cystic fibrosis, and their parents or relatives are donors. Once anastomosis is complete, the lung is gently reinflated, perfusion is reestablished, two chest tubes are placed, and the surgical incision is closed.

Postoperative Care

Early postoperative care includes ventilatory support, fluid and hemodynamic management, immunosuppression, nutritional support, detection of early rejection, and prevention or treatment of infection. Pulmonary clearance measures, including aerosolized bronchodilators, chest physiotherapy, and deep-breathing and coughing techniques, minimize potential complications. Maintenance of fluid balance is vital in the postoperative phase.

Lung transplant recipients are at high risk for bacterial, viral, fungal, and protozoal infections. Infections are the leading cause of death in the early period after the transplant. Bacterial pneumonia, the most common infection, occurs in more than 35% of patients within the first year posttransplant.[45] Cytomegalovirus (CMV), the second most common cause of pneumonia, is the most common opportunistic infection, usually occurring 1 to 4 months postoperatively. Infection by *Aspergillus* organisms is the most common fungal infection.

Immunosuppressive therapy usually includes a three-drug regimen of tacrolimus, mycophenolate mofetil (CellCept), and prednisone. (The mechanisms of action of these drugs are discussed in Table 14-16 and Fig. 14-13.) Drug levels are monitored on a regular basis. Lung transplant recipients usually receive higher levels of immunosuppressive therapy than other organ recipients.

Acute rejection is fairly common in lung transplantation, typically occurring in the first 5 to 10 days after surgery. Low-grade fever, fatigue, dyspnea, dry cough, and O_2 desaturation are signs of rejection. Accurate diagnosis of rejection is by transtracheal biopsy. Treatment is high doses of IV corticosteroids administered for 3 days, followed by high doses of oral prednisone. In patients with persistent or recurrent acute rejection, antilymphocyte therapy may be useful.

Bronchiolitis obliterans (BOS) is a manifestation of chronic rejection in lung transplant patients. BOS is characterized by airflow obstruction that progresses over time. The onset is often subacute, with gradual development of exertional dyspnea, nonproductive cough, wheezing, and/or low-grade fever. The airway obstruction is not responsive to bronchodilators and corticosteroid therapy. Although not proven effective, additional immunosuppressive agents are used in the treatment of chronic rejection. Because acute rejection is a major risk factor for BOS, prevention of acute rejection is key to decreasing the incidence of chronic rejection.

Before discharge, the patient needs to be able to perform self-care activities, including medication management and activities of daily living, and to accurately identify when to call the transplant team. Patients are placed in an outpatient rehabilitation program to improve physical endurance. Home spirometry is useful in monitoring trends in lung function. Teach patients to keep medication logs, laboratory results, and spirometry records.

After discharge, the transplant team follows patients for transplant-related issues. Patients return to their primary care team for health maintenance and routine illnesses. As transplant procedures become more frequent, transplant patients will return to hospitals for other routine procedures. Coordination of care between the transplant team, primary care team, and inpatient teams is essential for ongoing successful management of these patients. (Organ transplantation, histocompatibility, rejection, and immunosuppressive therapy are discussed in Chapter 14.)

CASE STUDY

Pneumonia and Lung Cancer

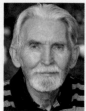

iStockphoto/Thinkstock

Patient Profile

J.H. is a 52-year-old white man who comes to the emergency department complaining of shortness of breath. He has not seen a health care provider for many years.

Subjective Data

- Has a 38 pack-year history of cigarette smoking
- States he has always been slender but has had 25-lb weight loss despite a normal appetite in the past few months
- Admits to a "smoker's cough" for the past 2 to 3 years; recently coughing up blood
- Is married and the father of three adult children

Objective Data

Physical Examination

- Thin, pale man looking older than stated age
- Height 6 ft; weight 135 lb (61.2 kg)
- Intermittently confused and anxious with rapid shallow respirations
- Vital signs: temperature 102.6° F (39.2° C), heart rate 120, respiratory rate 36
- Chest wall has limited excursion on right side; auscultation of left side reveals coarse crackles but clear with cough; right side has diminished breath sounds

Diagnostic Studies

- Arterial blood gases: pH 7.21, PaO_2 58 mm Hg, $PaCO_2$ 82 mm Hg, HCO_3^- 33 mEq/L, O_2 saturation 84%
- Chest x-ray: consolidation of the right lung, especially in the base with possible mass in the area of right bronchus; pleural effusion on the right side
- Bronchoscopy with biopsy of mass: small cell lung carcinoma

Collaborative Care

- Diagnosis: pneumonia with small cell lung cancer
- Follow-up with patient and family to consider treatment options

Discussion Questions

1. How would you classify J.H.'s pneumonia? Why is this important?
2. What is your analysis of J.H.'s arterial blood gas results?
3. ***Priority Decision:*** Based on the assessment data presented, what are the priority nursing diagnoses? Are there any collaborative problems?
4. ***Priority Decision:*** What are the priority nursing interventions for J.H.?
5. ***Delegation Decision:*** Identify activities that can be delegated to unlicensed assistive personnel (UAP).
6. You are planning a meeting with J.H. and his family to discuss their needs. The physician tells you that J.H. is terminally ill. Who will you include in this meeting?
7. ***Evidence-Based Practice:*** J.H.'s children tell you that they are worried they will get lung cancer, since their father has it and they grew up around his secondhand smoke. They want to know what kind of screening is available for them. How will you respond?
8. What is the goal if radiation therapy is used for J.H.?
9. What issues should be addressed in your teaching of J.H. and his wife as you prepare him for discharge and care at home?

evolve Answers available at *http://evolve.elsevier.com/Lewis/medsurg.*

BRIDGE TO NCLEX EXAMINATION

The number of the question corresponds to the same-numbered outcome at the beginning of the chapter.

1. When caring for a patient with acute bronchitis, the nurse will prioritize
   a. auscultating lung sounds.
   b. encouraging fluid restriction.
   c. administering antibiotic therapy.
   d. teaching the patient to avoid cough suppressants.
2. For which patients with pneumonia would the nurse suspect aspiration as the likely cause of pneumonia *(select all that apply)*?
   a. Patient with seizures
   b. Patient with head injury
   c. Patient who had thoracic surgery
   d. Patient who had a myocardial infarction
   e. Patient who is receiving nasogastric tube feeding

3. An appropriate nursing intervention for a patient with pneumonia with the nursing diagnosis of ineffective airway clearance related to thick secretions and fatigue would be to
   a. perform postural drainage every hour.
   b. provide analgesics as ordered to promote patient comfort.
   c. administer O_2 as prescribed to maintain optimal oxygen levels.
   d. teach the patient how to cough effectively to bring secretions to the mouth.
4. A patient with TB has been admitted to the hospital and is placed in an airborne infection isolation room. What should the patient be taught *(select all that apply)*?
   a. Expect routine TST to evaluate infection.
   b. Visitors will not be allowed while in airborne isolation.
   c. Take all medications for full length of time to prevent multidrug-resistant TB.
   d. Wear a standard isolation mask if leaving the airborne infection isolation room.
   e. Maintain precautions in airborne infection isolation room by coughing into a paper tissue.
5. A patient has been receiving high-dose corticosteroids and broad-spectrum antibiotics for treatment secondary to a traumatic injury and infection. The nurse plans care for the patient knowing that the patient is most susceptible to
   a. candidiasis.
   b. aspergillosis.
   c. histoplasmosis.
   d. coccidioidomycosis.
6. When caring for a patient with a lung abscess, what is the nurse's priority intervention?
   a. Postural drainage
   b. Antibiotic administration
   c. Obtaining a sputum specimen
   d. Patient teaching regarding home care
7. The emergency department nurse is caring for patients exposed to a chlorine leak from a local factory. The nurse would closely monitor these patients for
   a. pulmonary edema.
   b. anaphylactic shock.
   c. respiratory alkalosis.
   d. acute tubular necrosis.
8. The nurse receives an order for a patient with lung cancer to receive influenza vaccine and pneumococcal vaccines. The nurse will
   a. call the health care provider to question the order.
   b. administer both vaccines at the same time in different arms.
   c. administer the flu shot and tell the patient to come back 1 week later to receive the pneumococcal vaccine.
   d. administer the pneumococcal vaccine and suggest FluMist (nasal vaccine) instead of the influenza injection.
9. The nurse identifies a flail chest in a trauma patient when
   a. multiple rib fractures are determined by x-ray.
   b. a tracheal deviation to the unaffected side is present.
   c. paradoxic chest movement occurs during respiration.
   d. there is decreased movement of the involved chest wall.
10. The nurse notes tidaling of the water level in the tube submerged in the water-seal chamber in a patient with closed chest tube drainage. The nurse should
    a. continue to monitor the patient.
    b. check all connections for a leak in the system.
    c. lower the drainage collector further from the chest.
    d. clamp the tubing at progressively distal points away from the patient until the tidaling stops.
11. An appropriate nursing intervention for a patient postpneumonectomy is
    a. monitoring chest tube drainage and functioning.
    b. positioning the patient on the unaffected side or back.
    c. doing range-of-motion exercises on the affected upper limb.
    d. auscultating frequently for lung sounds on the affected side.
12. A priority nursing intervention for a patient who has just undergone a chemical pleurodesis for recurrent pleural effusion is
    a. administering ordered analgesia.
    b. monitoring chest tube drainage.
    c. sending pleural fluid for laboratory analysis.
    d. monitoring the patient's level of consciousness.
13. When planning care for a patient at risk for pulmonary embolism, the nurse prioritizes
    a. maintaining the patient on bed rest.
    b. using sequential compression devices.
    c. encouraging the patient to cough and deep breathe.
    d. teaching the patient how to use the incentive spirometer.
14. Which statement(s) describe(s) the management of a patient following lung transplantation *(select all that apply)*?
    a. The lung is biopsied using a transtracheal method if rejection is suspected.
    b. High doses of oxygen are administered around the clock.
    c. The use of a home spirometer will help to monitor lung function.
    d. Immunosuppressant therapy usually involves a three-drug regimen.
    e. Most patients experience an acute rejection episode in the first 3 days.

1. a, 2. a, b, e, 3. d, 4. c, d, e, 5. a, 6. b, 7. a, 8. b, 9. c, 10. a, 11. c, 12. a, 13. b, 14. a, c, d

evolve

For rationales to these answers and even more NCLEX review questions, visit *http://evolve.elsevier.com/Lewis/medsurg.*

REFERENCES

1. World Health Organization: WHO fact sheet, October 2008. Retrieved from *www.who.int/mediacentre/factsheets/fs310/en/index.html.*
2. US Department of Health and Human Services: National vital statistics reports, vol. 59, no. 4, March 16, 2011. Retrieved from *www.cdc.gov/nchs/data/nvsr/nvsr59/nvsr59_04.pdf.*

*3. Albert RH: Diagnosis and treatment of acute bronchitis, *Am Fam Physician* 82:1345, 2010.

*4. Hessen MT, Ferri FF, Pearson RL, et al: Pertussis latest updates: October 6, 2011. Retrieved from *www.mdconsult.com/das/pdxmd/body/308288232-3/0?type=med&eid=9-u1.0-_1_mt_1014575#Contributors.*

*Evidence-based information for clinical practice.

*5. Hessen MT, Thompson A, Murphy P, et al: Community-acquired pneumonia in adults. Retrieved from *www.mdconsult.com/das/pdxmd/body/308841038-3/0?type=med&eid=9-u1.0-_1_mt_5091406.*

*6. Thompson AB, Murphy PJ, Pearson RL, et al: Medical care–associated pneumonia. Retrieved from *www.mdconsult.com/das/pdxmd/body/308841038-4/1247664507?type=med&eid=9-u1.0-_1_mt_5091407.*

7. Ferri FF: *Ferri's clinical advisor*, St Louis, 2012, Mosby.

8. Vigil KJ, Adachi JA, Chemaly RF: Analytic review: viral pneumonias in immunocompromised adult hosts, *J Intens Care Med* 25:307, 2010.

9. US Department of Health and Human Services: How is pneumonia treated? Retrieved from *www.nhlbi.nih.gov/health/health-topics/topics/pnu/treatment.html.*

10. Waterer GW, Rello J, Wunderink RG: Community acquired pneumonia, *Am J Respir Crit Care Med* 183:157, 2010.

*11. Eisenstadt ES: Dysphagia and aspiration pneumonia in older adults, *J Am Acad Nurse Pract* 22:17, 2010.

*12. Vigil KJ, Adachi JA, Chemaly RF: Analytic review: viral pneumonias in immunocompromised adult hosts, *J Intens Care Med* 25:307, 2010.

*13. Pogorzelska M, Stone PW, Furuya EY, et al: Impact of the ventilator bundle on ventilator-associated pneumonia in intensive care unit, *Int J Qual Health Care* 1:7, 2011.

*14. Wren SM, Martin M, Yoon JK, et al: Postoperative pneumonia prevention program for the inpatient surgical ward, *J Am College Surg* 210:492, 2010.

*15. MDConsult: Tuberculosis. Retrieved from *www.mdconsult.com/das/pdxmd/body/310121351-3/0?type=med&eid=9-u1.0-_1_mt_1014609.*

16. Centers for Disease Control and Prevention: Tuberculosis fact sheet. Retrieved from *www.cdc.gov/tb/publications/factsheets/statistics/TBTrends.htm.*

17. Karim K: Tuberculosis and infection control, *Br J Nurs* 20:1128, 2011.

18. Gough A, Kaufman G: Pulmonary tuberculosis: clinical features and patient management, *Nurs Stand* 25:48, 2011.

*19. Centers for Disease Control and Prevention: Tuberculin skin testing. Retrieved from *www.cdc.gov/tb/publications/factsheets/testing/skintesting.htm.*

*20. Hargreaves JR, Boccia D, Evans CA, et al: The social determinants of tuberculosis: from evidence to action, *Am J Pub Health* 101:654, 2011.

21. Hsu LY, Ng ES, Koh LP: Common and emerging fungal pulmonary infections, *Infect Dis Clin North Am* 24:557, 2010.

*22. O'Hanlon KM, Choy E, Sisson SD, et al: Lung cancer. Retrieved from *www.mdconsult.com/das/pdxmd/body/312606682-3/0?type=med&eid=9-u1.0-_1_mt_1014666.*

23. Huethner SE, McCance KL: *Understanding pathophysiology*, ed 5, St Louis, 2012, Mosby.

24. Santacroce L, Harris JE: Paraneoplastic syndromes treatment and management. Retrieved from *http://emedicine.medscape.com/article/280744-treatment.*

25. Winston WD: Small cell lung cancer. Retrieved from *http://emedicine.medscape.com/article/280104-overview.*

*26. Jett JR, Midthun DE: Screening for lung cancer: for patients at increased risk for lung cancer, it works, *Ann Intern Med* 155:541, 2011.

27. American Cancer Society: Lung cancer (non-small cell). Retrieved from *www.cancer.org/acs/groups/cid/documents/webcontent/003115-pdf.*

28. American Cancer Society: Lung cancer (small cell). Retrieved from *www.cancer.org/acs/groups/cid/documents/webcontent/003116-pdf.*

*29. National Comprehensive Cancer Network: NCCN guidelines version 1:2012 lung cancer screening. Retrieved from *www.nccn.org/professionals/physician_gls/pdf/lung_screening.pdf.*

*30. Lehto RH: Identifying primary concerns in patients newly diagnosed with lung cancer, *Oncol Nurs Forum* 38:440, 2011.

31. Mancini MC: Blunt chest trauma. Retrieved from *http://emedicine.medscape.com/article/428723-overview.*

32. Mason RJ, Broaddus VC, Martin TR, et al: *Murray and Nadel's textbook of respiratory medicine*, ed 5, St Louis, 2010, Mosby.

*33. Wendling P: Study supports broader use of rib fixation in flail chest. Retrieved from *www.mdconsult.com/das/news/body/314081249-3/mnfp/1258119330/224596/1.html.*

34. American Association of Critical-Care Nurses: *Procedure manual for critical care*, ed 6, St Louis, 2010, Mosby.

*35. Phillips AM: Pigtail tube drainage as a safe and effective alternative to traditional chest tube thoracostomy in adults with spontaneous pneumothoraces: a systematic review, *School Phys Assist Stud*, paper 266. Retrieved from *http://commons.pacificu.edu/pa/266.*

*36. Cerfolio RJ, Bryant AY: The management of chest tubes after pulmonary resection, *Thorac Surg Clin* 20:399, 2010.

37. Domke MN: Get a positive outcome from negative pressure, *Nursing Made Incredibly Easy* 8:20, 2010.

38. Jarrar D: Video-assisted thoracoscopy. Retrieved from *http://emedicine.medscape.com/article/1970013.*

39. Kanaparthi LK: Restrictive lung disease. Retrieved from *http://emedicine.medscape.com/article/301760.*

*40. McGrath EE, Anderson PB: Diagnosis of pleural effusion: a systematic approach, *Am J Crit Care* 20:119, 2011.

41. Muduly DK, Subi TS, Kallianpur AA, et al: An update in the management of malignant pleural effusion, *Indian J Pall Care* 17:98, 2011.

*42. Lee JS, McLaughlin S, Collard HR: Comprehensive care of the patient with idiopathic pulmonary fibrosis, *Curr Opin Pulm Med* 17:348, 2011.

43. Ouellette DR: Pulmonary embolism. Retrieved from *http://emedicine.medscape.com/article/300901-overview.*

44. Oudiz RJ: Primary pulmonary hypertension. Retrieved from *http://emedicine.medscape.com/article/301450.*

45. Moffatt-Bruce SD: Lung transplantation. Retrieved from *http://emedicine.medscape.com/article/429499.*

RESOURCES

American Lung Association
www.lungusa.org

Centers for Disease Control and Prevention, Smoking and Tobacco Use
www.cdc.gov/tobacco

Pulmonary Fibrosis Foundation
www.pulmonaryfibrosis.org

Pulmonary Hypertension Association (PHA)
www.phassociation.org

CHAPTER 29

There's so much pollution in the air now that if it weren't for our lungs there'd be no place to put it all.
Robert Orben

Nursing Management
Obstructive Pulmonary Diseases

Jane Steinman Kaufman

evolve WEBSITE

http://evolve.elsevier.com/Lewis/medsurg

- NCLEX Review Questions
- Key Points
- Pre-Test
- Answer Guidelines for Case Study on p. 607
- Rationales for Bridge to NCLEX Examination Questions
- Case Studies
  - Patient With Asthma
  - Patient With Chronic Obstructive Pulmonary Disease (COPD)
  - Patient With Cystic Fibrosis
- Nursing Care Plans (Customizable)
  - NCP 29-1: Patient With Asthma
  - NCP 29-2: Patient With Chronic Obstructive Pulmonary Disease
- Concept Map Creator
- Concept Map for Case Study on p. 607
- Glossary
- Content Updates

eFigures
- eFig. 29-1: Postural drainage positions
- eFig. 29-2: Flutter mucus clearance device

eTables
- eTable 29-1: Drug Therapy: Asthma and Chronic Obstructive Pulmonary Disease (enhanced)
- eTable 29-2: Asthma Action Plan (Spanish)
- eTable 29-3: COPD Assessment Test (CAT)
- eTable 29-4: Modified Medical Research Council (mMRC) Dyspnea Scale
- eTable 29-5: Home Oxygen Delivery Systems

LEARNING OUTCOMES

1. Describe the etiology, pathophysiology, clinical manifestations, and collaborative care of asthma.
2. Describe the nursing management of the patient with asthma.
3. Describe the etiology, pathophysiology, clinical manifestations, and collaborative care of the patient with chronic obstructive pulmonary disease (COPD).
4. Describe the effects of cigarette smoking on the lungs.
5. Identify the indications for O_2 therapy, methods of delivery, and complications of O_2 administration.
6. Explain the nursing management of the patient with COPD.
7. Describe the pathophysiology, clinical manifestations, collaborative care, and nursing management of the patient with cystic fibrosis.
8. Describe the pathophysiology, clinical manifestations, collaborative care, and nursing management of the patient with bronchiectasis.

KEY TERMS

α_1-antitrypsin (AAT) deficiency, p. 582
asthma, p. 561
bronchiectasis, p. 606
chest physiotherapy (CPT), p. 594
chronic bronchitis, p. 580
chronic obstructive pulmonary disease (COPD), p. 580
cor pulmonale, p. 584
cystic fibrosis (CF), p. 601
emphysema, p. 580
O_2 toxicity, p. 592
postural drainage, p. 594
pursed-lip breathing (PLB), p. 593

Imagine needing to consciously think about every breath that you take for minutes, hours, or days. Many individuals with obstructive lung disease have this experience. Approximately 31.5 million adult Americans are living with asthma or chronic obstructive pulmonary disease (COPD).[1,2]

Obstructive pulmonary disease, the most common chronic lung disease, is characterized by increased resistance to airflow as a result of airway obstruction or airway narrowing. Types of obstructive lung diseases include asthma, COPD, cystic fibrosis (CF), and bronchiectasis. *Asthma* is a chronic inflammatory lung disease that results in variable episodes of airflow obstruction, but it is usually reversible. *COPD* is an obstructive pulmonary disease with progressive limitation in airflow that is not fully reversible. The patient with asthma has

Reviewed by Danese M. Boob, MSN/ED, RN-BC, Nursing Instructor, Pennsylvania State University, Hershey Campus, Hershey, Pennsylvania; Marianne Ferrin, MSN, ACNP-BC, Coordinator Penn Lung Center, Adult Cystic Fibrosis Program, Philadelphia, Pennsylvania; Mark R. Van Horn, BS, Respiratory Therapist, High Point Regional Hospital, High Point, North Carolina; and Karen M. Wood, RN, DNSc, CCRN, CNL, Associate Professor, Saint Xavier University, Evergreen Park, Illinois.

CULTURAL & ETHNIC HEALTH DISPARITIES

Obstructive Pulmonary Diseases

Asthma

- Asthma prevalence rates are more than 38% higher among African Americans than whites.
- Puerto Ricans have higher asthma prevalence rates and age-adjusted death rates than all other racial and ethnic subgroups.
- Female African Americans have the highest mortality rates from asthma among all ethnic/gender groups.

Chronic Obstructive Pulmonary Disease (COPD)

- Whites have the highest incidence of COPD in spite of higher rates of smoking among other ethnic groups.
- Hispanics have lower death rates related to COPD than other ethnic groups.

Cystic Fibrosis

- Whites have the highest incidence of cystic fibrosis.
- Cystic fibrosis is uncommon among African Americans, Hispanics, and Asian Americans.

variations in airflow over time, usually with normal lung function between exacerbations, whereas the limitation in expiratory airflow in the patient with COPD is generally more constant. The pathology of asthma and the response to therapy differ from those associated with COPD. However, the patient with a diagnosis of obstructive pulmonary disease may have features of both asthma and COPD. Patients with asthma who have less responsive reversible airflow obstruction are difficult to distinguish from COPD patients.

Cystic fibrosis, another form of obstructive pulmonary disease, is a genetic disorder that produces airway obstruction because of changes in exocrine glandular secretions, resulting in increased mucus production. *Bronchiectasis* is an obstructive disease characterized by dilated bronchioles. It most frequently results from untreated or poorly treated pulmonary infections that cause an increase in sputum production.

ASTHMA

Asthma is a chronic inflammatory disorder of the airways. The chronic inflammation leads to recurrent episodes of wheezing, breathlessness, chest tightness, and cough, particularly at night or in the early morning. These episodes are associated with widespread but variable airflow obstruction that is usually reversible, either spontaneously or with treatment. The clinical course of asthma is unpredictable, ranging from periods of adequate control to exacerbations with poor control of symptoms.[3]

GENDER DIFFERENCES

Asthma

Men	Women
• Before puberty, more boys are affected than girls.	• After puberty and into adulthood, more women are affected than men. • Women who are admitted to the emergency department are more likely to need hospitalization than men. • Death rate from asthma is greater in women than in men.

Asthma affects an estimated 18.8 million adult Americans. Among adults, women are 62% more likely to have asthma than men. Asthma is a public health concern, with more than 14.2 million lost workdays in adults. However, the good news is that after a long period of an increasing incidence of asthma, the mortality and use of health care services are continuing to plateau and/or decrease. Despite the decline in the number of deaths from asthma over the past 10 years, more than 3300 people still die from asthma yearly.[1]

Risk Factors for Asthma and Triggers of Asthma Attacks

Risk factors for asthma and triggers of asthma attacks can be related to the patient (e.g., genetic factors) or the environment (e.g., pollen) (Table 29-1). Male gender is a risk factor for asthma in children (but not adults). Obesity is also a risk factor for asthma.[4] Other factors and triggers are discussed in this section.

Genetics. Asthma has a component that is inherited, but the genetics are complex. Numerous genes may be involved in the development of asthma and a person's response to various asthma medications.[3,4] *Atopy,* the genetic predisposition to develop an allergic (immunoglobulin E [IgE]–mediated) response to common allergens, is a major risk factor for asthma.

TABLE 29-1 TRIGGERS OF ASTHMA ATTACKS

Allergen inhalation
- Animal dander (e.g., cats, mice, guinea pigs)
- House dust mite
- Cockroaches
- Pollens
- Molds

Air pollutants
- Exhaust fumes
- Perfumes
- Oxidants
- Sulfur dioxides
- Cigarette smoke
- Aerosol sprays

Inflammation and infection
- Viral upper respiratory tract infection
- Sinusitis, allergic rhinitis

Drugs
- Aspirin
- Nonsteroidal antiinflammatory drugs
- β-Adrenergic blockers

Occupational exposure
- Agriculture, farming
- Paints, solvents
- Laundry detergents
- Metal salts
- Wood and vegetable dusts
- Industrial chemicals and plastics
- Pharmaceutical agents

Food additives
- Sulfites (bisulfites and metabisulfites)
- Beer, wine, dried fruit, shrimp, processed potatoes
- Monosodium glutamate
- Tartrazine

Other factors
- Exercise and cold, dry air
- Stress
- Hormones, menses
- Gastroesophageal reflux disease (GERD)

Immune Response. The *hygiene hypothesis* suggests that a newborn baby's immune system must be educated so it will function properly during infancy and the rest of life. People who are exposed to certain infections early in life, use few antibiotics, are exposed to other children (e.g., siblings, day care), or live in the country or with pets have a lower incidence of asthma. People for whom these factors are not present in childhood have a higher incidence of asthma.[3]

Allergens. Indoor and outdoor allergens, such as cockroaches, furry animals, fungi, and molds, can trigger asthma attacks. However, their role in the actual development of asthma is not as clear.[3,4]

Exercise. Asthma that is induced or exacerbated during physical exertion is called *exercise-induced asthma* (EIA). Typically, EIA occurs after vigorous exercise, not during it (e.g., jogging, aerobics, walking briskly, climbing stairs). Symptoms of EIA are pronounced during activities where there is exposure to cold, dry air. For example, swimming in an indoor heated pool is less likely to produce symptoms than downhill skiing. Airway obstruction may occur due to changes in the airway mucosa caused by hyperventilation during exercise, with either cooling or rewarming of air and capillary leakage in the airway wall.

Air Pollutants. Various air pollutants, such as cigarette or wood smoke or vehicle exhaust, can trigger asthma attacks. In heavily industrialized or densely populated areas, climatic conditions often lead to concentrated pollution in the atmosphere, especially with thermal inversions and stagnant air masses. Ozone alert days are regularly noted on the news reports, and patients should minimize outdoor activity during these times. Cigarette smoking is associated with an accelerated decline of lung functioning in a person with asthma, increases the severity of the disease, may cause the patient to be less responsive to treatment, and reduces the chance of the asthma being controlled. Despite the relationship of pollutants in triggering asthma attacks, the role of outdoor air pollution as a cause of asthma development remains controversial.[4]

Occupational Factors. *Occupational asthma* is the most common occupational respiratory disorder, with up to 15% of new asthma cases arising from job-related exposures to more than 300 agents.[4,5] Irritants cause a change in the responsiveness of the airways. However, the development of symptoms from this alteration may not occur until the patient has had months to years of exposure. Agricultural worker, baker, hospital worker, plastics manufacturer, and beautician are occupations with a high risk of occupational asthma. Characteristically people with occupational asthma give a history of arriving at work feeling well but gradually develop symptoms by the end of the day.

Respiratory Tract Infections. Respiratory tract infections (i.e., viral and not bacterial) are often the major precipitating factor of an acute asthma attack. Acute infection can increase airway narrowing and airway hyperresponsiveness. Viral-induced alterations of epithelial cells, increased inflammatory cell accumulation, edema of airway walls, and exposure of airway nerve endings contribute to altered airway function. These alterations in airway function may exacerbate asthma.

Nose and Sinus Problems. Most patients with asthma have a history of allergic rhinitis. Treatment of allergic rhinitis usually improves the symptoms of asthma. Additional information on the relationship of rhinitis and asthma can be found at *www.whiar.org.*

Acute and chronic sinusitis may worsen asthma. Some patients with asthma have chronic sinus problems that cause inflammation of the mucous membranes. Sinusitis must be treated and large nasal polyps removed for an asthma patient to have good control. (Sinusitis is discussed in Chapter 27.)

Drugs and Food Additives. Sensitivity to specific drugs may occur in some people, especially those with nasal polyps and sinusitis. Some people with asthma have what is termed the *asthma triad:* nasal polyps, asthma, and sensitivity to aspirin and nonsteroidal antiinflammatory drugs (NSAIDs). Salicylic acid can be found in many over-the-counter (OTC) drugs and some foods, beverages, and flavorings. Some asthmatics who use aspirin or NSAIDs (e.g., ibuprofen [Motrin]) develop wheezing within 2 hours. In addition, there is usually profound rhinorrhea, congestion, tearing, and even angioedema. Avoidance of aspirin and NSAIDs is required. However, patients with aspirin sensitivity under the care of an allergist can be desensitized by daily administration of the drug.

β-Adrenergic blockers in oral form (e.g., metoprolol [Toprol]) or topical eyedrops (e.g., timolol) may trigger asthma because they can cause bronchospasm. Angiotensin-converting enzyme (ACE) inhibitors (e.g., lisinopril [Prinivil]) may produce cough in susceptible individuals, thus making asthma symptoms worse.

Other agents that may precipitate asthma in the susceptible patient are tartrazine (yellow dye no. 5, found in many foods) and sulfiting agents widely used in the food and pharmaceutical industries as preservatives and sanitizing agents. Sulfiting agents are commonly found in fruits, beer, and wine and used extensively in salad bars to protect vegetables from oxidation. Asthma exacerbations have been reported after the use of sulfite-containing preservatives found in topical ophthalmic solutions, IV corticosteroids, and some inhaled bronchodilator solutions.

Food allergies triggering asthma reactions in adults are rare. Avoidance diets are not recommended until an allergy has been demonstrated, usually by oral challenges.

Gastroesophageal Reflux Disease. Gastroesophageal reflux disease (GERD) is more common in people with asthma than in the general population. GERD may worsen asthma symptoms. Reflux may trigger bronchoconstriction and cause aspiration. On the other hand, asthma medications may worsen GERD symptoms. β_2-Agonists (especially given orally), which are used to treat asthma, relax the lower esophageal sphincter, thus allowing stomach contents to reflux into the esophagus and possibly be aspirated into the lungs. Medications used to treat GERD usually do not reduce asthma symptoms in most people.[4,6] (GERD is discussed in Chapter 42.)

Psychologic Factors. Asthma is not a psychosomatic disease. However, many people with asthma report that symptoms worsen with stress. Certainly psychologic factors cause bronchoconstriction via stimulation of the cholinergic reflex pathways. Extreme emotional expressions (e.g., crying, laughing, anger, fear) can lead to hyperventilation and hypocapnia, which can cause airway narrowing.[4]

An asthma attack caused by any triggering event can produce panic, stress, and anxiety. However, it varies from patient to patient and in the same patient from episode to episode.

Pathophysiology

The primary pathophysiologic process in asthma is persistent but variable inflammation of the airways. The airflow is limited

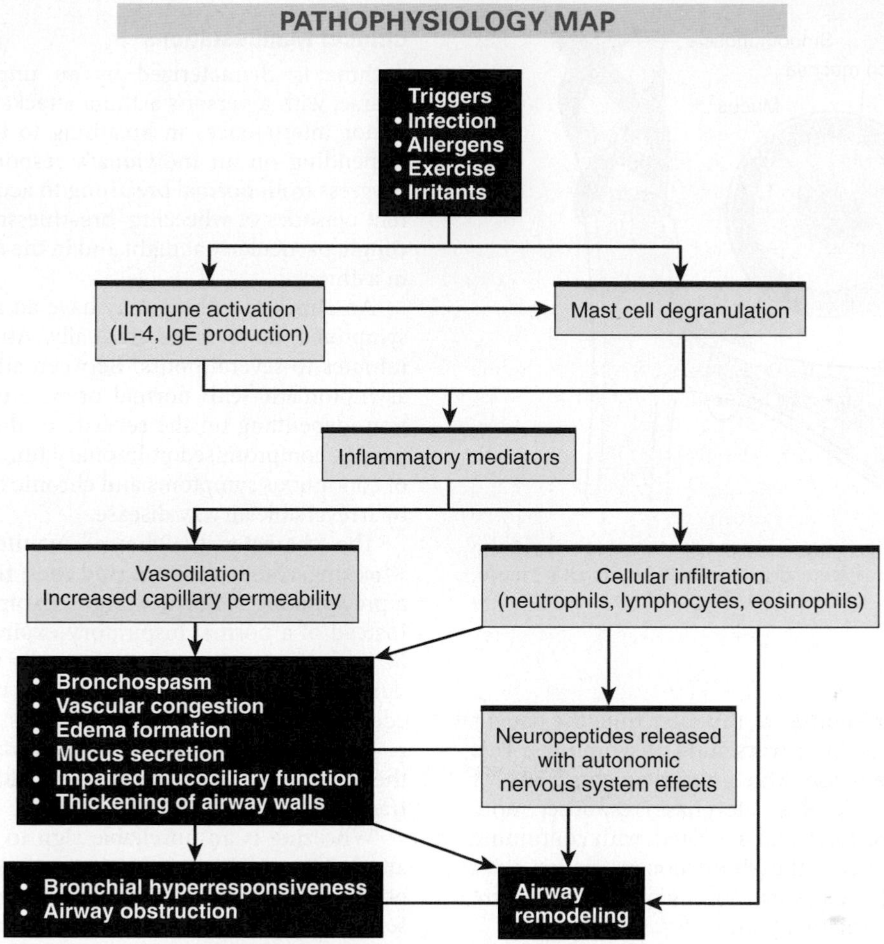

FIG. 29-1 Pathophysiology of asthma. *IL,* Interleukin.

because the inflammation results in bronchoconstriction, airway hyperresponsiveness (hyperreactivity), and edema of the airways. Exposure to allergens or irritants initiates the inflammatory cascade (Fig. 29-1). A variety of inflammatory cells are involved, including mast cells, macrophages, eosinophils, neutrophils, T and B lymphocytes, and epithelial cells of the airways.[3]

As the inflammatory process begins, mast cells (found beneath the basement membrane of the bronchial wall) degranulate and release multiple inflammatory mediators (Fig. 29-2). IgE antibodies are linked to mast cells, and the allergen cross-links the IgE. Then inflammatory mediators such as leukotrienes, histamine, cytokines, prostaglandins, and nitric oxide are released. Some inflammatory mediators have effects on the blood vessels, causing vasodilation and increasing capillary permeability. Some mediators result in the airways being infiltrated by eosinophils, lymphocytes, and neutrophils. The resulting inflammatory process causes vascular congestion, edema, production of thick and tenacious mucus, bronchial muscle spasm, thickening of airway walls, and increased bronchial hyperresponsiveness (Fig. 29-3). This whole process is sometimes referred to as the *early-phase response* in asthma. Clinically it can occur within 30 to 60 minutes after exposure to an allergen or irritant.

Symptoms can recur 4 to 6 hours after the early response because of the influx of many inflammatory cells, which are set

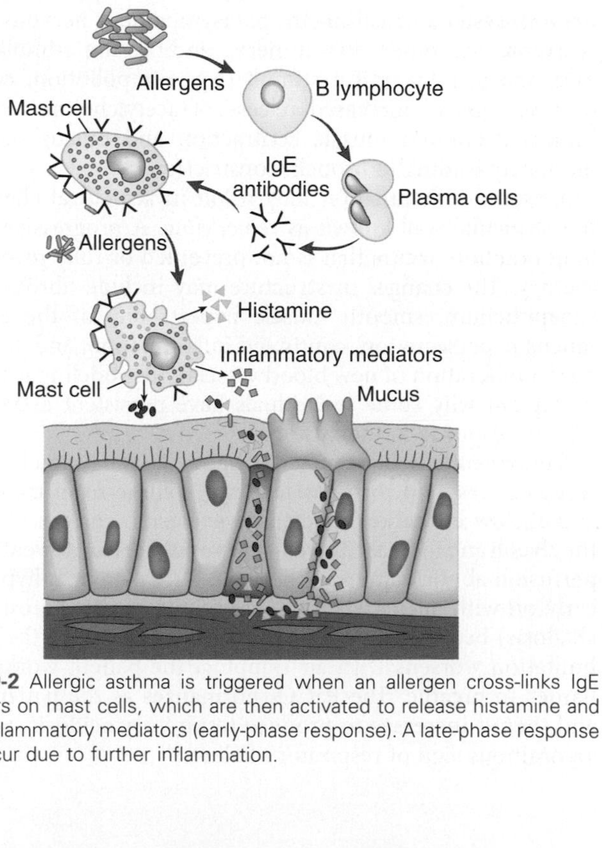

FIG. 29-2 Allergic asthma is triggered when an allergen cross-links IgE receptors on mast cells, which are then activated to release histamine and other inflammatory mediators (early-phase response). A late-phase response may occur due to further inflammation.

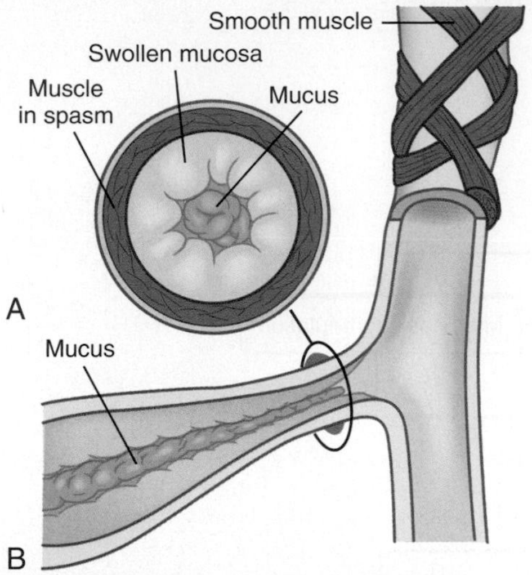

FIG. 29-3 Factors causing obstruction (especially expiratory obstruction) in asthma. **A,** Cross section of a bronchiole occluded by muscle spasm, swollen mucosa, and mucus in the lumen. **B,** Longitudinal section of a bronchiole.

in motion by the initial response. At this later time the patient may develop symptoms again or worsening of symptoms. This is called the *late-phase response,* which occurs in about 50% of individuals with asthma. In this late-phase response, more inflammatory cells are recruited and activated, with continuing inflammation of the airways. Thus bronchoconstriction with symptoms persists for 24 hours or more. Corticosteroids are effective in treating this inflammation.

Alterations in the neural control of the airways also occur in asthma. The autonomic nervous system, consisting of the parasympathetic and sympathetic systems, innervates the bronchi. Airway smooth muscle tone is regulated by the parasympathetic nervous system. In asthma the parasympathetic nervous system is overactive. When airway nerve endings are stimulated by mechanical or chemical stimuli (e.g., air pollution, cold air, dust, allergens), increased release of acetylcholine results in increased smooth muscle contraction and mucus secretion, ultimately leading to bronchoconstriction.

Chronic inflammation may result in structural changes in the bronchial wall known as *remodeling.* A progressive loss of lung function occurs that is not prevented or fully reversed by therapy. The changes in structure may include fibrosis of the subepithelium, smooth muscle hypertrophy of the airways, mucus hypersecretion, continued inflammation, and *angiogenesis* (proliferation of new blood vessels). Remodeling is thought to explain why some individuals have persistent asthma and limited response to therapy.[3,4]

Hyperventilation occurs during an asthma attack as lung receptors respond to increased lung volume from trapped air and airflow limitation. Decreased perfusion and ventilation of the alveoli and increased alveolar gas pressure lead to ventilation-perfusion abnormalities in the lungs. The patient is hypoxemic early on with decreased $PaCO_2$ and increased pH (respiratory alkalosis) because he or she is hyperventilating. As the airflow limitation worsens with air trapping, the patient works much harder to breathe. The $PaCO_2$ normalizes as the patient tires, and then it increases to produce respiratory acidosis, which is an ominous sign of respiratory failure.[6]

Clinical Manifestations

Asthma is characterized by an unpredictable and variable course, with a person's asthma attacks ranging from seemingly minor interferences in breathing to life-threatening episodes. Depending on an individual's response, asthma can rapidly progress from normal breathing to acute severe asthma. Recurrent episodes of wheezing, breathlessness, chest tightness, and cough, particularly at night and in the early morning, are typical in asthma.

An attack of asthma may have an abrupt onset, but usually symptoms occur more gradually. Attacks may last for a few minutes to several hours. Between attacks the patient may be asymptomatic with normal or near-normal pulmonary function, depending on the severity of disease. However, in some people, compromised pulmonary function may result in a state of continuous symptoms and chronic debilitation characterized by irreversible airway disease.

The characteristic clinical manifestations of asthma are wheezing, cough, dyspnea, and chest tightness after exposure to a precipitating factor or trigger. Expiration may be prolonged. Instead of a normal inspiratory-expiratory ratio of 1:2, it may be prolonged to 1:3 or 1:4. Normally the bronchioles constrict during expiration. However, as a result of bronchospasm, edema, and mucus in the bronchioles, the airways become narrower than usual. Thus it takes longer for the air to move out of the bronchioles. This produces the characteristic wheezing, air trapping, and hyperinflation.

Wheezing is an unreliable sign to gauge the severity of an attack. Many patients with minor attacks wheeze loudly, whereas others with severe attacks do not wheeze. The patient with severe asthma attacks may have no audible wheezing because of the marked reduction in airflow. For wheezing to occur, the patient must be able to move enough air to produce the sound. Wheezing usually occurs first on exhalation. As asthma progresses, the patient may wheeze during inspiration and expiration. The term *wheezing* may also be used to describe sounds arising from the nose and upper airways.[7]

In some patients with asthma, cough is the only symptom, and this is termed *cough variant asthma.* The bronchospasm may not be severe enough to cause airflow obstruction, but it can increase bronchial tone and cause irritation with stimulation of the cough receptors. The cough may be nonproductive. Secretions may be thick, tenacious, white, gelatinous mucus, which makes their removal difficult.

The person with asthma has difficulty with air movement in and out of the lungs, which creates a feeling of suffocation. Patients may express, "I can't get a deep breath." Therefore during an acute attack, the person with asthma usually sits upright or slightly bent forward using the accessory muscles of respiration to try to get enough air. The more difficult the breathing becomes, the more anxious the patient feels.

Examination of the patient during an acute attack usually reveals signs of hypoxemia, which may include restlessness, anxiety, inappropriate behavior, and increased pulse and blood pressure (BP). As the patient worsens, it becomes difficult to speak in complete sentences. The respiratory rate is significantly increased (greater than 30 breaths/minute) with the use of accessory muscles. Percussion of the lungs indicates hyperresonance, and auscultation indicates inspiratory or expiratory wheezing. As the episode resolves, coughing produces thick, stringy mucus.

TABLE 29-2 CLASSIFICATION OF ASTHMA SEVERITY

	Asthma Severity			
		Persistent		
Components of Severity	**Intermittent**	**Mild**	**Moderate**	**Severe**
Impairment				
Symptoms	≤2 days/wk	>2 days/wk, not daily	Daily	Continuous
Nighttime awakenings	≤2/mo	3-4/mo	>1/wk, not nightly	Often, 7/wk
SABA use for symptoms	≤2 days/wk	>2 days/wk, not daily	Daily	Several times per day
Interference with normal activity	None	Minor limitation	Some limitation	Extremely limited
Lung function*	Normal FEV_1 between exacerbations FEV_1 >80% FEV_1/FVC normal	FEV_1 >80% predicted FEV_1/FVC normal	FEV_1 60%-80% predicted FEV_1/FVC reduced by 5%	FEV_1 <60% predicted FEV_1/FVC reduced by 5%
Risk				
Exacerbations requiring oral corticosteroids	0-1/yr	≥2/yr even in the absence of impairment →		
	Consider severity and interval since last exacerbation →			
	Frequency and severity may fluctuate over time →			
	Relative annual risk of exacerbation may be related to FEV_1 →			
Recommended Step for Initiating Treatment	Step 1	Step 2	Step 3†	Step 4 or 5†
	Reevaluate asthma control in 2-6 wk and adjust therapy accordingly			

Guidelines for Using Table

- Patients should be assigned to the most severe step in which any feature occurs. Clinical features for individual patients may overlap across steps. Determine level of severity by assessment of both impairment and risk. Assess impairment by patient's recall of previous 2-4 wk and spirometry results.
- An individual's classification should change over time as treatment is initiated. After treatment, the focus switches to level of control, not the classification of severity.
- Patients at any level of severity of chronic asthma can have mild, moderate, or severe exacerbations of asthma. Some patients with intermittent asthma experience severe and life-threatening exacerbations separated by long periods of normal lung function and no symptoms.

Source: Adapted from National Asthma Education and Prevention Program, National Heart, Lung, and Blood Institute: *Expert Panel Report 3: guidelines for the diagnosis and management of asthma*, NIH pub no 08-4051, Bethesda, Md, 2007, National Institutes of Health. Retrieved from *www.nhlbi.nih.gov/guidelines*.

*Percent predicted values for FEV_1 or ratio of FEV_1/FVC. Normal FEV_1/FVC: 8-19 yr, 85%; 20-39 yr, 80%; 40-59 yr, 75%; 60-80 yr, 70%.

†Consider short-term corticosteroid therapy.

FEV_1, Forced expiratory volume in 1 sec; *FVC*, forced vital capacity; *SABA*, short-acting β_2-adrenergic agonist.

Diminished or absent breath sounds may indicate a significant decrease in air movement resulting from exhaustion and an inability to generate enough muscle force to ventilate. Severely diminished breath sounds, often referred to as the "silent chest," are an ominous sign, indicating severe obstruction and impending respiratory failure.

Classification of Asthma

Asthma can be classified as intermittent, mild persistent, moderate persistent, or severe persistent (Table 29-2). The classification system is used to determine the treatment. Patients may move to different asthma classifications over the course of their disease.

Complications

Severe and Life-Threatening Asthma Exacerbations. Severe asthma exacerbations occur when the patient is dyspneic at rest and the patient speaks in words, not sentences, because of the difficulty of breathing. The patient is usually sitting forward to maximize the diaphragmatic movement with prominent wheezing, a respiratory rate higher than 30 breaths/minute, and pulse greater than 120 beats/minute. Accessory muscles in the neck are straining to lift the chest wall, and the patient is often agitated. The peak flow (peak expiratory flow rate [PEFR]) is 40% of the personal best or less than 150 L/minute. Arterial blood gas (ABG) changes are listed in Table 29-3. Neck vein distention may result. These patients usually are seen in emergency departments (EDs) or hospitalized.[6]

A few patients perceive asthma symptoms poorly and may have a significant decrease in lung function without any change in symptoms. Patients with life-threatening asthma are typically too dyspneic to speak and perspire profusely. They may even be drowsy or confused as the ABGs further deteriorate. The breath sounds may be difficult to hear, and no wheezing is apparent because the airflow is exceptionally limited. Peak flow is less than 25% of the personal best. They become bradycardic and are close to respiratory arrest. These patients require ED or hospital care and are often admitted to an intensive care unit.

SAFETY ALERT

- If the patient has been wheezing and then there is an absence of a wheeze (i.e., silent chest) and the patient is obviously struggling, this is a life-threatening situation that may require mechanical ventilation.

Diagnostic Studies

Underdiagnosis of asthma is common. A detailed history is important to determine if a person has had similar attacks, which are often precipitated by a known trigger. (Triggers are discussed on pp. 561-562.) Because wheezing and cough are seen with a variety of disorders (e.g., COPD, GERD, vocal cord dysfunction, heart failure), it is important to determine if asthma is the cause of these problems.

TABLE 29-3 COMPARISON OF ASTHMA AND COPD*

	Asthma	COPD
Clinical Features		
Age	Usually <40 yr (onset).	Usually 40-50 yr (onset).
Smoking history	Not causal.	Often long history (>10-20 pack-years).
Health and family history	Presence of allergy, rhinitis, eczema. Family history of asthma.	Infrequent allergies. May have exposure to environmental pollutants. With α_1-antitrypsin deficiency, family history of lung or liver disease without smoking history.
Clinical symptoms	Intermittent, vary day to day, at night or early morning.	Slowly progressive and persistent.
Dyspnea	Absent except in exacerbations or poor control.	Dyspnea during exercise.
Sputum	Infrequent.	Often.
Disease course	Stable (with exacerbations).	Progressive worsening (with exacerbations).
Diagnostic Study Results		
ABGs	Normal between exacerbations.	Between exacerbations in advanced COPD • Often low-normal pH and PaO_2 • High-normal $PaCO_2$ with high HCO_3^- (compensated respiratory acidosis)
pH	↑ Early in exacerbation, then ↓ if prolonged or severe exacerbation.	N→↓
PaO_2	↓	N→↓
$PaCO_2$	↓ Early in exacerbation, then ↑ if prolonged or severe exacerbation.	N→↑
Chest x-ray	May reveal hyperinflation.	Hyperinflation. May have cardiac enlargement, flattened diaphragm.
Lung volumes	Often normalizes.	Never normalizes.
• Total lung capacity	Increased.	Increased.
• Residual volume	Increased.	Increased.
• FEV_1	Decreased.	Decreased.
• FEV_1/FVC	Normal to decreased.	Decreased (<70%).

*Individuals may have features of both asthma and COPD.
ABGs, Arterial blood gases; *FEV_1*, forced expiratory volume in 1 sec; *FVC*, forced vital capacity.

Some controversy exists about how to best diagnose asthma. Common diagnostic measures are presented in Table 29-4. In general, the health care provider should consider the diagnosis of asthma if various indicators (i.e., clinical manifestations, health history, peak flow variability or spirometry) are positive. Pulmonary function tests (PFTs) can be used to determine the reversibility of bronchoconstriction (using bronchodilators) and thus establish the diagnosis of asthma.

The peak expiratory flow rate (PEFR) measured by the peak flow meter is an aid to diagnose and monitor asthma. However, PEFR measurements are not interchangeable with other lung measurements of lung function (e.g., forced expiratory volume in 1 second [FEV_1]). PEFR should be compared with patients' own previous best measurements using their own meter, since types of peak flow meters vary.

TABLE 29-4 COLLABORATIVE CARE

Asthma

Diagnostic
- History and physical examination
- Pulmonary function studies, including response to bronchodilator therapy
- Peak expiratory flow rate (PEFR)
- Chest x-ray
- Measurement of oximetry
- Allergy skin testing (if indicated)
- Blood level of eosinophils and IgE (if indicated)

Collaborative Therapy

Intermittent or Persistent Asthma
- Identification and avoidance or elimination of triggers
- Patient and caregiver teaching
- Drug therapy (see Tables 29-6 and 29-7 and Fig. 29-4)
- Asthma action plan (see Table 29-12)
- Desensitization (immunotherapy) if indicated
- Assess for control (e.g., Asthma Control Test [ACT])*

Severe or Life-Threatening Asthma Exacerbation
- SaO_2 monitoring
- ABGs
- Inhaled β_2-adrenergic agonists
- Inhaled anticholinergic agents (only in the initial treatment)
- O_2 by mask or nasal prongs
- IV or oral corticosteroids
- IV fluids
- IV magnesium and/or heliox
- Intubation and assisted ventilation

*See *www.qualitymetric.com/demos/TP_Launch.aspx?SID=52461*.
ABGs, Arterial blood gases; *IgE*, immunoglobulin E; *SaO_2*, O_2 saturation.

PFTs are usually normal between asthma attacks if the patient has no other underlying pulmonary disease. However, the patient with asthma may show an obstructive pattern with asthma, including a decrease in forced vital capacity (FVC), FEV_1, PEFR, and FEV_1 to FVC ratio (FEV_1/FVC). (The normal values for PFTs are discussed in Chapter 26.)

When PFTs are scheduled, ask the patient to stop taking any bronchodilator medications for 6 to 12 hours before the tests. PFTs can be done before and after the administration of a bronchodilator to determine the degree of the response. This may help determine reversibility of airway obstruction, which is critical information for diagnosing asthma. A positive response to the bronchodilator is an increase of more than 200 mL and an increase of more than 12% between preadministration and postadministration values.

During an exacerbation of asthma, lung function parameters fall from their baseline levels. Some patients with symptoms of asthma have normal lung function. Therefore measures of airway responsiveness to known bronchial irritants (e.g., methacholine, histamine, exercise) may help establish a diagnosis of asthma.

An elevated serum eosinophil count and elevated serum IgE levels are highly suggestive of *atopy* (genetic predisposition to develop an allergic response), which may be a risk factor for asthma. Allergy skin testing may be of some value to determine sensitivity to specific allergens. However, a positive skin test does not necessarily mean that the allergen is causing the

TABLE 29-5 **COMPONENTS OF ASTHMA CONTROL**

Components of Control	Classification of Asthma Control: Well Controlled	Not Well Controlled	Very Poorly Controlled
Impairment			
Symptoms	≤2 days/wk	>2 days/wk	Throughout the day
Nighttime awakenings	≤2/mo	1-3/wk	≥4/wk
Interference with normal activity	None	Some limitation	Extremely limited
SABA use	≤2 days/wk	>2 days/wk	Several times/day
FEV_1 or peak flow	>80% predicted/personal best	60%-80% predicted/personal best	<60% predicted/personal best
Risk			
Exacerbations requiring oral corticosteroids	0-1/yr	≥2/yr	≥2/yr
	Consider severity and interval since last exacerbation. →		
Progressive loss of lung function	Evaluation requires long-term follow-up. →		
Treatment-related adverse effects	Can vary in intensity from none to very troublesome and worrisome. Level of intensity does not correlate to specific levels of control but should be considered in the overall assessment of risk. →		
Recommended Action for Treatment			
(Based on assessment of control)	• Maintain current step. • Regular follow-up every 1-6 mo to maintain control. • Consider step down if well controlled for at least 3 mo.	• Step up one step. • Reevaluate in 2-6 wk. • For side effects, consider alternative treatment options.	• Consider oral corticosteroids. • Step up one or two steps and reevaluate in 2 wk. • For side effects, consider alternative treatment options.

Source: Adapted from National Asthma Education and Prevention Program, National Heart, Lung, and Blood Institute: *Expert Panel Report 3: guidelines for the diagnosis and management of asthma*, NIH pub no 08-4051, Bethesda, Md, 2007, National Institutes of Health. Retrieved from *www.nhlbi.nih.gov/guidelines*.
FEV_1, Forced expiratory volume in 1 sec; *SABA*, short-acting β_2-adrenergic agonist.

asthma attack. On the other hand, a negative allergy test does not mean that the asthma is not allergy related. (Allergy testing is discussed in Chapter 14.)

A chest x-ray in an asymptomatic patient with asthma is usually normal, but needs to be obtained as a baseline on initial diagnosis. A chest x-ray obtained during an acute attack usually shows hyperinflation and may reveal other complications of asthma such as mucoid impaction, pneumothorax, or atelectasis.

If the patient has wheezing and acute distress, it is not feasible to obtain a detailed health history (although a family member may supply some pertinent information). During an acute attack of asthma, bedside spirometry (specifically FEV_1 or FVC, but usually PEFR) may be used to monitor obstruction. PFT results, serial spirometric parameters, oximetry, and measurement of ABGs provide information about the severity of the attack and the response to therapy. A complete blood cell count (CBC) and serum electrolytes are also obtained to help monitor the course of therapy.

A sputum specimen for culture and sensitivity may be obtained to rule out bacterial infection, especially if the patient has purulent sputum, a history of upper respiratory tract infection, a fever, or an elevated white blood cell (WBC) count. However, the vast majority of asthma exacerbations are viral, and sputum cultures are rarely done on an outpatient basis.

A hand-held, point-of-care device, called Niox Mino, measures airway inflammation related to asthma. It measures fractional exhaled nitric oxide (FENO). Nitric oxide levels are increased in the breath of people with asthma and decreased with oral and inhaled corticosteroid and leukotriene treatment. This allows the health care provider to rely on FENO measures versus a patient's symptoms and lung function. FENO may be used to assess a patient's' adherence to therapy or to determine if he or she needs more antiinflammatory medication. FENO is also a predictor of loss of asthma control and exacerbations.[8]

Collaborative Care

The National Asthma Education and Prevention Program (NAEPP) of the National Heart, Lung, and Blood Institute (NHLBI) convened expert panels to prepare guidelines for the diagnosis and management of asthma.[3] The first NAEPP report served as a basis for the development of reports prepared by asthma experts worldwide, and the Global Initiative for Asthma (GINA) was created. The goals of GINA are to decrease asthma morbidity and mortality rates and improve the management of asthma worldwide.[4] Although the reports of NAEPP and GINA are similar, GINA is updated every year. The NAEPP guidelines are presented in this chapter (e.g., Tables 29-2 and 29-5 and Fig. 29-4).

The goal of asthma treatment is to achieve and maintain control of the disease. Once the patient is diagnosed, the guidelines provide direction on classification of asthma severity (see Table 29-2) and which medications (based on steps 1 through 6) the patient requires (Table 29-5 and Fig. 29-4). The current guidelines focus on (1) assessing the severity of the disease at diagnosis and initial treatment and then (2) monitoring periodically to control the disease.

At the initial diagnosis a patient may have severe asthma and require step 4 or 5 of asthma medication. After treatment the patient's level of control is assessed (i.e., well controlled, not well controlled, or very poorly controlled) (see Table 29-5). The health care provider steps down the medication as the patient achieves control of the symptoms, or steps it up if the symptoms worsen. Achieving rapid control of the symptoms is the goal to return the patient to his or her daily functioning at the best possible level (see Fig. 29-4).

Validated questionnaires (e.g., Asthma Control Test [ACT], *www.qualitymetric.com/demos/TP_Launch.aspx?SID=52461*) can be used to assess quality-of-life issues in asthma patients. The level of control is determined by the patient's current peak

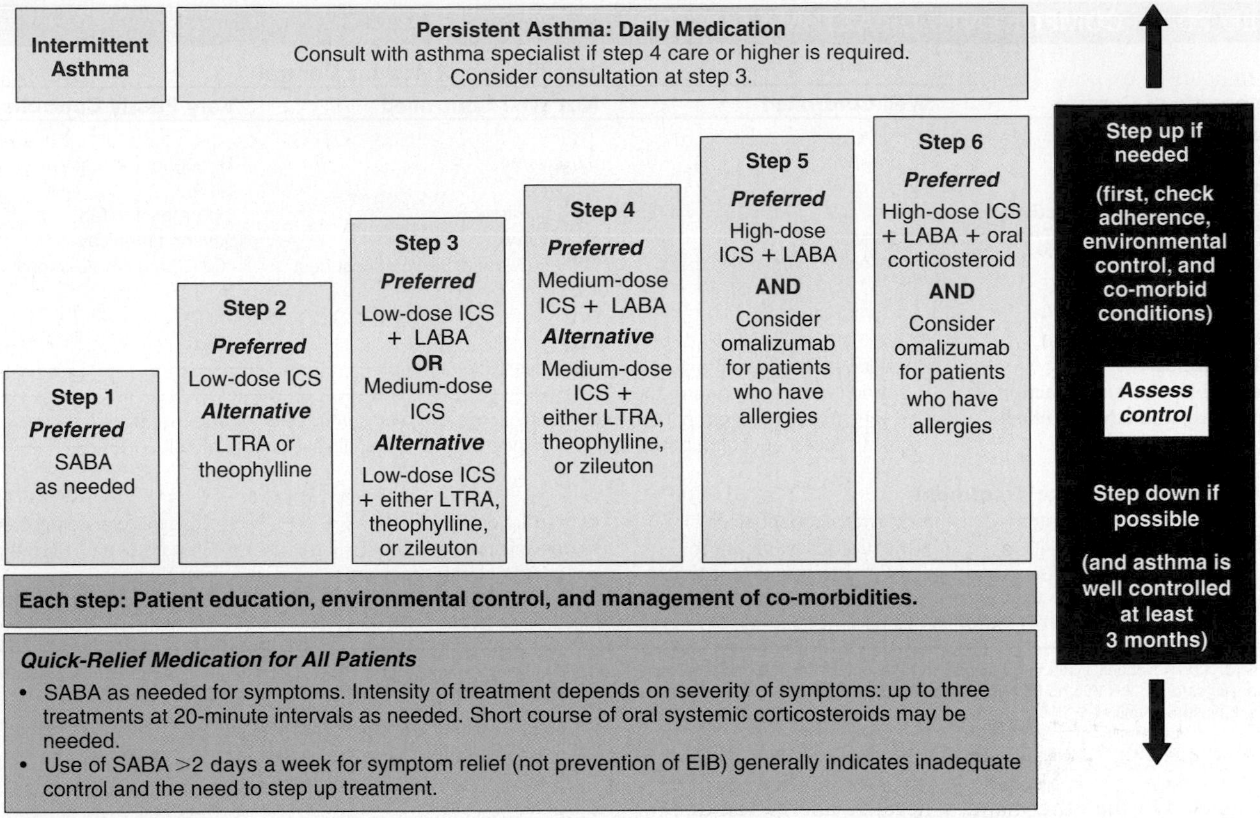

Key: *EIB,* Exercise-induced bronchospasm; *ICS,* inhaled corticosteroid; *LABA,* long-acting inhaled β_2-agonist; *LTRA,* leukotriene receptor antagonist; *SABA,* short-acting inhaled β_2-agonist.

FIG. 29-4 Drug therapy: stepwise approach for managing asthma. Modified from *Expert Panel Report 3: Guidelines for the Diagnosis and Management of Asthma.* Bethesda, Md, 2007, National Asthma Education and Prevention Program, National Heart, Lung, and Blood Institute.

TABLE 29-6 DRUG THERAPY

Long-Term Control Versus Quick Relief of Asthma

Long-Term Control Medications

Antiinflammatory Drugs

Corticosteroids
- Inhaled (e.g., fluticasone [Flovent Diskus or HFA])
- Oral (e.g., prednisone)

Leukotriene modifiers (e.g., montelukast [Singulair])

Anti-IgE (omalizumab [Xolair])

Bronchodilators

Long-acting inhaled β_2-adrenergic agonists (e.g., salmeterol [Serevent])

Long-acting oral β_2-adrenergic agonists (e.g., albuterol [VoSpire ER])

Methylxanthines (e.g., theophylline [Theo-24)

Quick-Relief Medications

Bronchodilators

Short-acting inhaled β_2-adrenergic agonists (e.g., albuterol [Proventil HFA])

Anticholinergics (inhaled) (e.g., ipratropium [Atrovent HFA])*

Antiinflammatory Drugs

Corticosteroids (systemic) (e.g., prednisone)†

*Used as alternative if patient has intolerable side effects to albuterol or in emergency department for moderate to severe exacerbations.

†Considered quick-relief drugs when used in a short burst (3-10 days) at the start of therapy or during a period of gradual deterioration. Corticosteroids are not used for immediate relief of an ongoing attack.

flow or FEV_1. In addition, any exacerbations or adverse effects of treatment will determine the level of control.

Intermittent and Persistent Asthma. The classification of severity of asthma at initial diagnosis helps determine which types of drugs are best suited to control the asthma symptoms (see Tables 29-2 and 29-5). Patients in all classifications of asthma require a short-term (rescue or reliever) medication. The most effective ones are the short-acting β_2-adrenergic agonists (SABAs) (e.g., albuterol [ProAir HFA, Proventil HFA, Ventolin HFA]). Patients with persistent asthma must also be on a long-term or controller medication (Table 29-6). Inhaled corticosteroids (ICSs) (e.g., fluticasone [Flovent Diskus or HFA]) are the most effective class of drugs to treat the inflammation. (See later section on drug therapy in this chapter.)

Acute Asthma Exacerbations. Asthma exacerbations may be mild to life threatening. With *mild exacerbations* the patient has difficulty breathing only with activity and may feel that he or she "can't get enough air." The peak flow is greater than 70% of the patient's personal best, and usually the symptoms are relieved at home promptly with an SABA such as albuterol delivered via a nebulizer or metered-dose inhaler (MDI) with a spacer. For any classification of asthma in a "rescue plan," patients are instructed to take 2 to 4 puffs of albuterol every 20 minutes three times to gain rapid control of symptoms. Occasionally a short course of oral corticosteroids is needed to decrease airway inflammation.

With a *moderate exacerbation,* dyspnea interferes with usual activities and peak flow is 40% to 60% of personal best. In this situation the patient usually comes to the ED or a health care provider's office to get help. Relief is provided with the SABA delivered as in the mild exacerbation, and oral corticosteroids are needed. Oral routes are usually as effective as IV routes, as well as being less invasive and less expensive. The patient's symptoms may persist for several days even after the corticosteroids are started. Oxygen can be used with both mild and moderate exacerbations to maintain SpO_2 at 90% or greater. The patient's symptoms and peak flow are monitored and lung auscultation is done to ensure the patient is moving air. A good response would be measured by the peak flow (or FEV_1) returning to 70% of personal best, normal airflow on physical examination, alleviation of patient's distress, and findings sustained more than 1 hour after the last treatment.[3]

Severe and Life-Threatening Asthma Exacerbations. Severe and life-threatening asthma exacerbations are discussed on p. 565. Management of the patient with severe and life-threatening asthma focuses on correcting hypoxemia and improving ventilation. The goal is to keep the O_2 saturation at 90% or greater. Continuous monitoring of the patient is critical. Obtaining a peak flow reading during a severe asthma attack is usually not possible. However, if it can be obtained and it is less than 200 L/min, it indicates severe obstruction in all but very small adults.

Many of the therapeutic measures are the same as those for acute asthma. Repetitive or continuous SABA administration is provided in the ED. Initially three treatments of SABA are given, 20 to 30 minutes apart. Then more SABA is given depending on the patient's airflow, improvement, and side effects from the SABA. The person with a severe asthma exacerbation usually has partial relief from the SABA plus ipratropium (Atrovent). However, the patient with life-threatening asthma has minimal if any relief from the same medications.

After the initial treatment, ipratropium is not given during the inpatient stay, since it has not been found to deliver any added benefit. Nebulized SABAs are continued for several days even after clinical improvement is noted.

In severe asthma, oral systemic corticosteroids are given to patients who do not respond to the initial SABA. In life-threatening asthma, IV corticosteroids are administered and are usually tapered rapidly. IV corticosteroids (e.g., methylprednisolone) are administered every 4 to 6 hours, although their peak effect is not apparent for 4 to 12 hours. Then the patient is started on oral corticosteroids. The length of oral prednisone treatment for both severe and life-threatening asthma is usually about 10 days after discharge. ICSs are usually added while the patient is still in the hospital. High-dose ICSs prevent asthma relapse and may be prescribed until the patient can step down to lower doses.

In severe and life-threatening asthma, adjunctive medications such as IV magnesium sulfate may be administered to adults with a very low FEV_1 or peak flow (less than 40% of predicted or personal best) or those who fail to respond to initial treatment. In addition, for hospitalized patients who do not respond to the usual therapy, heliox (a mixture of helium and oxygen) may be used to deliver the nebulized albuterol. Helium has a low density and may improve the bronchodilation effect of albuterol.

Supplemental O_2 is given by mask or nasal prongs to achieve a PaO_2 of at least 60 mm Hg or O_2 saturation greater than 90%. An arterial catheter may be inserted to facilitate frequent ABG monitoring. Because the patient's insensible loss of fluids and metabolic rate are increased, moderate rates of IV fluids are given to provide optimal hydration.

Sodium bicarbonate administration is usually limited to treatment of severe metabolic or respiratory acidosis (pH less than 7.29) in the mechanically ventilated patient because effective bronchodilation by β-adrenergic agonists is not possible if the patient has extreme acidosis. Bronchoscopy, although rarely performed during an acute attack, may be necessary to remove thick mucus plugs.

Occasionally, asthma exacerbations are life threatening and respiratory arrest is pending or actually occurring. The patient requires intubation and mechanical ventilation if there is no response to treatment. The patient is provided with 100% oxygen, hourly or continuously nebulized SABA, IV corticosteroids, and possibly other adjunctive therapies as noted previously.

Theophylline, mucolytics, and sedatives are no longer recommended for asthma exacerbations. Sedatives can result in depression of the respiratory drive and possible death. Antibiotics are not recommended for asthma treatment unless there are signs of pneumonia, fever, and purulent sputum, suggesting bacterial infections. Chest physiotherapy is generally not recommended for asthma because it is too stressful for the breathless patient.[3]

Epinephrine is not routinely indicated for treatment in asthma exacerbations. However, a subcutaneous or intramuscular (IM) injection of epinephrine may be indicated for acute treatment of anaphylaxis. If epinephrine is administered, patients need their BP and electrocardiogram (ECG) monitored closely.

Bronchial thermoplasty is a novel approach that may be used in addition to traditional therapy in those with severe asthma. Via a fiberoptic bronchoscope, a catheter directly applies heat and reduces the muscle mass in the bronchial wall. This benefits the patient by reversing the accumulation of excessive tissue that is part of the remodeling process that causes narrowing of the airway size and adds to bronchoconstriction.[9]

Drug Therapy

A stepwise approach to drug therapy is based initially on the asthma severity and then on the level of control. Persistent asthma requires daily long-term therapy in addition to appropriate medications to manage acute symptoms. Medications are divided into two general classifications: (1) *quick-relief* or *rescue medications* to treat symptoms and exacerbations, such as SABAs; and (2) *long-term control medications* to achieve and maintain control of persistent asthma, such as ICSs (see Table 29-6). Some of the controllers are used in combination to gain better asthma control (e.g., fluticasone and salmeterol [Advair]) (Table 29-7).

Antiinflammatory Drugs

Corticosteroids. Chronic inflammation is a primary component of asthma. Corticosteroids are antiinflammatory medications that reduce bronchial hyperresponsiveness, block the late-phase response, and inhibit migration of inflammatory cells. Corticosteroids are more effective in improving asthma control than any other long-term drug. ICSs are first-line therapy for patients with persistent asthma requiring step 2 through 6 therapies (see Fig. 29-4). Usually, ICSs must be administered for 1 to 2 weeks before maximum therapeutic effects can be seen. Some ICSs (e.g., fluticasone, budesonide [Pulmicort]) begin to have a therapeutic effect

TABLE 29-7 DRUG THERAPY

*Asthma and Chronic Obstructive Pulmonary Disease (COPD)**

Drug	Route of Administration	Comments†
Antiinflammatory Agents		
Corticosteroids		
hydrocortisone (Solu-Cortef) methylprednisolone (Medrol, Solu-Medrol) prednisone	IV Oral, IV Oral	Alternate-day therapy minimizes side effects. Oral dose should be taken in morning with food or milk. When given in high dosages, observe for epigastric distress. Long-term corticosteroid therapy requires supplementation with vitamin D and calcium to prevent osteoporosis. Discontinue gradually over time to prevent adrenal insufficiency. If symptoms recur during tapering, notify health care provider.
fluticasone (Flovent HFA, Flovent Diskus)	MDI, DPI	Not recommended for acute asthma attack. Rinse mouth with water or mouthwash after use to prevent oral fungal infections. Use of spacer device with MDI may decrease incidence of oral candidiasis. With ICSs, may not see effects until after at least 2 wk of regular treatment.
beclomethasone (Qvar)	MDI	Same as fluticasone except less oral candidiasis because of very small particle size, which is deposited deeper in the airways.
budesonide (Pulmicort Flexhaler)	DPI	Same as above.
mometasone (Asmanex Twisthaler)	DPI	Same as above.
ciclesonide (Alvesco)	MDI	Oral candidiasis and other localized oropharyngeal effects (e.g., hoarseness). Fewer side effects than other ICSs because of small particle size with minimal activation in oropharynx.
Phosphodiesterase Inhibitor Type 4 (PDE-4)		
roflumilast (Daliresp)	Oral	Only used in severe COPD to reduce exacerbation frequency. Not to be used for acute bronchospasm. GI symptoms occur within 6 mo of initiating medication. Patients to report any psychiatric symptoms (e.g., anxiety, depression, suicidal thoughts). Not to be used with theophylline.
Anticholinergics		
Short Acting		
ipratropium (Atrovent HFA)	Nebulizer, MDI	Approved for COPD. May provide additive benefit to SABA in moderate to severe asthma exacerbations (used in emergency department with no benefit beyond that). Use in asthma as alternative for patients with intolerable side effects with SABA. Temporary blurred vision if sprayed in eyes. Use cautiously in patients with narrow-angle glaucoma or prostatic enlargement.
aclidinium bromide (Tudorza, Pressair)	DPI	Only approved for COPD. Do not administer with other anticholinergics. Not for acute relief of bronchospasm.
Long Acting		
tiotropium (Spiriva HandiHaler)	DPI	Only approved for COPD. Blurred vision if powder comes in contact with eyes. Must discontinue use of ipratropium while on tiotropium. Patients with COPD must use SABA or short-acting anticholinergics for quick-relief medication. Maximum effect 1 wk after initiation of drug.
Anti-IgE		
omalizumab (Xolair)	Subcutaneous injection	Only for moderate to severe persistent allergic asthma with symptoms not adequately controlled by ICSs. Not for acute bronchospasm. Administer only under direct medical supervision and observe patient for a minimum of 2 hr after administration, since anaphylaxis has been reported with use.
Leukotriene Modifiers		
Leukotriene Receptor Blocker		
zafirlukast (Accolate)	Oral tablets	Take at least 1 hr before or 2 hr after meals. Affects metabolism of erythromycin and theophylline. Not used to treat acute asthma episodes.
montelukast (Singulair)	Oral tablets, chewable tablets, oral granules	Not used to treat acute asthma episodes.
Leukotriene Inhibitor		
zileuton (Zyflo, Zyflo CR)	Oral tablets	Monitor liver enzymes. May interfere with metabolism of warfarin (Coumadin) and theophylline. Not used to treat acute asthma episodes.
β_2-Adrenergic Agonists		
Inhaled: Short Acting (SABA)		
albuterol (Proventil HFA, Ventolin HFA, ProAir HFA, AccuNeb, VoSpire ER [oral only])	Nebulizer, MDI, oral tablets, including extended release NOTE: Oral tablets not for acute use, only long acting	Use with caution in patients with cardiac disorders, since β-agonists may cause ↑ BP and heart rate, CNS stimulation/excitation, and ↑ risk of dysrhythmias. Has rapid onset of action (1-3 min). Duration of action is 4-8 hr. Ventolin HFA is the only albuterol MDI with a counter.
levalbuterol (Xopenex, Xopenex HFA)	Nebulizer, MDI	Too frequent use can result in loss of effectiveness. Efficacy no better than other SABA.

*An enhanced version of this table listing side effects of drugs (eTable 29-1) is available on the website.

TABLE 29-7 **DRUG THERAPY—cont'd**

Asthma and Chronic Obstructive Pulmonary Disease (COPD)*

Drug	Route of Administration	Comments†
Inhaled: Long Acting (LABA)		*In asthma:* Never use as monotherapy. Use in combination with ICSs. *In COPD:* Can be used as monotherapy. Not used for rapid relief of dyspnea.
salmeterol (Serevent Diskus)	DPI	Not to exceed 2 puffs q12hr. Not used for acute exacerbations. Has a counter.
formoterol (Foradil Aerolizer, Perforomist)	DPI, nebulizer (Perforomist)	Can affect blood glucose levels. Use with caution in patients with diabetes.
arformoterol (Brovana)	Nebulizer	See formoterol. For chronic COPD use.
indacaterol (Arcapta Neohaler)	DPI	Only once-daily LABA. For chronic COPD use. Not intended to treat asthma.
Methylxanthines		
IV agent: aminophylline (second-line therapy) *Oral:* theophylline	Oral tablets, IV, elixir, sustained-release tablets	Wide variety of response to drug metabolism exists. Half-life is ↓ by smoking and ↑ by heart failure and liver disease. Cimetidine, ciprofloxacin, erythromycin, and other drugs may rapidly ↑ theophylline levels. Taking drug with food or antacids may help GI effects. Use usually limited to situations when other long-term bronchodilation not available or not affordable.
Combination Agents		Also see each component of medications for SE.
ipratropium/albuterol (Combivent Respimat, DuoNeb)	Nebulizer (DuoNeb), inhalation spray (Combivent Respimat)	Patients must be careful not to overuse. Respimat is an inhaler, but propellant free, unlike an MDI. Respimat is independent of inspiratory flow. Has dose indicator.
fluticasone/salmeterol (Advair Diskus or HFA)	DPI, MDI	See salmeterol and fluticasone. Has a counter. Comes in three different strengths.
budesonide/formoterol (Symbicort)	MDI	See budesonide and formoterol. Has a counter.
mometasone furoate/formoterol fumarate (Dulera)	MDI	
fluticasone/vilanterol (Breo Ellipta)	DPI	Vilanterol is an LABA.

†For patient instructions in English and Spanish for the devices, see *www.chestnet.org/accp/patient-guides/patient-instructions-inhaled-devices-english-and-spanish.*
DPI, Dry powder inhaler; *HFA,* hydrofluoroalkane (propellant); *ICSs,* inhaled corticosteroids; *MDI,* metered-dose inhaler.

in 24 hours. These drugs need to be administered on a fixed schedule.

When ICSs are administered, asthma can usually be controlled without significant systemic side effects, since little systemic drug absorption occurs from these devices. However, ICSs at the highest dosage levels have been associated with side effects (e.g., easy bruising, decreased bone mineral density).[4] Oropharyngeal candidiasis, hoarseness, and dry cough are local side effects caused by inhalation of corticosteroids. These problems can be reduced or prevented by using a spacer (Fig. 29-5) with the MDI and by gargling with water or mouthwash after each use. Using a spacer or holding device for inhalation of corticosteroids can be helpful in getting more medication into the lungs. However, drugs that are activated in the lungs (not the pharynx) (e.g., ciclesonide [Alvesco]) appear to minimize these side effects without the need for a spacer or mouth rinsing.[4]

To gain prompt control, short courses of orally administered corticosteroids are indicated for acute exacerbations of asthma. Maintenance doses of oral corticosteroids may be necessary to control asthma in a minority of patients with severe chronic asthma when long-term therapy is required. A single dose in the morning to coincide with endogenous cortisol production and alternate-day dosing are associated with fewer side effects. (Side effects of long-term corticosteroid therapy are discussed in Chapter 50.)

Women, especially postmenopausal women, who have asthma and who use corticosteroids should take adequate amounts of calcium and vitamin D and participate in regular weight-bearing exercise. (Osteoporosis is discussed in Chapter 64.)

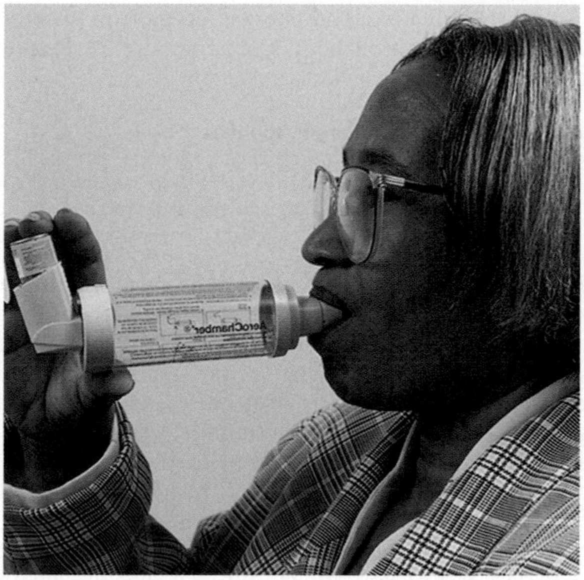

FIG. 29-5 Example of an AeroChamber spacer used with a metered-dose inhaler.

Leukotriene Modifiers. Leukotriene modifiers include leukotriene receptor blockers (antagonists) (zafirlukast [Accolate], montelukast [Singulair]) and leukotriene synthesis inhibitors (zileuton [Zyflo CR]). These drugs interfere with the synthesis or block the action of leukotrienes. Leukotrienes are inflammatory mediators produced from arachidonic acid metabolism (see Fig. 12-2). Leukotrienes are potent bronchoconstrictors, and some also cause airway edema and inflammation, thus contributing to the symptoms of asthma. Because these drugs block the release of some substances from mast cells and eosinophils, they have both bronchodilator and antiinflammatory effects.

These drugs are not indicated for use in the reversal of bronchospasm in acute asthma attacks. They are used for prophylactic and maintenance therapy. One advantage of leukotriene modifiers is that they are administered orally.

Anti-IgE. Omalizumab (Xolair) is a monoclonal antibody to IgE that decreases circulating free IgE levels. Omalizumab prevents IgE from attaching to mast cells, thus preventing the release of chemical mediators. This drug is indicated for patients with moderate to severe persistent, allergic asthma or those requiring step 5 or 6 care with persistent asthma that cannot be controlled with ICSs. Omalizumab is administered subcutaneously every 2 to 4 weeks. The drug has a risk of anaphylaxis, and patients must receive the medication in a health care provider's office where this potential emergency problem can be handled.

Bronchodilators. Three classes of bronchodilator drugs currently used in asthma therapy are β_2-adrenergic agonists (also referred to as β_2-agonists), methylxanthines and derivatives, and anticholinergics (see Table 29-7).

β_2-Adrenergic Agonist Drugs. These drugs may be short-acting β_2-adrenergic agonists (SABAs) or long-acting β_2-adrenergic agonists (LABAs). Because inhaled SABAs are the most effective drugs for relieving acute bronchospasm (as seen in acute exacerbations of asthma), they are known as rescue medications. Examples of these drugs include albuterol and pirbuterol (Maxair Autohaler). These drugs have an onset of action within minutes and are effective for 4 to 8 hours. These drugs act by stimulating β-adrenergic receptors in the bronchioles, thus producing bronchodilation. They also increase mucociliary clearance.

DRUG ALERT: β_2-Adrenergic Agonists
- Use with caution in patients with cardiac disorders, since both SABAs and LABAs may cause elevated BP and heart rate, central nervous system stimulation or excitation, and increased risk of dysrhythmias.
- Overuse of SABAs may cause rebound bronchospasms.

β_2-Adrenergic agonists are also useful in preventing bronchospasm precipitated by exercise and other stimuli because they prevent the release of inflammatory mediators from mast cells. They do not inhibit the late-phase response of asthma or have antiinflammatory effects. If used frequently, inhaled β_2-adrenergic agonists may produce tremors, anxiety, tachycardia, palpitations, and nausea. Too frequent use of β_2-adrenergic agonists indicates poor asthma control, may mask asthma severity, and may lead to reduced drug effectiveness. The goal in asthma therapy is that the patient with persistent asthma will never need to use SABAs for rescue, but that effective control is achieved with a long-term controller medication.

SABAs are not used for long-term control, and they should not be used alone for persistent asthma. They are used in any stage of asthma for quick relief and should be with the patient at all times for that purpose. Oral β_2-agonists are rarely used because of the cardiovascular side effects, skeletal muscle tremor, and anxiety. However, they may be used for long-term control, but they should not be used alone or as first-line therapy in treating asthma.

LABAs, including salmeterol (Serevent Diskus) and formoterol (Foradil), are effective for 12 hours. LABAs are added to a daily dose of ICSs for long-term control of moderate to severe persistent asthma (i.e., step 3 or higher for long-term control) and prevention of symptoms, particularly at night. When LABAs are added to a patient's daily regimen of corticosteroids, they decrease the need for SABAs and allow patients to achieve better asthma control with a lower dosage of ICSs.[3,4]

LABAs should never be used as monotherapy for asthma, and should only be used if the patient is on ICS. Tell patients that these drugs should not be used to treat acute symptoms or to obtain quick relief from bronchospasm. Teach the patient that these drugs are used only once every 12 hours.

DRUG ALERT: Long-Acting β_2-Adrenergic Agonists (LABAs)
- Should not be the first medicine used to treat asthma.
- Should never be used as the only medication to treat asthma but should be added to the treatment plan only if other controller medicines do not control asthma.
- Should not be used to treat wheezing that is getting worse.
- Always use a SABA to treat sudden wheezing.

Combination therapy using an ICS and LABA is available in several inhalers (e.g., Advair and budesonide/formoterol [Symbicort]). The combinations are more convenient, improve adherence, and ensure that patients receive the LABA together with an ICS.

Methylxanthines. Sustained-release methylxanthine (theophylline) preparations are not a first-line controller medication. They are used only as an alternative therapy for step 2 care in mild persistent asthma. Methylxanthine is a bronchodilator with mild antiinflammatory effects, but the exact mechanism of action is unknown.

DRUG ALERT: Theophylline
- Instruct patient to report signs of toxicity: nausea, vomiting, seizures, insomnia.
- Avoid caffeine to prevent intensifying adverse effects.

The main problems with theophylline are the relatively high incidence of interaction with other drugs and the side effects, which include nausea, headache, insomnia, gastrointestinal distress, tachycardia, dysrhythmias, and seizures. Because theophylline has a narrow margin of safety, monitor serum blood levels regularly to determine if the drug is within therapeutic range.

Anticholinergic Drugs. Anticholinergic agents (e.g., ipratropium) block the bronchoconstricting effect of the parasympathetic nervous system. These drugs are less effective than β_2-adrenergic agonists. Anticholinergic drugs are used for quick relief in those patients unable to tolerate SABAs. In addition, they are used for the patient in severe asthma exacerbation in emergency situations, often nebulized with an SABA. Other than these indications, they have no role in the treatment of asthma.

The onset of action of ipratropium is slower than that of β_2-adrenergic agonists, peaking at 30 minutes to 1 hour and lasting up to 4 to 6 hours. Systemic side effects of inhaled anticholinergics are uncommon because they are poorly absorbed. The most common side effect is a dry mouth.

Inhalation Devices for Drug Delivery. The multiple devices for asthma drug administration can be confusing. The majority of asthma drugs are administered only or preferably by inhalation because systemic side effects are reduced and the onset of action is faster. Inhalation devices include metered-dose inhalers (MDIs), dry powder inhalers (DPIs), and nebulizers.

Inhalers. MDIs are small, hand-held, pressurized devices that deliver a measured dose of drug with each activation.

Dosing is usually accomplished with one or two puffs. Depending on the specific MDI, a spacer or holding chamber (e.g. AeroChamber or InspirEase [see Fig. 29-5]) is used to reduce the amount of drug delivered to the oropharynx and improve the amount of drug delivered to the lungs. In addition, spacers assist people who have hand-breath coordination problems.[10]

All MDIs are mandated by international law to have an ozone-friendly propellant, which is a hydrofluoroalkane (HFA). This propellant is nontoxic, evaporates almost instantly once it forces medicine out of the MDI canister, and is not harmful to the patient. The number of times an MDI needs to be primed and the frequency of priming vary widely, so read the package insert with the patient.[10]

The MDI should be cleaned by removing the dust cap and rinsing the holder (not the medication chamber) in warm water at least two times per week (Fig. 29-6). The patient who needs to use several MDIs is often unclear about the order in which to take the medications. Historically it had been recommended that SABAs should be used first to open up the airway and improve the delivery of subsequent medications. However, this technique is not evidence based. It is a potential source of confusion to patients because the SABAs are usually used on an as-needed (PRN) basis.

One of the major problems with metered-dose drugs is the potential for overuse (more than two canisters per month) rather than seeking needed medical care (Table 29-8). As a patient develops additional asthmatic symptoms, he or she may use the β_2-adrenergic agonist MDI repeatedly. β_2-Adrenergic agonists help by relieving bronchospasm. They do not treat the inflammatory response. Therefore teach the patient the correct therapeutic use of these drugs. The patient also needs to know the correct way to determine whether the MDI is empty (see

Using an inhaler seems simple, but most patients do not use it the right way. When you use your inhaler the wrong way, less medicine gets to your lungs. (Your physician may give you other types of inhalers.)

For the next 2 weeks, read these steps aloud as you do them or ask someone to read them to you. Ask your physician or nurse to check how well you are using your inhaler.

Use your inhaler in one of the three ways pictured below (**A** or **B** is best, but **C** can be used if you have trouble with **A** or **B**).

Steps for Using Your Inhaler

Getting ready
1. Take off the cap and shake the inhaler.
2. Breathe out all the way.
3. Hold your inhaler the way your doctor said (**A, B,** or **C** below).

Breathe in slowly
4. As you start breathing in **slowly** through your mouth, press down on the inhaler **one** time. (If you use a holding chamber, first press down on the inhaler. Within 5 seconds, begin to breathe in slowly.)
5. Keep breathing in **slowly,** as deeply as you can.

Hold your breath
6. Hold your breath as you count to 10 slowly, if you can.
7. For inhaled quick-relief medicine (β_2-agonists), wait about 1 minute between puffs. There is no need to wait between puffs for other medicines.

A. Hold inhaler 1 to 2 inches in front of your mouth (about the width of two fingers).

B. Use a spacer/holding chamber. These come in many shapes and can be useful to any patient.

C. Put the inhaler in your mouth.

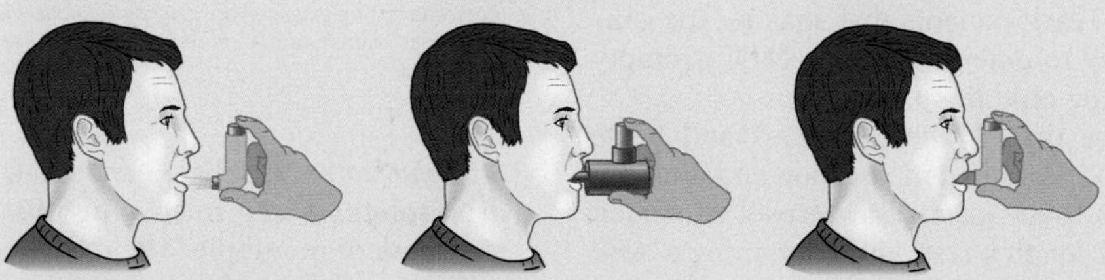

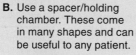

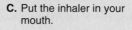

Clean Your Inhaler as Needed

Look at the hole where the medicine sprays out from your inhaler. If you see "powder" in or around the hole, clean the inhaler. Remove the metal canister from the L-shaped plastic mouthpiece. Rinse only the mouthpiece and cap in warm water. Let them dry over night. In the morning, put the canister back inside. Put the cap on.

Know When to Replace Your Inhaler

For medicines you take each day (an example): Say your new canister has 200 puffs (number of puffs is listed on canister) and you are told to take 8 puffs per day.

$$\text{8 puffs per day}\,\overline{\smash{)}\,\text{200 puffs in canister}}\quad = \text{25 days}$$

So this canister will last 25 days. If you started using this inhaler on May 1, replace it on or before May 25.

You can write the date on your canister.

For **quick-relief medicine take as needed** and count each puff.

Do not put your canister in water to see if it is empty as water may enter MDI and impair inhaler.

FIG. 29-6 How to use your metered-dose inhaler correctly.

TABLE 29-8 PROBLEMS USING A METERED-DOSE INHALER (MDI)

- Failing to coordinate activation with inspiration
- Activating MDI in the mouth while breathing through nose
- Inspiring too rapidly
- Not holding the breath for 10 sec (or as close to 10 sec as possible)
- Holding MDI upside down or sideways
- Inhaling more than 1 puff with each inspiration
- Not shaking MDI before use
- Not waiting a sufficient amount of time between each puff
- Not opening mouth wide enough, causing medication to bounce off teeth, tongue, or palate
- Not having adequate strength to activate MDI
- Being unable to understand and follow directions

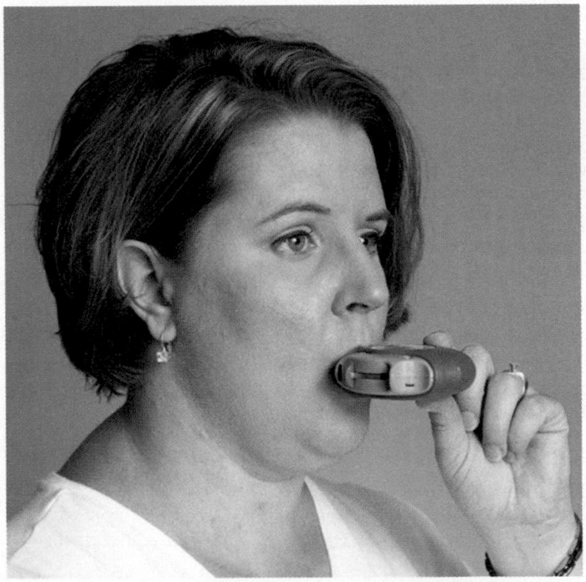

FIG. 29-7 Example of a dry powder inhaler (DPI).

Fig. 29-6). In the past, floating the MDI in water was an appropriate way to determine if medication remained in the MDI. Now this is not recommended because it is not accurate and water can enter the MDI. Teach patients that shaking the canister is not an accurate way to determine if the MDI is empty because they may be hearing only the propellant.

DPIs are simpler to use than MDIs (Fig. 29-7 and Table 29-9). The DPI contains dry, powdered medication and is breath activated. No propellant is used. Instead an aerosol is created when the patient inhales through a reservoir containing a dose of powder. The convenient-to-carry diskus has several advantages over MDIs: (1) less manual dexterity is needed, (2) there is no need to coordinate device puffs with inhalation, (3) an easily visible color or number system indicates the number of doses left in the diskus, and (4) no spacer is required. Disadvantages are that commonly prescribed drugs are not yet available in DPIs and the medication may clump if exposed to humidity. Since the medicine is delivered only by the patient's inspiratory effort, patients with a low FEV_1 (less than 1 L) may not be able to inspire the medication adequately.

Differences between MDIs and DPIs are presented in Table 29-10. Aerosolized medication delivery systems, when used with comparable drug doses, provide equivalent efficacy. Therefore patients should use the device best suited to their needs.

TABLE 29-9 PATIENT TEACHING GUIDE

How to Use a Dry Powder Inhaler (DPI)

Include the following instructions when teaching a patient to use a DPI.

1. Remove mouthpiece cap or open the device according to manufacturer's instructions. Check for dust or dirt. If there is an external counter, note the number of doses remaining.
2. Load the medicine into the inhaler or engage the lever to allow the medicine to become available. Some DPIs should be held upright while loading. Others should be held sideways or in a horizontal position.
3. Do not shake your medicine.
4. Tilt your head back slightly and breathe out, getting as much air out of your lungs as you can. Do not breathe into your inhaler because this could affect the dose.
5. Close your lips tightly around the mouthpiece of the inhaler.
6. Breathe in deeply and quickly. This will ensure that the medicine moves down deeply into your lungs. You may not taste or sense the medicine going into your lungs.
7. Hold your breath for 10 seconds or as long as you can to disperse the medicine into your lungs.
8. If there is an external counter, note the number of doses remaining. It should be one less than the number in step 1 above.
9. Do not keep your DPI in a humid place such as a shower room because the medicine may clump.

TABLE 29-10 COMPARISON OF METERED-DOSE AND DRY POWDER INHALERS

	Metered-Dose Inhaler (MDI)	Dry Powder Inhaler (DPI)
Shake before use	Yes, shake well*	No
Inspiration	Slow	Rapid
Spacer	Yes, at least with inhaled corticosteroids*	None permitted
Counting device	Few have external device	Most preloaded forms include counter
Inhalations/dose	Often 2/dose	Often 1/dose
Cleaning	Use water for plastic case	Avoid moisture

Source: National Jewish Health: Inhaled medication instructional videos: asthma and general lung diseases. Retrieved from *www.nationaljewish.org/healthinfo/medications/lung-diseases/devices/instructional-videos*.

*MDIs use hydrofluoroalkane (HFA) as a propellant, and shaking or a spacer may not be needed.

Nebulizers. Nebulizers are small machines used to convert drug solutions into mists. The mist can be inhaled through a face mask or mouthpiece held between the teeth. Nebulizers are usually used for individuals who have severe asthma or difficulty with the MDI inhalation.

Nebulizers are usually powered by a compressed air or O_2 generator. At home the patient may have an air-powered compressor. In the hospital, wall O_2 or compressed air is used to power the nebulizer.

Aerosolized medication orders must include the medication, dose, diluent, and whether it is to be nebulized with O_2 or compressed air. The advantage of nebulization therapy is that it is easy to use. Medications that are routinely nebulized include albuterol and ipratropium.

The patient is placed in an upright position that allows for most efficient breathing to ensure adequate penetration and deposition of the aerosolized medication. The patient must

INFORMATICS IN PRACTICE

Home Monitoring of Asthma

- To reduce the rate of readmission to hospital, the patient with asthma may be discharged with a home monitoring system. These systems provide an easy and inexpensive approach to remotely monitoring patients' lung functions.
- Asthma home monitoring usually consists of peak flow rate, pulse oximetry, vital signs, and lung sounds. This information is sent to the health care provider so that problems are quickly detected.
- As part of your discharge planning, assist the patient with receiving a system and reviewing its proper use.

breathe slowly and deeply through the mouth and hold inspirations for 2 or 3 seconds. Deep diaphragmatic breathing helps ensure deposition of the medication. Instruct the patient to breathe normally in between these large forced breaths to prevent alveolar hypoventilation and dizziness. After the treatment instruct the patient to cough effectively.

A disadvantage of nebulizer equipment use is the potential for bacterial growth. Review cleaning procedures for home respiratory equipment with the patient. A frequently used, effective home-cleaning method is to wash the nebulizer daily in soap and water, rinse it with water, and soak it for 20 to 30 minutes in a 1:1 white vinegar–water solution, followed by a water rinse and air drying. Commercial respiratory cleaning agents may also be used if directions are followed carefully. Cleaning the nebulizer in the top shelf of an automatic dishwasher saves time, and the hot water destroys most organisms.

Patient Teaching Related to Drug Therapy. Information about medications should include the name, purpose, dosage, method of administration, and schedule, taking into consideration activities of daily living (ADLs) that require energy expenditure and thus oxygen (e.g., bathing). Teaching should also include side effects, appropriate action if side effects occur, how to properly use and clean devices, how to prime and the frequency, and consequences of not taking medications as prescribed. One of the major factors determining success in asthma management is the correct administration of drugs.

Several factors can affect the correct use of these devices. These include advanced age, alterations in physical dexterity (e.g., arthritis in hands, coordination), psychologic state (e.g., cognition), affordability, convenience, and administration time and preference.[10]

Poor adherence with asthma therapy is a major challenge in the long-term management of chronic asthma. Lack of adherence often occurs in chronic asthma because the patient is symptom free and does not use the long-term therapy (e.g., ICS) regularly because no immediate benefit is felt. The patient does not realize that ICSs are needed to treat the ongoing inflammatory process.

Explain to the patient the importance and purpose of taking the long-term therapy regularly, emphasizing that maximum improvement may take longer than 1 week. Tell the patient that, without regular use, the swelling in the airways may progress and the asthma will likely worsen over time. Become familiar with the vast array of compassionate use programs offered by pharmaceutical companies to help lower-income patients obtain medications (e.g., *www.needymeds.com*).

In addition to the typical MDI and DPI devices, a variety of other devices are used to deliver inhalant pulmonary medications. Be certain that patients understand exactly how to use the device, and give them printed instructions. (For instructions, see *www.nationaljewish.org/healthinfo/medications/lung-diseases/devices.*) Most inhalant drugs have clear patient instructions, but you need to either use a placebo device or the actual drug to assess the patient's ability to deliver the medication. At every clinic visit or hospitalization reassess the patient's inhaler technique.

New drug delivery devices are becoming available at a rapid pace, and you must keep informed of the correct operation of these. If package inserts are available, you can review them before teaching the patient. The drug company websites have numerous excellent teaching videos available.

Nonprescription Combination Drugs. Several nonprescription combination drugs are available OTC. They are usually combinations of a bronchodilator (ephedrine) and an expectorant (guaifenesin). Inhalers containing epinephrine are also available.[11] These agents are advertised as medications to relieve bronchospasm. Often patients seek OTC drugs because they are less expensive than prescription medication. Many people consider these drugs safe because they can be obtained without a prescription. In general, they should be avoided.

Drugs containing ephedrine and epinephrine are dangerous because they stimulate the central nervous and cardiovascular systems, causing nervousness, heart palpitations and dysrhythmias, tremors, insomnia, and increases in BP. Many respiratory products containing ephedrine are located behind the counter at pharmacies or require a prescription. This limited access is to prevent the diversion of ephedrine to the production of methamphetamine. Also many of the OTC products have been reformulated with phenylephrine, instead of ephedrine, which works well topically but has modest effects in the oral form.

An important teaching responsibility is to warn patients about the dangers associated with nonprescription combination drugs. These drugs are especially dangerous to a patient with underlying cardiac problems because elevated BP and tachycardia often occur. Caution the patient who persists in taking these medications to read and follow the directions on the label.

NURSING MANAGEMENT ASTHMA

NURSING ASSESSMENT

If a patient can speak and is not in acute distress, take a detailed health history, including identification of any precipitating factors and what has helped alleviate attacks in the past. The patient may be using herbs and supplements to treat asthma.[12] When doing the health history, ask about specific herbs or supplements that a patient may be using.

Subjective and objective data that should be obtained from a patient with asthma are presented in Table 29-11. You may also assess the patient's asthma control using one of the validated self-administered questionnaires (e.g., ACT at *www.qualitymetric.com/demos/TP_Launch.aspx?SID=52461*).

NURSING DIAGNOSES

Nursing diagnoses for the patient with asthma may include, but are not limited to, those presented in Nursing Care Plan 29-1.

PLANNING

The overall goals are that the patient with asthma will have asthma control as evidenced by (1) minimal symptoms during the day and night, (2) acceptable activity levels (including

NURSING CARE PLAN 29-1

Patient With Asthma

NURSING DIAGNOSIS* **Ineffective airway clearance** *related to* bronchospasm, excessive mucus production, tenacious secretions, and fatigue *as evidenced by* ineffective cough, inability to raise secretions, and/or adventitious breath sounds

PATIENT GOALS
1. Maintains clear airway with removal of excessive secretions
2. Experiences normal breath sounds and respiratory rate

Outcomes (NOC)	Interventions (NIC) and *Rationales*
Respiratory Status: Airway Patency • Respiratory rate ____ • Respiratory rhythm ____ • Ability to clear secretions ____ **Measurement Scale** 1 = Severe deviation from normal range 2 = Substantial deviation from normal range 3 = Moderate deviation from normal range 4 = Mild deviation from normal range 5 = No deviation from normal range	***Asthma Management*** • Determine baseline respiratory status *to use as a comparison point.* • Monitor rate, rhythm, depth, and effort of respiration *to determine need for intervention and evaluate effectiveness of interventions.* • Observe chest movement, including symmetry, use of accessory muscles, and supraclavicular and intercostal muscle retractions, *to evaluate respiratory status.* • Auscultate breath sounds, noting areas of decreased or absent ventilation and adventitious sounds, *to evaluate respiratory status.* • Administer medication as appropriate and/or per policy and procedural guidelines *to improve respiratory function.* • Coach in breathing and relaxation techniques *to improve respiratory rhythm and rate.* • Offer warm fluids to drink *to liquefy secretions and promote bronchodilation.*

NURSING DIAGNOSIS **Anxiety** *related to* difficulty breathing, perceived or actual loss of control, and fear of suffocation *as evidenced by* restlessness and elevated pulse, respiratory rate, and blood pressure

PATIENT GOALS
1. Reports decreased anxiety with increased control of respirations
2. Experiences vital signs within normal limits

Outcomes (NOC)	Interventions (NIC) and *Rationales*
Anxiety Level • Restlessness ____ • Increased blood pressure ____ • Increased pulse rate ____ • Increased respiratory rate ____ • Verbalized anxiety ____ • Facial tension ____ **Measurement Scale** 1 = Severe 2 = Substantial 3 = Moderate 4 = Mild 5 = None	***Anxiety Reduction*** • Identify when level of anxiety changes *to determine possible precipitating factors.* • Use calm, reassuring approach *to provide reassurance.* • Stay with patient *to promote safety and reduce fear.* • Encourage verbalization of feelings, perceptions, and fears *to identify problem areas so appropriate planning can take place.* • Provide factual information concerning diagnosis, treatment, and prognosis *to help patient know what to expect.* • Instruct patient in the use of relaxation techniques *to relieve tension and to promote ease of respirations.*

NURSING DIAGNOSIS **Deficient knowledge** *related to* lack of information and education about asthma and its treatment *as evidenced by* frequent questioning regarding all aspects of long-term management

PATIENT GOALS
1. Describes the disease process and treatment regimen
2. Demonstrates correct administration of aerosol medications
3. Expresses confidence in ability for long-term management of asthma

Outcomes (NOC)	Interventions (NIC) and *Rationales*
Asthma Self-Management • Describes causal factors ____ • Initiates action to avoid and manage personal triggers ____ • Seeks early treatment of infections ____ • Monitors peak flow routinely ____ • Monitors peak flow when symptoms occur ____ • Makes appropriate medication choices ____ • Demonstrates appropriate use of inhalers, spacers, and nebulizers ____ • Self-manages exacerbations ____ • Reports uncontrolled symptoms to health care provider ____ **Measurement Scale** 1 = Never demonstrated 2 = Rarely demonstrated 3 = Sometimes demonstrated 4 = Often demonstrated 5 = Consistently demonstrated	***Asthma Management*** • Determine patient and family understanding of disease and management *to assess learning needs.* • Teach patient to identify and avoid triggers if possible *to prevent asthma attacks.* • Encourage verbalization of feelings about diagnosis, treatment, and impact on lifestyle *to offer support and increase adherence with treatment.* • Teach patient about the use of the peak expiratory flow rate (PEFR) meter at home *to promote self-management of symptoms.* • Instruct patient and family on antiinflammatory and bronchodilator medications and their appropriate use *to promote understanding of effects.* • Teach proper techniques for using medication and equipment (e.g., inhaler, nebulizer, peak flow meter) *to promote self-care.* • Assist in the recognition of signs and symptoms of impending asthmatic reaction and implementation of appropriate response measures *to prevent escalation of attacks.* • Establish a written plan with the patient for managing exacerbations *to plan adequate treatment of future exacerbations.*

*Nursing diagnoses listed in order of priority.

TABLE 29-11 NURSING ASSESSMENT

Asthma

Subjective Data

Important Health Information

Past health history: Allergic rhinitis, sinusitis, or skin allergies; previous asthma attack and hospitalization or intubation; symptoms worsened by triggers in the environment; gastroesophageal reflux disease (GERD); occupational exposure to chemical irritants (e.g., paints, dust)

Medications: Adherence to medication, inhaler technique; use of antibiotics; pattern and amount of short-acting β_2-adrenergic agonist used per week; medications that may precipitate an attack in susceptible asthmatics such as aspirin, nonsteroidal antiinflammatory drugs, β-adrenergic blockers

Functional Health Patterns

Health perception–health management: Family history of allergies or asthma; recent upper respiratory tract or sinus infection

Activity-exercise: Fatigue, decreased or absent exercise tolerance; dyspnea, cough (especially at night), productive cough with yellow or green sputum or sticky sputum; chest tightness, feelings of suffocation, air hunger, talking in short sentences or words or phrases, sitting upright to breathe

Sleep-rest: Awakened from sleep because of cough or breathing difficulties, insomnia

Coping–stress tolerance: Emotional distress, stress in work environment or home

Objective Data

General

Restlessness or exhaustion, confusion, upright or forward-leaning body position

Integumentary

Diaphoresis, cyanosis (circumoral, nail bed), eczema

Respiratory

Nasal discharge, nasal polyps, mucosal swelling; wheezing, crackles, diminished or absent breath sounds, and rhonchi on auscultation; hyperresonance on percussion; sputum (thick, white, tenacious), ↑ work of breathing with use of accessory muscles; intercostal and supraclavicular retractions; tachypnea with hyperventilation; prolonged expiration

Cardiovascular

Tachycardia, pulsus paradoxus, jugular venous distention, hypertension or hypotension, premature ventricular contractions

Possible Diagnostic Findings

Abnormal ABGs during attacks, ↓ O_2 saturation, serum and sputum eosinophilia, ↑ serum IgE, positive skin tests for allergens, chest x-ray demonstrating hyperinflation with attacks, abnormal pulmonary function tests showing ↓ flow rates; FVC, FEV_1, PEFR, and FEV_1/FVC ratio that improve between attacks and with bronchodilators

ABGs, Arterial blood gases; *FEV_1,* forced expiratory volume in 1 sec; *FVC,* forced vital capacity; *IgE,* immunoglobulin E; *PEFR,* peak expiratory flow rate.

exercise and other physical activity), (3) maintenance of greater than 80% of personal best PEFR or FEV_1, (4) few or no adverse effects of therapy, (5) no recurrent exacerbations of asthma, and (6) adequate knowledge to participate in and carry out management.

NURSING IMPLEMENTATION

HEALTH PROMOTION. Your role in preventing asthma attacks or decreasing their severity focuses primarily on teaching the patient and caregiver. Teach the patient to identify and avoid known personal triggers for asthma (e.g., cigarette smoke, pet dander) and irritants (e.g., cold air, aspirin, foods, cats, indoor air pollution) (see Table 29-1). Although special dust covers on mattresses and pillows may reduce exposure to dust mites and improve symptoms, the evidence does not support making this a definitive recommendation.[13] Washing bedclothes in hot water or cooler water with detergent and bleach has some effect on allergen levels. Avoidance of furred animals is suggested, but the allergen of pets is nearly impossible to avoid. Pet allergen can be found in many public areas for months even after removal of the animal. Many people are allergic to cockroach remains and the dried droppings, so measures to avoid or control cockroaches are partly effective in removing allergens.

If cold air cannot be avoided, dressing properly with scarves or using a mask helps reduce the risk of an asthma attack. Aspirin and NSAIDs should be avoided if they are known to precipitate an attack. Many OTC drugs contain aspirin. Therefore teach the patient to read the labels carefully. Nonselective β-blockers (e.g., propranolol [Inderal]) are contraindicated because they inhibit bronchodilation. Selective β-blockers (e.g., atenolol [Tenormin]) should be used with caution. Desensitization (immunotherapy) may be partially effective in decreasing the patient's sensitivity to known allergens (see Chapter 14).

Prompt diagnosis and treatment of upper respiratory tract infections and sinusitis may prevent an exacerbation of asthma. If occupational irritants are involved as etiologic factors, the patient may need to consider changing jobs. Individuals who are obese often find that weight loss improves control of asthma. Encourage the patient to maintain a fluid intake of 2 to 3 L/day, good nutrition, and adequate rest. If exercise is planned or if the patient has asthma only with exercise, the health care provider can suggest a medication regimen for pretreatment or long-term control of symptoms to prevent bronchospasm.

ACUTE INTERVENTION. A goal in asthma care is to maximize the patient's ability to safely manage acute asthma exacerbations using an asthma action plan developed in conjunction with the health care provider (Table 29-12). Action plans are particularly important for individuals with moderate to severe persistent asthma or severe exacerbations. The action plan dictates what symptoms or peak flow reading necessitates a change in asthma care to gain control.

The patient can take 2 to 4 puffs of an SABA every 20 minutes three times as a rescue plan. Depending on the response with alleviation of symptoms or improved peak flow, continued SABA use and/or oral corticosteroids may be a part of the home management plan at this point. If symptoms persist or if the patient's peak flow is less than 50% of the personal best, the health care provider or emergency medical services (EMS) needs to be immediately contacted.

When the patient is in the health care facility with an acute exacerbation, it is important to monitor the patient's respiratory and cardiovascular systems. This includes auscultating lung sounds; taking the heart and respiratory rates and BP; and monitoring ABGs, pulse oximetry, and peak flow.

Louder wheezing may actually occur in airways that are responding to the therapy as airflow increases. As improvement continues and airflow increases, breath sounds increase and wheezing decreases. Remember that, despite the disappearance of most of the bronchospasms, the edema and cellular infiltration of the airway mucosa and the viscous mucous plugs may take several days to improve. Thus intensive therapy must be continued even after clinical improvement.

An important nursing goal during an acute attack is to decrease the patient's sense of panic. A calm, quiet, reassuring attitude may help the patient relax. Position the patient comfortably (usually sitting) to maximize chest expansion. Stay with the patient and be available to provide additional comfort. A technique called "talking down" can help the patient remain calm. In talking down, you gain eye contact with the patient. In a firm, calm voice coach the patient to use pursed-lip breathing, which keeps the airways open by maintaining positive pressure (Table 29-13), and abdominal breathing, which slows the respiratory rate and encourages deeper breaths (see Table 7-5). You or the caregiver should stay with the patient until the respiratory rate (with the assistance of the medications) has slowed.

When the acute attack subsides, provide rest and a quiet, calm environment for the patient. When the patient has recovered from exhaustion, try to obtain the health history and pattern of asthma along with a physical assessment. If the caregiver and other family members are present, they may be able to provide information about the patient's health history (see Table 29-11). This information, which is important in planning an individualized nursing care plan, helps the patient with the goal of control.

AMBULATORY AND HOME CARE. Control of symptoms can also be achieved by teaching the patient about medications. The drug regimen itself can be confusing and complex. Teach patients the importance of monitoring their response to medication. It is easy to undermedicate or overmedicate unless careful monitoring is ongoing. Some patients may benefit from keeping a diary to record medication use, wheezing or coughing, peak flow, the drug's side effects, and activity level. This information will help the health care provider adjust the medication.

TABLE 29-12 ASTHMA ACTION PLAN*

General Information

- Name _____
- Emergency contact _____ Phone numbers _____
- Physician/health care provider _____ Phone numbers _____
- Physician signature _____ Date _____

Severity Classification	Triggers			Exercise
❍ Intermittent	❍ Colds	❍ Smoke	❍ Weather	1. Premedication (how much and when) _____
❍ Mild persistent	❍ Exercise	❍ Dust	❍ Air pollution	_____
❍ Moderate persistent	❍ Animals	❍ Food		2. Exercise modifications _____
❍ Severe persistent	❍ Other _____			_____

Green Zone: Doing Well
Symptoms
- Breathing is good
- No cough or wheeze
- Can work and play
- Sleeps all night

Peak Flow Meter
More than 80% of personal best or _____

Peak Flow Meter Personal Best =
Control Medications:

Medicine	How Much to Take	When to Take It
_____	_____	_____
_____	_____	_____
_____	_____	_____

Yellow Zone: Getting Worse
Symptoms
- Some problems breathing
- Cough, wheeze, or chest tight
- Problems working or playing
- Wake at night

Peak Flow Meter
Between 50% and 80% of personal best or _____ and _____

Contact Physician If Using Quick Relief More Than 2 Times per Week
Continue Control Medicines and Add:

Medicine	How Much to Take	When to Take It
_____	_____	_____
_____	_____	_____
_____	_____	_____

IF your symptoms (and peak flow, if used) return to Green Zone after 1 hour of the quick-relief treatment, THEN
- ❍ Take quick-relief medication every 4 hours for 1 to 2 days
- ❍ Change your long-term control medicines by _____
- ❍ Contact your physician for follow-up care

IF your symptoms (and peak flow, if used) DO NOT return to the Green Zone after 1 hour of the quick-relief treatment, THEN
- ❍ Take quick-relief treatment again
- ❍ Change your long-term control medicines by _____
- ❍ Call your physician/health care provider within _____ hours of modifying your medication routine

Red Zone: Medical Alert
Symptoms
- Lots of problems breathing
- Cannot work or play
- Getting worse instead of better
- Medicine is not helping

Peak Flow Meter
Between 0% and 50% of personal best or _____ and _____

Ambulance/Emergency Phone Number:
Continue Control Medicines and Add:

Medicine	How Much to Take	When to Take It
_____	_____	_____
_____	_____	_____
_____	_____	_____

Go to the hospital or call for an ambulance if
- ❍ Still in the red zone after 15 minutes
- ❍ You have not been able to reach your physician/health care provider for help

Call an ambulance immediately if the following danger signs are present
- ❍ Trouble walking/talking due to shortness of breath
- ❍ Lips or fingernails are blue

Source: American Lung Association. Retrieved from *www.lungusa.org*.
*Available in Spanish (eTable 29-2) on the website for this chapter.

TABLE 29-13 PATIENT TEACHING GUIDE

Pursed-Lip Breathing (PLB)

Teach the patient how to do PLB using the following guidelines.

1. Use PLB before, during, and after any activity causing you to be short of breath.
2. Inhale slowly and deeply through the nose.
3. Exhale slowly through pursed lips, almost as if whistling.
4. Relax your facial muscles without puffing your cheeks—like whistling—while you are exhaling.
5. Make breathing out (exhalation) three times as long as breathing in (inhalation).
6. The following activities can help you get the "feel" of PLB:
   - Blow through a straw in a glass of water with the intent of forming small bubbles.
   - Blow a lit candle enough to bend the flame without blowing it out.
   - Steadily blow a table-tennis ball across a table.
   - Blow a tissue held in the hand until it gently flaps.
7. Practice 8-10 repetitions of PLB three or four times a day.

Good nutrition is important. Physical exercise (e.g., swimming, walking, stationary cycling) within the patient's limit of tolerance is also beneficial and may require pretreatment with an SABA, as noted previously. Sleep that is uninterrupted by asthma symptoms is an important goal. If patients with asthma wake up because of asthma symptoms, their asthma is not under good control and their therapeutic plan should be reevaluated.

Together with the patient and caregiver, develop written asthma action plans (see Table 29-12). Base these plans on the patient's asthma symptoms and PEFR. To follow the management plan, the patient must measure his or her peak flow at least daily. Some patients may want to just monitor symptoms for self-management. Patients with asthma frequently do not perceive changes in their breathing. Therefore peak flow monitoring, when done correctly, can be a reliable, objective measurement of asthma control (Table 29-14).

TABLE 29-14 PATIENT TEACHING GUIDE

How to Use Your Peak Flow Meter

Include the following instructions when teaching the patient to use a peak flow meter.

Why Use a Peak Flow Meter?

- Peak flow meters are used to check your asthma the way that blood pressure cuffs are used to check blood pressure. A peak flow meter is a device that measures how well air moves out of your lungs.
- During an asthma episode, the airways of the lungs usually begin to narrow slowly. The peak flow meter may tell you if there is narrowing in the airways hours, sometimes even days, before you have any asthma symptoms.
- By taking your medicines early (before symptoms), you may be able to stop the episode quickly and avoid a severe asthma episode.
- The peak flow meter also can be used to help you and your health care provider:
  - Learn what makes your asthma worse.
  - Decide if your treatment plan is working well.
  - Decide when to add or stop medicine.
  - Decide when to seek emergency care.

How to Use Your Peak Flow Meter

- Do the following five steps with your peak flow meter:
  1. Move the indicator to the bottom of the numbered scale.
  2. Stand up.
  3. Take a deep breath, filling your lungs completely.
  4. Place the mouthpiece in your mouth and close your lips around it. Do not put your tongue inside the hole.
  5. Blow out as hard and fast as you can in a single blow.
- Write down the number you get. But if you cough or make a mistake, do not write down the number. Do it over again.
- Repeat steps 1 through 5 two more times, and write down the best of the three blows in your asthma diary.

Find Your Personal Best Peak Flow Number

- Your personal best peak flow number is the highest peak flow number you can achieve over a 2-week period when your asthma is under good control. Good control is when you feel good and do not have any asthma symptoms.
- Each patient's asthma is different, and your best peak expiratory flow (PEF) may be higher or lower than the peak flow of someone of your same height, weight, and gender. This means that it is important for you to find your own personal best peak flow number, which is the basis for your treatment plan.
- To find your personal best peak flow number, take peak flow readings:
  - At least twice a day for 2-3 wk, between 12 noon and 2 PM when your peak flow is the highest
  - 15-20 min after taking inhaled short-acting β_2-agonist (SABA) for quick relief
  - As instructed by your health care provider

The Peak Flow Zone System

Once you know your personal best peak flow number, your health care provider will put the peak flow numbers into zones that are set up like a traffic light. This will help you know what to do when your peak flow number changes. For example:

- Green Zone (more than __L/min [80% of your personal best number]) signals good control. No asthma symptoms are present. Take your medicines as usual.
- Yellow Zone (between __ and __L/min [50% to <80% of your personal best number]) signals caution. If you remain in the yellow zone after several measures of peak flow, take an inhaled SABA. If you continue to register peak flow readings in the yellow zone, your asthma may not be under good control. Ask your physician if you need to change or increase your daily medicines.
- Red Zone (<__L/min [<50% of your personal best number]) signals a medical alert. Take an inhaled SABA (quick-relief medicine) right away. Call your health care provider or the emergency department and ask what to do, or go directly to the emergency department.

Use the Diary to Keep Track of Your Peak Flow

- Record your personal best peak flow number and peak flow zones in your asthma diary.
- Measure your peak flow when you wake up, *before* taking medicine. Write down your peak flow number in the diary every day, or as instructed by your health care provider.

Actions to Take When Peak Flow Numbers Change

- PEF goes between __ and __L/min (50% to <80% of personal best, yellow zone).
  ACTION: Take an inhaled SABA (quick-relief medicine) as prescribed by your health care provider.
- PEF increases ≥20% when measured before and after taking an inhaled SABA (quick-relief medicine).
  ACTION: Talk to your physician about adding more medicine to control your asthma better (e.g., an antiinflammatory medication).

Source: Adapted from National Asthma Education and Prevention Program, National Heart, Lung, and Blood Institute: *Expert Panel Report 3: guidelines for the diagnosis and management of asthma*, NIH pub no 08-4051, Bethesda, Md, 2007, National Institutes of Health. Retrieved from *www.nhlbi.nih.gov/guidelines*.

If a patient's PEFR is within the green zone (usually 80% to 100% of the person's personal best), the patient should remain on her or his usual medications. If the PEFR is within the yellow zone (usually 50% to 80% of personal best), it indicates caution. Something is triggering the patient's asthma (e.g., viral infection).

The patient should have a written asthma action plan that prescribes a step increase in medications during the acute phase of the infection. The dose is stepped down once the viral infection symptoms subside. Based on the asthma management plan, the patient can use different strategies, such as using the SABA more frequently.

If the PEFR is in the red zone (50% or less of personal best), it indicates a serious problem. A rescue plan should be a part of the asthma action plan. Teach the patient and caregiver to take definitive action, as noted previously. Emphasize to the patient the need to monitor PEFR daily or several times a day to have an objective measure that can be correlated with symptoms. Although it may happen, it is unusual for a patient's PEFR to drop from the green zone to the red zone quickly. Usually the patient has time to make changes in medications, avoid triggers, and notify the health care provider.

It is important to involve the patient's caregiver or family. They should know where the patient's inhalers, oral medications, and emergency phone numbers are located. Instruct the caregiver or family on how to decrease the patient's anxiety if an asthma attack occurs. When the patient is stabilized or controlled, the caregiver can gently remind the patient about doing daily PEFR by asking questions such as, "What zone are you in? How's your peak flow today?" A patient and caregiver teaching guide for the patient with asthma is presented in Table 29-15.

An increased number of older adults are diagnosed with asthma. This is a special concern because they have more complicated health issues than younger patients with asthma. Issues that face older adults (especially urban and minority people) are costly medications, nonadherence to medical regimen, and difficulty accessing the health system. Keep these factors in mind when implementing a management plan for older adults.

A variety of factors may contribute to African Americans and Hispanics (especially those from Puerto Rico) having higher rates of poorly controlled asthma and deaths compared with whites. Some factors may be disparities in socioeconomic status and access to proper health care, cultural beliefs about the management of asthma, and underutilization of the long-term controller medications because of high costs. Seek to explore and eliminate any barriers to health care. Also seek out culturally appropriate resources and educational material in languages other than English to improve the asthma control of these individuals.

Relaxation therapies (e.g., yoga, meditation, relaxation techniques, breathing techniques) may help a patient relax respiratory muscles and decrease the respiratory rate. (Chapter 7 discusses relaxation breathing and other relaxation strategies.) A healthy emotional outlook can also be important in preventing future asthma attacks.[14] A variety of websites have excellent resources for patient teaching (see Resources at the end of the chapter). Some communities have asthma support groups.

EVALUATION

The expected outcomes for the patient with asthma are presented in Nursing Care Plan 29-1.

CHRONIC OBSTRUCTIVE PULMONARY DISEASE

Chronic obstructive pulmonary disease (COPD) is a preventable and treatable disease characterized by persistent airflow limitation that is slowly progressive. COPD is associated with an enhanced chronic inflammatory response of the airways and lungs to noxious particles or gases, primarily caused by cigarette smoking. COPD exacerbations and other coexisting illnesses contribute to the overall severity of the disease.[15,16]

Previous definitions of COPD encompassed two types of obstructive airway diseases: chronic bronchitis and emphysema. **Chronic bronchitis** is the presence of chronic productive cough for 3 months in each of 2 consecutive years in a patient in whom other causes of chronic cough have been excluded. **Emphysema** is an abnormal permanent enlargement of the air spaces distal to the terminal bronchioles, accompanied by destruction of their walls and without obvious fibrosis. Only about 10% of patients with COPD have pure emphysema. Patients may have a predominance of chronic bronchitis or emphysema, but it is often difficult to determine because the conditions usually coexist. COPD is discussed in this section as one disease state from the viewpoint of pathophysiology and management.[16]

Patients with COPD may have asthma. Although the evidence is not conclusive, asthma may be a risk factor for COPD development. An estimated 12.7 million adults in the United States over age 18 have COPD.[2,15] An additional 24 million people have evidence of impaired lung function. The number of people with COPD is greatly underestimated because the disease is usually not diagnosed until it is moderately advanced. COPD is the third leading cause of death in the United States, killing more than 133,000 Americans each year.[17,18]

Etiology

The many factors involved in the etiology of COPD are discussed in this section.

Cigarette Smoking. Worldwide the major risk factor for developing COPD is cigarette smoking.[18,19] COPD affects about 15% of smokers.[20] An intriguing question is why some smokers develop COPD and others do not. In people over age 40 with a smoking history of 10 or more pack-years, COPD should be considered.[21]

GENDER DIFFERENCES

Chronic Obstructive Pulmonary Disease (COPD)

Men	Women
• COPD is more common in men than in women, but the incidence is not increasing in men. • Fewer men die from COPD than women.	• The number of women with COPD is increasing. • Increase is probably due to increased number of women smoking cigarettes and increased susceptibility (e.g., smaller lungs and airways, lower elastic recoil). • Women with COPD have lower quality of life, more exacerbations, increased dyspnea, and better response to O_2 therapy compared with men.

TABLE 29-15 PATIENT & CAREGIVER TEACHING GUIDE

Asthma

Include the following information in a teaching plan for the patient with asthma and the caregiver. It will help to improve the patient's quality of life and promote lifestyle changes that support successful living with asthma.

Teaching Topic	Resources
What Is Asthma? • Basic anatomy and physiology of lung • Pathophysiology of asthma • Relationship of pathophysiology to signs and symptoms • Measurement and correlation of pulmonary function tests and peak expiratory flow rate	*What Is Asthma?* (National Heart, Lung, and Blood Institute) Retrieved from *www.nhlbi.nih.gov/health/dci/Diseases/Asthma/Asthma_WhatIs.html.* *What Is Asthma?* (Global Initiative for Asthma). Retrieved from *www.ginasthma.org/q-a-general-information-about-asthma.html.* *Asthma: Overview* (National Jewish Health). Retrieved from *www.njhealth.org/healthinfo/conditions/asthma/index.aspx.*
What Is Good Asthma Control?	Resource for patient on personal ideas of good control. *Asthma Control Test.* Retrieved from *www.qualitymetric.com/demos/TP_Launch.aspx?SID=52461.*
Hindrances to Asthma Treatment and Control • Intermittent nature of symptoms • Role of denial • Poor perception of asthma severity by patient	Discussion with patient and caregiver about possible hindrances.
Environmental and Trigger Control • Identifications of possible triggers and possible preventive measures • Avoidance of allergens and other triggers • Need to maintain good hydration	*Environmental Management* (National Jewish Health). Retrieved from *www.nationaljewish.org/healthinfo/conditions/asthma/lifestyle-management/environmental.* *Pollen Count Report* (sign up for daily notification about a particular area) (American Academy of Asthma Allergy and Immunology). Retrieved from *www.aaaai.org/nab.* Trigger diary kept by patient.
Medications Types (include mechanism of action) • β_2-Agonists • Corticosteroids • Methylxanthines • Anti-IgE • Leukotriene modifiers • Combination drugs Establishing medication schedule Use of preventive and maintenance agents (e.g., antiinflammatory agents)	*Asthma: Treatment* (National Jewish Health). Available at *www.nationaljewish.org/healthinfo/conditions/asthma/treatment.* Asthma Action Plan (see Table 29-12). Write out medication list and schedule.
Correct Use of Inhalers, Spacer, and Nebulizer	Demonstration–return demonstration with placebo devices (see Figs. 29-5 to 29-7 and Tables 29-8 to 29-10). *Inhaled Medication Instructional Videos: Asthma and General Lung Disease* (National Jewish Health). Retrieved from *www.nationaljewish.org/healthinfo/medications/lung-diseases/devices/instructional-videos.* Patient instructions for inhaled devices in English and Spanish (American College of Chest Physicians). Retrieved from *www.chestnet.org/accp/patient-guides/patient-instructions-inhaled-devices-english-and-spanish.*
Breathing Techniques • Pursed-lip breathing	See Table 29-13.
Correct Use of Peak Flow Meter	See Table 29-14. *Measuring Your Peak Flow Rate (text and video)* (American Lung Association). Retrieved from *www.lung.org/lung-disease/asthma/living-with-asthma/take-control-of-your-asthma/measuring-your-peak-flow-rate.html.*
Asthma Action Plan • Peak flow zones • Individualize plan • Early recognition of infection • Building a partnership with your health care provider • Questions patients may have about asthma, but patient cannot reach the provider	See Table 29-12. Patient completes asthma action plan and discusses it with health care provider. *Asthma Clinical Research Centers* (American Lung Association). Retrieved from *www.lung.org/finding-cures/our-research/acrc.* *My Asthma Wallet Card* (National Heart, Lung, and Blood Institute). Retrieved from *www.nhlbi.nih.gov/health/public/lung/asthma/asthma_walletcard.htm.* *Asthma Profiler* (online decision support tool to assist patients in understanding treatment options and side effects; includes personalized questions to ask the provider and research reports) (American Lung Association). Retrieved from *www.lung.org/lung-disease/asthma/living-with-asthma/making-treatment-decisions.* *Lung Line* (ask a specialized nurse questions about early detection, care, and prevention of respiratory diseases) (National Jewish Health). Telephone: 800-222-LUNG or *www.njhealth.org/about/contact/lung-line.aspx.*

Cigarette smoke has several direct effects on the respiratory tract (Table 29-16). The irritating effect of the smoke causes hyperplasia of cells, including goblet cells, thereby increasing the production of mucus. Hyperplasia reduces airway diameter and increases the difficulty in clearing secretions. Smoking reduces the ciliary activity and may cause actual loss of cilia. Smoking also produces abnormal dilation of the distal air space with destruction of alveolar walls. Many cells develop large, atypical nuclei, which are considered a precancerous condition. Smoking causes chronic, enhanced inflammation of various parts of the lung with structural changes and repair (called remodeling). The reasons for the inflammatory response are not clearly understood, but may be genetically determined, since patients who have never smoked can develop COPD.

Cigarette smoking causes oxidative stress, as well as an imbalance between proteases that break down connective tissue in the lung and antiproteases that protect the lungs.[16] These changes resulting from cigarette smoking increase with more severe disease and even persist with smoking cessation. (See Chapter 11 for more detail about cigarette smoking.)

Passive smoking is the exposure of nonsmokers to cigarette smoke, also known as *environmental tobacco smoke* (ETS) or secondhand smoke. In adults, involuntary smoke exposure is associated with decreased pulmonary function, increased respiratory symptoms, and severe lower respiratory tract infections (e.g., pneumonia). ETS is also associated with increased risk for lung cancer and nasal sinus cancer.

Occupational Chemicals and Dusts. If a person has intense or prolonged exposure to various dusts, vapors, irritants, or fumes in the workplace, symptoms of lung impairment consistent with COPD can develop. If a person has occupational exposure and smokes, the risk of COPD increases.[16]

Air Pollution. High levels of urban air pollution are harmful to people with existing lung disease. However, the effect of outdoor air pollution as a risk factor for the development of COPD is unclear. Another risk factor for COPD development is coal and other biomass fuels that are used for indoor heating and cooking. Many people who have never smoked are at significant risk for developing COPD because of cooking with these fuels in poorly ventilated areas.[16]

Infection. Infections are a risk factor for developing COPD. Severe recurring respiratory tract infections in childhood have been associated with reduced lung function and increased respiratory symptoms in adulthood. It is unclear whether the development of COPD can be related to recurrent infections in adults. People who smoke and also have human immunodeficiency virus (HIV) have an accelerated development of COPD. Tuberculosis is also a risk factor for COPD development.

Genetics. The fact that a relatively small percentage of smokers get COPD strongly suggests that genetic factors influence which smokers get the disease. Because of the genetic-environmental interaction, two people may have the same smoking history, but only one develops COPD. To date, one genetic factor has been clearly identified (see next section).[16]

α_1-Antitrypsin (AAT) Deficiency. **α_1-Antitrypsin (AAT) deficiency** is an autosomal recessive disorder that may affect the lungs or liver. AAT deficiency is a genetic risk factor for COPD. Approximately 3% of all people diagnosed with COPD may have undetected AAT deficiency. AAT is a serum protein produced by the liver and normally found in the lungs. The main function of AAT, an α_1-protease inhibitor, is to protect normal lung tissue from attack by proteases during inflammation related to cigarette smoking and infections. Severe AAT deficiency leads to premature bullous emphysema in the lungs found on x-ray. Smoking greatly exacerbates the disease process in these patients.[22]

Genetic Link

AAT deficiency is an autosomal recessive disorder (see Figs. 13-4 and 13-5 and the Genetics in Clinical Practice box). The

TABLE 29-16 EFFECTS OF TOBACCO SMOKE ON RESPIRATORY SYSTEM

Area of Defect	Acute Effects	Long-Term Effects
Respiratory mucosa		
• Nasopharyngeal	↓ Sense of smell	Cancer
• Tongue	↓ Sense of taste	Cancer
• Vocal cords	Hoarseness	Chronic cough, cancer
• Bronchus and bronchioles	Bronchospasm, cough	Chronic bronchitis, asthma, cancer
Cilia	Paralysis, sputum accumulation, cough	Chronic bronchitis, cancer
Mucous glands	↑ Secretions, ↑ cough	Hyperplasia and hypertrophy of glands, chronic bronchitis
Alveolar macrophages	↓ Function	↑ Incidence of infection
Elastin and collagen fibers	↑ Destruction by proteases ↓ Function of antiproteases (α_1-antitrypsin) ↓ Synthesis and repair of elastin	Emphysema

GENETICS IN CLINICAL PRACTICE

α_1-Antitrypsin (AAT) Deficiency

Genetic Basis
- Autosomal recessive disorder.
- Mutations in *SERPINA1* gene (located on chromosome 14) cause AAT deficiency.
- Gene provides instructions for the liver to make the protein AAT, which protects the lungs and liver from powerful proteolytic enzymes.
- Without enough functional AAT, proteolytic enzymes destroy alveoli and cause lung disease.

Incidence
- Occurs in 1 in 1700 to 3500 live births in the United States.
- People of northern European descent most affected.

Genetic Testing
- DNA testing is available.
- Screening of siblings is useful.
- Serum assay is available to measure the amount of AAT.

Clinical Implications
- AAT deficiency can cause lung and liver disease.
- Onset of disease is between ages 20 and 40 yr.
- Treatment includes AAT replacement (Prolastin).
- Disease predisposes to early-onset emphysema.

severity of AAT deficiency depends on which forms of the gene are inherited. The most common abnormal genes are the S and Z alleles. The normal genotype is MM. The most common genotype associated with AAT disease is ZZ (also referred to as PI-ZZ). Other variations include MZ (slightly increased risk of poor lung function) and SZ (higher risk of lung and liver problems in smokers). Some individuals with MZ and SZ genotypes may never seek health care because they have minimal manifestations of the disorder.[22]

Although 100,000 people in the United States are suspected of having the ZZ phenotype, fewer than 10% have been detected. Clues to AAT deficiencies are the onset of symptoms often occurring by age 40, minimal to no tobacco use, and family history of emphysema and/or liver disease.[23] Chronic liver disease as an infant or adult with increased liver enzyme levels may also be seen. Individuals with this type of emphysema are primarily of northern European origin.

A simple blood test can determine low levels of AAT. Those with borderline or low levels can then be genetically tested.

IV-administered AAT (e.g., Prolastin-C) augmentation therapy is used for people with AAT deficiency. The infusions are usually administered weekly. Its effectiveness in slowing the progression of the disease and the results of this treatment continue to be evaluated.

Aging. Although aging is often considered a risk factor for COPD, the evidence is unclear. Does the aging process lead to COPD, or is COPD a result of the cumulative exposures that occur over a long life?[16] Normal aging results in loss of elastic recoil, stiffening of the chest wall, gas exchange alteration, and decrease in exercise tolerance. As people age, the lungs gradually lose their elastic recoil. Thoracic cage changes result from osteoporosis and calcification of the costal cartilages. The thoracic cage becomes stiff and rigid, and the ribs are less mobile. The shape of the rib cage gradually changes because of the increased residual volume (RV), causing it to expand and become rounded. Decreased chest compliance and elastic recoil of the lungs caused by aging affect the mechanical aspects of ventilation and increase the work of breathing.[24]

As one ages, the number of functional alveoli decreases as peripheral airways lose supporting tissues. The surface area for gas exchange decreases, and the PaO_2 decreases. Changes in the elasticity of the lungs reduce the ventilatory reserve.[24] These changes are similar to those seen in the patient with emphysema.

Pathophysiology

COPD is characterized by chronic inflammation of the airways, lung parenchyma (respiratory bronchioles and alveoli), and pulmonary blood vessels (Fig. 29-8). The pathogenesis of COPD is complex and involves many mechanisms. The defining feature of COPD is not fully reversible airflow limitation during forced exhalation. This is caused by loss of elastic recoil and airflow obstruction caused by mucus hypersecretion, mucosal edema, and bronchospasm.

In COPD various processes occur such as airflow limitation, air trapping, gas exchange abnormalities, and mucus hyperse-

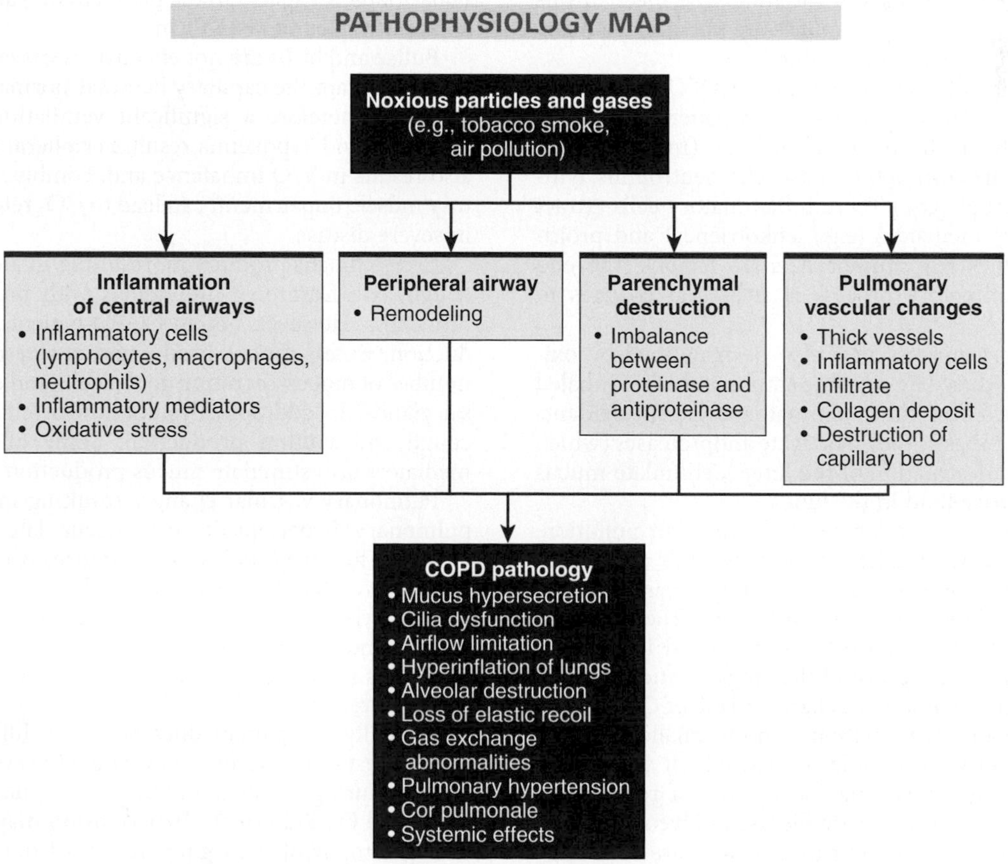

FIG. 29-8 Pathophysiology of chronic obstructive pulmonary disease *(COPD).*

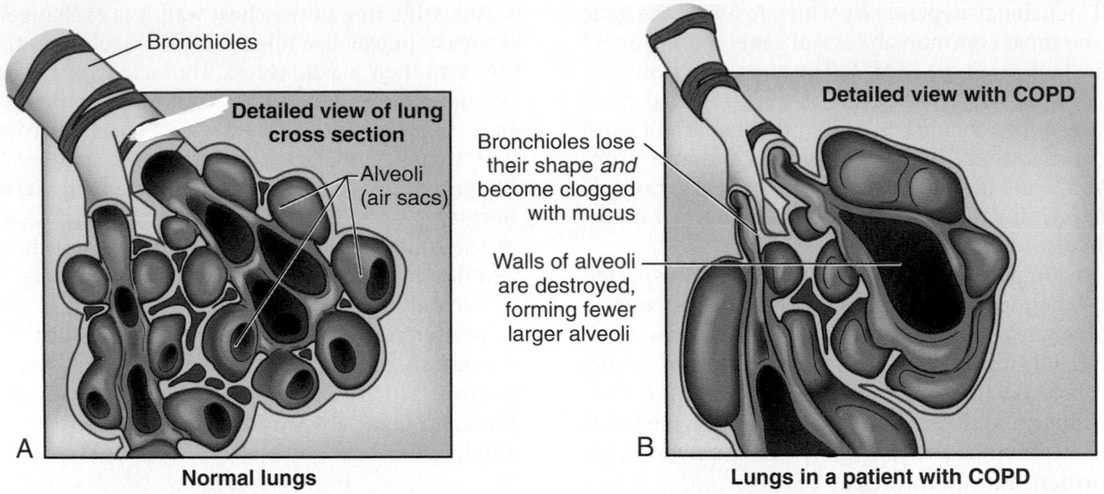

FIG. 29-9 A, Normal lungs showing bronchioles and alveoli. **B,** Changes in the bronchioles and alveoli in the lungs of a patient with chronic obstructive pulmonary disease *(COPD).*

cretion. In severe disease, pulmonary hypertension and systemic manifestations occur (see Fig. 29-8). COPD has an uneven distribution of pathologic changes, with severely destroyed lung areas existing together with areas of relatively normal lung.

The inflammatory process starts with inhalation of noxious particles and gases (e.g., cigarette smoke), but is magnified in the person with COPD. The abnormal inflammatory process causes tissue destruction and disrupts the normal defense mechanisms and repair process of the lung. The mechanisms for the enhanced inflammatory response are not clearly understood, but may be genetically determined.[16]

The predominant inflammatory cells in COPD are neutrophils, macrophages, and lymphocytes. This pattern of inflammatory cells is different from that in asthma. (In asthma the inflammatory cells are eosinophils, mast cells, neutrophils, lymphocytes, and macrophages.) These inflammatory cells attract other inflammatory mediators (e.g., leukotrienes) and proinflammatory cytokines (e.g., tumor necrosis factor). The end result of the inflammatory process is structural changes in the lungs.[16]

The inflammatory process may also be magnified by oxidants, which are produced by cigarette smoke and other inhaled particles and released from the inflammatory cells. The oxidants adversely affect the lungs as they inactivate antiproteases (which prevent the natural destruction of the lungs), stimulate mucus secretion, and increase fluid in the lungs.

After the inhalation of oxidants in tobacco or air pollution, the activity of proteases (which break down the connective tissue of the lungs) increases and the antiproteases (which protect against the breakdown) are inhibited. Therefore the natural balance of protease/antiprotease is tipped in favor of destruction of the alveoli and loss of the lungs' elastic recoil.[16,24]

Inability to expire air is a main characteristic of COPD. The primary site of the airflow limitation is in the smaller airways. As the peripheral airways become obstructed, air is progressively trapped during expiration. The volume of residual air becomes greatly increased in severe disease as alveolar attachments to small airways (similar to rubber bands) are destroyed. The residual air, combined with the loss of elastic recoil, makes passive expiration of air difficult. As air is trapped in the lungs, the chest hyperexpands and becomes barrel shaped, since the respiratory muscles are not able to function effectively. The functional residual capacity is increased. The patient is now trying to breathe in when the lungs are in an "overinflated" state; thus the patient appears dyspneic and exercise capacity is limited.

Gas exchange abnormalities result in hypoxemia and hypercapnia (increased CO_2) as the disease worsens. As the air trapping increases, walls of alveoli are destroyed (Fig. 29-9), and bullae (large air spaces in the parenchyma) and blebs (air spaces adjacent to pleurae) can form.

Bullae and blebs are not effective in gas exchange, since they do not contain the capillary bed that normally surrounds each alveolus. Therefore a significant ventilation-perfusion (V/Q) mismatch and hypoxemia result. Peripheral airway obstruction also results in V/Q imbalance and, combined with the respiratory muscle impairment, can lead to CO_2 retention, particularly in severe disease.

Excess mucus production, resulting in a chronic productive cough, is a feature of individuals with predominant chronic bronchitis. However, not all COPD patients have sputum production. Excess mucus production is a result of an increased number of mucus-secreting goblet cells and enlarged submucosal glands. In addition, dysfunction of cilia leads to chronic cough and sputum production. Some of the inflammatory mediators also stimulate mucus production.

Pulmonary vascular changes resulting in mild to moderate pulmonary hypertension may occur late in the course of COPD. The small pulmonary arteries vasoconstrict due to hypoxia. As the disease advances, the structure of the pulmonary arteries changes, resulting in thickening of the vascular smooth muscle. Because of the loss of alveolar walls and the capillaries surrounding them, pressure in the pulmonary circulation increases.

Typically, the patient does not have difficulty with hypoxemia at rest until late in the disease. However, hypoxemia may develop during exercise, and the patient may benefit from supplemental O_2. Pulmonary hypertension may progress and lead to hypertrophy of the right ventricle of the heart **(cor pulmonale).** The right ventricle dilates and may eventually lead to right-sided heart failure.[25]

In addition to lung disease, COPD is a systemic disease. Chronic inflammation is an underlying etiology for these systemic effects. Cardiovascular diseases commonly exist in COPD (smoking is a primary risk factor for both of them). Other common systemic diseases include cachexia (skeletal muscle wasting), osteoporosis, diabetes, and metabolic syndrome, which cannot be readily related to smoking.[16,26]

Clinical Manifestations

Clinical manifestations of COPD typically develop slowly, but COPD should be considered in all patients over age 40 with 10 or more pack-years of cigarette smoking.[21] A diagnosis of COPD should be considered in any patient who has symptoms of cough, sputum production, or dyspnea and/or a history of exposure to risk factors for the disease.

A chronic intermittent cough, which is often the first symptom to develop, may later be present every day as the disease progresses. The cough is often dismissed by patients as they expect it with smoking or environmental exposures. The cough may be unproductive of mucus. However, significant airflow limitation may exist without sputum or cough.[16] Typically dyspnea is progressive, usually occurs with exertion, and is present every day.

Patients may complain of not being able to take a deep breath, heaviness in the chest, gasping, increased effort to breathe, and air hunger. Patients usually ignore the symptoms and rationalize that "I'm getting older" and "I'm out of shape." They change behaviors to avoid dyspnea, such as taking the elevator. Gradually the dyspnea interferes with daily activities, such as carrying grocery bags. They cannot walk as fast as their partner or peers. However, as symptoms worsen and interfere with daily activity or they have their first COPD exacerbation, patients usually seek medical care.

In late stages of COPD, dyspnea may be present at rest. As more alveoli become overdistended, increasing amounts of air are trapped. This causes a flattened diaphragm, and the patient must breathe from partially inflated lungs. Effective abdominal breathing is decreased because of the flattened diaphragm from the overinflated lungs. The person becomes more of a chest breather, relying on the intercostal and accessory muscles. However, chest breathing is not efficient.

Wheezing and chest tightness may be present, but may vary by time of the day or from day to day, especially in patients with more severe disease. Wheezes may arise from the laryngeal area, or wheezes may not be present on auscultation. Chest tightness, which often follows activity, may feel similar to muscular contraction.

The person with advanced COPD frequently experiences fatigue, weight loss, and anorexia. Even with adequate caloric intake, the patient still loses weight. Fatigue is a highly prevalent symptom that affects the patient's activities of daily living. Paroxysms of coughing may be so severe the patient faints or fractures a rib.

During physical examination a prolonged expiratory respiratory phase, wheezes, or decreased breath sounds are noted in all lung fields. The patient may need to breathe louder than normal for auscultated breath sounds to be heard. The anteroposterior diameter of the chest is increased ("barrel chest") from the chronic air trapping. The patient may sit upright with arms supported on a fixed surface such as an overbed table *(tripod position)*. The patient may naturally purse lips on expiration (pursed-lip breathing) and use accessory muscles, such as those in the neck, to aid with inspiration. Edema in the ankles may be the only clue to right-sided heart involvement (cor pulmonale).

Over time, hypoxemia (PaO_2 less than 60 mm Hg or O_2 saturation less than 88%) may develop with hypercapnia ($PaCO_2$ over 45 mm Hg). The bluish red color of the skin results from polycythemia and cyanosis. Polycythemia develops as a result of increased production of red blood cells as the body attempts to compensate for chronic hypoxemia. Hemoglobin concentrations may reach 20 g/dL (200 g/L) or more. However, the person may also have lowered hemoglobin and hematocrit because of chronic anemia.

Clinically it is common for a person to have a combination of emphysema and chronic bronchitis, often with one condition predominating. It is sometimes difficult to distinguish COPD from asthma, especially if the individual has a history of cigarette smoking. However, some clinical features are different (see Table 29-3).

Classification of COPD. COPD should be considered in any person with a chronic cough and dyspnea who has smoked cigarettes or been exposed to environmental or occupational pollutants. The diagnosis is confirmed by spirometry.

COPD can be classified as mild, moderate, severe, and very severe (Table 29-17). An FEV_1/FVC ratio of less than 70% establishes the diagnosis of COPD, and the severity of obstruction (as indicated by FEV_1) determines the stage of COPD. The management of COPD is based on the patient's symptoms, classification, and exacerbation history.

Complications

Cor Pulmonale. *Cor pulmonale* results from pulmonary hypertension, which is caused by diseases affecting the lungs or pulmonary blood vessels (Fig. 29-10). In North America 50% of the cases of cor pulmonale are due to COPD. Cor pulmonale is a late manifestation of COPD, yet not all patients with COPD develop cor pulmonale. Once the patient develops cor pulmonale, the prognosis worsens.[27]

In COPD, pulmonary hypertension is caused primarily by constriction of the pulmonary vessels in response to alveolar hypoxia, with acidosis further potentiating the vasoconstriction. Chronic alveolar hypoxia causes vascular remodeling. Chronic hypoxia also stimulates erythropoiesis, which causes polycythemia. This results in increased viscosity of the blood. An anatomic reduction of the pulmonary vascular bed, as seen in emphysema with bullae, may occur. These patients have increased pulmonary vascular resistance and thus develop pulmonary hypertension.

TABLE 29-17 CLASSIFICATION OF COPD SEVERITY*

The following classification is based on postbronchodilator FEV_1.

Classification	Level of Severity	FEV_1 Results
GOLD 1	Mild	FEV_1 ≥80% predicted
GOLD 2	Moderate	FEV_1 50%-80% predicted
GOLD 3	Severe	FEV_1 30%-50% predicted
GOLD 4	Very severe	FEV_1 <30% predicted

Adapted from Global Initiative for Chronic Obstructive Lung Disease: Global strategy for the diagnosis, management, and prevention of chronic obstructive pulmonary disease (updated 2013). Retrieved from *www.goldcopd.org*.

*A diagnosis of COPD is made when a patient has a FEV_1/FVC <0.70.

COPD, Chronic obstructive pulmonary disease; *FEV_1,* forced expiratory volume in 1 sec; *FVC,* forced vital capacity.

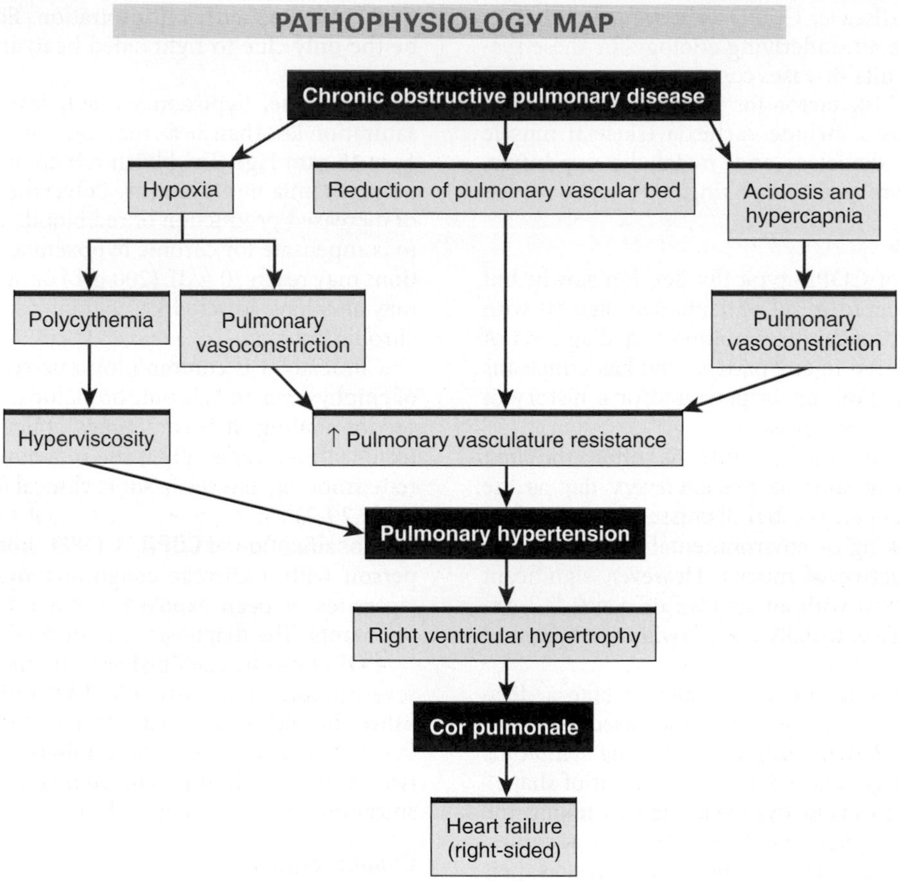

FIG. 29-10 Mechanisms involved in the pathophysiology of pulmonary hypertension and cor pulmonale secondary to chronic obstructive pulmonary disease.

Normally the right ventricle and pulmonary circulatory system are low-pressure systems compared with the left ventricle and systemic circulation. When pulmonary hypertension develops, the pressures on the right side of the heart must increase to push blood into the lungs. Eventually, right-sided heart failure develops.

Dyspnea is the most common symptom of chronic cor pulmonale. Lung sounds are normal, or crackles may be heard in the bases of the lungs bilaterally. Heart sound changes occur but are usually masked by the underlying lung disease. Other manifestations of right-sided heart failure may develop, including distended neck veins (jugular venous distention), hepatomegaly with right upper quadrant tenderness, peripheral edema, and weight gain.

ECG changes indicating right ventricular hypertrophy may be seen in severe cases. Typically the patient has large pulmonary vessels on chest x-ray and increased pressure on a right-sided heart cardiac catheterization. Echocardiogram may reflect right-sided heart enlargement. B-type natriuretic peptide (BNP) levels, which are used to diagnose heart failure, may be elevated in cor pulmonale secondary to the stretching of the right ventricle. Normally BNP levels are used to distinguish cardiac from respiratory causes of dyspnea, but in cor pulmonale the cause of the heart failure is the lung disease.[27]

Treatment of cor pulmonale is initially targeted at managing the COPD (e.g., bronchodilation). Continuous low-flow, long-term O_2 therapy (for more than 15 hr/day) improves survival.[28] Diuretics are generally used, similar to their use with chronic heart failure. (Cor pulmonale is also discussed in Chapter 28.)

COPD Exacerbations. According to the Global Initiative for Chronic Obstructive Lung Disease (GOLD) guidelines, a *COPD exacerbation* is an acute event in the natural course of the disease. The primary causes of exacerbations are bacterial or viral infections.[16,29] Exacerbations are signaled by an acute change in the patient's usual dyspnea, cough, and/or sputum (i.e., something different from the usual daily patterns). Exacerbations of COPD are typical and increase in frequency (average one or two a year) as the disease progresses. It may take several weeks for a patient to recover from an exacerbation.

Assess patients for the classic signs of exacerbation such as an increase in dyspnea, sputum volume, or sputum purulence. They may also have nonspecific complaints of malaise, insomnia, fatigue, depression, confusion, decreased exercise tolerance, increased wheezing, or fever without other causes.[30]

As the severity of COPD increases, exacerbations of COPD are associated with poorer outcomes. Exacerbations may be treated at home or in the hospital, depending on the severity. The severity is determined by the patient's medical history before the exacerbation, the presence of other diseases, symptoms, ABGs, and other laboratory tests. Typically in the later stages of COPD the patient has a low-normal pH, high-normal or above-normal $PaCO_2$, and high-normal bicarbonate (HCO_3^-). This indicates compensated respiratory acidosis as the patient has chronically retained CO_2 and the kidneys have conserved HCO_3^- to increase the pH to within the normal range (see Table 29-3).

Carefully assess the patient's ABGs for any movement toward respiratory acidosis and further hypoxemia, indicating respiratory failure. Also assess the patient's medical history for the stage of COPD as noted by the level of FEV_1. Assess for new symptoms or worsening of usual symptoms. Determine the number of previous exacerbations per year and if treatment occurred in the home or hospital. The presence of other co-morbid conditions complicates the exacerbation. In addition, the current treatment affects its management. Be alert for signs of severity such as use of accessory muscles, central cyanosis, edema in the lower extremities, unstable BP, right-sided heart failure, and altered alertness. These manifestations affect whether the patient is treated as an inpatient or outpatient.

Short-acting bronchodilators, oral systemic corticosteroids, and antibiotics are the typical therapies for exacerbations. SABAs with or without short-acting anticholinergics are preferred for those who are breathless. Drug administration via MDI or nebulizer works equally well, although sicker patients often prefer the nebulizer. Antibiotic use remains somewhat controversial. However, the presence of green or purulent sputum (as opposed to white sputum) is one of the best ways to determine if antibiotics are needed.[16,29]

Therapies used to treat exacerbations of COPD in the hospital are similar to home management, except supplemental O_2 therapy titrated by ABG measurement may be used. Attempts are made to use noninvasive mechanical methods (e.g., continuous positive airway pressure [CPAP] to support ventilation rather than invasive ventilatory support [e.g., intubation and mechanical ventilation]). Teach the patient and the caregiver early recognition of the three cardinal symptoms of exacerbations (increase in dyspnea, sputum volume, or sputum purulence) to promote early treatment and thus prevent hospitalization and possible respiratory failure.

Acute Respiratory Failure. Patients with severe COPD who have exacerbations are at risk for respiratory failure. Frequently, COPD patients wait too long to contact their health care provider when they first develop symptoms suggestive of exacerbation. Discontinuing bronchodilator or corticosteroid medication may also precipitate respiratory failure.

Cardioselective β-adrenergic blockers (e.g., atenolol, metoprolol) can be safely used. Chronic treatment with β-blockers may improve survival and reduce the risk of exacerbations of COPD.[16,31]

Indiscriminate use of sedatives, benzodiazepines, and opioids, especially in the preoperative or postoperative patient who retains CO_2, may suppress the ventilatory drive and lead to respiratory failure. The person with COPD who retains CO_2 is usually treated with low-flow rates of O_2 with careful monitoring of ABGs to avoid hypercapnia. It is vital to provide adequate O_2 while assessing the ABGs, rather than risk not providing O_2 because of the fear of CO_2 narcosis (discussed on p. 592).

In patients with COPD, surgery or severe, painful illness involving the chest or abdominal organs may lead to splinting and ineffective ventilation and respiratory failure. To prevent postoperative pulmonary complications, careful preoperative screening, which includes PFTs and ABG assessment, is important in the patient with a heavy smoking history and/or COPD. (Respiratory failure is discussed in Chapter 68.)

Depression and Anxiety. Patients with COPD experience many losses as the disease progresses. Because many patients with COPD experience depression and anxiety, assess for both. Ask patients if they "feel down or blue" most of the time. Do they appear anxious about being able to control their breathlessness or know what to do if they have an exacerbation? Are they exhibiting concern over more difficulty in self-care activities such as bathing? How is the family coping with the patient's disease?

Help the patient with muscle relaxation exercises that can reduce anxiety (see Chapter 7). In addition, teach patients about the treatment and disease, which can give them a sense of control of their disease and complex treatment regimens. It is important to include the patient's caregiver in the teaching so he or she can help the patient cope physically and emotionally.

A consultation with a mental health specialist may be needed for proper screening and diagnosis of depression or other mental health problems. Cognitive and behavioral therapy along with COPD teaching may improve the quality of life. Medications may be used to treat both depression and anxiety. Buspirone (BuSpar), which is used to treat anxiety, has few if any respiratory depression effects. Benzodiazepines should be avoided because they may depress the respiratory drive and may be habit forming. When the patient becomes anxious because of dyspnea, the use of pursed-lip breathing (see Table 29-13) and short-acting bronchodilators may be appropriate.

Diagnostic Studies

Spirometry is required to confirm the diagnosis in individuals suspected of having COPD. Spirometry confirms the presence of airflow obstruction and determines the severity of COPD. The patient is given a short-acting bronchodilator, and post-bronchodilator values are compared with a normal reference value.

A diagnosis of COPD is made when the FEV_1/FVC ratio is less than 70% along with the appropriate symptoms. The value of FEV_1 provides a guideline for the degree of severity of COPD. FEV_1 can be expressed as a percentage compared with a normal reference value (percent predicted). The lower the FEV_1, the sicker the patient.

In addition to spirometry, other diagnostic studies are performed (Table 29-18). Chest x-rays are not diagnostic but may show a flat diaphragm because of the hyperinflated lungs. Computed tomography (CT) scans are not routinely used to diagnose COPD. However, in individuals with predominant emphysema, enlarged air spaces in the apices may be seen on the CT scan.

Other tests may be used to assess the response to therapy, disease severity, and quality of life. Two validated questionnaires are the COPD Assessment Test (CAT) and modified Medical Research Council (mMRC) Dyspnea Scale. The CAT (see eTable 29-3 on the website for this chapter) measures the daily impact of COPD on a person's life and can help the health care team make better management decisions.[32] This test is found online in more than 50 languages with scoring and easy to understand guidelines *(www.catestonline.org)*. The mMRC measures the patient's level of dyspnea (see eTable 29-4).

Patients often have exercise-induced hypoxemia, and thus a 6-minute walk test should be done by a physical or respiratory therapist, with pulse oximetry readings taken when the patient is walking and at rest. If values of O_2 saturation are 88% or lower when at rest and the patient is breathing room air, he or she qualifies for supplemental O_2.[16] Later in the disease the findings presented in Table 29-3 may be present.

A history and physical examination are extremely important in a diagnostic workup.

The BODE index can be used to assess not only the risk of death from COPD, but also the pulmonary and systemic mani-

TABLE 29-18 COLLABORATIVE CARE

Chronic Obstructive Pulmonary Disease (COPD)

Diagnostic
- History and physical examination
- Pulmonary function tests
- Chest x-ray
- Serum α_1-antitrypsin levels
- ABGs
- Six-minute walk test
- COPD Assessment Test (CAT)* or modified Medical Research Council (mMRC) Dyspnea Scale†
- BODE Index‡

Collaborative Therapy
- Cessation of cigarette smoking
- Treatment of exacerbations
- Drug therapies (see Tables 29-7 and 29-19)
- Airway clearance techniques
- Breathing exercises and retraining
- Hydration of 3 L/day (if not contraindicated)
- Patient and caregiver teaching
- Influenza immunization yearly
- Pneumovax immunization
- Long-term O_2 (if indicated)
- Progressive plan of exercise, especially walking and upper body strengthening
- Pulmonary rehabilitation program
- Nutritional supplementation if low BMI
- Surgery
  - Lung volume reduction
  - Lung transplantation

*See eTable 29-3 or *www.catestonline.org*.
†See eTable 29-4 or *copd.about.com/od/copdbasics/a/MMRCdyspneascale.htm*.
‡See *www.qxmd.com/calculate-online/respirology/bode-index*. Index is a tool to help predict COPD mortality after diagnosis.
ABGs, Arterial blood gases; *BMI*, body mass index.

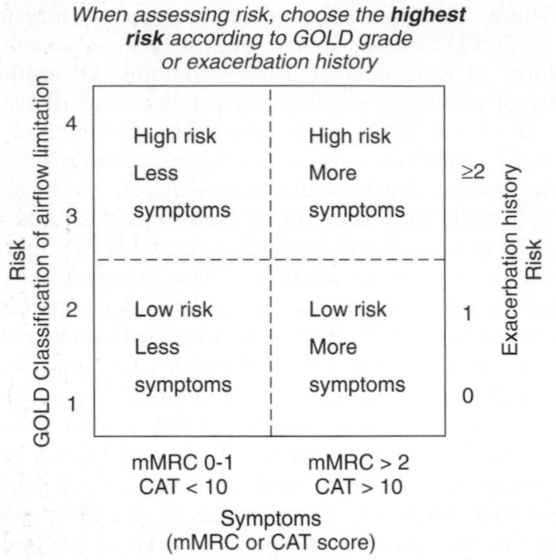

FIG. 29-11 Rubric for chronic obstructive pulmonary disease *(COPD)* showing the association between symptoms, spirometric classification, and future risk of exacerbations. The following factors are considered in the rubric: (1) current level of patient's symptoms as measured by one of two validated questionnaires (modified Medical Research Council *[mMRC]* Dyspnea Scale [see eTable 29-4] or the COPD Assessment Test *[CAT]* [see eTable 29-3]); (2) severity of the disease as measured by the FEV_1; (3) exacerbation risk as reflected in the spirometric classification or patient's history of exacerbations; and (4) presence of co-morbidities. Source: Global Initiative for Chronic Obstructive Lung Disease: Global strategy for the diagnosis, management, and prevention of chronic obstructive pulmonary disease (updated 2013). Retrieved from *www.goldcopd.org*.

festations (see *www.qxmd.com/calculate-online/respirology/bode-index*).

ABGs are usually assessed in the severe stages (FEV_1 less than 50%) and monitored in patients hospitalized with acute exacerbations. In the later stages of COPD, typical findings are low PaO_2, elevated $PaCO_2$, decreased or low-normal pH, and increased HCO_3^- levels. In early stages, there may be a normal or only slightly decreased PaO_2 and a normal $PaCO_2$. An ECG may be normal or show signs of right ventricular failure. An echocardiogram or multigated acquisition (MUGA) (cardiac blood pool) scan (see Table 32-6) can be used to evaluate right- and left-sided ventricular function. Sputum for culture and sensitivity may be obtained if the patient is hospitalized for an acute exacerbation and has not responded to empiric therapy with antibiotics.

Collaborative Care

Two major evidence-based references related to the care of COPD patients are (1) GOLD *(www.goldcopd.org)* and (2) clinical guidelines from the American College of Physicians.[15,16] Most patients are treated as outpatients. They are hospitalized for exacerbations and potential complications when respiratory failure, pneumonia, and cor pulmonale occur.

The GOLD guidelines present a rubric for assessing and diagnosing COPD (Fig. 29-11). You may be a part of the health care team that administers the mMRC or CAT and inquires about exacerbations. This information is used to detect COPD patients who are at risk for problems.[16]

Evaluate the patient's exposure to environmental or occupational irritants, and determine ways to control or avoid them. For example, teach the patient to avoid aerosol hair sprays and smoke-filled rooms. The patient with COPD is extremely susceptible to pulmonary infections. The patient with COPD and anyone who smokes should receive an influenza virus vaccine yearly. The pneumococcal vaccine (Pneumovax) is recommended for all smokers ages 19 or older and all patients with COPD.[21,33] (The guidelines for Pneumovax are presented in Table 28-5.)

Exacerbations of COPD should be treated as soon as possible, especially if the patient is in the severe stages. Some patients are given a prescription for antibiotics and are instructed to begin taking them when the first symptoms or signs of an exacerbation occur.[34]

Smoking Cessation. Cessation of cigarette smoking in any person with COPD at any level of severity is the most important intervention that can impact the natural history of COPD.[16] After a person discontinues smoking, the accelerated decline in pulmonary function found with smoking slows to almost nonsmoking levels.[21,29] Thus the sooner the smoker stops, the less pulmonary function is lost and the sooner the symptoms decrease, especially cough and sputum production. (Smoking cessation techniques are discussed in Chapter 11 and in Tables 11-4 to 11-6.)

Drug Therapy. Medications for COPD can reduce symptoms, increase exercise capacity, improve overall health, and reduce the number and severity of exacerbations. Bronchodilator drug therapy relaxes smooth muscles in the airway and improves the ventilation of the lungs, thus reducing the degree of breathlessness. Patients with COPD do not respond as dra-

TABLE 29-19 **DRUG THERAPY**

Medication Guidelines for Stable COPD

The treatment guidelines are based on the FEV_1 results.

FEV_1 Results	Treatment Guidelines*
FEV_1 60%-80% predicted (with respiratory symptoms)	Treatment with inhaled bronchodilators may be used.
FEV_1 <60% predicted (with respiratory symptoms)	Treat with inhaled bronchodilators: anticholinergics or long-acting β_2-agonist OR Monotherapy with long-acting inhaled anticholinergics or long-acting β_2-agonist OR Combination therapy with long-acting inhaled anticholinergics, long-acting β_2-agonist, or inhaled corticosteroids

*NOTE: Occasional use of short-acting inhaled bronchodilator for acute symptoms are not addressed in these recommendations.
Source: Qaseem A, Wilt T, Weinberger S, et al: Diagnosis and management of stable chronic obstructive pulmonary disease: a clinical practice guideline update from the American College of Physicians, American College of Chest Physicians, American Thoracic Society, and European Respiratory Society, *Ann Intern Med* 155:179, 2011.
FEV_1, Forced expiratory volume in 1 sec.

matically to bronchodilator therapy as those with asthma. However, bronchodilator therapy reduces dyspnea and increases FEV_1. The inhaled route of medication is preferred and given on a PRN or regular basis.

Patients commonly do not properly administer inhaled medications. Therefore it is important for you to demonstrate and talk with patients about inhaler use. Give the patient clear, readable instructions.[10]

Medications are given in a stepwise fashion according to the level of airflow obstruction determined from spirometry (FEV_1) and symptoms (see Fig. 29-11). Medications are stepped up but usually not stepped down, as in asthma, because in COPD continual symptoms are probably present (Table 29-19).

Bronchodilator medications commonly used are β_2-adrenergic agonists; anticholinergic agents; and, to a much lesser extent, methylxanthines (see Table 29-7). The choice of a bronchodilator depends on the patient's response. These medications are given on a PRN or scheduled basis. When the patient has mild COPD or fewer symptoms, a short-acting bronchodilator is used.[21] Albuterol or ipratropium may be used as single agents, but combining bronchodilators improves their effect and decreases the risk of adverse effects.[29] Albuterol and ipratropium can be nebulized together (DuoNeb) or delivered by inhalation spray (Combivent Respimat).

In the moderate stage of COPD (FEV_1 less than 60%), a long-acting bronchodilator may be used (see Tables 29-7 and 29-19). A short-acting bronchodilator may still be used PRN as a "rescue" for dyspnea. Salmeterol and formoterol are widely used LABAs, and they can be used in COPD as monotherapy (unlike drug therapy for asthma).[21] Indacaterol (Arcapta Neohaler) is the newest LABA with a duration of action of 24 hours, and thus it can be used just once a day.[16] Tiotropium (Spiriva), a long-acting anticholinergic, is used once a day.

The addition of an ICS to long-acting bronchodilator therapy is often prescribed in COPD patients with FEV_1 of less than 60%. Examples of combinations of ICSs with LABAs are fluticasone/salmeterol (Advair) and budesonide/formoterol (Symbicort). Inhaled long-acting anticholinergics, LABAs, or ICSs all reduce COPD exacerbations. However, in COPD, unlike asthma, ICSs are not used as monotherapy because of the concerns about side effects. Some patients are on triple therapy with Advair and tiotropium.[21] Oral corticosteroids should not be used for long-term therapy in COPD, but are effective for short-term use to treat exacerbations.

The use of long-acting theophylline in the treatment of COPD is controversial because it interacts with many drugs. A low dose of theophylline with an ICS may benefit a few patients with COPD who do not respond to other inhaled medications.

Roflumilast (Daliresp) is an oral medication used to decrease the frequency of exacerbations in severe COPD. This drug is a phosphodiesterase inhibitor, which is an antiinflammatory drug that suppresses the release of cytokines and other inflammatory mediators, and inhibits the production of reactive oxygen radicals.[21,35]

New drug delivery devices are becoming available at a rapid pace. One example is Respimat, which is an easy-to-use handheld device that provides a high deposition of drug to the lungs and low mouth and throat deposition. Respimat simplifies coordination between activation of the medication and inhalation without propellant, and it is independent of inspiratory flow. It also has a dose indicator. Combivent Respimat (ipratropium and albuterol) inhalation aerosol is now available.[36]

Oxygen Therapy. O_2 therapy is frequently used in the treatment of COPD and other problems associated with hypoxemia. Long-term continuous (more than 15 hr/day) O_2 therapy (LTOT) increases survival and improves exercise capacity and mental status in hypoxemic patients.[15,21]

Oxygen is a colorless, odorless, tasteless gas that constitutes 21% of the atmosphere. Administering supplemental O_2 increases the partial pressure of O_2 (PO_2) in inspired air. Used clinically, it is considered a drug. For reimbursement purposes, Medicare pays for oxygen when certain clinical criteria are met (i.e., the patient's O_2 saturation is 88% or less, and PaO_2 is 55 mm Hg or less).

Indications for Use. Goals for O_2 therapy are to keep the SaO_2 greater than 90% during rest, sleep, and exertion, or the PaO_2 greater than 60 mm Hg. O_2 is usually administered to treat hypoxemia caused by a variety of problems such as (1) respiratory disorders (e.g., COPD, pulmonary hypertension, cor pulmonale, pneumonia, lung cancer, pulmonary emboli); (2) cardiovascular disorders (e.g., myocardial infarction, dysrhythmias, angina pectoris, and cardiogenic shock); and (3) central nervous system disorders (e.g., overdose of opioids, head injury, sleep disorders [sleep apnea]).

Methods of Administration. The goal of O_2 administration is to supply the patient with adequate O_2 to maximize the oxygen-carrying ability of the blood. There are various methods of O_2 administration (Table 29-20 and Fig. 29-12). The method selected depends on factors such as the fraction of inspired O_2 (FIO_2) required by the patient and delivered by the device, the patient's mobility, humidification required, patient cooperation, comfort, cost, and financial resources.

O_2 delivery systems are classified as low- or high-flow systems. Most methods of O_2 administration are low-flow devices that deliver O_2 in concentrations that vary with the person's respiratory pattern. In contrast, the Venturi mask is a high-flow device that delivers fixed concentrations of O_2 (e.g., 24%, 28%) independent of the patient's respiratory pattern.

TABLE 29-20 METHODS OF OXYGEN ADMINISTRATION

Description	Nursing Interventions	
Low-Flow Delivery Devices		
Nasal Cannula		
• Most commonly used device. • O_2 delivered via plastic nasal prongs. • Safe and simple method that allows some freedom of movement. Patient can eat, talk, or cough while wearing device. • Useful for a patient requiring low O_2 concentrations. • O_2 concentrations of 24% (at 1 L/min) to 44% (at 6 L/min) can be obtained.	• Stabilize nasal cannula when caring for a restless patient. • Amount of O_2 inhaled depends on room air and patient's breathing pattern. • Most patients with COPD can tolerate 2 L/min via cannula. • Assess patient's nares and ears for skin breakdown. May need to pad cannula where it sits on ears. • If flow rates are >5 L/min, nasal membranes may dry and may cause pain in frontal sinuses.	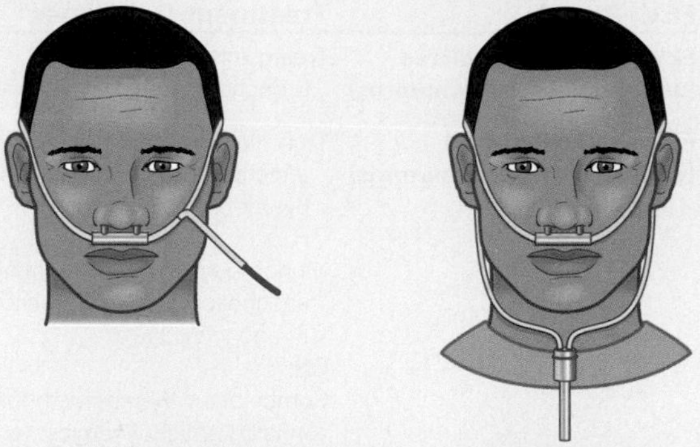
Simple Face Mask		
• Covers patient's nose and mouth. • Used only for short periods, especially when transporting patients. • Longer use is typically not tolerated because of tight seal and heat generated around nose and mouth from mask. • O_2 concentrations of 35%-50% can be achieved with flow rates of 6-12 L/min. • Mask provides adequate humidification of inspired air.	• Wash and dry under mask q2hr. • Mask must fit snugly. • Nasal cannula may be provided while patient is eating. • Watch for pressure necrosis at top of ears from elastic straps if patient wears for a longer time. (Gauze or other padding may alleviate this problem.)	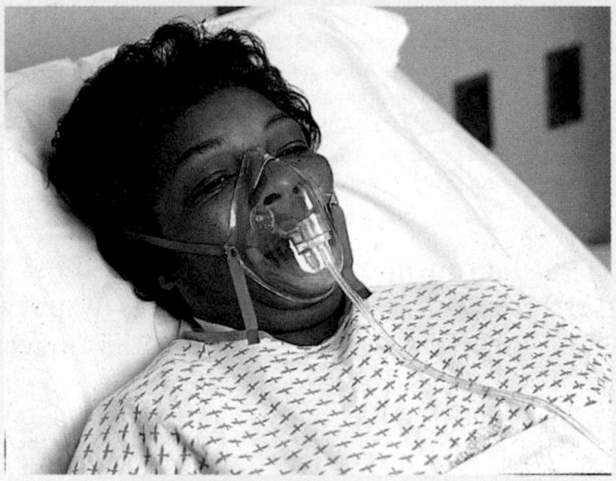
Partial and Non-Rebreather Masks		
• Useful for short-term (24 hr) therapy for patients needing higher O_2 concentrations (60%-90% at 10-15 L/min). • O_2 flows into reservoir bag and mask during inhalation. • This bag allows patient to rebreathe about first third of exhaled air (rich in O_2) in conjunction with flowing O_2. • Vents remain open on partial mask only. Some facilities prefer this over non-rebreather as a safety issue.	• O_2 flow rate must be sufficient to keep bag from collapsing during inspiration to avoid CO_2 buildup. • If deflation occurs, increase liter flow to keep bag inflated. • Mask should fit snugly. • With non-rebreather masks, make sure valves are open during expiration and closed during inhalation to prevent drastic decrease in FIO_2. • Monitor patient closely, since more advanced interventions may be required such as CPAP, BiPAP, or intubation with mechanical ventilation.	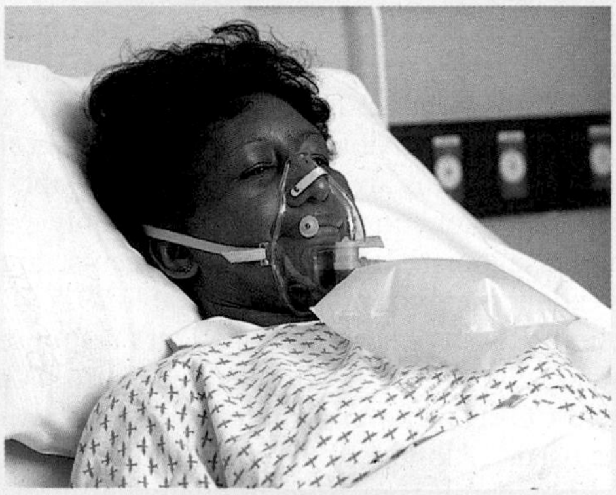
Oxygen-Conserving Cannula		
• Generally indicated for long-term O_2 therapy at home vs. during hospitalization (e.g., pulmonary fibrosis, pulmonary hypertension). • May be "moustache" (Oxymizer) or "pendant" type. • Cannula has a built-in reservoir that ↑ O_2 concentration and allows patient to use lower flow, usually 30%-50%, which increases comfort, lowers cost, and can be increased with activities. • Can deliver up to 8 L/min O_2.	• May cause necrosis over tops of ears. Can be padded. • Cannula cannot be cleaned. Manufacturer recommends changing cannula every week. • It is more expensive than standard cannulas and requires evaluation with ABGs and oximetry to determine correct flow for patient. • Cannula is highly visible.	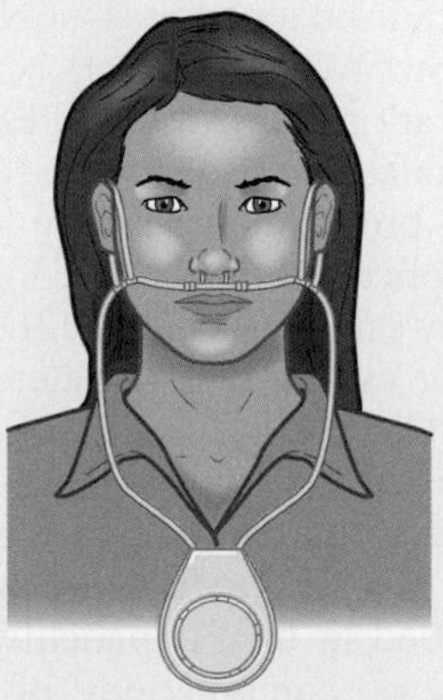 Pendant-type O_2-conserving cannula.

TABLE 29-20 METHODS OF OXYGEN ADMINISTRATION—cont'd

Description	Nursing Interventions
High-Flow Delivery Devices	
Tracheostomy Collar	
• Collar attaches to neck with elastic strap and can deliver high humidity and O_2 via tracheostomy. • O_2 concentration is lost into atmosphere because collar does not fit tightly. • Venturi device can be attached to flow meter and thus can deliver exact amounts of O_2 via collar.	• Secretions collect inside collar and around tracheostomy. Remove collar and clean at least q4hr to prevent aspiration of fluid and infection. • Because condensation occurs in tubing, periodically drain distally to tracheostomy.
Tracheostomy T Bar	
• Almost identical to tracheostomy collar, but it has a vent and a T connector that allow an inline catheter (e.g., Ballard catheter) to be connected for suctioning. • Tight fit allows better O_2 and humidity delivery than tracheostomy collar.	• Empty as necessary. • Because T bars disconnect easily, monitor closely. • T bar may pull on a patient's tracheostomy tube, causing irritation and potential tissue damage. Monitor this closely. • See tracheostomy collar above.
Venturi Mask	
• Mask can deliver precise, high-flow rates of O_2. • Lightweight plastic, cone-shaped device is fitted to face. • Masks are available for delivery of 24%, 28%, 31%, 35%, 40%, and 50% O_2. • Method is especially helpful for administering low, constant O_2 concentrations to patients with COPD. • Adaptors can be applied to increase humidification.	• Entrainment device on mask must be changed to deliver higher concentrations of O_2. • Air entrainment ports must not be occluded. • Mask is uncomfortable. Remove when patient eats. • Patient can talk but voice may be muffled. • See other applicable nursing interventions under simple face mask above.

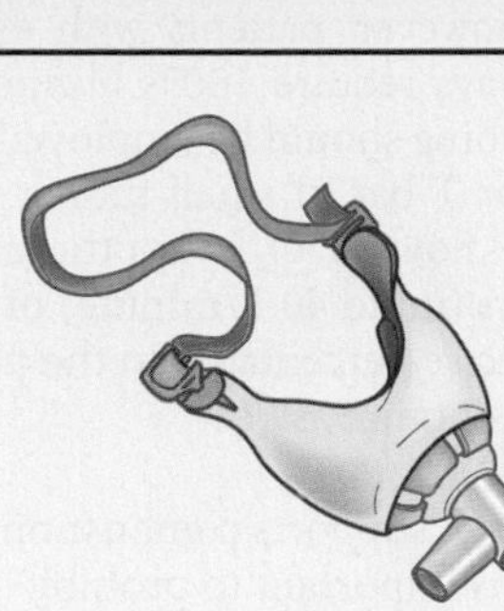

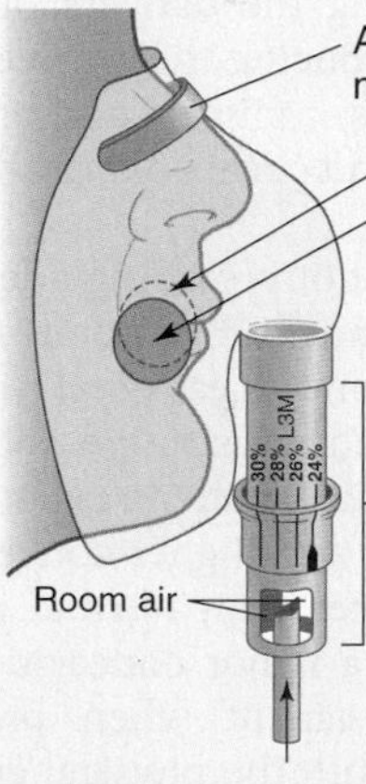

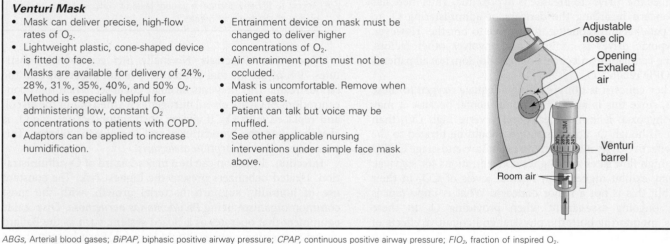

ABGs, Arterial blood gases; *BiPAP*, biphasic positive airway pressure; *CPAP*, continuous positive airway pressure; *FIO₂*, fraction of inspired O_2.

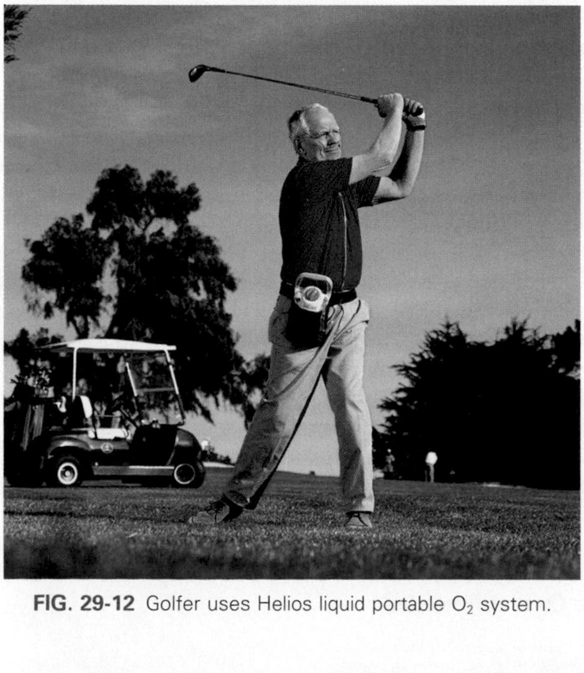

FIG. 29-12 Golfer uses Helios liquid portable O_2 system.

Mechanical ventilators are another example of a high-flow O_2 delivery system. Because room air is mixed with O_2, in low-flow systems the percentage of O_2 delivered to the patient is not as precise as with high-flow systems.

Humidification and Nebulization. O_2 obtained from cylinders or wall systems is dry. Dry O_2 has an irritating effect on mucous membranes and dries secretions. Therefore it is important that a high liter flow of O_2, delivering more than 35% to 50% O_2, be humidified, either by humidification or nebulization. A common device used for humidification when the patient has a cannula or a mask is a bubble-through humidifier. It is a small plastic jar filled with sterile distilled water that is attached to the O_2 source by means of a flow meter. O_2 passes into the jar, bubbles through the water, and then goes through tubing to the patient's cannula or mask. The purpose of the bubble-through humidifier is to restore the humidity conditions of room air. However, the need for bubble-through humidifiers at flow rates between 1 and 4 L/minute is based on the patient's comfort.

Another means of administering humidified O_2 is via a nebulizer. It delivers particulate water mist (aerosols) with nearly 100% humidity. The humidity can be increased by heating the water, which increases the gas's ability to hold moisture. Humidified (100%) gas is required when the upper airway is bypassed in acute care. However, patients with established tracheostomies do not always require 100% humidity. When nebulizers are used, large tubing should be employed to connect the device to a face mask or T bar. If small tubing is used, condensation can occlude the flow of O_2. Vapotherm Precision Flow can deliver high flows (up to 40 L/minute) of warm humidified gas (air/O_2) with precise percentages to the patient through a nasal cannula, and it is noninvasive.[37]

Complications

Combustion. O_2 supports combustion and increases the rate of burning, so it is important to prohibit smoking in the area in which O_2 is being used. A "No Smoking" sign should be prominently displayed on the patient's door. Also caution the patient against smoking cigarettes with an O_2 cannula in place.

Carbon Dioxide Narcosis. The chemoreceptors in the respiratory center that control the drive to breathe respond to CO_2 and O_2. Normally, CO_2 accumulation is the major stimulant of the respiratory center. Over time some COPD patients develop a tolerance for high CO_2 levels (the respiratory center loses its sensitivity to the elevated CO_2 levels). Theoretically, for these individuals the "drive" to breathe is hypoxemia. Thus there has been concern regarding the dangers of administering O_2 to COPD patients and reducing their drive to breathe. However, the "hypoxic drive" is complex and involves other factors, including ventilation and perfusion. In addition, not all patients with COPD retain CO_2.

The key concern is not providing adequate oxygen to these patients, since this is much more detrimental because it may lead to hypoxia. It is much easier to reverse high CO_2 than low O_2. Although O_2 administration should be titrated to the lowest effective dose, many patients who have end-stage COPD require high flow rates and higher concentrations for survival. They may exhibit higher than normal levels of CO_2 in their blood, but this is not a major concern. What is important is careful, ongoing assessment when providing O_2 to these patients, monitoring both the physical and cognitive effects of O_2 levels.

It is critical to start O_2 at low flow rates until ABGs can be obtained. ABGs are used as a guide to determine what FIO_2 level is sufficient and can be tolerated. Assess the patient's mental status and vital signs before starting O_2 therapy and frequently thereafter.

Oxygen Toxicity. Pulmonary **O_2 toxicity** may result from prolonged exposure to a high level of O_2 (PaO_2). High concentrations of oxygen can result in a severe inflammatory response because of oxygen radicals and damage to alveolar-capillary membranes resulting in severe pulmonary edema, shunting of blood, and hypoxemia. These individuals develop acute respiratory distress syndrome (ARDS) (see Chapter 68). Fortunately, O_2 toxicity is relatively rare.

Prevention of O_2 toxicity is important for the patient who is receiving O_2. The amount of O_2 administered should be just enough to maintain the PaO_2 within a normal or acceptable range for the patient. Monitor ABGs frequently to evaluate the effectiveness of therapy and to guide the tapering of supplemental O_2. A safe limit of O_2 concentrations has not yet been established. All levels above 50% and O_2 used for longer than 24 hours should be considered potentially toxic. Levels of 40% and below used for short periods may be regarded as relatively nontoxic and probably will not result in significant O_2 toxicity.

DELEGATION DECISIONS

Oxygen Administration

All members of the health care team should be alert to possible problems with gas exchange in patients who are receiving oxygenation. Patients who are hypoxemic should be cared for by the registered nurse (RN) until they consistently have O_2 saturations ≥90%.

Role of Registered Nurse (RN)

- Assess need for adjustments in O_2 flow rate.
- Evaluate response to O_2 therapy.
- Monitor patient for signs of adverse effects of O_2 therapy.
- In many cases, choose the optimal O_2 delivery device (e.g., a nasal cannula or simple face mask).
- Teach patient and caregivers about home O_2 use.

Role of Licensed Practical/Vocational Nurse (LPN/LVN)

- For stable patients, adjust O_2 flow rate depending on desired O_2 saturation level.

Role of Unlicensed Assistive Personnel (UAP)

- Use pulse oximetry to measure O_2 saturation.
- Report O_2 saturation level to RN.
- Assist patient with adjustment of O_2 delivery devices (e.g., nasal cannula, face mask).
- Report to RN any change in patient level of consciousness or complaints of shortness of breath.

Absorption Atelectasis. Normally, nitrogen (which constitutes 79% of the air that is breathed) is not absorbed into the bloodstream. This prevents alveolar collapse. When high concentrations of O_2 are given, nitrogen is washed out of the alveoli and replaced with O_2. If airway obstruction occurs, the O_2 is absorbed into the bloodstream and the alveoli collapse. This process is called *absorption atelectasis.*

Infection. Infection can be a major hazard of O_2 administration. Heated nebulizers present the highest risk. The constant use of humidity supports bacterial growth, with the most common organism being *Pseudomonas aeruginosa.* Disposable equipment that operates as a closed system, such as the Ballard closed suctioning system, should be used. Each hospital has a policy on the required frequency of equipment changes based on the type of equipment used.

Chronic Oxygen Therapy at Home. Improved survival occurs in patients with COPD who receive long-term O_2 therapy (LTOT) (more than 15 hr/day) to treat hypoxemia.[16,21] The improved prognosis results from preventing progression of the disease and subsequent cor pulmonale. The benefits of LTOT include improved mental acuity, sleep, and exercise tolerance; decreased hematocrit; and reduced pulmonary hypertension.

Some patients fear becoming "addicted" to O_2 and are reluctant to use it. Tell them that it is not "addicting" and that it needs to be used because of the positive effects on the heart, lungs, and brain. Evaluate the need for LTOT when the patient's condition has stabilized. The goal of O_2 therapy is to maintain SaO_2 greater than 90% during rest, sleep, and exertion.

Short-term home O_2 therapy (1 to 30 days) may be indicated for the patient in whom hypoxemia persists after discharge from the hospital. For example, a patient with underlying COPD who develops a serious respiratory tract infection may need continued O_2 therapy to treat hypoxemia for 4 to 6 weeks after discharge from the hospital. Measure the patient's oxygenation status by SaO_2 30 to 90 days after an acute episode to determine if the O_2 is still needed.

TABLE 29-21 HOME OXYGEN DELIVERY SYSTEMS*

- Liquid O_2
- Compressed O_2 cylinders
- Concentrator or extractor
- Portable O_2 concentrator
- O_2 conserving or pulsed devices

*Detailed descriptions of these delivery systems are presented in eTable 29-5 (available on the website for this chapter).

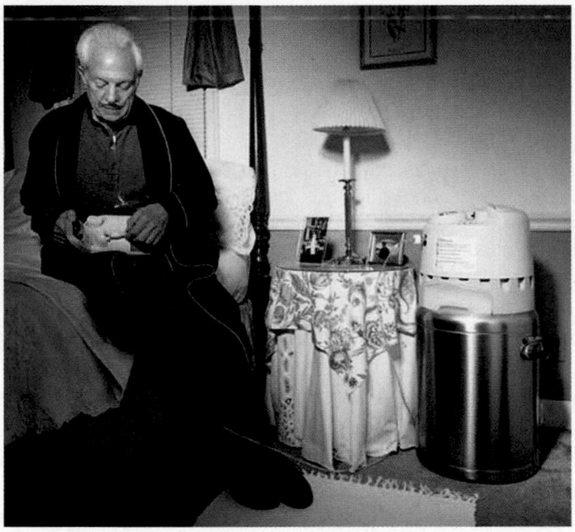

FIG. 29-13 A portable liquid O_2 unit can be refilled from a liquid O_2 reservoir unit.

Patients may receive O_2 only during exercise and/or sleep. Evaluate the need for O_2 during these periods with a 6-minute walk test or overnight oximetry. (Pulse oximetry is discussed in Chapter 26.)

Periodic reevaluations are necessary for the patient who is using chronic supplemental O_2. Generally, the patient should be reevaluated every 30 to 90 days during the first year of therapy and annually after that, as long as the patient remains stable.

Nasal cannulas, either regular or the O_2-conserving type (see Table 29-20), are usually used to deliver O_2 from a central source in the home. The source may be a liquid O_2 storage system, compressed O_2 in tanks, or an O_2 concentrator or extractor, depending on the patient's home environment, insurance coverage, activity level, and proximity to an O_2 supply company (Table 29-21). To increase mobility in the home, the patient can use extension tubing (up to 50 ft) without adversely affecting the O_2 flow delivery. Small, portable systems, such as liquid O_2, may be provided for the patient who remains active outside the home (see Fig. 29-12).

Home O_2 systems are usually rented from a company that sends a respiratory therapist to the patient's home (Fig. 29-13). The therapist teaches the patient and caregiver how to use the O_2 system, how to care for it, and how to recognize when the supply is running low and needs to be reordered. A patient and caregiver teaching guide for the use of O_2 at home is presented in Table 29-22.

Encourage the patient who uses home O_2 to remain active and travel normally. If travel is by automobile, arrangements can be made for O_2 to be available at the destination point. O_2 supply companies can often assist in these arrangements. If a patient wishes to travel by bus, train, or airplane, the patient should inform the appropriate people when reservations are made that O_2 will be needed for travel. If there is a potential for the patient to become hypoxic, O_2 needs for flying can be determined via a hypoxia inhalation test or through a mathematical formula. Portable oxygen concentrators are a ready source of renewable O_2 and can be available by recharging at home or with a DC (e.g., auto) power supply. These systems are widely approved by airlines for in-flight use. The patient should contact the airline to determine the particular accommodations and policies for in-flight O_2.

TABLE 29-22 PATIENT & CAREGIVER TEACHING GUIDE

Home Oxygen Use

The company that provides the prescribed O_2 therapy equipment will instruct the patient on equipment care. The following are some general instructions that you may include when teaching the patient and caregiver about the use of home O_2.

Decreasing Risk for Infection

- Brush teeth or use mouthwash several times a day.
- Wash nasal cannula (prongs) with a liquid soap and thoroughly rinse once or twice a week.
- Replace cannula every 2-4 wk.
- If you have a cold, replace the cannula after your symptoms pass.
- Always remove secretions that are coughed out.
- If you use an O_2 concentrator, every day unplug the unit and wipe down the cabinet with a damp cloth and dry it.
- Ask the company providing the equipment how often to change the filter.

Safety Issues

- Post "No Smoking" warning signs outside the home.
- O_2 will not "blow up," but it will increase the rate of burning, since it is a fuel for the fire.
- Do not allow smoking in the home, and do not smoke yourself while wearing O_2. Nasal cannulas and masks can catch fire and cause serious burns to face and airways.
- Do not use flammable liquids such as paint thinners, cleaning fluids, gasoline, kerosene, oil-based paints, or aerosol sprays while using O_2.
- Do not use blankets or fabrics that carry a static charge, such as wool or synthetics.
- Inform your electric company if you are using a concentrator. In case of a power failure, it will know the medical urgency of restoring your power.

Adapted from *www.YourLungHealth.org*.

Breathing Retraining. The patient with COPD has dyspnea with an increased respiratory rate. In addition, the accessory muscles of breathing in the neck and upper part of the chest are used excessively to promote chest wall movement. These muscles are not designed for long-term use, and as a result, the patient experiences increased fatigue.

The main types of breathing retraining exercises are (1) pursed-lip breathing and (2) diaphragmatic breathing. The purpose of **pursed-lip breathing (PLB)** is to prolong exhalation and thereby prevent bronchiolar collapse and air trapping. PLB is simple and easy to teach and learn, and it gives the patient more control over breathing, especially during exercise and periods of dyspnea[38] (see Table 29-13). Patients should be taught to use "just enough" positive pressure with the pursed lips because excessive resistance may increase the work of breathing.

Diaphragmatic (abdominal) breathing focuses on using the diaphragm instead of the accessory muscles of the chest to (1) achieve maximum inhalation and (2) slow the respiratory rate.[39] However, the use of diaphragmatic breathing in patients with COPD may increase the work of breathing and dyspnea. Patients with moderate to severe COPD with marked hyperinflation may be poor candidates for diaphragmatic breathing.[40]

PLB slows the respiratory rate and is easier to learn than diaphragmatic breathing. In the setting of extreme acute dyspnea, it is most important to focus on helping the patient slow the respiratory rate by using the principles of PLB. Other techniques that decrease breathing frequency, such as yoga, may also be used to reduce dyspnea.[40]

Airway Clearance Techniques. Many patients with COPD or other conditions (e.g., cystic fibrosis, bronchiectasis) who retain secretions require help to adequately clear their airways. Airway clearance techniques (ACTs) loosen mucus and secretions so they can be cleared by coughing. A variety of safe techniques can be used to achieve airway clearance. When ACTs are compared, it is primarily patient preference that determines which one is used.[41]

ACTs are especially beneficial in patients who have a COPD exacerbation.[42] Respiratory therapists, physical therapists, and nurses are involved in performing these techniques. ACTs are often used with other treatments. Typically the patient receives bronchodilator therapy via an inhaled device (e.g., nebulization) before ACT. Then the ACT is used, followed by effective coughing (e.g., huff coughing). ACTs include effective coughing, chest physiotherapy, airway clearance devices, and high-frequency chest ventilation.

Effective Coughing. Many patients with COPD have developed ineffective coughing patterns that do not adequately clear their airways of sputum. They also fear developing spastic coughing, resulting in increased dyspnea. Although other techniques (e.g., chest physiotherapy) are used to loosen secretions and mucus, the patient must cough effectively to bring the secretions to the central airways to expectorate them.

Huff coughing is an effective forced expiratory technique that you can easily teach the patient. Before starting, ensure that the patient is breathing deeply from the diaphragm. Place the patient's hands on the lower lateral chest wall, and then ask the patient to breathe deeply through the nose. You should feel the patient's hands move outward, which represents a breath from the diaphragm. Guidelines for effective huff coughing are presented in Table 29-23.

Chest Physiotherapy. **Chest physiotherapy (CPT)** is primarily used for patients with excessive bronchial secretions who have difficulty clearing them (e.g., cystic fibrosis, bronchiectasis). CPT consists of postural drainage, percussion, and vibration. CPT should be performed by an individual who has been properly trained.

Percussion and *vibration* are manual or mechanical techniques used to augment postural drainage. These techniques are used after the patient has assumed a postural drainage position to assist in loosening the mobilized secretions (see eFig. 29-1 on the website for this chapter). Percussion, vibration, and postural drainage assist in bringing secretions into larger, more central airways. Effective coughing (huff coughing) is then necessary to help raise these secretions.

Complications associated with improperly performed CPT include fractured ribs, bruising, hypoxemia, and discomfort.

TABLE 29-23 PATIENT & CAREGIVER TEACHING GUIDE

Effective Huff Coughing

When teaching effective huff coughing:

1. Help the patient assume a sitting position with head slightly flexed, shoulders relaxed, knees flexed, forearms supported by pillow, and, if possible, feet on the floor.

Then you should instruct the patient to:

2. Inhale slowly through the mouth while breathing deeply from the diaphragm.
3. Hold the breath for 2-3 seconds.
4. Forcefully exhale quickly as if one is fogging up a mirror with one's breath (thus creating a "huff"). (This moves the secretions to larger airways.)
5. Repeat the "huff" one or two more times while refraining from a "regular" cough.
6. Cough when mucus is felt in the breathing tubes.
7. Rest for five to ten regular breaths.
8. Repeat the huffs (three to five cycles) until you feel you have cleared mucus or you become tired.

CPT may be stressful for some patients, and some may develop hypoxemia and bronchospasms.

Postural Drainage. **Postural drainage** is the use of positioning techniques that drain secretions from specific segments of the lungs and bronchi into the trachea. The postural drainage positions used depend on the areas of lung that are involved. This is determined by patient assessment (including the patient's preference), chest x-rays, and chest auscultation. For example, some patients with left lower lobe involvement require postural drainage of only the affected region, whereas a person with cystic fibrosis may require postural drainage of all segments.

The purpose of various positions in postural drainage is to drain each segment toward the larger airways. A side-lying position can be used for the patient who cannot tolerate a head-down position. Aerosolized bronchodilators and hydration therapy are usually administered before postural drainage. The chosen postural drainage position is maintained for about 5 minutes during percussion and vibration. A common order is two to four times a day. In acute situations, postural drainage may be performed as frequently as every 4 hours. Schedule the procedure to be completed at least 1 hour before meals or 3 hours after meals.

Beds are available that can rotate and percuss in various postural drainage positions, and these are quite effective. Some positions for postural drainage (e.g., Trendelenburg) should not be performed on the patient with chest trauma, hemoptysis, heart disease, pulmonary embolus, or head injury, and in other situations where the patient's condition is not stable.

Percussion. *Percussion* is performed in the appropriate postural drainage position with the hands in a cuplike position, with the fingers and thumbs closed (Fig. 29-14). The cupped hand should create an air pocket between the patient's chest and the hand. Both hands are cupped and used in an alternating rhythmic fashion. Percussion is accomplished with flexion and extension of the wrists. If it is performed correctly, a hollow sound should be heard. The air-cushion impact facilitates the movement of thick mucus. Place a thin towel over the area to be percussed, or the patient may choose to wear a T-shirt or hospital gown.

Vibration. *Vibration* is accomplished by tensing the hand and arm muscles repeatedly and pressing mildly with the flat of

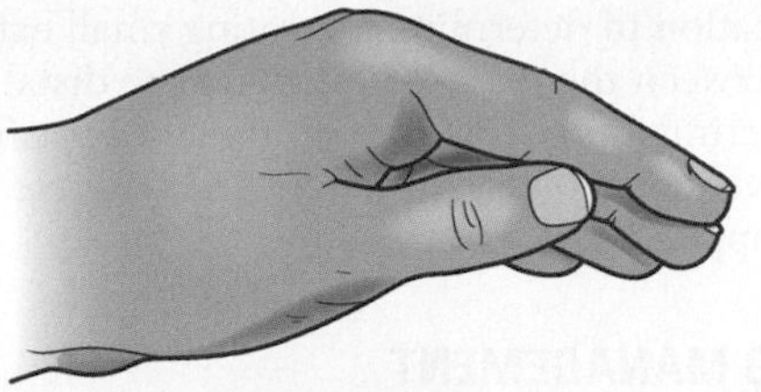

FIG. 29-14 Cupped-hand position for percussion. The hand should be cupped as though scooping up water.

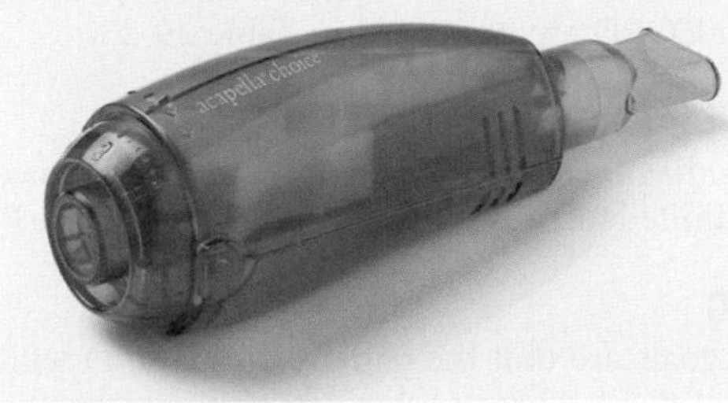

FIG. 29-15 Acapella airway clearance device.

the hand on the affected area while the patient slowly exhales a deep breath. The vibrations facilitate movement of secretions to larger airways. Mild vibration is tolerated better than percussion and can be used in situations where percussion may be contraindicated. Commercial vibrators are available for hospital and home use.

Airway Clearance Devices. Various *airway clearance devices* are available to mobilize secretions, are easier to tolerate than CPT, and take less time than conventional CPT sessions. These devices include the Flutter, Acapella, and TheraPEP Therapy System. These devices use the principle of positive expiratory pressure (PEP) and may provide greater benefit to patients with COPD than other ACTs.[42]

The Flutter mucus clearance device is a hand-held device that is shaped like a small, fat pipe (see eFig. 29-2 available on the website for this chapter). It provides PEP treatment for patients with mucus-producing conditions. The Flutter has a mouthpiece, a high-density stainless steel ball, and a cone that holds the ball. When the patient exhales through the Flutter, the steel ball moves, which causes oscillations (vibrations) in the airways and loosens mucus. It helps move mucus up through the airways to the mouth where the mucus can be expectorated. The patient must be upright, and the angle at which the Flutter is held is critical. The Acapella is another small hand-held device (Fig. 29-15) that combines the benefits of both PEP therapy and airway vibrations to mobilize pulmonary secretions. It can be used in virtually any setting, since patients are free to sit, stand, or recline. The patient may also inhale through the Acapella, and nebulizers can be attached to it. This saves time because the treatment does not have to be preceded by the nebulizer.

TheraPEP Therapy System can also provide sustained PEP and can simultaneously deliver aerosols so the patient can inhale and exhale through it. TheraPEP has a mouthpiece attached to tubing connected to a small cylindric resistor and a pressure indicator. The pressure indicator provides visual feedback about the pressure that the patient needs to hold in an exhalation to receive the PEP. The therapist initially determines the pressure, and you can reinforce the treatment. (A description and photo of this system are available at *www.smiths-medical.com/catalog/bronchial-hygiene/therapep/therapep-system.html.*)

High-Frequency Chest Wall Oscillation. High-frequency chest wall oscillation uses an inflatable vest (e.g., the Vest Airway system or the SmartVest) with hoses connected to a high-frequency pulse generator. (A description and photo are available at *www.thevest.com/products.*) The pulse generator delivers air to the vest, which vibrates the chest. The high-frequency airwaves dislodge mucus from the airways, mobilize the mucus, and move it toward larger airways. The vest can be used without the aid of another person. The units weigh 23 to 30 lb and are quiet. They come in a suitcase and are portable.

Nutritional Therapy. Many COPD patients in the advanced stages are underweight with loss of muscle mass and cachexia. Weight loss is a predictor of a poor prognosis and increased frequency of COPD exacerbations. Weight gain after nutritional support can decrease the risk of mortality.

The cause of weight loss is not entirely known. To some extent, loss of muscle mass is associated with aging. (Most people with COPD are older.) If the patient is on high doses of corticosteroids, the net effect is protein catabolism and loss of muscle mass. Eating becomes an effort because of the dyspnea related to the energy expended to chew, the reduction of airflow while swallowing, and O_2 desaturation.

Decreased appetite and weight loss also occur because of the systemic inflammatory process in COPD. The inflammation results in increased metabolism, which could explain why some individuals with COPD lose weight despite adequate nutritional intake.[43] Other factors that contribute to malnutrition in COPD include altered taste caused by chronic mouth breathing, excessive sputum, fatigue, anxiety, depression, increased energy needs, numerous infections, and side effects of polypharmacy.[44]

To decrease dyspnea and conserve energy, the patient should rest for at least 30 minutes before eating and use a bronchodilator before meals. Teach the patient to avoid exercise and treatments for at least 1 hour before and after eating. If a patient has O_2 therapy prescribed, use of supplemental O_2 by nasal cannula while eating may be beneficial. Assess the patient's dentition because broken or missing teeth or loose dentures make eating more difficult. Activity such as walking or getting out of bed during the day can stimulate the appetite and promote weight gain. Sensations of bloating and early satiety when eating can be attributed to swallowing air while eating, side effects of medication (especially corticosteroids and theophylline), and the abnormal position of the diaphragm relative to the stomach in association with hyperinflation of the lungs.

Fluid intake should be at least 3 L/day unless contraindicated by other medical conditions. Fluids should be taken between meals (rather than with them) to prevent excess stomach distention and to decrease pressure on the diaphragm. Sodium restriction may be indicated if there is accompanying heart failure.

Getting the patient to eat adequate amounts of nutritionally sound foods may be difficult even though well-balanced meals are available. Give the patient or meal preparer printed information that can make mealtime easier and more nutritious (Table 29-24).

Underweight patients with COPD need extra protein and calories. They may need 25 to 45 kcal/kg body weight and more than 1.5 g of protein/kg body weight to maintain their weight.[45] The patient with excessive malnutrition may need up to 2.5 g of protein/kg of body weight to restore muscle mass.

TABLE 29-24 NUTRITIONAL THERAPY

Maximizing Food Intake in COPD

Sometimes it is difficult for patients with COPD to consume adequate amounts of nutrients. Teach the patients to make mealtimes easier and more nutritious by increasing calories and protein without increasing the amount of food eaten.

- Eat high-calorie foods first.
- Limit liquids at mealtimes.
- Rest before meals.
- Try more frequent meals and snacks.
- Increase calories by adding margarine, butter, mayonnaise, sauces, gravies, and peanut butter to foods.
- Keep favorite foods and snacks on hand.
- Try cold foods, which can make you feel less full than hot foods.
- Keep ready-prepared meals available for times when you have increased shortness of breath.
- Eat larger meals when you are not as tired.
- Avoid foods that you know cause gas (e.g., cabbage, beans, cauliflower).
- Add skim milk powder (2 tbs) to regular milk (8 oz) to add protein and calories.
- Use milk or half-and-half instead of water when making soups, cereals, instant puddings, cocoa, or canned soups.
- Add grated cheese to sauces, vegetables, soups, and casseroles.
- Choose dessert recipes that contain egg (e.g., sponge cake, angel food cake, egg custard, bread pudding, rice pudding).

Source: Grodner M, Roth S, Walkingshaw B: *Nutritional foundations and clinical applications: a nursing approach,* ed 5, St Louis, 2011, Mosby.

A diet high in calories and protein, moderate in carbohydrate, and moderate to high in fat is recommended and can be divided into five or six small meals a day.[46] High-protein, high-calorie nutritional supplements can be offered between meals. Nonprotein calories should be divided evenly between fat and carbohydrate, but avoid overfeeding the patient (see Table 29-24).

The dietitian is the best resource to determine what combination of nutrients and what supplements are best for the patient.[44] (Nutritional supplements are discussed in Chapter 40.)

Surgical Therapy for COPD. Three different surgical procedures have been used in severe COPD. One type of surgery is *lung volume reduction surgery* (LVRS). The goal of this surgery is to reduce the size of the lungs by removing the most diseased lung tissue so the remaining healthy lung tissue can perform better. The rationale for LVRS is that reducing the size of the hyperinflated emphysematous lungs results in decreased airway obstruction and increased room for the remaining normal alveoli to expand and function. The procedure reduces lung volume and improves lung and chest wall mechanics. LVRS is being explored as a therapy that can be performed via a bronchoscope (BLVR).[16]

The second surgical procedure is *bullectomy.* This procedure is used for carefully selected patients with emphysematous COPD who have large bullae (larger than 1 cm). The bullae are usually resected via thoracoscope.

The third surgical procedure is *lung transplantation,* which benefits carefully selected patients with advanced COPD. Although single-lung transplant is the most commonly used technique because of a shortage of donors, bilateral transplantation can be performed. (Lung transplantation is discussed in Chapters 14 and 28.)

A novel approach is being explored for patients with emphysema. Airway bypass is a bronchoscopic procedure currently under evaluation to determine if creating small extra-anatomic openings between the diseased lung and the distal bronchi can reduce hyperinflation. This is a minimally invasive treatment that improves pulmonary function and reduces dyspnea by enabling trapped air to exit the lungs.[47]

NURSING MANAGEMENT CHRONIC OBSTRUCTIVE PULMONARY DISEASE

NURSING ASSESSMENT

Subjective and objective data that should be obtained from a person with COPD are presented in Table 29-25.

NURSING DIAGNOSES

The nursing diagnoses for the patient with COPD may include, but are not limited to, those presented in Nursing Care Plan 29-2.

PLANNING

The overall goals are that the patient with COPD will have (1) prevention of disease progression, (2) ability to perform ADLs and improved exercise tolerance, (3) relief from symptoms, (4) no complications related to COPD, (5) knowledge and ability to implement a long-term treatment regimen, and (6) overall improved quality of life.

NURSING IMPLEMENTATION

HEALTH PROMOTION. The incidence of COPD would decrease dramatically if people would not begin smoking or would stop smoking. (Techniques to help patients stop smoking are discussed in Chapter 11 and Tables 11-4 to 11-6.) Avoiding or controlling exposure to occupational and environmental pollutants and irritants is another preventive measure to maintain healthy lungs. (These factors are discussed in the section on nursing management of lung cancer in Chapter 28.)

Counseling the patient in smoking cessation is vital, because it is the only way to slow the progression of COPD. As health care professionals, nurses who smoke should reevaluate their own smoking behavior and its relationship to their health. Nurses and other health care providers who smoke should be aware that the odor of smoke is obvious on their clothes, and it can be offensive or tempting to patients.

Early diagnosis and treatment of respiratory tract infections and exacerbations of COPD help prevent progression of the disease. People with COPD should avoid others who are sick, practice good hand-washing techniques, take medications as prescribed, exercise regularly, and maintain a healthy weight. Influenza and pneumococcal pneumonia vaccines are recommended for patients with COPD.

Families with a history of COPD, as well as AAT deficiency, should be aware of the genetic nature of the disease. These individuals should consult a pulmonologist about regular spirometry screening even though they do not have symptoms. Genetic counseling is appropriate for the patient with AAT deficiency who is planning to have children.

ACUTE INTERVENTION. The patient with COPD requires acute intervention for complications such as exacerbations of COPD, pneumonia, cor pulmonale, and acute respiratory failure. (The nursing care for these conditions is discussed in Chapters 28 and 68.) Once the crisis in these situations has been resolved, assess the degree and severity of the underlying respiratory problem. The information obtained will help in planning the nursing care.

TABLE 29-25 **NURSING ASSESSMENT**

Chronic Obstructive Pulmonary Disease

Subjective Data	Objective Data
Important Health Information	**General**
Past health history: Long-term exposure to chemical pollutants, respiratory irritants, occupational fumes, dust; recurrent respiratory tract infections; previous hospitalizations	Debilitation, restlessness, assumption of upright position
Medications: Use of O_2 and duration of O_2 use, bronchodilators, corticosteroids, antibiotics, anticholinergics, OTC drugs, herbs, medications purchased outside United States	**Integumentary** Cyanosis (bronchitis), pallor or ruddy color, poor skin turgor, thin skin, digital clubbing, easy bruising; peripheral edema (cor pulmonale)
Functional Health Patterns	**Respiratory**
Health perception–health management: Smoking (pack-years, including passive smoking, willingness to stop smoking, and previous attempts); family history of respiratory disease (especially α_1-antitrypsin deficiency)	Rapid, shallow breathing; inability to speak; prolonged expiratory phase; pursed-lip breathing; wheezing; rhonchi, crackles, diminished or bronchial breath sounds; ↓ chest excursion and diaphragm movement; use of accessory muscles; hyperresonant or dull chest sounds on percussion
Nutritional-metabolic: Anorexia, weight loss or gain	
Activity-exercise: Increasing dyspnea and/or increase in sputum volume or purulence (to detect exacerbation); fatigue, ability to perform ADLs; swelling of feet; progressive dyspnea, especially on exertion; ability to walk up one flight of stairs without stopping; wheezing; recurrent cough; sputum production (especially in the morning); orthopnea	**Cardiovascular** Tachycardia, dysrhythmias, jugular venous distention, distant heart tones, right-sided S_3 (cor pulmonale), edema (especially in feet)
Elimination: Constipation, gas, bloating	**Gastrointestinal** Ascites, hepatomegaly (cor pulmonale)
Sleep-rest: Insomnia; sitting up position for sleeping, paroxysmal nocturnal dyspnea	**Musculoskeletal** Muscle atrophy, ↑ anteroposterior diameter (barrel chest)
Cognitive-perceptual: Headache, chest or abdominal soreness	
Coping–stress tolerance: Anxiety, depression	**Possible Diagnostic Findings** Abnormal ABGs (compensated respiratory acidosis, ↓ PaO_2 or SaO_2, ↑ $PaCO_2$), polycythemia, pulmonary function tests showing expiratory airflow obstruction (e.g., low FEV_1, low FEV_1/FVC, large RV), chest x-ray showing flattened diaphragm and hyperinflation or infiltrates

ABGs, Arterial blood gases; *FEV_1,* forced expiratory volume in 1 sec; *FVC,* forced vital capacity; *RV,* residual volume.

AMBULATORY AND HOME CARE. By far the most important aspect in the long-term care of the patient with COPD is teaching. (A patient and caregiver teaching guide is presented in Table 29-26.)

Pulmonary Rehabilitation. Pulmonary rehabilitation (PR) is an evidence-based intervention that includes many disciplines working together to individualize treatment of the symptomatic COPD patient. PR is designed to reduce symptoms and improve quality of life. PR is an effective intervention to improve exercise capacity and decrease hospitalizations, anxiety, and depression.[48,49] PR should no longer be viewed as a "last ditch" effort for patients with severe COPD.

PR can be done in an inpatient or outpatient setting or in the home. Components of PR vary, but usually include exercise training, smoking cessation, nutrition counseling, and education. A mandatory component of any PR program is exercise that focuses on the muscles used in ambulation, but upper limb exercises may be included also. Smoking cessation is critical to the patient's success. Some rehabilitation programs do not accept patients who are current smokers and not committed to quitting. Physical therapists or nurses who have experience in pulmonary care are often responsible for the management of pulmonary rehabilitation centers. A large part of your role is to teach patients self-management of their disease.

The minimum length of an effective program is 6 weeks with many insurance plans paying for it, but the longer the program, the more effective the results. Other important topics include health promotion, psychologic counseling, and vocational rehabilitation. One benefit of group PR appears to be the development of social relationships and support from peers and health care providers that boost patient's' self-confidence, coping, and motivation for self-care.[50]

PR groups may be inaccessible to many because of cost, disability, transportation, or geographic location. One alternative program uses the Internet to deliver daily motivational messages that are linked with individualized walking goals and feedback related to pedometer use.[51] Another program uses telehealth for homebound older adults with COPD with daily objective measures of health (e.g., weight, O_2 saturation). This information is received centrally by a nurse who calls back the patient for further evaluation if parameters are abnormal.[52]

Activity Considerations. Exercise training leads to energy conservation, which is an important component in COPD rehabilitation. The patient with severe COPD typically uses upper thoracic and neck muscles to breathe rather than the diaphragm. Thus the patient has difficulty performing upper-extremity

INFORMATICS IN PRACTICE

Texting for Chronic Obstructive Pulmonary Disease (COPD) Patients

- Sometimes patients with COPD or those requiring O_2 therapy experience difficulty speaking because of shortness of breath.
- Encourage your patient to use typed messages displayed on a monitor to communicate.
- Texting and instant messaging family and friends are good alternatives to having phone conversations.

NURSING CARE PLAN 29-2

Patient With Chronic Obstructive Pulmonary Disease

NURSING DIAGNOSIS* **Ineffective breathing pattern** *related to* alveolar hypoventilation, anxiety, chest wall alterations, and hyperventilation *as evidenced by* assumption of three-point position, dyspnea, increased anteroposterior diameter of chest, nasal flaring, orthopnea, prolonged expiration, pursed-lip breathing, use of accessory muscles to breathe

PATIENT GOALS
1. Returns to baseline respiratory function
2. Demonstrates an effective rate, rhythm, and depth of respirations

Outcomes (NOC)

Respiratory Status: Ventilation
- Respiratory rate ____
- Respiratory rhythm ____
- Depth of inspiration ____
- Pulmonary function tests ____

Measurement Scale
1 = Severe deviation from normal range
2 = Substantial deviation from normal range
3 = Moderate deviation from normal range
4 = Mild deviation from normal range
5 = No deviation from normal range

- Accessory muscle use ____
- Pursed-lip breathing ____
- Orthopnea ____
- Impaired expiration ____

Measurement Scale
1 = Severe
2 = Substantial
3 = Moderate
4 = Mild
5 = None

Interventions (NIC) and *Rationales*

Ventilation Assistance
- Monitor respiratory and oxygenation status *to assess need for intervention.*
- Auscultate breath sounds, noting areas of decreased or absent ventilation and presence of adventitious sounds *to obtain ongoing data on patient's response to therapy.*
- Encourage slow, deep breathing; turning; and coughing *to promote effective breathing techniques and secretion mobilization.*
- Administer medications (e.g., bronchodilators and inhalers) that promote airway patency and gas exchange.
- Position to minimize respiratory efforts (e.g., elevate head of the bed and provide overbed table for patient to lean on) *to save energy for breathing.*
- Monitor for respiratory muscle fatigue *to determine a need for ventilatory assistance.*
- Initiate a program of respiratory muscle strength and/or endurance training *to establish effective breathing patterns and techniques.*

NURSING DIAGNOSIS **Ineffective airway clearance** *related to* expiratory airflow obstruction, ineffective cough, decreased airway humidity, and tenacious secretions *as evidenced by* ineffective or absent cough, presence of abnormal breath sounds, or absence of breath sounds

PATIENT GOALS
1. Maintains clear airway by effectively coughing
2. Experiences clear breath sounds

Outcomes (NOC)

Respiratory Status: Airway Patency
- Adventitious breath sounds ____
- Anxiety ____
- Gasping ____
- Choking ____

Measurement Scale
1 = Severe
2 = Substantial
3 = Moderate
4 = Mild
5 = None

Interventions (NIC) and *Rationales*

Cough Enhancement
- Assist patient to sitting position with head slightly flexed, shoulders relaxed, and knees flexed *to allow for adequate chest expansion.*
- Instruct patient to inhale deeply, bend forward slightly, and perform three or four huffs (against an open glottis) *to prevent airway collapse during exhalation.*†
- Instruct patient to inhale deeply several times, exhale slowly, and cough at the end of exhalation *to loosen secretions before coughing.*
- Instruct the patient to follow coughing with several maximal inhalation breaths *to reoxygenate the lungs.*

Airway Management
- Encourage slow, deep breathing; turning; and coughing *to mobilize pulmonary secretions.*
- Position patient *to maximize ventilation potential.*
- Regulate fluid intake to optimize fluid balance *to liquefy secretions for easier expectoration.*
- Perform endotracheal or nasotracheal suctioning as appropriate *to clear the airway.*
- Administer bronchodilators and use airway clearance devices *to facilitate clearance of retained secretions and increase ease of breathing.*

NURSING DIAGNOSIS **Impaired gas exchange** *related to* alveolar hypoventilation *as evidenced by* headache on awakening, $PaCO_2 \geq 45$ mm Hg, $PaO_2 < 60$ mm Hg, or $SaO_2 < 90\%$ at rest

PATIENT GOALS
1. Returns to baseline respiratory function
2. $PaCO_2$ and PaO_2 return to levels normal for patient

Outcomes (NOC)

Respiratory Status: Gas Exchange
- PaO_2 ____
- $PaCO_2$ ____
- Arterial pH ____
- Chest x-ray findings ____

Measurement Scale
1 = Severe deviation from normal range
2 = Substantial deviation from normal range
3 = Moderate deviation from normal range
4 = Mild deviation from normal range
5 = No deviation from normal range

Interventions (NIC) and *Rationales*

Oxygen Therapy
- Administer supplemental O_2 as ordered.
- Set up O_2 equipment and administer through a heated, humidified system to provide moist O_2.
- Periodically check O_2 delivery device *to ensure that the prescribed concentration is being delivered.*
- Monitor the effectiveness of O_2 therapy (e.g., pulse oximetry, ABGs) *to evaluate patient response to therapy.*
- Observe for signs of O_2-induced hypoventilation *because this occurs with CO_2 narcosis.*
- Instruct patient and family about use of O_2 at home *to promote safe long-term O_2 therapy.*

*Nursing diagnoses listed in order of priority.
†Guidelines for effective huff coughing are presented in Table 29-23.

TABLE 29-26 PATIENT & CAREGIVER TEACHING GUIDE

Chronic Obstructive Pulmonary Disease

Include the following information in the teaching plan to assist the patient and caregiver to improve quality of life through teaching and promotion of lifestyle practices that support successful living with chronic obstructive pulmonary disease (COPD).

Teaching Topic	Resources
Overall Guide	*Patient Guide: What You Can Do About a Lung Disease Called COPD* (Global Initiative for Lung Disease). Retrieved from *www.goldcopd.org/uploads/users/files/GOLD_Patient_RevJan10.pdf.* (Also available in other languages.)
What Is COPD? • Basic anatomy and physiology of lung • Basic pathophysiology of COPD • Signs and symptoms of COPD, exacerbation, cold, flu, pneumonia • Tests to assess breathing	*COPD Statement: Patient Education Section* (American Thoracic Society [ATS]). Retrieved from *www.thoracic.org.* (Also available in Spanish.) *How Lungs Work* (American Lung Association [ALA]). Available under "Your Lungs" at *www.lung.org/your-lungs.*
Breathing and Airway Clearance Exercises • Pursed-lip breathing • Airway clearance technique—huff cough	 See Table 29-13. See Table 29-23.
Energy Conservation Techniques • Daily activities (e.g., waking up, bathing, grooming, shopping, traveling)	Consult with physical therapist and occupational therapist. *COPD: Lifestyle Management* (National Jewish Health). Retrieved from *www.nationaljewish.org/healthinfo/conditions/copd-chronic-obstructive-pulmonary-disease/lifestyle-management.*
Medications Types (include mechanism of action and types of devices) • Methylxanthines • β_2-Adrenergic agonists • Corticosteroids • Anticholinergics • Antibiotics • Other medications Establishing medication schedule	*COPD Statement: Patient Education Section: Medications and Other Treatments OR Patient Information Series: Medicines to Treat COPD* (ATS). Retrieved from *www.thoracic.org.* OR *COPD Medicines* (ALA). Retrieved from *www.lungusa.org.* OR *COPD Medications* (National Jewish Health). Search "COPD medications." Also has link to medication chart to take to provider. Retrieved from *www.nationaljewish.org/healthinfo.*
Correct Use of Inhalers, Spacer, and Nebulizer	See Figs. 29-5 to 29-7. See Tables 29-8 to 29-10. See Table 29-15 for links to videos on medication devices.
Home Oxygen • Explanation of rationale for use • Guide for home O_2 use and equipment	*Oxygen Therapy* (National Jewish Health). Retrieved from *www.nationaljewish.org/healthinfo/medications/lung-diseases/treatments/oxygen-therapy.* *Traveling With Oxygen* (American College of Chest Physicians). Retrieved from *www.chestnet.org/accp/patient-guides/traveling-oxygen.*
Psychosocial/Emotional Issues Concerns about interpersonal relationships • Dependency • Intimacy Problems with emotions • Depression, anxiety, panic Treatment decisions • Support and rehabilitation groups End-of-life issues	Open discussion (sharing with patient, significant other, and family). *Living With COPD: Get Social Support* (ALA help line, Better Breathers Club, and printed materials). Retrieved from *www.lung.org/lung-disease/copd/living-with-copd/get-social-support.html.* *Questions About Pulmonary Rehabilitation* (ATS). Retrieved from *patients.thoracic.org/materials/index.php.* (Available in English and Spanish.)
COPD Management Plan • Focus on self-management • Need to report changes • Cause of flare-ups or exacerbation • Recognition of signs and symptoms of respiratory infection, heart failure • Reduce risk factors, especially smoking cessation • Exercise program of walking and arm strengthening • Yearly follow-up	Nurse and patient develop and write up COPD management plan that meets individual needs. *COPD Management Tools* (ALA). Retrieved from *www.lung.org/lung-disease/copd/living-with-copd/copd-management-tools.html.*
Healthy Nutrition • Strategies to lose weight (if overweight) • Strategies to gain weight (if underweight)	Consultation with dietitian. See Table 29-24. *Nutrition* (ALA). Retrieved from *www.lung.org/lung-disease/copd/living-with-copd/nutrition.html.*

activities, particularly those that require raising the arm above the head. Exercise training of the upper extremities may improve muscle function and help to reduce dyspnea.

Frequently the patient has already adapted alternative energy-saving practices for ADLs. Alternative methods of hair care, shaving, showering, and reaching may need to be explored. An occupational therapist may help with ideas in these areas. Assuming a tripod posture (elbows supported on a table, chest in fixed position) and placing a mirror on the table while using an electric razor or hair dryer conserve much more energy than when the patient stands in front of a mirror to shave or blow-dry hair.

If the patient uses home O_2 therapy, O_2 should be used during activities of hygiene because these are energy consuming. Encourage the patient to make a schedule and plan daily and weekly activities to leave plenty of time for rest periods. The patient should also try to sit as much as possible when performing activities. Another energy-saving tip is to exhale when pushing, pulling, or exerting effort during an activity and inhale during rest.

Regular physical exercise is important for patients with COPD. To ensure long-term adherence, the exercise must be individualized and easy to perform. Walking or other endurance exercises (e.g., cycling) combined with strength training are likely the best interventions to strengthen muscles and improve the patient's endurance. Teach the patient coordinated walking with slow, pursed-lip breathing—breathing in through the nose while taking one step, then breathing out through pursed lips while taking two to four steps.

When patients are home, the adherence to exercise may wane. A simple but effective way to sustain optimal exercise intensity with positive outcomes (i.e., no exacerbations) in home settings is to use a metronome. The level of exercise intensity is established on a treadmill by the appropriate health care provider using a metronome. The patient then uses the clip-on metronome to maintain the rate and intensity of walking (instead of trying to walk a certain amount of time).[48]

At times patients may need rest periods and sit or lean against an object such as a tree or post. The patient may need to ambulate using O_2. Walk with the patient, giving verbal reminders when necessary regarding breathing (inhalation and exhalation) and steps. Walking with the patient helps decrease anxiety and helps maintain a slow pace. It also enables you to observe the patient's actions and physiologic responses to the activity. Many patients with moderate or severe COPD are anxious and fearful of walking or performing exercise. These patients and their caregivers require support while they build the confidence they need to walk or to perform daily exercises.

In many situations PR programs are not an option, and patients are advised to exercise on their own. If possible, arrange a one-time consult with the physical therapist to outline an exercise program for the patient that can be followed at home and that you can reinforce in the outpatient setting. Encourage the patient to walk 15 to 20 minutes a day at least three times a week with gradual increases. Severely disabled patients can begin at a slow pace by walking for 2 to 5 minutes three times a day and slowly building up to 20 minutes a day, if possible.

Some patients benefit from using their β_2-adrenergic agonist approximately 10 minutes before exercise. Parameters that may be monitored in the patient with mild COPD are resting pulse and pulse rate after walking. Pulse rate after walking should not exceed 75% to 80% of the maximum heart rate (maximum heart rate is age in years subtracted from 220). In some patients, exercise is limited by dyspnea and the limitation in breathing, rather than increased heart rate. Thus it is better to use the patient's perceived sense of dyspnea as an indication of exercise tolerance.

Tell the patient that shortness of breath will probably increase during exercise (as it does for a healthy individual) but that the activity is not being overdone if this increased shortness of breath returns to baseline within 5 minutes after cessation of exercise. Instruct the patient to wait 5 minutes after completion of exercise before using the β_2-adrenergic agonist to allow a chance to recover. During this time, slow, pursed-lip breathing should be used. If it takes longer than 5 minutes to return to baseline, the patient most likely has overdone it and should proceed at a slower pace during the next exercise period. The patient may benefit from keeping a diary or log of the exercise program. The diary can help provide a realistic evaluation of the patient's progress. In addition, the diary can help motivate the patient and add to the patient's sense of accomplishment. Stationary cycling can also be used either alone or with walking. Cycles and treadmills are particularly good when weather prevents walking outside.

Fatigue, sleep disturbances, and dyspnea are common complaints of patients with COPD. Of these symptoms, dyspnea appears to be the only one that affects the patient's ability to carry out daily activities. Therefore you and other health team members should focus your interventions on improving dyspnea, which would then improve the patient's functional performance. Nutritional counseling (discussed previously) is integral to a PR program. Teaching is an important component of PR and should include information on self-management and prevention and treatment of exacerbations (see Table 29-26).

Sexuality and Sexual Activity. Modifying but not abstaining from sexual activity can also contribute to a healthy psychologic well-being. Most patients with COPD are older. Assess and reflect on your own attitudes and feelings about sexuality, sexual functioning, and aging before exploring sexual issues with the older COPD patient. First assess the patient's concerns related to sexuality and functioning. Ask open-ended questions to determine if the patient wants to discuss any of these concerns. You could ask, "How has your breathing problem affected how you see yourself as a woman or man?" Another question could be, "How does your shortness of breath affect your desire for intimacy with your partner?" These types of questions give the person an opening to discuss concerns. Much of the sexual performance issues experienced by the patient with COPD are changes related to aging, and if you are aware of these changes, you can teach the patient the "normalcy" of the changes.

Dyspnea, the predominant symptom in COPD, should not be a major problem with success in sexual functioning, except for those patients in severe stages. If the patient can walk up two flights of stairs or walk briskly, he or she likely has sufficient energy for sexual activity. Erectile dysfunction can occur with COPD as with many chronic diseases. Using an inhaled bronchodilator before sexual activity can help ventilation. The patient with COPD may also find these suggestions helpful: (1) plan sexual activity during the part of the day when breathing is best, which is usually late morning or early afternoon (plus older men often achieve an erection more easily in the morning); (2) use slow pursed-lip breathing; (3) refrain from sexual activity after eating or drinking alcohol; (4) choose less stressful positions during intercourse (missionary position for men is the worst); (5) use O_2 if prescribed; and (6) understand that cigarettes can increase male impotence. Often the patient has coexisting cardiac disease and should obtain advice from a health care provider related to appropriate levels of activity. These aspects of sexual activity require open communication between partners regarding their needs and expectations and the changes that may be necessary as the result of a chronic disease (e.g., changes in body image, role reversal).[53,54]

Sleep. Adequate sleep is extremely important to maintain quality of life and productivity. Patients with COPD have an increased prevalence of sleep disorders. The hyperinflation of the lungs and the reduction in ventilation can result in severe drops in O_2 saturation (down to 60% or less) during sleep. This leads to a strain on the heart. In addition, hypercapnia may develop with more frequent awakening. The net result is sleeping poorly and awakening unrefreshed and fatigued.

Current tobacco use, depression, and anxiety are all common in COPD and lead to more trouble sleeping. β_2-Agonists may

ETHICAL/LEGAL DILEMMAS

Advance Directives

Situation

L.H., a 79-year-old man with COPD, is in respiratory failure when he is admitted to the hospital. He is placed on a ventilator and responds occasionally by opening his eyes. His advance directives (ADs) were drawn up 5 years ago, and copies were given to his wife and health care provider at that time. The patient's wife brings the documents to the intensive care unit and tells you that the hospital must stop treating her husband and allow him to die as he requested. However, the patient's oldest son is threatening the hospital with a lawsuit if the staff does not provide full care to his father.

Ethical/Legal Points for Consideration

- A Living Will, one form of AD, permits individuals to state their own preferences and refusals should the individual become terminally ill or be in a situation where there is no hope of recovery, and the person is not able to speak for himself or herself.*
- The Durable Power Attorney for Health Care, another form of AD, permits individuals to identify a proxy to make health care decisions in the event the individual is incapacitated.
- AD laws vary from state to state concerning the need for witnesses and who the proxy is.
- Some families are deeply divided about decisions for their loved ones, and conflicts often arise when money and property are involved.
- Health care providers are obligated to follow the patient's ADs when a patient is no longer able to speak for himself or herself.
- In your scope of nursing practice, you need to (1) be informed about the decision-making laws and regulations in your state, (2) make AD documents available to patients, (3) teach patients and their families about ADs, (4) determine if all involved health care providers are aware of the existence of ADs, (5) assist the patient and the family in communicating with the health care providers when a "no code" order is requested, and (6) assist the conflicted family in obtaining appropriate counseling whenever necessary.

Discussion Questions

1. What should you do next with the information provided by L.H.'s wife?
2. How should you address the needs of each member of this family in L.H.'s plan of care?
3. What resources can you use to facilitate decision making in this situation?

*Advance directives are listed in Table 10-6.

cause restlessness and insomnia. Many patients with COPD have postnasal drip or nasal congestion that may cause coughing and wheezing at night. Nasal saline sprays or rinses before sleep and in the morning may help. If the patient is prescribed O_2 therapy, using it at night will decrease insomnia. If the patient is a restless sleeper, snores, stops breathing while asleep, and has a tendency to fall asleep during the day, the patient may need to be tested for sleep apnea[55] (see Chapter 8).

Psychosocial Considerations. Healthy coping is a challenge for the COPD patient and the family. People with COPD frequently have to deal with many lifestyle changes that may involve decreased ability to care for themselves, decreased energy for social activities, and loss or change in a job.

When a patient with COPD is first diagnosed or has complications that require hospitalization, expect a variety of emotional responses. Emotions frequently encountered include guilt, loneliness from social isolation, denial, and frustration from increased dependence. Guilt may result from the knowledge that the disease was caused largely by cigarette smoking. Many patients struggle with depression and anxiety. It is important to convey a sense of understanding and caring to the patient. The patient with COPD may benefit from stress management techniques (e.g., massage, muscle relaxation) and referral to a therapist[16] (see Chapter 7). Support groups at local American Lung Association chapters (such as the Better Breathers Club), hospitals, and clinics can also be helpful.

Patients frequently ask whether moving to a warmer or drier climate will help. In general, such a move is not significantly beneficial. Discourage moves to places with an elevation of 4000 ft or more because of the lower partial pressure of O_2 found in the air at higher elevations. A disadvantage of moving may be that a person leaves a job, friends, and familiar environment, which could be psychologically stressful. Any advantage gained from a different climate may be outweighed by the psychologic effects of the move.

Patients need to know that symptoms can be managed, but COPD cannot be cured. End-of-life issues and advance directives are important topics for discussion in the terminal stages of COPD. However, this may be difficult for the patient and family to consider because of the uncertainty of the disease. (Palliative care and end-of-life care are discussed in Chapter 10.)

EVALUATION

The expected outcomes for the patient with COPD are presented in Nursing Care Plan 29-2.

CYSTIC FIBROSIS

Cystic fibrosis (CF) is an autosomal recessive, multisystem disease characterized by altered transport of sodium and chloride ions in and out of epithelial cells. This defect primarily affects the lungs, gastrointestinal tract (pancreas and biliary tract), and reproductive tract.[56]

CF was first described in 1938 when autopsies of young children revealed multiple cysts in the pancreas, so the disease was called "cystic fibrosis of the pancreas."[57] Once advances in care allowed children to live into later childhood, the lung disease became the more significant problem.

Approximately 30,000 children and adults in the United States have CF. About 10 million (about 1 in every 31) Americans are carriers of the CF gene but do not have the disease. Of the CF patients in the Cystic Fibrosis Patient Registry, more than 48% are 18 years of age or older. The first signs and symptoms typically occur in children, but some patients are not diagnosed until they are adults; some live to over 80 years old. The severity and progression of the disease vary. With early diagnosis and improvements in therapy, the prognosis of patients with CF has significantly improved. The median predicted survival was 16 years in 1970, but has increased to more than 37 years.[58] Nurses who work in adult care settings increasingly manage patients with CF.

Etiology and Pathophysiology

Genetic Link

CF is an autosomal recessive disorder (see Figs. 13-4 and 13-5 and the Genetics in Clinical Practice box). The CF gene is located on chromosome 7 and produces a protein called CF transmembrane regulator (CFTR). The CFTR protein localizes to the epithelial surface of the airways, gastrointestinal tract, and ducts of the liver, pancreas, and sweat glands. CFTR regulates sodium and chloride channels. Mutations in the *CFTR*

GENETICS IN CLINICAL PRACTICE

Cystic Fibrosis (CF)

Genetic Basis

- Autosomal recessive disorder.
- Caused by mutations in CF transmembrane regulator *(CFTR)* gene on chromosome 7.
- Many different mutations of *CFTR* gene have been identified.
- *CFTR* gene provides instructions for making protein that controls the channel that transports sodium and chloride.
- Mutations in the *CFTR* gene disrupt the function of the channels, preventing them from regulating the flow of sodium, chloride, and water across cell membranes.

Incidence

- In the United States 1 in 3000 white births.
- Less common in other ethnic populations (1 in 17,000 African Americans and 1 in 31,000 Asian Americans).
- One in 20-25 whites are carriers of the gene.
- If both parents carry the affected gene, there is a 25% chance each offspring will have the disease (see Figs. 13-4 and 13-5).

Genetic Testing

- Blood-based DNA testing is available for disease and carrier states.
- All 50 states have passed legislation requiring that all newborns be screened for CF.
- Testing is usually done in children if CF is suspected or if parents are possible carriers.
- In parents who are known carriers, amniocentesis or chorionic villus sampling in pregnant women may be useful for prenatal testing.

Clinical Implications

- CF is the most common autosomal recessive disease in whites.
- CF has a wide range of clinical expression of disease.
- CF requires long-term medical management.
- Advances in medical care have improved life expectancy.
- Most people who have a child with CF are not aware of a family history of disease.
- CF screening should be offered to all individuals of reproductive age regardless of family history.

gene alter this protein in such a way that the channels are blocked. As a result, cells that line the passageways of the lungs, pancreas, intestines, and other organs produce secretions that are low in sodium chloride content (thus low in water content), making mucus abnormally thick and sticky (Fig. 29-16). This mucus fills (plugs up) the glands in these organs and causes the glands to atrophy, ultimately resulting in organ failure. The high concentrations of sodium and chloride in the sweat of the patient with CF result from decreased chloride reabsorption in the sweat duct.[59]

In the respiratory system, both the upper and lower respiratory tracts can be affected. Upper respiratory tract manifestations may include chronic sinusitis and nasal polyposis. The hallmark of respiratory involvement in CF is its effect on the airways. The disease progresses from being a disease of the small airways *(chronic bronchiolitis)* to involvement of the larger airways, and finally causes destruction of lung tissue. The mucus becomes dehydrated and tenacious due to the defect in the chloride secretion and excess sodium absorption. Cilia motility is decreased, thus allowing mucus to adhere to the airways. The bronchioles become obstructed with thick mucus, leading to air trapping and hyperinflation of the lungs.

CF is characterized by chronic airway infection that cannot be eradicated. Organisms commonly cultured from the sputum

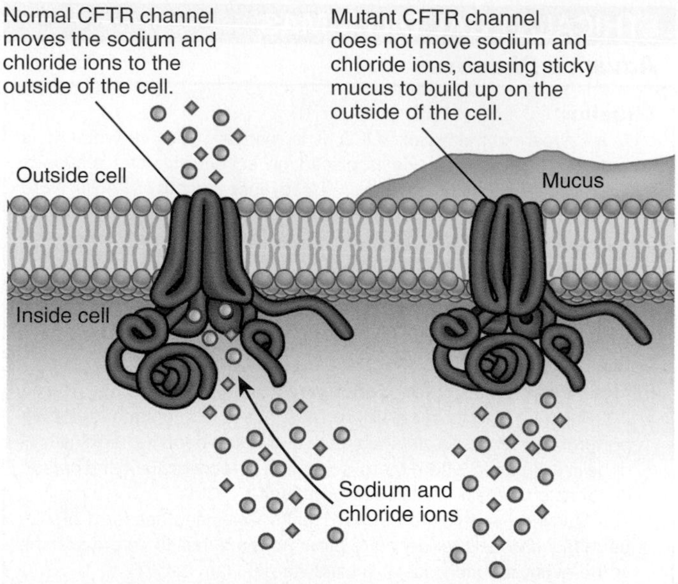

FIG. 29-16 People with cystic fibrosis inherit a defective gene on chromosome 7 called cystic fibrosis transmembrane regulator *(CFTR)*. The protein produced by this gene normally helps sodium and chloride move in and out of cells. If the protein does not work correctly, then the movement of sodium and chloride is blocked and an abnormally thick sticky mucus is produced on the outside of the cell.

of a patient with CF are *Staphylococcus aureus, Haemophilus influenzae,* and *Pseudomonas aeruginosa,* and less commonly but more seriously, *Burkholderia cepacia. Pseudomonas* is by far the most common organism. Antibiotic resistance often develops. Pulmonary inflammation may precede the chronic infection and can cause a decrease in respiratory function. Inflammatory mediators (e.g., interleukins, oxidants, proteases released by neutrophils) are increased and contribute to the progression of lung disease.

Lung disorders that initially occur are chronic bronchiolitis and bronchitis. However, after months or years, changes in the bronchial walls lead to bronchiectasis (Fig. 29-17). Over a long period, pulmonary vascular remodeling occurs because of local hypoxia and arteriolar vasoconstriction; pulmonary hypertension and cor pulmonale result in the later phases of the disease. Blebs and large cysts in the lung are also severe manifestations of lung destruction, and pneumothorax may develop. Other pulmonary complications include hemoptysis caused by erosion of enlarged pulmonary arteries. Hemoptysis may range from scant streaking to major bleeding, which can sometimes be fatal.

The sweat glands of CF patients secrete normal volumes of sweat, but sodium chloride cannot be absorbed from sweat as it moves through the sweat duct. Therefore four times the normal amount of sodium and chloride is excreted in sweat. This abnormality usually does not affect the person's general health, but it is the main diagnostic test for CF (explained later in the diagnostic studies section).

Pancreatic insufficiency is caused primarily by mucous plugging of the pancreatic exocrine ducts, which results in atrophy of the gland and progressive fibrotic cyst formation. The pancreas's exocrine function may be completely lost. Because of the exocrine dysfunction, pancreatic enzymes such as lipase, amylase, and the proteases (trypsin, chemotrypsin) are not made in sufficient amounts to allow for absorption of nutrients.

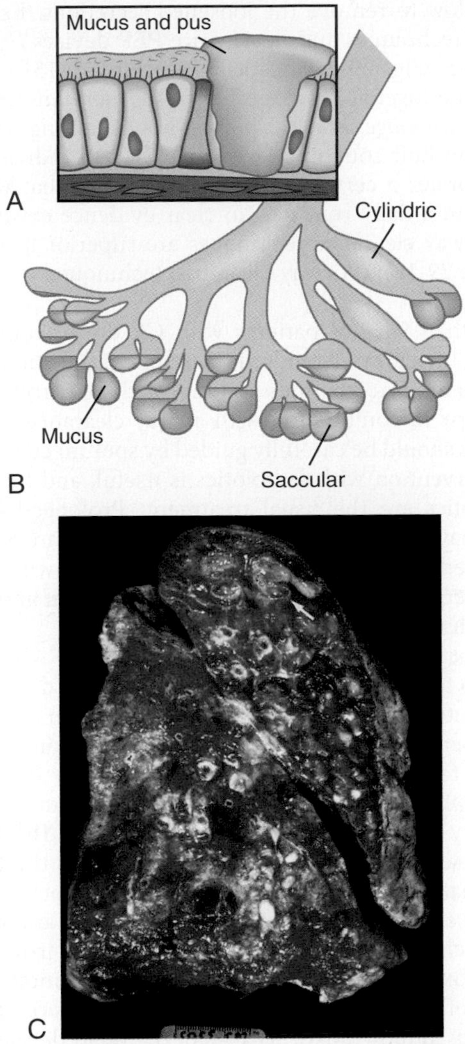

FIG. 29-17 Pathologic changes in bronchiectasis. **A,** Longitudinal section of bronchial wall where chronic infection has caused damage. **B,** Collection of purulent material in dilated bronchioles, leading to persistent infection. **C,** Bronchiectasis in a patient with cystic fibrosis who underwent lung transplantation. Cut surfaces of lung show markedly distended peripheral bronchi filled with mucopurulent secretions.

Malabsorption of fat, protein, and fat-soluble vitamins (A, D, E, and K) occurs. Fat malabsorption results in steatorrhea, and protein malabsorption results in failure to grow and gain weight.

CF-related diabetes mellitus (CFRD) is thought to be related to destruction of islet cells in the pancreas.[58] CFRD is a unique type of diabetes with characteristics of both type 1 and type 2 diabetes. The pancreas in people with CF produces insulin, but too late to fully respond to carbohydrate intake.

Other common disorders that develop in CF include osteopenia and osteoporosis. These disorders are related to malnutrition, malabsorption of vitamin D, insufficient testosterone levels, chronically elevated inflammatory cytokines, and the direct effect of the *CFTR* mutation on the development of bone.

Individuals with CF often have other gastrointestinal problems, including abdominal pain, which may be caused by conditions such as GERD. The liver and gallbladder can be damaged by mucus deposits. The liver enzymes may become chronically elevated, with cirrhosis developing over time. Gallstones, pancreatitis, and portal hypertension can also occur.[56] Distal intestinal obstruction syndrome (DIOS) results from intermittent obstruction commonly occurring in the terminal ileum. It is usually caused by thickened, dehydrated stool and mucus. The patient may appear to have a small bowel obstruction. DIOS develops because of chronic malabsorption related to exocrine dysfunction, nonadherence to enzyme supplementation, dehydration, swallowing of mucus, and use of opioids.

Clinical Manifestations

The clinical manifestations of CF vary depending on the severity of the disease. Carriers are not affected by the mutation. The disease severity may vary greatly, both within families and among different families.

The median age of diagnosis of CF is 5 months of age.[58] An initial finding of meconium ileus in the newborn infant prompts the diagnosis in 20% of people with CF. Other signs that suggest a CF diagnosis are acute or persistent respiratory symptoms (wheezing, coughing, frequent pneumonia), failure to thrive or malnutrition, steatorrhea (large, oily, frequent bowel movements), and family history. Without treatment, a large, protuberant abdomen may develop with an emaciated appearance of the extremities. A diagnosis may also be prompted by findings of bronchiectasis.

One of the most common symptoms of CF in the adult is frequent cough. With time, the cough becomes persistent and produces viscous, purulent, often yellow or greenish sputum. Although the most common bacteria in the airways in childhood is *S. aureus*, as the patient ages, the prevalence of *Pseudomonas* organisms increases. Other respiratory problems are recurring lung infections such as bronchiolitis, bronchitis, and pneumonia. As the disease progresses, periods of clinical stability are interrupted by exacerbations characterized by increased cough, weight loss, increased sputum, and decreased pulmonary function. Over time the exacerbations become more frequent, bronchiectasis worsens, and the recovery of lost lung function is less complete, which may ultimately lead to respiratory failure.

If the patient with CF develops DIOS, he or she may have right lower quadrant pain (the area of the ileocecal valve), loss of appetite, nausea, emesis, and often a palpable mass. Insufficient pancreatic enzyme release causes the typical pattern of protein and fat malabsorption with a person being thin with a low body mass index (BMI) and frequent, bulky, foul-smelling stools.

Both males and females have delayed puberty. Nearly all men with CF have reproductive issues because their vas deferens fails to develop in utero, so there is no transport of sperm from storage in the testes to the penile urethra. However, they make sperm normally, and with assisted reproductive technology are capable of fathering a child.

Some women with CF have difficulty conceiving; the cervical mucus is thought to be thickened. During exacerbations, menstrual irregularities and secondary amenorrhea are common. A majority of women with CF are able to become pregnant. Most pregnancies result in viable infants with mothers who are able to breastfeed normally.[60]

Complications

Complications in CF include CFRD, bone disease, sinus disease, and liver disease. Pneumothorax, a relatively uncommon but serious complication, is caused by the formation of bullae and blebs. A small amount of blood in sputum is common in the

CF patient because of chronic lung infection. Massive hemoptysis, which is relatively uncommon, can be life threatening.[58] With advanced lung disease, digital clubbing occurs. Respiratory failure and cor pulmonale caused by pulmonary hypertension are late complications of CF.

Diagnostic Studies

The diagnostic criteria for CF include a combination of clinical presentation, family history, laboratory testing, and genetic testing. The sweat chloride test is considered the gold standard for the diagnosis of CF. However, the diagnosis is not clear-cut in all individuals, especially in adults. The sweat chloride test is performed with the pilocarpine iontophoresis method. Pilocarpine is placed on the skin and carried by a small electric current to stimulate sweat production. This part of the process takes about 5 minutes, and the patient feels a slight tingling or warmth. The sweat is collected on filter paper or gauze and then analyzed for sweat chloride concentrations. The test takes approximately 1 hour. Sweat chloride values above 60 mmol/L are considered positive for the diagnosis of CF. Usually a second sweat chloride test is obtained at the same time (one test in each arm) to confirm the diagnosis.

A genetic test is often used if the results from a sweat chloride test are unclear. A blood sample or cells taken inside the cheek (buccal smear) are sent to a laboratory that specializes in genetic testing. Most laboratories test for only the most common mutations of the CF gene. Because more than 1700 mutations cause CF, screening for all mutations is difficult and is performed in a specialty laboratory.

Collaborative Care

A multidisciplinary team should be involved in the care of a patient with CF. The Cystic Fibrosis Foundation provides funding for and accredits more than 100 CF care centers nationwide. The high quality of specialized care available throughout the care center network has led to the improved length and quality of life for people with CF. These care centers offer the best care, treatments, and support for those with CF (see *www.cff.org/LivingWithCF/CareCenterNetwork/CFFoundation-accreditedCareCenters*). The teams at these care centers include a nurse, physician, respiratory therapist, physical therapist, dietitian, social worker, and often a nurse practitioner.

Management of pulmonary problems in CF aims at relieving airway obstruction and controlling infection. Drainage of thick bronchial mucus is assisted by aerosol and nebulization treatments of medications used to dilate the airways, liquefy mucus, and facilitate clearance. The abnormal viscosity of CF secretions is increased by concentrated deoxyribonucleic acid (DNA) from neutrophils involved in chronic infection. Agents that degrade the DNA in CF sputum (e.g., dornase alfa [Pulmozyme]) increase airflow and reduce the number of acute pulmonary exacerbations. Inhaled hypertonic saline (7%) is effective in clearing mucus and also decreases the frequency of exacerbations. Hypertonic saline is safe, but some patients require concomitant bronchodilators to avoid bronchospasm. Bronchodilators (e.g., β_2-adrenergic agonists) may be used to control bronchospasm, but the long-term benefit is not proven.

Airway clearance techniques are critical, since the normal ciliary motion in CF airways is impaired. CPT (including postural drainage with percussion and vibration) and high-frequency chest wall oscillation loosen mucus. Clearance is achieved by the specialized expiratory techniques aimed at using airflow to remove the loosened secretions. Examples of clearance techniques and devices are PEP devices (e.g., Flutter device [see eFig. 29-2], Acapella [see Fig. 29-15]), breathing exercises (autogenic drainage [see *http://hospitals.unm.edu/cf/autogenic_drainage.shtml*]), pursed-lip breathing (see Table 29-13), and huff coughing (see Table 29-23). Individuals with CF may prefer a certain technique or device that works well for them in a daily routine. No clear evidence exists that any of the airway clearance techniques are superior to the others (see Table 29-18). (Airway clearance techniques are discussed on p. 594.)

More than 95% of patients with CF die of complications from lung infection.[60] Standard treatment of infections includes antibiotics for exacerbations and may include chronic suppressive therapy in conjunction with airway clearance. The use of antibiotics should be carefully guided by sputum culture results. Early intervention with antibiotics is useful, and long courses of antibiotics are the usual treatment. Prolonged high-dose therapy may be necessary because many drugs are abnormally metabolized and rapidly excreted in the patient with CF. There is no evidence to support the chronic use of oral antibiotics in adults with CF.

Most patients have *Pseudomonas* infection, which can be difficult to treat because over time the organism develops resistance to antibiotics. It also has the ability to form a biofilm that must be penetrated to kill the organism. One commonly used antibiotic to treat patients who are chronically infected with *Pseudomonas* organisms is aerosolized tobramycin (TOBI) given every other month, every day, twice a day. This treatment regimen increases lung function and decreases the frequency of exacerbations. Oral agents commonly used for mild exacerbations (i.e., increased cough and sputum) are oral antibiotics such as a semisynthetic penicillin or trimethoprim/sulfamethoxazole (to treat *S. aureus*) or oral quinolones, especially ciprofloxacin (Cipro) (to treat *P. aeruginosa*). The quinolones are used judiciously because of the rapid development of resistant strains. More severe exacerbations require a 2- to 4-week course of IV antimicrobial therapy. Azithromycin, used chronically (longer than 6 months), decreases the frequency of pulmonary exacerbations in CF, especially in those infected with *Pseudomonas*. The effectiveness of this drug is probably related to its antiinflammatory effect.[61]

If home support and resources are adequate, the CF patient and caregiver may choose to continue IV antibiotic therapy at home.[62] The usual treatment is two antibiotics with different mechanisms of action (e.g., cephalosporin and an aminoglycoside). The patient with cor pulmonale or hypoxemia may require home O_2 therapy. (O_2 therapy is discussed on p. 589.) Patients with a large pneumothorax require chest tube drainage, perhaps repeatedly. Sclerosing of the pleural space or partial pleural stripping and pleural abrasion performed surgically may be indicated for recurrent episodes of pneumothorax. With massive hemoptysis, bronchial artery embolization is performed. CF has become a leading indication for lung transplantation.[58] (Lung transplants are discussed in Chapter 28.)

The management of pancreatic insufficiency includes pancreatic enzyme replacement of lipase, protease, and amylase (e.g., pancrelipase [Pancreaze, Creon, Ultresa, Viokase, Zenpep]) administered before each meal and snack. Adequate intake of fat, calories, protein, and vitamins is important. Fat-soluble vitamins (A, D, E, and K) must be supplemented, since they are malabsorbed. Use of caloric supplements improves nutritional status. Added dietary salt is indicated whenever sweating is excessive, such as during hot weather, when fever is present, or from intense physical activity. Hyperglycemia may require insulin treatment.

If the patient develops DIOS with complete bowel obstruction, gastric decompression may be needed. This complication is most often managed medically. If DIOS does not resolve with medical treatment, surgery may be needed to prevent the development of ischemic bowel. Partial and uncomplicated episodes of DIOS are treated with ingestion of a balanced polyethylene glycol (PEG) electrolyte solution (MiraLax, GoLYTELY) used to hydrate bowel contents. In addition, water-soluble contrast enemas may be used.[50] Careful monitoring of bowel habits and patterns is essential for CF patients.

Ivacaftor (Kalydeco) is used to treat patients who have a specific *G551D* mutation in the *CFTR* gene. About 4% of those with CF, or roughly 1200 people, have the *G551D* mutation. Ivacaftor is effective only in patients with CF who have this mutation. It is not effective in patients with CF who have two copies of the *F508* mutation in the *CFTR* gene, which is the most common mutation that results in CF. If a patient's mutation status is not known, a CF mutation test should be done to determine whether the *G551D* mutation is present. Ivacaftor, rather than treating the effects of the basic chloride ion channel defect (e.g., pancreatic insufficiency), targets the function of the gene itself, assisting this mutation to open the chloride channel. This drug proves that it is possible to alter the function of a mutation. Further research is ongoing to develop a drug that targets a more common mutation.[63]

Aerobic exercise is effective in clearing the airways. Important needs to consider when planning an aerobic exercise program for the patient with CF are (1) meeting increased nutritional demands of exercise, (2) observing for dehydration, and (3) drinking large amounts of fluid and replacing salt losses.

There is a higher incidence of depression among individuals with CF than their unaffected peers. CF imposes a significant burden on the individual and family. Issues related to fertility, decreased life expectancy, costs of health care, and career choices may lead to depression.[58]

NURSING MANAGEMENT CYSTIC FIBROSIS

NURSING ASSESSMENT

Subjective and objective data that should be obtained from the patient with CF are presented in Table 29-27.

NURSING DIAGNOSES

Nursing diagnoses for the patient with CF may include, but are not limited to, the following:

- Ineffective airway clearance *related to* abundant, thick bronchial mucus, weakness, and fatigue
- Ineffective breathing pattern *related to* bronchoconstriction, anxiety, and airway obstruction
- Impaired gas exchange *related to* recurring lung infections
- Imbalanced nutrition: less than body requirements *related to* dietary intolerances, intestinal gas, and altered pancreatic enzyme production
- Ineffective coping *related to* multiple life stressors such as decreased life expectancy, cost of treatment, and limitation on career choices

TABLE 29-27 NURSING ASSESSMENT
Cystic Fibrosis

Subjective Data

Important Health Information

Past health history: Recurrent respiratory and sinus infections, persistent cough with excessive sputum production

Medications: Use of and compliance with bronchodilators, antibiotics, herbs

Functional Health Patterns

Health perception–health maintenance: Family history of cystic fibrosis; diagnosis of cystic fibrosis in childhood, genetic testing in offspring

Nutritional-metabolic: Dietary intolerances, voracious appetite, weight loss, heartburn

Elimination: Intestinal gas; large, frequent bowel movements, constipation

Activity-exercise: Fatigue, ↓ exercise tolerance, amount and type of exercise; dyspnea, cough, excessive mucus or sputum production, coughing up blood, airway clearance techniques

Cognitive-perceptual: Abdominal pain

Sexuality-reproductive: Delayed menarche, menstrual irregularities, problems conceiving or fathering a child

Coping–stress tolerance: Anxiety, depression, problems adapting to diagnosis

Objective Data

General

Restlessness; failure to thrive

Integumentary

Cyanosis (circumoral, nail bed), digital clubbing; salty skin

Eyes

Scleral icterus

Respiratory

Sinus difficulties; persistent runny nose; diminished breath sounds, sputum (thick, white or green, tenacious), hemoptysis, ↑ work of breathing, use of accessory muscles of respiration, barrel chest

Cardiovascular

Tachycardia

Gastrointestinal

Protuberant abdomen; abdominal distention; foul, fatty stools

Possible Diagnostic Findings

Abnormal ABGs and pulmonary function tests; abnormal sweat chloride test, chest x-ray, fecal fat analysis

ABGs, Arterial blood gases.

PLANNING

The overall goals are that the patient with CF will have (1) adequate airway clearance, (2) reduced risk factors associated with respiratory infections, (3) adequate nutritional support to maintain appropriate BMI, (4) ability to perform ADLs, (5) recognition and treatment of complications related to CF, and (6) active participation in planning and implementing a therapeutic regimen.

NURSING IMPLEMENTATION

Assist young adults in gaining independence by helping them assume responsibility for their care and for their vocational or school goals. An important issue to discuss is sexuality. Delayed or irregular menstruation is not uncommon. There may be delayed development of secondary sex characteristics such as breasts in girls. The person with CF may use the illness to avoid certain events or relationships. Other crises and life transitions that must be dealt with in the young adult include building confidence and self-respect on the basis of achievements, persevering with employment goals, developing motivation to achieve, learning to cope with the treatment program, and adjusting to the need for dependence if health fails. Disclosing the CF diagnosis to friends, potential spouses, or employers may pose emotional and financial challenges.

The issue of marrying and having children is difficult. Genetic counseling may be an appropriate suggestion for the couple considering having children. Another concern is the uncertainty surrounding the shortened life span of the parent with CF. In addition, the parent's ability to care for the child must be taken into consideration.

Acute intervention for the patient with CF includes relief of bronchoconstriction, airway obstruction, and airflow limitation. Interventions include aggressive CPT, antibiotics, and O_2 therapy in severe disease. Good nutrition is important. Advances in long-term vascular access (e.g., implanted ports) and inhaled antibiotics have made administration of medication much easier. This has also eased the transition for treatment at home.

The family and the person with CF have a great financial and emotional burden. The cost of drugs, special equipment, and health care is often a financial hardship. Because most CF patients now live to childbearing age, family planning and genetic counseling are important. The burden of living with a chronic disease at a young age can be emotionally overwhelming. Community resources are often available to help the family. In addition, the Cystic Fibrosis Foundation can be of assistance. As the person continues toward and into adulthood, you and other skilled health professionals should be available to help the patient and the family cope with complications resulting from the disease.

BRONCHIECTASIS

Etiology and Pathophysiology

Bronchiectasis is characterized by permanent, abnormal dilation of medium-sized bronchi that is a result of inflammatory changes that destroy elastic and muscular structures supporting the bronchial wall. Infection is the primary reason for the continuing cycle of inflammation, airway damage, and remodeling. Bronchiectasis can follow a single episode of severe pneumonia, with a wide variety of infectious agents initiating the condition. Airways can become colonized with microorganisms (e.g., *Pseudomonas* species), which cause the bronchial walls to weaken, and pockets of infection begin to form (see Fig. 29-17).

When the walls of the bronchial system are injured, the mucociliary mechanism is damaged, allowing bacteria and mucus to accumulate within the pockets. Stasis of thickened mucus occurs due to impaired clearance of mucus by the cilia. This results in a reduced ability to clear mucus from the lungs and decreased expiratory airflow. Thus bronchiectasis is classified as an obstructive lung disease. Large connections (anastomoses) develop between the blood vessels in the lungs, and hemoptysis is often the result.[59]

A variety of pathophysiologic processes can result in bronchiectasis.[64] CF is the main cause of bronchiectasis in children. In adults the main cause is bacterial infections of the lungs that are either not treated or receive delayed treatment. Other causes of bronchiectasis are obstruction of an airway with mucus plugs or generalized impairment of pulmonary defenses. A number of systemic diseases such as inflammatory bowel disease, rheumatoid arthritis, or immune disorders (e.g., acquired immunodeficiency syndrome [AIDS]) may be associated with bronchiectasis.[25]

Clinical Manifestations

The hallmark of bronchiectasis is persistent cough with consistent production of thick, tenacious, purulent sputum. However, some patients with severe disease and upper lobe involvement may have no sputum production and little cough. Recurrent infections injure blood vessels, and hemoptysis occurs. In severe cases it may be life threatening. The other manifestations of bronchiectasis are pleuritic chest pain, dyspnea, wheezing, clubbing of digits, weight loss, and anemia. On auscultation of the lungs, a variety of adventitious sounds can be heard (e.g., crackles, wheezes, rhonchi).[65,66]

Diagnostic Studies

An individual with a chronic productive cough with copious purulent sputum (which may be blood streaked) should be suspected of having bronchiectasis. Chest x-rays may show some nonspecific abnormalities. A high-resolution CT (HRCT) scan of the chest is the preferred method for diagnosing bronchiectasis.

Sputum may provide additional information regarding the severity of impairment and the presence of active infection. Patients are frequently found to have *H. influenzae, Streptococcus pneumoniae, S. aureus,* or *P. aeruginosa,* with the latter leading to more frequent exacerbations and rapid decline in lung function. PFTs usually show an obstructive pattern, including a decrease in FEV_1 and FEV_1/FVC.[65,66]

Collaborative Care

Bronchiectasis is difficult to treat. Therapy is aimed at treating acute flare-ups and preventing a decline in lung function. Antibiotics are the mainstay of treatment and are often given empirically, but attempts are made to culture the sputum. Long-term suppressive therapy with antibiotics is reserved for those patients who have symptoms that recur a few days after stopping antibiotics. Antibiotics may be given orally, IV, or inhaled. Inhaled tobramycin is effective in treating patients with *P. aeruginosa.*

Concurrent bronchodilator therapy with LABAs, SABAs, or anticholinergics is given to prevent bronchospasm and stimulate mucociliary clearance. Hyperosmolar agents (e.g., hypertonic saline) may be given via a nebulizer to liquefy secretions. In addition, oral and inhaled corticosteroids may be used.

Maintaining good hydration is important to liquefy secretions. CPT and other airway clearance techniques are important to facilitate expectoration of sputum. Teach the patient to reduce exposure to excessive air pollutants and irritants, avoid cigarette smoking, and obtain pneumococcal and influenza vaccinations.

Surgical resection of parts of the lungs, which was common in the past, has largely been replaced by more effective supportive and antibiotic therapy. For selected patients who are disabled in spite of maximal therapy, lung transplantation is an option. Massive hemoptysis may require surgical resection or embolization of the bronchial artery.[66]

NURSING MANAGEMENT BRONCHIECTASIS

Early detection and treatment of lower respiratory tract infections helps prevent complications such as bronchiectasis. Any obstructing lesion or foreign body should be removed promptly.

An important nursing goal is to promote drainage and removal of mucus. Various airway clearance techniques can be effectively used to facilitate secretion removal. CPT with postural drainage is widely used.

Administration of the prescribed medications is important. The patient needs to understand the importance of taking the prescribed regimen of drugs to obtain maximum effectiveness. Rest is important to prevent overexertion.

If hemoptysis occurs, patients should be given explicit instructions on when they should contact the health care provider. Some patients may periodically expectorate a "spot" of blood that is usual for them. In the acute care setting, if the patient has hemoptysis, contact the health care provider immediately, elevate the head of the bed, and place the patient in a side-lying position with the suspected bleeding side down.

Good nutrition is important and may be difficult to maintain because the patient is often anorexic. Oral hygiene to cleanse the mouth and remove dried sputum crusts may improve the patient's appetite. Offer foods that are appealing, since they may increase the patient's desire to eat.

Adequate hydration to help liquefy secretions and thus make it easier to remove them is extremely important. Unless there are contraindications, instruct the patient to drink at least 3 L of fluid daily. To accomplish this, advise the patient to increase fluid consumption by increasing intake by one glass per day until the goal is reached. Generally, the patient should be counseled to use low-sodium fluids to avoid systemic fluid retention.

Direct hydration of the respiratory system may also prove beneficial in the expectoration of secretions. Often nebulized hypertonic saline may be ordered for a more aggressive effect. At home, a steamy shower can prove effective. Expensive equipment that requires frequent cleaning is usually unnecessary. Teach the patient and caregiver to recognize significant clinical manifestations to report to the health care provider. These manifestations include increased sputum production, bloody sputum, increasing dyspnea, fever, chills, and chest pain.

CASE STUDY

Chronic Obstructive Pulmonary Disease

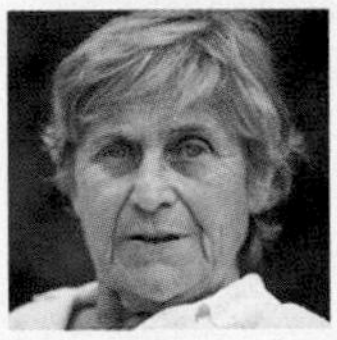
iStockphoto/Thinkstock

Patient Profile

H.M. is a 68-year-old white, married, female, retired traffic police officer. She has been in the hospital for 3 days with a COPD exacerbation and will be discharged tomorrow.

Subjective Data

- Before admission had 7 days of exceptional shortness of breath and increased volume of sputum, which turned greenish
- Had increased Ventolin HFA use at home to five or six times a day for dyspnea
- Had jitters and racing heart
- Had three or four bouts of bronchitis in the past year that she treated at home
- Thirty pack-year history of smoking; smokes half a pack per day now to "clear out lungs" in the morning
- Eats a regular diet but "gets full fast"
- Cannot climb one flight of stairs without stopping; walks down the flat driveway 10 yards without difficulty
- Awakens two or three times per night coughing and short of breath

Objective Data

Physical Examination

- Weight 129 lb, height 5 ft 8 in, BMI 20 kg/m^2
- BP 136/76 mm Hg, pulse 86, respiratory rate 28
- Increased anteroposterior diameter of chest (barrel shaped)
- Slight use of accessory (neck) muscles with breathing
- Distant breath sounds with occasional rhonchi
- No peripheral edema

Diagnostic Studies

- Last PFT: decreased FEV_1 (48%) and FEV_1/FVC (62%)
- ABGs on admission: pH 7.34, $PaCO_2$ 49 mm Hg, HCO_3^- 27 mEq/L, PaO_2 70 mm Hg
- WBC: 14,000/μL on admission
- Chest x-ray: hyperinflation, flat diaphragm, no sign of pneumonia

Collaborative Care

- GOLD 3 (severe) COPD with acute exacerbation
- O_2 2 L via nasal catheter while in hospital
- Prednisone 30 mg daily PO for 3 days, 20 mg for 3 days, 10 mg for 10 days
- Azithromycin 250 mg PO: take two tablets day 1, then take one tablet days 2 through 4
- Ipratropium HFA MDI 2 puffs four times a day
- At discharge: Advair Diskus 250/50 one inhalation q12hr

Discussion Questions

1. What classic manifestations indicate the patient had a COPD exacerbation?
2. What are some likely causes of her COPD?
3. What symptoms indicate the overuse of inhalers, and which drug would cause the symptoms described?
4. What is the only way H.M. can halt the progression of her lung disease?
5. Why would H.M. "feel full fast" when eating? What could you do to minimize this issue?
6. Interpret the ABGs. What pattern do you see?
7. ***Priority Decision:*** What are nursing priorities for discharge planning and teaching?
8. ***Priority Decision:*** Based on the assessment data presented, what are the priority nursing diagnoses? Are there any collaborative problems?
9. ***Evidence-Based Practice:*** H.M.'s son has been trying to convince his mother to quit smoking for many years without success. He asks you to tell his mother the results of her PFTs to convince her it is time to quit. Will this approach work?

evolve Answers available at *http://evolve.elsevier.com/Lewis/medsurg.*

BRIDGE TO NCLEX EXAMINATION

The number of the question corresponds to the same-numbered outcome at the beginning of the chapter.

1. A patient is concerned that he may have asthma. Of the symptoms that he relates to the nurse, which ones suggest asthma or risk factors for asthma *(select all that apply)*?
   a. Allergic rhinitis
   b. Prolonged inhalation
   c. History of skin allergies
   d. Cough, especially at night
   e. Gastric reflux or heartburn
2. In evaluating an asthmatic patient's knowledge of self-care, the nurse recognizes that additional instruction is needed when the patient says,
   a. "I use my corticosteroid inhaler when I feel short of breath."
   b. "I get a flu shot every year and see my health care provider if I have an upper respiratory tract infection."
   c. "I use my inhaler before I visit my aunt who has a cat, but I only visit for a few minutes because of my allergies."
   d. "I walk 30 minutes every day but sometimes I have to use my bronchodilator inhaler before walking to prevent me from getting short of breath."
3. A plan of care for the patient with COPD could include *(select all that apply)*
   a. exercise such as walking.
   b. high flow rate of O_2 administration.
   c. low-dose chronic oral corticosteroid therapy.
   d. use of peak flow meter to monitor the progression of COPD.
   e. breathing exercises such as pursed-lip breathing that focus on exhalation.
4. The effects of cigarette smoking on the respiratory system include
   a. hypertrophy of capillaries causing hemoptysis.
   b. hyperplasia of goblet cells and increased production of mucus.
   c. increased proliferation of cilia and decreased clearance of mucus.
   d. proliferation of alveolar macrophages to decrease the risk for infection.
5. The major advantage of a Venturi mask is that it can
   a. deliver up to 80% O_2.
   b. provide continuous 100% humidity.
   c. deliver a precise concentration of O_2.
   d. be used while a patient eats and sleeps.
6. Which guideline would be a part of teaching patients how to use a metered-dose inhaler (MDI)?
   a. After activating the MDI, breathe in as quickly as you can.
   b. Estimate the amount of remaining medicine in the MDI by floating the canister in water.
   c. Disassemble the plastic canister from the inhaler and rinse both pieces under running water every week.
   d. To determine how long the canister will last, divide the total number of puffs in the canister by the puffs needed per day.
7. Which treatments in CF would the nurse expect to implement in the management plan of patients with CF *(select all that apply)*?
   a. Sperm banking
   b. IV corticosteroids on a chronic basis
   c. Airway clearance techniques (e.g., Acapella)
   d. GoLYTELY given PRN for severe constipation
   e. Inhaled tobramycin to combat *Pseudomonas* infection
8. A patient who has bronchiectasis asks the nurse, "What conditions would warrant a call to the clinic?"
   a. Blood clots in the sputum
   b. Sticky sputum on a hot day
   c. Increased shortness of breath after eating a large meal
   d. Production of large amounts of sputum on a daily basis

1. a, c, d, e, 2. a, 3. a, e, 4. b, 5. c, 6. d, 7. a, c, d, e, 8. a

evolve

For rationales to these answers and even more NCLEX review questions, visit *http://evolve.elsevier.com/Lewis/medsurg.*

REFERENCES

1. American Lung Association: Trends in asthma morbidity and mortality, Epidemiology and Statistics Unit, Research and Health Education Division, Sept. 2012. Retrieved from *www.lungusa.org.*
2. American Lung Association: Trends in COPD (chronic bronchitis and emphysema): morbidity and mortality, Epidemiology and Statistics Unit, Research and Health Education Division, March 2013. Retrieved from *www.lungusa.org.*

*3. National Heart, Lung, and Blood Institute and National Asthma Education and Prevention Program: *Expert Panel Report 3: guidelines for the diagnosis and management of asthma*, NIH pub no 08-4051, Bethesda, Md, 2007, National Institutes of Health. Retrieved from *www.nhlbi.nih.gov/guidelines.*

*4. Global Initiative for Asthma: Global strategy for asthma management and prevention, 2012. Retrieved from *www.ginasthma.org.*

5. American Academy of Allergy, Asthma, and Immunology: Tips to remember: occupational asthma. Retrieved from *www.aaaai.org/patients/publicedmat/tips/occupationalasthma.stm.*

*6. Barnes P: Asthma. In Longo D, Fauci A, Kasper A, et al, editors: *Harrison's principles of internal medicine*, ed 18, New York, 2012, McGraw-Hill.

*7. Fanta C, Fletcher S: Diagnosis of asthma in adolescents and adults, 2011. Retrieved from *www.uptodate.com.*

*8. Sandrini A, Taylor D, Thomas P, et al: Fractional exhaled nitric oxide in asthma: an update, *Respirology* 13:57, 2010.

*9. Cox G: Bronchial thermoplasty for severe asthma, *Curr Opin Pulm Med* 17:34, 2011.

*10. Lareau SC, Hodder R: Teaching inhaler use in chronic obstructive pulmonary disease patients, *J Am Acad Nurs Pract* 24:113, 2012.

11. US Food and Drug Administration: Epinephrine cfc metered-dose inhalers: questions and answers. Retrieved from *www.fda.gov/Drugs/DrugSafety/InformationbyDrugClass/ucm080427.htm.*

*12. Zayas L, Wisniewski A, Cadzow R, et al: Knowledge and use of ethnomedical treatments for asthma among Puerto Ricans in

*Evidence-based information for clinical practice.

an urban community, *Ann Fam Med* 9: 2011. Retrieved from *www.annfammed.org*.

*13. Gøtzsche PC, Johansen HK: House dust mite control measures for asthma, *Cochrane Database Syst Rev* 3:CD001187, 2008.

*14. Moerman D: Meaningful placebos—controlling the uncontrollable, *N Engl J Med* 365:171, 2012.

*15. Qaseem A, Wilt T, Weinberger S, et al: Diagnosis and management of stable chronic obstructive pulmonary disease: a clinical practice guideline update from the American College of Physicians, American College of Chest Physicians, American Thoracic Society, and European Respiratory Society, *Ann Intern Med* 155:179, 2011.

*16. Global Initiative for Chronic Obstructive Lung Disease: Global strategy for the diagnosis, management, and prevention of chronic obstructive pulmonary disease (updated 2013). Retrieved from *www.goldcopd.org*.

17. Murphy S, Xu J, Kochanek M: Deaths: preliminary data for 2010, *Natl Vital Stat Rep* 60(4), 2012. Retrieved from *www.cdc.gov/nchs/data/nvsr/nvsr60/nvsr60_04.pdf*.

18. National Heart, Lung, and Blood Institute: COPD: are you at risk? Retrieved from *www.nhlbi.nih.gov/health/public/lung/copd/campaign-materials/html/copd-atrisk.htm*.

19. National Institute on Drug Abuse: Info facts: cigarettes and other tobacco products. Retrieved from *www.drugabuse.gov/publications/infofacts/cigarettes-other-tobacco-products*.

20. Health 24: How many smokers develop COPD? Retrieved from: *www.health24.com/medical/Condition_centres/777-792-805-1535,28674.asp*.

*21. Corbridge S, Wilken L, Kapella M, et al: An evidence-based approach to COPD, *Am J Nurs* 112:46, 2012.

22. Alpha-1 Foundation: Healthcare providers: what is alpha-1? Retrieved from *www.alphaone.org*.

*23. Stoller J: Clinical manifestations, diagnosis, and natural history of alpha-1 antitrypsin deficiency, 2011, *UpToDate*. Retrieved from *www.uptodate.com*.

24. Brashers V: Structure and function of the pulmonary system. In Huether S, McCance K, editors: *Understanding pathophysiology*, ed 5, St Louis, 2012, Mosby.

25. Brashers V: Alterations of pulmonary function. In McCance K, Huether S, Brashers V, et al, editors: *Pathophysiology: the biologic basis for disease in adults and children*, ed 6, St Louis, 2010, Mosby.

*26. Nussbaumer-Ochsner Y, Rabe K: Systemic manifestations and comorbidities of COPD, *Chest* 139:165, 2011.

27. Mann DL, Chakinala M: Heart failure and cor pulmonale. In Longo C, Fauci A, Kasper D, et al, editors: *Harrison's principles of internal medicine*, ed 18, New York, 2012, McGraw-Hill.

*28. Stoller J, Panos R, Krachman S, et al: Oxygen therapy for patients with COPD: current evidence and the long-term oxygen treatment trial, *Chest* 138:179, 2010.

*29. Decramer M, Janssens W, Miravitlles M: Chronic obstructive pulmonary disease, *Lancet* 379(9823:7-13):1341-1351, 2012. Retrieved from *www.sciencedirect.com/science/article/pii/S0140673611609689*.

*30. Anthonisen N, Manfreda F, Warren C, et al: Antibiotic therapy in exacerbations of chronic obstructive pulmonary disease, *Ann Intern Med* 106:196, 1987. (Classic)

*31. Rutten F, Zuithoff N, Hak E, et al: β-Blockers may reduce mortality and risk of exacerbations in patients with chronic obstructive pulmonary disease, *Arch Intern Med* 170:880, 2010.

32. GlaxoSmithKline: CAT: COPD assessment test: healthcare professional user guide. Retrieved from *www.catestonline.org/images/UserGuides/CATHCPUser%20guideEn.pdf*.

33. Centers for Disease Control and Prevention: Recommended adult immunization schedule—quickguide 2012, *MMWR* 61(4), 2012. Retrieved from *www.cdc.gov/vaccines/recs/schedules/downloads/adult/mmwr-adult-schedule.pdf*.

*34. Bartlett J, Sethi S: Management of infection in acute exacerbation of COPD, 2012, *UpToDate*. Retrieved from *www.uptodate.com*.

35. US Food and Drug Administration: FDA approves new drug to treat chronic obstructive pulmonary disease (news release), 2011. Retrieved from *www.fda.gov/NewsEvents/newsroom/PressAnnouncements/ucm244989.htm*.

36. Boehringer Ingelheim Pharmaceuticals: FDA approves Combivent Respimat (ipratropium bromide and albuterol) inhalation spray for the treatment of patients with chronic obstructive pulmonary disease. Retrieved from *www.prnewswire.com/news-releases/fda-approves-combivent-respimat-ipratropium-bromide-and-albuterol-inhalation-spray-for-the-treatment-of-patients-with-chronic-obstructive-pulmonary-disease-131368648.html*.

37. Vapotherm: Clinical resources. Retrieved from *www.vtherm.com/forclinicians*.

*38. Facchiano L, Snyder C, Nuñez D: A literature review on breathing retraining as a self-management strategy operationalized through Rosswurm and Larrabee's evidence based practice model, *J Am Acad Nurs Pract* 23:421, 2011.

39. Canadian Lung Association: COPD breathing techniques. Retrieved from *www.lung.ca/diseases-maladies/copd-mpoc/breathing-respiration/index_e.php*.

*40. Celli B, Stoller J: Pulmonary rehabilitation in COPD, 2012, *UpToDate*. Retrieved from *www.uptodate.com*.

*41. Main E, Prasad A, van der Schans C: Conventional chest physiotherapy compared to other airway clearance techniques for cystic fibrosis, *Cochrane Database Syst Rev* 2:CD002011, 2009.

*42. Osadnik CR, McDonald CF, Jones AP, et al: Airway clearance techniques for chronic obstructive pulmonary disease, *Cochrane Database Syst Rev* 2:CD008328, 2012.

*43. Bellini L: Nutritional support in advanced lung disease, 2012, *UpToDate*. Retrieved from *www.uptodate.com*.

44. Grodner M, Roth S, Walkingshaw B: *Nutritional foundations and clinical applications: a nursing approach*, ed 5, St Louis, 2012, Mosby.

*45. Burtin C, Decramer M, Gosselink R, et al: Rehabilitation and acute exacerbations, *Eur Respir J* 38:702, 2011.

*46. Payne C, Wiffen PJ, Martin S: Interventions for fatigue and weight loss in adults with advanced progressive illness, *Cochrane Database Syst Rev* 2:CD008427, 2012.

*47. Shah P, Slebos D, Cardoso P, et al: Design of the exhale airway stents for emphysema (EASE) trial: an endoscopic procedure for reducing hyperinflation, *BMC Pulm Med* 11:1, 2011.

*48. Pomidori L, Contoli M, Mandolesi G, et al: A simple method for home exercise training in patients with chronic obstructive pulmonary disease: 1 year study, *J Cardiopulm Rehabil Prev* 32:53, 2012.

*49. Harrison S, Greening N, Williams J, et al: Have we underestimated the efficacy of pulmonary rehabilitation in improving mood? *Respir Med* 106:838, 2012.

*50. Halding A, Wahl A, Heggdal K: "Belonging": patients' experiences of social relationships during pulmonary rehabilitation, *Disabil Rehabil* 32:1272, 2010.

*51. Moy M, Janney A, Nguyen H, et al: Use of pedometer and internet-mediated walking program in patients with chronic obstructive pulmonary disease, *J Rehabil Res Devel* 47:485, 2010.

*52. Gellis Z, Kenaley B, McGinty J, et al: Outcomes of a telehealth intervention for homebound older adults with heart or chronic respiratory failure: a randomized controlled trial, *Gerontologist* 52:541, 2012.

53. Leader D: Sex and COPD, 2010. Retrieved from *copd.about.com/od/livingwithcopd/a/sexandcopd.htm*.

54. Kam K: COPD and sex: nine tips for better sex and intimacy when you have COPD, 2010. Retrieved from *www.webmd.com/lung/copd/features/copd-sex*.

*55. Budhiraja R, Parthasarathy S, Budhiraja P, et al: Insomnia in patients with COPD, *Sleep* 35:369, 2012.

56. Gott K, Froh D: Alterations of pulmonary function in children. In McCance K, Huether S, Brashers V, et al, editors: *Pathophysiology: the biologic basis for disease in adults and children*, ed 6, St Louis, 2010, Mosby.

*57. Andersen D: Cystic fibrosis of the pancreas and its relation to celiac disease, *Am J Dis Child* 56:344, 1938. (Classic)

58. Cystic Fibrosis Foundation Patient Registry: *2011 annual data report,* Bethesda, Md, 2012, Cystic Fibrosis Foundation. Retrieved from *www.cff.org*.

59. Gott K, Brashers V: Alterations of pulmonary function in children. In Huether S, McCance K, editors: *Understanding pathophysiology*. ed 5, St Louis, 2012, Mosby.

60. Boucher R: Cystic fibrosis. In Longo D, Fauci A, Kasper D, et al, editors: *Harrison's principles of internal medicine*, ed 18, New York, 2012, McGraw-Hill.

*61. Sanders D, Farrell P: Transformative mutation specific pharmacotherapy for cystic fibrosis, *Br Med J* 344:e79, 2012.

*62. Yousef AA, Jaffe A: The role of azithromycin in patients with cystic fibrosis, *Paediatr Respir Rev* 11:108, 2010.

63. Ramsey B, Davies J, McElvaney NG, et al: A CFTR potentiator in patients with cystic fibrosis and the *G551D* mutation, *N Engl J Med* 365:1663, 2011.

64. Barker A: Clinical manifestations and diagnosis of bronchiectasis in adults, 2011, *UpToDate*. Retrieved from *www.uptodate.com*.

*65. Chesnutt M, Prendergast T: Pulmonary disorders. In McPhee S, Papadakis M, Rabow M, editors: *Current medical diagnosis and treatment*, ed 51, New York, 2012, McGraw-Hill.

66. Baron R, Bartlett J: Bronchiectasis and lung abscess. In Longo D, Fauci A, Kasper D, et al, editors: *Harrison's principles of internal medicine*, ed 18, New York, 2012, McGraw-Hill.

RESOURCES

American Lung Association
www.lung.org

Cystic Fibrosis Foundation
www.cff.org

Global Initiative for Asthma (GINA)
www.ginasthma.com

Global Initiative for Chronic Obstructive Lung Disease (GOLD)
www.goldcopd.com

CASE STUDY
Managing Multiple Patients

Introduction

You are assigned to care for the following four patients on a medical-surgical unit. You are sharing one unlicensed assistive personnel (UAP) assigned with another RN.

Patients

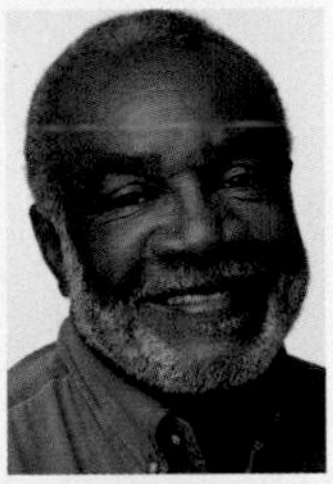

Kevin Peterson/ Photodisc/Thinkstock

F.T. is a 70-year-old man admitted yesterday with left-lower lobe pneumonia. He is receiving oxygen at 2 L/min via nasal cannula and IV antibiotics. His last pulse oximetry reading was 92%.

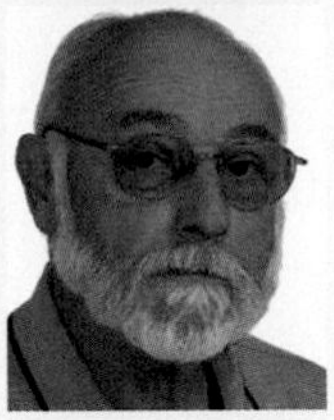

iStockphoto/Thinkstock

M.R. is a 60-year-old man who is 4 days postoperative following a total laryngectomy with tracheostomy for treatment of laryngeal cancer. He is receiving intermittent tube feeding via a percutaneous gastrostomy (PEG) tube and last received pain medication 4 hours ago.

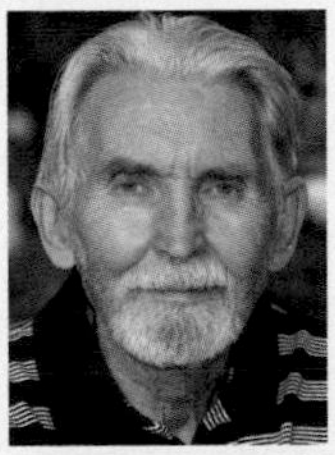

iStockphoto/Thinkstock

J.H. is a 52-year-old man admitted with right lower lobe pneumonia. A bronchoscopy with biopsy done on admission revealed small cell lung carcinoma. He is intermittently confused and anxious with rapid, shallow respirations. He is currently considering his treatment options.

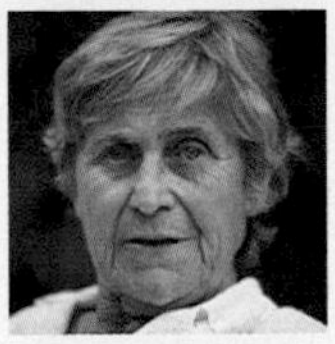

iStockphoto/Thinkstock

H.M. is a 68-year-old white woman admitted 3 days ago with a COPD exacerbation who is anticipating discharge later today. She is on oral prednisone and had been given a new inhaler to use. She will also be started on home oxygen.

Management Discussion Questions

1. ***Priority Decision:*** After receiving report, which patient should you see first? Provide a rationale for your decision.
2. ***Delegation Decision:*** Which morning tasks can you delegate to the UAP *(select all that apply)?*
   a. Take a pulse oximetry reading on F.T.
   b. Assess M.R.'s pain level and show him how to administer his tube feeding.
   c. Assist H.M. with AM care and gather belongings in anticipation of discharge.
   d. Teach F.T. how to use the incentive spirometer and titrate oxygen to obtain pulse oximetry >95%.
   e. Provide coffee and emotional support for J.H.'s family as they await a family meeting with the physician.
3. ***Priority and Delegation Decision:*** While you are assessing J.H., the UAP tells you that H.M. is complaining of chest pain and worsening shortness of breath. M.R. is also requesting pain medication. What should you do first?
   a. Ask the UAP to get H.M.'s vital signs while you give M.R. pain medication.
   b. Ask the UAP to increase H.M.'s oxygen to 4L/minute while you assess M.R.'s pain.
   c. Ask the UAP to obtain a stat 12-lead ECG on H.M. while you perform a focused assessment.
   d. Ask the UAP to have another RN give M.R. his pain medication while you go directly to H.M.'s room.

Case Study Progression

After assessing H.M., you notify her health care provider. A stat 12-lead ECG is obtained and a blood sample is drawn to check cardiac enzymes. H.M.'s chest pain is not relieved by sublingual nitroglycerin. You then administer 4 mg IV morphine. H.M. states that her pain is "a little better" but continues to complain of dyspnea. The 12-lead ECG and cardiac enzyme results are all within normal limits.

4. Because of H.M.'s reduced mobility, you recognize that she is at risk for pulmonary emboli and anticipate the health care provider will order which tests to determine the cause of her current symptoms?
   a. BNP and echocardiogram
   b. D-dimer and spiral CT scan
   c. CBC and abdominal flat-plate
   d. Serum electrolytes and renal ultrasound
5. While the charge nurse accompanies H.M. to radiology, you turn your attention back to your remaining three patients. Prior to administering M.R.'s 8 AM tube feeding, you aspirate 300 mL of gastric contents from his PEG tube. Which action should you take next?
   a. Discard the aspirated contents and administer the tube feeding as ordered.
   b. Replace the aspirated contents and administer half of ordered tube feeding volume.
   c. Discard the aspirated contents and withhold the next two scheduled tube feedings.
   d. Replace the aspirated contents and notify the health care provider prior to administering any further tube feedings.
6. When preparing F.T.'s AM medications, you note that he is scheduled to receive the following antibiotics at 8 AM: levofloxacin (Levaquin) 750 mg in 150 mL normal saline over 90 minutes (give once every 24 hours) and cefazolin (Kefzol) 1 g in 100 mL normal saline over 30 minutes (give q8hr). He has only one IV site. Which action is most appropriate?
   a. Obtain a second peripheral IV site.
   b. Call the health care provider to change the administration times.
   c. Check with pharmacy to see if they can be mixed together in the same IV bag.
   d. Administer the cefazolin first because it takes the least amount of time to infuse.
7. ***Management Decision:*** J.H.'s son calls you on the telephone to inquire about his father's current condition and long-term prognosis. Which initial response would be most appropriate?
   a. Ask the person calling what the code word is to identify themselves as family.
   b. Tell the caller that you are not allowed to discuss any information over the telephone.
   c. Ask J.H. what the physician has explained to him in order to clarify his current understanding of the situation.
   d. Empathize with J.H.'s son's need to know his father's prognosis while acknowledging that no one really knows.

evolve Answers available at *http://evolve.elsevier.com/Lewis/medsurg.*

SECTION 6

Problems of Oxygenation: Transport

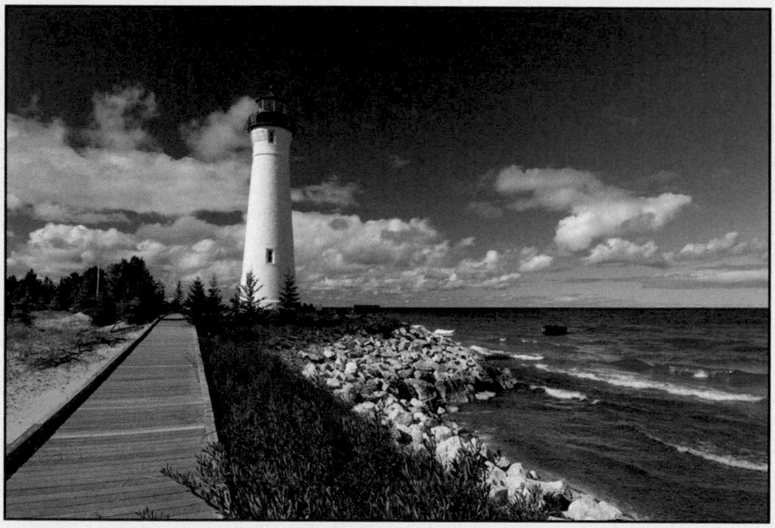

iStockphoto

There are only two mistakes one can make along the road to truth; not going all the way, and not starting.
Buddha

CHAPTER

30

All the soarings of my mind begin in my blood.
Rainer Maria Rilke

Nursing Assessment Hematologic System

Sandra Irene Rome

evolve WEBSITE

http://evolve.elsevier.com/Lewis/medsurg

- NCLEX Review Questions
- Key Points
- Pre-Test
- Answer Guidelines for Case Study in this chapter
- Rationales for Bridge to NCLEX Examination Questions
- Concept Map Creator
- Glossary
- Videos
  - Physical Examination: Abdominal Reflexes, Abdominal Muscles, and Inguinal Area
  - Physical Examination: Anterior Chest
  - Physical Examination: Neck
  - Physical Examination: Precordium and Jugular Veins
  - Physical Examination: Upper Extremities
- Content Updates

eFigure
- eFig. 30-1: Lymphatic drainage

eTable
- eTable 30-1: Drugs Affecting Hematologic Function

LEARNING OUTCOMES

1. Describe the structures and functions of the hematologic system.
2. Differentiate among the different types of blood cells and their functions.
3. Explain the process of hemostasis.
4. Link the age-related changes in the hematologic system to differences in findings of hematologic studies.
5. Select the significant subjective and objective assessment data related to the hematologic system that should be obtained from a patient.
6. Describe the components of a physical assessment of the hematologic system.
7. Differentiate normal from common abnormal findings of a physical assessment of the hematologic system.
8. Describe the purpose, significance of results, and nursing responsibilities related to diagnostic studies of the hematologic system.

KEY TERMS

ecchymoses, p. 625
erythropoiesis, p. 615
fibrinolysis, p. 618
hematopoiesis, p. 613
hemolysis, p. 615
leukopenia, p. 626
neutropenia, p. 626
pancytopenia, p. 625
petechiae, p. 625
reticulocyte, p. 615
thrombocytopenia, p. 626
thrombocytosis, p. 626

Hematology is the study of blood and blood-forming tissues. This includes bone marrow, blood, spleen, and lymph system. A basic knowledge of hematology is useful in clinical settings to evaluate the patient's ability to transport oxygen and carbon dioxide, maintain intravascular volume, coagulate blood, and combat infections. Assessment of the hematologic system is based on the patient's health history, physical examination, and results of diagnostic studies.

STRUCTURES AND FUNCTIONS OF HEMATOLOGIC SYSTEM

Bone Marrow

Blood cell production **(hematopoiesis)** occurs within the bone marrow. *Bone marrow* is the soft material that fills the central core of bones. Although there are two types of bone marrow (yellow [adipose] and red [hematopoietic]), it is the red marrow that actively produces blood cells. In the adult the red marrow is found primarily in the flat and irregular bones, such as the ends of long bones, pelvic bones, vertebrae, sacrum, sternum, ribs, flat cranial bones, and scapulae.

All three types of blood cells (red blood cells [RBCs], white blood cells [WBCs], and platelets) develop from a common hematopoietic stem cell within the bone marrow. The hematopoietic *stem cell* is best described as an immature blood cell that is able to self-renew and to differentiate into hematopoietic progenitor cells. As the cells mature and differentiate, several different types of blood cells are formed (Fig. 30-1). The marrow responds to increased demands for various types of blood cells by increasing production via a negative feedback

Reviewed by Katrina Allen, RN, MSN, CCRN, Nursing Instructor, Faulkner State Community College, Division of Nursing, Fairhope and Bay Minette, Alabama; and Mimi Haskins, RN, MS, CMSRN, Nursing Staff Development Instructor, Roswell Park Cancer Institute, Buffalo, New York.

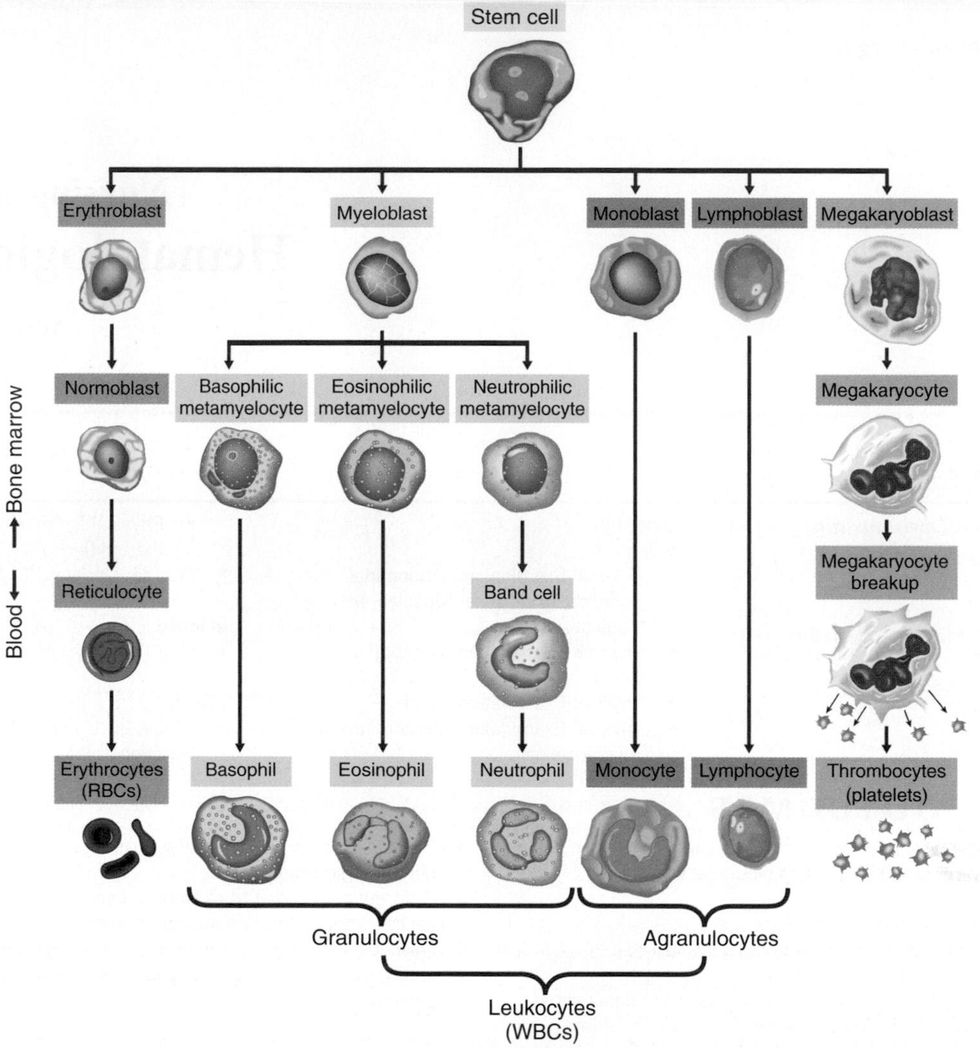

FIG. 30-1 Development of blood cells. *RBCs,* Red blood cells; *WBCs,* white blood cells.

system. The bone marrow is stimulated by various factors or cytokines (e.g., erythropoietin, granulocyte colony-stimulating factor [G-CSF], stem cell factor, thrombopoietin) that cause differentiation of the stem cells into one of the committed hematopoietic cells (e.g., RBC). For example, when tissue hypoxia occurs, erythropoietin is secreted by the kidney and liver. It circulates to the bone marrow and causes differentiation of proerythroblasts in the bone marrow.[1]

Blood

Blood is a type of connective tissue that performs three major functions: transportation, regulation, and protection (Table 30-1). Blood has two major components: plasma and blood cells. In an adult weighing between 150 and 180 lb, the volume of blood is usually between 4.7 and 5.5 L (5 to 6 quarts).

Plasma. Approximately 55% of blood is plasma (Fig. 30-2). Plasma is composed primarily of water, but it also contains proteins, electrolytes, gases, nutrients (e.g., glucose, amino acids, lipids), and waste. The term *serum* refers to plasma minus its clotting factors. Plasma proteins include albumin, globulin, and clotting factors (mostly fibrinogen). Most plasma proteins are produced by the liver, except for antibodies (immunoglobulins), which are produced by plasma cells. Albumin is a protein that helps maintain oncotic pressure in the blood.[1]

TABLE 30-1 FUNCTIONS OF BLOOD

Function	Examples
Transportation	• O_2 from lungs to cells • Nutrients from gastrointestinal tract to cells • Hormones from endocrine glands to tissues and cells • Metabolic waste products (e.g., CO_2, NH_3, urea) from cells to lungs, liver, and kidneys
Regulation	• Fluid and electrolyte balance • Acid-base balance • Body temperature • Maintaining intravascular oncotic pressure
Protection	• Maintaining homeostasis of blood coagulation • Combating invasion of pathogens and other foreign substances

Blood Cells. About 45% of the blood (see Fig. 30-2) is composed of formed elements, or blood cells. The three types of blood cells are *erythrocytes* (RBCs), *leukocytes* (WBCs), and *thrombocytes* (platelets). The primary function of erythrocytes is oxygen transportation, whereas the leukocytes are involved in protecting the body from infection. Platelets promote blood coagulation.

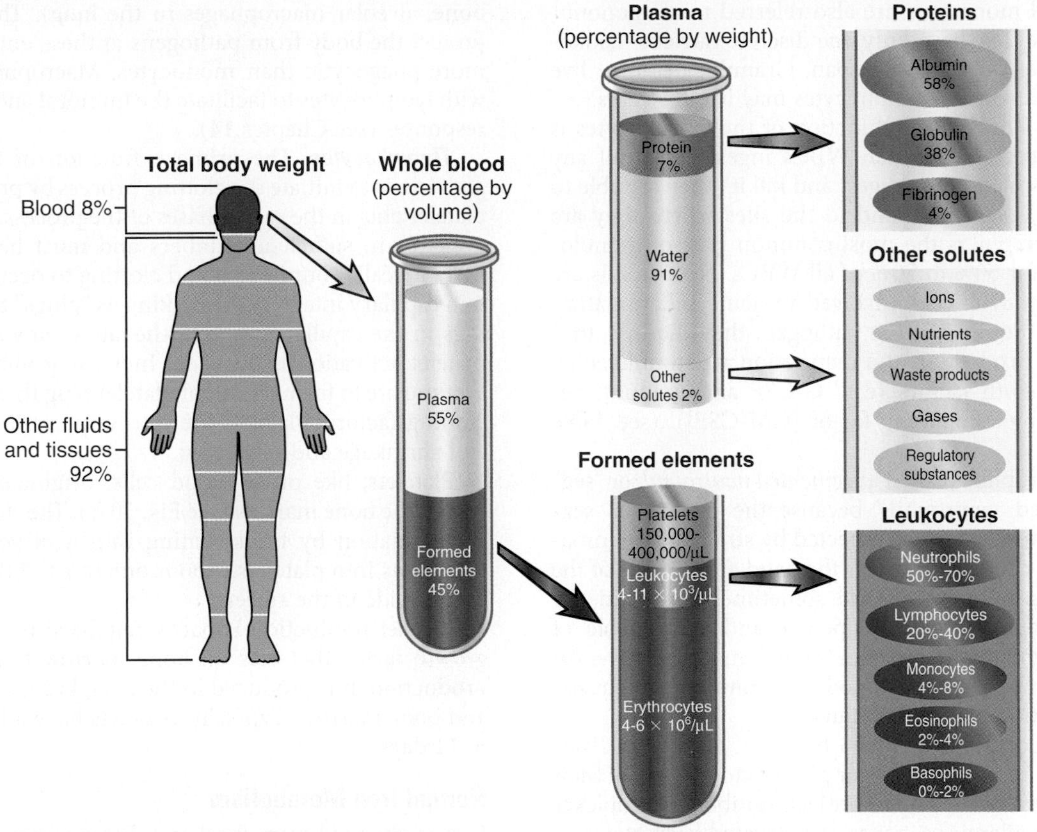

FIG. 30-2 Approximate values for the components of blood in the adult. Normally, 45% of the blood is composed of blood cells and 55% is composed of plasma.

Erythrocytes. The primary functions of RBCs include transport of gases (both oxygen and carbon dioxide) and assistance in maintaining acid-base balance. RBCs are flexible cells with a unique biconcave shape. Flexibility enables the cell to alter its shape so that it can easily pass through tiny capillaries. The cell membrane is thin to facilitate diffusion of gases.

Erythrocytes are primarily composed of a large molecule called hemoglobin. *Hemoglobin,* a complex protein-iron compound composed of heme (an iron compound) and globin (a simple protein), binds with oxygen and carbon dioxide. As RBCs circulate through the capillaries surrounding alveoli within the lung, oxygen attaches to the iron on the hemoglobin. The oxygen-bound hemoglobin is referred to as *oxyhemoglobin* and is responsible for giving arterial blood its bright red appearance. As RBCs flow to body tissues, oxygen detaches from the hemoglobin and diffuses from the capillary into tissue cells. Carbon dioxide diffuses from tissue cells into the capillary, attaches to the globin portion of hemoglobin, and is transported to the lungs for removal. Hemoglobin also acts as a buffer and plays a role in maintaining acid-base balance. This buffering function is described further in Chapter 17.

Erythropoiesis (the process of RBC production) is regulated by cellular oxygen requirements and general metabolic activity. Erythropoiesis is stimulated by hypoxia and controlled by *erythropoietin,* a glycoprotein growth factor synthesized and released primarily by the kidney. Erythropoietin stimulates the bone marrow to increase erythrocyte production. Normally the bone marrow releases 3×10^9 RBC/kg of body weight/day. The normal life span of an erythrocyte is about 120 days. Erythropoiesis is also influenced by the availability of nutrients. Many essential nutrients are necessary for erythropoiesis, including protein, iron, folate (folic acid), cobalamin (vitamin B_{12}), riboflavin (vitamin B_2), pyridoxine (vitamin B_6), pantothenic acid, niacin, ascorbic acid, and vitamin E.[1] Erythrocyte production is also affected by endocrine hormones, such as thyroxine, corticosteroids, and testosterone. For example, hypothyroidism is often associated with anemia.[2]

Several distinct cell types evolve during erythrocyte maturation (see Fig. 30-1). The **reticulocyte** is an immature erythrocyte. The reticulocyte count measures the rate at which new RBCs appear in the circulation. Reticulocytes can develop into mature RBCs within 48 hours of release into the circulation. Therefore assessing the number of reticulocytes is a useful means of evaluating the rate and adequacy of erythrocyte production.

Hemolysis (destruction of RBCs) by monocytes and macrophages removes abnormal, defective, damaged, and old RBCs from circulation. Hemolysis normally occurs in the bone marrow, liver, and spleen. Because one of the components of RBCs is bilirubin, hemolysis of these cells results in increased bilirubin to be processed by the body. When hemolysis occurs via normal mechanisms, the liver is able to conjugate and excrete all bilirubin that is released (see Fig. 31-2).

Leukocytes. *Leukocytes* (WBCs) appear white when separated from blood. Like the RBCs, leukocytes originate from stem cells within the bone marrow (see Fig. 30-1). There are different types of leukocytes, each with a different function. Leukocytes containing granules within the cytoplasm are called *granulocytes* (also known as polymorphonuclear leukocytes). Granulocytes include three types: neutrophils, basophils, and eosinophils. Leukocytes that do not have granules within the cytoplasm are called *agranulocytes* and include lymphocytes and monocytes.

Lymphocytes and monocytes are also referred to as mononuclear cells because they have only one discrete nucleus. Leukocytes have a widely variable life span. Granulocytes may live only for hours, yet some T lymphocytes may live for years.

Granulocytes. The primary function of the granulocytes is *phagocytosis,* a process by which WBCs ingest or engulf any unwanted organism and then digest and kill it. They are able to migrate through vessel walls and to the sites where they are needed. The *neutrophil* is the most common type of granulocyte, accounting for 50% to 70% of all WBCs. Neutrophils are the primary phagocytic cells involved in acute inflammatory responses. Once they engulf the pathogen, they die in 1 to 2 days.[1] Neutrophil production and maturation are stimulated by hematopoietic growth factors (e.g., G-CSF and granulocyte-macrophage colony-stimulating factor [GM-CSF])[1] (see Table 14-3).

A mature neutrophil is called a *segmented neutrophil,* or "seg" or "polysegmented neutrophil," because the nucleus is segmented into two to five lobes connected by strands. An immature neutrophil is called a *band* (for the band appearance of the nucleus). Although band cells are sometimes found in the peripheral circulation of normal people and are capable of phagocytosis, the mature neutrophil is much more effective. An increase in neutrophils in the blood is a common diagnostic indicator of infection and tissue injury.

Eosinophils account for only 2% to 4% of all WBCs. They have a similar but reduced ability for phagocytosis. One of their primary functions is to engulf antigen-antibody complexes formed during an allergic response. An elevated level of eosinophils is also seen in some neoplastic disorders, such as Hodgkin's lymphoma, and in various skin diseases and connective tissue disorders.[3] Eosinophils are also able to defend against parasitic infections.

Basophils make up less than 2% of all leukocytes. These cells have cytoplasmic granules that contain chemical mediators, such as heparin and histamine. If a basophil is stimulated by an antigen or by tissue injury, it responds by releasing substances within the granules. This is part of the response seen in allergic and inflammatory reactions. *Mast cells* are similar to basophils, but they reside in connective tissues and play a central role in inflammation, permeability of blood vessels, and smooth muscle contraction.

Lymphocytes. Lymphocytes, one of the agranular leukocytes, constitute 20% to 40% of the WBCs. Lymphocytes form the basis of the cellular and humoral immune responses (see Chapter 14). Two lymphocyte subtypes are B cells and T cells. Although T cell precursors originate in the bone marrow, these cells migrate to the thymus gland for further differentiation into T cells. *Natural killer (NK) cells* are lymphocytes that do not require prior exposure to antigens to kill virus-infected cells and activate T cells and phagocytes. Most lymphocytes transiently circulate in the blood and also reside in lymphoid tissues. (Details of lymphocyte function are presented in Chapter 14.)

Monocytes. Monocytes, the other type of agranular leukocytes, account for approximately 4% to 8% of the total WBCs. Monocytes are potent phagocytic cells that ingest small or large masses of matter, such as bacteria, dead cells, tissue debris, and old or defective RBCs. These cells are only present in the blood for a short time before they migrate into the tissues and become macrophages (see Chapter 13). In addition to macrophages that have differentiated from monocytes, tissues also contain resident macrophages. These resident macrophages are given special names (e.g., Kupffer cells in the liver, osteoclasts in the bone, alveolar macrophages in the lung). These macrophages protect the body from pathogens at these entry points and are more phagocytic than monocytes. Macrophages also interact with lymphocytes to facilitate the humoral and cellular immune responses (see Chapter 14).

Thrombocytes. The primary function of thrombocytes, or *platelets,* is to initiate the clotting process by producing an initial platelet plug in the early phases of the process. Platelets must be available in sufficient numbers and must be structurally and metabolically sound for blood clotting to occur. Platelets maintain capillary integrity by working as "plugs" to close any openings in the capillary wall. At the site of any capillary damage, platelet activation is initiated. Increasing numbers of platelets accumulate to form an initial platelet plug that is stabilized with clotting factors. Platelets are also important in the process of clot shrinkage and retraction.

Platelets, like other blood cells, originate from stem cells within the bone marrow (see Fig. 30-1). The stem cell undergoes differentiation by transforming into a *megakaryocyte,* which fragments into platelets. About one third of the platelets in the body reside in the spleen.

Platelet production is partly regulated by *thrombopoietin,* a growth factor that acts on bone marrow to stimulate platelet production. It is produced in the liver, kidneys, smooth muscle, and bone marrow. Typically, platelets have a life span of only 8 to 11 days.

Normal Iron Metabolism

Iron is obtained from food and dietary supplements. Approximately 1 mg of every 10 to 20 mg of iron ingested is absorbed in the duodenum and upper jejunum. Therefore only 5% to 10% of ingested iron is absorbed. About two thirds of total body iron is bound to heme in erythrocytes (hemoglobin) and muscle cells (myoglobin).

The other one third of iron is stored as ferritin and hemosiderin (degraded form of ferritin) in the bone marrow, spleen, liver, and macrophages (Fig. 30-3).When the stored iron is not replaced, hemoglobin production is reduced.

Transferrin, which is synthesized in the liver, serves as a carrier plasma protein for iron. The degree to which transferrin is saturated with iron is a reliable indicator of the iron supply for developing RBCs.

As part of normal iron metabolism, iron is recycled after macrophages in the liver and spleen phagocytize, or ingest and destroy, old and damaged RBCs. Iron binds to transferrin in the plasma or is stored as ferritin or hemosiderin (see Fig. 30-3). Only about 3% is lost daily in urine, sweat, bile, and epithelial cells in the gastrointestinal (GI) tract. Therefore there is normally very little iron loss except from blood loss.

Normal Clotting Mechanisms

Hemostasis is a term used to describe the arrest of bleeding. This process is important in minimizing blood loss when various body structures are injured. Four components contribute to normal hemostasis: vascular response, platelet plug formation, the development of the fibrin clot on the platelet plug by plasma clotting factors, and the ultimate lysis of the clot.

Vascular Response. When a blood vessel is injured, an immediate local vasoconstrictive response occurs. Vasoconstriction reduces the leakage of blood from the vessel not only by restricting the vessel size but also by pressing the endothelial surfaces together. The latter reaction enhances vessel wall stickiness and maintains closure of the vessel even after vasocon-

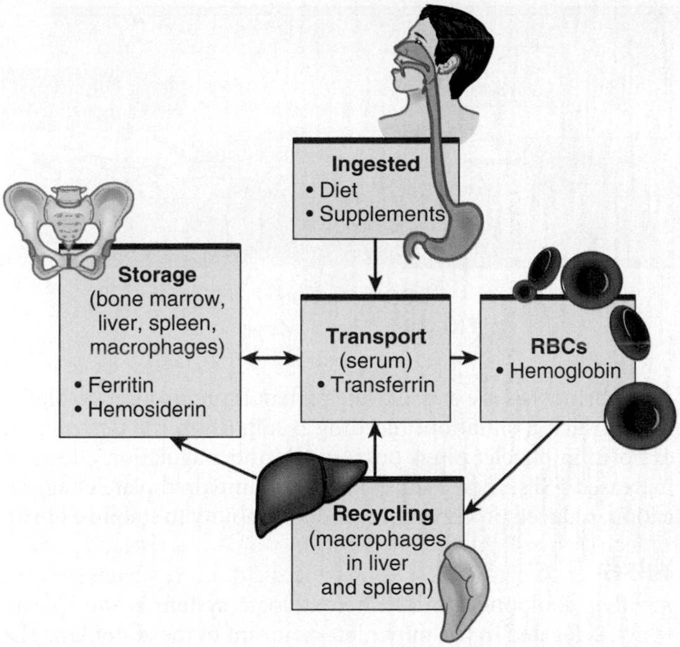

FIG. 30-3 Normal iron metabolism. Iron is ingested in the diet or from supplements. Macrophages break down ingested red blood cells *(RBCs)*. Iron is returned to blood bound to transferrin or stored as ferritin or hemosiderin.

striction subsides. Vascular spasm may last for 20 to 30 minutes, allowing time for the platelet response and plasma clotting factors to be activated. The platelet response and plasma clotting factors are triggered by endothelial injury and the release of substances such as tissue factor (TF).[1]

Platelet Plug Formation. Platelets are activated when they are exposed to interstitial collagen from an injured blood vessel. Platelets stick to one another and form clumps. The stickiness is termed *adhesiveness,* and the formation of clumps is termed *aggregation* or *agglutination.* This interaction causes the platelets to release substances such as platelet factor 3 and serotonin, which facilitate coagulation. At the same time, platelets release adenosine diphosphate, which increases platelet adhesiveness and aggregation, thereby enhancing the formation of a platelet plug. In addition, von Willebrand factor (vWF) is important in forming an adhesive bridge between platelets and vascular subendothelial structures. It is synthesized in endothelial cells and megakaryocytes and acts as a carrier for factor VIII.

In addition to their independent contribution to clotting, platelets also facilitate the reactions of the plasma clotting factors. As Fig. 30-4 shows, platelet lipoproteins stimulate necessary conversions in the clotting process.

Plasma Clotting Factors. The formation of a visible fibrin clot on the platelet plug is the conclusion of a complex series of reactions involving different clotting (coagulation) factors. The plasma clotting factors are labeled with both names and Roman

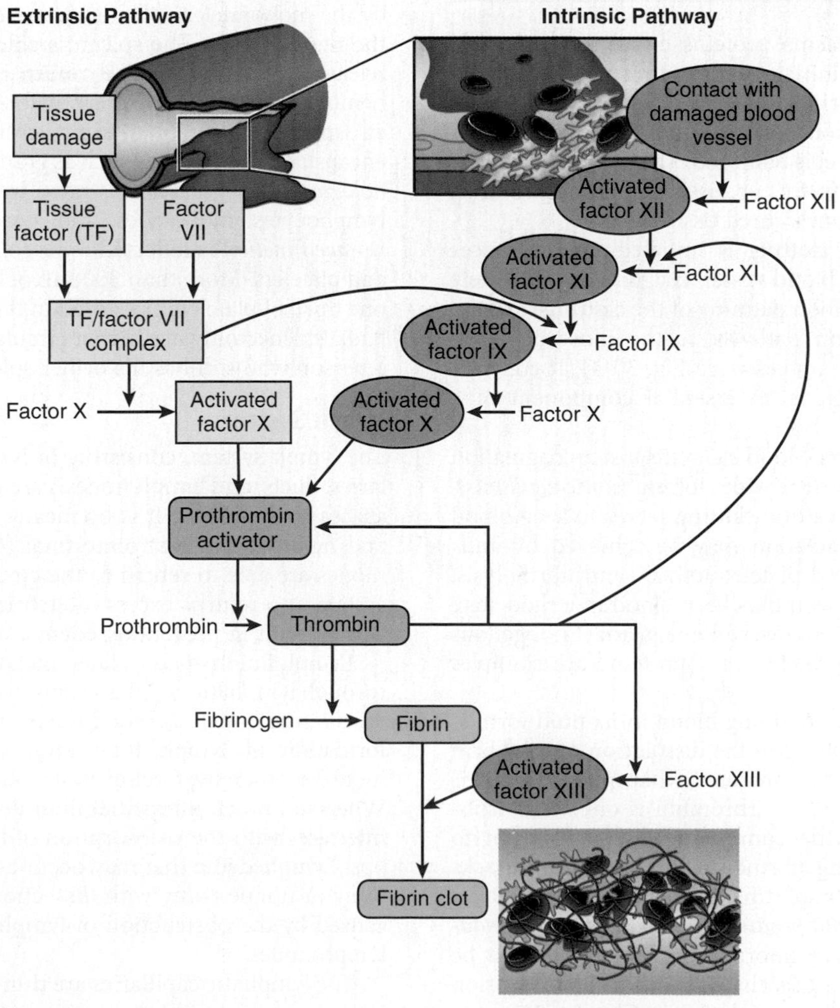

FIG. 30-4 Coagulation mechanism showing steps in the intrinsic pathway and extrinsic pathway as they would occur in the test tube.

TABLE 30-2 **COAGULATION FACTORS**

Coagulation Factor		Action
I	Fibrinogen	Source of fibrin to form a clot. Made in liver.
II	Prothrombin	Converted to thrombin, which then activates fibrinogen into fibrin.
III	Tissue factor, tissue thromboplastin	Released from damaged endothelial cells and activates the extrinsic pathway by reacting with factor VII.
IV	Calcium	Required cofactor at several points in the coagulation cascade.
V	Labile factor, proaccelerin	Binds with factor X to activate prothrombin.
VI		Not in use (now obsolete).
VII	Stable factor, proconvertin	Forms a complex with factor III and activates factors IX and X.
VIII	Antihemophilic factor	Works with factor IX and calcium to activate factor X.
IX	Christmas factor, plasma thromboplastin component	Together with factor VIII, activates factor X.
X	Stuart-Prower factor, Stuart factor	Activates conversion of factor II (prothrombin) to thrombin.
XI	Plasma thromboplastin antecedent	Activates factor IX when calcium is present.
XII	Hageman factor	Activates factor XI, which starts the intrinsic pathway.
XIII	Fibrin-stabilizing factor	Cross-links fibrin strands and stabilizes fibrin clot.

numerals (Table 30-2). Plasma proteins circulate in inactive forms until stimulated to initiate clotting through one of two pathways, intrinsic or extrinsic (see Fig. 30-4). The *intrinsic pathway* is activated by collagen exposure from endothelial injury when the blood vessel is damaged. The *extrinsic pathway* is initiated when tissue factor or tissue thromboplastin is released extravascularly from injured tissues.

Regardless of whether clotting is initiated by substances internal or external to the blood vessel, coagulation ultimately follows the same final common pathway of the clotting cascade. Thrombin, in the common pathway, is the most powerful enzyme in the coagulation process (see Fig. 30-4). It converts fibrinogen to fibrin, which is an essential component of a blood clot.

Lysis of Clot. Just as some blood elements foster coagulation *(procoagulants)*, others interfere with clotting *(anticoagulants)*. This counter mechanism to blood clotting serves to keep blood in its fluid state. Anticoagulation may be achieved by antithrombin activity, vessel and platelet activity, and fibrinolysis. As the name implies, antithrombins keep blood in a fluid state by antagonizing thrombin, a powerful coagulant. Endogenous heparin, antithrombin III, protein C, and protein S are examples of anticoagulants.

The second means of maintaining blood in its fluid form is **fibrinolysis,** a process resulting in the dissolution of the fibrin clot. The fibrinolytic system is initiated when plasminogen is activated to plasmin (Fig. 30-5). Thrombin is one of the substances that can activate the conversion of plasminogen to plasmin, thereby promoting fibrinolysis. The plasmin attacks either fibrin or fibrinogen by splitting the molecules into smaller elements known as *fibrin split products* (FSPs) or *fibrin degradation products* (FDPs). (More information about FSPs can be found in Table 30-7 later in this chapter and in the discussion of disseminated intravascular coagulation in Chapter 31.)

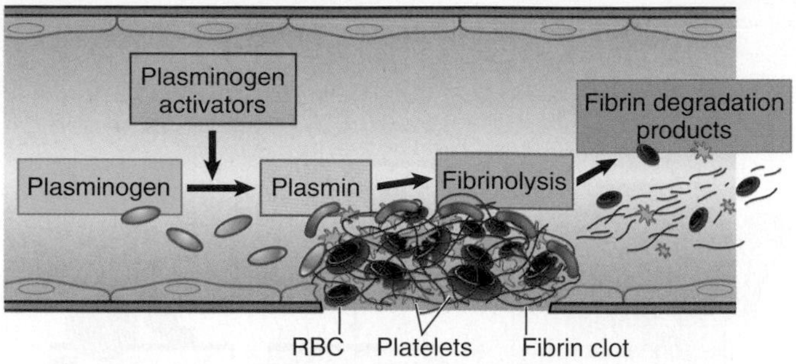

FIG. 30-5 Fibrinolytic system.

If fibrinolysis is excessive, the patient is predisposed to bleeding. In such a situation, bleeding results from the destruction of fibrin in platelet plugs or from the anticoagulation effects of increased FSPs. Increased FSPs lead to impaired platelet aggregation, reduced prothrombin, and an inability to stabilize fibrin.

Spleen

Another component of the hematologic system is the spleen, which is located in the upper left quadrant of the abdomen. The spleen has four major functions: hematopoietic, filtration, immunologic, and storage. *Hematopoietic function* is manifested by the spleen's ability to produce RBCs during fetal development. The *filtration function* is demonstrated by the spleen's ability to remove old and defective RBCs from the circulation by the mononuclear phagocyte system. Filtration also involves the reuse of iron. The spleen is able to catabolize hemoglobin released by hemolysis and return the iron component of the hemoglobin to the bone marrow for reuse. The spleen also plays an important role in filtering circulating bacteria, especially encapsulated organisms such as gram-positive cocci. The *immunologic function* is demonstrated by the spleen's rich supply of lymphocytes, monocytes, and stored immunoglobulins. The *storage function* is reflected in its role as a storage site for RBCs and platelets. More than 300 mL of blood can be stored. About one third of platelets are stored in the spleen. A person who has had a splenectomy has higher circulating levels of platelets than a person who still has his or her spleen.

Lymph System

The lymph system, consisting of lymph fluid, lymphatic capillaries, ducts, and lymph nodes, carries fluid from the interstitial spaces to the blood. It is by means of the lymph that proteins and fat from the gastrointestinal (GI) tract and certain hormones are able to return to the circulatory system. The lymph system also returns excess interstitial fluid to the blood, which is important in preventing edema.

Lymph fluid is pale yellow interstitial fluid that has diffused through lymphatic capillary walls. It circulates through a special vasculature, much as blood moves through blood vessels. The formation of lymph fluid increases when interstitial fluid increases, thereby forcing more fluid into the lymph system. When too much interstitial fluid develops or when something interferes with the reabsorption of lymph, lymphedema develops. Lymphedema that may occur as a complication of mastectomy or lumpectomy with dissection of axillary nodes is often caused by the obstruction of lymph flow from the removal of lymph nodes.

The lymphatic capillaries are thin-walled vessels that have an irregular diameter. They are somewhat larger than blood capillaries and do not contain valves. (eFig. 30-1 shows the lymph drainage throughout the body and is available on the website for this chapter.)

The *lymph nodes,* which are also a part of the lymphatic system, are round, oval, or bean shaped and vary in size according to their location. Structurally, the nodes are small clumps of lymphatic tissue and are found in groups along lymph vessels at various sites. More than 200 lymph nodes are found throughout the body, with the greatest number being in the abdomen surrounding the GI tract. Lymph nodes are situated both superficially and deep. The superficial nodes can be palpated, but evaluation of the deep nodes requires radiologic examination.[4] A primary function of lymph nodes is filtration of pathogens and foreign particles that are carried by lymph to the nodes.

Liver

The liver functions as a filter. It also produces all the procoagulants that are essential to hemostasis and blood coagulation. Additionally, it stores iron that is in excess of tissue needs, which can occur with frequent blood transfusions or diseases that cause iron overload. *Hepcidin,* produced by the liver, is a key regulator of iron balance. The synthesis of hepcidin is stimulated by iron overload or inflammation. Hepcidin reduces the release of stored iron from enterocytes (in the intestines) and macrophages.[5] Thus when iron is deficient, hepatocytes produce less hepcidin. Other functions of the liver are described in Chapters 39 and 44.

GERONTOLOGIC CONSIDERATIONS

HEMATOLOGIC SYSTEM

Physiologic aging is a gradual process that involves cell loss and organ atrophy. Aging leads to a decrease in bone marrow mass and cellularity and an increase in bone marrow fat.[6] However, peripheral blood cell concentrations in healthy older adults are similar to those of younger adults.[7] Although the older adult is still capable of maintaining adequate blood cell levels, the reserve capacity leaves the older adult more vulnerable to possible problems with clotting, transporting oxygen, and fighting infection, especially during periods of increased demand. This results in a diminished ability of an older adult to compensate for an acute or chronic illness.[6,7]

Hemoglobin levels begin to decrease in both men and women after middle age, with the low-normal levels seen in most older people. Total serum iron, total iron-binding capacity, and intestinal iron absorption are all decreased in older adults. Iron deficiency is usually responsible for the low hemoglobin levels. Healthy older patients are not able to produce reticulocytes in response to hemorrhage or hypoxemia as well as younger adults.[1]

The RBC plasma membranes are more fragile in the older person. This may account for a slight increase in mean corpuscular volume (MCV) and a slight decrease in mean corpuscular hemoglobin concentration (MCHC) of RBCs in some older individuals. It is essential to assess for signs of disease processes such as GI bleeding before concluding that decreased hemoglobin levels are caused solely by aging. Thus iron-deficiency anemia is a diagnosis that should be made after other causes have been ruled out.

The total WBC count and differential are generally not affected by aging. However, decreases in humoral antibody response and T cell function may occur.[6,8] During an infection, the older adult may have only a minimal elevation in the total WBC count. These laboratory findings suggest a diminished bone marrow reserve of granulocytes in older adults and reflect the possible impaired stimulation of hematopoiesis. The number of platelets is unaffected by the aging process, but functionally they may have increased adhesiveness.[9] Changes in vascular integrity related to aging can manifest as easy bruising.

The effects of aging on hematologic studies[9-11] are presented in Table 30-3. Immune changes related to aging are presented in Chapter 14.

TABLE 30-3 GERONTOLOGIC ASSESSMENT DIFFERENCES

Effects of Aging on Hematologic Studies

Study	Changes
CBC Studies	
Hgb	Normal; possibly slight decrease in men
MCV	May be slightly increased
MCHC	May be slightly decreased
WBC count	Diminished response to infection
Platelets	Unchanged but possible increase in adhesiveness
Clotting Studies	
Partial thromboplastin time	Decreased
Fibrinogen	May be elevated
Factors V, VII, IX	May be elevated
ESR	Increased significantly
D-dimers	Increased
Iron Studies	
Serum iron	Decreased
Total iron-binding capacity	Decreased
Ferritin	Increased
Erythropoietin	May be decreased

MCHC, Mean corpuscular hemoglobin concentration; *MCV,* mean corpuscular volume.

ASSESSMENT OF HEMATOLOGIC SYSTEM

Much of the evaluation of the hematologic system is based on a thorough health history. Consequently, you need to be knowledgeable about what to include in the health history so that you can phrase questions to elicit the most information.

Subjective Data

Important Health Information

Past Health History. It is important to learn whether the patient has had prior hematologic problems. Specifically ask about previous problems with anemia, bleeding disorders, and blood diseases such as leukemia. Also document other related medical conditions such as malabsorption or liver (e.g., hepatitis, cirrhosis), kidney, or spleen disorders. Patients may have received a kidney transplant, may have lost a spleen to traumatic injury, or may have a history of IV drug or alcohol use that affects their risk for hematologic disorders. A history of recent or recurrent infections or problems with blood clotting is also important to note.

Medications. A complete medication history of prescription and over-the-counter drugs is an important component of a hematologic assessment. Specifically address the use of vitamins, herbal products, or dietary supplements because many patients may not consider them to be drugs. Many drugs may

CASE STUDY

Patient Introduction

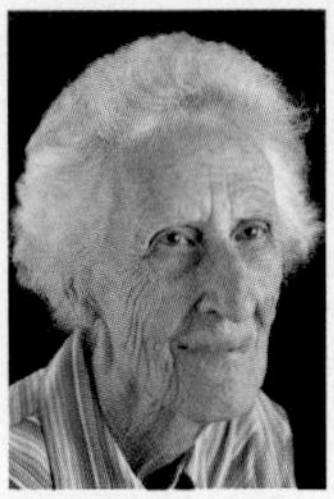

iStockphoto/Thinkstock

A.J. is a 90-year-old white woman who is brought to the emergency department by her son. He came from out of town for a visit and found his mother at home, weak and lying in bed. She says she has been slowly getting more and more "cold and tired" but "that is what happens when you live as long as I do." Her son had not seen her for 6 months and was concerned with how pale and frail she looked. He got scared when he noticed that his mother could not even walk to the bathroom without having to stop to catch her breath.

Critical Thinking

As you read through this assessment chapter, think about A.J. with the following questions in mind:

1. What are the possible causes of A.J.'s weakness, pallor, and shortness of breath?
2. What would be your priority assessment of A.J.?
3. What questions would you ask A.J.?
4. What should be included in the physical assessment? What would you be looking for?
5. What diagnostic studies might you expect to be ordered?

evolve Answers available at *http://evolve.elsevier.com/Lewis/medsurg.*

interfere with normal hematologic function (see eTable 30-1 available on the website for this chapter).[12-14] Herbal therapy can interfere with clotting (see Complementary & Alternative Therapies box in Chapter 38 on p. 851). Antineoplastic agents used to treat malignant disorders (see Chapter 16) and antiretroviral agents used to treat human immunodeficiency virus (HIV) infection (see Chapter 15) may cause bone marrow depression. A patient previously treated with chemotherapy agents, particularly alkylating agents, has a higher risk of developing a secondary malignancy of leukemia or lymphoma. A patient on long-term anticoagulant therapy such as warfarin (Coumadin) could be at risk for bleeding problems.

Surgery or Other Treatments. Ask the patient about specific past surgical procedures, including splenectomy, tumor removal, prosthetic heart valve placement, surgical excision of the duodenum (where iron absorption occurs), partial or total gastrectomy (which removes parietal cells, thus reducing intrinsic factor needed for the absorption of cobalamin [vitamin B_{12}]), gastric bypass (where the duodenum may be bypassed and parietal cell surface area decreased), and ileal resection (where cobalamin absorption takes place). Also assess how wound healing progressed postoperatively and if and when any bleeding problems occurred in relation to the surgery. Discuss wound healing and bleeding as responses to past injuries (including minor trauma) and to dental extractions. Also determine the number of previous blood transfusions and possible complications during administration, since the risk of transfusion reactions and iron overload increases with the number of blood transfusions.

Functional Health Patterns. Key questions to ask a patient with a hematologic problem are presented in Table 30-4.

Health Perception–Health Management Pattern. Ask the patient to describe the usual and present state of health. Gather complete demographic data, including age, gender, race, and ethnic background. Ask if there is any family history of hematologic problems.

GENETIC RISK ALERT

- Hematologic problems that have a strong genetic link include sickle cell anemia, hemophilia, thalassemia, and hemochromatosis.
- People with a family history of these hematologic problems have a much greater risk of developing them.
- Other hematologic problems, such as leukemia, pernicious anemia, and clotting disorders, may have a genetic predisposition.

When taking a family health history, explore the following health problems: jaundice, anemia, malignancies, RBC disorders such as sickle cell disease, bleeding disorders such as hemophilia, and clotting disorders.

Assess risk factors such as alcohol and cigarette use that might disrupt the hematologic system. Explore alcohol use tactfully. Alcohol is a caustic agent to the GI mucosa and can cause damage that results in GI bleeding, esophageal varices, and decreased absorption of cobalamin and other nutrients. Chronic alcohol abusers frequently have vitamin deficiencies. Alcohol also exerts a damaging effect on platelet function and the liver, where clotting factors are produced. Consequently, bleeding problems can develop and should be anticipated in cases of known alcohol abuse. Illicit drug use is also important to document, since many of these drugs may affect hematopoiesis.

Cigarette smoking increases low-density lipoprotein (LDL) cholesterol and levels of CO_2, leading to hypoxia and altering the anticoagulant properties of the endothelium. Smoking increases platelet reactivity, plasma fibrinogen, hematocrit, and blood viscosity.

Nutritional-Metabolic Pattern. Obtain the patient's weight and determine if the patient has experienced anorexia, nausea, vomiting, or oral discomfort. A dietary history may provide clues about the cause of anemia. Iron, cobalamin, and folic acid are necessary for the development of RBCs. Iron and folic acid deficiencies are associated with inadequate intake of foods such as liver, meat, eggs, whole-grain and enriched breads and cereals, potatoes, leafy green vegetables, dried fruits, legumes, and citrus fruits. Folic acid deficiencies may be offset by a diet including foods that are also high in iron.[15]

Hematemesis (bright red, brown, or black vomitus) is a symptom of an underlying problem and should always be investigated. Peptic ulcer disease is a common cause of hematemesis.

Explore any changes in the skin's texture or color. Ask about bleeding of gum tissue. Note any *petechiae* or *ecchymotic* areas on the skin and, if present, document the frequency, size, and cause. The location of petechiae can indicate an accumulation of blood in the skin or mucous membranes. Small vessels leak under pressure, and the platelet numbers are insufficient to stop the bleeding. Petechiae are more likely to occur where clothing constricts the circulation.

Also ask about any lumps or swelling in the neck, armpits, or groin. Specifically, ask what the lumps feel like (i.e., hard or soft, tender or nontender) and if they are mobile or fixed. Primary lymph tumors are usually not painful. A nontender, consistently swollen lymph node may be a sign of a malignancy, such as Hodgkin's or non-Hodgkin's lymphoma. Lymph nodes that are enlarged and tender are usually associated with an acute infection.[16] Explore any reports of fever. Determine if the patient currently has a fever, recurring fevers, chills, or night sweats.

Ask patients if they have a history of cardiac or pulmonary diseases. Cardiovascular disorders such as valvular disease or hypertension may predispose patients to hemolysis. Many of the medications used to treat cardiovascular disease can also cause abnormalities in hematopoietic cell production or coagulation.

TABLE 30-4 HEALTH HISTORY

Hematologic System

Health Perception–Health Management
- Do you have any difficulty performing daily activities because of a lack of energy?*
- Do you smoke cigarettes or drink alcohol?*
- Do you take any prescribed or over-the-counter medications?*
- Are you taking any herbal products?* Home remedies?*
- Have you in the past or are you currently consuming illegal drugs? What agents? What route? How frequently? When did you last use?
- Have you ever received a blood transfusion?*
- Is there any family history of anemia, cancer, bleeding, or clotting problems?*
- Have you had any surgeries?*

Nutritional-Metabolic
- Do you have any difficulties with eating, chewing, or swallowing?*
- Have you had any mouth sores, sore tongue, swollen or sore gums, excessive oral bleeding?*
- What kind of diet do you follow? If a vegetarian, do you eat eggs, milk products, fish, chicken?
- How has your appetite been?
- Have you had any changes in your weight in the past year?*
- Do you take any vitamins, nutritional supplements, or iron?*
- Is nausea and vomiting a problem for you?*
- Have you ever experienced any unusual bleeding or bruising?*
- Have there been recent changes in the condition or color of your skin?*
- Have you experienced night sweats or cold intolerance?*
- Have you noticed any swelling in your armpits, neck, or groin?*

Elimination
- Have you had black or tarry stools?* Have you had light, clay-colored stools?*
- Have you noticed any blood or dark "tea color" in your urine?*
- Has your urine had a foul odor or cloudiness?
- Have you had any decrease in urine output?*
- Do you ever have diarrhea or change in bowel patterns?*

Activity-Exercise
- Do you have any shortness of breath at rest? With activity?*
- Do you have any limitations in joint motion?* Have any of your joints been swollen?*
- Do you have a problem with unsteady gait? Have you fallen recently?*
- After activity, do you ever notice bleeding or bruising?*

Sleep-Rest
- Have you experienced excessive fatigue recently?*
- Are you more fatigued than usual?*
- Do you feel rested on awakening? If no, explain.

Cognitive-Perceptual
- Have you experienced any numbness or tingling?*
- Have you had any problems with your vision, hearing, or taste?*
- Have you noticed any changes in your mental function?*
- Do you have any pain, such as bone, joint, or abdominal pain, or abdominal fullness?*
- Do you have pain when moving your joints?*
- Have your muscles been sore or achy recently?*

Self-Perception–Self-Concept
- Does your health problem make you feel differently about yourself?*
- Do you have any physical changes that cause you distress?*

Role-Relationship
- Does your occupation bring you into contact with hazardous substances?*
- Has your present illness caused a change in your roles and relationships?*

Sexuality-Reproductive
- Has your hematologic problem caused any sexual problems that concern you?*
- *Women*: When was your last menses? Do you consider your cycle normal? How long does your bleeding usually last? Have you had any increase in cramping or clotting?* Have there been any changes in the amount of flow?*
- *Men*: Do you experience impotence?*
- Have you had unprotected sex in the past 6 months?* Was your partner someone new or a person with whom you have had a long-term sexual relationship?

Coping–Stress Tolerance
- Do you have a support system to assist you when needed?
- What coping strategies do you use during exacerbation of symptoms?
- Do you experience any specific symptoms when you feel stressed?*

Value-Belief
- Do you have any personal or religious objection to receiving blood or blood products?*
- Do you have any conflicts between your planned therapy and your value-belief system?*

*If yes, describe.

Pulmonary disorders that lead to hypoxemia may cause chronic stimulation of erythropoietin and result in *polycythemia* (excessive RBCs).

Elimination Pattern. Ask if blood has been noted in the urine or stool or if black, tarry stools have occurred. Ask the patient if he or she has had a recent stool Hemoccult (blood) test or colonoscopy. Document any decrease in urine output or diarrhea.

Activity-Exercise Pattern. Because fatigue is a prominent symptom in many hematologic disorders, ask about feelings of tiredness. Also determine any weakness or complaints of heavy extremities. Document symptoms of apathy, malaise, dyspnea, or palpitations. Note any change in the patient's ability to perform activities of daily living (ADLs), especially as they relate to patient safety and a history of falling.

Sleep-Rest Pattern. Determine whether the patient feels rested after a night's sleep. Fatigue secondary to a hematologic problem often does not resolve after sleep.

Cognitive-Perceptual Pattern. *Arthralgia* (joint pain) may be caused by a hematologic problem and should be assessed. Pain in the joint may indicate an autoimmune disorder, such as rheumatoid arthritis, or may be caused by gout secondary to increased uric acid production as a result of a hematologic malignancy or hemolytic anemia. Aching bones may result from pressure of expanding bone marrow with diseases such as leukemia. *Hemarthrosis* (blood in a joint) occurs in the patient with bleeding disorders and can be painful.

Paresthesias, numbness, and tingling may be related to a hematologic disorder and should be noted. Also assess any changes in vision, hearing, taste, or mental status.

Self-Perception–Self-Concept Pattern. Determine the effect of the health problem on the patient's perception of self and personal abilities. Also assess the effect of certain problems, such as bruising, petechiae, and lymph node swelling, on the patient's personal appearance.

Role-Relationship Pattern. Question the patient about any past or present occupational or household exposures to radiation or chemicals. If such exposure has occurred, determine the type, amount, and duration of the exposure.

A person who has been exposed to radiation, as a treatment modality or by accident, has a higher incidence of certain hematologic problems. The same is true of a person who has been exposed to certain chemicals (e.g., benzene, lead, naphthalene, phenylbutazone). These chemicals are commonly used by potters, dry cleaners, and individuals involved with occupations that use adhesives. Ask the patient about a history in the military. Many Vietnam War veterans were exposed to a dioxin-containing defoliant (Agent Orange), which has been linked with leukemia and lymphoma. Also assess the effect of the present illness on the patient's usual roles and responsibilities.

Sexuality-Reproductive Pattern. Obtain a careful menstrual history from women, including the age at which menarche and menopause began, duration and amount of bleeding, incidence of clotting and cramping, and any associated problems. Ask men if they have any problems related to impotence, since this is common in men with hematologic problems. Also question the patient about sexual behavior because HIV infection is potentially a concern, particularly among high-risk groups.

CASE STUDY

Subjective Data

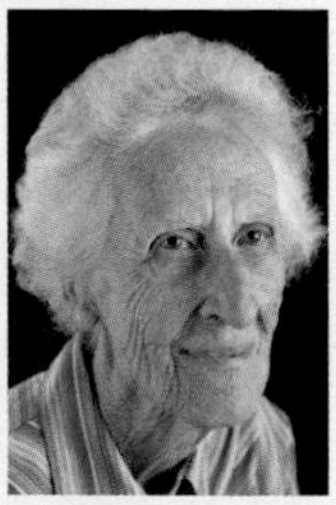

iStockphoto/Thinkstock

A focused subjective assessment of A.J. revealed the following information:

PMH: History of osteoarthritis. No surgical history. Prefers to take care of self with "natural therapy" and has not seen a health care provider for 10 years.

Medications: Metamucil 1 tbs PO daily; vitamins C, E, and D with calcium.

Health Perception–Health Management: A.J. denies family or personal history of anemia, cancer, or bleeding disorders. She believes she comes from a family with great genes for longevity because they "live off the land." She admits to drinking one glass of red wine with her evening meal "because it's good for your heart." She is a nonsmoker and just can't understand her gradual increase in shortness of breath with exertion. She states she really can't do anything anymore without having to stop and catch her breath. She says "it's tough getting old."

Nutritional-Metabolic: A.J. is living on a fixed income and therefore eats a lot of pasta "because it is cheap." She uses a lot of garlic for flavoring and the "health benefit of it." Although not a vegetarian, she states that she eats little meat.

Elimination: Denies black tarry stool. Occasional constipation. No problems with urination. Urine without odor.

Activity-Exercise: As noted above, A.J. is having difficulty performing ADLs without having to stop and catch her breath. Denies dyspnea at rest. States joints are stiff on arising in morning and after sitting but able to get around OK. States her walking is steady but weak. No history of falling.

Sleep-Rest: Typically sleeps 8-9 hr/night with no difficulty falling asleep. However, she still feels tired and needs to nap on and off during the day.

Cognitive-Perceptual: Denies any numbness or tingling. Admits to being a little hard-of-hearing but can still see "pretty good."

Value-Belief: Prefers natural therapies over traditional medication.

Coping–Stress Tolerance Pattern. The patient with a hematologic problem often needs assistance with ADLs. Ask the patient if adequate support is available to meet daily needs. Determine the patient's usual methods of handling stress. In the patient with platelet disorders or hemophilia, the potential for hemorrhage can be so frightening that usual life patterns may be drastically curtailed, affecting the person's quality of life. Explore the patient's understanding of the problem and provide teaching.

Value-Belief Pattern. Some hematologic problems are treated with blood transfusions or a bone marrow transplant. Determine if these types of treatments conflict with the patient's value-belief system, including the patient's cultural and religious beliefs related to blood and blood transfusions. If conflicts are identified, notify the health care provider.

Objective Data

Physical Examination. A complete physical examination is necessary to accurately examine all systems that affect or are affected by the hematologic system (see Chapter 3). Be aware that disorders of the hematologic system can manifest in various ways. Thus a patient's presenting symptoms may not immediately point to a hematologic problem (Table 30-5). For example, paresthesias of the lower extremities may not immediately appear to reflect a hematologic problem, but when combined with other clinical findings or risk factors, they may indicate cobalamin deficiency and resulting pernicious anemia. Although a full examination should be performed on patients suspected of a hematologic disorder, certain aspects of the physical examination are specifically relevant. These include skin, lymph nodes, spleen, and liver. Examination of the skin is discussed in Chapter 23; spleen and liver examination is found in Chapter 39.

Lymph Node Assessment. Lymph nodes are distributed throughout the body. Superficial lymph nodes can be evaluated by light palpation (Fig. 30-6). Deep lymph nodes cannot be

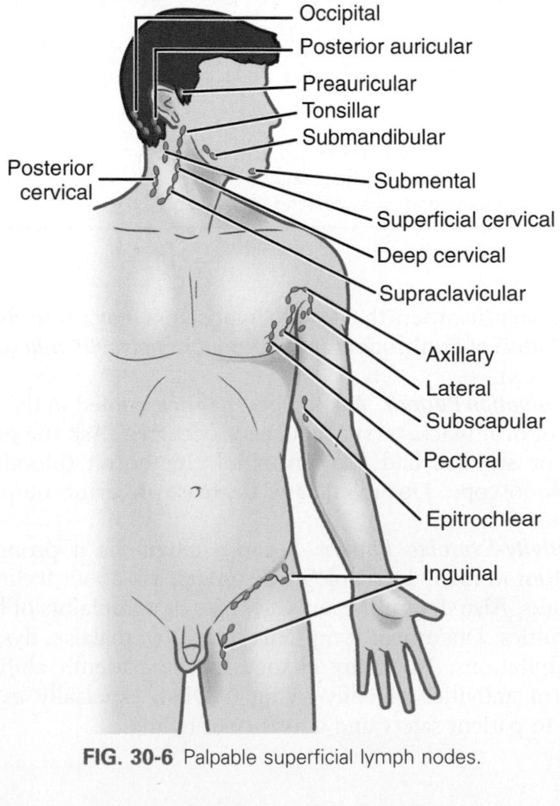

FIG. 30-6 Palpable superficial lymph nodes.

TABLE 30-5 ASSESSMENT ABNORMALITIES

Hematologic System

Finding	Description	Possible Etiology and Significance
Skin		
Pallor of skin or nail beds	Paleness. Decreased or absence of skin coloration.	Low Hgb level (anemia).
Flushing	Transient, episodic redness of skin (usually around face and neck).	Increase in Hgb (polycythemia), congestion of capillaries. Flushing of the palms of the hands or soles of the feet possible indication of anemia.
Jaundice	Yellow appearance of skin and mucous membranes.	Accumulation of bile pigment caused by rapid or excessive hemolysis or liver damage.
Cyanosis	Bluish discoloration of skin and mucous membranes.	Reduced Hgb, excessive concentration of deoxyhemoglobin in blood.
Excoriation	Scratch or abrasion of skin.	Scratching from intense pruritus.
Pruritus	Unpleasant cutaneous sensation that provokes the desire to rub or scratch the skin.	Hodgkin's lymphoma, cutaneous lymphomas, infiltrative leukemias, increased bilirubin.
Leg ulcers	Prominent on the malleoli on the ankles.	Sickle cell disease.
Angioma	Benign tumor consisting of blood or lymph vessels.	Most are congenital. Some may disappear spontaneously.
Telangiectasia	Small angioma with tendency to bleed. Focal red lesions, coarse or fine red lines.	Dilation of small vessels.
Spider nevus	Form of telangiectasia characterized by a round red central portion and branching radiations resembling the profile of a spider. Usually develop on face, neck, or chest.	Elevated estrogen levels as in pregnancy or liver disease.
Purpura	Any of a small group of conditions characterized by ecchymosis or other small hemorrhages in skin and mucous membranes.	Decreased platelets or clotting factors resulting in hemorrhage into the skin. Vascular abnormalities. Break in blood vessel walls resulting from trauma.
Petechiae	Pinpoint, nonraised, perfectly round area >2 mm. Purple, dark red, or brown.	Same as above.
Ecchymosis (bruise)	Small hemorrhagic spot, larger than petechiae; nonelevated. Round or irregular.	Same as above.
Hematoma	A localized collection of blood, usually clotted.	Same as above.
Chloroma	A tumor arising from myeloid tissue and containing a pale green pigment.	Acute myelogenous leukemia that has infiltrated the skin.
Plasmacytoma	A tumor arising from abnormal plasma cells.	Multiple myeloma that has infiltrated tissue.
Eyes		
Jaundiced sclera	Yellow appearance of the sclera.	Accumulation of bile pigment resulting from rapid or excessive hemolysis or liver disease or infiltration.
Conjunctival pallor	Paleness. Decreased or absence of coloration in the conjunctiva.	Low Hgb level (anemia).
Blurred vision, diplopia, visual field cuts	Decreased visual acuity or areas of blindness (field cuts).	Anemia, extreme leukocytosis, polycythemia may cause visual abnormalities. Thrombocytopenia may cause intraocular hemorrhage with visual abnormalities. Excessive clotting may cause thromboses in the circulation to the brain that cause visual field cuts.
Nose		
Epistaxis	Spontaneous bleeding from the nares.	May occur with low platelet counts, especially if the patient bends down for a long time, tries to lift a heavy item, or performs an intense Valsalva maneuver.
Mouth		
Gingival and mucous membrane changes	Pallor. Gingival and mucosal ulceration, swelling, or bleeding.	Low Hgb level (anemia). Neutropenia. Inability of impaired leukocytes to combat oral infections. Thrombocytopenia. Gingival hyperplasia may be present with some types of leukemia.
Smooth tongue	Tongue surface smooth and shiny. Mucosa thin and red from decreased papillae.	Pernicious anemia, iron-deficiency anemia.
Musculoskeletal System		
Bone pain	Pain in pelvis, ribs, spine, sternum.	Multiple myeloma related to enlarged tumors that stretch periosteum; bone invasion by leukemia cells. Bone demineralization resulting from various malignancies. Sickle cell disease.
Joint swelling	Fluid-filled spaces surrounding the joints.	Occurs with hemophilia and sickle cell anemia as bleeding occurs into the joint (hemarthria) causing inflammation.
Arthralgia	Joint pain.	Sickle cell disease from hemarthrosis.

Continued

TABLE 30-5 ASSESSMENT ABNORMALITIES—cont'd

Hematologic System

Finding	Description	Possible Etiology and Significance
Lymph Nodes		
Lymphadenopathy	Lymph nodes enlarged (>1 cm). May be tender to touch.	Infection; foreign infiltrations. Systemic disease such as leukemia, lymphoma, Hodgkin's lymphoma, and metastatic cancer.
Heart and Chest		
Tachycardia	Heart rate >100 beats/min.	Compensatory mechanism in anemia to increase cardiac output.
Palpitations	Feeling the heartbeat, flutter, or pound in the chest.	Anemia, fluid volume overload, hypotension with impending syncope, hypertension, dysrhythmias.
Altered blood pressure	*Orthostasis:* heart rate >20 beats/min increase or blood pressure >20 mm Hg decrease from baseline when moving from a lying position to either sitting or standing.	Orthostasis is a common manifestation in anemia, especially if also accompanied by low blood volume.
	Hypotension: <90 mm Hg systolic or >40 mm Hg drop from baseline.	Hypotension may indicate an infectious process, blood loss, or compromised cardiovascular compensatory mechanisms.
	Hypertension: >140/90 mm Hg.	Hypertension may occur initially as a compensatory mechanism for anemia.
Sternal tenderness	Abnormal sensitivity to touch or pressure on sternum.	Leukemia resulting from increased bone marrow cellularity, causing increase in pressure and bone erosion. Multiple myeloma as a result of stretching of periosteum.
Low O_2 saturation	O_2-carrying capacity as reflected by the O_2 saturation by pulse oximetry.	O_2 saturation may be decreased in cases of severe anemia.
Abdomen		
Hepatomegaly	Palpable liver.	Leukemia, cirrhosis, or fibrosis secondary to iron overload from sickle cell disease or thalassemia.
Splenomegaly	Palpable spleen.	Anemia, thrombocytopenia, leukemia, lymphomas, leukopenia, mononucleosis, malaria, cirrhosis, trauma, portal hypertension.
Distended abdomen	A larger than normal abdominal profile. May be soft or firm, tender or nontender, and accompanied by other symptoms such as nausea, vomiting, or rebound tenderness.	Lymphoma may manifest as abdominal adenopathy, mass(es), or bowel obstruction.
Nervous System		
Paresthesias of feet and hands; ataxia	Numbness sensation and extreme sensitivity experienced in central and peripheral nerves. Impaired muscle movement.	Cobalamin (vitamin B_{12}) deficiency or folate deficiency.
Weakness	Lacking physical strength or energy.	Low Hgb level (anemia).
Headache, nuchal rigidity	Pain in the cranium, potentially involving one area or extending from the frontal area to the back of the neck.	Generalized headache is a common manifestation of mild to moderate anemia. Severe headache with or without visual disturbances may signal intracranial hemorrhage due to thrombocytopenia.

palpated and are best evaluated by radiologic examination. Assess lymph nodes symmetrically and take note of location, size (in centimeters), degree of fixation (e.g., movable, fixed), tenderness, and texture. To assess superficial lymph nodes, lightly palpate the nodes using the pads of the fingers. Then gently roll the skin over the area and concentrate on feeling for possible lymph node enlargement. Ordinarily, lymph nodes are not palpable in adults. If a node is palpable, it should be small (0.5 to 1 cm), mobile, firm, and nontender to be considered a normal finding. A node that is tender, hard, fixed, or enlarged (regardless if it is tender or not) is an abnormal finding and warrants further investigation. Tender nodes are usually a result of inflammation, whereas hard or fixed nodes suggest malignancy.[16]

Develop a sequence when examining the lymph nodes. A convenient sequence is to start at the head and neck. First, palpate the preauricular, posterior auricular, occipital, tonsillar, submandibular, submental, superficial cervical, posterior cervical chain, deep cervical chain, and supraclavicular nodes. Next, palpate the axillary lymph nodes and pectoral, subscapular, and lateral groups of nodes. Then examine the epitrochlear nodes, located in the antecubital fossa between the biceps and triceps muscles. Last, palpate the inguinal lymph nodes, found in the groin.

Palpation of Liver or Spleen. Both the liver and spleen are normally not detectable by palpating the abdomen. When they are enlarged, they may be detectable by percussion or palpation. Measure the degree of enlargement of the liver by the number of fingerbreadths it extends below the rib border. The spleen may be more difficult to detect because of its deep location in the left abdomen. Specific techniques for palpating the liver and spleen are described in Chapter 39.

Skin Assessment. In hematologic disorders, assessment of the skin may be a valuable source of information about the hematologic system. Examine the skin over the entire body in a systematic manner (e.g., starting with the face and oral cavity

FOCUSED ASSESSMENT
Hematologic System

Use this checklist to make sure the key assessment steps have been done.

Subjective

Ask the patient about any of the following and note responses.

Unusual bleeding or bruising	Y	N
Black, tarry stool	Y	N
Blood in vomitus	Y	N
Swelling in neck, armpits, or groin	Y	N
Dark-colored urine	Y	N
Fatigue	Y	N
Heart palpitations	Y	N

Objective: Diagnostic

Check the following laboratory results for critical values.

CBC	✓
White blood cell count with differential	✓
Clotting: PT, INR, aPTT, platelets	✓
Hgb, Hct	✓

Objective: Physical Examination

Inspect

Skin for lesions or color changes	✓

Auscultate

BP for alteration or orthostasis	✓

Palpate

Pulse for tachycardia	✓
Liver and spleen for enlargement	✓
Lymph nodes for lymphadenopathy	✓

aPTT, Activated partial thromboplastin time; *INR,* international normalized ratio; *PT,* prothrombin time.

and moving downward over the body). In patients with RBC disorders the skin may be pale or pasty, or it may have a cyanotic tinge in severe anemia. Erythrocytosis often produces small vessel occlusions causing a purple, mottled appearance of the face, nose, fingers, or toes. Clubbing of the fingers can be seen with chronic anemia such as in patients with sickle cell disease. Leukocyte disorders may cause infectious skin lesions or malignant nodular lesions. These may occur anywhere and have a variable distribution pattern. During the physical assessment of the skin, look carefully for **petechiae** (small purplish red pinpoint lesions), **ecchymoses** (bruising), and *spider nevus* (a form of *telangiectasia*) (see Table 30-5) because these can indicate bleeding disorders. In general, skin and mucosal bleeding indicates a platelet disorder, whereas spontaneous bleeding into joints or muscles indicates a coagulation factor problem. Excessive bleeding from trauma can be due to either or both.[17]

A *focused assessment* is used to evaluate the status of previously identified hematologic problems and to monitor for signs of new problems (see Table 3-6). A focused assessment of the hematologic system is presented in the box above.

DIAGNOSTIC STUDIES OF HEMATOLOGIC SYSTEM

The most direct means of evaluating the hematologic system is through laboratory analysis and other diagnostic studies. Diagnostic tests of the hematologic system are presented in Tables 30-6, 30-7, 30-9, and 30-10.

CASE STUDY
Objective Data: Physical Examination

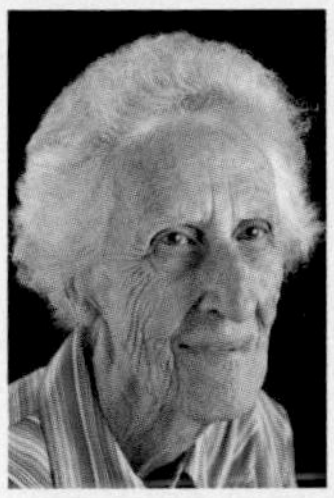

iStockphoto/Thinkstock

Physical examination findings of A.J. are as follows: BP 100/70 (lying), 88/60 (standing); apical pulse 110 (lying), 124 (standing), but regular in rhythm. Respiratory rate 26, temperature 96.8° F (36° C), O_2 saturation 90% on room air. No jugular venous distention. Weight: 106 lb (48 kg). Height: 5 ft 1 in. Skin pale. No jaundice noted. Conjunctiva pale. Tongue smooth and shiny. Lungs clear but diminished breath sounds in the bases bilaterally. No visible bleeding. No enlarged lymph nodes, spleen, or liver noted. General weakness with dyspnea on exertion. No numbness or tingling or peripheral edema.

As you continue to read this chapter, consider diagnostic studies you would anticipate being performed for A.J.

Laboratory Studies

Complete Blood Count. The complete blood count (CBC) involves several laboratory tests (Table 30-6). In addition to the CBC, a *peripheral smear* may be ordered. The smear is used to look at the *morphology* (shape and appearance) of the blood cells and may assist with the diagnosis. For example, a large number of immature *blast* WBCs may indicate acute leukemia.

Although the status of each cell type is important, the entire system may be disrupted by diseases or by treatment of diseases. When the entire CBC is suppressed, a condition termed **pancytopenia** (marked decrease in the number of RBCs, WBCs, and platelets) exists. The effects of aging on hematologic studies are presented in Table 30-4.

Red Blood Cells. Normal values of some RBC tests are reported separately for men and for women because normal values are based on body mass, and men usually have a larger body mass than women.

The *hemoglobin (Hgb) value* is reduced in cases of anemia, hemorrhage, and hemodilution, such as that occurring when the fluid volume is excessive. Increases in hemoglobin are found in polycythemia or in states of hemoconcentration, which can develop from volume depletion (dehydration).

The *hematocrit (Hct) value* is determined by spinning blood in a centrifuge, which causes RBCs and plasma to separate. The RBCs, being the heavier elements, settle to the bottom. The hematocrit value represents the percentage of RBCs compared with the total blood volume. Reductions and elevations of the hematocrit value are seen in the same conditions that raise and lower the hemoglobin value. The hematocrit value generally is three times the hemoglobin value.

The total RBC count is reported as RBC $\times 10^6/\mu L$. However, the total RBC count is not always reliable in determining the adequacy of RBC function. Consequently, other data, such as hemoglobin, hematocrit, and RBC indices, must also be evaluated. The RBC count is altered by the same conditions that raise and lower the hemoglobin and hematocrit values.

RBC indices are special indicators that reflect RBC volume, color, and hemoglobin saturation (see Table 30-6). These parameters may provide insight into the cause of anemia. (The significance of these parameters is discussed further in Chapter 31.)

White Blood Cells. The WBC count provides two different sets of information. The first is a total count of WBCs in 1 μL of peripheral blood. Elevations in WBC count over 11,000/μL are associated with infection, inflammation, tissue injury or death,

TABLE 30-6 **DIAGNOSTIC STUDIES**

Complete Blood Count Studies

Study	Description and Purpose	Reference Intervals
Hemoglobin (Hgb)	Measurement of gas-carrying capacity of RBC.	*Female:* 11.7-16.0 g/dL (117-160 g/L) *Male:* 13.2-17.3 g/dL (132-173 g/L)
Hematocrit (Hct)	Measure of packed cell volume of RBCs expressed as a percentage of the total blood volume.	*Female:* 35%-47% (0.35-0.47) *Male:* 39%-50% (0.39-0.50)
Total RBC count	Number of circulating RBCs.	*Female:* 3.8-5.1 × 10^6/μL (3.8-5.1 × 10^{12}/L) *Male:* 4.3-5.7 × 10^6/μL (4.3-5.7 × 10^{12}/L)
Red cell indices		
$MCV = \frac{Hct \times 10}{RBC \times 10^6}$	Determination of relative size of RBCs. Low MCV reflection of microcytosis, high MCV reflection of macrocytosis.	80-100 fL
$MCH = \frac{Hgb \times 10}{RBC \times 10^6}$	Measurement of average weight of Hgb/RBCs. Low MCH indication of microcytosis or hypochromia, high MCH indication of macrocytosis.	27-34 pg
$MCHC = \frac{Hgb \times 100}{Hct}$	Evaluation of RBC saturation with Hgb. Low MCHC indication of hypochromia, high MCHC evident in spherocytosis.	32%-37% (0.32-0.37)
RBC morphology	Examination of the shape and size of RBCs.	No variation in RBC morphology
WBC count	Measurement of total number of leukocytes.	4000-11,000/μL (4-11 × 10^9/L)
WBC differential	Determination of whether each kind of WBC is present in proper proportion. Absolute value of each type of WBC can be determined by multiplying the percentage of cell type by total WBC count and dividing by 100.	*Neutrophils:* 50%-70% (0.50-0.70) *Eosinophils:* 0%-4% (0-0.04) *Basophils:* 0%-2% (0-0.02) *Lymphocytes:* 20%-40% (0.20-0.40) *Monocytes:* 4%-8% (0.04-0.08)
Platelet count	Number of platelets available to maintain platelet clotting functions (not measurement of quality of platelet function).	150,000-400,000/μL (150-400 × 10^9/L)

MCH, Mean corpuscular hemoglobin; *MCHC,* mean corpuscular hemoglobin concentration; *MCV,* mean corpuscular volume.

and malignancies (e.g., leukemia, lymphoma). Although the degree of WBC elevation does not necessarily predict the severity of illness, it can provide clues to the etiology. Certain types of leukemias are more likely to produce extremely high WBC counts (e.g., greater than 25,000/μL). A WBC count less than 4000/μL **(leukopenia)** is associated with bone marrow depression, severe or chronic illness, and some types of leukemia.

The second aspect of the WBC count, the *differential count,* measures the percentage of each type of leukocyte. The WBC differential provides valuable clues in determining the cause of illness. When infections are severe, more granulocytes are released from the bone marrow as a compensatory mechanism. To meet the increased demand, many young, immature polymorphonuclear neutrophils (bands) are released into circulation. The usual laboratory procedure is to report the WBCs in order of maturity, with the less mature forms on the left side of the written report. Consequently, the existence of many immature cells is termed a *"shift to the left."*

The WBC differential is of considerable significance because it is possible for the total WBC count to remain essentially normal despite a marked change in one type of leukocyte. For example, a patient may have a normal WBC count of 8800/μL, but the differential count may show that the proportion of lymphocytes is reduced to 10%. This is an abnormal finding that warrants further investigation.

When the lymphocyte count is low, an absolute lymphocyte count (ALC) may be tabulated. If the ALC is low, other diagnostic tests may be performed to look for an underlying reason.

When the bone marrow does not produce enough neutrophils, neutropenia occurs. **Neutropenia** is a condition in which the absolute neutrophil count (ANC) is less than 1000 cells/μL; severe neutropenia is associated with an ANC of less than 500 cells/μL. The ANC is determined by multiplying the total WBC count by the percentage of neutrophils. Neutropenia results from a number of disease processes, such as leukemia, or from bone marrow depression (see Chapter 31), and is associated with a high risk of infection and death from sepsis.

Platelet Count. The platelet count is the number of platelets per microliter of blood. Normal platelet counts are between 150,000 and 400,000/μL. Counts below 100,000/μL signify a condition termed **thrombocytopenia.** Bleeding may occur with thrombocytopenia. Spontaneous hemorrhage is possible once platelet counts fall below 10,000/μL.[18] A more extensive description of clotting studies is presented in Table 30-7.

Thrombocytosis is defined as excessive platelets, a disorder that occurs with inflammation and some malignant disorders (see Chapter 31). The most likely complication related to thrombocytosis is excessive clotting.

Blood Typing and Rh Factor. Blood group antigens (A and B) are found only on RBC membranes and form the basis for the ABO blood typing system. The presence or absence of one or both of the two inherited antigens is the basis for the four blood groups: A, B, AB, and O. Blood group A has A antigens, group B has B antigens, group AB has both antigens, and group O has neither A nor B antigens. Each person has antibodies in the serum termed *anti-A* and *anti-B* that react with A or B antigens. These antibodies are found when the corresponding antigen is absent from the RBC surface. For example, B antibodies are found in the serum of people with blood group A (Table 30-8).

Blood reactions based on ABO incompatibilities result from intravascular hemolysis of the RBCs. RBCs *agglutinate* (or clump) when a serum antibody is present to react with the antigens on the RBC membrane. For example, agglutination would occur in the blood of a person with type A blood when he or she receives blood transfused from a person with B antigens (i.e., type B or AB). The anti-B antibodies in the type A

TABLE 30-7 DIAGNOSTIC STUDIES

Clotting Studies

Study	Description and Purpose	Reference Intervals
Activated clotting time (ACT)	Evaluation of intrinsic coagulation status. More accurate than aPTT. Used during dialysis, coronary artery bypass procedure, arteriograms.	70-120 sec
Activated partial thromboplastin time (aPTT)	Assessment of intrinsic coagulation by measuring factors I, II, V, VIII, IX, X, XI, XII. Longer in patients using heparin.	25-35 sec
Antithrombin	Naturally occurring protein synthesized by liver that inhibits coagulation through inactivation of thrombin and other factors. Depleted in DIC.	21-30 mg/dL (210-300 mg/L) or 80%-120% of standard
Bleeding time	Measurement of timed, small skin incision bleeds. Reflection of ability of small blood vessels to constrict.	2-7 min
Capillary fragility test (tourniquet test, Rumpel-Leede test)	Reflection of capillary integrity when positive or negative pressure is applied to various areas of the body. Positive test indication of thrombocytopenia, toxic vascular reactions.	No petechiae or negative
Clot retraction	Reflection of clot shrinkage or retraction from sides of test tube after 24 hr. Used to confirm a platelet problem.	Begins in 1 hr. Maximum by 24 hr
D-dimer	Assay to measure a fragment of fibrin that is formed as a result of fibrin degradation and clot lysis. Used as an adjunctive measure in diagnosis of hypercoagulable conditions (e.g., DIC, pulmonary embolism).	<250 ng/mL (<250 mcg/L)
Fibrin split products (FSPs), or fibrin degradation products (FDPs)	Reflection of degree of fibrinolysis and predisposition to bleed (if present). Screening test for DIC. Elevated levels associated with DIC, advanced malignancy, severe inflammation.	<10 mcg/mL (<10 mg/L)
Fibrinogen	Reflection of level of fibrinogen. Increase in fibrinogen possible indication of enhancement of fibrin formation, making patient hypercoagulable. Decrease in fibrinogen indicates that patient possibly predisposed to bleeding.	200-400 mg/dL (2-4 g/L)
International normalized ratio (INR)	Standardized system of reporting PT based on a reference calibration model and calculated by comparing the patient's PT with a control value.	2-3*
Platelet count	Number of circulating platelets.	150,000-400,000/μL
Prothrombin time (PT)	Assessment of extrinsic coagulation by measurement of factors I, II, V, VII, X.	11-16 sec
Thrombin time	Reflection of adequacy of thrombin. Prolonged thrombin time indicates that coagulation is inadequate secondary to decreased thrombin activity.	17-23 sec

*Desired therapeutic level with warfarin (Coumadin).
DIC, Disseminated intravascular coagulation.

blood would react with the B antigens, thus initiating the process that results in RBC hemolysis.

The *Rh system* is based on a third antigen, D, which is also on the RBC membrane. Rh-positive people have the D antigen, whereas Rh-negative people do not. Rh-positive blood is indicated with a "+" after the ABO group (e.g., AB+). A Coombs test is used to evaluate the person's Rh status (Table 30-9).

As a result of transfusion therapy or during childbirth, an Rh-negative person may be exposed to Rh-positive blood. After exposure during childbirth the mother forms an antibody, anti-D, which acts against Rh antigens. (Rh-positive people normally have no anti-D.) In subsequent pregnancies the mother's anti-D antibodies can cross the placenta and attack the RBCs of a fetus who is Rh-positive, thus causing hemolysis of the RBCs. A pregnant Rh-negative woman should receive Rho(D) immune globulin (RhoGAM) injections to prevent anti-D antibodies from forming.

Iron Metabolism. The laboratory tests used to evaluate iron metabolism include serum iron, total iron-binding capacity (TIBC), serum ferritin, and transferrin saturation. Additional tests for nutritional deficiencies leading to defective RBC production may also be done (see Table 30-9).

Serum iron is a measurement of the amount of protein-bound iron circulating in the serum. TIBC provides a measurement of all proteins that act to bind or transport iron between the tissues and bone marrow. Although this indirect measurement is a general reflection of the amount of transferrin present in the circulation, it overestimates transferrin levels by 16% to 20% because it also measures other proteins that can bind iron. These alternative proteins bind iron only when transferrin is

TABLE 30-8 ABO BLOOD GROUPS AND COMPATIBILITIES*

Recipient's Blood Group	A	B	AB (Universal Recipient)	O (Universal Donor)
RBC antigen	A	B	A and B	Neither
Plasma or serum antibody	Anti-B	Anti-A	Neither anti-A nor anti-B	Anti-A and anti-B
Compatible donor for RBC transfusions	A and O	B and O	A, B, AB, and O	O
Compatible donor for plasma transfusions	A and AB	B and AB	AB	A, B, AB, and O
Percent of population	42%	10%	6%	42%

*ABO blood groups are named for the antigen found on the RBCs. Compatibility is based on the antibodies present in the serum.

TABLE 30-9 DIAGNOSTIC STUDIES

Miscellaneous Blood Studies

Study	Description and Purpose	Normal Values
Bilirubin	Measurement of degree of RBC hemolysis or liver's inability to excrete normal quantities of bilirubin. Increase in indirect bilirubin with hemolytic problems.	*Total:* 0.2-1.2 mg/dL (3.0-21.0 μmol/L) *Direct:* 0.1-0.3 mg/dL (1.7-5.1 μmol/L) *Indirect:* 0.1-1.0 mg/dL (1.7-17.0 μmol/L)
Coombs test	Differentiation among types of hemolytic anemias. Detection of immune antibodies and Rh factor.	Negative
• Direct	Detection of antibodies that are attached to RBCs.	Negative
• Indirect	Detection of antibodies in serum.	Negative
Cobalamin (vitamin B_{12})	Level of cobalamin available for production of new RBCs.	200-835 pg/mL (148-616 pmol/L)
Erythropoietin	Measurement of degree of hormonal stimulation to the bone marrow to stimulate the release of RBCs.	5-30 mU/mL (5-30 U/L)
Erythrocyte sedimentation rate (ESR)	Measurement of sedimentation or settling of RBCs in 1 hr. Inflammatory process causes an alteration in plasma proteins, resulting in aggregation of RBCs and making them heavier. The faster the sedimentation rate, the higher the ESR.	<30 mm/hr (some gender variation)
Ferritin	Major iron storage protein. Is normally present in blood in concentrations directly related to iron storage.	10-250 ng/mL (10-250 mcg/L)
Folic acid (folate)	Amount of folic acid (folate) available for RBC production.	3-16 ng/mL (7-36 nmol/L)
Hemoglobin (Hgb) electrophoresis	Proteins involved in development of the Hgb molecule have a definitive pattern of separation on electrophoresis. This pattern is altered with abnormal Hgb synthesis (e.g., thalassemia) or sickle cell anemia (where Hgb S is increased).	*Normal Hb A1:* >95% *Hb A2:* 1.5%-3.7% *Hb F:* <2% *Hb S:* 0% *Hb C:* 0%
Homocysteine	An amino acid formed from methionine. Rapidly metabolized through pathways that require cobalamin (vitamin B_{12}) and folic acid. Increased in cobalamin and folic acid deficiency.	*Male:* 5.2-12.9 μmol/L *Female:* 3.7-10.4 μmol/L
Iron		
• Serum iron	Reflection of amount of iron combined with proteins in serum. Accurate indication of status of iron storage and use.	50-175 mcg/dL (9-31.3 μmol/L)
• Total iron-binding capacity (TIBC)	Measurement of all proteins available for binding iron. Transferrin represents the largest quantity of iron-binding proteins. Therefore TIBC is an indirect measure of transferrin, an evaluation of amount of extra iron that can be carried.	250-425 mcg/dL (45-76 μmol/L)
Methylmalonic acid (MMA)	Indirect test for cobalamin. MMA metabolism requires cobalamin. Helps differentiate cobalamin deficiency from folic acid deficiency.	<0.2 μmol/L (<2.4 mcg/dL)
Reticulocyte count	Measurement of immature RBCs, a reflection of bone marrow activity in producing RBCs.	0.5%-1.5% of RBC count (0.005-0.015 of RBC count)
Serum protein electrophoresis (SPEP)	Separates proteins in the blood on basis of electric charge. Helps detect hyperglobulinemic states, such as in multiple myeloma or some lymphomas.	Normal banding pattern of albumin and globulins. Increase in any protein ("protein spike") is abnormal.
Transferrin	The largest of proteins that bind to iron. Increased in most people with iron-deficiency anemia.	190-380 mg/dL (1.9-3.8 g/L)
Transferrin saturation (%)	Decreased in iron-deficiency anemia and increased in hemolytic and megaloblastic anemia.	15%-50%

more than half saturated. Also, TIBC varies inversely with tissue iron stores; it is higher when iron stores are low and lower when iron stores are high.

Transferrin saturation is a better indicator of the availability of iron for erythropoiesis than serum iron because, unlike serum iron, the iron bound to transferrin is readily available for the body to use. Transferrin saturation is calculated by dividing serum iron by TIBC and multiplying by 100. For example, a patient with a serum iron level of 100 mcg/dL and a TIBC of 300 mcg/dL would have a transferrin saturation of about 33%.

Under normal conditions, the serum ferritin concentration correlates closely with body iron stores. In normal patients, 1 ng/mL of ferritin corresponds to 8 to 10 mg of stored iron.

Radiologic Studies

Radiologic studies for the hematology system involve primarily the use of computed tomography (CT) or magnetic resonance imaging (MRI) for evaluating the spleen, liver, and lymph nodes. Nursing responsibilities related to these studies are presented in Table 30-10.

Biopsies

Biopsy procedures specific to hematologic assessment are bone marrow examination and lymph node biopsy. In general, these procedures are done because a peripheral blood smear is nonspecific and usually a diagnosis cannot be established from a peripheral blood smear. Furthermore, a biopsy provides additional information about a hematologic problem that is needed for diagnosis and treatment planning.

Bone Marrow Examination. Bone marrow examination is important in the evaluation of many hematologic disorders. The examination of the marrow may involve aspiration only or aspiration with biopsy. The benefits gained from bone marrow examination are (1) a full evaluation of hematopoiesis and (2)

TABLE 30-10 **DIAGNOSTIC STUDIES**

Hematologic System

Study	Description and Purpose	Nursing Responsibility
Blood Studies	See Tables 30-6, 30-7, and 30-9.	
Urine Studies		
Bence Jones protein	An electrophoretic measurement is used to detect the Bence Jones protein, which is found in most cases of multiple myeloma. Negative finding is considered normal.	Acquire random urine specimen.
Radioisotope Studies		
Liver and spleen scan	Radioactive isotope is injected IV. Images from the radioactive emissions are used to evaluate the structure of spleen and liver. Patient is not a source of radioactivity.	No specific nursing responsibilities.
Bone scan	Same procedure as for the spleen scan except used for evaluating the structure of the bones.	Patient needs to lie still during the imaging. Patient may be asked to drink 4-6 glasses of water and then void before the imaging (to see pelvic bones).
Radiologic Studies		
Skeletal x-ray	X-rays done as a bone survey to detect lytic lesions associated with multiple myeloma. Bone scans do not identify lesions in this condition because there is no uptake of radioactive isotopes due to lack of blood supply.	No specific nursing responsibilities.
Liver, spleen, or abdominal ultrasound	Noninvasive probe is lubricated and slid across the abdomen to detect the density and borders of the abdominal organs. Can detect irregular borders, masses, vascular structure, and biliary tree.	Patients must be comfortable lying flat and having the probe compress the abdomen.
Positron emission tomography (PET)	A nuclear tracer substance is injected and is taken up by metabolically active cells. The follow-up scan shows different-colored tissues based on the metabolic rate. "Hot spots" reflect increased glucose consumption that is typical of tumors. A valuable diagnostic tool to detect active malignancy because it highlights areas with increased metabolism. PET or CT scanning may also be used.	IV access is required for injection of the tracer substance. Patients should have nothing by mouth, except water and medications, for at least 4 hr before the test. IV solutions containing glucose may be held. Patients who are glucose intolerant or diabetic may need adjustments in their medications. Bowel preparation may also be needed, depending on the area being studied.
Computed tomography (CT)	Noninvasive radiologic examination using computer-assisted x-ray evaluates the lymph nodes. Contrast medium often is used in abdominal studies of liver or spleen. Spiral (helical) CT scans are used to evaluate lymph nodes.	Investigate iodine sensitivity if contrast medium used.
Magnetic resonance imaging (MRI)	Noninvasive procedure produces sensitive images of soft tissue without using contrast media. No ionizing radiation is required. Technique is used to evaluate spleen, liver, and lymph nodes.	Instruct patient to remove all metal objects and ask about any history of surgical insertion of staples, plates, or other metal appliances. Inform patient of need to lie still in small chamber.
Biopsies		
Bone marrow	Technique involves removal of bone marrow through a locally anesthetized site to evaluate the status of the blood-forming tissue. It is used to diagnose multiple myeloma, all types of leukemia, and some lymphomas and to stage some solid tumors (e.g., breast cancer). It is also done to assess efficacy of leukemia therapy (see Chapter 31).	Explain procedure to patient. Obtain signed consent form. Ensure that a *time-out** is done before procedure. Consider preprocedure analgesic administration to enhance patient comfort and cooperation. Apply pressure dressing after procedure. Assess biopsy site for bleeding.
Lymph node biopsy	Purpose is to obtain lymph tissue for histologic examination to determine diagnosis and therapy.	Explain procedure to patient. Obtain signed consent form. Use sterile technique in dressing changes after procedure.
• Open	Performed in the operating room or procedure area using either local or general anesthesia. An incision is made, and the lymph node and surrounding tissue are dissected (excised) whenever possible.	Apply direct pressure to the area after the biopsy procedure to achieve hemostasis. Observe site for bleeding and monitor vital signs, especially if the platelet count is low. The sterile dressing should be changed as ordered, and the wound should be inspected for healing and infection.
• Closed (needle) or fine needle	Performed by a physician at the bedside or in an outpatient area. An extremely small needle is used to reduce the risk of tracking malignant cells through normal subcutaneous tissue.	
Molecular, Cytogenetic, and Gene Analysis Studies		
Fluorescence in situ hybridization (FISH) **Comparative genomic hybridization (CGH)** **Spectral karyotyping (SKY)**	Tests are performed on malignant cells, either peripheral blood (e.g., leukemia) or biopsy specimen (bone marrow, lymph node) to assess genetic or chromosomal abnormalities of cancer cells. May be useful in confirming diagnosis and determining treatment modalities and prognosis.	No specific nursing responsibilities. Explain purpose of testing to patient.

*Time-out is done just before the procedure starts to verify patient identification, surgical procedure, and surgical site.

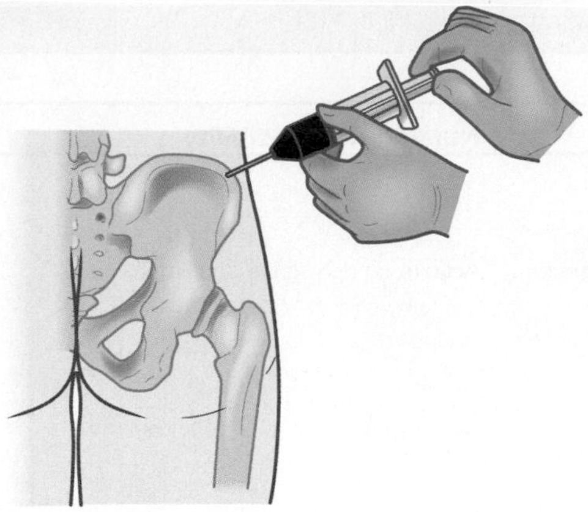

FIG. 30-7 Bone marrow aspiration from the posterior iliac crest.

the ability to obtain specimens for cytopathologic and chromosomal abnormalities. The preferred site for both aspiration and biopsy of bone marrow is the posterior iliac crest.[19] The anterior iliac crest and sternum are alternative sites. However, the sternum is usually used only for aspiration. Bone marrow aspiration and biopsy are performed by a physician or specially credentialed nurse. Local anesthesia and sedation may be used to minimize anxiety and pain that the patient may experience.

For bone marrow aspiration, the skin over the puncture site is cleansed with a bactericidal agent. The skin, subcutaneous tissue, and periosteum are infiltrated with a local anesthetic agent. The patient may be uncomfortable when the periosteum is penetrated. Once the area is anesthetized, a bone marrow needle is inserted through the cortex of the bone. The stylet of the needle is then removed, the hub is attached to a 10-mL syringe, and 0.2 to 0.5 mL of the fluid marrow is aspirated (Fig. 30-7). The patient experiences pain with aspiration. Although it lasts only a few seconds, the pain may be quite uncomfortable. After the marrow aspiration, the needle is removed. Pressure is applied over the aspiration site to ensure hemostasis.

Although complications of bone marrow aspiration are minimal, there is a possibility of damaging underlying structures. This hazard is greatest in aspiration procedures involving the sternum.[20] Other complications include hemorrhage (especially if the patient is thrombocytopenic) and infection (especially if the patient is leukopenic).

The needle aspiration or biopsy site is covered with a sterile pressure dressing. Monitor the patient's vital signs until stable, and assess the site for excess drainage or bleeding. If bleeding is present, advise the patient to lie on the side for 30 to 60 minutes to maintain pressure on the site. If the bed is too soft, have the patient lie on a rolled towel to provide additional pressure. Analgesics for postprocedure pain may be administered. Soreness over the puncture site for 3 to 4 days after the procedure is normal.[20]

CASE STUDY

Objective Data: Diagnostic Studies

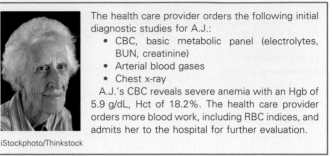

iStockphoto/Thinkstock

The health care provider orders the following initial diagnostic studies for A.J.:

- CBC, basic metabolic panel (electrolytes, BUN, creatinine)
- Arterial blood gases
- Chest x-ray

A.J.'s CBC reveals severe anemia with an Hgb of 5.9 g/dL, Hct of 18.2%. The health care provider orders more blood work, including RBC indices, and admits her to the hospital for further evaluation.

Lymph Node Biopsy. Lymph node biopsy involves obtaining lymph tissue for histologic examination to determine the diagnosis and help plan therapy. This may be accomplished by either an open biopsy or a closed (needle) biopsy.

If the results from a needle biopsy are negative, it may only indicate that the cancer cells were not part of the tissue in the biopsy specimen. However, a positive finding is sufficient evidence for confirming a diagnosis. This technique is rarely used to confirm an initial diagnosis because larger specimens are usually required to perform cytopathologic tests, but it may be used to validate disease recurrence or a new site of disease.

Molecular Cytogenetics and Gene Analysis

Testing for specific genetic or chromosomal variations in hematologic conditions is often helpful in diagnosis and staging. These results also help determine the treatment options and prognosis. If a large number of abnormal cells are circulating in the blood, such as in acute leukemia, these tests may be done by obtaining peripheral blood. However, testing is usually done on samples from bone marrow and lymph node biopsies. For example, fluorescence in situ hybridization (FISH) can identify specific areas by attaching a probe to a targeted region of deoxyribonucleic acid (DNA). It may be used to illuminate an abnormal extra chromosome 8, which is common in certain leukemias. Spectral karyotyping (SKY) allows each set of chromosomes to be painted different colors. It can be used to identify the chromosomal translocation of 22 to 9 in the Philadelphia chromosome of chronic myelogenous leukemia. More information on genetics is in Chapter 13.

BRIDGE TO NCLEX EXAMINATION

The number of the question corresponds to the same-numbered outcome at the beginning of the chapter.

1. An individual who lives at a high altitude may normally have an increased RBC count because
   a. high altitudes cause vascular fluid loss, leading to hemoconcentration.
   b. hypoxia caused by decreased atmospheric oxygen stimulates erythropoiesis.
   c. the function of the spleen in removing old RBCs is impaired at high altitudes.
   d. impaired production of leukocytes and platelets leads to proportionally higher red cell counts.
2. Malignant disorders that arise from granulocytic cells in the bone marrow will have the primary effect of causing
   a. risk for hemorrhage.
   b. altered oxygenation.
   c. decreased production of antibodies.
   d. decreased phagocytosis of bacteria.
3. An anticoagulant such as warfarin (Coumadin) that interferes with prothrombin production will alter the clotting mechanism during
   a. platelet aggregation.
   b. activation of thrombin.
   c. the release of tissue thromboplastin.
   d. stimulation of factor activation complex.

4. When reviewing laboratory results of an 83-year-old patient with an infection, the nurse would expect to find
   a. minimal leukocytosis.
   b. decreased platelet count.
   c. increased hemoglobin and hematocrit levels.
   d. decreased erythrocyte sedimentation rate (ESR).
5. Significant information obtained from the patient's health history that relates to the hematologic system includes
   a. jaundice.
   b. bladder surgery.
   c. early menopause.
   d. multiple pregnancies.
6. While assessing the lymph nodes, the nurse should
   a. apply gentle, firm pressure to deep lymph nodes.
   b. palpate the deep cervical and supraclavicular nodes last.
   c. lightly palpate superficial lymph nodes with the pads of the fingers.
   d. use the tips of the second, third, and fourth fingers to apply deep palpation.
7. If a lymph node is palpated, what is a normal finding?
   a. Hard, fixed nodes
   b. Firm, mobile nodes
   c. Enlarged, tender nodes
   d. Hard, nontender nodes
8. Nursing care for a patient immediately after a bone marrow biopsy and aspiration includes *(select all that apply)*
   a. administering analgesics as necessary.
   b. preparing to administer a blood transfusion.
   c. instructing on need to lie still with a sterile pressure dressing intact.
   d. monitoring vital signs and assessing the site for excess drainage or bleeding.
   e. instructing on the need for preprocedure and postprocedure antibiotic medications.
9. You are taking care of a male patient who has the following laboratory values from his CBC: WBC $6.5 \times 10^3/\mu L$, Hgb 13.4 g/dL, Hct 40%, platelets $50 \times 10^3/\mu L$. What are you most concerned about?
   a. Your patient is neutropenic.
   b. Your patient has an infection.
   c. Your patient is at risk for bleeding.
   d. Your patient is at fall risk due to his anemia.

1. b, 2. d, 3. b, 4. a, 5. a, 6. c, 7. b, 8. a, c, d, 9. c

evolve

For rationales to these answers and even more NCLEX review questions, visit *http://evolve.elsevier.com/Lewis/medsurg.*

REFERENCES

1. McCance KL, Huether SE: *Pathophysiology: the biologic basis for disease in adults and children*, ed 6, St Louis, 2010, Mosby.
2. Porter RS, Kaplan JL: *The Merck manual*, Whitehouse Station, NJ, 2011, Merck.
3. Kumar V, Abbas AK: *Pathologic basis of disease*, ed 8, Philadelphia, 2010, Saunders.
4. Monahan FD: *Mosby's expert physician exam handbook*, ed 3, St Louis, 2009, Mosby.
5. Ganz T, Nemeth E: Hepcidin and disorders of iron metabolism, *Ann Rev Med* 62:347, 2011.
6. Beerman I, Maloney WJ, Weissman IL, et al: Stem cells and the aging hematopoietic system, *Curr Opin Immunol* 22:500, 2010.
7. Hurria A, Muss HB, Cohen HG: Cancer and aging. In Hong WK, Bast RC, Hait WN, and Kufe DW, editors: *Holland-Frei cancer medicine*, ed 8, Shelton, Conn, 2010, People's Medical Publishing House.
8. Malaguarnera L, Cristald E, Malaguarnera M: The role of immunity in elderly cancer, *Crit Rev Oncol Hematol* 74:40, 2010.
9. Taffet GE: Normal aging. Retrieved from *www.uptodate.com/contents/normal aging.*
10. Balducci L: Anemia, fatigue, and aging, *Transf Clin Biol* 17:375, 2010.
11. Tita-Nwa F, Bos A, Adjei A, et al: Correlates of D-dimer in older people, *Aging Clin Exper Res* 22(1):20, 2010.
12. Sivilotti MLA: Hematologic principles. In Nelson LS, Lewin NA, Howland MA, et al, editors: *Goldfrank's toxicologic emergencies*, ed 9, New York, 2009, McGraw-Hill.
13. Lopez JA, Lockhart E: Acquired disorders of platelet dysfunction. In Hoffman R, Benz R, Shattil S, et al, editors: *Hematology: basic principles and practice*, ed 5, Philadelphia, 2009, Saunders.
14. Hodgson BB, Kizior RJ: *Saunders nursing drug handbook*, St Louis, 2012, Saunders.
15. American Dietetic Association: Health benefits of folate. Retrieved from *www.eatright.org.*
16. Jarvis C: *Physical examination and health assessment*, ed 6, St Louis, 2012, Saunders.
17. Collar BS, Schneiderman PI: Clinical evaluation of hemorrhagic disorders: the bleeding history and differential diagnosis of purpura. In Hoffman R, Benz R, Shattil S, et al, editors: *Hematology: basic principles and practice*, ed 5, Philadelphia, 2009, Saunders.
18. Babic A, Kaufman RM: Principles of platelet transfusion therapy. In Hoffman R, Benz R, Shattil S, et al, editors: *Hematology: basic principles and practice*, ed 5, Philadelphia, 2009, Saunders.
19. Venes D: *Taber's cyclopedic medical dictionary*, ed 21, Philadelphia, 2009, FA Davis.
20. Fischbach FT, Dunning MB: A manual of laboratory and diagnostic tests, ed 8, Philadelphia, 2009, Lippincott Williams & Wilkins.

RESOURCES

Resources for this chapter are listed in Chapter 31 on p. 683.

CHAPTER

31

I have nothing to offer but blood, toil, tears, and sweat.
Winston Churchill

Nursing Management
Hematologic Problems

Sandra Irene Rome

evolve WEBSITE

http://evolve.elsevier.com/Lewis/medsurg

- NCLEX Review Questions
- Key Points
- Pre-Test
- Answer Guidelines for Case Study on p. 680
- Rationales for Bridge to NCLEX Examination Questions
- Case Studies
  - Patient With Chronic Myelogenous Leukemia Including End-of-life Care
  - Patient With Sickle Cell Anemia
- Concept Map Creator
- Concept Map for Case Study on p. 680
- Nursing Care Plans (Customizable)
  - NCP 31-1: Patient With Anemia
  - eNCP 31-1: Patient With Thrombocytopenia
  - eNCP 31-2: Patient With Neutropenia
- Glossary
- Content Updates

LEARNING OUTCOMES

1. Describe the general clinical manifestations and complications of anemia.
2. Differentiate the etiologies, clinical manifestations, diagnostic findings, and nursing and collaborative management of iron-deficiency, megaloblastic, and aplastic anemias and anemia of chronic disease.
3. Explain the nursing management of anemia secondary to blood loss.
4. Describe the pathophysiology, clinical manifestations, and nursing and collaborative management of anemia caused by increased erythrocyte destruction, including sickle cell disease and acquired hemolytic anemias.
5. Describe the pathophysiology and nursing and collaborative management of polycythemia.
6. Explain the pathophysiology, clinical manifestations, and nursing and collaborative management of various types of thrombocytopenia.
7. Describe the types, clinical manifestations, diagnostic findings, and nursing and collaborative management of hemophilia and von Willebrand disease.
8. Explain the pathophysiology, diagnostic findings, and nursing and collaborative management of disseminated intravascular coagulation.
9. Describe the etiology, clinical manifestations, and nursing and collaborative management of neutropenia.
10. Describe the pathophysiology, clinical manifestations, and nursing and collaborative management of myelodysplastic syndrome.
11. Compare and contrast the major types of leukemia regarding distinguishing clinical and laboratory findings.
12. Explain the nursing and collaborative management of acute and chronic leukemias.
13. Compare Hodgkin's lymphoma and non-Hodgkin's lymphomas in terms of clinical manifestations, staging, and nursing and collaborative management.
14. Describe the pathophysiology, clinical manifestations, and nursing and collaborative management of multiple myeloma.
15. Describe the spleen disorders and related collaborative care.
16. Describe the nursing management of the patient receiving transfusions of blood and blood components.

KEY TERMS

anemia, p. 633
aplastic anemia, p. 642
disseminated intravascular coagulation (DIC), p. 657
hemochromatosis, p. 647
hemolytic anemia, p. 643
hemophilia, p. 655
Hodgkin's lymphoma, p. 669
iron-deficiency anemia, p. 637
leukemia, p. 664
lymphomas, p. 669
megaloblastic anemias, p. 640
multiple myeloma, p. 673
myelodysplastic syndrome (MDS), p. 663
neutropenia, p. 660
non-Hodgkin's lymphomas (NHLs), p. 671
pernicious anemia, p. 640
polycythemia, p. 648
sickle cell disease (SCD), p. 644
thalassemia, p. 639
thrombocytopenia, p. 650

Reviewed by Mimi Haskins, RN, MS, CMSRN, Nursing Staff Development Instructor, Roswell Park Cancer Institute, Buffalo, New York.

CULTURAL & ETHNIC HEALTH DISPARITIES

Hematologic Problems

- Sickle cell disease has a high incidence among African Americans.
- Thalassemia has a high incidence among African Americans and people of Mediterranean origin.
- Tay-Sachs disease has the highest incidence in families of Eastern European Jewish origin, especially the Ashkenazi Jews.
- Pernicious anemia has a high incidence among Scandinavians and African Americans.

ANEMIA

Definition and Classification

Anemia is a deficiency in the number of erythrocytes (red blood cells [RBCs]), the quantity or quality of hemoglobin, and/or the volume of packed RBCs (hematocrit). It is a prevalent condition with many diverse causes such as blood loss, impaired production of erythrocytes, or increased destruction of erythrocytes (Fig. 31-1). Because RBCs transport oxygen (O_2), erythrocyte disorders can lead to tissue hypoxia. This hypoxia accounts for many of the signs and symptoms of anemia. Anemia is not a specific disease. It is a manifestation of a pathologic process.

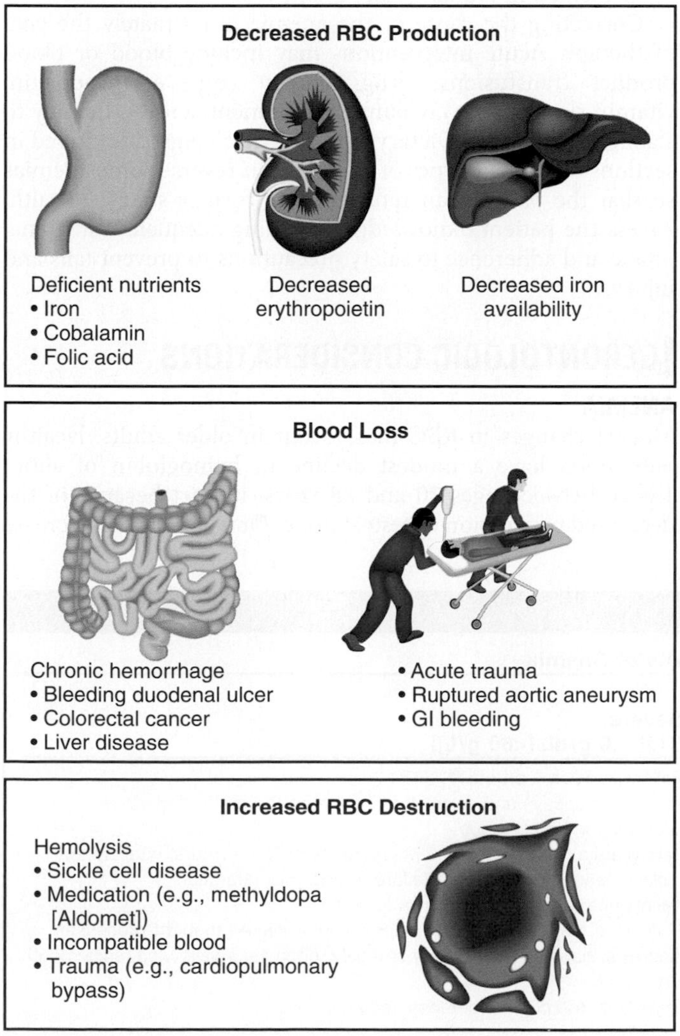

FIG. 31-1 Causes of anemia.

Anemia is classified by review of the complete blood count (CBC), reticulocyte count, and peripheral blood smear. Once anemia is identified, further investigation is done to determine its specific cause.[1]

Anemia can result from primary hematologic problems or can develop as a secondary consequence of diseases or disorders of other body systems. The various types of anemia can be classified according to either *morphology* (cellular characteristic) or *etiology* (cause). Morphologic classification is based on erythrocyte size and color (Table 31-1). Etiologic classification is related to the clinical conditions causing the anemia[2,3] (Table 31-2). Although the morphologic system is the most accurate means of classifying anemias, it is easier to discuss patient care by focusing on the etiology of the anemia.

Clinical Manifestations

The clinical manifestations of anemia are caused by the body's response to tissue hypoxia. Specific manifestations vary depending on the rate at which the anemia has evolved, its severity, and any coexisting disease. Hemoglobin (Hgb) levels are often used to determine the severity of anemia.

Mild states of anemia (Hgb 10 to 12 g/dL [100 to 120 g/L]) may exist without causing symptoms. If symptoms develop, it is because the patient has an underlying disease or is experiencing a compensatory response to heavy exercise. Symptoms include palpitations, dyspnea, and mild fatigue.[2,3]

In moderate anemia (Hgb 6 to 10 g/dL [60 to 100 g/L]) the cardiopulmonary symptoms are increased. The patient may experience them while resting, as well as with activity.

In severe anemia (Hgb less than 6 g/dL [60 g/L]) the patient has many clinical manifestations involving multiple body systems (Table 31-3).

Integumentary Changes. Integumentary changes include pallor, jaundice, and pruritus. Pallor results from reduced amounts of hemoglobin and reduced blood flow to the skin. Jaundice occurs when hemolysis of RBCs results in an increased concentration of serum bilirubin. Pruritus occurs because of increased serum and skin bile salt concentrations. In addition to the skin, the sclera of the eyes and mucous membranes should be evaluated for jaundice because they reflect the integumentary changes more accurately, especially in a dark-skinned individual.

Cardiopulmonary Manifestations. Cardiopulmonary manifestations of severe anemia result from additional attempts by

TABLE 31-1 MORPHOLOGY AND ETIOLOGY OF ANEMIA

Morphology	Etiology
Normocytic, normochromic (normal size and color) MCV 80-100 fL, MCH 27-34 pg	Acute blood loss, hemolysis, chronic kidney disease, chronic disease, cancers, sideroblastic anemia, endocrine disorders, starvation, aplastic anemia, sickle cell anemia, pregnancy
Microcytic, hypochromic (small size, pale color) MCV <80 fL, MCH <27 pg	Iron-deficiency anemia, vitamin B_6 deficiency, copper deficiency, thalassemia, lead poisoning
Macrocytic (megaloblastic), normochromic (large size, normal color) MCV >100 fL, MCH >34 pg	Cobalamin (vitamin B_{12}) deficiency, folic acid deficiency, liver disease (including effects of alcohol abuse), postsplenectomy

MCH, Mean corpuscular hemoglobin; *MCV,* mean corpuscular volume.

the heart and lungs to provide adequate amounts of oxygen to the tissues. Cardiac output is maintained by increasing the heart rate and stroke volume. The low viscosity of the blood contributes to the development of systolic murmurs and bruits. In extreme cases or when concomitant heart disease is present, angina pectoris and myocardial infarction (MI) may occur if myocardial O_2 needs cannot be met. Heart failure (HF), cardiomegaly, pulmonary and systemic congestion, ascites, and peripheral edema may develop if the heart is overworked for an extended period.

TABLE 31-2 CLASSIFICATION OF ANEMIA

Decreased RBC Production	Blood Loss
Decreased Hemoglobin Synthesis • Iron deficiency • Thalassemias (decreased globin synthesis) • Sideroblastic anemia (decreased porphyrin) ***Defective DNA Synthesis*** • Cobalamin (vitamin B_{12}) deficiency • Folic acid deficiency ***Decreased Number of RBC Precursors*** • Aplastic anemia and inherited disorders (e.g., Fanconi syndrome) • Anemia of myeloproliferative diseases (e.g., leukemia) and myelodysplasia • Chronic diseases or disorders • Medications and chemicals (e.g., chemotherapy, lead) • Radiation	***Acute*** • Trauma • Blood vessel rupture • Splenic sequestration crisis ***Chronic*** • Gastritis • Menstrual flow • Hemorrhoids **Increased RBC Destruction (Hemolytic Anemias)** ***Hereditary (Intrinsic)*** • Abnormal hemoglobin (sickle cell disease) • Enzyme deficiency (G6PD) • Membrane abnormalities (paroxysmal nocturnal hemoglobinuria, hereditary spherocytosis) ***Acquired (Extrinsic)*** • Macroangiopathic: physical trauma (prosthetic heart valves, extracorporeal circulation) • Microangiopathic: disseminated intravascular coagulopathy (DIC), thrombotic thrombocytopenic purpura (TTP) • Antibodies (isoimmune and autoimmune) • Infectious agents (e.g., malaria) and toxins

G6PD, Glucose-6-phosphate dehydrogenase.

NURSING MANAGEMENT ANEMIA

This section discusses general nursing management of anemia. Specific care related to various types of anemia is discussed later in this chapter.

NURSING ASSESSMENT

Subjective and objective data that should be obtained from a patient with anemia are presented in Table 31-4.

NURSING DIAGNOSES

Nursing diagnoses for the patient with anemia include, but are not limited to, those presented in Nursing Care Plan 31-1.

PLANNING

The overall goals are that the patient with anemia will (1) assume normal activities of daily living, (2) maintain adequate nutrition, and (3) develop no complications related to anemia.

NURSING IMPLEMENTATION

The numerous causes of anemia necessitate different nursing interventions specific to the patient's needs. Nevertheless, certain general components of care for all patients with anemia are presented in Nursing Care Plan 31-1.

Correcting the cause of the anemia is ultimately the goal of therapy. Acute interventions may include blood or blood product transfusions, drug therapy (e.g., erythropoietin, vitamin supplements), volume replacement, and O_2 therapy to stabilize the patient. Dietary and lifestyle changes (described in sections on specific types of anemia) can reverse some anemias so that the patient can return to the former state of health. Assess the patient's knowledge regarding adequate nutritional intake and adherence to safety precautions to prevent falls and injury.

GERONTOLOGIC CONSIDERATIONS

ANEMIA

Modest changes in RBC mass occur in older adults. Healthy older men have a modest decline in hemoglobin of about 1 g/dL between ages 70 and 88 years, in part because of the decreased production of testosterone. Only a minimal decrease

TABLE 31-3 MANIFESTATIONS OF ANEMIA

Body System	Severity of Anemia: Mild (Hgb 10-12 g/dL [100-120 g/L])	Moderate (Hgb 6-10 g/dL [60-100 g/L])	Severe (Hgb <6 g/dL [<60 g/L])
Integument	None	None	Pallor, jaundice,* pruritus*
Eyes	None	None	Icteric conjunctiva and sclera,* retinal hemorrhage, blurred vision
Mouth	None	None	Glossitis, smooth tongue
Cardiovascular	Palpitations	Increased palpitations, "bounding pulse"	Tachycardia, increased pulse pressure, systolic murmurs, intermittent claudication, angina, heart failure, myocardial infarction
Pulmonary	Exertional dyspnea	Dyspnea	Tachypnea, orthopnea, dyspnea at rest
Neurologic	None	"Roaring in the ears"	Headache, vertigo, irritability, depression, impaired thought processes
Gastrointestinal	None	None	Anorexia, hepatomegaly, splenomegaly, difficulty swallowing, sore mouth
Musculoskeletal	None	None	Bone pain
General	None or mild fatigue	Fatigue	Sensitivity to cold, weight loss, lethargy

*Caused by hemolysis.

TABLE 31-4 NURSING ASSESSMENT

Anemia

Subjective Data

Important Health Information

Past health history: Recent blood loss or trauma; chronic liver, endocrine, or renal disease (including dialysis); GI disease (malabsorption syndrome, ulcers, gastritis, or hemorrhoids); inflammatory disorders (especially Crohn's disease); smoking, exposure to radiation or chemical toxins (arsenic, lead, benzenes, copper); infectious diseases (HIV) or recent travel with possible exposure to infection; angina, myocardial infarction; history of falling

Medications: Use of vitamin and iron supplements; aspirin, anticoagulants, oral contraceptives, phenobarbital, penicillins, nonsteroidal antiinflammatory drugs, omeprazole, phenacetin, phenytoin (Dilantin), sulfonamides, herbal products

Surgery or other treatments: Recent surgery, small bowel resection, gastrectomy, prosthetic heart valves, chemotherapy, radiation therapy

Dietary history: General dietary patterns, consumption of alcohol

Functional Health Patterns

Health perception–health management: Family history of anemia; malaise

Nutritional-metabolic: Nausea, vomiting, anorexia, weight loss; dysphagia, dyspepsia, heartburn; night sweats, cold intolerance

Elimination: Hematuria, decreased urine output; diarrhea, constipation, flatulence, tarry stools, bloody stools

Activity-exercise: Fatigue, muscle weakness and decreased strength; dyspnea, orthopnea, cough, hemoptysis; palpitations; shortness of breath with activity

Cognitive-perceptual: Headache; abdominal, chest, and bone pain; painful tongue; paresthesias of feet and hands; pruritus; disturbances in vision, taste, or hearing; vertigo; hypersensitivity to cold; dizziness

Sexuality-reproductive: Menorrhagia, metrorrhagia; recent or current pregnancy; male impotence

Objective Data

General

Lethargy, apathy, general lymphadenopathy, fever

Integumentary

Pale skin and mucous membranes; blue, pale white, or icteric sclera; cheilitis (inflammation of the lips); poor skin turgor; brittle, spoon-shaped fingernails; jaundice; petechiae; ecchymoses; nose or gingival bleeding; poor healing; dry, brittle, thinning hair

Respiratory

Tachypnea

Cardiovascular

Tachycardia, systolic murmur, dysrhythmias; postural hypotension, widened pulse pressure, bruits (especially carotid); intermittent claudication, ankle edema

Gastrointestinal

Hepatosplenomegaly; glossitis; beefy, red tongue; stomatitis; abdominal distention; anorexia

Neurologic

Headache, roaring in the ears, confusion, impaired judgment, irritability, ataxia, unsteady gait, paralysis, loss of vibration sense

Possible Diagnostic Findings

↓ RBCs, ↓ Hgb; ↓ Hct; ↑ or ↓ reticulocytes, MCV, serum iron, ferritin, folate, or cobalamin (vitamin B_{12}); heme (guaiac)–positive stools; ↓ serum erythropoietin level; ↑ or ↓ LDH, bilirubin, transferrin (see Table 31-6)

LDH, Lactate dehydrogenase; *MCV,* mean corpuscular volume.

NURSING CARE PLAN 31-1

Patient With Anemia

NURSING DIAGNOSIS* **Fatigue** *related to* inadequate oxygenation of the blood *as evidenced by* increased pulse and blood pressure in response to activity, anorexia, impaired concentration, and/or patient verbalization of an overwhelming lack of energy

PATIENT GOALS
1. Participates in activities of daily living without abnormal increases in blood pressure and pulse
2. Reports increased endurance for activity

Outcomes (NOC)

Fatigue Level

- Exhaustion _____
- Loss of appetite _____
- Decreased motivation _____
- Lassitude _____

Measurement Scale

1 = Severe
2 = Substantial
3 = Moderate
4 = Mild
5 = None

Energy Conservation

- Recognizes energy limitations _____
- Balances activity and rest _____
- Uses energy conservation techniques _____
- Organizes activities to conserve energy _____
- Maintains adequate nutrition _____

Measurement Scale

1 = Never demonstrated
2 = Rarely demonstrated
3 = Sometimes demonstrated
4 = Often demonstrated
5 = Consistently demonstrated

Interventions (NIC) and *Rationales*

Energy Management

- Correct physiologic status deficits (e.g., chemotherapy-induced anemia) as priority items.
- Encourage alternate rest and activity periods *to provide activity without tiring the patient.*
- Monitor cardiorespiratory response to activity (e.g., tachycardia, dysrhythmias, dyspnea, diaphoresis, pallor, respiratory rate) *to evaluate activity intolerance.*
- Limit number of visitors and interruptions by visitors *to provide rest periods.*
- Assist the patient in assigning priority to activities to accommodate energy levels *to promote tolerance for important activities.*
- Arrange physical activities (e.g., avoid activity immediately after meals) *to reduce competition for O_2 supply to vital functions.*
- Assist with regular physical activities (e.g., ambulation, transfers, personal care) *to minimize fatigue and risk of injury from falls.*
- Instruct patient and caregiver to recognize signs and symptoms of fatigue that require reduction in activity *to promote self-care.*
- Instruct patient and caregiver to notify health care provider if signs and symptoms of fatigue persist *to review treatment plan.*

*Nursing diagnoses listed in order of priority.

Continued

NURSING CARE PLAN 31-1—cont'd

Patient With Anemia

NURSING DIAGNOSIS **Imbalanced nutrition: less than body requirements** *related to* inadequate nutritional intake and anorexia *as evidenced by* weight loss, low serum albumin, decreased iron level, vitamin deficiencies

PATIENT GOALS
1. Maintains dietary intake that provides minimum daily requirements of nutrients
2. Attains normal blood values of nutrients necessary to prevent anemia

Outcomes (NOC)	Interventions (NIC) and *Rationales*
Nutritional Status • Nutrient intake ____ • Weight/height ratio ____ ***Nutritional Status: Biochemical Measures*** • Serum albumin ____ • Serum transferrin ____ • Hemoglobin ____ • Hematocrit ____ • Total iron-binding capacity ____ **Measurement Scale** 1 = Severe deviation from normal range 2 = Substantial deviation from normal range 3 = Moderate deviation from normal range 4 = Mild deviation from normal range 5 = No deviation from normal range	***Nutrition Management*** • Determine, in collaboration with dietitian, number of calories and type of nutrients needed to meet nutritional requirements *to plan interventions.* • Teach patient how to keep a food diary *to help evaluate nutritional intake.* • Monitor recorded intake for nutritional content and calories *to evaluate nutritional status.* • Provide appropriate information about nutritional needs and how to meet them *to increase intake of essential nutrients needed.* • Encourage increased intake of protein, iron, and vitamin C *to provide nutrients needed for maximum iron absorption and hemoglobin production.* • Encourage increased intake of foods high in iron *to provide nutrient needed for hemoglobin production.*

NURSING DIAGNOSIS **Ineffective self-health management** *related to* lack of knowledge about appropriate nutrition and medication regimen *as evidenced by* questioning about lifestyle adjustments, diet, medications

PATIENT GOAL Verbalizes knowledge necessary to maintain adequate nutrition and management of medication regimen

Outcomes (NOC)	Interventions (NIC) and *Rationales*
Knowledge: Diet • Recommended diet ____ • Dietary goals ____ • Healthy nutritional practices ____ • Potential food and medication interactions ____ ***Knowledge: Medication*** • Identification of correct name of medication(s) ____ • Medication therapeutic effects ____ • Medication adverse effects ____ • Correct use of prescribed medication ____ • Required laboratory tests for monitoring medication ____ **Measurement Scale** 1 = No knowledge 2 = Limited knowledge 3 = Moderate knowledge 4 = Substantial knowledge 5 = Extensive knowledge	***Nutritional Counseling*** • Facilitate identification of eating behaviors to be changed. • Use accepted nutritional standards to assist patient in evaluating adequacy of dietary intake *to evaluate adequacy.* • Discuss nutritional requirements and patient's perceptions of prescribed or recommended diet. • Provide referral or consultation with other members of the health care team *to help patient maintain gains and adjustments throughout recovery.* • Review with patient measurements of hemoglobin values *to evaluate response to therapeutic plan.* ***Teaching: Prescribed Medication*** • Instruct the patient on the purpose and action of each medication. • Instruct the patient on dosage, route, and duration of each medication *to improve adherence.* • Instruct the patient on possible adverse effects of each medication *to ensure early detection of untoward responses to medication.*

in hemoglobin (about 0.2 g/dL) occurs between these ages in healthy women.

For older adults with anemia, about one third have a nutritional type of anemia (e.g., iron, folate, cobalamin). About another third have renal insufficiency and/or chronic inflammation, and the other third have anemia that is unexplained.

Cobalamin (vitamin B_{12}) and folate deficiency may occur in about 14% of older adults because of pernicious anemia, insufficient dietary intake, and malabsorption caused by low stomach acidity.[4] Multiple co-morbid conditions in older adults increase the likelihood of many types of anemia occurring.

Clinical manifestations of anemia in older adults may include pallor, confusion, ataxia, fatigue, worsening angina, and heart failure.[2] Unfortunately, anemia may go unrecognized in older adults because these manifestations may be mistaken for normal aging changes or overlooked because of another health problem. By recognizing signs of anemia, you can play a pivotal role in health assessment and related interventions for older adults.

ANEMIA CAUSED BY DECREASED ERYTHROCYTE PRODUCTION

Normally RBC production (termed *erythropoiesis*) is in equilibrium with RBC destruction and loss. This balance ensures that an adequate number of erythrocytes is available at all times. The normal life span of an RBC is 120 days. Three alterations in erythropoiesis may occur that decrease RBC production: (1) decreased hemoglobin synthesis may lead to iron-deficiency anemia, thalassemia, and sideroblastic anemia; (2) defective deoxyribonucleic acid (DNA) synthesis in RBCs (e.g., cobalamin deficiency, folic acid deficiency) may lead to megaloblastic anemias; and (3) diminished availability of erythrocyte precursors may result in aplastic anemia and anemia of chronic disease (see Table 31-2).

IRON-DEFICIENCY ANEMIA

Iron-deficiency anemia, one of the most common chronic hematologic disorders, is found in 2% to 5% of adult men and postmenopausal women in developed countries. Those most susceptible to iron-deficiency anemia are the very young, those on poor diets, and women in their reproductive years.[5,6] Normally, 1 mg of iron is lost daily through feces, sweat, and urine.[7]

Etiology

Iron-deficiency anemia may develop as a result of inadequate dietary intake, malabsorption, blood loss, or hemolysis. (Normal iron metabolism is discussed in Chapter 30 on p. 616.) Normal dietary iron intake is usually sufficient to meet the needs of men and older women, but it may be inadequate for those individuals who have higher iron needs (e.g., menstruating or pregnant women). Table 31-5 lists nutrients needed for erythropoiesis.[8,9]

Malabsorption of iron may occur after certain types of gastrointestinal (GI) surgery and in malabsorption syndromes. Surgical procedures may involve removal or bypass of the duodenum (see Chapter 42). As iron absorption occurs in the duodenum, malabsorption syndromes may involve disease of the duodenum in which the absorption surface is altered or destroyed.

Blood loss is a major cause of iron deficiency in adults. Two milliliters of whole blood contain 1 mg of iron. The major sources of chronic blood loss are from the GI and genitourinary (GU) systems. GI bleeding is often not apparent and therefore may exist for a considerable time before the problem is identified. Loss of 50 to 75 mL of blood from the upper GI tract is required for stools to appear black *(melena)*. The black color results from the iron in the RBCs. Common causes of GI blood loss are peptic ulcer, gastritis, esophagitis, diverticuli, hemorrhoids, and neoplasia. GU blood loss occurs primarily from menstrual bleeding. The average monthly menstrual blood loss is about 45 mL and causes the loss of about 22 mg of iron. Postmenopausal bleeding can contribute to anemia in a susceptible older woman. In addition to anemia of chronic kidney disease, dialysis treatment may induce iron-deficiency anemia because of the blood lost in the dialysis equipment and frequent blood sampling.

Clinical Manifestations

In the early course of iron-deficiency anemia the patient may not have any symptoms. As the disease becomes chronic, any of the general manifestations of anemia may develop (see Table 31-3). In addition, specific clinical manifestations may occur related to iron-deficiency anemia. Pallor is the most common finding, and *glossitis* (inflammation of the tongue) is the second most common. Another finding is *cheilitis* (inflammation of the lips). In addition, the patient may report headache, paresthesias, and a burning sensation of the tongue, all of which are caused by lack of iron in the tissues.

TABLE 31-5 NUTRITIONAL THERAPY

Nutrients for Erythropoiesis

Role in Erythropoiesis	Food Sources
Cobalamin (Vitamin B_{12})	
RBC maturation	Red meats, especially liver, eggs, enriched grain products, milk and dairy foods, fish
Copper	
Mobilization of iron from tissues to plasma*	Shellfish, whole grains, beans, nuts, potatoes, organ meats, dark green leafy vegetables, dried prunes
Folic Acid	
RBC maturation	Green leafy vegetables, liver, meat, fish, legumes, whole grains, orange juice, peanuts
Iron	
Hemoglobin synthesis	Liver and muscle meats, eggs, dried fruits, legumes, dark green leafy vegetables, whole-grain and enriched bread and cereals, potatoes
Niacin	
Needed for maturation of RBC	High-protein foods such as peanut butter, beans, meats, avocado; enriched and fortified grains
Pantothenic Acid (Vitamin B_5)	
Heme synthesis	Meats, vegetables, cereal grains, legumes, eggs, milk
Pyridoxine (Vitamin B_6)	
Hemoglobin synthesis	Meats, fortified cereals, whole grains, legumes, potatoes, cornmeal, bananas, nuts
Riboflavin (Vitamin B_2)	
Oxidative reactions	Milk and dairy foods, enriched bread and other grain products, salmon, chicken, eggs, leafy green vegetables
Vitamin E	
Possible role in heme synthesis. Protection against oxidative damage to RBCs	Vegetable oils, salad dressings, margarine, wheat germ, whole-grain products, seeds, nuts, peanut butter
Amino Acids	
Synthesis of nucleoproteins	Eggs, meat, milk and milk products (cheese, ice cream), poultry, fish, legumes, nuts
Ascorbic Acid (Vitamin C)	
Conversion of folic acid to its active forms, aids in iron absorption	Citrus fruits, green leafy vegetables, strawberries, cantaloupe

*Supplementation rarely needed and large amounts of copper are poisonous.

Diagnostic Studies

Laboratory abnormalities characteristic of iron-deficiency anemia are presented in Table 31-6. Other diagnostic studies (e.g., stool guaiac test) are done to determine the cause of the

TABLE 31-6 LABORATORY STUDY FINDINGS IN ANEMIAS

Etiology of Anemia	Hgb/ Hct	MCV	Reticulocytes	Serum Iron	TIBC	Transferrin	Ferritin	Bilirubin	Serum B_{12}	Folate
Iron deficiency	↓	↓	N or slight ↓ or ↑	↓	↑	N or ↓	↓	N or ↓	N	N
Thalassemia major	↓	N or ↓	↑	↑	↓	↓	N or ↑	↑	N	↓
Cobalamin deficiency	↓	↑	N or ↓	N or ↑	N	Slight ↑	↑	N or slight ↑	↓	N
Folic acid deficiency	↓	↑	N or ↓	N or ↑	N	Slight ↑	↑	N or slight ↑	N	↓
Aplastic anemia	↓	N or slight ↑	↓	N or ↑	N or ↑	N	N	N	N	N
Chronic disease	↓	N or ↓	N or ↓	N or ↓	↓	N or ↓	N or ↑	N	N	N
Acute blood loss	↓	N or ↓	N or ↑	N	N	N	N	N	N	N
Chronic blood loss	↓	↓	N or ↑	↓	↓	N	N	N or ↓	N	N
Sickle cell anemia	↓	N	↓	N or ↑	N or ↓	N	N	↑	N	↓
Hemolytic anemia	↓	N or ↑	↑	N or ↑	N or ↓	N	N or ↑	↑	N	N

MCV, Mean corpuscular volume; *N,* normal; *TIBC,* total iron-binding capacity.

TABLE 31-7 COLLABORATIVE CARE

Iron-Deficiency Anemia

Diagnostic	Collaborative Therapy
• History and physical examination • Hct and Hgb levels • RBC count, including morphology • Reticulocyte count • Serum iron • Serum ferritin • Serum transferrin • Total iron-binding capacity (TIBC) • Stool examination for occult blood	• Identification and treatment of underlying cause • Ferrous sulfate or ferrous gluconate • Iron dextran, sodium ferrous gluconate, iron sucrose IM or IV • Nutritional and diet therapy (see Table 31-5) • Transfusion of packed RBCs (symptomatic patient only)

iron deficiency. Endoscopy and colonoscopy may be used to detect GI bleeding. A bone marrow biopsy may be done if other tests are inconclusive.

Collaborative Care

The main goal is to treat the underlying disease that is causing reduced intake (e.g., malnutrition, alcoholism) or absorption of iron. In addition, efforts are directed toward replacing iron (Table 31-7). Teach the patient which foods are good sources of iron (see Table 31-5). If nutrition is already adequate, increasing iron intake by dietary means may not be practical. Consequently, oral or occasionally parenteral iron supplements are used. If the iron deficiency is from acute blood loss, the patient may require a transfusion of packed RBCs.

Drug Therapy. Oral iron should be used whenever possible because it is inexpensive and convenient. Many iron preparations are available. When administering iron, consider the following five factors:

1. Iron is absorbed best from the duodenum and proximal jejunum. Therefore enteric-coated or sustained-release capsules, which release iron farther down in the GI tract, are counterproductive and expensive.
2. The daily dose should provide 150 to 200 mg of elemental iron. This can be ingested in three or four daily doses, with each tablet or capsule of the iron preparation containing between 50 and 100 mg of iron (e.g., a 300-mg tablet of ferrous sulfate contains 60 mg of elemental iron).
3. Iron is best absorbed as ferrous sulfate (Fe^{2+}) in an acidic environment. For this reason and to avoid binding the iron with food, iron should be taken about an hour before meals, when the duodenal mucosa is most acidic. Taking iron with vitamin C (ascorbic acid) or orange juice, which contains ascorbic acid, enhances iron absorption. Gastric side effects, however, may necessitate ingesting iron with meals.
4. Undiluted liquid iron may stain the patient's teeth. Therefore it should be diluted and ingested through a straw.
5. GI side effects of iron administration may occur, including heartburn, constipation, and diarrhea. If side effects develop, the dose and type of iron supplement may be adjusted. For example, many individuals who need supplemental iron cannot tolerate ferrous sulfate because of the effects of the sulfate base. However, ferrous gluconate may be an acceptable substitute. Tell patients that the use of iron preparations will cause their stools to become black because the GI tract excretes excess iron. Constipation is common, and the patient should be started on stool softeners and laxatives, if needed, when started on iron.

DRUG ALERT: Iron

- Some preparations of IV iron have a risk of an allergic reaction, and the patient should be monitored accordingly.
- Oral iron should be taken about 1 hr before meals.
- Vitamin C (ascorbic acid) enhances iron absorption.

In some situations it may be necessary to administer iron parenterally. Parenteral use of iron is indicated for malabsorption, intolerance of oral iron, a need for iron beyond oral limits, or poor patient adherence in taking the oral preparations of iron. Parenteral iron can be given intramuscularly (IM) or IV. An iron-dextran complex (INFeD) contains 50 mg/mL of elemental iron available in 2-mL single-dose vials. Sodium ferrous gluconate and iron sucrose are alternatives and may carry less risk of life-threatening anaphylaxis.[10]

Because IM iron solutions may stain the skin, separate needles should be used for withdrawing the solution and for injecting the medication. Use a Z-track injection technique.

NURSING MANAGEMENT IRON-DEFICIENCY ANEMIA

Certain groups of individuals are at an increased risk for the development of iron-deficiency anemia. These include premenopausal and pregnant women, persons from low socioeco-

EVIDENCE-BASED PRACTICE

Translating Research Into Practice

Does Intermittent Iron Supplementation Improve Anemia?

Clinical Question

In menstruating women (P) does intermittent iron supplementation (I) compared to no iron, placebo, or daily use (C) reduce anemia (O)?

Best Available Evidence

Randomized and quasi-randomized controlled trials

Critical Appraisal and Synthesis of Evidence

- Twenty-one trials (*n* = 10,258) of menstruating women taking iron supplements intermittently compared with no intervention, placebo, or use of the same supplements on a daily basis.
- Intermittent iron supplementation reduced the risk of anemia and improved hemoglobin and ferritin concentrations. However, women using supplements intermittently had anemia more frequently than women who were taking daily supplementation.
- Frequency of use of intermittent supplements (one, two, or three times per week) did not affect findings.

Conclusion

- Intermittent iron supplementation in menstruating women is beneficial and an effective alternative when daily supplementation is not done.

Implications for Nursing Practice

- Many people who need iron supplementation do not take iron on a regular basis. The reasons include not liking the side effects or forgetting to take it.
- Encourage intermittent iron supplementation if usage is recommended and daily use is not feasible for the patient. It is better to take iron once in awhile than not at all.
- Inform women that side effects of iron, including nausea, constipation, and teeth staining, decrease with intermittent use as compared to daily supplementation.

Reference for Evidence

Fernández-Gaxiola A, De-Regil L: Intermittent iron supplementation for reducing anaemia and its associated impairments in menstruating women, *Cochrane Database Syst Rev* 12:CD009218, 2011.

P, Patient population of interest; *I*, intervention or area of interest; *C*, comparison of interest or comparison group; *O*, outcomes of interest (see p. 12).

nomic backgrounds, older adults, and individuals experiencing blood loss. Diet teaching, with an emphasis on foods high in iron and ways to maximize absorption, is important for these groups.

Appropriate nursing measures are presented in Nursing Care Plan 31-1. Discuss with the patient the need for diagnostic studies to identify the cause. Reassess the hemoglobin and RBC counts to evaluate the response to therapy. Emphasize adherence with dietary and drug therapy. To replenish the body's iron stores, the patient needs to take iron therapy for 2 to 3 months after the hemoglobin level returns to normal. Patients who require lifelong iron supplementation should be monitored for potential liver problems related to the iron storage.

THALASSEMIA

Etiology

Thalassemia is a group of diseases involving inadequate production of normal hemoglobin, and therefore decreased erythrocyte production. Thalassemia is due to an absent or reduced globulin protein. α-Globin chains are absent or reduced in α-thalassemia, and β-globin chains are absent or reduced in β-thalassemia. Hemolysis also occurs in thalassemia, but insufficient production of normal hemoglobin is the predominant problem. Thalassemia is commonly found in members of ethnic groups whose origins are near the Mediterranean Sea and equatorial or near-equatorial regions of Asia, the Middle East, and Africa.

Genetic Link

Thalassemia has an autosomal recessive genetic basis (see Table 13-2). An individual with thalassemia may have a heterozygous or homozygous form of the disease. A person who is heterozygous has one thalassemic gene and one normal gene and is said to have *thalassemia minor* (or thalassemic trait), which is a mild form of the disease. A homozygous person has two thalassemic genes, causing a severe condition known as *thalassemia major.*[11]

Clinical Manifestations

The patient with thalassemia minor is frequently asymptomatic. The patient has mild to moderate anemia with *microcytosis* (small cells) and *hypochromia* (pale cells).

Thalassemia major is a life-threatening disease in which growth, both physical and mental, is often retarded. The person who has thalassemia major is pale and displays other general symptoms of anemia (see Table 31-3). The symptoms develop in childhood by 2 years of age and can cause growth and developmental deficits. Jaundice from the hemolysis of RBCs is prominent. In addition, the person has pronounced splenomegaly, since the spleen continuously tries to remove the damaged red cells. Hepatomegaly and cardiomyopathy may occur from iron deposition. As the bone marrow responds to the reduced oxygen-carrying capacity of the blood, RBC production is stimulated and the marrow becomes packed with immature erythroid precursors that die. This stimulates further erythropoiesis, leading to chronic bone marrow hyperplasia and expansion of the marrow space. This may cause thickening of the cranium and maxillary cavity. Thrombocytosis after spleen dysfunction and/or removal may occur.

Patients with thalassemia may have hepatitis C because of having received blood transfusions before donated blood was screened for hepatitis C virus (screening started in 1992). Hepatitis C may result in cirrhosis and hepatocellular carcinoma. Cardiac complications from iron overload, pulmonary disease, and hypertension also contribute to early death. Endocrinopathies (hypogonadotrophic hypogonadism) and thrombosis may also be complications of the disease.

Collaborative Care

The laboratory abnormalities of thalassemia major are summarized in Table 31-6. No specific drug or diet therapies are effective in treating thalassemia. Thalassemia minor requires no treatment because the body adapts to the reduction of normal hemoglobin.

Thalassemia major is managed with blood transfusions or exchange transfusions in conjunction with oral deferasirox (Exjade), or deferiprone (Ferriprox) or deferoxamine (Desferal) (chelating agents that bind to iron) is given IV or subcutaneously to reduce the iron overloading (hemochromatosis) that occurs with chronic transfusion therapy.[11] Folic acid is given if there is evidence of hemolysis. Transfusions are administered to keep the hemoglobin level at approximately 10 g/dL (100 g/L) to maintain the patient's own erythropoiesis without causing the spleen to enlarge. Zinc supplementation may be needed, since zinc is reduced with chelation therapy. Ascorbic acid supplementation may be needed during chelation therapy, since it increases urine excretion of iron. Other than during chelation therapy, ascorbic acid should not be taken because it increases the absorption of dietary iron. Iron supplements should not be given.

Because RBCs are sequestered in the enlarged spleen, thalassemia major may be treated by splenectomy. Hepatic, cardiac, and pulmonary organ function should be monitored and treated as appropriate.

Although hematopoietic stem cell transplantation (HSCT) remains the only cure for patients with thalassemia, the risk of this procedure may outweigh its benefits. With proper iron chelation therapy, patients are living longer.

MEGALOBLASTIC ANEMIAS

Megaloblastic anemias are a group of disorders caused by impaired DNA synthesis and characterized by the presence of large RBCs. When DNA synthesis is impaired, defective RBC maturation results. The RBCs are large *(macrocytic)* and abnormal and are referred to as *megaloblasts.* Macrocytic RBCs are easily destroyed because they have fragile cell membranes. Although the overwhelming majority of megaloblastic anemias result from cobalamin (vitamin B_{12}) and folic acid deficiencies, this type of RBC deformity can also occur from suppression of DNA synthesis by drugs, inborn errors of cobalamin and folic acid metabolism, and *erythroleukemia* (malignant blood disorder characterized by a proliferation of erythropoietic cells in bone marrow) (Table 31-8).

TABLE 31-8 CLASSIFICATION OF MEGALOBLASTIC ANEMIA

Cobalamin (Vitamin B_{12}) Deficiency
- Dietary deficiency
- Deficiency of gastric intrinsic factor
  - Pernicious anemia
  - Gastrectomy
- Intestinal malabsorption
- Increased requirement
- Chronic alcoholism

Folic Acid Deficiency
- Dietary deficiency (e.g., leafy green vegetables, citrus fruits)
- Malabsorption syndromes
- Drugs interfering with absorption or use of folic acid
  - Methotrexate
  - Antiseizure drugs (e.g., phenobarbital, phenytoin [Dilantin])
- Increased requirement
- Alcohol abuse
- Anorexia
- Hemodialysis patients (folic acid lost during dialysis)

Drug-Induced Suppression of DNA Synthesis
- Folate antagonists
- Metabolic inhibitors
- Alkylating agents

Inborn Errors
- Defective folate metabolism
- Defective transport of cobalamin

Erythroleukemia

Cobalamin (Vitamin B_{12}) Deficiency

Normally, a protein termed *intrinsic factor* (IF) is secreted by the parietal cells of the gastric mucosa. IF is required for cobalamin (extrinsic factor) absorption. (Cobalamin is normally absorbed in the distal ileum.) Therefore if IF is not secreted, cobalamin will not be absorbed.

Etiology

Pernicious Anemia. The most common cause of cobalamin deficiency is **pernicious anemia,** which is caused by an absence of IF. In pernicious anemia the gastric mucosa is not secreting IF because of either gastric mucosal atrophy or autoimmune destruction of parietal cells. In the autoimmune process antibodies are directed against the gastric parietal cells and/or IF itself. Because parietal cells also secrete hydrochloric acid (HCl), in pernicious anemia there is a decrease in HCl in the stomach. An acid environment in the stomach is required for the secretion of IF.

Pernicious anemia is a disease of insidious onset that begins in middle age or later (usually after age 40), with 60 years being the most common age at diagnosis. Pernicious anemia occurs frequently in persons of Northern European ancestry (particularly Scandinavians) and African Americans. In African Americans the disease tends to begin early, occurs with higher frequency in women, and is often severe.

Other Causes of Cobalamin Deficiency. Cobalamin deficiency can also occur in patients who have had GI surgery (e.g., gastrectomy, gastric bypass); patients who have had a small bowel resection involving the ileum; and patients with Crohn's disease, ileitis, celiac disease, diverticuli of the small intestine, or chronic atrophic gastritis (see Table 31-8). In these cases, cobalamin deficiency results from the loss of IF-secreting gastric mucosal cells or impaired absorption of cobalamin in the distal ileum. Cobalamin deficiency is also found in chronic alcoholics, long-term users of H_2-histamine receptor blockers and proton pump inhibitors, and those who are strict vegetarians.[2,3]

Clinical Manifestations

General manifestations of anemia related to cobalamin deficiency develop because of tissue hypoxia (see Table 31-3). GI manifestations include a sore, red, beefy, and shiny tongue; anorexia, nausea, and vomiting; and abdominal pain. Typical neuromuscular manifestations include weakness, paresthesias of the feet and hands, reduced vibratory and position senses, ataxia, muscle weakness, and impaired thought processes ranging from confusion to dementia. Because cobalamin deficiency–related anemia has an insidious onset, it may take several months for these manifestations to develop.

Diagnostic Studies

Laboratory data reflective of cobalamin deficiency anemia are presented in Table 31-6. The RBCs appear large (macrocytic) and have abnormal shapes. This structure contributes to erythrocyte destruction because the cell membrane is fragile. Serum cobalamin levels are reduced.

Serum folate levels are also obtained. If they are normal and cobalamin levels are low, it suggests that megaloblastic anemia is due to a cobalamin deficiency. A serum test for anti-IF antibodies may be done that is specific for pernicious anemia. Because the potential for gastric cancer is increased in patients with pernicious anemia, an upper GI endoscopy and biopsy of the gastric mucosa may also be done.

Testing of serum methylmalonic acid (MMA) (elevated mainly in cobalamin deficiency) and serum homocysteine (elevated in both cobalamin and folic acid deficiencies) helps determine the cause of this type of anemia.

Collaborative Care

Regardless of how much is ingested, the patient is not able to absorb cobalamin if IF is lacking or if absorption in the ileum is impaired. For this reason, increasing dietary cobalamin does not correct this anemia. However, instruct the patient on adequate dietary intake to maintain good nutrition (see Table 31-5).

Parenteral vitamin B_{12} (cyanocobalamin or hydroxocobalamin) or intranasal cyanocobalamin (Nascobal, CaloMist) is the treatment of choice. Without cobalamin administration, these individuals will die in 1 to 3 years. A typical treatment schedule consists of 1000 mcg/day of cobalamin IM for 2 weeks and then weekly until the hemoglobin is normal, and then monthly for life. High-dose oral cobalamin and sublingual cobalamin are also available for those in whom GI absorption is intact. As long as supplemental cobalamin is used, the anemia can be reversed. However, if the person has had long-standing neuromuscular complications, they may not be reversible.

Folic Acid Deficiency

Folic acid (folate) deficiency also causes megaloblastic anemia. Folic acid is required for DNA synthesis leading to RBC formation and maturation. Common causes of folic acid deficiency are listed in Table 31-8.

The clinical manifestations of folic acid deficiency are similar to those of cobalamin deficiency. The disease develops insidiously, and the patient's symptoms may be attributed to other coexisting problems (e.g., cirrhosis, esophageal varices). GI disturbances include dyspepsia and a smooth, beefy red tongue. The absence of neurologic problems is an important diagnostic finding and differentiates folic acid deficiency from cobalamin deficiency.

The diagnostic findings for folic acid deficiency are presented in Table 31-6. In addition, the serum folate level is low (normal is 3 to 25 mg/mL [7 to 57 mol/L]) and the serum cobalamin level is normal.

Folic acid deficiency is treated by replacement therapy. The usual dosage is 1 mg/day by mouth. In malabsorption states or with chronic alcoholism, up to 5 mg/day may be required. The duration of treatment depends on the reason for the deficiency. Encourage the patient to eat foods containing large amounts of folic acid (see Table 31-5).

NURSING MANAGEMENT MEGALOBLASTIC ANEMIA

Because of the familial predisposition for pernicious anemia, the most common type of cobalamin deficiency, patients who have a positive family history of pernicious anemia should be evaluated for symptoms. Although the disease cannot be prevented, early detection and treatment can lead to reversal of symptoms. Also consider signs and symptoms of other possible megaloblastic anemias and bring them to the attention of the health care provider.

The nursing measures presented in Nursing Care Plan 31-1, for the patient with anemia, are appropriate for the patient with cobalamin or folic acid deficiency anemia. In addition to these measures, ensure that injuries are not sustained because of the diminished sensitivity to heat and pain resulting from the neurologic impairment. Protect the patient from falling, burns, and trauma. If heat therapy is required, evaluate the patient's skin at frequent intervals to detect redness.

Ongoing care focuses on ensuring good patient adherence with treatment. Carefully assess for neurologic difficulties that were not fully corrected by adequate replacement therapy. Because the potential for gastric cancer may be increased in patients with atrophic gastritis-related pernicious anemia, the patient should have frequent and careful appropriate screenings.

ANEMIA OF CHRONIC DISEASE

Anemia of chronic disease (also called anemia of inflammation) can be caused by chronic inflammation, autoimmune and infectious disorders (human immunodeficiency virus [HIV], hepatitis, malaria), HF, or malignant diseases. Bleeding episodes can also contribute to anemia of chronic disease.

Anemia of chronic disease is associated with an underproduction of RBCs and mild shortening of RBC survival. The RBCs are usually normocytic, normochromic, and hypoproliferative. The anemia is usually mild, but it can become more severe if the underlying disorder is not treated.

This type of anemia, which usually develops after 1 to 2 months of disease activity, has an immune basis. The cytokines released in these conditions, particularly interleukin 6 (IL-6), cause an increased uptake and retention of iron within macrophages (see Fig. 30-3). This leads to a diversion of iron from circulation into storage sites with subsequent limited iron available for erythropoiesis. There is also reduced RBC life span, suppressed production of erythropoietin, and an ineffective bone marrow response to erythropoietin.[12]

For any chronic disease, additional factors may contribute to the anemia. For example, with renal disease, the primary factor causing anemia is decreased erythropoietin, a hormone made in the kidneys that stimulates erythropoiesis. With impaired renal function, erythropoietin production is decreased (see Chapter 47).

Anemia of chronic disease must first be recognized and differentiated from anemia of other etiologies. Findings of elevated serum ferritin and increased iron stores distinguish it from iron-deficiency anemia. Normal folate and cobalamin blood levels distinguish it from those types of anemias. The best treatment of anemia of chronic disease is correction of the underlying disorder. If the anemia is severe, blood transfusions may be indicated, but they are not recommended for long-term treatment. Erythropoietin therapy (epoetin alfa [Epogen], darbepoetin) is used for anemia related to renal disease (see Chapter 47) and may be used for anemia related to cancer and its therapies (see Chapter 16 and Table 16-14). However, erythropoietin therapy needs to be used conservatively because of the increased risk of thromboembolism and death in some patients.[12,13] IV iron may be administered, if necessary, to improve the response to therapy with erythropoietin.

APLASTIC ANEMIA

Aplastic anemia is a disease in which the patient has peripheral blood *pancytopenia* (decrease of all blood cell types—RBCs, white blood cells [WBCs], and platelets) and hypocellular bone marrow. The spectrum of the anemia can range from a chronic condition managed with erythropoietin or blood transfusions to a critical condition with hemorrhage and sepsis. The incidence of aplastic anemia is low, affecting approximately 2 of every 1 million persons per year.[14]

Etiology

Aplastic anemia has various etiologic classifications, but is divided into two major groups: *congenital* or *acquired* (Table 31-9). Approximately 75% of the acquired aplastic anemias are idiopathic and thought to have an autoimmune basis.

Clinical Manifestations

Aplastic anemia can manifest abruptly (over days) or insidiously over weeks to months and can vary from mild to severe. Clinically the patient may have symptoms caused by suppression of any or all bone marrow elements. General manifestations of anemia such as fatigue and dyspnea, as well as cardiovascular and cerebral responses, may be seen (see Table 31-3). The patient with neutropenia (low neutrophil count) is susceptible to infection and is at risk for septic shock and death. Even a low-grade fever (above 100.4° F [38° C]) should be considered a medical emergency. Thrombocytopenia is manifested by a predisposition to bleeding (e.g., petechiae, ecchymosis, epistaxis).

Diagnostic Studies

The diagnosis is confirmed by laboratory studies. Because all marrow elements are affected, hemoglobin, WBC, and platelet values are often decreased in aplastic anemia. Other RBC indices are generally normal (see Table 31-6). The condition is therefore classified as a normocytic, normochromic anemia. The reticulocyte count is low. Bleeding time is prolonged.

Aplastic anemia can be further evaluated by assessing various iron studies. The serum iron and total iron-binding capacity (TIBC) may be elevated as initial signs of erythropoiesis suppression. Bone marrow biopsy, aspiration, and pathologic examination may be done for any anemic state. However, the findings are especially important in aplastic anemia because the marrow is hypocellular with increased yellow marrow (fat content).

TABLE 31-9 CAUSES OF APLASTIC ANEMIA

Congenital (Chromosomal Alterations)	Acquired
• Fanconi syndrome • Congenital dyskeratosis • Amegakaryocytic thrombocytopenia • Shwachman-Diamond syndrome	• Idiopathic or autoimmune • Chemical agents and toxins (e.g., benzene, insecticides, arsenic, alcohol) • Drugs (e.g., alkylating agents, antiseizure drugs, antimetabolites, antimicrobials, gold) • Radiation • Viral and bacterial infections (e.g., hepatitis, parvovirus)

NURSING AND COLLABORATIVE MANAGEMENT APLASTIC ANEMIA

Management of aplastic anemia is based on identifying and removing the causative agent (when possible) and providing supportive care until the pancytopenia reverses. Nursing interventions appropriate for the patient with pancytopenia from aplastic anemia are presented in Nursing Care Plan 31-1 for anemia and in eNursing Care Plan 31-1 for thrombocytopenia and eNursing Care Plan 31-2 for neutropenia (available on the website for this chapter). Nursing actions are directed at preventing complications from infection and hemorrhage.

The prognosis of severe untreated aplastic anemia is poor. The median survival of untreated severe aplastic anemia is 3 to 6 months (20% survive longer than 1 year).[3] However, advances in medical management, including HSCT and immunosuppressive therapy with antithymocyte globulin (ATG) and cyclosporine or high-dose cyclophosphamide (Cytoxan), have improved outcomes significantly. ATG is a horse serum that contains polyclonal antibodies against human T cells. It can cause anaphylaxis and a serum sickness. The rationale for this therapy is that idiopathic aplastic anemia is considered an autoimmune disorder resulting from activated cytotoxic T cells that target and destroy the patient's own hematopoietic stem cells. (ATG and cyclosporine are discussed in Chapter 14 and Table 14-16.)

The treatment of choice for adults less than 55 years of age who do not respond to the immunosuppressive therapy and who have a human leukocyte antigen (HLA)–matched donor is an HSCT. The best results occur in younger patients who have not had previous blood transfusions. Prior transfusions increase the risk of graft rejection. (HSCT is discussed in Chapter 16.)

For older adults without an HLA-matched donor, the treatment of choice is immunosuppression with ATG or cyclosporine or high-dose cyclophosphamide. High-dose corticosteroids may also be used. However, this therapy may be only partially beneficial. Patients who need ongoing supportive blood transfusion should be on an iron-binding agent to prevent iron overload.

ANEMIA CAUSED BY BLOOD LOSS

Anemia resulting from blood loss may be caused by either acute or chronic problems.

ACUTE BLOOD LOSS

Acute blood loss occurs as a result of sudden hemorrhage. Causes of acute blood loss include trauma, complications of surgery, and conditions or diseases that disrupt vascular integrity. There are two clinical concerns in such situations. First, a sudden reduction in the total blood volume can lead to hypovolemic shock. Second, if the acute loss is more gradual, the body maintains its blood volume by slowly increasing the plasma volume. Although the circulating fluid volume is preserved, the number of RBCs available to carry oxygen is significantly diminished.

Clinical Manifestations

The clinical manifestations of anemia from acute blood loss are caused by the body's attempts to maintain an adequate blood

TABLE 31-10 MANIFESTATIONS OF ACUTE BLOOD LOSS

Volume Lost* %	mL	Manifestations
10	500	None or rare vasovagal syncope.
20	1000	No detectable signs or symptoms at rest. Tachycardia with exercise and slight postural hypotension.
30	1500	Normal supine blood pressure and pulse at rest. Postural hypotension and tachycardia with exercise.
40	2000	Blood pressure, central venous pressure, and cardiac output below normal at rest; air hunger; rapid, thready pulse and cold, clammy skin.
50	2500	Shock, lactic acidosis, and potential death.

*Based on an adult with a total blood volume of 5 L.

volume and meet oxygen requirements. Table 31-10 summarizes the clinical manifestations of patients with varying degrees of blood volume loss. It is essential to understand that the clinical signs and symptoms the patient is experiencing are more important than the laboratory values. For example, an adult with a bleeding peptic ulcer who had a 750-mL hematemesis (15% of a normal total blood volume) within the past 30 minutes may have postural hypotension, but have normal values for hemoglobin and hematocrit. Over the next 36 to 48 hours, most of the blood volume deficit will be replaced by the movement of fluid from the extravascular into the intravascular space. Only then will the hemoglobin and hematocrit reflect the blood loss.

Assess the patient's expression of pain. Internal hemorrhage may cause pain because of tissue distention, organ displacement, and nerve compression. Pain may be localized or referred. In the case of retroperitoneal bleeding, the patient may not experience abdominal pain. Instead the patient may have numbness and pain in a lower extremity secondary to compression of the lateral cutaneous nerve, which is located in the region of the first to third lumbar vertebrae. The major complication of acute blood loss is shock (see Chapter 67).

Diagnostic Studies

When blood volume loss is sudden, plasma volume has not yet had a chance to increase, the loss of RBCs is not reflected in laboratory data, and values may seem normal or high for 2 to 3 days. However, once the plasma volume is replaced, the RBC mass is less concentrated. At this time, RBC, hemoglobin, and hematocrit levels are low and reflect the actual blood loss.

Collaborative Care

Collaborative care is initially concerned with (1) replacing blood volume to prevent shock and (2) identifying the source of the hemorrhage and stopping the blood loss. IV fluids used in emergencies include dextran, hetastarch, albumin, and crystalloid electrolyte solutions such as lactated Ringer's solution. The amount of infusion varies with the solution used. (Management of shock is discussed in Chapter 67.)

Once volume replacement is established, attention can be directed to correcting the RBC loss. The body needs 2 to 5 days to manufacture more RBCs in response to increased erythropoietin. Consequently, blood transfusions (packed RBCs) may be needed if the blood loss is significant. In addition, if the bleeding is related to a platelet or clotting disorder, replacement of that deficiency is addressed.

The patient may also need supplemental iron because the availability of iron affects the marrow production of erythrocytes. When anemia exists after acute blood loss, dietary sources of iron will probably not be adequate to maintain iron stores. Therefore oral or parenteral iron preparations are administered.

NURSING MANAGEMENT ACUTE BLOOD LOSS

In the case of trauma it may be impossible to prevent the loss of blood. For the postoperative patient, carefully monitor the blood loss from various drainage tubes and dressings and implement appropriate actions. The nursing care for the patient with anemia resulting from acute blood loss most likely includes administration of blood products (described at the end of this chapter).

The anemia should begin to correct itself once the source of hemorrhage is identified, blood loss is controlled, and fluid and blood volumes are replaced. There should be no need for long-term treatment of this type of anemia.

CHRONIC BLOOD LOSS

The sources of chronic blood loss are similar to those of iron-deficiency anemia (e.g., bleeding ulcer, hemorrhoids, menstrual and postmenopausal blood loss). The effects of chronic blood loss are usually related to the depletion of iron stores and considered as iron-deficiency anemia. Management of chronic blood loss anemia involves identifying the source and stopping the bleeding. Supplemental iron may be required.

ANEMIA CAUSED BY INCREASED ERYTHROCYTE DESTRUCTION

The third major cause of anemia is termed **hemolytic anemia,** a condition caused by the destruction or hemolysis of RBCs at a rate that exceeds production. Hemolysis can occur because of problems intrinsic or extrinsic to the RBCs. *Intrinsic hemolytic anemias,* which are usually hereditary, result from defects in the RBCs themselves (see Table 31-2).

More common are the *acquired hemolytic anemias.* In this type of anemia the RBCs are normal, but damage is caused by external factors (see Table 31-2). The spleen is the primary site of the destruction of RBCs that are old, defective, or moderately damaged. Fig. 31-2 indicates the sequence of events involved in extravascular hemolysis.

The patient with hemolytic anemia has the general manifestations of anemia and specific manifestations related to this type of anemia (see Table 31-3). Jaundice is likely because the increased destruction of RBCs causes an elevation in bilirubin levels. The spleen and liver may enlarge because of their hyperactivity, which is related to macrophage phagocytosis of the defective erythrocytes.

In all causes of hemolysis, a major focus of treatment is to maintain renal function. When RBCs are hemolyzed, the hemoglobin molecule is released and filtered by the kidneys. The accumulation of hemoglobin molecules can obstruct the renal tubules and lead to acute tubular necrosis (see Chapter 47).

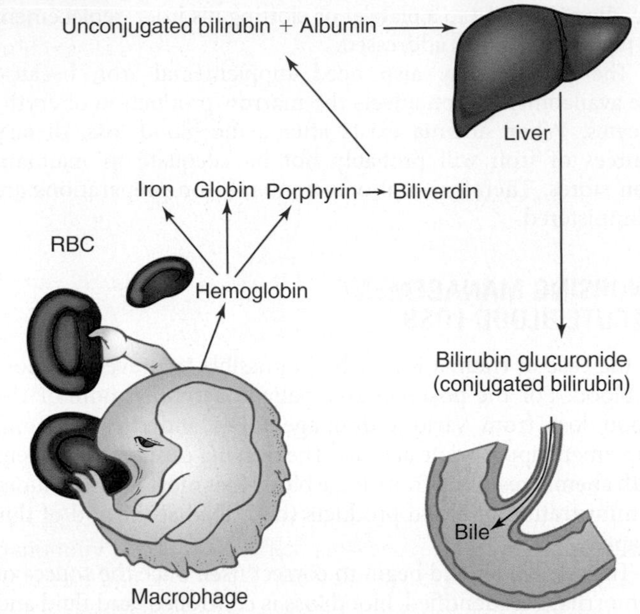

FIG. 31-2 Sequence of events in extravascular hemolysis.

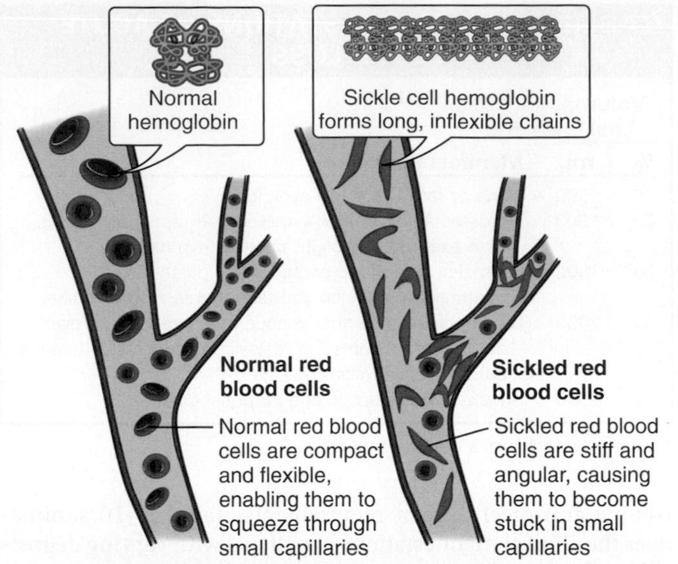

FIG. 31-3 In sickle cell, the hemoglobin forms long inflexible chains and alters the shape of the red blood cells (RBCs). The sickled RBCs can become stuck in the capillaries and occlude the blood flow.

SICKLE CELL DISEASE

Sickle cell disease (SCD) is a group of inherited, autosomal recessive disorders characterized by an abnormal form of hemoglobin in the RBC. (Autosomal recessive genetic disorders are discussed in Chapter 13 and Table 13-2.) Because this is a genetic disorder, SCD is usually identified during infancy or early childhood. It is an incurable disease that is often fatal by middle age because of renal failure, infection, pulmonary failure, and/or stroke.[3]

SCD affects about 100,000 Americans and is predominant in African Americans, occurring in an estimated 1 in about 500 live births. It can also affect people of Mediterranean, Caribbean, South and Central American, Arabian, or East Indian ancestry.[15]

Etiology and Pathophysiology

Genetic Link

In SCD the abnormal hemoglobin, *hemoglobin S* (Hgb S), results from the substitution of valine for glutamic acid on the β-globin chain of hemoglobin (see Fig. 13-3). Hgb S causes the erythrocyte to stiffen and elongate, taking on a sickle shape in response to low oxygen levels (Fig. 31-3).

Types of SCD disorders include sickle cell anemia, sickle cell–thalassemia, sickle cell Hgb C disease, and sickle cell trait. *Sickle cell anemia,* the most severe of the SCD syndromes, occurs when a person is homozygous for hemoglobin S (Hgb SS); the person has inherited Hgb S from both parents. *Sickle cell–thalassemia* and *sickle cell Hgb C* occur when a person inherits Hgb S from one parent and another type of abnormal hemoglobin (such as thalassemia or hemoglobin C) from the other parent. Both of these forms of SCD are less common and less severe than sickle cell anemia. *Sickle cell trait* occurs when a person is heterozygous for hemoglobin S (Hgb AS); the person has inherited hemoglobin S from one parent and normal hemoglobin (Hgb A) from the other parent. Sickle cell trait is typically a mild to asymptomatic condition.

Sickling Episodes. The major pathophysiologic event of SCD is the sickling of RBCs (see Fig. 31-3). Sickling episodes are most commonly triggered by low oxygen tension in the blood. Hypoxia or deoxygenation of the RBCs can be caused by viral or bacterial infection, high altitude, emotional or physical stress, surgery, and blood loss. Infection is the most common precipitating factor. Other events that can trigger or sustain a sickling episode include dehydration, increased hydrogen ion concentration (acidosis), increased plasma osmolality, decreased plasma volume, and low body temperature. A sickling episode can also occur without an obvious cause.

Sickled RBCs become rigid and take on an elongated, crescent shape (see Fig. 31-3). Sickled cells cannot easily pass through capillaries or other small vessels and can cause vascular occlusion, leading to acute or chronic tissue injury. The resulting hemostasis promotes a self-perpetuating cycle of local hypoxia, deoxygenation of more erythrocytes, and more sickling. Circulating sickled cells are hemolyzed by the spleen, leading to anemia. Initially the sickling of cells is reversible with reoxygenation, but it eventually becomes irreversible because of cell membrane damage from recurrent sickling. Thus vaso-occlusive phenomena and hemolysis are the clinical hallmarks of SCD.

Sickle cell crisis is a severe, painful, acute exacerbation of RBC sickling causing a vaso-occlusive crisis. As blood flow is impaired by sickled cells, vasospasm occurs, further restricting blood flow. Severe capillary hypoxia causes changes in membrane permeability, leading to plasma loss, hemoconcentration, thrombi, and further circulatory stagnation. Tissue ischemia, infarction, and necrosis eventually occur from lack of oxygen. Shock is a possible life-threatening consequence of sickle cell crisis because of severe oxygen depletion of the tissues and a reduction of the circulating fluid volume. Sickle cell crisis can begin suddenly and persist for days to weeks.

The frequency, extent, and severity of sickling episodes are highly variable and unpredictable, but largely depend on the percentage of Hgb S present. Individuals with sickle cell anemia have the most severe form because the erythrocytes contain a high percentage of Hgb S.

GENETICS IN CLINICAL PRACTICE

Sickle Cell Disease

Genetic Basis

- Autosomal recessive disorder.
- Mutation in β-globin *(HBB)* gene located on chromosome 11.
- Various versions of β-globin result from different mutations in the *HBB* gene.
- Hgb S variant involves substitution of valine for glutamic acid in the β-globin gene in sickle cell anemia.

Incidence

- Most common inherited blood disorder in the United States.
- Affects 8 of every 100,000 people.
- Affects 1 in 350 to 500 African Americans.
- Affects 1 in 1000 to 1400 Hispanic Americans.
- Also affects people of Mediterranean, Caribbean, Arabian, and East Indian descent.

Genetic Testing

- DNA testing is available.
- Electrophoresis of hemoglobin and sickling screening test are more commonly used.

Clinical Implications

- Requires ongoing continuity of care and extensive patient teaching.
- Sickle cell trait is the carrier state for sickle cell disease and represents a mild type of sickle cell disease; 1 in 10 to 12 African Americans and 1 in 25 Hispanics have sickle cell trait.
- If both parents have the trait, there is a 1 in 4 chance that their baby will have sickle cell disease.
- Management of sickle cell disease should focus on the prevention of sickle cell crisis (e.g., prevention of dehydration and infection).
- Genetic counseling is recommended for individuals with a family history of sickle cell disease. Individuals should understand the risks of transmitting the genetic mutation.

Clinical Manifestations

The effects of SCD vary greatly from person to person, the severity of which may be due to genetic polymorphisms. Many people with sickle cell anemia are in reasonably good health the majority of the time. However, they may have chronic health problems and pain because of organ tissue hypoxia and damage (e.g., involving the kidneys or liver).

The typical patient is anemic but asymptomatic except during sickling episodes. Because most individuals with sickle cell anemia have dark skin, pallor is more readily detected by examining the mucous membranes. The skin may have a grayish cast. Because of the hemolysis, jaundice is common and patients are prone to gallstones (cholelithiasis).

The primary symptom associated with sickling is pain. The pain severity can range from trivial to excruciating. During sickle cell crisis the pain is severe because of ischemia of tissue. The episodes can affect any area of the body or several sites simultaneously, with the back, chest, extremities, and abdomen being most commonly affected. Pain episodes are often accompanied by clinical manifestations such as fever, swelling, tenderness, tachypnea, hypertension, nausea, and vomiting.

Complications

With repeated episodes of sickling, there is gradual involvement of all body systems, especially the spleen, lungs, kidneys, and brain. Organs that have a high need for oxygen are most often affected and form the basis for many of the complications of SCD (Fig. 31-4). Infection is a major cause of morbidity and mortality in patients with SCD. One reason for this is the failure of the spleen to phagocytize foreign substances as it becomes infarcted and dysfunctional (usually by 2 to 4 years of age) from the sickled RBCs. The spleen becomes small because of repeated scarring, a phenomenon termed *autosplenectomy.*

Pneumonia is the most common infection and often is of pneumococcal origin. Infections can be so severe that they cause an aplastic and hemolytic crisis and gallstones. *Aplastic crisis* can be so severe that it causes a temporary shutdown of RBC production in the bone marrow.

Acute chest syndrome is a term used to describe acute pulmonary complications that include pneumonia, tissue infarction, and fat embolism. It is characterized by fever, chest pain, cough, pulmonary infiltrates, and dyspnea. Pulmonary infarctions may cause pulmonary hypertension, MI, HF, and ultimately cor pulmonale. The heart may become ischemic and enlarged, leading to HF. Retinal vessel obstruction may result in hemorrhage, scarring, retinal detachment, and blindness. The kidneys may be injured from the increased blood viscosity and the lack of oxygen, and renal failure may occur. Pulmonary embolism or stroke can result from thrombosis and infarction of cerebral blood vessels. Bone changes may include osteoporosis and osteosclerosis after infarction. Chronic leg ulcers can result from the hypoxia and are especially prevalent around the ankles. *Priapism* (persistent penile erection) may occur if penile veins become occluded.

Diagnostic Studies

A peripheral blood smear may reveal sickled cells and abnormal reticulocytes. The presence of Hgb S can be diagnosed by the sickling test, which uses RBCs (in vitro) and exposes them to a deoxygenation agent.

As a result of the accelerated RBC breakdown, the patient has characteristic clinical findings of hemolysis (jaundice, elevated serum bilirubin levels) and abnormal laboratory test results (see Table 31-6). Hemoglobin electrophoresis may be done to determine the amount of hemoglobin S. Skeletal x-rays demonstrate bone and joint deformities and flattening. Magnetic resonance imaging (MRI) may be used to diagnose a stroke caused by blocked cerebral vessels from sickled cells. Doppler studies may be used to assess for deep vein thromboses. Other tests may be indicated, such as a chest x-ray, to diagnose infection or organ malfunction.

NURSING AND COLLABORATIVE MANAGEMENT SICKLE CELL DISEASE

Collaborative care for a patient with SCD is directed toward (1) alleviating the symptoms from the complications of the disease; (2) minimizing end-organ damage; and (3) promptly treating serious sequelae, such as acute chest syndrome, that can lead to immediate death. Teach patients with SCD to avoid high altitudes, maintain adequate fluid intake, and treat infections promptly. Pneumovax, *Haemophilus influenzae,* influenza, and hepatitis immunizations should be administered. Chronic leg ulcers may be treated with rest, antibiotics, warm saline soaks, mechanical or enzyme debridement, and grafting if necessary.

Priapism is managed with pain medication, fluids, and nifedipine (Procardia). If it does not resolve within a few hours, a urologist can be called to inject the corpus cavernosum with a dilute solution of epinephrine to preserve penile function.

Sickle cell crises may require hospitalization. Oxygen may be administered to treat hypoxia and control sickling. Because

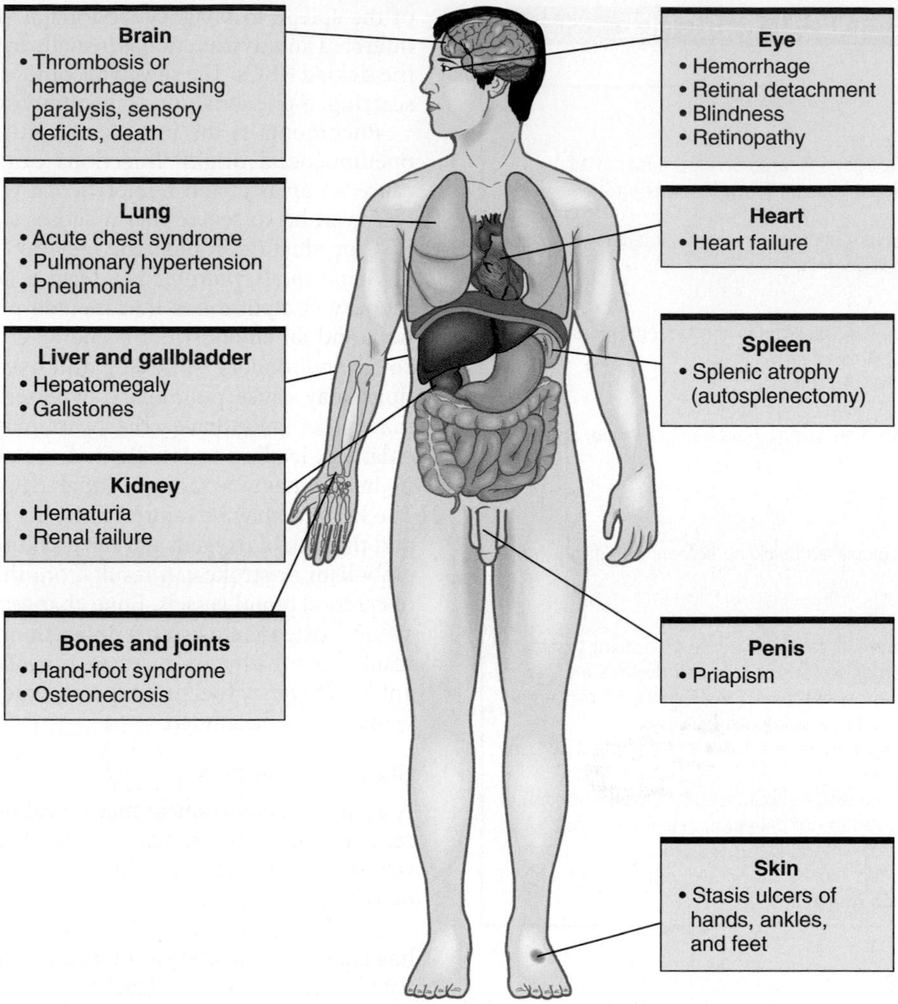

FIG. 31-4 Clinical manifestations and complications of sickle cell disease.

respiratory failure is the most common cause of death, vigilantly assess for any changes in respiratory status.[16] Rest may be instituted to reduce metabolic requirements, and deep vein thrombosis prophylaxis (using anticoagulants) should be prescribed. Fluids and electrolytes are administered to reduce blood viscosity and maintain renal function. Transfusion therapy is indicated when an aplastic crisis occurs. Aggressive total RBC exchange transfusion programs may be implemented for patients who have frequent crises or serious complications such as acute chest syndrome. These patients, like those with thalassemia major, may require iron chelation therapy to reduce transfusion-produced iron overload.

Undertreatment of sickle cell pain is a major problem. Lack of understanding can lead health care professionals to underestimate how much pain these patients suffer. Patients, because of their prior opioid treatment, may be tolerant, and thus large doses may be needed to reduce the pain to a tolerable level. During an acute crisis, optimal pain control usually includes large doses of continuous (rather than as-needed [PRN]) opioid analgesics along with breakthrough analgesia, often in the form of patient-controlled analgesia (PCA) (PCA is discussed in Chapter 9). Morphine and hydromorphone are the drugs of choice. Meperidine (Demerol) is contraindicated because high doses can lead to the accumulation of a toxic metabolite, normeperidine, which can cause seizures.

Because patients may be experiencing different types and sites of pain, a multimodal and interdisciplinary approach should be used that incorporates emotional aspects of pain (see Chapter 9). Adjunctive measures, such as nonsteroidal anti-inflammatory agents, antineuropathic pain medications (e.g., tricyclic antidepressants, antiseizure medications), local anesthetics, or nerve blocks may be used.

Although pain is the most common symptom of patients with SCD seeking medical care, infection is a frequent complication and must be treated. Patients with acute chest syndrome are treated with broad-spectrum antibiotics, O_2 therapy, fluid therapy, and possibly exchange transfusion. Blood transfusions have little if any role in the treatment between crises, since patients develop antibodies to RBCs and iron overload. However, because chronic hemolysis results in increased use of folic acid stores, routine oral folic acid should be taken.

Although many antisickling agents have been tried, hydroxyurea (Hydrea), which is a chemotherapy drug, is the only one that has been shown to be clinically beneficial.[17] This drug increases the production of hemoglobin F (fetal hemoglobin), decreases the reactive neutrophil count, increases RBC volume and hydration, and alters the adhesion of sickle RBCs to the endothelium. The increase in Hgb F is accompanied by a reduction in hemolysis, an increase in hemoglobin concentration, and a decrease in sickled cells and painful crises.[11]

ETHICAL/LEGAL DILEMMAS

Pain Management

Situation

N.C., a 21-year-old African American man, is admitted to the emergency department (ED) in sickle cell crisis with complaints of excruciating pain. He is known to several of the nurses and physicians in the ED. One of the nurses remarks to you that it must be time for his "fix" of pain drugs.

Ethical/Legal Points for Consideration

- The standard of care for pain requires that (1) a pain assessment is done based on the patient's self-report, (2) the best possible relief of pain is provided under the circumstances, and (3) competent and compassionate care is provided to all patients.
- The pain assessment also includes reviewing the patient's medical record to determine if there are health care issues or conditions (e.g., frequent ED visits to request pain medication) that may affect the patient's response to pain and pain management.
- As a nurse, you have a duty to notify the health care professional of those issues or conditions. You also need to document behaviors exhibited by the patient related to pain management. Make sure that the documentation is objective (factual observations) rather than labeling (the patient was in withdrawal).
- When pain relief is inadequate, as a nurse, you are responsible for notifying the health care professional. Efforts to notify must continue and be appropriately documented until the managing health care professional has assessed the patient and made a plan of care based on that assessment.

Discussion Questions

1. How can you educate your colleagues regarding pain assessment and management?
2. What important factors would need to be included in your assessment and management of N.C.?

Hematopoietic stem cell transplantation (HSCT) is the only available treatment that can cure some patients with SCD. The selection of appropriate recipients, scarcity of appropriate donors, risk, and cost-effectiveness limit the use of HSCT for SCD. (HSCT is discussed in Chapter 16.)

Patient teaching and support are important in the long-term care of the patient with SCD. The patient and caregiver must understand the basis of the disease and the reasons for supportive care and ongoing pertinent screening tailored to SCD manifestations, such as eye examinations. Teach the patient ways to avoid crises, including taking steps to avoid dehydration and hypoxia, such as avoiding high altitudes and seeking medical attention quickly to counteract problems such as upper respiratory tract infections. Teaching about pain control is also needed because the pain during a crisis may be severe and often requires considerable analgesia. Minor pain episodes that are not associated with infection or other symptoms warranting medical attention can sometimes be managed at home.

Recurrent episodes of severe acute pain and unrelenting chronic pain can be disabling and depressing. The quality of life of patients with SCD can be profoundly affected. Occupational and physical therapists can help the patient achieve optimum physical functioning and independence. Cognitive behavioral therapy may help patients with SCD cope with anxiety and depression. Support groups may also be helpful.

ACQUIRED HEMOLYTIC ANEMIA

Acquired hemolytic anemia results from hemolysis of RBCs from extrinsic factors. These factors can be separated into four categories: (1) macroangiopathic (physical trauma), (2) microangiopathic, (3) antibody reactions, and (4) infectious agents and toxins (see Table 31-2).

Macroangiopathic or physical destruction of RBCs results from the exertion of extreme force on the cells. Traumatic events causing disruption of the RBC membrane include hemodialysis, extracorporeal circulation used in cardiopulmonary bypass, and prosthetic heart valves. In addition, the force needed to push blood through abnormal vessels, such as those that have been burned, irradiated, or affected by vascular disease (e.g., diabetes mellitus), may also physically damage RBCs.

Microangiopathic destruction of RBCs is a result of fragmentation of the cells as they try to pass by abnormal arterial or venous microcirculation. The RBCs are sheared as they try to pass by excessive platelet aggregation and/or fibrin polymer formation, such as is seen in thrombotic thrombocytopenic purpura (TTP) and disseminated intravascular coagulation (DIC) (discussed later in this chapter).

Antibodies may destroy RBCs by the mechanisms involved in antigen-antibody reactions. The reactions may be of an isoimmune or autoimmune type. *Isoimmune reactions* occur when antibodies develop against antigens from another person of the same species. In blood transfusion reactions the recipient's antibodies hemolyze donor cells. *Autoimmune reactions* result when individuals develop antibodies against their own RBCs. Autoimmune hemolytic reactions may be idiopathic, developing with no prior hemolytic history as a result of immunoglobulin G (IgG) covering the RBCs, or secondary to other autoimmune diseases (e.g., systemic lupus erythematosus), leukemia, lymphoma, or medications (penicillin, ibuprofen, metformin, chlorpromazine, procainamide).

Infectious agents and toxins cause the fourth type of acquired hemolytic disorder. Infectious agents cause hemolysis in three ways: (1) by invading the RBC and destroying its contents (e.g., parasites such as in malaria), (2) by releasing hemolytic substances (e.g., *Clostridium perfringens*), and (3) by generating an antigen-antibody reaction (e.g., *Mycoplasma pneumoniae*). Various agents may be toxic to RBCs and cause hemolysis. These hemolytic toxins involve chemicals such as oxidative drugs, arsenic, lead, copper, and bee stings or spider bites.

Laboratory findings in hemolytic anemia are presented in Table 31-6. Treatment and management of acquired hemolytic anemias involve general supportive care until the causative agent can be eliminated or at least made less injurious to the RBCs. Because a hemolytic crisis is a potential consequence, be ready to institute appropriate emergency therapy. This includes aggressive hydration and electrolyte replacement to reduce the risk of kidney injury caused by hemoglobin (from RBC lysis) clogging the kidney tubules and subsequent shock. Additional supportive care may include administering corticosteroids and blood products or removing the spleen.

For chronic hemolytic anemia, folate may need to be replaced. To suppress the RBC destruction, immunosuppressive agents may be used, such as rituximab (Rituxan), a monoclonal antibody to B-cell CD20, and eculizumab (Soliris), a monoclonal antibody to complement protein C5.

OTHER RED BLOOD CELL DISORDERS

HEMOCHROMATOSIS

Hemochromatosis is an iron overload disorder. Although it is primarily caused by a genetic defect, hemochromatosis may

GENETICS IN CLINICAL PRACTICE

Hemochromatosis

Genetic Basis
- Autosomal recessive disorder.
- Caused by mutations in the *HAMP, HFE, HFE2, SLC40A1*, and *TFR2* genes.
- These genes play an important role in regulating the absorption, transport, and storage of iron.
- Mutations in these genes impair the control of iron absorption during digestion and alter the distribution of iron to other parts of the body. As a result, iron accumulates in tissues and organs.

Incidence
- Most common genetic disease in people of European ancestry.
- One in 8 are carriers of the single HH gene mutation.
- Affects 1 in 200 to 500 in the United States.
- Very low prevalence in other ethnic populations.

Genetic Testing
- DNA testing is available and recommended for all first-degree relatives of people with the disease.
- American Hemochromatosis Society recommends genetic testing regardless of family history.
- Useful diagnostic tests include serum iron concentration, total iron-binding capacity, and transferrin saturation.

Clinical Implications
- Most of the 33 million Americans who have the gene mutation do not know it.
- Clinical expression is variable depending on dietary iron, blood loss, and other modifying factors.
- Early treatment can prevent serious complications.
- If untreated, progressive iron deposits can lead to multiple organ failure.

occur secondary to diseases such as sideroblastic anemia. It may also be caused by liver disease and chronic blood transfusions that are used to treat thalassemia and SCD.[18]

Genetic Link

The genetic disorder *(hereditary hemochromatosis)* is an autosomal recessive disorder characterized by increased intestinal iron absorption and, as a result, increased tissue iron deposition.[18] (Autosomal recessive disorders are discussed in Chapter 13 and Table 13-2.) It is the most common genetic disorder among whites, with an incidence of about 5 per 1000 whites of European ancestry.[19]

The normal range for total body iron is 2 to 6 g. Individuals with hemochromatosis accumulate iron at a rate of 0.5 to 1.0 g/yr and may exceed total iron concentrations of 50 g. Symptoms of hemochromatosis usually develop between 40 and 60 years of age.

Early symptoms are nonspecific and include fatigue, arthralgia, impotence, abdominal pain, and weight loss. Later, the excess iron accumulates in the liver and causes liver enlargement and eventually cirrhosis. Then other organs become affected, resulting in diabetes mellitus, skin pigment changes (bronzing), cardiac changes (e.g., cardiomyopathy), arthritis, and testicular atrophy. Physical examination reveals an enlarged liver and spleen and pigmentation changes in the skin.

Laboratory values demonstrate an elevated serum iron, TIBC, and serum ferritin. Testing for known genetic mutations confirms the diagnosis. Liver biopsy can quantify the amount of iron and establish the degree of organ damage.

The goal of treatment is to remove excess iron from the body and minimize any symptoms the patient may have. Iron removal is achieved by removing 500 mL of blood each week for 2 to 3 years until the iron stores in the body are depleted. Then blood is removed less frequently to maintain iron levels within normal limits.

Iron chelating agents may be used. Deferoxamine, which chelates and removes accumulated iron via the kidneys, can be administered IV or subcutaneously. Deferasirox and deferiprone are oral agents that chelate iron. Chelating agents form a complex with iron and promote its excretion from the body.[20]

Management of organ involvement (e.g., diabetes mellitus, HF) is the same as conventional treatment for these problems. Iron accumulation can also be reduced by dietary modifications such as avoidance of vitamin C and iron supplements, uncooked seafood, and iron-rich foods. The most common causes of death are cirrhosis, liver failure, hepatocellular cancer, and cardiac failure. With early diagnosis and treatment, life expectancy is normal. However, many cases go undetected and untreated.

POLYCYTHEMIA

Polycythemia is the production and presence of increased numbers of RBCs. The increase in RBCs can be so great that blood circulation is impaired as a result of the increased blood viscosity *(hyperviscosity)* and volume *(hypervolemia).*

Etiology and Pathophysiology

The two types of polycythemia are primary polycythemia, or polycythemia vera, and secondary polycythemia (Fig. 31-5). Their etiologies and pathogenesis differ, although their complications and clinical manifestations are similar.

Primary Polycythemia. *Polycythemia vera* is a chronic myeloproliferative disorder. Therefore not only are RBCs involved, but also WBCs and platelets, leading to increased production of each of these blood cells. The disease develops insidiously and follows a chronic, vacillating course. The median age at diagnosis is 60 years old, with a slight male predominance. In polycythemia vera there is enhanced blood viscosity and blood volume and congestion of organs and tissues with blood. Splenomegaly (which occurs in 90% of patients) and hepatomegaly are common. These patients have hypercoagulopathies that predispose them to clotting.

Genetic Link

Polycythemia vera is associated with mutations in the *Janus kinase-2 (JAK2)* gene. The *JAK2* gene provides instructions for making a protein that promotes proliferation of cells, especially blood cells from hematopoietic stem cells. Polycythemia vera begins with one or more DNA mutations of a single hematopoietic stem cell. Most cases of polycythemia vera are not inherited. This condition is associated with genetic changes that are somatic, which means they are acquired during a person's lifetime and are present only in certain cells.

Secondary Polycythemia. *Secondary polycythemia* can be either hypoxia driven or hypoxia independent. In hypoxia-driven secondary polycythemia, hypoxia stimulates erythropoietin (EPO) production in the kidney, which in turn stimulates RBC production. The need for oxygen may result from high altitude, pulmonary disease, cardiovascular disease, alveolar hypoventilation, defective oxygen transport, or tissue hypoxia. EPO levels may return to normal once the hemoglobin is

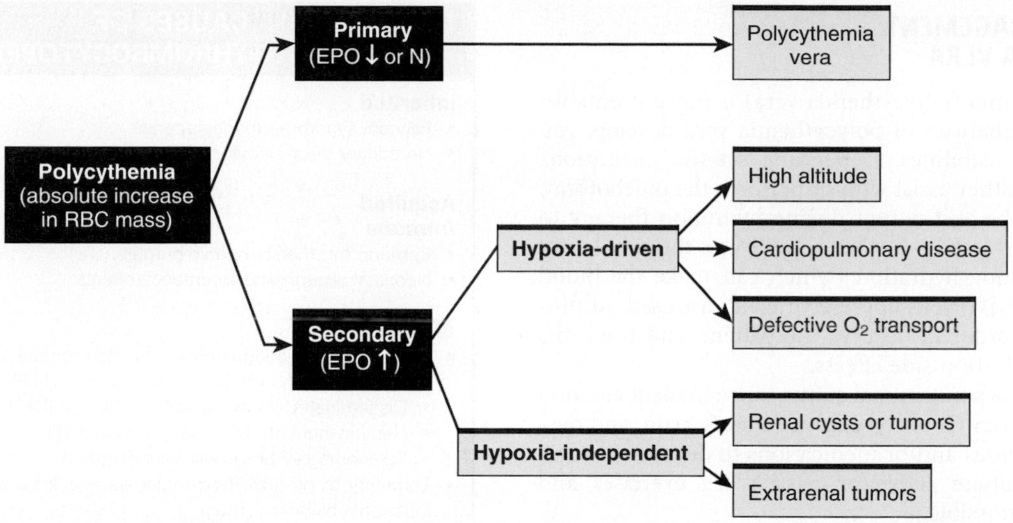

FIG. 31-5 Differentiating between primary and secondary polycythemia. *EPO,* Erythropoietin; *N,* normal.

stabilized at a higher level. In this situation, secondary polycythemia is a physiologic response in which the body tries to compensate for a problem, rather than a pathologic response. (Hypoxia-driven secondary polycythemia is discussed in the section on chronic obstructive pulmonary disease in Chapter 29.)

In hypoxia-independent secondary polycythemia, EPO is produced by a malignant or benign tumor tissue. Serum EPO levels often remain elevated in these situations. Splenomegaly does not accompany secondary polycythemia.

Clinical Manifestations and Complications

Circulatory manifestations of polycythemia vera occur because of the hypertension caused by hypervolemia and hyperviscosity. They are often the first manifestations and include subjective complaints of headache, vertigo, dizziness, tinnitus, and visual disturbances. Generalized pruritus (often exacerbated by a hot bath) may be a striking symptom and is related to histamine release from an increased number of basophils. Paresthesias and *erythromelalgia* (painful burning and redness of the hands and feet) may also be present. In addition, the patient may experience angina, HF, intermittent claudication, and thrombophlebitis, which may be complicated by embolization. These manifestations are caused by blood vessel distention, impaired blood flow, circulatory stasis, thrombosis, and tissue hypoxia caused by the hypervolemia and hyperviscosity. The most common serious acute complication is stroke secondary to thrombosis.

Hemorrhagic phenomena caused by either vessel rupture from overdistention or inadequate platelet function may result in petechiae, ecchymoses, epistaxis, or GI bleeding. Hemorrhage can be acute and catastrophic. Hepatomegaly and splenomegaly from organ engorgement may contribute to patient complaints of satiety and fullness. The patient may also experience pain from peptic ulcer caused either by increased gastric secretions or by liver and spleen engorgement. *Plethora* (ruddy complexion) may also be present. Hyperuricemia is caused by the increase in RBC destruction that accompanies excessive RBC production. Uric acid is one of the products of cell destruction. As RBC destruction increases, uric acid production also increases, thus leading to hyperuricemia and possible gout.

Although the incidence is low, myelofibrosis and leukemia develop in some patients with polycythemia vera. These disorders may be caused by the chemotherapeutic drugs used to treat the disease, or they may be secondary to a disorder in the stem cells that progresses to erythroleukemia. The major cause of morbidity and mortality from polycythemia vera is related to thrombosis (e.g., stroke).

Diagnostic Studies

The following laboratory manifestations are seen in a patient with polycythemia vera: (1) elevated hemoglobin and RBC count with microcytosis; (2) low to normal EPO level (secondary polycythemia has a high level); (3) elevated WBC count with basophilia; (4) elevated platelet count (thrombocytosis) and platelet dysfunction; (5) elevated leukocyte alkaline phosphatase, uric acid, and cobalamin levels; and (6) elevated histamine levels. Bone marrow examination in polycythemia vera shows hypercellularity of RBCs, WBCs, and platelets.

Collaborative Care

Treatment is directed toward reducing blood volume and viscosity and bone marrow activity. Phlebotomy is the mainstay of treatment. The aim of phlebotomy is to reduce the hematocrit and keep it less than 45% to 48%. Generally, at the time of diagnosis 300 to 500 mL of blood may be removed every other day until the hematocrit is reduced to normal levels. An individual managed with repeated phlebotomies eventually becomes deficient in iron, although this effect is rarely symptomatic. Avoid iron supplementation. Hydration therapy is used to reduce the blood's viscosity. Myelosuppressive agents such as hydroxyurea, busulfan (Myleran), and chlorambucil are used.

Ruxolitinib (Jakafi), which is a new drug inhibiting the expression of the *JAK2* mutation, is used for patients who have polycythemia-related myelofibrosis. Low-dose aspirin is used to prevent clotting. α-Interferon (α-IFN) is of particular use in women of childbearing age or those with intractable pruritus. Anagrelide (Agrylin) may be used to reduce the platelet count and inhibit platelet aggregation. Allopurinol (Zyloprim) may reduce the number of acute gouty attacks.[21]

NURSING MANAGEMENT POLYCYTHEMIA VERA

Primary polycythemia (polycythemia vera) is not preventable. When acute exacerbations of polycythemia vera develop, you have several responsibilities. Depending on the institution's policies, you may either assist with or perform the phlebotomy. Evaluate fluid intake and output during hydration therapy to avoid fluid overload (which further complicates the circulatory congestion) and underhydration (which can make the blood even more viscous). If myelosuppressive agents are used, administer the drugs as ordered, observe the patient, and teach the patient about medication side effects.

Assess the patient's nutritional status, since inadequate food intake can result from GI symptoms of fullness, pain, and dyspepsia. Begin activities and/or medications to decrease thrombus formation. Initiate active or passive leg exercises and ambulation when possible.

Because of its chronic nature, polycythemia vera requires ongoing evaluation. Phlebotomy may need to be done every 2 to 3 months, reducing the blood volume by about 500 mL each time. Evaluate the patient for complications.

PROBLEMS OF HEMOSTASIS

Hemostasis involves the vascular endothelium, platelets, and coagulation factors, which normally function together to stop hemorrhage and repair vascular injury. (These mechanisms are described in Chapter 30.) Disruption in any of these components may result in bleeding or thrombotic disorders.

Three major disorders of hemostasis discussed in this section are (1) thrombocytopenia (low platelet count), (2) hemophilia and von Willebrand disease (inherited disorders of specific clotting factors), and (3) disseminated intravascular coagulation (DIC).

THROMBOCYTOPENIA

Etiology and Pathophysiology

Thrombocytopenia is a reduction of platelets below 150,000/μL (150×10^9/L). Acute, severe, or prolonged decreases from this normal range can result in abnormal hemostasis that manifests as prolonged bleeding from minor trauma or spontaneous bleeding without injury.

Platelet disorders can be inherited (e.g., Wiskott-Aldrich syndrome), but the vast majority are acquired (Table 31-11). A common cause of acquired disorders is the ingestion of certain herbs or drugs[22,23] (Table 31-12). Although some agents are directly myelosuppressive (e.g., chemotherapy, ganciclovir [Cytovene]), the usual mechanism of thrombocytopenia caused by herbs or drugs is accelerated platelet destruction caused by drug-dependent antibodies. Antibodies attack the platelets when the offending agent binds to the platelet surface.

A careful review of the patient's history helps to identify the cause of thrombocytopenia. For example, quinine is in tonic water and in many herbal preparations. In addition, some drugs can affect platelet aggregation. Aspirin doses as low as 81 mg (baby aspirin) can alter platelet aggregation. Normal function is restored when new platelets are formed.

Immune Thrombocytopenic Purpura. The most common acquired thrombocytopenia is a syndrome of abnormal destruction of circulating platelets termed *immune thrombocytopenic purpura* (ITP). It was originally termed *idiopathic thrombocytopenic purpura* because its cause was unknown. However, it is now known that ITP is primarily an autoimmune disease. In ITP, platelets are coated with antibodies. Although these platelets function normally, when they reach the spleen, the antibody-coated platelets are recognized as foreign and are destroyed by macrophages. Decreased platelet production contributes to ITP.

TABLE 31-11 CAUSES OF THROMBOCYTOPENIA

Inherited
- Fanconi syndrome (pancytopenia)
- Hereditary thrombocytopenia

Acquired
Immune
- Immune thrombocytopenic purpura (ITP)
- Neonatal alloimmune thrombocytopenia

Nonimmune
- Shortened circulation (increased consumption)
  - Thrombotic thrombocytopenic purpura (TTP)
  - Disseminated intravascular coagulation (DIC)
  - Heparin-induced thrombocytopenia (HIT)
  - Splenomegaly or splenic sequestration
- Turbulent blood flow (hemangiomas, abnormal cardiac valves, intraaortic balloon pumps)
- Decreased production
  - Drug-induced marrow suppression
  - Chemotherapy
  - Viral infection (hepatitis C virus, HIV, cytomegalovirus)
  - Bacterial infection (sepsis)
  - Alcoholism, bone marrow suppression
  - Myelodysplastic syndrome (MDS)
  - Myelofibrosis
  - Aplastic anemia
  - Hematologic malignancy (leukemias, lymphomas, myeloma)
  - Solid tumor infiltrating bone marrow
  - Radiation to the bone

TABLE 31-12 DRUG AND HERBAL CAUSES OF THROMBOCYTOPENIA*

- Thiazide diuretics
- Alcohol
- Chemotherapeutic drugs
- Digoxin
- Nonsteroidal antiinflammatory drugs: ibuprofen (Advil, Motrin), indomethacin (Indocin), naproxen (Naproxyn, Aleve)
- Antibiotics: penicillins, cephalosporins, sulfonamides
- Other antiinfectives: rifampin (Rifadin), ganciclovir (Cytovene), amphotericin B
- Analgesics: aspirin and aspirin-containing drugs, acetaminophen
- Antipsychotic and antiseizure agents: haloperidol (Haldol), valproate (Depakene), lithium
- Platelet glycoprotein inhibitors: abciximab (ReoPro), tirofiban (Aggrastat), eptifibatide (Integrilin), clopidogrel (Plavix)
- H_2-receptor antagonists: cimetidine (Tagamet), ranitidine (Zantac)
- Gold compounds: auranofin (Ridaura)
- Spices: ginger, cumin, turmeric, cloves
- Vitamins: vitamin C, vitamin E
- Heparin
- Herbs: angelica, bilberry, feverfew, garlic, ginkgo biloba, ginseng
- Quinine compounds: tonic water

*List is not all-inclusive.

Sometimes infection, such as *Helicobacter pylori* or viral infection, contributes to this disorder.[23]

Platelets normally survive 8 to 10 days. However, in ITP survival of platelets is shortened. The clinical syndrome manifests as an acute condition in children and a chronic condition in adults. Chronic ITP may occur in women between 15 and 40 years of age or older individuals. Chronic ITP has a gradual onset, and transient remissions may occur.[23]

Thrombotic Thrombocytopenic Purpura. *Thrombotic thrombocytopenic purpura* (TTP) is an uncommon syndrome characterized by hemolytic anemia, thrombocytopenia, neurologic abnormalities, fever (in the absence of infection), and renal abnormalities; not all features are present in all patients. Because it is almost always associated with hemolytic-uremic syndrome (HUS), it is often referred to as TTP-HUS. The disease is associated with enhanced aggregation of platelets, which form microthrombi that deposit in arterioles and capillaries.

In most cases the syndrome is caused by the deficiency of a plasma enzyme (ADAMTS13) that usually breaks down the von Willebrand clotting factor (vWF) into normal size. (vWF is the most important protein mediating platelet adhesion to damaged endothelial cells.) Without the enzyme, unusually large amounts of vWF attach to activated platelets, thereby promoting platelet aggregation.

TTP is seen primarily in adults between 20 and 50 years of age, with a slight female predominance. The syndrome may be idiopathic (thought to be due to an autoimmune disorder against ADAMTS13), but it may be due to certain drug toxicities (e.g., chemotherapy, cyclosporine, quinine, oral contraceptives, valacyclovir [Valtrex], clopidogrel [Plavix]), pregnancy or preeclampsia, infection, or a known autoimmune disorder such as systemic lupus erythematosus or scleroderma. TTP is a medical emergency because bleeding and clotting occur simultaneously.[24]

Heparin-Induced Thrombocytopenia. One of the risks associated with the broad and increasing use of heparin is the development of the life-threatening condition called *heparin-induced thrombocytopenia* (HIT), also called *heparin-induced thrombocytopenia and thrombosis syndrome* (HITTS). Typically, patients develop thrombocytopenia 5 to 10 days after the onset of heparin therapy. HIT should be suspected if the platelet count falls by more than 50% or falls to below 150,000/μL. As many as 5% of patients on heparin therapy develop HIT.[24]

The major clinical problem of HIT is venous thrombosis; arterial thrombosis can also develop. Deep vein thromboses and pulmonary emboli most commonly result as a complication of the thromboses. Additional complications may include arterial vascular infarcts resulting in skin necrosis, stroke, and end-organ damage (e.g., kidneys). Symptoms of bleeding are unusual because the platelet count rarely drops below 60,000/μL.

In HIT, platelet destruction and vascular endothelial injury are the two major responses to an immune-mediated response to heparin. Platelet factor 4 (PF4) binds to heparin (this protein is made and released by platelets). This complex then binds to the platelet surface, leading to further platelet activation and release of more PF4, thus creating a positive feedback loop. Antibodies are created against this complex, and they are removed prematurely from circulation, leading to thrombocytopenia and platelet-fibrin thrombi. Platelet aggregation also induces heparin to be neutralized. Thus more heparin is required to maintain therapeutic activated partial thromboplastin times (aPTT).

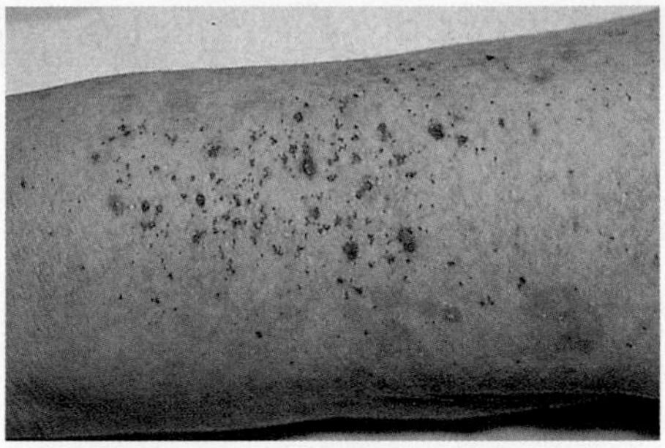

FIG. 31-6 Acute idiopathic thrombocytopenic purpura commonly manifests with purpuric lesions of this kind, although they may often be widespread by the time medical attention is sought.

Clinical Manifestations

Many patients with thrombocytopenia are usually asymptomatic. The most common symptom is bleeding, usually mucosal or cutaneous. Mucosal bleeding may manifest as epistaxis and gingival bleeding, and large bullous hemorrhages may appear on the buccal mucosa because of the lack of vessel protection by the submucosal tissue.

Bleeding into the skin is manifested as petechiae, purpura, or superficial ecchymoses (Fig. 31-6). *Petechiae* are small, flat, pinpoint, red or reddish brown microhemorrhages. When the platelet count is low, RBCs may leak out of the blood vessels and into the skin to cause petechiae. When petechiae are numerous, the resulting reddish skin bruise is called *purpura.* Larger purplish lesions caused by hemorrhage are termed *ecchymoses.* Ecchymoses may be flat or raised; pain and tenderness sometimes are present.

Prolonged bleeding after routine procedures such as venipuncture or IM injection may indicate thrombocytopenia. Because the bleeding may be internal, be aware of manifestations that reflect this type of blood loss, including weakness, fainting, dizziness, tachycardia, abdominal pain, and hypotension.

The major complication of thrombocytopenia is hemorrhage. The hemorrhage may be insidious or acute, and internal or external. It may occur in any area of the body, including the joints, retina, and brain. Cerebral hemorrhage may be fatal. Insidious hemorrhage may first be detected by discovering the anemia that accompanies blood loss.

Because thrombocytopenia can be accompanied by vascular thromboses in some of these disorders, signs and symptoms of vascular ischemic problems can manifest (see Chapter 38). For example, subtle confusion, headache, or even serious manifestations such as seizures and coma due to TTP-related thrombosis may be seen. Because signs and symptoms may be subtle, astute and thorough assessment of the patient is essential.

Diagnostic Studies

The platelet count is decreased in thrombocytopenia. Any reduction below 150,000/μL (150×10^9/L) may be termed *thrombocytopenia.* However, prolonged bleeding from trauma or injury does not usually occur until platelet counts are less than 50,000/μL (50×10^9/L). When the count drops below 20,000/μL (20×10^9/L), spontaneous, life-threatening hemorrhages (e.g., intracranial bleeding) can occur. Platelet transfusions are generally not recommended until the count is below 10,000/μL (10×10^9/L) unless the patient is actively bleeding.

TABLE 31-13 LABORATORY RESULTS IN THROMBOCYTOPENIA

Laboratory Test	Immune Thrombocytopenic Purpura	Thrombotic Thrombocytopenic Purpura	Heparin-Induced Thrombocytopenia	Disseminated Intravascular Coagulation
Platelets	↓↓↓	↓↓↓	↓↓	↓↓↓
Hemolysis				
Hgb	N	↓↓	N	N or ↓
LDH	N	↑↑↑	N	↑
Reticulocytes	N	↑	N	N or ↑
Haptoglobin	N	↓	N	↓
Indirect bilirubin	N	↑	N	N or ↑
Schistocytes	N	↑↑↑	N or ↑	N or ↑
Coagulopathy				
PT	N	N	N	↑
aPTT	N	N	N	↑
D-dimer	N	N or ↑	↑	↑↑
Other Tests	ITP platelet antigen-specific assay, ^{14}C-serotonin release assay, *Helicobacter pylori*, bone marrow biopsy	ADAMTS13	^{14}C-serotonin release assay, PF4-heparin complex	

aPTT, Activated partial thromboplastin time; *ITP*, idiopathic thrombocytopenic purpura; *LDH*, lactate dehydrogenase; *N*, normal; *PF4*, platelet factor 4; *PT*, prothrombin time.

Examination of the peripheral blood smear may help distinguish acquired disorders such as ITP and TTP from congenital disorders, which may be indicated by abnormally sized platelets. The patient's medical history and clinical examination, along with comparisons of laboratory parameters, help to determine the etiology of the thrombocytopenia. Table 31-13 compares the types of thrombocytopenia.[23,24]

Laboratory tests that assess secondary hemostasis or coagulation, such as the prothrombin time (PT) and aPTT, can be normal even in severe thrombocytopenia. If they are elevated, this may point toward DIC. Bone marrow examination is done to rule out production problems as the cause of thrombocytopenia (e.g., leukemia, aplastic anemia, other myeloproliferative disorders).

Specific assays, such as ITP antigen-specific assay, ^{14}C-serotonin release assay, or enzyme-linked immunosorbent assay (ELISA) for PF4-heparin complex for HIT, can be done to assist with the diagnosis. In TTP, testing for deficiency of ADAMTS13 is not always diagnostic, so an increase of lactate dehydrogenase (LDH) may help establish the diagnosis.[23,24] When thrombocytopenia occurs with anemia characterized by altered RBC morphology, including *spherocytes* (small, globular, completely hemoglobinated erythrocytes), fragmented cells (schistocytes), and pronounced reticulocytosis, a diagnosis of TTP should be suspected. These findings are partially a result of intravascular fibrin deposition causing a "slicing" of RBCs. In TTP, thrombocytopenia may be severe, but coagulation studies are normal.

Bone marrow analysis is performed if other test results are inconclusive, especially in older patients because of a higher suspicion of an underlying bone marrow disorder. When destruction of circulating platelets is the cause, bone marrow analysis shows *megakaryocytes* (precursors of platelets) to be normal or increased, even though circulating platelets are reduced. The absence or decreased number of megakaryocytes on bone marrow biopsy is consistent with thrombocytopenia caused by decreased bone marrow production (e.g., aplastic anemia). Special blood analyses using flow cytometry and other techniques can detect antiplatelet antibodies as the source of destruction.

Collaborative Care

Collaborative care of thrombocytopenia differs based on the etiology. Removal or treatment of the underlying cause or disorder is sometimes sufficient. The patient with thrombocytopenia should avoid aspirin and other medications that affect platelet function or production. The following sections discuss management strategies for the different causes of thrombocytopenia (Table 31-14).

Immune Thrombocytopenic Purpura. Multiple therapies are used to manage the patient with ITP.[25] If the patient is asymptomatic, therapy may not be used unless the patient's platelet count is below 30,000/μL. Corticosteroids (e.g., prednisone, methylprednisolone) are used initially to treat ITP because of their ability to suppress the phagocytic response of splenic macrophages. This alters the spleen's recognition of platelets and increases the life span of the platelets. In addition, corticosteroids depress antibody formation and reduce capillary leakage.

High doses of IV immunoglobulin (IVIG) and a component of IVIG, anti-Rh_o(D) (anti-D, WinRho), may be used in the patient who is unresponsive to corticosteroids or splenectomy, or for whom splenectomy is not an option. It is believed that one way these agents work is by competing with the antiplatelet antibodies for macrophage receptors in the spleen. Rituximab may be used for its ability to lyse activated B cells, therapy reducing the immune recognition of platelets.

Splenectomy may be indicated if the patient does not respond to the above treatments. Splenectomy can usually be done laparoscopically, and 60% to 70% of patients benefit from splenectomy, resulting in a complete or partial remission.[26] The effectiveness of splenectomy is based on four factors. First, the spleen contains an abundance of the macrophages that sequester and destroy platelets. Second, structural features of the spleen enhance the interaction between antibody-coated platelets and macrophages. Third, some antibody synthesis occurs in the spleen; thus antiplatelet antibodies decrease after splenec-

TABLE 31-14 COLLABORATIVE CARE

Thrombocytopenia

Diagnostic
- History and physical examination
- Bone marrow aspiration and biopsy
- CBC, including platelet count
- Specific studies (see Table 31-13)

Collaborative Therapy

Immune Thrombocytopenic Purpura
- Corticosteroids
- IV immunoglobulin (IVIG)
- Anti-Rh_0(D)
- Rituximab
- Splenectomy
- Romiplostim (Nplate)
- Eltrombopag (Promacta)
- Danazol
- Immunosuppressives (e.g., cyclosporine, cyclophosphamide [Cytoxan], azathioprine [Imuran], mycophenolate mofetil [CellCept])
- High-dose cyclophosphamide or combination chemotherapy
- Platelet transfusions

Thrombotic Thrombocytopenic Purpura
- Identification and treatment of cause
- Plasmapheresis (plasma exchange)
- High-dose prednisone
- Dextran
- Chemotherapy (vincristine [Oncovin], vinblastine [Velban])
- Immunosuppressives (cyclophosphamide, rituximab [Rituxan])
- Splenectomy

Heparin-Induced Thrombocytopenia
- Direct thrombin inhibitor (lepirudin [Refludan], argatroban [Acova])
- Indirect thrombin inhibitor (fondaparinux [Arixtra])
- Warfarin (Coumadin)
- Plasmapheresis (plasma exchange)
- Protamine sulfate
- Thrombolytic agents

Decreased Platelet Production
- Identification and treatment or removal of cause
- Corticosteroids
- Platelet transfusions

tomy. Fourth, the spleen normally sequesters approximately one third of the platelets, so its removal increases the number of platelets in circulation.

Romiplostim (Nplate) and eltrombopag (Promacta) are used for patients with chronic ITP who have had an insufficient response to the other treatments or who have a contraindication to splenectomy. These drugs are thrombopoietin receptor agonists, thus increasing platelet production.[27] Danazol (Danocrine), an androgen, may be used along with corticosteroids in some patients. Although the mechanism is not totally understood, danazol increases $CD4^+$ T cells, thereby decreasing the immune response. Immunosuppressive therapy may be used in refractory cases[23] (see Table 31-14).

Platelet transfusions may be used to increase platelet counts in cases of life-threatening hemorrhage. Platelets should not be administered prophylactically because of the possibility of antibody formation. The usual indication for administering platelets is for a platelet count less than 10,000/μL or if there is anticipated bleeding before a procedure. Epsilon-aminocaproic acid (EACA, Amicar), an antifibrinolytic agent, may be used for severe bleeding.

Thrombotic Thrombocytopenic Purpura. TTP may be treated in a variety of ways. The first step is to treat the underlying disorder (e.g., infection) or remove the causative agent, if identified. If untreated, TTP usually results in irreversible renal failure and death. Plasma exchange (plasmapheresis) (see Chapter 14) is used to aggressively reverse platelet consumption by supplying the appropriate vWF and enzyme (ADAMTS13) and removing the large vWF molecules that bind with platelets. Treatment should be continued daily until the patient's platelet counts normalize and hemolysis has ceased. Corticosteroids may be added to this treatment. Recently, rituximab has been used for patients refractory to plasma exchange; it decreases the level of inhibitory ADAMTS13 IgG antibodies. Other immunosuppressants such as cyclosporine or cyclophosphamide may also be used. Splenectomy may be considered in patients refractory to plasma exchange or immunosuppression. The administration of platelets is generally contraindicated because this may lead to new vWF-platelet complexes and increased clotting.

Heparin-Induced Thrombocytopenia. Heparin must be discontinued when HIT is first recognized. Heparin flushes for vascular catheters should also be stopped.

To maintain anticoagulation, the patient should be started on a direct thrombin inhibitor, such as lepirudin (Refludan) or argatroban (Acova). Fondaparinux (Arixtra), a factor Xa inhibitor (indirect thrombin inhibitor), may be used. Warfarin should be started only when the platelet count has reached 150,000/μL. If the clotting is severe, the most commonly used treatment modalities are plasmapheresis to clear the platelet-aggregating IgG from the blood, protamine sulfate to interrupt the circulating heparin, thrombolytic agents to treat the thromboembolic events, and surgery to remove clots. Platelet transfusions are not effective because they may enhance thromboembolic events.

Patients who have had HIT should never be given heparin or low-molecular-weight heparin (LMWH). This should be clearly marked on the patient's medical record.

Acquired Thrombocytopenia From Decreased Platelet Production. The management of acquired thrombocytopenia is based on identifying the cause and treating the disease or removing the causative agent. If the precipitating factor is unknown, the patient may receive corticosteroids. Platelet transfusions are given if life-threatening hemorrhage develops.

Often acquired thrombocytopenia is caused by another underlying condition (e.g., aplastic anemia, leukemia) or therapy used to treat another problem. For example, in acute leukemia all blood cell types may be depressed. Additionally, the patient may receive chemotherapeutic drugs that cause bone marrow suppression. If the patient can be adequately supported throughout the course of chemotherapy-induced thrombocytopenia, the thrombocytopenia will also resolve.

NURSING MANAGEMENT THROMBOCYTOPENIA

NURSING ASSESSMENT

Subjective and objective data that should be obtained from a patient with thrombocytopenia are presented in Table 31-15.

NURSING DIAGNOSES

Nursing diagnoses for the patient with thrombocytopenia may include, but are not limited to, the following.

TABLE 31-15 NURSING ASSESSMENT

Thrombocytopenia

Subjective Data

Important Health Information

Past health history: Recent hemorrhage, excessive bleeding, or viral illness; HIV infection; cancer (especially leukemia or lymphoma); aplastic anemia; systemic lupus erythematosus; cirrhosis; exposure to radiation or toxic chemicals; disseminated intravascular coagulation

Medications: See Table 31-12

Functional Health Patterns

Health perception–health management: Family history of bleeding problems; malaise

Nutritional-metabolic: Bleeding gingiva; coffee-ground or bloody vomitus; easy bruising

Elimination: Hematuria, dark or bloody stools

Activity-exercise: Fatigue, weakness, fainting; epistaxis, hemoptysis; dyspnea

Cognitive-perceptual: Pain and tenderness in bleeding areas (e.g., abdomen, head, extremities); headache

Sexuality-reproductive: Menorrhagia, metrorrhagia

Objective Data

General

Fever, lethargy

Integumentary

Petechiae, ecchymoses, purpura

Gastrointestinal

Splenomegaly, abdominal distention; guaiac-positive stools

Possible Diagnostic Findings

Platelet count <150,000/μL (150×10^9/L), prolonged bleeding time, ↓ hemoglobin and hematocrit; normal or ↑ megakaryocytes in bone marrow examination

- Impaired oral mucous membrane *related to* low platelet counts and/or effects of pathologic conditions and treatment
- Risk for bleeding *related to* decreased platelets
- Deficient knowledge *related to* lack of information regarding the disease process and treatment

PLANNING

The overall goals are that the patient with thrombocytopenia will (1) have no gross or occult bleeding, (2) maintain vascular integrity, and (3) manage home care to prevent any complications related to an increased risk for bleeding.

NURSING IMPLEMENTATION

HEALTH PROMOTION. Discourage excessive use of over-the-counter (OTC) medications known to be possible causes of acquired thrombocytopenia. Many medications contain aspirin as an ingredient. Aspirin reduces platelet adhesiveness, thus contributing to bleeding.

Encourage persons to have a complete medical evaluation if manifestations of bleeding tendencies (e.g., prolonged epistaxis, petechiae) develop. Observe for early signs of thrombocytopenia in the patient receiving cancer chemotherapy drugs.

ACUTE INTERVENTION. The goal during acute episodes of thrombocytopenia is to prevent or control hemorrhage (see eNursing Care Plan 31-1 on the website for this chapter). In the patient with thrombocytopenia, bleeding is usually from superficial sites. Deep bleeding (into muscles, joints, and abdomen) usually occurs only when clotting factors are diminished. Emphasize that a seemingly minor nosebleed or new petechiae may indicate potential hemorrhage and the health care provider should be notified.

Bleeding from the posterior nasopharynx may be difficult to detect because the blood may be swallowed. If a subcutaneous injection is unavoidable, the use of a small-gauge needle and application of direct pressure for at least 5 to 10 minutes after injection is indicated, or application of an ice pack may be helpful. Avoid IM injections. Help the patient understand the importance of adherence to self-care measures that reduce the risk of bleeding (Table 31-16).

Note that many of these disorders may be accompanied by vascular clotting, and appropriate assessment and management should be taken (see Chapter 38). As bleeding occurs, red blood cell and coagulation factors are consumed along with platelets, so it is important to monitor all blood cell and coagulation studies.

TABLE 31-16 PATIENT & CAREGIVER TEACHING GUIDE

Thrombocytopenia

Include the following instructions when teaching a patient or caregiver the precautions to take when the platelet count is low.

1. Notify your health care provider of any manifestations of bleeding. These include the following:
   - Black, tarry, or bloody bowel movements
   - Black or bloody vomit, sputum, or urine
   - Bruising or small red or purple spots on the skin
   - Bleeding from the mouth or anywhere in the body
   - Headache or changes in how well you can see
   - Difficulty talking, sudden weakness of an arm or leg, confusion
2. Ask your health care provider regarding restrictions in your normal activities, such as vigorous exercise, lifting weights. Generally, walking can be done safely and should be done with sturdy shoes or slippers. If you are weak and at risk for falling, get help or supervision when getting out of bed or chair.
3. Do not blow your nose forcefully; gently pat it with a tissue if needed. For a nosebleed, keep your head up and apply firm pressure to the nostrils and bridge of your nose. If bleeding continues, place an ice bag over the bridge of your nose and the nape of your neck. If you are unable to stop a nosebleed after 10 min, call your health care provider.
4. Do not bend down with your head lower than your waist.
5. Prevent constipation by drinking plenty of fluids. Do not strain when having a bowel movement. Your health care provider may prescribe a stool softener. Do not use a suppository, an enema, or a rectal thermometer without the permission of your health care provider.
6. Shave only with an electric razor; do not use blades.
7. Do not pluck your eyebrows or other body hair.
8. Do not puncture your skin, such as getting tattoos or body piercing.
9. Avoid using any medication that can prolong bleeding, such as aspirin. Other medications and herbs can have similar effects. If you are unsure about any medication, ask your health care provider or pharmacist about it in relation to your thrombocytopenia.
10. Use a soft-bristle toothbrush to prevent injuring the gums. Flossing is usually safe if it is done gently using the thin tape floss. Do not use alcohol-based mouthwashes, since they can dry your gums and increase bleeding.
11. Women who are menstruating should keep track of the number of pads that are used per day. When you start using more pads per day than usual or bleed more days, notify your health care provider. Do not use tampons; use sanitary pads only.
12. Ask your health care provider before you have any invasive procedures done, such as a dental cleaning, manicure, or pedicure.

In a woman with thrombocytopenia, menstrual blood loss may exceed the usual amount and duration. Counting sanitary napkins used during menses is another important intervention to detect excess blood loss. Blood loss of 50 mL will completely soak a sanitary napkin. Suppression of menses with hormonal agents may be indicated during predictable periods of thrombocytopenia (e.g., during chemotherapy and HSCT) to reduce blood loss from menses.

Closely monitor the platelet count, coagulation studies, hemoglobin, and hematocrit. Together these provide important information regarding potential or actual bleeding.

The proper administration of platelet transfusions is an important nursing responsibility. This is discussed under Blood Component Therapy later in this chapter.

AMBULATORY AND HOME CARE. Monitor the patient with ITP who is receiving treatment for the response to therapy. Teach the person with acquired thrombocytopenia to avoid causative agents when possible (see Table 31-12). If the causative agents cannot be avoided (e.g., chemotherapy), teach the patient to avoid injury or trauma during these periods and to be aware of the clinical signs and symptoms of bleeding caused by thrombocytopenia (see Table 31-16).

Patients with either ITP or acquired thrombocytopenia should have planned periodic medical evaluations to assess their status. These regular evaluations can be used to assess and treat situations in which exacerbations and bleeding are likely to occur. The impact of either an acute or a chronic condition on the patient's quality of life should also be addressed appropriately.

EVALUATION

The expected outcomes are that the patient with thrombocytopenia will

- Have no evidence of bleeding or bruising
- Verbalize required knowledge and skills to manage disease process at home

HEMOPHILIA AND VON WILLEBRAND DISEASE

Hemophilia is an X-linked recessive genetic disorder caused by a defective or deficient coagulation factor. The two major types of hemophilia, which can occur in mild to severe forms, are *hemophilia A* (classic hemophilia, factor VIII deficiency) and *hemophilia B* (Christmas disease, factor IX deficiency). *von Willebrand disease* is a related disorder involving a deficiency of the von Willebrand coagulation protein. Factor VIII is synthesized in the liver and circulates as a complex with von Willebrand factor (vWF).

Hemophilia A is the most common form of hemophilia, accounting for about 85% to 90% of all cases. Hemophilia B accounts for about 10% to 15% of all cases. von Willebrand disease is considered the most common congenital bleeding disorder, with estimates as high as 1 or 2 in 100.[28]

Genetic Link

The inheritance patterns of hemophilia and von Willebrand disease are compared in Table 31-17. (X-linked genetic disorders are discussed in Chapter 13 and Table 13-2.)

Clinical Manifestations and Complications

All clinical manifestations relate to bleeding, and any bleeding episode in persons with hemophilia may lead to a life-threatening hemorrhage. Clinical manifestations and complications related to hemophilia include (1) slow, persistent, prolonged bleeding from minor trauma and small cuts; (2) delayed bleeding after minor injuries (the delay may be several hours or days); (3) uncontrollable hemorrhage after dental extractions or irritation of the gingiva with a hard-bristle toothbrush; (4) epistaxis, especially after a blow to the face; (5) GI bleeding from ulcers and gastritis; (6) hematuria and potential renal failure from GU trauma and splenic rupture resulting from falls or abdominal trauma; (7) ecchymoses and subcutaneous hematomas (Fig. 31-7); (8) neurologic signs, such as pain, anesthesia, and paralysis, which may develop from nerve compression caused by hematoma formation; and (9) hemarthrosis (bleeding into the joints) (Fig. 31-8), which may lead to joint injury and deformity severe enough to cause crippling (most commonly in knees, elbows, shoulders, hips, and ankles).

TABLE 31-17 TYPES OF HEMOPHILIA

Type	Inheritance Pattern
Hemophilia A	
Factor VIII	Recessive sex-linked (transmitted by female carriers, displayed almost exclusively in men)
Hemophilia B	
Factor IX	Recessive sex-linked (transmitted by female carriers, displayed almost exclusively in men)
von Willebrand Disease	
vWF, variable factor VIII deficiencies and platelet dysfunction	Autosomal dominant, seen in both genders Recessive (in severe forms of the disease)

vWF, von Willebrand factor.

GENETICS IN CLINICAL PRACTICE

Hemophilia A and B

Genetic Basis

- X-linked recessive disorder.
- *Hemophilia A:* Caused by mutations in the *F8* gene that provides instructions for making coagulation factor VIII.
- *Hemophilia B:* Caused by mutations in the *F9* gene that provides instructions for making coagulation factor IX.
- Mutations in the *F8* or *F9* gene lead to the production of an abnormal version or reduced amounts of these coagulation factors.

Incidence

- *Hemophilia A:* 1 in 5000 to 10,000 male births.
- *Hemophilia B:* 1 in 30,000 to 50,000 male births.

Genetic Testing

- DNA testing is available.

Clinical Implications

- Female carriers transmit the genetic defect to 50% of their sons, and 50% of their daughters are carriers.
- Males with hemophilia do not transmit the genetic defect to their sons, but all of their daughters are carriers.
- Female hemophilia can occur if a male with hemophilia mates with a female carrier. However, this is a rare situation.
- Clinical manifestations of hemophilia A and B are similar.
- Replacement therapy is available for factors VIII and IX (see Table 31-19).

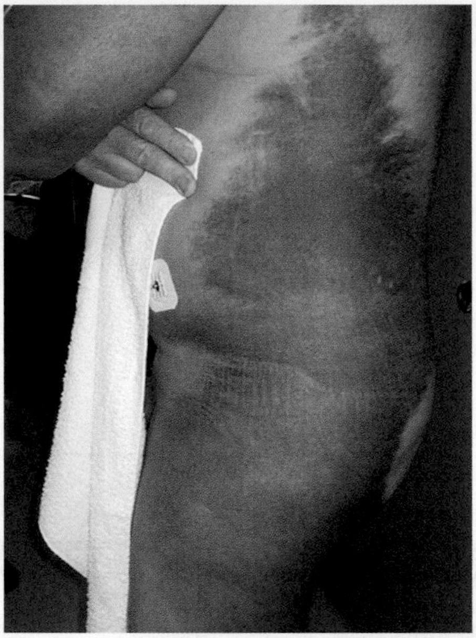

FIG. 31-7 Severe ecchymoses in a person with hemophilia after a fall.

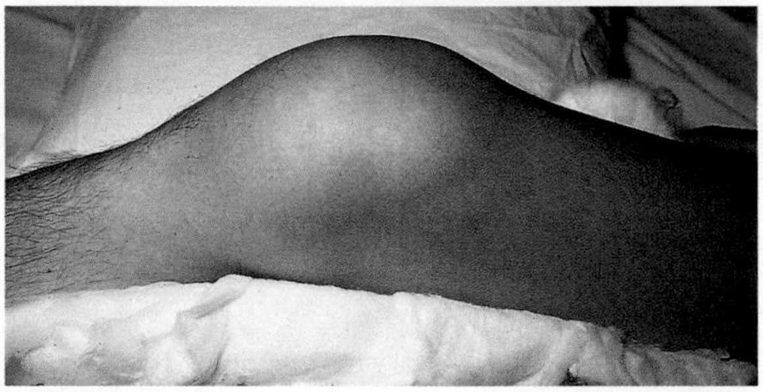

FIG. 31-8 Acute hemarthrosis of the knee is a common complication of hemophilia.

TABLE 31-18 LABORATORY RESULTS IN HEMOPHILIA

Test	Results
Prothrombin time	Normal. No involvement of extrinsic system.
Thrombin time	Normal. No impairment of thrombin-fibrinogen reaction.
Platelet count	Normal. Adequate platelet production.
Partial thromboplastin time	Prolonged because of deficiency in intrinsic clotting system factor.
Bleeding time	Prolonged in von Willebrand disease because of structurally defective platelets. Normal in hemophilia A and B because platelets not affected.
Factor assays	Reductions of factor VIII in hemophilia A, factor IX in hemophilia B, vWF in von Willebrand disease.

vWF, von Willebrand factor.

TABLE 31-19 DRUG THERAPY

Replacement Factors for Hemophilia

Factor VIII	Factor IX	For Patients Who Have Inhibitors
Advate	AlphaNine SD	NovoSeven (factor VIIa)
Alphanate	Bebulin VH	Autoplex T
Helixate FS	Benefix	FEIBA (factor VIII inhibitor bypassing activity)
Hemofil M	Mononine	
Humate-P	Profilnine SD	
Koāte-DVI		
Kogenate FS		
Monoclate P		
Recombinate		
Xyntha		

In children these manifestations may lead to the diagnosis. In adults these developments may be the first sign of a newly diagnosed mild form of the disease that escaped detection through a childhood free of major injuries, dental procedures, or surgeries.

Diagnostic Studies

Laboratory studies are used to determine the type of hemophilia present. Any factor deficiency within the intrinsic system (factor VIII, IX, XI, or XII or vWF) will yield the laboratory results presented in Table 31-18.

Collaborative Care

The goals of collaborative care are to prevent and treat bleeding. Collaborative care for persons with hemophilia or von Willebrand disease requires (1) preventive care, (2) the use of replacement therapy during acute bleeding episodes and as prophylaxis, and (3) the treatment of the complications of the disease and its therapy. Today most patients can expect almost normal life spans free of bloodborne illnesses because of improved preparation of replacement products, improved screening of blood donor populations, and use of recombinant replacement factors.[29]

Replacement of deficient clotting factors is the primary means of supporting a patient with hemophilia. In addition to treating acute crises, replacement therapy may be given before surgery and dental care as a prophylactic measure.[30] Examples of replacement therapy are listed in Table 31-19. Fresh frozen plasma, once commonly used for replacement therapy, is rarely used today.

For mild hemophilia A and certain subtypes of von Willebrand disease, desmopressin acetate (also known as DDAVP), a synthetic analog of vasopressin, may be used to stimulate an increase in factor VIII and vWF. This drug acts on platelets and endothelial cells to cause the release of vWF, which subsequently binds with factor VIII, thus increasing their concentration. It can be administered IV, subcutaneously, or by intranasal spray. Beneficial effects (e.g., decreased bleeding time) of DDAVP, when administered IV, are seen within 30 minutes and can last for more than 12 hours. Because the effect of DDAVP is relatively short lived, the patient must be closely monitored and repeated doses may be necessary. It is an appropriate therapy for minor bleeding episodes and dental procedures. The intranasal form may be indicated for home therapy for some patients with mild to moderate forms of the disease.

Antifibrinolytic therapy (tranexamic acid [Cyklokapron] and epsilon-aminocaproic acid) inhibits fibrinolysis by inhibiting plasminogen activation in the fibrin clot, thereby enhancing clot stability. These agents are used to stabilize clots in areas of increased fibrinolysis, such as the oral cavity, and in patients with difficult episodes of epistaxis and menorrhagia.[31]

Complications of the treatment of hemophilia include development of inhibitors to factors VIII or IX, transfusion-transmitted infectious disorders (hepatitis, HIV), allergic reactions, and thrombotic complications with the use of factor IX because it contains activated coagulation factors. Patients with vWF may also develop alloantibodies against vWF concentrates, the infusion of which could cause life-threatening anaphylaxis. Thus replacement factors for these patients should not contain vWF.

The most common difficulties with acute management are starting factor replacement therapy too late and stopping it too soon. Generally, minor bleeding episodes should be treated for at least 72 hours. Surgery and traumatic injuries may need more prolonged therapy. Chronically, development of inhibitors to the factor products has occurred and requires individualized expert patient management. Designated treatment centers in the United States and many other countries provide interdisciplinary care of hemophilia and related disorders. Gene therapy has been used on an experimental basis to treat hemophilia.[32]

NURSING MANAGEMENT HEMOPHILIA

NURSING IMPLEMENTATION

HEALTH PROMOTION. Because of the hereditary nature of hemophilia, referral of affected persons for genetic counseling before reproduction is an important measure. This is especially important because many persons with hemophilia live into adulthood. Reproductive concerns and long-term effects are issues that you should include in the patient's care plan.

ACUTE INTERVENTION. Interventions are related primarily to controlling bleeding and include the following:

1. Stop the topical bleeding as quickly as possible by applying direct pressure or ice, packing the area with Gelfoam or fibrin foam, and applying topical hemostatic agents such as thrombin.
2. Administer the specific coagulation factor to raise the patient's level of the deficient coagulation factor. Monitor the patient for signs and symptoms, such as hypersensitivity.
3. When joint bleeding occurs, in addition to administering replacement factors, it is important to totally rest the involved joint to prevent crippling deformities from hemarthrosis. Pack the joint in ice. Give analgesics (e.g., acetaminophen, codeine) to reduce severe pain. Aspirin and aspirin-containing compounds should never be used. As soon as bleeding ceases, encourage mobilization of the affected area through range-of-motion exercises and physical therapy. Weight bearing is avoided until all swelling has resolved and muscle strength has returned.
4. Manage any life-threatening complications that may develop as a result of hemorrhage or side effects from coagulation factors. Examples include nursing interventions to prevent or treat airway obstruction from hemorrhage into the neck and pharynx, recognition of compartment syndrome in an extremity, and early assessment and treatment of intracranial bleeding.

AMBULATORY AND HOME CARE. Home management is a primary consideration for the patient with hemophilia because the disease follows a progressive, chronic course. The quality and the length of life may be significantly affected by the patient's knowledge of the illness and how to live with it. The patient and caregiver can be referred to a local chapter of the Hemophilia Federation of America to encourage associations with other individuals who are dealing with the problems of hemophilia. Provide ongoing assessment of the patient's adaptation to the illness. Psychosocial support and assistance should be readily available as needed.

Most of the long-term care measures are related to patient teaching. Teach the patient to recognize disease-related problems and to learn which problems can be resolved at home and which require hospitalization. Immediate medical attention is required for severe pain or swelling of a muscle or joint that restricts movement or inhibits sleep and for a head injury, swelling in the neck or mouth, abdominal pain, hematuria, melena, and skin wounds in need of suturing.

Teach the patient to perform daily oral hygiene without causing trauma. Understanding how to prevent injuries is another consideration. Advise the patient to participate only in noncontact sports (e.g., golf) and to wear gloves when doing household chores to prevent cuts or abrasions from knives, hammers, and other tools. The patient should wear a Medic Alert tag to ensure that health care providers know about the hemophilia in case of an accident. Many patients or their caregivers can be taught to self-administer the factor replacement therapies at home.

EVALUATION

The overall expected outcomes are similar to those for the patient with thrombocytopenia (see p. 655).

DISSEMINATED INTRAVASCULAR COAGULATION

Disseminated intravascular coagulation (DIC) is a serious bleeding and thrombotic disorder that results from abnormally initiated and accelerated clotting. Subsequent decreases in clotting factors and platelets ensue, which may lead to uncontrollable hemorrhage. The term *disseminated intravascular coagulation* can be misleading because it suggests that blood is clotting. However, this condition is characterized by the profuse bleeding that results from the depletion of platelets and clotting factors. DIC is always caused by an underlying disease or condition. The underlying problem must be treated for the DIC to resolve.

Etiology and Pathophysiology

DIC is not a disease. It is an abnormal response of the normal clotting cascade stimulated by a disease process or disorder.[33] The diseases and disorders known to predispose a patient to DIC are listed in Table 31-20. DIC can occur as an acute, catastrophic condition or it may exist at a subacute or chronic level. Each condition may have one or multiple triggering mechanisms to start the clotting cascade. For example, tumors and traumatized or necrotic tissue release tissue factors into circulation. Endotoxin from gram-negative bacteria activates several steps in the coagulation cascade.

Tissue factor is released at the site of tissue injury and by some malignancies, such as leukemia, and enhances normal coagulation mechanisms. Abundant intravascular thrombin, the most powerful coagulant, is produced (Fig. 31-9). It catalyzes the conversion of fibrinogen to fibrin and enhances platelet aggregation. There is widespread fibrin and platelet deposition in capillaries and arterioles, resulting in thrombosis. This process can lead to multiorgan failure.

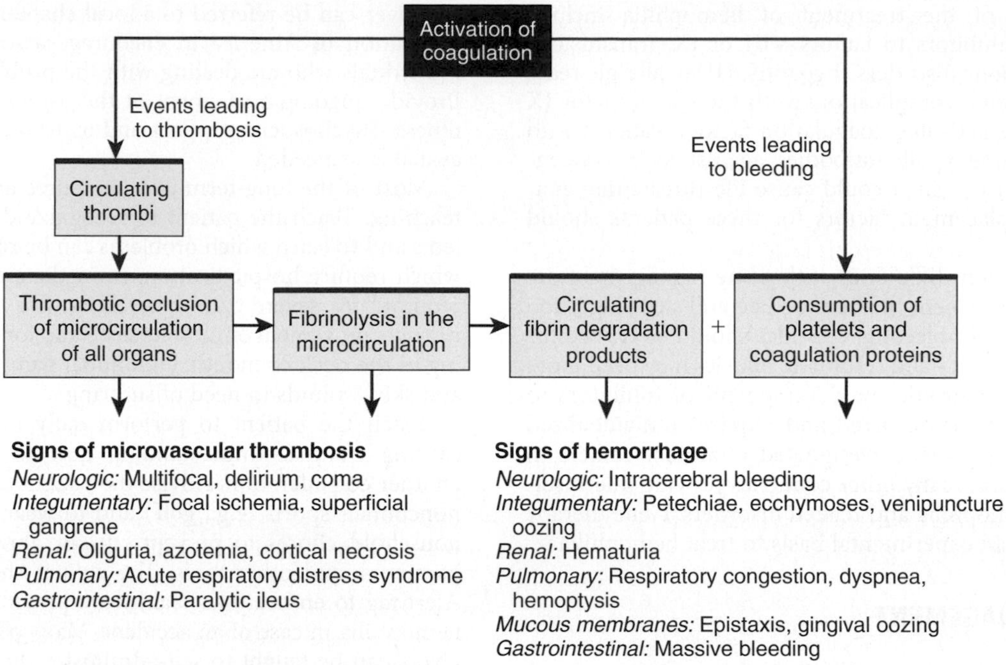

FIG. 31-9 The sequence of events that occur during disseminated intravascular coagulation (DIC).

In addition, clotting inhibitory mechanisms, such as antithrombin III (AT III) and protein C, are depressed. Excessive clotting activates the fibrinolytic system, which in turn breaks down the newly formed clot, creating fibrin split products (FSPs). These products have anticoagulant properties and inhibit normal blood clotting. Ultimately, as FSPs accumulate and clotting factors are depleted, the blood loses its ability to clot. Therefore a stable clot cannot be formed at injury sites, which predisposes the patient to hemorrhage.

Chronic and subacute DIC is most commonly seen in patients with long-standing illnesses such as malignant disorders or autoimmune diseases. Occasionally these patients have subclinical disease manifested only by laboratory abnormalities. However, the clinical spectrum ranges from easy bruising to hemorrhage, and from hypercoagulability to thrombosis.

TABLE 31-20 RISK FACTORS FOR DIC

Acute DIC

Shock
- Hemorrhagic
- Cardiogenic
- Anaphylactic

Septicemia (bacterial, viral, fungal, parasitic)

Hemolytic processes
- Transfusion of mismatched blood
- Acute hemolysis from infection or immunologic disorders

Obstetric conditions
- Abruptio placentae
- Amniotic fluid embolism
- Septic abortion
- HELLP syndrome

Malignancies
- Acute leukemia
- Lymphoma
- Tumor lysis syndrome

Tissue damage
- Extensive burns and trauma
- Heatstroke
- Severe head injury
- Transplant rejections
- Postoperative damage, especially after extracorporeal membrane oxygenation
- Fat and pulmonary emboli
- Snakebites
- Glomerulonephritis
- Acute anoxia (e.g., after cardiac arrest)
- Prosthetic devices
- Fulminant hepatitis

Subacute DIC

Malignancy
- Myeloproliferative/ lymphoproliferative malignancies
- Metastatic cancer

Obstetric
- Retained dead fetus

Chronic DIC

Liver disease

Systemic lupus erythematosus

Malignancy

DIC, Disseminated intravascular coagulation; *HELLP syndrome,* a life-threatening liver disorder thought to be a type of severe preeclampsia, it is characterized by **H**emolysis (destruction of red blood cells), **E**levated **L**iver enzymes (which indicate liver damage), and **L**ow **P**latelet count.

Clinical Manifestations

DIC has both bleeding and thrombotic manifestations. Multiple factors cause bleeding manifestations of DIC (see Fig. 31-9) and result from consumption and depletion of platelets and coagulation factors, as well as clot lysis and formation of FSPs that have anticoagulant properties. Bleeding in a person with no previous history or obvious cause should be questioned because it may be one of the first manifestations of acute DIC.

Bleeding manifestations include (1) *integumentary manifestations* such as pallor, petechiae, purpura (Fig. 31-10), oozing

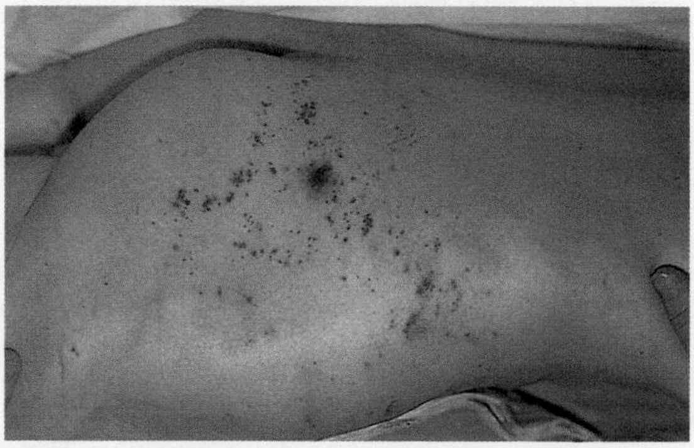

FIG. 31-10 Disseminated intravascular coagulation (DIC) resulting from staphylococcal septicemia. Note the characteristic skin hemorrhage ranging from small purpuric lesions to larger ecchymoses.

blood, venipuncture site bleeding, hematomas, and occult hemorrhage; (2) respiratory manifestations such as tachypnea, hemoptysis, and orthopnea; (3) cardiovascular manifestations such as tachycardia and hypotension; (4) GI manifestations such as upper and lower GI bleeding, abdominal distention, and bloody stools; (5) urinary manifestations such as hematuria; (6) neurologic manifestations such as vision changes, dizziness, headache, changes in mental status, and irritability; and (7) musculoskeletal complaints such as bone and joint pain.

Thrombotic manifestations are a result of fibrin or platelet deposition in the microvasculature (see Fig. 31-9). They include (1) integumentary manifestations, such as cyanosis, ischemic tissue necrosis (e.g., gangrene), and hemorrhagic necrosis; (2) respiratory manifestations, such as tachypnea, dyspnea, pulmonary emboli, and acute respiratory distress syndrome (ARDS); (3) cardiovascular manifestations, such as electrocardiogram (ECG) changes and venous distention; (4) GI manifestations, such as abdominal pain and paralytic ileus; and (5) kidney damage and oliguria, leading to failure.

Diagnostic Studies

Tests to diagnose acute DIC are listed in Table 31-21. As more clots are made in the body, more breakdown products from fibrinogen and fibrin are also formed. These are termed *fibrin split products* (FSPs), and they interfere with blood coagulation by (1) coating the platelets and interfering with platelet function; (2) interfering with thrombin and thus disrupting coagulation; and (3) attaching to fibrinogen, which interferes with the polymerization process necessary to form a stable clot. D-dimer, a polymer resulting from the breakdown of fibrin (and not fibrinogen), is a specific marker for the degree of fibrinolysis. In general, tests that measure raw materials needed for coagulation (e.g., platelets, fibrinogen) are reduced, and values that measure times to clot are prolonged. Fragmented erythrocytes (schistocytes), indicative of partial occlusion of small vessels by fibrin thrombi, may be found on blood smears.

TABLE 31-21 LABORATORY RESULTS IN ACUTE DIC

Test	Finding in Acute DIC
Screening Tests	
Prothrombin time (PT)	Prolonged
Partial thromboplastin time (PTT)	Prolonged
Activated partial thromboplastin time (aPTT)	Prolonged
Thrombin time	Prolonged
Fibrinogen	Reduced
Platelets	Reduced
Special Tests	
Fibrin split products (FSPs)	Elevated
Factor assays (prothrombin and factors V, VIII, X, XIII)	Reduced but may give misleading results, since V and VIII rise with inflammation
D-dimers (cross-linked fibrin fragments)	Elevated
Antithrombin III (AT III)	Reduced
Proteins C and S	Reduced
Plasminogen, tissue plasminogen activator	Reduced
Peripheral blood smear	Schistocytes present
Soluble fibrin monomer	Positive

DIC, Disseminated intravascular coagulation.

Collaborative Care

It is important to diagnose DIC quickly, stabilize the patient if needed (e.g., oxygenation, volume replacement), treat the underlying causative disease or problem, and control the ongoing thrombosis and bleeding. Depending on its severity, a variety of different methods are used to manage DIC (Fig. 31-11). First, if chronic DIC is diagnosed in a patient who is not bleeding, no therapy for DIC is necessary. Treatment of the underlying disease may be sufficient to reverse the DIC (e.g., chemotherapy when DIC is caused by malignancy). Second, when the patient with DIC is bleeding, therapy is directed toward providing support with necessary blood products while treating the primary disorder.

The blood products are administered cautiously based on specific component deficiencies to patients who have serious bleeding, are at high risk for bleeding (e.g., surgery), or require invasive procedures. Blood product support with platelets, cryoprecipitate, and fresh frozen plasma (FFP) is usually reserved for a patient with life-threatening hemorrhage. Therapy stabilizes a patient, prevents exsanguination or massive thrombosis, and permits institution of definitive therapy to treat the underlying cause. In general, platelets are given to correct thrombocytopenia if the platelet count is less than 20,000/μL or less than 50,000/μL with bleeding. Cryoprecipitate replaces factor VIII and fibrinogen and is given if the fibrinogen level is below 100 mg/dL. Fresh frozen plasma replaces all clotting factors except platelets and provides a source of antithrombin.

A patient with manifestations of thrombosis is often treated by anticoagulation with heparin or low-molecular-weight heparin. Heparin is used in the treatment of DIC only when the benefit (reduce clotting) outweighs the risk (further bleeding). Antithrombin III (ATnativ) may be useful in fulminant DIC, although it increases the risk of bleeding. Chronic DIC does not respond to oral anticoagulants, but it can be controlled with long-term use of heparin.

NURSING MANAGEMENT DISSEMINATED INTRAVASCULAR COAGULATION

NURSING DIAGNOSES

Nursing diagnoses for the patient with DIC may include, but are not limited to, the following:

- Ineffective peripheral tissue perfusion *related to* bleeding and sluggish or diminished blood flow secondary to thrombosis
- Acute pain *related to* bleeding into tissues and diagnostic procedures
- Decreased cardiac output *related to* fluid volume deficit
- Anxiety *related to* fear of the unknown, disease process, diagnostic procedures, and therapy

NURSING IMPLEMENTATION

Be alert to the possible development of DIC and especially to the precipitating factors listed in Table 31-20. Remember that because DIC is secondary to an underlying disease, the causative problem needs to be managed while providing supportive care for the manifestations of DIC.

Appropriate nursing interventions are essential to the survival of a patient with acute DIC. Astute ongoing assessment, active attention to manifestations of DIC, and prompt administration of prescribed therapies are crucial. Table 31-15 and

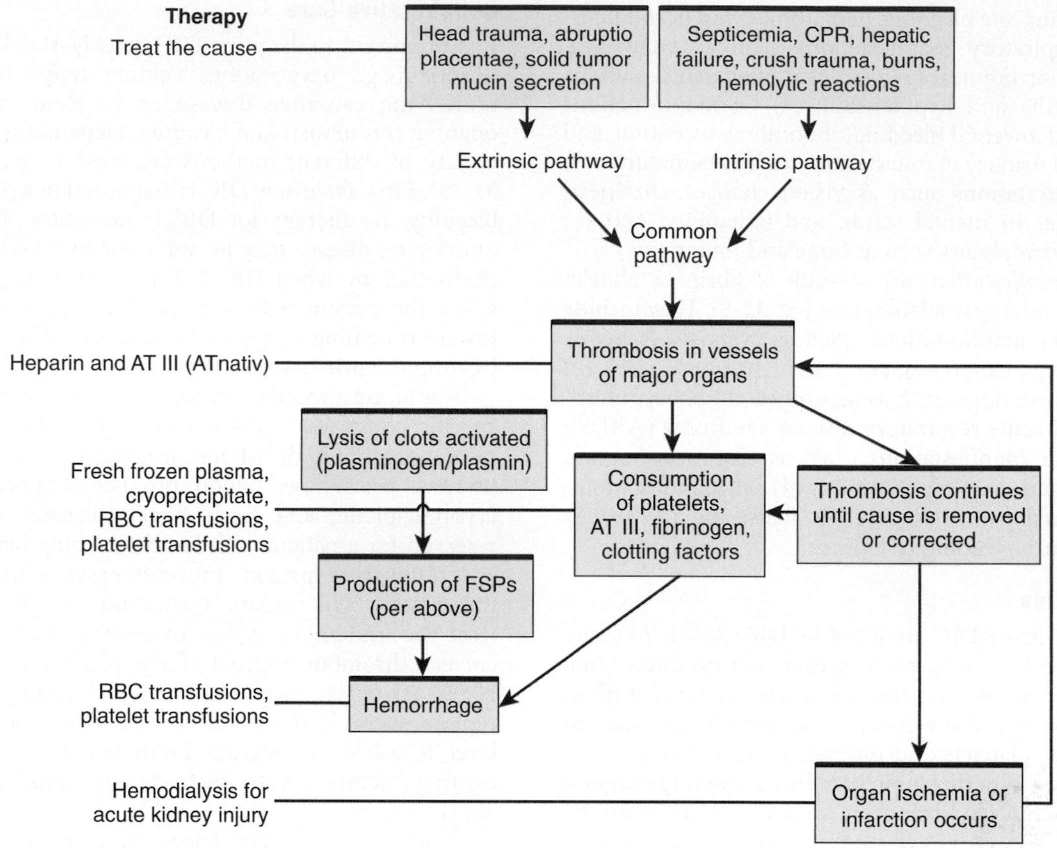

FIG. 31-11 Intended sites of action for therapies in disseminated intravascular coagulation (DIC). *AT III,* Antithrombin III; *FSPs,* fibrin split products.

eNursing Care Plan 31-1 (available on the website for this chapter) provide assessments and interventions appropriate for the patient with DIC.

Early detection of bleeding, both occult and overt, must be a primary goal. Assess for signs of external bleeding (e.g., petechiae, oozing at IV or injection sites), signs of internal bleeding (e.g., increased heart rate, changes in mental status, increasing abdominal girth, pain), and any indications that microthrombi may be causing clinically significant organ damage (e.g., decreased renal output). Minimize tissue damage and protect the patient from additional foci of bleeding.

An additional nursing responsibility is to administer blood products and medications correctly. (Blood product transfusion is discussed later in this chapter.)

NEUTROPENIA

Leukopenia refers to a decrease in the total WBC count (granulocytes, monocytes, and lymphocytes). *Granulocytopenia* is a deficiency of granulocytes, which include neutrophils, eosinophils, and basophils. The neutrophilic granulocytes, which play a major role in phagocytizing pathogenic microbes, are closely monitored in clinical practice as an indicator of a patient's risk for infection. A reduction in neutrophils is termed **neutropenia.** (Some clinicians use the terms *granulocytopenia* and *neutropenia* interchangeably because the largest constituency of granulocytes is the neutrophils.) The *absolute neutrophil count* (ANC) is determined by multiplying the total WBC count by the percentage of neutrophils. *Neutropenia* is defined as ANC less than 1000 cells/µL (1×10^9/L). (Normally, neutrophils range from 2200 to 7700 cells/µL.) *Severe neutropenia* is defined as an ANC less than 500 cells/µL.

In considering the clinical significance of neutropenia, it is important to know whether the decrease in the neutrophil count was gradual or rapid, the degree of neutropenia, and the duration. The faster the drop and the longer the duration, the greater the likelihood of life-threatening infection, sepsis, or death. Other factors and co-morbid conditions, such as being older than 60, having an existing infection, being in the hospital, and having diabetes, can increase the risk of a serious infection.

Neutropenia is a clinical consequence that occurs with a variety of conditions or diseases[34,35] (Table 31-22). It can also be an expected effect, a side effect, or an unintentional effect of taking certain drugs. The most common cause of neutropenia is the use of chemotherapy and immunosuppressive therapy in the treatment of malignancies and autoimmune diseases. A term that is often used to describe the lowest point of neutropenia (and other blood cells) in a patient treated with chemotherapy is *nadir.*

Clinical Manifestations

The patient with neutropenia is predisposed to infection with opportunistic pathogens and nonpathogenic organisms from the normal body flora. When the WBC count is depressed or immature WBCs are present, normal phagocytic mechanisms are impaired. Also the classic signs of inflammation—redness, heat, and swelling—may not occur. WBCs are the major component of pus. Therefore in the patient with neutropenia, pus formation (e.g., as a visible skin lesion or as pulmonary infiltrates on a chest x-ray) is also absent.

TABLE 31-22 CAUSES OF NEUTROPENIA

Drugs*
- Antitumor antibiotics (daunorubicin [Cerubidine], doxorubicin [Adriamycin])
- Alkylating agents (nitrogen mustards, busulfan [Myleran])
- Antimetabolites (methotrexate, 6-mercaptopurine [6-MP])
- Antiinflammatory drugs (phenylbutazone)
- Cardiovascular drugs (captopril [Capoten], procainamide [Pronestyl])
- Diuretics (thiazides, furosemide [Lasix])
- Psychotropic and antidepressant agents (clozapine)
- Miscellaneous (gold, penicillamine)
- Antimicrobial agents (ganciclovir, penicillin G, amphotericin B, vancomycin, trimethoprim/sulfamethoxazole [Bactrim])

Hematologic Disorders
- Idiopathic neutropenia
- Congenital (cyclic neutropenia)
- Aplastic anemia
- Fanconi syndrome
- Leukemia
- Myelodysplastic syndrome

Autoimmune Disorders
- Systemic lupus erythematosus
- Felty syndrome
- Rheumatoid arthritis

Infections
- Viral (e.g., hepatitis, influenza, HIV, measles)
- Fulminant bacterial infection (e.g., typhoid fever, miliary tuberculosis)
- Parasitic
- Rickettsial

Others
- Severe sepsis
- Bone marrow infiltration (e.g., carcinoma, tuberculosis, lymphoma)
- Hypersplenism (e.g., portal hypertension, Felty syndrome, storage diseases [e.g., Gaucher disease])
- Nutritional deficiencies (cobalamin, folic acid)
- Transfusion reaction
- Hemodialysis

*Not all inclusive.

SAFETY ALERT
- A low-grade fever in neutropenic patients is of great significance because it may indicate infection and lead to septic shock and death unless treated promptly.
- Neutropenic fever (≥100.4°F [38°C] and a neutrophil count <500/μL) is a medical emergency.
- Blood cultures should be drawn STAT and antibiotics started within 1 hr.

When fever occurs in a neutropenic patient, it is assumed to be caused by infection and requires immediate attention. The immunocompromised, neutropenic patient has little or no ability to fight infection. Thus minor infections can lead rapidly to sepsis. The mucous membranes of the throat and mouth, the skin, the perineal area, and the pulmonary system are common entry points for pathogenic organisms in susceptible hosts.

Clinical manifestations related to infection at these sites include complaints of sore throat and dysphagia, ulcerative lesions of the pharyngeal and buccal mucosa, diarrhea, rectal tenderness, vaginal itching or discharge, shortness of breath, and nonproductive cough. Seriously consider any minor complaint of pain or any other symptom by the patient, and report it to the physician immediately. These seemingly minor complaints can progress to fever, chills, sepsis, and septic shock if not recognized and treated early.

DELEGATION DECISIONS

Caring for the Patient With Neutropenia

All members of the health care team have important roles in preventing infection in the patient with neutropenia. Careful hand washing is an important preventive measure and should be done before, during, and after patient care by everyone caring for the patient.

Role of Registered Nurse (RN)
- Determine the type of isolation precautions that need to be initiated, if any.
- Assess patient for subtle signs of infection such as confusion or fatigue.
- Screen visitors for infectious diseases.
- Communicate with nutrition services to eliminate undercooked meats from the patient diet.
- Instruct patient and visitors about hand washing.
- Teach patient and caregivers about how to avoid infection, including the need for skin care and oral hygiene.
- If the patient is managed as an outpatient, teach the patient and the caregivers about signs and symptoms of infection and to report promptly to a health care facility if they occur.

Role of Licensed Practical/Vocational Nurse (LPN/LVN)
- Administer antibiotics and hematopoietic growth factors (consider state nurse practice act and agency policy for IV medications).
- Check the skin, oral mucosa, and perineal area for signs of infection.
- Monitor for signs and symptoms of infection and report them to the RN.

Role of Unlicensed Assistive Personnel (UAP)
- Obtain vital signs and report changes to the RN.
- Assist the patient with oral care and personal hygiene.

Systemic infections caused by bacterial, fungal, and viral organisms are common in patients with neutropenia. The patient's own flora (normally nonpathogenic) contributes significantly to life-threatening infections such as pneumonia. Organisms known to be common sources of infection include gram-positive coagulase-negative staphylococci and *Staphylococcus aureus* and gram-negative organisms such as *Escherichia coli* and *Pseudomonas aeruginosa*.[36,37] Fungi involved include *Candida* (usually *C. albicans*) and *Aspergillus* organisms. Viral infections caused by reactivation of herpes simplex and zoster are common after prolonged periods of neutropenia, such as in HSCT patients.

Diagnostic Studies

The primary diagnostic tests for assessing neutropenia are the peripheral WBC count and bone marrow aspiration and biopsy (Table 31-23). A total WBC count of less than 4000/μL (4×10^9/L) reflects leukopenia. However, only a differential count can confirm the presence of neutropenia (neutrophil count less than 1000/μL [1×10^9/L]). If the differential WBC count reflects an absolute neutropenia of 500 to 1000/μL (0.5 to 1.0×10^9/L), the patient is at moderate risk for a bacterial infection. An absolute neutropenia of less than 500/μL (0.5×10^9/L) places the patient at severe risk.

A peripheral blood smear is used to assess for immature forms of WBCs (e.g., bands). The hematocrit level, reticulocyte count, and platelet count are done to evaluate bone marrow function. Also review the patient's recent past and current drug

TABLE 31-23 COLLABORATIVE CARE
Neutropenia

Diagnostic
- History and physical examination
- WBC count with differential count
- WBC morphology
- Hct and Hgb values
- Reticulocyte and platelet count
- Bone marrow aspiration or biopsy
- Cultures of nose, throat, sputum, urine, stool, obvious lesions, blood (as indicated)
- Chest x-ray

Collaborative Therapy
- Identification and removal of cause of neutropenia (if possible)
- Identification of site of infection (if present) and causative organism
- Antibiotic therapy*
- Blood cultures drawn STAT, immediately before antibiotics
- Hematopoietic growth factors (G-CSF, GM-CSF, pegfilgrastim [Neulasta])
- Strict hand washing and patient hygiene (skin and oral care)
- Single-patient room, positive-pressure or high-efficiency particulate air (HEPA) filtration, depending on risk
- Community isolation and home precautions if outpatient

*Prompt initiation of empiric broad-spectrum antibiotic therapy at any sign of infection, even a low-grade fever (100.4° F [38° C]), is essential.
G-CSF, Granulocyte colony-stimulating factor; *GM-CSF*, granulocyte-macrophage colony-stimulating factor.

history. If the cause of neutropenia is unknown, bone marrow aspirations and biopsies are done to examine cellularity and cell morphology. Additional studies may be done as indicated to assess spleen and liver function.

NURSING AND COLLABORATIVE MANAGEMENT NEUTROPENIA

The factors involved in the nursing and collaborative care of neutropenia include (1) determining the cause of the neutropenia, (2) identifying the offending organisms if an infection has developed, (3) instituting antibiotic therapy, (4) administering hematopoietic growth factors, and (5) implementing protective environmental practices (e.g., strict hand washing)[38] (see Table 31-23).

Occasionally the cause of the neutropenia can be easily treated (e.g., nutritional deficiencies). However, neutropenia can also be a side effect that must be tolerated as a necessary step in therapy (e.g., chemotherapy, radiation therapy). In some situations the neutropenia resolves when the primary disease (e.g., tuberculosis) is treated.

Monitor the neutropenic patient for signs and symptoms of infection (e.g., any fever 100.4° F [38° C] or greater) and early septic shock. Early identification of a potentially infective organism depends on acquiring cultures from various sites. Serial blood cultures (at least two) or one from a peripheral site and one from a venous access device should be done promptly and antibiotics started immediately (within 1 hour). Communicate with the pharmacy regarding the urgency required for dispensing the medication. Cultures of sputum, throat, lesions, wounds, urine, and feces may also be ordered in the surveillance of the patient. Depending on the clinical situation, it may also be necessary to do a tracheal aspiration, bronchoscopy with bronchial brushings, or lung biopsy to diagnose the cause of pneumonic infiltrates. Invasive diagnostic studies are often contraindicated because of the concern of introducing infection and the fact that these patients are also often thrombocytopenic. Despite these many tests, the causative organism is identified in only approximately one half of neutropenic patients. Thus the priority is to obtain the blood cultures and administer the antibiotic STAT.

When a febrile episode occurs in a neutropenic patient, antibiotic therapy must be initiated immediately (within 1 hour) even before the determination of a specific causative organism by culture. Administration of broad-spectrum antibiotics is usually by the IV route because of the rapidly lethal effects of infection. However, some oral antibiotics are highly effective and routinely used for prophylaxis against infection in some neutropenic patients. The use of a third- or fourth-generation cephalosporin (e.g., cefepime [Maxipime], ceftazidime [Ceptaz]), a carbapenem (e.g., imipenem/cilastatin [Primaxin]), or a combination of an aminoglycoside plus an antipseudomonal offers broad-spectrum coverage for initial management.[37]

Regardless of the combination, you must initiate therapy promptly and observe the patient for side effects of antimicrobial agents. Side effects common to aminoglycosides include nephrotoxicity and ototoxicity. Side effects common to cephalosporins include rashes, fever, and pruritus. Additionally, ongoing febrile episodes or a change in the patient's assessment requires a call to the physician for additional cultures, diagnostic tests, or additional antimicrobial therapies.

The duration of the neutropenia also increases the patient's infection risk. The longer the neutropenia, the greater the risk of a fungal infection. Antifungal therapy is initiated whenever a culture is positive, or in patients who do not become afebrile with broad-spectrum antibiotic coverage.

Granulocyte colony-stimulating factor (G-CSF) (filgrastim [Neupogen], pegfilgrastim [Neulasta]), and granulocyte-macrophage colony-stimulating factor (GM-CSF) (sargramostim [Leukine, Prokine]) (see Table 16-14) can be used to prevent neutropenia or to reduce its severity and duration.[37] Once neutropenia has occurred, these agents are generally not as effective. G-CSF stimulates the production and function of neutrophils. GM-CSF stimulates the production and function of neutrophils and monocytes. These agents can be given IV or subcutaneously. Keratinocyte growth factor (palifermin [Kepivance]) may also be used to reduce the duration and severity of mucositis that may contribute to infection. (G-CSF, GM-CSF, and palifermin are discussed in Chapter 16.)

Determine the best means to protect the patient whose own defenses against infection are compromised. Keep the following principles in mind: (1) the patient's normal flora is the most common source of microbial colonization and infection; (2) transmission of organisms from humans most commonly occurs by direct contact with the hands; (3) air, food, water, and equipment provide additional opportunities for infection transmission; and (4) health care providers with transmissible illnesses and other patients with infections can also be sources of infection transmission under certain conditions.

Hand washing is the single most important preventive measure to minimize the risk of infection in the neutropenic patient. Strict hand washing by staff and visitors using an antiseptic hand wash, before and after contact, is the major method to prevent transmission of harmful pathogens.

TABLE 31-24 PATIENT & CAREGIVER TEACHING GUIDE

Neutropenia

Include the following instructions when teaching a patient or caregiver the precautions to take when the neutrophil count is low.

1. WASH YOUR HANDS frequently and make sure those around you wash their hands frequently, particularly if they help with your care. An antibacterial hand gel may also be used.
2. Notify your nurse or health care provider if you have any of the following:
   - Fever ≥100.4°F (38°C)*
   - Chills or feeling hot
   - Redness, swelling, discharge, or new pain on or in your body
   - Changes in urination or bowel movements
   - Cough, sore throat, mouth sores, or blisters
3. If you are at home, take your temperature as directed and follow instructions on what to do if you have a fever.
4. Avoid crowds and people with colds, flu, or infections. If you are in a public area, wear a mask and use hand sanitizing gel frequently.
5. Avoid uncooked meats, seafood, or eggs and unwashed fruits and vegetables. Ask your health care provider about specific dietary guidelines for you.
6. Bathe or shower daily. A moisturizer may be used to prevent skin from drying and cracking.
7. Brush your teeth with a soft toothbrush four times daily. You may floss once daily if it does not cause excessive pain or bleeding. Avoid alcohol-based mouthwashes.
8. Do not perform gardening or clean up after pets. Feeding and petting your dog or cat are fine as long as you wash your hands well after handling.

*Need to verify cut-off temperature with health care provider.

Separate immunocompromised patients from those who are infected or have conditions that increase the probability of transmitting infections (e.g., poor hygiene caused by lack of understanding or cognitive dysfunction). Often, patients can be managed on an outpatient basis if the patient and caregiver can astutely monitor for fevers and other signs of infection and then report promptly to a nearby health care facility (Table 31-24). If the patient is hospitalized, a private room should be used. High-efficiency particulate air (HEPA) filtration is an air-handling method with a high-flow filtering system that can reduce or eliminate the number of aerosolized pathogens in the environment. Although it is expensive to install, it is often used for a patient with severe prolonged neutropenia (e.g., bone marrow transplant patients). Care routines in a HEPA environment are essentially the same as care in any other private room. Additional neutropenic precaution guidelines may also be employed, such as prophylactic antibiotics and antifungals or the avoidance of uncooked meat. The nursing measures presented in eNursing Care Plan 31-2 (available on the website for this chapter) are important in the treatment of the patient with neutropenia.

Quality-of-life issues for the patient with neutropenia should not be overlooked. Fatigue, malaise, a decrease in functioning, and social isolation require appropriate interventions.

MYELODYSPLASTIC SYNDROME

Myelodysplastic syndrome (MDS) is a group of related hematologic disorders characterized by peripheral blood cytopenias (from ineffective blood cell production) and changes in the cellularity of the bone marrow with dysplastic changes. In MDS, *hematopoiesis* is disorderly and ineffective. It is estimated that 11,000 new cases of MDS are diagnosed each year in the United States. Although it can occur in all age-groups, the highest prevalence is in men over 80 years of age.[39,40]

INFORMATICS IN PRACTICE

Use of Internet to Access Information on Unfamiliar Diseases

- If you are assigned to take care of a patient with a disease or disorder that you are not familiar with, such as thalassemia, access the Internet and perform a quick search.
- Within minutes, you can learn the pathophysiology of thalassemia, treatment options, possible complications that you will need to monitor, and recommended medical and nursing interventions.
- Using this readily available information will help you deliver high-quality, evidence-based care.

Etiology and Pathophysiology

The etiology of MDS is unknown. People who have received radiation therapy, had chemotherapy with alkylating agents (e.g., chlorambucil, cyclophosphamide, melphalan), or been exposed to industrial solvents (e.g., benzene) have a higher risk of developing MDS than people who have not had these exposures. Rarely, genetic disorders are responsible for the disease. Nevertheless, in 60% to 70% of MDS patients, no specific cause can be identified.

MDS is referred to as a *clonal disorder* because some bone marrow stem cells continue to function normally, whereas others (a specific clone) do not. The abnormal clone of the stem cells is usually found in the bone marrow but eventually may be found in the circulation.

Occasionally one type of MDS transforms into another. In about 30% of cases, MDS progresses to acute myelogenous leukemia (AML).[41,42] In contrast to AML, in which the leukemic cells show little normal maturation, the clonal cells in MDS always display some degree of maturity. Disease progression is slower than in AML, and sometimes treatment is not required.

Clinical Manifestations

Manifestations result from neoplastic transformation of the pluripotent hematopoietic stem cells in the bone marrow. MDS commonly manifests as infection and bleeding caused by inadequate numbers of ineffectively functioning circulating granulocytes or platelets. MDS is often discovered in the older adult during testing for the symptoms of anemia, thrombocytopenia, or neutropenia. It may also be diagnosed incidentally from a routine CBC. During the advanced stage of MDS, life-threatening anemia, thrombocytopenia, and neutropenia occur.

Diagnostic Studies

Bone marrow biopsy with aspirate analysis is essential for both the diagnosis and the classification of the specific type of myelodysplasia. In MDS the patient has peripheral cytopenia and changes in the bone marrow (hypocellular or hypercellular). Laboratory data and bone marrow studies help rule out other causes of the dysplasia, such as nonmalignant disorders, cobalamin and folate deficiencies, and infections.[42,43]

NURSING AND COLLABORATIVE MANAGEMENT MYELODYSPLASTIC SYNDROME

Supportive treatment of MDS is based on the premise that the aggressiveness of treatment should match the aggressiveness of the disease. Supportive treatment consists of hematologic monitoring (serial bone marrow and peripheral blood examinations); antibiotic therapy; or transfusions with blood products, along with iron chelators to prevent iron overload.

Low-risk patients can often be treated with erythropoietin and G-CSF. Only about one third of high-risk patients are treated with intensive chemotherapy and/or HSCT. Azacitidine (Vidaza) and decitabine (Dacogen) are drugs that help restore normal growth control and differentiation of hematopoietic cells and reduce the frequency of transformation of MDS to acute leukemia. Side effects include myelosuppression, nausea, vomiting, constipation or diarrhea, renal dysfunction, and injection site erythema.

Lenalidomide (Revlimid) or thalidomide may also be used. Other treatments for MDS include cytarabine (Cytosar, Ara-C) with or without antitumor antibiotics (anthracyclines), antithymocyte globulin, and cyclosporine. High-dose chemotherapy and allogeneic HSCT have been used in an attempt to treat bone marrow dysfunction of MDS and restore it with normal hematopoiesis. However, because of the aggressiveness of this treatment, it is generally recommended for patients less than 55 years old.

Nursing care of a patient with MDS is similar to that of a patient with manifestations of anemia, thrombocytopenia, and neutropenia (see Nursing Care Plan 31-1 for the patient with anemia, and eNursing Care Plan 31-1 for the patient with thrombocytopenia, and eNursing Care Plan 31-2 for the patient with neutropenia. The eNCPs are available on the website for this chapter.)

LEUKEMIA

Leukemia is the general term used to describe a group of malignant disorders affecting the blood and blood-forming tissues of the bone marrow, lymph system, and spleen. Leukemia occurs in all age-groups. It results in an accumulation of dysfunctional cells because of a loss of regulation in cell division. It follows a progressive course that is eventually fatal if untreated. An estimated 43,000 new cases are diagnosed each year. Although often thought of as a disease of children, leukemia affects approximately 10 times more adults than children.[44]

Etiology and Pathophysiology

Regardless of the specific type, leukemia has no single cause. It is now known that all cancers, including leukemia, begin as a mutation in the DNA of certain cells. Most leukemias result from a combination of factors, including genetic and environmental influences. Abnormal genes *(oncogenes)* are capable of causing many types of cancers, including leukemias (see Chapter 16). Chemical agents (e.g., benzene), chemotherapeutic agents (e.g., alkylating agents), viruses, radiation, and immunologic deficiencies have all been associated with the development of leukemia. The incidence of leukemia is increased in radiologists, persons who have lived near nuclear bomb test sites or nuclear reactor accidents (e.g., Chernobyl), and persons previously treated with radiation therapy or chemotherapy.

Although ribonucleic acid (RNA) retroviruses cause a number of leukemias in animals, a viral cause for a human leukemia has been established only for some patients with adult T-cell leukemia. This form of leukemia is endemic in southwestern Japan and parts of the Caribbean and central Africa and is caused by the human T-cell leukemia virus type 1 (HTLV-1).[45]

Classification

Leukemia can be classified based on acute versus chronic disease and on the type of WBC involved. The terms *acute* and *chronic* refer to cell maturity and nature of disease onset. Acute leukemia is characterized by the clonal proliferation of immature hematopoietic cells. The leukemia develops after malignant transformation of a single type of immature hematopoietic cell, followed by cellular replication and expansion of that malignant clone. Chronic leukemias involve more mature forms of the WBC, and the disease onset is more gradual.

Leukemia can also be classified by identifying the type of leukocyte involved, whether it is of myelogenous or lymphocytic origin. By combining the acute and chronic categories with the cell type involved, one can identify four major types of leukemia: acute lymphocytic leukemia (ALL), acute myelogenous leukemia (AML), chronic myelogenous (granulocytic) leukemia (CML), and chronic lymphocytic leukemia (CLL). Other defining features of these leukemic subtypes are presented in Table 31-25.

Acute Myelogenous Leukemia. AML represents only one fourth of all leukemias, but it makes up approximately 80% of the acute leukemias in adults. Its onset is often abrupt and dramatic. A patient may have serious infections and abnormal bleeding from the onset of the disease.[44]

AML is characterized by uncontrolled proliferation of myeloblasts, the precursors of granulocytes. There is hyperplasia of the bone marrow. The clinical manifestations are usually related to replacement of normal hematopoietic cells in the marrow by leukemic myeloblasts and, to a lesser extent, to infiltration of other organs and tissue (see Table 31-25).

Acute Lymphocytic Leukemia. ALL is the most common type of leukemia in children and accounts for about 20% of acute leukemia cases in adults.[44] In ALL, immature small lymphocytes proliferate in the bone marrow; most are of B-cell origin. The majority of patients have fever at the time of diagnosis. Signs and symptoms may appear abruptly with bleeding or fever, or they may be insidious with progressive weakness, fatigue, bone and/or joint pain, and bleeding tendencies.

Central nervous system (CNS) manifestations are especially common in ALL and represent a serious problem. Leukemic meningitis caused by arachnoid infiltration occurs in many patients with ALL.

Chronic Myelogenous Leukemia. CML is caused by excessive development of mature neoplastic granulocytes in the bone marrow. The excess neoplastic granulocytes move into the peripheral blood in massive numbers and ultimately infiltrate the liver and spleen.

The natural history of CML is a chronic stable phase, followed by the development of a more acute, aggressive phase referred to as the *blastic phase*. The chronic phase of CML can last for several years and can usually be well controlled with treatment. Even with treatment, the chronic phase of the disease eventually progresses to the accelerated phase, ending in a blastic phase. Once CML transforms to an acute or blastic

TABLE 31-25 **TYPES OF LEUKEMIA**

Age of Onset	Clinical Manifestations	Diagnostic Findings
Acute Myelogenous Leukemia (AML)		
Most common cancer in children ages 0-7 yr. Increase in incidence with advancing age after 55 yr.	Fatigue and weakness, headache, mouth sores, anemia, bleeding, fever, infection, sternal tenderness, gingival hyperplasia, mild hepatosplenomegaly (one third of patients).	Low RBC count, Hgb, Hct, platelet count. Low to high WBC count with myeloblasts. High LDH. Hypercellular bone marrow with myeloblasts.
Acute Lymphocytic Leukemia (ALL)		
In children median age at diagnosis is 13 yr. Increases in incidence with advancing age after 60 yr.	Fever, pallor, bleeding, anorexia, fatigue and weakness. Bone, joint, and abdominal pain. Generalized lymphadenopathy, infections, weight loss, hepatosplenomegaly, headache, mouth sores, neurologic manifestations: CNS involvement, increased intracranial pressure (nausea, vomiting, lethargy, cranial nerve dysfunction) secondary to meningeal infiltration.	Low RBC count, Hgb, Hct, platelet count. Low, normal, or high WBC count. High LDH. Transverse lines of rarefaction at ends of metaphysis of long bones on x-ray. Hypercellular bone marrow with lymphoblasts. Lymphoblasts also possible in cerebrospinal fluid. Presence of Philadelphia chromosome (20%-25% of patients).
Chronic Myelogenous Leukemia (CML)		
Increase in incidence with advancing age after 55 yr.	No symptoms early in disease. Fatigue and weakness, fever, sternal tenderness, weight loss, joint pain, bone pain, massive splenomegaly, increase in sweating.	Low RBC count, Hgb, Hct. High platelet count early, lower count later. ↑ Neutrophils, normal number of lymphocytes, and normal or low number of monocytes. Low leukocyte alkaline phosphatase. Presence of Philadelphia chromosome in 90% of patients.
Chronic Lymphocytic Leukemia (CLL)		
Increase in incidence with advancing age after 50 yr, with predominance in men.	Frequently no symptoms. Detection of disease often during examination for unrelated condition, chronic fatigue, anorexia, splenomegaly and lymphadenopathy, hepatomegaly. May progress to fever, night sweats, weight loss, fatigue, and frequent infections.	Mild anemia and thrombocytopenia with disease progression. Total WBC count >100,000/μL. Increase in peripheral lymphocytes and lymphocytes in bone marrow. Hypogammaglobulinemia. May have autoimmune hemolytic anemia, idiopathic thrombocytopenic purpura.

LDH, Lactate dehydrogenase.

phase, it needs to be treated more aggressively, similar to an acute leukemia.

Genetic Link

The *Philadelphia chromosome* originates from the translocation between the *BCR* gene on chromosome 22 and the *ABL* gene on chromosome 9. The protein that is encoded by the newly created *BCR-ABL* gene on the Philadelphia chromosome interferes with normal cell cycle events, such as the regulation of cell proliferation.

The Philadelphia chromosome, which is present in 90% to 95% of patients with CML, is a diagnostic hallmark of CML. In addition, its presence is an important indicator of residual disease or relapse after treatment. However, the presence of the Philadelphia chromosome is not *specific* to diagnose CML, since it is also found in ALL and occasionally in AML.

Chronic Lymphocytic Leukemia. CLL is the most common leukemia in adults. CLL is characterized by the production and accumulation of functionally inactive but long-lived, small, mature-appearing lymphocytes. B cells are usually involved. The lymphocytes infiltrate the bone marrow, spleen, and liver. Lymph node enlargement (lymphadenopathy) is present throughout the body.

Complications are rare in early-stage CLL but may develop as the disease advances. Pressure on nerves from enlarged lymph nodes causes pain and even paralysis. Mediastinal node enlargement leads to pulmonary symptoms. Because CLL is usually a disease of older adults, treatment decisions must be made by considering the progression of the disease and the side effects of treatment. Many individuals in the early stages of CLL require no treatment. Others may be followed closely and receive treatment only when the disease progresses. Approximately one third require immediate intervention at the time of diagnosis.

Other Leukemias. Occasionally the subtype of leukemia cannot be identified. The malignant leukemic cells may have lymphoid, myeloid, or mixed characteristics. Frequently these patients do not respond to treatment and have a poor prognosis. Other rare types include hairy cell and biphenotypic (both abnormal myeloid and lymphoid clones) leukemias.

Overlap Between Leukemia and Lymphoma. Overlap exists between leukemia and non-Hodgkin's lymphoma (NHL) because both involve proliferation of lymphocytes or their precursors. A leukemia-like picture with peripheral lymphocytosis and bone marrow involvement may be present in about 20% of adults with some types of NHL. Although differentiation can be difficult, generally patients with more extensive nodal involvement (especially mediastinal), fewer circulating abnormal cells, and fewer blast forms in the marrow are considered to have lymphoma. A prominent leukemic phase is less common in aggressive lymphomas, except Burkitt's and lymphoblastic lymphomas.[45]

Clinical Manifestations

Although the clinical manifestations of leukemia are varied (see Table 31-25), they relate to problems caused by bone marrow failure and the formation of leukemic infiltrates (Fig. 31-12). Bone marrow failure results from (1) bone marrow overcrowding by abnormal cells and (2) inadequate production of normal marrow elements. The patient is predisposed to anemia, thrombocytopenia, and decreased number and function of WBCs.

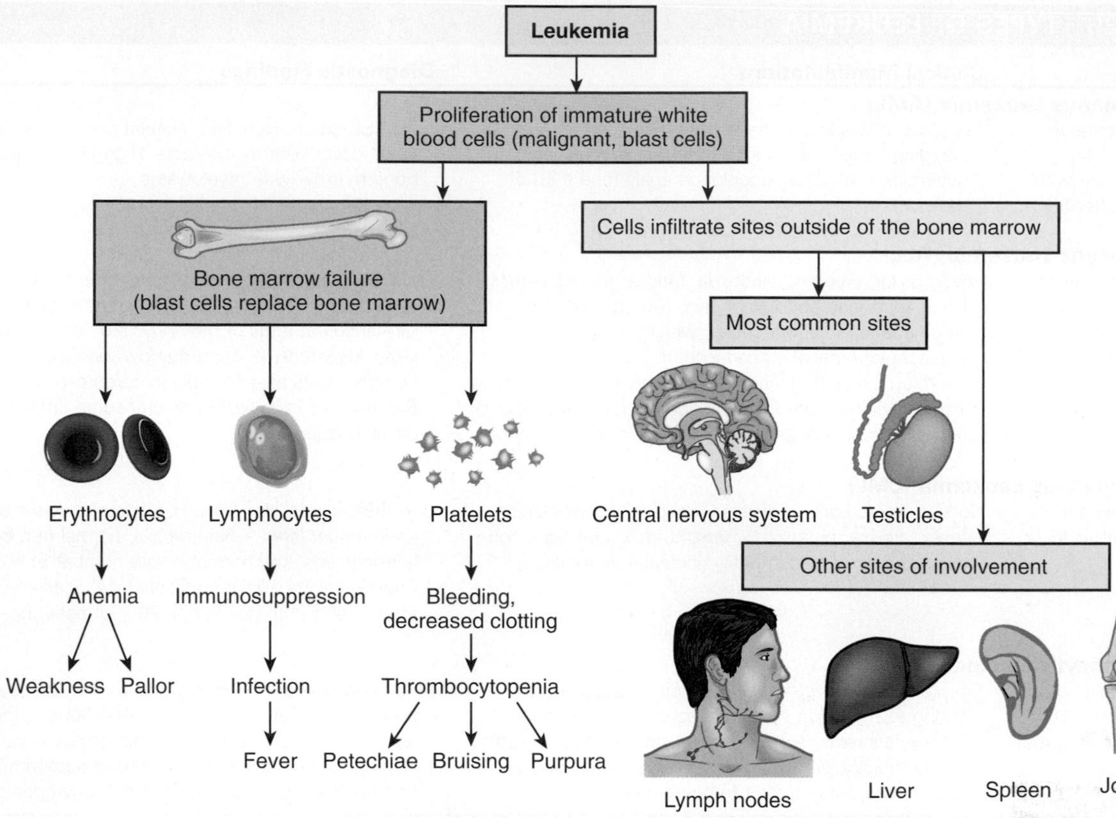

FIG. 31-12 Pathophysiology of leukemia.

As leukemia progresses, fewer normal blood cells are produced. The abnormal WBCs continue to accumulate because they do not go through the normal cell life cycle to death *(apoptosis).* The leukemic cells may infiltrate the patient's organs, leading to problems such as splenomegaly, hepatomegaly, lymphadenopathy, bone pain, meningeal irritation, and oral lesions. Solid masses resulting from collections of leukemic cells called *chloromas* can also occur. A high leukemic white count in the peripheral blood (more than 100,000 cells/μL) can cause the blood to thicken and potentially block circulatory pathways. This is called *leukostasis* and can be life threatening.

Diagnostic Studies

Peripheral blood evaluation and bone marrow examination are the primary methods of diagnosing and classifying the types of leukemia. Morphologic, histochemical, immunologic, and cytogenetic methods are all used to identify leukemic cell types and stage of development. Identifying the type of leukemia is important because the various types have different prognoses and chemotherapeutic regimens. Other studies such as lumbar puncture and computed tomography (CT) scan can detect leukemic cells outside of the blood and bone marrow.

The malignant cells in most patients with leukemia have specific cytogenetic abnormalities that are associated with distinct subsets of the disease. These cytogenetic abnormalities have diagnostic, prognostic, and therapeutic importance. For example, in CML, the finding of the Philadelphia chromosome has a good prognostic significance, but not so in ALL.

Collaborative Care

Once a diagnosis of leukemia has been made, collaborative care is focused on the initial goal of attaining remission. Age and cytogenetic analysis often help form the basis of important treatment decisions. Because cytotoxic chemotherapy is the mainstay of the treatment, you need to understand the principles of cancer chemotherapy, including cellular kinetics, the use of multiple drugs rather than single agents, and the cell cycle. (See the section on chemotherapy in Chapter 16.)

In some cases, such as nonsymptomatic patients with CLL, watchful waiting with active supportive care may be appropriate. Although a patient may not be cured, attaining remission or disease control is a realistic option for the majority of patients. In some cases, cure is a realistic goal. In *complete remission* there is no evidence of overt disease on physical examination, and the bone marrow and peripheral blood appear normal. A lesser state of control is known as partial remission. *Minimal residual disease* is defined as tumor cells that cannot be detected by morphologic examination, but can be identified by molecular testing. *Partial remission* is characterized by a lack of symptoms and a normal peripheral blood smear, but still evidence of disease in the bone marrow. *Molecular remission* indicates that all molecular studies are negative for residual leukemia. The patient's prognosis is directly related to the ability to maintain a remission. The patient's prognosis becomes more unfavorable with each relapse. After each relapse, the succeeding remission may be more difficult to achieve and shorter in duration.

Sometimes patients have such a high WBC count (e.g., 100,000 cells/μL or more) that initial emergent treatment may include leukapheresis and hydroxyurea. The purpose of these treatments is to reduce the WBC count and risk of leukemia cell–induced thrombosis.

Stages of Chemotherapy. Chemotherapy is often divided into stages: induction, postinduction or postremission, and maintenance.

Induction Therapy. The first stage, *induction therapy,* is the attempt to bring about a remission. Induction is aggressive treatment that seeks to destroy leukemic cells in the tissues, peripheral blood, and bone marrow to eventually restore normal hematopoiesis on bone marrow recovery. During induction therapy, a patient may become critically ill because the bone marrow is severely depressed by the chemotherapeutic agents. Throughout the induction phase, nursing interventions focus on neutropenia, thrombocytopenia, and anemia, as well as providing psychosocial support to the patient and family. Common chemotherapy agents for induction of AML include cytarabine and an antitumor antibiotic (anthracycline) such as daunorubicin (Cerubidine), idarubicin (Idamycin), or mitoxantrone (Novantrone). After one course of induction therapy, approximately 70% of newly diagnosed patients achieve complete remission. It is generally assumed that leukemic cells persist undetected after induction therapy. This could lead to relapse within a few months if no further therapy is administered.[46]

Postinduction or Postremission Therapy. Terms used to describe postinduction or postremission chemotherapy include *intensification* and *consolidation. Intensification therapy,* or high-dose therapy, may be given immediately after induction therapy for several months. Other drugs that target the cell in a different way than those administered during induction may also be added.

Consolidation therapy is started after a remission is achieved. It may consist of one or two additional courses of the same drugs given during induction or involve high-dose therapy (intensive consolidation). The purpose of consolidation therapy is to eliminate remaining leukemic cells that may not be clinically or pathologically evident.

Maintenance Therapy. *Maintenance therapy* is treatment with lower doses of the same drugs used in induction or other drugs given every 3 to 4 weeks for a prolonged period. Like consolidation or intensification, the goal is to keep the body free of leukemic cells. Each type of leukemia requires different maintenance therapy. In AML, maintenance therapy is rarely effective and therefore rarely administered.

Drug Therapy Regimens. The therapeutic agents used to treat leukemia vary. Table 31-26 gives examples of treatment regimens used in various types of leukemia.[45-48]

Combination therapy is the mainstay of treatment for leukemia. The three purposes for using multiple drugs are to (1) decrease drug resistance, (2) minimize the drug toxicity to the patient by using multiple drugs with varying toxicities, and (3) interrupt cell growth at multiple points in the cell cycle.

Newer therapeutic drugs are aimed at small molecules that promote the growth and differentiation of leukemic cells. For example, arsenic trioxide (Trisenox), which is used to treat acute promyelocytic leukemia (a type of AML), causes DNA fragmentation and cell death. In addition, it inhibits cell proliferation and angiogenesis (new blood vessel growth). Imatinib targets the *BCR-ABL* protein (discussed above) that is present in nearly all patients with CML. Thus this drug kills only cancer cells, leaving healthy cells alone. (Targeted therapy is discussed in Chapter 16.)

The use of specific targeted therapy in the form of monoclonal antibodies is an important treatment modality in hematopoietic malignancies, but cures with these therapies alone are rare (see Table 16-13 and Fig. 16-16). Rituximab binds to the B-cell antigen (CD20) and has been used with CLL. Alemtuzumab (Campath) binds to CD52, a panlymphocyte antigen present on both T and B cells, and is used to treat CLL.

TABLE 31-26 DRUG THERAPY

Leukemia*

Drug Therapy	Other Therapy
Acute Myelogenous Leukemia	
cytarabine (Cytosar, Ara-C),† daunorubicin (Cerubidine),† idarubicin (Idamycin), 6-thioguanine (6-TG), mitoxantrone (Novantrone), arsenic trioxide (Trisenox),† tretinoin (Vesanoid),† etoposide (VePesid), clofarabine (Clolar), decitabine (Dacogen), fludarabine (Fludara)	Autologous or allogeneic hematopoietic stem cell transplant (HSCT) (see Chapter 16)
Combination chemotherapy of cytarabine and antitumor antibiotic (most common)	
Acute Lymphocytic Leukemia	
daunorubicin, doxorubicin (Adriamycin), vincristine (Oncovin), prednisone, dexamethasone (Decadron), L-asparaginase (Elspar), ponatinib (Iclusig), pegaspargase (Oncaspar), dasatinib (Sprycel), cyclophosphamide (Cytoxan), methotrexate, 6-mercaptopurine (Purinethol), cytarabine, nelarabine (Arranon), imatinib (Gleevec), clofarabine	Cranial radiation therapy, intrathecal methotrexate or cytarabine, allogeneic HSCT (see Chapter 16)
Combination chemotherapy of several agents is common over a prolonged time	
Chronic Myelogenous Leukemia	
bosutinib (Bosulif), imatinib, dasatinib, nilotinib (Tasigna), omacetaxine (Synribo), ponatinib, hydroxyurea (Hydrea)	Radiation, HSCT, α-interferon, leukapheresis
Combination chemotherapy including any of the following: cytarabine, thioguanine, daunorubicin, methotrexate, prednisone, vincristine, L-asparaginase, carmustine (BCNU), 6-mercaptopurine	
Chronic Lymphocytic Leukemia	
chlorambucil (Leukeran), cyclophosphamide, prednisone, vincristine, fludarabine, rituximab (Rituxan), alemtuzumab (Campath), pentostatin (Nipent), bendamustine (Treanda), oxaliplatin (Eloxatin), methotrexate, ofatumumab (Arzerra)	Radiation, splenectomy, colony-stimulating factors, allogeneic HSCT

*The classification and mechanisms of action of these drugs are presented in Table 16-7.
†Used for acute promyelocytic leukemia.

Other Treatments. In addition to chemotherapy, corticosteroids and radiation therapy can also have a role in the treatment of the patient with leukemia. Total body radiation may be used to prepare a patient for bone marrow transplantation, or radiation may be restricted to certain areas (fields) such as the liver and spleen or other organs affected by infiltrates. In ALL, prophylactic intrathecal methotrexate or cytarabine is given to decrease the chance of CNS involvement, which is common in this type of leukemia. When CNS leukemia does occur, cranial radiation may be given. Biologic and targeted therapy may be indicated for specific leukemias. (Biologic and targeted therapy is discussed in Chapter 16 and Table 16-13.)

Hematopoietic Stem Cell Transplantation. HSCT is another type of therapy used for patients with different forms of leukemia. The goal of HSCT is to totally eliminate leukemic cells from the body using combinations of chemotherapy with or without total body irradiation. This treatment also eradicates the patient's hematopoietic stem cells, which are then replaced with those of an HLA-matched sibling or volunteer donor *(allogeneic)* or an identical twin *(syngeneic)*, or with the patient's own *(autologous)* stem cells that were removed (harvested) before the intensive therapy. (HSCT is discussed in Chapter 16.)

The primary complications for patients with allogeneic HSCT are graft-versus-host disease (GVHD), relapse of leukemia (especially ALL), and infection (especially interstitial pneumonia). GVHD is discussed in Chapter 14. Because HSCT has serious associated risks, the patient must weigh the significant risks of treatment-related death or treatment failure (relapse) with the hope of cure.

NURSING MANAGEMENT LEUKEMIA

NURSING ASSESSMENT

Subjective and objective data that should be obtained from a patient with leukemia are presented in Table 31-27.

NURSING DIAGNOSES

Nursing diagnoses for the patient with leukemia include those for anemia (see Nursing Care Plan 31-1), thrombocytopenia (eNursing Care Plan 31-1), and neutropenia (see eNursing Care Plan 31-2, available on the website for this chapter).

PLANNING

The overall goals are that the patient with leukemia will (1) understand and cooperate with the treatment plan; (2) experience minimal side effects and complications associated with both the disease and its treatment; and (3) feel hopeful and supported during periods of treatment, relapse, or remission.

NURSING IMPLEMENTATION

ACUTE INTERVENTION. The nursing role during acute phases of leukemia is extremely challenging because the patient has many physical and psychosocial needs. As with other forms of cancer, the diagnosis of leukemia can evoke great fear and be equated with death. It may be viewed as a hopeless, horrible disease with many painful and undesirable consequences. The treatment and prognosis of each patient with leukemia are driven by many factors, such as age and type of leukemia. Patients are not the same. Therefore it is important that you understand the patient's type of leukemia, the prognosis, the treatment plan, and the goals. By doing this, you can help the patient realize that, although the future may be uncertain, one can have a meaningful quality of life while in remission or with disease control, and that, in some cases, there is reasonable hope for cure.

The family also needs help adjusting to the stress of this abrupt onset of serious illness and the losses imposed by the sick role (e.g., dependence, withdrawal, changes in role responsibilities, alterations in body image). The diagnosis of leukemia often brings with it the need to make difficult decisions at a time of profound stress for the patient and family.

Patients may have co-morbid conditions that affect treatment decisions. Important nursing interventions include (1) maximizing the patient's physical functioning, (2) teaching patients that acute side effects of treatment are usually temporary, and (3) encouraging patients to discuss their quality-of-life issues. You are an important advocate in helping the patient and family understand the complexities of treatment decisions and manage the side effects and toxicities. A patient may require hospitalization or may need to temporarily relocate to an appropriate treatment center. This situation can lead a patient to feel deserted and isolated at a time when support is most needed. You have contact with a patient many hours a day and can help reverse feelings of abandonment and loneliness by balancing

TABLE 31-27 NURSING ASSESSMENT
Leukemia

Subjective Data
Important Health Information
Past health history: Exposure to chemical toxins (e.g., benzene, arsenic), radiation, or viruses (Epstein-Barr, HTLV-1); chromosome abnormalities (Down syndrome, Klinefelter syndrome, Fanconi syndrome), immunologic deficiencies; organ transplantation; frequent infections; bleeding tendencies
Medications: Use of phenylbutazone (Butazolidin), chloramphenicol, chemotherapy
Surgery or other treatments: Radiation exposure; prior radiation and chemotherapy for cancer

Functional Health Patterns
Health perception–health management: Family history of leukemia; malaise
Nutritional-metabolic: Mouth sores, weight loss; chills, night sweats; nausea, vomiting, anorexia, dysphagia, early satiety; easy bruising
Elimination: Hematuria, decreased urine output; diarrhea, dark or bloody stools
Activity-exercise: Fatigue with progressive weakness; dyspnea, epistaxis, cough
Cognitive-perceptual: Headache; muscle cramps; sore throat; generalized sternal tenderness, bone, joint, abdominal pain; paresthesias, numbness, tingling, visual disturbances
Sexuality-reproductive: Prolonged menses, menorrhagia, impotence

Objective Data
General
Fever, generalized lymphadenopathy, lethargy

Integumentary
Pallor or jaundice; petechiae, ecchymoses, purpura, reddish brown to purple cutaneous infiltrates, macules, and papules

Cardiovascular
Tachycardia, systolic murmurs

Gastrointestinal
Gingival bleeding and hyperplasia; oral ulcerations, herpes and Candida infections; perirectal irritation and infection; hepatomegaly, splenomegaly

Neurologic
Seizures, disorientation, confusion, decreased coordination, cranial nerve palsies, papilledema

Musculoskeletal
Muscle wasting, bone pain, joint pain

Possible Diagnostic Findings
Low, normal, or high WBC count with shift to the left (↑ blast cells); anemia, ↓ hematocrit and hemoglobin, thrombocytopenia, Philadelphia chromosome; hypercellular bone marrow aspirate or biopsy with myeloblasts, lymphoblasts, and markedly ↓ normal cells

HTLV-1, Human T-cell leukemia virus, type 1.

the demanding technical needs with a humanistic, caring approach. The needs of the patient with leukemia are best met by an interdisciplinary team (e.g., psychiatric and oncology clinical nurse specialists, case managers, dietitians, chaplains, and social workers).

From a physical care perspective, you are challenged to make astute assessments and plan care to help the patient manage the severe side effects of chemotherapy. The life-threatening results of bone marrow suppression (neutropenia, thrombocytopenia, and anemia) require aggressive nursing interventions. These patients may be at risk for oncologic emergencies such as tumor lysis syndrome, DIC, and leukostasis. Additional complications of chemotherapy may affect the patient's GI tract, nutritional status, skin and mucosa, cardiopulmonary status, liver, kidneys, and neurologic system. (Nursing interventions related to chemotherapy are discussed in Chapter 16.)

Review all drugs being administered, including the mechanism of action, purpose, routes of administration, usual doses, potential side effects, safe-handling considerations, and toxic effects. Assess laboratory data reflecting the effects of the drugs and sequelae of the disease. Unlike treatments for solid tumors, chemotherapy is administered to patients with leukemia even if they have severe myelosuppression, since the underlying disorder is causing the problem and will not resolve unless treated. Patient survival and comfort during aggressive chemotherapy are significantly affected by the quality of nursing care.

AMBULATORY AND HOME CARE. Ongoing care for the patient with leukemia is necessary to monitor for signs and symptoms of disease control or relapse. For a patient requiring long-term or maintenance chemotherapy, the fatigue of long-term chronic disease management can become arduous and discouraging. Therefore teach the patient and caregiver to understand the importance of continued diligence in disease management and the need for follow-up care. Also teach them about the drugs, self-care measures, and when to seek medical attention.

The goals of rehabilitation for long-term survivors of leukemia are to manage the physical, psychologic, social, and spiritual consequences and delayed effects from the disease and its treatment. (Delayed effects are discussed in Chapter 16.) Assistance may be needed to reestablish the various relationships that are a part of the patient's life. Involving the patient in survivor networks and support groups or services may help the patient adapt to living after a life-threatening illness. Exploring resources in the community (e.g., American Cancer Society, Leukemia & Lymphoma Society) may reduce the financial burden and the feelings of dependence. Also provide the resources for spiritual support.

Vigilant follow-up care helps to ensure that the cancer survivor's unique needs are recognized and treated. Often these needs may require a referral or consultation. For example, physical therapy personnel may be asked to develop an exercise program to prevent posttreatment deficits caused by drug-induced peripheral neuropathy. Most patients should receive the pneumococcal vaccine (Pneumovax) at diagnosis and every 5 years, and an annual influenza vaccine. These needs can also include other concerns such as vocational retraining and reproductive concerns for a patient of childbearing age.

EVALUATION

The expected outcomes are that the patient with leukemia will

- Cope effectively with the diagnosis, treatment regimen, and prognosis
- Experience no complications related to the disease or its treatment
- Feel comfortable and supported throughout treatment

TABLE 31-28 COMPARISON OF HODGKIN'S AND NON-HODGKIN'S LYMPHOMA

	Hodgkin's Lymphoma	Non-Hodgkin's Lymphoma
Cellular origin	B lymphocytes	B lymphocytes (85%) T or natural killer lymphocytes (15%)
Extent of disease	Localized to regional, but may be more widespread	Disseminated
B symptoms*	Common	40%
Extranodal involvement	Rare	Common

*B symptoms include fever (>100.4°F [38°C]), drenching night sweats, and weight loss (>10% from baseline within 6 mo).

LYMPHOMAS

Lymphomas are malignant neoplasms originating in the bone marrow and lymphatic structures resulting in the proliferation of lymphocytes. Lymphomas are the fifth most common type of cancer in the United States.[49] Two major types of lymphoma are Hodgkin's lymphoma and non-Hodgkin's lymphoma (NHL). A comparison of these two types of lymphoma is presented in Table 31-28.

HODGKIN'S LYMPHOMA

Hodgkin's lymphoma, also called Hodgkin's disease, makes up about 11% of all lymphomas. It is a malignant condition characterized by proliferation of abnormal giant, multinucleated cells, called *Reed-Sternberg cells,* which are located in lymph nodes. The disease has a bimodal age-specific incidence, occurring most frequently in persons from 15 to 35 years of age and above 50 years of age. In adults, it is twice as prevalent in men as in women. Each year, approximately 9060 new cases of Hodgkin's lymphoma are diagnosed and approximately 1200 deaths occur. However, long-term survival exceeds 85% for all stages.[50]

Etiology and Pathophysiology

Although the cause of Hodgkin's lymphoma remains unknown, several key factors are thought to play a role in its development. The main interacting factors include infection with Epstein-Barr virus (EBV), genetic predisposition, and exposure to occupational toxins. The incidence of Hodgkin's lymphoma is increased among patients who have HIV infection.[50]

Normally, the lymph nodes are composed of connective tissues that surround a fine mesh of reticular fibers and cells. In Hodgkin's lymphoma the normal structure of lymph nodes is destroyed by hyperplasia of monocytes and macrophages. The main diagnostic feature of Hodgkin's lymphoma is the presence of Reed-Sternberg cells in lymph node biopsy specimens. The disease is believed to arise in a single location (it originates in cervical lymph nodes in 70% of patients) and then spreads along adjacent lymphatics. However, in recurrent disease, it may be more diffuse and not necessarily contiguous. It eventually infiltrates other organs, especially lungs, spleen, and liver. When the

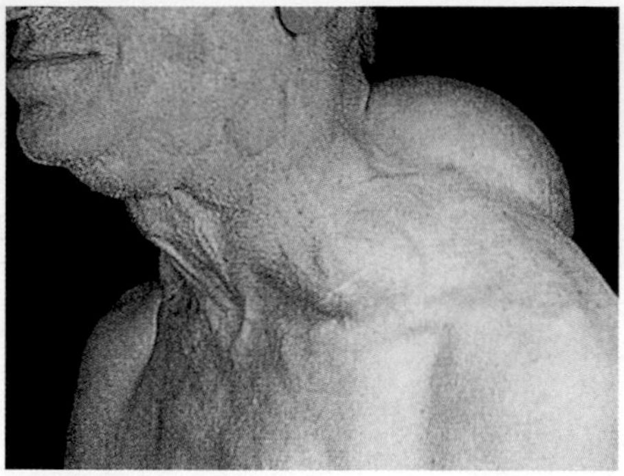

FIG. 31-13 Hodgkin's lymphoma (stage IIA). This patient has enlargement of the cervical lymph nodes.

disease begins above the diaphragm, it remains confined to lymph nodes for a variable time. Disease originating below the diaphragm frequently spreads to extralymphoid sites such as the liver.

Clinical Manifestations

The onset of symptoms in Hodgkin's lymphoma is usually insidious. The initial development is most often enlargement of cervical, axillary, or inguinal lymph nodes (Fig. 31-13); a mediastinal node mass is the second most common location. This lymphadenopathy affects discrete nodes that remain movable and nontender. The enlarged nodes are not painful unless they exert pressure on adjacent nerves.

The patient may notice weight loss, fatigue, weakness, fever, chills, tachycardia, or night sweats. A group of initial findings including fever (in excess of 100.4° F [38° C]), drenching night sweats, and weight loss (exceeding 10% in 6 months) are termed *B symptoms* and correlate with a worse prognosis. After the ingestion of even small amounts of alcohol, individuals with Hodgkin's lymphoma may complain of a rapid onset of pain at the site of disease. The cause for the alcohol-induced pain is unknown. Generalized pruritus without skin lesions may develop. Cough, dyspnea, stridor, and dysphagia may all reflect mediastinal node involvement.

In more advanced disease, there may be hepatomegaly and splenomegaly. Anemia results from increased destruction and decreased production of erythrocytes. Other physical signs vary depending on where the disease is located. For example, intrathoracic involvement may lead to superior vena cava syndrome, enlarged retroperitoneal nodes may cause palpable abdominal masses or interfere with renal function, jaundice may occur from liver involvement, spinal cord compression leading to paraplegia may occur with extradural involvement, and bone pain occurs as a result of bone involvement.

Diagnostic and Staging Studies

Peripheral blood analysis, excisional lymph node biopsy, bone marrow examination, and radiologic studies are important means of evaluating Hodgkin's lymphoma. Abnormalities in the CBC, such as a microcytic hypochromic anemia, are variable and not diagnostic. Leukopenia and thrombocytopenia may develop, but they are usually a consequence of treatment, advanced disease, or superimposed hypersplenism. Other blood studies may show hypoferremia caused by excessive iron uptake by the liver and the spleen, elevated leukocyte alkaline phosphatase from liver and bone involvement, hypercalcemia from bone involvement, and hypoalbuminemia from liver involvement.

Radiologic evaluation can help define all sites and determine the clinical stage of the disease. Positron emission tomography (PET) with or without CT scan is used to stage and then assess the response to therapy and to differentiate residual tumor from fibrotic masses after treatment. These scans may show increased uptake (by PET) and masses (by CT) such as mediastinal lymphadenopathy; renal displacement caused by retroperitoneal node enlargement; abdominal lymph node enlargement; and liver, spleen, bone, and brain infiltration.[50]

NURSING AND COLLABORATIVE MANAGEMENT HODGKIN'S LYMPHOMA

Using all of the information from the various diagnostic studies, one can determine a clinical stage of disease[50,51] (Fig. 31-14). The final staging is based on the clinical stage (extent of the disease) and the presence of B symptoms. Treatment depends on the nature and extent of the disease. The nomenclature used in staging involves an A or B classification, depending on whether symptoms are present when the disease is found, and a Roman numeral (I to IV) that reflects the location and extent of the disease. Additional features that may move an early stage (I or II) to an unfavorable prognosis, warranting more aggressive therapy, include an elevated sedimentation rate; age of 45 years or older; male gender; and the presence of a large mediastinal mass and low serum albumin, hemoglobin, and low or high lymphocyte counts.[51]

Once the stage of Hodgkin's lymphoma is established, management focuses on selecting a treatment plan. The standard for chemotherapy is the ABVD regimen: doxorubicin (**A**driamycin), **b**leomycin, **v**inblastine, and **d**acarbazine. Patients with favorable early-stage disease receive two to four cycles of chemotherapy. Patients with early-stage disease but unfavorable prognostic features (e.g., B symptoms) or intermediate-stage disease are treated with four to six cycles of chemotherapy. Advanced-stage Hodgkin's lymphoma is treated more aggressively using six to eight cycles of chemotherapy. A common regimen is BEACOPP (**b**leomycin, **e**toposide, doxorubicin (**A**driamycin), **c**yclophosphamide, vincristine (**O**ncovin), **pro**carbazine, and **p**rednisone).[51] The role of radiation as a supplement to chemotherapy varies depending on sites of disease and the presence of resistant disease after chemotherapy. Response to therapy is determined by CT and PET scans and other diagnostic tests (e.g., bone marrow biopsy).

A variety of chemotherapy regimens and newer agents, such as brentuximab vedotin (Adcetris), are used to treat patients who have relapsed or refractory disease. Ideally, once remission is obtained, a hope for curative option may be intensive chemotherapy with the use of autologous or allogeneic HSCT.[51] HSCT has allowed patients to receive higher, potentially curative doses of chemotherapy while reducing life-threatening leukopenia (see Chapter 16). Combination chemotherapy works well because, as in leukemia, the drugs used have an additive antitumor effect without increasing side effects. As with leukemia, therapy must be aggressive. Therefore potentially life-threatening problems are encountered in an attempt to achieve a remission.

Maintenance chemotherapy does not contribute to increased survival once a complete remission is achieved. Occasionally, single drugs may be administered palliatively to patients who cannot tolerate intensive combination therapy. A serious consequence of the treatment for Hodgkin's lymphoma is the later

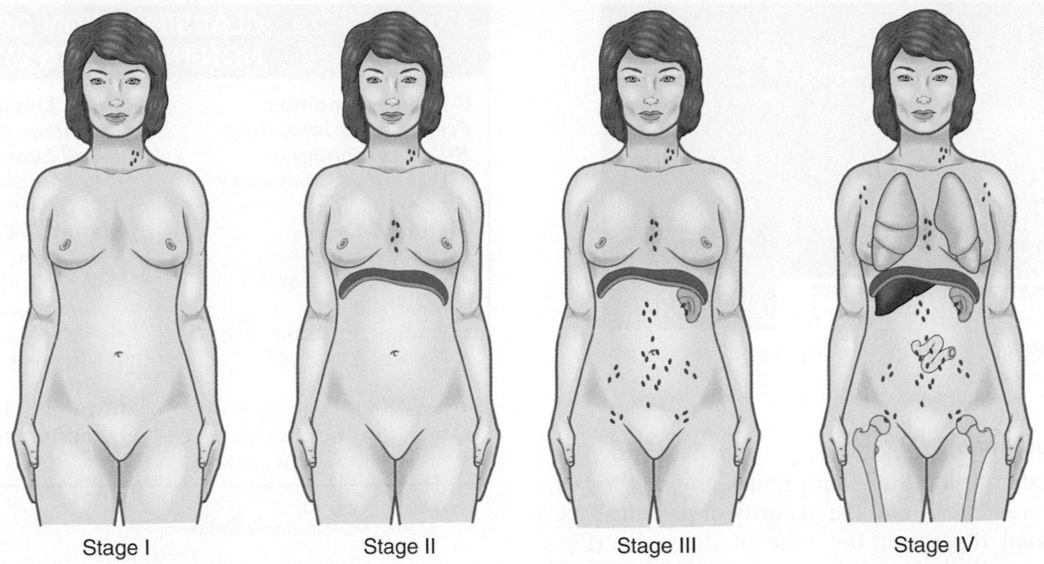

FIG. 31-14 Staging system for Hodgkin's lymphoma and non-Hodgkin's lymphoma. *Stage I,* involvement of single lymph node (e.g., cervical node). *Stage II,* involvement of two or more lymph nodes on one side of diaphragm. *Stage III,* lymph node involvement above and below the diaphragm. *Stage IV,* involvement outside of diaphragm (e.g., liver, bone marrow). The stage is followed by the letter *A* (absence) or *B* (presence) to indicate significant systemic symptoms (e.g., fever, night sweats, weight loss).

development of secondary malignancies (see Chapter 16), as well as potential long-term toxicities from the treatment, such as endocrine, cardiac, and pulmonary dysfunction.[50,51] The estimated risk of a secondary cancer is about 5% and generally occurs within the first 10 years after treatment for Hodgkin's lymphoma.[50] The most common secondary malignancies are AML, NHL, and solid tumors.

The nursing care for Hodgkin's lymphoma is largely based on managing problems related to the disease (e.g., pain caused by a tumor, superior vena cava syndrome), pancytopenia, and other side effects of therapy. Because the survival of patients with Hodgkin's lymphoma depends on their response to treatment, supporting the patient through the consequences of treatment is extremely important.

Psychosocial considerations are as important as they are with leukemia. However, the prognosis for Hodgkin's lymphoma is better than that for many forms of cancer or leukemia. The physical, psychologic, social, and spiritual consequences of the patient's disease must be addressed. Fertility issues may be of particular concern because this disease is frequently seen in adolescents and young adults. Help to ensure that these issues have been addressed soon after diagnosis. Evaluation of patients for long-term effects of therapy is important because delayed consequences of disease and treatment may not be apparent for many years. (Secondary malignancies and delayed effects are discussed in Chapter 16.)

NON-HODGKIN'S LYMPHOMA

Non-Hodgkin's lymphomas (NHLs) are a heterogeneous group of malignant neoplasms of primarily B-, T-, or natural killer (NK) cell origin affecting all ages. B-cell lymphomas constitute about 85% of all NHLs. They are categorized by the level of differentiation, cell of origin, and rate of cellular proliferation.[26] A variety of clinical presentations and courses are recognized, from indolent (slowly developing) to rapidly progressive disease. NHL is the most commonly occurring hematologic cancer and the fifth leading cause of cancer death. Each year approximately 66,360 new cases of NHL are diagnosed and approximately 19,320 deaths occur.[49]

Etiology and Pathophysiology

As with Hodgkin's lymphoma, the cause of NHL is usually unknown. NHLs may result from chromosomal translocations, infections, environmental factors, and immunodeficiency states. Chromosomal translocations have an important role in the pathogenesis of many NHLs. Some viruses and bacteria are implicated in the pathogenesis of NHL, including HTLV-1, EBV, human herpesvirus 8, hepatitis B and C, *Helicobacter pylori, Chlamydophila psittaci, Campylobacter jejuni,* and *Borrelia burgdorferi.* Environmental factors linked to the development of NHL include chemicals (e.g., pesticides, herbicides, solvents, organic chemicals, wood preservatives). NHL is also more common in individuals who have inherited immunodeficiency syndromes and who have used immunosuppressive medications (e.g., to prevent rejection after an organ transplant or to treat autoimmune disorders) or received chemotherapy or radiation therapy.

NHL does not have a hallmark feature that parallels the Reed-Sternberg cell of Hodgkin's lymphoma. However, all NHLs involve lymphocytes arrested in various stages of development and may mimic a leukemia. For example, small lymphocytic lymphoma (SLL) and chronic lymphocytic leukemia (CLL) result from malignant proliferation of small B lymphocytes, with CLL having the majority of disease within the bone marrow (versus the lymph nodes).[45] (The overlap among leukemia and NHLs is discussed on p. 665.) Diffuse large B-cell lymphoma, the most common aggressive lymphoma, is a neoplasm that originates in the lymph nodes, usually in the neck or abdomen. Burkitt's lymphoma is the most highly aggressive disease and is thought to originate from B-cell blasts in the lymph nodes.

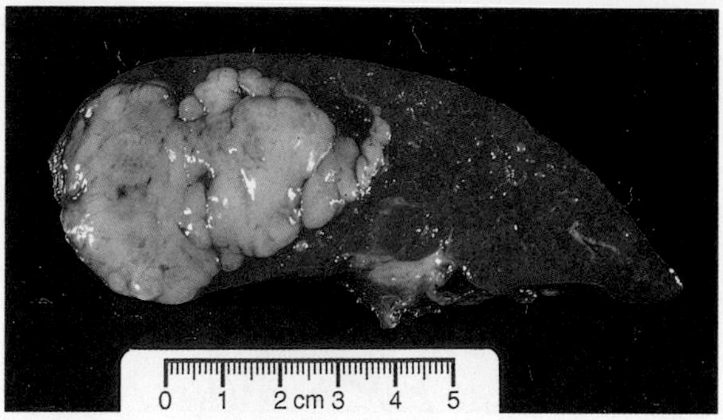

FIG. 31-15 Non-Hodgkin's lymphoma involving the spleen. The presence of an isolated mass is typical.

Clinical Manifestations

NHLs can originate outside the lymph nodes, the method of spread can be unpredictable, and the majority of patients have widely disseminated disease at the time of diagnosis (Fig. 31-15). The primary clinical manifestation is painless lymph node enlargement. The lymphadenopathy can wax and wane in indolent disease. Because the disease is usually disseminated when it is diagnosed, other symptoms are present depending on where the disease has spread (e.g., hepatomegaly with liver involvement, neurologic symptoms with CNS disease). NHL can also manifest in nonspecific ways, such as an airway obstruction, hyperuricemia and renal failure from tumor lysis syndrome, pericardial tamponade, and GI complaints.

Patients with high-grade lymphomas may have lymphadenopathy and constitutional symptoms (B symptoms) such as fever, night sweats, and weight loss. The peripheral blood is usually normal, but some lymphomas manifest in a "leukemic" phase.

Diagnostic and Staging Studies

Diagnostic studies used for NHL resemble those used for Hodgkin's lymphoma. However, because NHL is more often in extranodal sites, more diagnostic studies may be done, such as an MRI to rule out CNS or bone marrow infiltration, or a barium enema, upper endoscopy, or CT to visualize suspected GI involvement. Clinical staging, as described for Hodgkin's lymphoma, is used to help guide therapy (see Fig. 31-14), but establishment of the precise histologic subtype is extremely important. Lymph node excisional biopsy establishes the cell type and pattern. NHL is classified based on morphologic, genetic, immunophenotypic (cell surface antigens, CD20, CD52), and clinical features.

The World Health Organization has categorized more than 30 unique types of NHL. However, clinical studies have verified that different disease categories can be divided into one of two major categories: *indolent* (low grade) and *aggressive* (high grade), which is useful, along with gene expression patterns, in determining therapy[52] (Table 31-29). Additional factors, known as the International Prognostic Index (IPI), may be considered for each subtype to help select the appropriate treatment for these patients. Factors considered may include the clinical stage, number of extranodal sites, serum LDH, WBC count, hemoglobin, and patient's age and performance status. Immunologic, cytogenetic, and molecular studies are also useful for making therapeutic decisions and assessing prognosis. Other studies might include blood tests for tumor lysis (see Chapter 16); screening for hepatitis, HIV, and *H. pylori*; skin biopsies; bone marrow biopsies; and lumbar punctures. The prognosis for NHL is based on the histopathology.

TABLE 31-29 CLASSIFICATION OF NON-HODGKIN'S LYMPHOMA*

B-Cell Lymphomas	T-Cell Lymphomas
Precursor or Immature B-Cell Lymphomas	***Precursor or Immature T-Cell Lymphomas***
• Lymphoblastic lymphoma	• Lymphoblastic lymphoma
Mature B-Cell Lymphomas	***Mature T-Cell Lymphomas***
• Diffuse large B-cell lymphoma	• Peripheral T-cell lymphoma
• Follicular lymphoma	• Mycosis fungoides and Sézary syndrome
• Marginal zone B-cell lymphoma (MALT)	• Anaplastic large T-cell lymphoma
• Small lymphocytic lymphoma	**Natural Killer Cell Lymphomas**
• Mantle cell lymphoma	
• Burkitt's lymphoma	

*This is only a partial list.
MALT, Mucosa-associated lymphoid tissue.

NURSING AND COLLABORATIVE MANAGEMENT NON-HODGKIN'S LYMPHOMA

Treatment for NHL involves chemotherapy and sometimes radiation therapy (Table 31-30). Ironically, more aggressive lymphomas are more responsive to treatment and more likely to be cured. In contrast, indolent lymphomas have a naturally long course but are difficult to effectively treat.[52]

Patients with low-grade (indolent) lymphoma may live 10 years or more without treatment. However, some initial therapies can be well tolerated and have been shown to reduce the time to progression of the disease. Lymphomas that are infectious driven, such as *H. pylori* gastric lymphomas, may be treated with antibiotic or antiviral therapy. HSCT may have some benefit in certain subtypes of aggressive or refractory lymphomas.[45]

Rituximab, a monoclonal antibody against the CD20 antigen on the surface of normal and malignant B cells, is used to treat NHL. Once bound to the cells, rituximab causes lysis and cell death. Numerous chemotherapy combinations have been used to try to overcome the resistant nature of this disease (see Table 31-30). Complete remissions are uncommon, but the majority of patients respond with improvement in symptoms.

DRUG ALERT: Rituximab (Rituxan)
- Monitor patient for signs of severe hypersensitivity infusion reactions, especially with first infusion.
- Manifestations may include hypotension, bronchospasm, dysrhythmias, angioedema, and cardiogenic shock.
- Screen for history of hepatitis because the drug may reactivate hepatitis.

Other therapies for some types of NHL include the monoclonal antibodies ibritumomab tiuxetan (Zevalin) and tositumomab (Bexxar). These antibodies are linked to a radioactive isotope (yttrium-90 and iodine-131, respectively) (see Table 16-13). The monoclonal antibody targets the CD20 antigen, which is on the surface of mature B cells and B-cell tumors. This targeting allows for the delivery of radiation directly to the malignant cells. Side effects of this type of treatment include pancytopenia. Use radiation precautions in caring for these

TABLE 31-30 **TREATMENT OF NON-HODGKIN'S LYMPHOMA***

Recommended Therapies	Common Chemotherapy Combinations
Indolent (Low Grade) (e.g., follicular lymphoma, marginal zone B-cell lymphoma [MALT])	
Observation until disease progression for asymptomatic patients with low-volume tumors and normal blood counts	**R-CHOP:** rituximab, cyclophosphamide, doxorubicin hydrochloride, vincristine (Oncovin), prednisone
External beam irradiation for local, limited disease	**FMC:** fludarabine, mitoxantrone, cyclophosphamide
Single-agent rituximab (Rituxan)	**R-CVP:** rituximab, cyclophosphamide, vincristine, prednisone
Single-agent chemotherapy (chlorambucil, cyclophosphamide, bendamustine) or alemtuzumab	**FND:** fludarabine, mitoxantrone [Novantrone], dexamethasone ± rituximab
Rituximab with another agent (bendamustine, cyclophosphamide, fludarabine, cladribine, pentostatin, chlorambucil, denileukin diftitox)	**FC:** fludarabine, cyclophosphamide
Combination chemotherapy (R-CHOP or other)	
Radioimmunotherapy	
Hematopoietic stem cell transplant (HSCT)	
Aggressive (Intermediate or High Grade) (e.g., mantle cell, diffuse large B-cell, Burkitt's, peripheral T-cell, natural killer cell lymphomas)	
Combination chemotherapy with localized radiation if needed	**R-CHOP** (see above)
Aggressive combination chemotherapy for 3-8 cycles with rituximab with local radiation if needed	**ICE** (or "RICE" with rituximab): ifosfamide, cyclophosphamide, etoposide
Intrathecal chemotherapy if needed	**R-EPOCH:** rituximab, etoposide, prednisone, vincristine (Oncovin), cyclophosphamide, doxorubicin hydrochloride
HSCT	**ESHAP ± R:** etoposide, methylprednisolone (Solu-Medrol), high-dose cytarabine (Ara-C), cisplatin (Platinol), with or without rituximab
	Hyper-CVAD ± R: hyperfractionated cyclophosphamide, vincristine, doxorubicin (Adriamycin), dexamethasone alternating with high-dose methotrexate and cytarabine with or without rituximab
	DHAP ± R: dexamethasone, high-dose cytarabine (Ara-C), cisplatin (Platinol), with our without rituximab
	CODOX-M: cyclophosphamide, vincristine (Oncovin), doxorubicin, high-dose methotrexate, with or without rituximab (includes intrathecal methotrexate)
	FCR: fludarabine, cyclophosphamide, rituximab
	SMILE: steroids, methotrexate, ifosfamide, L-asparaginase, etoposide
	High-dose cytarabine and high-dose methotrexate with leucovorin rescue

*Not all inclusive.
MALT, Mucosa-associated lymphoid tissue.

patients. Teach patients about safety issues and how to minimize the risk of radiation exposure to staff and others.

Peripheral T-cell lymphomas are treated similarly to intermediate-grade or high-grade B-cell lymphomas (without rituximab because they are generally not $CD20^+$). Cutaneous T-cell lymphomas may be treated with topical corticosteroids or topical chemotherapy for limited-stage disease. For more diffuse disease, treatment may include phototherapy, α-interferon, oral bexarotene (Targretin), vorinostat (Zolinza), or denileukin diftitox (Ontak), which is a fusion protein consisting of interleukin-2 and diphtheria toxin.[45,53] (Biologic and targeted therapy is discussed in Chapter 16.)

The nursing care for NHL is similar to that for Hodgkin's lymphoma. It is largely based on managing problems related to the disease (e.g., pain caused by the tumor, spinal cord compression, tumor lysis syndrome), pancytopenia, and other side effects of therapy. However, because NHL can be more extensive and involve specific organs (e.g., CNS, spleen, liver, GI tract, bone marrow), it is important to understand the subtype and extent of the disease. For example, a patient with known involvement of the colon may complain of acute abdominal pain. The patient most likely would have abdominal guarding and an enlarged and tympanic abdomen. This could indicate a bowel perforation and be considered a medical emergency. A patient with a Burkitt's NHL beginning chemotherapy would be at high risk for tumor lysis syndrome and would require frequent laboratory studies and monitoring, as well as strict documentation of intake and output. (Cancer-related therapies and side effects are discussed in Chapter 16.)

The patient undergoing external beam radiation therapy has special nursing needs. The skin in the radiation field requires attention. Concepts related to safety issues regarding radiation therapy are important in the plan of care (see Chapter 16).

Psychosocial considerations are important. Help the patient and family understand the disease, treatment, and expected and potential side effects. Fertility issues may be of concern in young patients. As in Hodgkin's lymphoma, evaluation of patients with NHL for long-term effects of therapy is important because the delayed consequences of disease and treatment may not become apparent for many years. (Secondary malignancies and delayed effects are discussed in Chapter 16.)

MULTIPLE MYELOMA

Multiple myeloma, or *plasma cell myeloma,* is a condition in which neoplastic plasma cells infiltrate the bone marrow and destroy bone. Multiple myeloma accounts for 1% of all malignancies and for about 10% of all hematologic malignancies.[49] The disease is twice as common in men as in women and usually develops after 40 years of age, with an average age of 65 years. Multiple myeloma occurs in African Americans more commonly than in whites. Although it was previously not considered curable, many patients are living 10 or more years because of the variety of treatments that can be provided throughout the course of the disease.[54]

Etiology and Pathophysiology

The cause of multiple myeloma is unknown. It is possible that exposure to radiation, organic chemicals (such as benzene), metals, herbicides, and insecticides may play a role. Genetic factors and viral infection may also influence the risk of developing multiple myeloma.

The disease process involves excessive production of plasma cells. Plasma cells are activated B cells, which produce immunoglobulins (antibodies) that normally serve to protect the body. However, in multiple myeloma instead of a variety of plasma cells producing antibodies to fight different infections, myeloma tumors produce monoclonal antibodies. *Monoclonal* means they are all of one kind, making them ineffective and even harmful. Not only do they not fight infections, but they also infiltrate the bone marrow. These monoclonal proteins (called M proteins) are made up of two light chains and two heavy chains. *Bence-Jones proteins* are the light chain part of these monoclonal antibodies. They show up in the urine in many patients with multiple myeloma.

Furthermore, plasma cell production of excessive and abnormal amounts of cytokines (interleukins [ILs]; IL-4, IL-5, and IL-6) also plays an important role in the pathologic process of bone destruction. As myeloma protein increases, normal plasma cells are reduced, which further compromises the body's normal immune response. Proliferation of malignant plasma cells and the overproduction of immunoglobulin and proteins result in the end-organ effects of myeloma on the bone marrow, bone, and kidneys and possibly the spleen, lymph nodes, liver, and even heart muscle.

Clinical Manifestations

Multiple myeloma develops slowly and insidiously. The patient often does not manifest symptoms until the disease is advanced, at which time skeletal pain is the major manifestation. Pain in the pelvis, spine, and ribs is particularly common and is triggered by movement. Diffuse osteoporosis develops as the myeloma protein destroys bone. Osteolytic lesions are seen in the skull, vertebrae, and ribs. Vertebral destruction can lead to collapse of vertebrae with ensuing compression of the spinal cord. Loss of bone integrity can lead to the development of pathologic fractures.

Bony degeneration also causes calcium to be lost from bones, eventually causing hypercalcemia. Hypercalcemia may cause renal, GI, or neurologic manifestations such as polyuria, anorexia, confusion, and ultimately seizures, coma, and cardiac problems. A serum "hyperviscosity syndrome" leading to cerebral, pulmonary, renal, and other organ dysfunction can occur in some patients. Even without hyperviscosity, high protein levels caused by the myeloma protein can result in renal tubular obstruction, interstitial nephritis, and renal failure. The patient may also display manifestations of anemia, thrombocytopenia, neutropenia, and immune dysfunction, all of which are related to the replacement of normal bone marrow with plasma cells. Neurologic abnormalities may be caused by regional myeloma cell growth compressing the spinal cord or cranial nerves, or by perineuronal or perivascular deposition.

Diagnostic Studies

Evaluating multiple myeloma involves laboratory, radiologic, and bone marrow examination. M protein is found in the blood and urine. Possible findings include pancytopenia, hypercalcemia, Bence Jones protein in the urine, and an elevated serum creatinine.

Skeletal bone surveys, MRI, and/or PET and CT scans show distinct lytic areas of bone erosions; generalized thinning of the bones; or fractures, especially in the vertebrae, ribs, pelvis, and bones of the thigh and upper arms. Bone marrow analysis shows significantly increased numbers of plasma cells in the bone marrow. The simplest measure of staging and prognosis in multiple myeloma is based on blood levels of two markers: β_2-microglobulin and albumin. In general, higher levels of β_2-microglobulin and lower levels of albumin are associated with a poorer prognosis.

Collaborative Care

Collaborative care involves managing both the disease and its symptoms. The current treatment options include watchful waiting (for early multiple myeloma, also called MGUS [monoclonal gammopathy of undetermined significance]), corticosteroids, chemotherapy, targeted therapy, and HSCT. Multiple myeloma is seldom cured, but treatment can relieve symptoms, produce remission, and prolong life. Ambulation and adequate hydration are used to treat hypercalcemia, dehydration, and potential renal damage. Weight bearing helps the bones resorb some calcium, and fluids dilute calcium and prevent protein precipitates from causing renal tubular obstruction. Control of pain and prevention of pathologic fractures are other goals of management. Analgesics, orthopedic supports, and localized radiation help reduce the skeletal pain.

Bisphosphonates, such as pamidronate (Aredia), zoledronic acid (Zometa), and etidronate (Didronel), inhibit bone breakdown and are used for the treatment of skeletal pain and hypercalcemia. They inhibit bone resorption without inhibiting bone formation and mineralization. They are given monthly by IV infusion. Radiation therapy is another important component of treatment, primarily because of its effect on localized lesions. Surgical procedures, such as vertebroplasty, may be done to support degenerative vertebrae.

DRUG ALERT: Zoledronic Acid (Zometa)

- Patient should be adequately rehydrated before administering drug.
- Renal toxicity may occur if IV infusion of drug is administered in less than 15 min.

Chemotherapy with corticosteroids is usually the first treatment recommended for multiple myeloma. It is used to reduce the number of plasma cells. Initial treatment depends on whether the patient is a future bone marrow transplant candidate and anticipated tolerance of therapy. The treatment usually includes a corticosteroid (dexamethasone or prednisone) plus one or two therapies, such as cyclophosphamide, lenalidomide, thalidomide, pomalidomide (Pomalyst), doxorubicin, or melphalan. High-dose chemotherapy followed by HSCT has evolved as the standard of care in eligible patients.[55]

Targeted therapy for multiple myeloma may include bortezomib (Velcade) and carfilzomib (Kyprolis). These drugs inhibit proteasomes, which are intracellular multienzyme complexes that degrade proteins. Proteasome inhibitors can cause these proteins to accumulate, thus leading to altered cell function. Normal cells are capable of recovering from proteasome inhibition, but cancer cells undergo death when proteasomes are inhibited.

Drugs may be used to treat complications of multiple myeloma. For example, allopurinol may be given to reduce hyperuricemia, and IV furosemide (Lasix) promotes renal excretion of calcium.

NURSING MANAGEMENT MULTIPLE MYELOMA

A major focus of care relates to the bone involvement and sequelae from bone breakdown. Maintaining adequate hydration is a primary nursing consideration to minimize problems from hypercalcemia. IV fluids may be administered to attain a urine output of 1.5 to 2 L/day. Although tumor lysis is rare, once chemotherapy is initiated, allopurinol may be given to prevent any renal damage from uric acid accumulation (from cell breakdown). Because of the myeloma proteins, the patient is at additional risk of renal dysfunction and electrolyte and fluid imbalances.

Because of the potential for pathologic fractures, use caution when moving and ambulating the patient. A slight twist or strain in the wrong area (e.g., a weak area in the patient's bones) may be sufficient to cause a fracture. In addition, the development of peripheral neuropathy is common with several therapies for multiple myeloma and can contribute to discomfort, the inability to perform basic activities of daily living, and the risk of injury from falling. Pain medications and therapies can also lead to severe constipation.

Pain management requires innovative and knowledgeable nursing interventions. Analgesics, such as nonsteroidal antiinflammatory drugs, acetaminophen, or an acetaminophen/opioid combination, may be more effective than opioids alone in diminishing bone pain. Braces, especially for the spine, may also help control pain. As in any pain management situation, assess the patient and implement necessary measures to alleviate the pain. (Pain management is discussed in Chapter 9.) Patients may also be at risk for deep vein thrombosis related to chemotherapy and immobility and should have appropriate preventive measures employed.[55]

Assessment and prompt treatment of infection are important in the care of patients with multiple myeloma. These recurrent infections may be due to a decrease in the production of normal immunoglobulins, the ineffectiveness of the overproduced and abnormal immunoglobulins, corticosteroids, and/or neutropenia as a result of the bone marrow infiltration or side effects of treatment.

The patient's psychosocial needs require sensitive, skilled management. Help the patient and significant others adapt to changes fostered by chronic sickness and adjust to the losses related to the disease process, while helping to maximize functioning and quality of life.[56] The patient with multiple myeloma may experience remissions and exacerbations. Patients may be on dialysis because of myeloma-induced renal failure. Consequently acute care is needed at various times during the course of the illness. The final, acute phase is unresponsive to treatment and usually short in duration. The way in which patients and families confront death may be affected by the manner in which they have learned to accept and live with the chronic disease.

DISORDERS OF THE SPLEEN

The spleen can be affected by many illnesses, most of which can cause some degree of *splenomegaly* (enlarged spleen) (Table 31-31). The term *hypersplenism* refers to the occurrence of splenomegaly and peripheral cytopenias (anemia, leukopenia, and thrombocytopenia). The degree of splenic enlargement varies with the disease. For example, massive splenic enlargement occurs with infectious mononucleosis, chronic myelogenous leukemia, and thalassemia major. Mild splenic enlargement occurs with HF and systemic lupus erythematosus. The normal spleen contains 350 mL of blood, and about one third of the platelet mass is sequestered in the spleen.[57]

TABLE 31-31 CAUSES OF SPLENOMEGALY

Hereditary Hemolytic Anemias
- Sickle cell disease
- Thalassemia

Autoimmune Cytopenias
- Acquired hemolytic anemia
- Immune thrombocytopenia

Infections and Inflammations
- Bacterial infections: endocarditis, salmonella
- Mycobacterial infections: tuberculosis
- Spirochetes: syphilis, Lyme disease
- Viral infections: hepatitis, human immunodeficiency virus, cytomegalovirus, mononucleosis
- Parasitic infections: malaria, trypanosomiasis, schistosomiasis, leishmaniasis, toxoplasmosis
- Rickettsial infections: Rocky Mountain spotted fever, typhoid fever
- Fungal infections: histoplasmosis
- Autoimmune diseases: systemic lupus erythematosus, rheumatoid arthritis

Infiltrative Diseases
- Acute and chronic leukemia
- Lymphomas
- Polycythemia vera
- Multiple myeloma, amyloidosis
- Other primary or secondary neoplasms and cysts
- Sarcoidosis
- Gaucher disease

Congestion
- Cirrhosis of the liver
- Heart failure (portal hypertension)
- Portal or splenic vein thrombosis

When the spleen enlarges, its normal filtering and sequestering capacity increases. Consequently, there is often a reduction in the number of circulating blood cells as they engorge the spleen. In addition, there are unusual findings in the peripheral smear, such as pitted or pocked erythrocytes or Howell-Jolly bodies. These findings assist in diagnosing a malfunctioning spleen. A slight to moderate enlargement of the spleen is usually asymptomatic and found during routine examination of the abdomen. Even massive splenomegaly can be well tolerated, but the patient may complain of abdominal discomfort and early satiety. In addition to physical examination, other techniques to assess the size of the spleen include radionuclide colloid liver-spleen scan, CT or PET scan, MRI, and ultrasound scan.

Occasionally laparoscopy or open laparotomy and splenectomy are indicated in the evaluation or treatment of splenomegaly. Another major indication for splenectomy is splenic rupture. The spleen may rupture from trauma; inadvertent tearing during other surgical procedures; and diseases such as mononucleosis, malaria, and lymphoid neoplasms. After a splenectomy, there can be a dramatic increase in peripheral RBC, WBC, and platelet counts.

Nursing responsibilities for the patient with spleen disorders vary depending on the problem. Splenomegaly may be painful and may require analgesic administration; care in moving, turning, and positioning; and evaluation of lung expansion because spleen enlargement may impair diaphragmatic excursion. If anemia, thrombocytopenia, or leukopenia develops from splenic enlargement, institute nursing measures to support the patient and prevent life-threatening complications. If splenectomy is performed, observe the patient for hemorrhage and shock.

After splenectomy, immunologic deficiencies may develop. IgM levels are reduced, while IgG and IgA values remain within normal limits. Postsplenectomy patients have a lifelong risk for infection, especially from encapsulated organisms such as *Pneumococcus* species. This risk is reduced by immunization with pneumococcal vaccine (e.g., Pneumovax).

BLOOD COMPONENT THERAPY

Blood component therapy is frequently used to manage hematologic diseases. Many therapeutic and surgical procedures depend on blood product support. However, blood component therapy only temporarily supports the patient until the underlying problem is resolved. Because transfusions are not free from hazards, they should be used only if necessary.

Avoid developing a complacent attitude about this common but potentially dangerous therapy. Make sure that the physician has discussed the risks, benefits, and alternatives with the patient and that this is documented in the patient's medical record.

Traditionally, the term *blood transfusion* meant the administration of whole blood. Blood transfusion now has a broader meaning because of the ability to administer specific components of blood such as platelets, packed red blood cells (PRBCs), or plasma. Usually a specific component is ordered, although whole blood may be rarely used with massive hemorrhage or for an exchange transfusion[58-60] (Table 31-32).

TABLE 31-32 BLOOD PRODUCTS*

Description	Special Considerations	Indications for Use
Packed RBCs		
Packed RBCs are prepared from whole blood by sedimentation or centrifugation. One unit contains 250-350 mL. They can be stored up to 35 days depending on processing.	Use of RBCs for treatment allows remaining components of blood (e.g., platelets, albumin, plasma) to be used for other purposes. There is less danger of fluid overload. Packed RBCs are preferred RBC source because they are more component specific. Leukocyte depletion (leukoreduction) by filtration, washing, or freezing frequently used. Decreases hemolytic febrile or mild allergic reactions in patients who receive frequent transfusions.	Severe or symptomatic anemia, acute blood loss. One unit of RBCs can be expected to increase Hgb by 1 g/dL or Hct by 3% in a typical adult. One unit of RBCs can replace a blood loss of 500 mL.
Frozen RBCs		
Frozen RBCs are prepared from RBCs using glycerol for protection and frozen. They can be stored for 10 yr.	Must be used within 24 hr of thawing. Successive washings with saline solution remove majority of WBCs and plasma proteins.	Autotransfusion. Stockpiling or rare donors for patients with alloantibodies.
Platelets		
Platelets are prepared from fresh whole blood. One donor unit contains 30-60 mL of platelet concentrate (from whole blood). Platelets also pooled from multiple donors. An apheresed single donation contains 200-400 mL of platelets.	Multiple units of platelets can be obtained from one donor by plateletpheresis. They can be kept at room temperature for 1-5 days depending on type of collection and storage bag used. Bag should be agitated periodically. For patients who receive frequent transfusions and become refractory, may give leukocyte reduced, HLA, or type specific to prevent alloimmunization to HLA antigens.	Bleeding caused by thrombocytopenia; may be contraindicated in thrombotic thrombocytopenic purpura and heparin-induced thrombocytopenia except in life-threatening hemorrhage. Expected increase is 10,000/µL/U. Failure to have an increase may be due to fever, sepsis, splenomegaly, or DIC or development of antibodies *(refractory).*
Fresh Frozen Plasma		
Liquid portion of whole blood is separated from cells and frozen. One unit contains 200-250 mL. Plasma is rich in clotting factors but contains no platelets. May be stored for ≥1 yr, depending on storage. Must be used within 24 hr after thawing.	Use of plasma in treating hypovolemic shock is being replaced by pure preparations such as albumin and plasma expanders.	Bleeding caused by deficiency in clotting factors (e.g., DIC, hemorrhage, massive transfusion, liver disease, vitamin K deficiency, excess warfarin).
Albumin		
Albumin is prepared from plasma. It can be stored for 5 yr. It is available in 5% or 25% solution.	Albumin 25 g/dL is osmotically equal to 500 mL of plasma. Hyperosmolar solution acts by moving water from extravascular to intravascular space. It is heat treated and does not transmit viruses.	Hypovolemic shock, hypoalbuminemia.
Cryoprecipitates and Commercial Concentrates		
Cryoprecipitate is prepared from fresh frozen plasma, with 10-20 mL/bag. It can be stored for 1 yr. Once thawed, must be used within 5 days.	See Table 31-19.	Replacement of clotting factors, especially factor VIII, von Willebrand factor, and fibrinogen.

*Component therapy has replaced the use of whole blood, which accounts for <10% of all transfusions. Granulocyte transfusions are not included here because they are rarely used.
DIC, Disseminated intravascular coagulation; *HLA,* human leukocyte antigen.

Administration Procedure

Blood components are usually administered with at least a 19-gauge needle, cannula, or catheter. Larger sizes (e.g., 18 or 16 gauge) may be preferred if rapid transfusions are given. Smaller needles can be used for platelets, albumin, and clotting factor replacement. Whatever type of venous access is used, verify its patency before requesting the blood component from the blood bank. Most blood product administration tubing is of a "Y type" with a microaggregate filter (filters out particulate), with one arm of the Y for the isotonic saline solution and the other arm of the Y for the blood product.

SAFETY ALERT

- Do not use dextrose solutions or lactated Ringer's solution for administering blood because they will cause RBC hemolysis.
- Do not give any additives (including medications) via the same tubing as the blood unless the tubing is first cleared with saline solution.

After obtaining the blood or blood components from the blood bank, make a positive identification of the donor blood and recipient. Improper product-to-patient identification is the most common cause of hemolytic transfusion reactions, thus placing a great responsibility on nurses to carry out the identification procedure appropriately. Follow the policy and procedures at your place of employment. Many institutions have implemented a dual-checking system with two licensed individuals checking the patient identification with the labeled blood component. The blood bank is responsible for typing and crossmatching the donor's blood with the recipient's blood. The result of the compatibility testing should be noted on the product bag or tag, if pertinent.

ABO compatibility is not a prerequisite for platelet transfusions. However, after multiple platelet transfusions, a patient may develop anti-HLA antibodies to the transfused platelets. With the use of lymphocyte typing to match HLA types of the donor and the recipient, multiple platelet transfusions can be given with fewer complications to those who develop antibodies to platelets. In addition, the patient may be premedicated with an antihistamine (e.g., diphenhydramine [Benadryl]) and hydrocortisone to decrease the possibility of reacting to platelet transfusions.

Take the patient's vital signs before beginning the transfusion so that you have a baseline measure. If the patient has abnormal vital signs (e.g., high fever), call the physician to clarify when the blood component may be administered. Administer the blood as soon as it is brought to the patient. Do not refrigerate it on the nursing unit. If the blood is not used within 30 minutes, return it to the blood bank. During the first 15 minutes or 50 mL of blood infusion, remain with the patient. If there are any untoward reactions, they are most likely to occur at this time. The rate of infusion during this period should be no more than 2 mL/minute. Do not infuse PRBCs quickly except in an emergency. Rapid infusion of cold blood may cause the patient to become chilled. If rapid replacement of large amounts of blood is necessary, a blood-warming device may be used. Other blood components, such as fresh frozen plasma and platelets, may be infused over 15 to 30 minutes. Refer to your institution's policy and procedure.

After the first 15 minutes, vital signs are usually retaken, and the rate of infusion is determined by the patient's clinical condition and the product being infused. Observe the patient periodically throughout the transfusion (e.g., every 30 minutes) and up to 1 hour after the transfusion. Most patients not in danger of fluid overload can tolerate the infusion of 1 unit of PRBCs over 2 hours. The transfusion should not take more than 4 hours to administer because of the increased risk of bacterial growth in the product once it is out of refrigeration. Blood that is unrefrigerated for 4 hours or longer should not be infused and should be returned to the blood bank.

ETHICAL/LEGAL DILEMMAS

Religious Beliefs

Situation

W.D., an 81-year-old woman with dementia, is transferred from a nursing home to a hospital because of gastrointestinal bleeding from an unknown cause. Some of her family members tell you that she is a Jehovah's Witness and must not receive blood products. If she does not have exploratory surgery and transfusions, the surgeon believes that she will die.

Ethical/Legal Points for Consideration

- Competent adults have the right to make health care decisions, including the right to refuse treatment, based on their religious beliefs.
- If the patient is determined to be incompetent and a guardian has been appointed, the guardian has the legal right to make the consent or refusal.
- If the health care professional believes that the treatment is essential to preserve life and health and there is no legal decision maker, a request is made for a legal determination of whether the patient is incapable of consent or refusal. If the judge agrees, the patient is made a ward of the court for this issue. Usually the physician is directed to make a decision based on the patient's best interests.
- Courts tend to defer to any past information coming directly from patients about their own personal desires, even if that information is not in valid advance directives.

Discussion Questions

1. What resources do you have available to consult about religious practices?
2. How could you make a determination if the family were acting in W.D.'s best interest or their own?
3. What nonblood alternatives are available for Jehovah's Witnesses?

DELEGATION DECISIONS

Blood Transfusions

Role of Registered Nurse (RN)

- Ensure that an IV line is being used with a large-bore needle, catheter, or cannula, preferably 19 gauge or larger.
- Double-check patient identification and blood product identification data with another licensed nurse (consider state nurse practice act and agency policy).
- Adjust infusion rate of transfusion according to patient needs.
- Evaluate patient for signs of transfusion reactions.
- Evaluate for therapeutic effect of blood product (improvement in complete blood count, increased blood pressure, improved patient color, decreased bleeding).
- Monitor for signs of circulatory overload (e.g., shortness of breath) if the transfusion must be given rapidly.

Role of Licensed Practical/Vocational Nurse (LPN/LVN)

- Assist with checking patient identification and blood product identification data with the RN (consider state nurse practice act and agency policy).
- Monitor blood transfusion rate (consider state nurse practice act and agency policy).

Role of Unlicensed Assistive Personnel (UAP)

- Obtain blood products from the blood bank as directed by the RN.
- Take vital signs before the transfusion and after the first 15 min.

Blood Transfusion Reactions

A *blood transfusion reaction* is an adverse reaction to blood transfusion therapy that can range in severity from mild symptoms to a life-threatening condition. Because complications of transfusion therapy may be significant, judicious evaluation of the patient is required. Blood transfusion reactions can be classified as acute or delayed (Tables 31-33 and 31-34).

If an acute transfusion reaction occurs, take the following steps: (1) stop the transfusion; (2) maintain a patent IV line with saline solution; (3) notify the blood bank and the health care provider immediately; (4) recheck identifying tags and numbers; (5) monitor vital signs and urine output; (6) treat symptoms per physician order; (7) save the blood bag and tubing and send them to the blood bank for examination;

TABLE 31-33 ACUTE TRANSFUSION REACTIONS

Cause	Manifestations	Management	Prevention
Acute Hemolytic Reaction			
Infusion of ABO-incompatible whole blood, RBCs, or components containing ≥10 mL of RBCs. Antibodies in the recipient's plasma attach to antigens on transfused RBCs, causing RBC destruction.	Reactions usually develop in first 15 min. Chills, fever, low back pain, flushing, tachycardia, dyspnea, tachypnea, hypotension, vascular collapse, hemoglobinuria, acute jaundice, dark urine, bleeding, acute kidney injury, shock, cardiac arrest, DIC, death.	Treat shock and DIC if present. Draw blood samples for serologic testing slowly to avoid hemolysis from the procedure. Send urine specimen to the laboratory. Maintain BP with IV colloid solutions. Give diuretics as prescribed to maintain urine flow. Insert indwelling urinary catheter or measure voided amounts to monitor hourly urine output. Dialysis may be required if renal failure occurs. Do not transfuse additional RBC-containing components until blood bank has provided newly crossmatched units.	Meticulously verify and document patient identification from sample collection to component infusion (e.g., visually compare label on sample collection and blood component with patient identification).
Febrile, Nonhemolytic Reaction (most common)			
Sensitization to donor WBCs (most common), platelets, or plasma proteins.	Sudden chills, rigors, and fever (rise in temperature of >1° C), headache, flushing, anxiety, vomiting, muscle pain.	Give antipyretics as prescribed (acetaminophen). Avoid aspirin in thrombocytopenic patients. Do not restart transfusion unless physician orders.	Consider leukocyte-reduced blood products (filtered, washed, or frozen) for patients with a history of two or more such reactions. Give acetaminophen or diphenhydramine (Benadryl) 30 min before transfusion.
Mild Allergic Reaction			
Sensitivity to foreign plasma proteins. More common in people with history of allergies.	Flushing, itching, pruritus, urticaria (hives).	Give antihistamine, corticosteroid, epinephrine, as ordered. If symptoms are mild and transient, transfusion may be restarted slowly with physician's order. Do not restart transfusion if fever or pulmonary symptoms develop.	Treat prophylactically with antihistamines. Consider washed RBCs and platelets.
Anaphylactic and Severe Allergic Reaction			
Sensitivity to donor plasma proteins. Infusion of IgA proteins to IgA-deficient recipient who has developed IgA antibody.	Anxiety, urticaria, dyspnea, wheezing, progressing to cyanosis, bronchospasm, hypotension, shock, and possible cardiac arrest.	Initiate CPR, if indicated. Have epinephrine ready for injection. Antihistamines, corticosteroids, β_2-agonists may also be prescribed. Do not restart transfusion.	Transfuse extensively washed RBC products from which all plasma has been removed. Use blood from IgA-deficient donor. Use autologous components.
Circulatory Overload Reaction			
Fluid administered faster than the circulation can accommodate. People with cardiac or renal disease at risk.	Cough, dyspnea, pulmonary congestion, adventitious breath sounds, headache, hypertension, tachycardia, distended neck veins.	Place patient upright with feet in dependent position. Obtain chest x-ray STAT if ordered. Administer prescribed diuretics, O_2, morphine. Phlebotomy may be indicated.	Adjust transfusion volume and flow rate based on patient size and clinical status. Have blood bank divide future units into smaller aliquots for better spacing of fluid input.
Sepsis Reaction			
Transfusion of bacterially infected blood components.	Rapid onset of chills, high fever, vomiting, diarrhea, marked hypotension, or shock.	Obtain culture of patient's blood and send bag with remaining blood and tubing to blood bank for further study. Treat septicemia as directed—antibiotics, IV fluids, vasopressors.	Collect, process, store, and transfuse blood products according to blood banking standards and infuse within 4 hr of starting time.

TABLE 31-33 ACUTE TRANSFUSION REACTIONS—cont'd

Cause	Manifestations	Management	Prevention
Transfusion-Related Acute Lung Injury (TRALI) Reaction			
Reaction between transfused antileukocyte antibodies and recipient's leukocytes, causing pulmonary inflammation and capillary leak.	Noncardiogenic pulmonary edema. Fever, hypotension, tachypnea, frothy sputum, dyspnea, hypoxemia, respiratory failure. Leading cause of transfusion-related deaths.	Send bag with remaining blood and tubing to blood bank. Draw blood for arterial blood gases and HLA or antileukocyte antibodies. Obtain chest x-ray STAT. Provide O_2 and administer corticosteroids (diuretics of no value) as ordered. Initiate CPR if needed, and provide ventilatory and BP support if needed.	Provide leukocyte-reduced products. Identify donors who are implicated in TRALI reactions and do not allow them to donate.
Massive Blood Transfusion Reaction			
Can occur when replacement of RBCs or blood exceeds the total blood volume within 24 hr. RBC transfusions do not contain clotting factors, albumin, and platelets.	Hypothermia and cardiac dysrhythmias (from rapid infusion of large quantities of cold blood). Citrate toxicity and hypocalcemia (from the use of citrate as a storage solution). Hypocalcemia (citrate binds calcium) manifested as muscle tremors and ECG changes. Hyperkalemia (from potassium leaking from stored RBCs). Manifested as muscle weakness, diarrhea, paresthesias, paralysis of the cardiac or respiratory muscles, and cardiac arrest.	When patients receive massive transfusions of blood products, monitor clotting status and electrolyte levels.	Use blood-warming equipment. Infusion of 10% calcium gluconate (10 mL with every 1 L of citrated blood).

DIC, Disseminated intravascular coagulation; *HLA,* human leukocyte antigen; *IgA,* immunoglobulin A.

TABLE 31-34 DELAYED TRANSFUSION REACTIONS

Manifestations	Prevention and Management	Manifestations	Prevention and Management
Delayed Hemolytic		**Iron Overload**	
Fever, mild jaundice, decreased hemoglobin. Occurs as early as 3 days or as late as several mo, but usually 5-10 days posttransfusion as the result of destruction of transfused RBCs by alloantibodies not detected during crossmatch.	Generally, no acute treatment is required. But hemolysis may be severe enough to warrant further transfusions.	Excess iron is deposited in heart, liver, pancreas, and joints, causing dysfunction. Heart failure, dysrhythmias, impaired thyroid and gonadal function, diabetes, arthritis, cirrhosis. Commonly occurs in patients receiving >100 units for chronic anemia (e.g., sickle cell anemia, β-thalassemia) over time.	Treat symptomatically. Deferoxamine (Desferal), which chelates and removes accumulated iron via the kidneys, administered IV or subcutaneously. Deferasirox (Exjade) and deferiprone (Ferriprox) are oral agents that chelate iron.
Hepatitis B*		**Other**	
Elevated liver enzymes (AST and ALT), anorexia, malaise, nausea and vomiting, fever, dark urine, jaundice. Usually resolves spontaneously within 4-6 wk. Chronic carrier state can develop and result in permanent damage to the liver.	Hepatitis B virus can be detected in donated blood by the presence of hepatitis B surface antigen (HBsAg). Treat symptomatically (see Chapter 44).	Cytomegalovirus (CMV), HIV, human herpesvirus type 6 (HSV-6), Epstein-Barr virus (EBV), human T cell leukemia virus, HTLV-1, and malaria. Most recent threats have been agents that primarily affect animals, but have been transmitted to the blood supply through the food supply, or vectors such as mosquitoes or ticks. These include *Plasmodium* species (malaria), dengue fever virus, West Nile virus, *Trypanosoma cruzi* (Chagas' disease), *Babesia* species (babesiosis), human herpesvirus 8 (KS virus), and variant Creutzfeldt-Jakob disease ("mad cow disease").	Treatment based on the cause. Ways of detecting some of these agents are now available and required, such as the nucleic acid test for West Nile virus and *T. cruzi.* Donor screening has been the only available method to reduce the risk of donor-contaminated blood for others.
Hepatitis C*			
Similar to hepatitis B, but symptoms are usually less severe. Chronic liver disease and cirrhosis may develop.	Before testing of anti-HCV in donated blood, accounted for 90%-95% of all posttransfusion hepatitis. Treat symptomatically (see Chapter 44).		

*New cases of transfusion-related hepatitis B and C are not common.
ALT, Alanine aminotransferase; *AST,* aspartate aminotransferase; *HCV,* hepatitis C virus; *HTLV-1,* human T-cell leukemia virus, type 1; *KS,* Kaposi sarcoma.

(8) collect required blood and urine specimens at intervals based on the hospital policy to evaluate for hemolysis; and (9) document on transfusion reaction form and patient chart. The blood bank and laboratory are responsible for identifying the type of reaction.

Acute Transfusion Reactions. The most common cause of hemolytic reactions is transfusion of ABO-incompatible blood (see Table 31-33). This is an example of a type II cytotoxic hypersensitivity reaction (see Chapter 14). Severe hemolytic reactions are rare. Mislabeling specimens and administering blood to the wrong individual cause most acute hemolytic reactions. This again points to the importance of using proper patient identifiers when drawing blood samples and when administering medications and blood products.

Delayed Transfusion Reactions. Delayed transfusion reactions include delayed hemolytic reactions (discussed previously), infections, and iron overload (see Table 31-34).

Autotransfusion

Autotransfusion, or autologous transfusion, involves removing whole blood from a person and transfusing that blood back into the same person. The problems of incompatibility, allergic reactions, and transmission of disease can be avoided. Methods of autotransfusion include the following:

- *Autologous donation* or *elective phlebotomy* (predeposit transfusion). A person donates blood before a planned surgical procedure. The blood can be frozen and stored for up to 10 years. Usually the blood is stored without being frozen and is given to the person within a few weeks of donation. This technique is especially beneficial to the patient with a rare blood type or for any patient who might be expected to require limited blood product support during a major surgical procedure (e.g., elective orthopedic surgery).
- *Autotransfusion.* A newer method for replacing blood volume involves safely and aseptically collecting, filtering, and returning the patient's own blood lost during a major surgical procedure or from a traumatic injury. This system was originally developed in response to patients' concerns about the safety of blood from blood products. However, today it provides an important way to safely replace volume and stabilize bleeding patients. Collection devices are most often used during surgeries. Some systems allow blood to be automatically and continuously reinfused. Others require collecting the blood for a time (usually no longer than 4 hours) and then reinfusing it.

Drainage after the first 24 hours or drainage that is suspected to contain pathogens should not be reinfused. Anticoagulants may or may not be added before reinfusion. Development of clots after blood is filtered through the collection system can sometimes prevent reinfusion of the blood. Sometimes blood that has been collected has become depleted of its normal coagulation factors. Therefore monitoring coagulation studies in the patient receiving an autotransfusion is important.

CASE STUDY

Leukemia

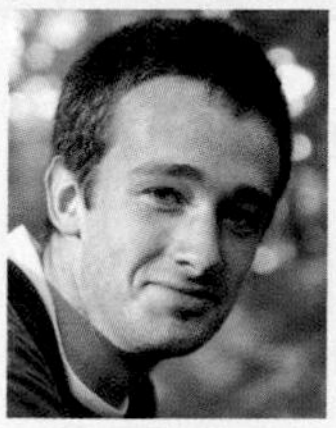

iStockphoto/Thinkstock

Patient Profile

J.J., a 28-year-old white man, had a bad fall while hiking in the nearby hills. He went to the emergency department because of severe bruising from the fall.

Subjective Data

- Complains of oral pain and white patches covering his tongue
- Has had a 2-month history of extreme fatigue, malaise, and flu symptoms
- Complains of shortness of breath and his heart bounding
- Has taken numerous prescribed antibiotics and increased rest and sleep in the past 2 months without relief of symptoms

Objective Data

Physical Examination

- Has bruises and ecchymoses from fall
- Gingiva has petechiae and patchy white spots
- Temperature 102.2° F (39° C), respiratory rate 26/min, pulse 110/min
- Has splenomegaly

Laboratory Results

- Hct 20%
- Hgb 6.9 g/dL
- WBC count 120,000/μL (120×10^9/L)
- Platelet count 25,000/μL (25×10^9/L)

Bone Marrow Biopsy

- Multiple myeloblasts (>50%)

Collaborative Care

- Consultation with a hematologist-oncologist
- Two units of packed red blood cells

Discussion Questions

1. What components of the laboratory test results suggest acute leukemia?
2. How is acute myelogenous leukemia treated?
3. What is J.J.'s prognosis?
4. What are the life-threatening problems that can occur as a result of this disease and treatment? How can you anticipate and assess for these problems?
5. ***Priority Decision:*** What are the priority nursing interventions?
6. ***Priority Decision:*** What are the priorities for patient teaching with a newly diagnosed young adult with leukemia?
7. ***Priority Decision:*** Based on the assessment data presented, what are the priority nursing diagnoses? Are there any collaborative problems?
8. ***Delegation Decision:*** What nursing interventions can the registered nurse (RN) delegate to unlicensed assistive personnel (UAP) while J.J. is getting his blood transfusions?
9. ***Evidence-Based Practice:*** J.J. becomes fatigued after starting chemotherapy. He wants to know if he can still exercise even if he is so fatigued. What is your best advice for him?

evolve Answers available at *http://evolve.elsevier.com/Lewis/medsurg.*

BRIDGE TO NCLEX EXAMINATION

The number of the question corresponds to the same-numbered outcome at the beginning of the chapter.

1. In a severely anemic patient, the nurse would expect to find
   a. dyspnea and tachycardia.
   b. cyanosis and pulmonary edema.
   c. cardiomegaly and pulmonary fibrosis.
   d. ventricular dysrhythmias and wheezing.
2. When obtaining assessment data from a patient with a microcytic, hypochromic anemia, the nurse would question the patient about
   a. folic acid intake.
   b. dietary intake of iron.
   c. a history of gastric surgery.
   d. a history of sickle cell anemia.
3. Nursing interventions for a patient with severe anemia related to peptic ulcer disease include *(select all that apply)*
   a. monitoring stools for guaiac.
   b. instructions for high-iron diet.
   c. taking vital signs every 8 hours.
   d. teaching self-injection of erythropoietin.
   e. administration of cobalamin (vitamin B_{12}) injections.
4. The nursing management of a patient in sickle cell crisis includes *(select all that apply)*
   a. monitoring CBC.
   b. optimal pain management and O_2 therapy.
   c. blood transfusions if required and iron chelation.
   d. rest as needed and deep vein thrombosis prophylaxis.
   e. administration of IV iron and diet high in iron content.
5. A complication of the hyperviscosity of polycythemia is
   a. thrombosis.
   b. cardiomyopathy.
   c. pulmonary edema.
   d. disseminated intravascular coagulation (DIC).
6. When caring for a patient with thrombocytopenia, the nurse instructs the patient to
   a. dab his or her nose instead of blowing.
   b. be careful when shaving with a safety razor.
   c. continue with physical activities to stimulate thrombopoiesis.
   d. avoid aspirin because it may mask the fever that occurs with thrombocytopenia.
7. The nurse would anticipate that a patient with von Willebrand disease undergoing surgery would be treated with administration of vWF and
   a. thrombin.
   b. factor VI.
   c. factor VII.
   d. factor VIII.
8. DIC is a disorder in which
   a. the coagulation pathway is genetically altered, leading to thrombus formation in all major blood vessels.
   b. an underlying disease depletes hemolytic factors in the blood, leading to diffuse thrombotic episodes and infarcts.
   c. a disease process stimulates coagulation processes with resultant thrombosis, as well as depletion of clotting factors, leading to diffuse clotting and hemorrhage.
   d. an inherited predisposition causes a deficiency of clotting factors that leads to overstimulation of coagulation processes in the vasculature.
9. Priority nursing actions when caring for a hospitalized patient with a new-onset temperature of 102.2° F and severe neutropenia include *(select all that apply)*
   a. administering the prescribed antibiotic STAT.
   b. drawing peripheral and central line blood cultures.
   c. ongoing monitoring of the patient's vital signs for septic shock.
   d. taking a full set of vital signs and notifying the physician immediately.
   e. administering transfusions of WBCs treated to decrease immunogenicity.
10. Because myelodysplastic syndrome arises from the pluripotent hematopoietic stem cell in the bone marrow, laboratory results the nurse would expect to find include a(n)
    a. excess of T cells.
    b. excess of platelets.
    c. deficiency of granulocytes.
    d. deficiency of all cellular blood components.
11. The most common type of leukemia in older adults is
    a. acute myelocytic leukemia.
    b. acute lymphocytic leukemia.
    c. chronic myelocytic leukemia.
    d. chronic lymphocytic leukemia.
12. Multiple drugs are often used in combinations to treat leukemia and lymphoma because
    a. there are fewer toxic and side effects.
    b. the chance that one drug will be effective is increased.
    c. the drugs are more effective without causing side effects.
    d. the drugs work by different mechanisms to maximize killing of malignant cells.
13. The nurse is aware that a major difference between Hodgkin's lymphoma and non-Hodgkin's lymphoma is that
    a. Hodgkin's lymphoma occurs only in young adults.
    b. Hodgkin's lymphoma is considered potentially curable.
    c. non-Hodgkin's lymphoma can manifest in multiple organs.
    d. non-Hodgkin's lymphoma is treated only with radiation therapy.
14. A patient with multiple myeloma becomes confused and lethargic. The nurse would expect that these clinical manifestations may be explained by diagnostic results that indicate
    a. hyperkalemia.
    b. hyperuricemia.
    c. hypercalcemia.
    d. CNS myeloma.
15. When reviewing the patient's hematologic laboratory values after a splenectomy, the nurse would expect to find
    a. leukopenia.
    b. RBC abnormalities.
    c. decreased hemoglobin.
    d. increased platelet count.
16. Complications of transfusions that can be decreased by the use of leukocyte depletion or reduction of RBC transfusion are
    a. chills and hemolysis.
    b. leukostasis and neutrophilia.
    c. fluid overload and pulmonary edema.
    d. transmission of cytomegalovirus and fever.

1. a, 2. b, 3. a, b, 4. a, b, c, d, 5. a, 6. a, 7. d, 8. c, 9. a, b, c, d, 10. d, 11. d, 12. d, 13. c, 14. c, 15. d, 16. d

evolve

For rationales to these answers and even more NCLEX review questions, visit *http://evolve.elsevier.com/Lewis/medsurg.*

REFERENCES

1. Marks PW, Glader B: Approach to anemia in the adult and child. In Hoffman R, Silberstein LE, Shattil SJ, et al, editors: *Hematology: basic principles and practice*, ed 5, Philadelphia, 2009, Churchill Livingstone.
2. Rote NS, McCance KL: Alterations of erythrocyte function. In McCance KL, Huether SE, Brashers VL, et al, editors: *Pathophysiology: the biologic basis for disease in adults and children*, ed 6, St Louis, 2010, Mosby.
3. Lichtman MA, Kaushansky K, Kipps TJ, et al: *Williams manual of hematology*, ed 8, New York, 2011, McGraw-Hill.
4. Balducci L: Anemia, fatigue, and aging, *Transf Clin Biol* 17:375, 2010.
5. Goddard AF, James MW, McIntyre AS, et al: Guidelines for the management of iron deficiency anemia, *Gut* 60:1309, 2011.
6. US Department of Health and Human Services, National Heart, Lung, and Blood Institute. Retrieved from *www.nhlbi.nih.gov*.
7. Rote NS, McCance KL: Structure and function of the hematologic system. In McCance KL, Huether SE, Brashers VL, et al, editors: *Pathophysiology: the biologic basis for disease in adults and children*, ed 6, St Louis, 2010, Mosby.
8. American Dietetic Association: B-vitamins and folate: thiamine, riboflavin, and niacin. Retrieved from *www.eatright.org*.
9. US National Library of Medicine, National Institutes of Health, Medline Plus: Copper in diet—pantothenic acid. Retrieved from *www.nlm.nih.gov/medlineplus*.
10. Beutler E: Disorders of iron metabolism. In Lichtman MA, Kipps TJ, Seligsohn U, et al, editors: *Williams hematology*, ed 8, New York, 2010, McGraw-Hill. Retrieved from *www.accessmedicine.com*.
11. Kline NE: Alterations in hematologic function in children. In McCance KL, Huether SE, Brashers VL, et al, editors: *Pathophysiology: the biologic basis for disease in adults and children*, ed 6, St Louis, 2010, Mosby.
12. Ganz T: Anemia of chronic disease. In Lichtman MA, Kipps TJ, Seligsohn U, et al, editors: *Williams hematology*, ed 8, New York, 2010, McGraw-Hill. Retrieved from *www.accessmedicine.com*.

*13. Rogers GM, Becker PS, Bennett CL, et al: Cancer- and chemotherapy-induced anemia, NCCN Clinical Practice Guidelines in Oncology, version 2, 2012. Retrieved from *www.nccn.org*.

14. American Cancer Society: Learn about cancer: aplastic anemia. Retrieved from *www.cancer.org/Cancer/Aplastic Anemia*.
15. Natarajan K, Townes TM, Kutlar A: Disorders of hemoglobin structure: sickle cell anemia and related abnormalities. In Lichtman MA, Kipps TJ, Seligsohn U, et al, editors: *Williams hematology*, ed 8, New York, 2010, McGraw-Hill. Retrieved from *www.accessmedicine.com*.
16. Williams-Johnson J, Williams E: Sickle cell disease and other hereditary hemolytic anemias. In Tintinalli JE, Stapczynski JS, Cline DM, et al, editors: *Tintinalli's emergency medicine: a comprehensives study guide*, ed 7, New York, 2011, McGraw-Hill.
17. Heeney MM, Ware RE: Hydroxyurea for children with sickle cell disease, *Hematol Oncol Clin North Am* 24:199, 2010.
18. Ganz T, Nemeth E: Hepcidin and disorders of iron metabolism, *Ann Rev Med* 62:347, 2011.
19. Doig K: Disorders of iron and heme metabolism. In Rodak BF, Fritsma GA, Keohane EM, editors: *Hematology: clinical principles and application*, ed 4, St Louis, 2012, Mosby.
20. Brittenham GM: Iron-chelating therapy for transfusional iron overload, *N Engl J Med* 364:146, 2011.
21. Prchal JT, Prchal JF: Polycythemia vera. In Lichtman MA, Kipps TJ, Seligsohn U, et al, editors: *Williams hematology*, ed 8, New York, 2010, McGraw-Hill. Retrieved from *www.accessmedicine.com*.
22. Konkle B: Acquired disorders of platelet function, *Hematol Am Soc Hematol Educ Program* 391:391, 2011.
23. Diz-Kucukkaya R, Chen J, Geddis A, et al: Thrombocytopenia. In Lichtman MA, Kipps TJ, Seligsohn U, et al, editors: *Williams hematology*, ed 8, New York, 2010, McGraw-Hill. Retrieved from *www.accessmedicine.com*.
24. Sadler J, Poncz M: Antibody-mediated thrombotic disorders: thrombotic thrombocytopenic purpura and heparin-induced thrombocytopenia. In Lichtman MA, Kipps TJ, Seligsohn U, et al, editors: *Williams hematology*, ed 8, New York, 2010. McGraw-Hill. Retrieved from *www.accessmedicine.com*.

*25. Neunert C, Lim W, Crowther M, et al: The American Society of Hematology 2011 evidence-based practice guidelines for immune thrombocytopenia, *Blood* 117:4190, 2011.

26. Rote NS, McCance KL: Alterations of leukocyte, lymphoid, and hemostatic function. In McCance KL, Huether SE, Brashers VL, et al, editors: *Pathophysiology: the biologic basis for disease in adults and children*, ed 6, St Louis, 2010, Mosby.
27. Imbach P, Crowther M: Thrombopoietin-receptor agonists for primary immune thrombocytopenia, *N Engl J Med* 365:734, 2011.
28. Hemophilia Federation of America: About bleeding disorders. Retrieved from *www.hemophliafed.org*.
29. Roberts HR, Key NS, Escobar MA: Hemophilia A and hemophilia B. In Lichtman MA, Kipps TJ, Seligsohn U, et al, editors: *Williams hematology*, ed 8, New York, 2010, McGraw-Hill. Retrieved from *www.accessmedicine.com*.
30. Fritsma GA: Hemorrhagic coagulation disorders. In Rodak BF, Fritsma GA, Keohane EM: *Hematology: clinical principles and application*, ed 4, St Louis, 2012, Mosby.
31. Chitlur M, Kulkarni R: Hemophilia and related bleeding disorders. In Bope ET, Kellerman RD, editors: *Bope and Kellerman: Conn's current therapy*, Philadelphia, 2012, Saunders.
32. Nathwani AC, Tuddenham EGD, Rangarajan S, et al: Adenovirus-associated virus vector–mediated gene transfer in hemophilia B, *N Engl J Med* 365:2357, 2011.
33. Fritsma GA: Thrombosis risk testing. In Rodak BF, Fritsma GA, Keohane EM, editors: *Hematology: clinical principles and application*, ed 4, St Louis, 2012, Mosby.
34. Baehner RL: Drug-induced neutropenia and agranulocytosis. Retrieved from *www.uptodate.com*.
35. Sivilotti MLA: Hematologic principles. In Nelson LS, Lewin NA, Howland MA, et al, editors: *Goldfrank's toxicologic emergencies*, ed 9, New York, 2011, McGraw-Hill.
36. Klastersky J, Awada A, Paesmans M, et al: Febrile neutropenia: a critical review of the initial management, *Crit Rev Oncol Hematol* 78:185, 2011.

*37. Baden LR, Bensinger W, Angarone M, et al: Prevention and treatment of cancer-related infections, NCCN Clinical Practice Guidelines in Oncology, version 2, 2011. Retrieved from *www.nccn.org*.

*Evidence-based information for clinical practice.

*38. Saria M: Preventing and managing infections in neutropenic stem cell transplantation recipients: evidence-based review, *Clin J Oncol Nurs* 15:133, 2011.
39. Goossen LH: Pediatric and geriatric hematology. In Rodak BF, Fritsma GA, Keohane EM, editors: *Hematology: clinical principles and application*, ed 4, St Louis, 2012, Mosby.
40. Leukemia and Lymphoma Society: Myelodysplastic syndromes. Retrieved from *www.lls.org*.
41. Lindsay M, Beavers J: Myelodysplastic syndromes in older adults, *Clin J Oncol Nurs* 14:545, 2010.
*42. Greenberg PL, Gordeuk V, Issaraqrisil S, et al: Myelodysplastic syndromes, NCCN Clinical Practice Guidelines in Oncology, version 1. 2011, 2012. Retrieved from *www.nccn.org*.
43. Kurtin S: Current approaches to the diagnosis and management of myelodysplastic syndromes, *J Adv Pract Oncol Suppl* 2:7, 2011.
44. Leukemia and Lymphoma Society: Leukemia. Retrieved from *www.lls.org*.
*45. Zelenetz AD, Abramson JS, Advani RH, et al: Non-Hodgkin's lymphomas, NCCN Clinical Practice Guidelines in Oncology, version 4, 2011. Retrieved from *www.nccn.org*.
*46. Estey EH: Acute myeloid leukemia: 2013 update on risk-stratification and management, *Am J Hematol* 88(4):318, 2013.
*47. Jabbour E, Kantarjian H: Chronic myeloid leukemia: 2012 update on diagnosis, monitoring, and management, *Am J Hematol* 87(11):1037, 2012.
48. Pui C: Acute lymphoblastic leukemia. In Lichtman MA, Kipps TJ, Seligsohn U, et al, editors: *Williams hematology*, ed 8, New York, 2010, McGraw-Hill. Retrieved from *www.accessmedicine.com*.
49. Siegel R, Ward E, Brawley O, et al: Cancer statistics, 2011, *CA Cancer J Clin* 61:212, 2011.
50. Horning SJ: Hodgkin lymphoma. In Lichtman MA, Kipps TJ, Seligsohn U, et al: *Williams hematology*, ed 8, New York, 2010, McGraw-Hill. Retrieved from *www.accessmedicine.com*.
*51. Hoppe RT, Advanti RH, Ai WZ, et al: Hodgkin lymphoma, NCCN Clinical Practice Guidelines in Oncology version 3, 2011. Retrieved from *www.nccn.org*.
52. Kipps TJ, Wang H: Acute lymphoblastic leukemia. In Lichtman MA, Kipps TJ, Seligsohn U, et al, editors: *Williams hematology*, ed 8, New York, 2010, McGraw-Hill. Retrieved from *www.accessmedicine.com*.
53. Bragalone DL: *Drug information handbook for oncology*, ed 9, Hudson, Ohio, 2011, Lexicomp.
54. Van Rhee F, Anaissie E, Angtuaco E, et al: Myeloma. In Lichtman MA, Kipps TJ, Seligsohn U, et al, editors: *Williams hematology*, ed 8, New York, 2010, McGraw-Hill. Retrieved from *www.accessmedicine.com*.
*55. Anderson KC, Becker PS, Bennett CL, et al: Multiple myeloma, NCCN Clinical Practice Guidelines in Oncology, version 1, 2012. Retrieved from *www.nccn.org*.
56. Rome SI: Mobility and safety in the multiple myeloma survivor: survivorship care plan of the International Myeloma Foundation Nurse Leadership Board, *Clin J Oncol Nurs* 15(Suppl):41, 2011.
57. Smith L: Hematopoiesis. In Rodak BF, Fritsma GA, Keohane EM, editors: *Hematology: clinical principles and application*, ed 4, St Louis, 2012, Mosby.
58. Nester T, AuBuchon JP: Hemotherapy decisions and their outcomes. In Rodak JD, Grossman BJ, Harris T, et al: *Technical manual: standards for blood banks and transfusion services*, ed 17, Bethesda, Md, 2011, AABB.
59. Lockwood WB, Leonard J, Liles SL: Storage, monitoring, pretransfusion processing, and distribution of blood components. In Rodak JD, Grossman BJ, Harris T, et al: *Technical manual: standards for blood banks and transfusion services*, ed 17, Bethesda, Md, 2011, AABB.
60. Lerner NB, Rafaai MA, Blumberg N: Red cell transfusion. In Lichtman MA, Kipps TJ, Seligsohn U, et al, editors: *Williams hematology*, ed 8, New York, 2010, McGraw-Hill.

RESOURCES

American Hemochromatosis Society
www.americanhs.org
American Sickle Cell Anemia Association
www.ascaa.org
American Society of Hematology
www.hematology.org
Aplastic Anemia & MDS International Foundation, Inc.
www.aamds.org
Hemophilia Federation of America
www.hemophiliafed.org
International Myeloma Foundation
www.myeloma.org
Leukemia and Lymphoma Society
www.lls.org
Managing Myeloma
www.ManagingMyeloma.com
Myelodysplastic Syndromes Foundation
www.mds-foundation.org
National Hemophilia Foundation
www.hemophilia.org
Platelet Disorder Support Association
www.pdsa.org
Sickle Cell Disease Association of America, Inc.
www.sicklecelldisease.org
World Federation of Hemophilia
www.wfh.org

CASE STUDY

Managing Multiple Patients

Introduction

You are working on the oncology unit and have been assigned to care for the following four patients. You have one UAP who is assigned to help you and there are two other RNs on your clinical unit.

Patients

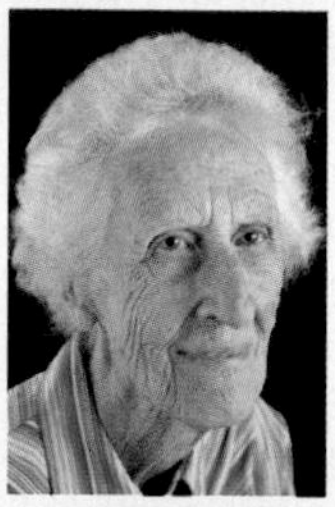

iStockphoto/Thinkstock

A.J. is a 90-year-old white woman who is admitted with severe anemia (Hgb 5.9 g/dL and Hct 18.2%). She prefers to take care of herself with "natural therapy" and has not seen a health care provider for 10 years. A.J. is having difficulty performing ADLs without having to stop and catch her breath. She received 2 units of RBCs and is undergoing further workup to determine the cause of her anemia.

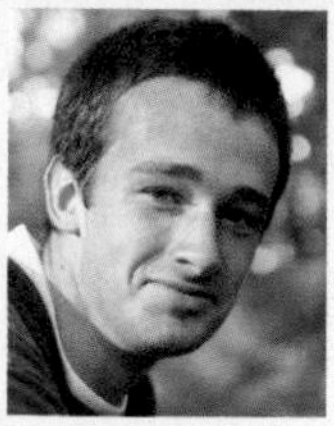

iStockphoto/Thinkstock

J.J. is a 28-year-old white man newly diagnosed with acute myeloblastic leukemia (AML). His most recent vital signs are BP 100/70, temperature 102.2°F (39°C), respiratory rate 26/min, pulse 110. Lab results reveal hematocrit 20%, Hgb 6.9 g/dL, WBC count 120,000/μL (120×10^9/L), and platelet count 25,000/μL (25×10^9/L). He is admitted for blood transfusions and induction therapy.

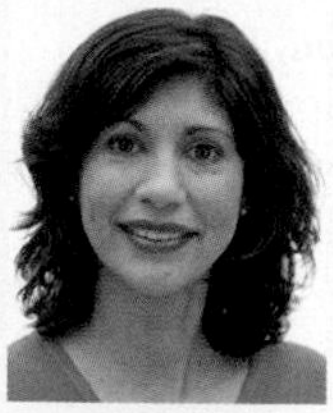

iStockphoto/Thinkstock

P.H. is a 45-year-old woman who is currently receiving chemotherapy for treatment of ovarian cancer. She is admitted with fever and chills. Her WBC count is 2200/μL (2.2×10^9/L) with an absolute neutrophil count of 400/μL (0.4×10^9/L). She is admitted for IV antibiotic therapy and is in protective isolation. Her most recent vital signs are BP 118/60, temperature 99.2°F (37.3°C), respiratory rate 20/min, pulse 98.

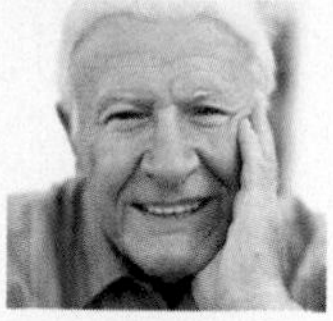

iStockphoto/Thinkstock

G.L. is a 70-year-old man who came to the emergency department yesterday evening with complaints of abdominal pain. A CT scan of the abdomen revealed several masses in his lymphatic system. The physician suspects non-Hodgkin's lymphoma and admits him for a diagnostic workup. He currently rates his pain as a 3 on a scale of 0-10.

Management Discussion Questions

1. ***Priority Decision:*** After receiving report, which patient should you see first? Provide a rationale for your decision.
2. ***Delegation Decision:*** Which task could you delegate to the UAP *(select all that apply)?*
   a. Assist A.J. to a chair after completing her AM care.
   b. Obtain the first unit of blood for J.J. from the blood bank.
   c. Explain the importance of protective isolation to P.H. and her family.
   d. Ask A.J. why she has not been willing to get any medical care for 10 years.
   e. Ask G.L. about the presence of additional clinical manifestations of non-Hodgkin's lymphoma.
3. ***Priority and Delegation Decision:*** When you enter J.J.'s room, you find him somewhat confused and lethargic. His family states he had just had a severe coughing episode. What initial action would be the most appropriate?
   a. Perform a focused neurologic examination.
   b. Call respiratory therapy to give him a breathing treatment.
   c. Ask his family members if they have a copy of his living will.
   d. Have the UAP stay with J.J. while you page the health care provider STAT.

Case Study Progression

J.J.'s health care provider orders a repeat CBC and an emergency CT scan of the head. Your supervisor makes arrangements for another RN to accompany J.J. to the CT scan while you prepare to administer the first unit of RBCs.

4. A.J. is diagnosed with iron-deficiency anemia. The physician orders ferrous sulfate 325 mg TID. You teach A.J. to take her iron *(select all that apply)*
   a. at breakfast time in the morning.
   b. with orange juice to increase absorption.
   c. 1 hour before meals to facilitate absorption.
   d. 2 hours after eating to minimize side effects.
   e. whenever she feels tired or is short of breath with activity.
5. When teaching P.H.'s family about neutropenic precautions, you emphasize that the most important intervention to prevent infection is
   a. hand washing.
   b. wearing a mask.
   c. keeping P.H. in a private room.
   d. limiting the number of visitors in her room.
6. G.L. asks you to explain the diagnostic testing he can expect to undergo related to the suspected lymphoma. Which tests will you explain to him *(select all that apply)?*
   a. PET scan
   b. Bone marrow biopsy
   c. Peripheral blood smear
   d. Excisional lymph node biopsy
   e. Lymphangiography of internal lymph nodes
7. ***Management Decision:*** An RN from the float pool arrives to accompany J.J. to CT scan at the same time the UAP arrives with his first unit of RBCs. Which intervention would be most appropriate?
   a. Put the unit of RBCs in the refrigerator to start when J.J. returns to the floor.
   b. Ask the RN to verify the correct unit of RBCs with you and start the infusion.
   c. Give the RN a SBAR report on J.J. and ask her to start the blood on route to CT scan.
   d. Ask the RN if she would prefer to give the blood or hold it for J.J.'s return to the unit.

evolve Answers available at *http://evolve.elsevier.com/Lewis/medsurg.*

SECTION 7

Problems of Oxygenation: Perfusion

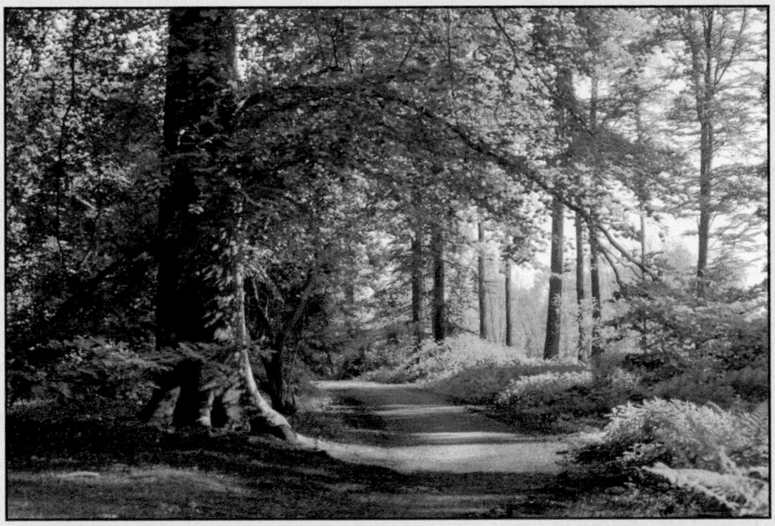

David De Lossy/Photodisc/Thinkstock

The trail is the thing, not the end of the trail.
Travel too fast and you miss all you are traveling for.
Louis L'Amour

CHAPTER 32

Let your heart guide you.
It whispers, so listen closely.
Author Unknown

Nursing Assessment
Cardiovascular System

Angela DiSabatino and Linda Bucher

evolve WEBSITE

http://evolve.elsevier.com/Lewis/medsurg

- NCLEX Review Questions
- Key Points
- Pre-Test
- Answer Guidelines for Case Study in this chapter
- Rationales for Bridge to NCLEX Examination Questions
- Concept Map Creator
- Glossary
- Animations
  - Auscultation of Heart Valves
  - Blood Flow: Circulatory System
  - Cardiac Cycle During Systole and Diastole
  - Pulse Variations
- Videos
  - Auscultation: Cardiac, With Bell
  - Auscultation: Cardiac, With Diaphragm
  - Auscultation: Cardiac, With Diaphragm and Bell
  - Auscultation: Carotid Artery
  - Inspection and Palpation: Cardiac Auscultatory Landmarks
  - Inspection and Palpation: Cardiac, Anterior Chest
  - Inspection and Palpation: Pulses, Lower Extremities
  - Physical Examination: Anterior Chest, Lungs, and Heart
  - Physical Examination: Breasts and Heart
  - Physical Examination: Neck
  - Physical Examination: Precordium and Jugular Veins
  - Physical Examination: Upper Extremities
- Content Updates
- Audio
  - Diastolic Murmur
  - Fourth Heart Sound (S_4)
  - Murmurs: Blowing, Harsh or Rough, and Rumble
  - Murmurs: High, Medium, and Low
  - S_1 at Various Locations
  - S_2 at Various Locations
  - Single S_1
  - Single S_2
  - Systolic Murmur
- Third Heart Sound (S_3)

eFigures
- eFig. 32-1: Types of serum lipids
- eFig. 32-2: Cholesterol delivery

LEARNING OUTCOMES

1. Differentiate the anatomic location and function of the following cardiac structures: pericardial layers, atria, ventricles, semilunar valves, and atrioventricular valves.
2. Relate the coronary circulation to the areas of heart muscle supplied by the major coronary arteries.
3. Differentiate the structure and function of arteries, veins, capillaries, and endothelium.
4. Describe the mechanisms involved in the regulation of blood pressure.
5. Relate the various waveforms on a normal electrocardiogram to the associated cardiac events.
6. Select essential assessment data related to the cardiovascular system that should be obtained from a patient and/or caregiver.
7. Select appropriate techniques to use in the physical assessment of the cardiovascular system.
8. Differentiate normal from abnormal findings of a physical assessment of the cardiovascular system.
9. Link the age-related changes of the cardiovascular system to the differences in assessment findings.
10. Describe the purpose, significance of results, and nursing responsibilities related to diagnostic studies of the cardiovascular system.

KEY TERMS

action potential, p. 687
afterload, p. 689
arterial blood pressure, p. 690
cardiac index (CI), p. 689
cardiac output (CO), p. 689
cardiac reserve, p. 689
coronary angiography, p. 706
diastole, p. 687
diastolic blood pressure (DBP), p. 690
ejection fraction (EF), p. 704
heaves, p. 697
Korotkoff sounds, p. 690
mean arterial pressure (MAP), p. 690
murmur, p. 691
point of maximal impulse (PMI), p. 697
preload, p. 689
pulse pressure, p. 690
systole, p. 689
systolic blood pressure (SBP), p. 690

Reviewed by Jennifer Saylor, RN, PhD, ACNS-BC, Assistant Professor, University of Delaware, Wilmington, Delaware; and Julie Willenbrink, RN, MSN, Assistant Professor of Nursing, Edison State Community College, Piqua, Ohio.

STRUCTURES AND FUNCTIONS OF CARDIOVASCULAR SYSTEM

Heart

Structure. The heart is a four-chambered hollow muscular organ normally about the size of a fist. It lies within the thorax in the mediastinal space that separates the right and left pleural cavities. The heart is composed of three layers: a thin inner lining, the *endocardium;* a layer of muscle, the *myocardium;* and an outer layer, the *epicardium.* The heart is covered by a fibroserous sac called the *pericardium.* This sac consists of two layers: the inside *(visceral)* layer of the pericardium (part of the epicardium) and the outer *(parietal)* layer. A small amount of pericardial fluid (approximately 10 to 15 mL) lubricates the space between the pericardial layers *(pericardial space)* and prevents friction between the surfaces as the heart contracts.[1]

The heart is divided vertically by the septum. The interatrial septum creates a right and left atrium, and the interventricular septum creates a right and left ventricle. The thickness of the wall of each chamber is different. The atrial myocardium is thinner than that of the ventricles, and the left ventricular wall is two or three times thicker than the right ventricular wall.[1] The thickness of the left ventricle is necessary to produce the force needed to pump the blood into the systemic circulation.

Blood Flow Through Heart. The blood flow through the heart is illustrated in Fig. 32-1.

Cardiac Valves. The four valves of the heart serve to keep blood flowing in a forward direction. The cusps of the mitral and tricuspid valves are attached to thin strands of fibrous tissue termed *chordae tendineae* (Fig. 32-2). Chordae are anchored in the papillary muscles of the ventricles. This support system prevents the eversion of the leaflets into the atria during ventricular contraction. The pulmonic and aortic valves (also known as *semilunar valves*) prevent blood from regurgitating into the ventricles at the end of each ventricular contraction.

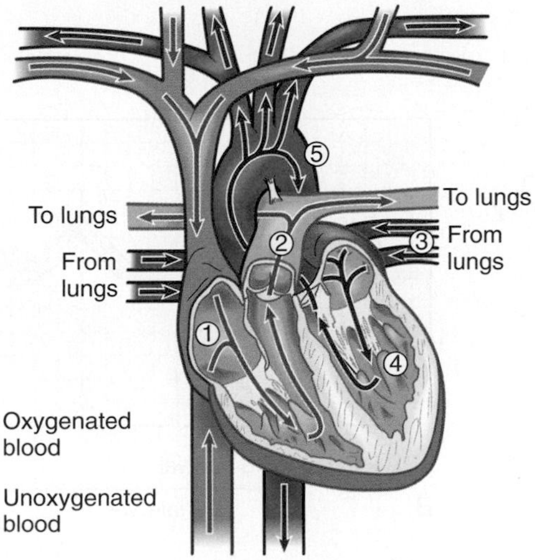

FIG. 32-1 Schematic representation of blood flow through the heart. *Arrows* indicate direction of flow. *1,* The right atrium receives venous blood from the inferior and superior venae cavae and the coronary sinus. The blood then passes through the tricuspid valve into the right ventricle. *2,* With each contraction, the right ventricle pumps blood through the pulmonic valve into the pulmonary artery and to the lungs. *3,* Oxygenated blood flows from the lungs to the left atrium by way of the pulmonary veins. *4,* It then passes through the mitral valve and into the left ventricle. *5,* As the heart contracts, blood is ejected through the aortic valve into the aorta and thus enters the systemic circulation.

Blood Supply to Myocardium. The myocardium has its own blood supply, the *coronary circulation* (Fig. 32-3). Blood flow into the two major coronary arteries occurs primarily during **diastole** (relaxation of the myocardium). The left coronary artery arises from the aorta and divides into two main branches: the left anterior descending artery and the left circumflex artery. These arteries supply the left atrium, the left ventricle, the interventricular septum, and a portion of the right ventricle. The right coronary artery also arises from the aorta, and its branches supply the right atrium, the right ventricle, and a portion of the posterior wall of the left ventricle. In 90% of people the atrioventricular (AV) node and the bundle of His receive blood supply from the right coronary artery. For this reason, blockage of this artery often causes serious defects in cardiac conduction.

The divisions of coronary veins parallel the coronary arteries. Most of the blood from the coronary system drains into the coronary sinus (a large channel), which empties into the right atrium near the entrance of the inferior vena cava.

Conduction System. The conduction system is specialized nerve tissue responsible for creating and transporting the electrical impulse, or **action potential.** This impulse starts depolarization and subsequently cardiac contraction (Fig. 32-4, *A*). The electrical impulse is normally started by the sinoatrial (SA) node (the pacemaker of the heart). Each impulse coming from the SA node travels through interatrial pathways to depolarize the atria, resulting in a contraction.

The electrical impulse travels from the atria to the AV node through internodal pathways. The excitation then moves through the bundle of His and the left and right bundle branches. The left bundle branch has two fascicles (divisions): anterior and posterior. The action potential moves through the walls of both ventricles by means of *Purkinje fibers.* The ventricular conduction system delivers the impulse within 0.12 second. This triggers a synchronized right and left ventricular contraction.

The result of the cardiac cycle is the ejection of blood into the pulmonary and systemic circulations. It ends with repolarization when the contractile fiber cells and the conduction pathway cells regain their resting polarized condition. Cardiac

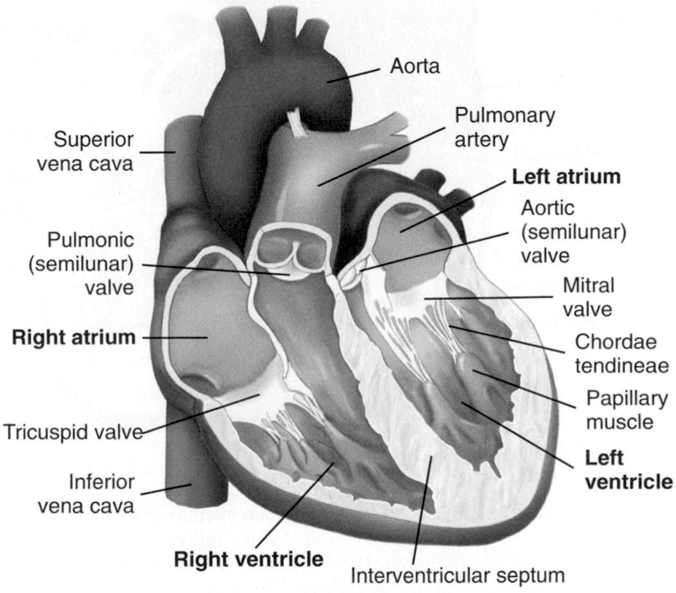

FIG. 32-2 Anatomic structures of the heart and heart valves.

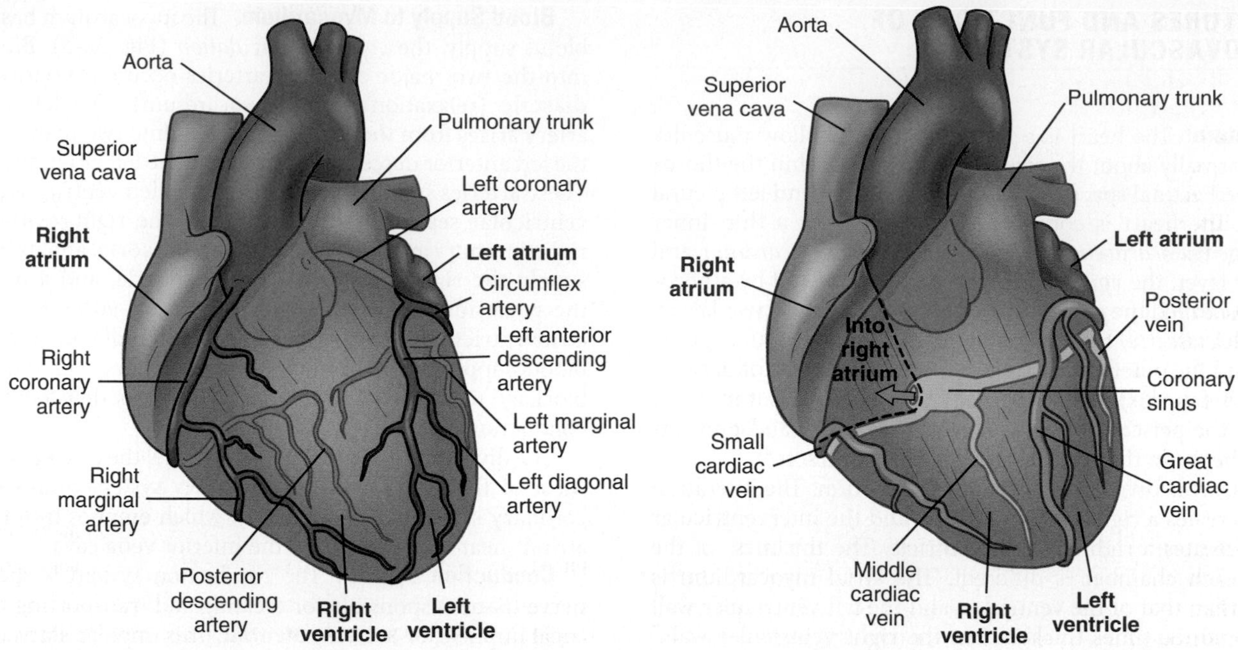

FIG. 32-3 Coronary arteries and veins.

muscle cells have a compensatory mechanism that makes them unresponsive or refractory to restimulation during the action potential. During ventricular contraction, there is an *absolute refractory period* during which cardiac muscle does not respond to any stimuli. After this period, cardiac muscle gradually recovers its excitability, and a *relative refractory period* occurs by early diastole.

Electrocardiogram. The electrical activity of the heart can be detected on the body surface using electrodes and is recorded on an electrocardiogram (ECG). The letters P, QRS, T, and U are used to identify the separate waveforms (Fig. 32-4, *B*). The first wave, P, begins with the firing of the SA node and represents depolarization of the atria. The QRS complex represents depolarization from the AV node throughout the ventricles. There is a delay of impulse transmission through the AV node that accounts for the time between the beginning of the P wave and the beginning of the QRS wave. The T wave represents repolarization of the ventricles. The U wave, if seen, may repre-

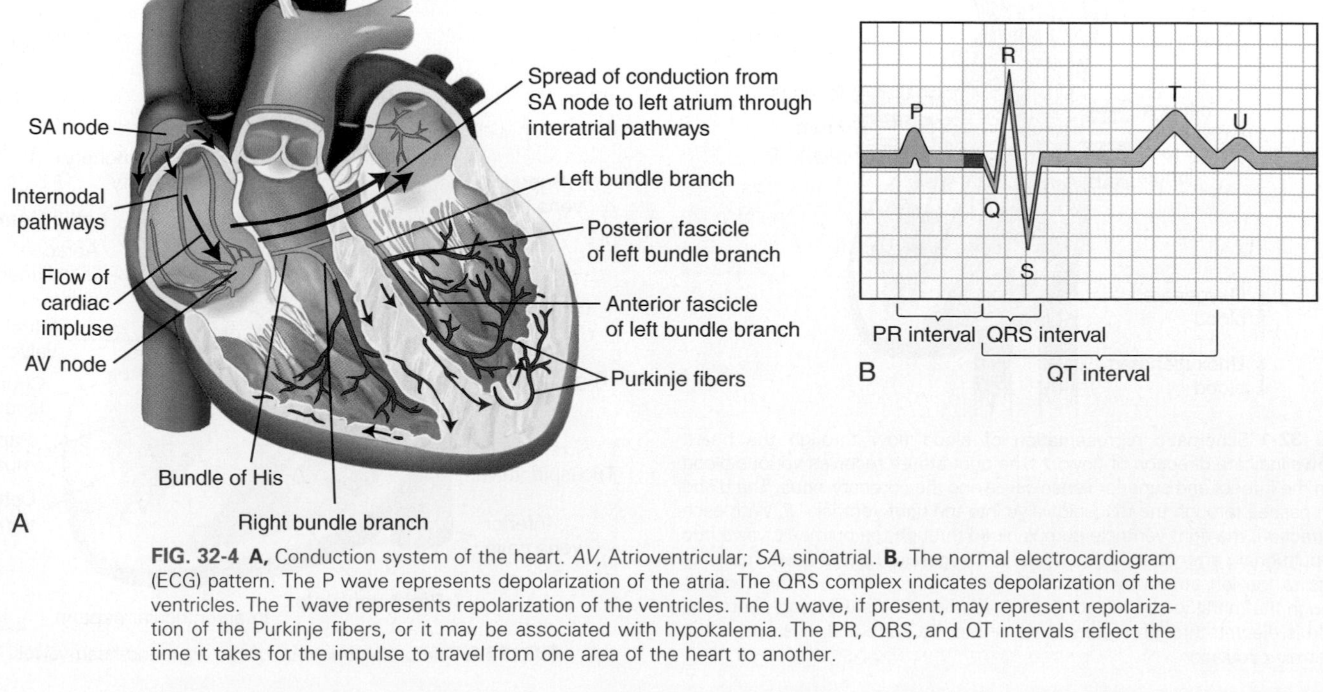

FIG. 32-4 A, Conduction system of the heart. *AV,* Atrioventricular; *SA,* sinoatrial. **B,** The normal electrocardiogram (ECG) pattern. The P wave represents depolarization of the atria. The QRS complex indicates depolarization of the ventricles. The T wave represents repolarization of the ventricles. The U wave, if present, may represent repolarization of the Purkinje fibers, or it may be associated with hypokalemia. The PR, QRS, and QT intervals reflect the time it takes for the impulse to travel from one area of the heart to another.

sent repolarization of the Purkinje fibers, or it may be associated with hypokalemia.[2]

Intervals between these waves (PR, QRS, and QT intervals) reflect the time it takes for the impulse to travel from one area of the heart to another. These time intervals can be measured, and changes from these time references often indicate pathologic conditions. (See Chapter 36 for a complete discussion of ECG monitoring.)

Mechanical System. *Depolarization* triggers mechanical activity. Systole, contraction of the myocardium, results in ejection of blood from the ventricles. Relaxation of the myocardium, *diastole,* allows for filling of the ventricles. Cardiac output (CO) is the amount of blood pumped by each ventricle in 1 minute. It is calculated by multiplying the amount of blood ejected from the ventricle with each heartbeat—the *stroke volume* (SV)—by the heart rate (HR) per minute:

$$CO = SV \times HR$$

For the normal adult at rest, CO is maintained in the range of 4 to 8 L/min. Cardiac index (CI) is the CO divided by the body surface area (BSA). The CI adjusts the CO to the body size. The normal CI is 2.8 to 4.2 L per minute per meter squared (L/min/m^2).

Factors Affecting Cardiac Output. Numerous factors can affect either the HR or the SV, and thus the CO. The HR, which is controlled primarily by the autonomic nervous system, can reach as high as 180 beats/minute for short periods without harmful effects. The factors affecting the SV are preload, contractility, and afterload. Increasing preload, contractility, and afterload increases the workload of the myocardium, resulting in increased oxygen demand.

Frank-Starling law states that, to a point, the more the myocardial fibers are stretched, the greater their force of contraction. The volume of blood in the ventricles at the end of diastole, before the next contraction, is called preload. Preload determines the amount of stretch placed on myocardial fibers. Preload can be increased by a number of conditions such as myocardial infarction, aortic stenosis, and hypervolemia.[3] Contractility can be increased by epinephrine and norepinephrine released by the sympathetic nervous system. Increasing contractility raises the SV by increasing ventricular emptying.

Afterload is the peripheral resistance against which the left ventricle must pump. Afterload is affected by the size of the ventricle, wall tension, and arterial blood pressure (BP). If the arterial BP is elevated, the ventricles meet increased resistance to ejection of blood, increasing the work demand. Eventually this results in *ventricular hypertrophy,* an enlargement of the cardiac muscle tissue without an increase in CO or the size of chambers (see Fig. 35-1, *B*).

Cardiac Reserve. The cardiovascular system must respond to numerous situations in health and illness (e.g., exercise, stress, hypovolemia). The ability to respond to these demands by altering CO is termed cardiac reserve.

Vascular System

Blood Vessels. The three major types of blood vessels in the vascular system are the arteries, veins, and capillaries. Arteries, except for the pulmonary artery, carry oxygenated blood away from the heart. Veins, except for the pulmonary veins, carry deoxygenated blood toward the heart. Small branches of arteries and veins are arterioles and venules, respectively. Blood circulates from the left side of the heart into arteries, arterioles, capillaries, venules, and veins, and then back to the right side of the heart.

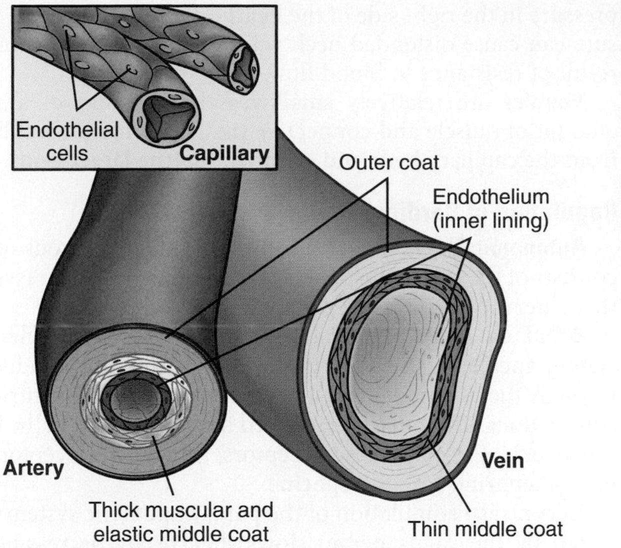

FIG. 32-5 Comparative thickness of layers of the artery, vein, and capillary.

Arteries and Arterioles. The arterial system differs from the venous system by the amount and type of tissue that make up arterial walls (Fig. 32-5). The large arteries have thick walls composed mainly of elastic tissue. This elastic property cushions the impact of the pressure created by ventricular contraction and provides recoil that propels blood forward into the circulation. Large arteries also contain some smooth muscle. Examples of large arteries are the aorta and the pulmonary artery.

Arterioles have relatively little elastic tissue and more smooth muscle. Arterioles serve as the major control of arterial BP and distribution of blood flow. They respond readily to local conditions such as low oxygen (O_2) and increasing levels of carbon dioxide (CO_2) by dilating or constricting.

The innermost lining of the arteries is the endothelium. The endothelium serves to maintain hemostasis, promote blood flow, and, under normal conditions, inhibit blood coagulation. When the endothelial surface is disrupted (e.g., rupture of an atherosclerotic plaque), the coagulation cascade is initiated and results in the formation of a fibrin clot.

Capillaries. The thin capillary wall is made up of endothelial cells, with no elastic or muscle tissue (see Fig. 32-5). The exchange of cellular nutrients and metabolic end products takes place through these thin-walled vessels. Capillaries connect the arterioles and venules.

Veins and Venules. Veins are large-diameter, thin-walled vessels that return blood to the right atrium (see Fig. 32-5). The venous system is a low-pressure, high-volume system. The larger veins contain semilunar valves at intervals to maintain the blood flow toward the heart and to prevent backward flow. The amount of blood in the venous system is affected by a number of factors, including arterial flow, compression of veins by skeletal muscles, alterations in thoracic and abdominal pressures, and right atrial pressure.

The largest veins are the *superior vena cava,* which returns blood to the heart from the head, neck, and arms, and the *inferior vena cava,* which returns blood to the heart from the lower part of the body. These large-diameter vessels are affected by the pressure in the right side of the heart. Elevated right atrial pressure can cause distended neck veins or liver engorgement as a result of resistance to blood flow.

Venules are relatively small vessels made up of a small amount of muscle and connective tissue. Venules collect blood from the capillary beds and channel it to the larger veins.

Regulation of Cardiovascular System

Autonomic Nervous System. The autonomic nervous system consists of the sympathetic nervous system and the parasympathetic nervous system (see Chapter 56).

Effect on Heart. Stimulation of the sympathetic nervous system increases the HR, the speed of impulse conduction through the AV node, and the force of atrial and ventricular contractions. This effect is mediated by specific sites in the heart called beta (β)-adrenergic receptors, which are receptors for norepinephrine and epinephrine.

In contrast, stimulation of the parasympathetic system (mediated by the vagus nerve) slows the HR by decreasing the impulses from the SA node, and thus conduction through the AV node.

Effect on Blood Vessels. The source of neural control of blood vessels is the sympathetic nervous system. The alpha$_1$ (α_1)-adrenergic receptors are located in vascular smooth muscles. Stimulation of α_1-adrenergic receptors results in vasoconstriction. Decreased stimulation to α_1-adrenergic receptors causes vasodilation. (Sympathetic nervous system receptors that influence BP are presented in Table 33-1.)

The parasympathetic nerves have selective distribution in the blood vessels. For example, blood vessels in skeletal muscle do not receive parasympathetic input.

Baroreceptors. *Baroreceptors* in the aortic arch and carotid sinus (at the origin of the internal carotid artery) are sensitive to stretch or pressure within the arterial system. Stimulation of these receptors (e.g., volume overload) sends information to the vasomotor center in the brainstem. This results in temporary inhibition of the sympathetic nervous system and enhancement of the parasympathetic influence, causing a decreased HR and peripheral vasodilation. Decreased arterial pressure causes the opposite effect.

Chemoreceptors. *Chemoreceptors* are located in the aortic and carotid bodies and the medulla. They are capable of causing changes in respiratory rate and BP in response to increased arterial CO_2 pressure (hypercapnia) and, to a lesser degree, decreased plasma pH (acidosis) and arterial O_2 pressure (hypoxia). When the chemoreceptors in the medulla are triggered, they stimulate the vasomotor center to increase BP.[4]

Blood Pressure

The **arterial blood pressure** is a measure of the pressure exerted by blood against the walls of the arterial system. The **systolic blood pressure (SBP)** is the peak pressure exerted against the arteries when the heart contracts. The **diastolic blood pressure (DBP)** is the residual pressure in the arterial system during ventricular relaxation (or filling). BP is usually expressed as the ratio of systolic to diastolic pressure.

The two main factors influencing BP are *cardiac output* (CO) and *systemic vascular resistance* (SVR):

$$BP = CO \times SVR$$

SVR is the force opposing the movement of blood. This force is created primarily in small arteries and arterioles. Normal blood pressure is SBP less than 120 mm Hg and DBP less than 80 mm Hg[5] (see Chapter 33).

Measurement of Arterial Blood Pressure. BP can be measured by invasive and noninvasive techniques. The invasive technique consists of catheter insertion into an artery. The catheter is attached to a transducer, and the pressure is measured directly (see Chapter 66).

Noninvasive, indirect measurement of BP can be done with a sphygmomanometer and a stethoscope. The sphygmomanometer consists of an inflatable cuff and a pressure gauge. The BP is measured by auscultating for sounds of turbulent blood flow through a compressed artery (termed **Korotkoff sounds**). The brachial artery is the recommended site for taking a BP.

After placing the appropriate size cuff on the upper arm, inflate the cuff to a pressure 20 to 30 mm Hg above the SBP. This causes blood flow in the artery to cease. If the SBP is not known, estimate the pressure by palpating the brachial pulse and inflating the cuff until the pulse ceases. The pressure noted at this time is the estimated SBP. Inflate the BP cuff 20 to 30 mm Hg above this number.

As the pressure in the cuff is lowered, auscultate the artery for Korotkoff sounds. There are five phases of Korotkoff sounds. The first phase is a tapping sound caused by the spurt of blood into the constricted artery as the pressure in the cuff is gradually deflated. This sound is noted as the SBP. The fifth phase occurs when the sound disappears, which is noted as the DBP.[6] BP is recorded as SBP/DBP (e.g., 120/80 mm Hg). Sometimes, an *auscultatory gap* occurs, which is a loss of sound between the SBP and the DBP. Proper BP technique (e.g., using the correct cuff size, positioning arm at heart level) is essential for accurate readings[6] (see Table 33-11).

Another noninvasive way to measure BP indirectly is an automated device that uses oscillometric measurements to assess BP. Though this method does not involve auscultation, the same attention to proper technique is essential for accuracy. Finally, SBP (and pulse) can be assessed using a Doppler ultrasonic flowmeter. The hand-held transducer is positioned over the artery (identified by audible, pulsatile sounds). The cuff is applied above the artery, inflated until the sounds disappear, and then another 20 to 30 mm Hg beyond that point. The cuff is then slowly deflated until sounds return. This point is the SBP.[6]

Pulse Pressure and Mean Arterial Pressure. **Pulse pressure** is the difference between the SBP and DBP. It is normally about one third of the SBP. If the BP is 120/80 mm Hg, the pulse pressure is 40 mm Hg. An increased pulse pressure due to an increased SBP may occur during exercise or in individuals with atherosclerosis of the larger arteries. A decreased pulse pressure may be found in heart failure or hypovolemia.

Another measurement related to BP is **mean arterial pressure (MAP)**. The MAP refers to the average pressure within the arterial system that is felt by organs in the body. It is not the average of the diastolic and systolic pressures because the length of diastole exceeds that of systole at normal HRs. MAP is calculated as follows:

$$MAP = (SBP + 2\,DBP) \div 3$$

A person with a BP of 120/60 mm Hg has an estimated MAP of 80 mm Hg. In patients with invasive BP monitoring, this value is automatically calculated and takes the patient's HR into consideration (see Chapter 66).

An MAP greater than 60 mm Hg is needed to adequately perfuse and sustain the vital organs of an average person under most conditions. When the MAP falls below this number for a period of time, vital organs are underperfused and will become ischemic.

GERONTOLOGIC CONSIDERATIONS

EFFECTS OF AGING ON THE CARDIOVASCULAR SYSTEM

One of the greatest risk factors for cardiovascular disease (CVD) is age. CVD remains the leading cause of death in adults older than age 85. It is the most common cause of hospitalization and the second leading cause of death in adults younger than age 85. The most common cardiovascular problem is coronary artery disease (CAD) secondary to atherosclerosis. It is difficult to separate normal aging changes from the pathophysiologic changes of atherosclerosis. Many of the physiologic changes in the cardiovascular system of older adults are a result of the combined effects of the aging process, disease, environmental factors, and lifetime health behaviors rather than just age alone.[7]

Age-related changes in the cardiovascular system and differences in assessment findings are presented in Table 32-1. With increased age, the amount of collagen in the heart increases and elastin decreases. These changes affect the myocardium's ability to stretch and contract. One of the major changes in the cardiovascular system is the response to physical or emotional stress. In times of increased stress, CO and SV decrease due to reduced contractility and HR response. The resting supine HR is not markedly affected by aging. When the patient changes positions (e.g., sits upright), the sympathetic nerve pathway may be affected by fibrous tissue and fatty deposits, resulting in a blunted HR response.[7]

Cardiac valves become thicker and stiffer from lipid accumulation, degeneration of collagen, and fibrosis. The aortic and mitral valves are most frequently affected. These changes result in either regurgitation of blood when the valve should be closed or narrowing of the orifice of the valve (stenosis) when the valve should be open. The turbulent blood flow across the affected valve results in a **murmur.**

The number of pacemaker cells in the SA node decreases with age. By age 75, a person may have only 10% of the normal number of pacemaker cells. Although this is compatible with adequate SA node function, it may account for the frequency of some sinus dysrhythmias in older adults. Similar decreases also occur in the number of conduction cells in the internodal tracts, bundle of His, and bundle branches. These changes contribute to the development of atrial dysrhythmias and heart blocks. About 50% of older adults have an abnormal resting ECG that shows increases in the PR, QRS, and/or QT intervals.[8]

The autonomic nervous system control of the cardiovascular system changes with aging. The number and function of β-adrenergic receptors in the heart decrease with age. So the older adult not only has a decreased response to physical and emotional stress, but also is less sensitive to β-adrenergic agonist drugs. The lower maximum HR during exercise results in only a twofold increase in CO compared with the three or four times increase seen in younger adults.

Arterial and venous blood vessels thicken and become less elastic with age.[9] Arteries increase their sensitivity to vasopressin (antidiuretic hormone). With aging both of these changes contribute to a progressive increase in SBP and a decrease or no change in DBP. Thus an increase in the pulse pressure is found. Hypertension is not a normal consequence of aging, and should be treated. Valves in the large veins in the lower extremities have a reduced ability to return the blood to the heart, often resulting in dependent edema.

Orthostatic hypotension, which is estimated to be present in more than 30% of patients over age 70 with systolic hypertension, may be related to medications and/or decreased baroreceptor function.[8] *Postprandial hypotension* (decrease in BP of at least 20 mm Hg that occurs within 75 minutes after eating) may also occur in about a third of otherwise healthy older adults. Both orthostatic and postprandial hypotension may be related to falls in older adults. Despite the changes associated with aging, the heart is able to function adequately under most circumstances.

TABLE 32-1 GERONTOLOGIC ASSESSMENT DIFFERENCES

Cardiovascular System

Changes	Differences in Assessment Findings
Chest Wall	
Kyphosis	Altered chest landmarks for palpation, percussion, and auscultation. Distant heart sounds.
Heart	
Myocardial hypertrophy, ↑ collagen and scarring, ↓ elastin	↓ Cardiac reserve, heart failure.
Downward displacement	Difficulty in isolating apical pulse
↓ CO, HR, SV in response to exercise or stress	↓ Response to exercise and stress. Slowed recovery from activity.
Cellular aging and fibrosis of conduction system	↓ Amplitude of QRS complex and slight. lengthening of PR, QRS, and QT intervals. Irregular cardiac rhythms, ↓ maximal HR, ↓ HR variability.
Valvular rigidity from calcification, sclerosis, or fibrosis, impeding complete closure of valves	Systolic murmur (aortic or mitral) possible without an indication of cardiovascular disease.
Blood Vessels	
Arterial stiffening caused by loss of elastin in arterial walls, thickening of intima of arteries, and progressive fibrosis of media	↑ In systolic BP and possible ↑ or ↓ in diastolic BP. Possible widened pulse pressure. Pedal pulses diminished. ↑ In intermittent claudication.
Venous tortuosity increased	Inflamed, painful, or cordlike varicosities. Dependent edema.

ASSESSMENT OF CARDIOVASCULAR SYSTEM

Subjective Data

A careful health history and physical examination will help you distinguish symptoms that reflect a cardiovascular problem from problems of other body systems. Explore and document all cues that alert you to the possibility of underlying cardiovascular problems.

Important Health Information

History of Present Illness. Ask the patient what problem has brought him or her to the health care facility or provider.

CASE STUDY

Patient Introduction

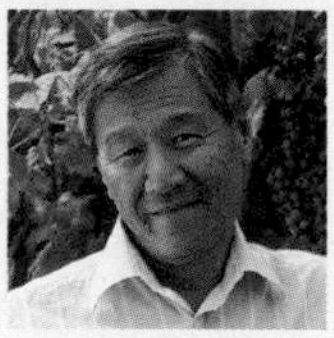

Jupiterimages/Banana-Stock/Thinkstock

L.P., a 63-year-old Asian American man, is brought to the emergency department by ambulance at 6 AM after calling 911 with complaints of chest pain, shortness of breath (SOB), palpitations, and dizziness. The paramedics have started an IV and oxygen at 2 L/min via nasal cannula. They also administered four chewable baby ASA and a nitroglycerin tablet, and they obtained a 12-lead ECG. L.P. is pain free on arrival but still complains of palpitations and dizziness.

Critical Thinking

As you read through this assessment chapter, think about L.P.'s symptoms with the following questions in mind:

1. What are the possible causes of L.P.'s chest pain, SOB, palpitations, and dizziness?
2. What would be your major focus when assessing L.P.?
3. What questions would you ask L.P.?
4. What should be included in the physical assessment? What would you be looking for?
5. What diagnostic studies would you expect to be ordered?

evolve Answers available at *http://evolve.elsevier.com/Lewis/medsurg.*

Fully explore all symptoms the patient is experiencing (see Table 32-1).

Past Health History. Many illnesses affect the cardiovascular system directly or indirectly. Ask the patient about a history of chest pain, shortness of breath, fatigue, alcohol and tobacco use, anemia, rheumatic fever, streptococcal throat infections, congenital heart disease, stroke, palpitations, dizziness with position changes, syncope, hypertension, thrombophlebitis, intermittent claudication, varicosities, and edema.

Medications. Assess the patient's current and past use of medications. This includes over-the-counter (OTC) drugs, herbal supplements, and prescription drugs. For example, aspirin prolongs the blood clotting time, and is found in many drugs used to treat cold symptoms. List all of the patient's drugs. Include dosage, time of last dose, and the patient's understanding of the drug's purpose and side effects. Many noncardiac drugs can adversely affect the cardiovascular system and should be assessed (Table 32-2).

Surgery or Other Treatments. Ask the patient about specific treatments, past surgeries, or hospital admissions related to cardiovascular problems. Explore any admissions or outpatient procedures for diagnostic workups or cardiovascular symptoms. Note whether an ECG or a chest x-ray has been done for baseline data.

Functional Health Patterns. The strong correlation between components of a patient's lifestyle and cardiovascular health supports the need to review each functional health pattern. Key questions to ask a person with a cardiovascular problem are listed in Table 32-3.

Health Perception–Health Management Pattern. Ask the patient about the presence of major cardiovascular risk factors. These include abnormal serum lipids, hypertension, sedentary lifestyle, diabetes mellitus, obesity, and tobacco use. If a patient uses tobacco, estimate the number of pack-years of tobacco use (number of packs smoked per day multiplied by the number of years the patient has smoked). Document the patient's attitude about tobacco use and attempts and methods used to stop. Record any alcohol use. This information should include type

TABLE 32-2 CARDIOVASCULAR EFFECTS OF NONCARDIAC DRUGS*

Drug Classification	Examples	Cardiovascular Effects
Anticancer agents	daunorubicin (Cerubidine) doxorubicin (Adriamycin)	Dysrhythmias, cardiomyopathy
Antipsychotics	chlorpromazine (Thorazine) haloperidol (Haldol)	Dysrhythmias, orthostatic hypotension
Corticosteroids	cortisone (Cortone) prednisone (Orasone)	Hypotension, edema, potassium depletion
Hormone therapy, oral contraceptives	estrogen + progestin (Ortho-Novum, Prempro, Tri-Norinyl)	Myocardial infarction, thromboembolism, stroke, hypertension
Nonsteroidal antiinflammatory drugs (NSAIDs) †	ibuprofen (Motrin) celecoxib (Celebrex)	Hypertension, myocardial infarction, stroke
Psychostimulants	cocaine amphetamines	Tachycardia, angina, myocardial infarction, hypertension, dysrhythmias
Tricyclic antidepressants	amitriptyline (Elavil) doxepin (Sinequan)	Dysrhythmias, orthostatic hypotension

*List is not all-inclusive.

†Second-generation NSAIDs, known as COX-2 inhibitors, have been linked to an increased risk of serious adverse cardiovascular events.

of alcohol, amount, frequency, and any changes in the reaction to it. Also note any use of habit-forming drugs, including recreational drugs.

Question the patient about any allergies, including food and environmental allergies. Determine whether the patient has ever experienced a drug reaction or an allergic or anaphylactic reaction. Ask specifically about any allergic reaction to contrast media if there is a chance that a cardiac catheterization may be needed.

GENETIC RISK ALERT

Coronary Artery Disease

- Specific genetic links, especially related to lipoprotein genes, have been identified for some families with CAD.
- The clustering of CAD in families is strong if there is early age of onset affecting several relatives.

Cardiomyopathy

- Hypertrophic cardiomyopathy can be caused by autosomal dominant mutations.
- Dilated cardiomyopathy can be caused by autosomal and X-linked dominant mutations.

Hypertension

- Hypertension results from a complex interplay between genetic and environmental factors.
- Lifestyle choices (e.g., smoking, lack of exercise) may trigger genetic tendencies to hypertension.

Confirmed illnesses of blood relatives can highlight any genetic or familial tendencies toward CAD, peripheral vascular disease, hypertension, bleeding, cardiac disorders, diabetes mellitus, atherosclerosis, and stroke. Note any family members who developed cardiac disease younger than age 55. In addition, disorders affecting the vascular system, such as intermittent claudication and varicosities, may be familial. Finally, assess any family health history of noncardiac problems such as asthma,

TABLE 32-3 HEALTH HISTORY

Cardiovascular System

Health Perception–Health Management
- Do you practice any preventive measures to decrease risk factors for heart disease?*
- Have you noticed an increase in heart symptoms such as chest pain or dyspnea?*
- Does your heart problem cause you to be less able to care for yourself?*
- Do you foresee any potential self-care problems because of your heart problem?*
- Have you ever used tobacco? If yes, in what form, how much, and for how long? Have you tried to quit? If yes, what methods have you tried? Are you interested in more information about quitting?
- How often and how much alcohol do you drink?

Nutritional-Metabolic
- Describe your usual daily diet, including salt, fat, and liquid intake.
- What is your present weight? What was your weight 1 year ago? If different, explain.
- Does eating cause fatigue or shortness of breath?*

Elimination
- Do your feet or ankles ever swell?* If yes, how far up your legs? Does it go away after sleeping all night?
- Have you ever taken medication to help you get rid of excess fluid or to relieve constipation?*
- Are you having any problems related to urination?*
- Do you ever strain to have a bowel movement?

Activity-Exercise
- Are your daily activities or exercise limited because of your heart problem?*
- When were you last able to comfortably perform your usual activities or exercise?
- Do you experience any discomfort or side effects as a result of exercise or any activity?*
- Can you comfortably walk and talk at the same time?
- How often do you attend activities outside your home?
- What was your most strenuous activity in the last few weeks compared with 6 months ago?

Sleep-Rest
- How many pillows do you sleep on at night? Has this changed recently?*
- Do you ever wake up suddenly and feel as if you cannot catch your breath?*
- Do you have a history of sleep apnea?*
- How many times a night do you awaken to urinate?

Cognitive-Perceptual
- Do you ever experience dizziness or fainting?*
- Do you ever find it difficult to verbally express yourself or to remember things?*
- Do you experience any pain (e.g., chest pain, leg pain with activity) as a result of your heart problem?*

Self-Perception–Self-Concept
- Have your perceptions of yourself changed since you were diagnosed with a heart disease?*
- How has your heart disease affected the quality of your life?

Role-Relationship
- Has this illness affected any of the roles that you play in your daily life?*
- How have your significant others been affected by your heart disease?

Sexuality-Reproductive
- Has your heart disease caused a change in your sexual activity?*
- Do you experience any heart-related symptoms during sexual activity?*
- Do any of your medications affect your ability to participate in sexual activities?*
- Females: Are you currently taking oral contraceptives, hormonal therapy, or drug therapy for breast cancer?

Coping–Stress Tolerance
- Describe your normal coping mechanisms during times of stress or anxiety.
- To whom or where would you turn during a time of stress? Are these people or services helping you now?*
- Do you practice any stress reduction techniques?*
- Do you have a history of depression?*
- Do you feel capable of handling your present health situation?
- Do you experience any heart symptoms (e.g., chest pain, palpitations) during times of stress or anger?*

Values-Beliefs
- What influence have your values or beliefs had during your illness?
- Do you feel any conflicts between your values or beliefs and the plan of care?*
- Describe any cultural or religious beliefs that may influence the management of your heart problem.

*If yes, describe.

renal disease, liver disease, and obesity because they can affect the cardiovascular system.

Nutritional-Metabolic Pattern. Being underweight or overweight may indicate potential cardiovascular problems. Thus it is important to assess the patient's weight history (e.g., over the past year) in relation to height. Determine the amount of salt and saturated fats in the patient's typical diet. In addition to actual food habits, which may be influenced by culture, investigate the patient's attitudes and plans relative to diet and weight management.

Elimination Pattern. The patient on diuretics may report increased voiding and/or nocturia. Investigate any history of incontinence or constipation, including any use of medications (prescribed and OTC) for constipation. Teach patients with cardiovascular problems to avoid straining during a bowel movement (Valsalva maneuver). Ask patients if they have any swelling of the lower extremities and if it resolves when their feet are elevated or after an overnight sleep.

Activity-Exercise Pattern. The benefit of exercise for cardiovascular health is clear, with aerobic exercise being most beneficial. Record the types of exercise done and the duration, intensity, and frequency of each. Ask about and note the occurrence of any symptoms during exercise (e.g., chest pain, shortness of breath, claudication) that may indicate a cardiovascular problem.

Sleep-Rest Pattern. Cardiovascular problems often disrupt sleep. *Paroxysmal nocturnal dyspnea* (attacks of shortness of breath, especially ones at night that awaken the patient) and Cheyne-Stokes respiration are associated with heart failure. Many patients with heart failure need to sleep with their head elevated on pillows or in a chair. Note the number of pillows needed to sleep or the need to sleep upright *(orthopnea)* and whether this has changed recently.

Sleep apnea has been associated with an increased risk of life-threatening dysrhythmias, especially in patients with heart failure. Nocturia, a common finding with cardiovascular patients, also interrupts normal sleep patterns. Fully explore both conditions.

Cognitive-Perceptual Pattern. It is important to ask both the patient and the caregiver about cognitive-perceptual problems. Cardiovascular problems such as dysrhythmias, hypertension, and stroke may cause problems with syncope, language, and memory. Report any pain associated with the cardiovascular system (e.g., chest pain, claudication).

Self-Perception–Self-Concept Pattern. If a cardiovascular event is acute, the patient's self-perception may be affected. Invasive diagnostic procedures often lead to body image concerns for the patient. When CVD is chronic, the patient may not be able to identify the cause but can often describe the inability to "keep up" previous levels of activity. This may also affect the patient's quality of life, so inquire about the effects of the illness on the patient.

Role-Relationship Pattern. The patient's gender, race, and age are all related to cardiovascular health. In addition, the patient's marital status, role in the household, employment status, number of children and their ages, living environment, and caregivers help you to identify strengths and support systems in the patient's life. Assess the patient's level of satisfaction or dissatisfaction with life roles, since this may alert you to possible areas of stress or conflict.

Sexuality-Reproductive Pattern. Ask the patient about the effect of the cardiovascular problem on sexual activity. Because older patients often fear sudden death during sexual intercourse, it may lead to changes in their sexual behavior. Fatigue, chest pain, or shortness of breath may also limit sexual activity. Erectile dysfunction (ED) may be a symptom of peripheral vascular disease and/or a side effect of some medications used to treat CVD (e.g., β-adrenergic blockers [beta blockers], diuretics). Ask about the use of drugs for ED (e.g., sildenafil [Viagra]). These drugs are contraindicated if the patient is also taking a nitrate because the combination of ED drugs and nitrates can cause significant hypotension.[10] Determine whether counseling may be helpful.

Ask female patients if they use oral contraceptives, hormone therapy (HT) for symptoms of menopause, or drug therapy for breast cancer. Women who smoke and use oral contraceptives are at increased risk for blood clots (e.g., venous thromboembolism). Similarly, there is an increased risk for CVD with the use of HT and selective estrogen-receptor modulators (e.g., tamoxifen [Novaldex]).[11]

Coping–Stress Tolerance Pattern. Ask the patient to identify areas that cause stress and the usual methods of coping with stress. Potentially stressful areas include health concerns, marital relationships, family and friends, occupation, and finances.

Work-related stress, depression, and inadequate social support are risk factors for CVD and cardiac events.[4] Ask the patient about each of these factors. Information about support systems such as family, extended family and friends, counselors, or religious groups can provide vital insight when planning care.

Values-Belief Pattern. Individual values and beliefs, which are greatly affected by culture, may play a significant role in the real or potential conflict a patient faces when dealing with a diagnosis of CVD. Some patients may attribute their illness to punishment from God; others may think that a "higher power" may assist them. Information about a patient's values and beliefs will help you intervene during periods of crisis.

CASE STUDY—cont'd

Subjective Data

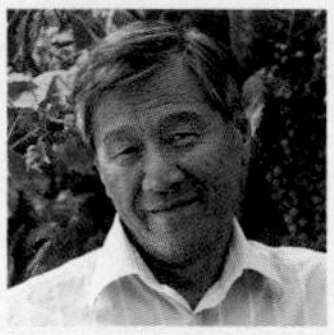

Jupiterimages/Banana-Stock/Thinkstock

A focused subjective assessment of L.P. revealed the following information:

- ***PMH:*** History of hypertension, mitral valve prolapse with mild regurgitation, heart failure, and type 2 diabetes mellitus.
- ***Medications:*** Lisinopril (Prinivil) 10 mg/day PO, metoprolol (Lopressor) 50 mg PO BID, ASA 325 mg/day PO, furosemide (Lasix) 40 mg/day PO, and glipizide (Glucotrol) 5 mg/day PO.
- ***Health Perception–Health Management:*** L.P. denies any previous history of chest pain or CAD. He was feeling fine until this morning when he awoke and experienced SOB, chest pain, palpitations, and dizziness while walking to the bathroom. He became frightened that he was having a heart attack so called 911. Denies smoking or alcohol intake. SOB and chest pain are now gone, but he continues to feel palpitations and dizziness when he sits up.
- ***Elimination:*** Denies any edema. States takes Lasix in the morning and typically "pees until lunchtime." Denies nocturia.

Objective Data

Physical Examination

Vital Signs. After you observe the patient's general appearance, obtain vital signs. Measure BP bilaterally. These readings normally vary from 5 to 15 mm Hg. Use the arm with the highest BP for subsequent BP measurements. Take orthostatic (postural) BPs and HRs while the patient is supine, sitting with legs dangling, and standing. SBP should not decrease more than 20 mm Hg from the supine to the standing position. HR should not increase more than 20 beats/minute from the supine to the standing position.

Peripheral Vascular System

Inspection. Inspect the skin for color, hair distribution, and venous pattern. Inspect the extremities for conditions such as edema, dependent rubor, clubbing of the nail beds, varicosities, and lesions such as stasis ulcers. Edema in the extremities can be caused by gravity, interruption of venous return, or right-sided heart failure.

Inspect the large veins in the neck (internal and external jugular) while the patient is gradually elevated from a supine position to an upright (30 to 45 degrees) position. Distention and prominent pulsations of these neck veins, referred to as *jugular venous distention,* can be caused by right-sided heart failure.

Palpation. Palpate the upper and lower extremities for temperature, moisture, pulses, and edema bilaterally to assess for symmetry. Look for edema by depressing the skin over the tibia or medial malleolus for 5 seconds. Normally, there is no depression after releasing pressure. If pitting edema is present, grade it from 1+ (mild pitting, slight brief indentation) to 4+ (very deep pitting, indentation that lasts a long time).[6]

Palpate the pulses in the neck and extremities for information on arterial blood flow. Assess the rhythm (e.g., regular, irregular) and force. It is important to palpate each carotid pulse separately to avoid vagal stimulation and possible dysrhythmias. Compare the characteristics of the arteries on the right and left extremities simultaneously to determine symmetry.

When palpating the arteries identified in Fig. 32-6, rate the force of the pulse using the following scale[6]:

0 = Absent
1+ = Weak
2+ = Normal
3+ = Increased, full, bounding

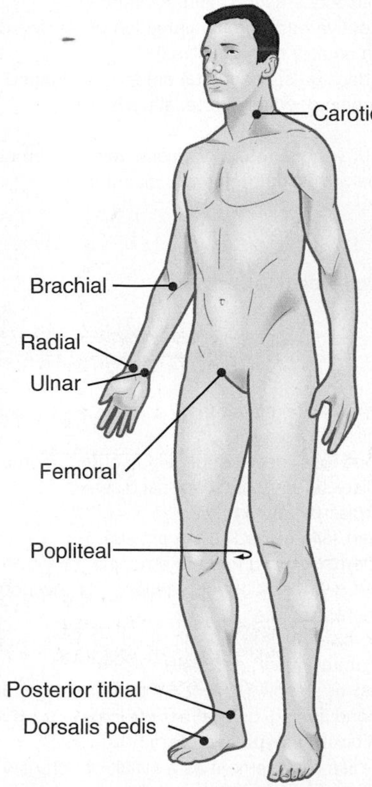

FIG. 32-6 Common sites for palpating arteries.

The rigidity (hardness) of the vessel should also be noted. The normal pulse feels like a tap, whereas a vessel wall that is narrowed or bulging vibrates. The term for a palpable vibration is *thrill.*

Capillary refill is used to assess arterial flow to the extremities. Position the patient's hands near the level of the heart and squeeze a nail bed to produce blanching. Observe for the return of color. This should occur in less than 2 seconds with normal peripheral perfusion and CO.

Auscultation. An artery that is narrowed or has a bulging wall may create turbulent blood flow. This abnormal flow can create a buzzing or humming termed a *bruit.* This is heard with a stethoscope placed over the vessel. Auscultation of major arteries such as the carotid arteries, abdominal aorta, and femoral arteries should be part of the initial cardiovascular assessment. Abnormalities of the cardiovascular system are described in Table 32-4.

Thorax

Inspection and Palpation. An overall inspection and palpation of the bony structures of the thorax are the initial steps in the examination. Next, inspect and palpate the areas where the cardiac valves project their sounds by identifying the intercostal spaces (ICSs). The raised notch, the *angle of Louis,* is where the manubrium and the body of the sternum are joined, and is located at the level of the second rib. It is palpable in the midline of the sternum. It is used to count ICSs and locate specific auscultatory areas (Fig. 32-7).

Locate the following auscultatory areas: the aortic area in the second ICS to the right of the sternum, the pulmonic area in the second ICS to the left of the sternum, the tricuspid area in the fifth left ICS close to the sternum, and the mitral area in the left midclavicular line at the fifth ICS. A fifth auscultatory area is *Erb's point,* located at the third left ICS near the sternum. Normally, no pulsations are felt in these areas unless the patient has a thin chest wall.

A valvular disorder may be suspected if abnormal pulsations or thrills are felt. Next, inspect and palpate the epigastric area, which lies on either side of the midline just below the xiphoid

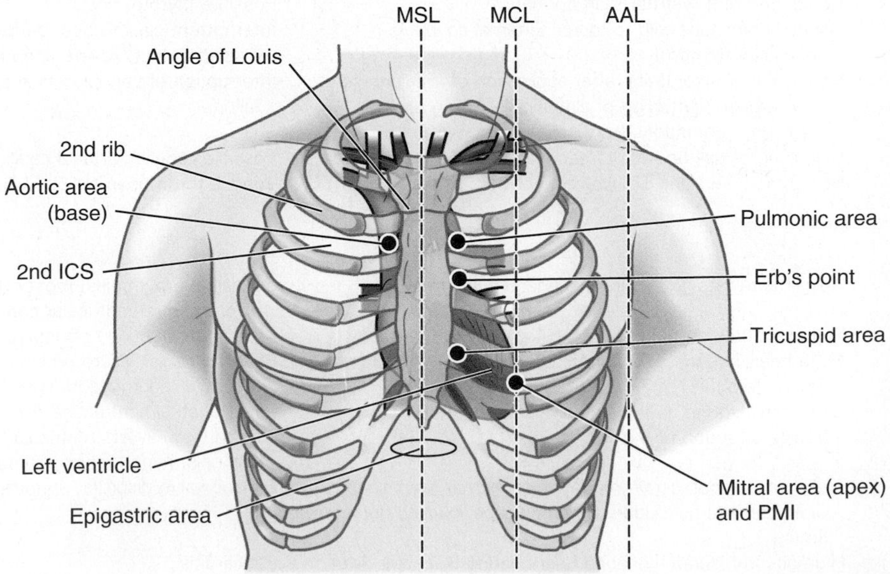

FIG. 32-7 Orientation of the heart within the thorax and cardiac auscultatory areas. *Red lines* indicate the midsternal line *(MSL),* midclavicular line *(MCL),* and anterior axillary line *(AAL). ICS,* Intercostal space; *PMI,* point of maximal impulse.

TABLE 32-4 ASSESSMENT ABNORMALITIES

Cardiovascular System

Finding*	Description	Possible Etiology* and Significance
Inspection		
Jugular venous distention	Distended neck (jugular) veins with patient sitting at 30- to 45-degree angle	Elevated right atrial pressure, right-sided heart failure
Central cyanosis	Bluish or purplish tinge in central areas such as tongue, conjunctivae, inner surface of lips	Inadequate O_2 saturation of arterial blood because of pulmonary or cardiac disorders (e.g., congenital defects)
Peripheral cyanosis	Bluish or purplish tinge in extremities or in nose and ears	Reduced blood flow because of heart failure, vasoconstriction, cold environment
Splinter hemorrhages	Small red to black streaks under fingernails	Infective endocarditis (infection of endocardium, usually in area of cardiac valves)
Clubbing of nail beds	Obliteration of normal angle between base of nail and skin	Endocarditis, congenital defects, prolonged O_2 deficiency
Color changes in extremities with postural change	Pallor, cyanosis, mottling of skin after limb elevation. Dependent rubor (reddish blue discoloration). Glossy skin	Chronic decreased arterial perfusion
Ulcers	*Venous:* Necrotic crater-like lesion usually found on lower leg at medial malleolus. Characterized by slow wound healing *Arterial:* Pale ischemic base, well-defined edges usually found on toes, heels, lateral malleoli	Poor venous return, varicose veins, incompetent venous valves. Arteriosclerosis, diabetes
Varicose veins	Visible dilated, discolored, tortuous vessels in lower extremities	Incompetent valves in vein
Palpation		
Pulse		
Bounding	Sharp, brisk, pounding pulse	Hyperkinetic states (e.g., anxiety, fever), anemia, hyperthyroidism
Thready	Weak, slowly rising pulse easily obliterated by pressure	Blood loss, decreased cardiac output, aortic valve disease, peripheral arterial disease
Irregular	Regularly irregular or irregularly irregular. Skipped beats	Cardiac dysrhythmias
Pulsus alternans	Regular rhythm, but strength of pulse varies with each beat	Heart failure, cardiac tamponade
Absent	Lack of pulse	Atherosclerosis, trauma, embolus
Thrill	Vibration of vessel or chest wall	Aneurysm, aortic regurgitation, arteriovenous fistula
Rigidity	Stiffness or inflexibility of vessel wall	Atherosclerosis
>100 beats/min	Tachycardia	Exercise, anxiety, shock, need for increased cardiac output, hyperthyroidism
<60 beats/min	Bradycardia	Rest or sleeping, SA or AV node damage, athletic conditioning, side effect of drugs (e.g., β-adrenergic blockers), hypothyroidism
Displaced point of maximal impulse (apical pulse)	Point of maximal impulse is palpated (or auscultated) below the fifth ICS and to the left of the MCL	Cardiac enlargement as a result of coronary artery disease, heart failure, cardiomyopathy
Extremities		
Unusually warm extremities	Hands and feet warmer than normal	Possible thyrotoxicosis
Cold extremities	Hands and/or feet cold to touch. External covering necessary for comfort	Intermittent claudication, peripheral arterial disease, low cardiac output, severe anemia
Pitting edema of lower extremities or sacral area	Visible finger indentation after application of firm pressure, weight gain, tightening of clothing, including shoes, marks or indentations from constricting garments	Interruption of venous return to heart, right-sided heart failure
Abnormal capillary refill	Blanching of nail bed for ≥2 sec after release of pressure	Possible reduced arterial capillary perfusion, anemia
Asymmetry in limb circumference	Measurable swelling of involved limb	Venous thromboembolism, varicose veins, lymphedema
Auscultation		
Pulse deficit	Apical heart rate exceeding peripheral pulse rate	Cardiac dysrhythmias, most often atrial fibrillation/flutter or premature ventricular contractions
Arterial bruit	Turbulent flow sound in peripheral artery	Arterial obstruction or aneurysm
Third heart sound (S_3)	Extra heart sound, low pitched, heard in early diastole. Similar to sound of a gallop	Left ventricular failure. Volume overload. Mitral, aortic, or tricuspid regurgitation. Hypertension (possible)
Fourth heart sound (S_4)	Extra heart sound, low pitched, heard in late diastole. Similar to sound of a gallop	Forceful atrial contraction from resistance to ventricular filling (e.g., in left ventricular hypertrophy, aortic stenosis, hypertension, coronary artery disease)
Cardiac murmurs	Turbulent sounds occurring between normal heart sounds. Characterized by loudness, pitch, shape, quality, duration, timing	Cardiac valve disorder, abnormal blood flow patterns
Pericardial friction rub	High-pitched, scratchy sound heard during S_1 and/or S_2 at the apex. Heard best with patient sitting and leaning forward, and at the end of expiration	Pericarditis

*Limited to common assessment findings and etiologic factors. (Further discussion of conditions listed may be found in Chapters 33 to 38, 66, and 67.)

of corticosteroids, sex hormones, and bile salts. In addition to being absorbed from food in the gastrointestinal tract, cholesterol can also be synthesized in the liver. Phospholipids contain glycerol, fatty acids, phosphates, and a nitrogenous compound. Although formed in most cells, phospholipids usually enter the circulation as lipoproteins synthesized by the liver. Apoproteins are water-soluble proteins that combine with most lipids to form lipoproteins.

Different classes of lipoproteins contain varying amounts of the naturally occurring lipids. These include the following:

1. *Chylomicrons:* primarily exogenous triglycerides from dietary fat
2. *Low-density lipoproteins (LDLs):* mostly cholesterol with moderate amounts of phospholipids
3. *High-density lipoproteins (HDLs):* about 50% protein and 50% phospholipids and cholesterol
4. *Very-low-density lipoproteins (VLDLs):* primarily endogenous triglycerides with moderate amounts of phospholipids and cholesterol

Text continued on p. 704

TABLE 32-6 DIAGNOSTIC STUDIES

Cardiovascular System

Study	Description and Purpose	Nursing Responsibility
Blood Studies*		
Troponin (cardiac)	Contractile proteins that are released after an MI. Both troponin T and troponin I are highly specific to cardiac tissue. *Reference intervals:* ***Troponin I (cTnI)*** Negative: <0.5 ng/mL (<0.5 mcg/L) Indeterminate or suspicious for injury to myocardium: 0.5-2.3 ng/mL (0.5-2.3 mcg/L) Positive for myocardial injury: >2.3 ng/mL (>2.3 mcg/L) ***Troponin T (cTnT)*** <0.1 ng/mL (<0.1 mcg/L)	Rapid point-of-care (bedside) assays are available. Explain to patient the purpose of serial sampling (e.g., q6-8hr × 3) in conjunction with CK-MB and serial ECGs.
CK-MB	Cardiospecific isozyme that is released in the presence of myocardial tissue injury. Concentrations >4%-6% of total creatine kinase (CK) are highly indicative of MI. Serum levels increase within 4-6 hr after MI.	Serial sampling often done in conjunction with troponin and ECGs.
Myoglobin	Low-molecular-weight protein that is 99%-100% sensitive for myocardial injury. Serum concentrations rise 30-60 min after MI. *Reference interval:* *Male:* 15.2-91.2 mcg/L *Female:* 11.1-57.5 mcg/L	Cleared from the circulation rapidly, limited use in the diagnosis of cardiac injury/infarction.
C-reactive protein (CRP)	Marker of inflammation that can predict risk of cardiac disease and cardiac events, even in patients with normal lipid values. High-sensitivity (hs) CRP assay used. *Lowest risk:* <1 mg/L *Moderate risk:* 1-3 mg/L *High risk:* >3 mg/L	Stable levels that can be measured nonfasting and any time during the day. May be more predictive risk factor of cardiovascular disease than LDLs for women. The average of two assays obtained 2 wk apart provides a more stable measurement than one single measurement.
Homocysteine	Amino acid produced during protein catabolism that has been identified as a risk factor for cardiovascular disease. Homocysteine may cause damage to the endothelium or have a role in formation of thrombi. *Reference interval:* *Male:* 5.2-12.9 μmol/L *Female:* 3.7-10.4 μmol/L	Hyperhomocysteinemia resulting from dietary deficiencies is treated with folic acid, vitamin B_6, and vitamin B_{12} supplements.
b-Type natriuretic peptide (BNP)	Peptide that causes natriuresis. Elevation helps to distinguish cardiac vs. respiratory cause of dyspnea. *Reference interval:* *BNP* (diagnostic for heart failure) >100 pg/mL (28.8 pmol/L)	Infusion of nesiritide (Natrecor) elevates levels temporarily.
NT-Pro-BNP	Aids in assessing the severity of heart failure in symptomatic and asymptomatic patients. *Reference interval:* *≤74 yr:* 124 pg/mL *>75 yr:* 449 pg/mL	In patients with renal insufficiency, NT-pro-BNP concentrations may increase and may not correlate with New York Heart Association functional classification of heart failure.
Serum Lipids		
Cholesterol	A blood lipid. Elevated cholesterol is considered a risk factor for cardiovascular heart disease. *Reference interval:* <200 mg/dL (<5.18 mmol/L) (varies with age and gender)	Cholesterol levels can be obtained in a nonfasting state.

*Reference ranges for the laboratory tests vary by institution because of differences in equipment and reagents used.

Continued

TABLE 32-6 DIAGNOSTIC STUDIES—cont'd

Cardiovascular System

Study	Description and Purpose	Nursing Responsibility
Serum Lipids—cont'd		
Triglycerides	Mixtures of fatty acids. Elevations are associated with cardiovascular disease and diabetes. *Reference interval:* <150 mg/dL (<1.7 mmol/L) (varies with age)	Triglyceride and lipoprotein levels must be obtained in a fasting state (at least 12 hr, except for water). Alcohol should be withheld for 24 hr before testing.
Lipoproteins† (HDL, LDL)	Electrophoresis is done to separate lipoproteins into HDL and LDL. There are marked day-to-day fluctuations in serum lipid levels. More than one determination is needed for accurate diagnosis and treatment. *Reference intervals* (vary with age): **HDL** *Recommended* *Male:* >40 mg/dL (>1.04 mmol/L) *Female:* >50 mg/dL (>1.3 mmol/L) *Low risk for CAD:* ≥60 mg/dL (>1.55 mmol/L) *High risk for CAD:* <40 mg/dL (<1.04 mmol/L) **LDL** *Recommended:* <100 mg/dL (<2.6 mmol/L) *Near optimal:* 100-129 mg/dL (2.6-3.34 mmol/L) *Moderate risk for CAD:* 130-159 mg/dL (3.37-4.12 mmol/L) *High risk for CAD:* >160 mg/dL (>4.14 mmol/L)	Risk for cardiac disease is assessed by dividing the total cholesterol level by the HDL level and obtaining a ratio. *Low risk:* Ratio <3 *Average risk:* Ratio 3-5 *Increased risk:* Ratio >5
Lipoprotein (a) [Lp(a)]	Increased levels are associated with an increased risk of premature CAD and stroke. *Reference interval:* <30 mg/dL (<0.3 g/L)	Lp(a) levels can be obtained in a nonfasting state.
Lipoprotein-associated phospholipase A_2 (Lp-PLA_2)	Elevated levels of Lp-PLA_2 are associated with vascular inflammation and increased risk for CAD. Serum levels of Lp-PLA_2 are measured by the PLAC test. *Reference interval:* *Male:* 131-376 ng/mL *Female:* 120-342 ng/mL	Lp-PLA_2 levels can be obtained in a nonfasting state.
Chest X-Ray	Patient is placed in two upright positions to examine the lung fields and heart size. The two common positions are posteroanterior (PA) and lateral. Normal heart size and contour for the individual's age, sex, and size are noted.	Inquire about frequency of recent x-rays and possibility of pregnancy. Provide lead shielding to areas not being viewed. Remove any jewelry or metal objects that may obstruct the view of the heart and lungs.
12-Lead ECG	Electrodes are placed on the chest and extremities, allowing the ECG machine to record cardiac electrical activity from 12 different views. A resting 12-lead ECG can identify conduction problems, dysrhythmias, position of heart, cardiac hypertrophy, pericarditis, myocardial ischemia or infarction, pacemaker activity, and effectiveness of drug therapy at one point in time.	Prepare skin and apply electrodes and leads. Position patient supine (or with head of bed elevated, if short of breath). Inform patient that no discomfort is involved and to lie still to decrease motion artifact.
Signal-averaged ECG (SAECG)	A high-resolution ECG that can identify electrical activity called late potentials, indicating a patient is at risk for developing ventricular dysrhythmias (e.g., ventricular tachycardia).	Same as for 12-lead ECG.
Ambulatory ECG Monitoring		
Holter monitoring	Recording of ECG rhythm for 24-48 hr and then correlating rhythm changes with symptoms and activities recorded in diary. Normal patient activity is encouraged to simulate conditions that produce symptoms. Electrodes are placed on chest, and a recorder is used to store information until it is recalled, printed, and analyzed for any rhythm disturbance. It can be performed on an inpatient or outpatient basis.	Prepare skin and apply electrodes and leads. Explain importance of keeping an accurate diary of activities and symptoms. Tell patient that no bath or shower can be taken during monitoring. Skin irritation may develop from electrodes.
Event monitor or loop recorder	Records rhythm disturbances that are not frequent enough to be recorded in one 24-hr period. It allows more freedom than a regular Holter monitor. Some units have electrodes that are attached to the chest and have a loop of memory that captures the onset and end of an event. Other types are placed directly on patient's wrist, chest, or fingers and have no loop of memory, but record the patient's ECG in real time. Recordings may be transmitted over the phone to a receiving unit.	Instruct in the use of equipment for recording and transmitting (if appropriate) of transient events. Teach patient about skin preparation for lead placement or steady skin contact for units not requiring electrodes. This will ensure the reception of optimal ECG tracings for analysis. Instruct patient to initiate recording as soon as symptoms begin or as soon thereafter as possible.

†Source: American Heart Association: What your cholesterol levels mean, 2009. Available at *www.americanheart.org/presenter.jhtml?identifier=183#HDL.*

TABLE 32-6 **DIAGNOSTIC STUDIES—cont'd**

Cardiovascular System

Study	Description and Purpose	Nursing Responsibility
Exercise or Stress Testing	Various protocols are used to evaluate the effect of exercise tolerance on cardiovascular function. A common protocol uses 3-min stages at set speeds and elevation of the treadmill belt. The patient can exercise to either predicted peak HR (calculated by subtracting the person's age from 220) or to peak exercise tolerance, at which time the test is terminated. The test is also terminated for chest discomfort, significant increase or decrease in vital signs from baseline, or significant ECG changes indicating cardiac ischemia. Vital signs and ECG are monitored. The ECG is monitored after exercise for rhythm disturbances or, if ECG changes occurred with exercise, for return to baseline. Continual monitoring of vital signs and ECG rhythms for ischemic changes is important in the diagnosis of CAD. An exercise bike may be used if the patient is unable to walk on the treadmill.	Instruct patient to wear comfortable clothes and shoes that can be used for walking and running. Instruct patient about procedure and importance of reporting any symptoms that occur. Monitor vital signs and obtain 12-lead ECG before exercise, during each stage of exercise, and after exercise until all vital signs and ECG changes have returned to normal. Monitor patient's response throughout procedure. Contraindications include any reasons patient is unable to reach peak exercise tolerance. β-Adrenergic blockers may be held 24 hr before the test because they blunt the HR and limit the patient's ability to achieve maximal HR. Caffeine-containing food and fluids are held for 24 hr. Patients must refrain from smoking and strenuous exercise for 3 hr before test.
6-Minute walk test	Distance patient is able to walk on a flat surface in 6 min. Used to measure response to treatments and determine functional capacity for activities of daily living. Useful in people who are unable to perform treadmill or exercise bike testing. May be a better measure of fitness for older adults than exercise testing.	Instruct patient to wear comfortable shoes. Inform patient to carry or pull oxygen if used routinely. Encourage patient to walk as quickly as possible.
Echocardiogram • Contrast • M-mode • Two-dimensional • Color-flow imaging (duplex) • Real-time three-dimensional	Transducer that emits and receives ultrasound waves is placed in four positions on the chest above the heart. Transducer records sound waves that are bounced off the heart. Also records direction and flow of blood through the heart and transforms it to audio and graphic data that measure valvular abnormalities, congenital cardiac defects, wall motion, EF, and cardiac function. IV contrast agent may be used to enhance images.	Place patient in a left side-lying position facing equipment. Instruct patient about procedure and sensations (pressure and mechanical movement from head of transducer). No contraindications to procedure exist.
Stress echocardiogram	Combination of exercise test and echocardiogram. Resting images of the heart are taken with ultrasound, and then the patient exercises. Postexercise images are taken within 1 min of stopping exercise. Differences in left ventricular wall motion and thickening before and after exercise are evaluated.	Instruct and prepare patient for treadmill or exercise bicycle. Inform patient of importance of timely return to examination table for imaging after exercise. Contraindications include any reasons patient is unable to reach peak exercise tolerance.
Pharmacologic echocardiogram	Used as a substitute for the exercise stress test in individuals unable to exercise. IV dobutamine or dipyridamole is infused, and dosage is increased in 5-min intervals while echocardiogram is performed to detect wall motion abnormalities at each stage.	Start IV infusion. Administer medication per protocol. Monitor vital signs before, during, and after test until baseline achieved. Monitor patient for signs and symptoms of distress during procedure. Observe patient for side effects (e.g., shortness of breath, dizziness, nausea). Aminophylline may be given to prevent or reverse side effects of dipyridamole. Contraindications include any known allergies to medications.
Transesophageal echocardiogram (TEE)	A probe with an ultrasound transducer at the tip is swallowed while the physician controls angle and depth. As it passes down the esophagus, it sends back clear images of heart size, wall motion, valvular abnormalities, endocarditis vegetation, and possible source of thrombi without interference from lungs or chest ribs. A contrast medium may be injected IV for evaluating direction of blood flow if an atrial or ventricular septal defect is suspected. Doppler ultrasound and color-flow imaging can also be used concurrently.	Instruct patient to be NPO for at least 6 hr before test. Remove dentures. IV sedation is administered and throat locally anesthetized. A bite block is placed in the mouth. A designated driver is needed if done in the outpatient department. Monitor vital signs and oxygen saturation levels and perform suctioning as needed during procedure. Assist patient to relax. Patient may not eat or drink until gag reflex returns. Sore throat is temporary.
Nuclear Cardiology	Study involves IV injection of radioactive isotopes (^{99m}technetium-sestamibi [Cardiolite]). Radioactive uptake is counted over the heart by scintillation camera. It supplies information about myocardial contractility, myocardial perfusion, and acute cell injury.	Explain procedure to patient. Women should not wear bras to decrease breast attenuation. Establish IV line for injection of isotopes. Explain that radioactive isotope used is a small, diagnostic amount and will lose most of its radioactivity in a few hours. Inform the patient that he or she will be lying still on back with arms extended overhead for 20 min. Repeat scans are performed within a few minutes to hours after the injection.

Continued

TABLE 32-6 **DIAGNOSTIC STUDIES—cont'd**

Cardiovascular System

Study	Description and Purpose	Nursing Responsibility
Multigated acquisition (MUGA) (cardiac blood pool) scan	A small amount of the patient's blood is removed, mixed with a radioactive isotope (e.g., ^{99m}technetium-sestamibi), and reinjected IV. With the ECG used for timing, images are acquired during the cardiac cycle. Indicated for patients with MI, heart failure, or valvular heart disease. Can be used to evaluate the effect of various cardiac or cardiotoxic medications on the heart.	Explain procedure to patient. Establish IV line for removal of blood sample and reinjection of isotope. Establish ECG monitoring. Inform patient that procedure involves little risk.
Single-photon emission computed tomography (SPECT)	Used to determine size or risk of infarction and to determine infarction size. Small amounts of a radioactive isotope (e.g., ^{99m}technetium-tetrofosmin [Myoview], thallium-201) are injected IV and recordings are made of the radioactivity emitted over a specific area of the body. Circulation of the isotope can be used to detect coronary artery blood flow, intracardiac shunts, motion of ventricles, EF, and size of the heart chambers.	Explain procedure to patient. Establish IV line for injection of isotope. Establish ECG monitoring. Inform patient that procedure involves little risk.
Exercise (stress) nuclear imaging	Nuclear imaging images are taken at rest and after exercise. The injection is given at maximum HR (usually 85% of age-predicted maximum) on bicycle or treadmill. Patient is then required to continue exercise for 1 min to circulate the radioactive isotope. Scanning is done 15-60 min after exercise. A resting scan is performed 60-90 min after initial infusion or 24 hr later.	Explain procedure to patient. Instruct patient to eat only a light meal between scans. Certain medications may need to be held for 1-2 days before the scan. Patients should not have caffeine 12 hr prior. If targeted maximum HR is not achieved with exercise, test may be changed to pharmacologic imaging.
Pharmacologic nuclear imaging	Dipyridamole or adenosine is used to produce vasodilation when patients are unable to tolerate exercise. Vasodilation increases blood flow to well-perfused coronary arteries. Scanning procedure is same. Aminophylline may be given to prevent or reverse side effects of dipyridamole (e.g., shortness of breath, dizziness, nausea). Dobutamine is used if vasodilators are contraindicated.	Explain procedure to patient. Instruct patient to hold all caffeine products for 12 hr before procedure. Calcium channel blockers and β-adrenergic blockers should be held 24 hr before the test. Observe patient for side effects (e.g., shortness of breath, dizziness, nausea).
Positron emission tomography (PET)	Highly sensitive in distinguishing viable and nonviable myocardial tissue. Uses two radionuclides. Nitrogen-13-ammonia is injected IV first and scanned to evaluate myocardial perfusion. A second radioactive isotope, fluoro-18-deoxyglucose, is then injected and scanned to show myocardial metabolic function. In the normal heart, both scans match, but in an ischemic or damaged heart, they differ. The patient may or may not be stressed. A baseline resting scan is usually obtained for comparison.	Instruct patient on procedure. Explain that patient will be scanned by a machine and will need to stay still for a time. Patient's glucose level must be between 60-140 mg/dL (3.3-7.8 μmol/L) for accurate glucose metabolic activity. If exercise is included as part of testing, patient needs to be NPO and refrain from tobacco and caffeine for 24 hr before test.
Cardiovascular Magnetic Resonance Imaging (CMRI)	Noninvasive imaging technique obtains information about cardiac tissue integrity, aneurysms, EF, cardiac output, and patency of proximal coronary arteries. It does not involve ionizing radiation and is an extremely safe procedure. It provides images in multiple planes with uniformly good resolution.	Explain procedure to patient. Inform patient that the small diameter of the cylinder, along with loud noise of the procedure, may cause panic or anxiety. Antianxiety drugs and distraction strategies (e.g., music) may be recommended. Patient must lie still during test. Contraindicated for persons with implanted metallic devices or other metal fragments unless noted to be MRI safe. Discuss any implants before scan.
Magnetic resonance angiography (MRA)	Used for imaging vascular occlusive disease and abdominal aortic aneurysms. Same as MRI but with use of gadolinium as IV contrast medium.	Contraindications include any known allergies to contrast medium and persons with implanted metallic devices or other metal fragments.
Cardiac Computed Tomography (CT)	Cardiac CT is heart-specific CT imaging technology with or without IV contrast medium used to visualize heart anatomy, coronary circulation, and blood vessels.	
Coronary CT angiography (CTA)	Use of CT with injected IV contrast medium to obtain images of blood vessels and diagnose CAD.	Explain procedure to patient. Metal objects should be removed before examination. Patients should have a regular heart rhythm to allow for accurate testing. A β-adrenergic blocker may need to be administered before the test to control HR. The patient may need to be NPO for several hours before the procedure.

TABLE 32-6 DIAGNOSTIC STUDIES—cont'd

Cardiovascular System

Study	Description and Purpose	Nursing Responsibility
Calcium-scoring CT scan • Electron beam computed tomography (EBCT)	EBCT, also known as ultrafast CT, uses a scanning electron beam to quantify calcification in coronary arteries and heart valves (see Fig. 32-11). Primarily used for risk assessment in asymptomatic patients and to assess for heart disease in patients with atypical symptoms potentially related to cardiac causes.	Explain procedure to patient. Inform patient that procedure is quick and involves little or no risk.
Cardiac Catheterization	Involves insertion of catheter into heart to obtain information about O_2 levels and pressure readings within heart chambers. Contrast medium is injected to assist in seeing structures and motion of heart. Procedure is done by insertion of catheter into a vein (for right side of heart) and/or an artery (for left side of heart).	Check for sensitivity to contrast media. Withhold food and fluids for 6-12 hr before procedure. Give sedative and other drugs, if ordered. Inform patient about use of local anesthesia, insertion of catheter, feeling of warmth when dye is injected, and possible fluttering sensation of heart as catheter is passed. Note that patient may be instructed to cough or take a deep breath when dye is injected and that patient is monitored by ECG throughout procedure. After procedure, frequently assess circulation to extremity used for catheter insertion. Check peripheral pulses, color, and sensation of extremity per agency protocol. Observe puncture site for hematoma and bleeding. Place compression device over arterial site to achieve hemostasis, if indicated. Monitor vital signs and ECG. Assess for hypotension or hypertension, dysrhythmias, and signs of pulmonary emboli (e.g., respiratory difficulty).
Coronary angiography	During a cardiac catheterization, contrast medium is injected directly into coronary arteries. Used to evaluate patency of coronary arteries and collateral circulation.	Same as for cardiac catheterization.
Intracoronary ultrasound (ISUS)	During cardiac catheterization a small ultrasound probe is introduced into coronary arteries. Data are used to assess size and consistency of plaque, arterial walls, and effectiveness of intracoronary artery treatment.	Same as for cardiac catheterization.
Fractional flow reserve (FFR)	During cardiac catheterization a special wire is inserted into coronary arteries to measure pressure and flow. Information is used to determine need for angioplasty or stenting on nonsignificant blockages.	Same as for cardiac catheterization.
Electrophysiology Study (EPS)	Invasive study used to record intracardiac electrical activity using catheters (with multiple electrodes) inserted via the femoral and jugular veins into the right side of the heart. The catheter electrodes record the electrical activity in different cardiac structures. In addition, dysrhythmias can be induced and terminated.	Antidysrhythmic medications may be discontinued several days before study. Keep patient NPO 6-8 hr before test. Give premedication to promote relaxation if ordered. IV sedation often used during procedure. Patient must have frequent vital signs and continuous ECG monitoring after the procedure.
Peripheral Arteriography and Venography	Peripheral vessel blood flow is assessed by injecting contrast media into the appropriate arteries or veins (arteriography and venography). Serial x-ray studies taken to detect and visualize any atherosclerotic plaques, occlusion, aneurysms, venous abnormalities, or traumatic injury.	Check for allergy to contrast media. Give mild sedative, if ordered. Check extremity with puncture site for pulsation, warmth, color, and motion after procedure. Inspect insertion site for bleeding or swelling. Observe patient for allergic reactions to contrast media. See Table 38-9 for additional peripheral vascular diagnostic studies.
Hemodynamic Monitoring	Invasive and minimally invasive bedside hemodynamic monitoring is done using intraarterial, pulmonary artery, and central vein catheters to monitor arterial BP, stroke volume variation, pulmonary artery pressure, pulmonary artery wedge pressure, cardiac output, and central venous pressure. Used to evaluate cardiovascular status and response to treatment.	Patients requiring hemodynamic monitoring are critically ill and are monitored in intensive care units. See Chapter 66 for complete information on hemodynamic monitoring.

A lipid panel usually measures cholesterol, triglyceride, LDL, and HDL. Elevations in triglycerides and LDL are strongly associated with CAD. An increased HDL level is associated with a decreased risk of CAD.[4] High levels of HDLs serve a protective role by mobilizing cholesterol from tissues. (This is shown in eFig. 32-2, available on the website for this chapter.)

Although an association exists between elevated serum cholesterol levels and CAD, a measure of total cholesterol alone is not sufficient for an assessment of CAD. A risk assessment is calculated by comparing the total cholesterol to HDL ratio over time. An increase in the ratio indicates increased risk. This provides more information than either value alone. The patient must fast before blood is drawn for a lipid panel so food intake does not affect the results.

Plasma levels of apolipoprotein A-I (apo A-I) (the major HDL protein) and the ratio of apo A-I to apolipoprotein B (apo B) (the major LDL protein) are stronger predictors of CAD than the HDL cholesterol level alone. Measurements of these lipoproteins can be useful in identifying patients at risk for CAD.[13]

Lipoprotein (a), or Lp(a), has been studied for its role as a risk factor for CAD. Increased levels of Lp(a), especially with increased levels of lactate dehydrogenase (LDH), have been linked with the progression of atherosclerosis, especially in women.[4]

Lipoprotein-Associated Phospholipase A_2. Lipoprotein-associated phospholipase A_2 (Lp-PLA_2) is an inflammatory enzyme expressed in atherosclerotic plaques. Elevated levels of Lp-PLA_2 are related to an increased risk of CAD.[16]

Chest X-Ray

A radiographic picture of the chest can show cardiac contours, heart size, and anatomic changes in individual chambers (Fig. 32-9). The chest x-ray records any displacement or enlargement of the heart, extra fluid around the heart (pericardial effusion), and pulmonary congestion.

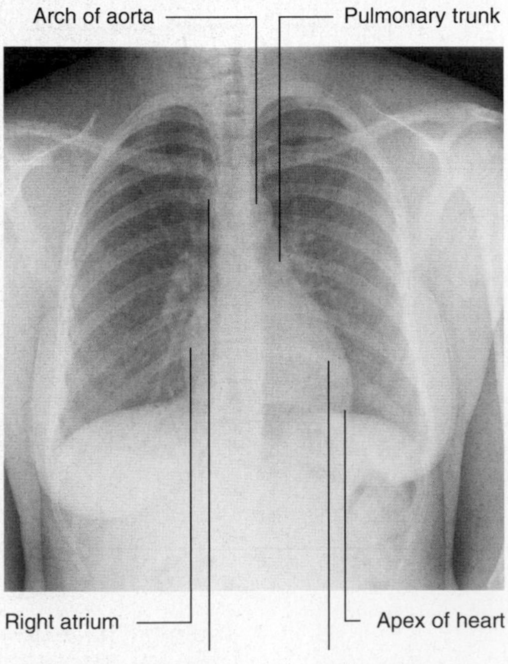

FIG. 32-9 Chest x-ray: standard posterior-anterior view.

Electrocardiogram

The basic P, QRS, and T waveforms (see Fig. 32-4, *B*) are used to assess cardiac activity. Deviations from the normal sinus rhythm can indicate problems in heart function. There are many types of ECG monitoring, including a resting 12-lead ECG, ambulatory ECG monitoring, and exercise or stress testing (see Table 32-6). Continuous ambulatory ECG (Holter monitoring) provides diagnostic information over a period of time. (See Chapter 36 for a complete discussion of ECG monitoring.)

Event Monitor or Loop Recorder. An event monitor or loop recorder is used to document less frequent ECG events. An event monitor is a portable unit that uses electrodes to store ECG data once triggered by the patient. A disadvantage of this type of monitoring is that, if symptoms occur for only a brief time, they may be over before the patient puts on the device and triggers it to record. Likewise, if patients are extremely symptomatic (e.g., syncopal), they may not be physically able to trigger the ECG recording. These devices can be used for routine pacemaker checks over the phone to the health care provider's office.[17]

An implantable loop recorder is used for patients who may have serious yet infrequent dysrhythmias. This small recorder is implanted though a small incision into the chest wall. It is activated to record either by the patient using a remote device or automatically if the HR exceeds or goes below a set rate. External loop recorders are worn for a month, and require electrodes continuously placed on the skin. This device only records when activated by the patient when symptoms occur.

Exercise or Stress Testing

Cardiac symptoms frequently occur only with activity because of the demand on the coronary arteries to provide more oxygen. Exercise testing is used to evaluate the heart's response to physical stress. This helps to assess CVD and set limits for exercise programs. Exercise testing is used for individuals who do not have restrictions related to walking or using a bicycle. It is also helpful for those with normal ECGs that limit diagnostic interpretation (e.g., pacemakers) (see Table 32-6).

Echocardiogram

The echocardiogram uses ultrasound (US) waves to record the movement of the structures of the heart. In the normal heart, ultrasonic sound waves directed at the heart are reflected back in typical configurations. *Contrast echocardiography* involves the addition of an IV contrast agent (e.g., albumin microbubbles, agitated saline) to assist in defining the images, especially in technically difficult patients (e.g., obese).

The echocardiogram provides information about abnormalities of (1) valvular structures and motion, (2) cardiac chamber size and contents, (3) ventricular and septal motion and thickness, (4) pericardial sac, and (5) ascending aorta. The **ejection fraction (EF)**, or the percentage of end-diastolic blood volume that is ejected during systole, can also be measured. The EF provides information about the function of the left ventricle during systole.

Two commonly used types of echocardiograms are the *motion-mode (M-mode) echocardiogram* and the *two-dimensional (2-D) echocardiogram.* In the M-mode type, a single ultrasound beam is directed toward the heart, recording the motion of the intracardiac structures and detecting wall thickness and chamber size. The 2-D echocardiogram sweeps

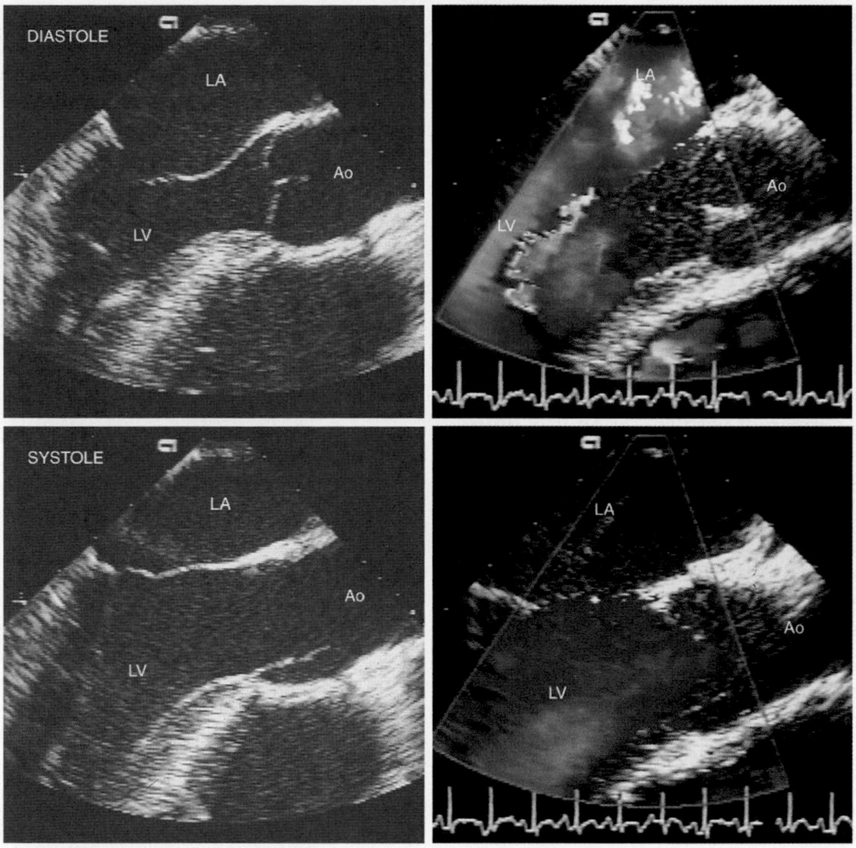

FIG. 32-10 Long-axis images of the aortic and mitral valve with the depth adjusted to optimize evaluation of valve anatomy and motion. The 2-D images *(left)* in diastole *(top)* and systole *(bottom)* show normal aortic and mitral opening and closure. The color flow images *(right)* show normal left ventricular inflow with no aortic regurgitation in diastole *(top)* and normal antegrade flow in the left ventricular outflow tract and no mitral regurgitation in systole *(bottom)*.

the ultrasound beam through an arc, producing a cross-sectional view. This shows correct spatial relationships among the structures.

Doppler technology allows for sound evaluation of the flow or motion of the scanned object (heart valves, ventricular walls, blood flow). *Color-flow imaging (duplex)* is the combination of 2-D echocardiography and Doppler technology (Fig. 32-10). It uses color changes to demonstrate the speed and direction of blood flow. Pathologic conditions, such as valvular leaks and congenital defects, can be diagnosed more effectively.

Real-time three-dimensional (3-D) ultrasound is a technology that uses multiple 2-D echo images with computer technology to provide a reconstruction of the heart. This technique produces information about the structures of the heart and how these structures change during the cardiac cycle.

Stress echocardiography, a combination of treadmill test and ultrasound images, evaluates wall motion abnormalities. By using a digital computer to compare images before and after exercise, wall motion and function are revealed. This test provides the information of an exercise stress test with the information from an echocardiogram. For those individuals unable to exercise, an IV drug (e.g., dobutamine [Dobutrex], dipyridamole [Persantine]) is used to produce pharmacologic stress on the heart while the patient is at rest.

Transesophageal echocardiography (TEE) provides more precise echocardiography of the heart than surface 2-D echocardiography by removing interference from the chest wall and lungs. The TEE uses a flexible endoscope probe with a ultrasound transducer in the tip for imaging of the heart and great vessels. The probe is passed into the esophagus to the level of the heart, and M-mode, 2-D, Doppler, and color-flow imaging can be obtained.

TEE is used frequently in an outpatient setting for evaluation of mitral valve disease and for identification of endocarditis vegetation, thrombus before cardioversion, or the source of cardiac emboli. In addition, TEE is used in the operating room to assess intraoperative cardiac function and in the emergency department to detect suspected aortic dissection.

The risks of TEE are low. However, complications may include perforation or tearing of the esophagus, hemorrhage, dysrhythmias, vasovagal reactions, and transient hypoxemia. TEE is contraindicated if the patient has a history of esophageal disorders, dysphagia, or radiation therapy to the chest wall. Patients require sedation during a TEE.

Nuclear Cardiology

One of the most common nuclear imaging tests is the multigated acquisition (MUGA) or cardiac blood pool scan. This test provides information on wall motion during systole and diastole, cardiac valves, and EF (see Table 32-6).

Perfusion imaging is also used with exercise testing to determine whether the coronary blood flow changes with increased activity. Stress perfusion imaging may show an abnormality even when a resting image is normal. This procedure is used to diagnose CAD, make a prognosis in existing CAD, differentiate viable myocardium from scar tissue, and determine the potential for success of various interventions (e.g., coronary artery bypass surgery, percutaneous coronary intervention)[18] (see Chapter 34).

Exercise stress perfusion imaging is always preferred but, if a patient cannot exercise, IV dipyridamole or adenosine (Adenocard) can be given to dilate the coronary arteries and simulate the effect of exercise. After the drug takes effect, the isotope is injected and the imaging is done.

Cardiovascular Magnetic Resonance Imaging

Cardiovascular magnetic resonance imaging (CMRI) can detect and find areas of MI in a 3-D view. It is sensitive enough to find even small MIs that are not apparent with single-photon emission computed tomography imaging. CMRI aids in the final diagnosis of MI and the assessment of EF. It also plays a role in prediction of recovery from MI and in the diagnosis of congenital heart and aortic disorders and CAD.[19]

One major advantage of CMRI is that it does not require any radiation to the patient. In general, the use of CMRI in patients with pacemakers and ICDs is discouraged because the magnets can alter the function of the devices. When there is a strong clinical need and the benefits outweigh the risks, CMRI should only be performed in these patients at experienced centers.[19] Some newer models of these devices are approved for use with MRI.

Cardiac Computed Tomography

Cardiac computed tomography (CT) is a heart-imaging test that uses CT technology with or without IV contrast (dye) to see the heart anatomy, coronary circulation, and great blood vessels (e.g., aorta, pulmonary veins, artery). This technology is often called multidetector CT (MDCT) scanning. Types of CT scans used to diagnosis heart disease include coronary CT angiography (CTA) and calcium-scoring CT scan (see Table 32-6).

Coronary CTA is a noninvasive test. It can be done faster than a cardiac catheterization with less risk and discomfort to the patient.[20] Although the use of coronary CTA is increasing, cardiac catheterization (discussed in the next section) remains the gold standard to diagnose coronary artery stenosis. Further, when a cardiac catheterization is done, interventions (e.g., angioplasty, stent placement) can be performed if coronary blockages are found.

The calcium-scoring CT scan is used to find calcium deposits in plaque in the coronary arteries. The most common method used is the electron beam CT (EBCT) (Fig. 32-11). It can detect early coronary calcification before symptoms develop. The amount of coronary calcium is a predictor of future cardiac events.

Cardiac Catheterization

Cardiac catheterization is a common outpatient procedure. It provides information about CAD, coronary spasm, congenital and valvular heart disease, and ventricular function. Cardiac catheterization is also used to measure intracardiac pressures and O_2 levels, as well as CO and EF. With injection of contrast media and fluoroscopy, the coronary arteries can be seen, chambers of the heart can be outlined, and wall motion can be observed.

Cardiac catheterization is done by inserting a radiopaque catheter into the right and/or left side of the heart. For the right side of the heart, a catheter is inserted through an arm vein (basilic or cephalic) or a leg vein (femoral). Pressures are recorded as the catheter is moved into the vena cava, the right atrium, the right ventricle, and the pulmonary artery. The catheter is then moved until it is wedged or lodged in position. This blocks the blood flow and pressure from the right side of the heart and looks ahead through the pulmonary capillary bed to the pressure in the left side of the heart *(pulmonary artery wedge pressure)*. This pressure is used to assess the function of the left side of the heart.

Left-sided heart catheterization is done by inserting a catheter into a femoral, brachial, or radial artery. The catheter is passed in a retrograde manner up to the aorta, across the aortic valve, and into the left ventricle.

Coronary angiography is done with a left-sided heart catheterization. The catheter is positioned at the origin of the coronary arteries (see Fig. 32-3), and contrast medium is injected into the arteries. Patients often feel a temporary flushed sensation with dye injection. The images identify the location and severity of any coronary blockages (see Figs. 32-12 and 34-7). Complications of cardiac catheterization include bleeding or hematoma at the puncture site; allergic reactions to the contrast

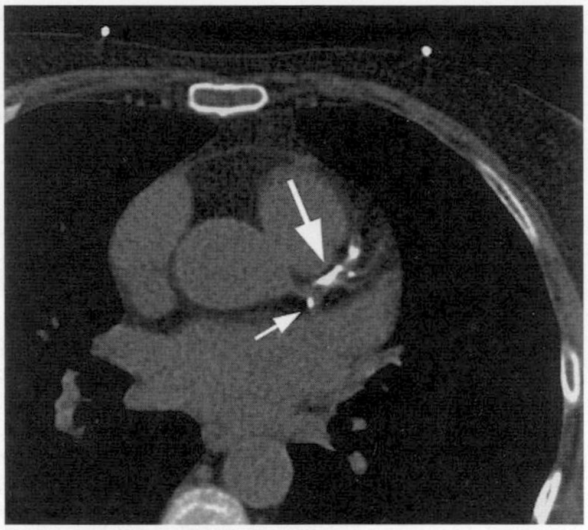

FIG. 32-11 Examples of coronary calcification of the left anterior descending coronary artery *(large arrow)* and left circumflex artery *(small arrow)* as seen on electron beam computed tomography.

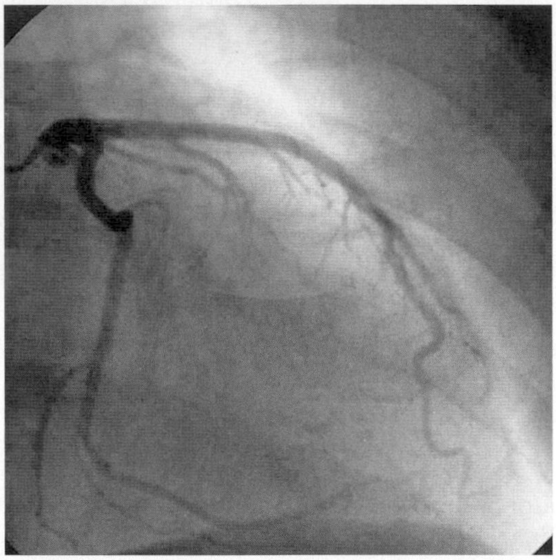

FIG. 32-12 Normal left coronary artery angiogram.

media; looping or kinking of the catheter; infection; thrombus formation; aortic dissection; dysrhythmias; MI; stroke; and puncture of the ventricles, cardiac septum, or lung tissue.

Intracoronary Ultrasound. Intracoronary ultrasound (ICUS), also known as intravascular ultrasound (IVUS), is an invasive procedure performed in the catheterization laboratory with coronary angiography. The 2-D or 3-D ultrasound images provide a cross-sectional view of the arterial walls of the coronary arteries. In this procedure a miniature transducer attached to a small catheter is moved to the artery to be studied. Once it is in the artery, ultrasound images are obtained. The health of the arterial layers is assessed, including the composition, location, and thickness of any plaque. ICUS can evaluate vessel response to treatments such as stent placement and atherectomy, as well as any complications that may have occurred during the procedure (see Chapter 34). Patients most often have ICUS in addition to angiography or a coronary intervention. Thus nursing care is similar to that following cardiac catheterization (see Table 32-6).

Fractional Flow Reserve. Fractional flow reserve (FFR) is a procedure that is done during a cardiac catheterization. It involves using a special wire that can measure pressure and flow in the coronary artery. FFR helps to determine the need to perform angioplasty or stenting on nonsignificant blockages.

Electrophysiology Study

The electrophysiology study (EPS) records and manipulates the heart's electrical activity using electrodes placed inside the heart chambers. It provides information on SA node, AV node, and ventricular conduction. It is particularly helpful in determining the source and treatment of dysrhythmias. Patients with symptomatic supraventricular or ventricular tachycardias may be at risk for sudden cardiac death. Information from an EPS helps to make an accurate diagnosis and guides treatment decisions.

In EPS, catheters are inserted in a manner similar to that used in a right-sided heart catheterization. These catheters are placed at specific anatomic sites within the heart to record electrical activity. Nursing care for patients after EPS is similar to the care of patients after cardiac catheterization. This includes continuous ECG monitoring and frequent assessment of vital signs and puncture site.

CASE STUDY—cont'd

Objective Data: Diagnostic Studies

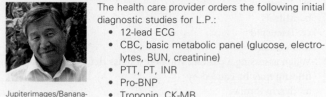

Jupiterimages/Banana-Stock/Thinkstock

The health care provider orders the following initial diagnostic studies for L.P.:

- 12-lead ECG
- CBC, basic metabolic panel (glucose, electrolytes, BUN, creatinine)
- PTT, PT, INR
- Pro-BNP
- Troponin, CK-MB
- TSH, free T_4
- Chest x-ray

L.P.'s initial troponin and CK-MB levels are within normal limits. The ECG demonstrates atrial fibrillation with a rapid ventricular response. Chest x-ray, CBC, basic metabolic panel, pro-BNP, and coagulation studies are all within normal limits. The health care provider orders IV diltiazem (Cardizem) and heparin to be started in the emergency department. L.P. will be admitted to the progressive care unit and will have a consult with a cardiologist.

BRIDGE TO NCLEX EXAMINATION

The number of the question corresponds to the same-numbered outcome at the beginning of the chapter.

1. A patient with a tricuspid valve disorder will have impaired blood flow between the
   a. vena cava and right atrium.
   b. left atrium and left ventricle.
   c. right atrium and right ventricle.
   d. right ventricle and pulmonary artery.
2. A patient has a severe blockage in his right coronary artery. Which cardiac structures are most likely to be affected by this blockage *(select all that apply)?*
   a. AV node
   b. Left ventricle
   c. Coronary sinus
   d. Right ventricle
   e. Pulmonic valve
3. The portion of the vascular system responsible for hemostasis is the
   a. thin capillary vessels.
   b. endothelial layer of the arteries.
   c. elastic middle layer of the veins.
   d. smooth muscle of the arterial wall.
4. When a person's blood pressure rises, the homeostatic mechanism to compensate for an elevation involves stimulation of
   a. baroreceptors that inhibit the sympathetic nervous system, causing vasodilation.
   b. chemoreceptors that inhibit the sympathetic nervous system, causing vasodilation.
   c. baroreceptors that inhibit the parasympathetic nervous system, causing vasodilation.
   d. chemoreceptors that stimulate the sympathetic nervous system, causing an increased heart rate.
5. A P wave on an ECG represents an impulse arising at the
   a. SA node and repolarizing the atria.
   b. SA node and depolarizing the atria.
   c. AV node and depolarizing the atria.
   d. AV node and spreading to the bundle of His.
6. When collecting subjective data related to the cardiovascular system, which information should be obtained from the patient *(select all that apply)?*
   a. Annual income
   b. Smoking history
   c. Religious preference
   d. Number of pillows used to sleep
   e. Blood for basic laboratory studies

7. The auscultatory area in the left midclavicular line at the level of the fifth ICS is the best location to hear sounds from which heart valve?
   a. Aortic
   b. Mitral
   c. Tricuspid
   d. Pulmonic
8. When assessing a patient, you note a pulse deficit of 23 beats. This finding may be caused by
   a. dysrhythmias.
   b. heart murmurs.
   c. gallop rhythms.
   d. pericardial friction rubs.
9. When assessing the cardiovascular system of a 79-year-old patient, you might expect to find
   a. a narrowed pulse pressure.
   b. diminished carotid artery pulses.
   c. difficulty in isolating the apical pulse.
   d. an increased heart rate in response to stress.
10. Which nursing responsibilities are priorities when caring for a patient returning from a cardiac catheterization *(select all that apply)?*
   a. Monitoring vital signs and ECG
   b. Checking the catheter insertion site and distal pulses
   c. Assisting the patient to ambulate to the bathroom to void
   d. Informing the patient that he will be sleepy from the general anesthesia
   e. Instructing the patient about the risks of the radioactive isotope injection

1. c, 2. a, b, d, 3. b, 4. a, 5. b, 6. b, c, d, 7. b, 8. a, 9. c, 10. a, b

evolve

For rationales to these answers and even more NCLEX review questions, visit http://evolve.elsevier.com/Lewis/medsurg.

REFERENCES

1. Patton KT, Thibodeau GA, Douglas MM: *Essentials of anatomy and physiology*, St Louis, 2012, Mosby.
2. Wesley K: *Huszar's basic dysrhythmias and acute coronary syndromes*, ed 4, St Louis, 2011, Mosby Jems.
3. Watson S, Gorski KA: *Invasive cardiology*, ed 3, Sudbury, Mass, 2011, Jones & Bartlett Learning.
4. Huether S, McCance K: *Understanding pathophysiology*, ed 5, St Louis, 2012, Mosby.
5. American Heart Association: Understand blood pressure readings, 2012. Retrieved from *www.heart.org/HEARTORG/Conditions/HighBloodPressure/AboutHighBloodPressure/Understanding-Blood-Pressure-Readings_UCM_301764_Article.jsp.*
6. Jarvis C: *Physical examination and health assessment*, ed 6, St Louis, 2012, Saunders.
7. Karavidas A, Lazaros G, Tsiachris D, et al: Aging and the cardiovascular system, *Hellenic J Cardiol* 51:421, 2010.
8. Carlson KK: *Advanced critical care nursing*, St Louis, 2009, Saunders.
9. National Institute on Aging: Aging heart and arteries: a scientific quest, 2011. Retrieved from *www.nia.nih.gov/health/publication/aging-hearts-and-arteries-scientific-quest/chapter-2-aging-heart.*
10. Hodgson BB, Kizior RJ: *Saunders nursing drug handbook 2012*, St Louis, 2012, Mosby.
*11. Mosca L, Benjamin EJ, Berry K, et al: Effectiveness-based guidelines for cardiovascular disease prevention in women: 2011 update, *Circulation* 123:1243, 2011.
12. Hughes S: One high-sensitivity troponin test rules out MI, 2011. Retrieved from *www.theheart.org/article/1277167.do.*
13. Malarkey LM, McMorrow ME: *Saunders nursing guide to laboratory and diagnostic tests*, ed 2, St Louis, 2012, Saunders.
14. The Emerging Risk Factors Collaboration: C-reactive protein concentration and risk of coronary heart disease, stroke, and mortality: an individual participant meta-analysis, *Lancet* 375:132, 2010. Original Text
15. American Heart Association: Homocysteine, folic acid and cardiovascular disease, 2012. Retrieved from *www.heart.org/HEARTORG/GettingHealthy/NutritionCenter/Homocysteine-Folic-Acid-and-Cardiovascular-Disease_UCM_305997_Article.jsp.*
*16. The Lp-PLA_2 Studies Collaboration: Lipoprotein-associated phospholipase A_2 and risk of coronary disease, stroke, and mortality: collaborative analysis of 32 prospective studies, *Lancet* 375:1536, 2010.
17. American Heart Association: Common tests for arrhythmia, 2011. Retrieved from *www.heart.org/HEARTORG/Conditions/Arrhythmia/SymptomsDiagnosisMonitoringofArrhythmia/Common-Tests-for-Arrhythmia_UCM_301988_Article.jsp.*
18. Zaret BL, Beller GA: *Clinical nuclear cardiology*, ed 4, St Louis, 2010, Mosby.
*19. Hundley WG, Bluemke DA, Finn JP, et al: ACCF/ACR/AHA/NASCI/SCMR 2010 expert consensus document on cardiovascular magnetic resonance: a report of the American College of Cardiology Foundation Task Force on Expert Consensus Documents, *Circulation* 121:2462, 2010.
*20. Mark DB, Berman DS, Budoff MJ, et al: ACCF/ACR/AHA/NASCI/SAIP/SCAI/SCCT 2010 expert consensus document on coronary computed tomographic angiography: a report of the American College of Cardiology Foundation Task Force on Expert Consensus Documents, *Circulation* 121:2509, 2010.

*Evidence-based information for clinical practice.

RESOURCES

Resources for this chapter are listed at the end of Chapter 33 on p. 729 and at the end of Chapter 34 on p. 765.

CHAPTER

33

One way to get high blood pressure is to go mountain climbing over molehills.
Earl Wilson

Nursing Management
Hypertension

Elisabeth G. Bradley

evolve WEBSITE

http://evolve.elsevier.com/Lewis/medsurg

- NCLEX Review Questions
- Key Points
- Pre-Test
- Answer Guidelines for Case Study on p. 727
- Rationales for Bridge to NCLEX Examination Questions
- Case Study
  - Patient With Hypertension and Stroke
- Concept Map Creator
- Glossary
- Content Updates

eTables

- eTable 33-1: Your Guide to Lowering Your Blood Pressure With DASH
- eTable 33-2: Drug Therapy: Hypertension (expanded)

LEARNING OUTCOMES

1. Relate the pathophysiologic mechanisms associated with primary hypertension to the clinical manifestations and complications.
2. Select appropriate strategies for the prevention of primary hypertension.
3. Describe the collaborative care for primary hypertension, including drug therapy and lifestyle modifications.
4. Explain the collaborative care of the older adult with primary hypertension.
5. Prioritize the nursing management of the patient with primary hypertension.
6. Describe the collaborative care of a patient with hypertensive crisis.

KEY TERMS

blood pressure (BP), p. 710
hypertension, p. 712
hypertensive crisis, p. 726
isolated systolic hypertension (ISH), p. 712
orthostatic hypotension, p. 723
prehypertension, p. 712
primary hypertension, p. 712
secondary hypertension, p. 712
systemic vascular resistance (SVR), p. 710

Hypertension, or high blood pressure (BP), is an important medical and public health problem. There is a direct relationship between hypertension and cardiovascular disease (CVD). As BP increases, so does the risk of myocardial infarction (MI), heart failure, stroke, and renal disease.[1] This chapter discusses the nursing care and collaborative management of patients at risk for or who have hypertension.

One in three adults in the United States has hypertension. Additionally, 30% of adults have prehypertension,[2] and approximately 8% have undiagnosed hypertension.[3] *Healthy People 2020* lists the number of adults with hypertension whose BP is under control as one of the 26 high-priority, leading health indicators for the coming decade.[4] The National Health and Nutrition Examination Survey (NHANES) tracks prevention, treatment, and control of hypertension. Data from NHANES show that most people 20 years of age and older with hypertension (82%) were aware that they had high BP, and 75% were being treated. However, 53% did not have their BP controlled.[2]

The American College of Cardiology Foundation and the American Heart Association (AHA) provide performance measures for hypertension management that address not only treatment, but also control of BP to target goals. To achieve the measures, patients with hypertension must have a BP of less than 140/90 mm Hg or, if their BP is higher, have at least two antihypertensive medications prescribed.[5]

National guidelines are designed to apply to all racial and ethnic groups. However, certain groups have a higher incidence of risk factors[2,6-8] (see boxes on Cultural & Ethnic Health Disparities and Gender Differences).

Reviewed by Susan J. Eisel, RN, MSEd, Associate Professor of Nursing, Mercy College of Ohio, Toledo, Ohio; Christina D. Keller, RN, MSN, Instructor, Radford University School of Nursing: Clinical Simulation Center, Radford, Virginia; Krista Krause, MSN, FNP-C, Faculty, St. Joseph's College of Nursing, Syracuse, New York; and Erin M. Loughery, MSN, APRN, Acute Care APN, William W. Backus Hospital, Norwich, Connecticut.

CULTURAL & ETHNIC HEALTH DISPARITIES

Hypertension

African Americans
- Have the highest prevalence of hypertension in the world.
- Develop hypertension at a younger age than whites.
- Have a higher incidence of hypertension among women than among men.
- Hypertension is more aggressive and results in more severe end-organ damage.
- Have a higher death rate resulting from hypertension than whites.
- Produce less renin and do not respond well to renin-inhibiting drugs. They respond better to calcium channel blockers and diuretics.
- Have a higher risk of angioedema with angiotensin-converting enzyme inhibitors than whites.

Mexican Americans
- Are less likely to receive treatment for hypertension than whites and African Americans.
- Have lower rates of BP control than whites and African Americans.
- Have lower levels of awareness of hypertension and its treatment than whites and African Americans.

GENDER DIFFERENCES

Hypertension

Men
- Before age 45, hypertension is more common in men than in women.

Women
- After age 64, hypertension is more common in women than in men.
- Part of the rise in BP in women is attributed to menopause-related factors such as estrogen withdrawal, overproduction of pituitary hormones, and weight gain.
- Older women (ages 70-79) have very poor control of hypertension compared with women ages 50-69, despite having similar rates of treatment.
- Hypertension is two to three times more common in women who take oral contraceptives than in women who do not.
- A history of preeclampsia may be an early sign of risk for cardiovascular disease.

NORMAL REGULATION OF BLOOD PRESSURE

Blood pressure (BP) is the force exerted by the blood against the walls of the blood vessel. It must be adequate to maintain tissue perfusion during activity and rest. The maintenance of normal BP and tissue perfusion requires the integration of both systemic factors and local peripheral vascular effects. BP is primarily a function of cardiac output (CO) and systemic vascular resistance (Fig. 33-1).

CO is the total blood flow through the systemic or pulmonary circulation per minute. It is described as the stroke volume (amount of blood pumped out of the left ventricle per beat [approximately 70 mL]) multiplied by the heart rate (HR) for 1 minute.

Systemic vascular resistance (SVR) is the force opposing the movement of blood within the blood vessels. The radius of the small arteries and arterioles is the principal factor determining vascular resistance. A small change in the radius of the arterioles creates a major change in the SVR. If SVR is increased and CO remains constant or increases, arterial BP will increase.

The mechanisms that regulate BP can affect either CO or SVR, or both. Regulation of BP is a complex process involving both short-term (seconds to hours) and long-term (days to weeks) mechanisms. Short-term mechanisms, including the sympathetic nervous system (SNS) and vascular endothelium, are active within a few seconds. Long-term mechanisms include renal and hormonal processes that regulate arteriolar resistance and blood volume. In a healthy person these regulatory mechanisms function in response to the body's demands.

Sympathetic Nervous System

The nervous system, which reacts within seconds after a drop in BP, increases BP primarily by activating the SNS. Increased SNS activity increases HR and cardiac contractility, produces widespread vasoconstriction in the peripheral arterioles, and promotes the release of renin from the kidneys. The net effect of SNS activation is to increase BP by increasing both CO and SVR.

Specialized nerve cells called *baroreceptors (pressoreceptors)* are located in the carotid arteries and the arch of the aorta. These cells sense changes in BP and transmit this information to the vasomotor centers in the brainstem. The brainstem sends

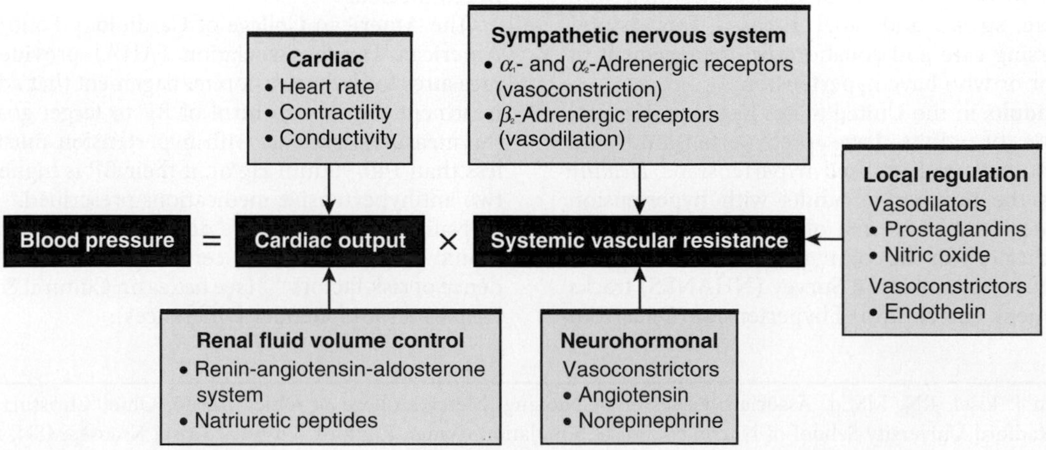

FIG. 33-1 Factors influencing blood pressure (BP). Hypertension develops when one or more of the BP-regulating mechanisms are defective.

this information through complex networks of neurons that excite or inhibit efferent nerves. SNS efferent nerves innervate cardiac and vascular smooth muscle cells. Under normal conditions, a low level of continuous SNS activity maintains vascular tone. BP may be reduced by withdrawal of SNS activity or by stimulation of the parasympathetic nervous system. This decreases the HR (via the vagus nerve) and thereby decreases CO.

The neurotransmitter norepinephrine (NE) is released from SNS nerve endings. NE activates receptors located in the sinoatrial node, myocardium, and vascular smooth muscle. The response to NE depends on the type of receptors present. SNS receptors are classified as α_1, α_2, β_1, and β_2 (Table 33-1). The smooth muscle of the blood vessels has α-adrenergic and β_2-adrenergic receptors. α-Adrenergic receptors located in the peripheral vasculature cause vasoconstriction when stimulated by NE. β_1-Adrenergic receptors in the heart respond to NE and epinephrine with increased HR *(chronotropic),* increased force of contraction *(inotropic),* and increased speed of conduction *(dromotropic).* β_2-Adrenergic receptors are activated primarily by epinephrine released from the adrenal medulla and cause vasodilation (see Fig. 33-1).

The sympathetic vasomotor center interacts with many areas of the brain to maintain normal BP under various conditions. It is activated during times of pain, stress, and exercise. The SNS response causes an appropriate increase in CO and BP to adjust to the body's increased oxygen demands. During postural change from lying to standing, there is a transient decrease in BP. The vasomotor center is stimulated, and the SNS response causes peripheral vasoconstriction and increased venous return to the heart. If this response did not occur, blood flow to the brain would be inadequate, resulting in dizziness or syncope.

Baroreceptors. Baroreceptors have an important role in the maintenance of BP stability during normal activities. They are sensitive to stretching and, when stimulated by an increase in BP, send inhibitory impulses to the sympathetic vasomotor center. Inhibition of the SNS results in decreased HR, decreased force of contraction, and vasodilation in peripheral arterioles.

When a fall in BP is sensed by the baroreceptors, the SNS is activated. The result is constriction of the peripheral arterioles, increased HR, and increased contractility of the heart. In long-standing hypertension the baroreceptors become adjusted to elevated levels of BP and recognize this level as "normal."

TABLE 33-1 SYMPATHETIC NERVOUS SYSTEM RECEPTORS AFFECTING BLOOD PRESSURE

Receptor	Location	Response When Activated
α_1	Vascular smooth muscle	Vasoconstriction
	Heart	Increased contractility (positive inotropic effect)
α_2	Presynaptic nerve terminals	Inhibition of norepinephrine release
	Vascular smooth muscle	Vasoconstriction
β_1	Heart	Increased contractility (positive inotropic effect) Increased heart rate (positive chronotropic effect) Increased conduction (positive dromotropic effect)
	Juxtaglomerular cells of the kidney	Increased renin secretion
β_2	Smooth muscle of blood vessels in heart (e.g., coronary arteries), lungs (e.g., bronchi), and skeletal muscle	Vasodilation
Dopamine receptors	Primarily renal blood vessels	Vasodilation

Vascular Endothelium

The vascular endothelium is a single-cell layer that lines the blood vessels. It produces several vasoactive substances and growth factors. Nitric oxide and prostacyclin help maintain low arterial tone, inhibit growth of the smooth muscle layer, and inhibit platelet aggregation. *Endothelin* (ET) is an extremely potent vasoconstrictor. It also causes adhesion and aggregation of neutrophils and stimulates smooth muscle growth (see Fig. 33-1).

Renal System

The kidneys contribute to BP regulation by controlling sodium excretion and extracellular fluid (ECF) volume (see Chapter 45). Sodium retention results in water retention, which causes an increased ECF volume. This increases the venous return to the heart and the stroke volume. Together, these increase CO and BP.

The renin-angiotensin-aldosterone system (RAAS) also plays an important role in BP regulation (see Fig. 33-1). The juxtaglomerular apparatus in the kidney secretes renin in response to SNS stimulation, decreased blood flow through the kidneys, or decreased serum sodium concentration. Renin is an enzyme that converts angiotensinogen to angiotensin I. Angiotensin-converting enzyme (ACE) converts angiotensin I into angiotensin II (A-II). A-II increases BP by two different mechanisms (see Fig. 45-4). First, A-II is a potent vasoconstrictor and increases SVR. This results in an immediate increase in BP. Second, over a period of hours or days, A-II increases BP indirectly by stimulating the adrenal cortex to secrete aldosterone (discussed below).

A-II also acts at a local level within the heart and blood vessels. These effects include vasoconstriction and tissue growth that results in remodeling of the vessel walls. These changes are linked to the development of primary hypertension and also the long-term effects of hypertension (e.g., atherosclerosis, renal disease, cardiac hypertrophy).

Prostaglandins (PGE_2 and PGI_2) secreted by the renal medulla have a vasodilator effect on the systemic circulation. This results in decreased SVR and lowering of BP. (Prostaglandins are discussed in Chapter 12.) The natriuretic peptides (atrial natriuretic peptide [ANP] and b-type natriuretic peptide [BNP]) are secreted by heart cells. They antagonize the effects of antidiuretic hormone (ADH) and aldosterone. This results in *natriuresis* (excretion of sodium in urine) and diuresis, resulting in reduced blood volume and BP.

Endocrine System

Stimulation of the SNS results in release of epinephrine along with a small fraction of NE by the adrenal medulla. Epinephrine increases the CO by increasing the HR and myocardial contractility. Epinephrine activates β_2-adrenergic receptors in peripheral arterioles of skeletal muscle, causing vasodilation. In

TABLE 33-2 **CLASSIFICATION OF HYPERTENSION**

Category	SBP (mm Hg)		DBP (mm Hg)
Normal	<120	and	<80
Prehypertension	120-139	or	80-89
Hypertension, stage 1	140-159	or	90-99
Hypertension, stage 2	≥160	or	≥100

From the National Heart, Lung, and Blood Institute: Seventh report of the Joint National Committee on Detection, Evaluation, and Treatment of High Blood Pressure (JNC-7), NIH Publication No. 04-5230, Bethesda, Md, 2004, The Institute. Retrieved from *www.nhlbi.nih.gov/guidelines/hypertension/jnc7full.pdf.*
DBP, Diastolic blood pressure; *SBP,* systolic blood pressure.

peripheral arterioles with only α_1-adrenergic receptors (skin and kidneys), epinephrine causes vasoconstriction.

A-II stimulates the adrenal cortex to release aldosterone. (Release of aldosterone is also regulated by other factors [see Chapters 48 and 50].) Aldosterone stimulates the kidneys to retain sodium and water. This increases blood volume and CO (see Fig. 45-4).

An increased blood sodium and osmolarity level stimulates the release of ADH from the posterior pituitary gland. ADH increases the ECF volume by promoting the reabsorption of water in the distal and collecting tubules of the kidneys. The resulting increase in blood volume causes an increase in CO and BP.

HYPERTENSION

Classification of Hypertension

Hypertension is defined as a persistent systolic BP (SBP) of 140 mm Hg or more, diastolic BP (DBP) of 90 mm Hg or more, or current use of antihypertensive medication.[1] **Prehypertension** is defined as SBP of 120 to 139 mm Hg or DBP of 80 to 89 mm Hg.

Isolated systolic hypertension (ISH) is defined as an average SBP of 140 mm Hg or more, coupled with an average DBP of less than 90 mm Hg.[9] SBP increases with aging. DBP rises until approximately age 55 and then declines. Control of ISH decreases the incidence of stroke, heart failure, and death.

The classification of BP is based on the average of two or more properly measured BP readings on two or more office visits. Table 33-2 presents the BP classification for people 18 years of age and older.

Etiology

Hypertension can be classified as either primary or secondary.

Primary Hypertension. **Primary** *(essential* or *idiopathic)* **hypertension** is elevated BP without an identified cause, and it accounts for 90% to 95% of all cases of hypertension. Although the exact cause of primary hypertension is unknown, there are several contributing factors. These include increased SNS activity, overproduction of sodium-retaining hormones and vasoconstricting substances, increased sodium intake, greater-than-ideal body weight, diabetes mellitus, tobacco use, and excessive alcohol consumption. Primary hypertension is the major focus of this chapter because of its prevalence and impact on health.

Secondary Hypertension. **Secondary hypertension** is elevated BP with a specific cause that often can be identified and corrected (Table 33-3). This type of hypertension accounts for 5% to 10% of hypertension in adults. Secondary hypertension should be suspected in people who suddenly develop high BP, especially if it is severe. Clinical findings that suggest secondary hypertension relate to the underlying cause. For example, an abdominal bruit heard over the renal arteries may indicate renal disease. Treatment of secondary hypertension is aimed at removing or treating the underlying cause. Secondary hypertension is a contributing factor to hypertensive crisis (discussed later in this chapter).

TABLE 33-3 **CAUSES OF SECONDARY HYPERTENSION***

- Cirrhosis
- Coarctation or congenital narrowing of the aorta
- Drug-related: estrogen replacement therapy, oral contraceptives, corticosteroids, nonsteroidal antiinflammatory drugs (e.g., cyclooxygenase-2 inhibitors), sympathetic stimulants (e.g., cocaine, monoamine oxidase)
- Endocrine disorders (e.g., pheochromocytoma, Cushing syndrome, thyroid disease)
- Neurologic disorders (e.g., brain tumors, quadriplegia, traumatic brain injury)
- Pregnancy-induced hypertension
- Renal disease (e.g., renal artery stenosis, glomerulonephritis)
- Sleep apnea

*List is not all inclusive.

Pathophysiology of Primary Hypertension

BP rises with any increase in CO or SVR. Increased CO is sometimes found in the person with prehypertension. Later in the course of hypertension, the SVR rises and the CO returns to normal. The hemodynamic hallmark of hypertension is persistently increased SVR. This persistent elevation in SVR may occur in various ways. Table 33-4 presents factors that relate to the development of primary hypertension or contribute to its consequences. Abnormalities of any of the mechanisms involved in the maintenance of normal BP can result in hypertension (see Fig. 33-1).

Genetic Link

Different sets of genes may regulate BP at different times throughout the life span.[2] Genetic abnormalities associated with a rare form of hypertension characterized by excess levels of potassium have been identified. To date, the known contribution of genetic factors to BP in the general population remains very small.[1]

The International Consortium for Blood Pressure Genome-Wide Association Studies is a network of researchers currently working to uncover genetic factors related to hypertension. In practice, you should screen children and siblings of persons with hypertension and strongly advise them to adopt healthy lifestyles to prevent hypertension.

Water and Sodium Retention. Excessive sodium intake is linked to the start of hypertension. Although most people consume a high-sodium diet, only one in three will develop hypertension. When sodium is restricted in many people with hypertension, their BP falls. This suggests that some degree of sodium sensitivity may exist for high sodium intake to trigger the development of hypertension. A high sodium intake may activate a number of pressor mechanisms and cause water retention.

TABLE 33-4 **RISK FACTORS FOR PRIMARY HYPERTENSION**

Risk Factor	Description
Age	• SBP rises progressively with increasing age. • After age 50, SBP >140 mm Hg is a more important cardiovascular risk factor than DBP.
Alcohol	• Excessive alcohol intake is strongly associated with hypertension. • Patients with hypertension should limit their daily intake to 1 oz of alcohol.
Tobacco use	• Smoking tobacco greatly ↑ risk of cardiovascular disease. • People with hypertension who smoke tobacco are at even greater risk for cardiovascular disease.
Diabetes mellitus	• Hypertension is more common in patients with diabetes. • When hypertension and diabetes coexist, complications (e.g., target organ disease) are more severe.
Elevated serum lipids	• ↑ Levels of cholesterol and triglycerides are primary risk factors in atherosclerosis. • Hyperlipidemia is more common in people with hypertension.

Excess dietary sodium	• High sodium intake can
	  • Contribute to hypertension in some patients
	  • Decrease the effectiveness of certain antihypertensive medications

Gender	• Hypertension is more prevalent in men in young adulthood and early middle age (<55 yr of age). • After age 64, hypertension is more prevalent in women. (See Gender Differences box on p. 710.)
Family history	• History of a close blood relative (e.g., parents, sibling) with hypertension is associated with an ↑ risk for developing hypertension.
Obesity	• Weight gain is associated with increased frequency of hypertension. • The risk is greatest with central abdominal obesity.
Ethnicity	• Incidence of hypertension is 2 times higher in African Americans than in whites. (See Cultural & Ethnic Health Disparities box on p. 710.)
Sedentary lifestyle	• Regular physical activity can help control weight and reduce cardiovascular risk. • Physical activity may ↓ BP.
Socioeconomic status	• Hypertension is more prevalent in lower socioeconomic groups and among the less educated.
Stress	• People exposed to repeated stress may develop hypertension more frequently than others. • People who develop hypertension may respond differently to stress than those who do not develop hypertension.

DBP, Diastolic blood pressure; *SBP,* systolic blood pressure.

In clinical practice, there is not an easy or simple test to identify individuals whose BP will rise with even a small increase in salt intake *(salt sensitive)* versus those who can ingest large amounts of sodium without much change in BP *(salt resistant)*. In general, the effect of sodium on BP is greater in African Americans and in middle-aged and older adults.[10]

Altered Renin-Angiotensin-Aldosterone Mechanism. High plasma renin activity (PRA) results in the increased conversion of angiotensinogen to angiotensin I (see Fig. 45-4). This alteration in the RAAS may contribute to the development of hypertension. Any rise in BP inhibits the release of renin from the renal juxtaglomerular cells. Based on this feedback loop, low levels of PRA would be expected in patients with primary hypertension. However, only about 30% have low PRA, 50% have normal levels, and 20% have high PRA. These normal or high PRA levels may be related to excess renin secretion from ischemic nephrons.

Stress and Increased Sympathetic Nervous System Activity. It has long been recognized that BP is influenced by factors such as anger, fear, and pain. Physiologic responses to stress, which are normally protective, may persist to a pathologic degree, resulting in a prolonged increase in SNS activity. Increased SNS stimulation produces increased vasoconstriction, increased HR, and increased renin release. Increased renin activates the RAAS, leading to elevated BP. People exposed to high levels of repeated psychologic stress develop hypertension to a greater extent than those who experience less stress.

Insulin Resistance and Hyperinsulinemia. Abnormalities of glucose, insulin, and lipoprotein metabolism are common in primary hypertension. They are not present in secondary hypertension and do not improve when hypertension is treated. Insulin resistance is a risk factor in the development of hypertension and CVD. High insulin levels stimulate SNS activity and impair nitric oxide–mediated vasodilation. Additional pressor effects of insulin include vascular hypertrophy and increased renal sodium reabsorption.

Endothelium Dysfunction. Endothelium dysfunction may contribute to atherosclerosis and primary hypertension. Some people with hypertension have a reduced vasodilator response to nitric oxide. Others have high levels of ET that produce a pronounced and prolonged vasoconstriction. The role of endothelium dysfunction in the pathogenesis and treatment of hypertension is an area of ongoing investigation.

Clinical Manifestations

Hypertension is often called the "silent killer" because it is frequently asymptomatic until it becomes severe and target organ disease occurs. A patient with severe hypertension may experience a variety of symptoms secondary to the effects on blood vessels in the various organs and tissues or to the increased workload of the heart. These secondary symptoms include fatigue, dizziness, palpitations, angina, and dyspnea. In the past, symptoms of hypertension were thought to include headache and nosebleeds. Unless BP is very high, these symptoms are no more frequent in people with hypertension than in the general population. However, patients with hypertensive crisis (discussed later in the chapter) may experience severe headaches, dyspnea, anxiety, and nosebleeds.[11]

Complications

The most common complications of hypertension are *target organ diseases* occurring in the heart (hypertensive heart disease), brain (cerebrovascular disease), peripheral vessels (peripheral vascular disease), kidneys (nephrosclerosis), and eyes (retinal damage) (Table 33-5).

Hypertensive Heart Disease

Coronary Artery Disease. Hypertension is a major risk factor for coronary artery disease (CAD). The mechanisms by which hypertension contributes to the development of atherosclerosis are not fully known. The "response-to-injury" theory of atherogenesis suggests that hypertension disrupts the coronary artery endothelium (see Fig. 34-1). This results in a stiff arterial wall with a narrowed lumen, and accounts for a high rate of CAD, angina, and MI.

TABLE 33-5 MANIFESTATIONS OF TARGET ORGAN DISEASE

Organ	Manifestations
Cardiac	• Clinical, electrocardiographic, or radiologic evidence of coronary artery disease (e.g., previous myocardial infarction, coronary revascularization) • Left ventricular hypertrophy by ECG or echocardiography • Left ventricular dysfunction or heart failure
Cerebrovascular	• Transient ischemic attack • Stroke
Peripheral vascular	• One or more major pulses in the extremities (except for dorsalis pedis) reduced or absent • Intermittent claudication • Abdominal or carotid bruits or thrills • Aneurysm
Renal	• Serum creatinine ≥1.5 mg/dL (130 μmol/L) • Proteinuria (≥1+) • Microalbuminuria
Retinopathy	• Generalized or focal narrowing of retinal arterioles • Arteriovenous nicking • Hemorrhages or exudates with or without papilledema

Source: National Heart, Lung, and Blood Institute: Seventh report of the Joint National Committee on Detection, Evaluation, and Treatment of High Blood Pressure (JNC-7), NIH Publication No. 04-5230, Bethesda, Md, 2004, The Institute. Retrieved from *www.nhlbi.nih.gov/guidelines/hypertension/jnc7full.pdf.*

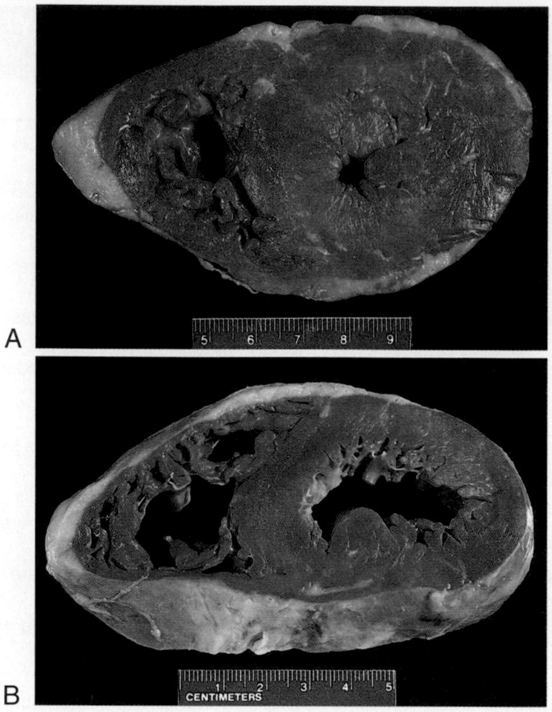

FIG. 33-2 **A,** Massively enlarged heart caused by hypertrophy of the muscle in the left ventricle. **B,** Compare with the thickness of the normal left ventricle. The patient suffered from severe hypertension.

Left Ventricular Hypertrophy. Sustained high BP increases the cardiac workload and produces left ventricular hypertrophy (LVH) (Fig. 33-2). Initially, LVH is a compensatory mechanism that strengthens cardiac contraction and increases CO. However, increased contractility increases myocardial work and oxygen demand. Progressive LVH, especially in the presence of CAD, is associated with the development of heart failure.

Heart Failure. Heart failure occurs when the heart's compensatory mechanisms are overwhelmed and the heart can no longer pump enough blood to meet the body's demands (see Chapter 35). Contractility is depressed, and stroke volume and CO are decreased. The patient may complain of shortness of breath on exertion, paroxysmal nocturnal dyspnea, and fatigue.

Cerebrovascular Disease. Atherosclerosis is the most common cause of cerebrovascular disease. Hypertension is a major risk factor for cerebral atherosclerosis and stroke. Even in mildly hypertensive people, the risk of stroke is four times higher than in normotensive people. Adequate control of BP diminishes the risk of stroke.

Atherosclerotic plaques are commonly found at the bifurcation of the common carotid artery and in the internal and external carotid arteries. Portions of the atherosclerotic plaque or the blood clot that forms with disruption of the plaque may break off and travel to cerebral vessels, producing a thromboembolism. The patient may experience transient ischemic attacks or a stroke. (These conditions are discussed in Chapter 58.)

Hypertensive encephalopathy may occur after a marked rise in BP if the cerebral blood flow is not decreased by autoregulation. Autoregulation is a physiologic process that maintains constant cerebral blood flow despite fluctuations in BP. Normally, as pressure in the cerebral blood vessels rises, the vessels constrict to maintain constant flow. When BP exceeds the body's ability to autoregulate, the cerebral vessels suddenly dilate, capillary permeability increases, and cerebral edema develops. This produces a rise in intracranial pressure. If left untreated, patients die quickly from brain damage. (Chapter 57 discusses cerebral blood flow and autoregulation.)

Peripheral Vascular Disease. Hypertension speeds up the process of atherosclerosis in the peripheral blood vessels. This leads to the development of peripheral vascular disease, aortic aneurysm, and aortic dissection (see Chapter 38). *Intermittent claudication* (ischemic leg pain precipitated by activity and relieved with rest) is a classic symptom of peripheral vascular disease.

Nephrosclerosis. Hypertension is one of the leading causes of chronic kidney disease, especially among African Americans. Some degree of renal disease is usually present in the hypertensive patient, even one with a minimally elevated BP. Renal disease results from ischemia caused by the narrowing of the renal blood vessels. This leads to atrophy of the tubules, destruction of the glomeruli, and eventual death of nephrons. Initially intact nephrons can compensate, but these changes may eventually lead to renal failure. Laboratory indications of renal disease are microalbuminuria, proteinuria, microscopic hematuria, and elevated serum creatinine and blood urea nitrogen (BUN) levels. The earliest manifestation of renal disease is usually nocturia (see Chapter 47).

Retinal Damage. The appearance of the retina provides important information about the severity and duration of hypertension. The blood vessels of the retina can be directly visualized with an ophthalmoscope. Damage to the retinal vessels provides an indication of related vessel damage in the heart, brain, and kidneys. Manifestations of severe retinal damage include blurring of vision, retinal hemorrhage, and loss of vision.

TABLE 33-6 COLLABORATIVE CARE

Hypertension

Diagnostic Studies

History and physical examination, including an ophthalmic examination
Routine urinalysis
Basic metabolic panel (serum glucose, sodium, potassium, chloride, carbon dioxide, BUN, and creatinine)
Complete blood count
Serum lipid profile (total lipids, triglycerides, HDL and LDL cholesterol, total-to-HDL cholesterol ratio)
Serum uric acid
12-lead electrocardiogram (ECG)
Optional:

- 24-hr urinary creatinine clearance
- Echocardiography
- Liver function studies
- Serum thyroid-stimulating hormone (TSH)

Collaborative Therapy

Periodic monitoring of BP

- Home BP monitoring
- Ambulatory BP monitoring (if indicated)
- Every 3-6 mo by health care provider once BP is stabilized

Nutritional therapy (see eTable 33-1)

- Restrict salt and sodium
- Restrict cholesterol and saturated fats
- Maintain adequate intake of potassium
- Maintain adequate intake of calcium and magnesium

Weight management
Regular, moderate physical activity
Tobacco cessation (see Tables 11-4 through 11-6)
Moderation of alcohol consumption
Management of psychosocial risk factors (see Chapter 7)
Antihypertensive drugs (see Tables 33-7 and 33-8)
Patient and caregiver teaching

HDL, High-density lipoprotein; *LDL*, low-density lipoprotein.

Diagnostic Studies

Chapter 32 and the Nursing Management section later in this chapter discuss BP measurement.

Some controversy exists over the diagnostic workup in the initial assessment of a person with hypertension. Because most hypertension is classified as primary hypertension, testing for secondary causes is not routinely done. Basic laboratory studies are performed to (1) identify or rule out causes of secondary hypertension, (2) evaluate target organ disease, (3) determine overall cardiovascular risk, or (4) establish baseline levels before initiating therapy.

Table 33-6 lists basic diagnostic studies performed in a person with hypertension. Routine urinalysis, BUN, and serum creatinine levels are used to screen for renal involvement and to provide baseline information about kidney function. Creatinine clearance reflects the glomerular filtration rate. Decreases in creatinine clearance indicate renal insufficiency. (Chapters 45 and 47 discuss serum creatinine and creatinine clearance.)

Measurement of serum electrolytes, especially potassium, is important to detect hyperaldosteronism, a cause of secondary hypertension. Blood glucose levels assist in the diagnosis of diabetes mellitus. A lipid profile provides information about additional risk factors related to atherosclerosis and CVD. Uric acid levels establish a baseline, since the levels often rise with diuretic therapy. An electrocardiogram (ECG) provides baseline information about cardiac status. It can identify the presence of LVH, cardiac ischemia, or previous MI. If LVH is suspected, echocardiography is often performed. If the patient's age, history, physical examination, or severity of hypertension points to a secondary cause, further diagnostic testing is indicated.

Ambulatory Blood Pressure Monitoring. Some patients have elevated BP readings in a clinical setting and normal readings when BP is measured elsewhere. This phenomenon is referred to as "white coat" hypertension. Self-monitoring of BP is an easy, cost-effective approach that may be chosen before ambulatory BP monitoring (ABPM). ABPM is a noninvasive, fully automated system that measures BP at preset intervals over a 24-hour period. The equipment includes a BP cuff and a microprocessing unit that fits into a pouch worn on a shoulder strap or belt. Tell patients to hold their arm still by their side when the device is taking a reading. Also ask them to maintain a diary of activities that may affect BP. Other potential applications for ABPM include suspected antihypertensive drug resistance, hypotensive symptoms with antihypertensive drugs, episodic hypertension, or SNS dysfunction.

BP demonstrates diurnal variability expressed as sleep-wakefulness difference. For day-active people, BP is highest in the early morning, decreases during the day, and is lowest at night. BP at night (during sleep) usually drops by 10% or more from daytime (awake) BP.[9] Some patients with hypertension do not show a normal nocturnal dip in BP and are referred to as "nondippers." The absence of diurnal variability has been associated with more target organ disease and an increased risk for CVD. The presence or absence of diurnal variability can be determined by ABPM.

Collaborative Care

Table 33-6 summarizes the collaborative care for a patient with hypertension. Goals include achieving and maintaining goal BP, and reducing cardiovascular risk and target organ disease. Lifestyle modifications are indicated for all patients with prehypertension and hypertension.

Lifestyle Modifications. Lifestyle modifications are directed toward reducing the patient's BP and overall cardiovascular risk. Modifications include (1) weight reduction, (2) Dietary Approaches to Stop Hypertension (DASH) eating plan, (3) dietary sodium reduction, (4) moderation of alcohol consumption, (5) regular physical activity, (6) avoidance of tobacco use (smoking and chewing), and (7) management of psychosocial risk factors.

Weight Reduction. Overweight persons have an increased incidence of hypertension and increased risk for CVD. Weight reduction has a significant effect on lowering BP in many people, and the effect is seen with even moderate weight loss. A weight loss of 22 lb (10 kg) may decrease SBP by approximately 5 to 20 mm Hg.[1] When a person decreases caloric intake, sodium and fat intake are usually also reduced. Although reducing the fat content of the diet has not been shown to produce sustained benefits in BP control, it may slow the progress of atherosclerosis and reduce overall CVD risk (see Chapter 34). Weight reduction through a combination of calorie restriction and moderate physical activity is recommended for overweight patients with hypertension (see Chapter 41).

DASH Eating Plan. The DASH eating plan emphasizes fruits, vegetables, fat-free or low-fat milk and milk products, whole grains, fish, poultry, beans, seeds, and nuts. Compared with the typical American diet, the plan contains less red meat, salt, sweets, added sugars, and sugar-containing beverages[12] (see eTable 33-1 on the website for this chapter). The DASH eating plan significantly lowers BP, and these decreases compare with those achieved with BP-lowering medication.[1] Additional benefits also include lowering of low-density lipoprotein (LDL) cholesterol.[12]

Dietary Sodium Reduction. Healthy adults should restrict sodium intake to less than or equal to 2300 mg/day. African Americans; people middle aged and older; and those with hypertension, diabetes mellitus, or chronic kidney disease should restrict sodium to less than or equal to 1500 mg/day.[10,12] This involves avoiding foods known to be high in sodium (e.g., canned soups, frozen dinners) and not adding salt in the preparation of foods or at meals (see Table 35-8).

Most adults exceed the recommended limits for sodium. Average sodium intake is approximately 4200 mg/day in men and 3300 mg/day in women.[12] The patient and caregiver, especially the person who prepares the meals, need to learn about sodium-restricted diets. Instruction should include reading labels of over-the-counter drugs, packaged foods, and health products (e.g., toothpaste containing baking soda) to identify hidden sources of sodium (see Fig. 35-5). Review the patient's normal diet to identify foods high in sodium.

Sodium restriction may be enough to control BP in some patients. If drug therapy is needed, a lower dosage may be effective if the patient also restricts sodium intake. Further, moderate sodium restriction lessens the risk of hypokalemia associated with diuretic therapy. However, the response differs between patients who are salt sensitive or salt resistant.

The significance of other dietary elements for the control of hypertension is not certain. There is some evidence that greater levels of dietary potassium, calcium, vitamin D, and omega-3 fatty acids are associated with lower BP in the general population and in those with hypertension. People with hypertension should maintain adequate potassium, calcium, and vitamin D intake from food sources. Calcium supplements are not recommended to lower BP. Omega-3 fatty acids found in certain fish oils can contribute to a reduction in BP and triglycerides (see Complementary & Alternative Therapies box).

Moderation of Alcohol Consumption. Excessive alcohol consumption is strongly associated with hypertension. Consumption of three or more alcoholic drinks daily is also a risk factor for CVD and stroke. Men should limit their intake of alcohol to no more than two drinks per day and women and lighter-weight men to no more than one drink per day. One drink is defined as 12 oz of regular beer, 5 oz of wine (12% alcohol), or 1.5 oz of 80-proof distilled spirits. Excessive alcohol consumption that results in cirrhosis is the most frequent cause of secondary hypertension.

Physical Activity. A physically active lifestyle is essential to promote and maintain good health. The AHA and American College of Sports Medicine recommend that adults perform moderate-intensity aerobic physical activity for at least 30 minutes most days (i.e., more than 5 days per week) or vigorous-intensity aerobic activity for at least 20 minutes 3 days a week. The 30-minute goal can be accomplished by performing shorter periods of exercise that last at least 10 minutes. Additionally, combinations of moderate and vigorous activity are acceptable (e.g., walking briskly for 30 minutes on 2 days of the week and jogging for 20 minutes on 2 other days).[13,14]

Separate physical activity guidelines exist for adults age 18 to 65 years, adults over 65 years, and adults age 50 to 64 years with functional limitations. The differences relate to the definition of moderate and vigorous aerobic activity. For adults ages 18 to 65, walking briskly at a pace that noticeably increases the pulse defines moderate-intensity aerobic activity. Jogging at a pace that substantially increases the pulse and causes rapid breathing is an example of vigorous activity for this age-group. For all other adults, individual fitness levels guide aerobic intensity.[13,14]

All adults should perform muscle-strengthening activities using the major muscles of the body at least twice a week. This helps to maintain or increase muscle strength and endurance. Additionally, flexibility and balance exercises are recommended at least twice a week for older adults, especially for those at risk for falls.[14] Moderate-intensity activities can lower BP, promote relaxation, and decrease or control body weight. Regular activity of this type can reduce SBP by approximately 4 to 9 mm Hg.[1]

Generally, physical activity is more likely to be done if it is safe and enjoyable, fits easily into one's daily schedule, and is inexpensive. Many shopping malls open early in the morning and provide a warm, safe, flat area for walking. Some health clubs offer special "off-peak" rates to encourage physical activity among older adults. Cardiac rehabilitation programs offer supervised exercise and education about cardiovascular risk factor reduction.

You can help people with hypertension increase their physical activity by explaining the need for physical activity, describing the different types of physical activities, and assisting in starting an exercise plan. Advise sedentary people to increase activity levels gradually. Individuals with CVD or other serious health problems need a thorough examination and possibly a stress test before beginning an exercise program.

Avoidance of Tobacco Products. Nicotine contained in tobacco causes vasoconstriction and increases BP, especially in people with hypertension. Smoking tobacco is also a major risk factor for CVD. The cardiovascular benefits of stopping tobacco use are seen within 1 year in all age-groups. Strongly encourage everyone, especially patients with hypertension, to avoid tobacco use. Advise those who continue to use tobacco products to monitor their BP during use. (Chapter 11 discusses tobacco use and smoking cessation.)

Management of Psychosocial Risk Factors. Psychosocial risk factors can contribute to the risk of developing CVD, and to a poorer prognosis and clinical course in patients with CVD.

COMPLEMENTARY & ALTERNATIVE THERAPIES

Fish Oil and Omega-3 Fatty Acids

Dietary sources of omega-3 fatty acids include fish oil and certain plant and nut oils. Fish oil contains both docosahexaenoic acid (DHA) and eicosapentaenoic acid (EPA). Some nuts and vegetable oils contain α-linolenic acid (ALA).

Scientific Evidence

- Reduce blood triglyceride levels
- May cause a small reduction in BP
- May reduce the risk of heart attack, stroke, and death among people with cardiovascular disease

Nursing Implications

- For healthy adults with no history of heart disease, the American Heart Association recommends eating fish at least two times per wk. Fatty fish such as anchovies, bluefish, carp, catfish, halibut, lake trout, mackerel, pompano, salmon, striped sea bass, albacore tuna, and whitefish are recommended.
- Fish oil is generally safe in recommended dosages. Higher doses may result in increased risk of bleeding.

Sources: *www.naturalstandard.com* and *http://nccam.nih.gov/health/omega3/introduction.htm.*

These risk factors include low socioeconomic status, social isolation and lack of support, stress at work and in family life, and negative emotions such as depression and hostility.[15] Frequently, these risk factors are clustered together. For example, rates of depression tend to be higher in individuals with job stress.

Psychosocial risk factors have direct effects on the cardiovascular system by activating the SNS and stress hormones. This can cause a wide variety of pathophysiologic responses, including hypertension and tachycardia, inflammation, endothelium dysfunction, increased platelet aggregation, insulin resistance, and central obesity.[16]

Psychosocial risk factors can contribute to CVD indirectly as well, simply by their impact on lifestyle behaviors and choices. Screening for psychosocial risk factors is important. Make appropriate referrals (e.g., counseling), when indicated. Suggest behavioral interventions such as relaxation training, stress management courses, support groups, and exercise training for individuals who are not in acute psychologic distress.[16]

Drug Therapy. The goal for treating hypertension is a BP less than 140/90 mm Hg. Persons with high risk for CVD (e.g., diabetes mellitus, kidney disease, tobacco use) have the greatest chance of having a cardiovascular event related to uncontrolled hypertension. For these individuals, a lower goal of 130/80 mm Hg may be appropriate. However, specific guidelines for BP goals for high-risk patients will be published when the Eighth Report of the Joint National Committee on Prevention, Detection, Evaluation, and Treatment of High Blood Pressure (JNC 8) is released.[5]

The drugs currently available for treating hypertension have two main actions: (1) they decrease the volume of circulating blood and (2) they reduce SVR (Table 33-7). The drugs used in the treatment of hypertension include diuretics,

TABLE 33-7 DRUG THERAPY*

Hypertension

Drug	Mechanism of Action	Nursing Considerations
Diuretics		
Thiazide and Related Diuretics		
bendroflumethiazide (Naturetin) chlorothiazide (Diuril) chlorthalidone (Hygroton) hydrochlorothiazide (Microzide, HydroDIURIL) indapamide (Lozol) metolazone (Zaroxolyn)	Inhibit NaCl reabsorption in the distal convoluted tubule. Increase excretion of Na^+ and Cl^-. Initial decrease in ECF. Sustained decrease in SVR. Lower BP moderately in 2-4 wk.	Monitor for orthostatic hypotension, hypokalemia, and alkalosis. Thiazides may potentiate cardiotoxicity of digoxin by producing hypokalemia. Dietary sodium restriction reduces the risk of hypokalemia. NSAIDs can decrease diuretic and antihypertensive effect of thiazide diuretics. Advise patient to supplement with potassium-rich foods.
Loop Diuretics		
bumetanide (Bumex) ethacrynic acid (Edecrin) furosemide (Lasix) torsemide (Demadex)	Inhibit NaCl reabsorption in the ascending limb of the loop of Henle. Increase excretion of Na^+ and Cl^-. More potent diuretic effect than thiazides, but shorter duration of action. Less effective for hypertension.	Monitor for orthostatic hypotension and electrolyte abnormalities. Loop diuretics remain effective despite renal insufficiency. Diuretic effect of drug increases at higher doses.
Potassium-Sparing Diuretics		
amiloride (Midamor) triamterene (Dyrenium)	Reduce K^+ and Na^+ exchange in the distal and collecting tubules. Reduce excretion of K^+, H^+, Ca^+, and Mg^+.	Monitor for orthostatic hypotension and hyperkalemia. Contraindicated in patients with renal failure. Use with caution in patients on ACE inhibitors or angiotensin II blockers. Avoid potassium supplements.
Aldosterone Receptor Blockers		
spironolactone (Aldactone) eplerenone (Inspra)	Inhibit the Na^+-retaining and K^+-excreting effects of aldosterone in the distal and collecting tubules.	Monitor for orthostatic hypotension and hyperkalemia. Do not combine with potassium-sparing diuretics or potassium supplements. Use with caution in patients on ACE inhibitors or angiotensin II blockers. These drugs are also classified as potassium-sparing diuretics.
Adrenergic Inhibitors		
Central-Acting α-Adrenergic Antagonists		
clonidine (Catapres) clonidine patch (Catapres-TTS)	Reduce sympathetic outflow from CNS. Reduce peripheral sympathetic tone, produces vasodilation, decreases SVR and BP.	Sudden discontinuation may cause withdrawal syndrome, including rebound hypertension, tachycardia, headache, tremors, apprehension, sweating. Chewing gum or hard candy may relieve dry mouth. Alcohol and sedatives increase sedation. Transdermal patch may be related to fewer side effects and better adherence.
guanabenz (Wytensin)	Same as clonidine.	Same as clonidine, but not available in transdermal formulation.
guanfacine (Tenex)	Same as clonidine.	Same as clonidine, but not available in transdermal formulation.
methyldopa (Aldomet)	Same as clonidine.	Instruct patient about daytime sedation and avoidance of hazardous activities. Administration of a single daily dose at bedtime minimizes sedative effect.

*An expanded version of this table (eTable 33-2) is available on the website for this chapter.

ACE, Angiotensin-converting enzyme; *AV*, atrioventricular; *CO*, cardiac output; *DBP*, diastolic blood pressure; *ECF*, extracellular fluid; *HDL*, high-density lipoprotein; *LDL*, low-density lipoprotein; *SBP*, systolic blood pressure; *SVR*, systemic vascular resistance.

Continued

TABLE 33-7 DRUG THERAPY—cont'd

Hypertension

Drug	Mechanism of Action	Nursing Considerations
Adrenergic Inhibitors—cont'd		
Peripheral-Acting α-Adrenergic Antagonists		
guanethidine (Ismelin)	Prevents peripheral release of norepinephrine, resulting in vasodilation. Lowers CO and reduces SBP more than DBP.	May cause severe orthostatic hypotension. Not recommended for use in patients with cerebrovascular or coronary insufficiency or in older adults. Advise patient to rise slowly and wear support stockings. Hypotensive effect is delayed for 2-3 days and lasts 7-10 days after withdrawal.
guanadrel (Hylorel)	Same as guanethidine	Must be given twice daily. Contraindicated in patients with history of depression. Monitor mood and mental status regularly. Advise patient to avoid barbiturates, alcohol, opioids.
reserpine (Serpasil)	Depletes central and peripheral stores of norepinephrine. Results in peripheral vasodilation (decreases SVR and BP).	
α_1-Adrenergic Blockers		
doxazosin (Cardura) prazosin (Minipress) terazosin (Hytrin)	Block α_1-adrenergic effects, producing peripheral vasodilation (decreases SVR and BP). Beneficial effects on lipid profile.	Reduced resistance to the outflow of urine in benign prostatic hyperplasia. Taking drug at bedtime reduces risks associated with orthostatic hypotension.
phentolamine (Regitine)	Blocks α_1-adrenergic receptors, resulting in peripheral vasodilation (decreases SVR and BP).	Used in short-term management of pheochromocytoma. Also used locally to prevent necrosis of skin and subcutaneous tissue after extravasation of adrenergic drug. No oral formulation.
β-Adrenergic Blockers		
Cardioselective Blockers acebutolol (Sectral) atenolol (Tenormin) betaxolol (Kerlone) bisoprolol (Zebeta) esmolol (Brevibloc) metoprolol (Lopressor) nebivolol (Bystolic)	Cardioselective agents block β_1-adrenergic receptors (see Table 33-1). Reduce BP by blocking β-adrenergic effects. Decrease CO and reduce sympathetic vasoconstrictor tone. Decrease renin secretion by kidneys.	Monitor pulse and BP regularly. Use with caution in patients with diabetes mellitus because drug may depress the tachycardia associated with hypoglycemia. Esmolol is for IV use only. Cardioselective agents lose cardioselectivity at higher doses.
Nonselective Blockers carteolol (Cartrol) nadolol (Corgard) penbutolol (Levatol) pindolol (Visken) propranolol (Inderal) timolol (Blocadren)	Nonselective agents block β_1- and β_2-adrenergic receptors (see Table 33-1). Reduce BP by blocking β_1- and β_2-adrenergic effects.	Same as cardioselective, except nonselective agents may cause bronchospasm, especially in patients with a history of asthma.
Mixed α- and β-Blockers		
carvedilol (Coreg) labetalol (Normodyne, Trandate)	α_1-, β_1-, and β_2-adrenergic blocking properties producing peripheral vasodilation and decreased heart rate (see Table 33-1). Reduce CO, SVR, and BP.	Same as β-adrenergic blockers. IV form available for hypertensive crisis in hospitalized patients. Patients must be kept supine during IV administration. Assess patient tolerance of upright position (severe orthostatic hypotension) before allowing upright activities (e.g., commode).
Direct Vasodilators		
fenoldopam (Corlopam)	Activates dopamine receptors, resulting in systemic and renal vasodilation.	IV use only for hypertensive crisis in hospitalized patients. Use cautiously in patients with glaucoma. Patient should remain supine for 1 hr after administration.
hydralazine (Apresoline)	Reduces SVR and BP by direct arterial vasodilation.	IV use for hypertensive crisis in hospitalized patients. Twice-daily oral dosage. Not used as monotherapy because of side effects. Contraindicated in patients with coronary artery disease.
minoxidil (Loniten)	Reduces SVR and BP by direct arterial vasodilation.	Reserved for treatment of severe hypertension associated with renal failure and resistant to other therapy. Once- or twice-daily dosage.
nitroglycerin (Tridil)	Relaxes arterial and venous smooth muscle, reducing preload and SVR. At low dose, venous dilation predominates; at higher dose, arterial dilation is present.	IV use for hypertensive crisis in hospitalized patients with myocardial ischemia. Administered by continuous IV infusion with pump or control device.

TABLE 33-7 **DRUG THERAPY—cont'd**

Hypertension

Drug	Mechanism of Action	Nursing Considerations
Direct Vasodilators—cont'd		
sodium nitroprusside (Nipride)	Direct arterial vasodilation reduces SVR and BP.	IV use for hypertensive crisis in hospitalized patients. Administered by continuous IV infusion with pump or control device. Intraarterial monitoring of BP recommended. Wrap IV solutions with an opaque material to protect from light. Stable for 24 hr. Metabolized to cyanide, then thiocyanate. Monitor thiocyanate levels with prolonged use (>3 days) or doses (≥4 mcg/kg/min).
Ganglionic Blockers		
trimethaphan (Arfonad)	Interrupts adrenergic control of arteries, results in vasodilation, and reduces SVR and BP.	IV use for initial control of BP in patient with dissecting aortic aneurysm. Administered by continuous IV infusion with pump or control device.
Angiotensin Inhibitors		
Angiotensin-Converting Enzyme Inhibitors		
benazepril (Lotensin) captopril (Capoten) enalapril (Vasotec) fosinopril (Monopril) lisinopril (Prinivil, Zestril) moexipril (Univasc) perindopril (Aceon) quinapril (Accupril) ramipril (Altace) trandolapril (Mavik)	Inhibit ACE, reduce conversion of angiotensin I to angiotensin II (A-II). Inhibit A-II–mediated vasoconstriction.	Aspirin and NSAIDs may reduce drug effectiveness. Addition of diuretic enhances drug effect. Should not be used with potassium-sparing diuretics. Inhibit breakdown of bradykinin, which may cause a dry, hacking cough. Captopril may be given orally for hypertensive crisis.
enalapril (Vasotec IV)	Inhibits ACE when oral agents not appropriate.	Given IV over 5 min. Monitor BP.
Angiotensin II Receptor Blockers		
candesartan (Atacand) eprosartan (Teveten) irbesartan (Avapro) losartan (Cozaar) olmesartan (Benicar) telmisartan (Micardis) valsartan (Diovan)	Prevent action of A-II and produce vasodilation and increased Na^+ and water excretion.	Full effect on BP may not be seen for 3-6 wk. Do not affect bradykinin levels, therefore acceptable alternative to ACE inhibitors in people who develop dry cough.
Renin Inhibitors		
aliskiren (Tekturna)	Directly inhibits renin, thus reducing conversion of angiotensinogen to angiotensin I.	May cause angioedema of the face, extremities, lips, tongue, glottis, and/or larynx. Not to be used in pregnancy.
Calcium Channel Blockers		
Non-Dihydropyridines		
diltiazem extended release (Cardizem LA, Dilacor XR) verapamil intermediate release (Isoptin, Calan) verapamil long-acting (Covera-HS, Calan SR) verapamil timed-release (Verelan PM)	Inhibit movement of Ca^{2+} across cell membrane, resulting in vasodilation. Cardioselective resulting in decrease in heart rate and slowing of AV conduction.	Use with caution in patients with heart failure. Serum concentrations and toxicity of certain calcium channel blockers may be increased by grapefruit juice; avoid concurrent use. Used for supraventricular tachydysrhythmias. Avoid in patients with second- or third-degree AV block or left ventricular systolic dysfunction.
Dihydropyridines		
amlodipine (Norvasc) clevidipine (Cleviprex) felodipine (Plendil) isradipine (DynaCirc CR) nicardipine sustained release (Cardene SR) nifedipine long acting (Adalat CC, Procardia XL) nisoldipine (Sular)	Cause vascular smooth muscle relaxation resulting in decreased SVR and arterial BP.	More potent peripheral vasodilators. Clevidipine is for IV use only. Use of sublingual short-acting nifedipine in hypertensive emergencies is unsafe and not effective. Serious adverse events (e.g., stroke, acute MI) have been reported. IV nicardipine available for hypertensive crisis in hospitalized patients. Change peripheral IV infusion sites every 12 hr.

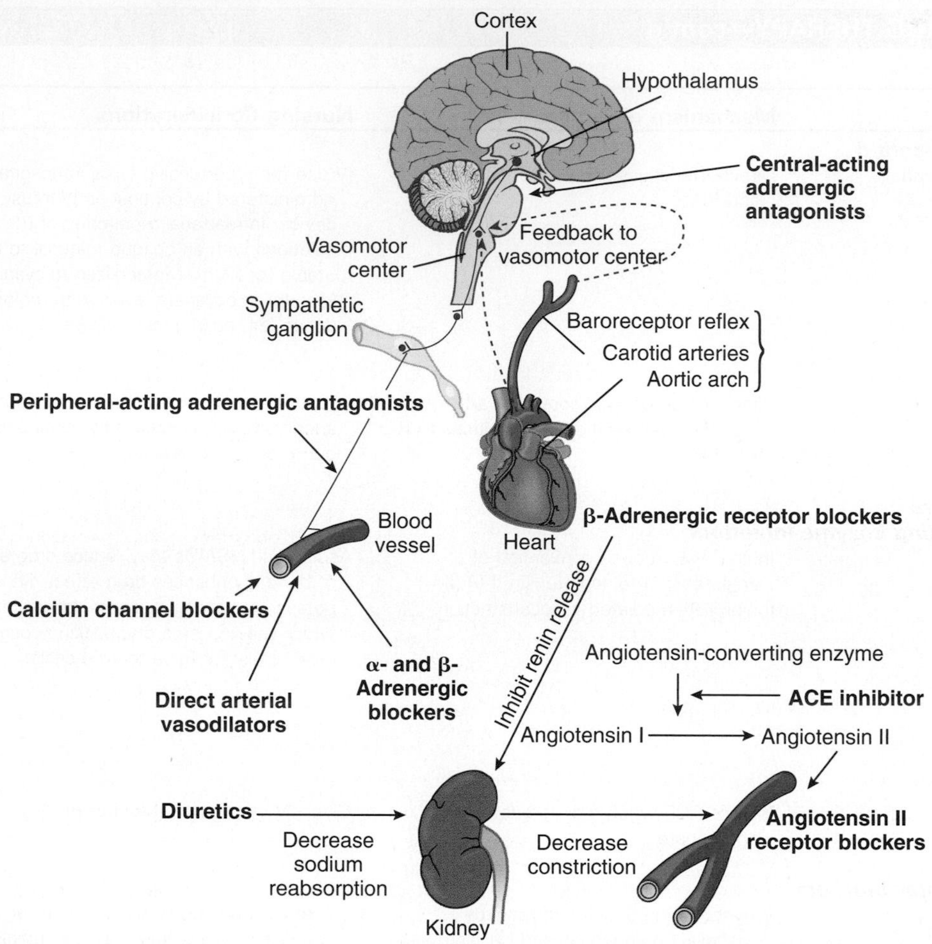

FIG. 33-3 Site and method of action of various antihypertensive drugs *(bold type)*. *ACE,* Angiotensin-converting enzyme.

adrenergic (SNS) inhibitors, direct vasodilators, angiotensin and renin inhibitors, and calcium channel blockers.[17,18] Fig. 33-3 presents the various sites and methods of action of antihypertensive drugs.

Although the precise action of diuretics in the reduction of BP is unclear, it is known that they promote sodium and water excretion, reduce plasma volume, and reduce the vascular response to catecholamines. Adrenergic-inhibiting agents act by decreasing the SNS effects that increase BP. Adrenergic inhibitors include drugs that act centrally on the vasomotor center and peripherally to inhibit NE release or to block the adrenergic receptors on blood vessels. Direct vasodilators decrease the BP by relaxing vascular smooth muscle and reducing SVR. Calcium channel blockers increase sodium excretion and cause vasodilation by preventing the movement of extracellular calcium into cells.

There are two types of angiotensin inhibitors. The first type is angiotensin-converting enzyme (ACE) inhibitors. These prevent the conversion of angiotensin I to A-II and thus reduce A-II-mediated vasoconstriction and sodium and water retention. The second type is A-II receptor blockers (ARBs). These prevent A-II from binding to its receptors in the blood vessel walls.

Most patients who are hypertensive require two or more antihypertensive medications to achieve their goal BP. The addition of a second drug from a different class is started when use of a single drug in adequate doses fails to achieve the goal BP. These can be separate prescriptions or combination therapy (Table 33-8). If a drug is not tolerated or is contraindicated, then a drug from another class is used.

Once antihypertensive therapy is started, patients should return for follow-up and adjustment of medications at monthly intervals until the goal BP is reached. More frequent visits are necessary for patients with stage 2 hypertension or with co-morbidities. After BP is at goal and stable, follow-up visits can usually be at 3- to 6-month intervals. Co-morbidities (e.g., heart failure), associated diseases (e.g., diabetes mellitus), and the need for ongoing monitoring (e.g., laboratory testing) influence the frequency of visits.

Patient and Caregiver Teaching Related to Drug Therapy. Side effects of antihypertensive drugs are common and may be so severe or undesirable that the patient does not adhere to the therapy[17,18] (see Table 33-7). Patient and caregiver teaching related to drug therapy helps them identify and minimize side effects. This may help the patient adhere to therapy. Side effects may be an initial response to a drug and may decrease over time. Informing the patient about side effects that may decrease with time may enable the person to continue taking the drug. The number or severity of side effects may relate to the dosage. It may be necessary to change the drug or decrease the dosage. Advise the patient to report all side effects to the health care provider who prescribes the medication.

A common side effect of several of these drugs is orthostatic hypotension. This condition results from an alteration of the

TABLE 33-8 **DRUG THERAPY**

Combination Therapy for Hypertension

Combinations	Trade Names
Angiotensin-Converting Enzyme Inhibitors and Diuretics	
benazepril/hydrochlorothiazide	Lotensin HCT
captopril/hydrochlorothiazide	Capozide
enalapril/hydrochlorothiazide	Vaseretic
fosinopril/hydrochlorothiazide	Monopril-HCT
lisinopril/hydrochlorothiazide	Prinzide, Zestoretic
moexipril/hydrochlorothiazide	Uniretic
quinapril/hydrochlorothiazide	Accuretic
Angiotensin II Receptor Blockers and Diuretics	
azilsartan/chlorthalidone	Edarbyclor
candesartan/hydrochlorothiazide	Atacand HCT
eprosartan/hydrochlorothiazide	Teveten HCT
irbesartan/hydrochlorothiazide	Avalide
losartan/hydrochlorothiazide	Hyzaar
olmesartan medoxomil/hydrochlorothiazide	Benicar HCT
telmisartan/hydrochlorothiazide	Micardis HCT
valsartan/hydrochlorothiazide	Diovan HCT
β-Adrenergic Blockers and Diuretics	
atenolol/chlorthalidone	Tenoretic
bisoprolol/hydrochlorothiazide	Ziac
metoprolol/hydrochlorothiazide	Lopressor HCT
nadolol/bendroflumethiazide	Corzide
propranolol/hydrochlorothiazide	Inderide
timolol/hydrochlorothiazide	Timolide
Centrally Acting Drugs and Diuretics	
methyldopa/hydrochlorothiazide	Aldoril
reserpine/chlorthalidone	Demi-Regroton
reserpine/hydrochlorothiazide	Hydropres
prazosin/polythiazide	Minizide
guanethidine/hydrochlorothiazide	Esimil
clonidine/chlorthalidone	Combipres
Angiotensin-Converting Enzyme Inhibitors and Calcium Channel Blockers	
amlodipine/benazepril	Lotrel
enalapril/felodipine	Lexxel
enalapril/diltiazem	Teczem
trandolapril/verapamil	Tarka
Angiotensin II Receptor Blockers and Calcium Channel Blockers	
telmisartan/amlodipine	Twynsta
valsartan/amlodipine	Exforge
olmesartan/amlodipine	Azor
Diuretics and Diuretics	
amiloride/hydrochlorothiazide	Moduretic
spironolactone/hydrochlorothiazide	Aldactazide
triamterene/hydrochlorothiazide	Dyazide, Maxzide
Angiotensin II Receptor Blocker, Calcium Channel Blocker, and Diuretic	
olmesartan medoxomil/amlodipine/hydrochlorothiazide	Tribenzor

autonomic nervous system's mechanisms for regulating BP, which are required for position changes. Consequently, the patient may feel dizzy and faint when assuming an upright position after sitting or lying down. Table 33-12 (later in this chapter) presents specific measures to control or decrease orthostatic hypotension.

EVIDENCE-BASED PRACTICE

Applying the Evidence

You are caring for P.N., a 46-year-old man with a history of poorly controlled hypertension and chronic kidney disease. You note that he is taking three antihypertensive medications. He tells you that he can no longer live with the side effects of these drugs (e.g., fatigue, dry mouth, erectile dysfunction). He states that he wants to stop taking the medications. He believes that if he changes his lifestyle by reducing salt from his diet, losing weight, and beginning exercise, he can control his hypertension.

Best Available Evidence	Clinician Expertise	Patient Preferences and Values
Uncontrolled BP places persons with concurrent risk for cardiovascular disease (e.g., diabetes, kidney disease) at highest risk for a cardiovascular event (e.g., stroke). Most hypertensive patients will need two or more medications to achieve their goal BP in addition to lifestyle changes.	You know that lifestyle changes can help reduce and control BP in many patients. However, patients with poorly controlled hypertension and target organ disease require medications to control BP and prevent further complications.	P.N. wishes to eliminate antihypertensive medications because of unpleasant and unacceptable side effects that are interfering with his quality of life.

Your Decision and Actions

You discuss the role of lifestyle changes and medications in the treatment of hypertension and prevention of (further) target organ disease with P.N. You support his intention to make lifestyle changes and validate his concerns regarding the side effects of the medications. You discuss the side effects that he is experiencing and explain that it may be possible to change some of his medications to eliminate or reduce the unpleasant side effects. However, given the severity of his hypertension and the chronic kidney disease, he will need to be on medications on a long-term basis. Any of his plans to discontinue medications need to be discussed with his physician.

Reference for Evidence

National Heart, Lung, and Blood Institute: Seventh report of the Joint National Committee on Detection, Evaluation, and Treatment of High Blood Pressure (JNC-7), NIH Publication No. 04-5230, Bethesda, Md, 2004, The Institute. Retrieved from *www.nhlbi.nih.gov/guidelines/hypertension/jnc7full.pdf*.

Sexual problems may occur with many of the antihypertensive drugs and can be a major reason that patients do not adhere to the treatment plan. Problems can range from reduced libido to erectile dysfunction. Rather than discussing a sexual problem with a health care provider, the patient may decide just to stop taking the drug. Approach the patient on this sensitive subject and encourage discussion of any sexual problem that may be experienced. The sexual problems may be easier for the patient to discuss once you explain that the drug may be the source of the problem. Changing to another antihypertensive drug can decrease or remove these side effects. Encourage the patient to discuss sexual issues with the health care provider. If the patient is reluctant to do so, offer to alert the health care provider to the side effects that the patient is experiencing. There are many drug options in treating hypertension. A plan that is acceptable to the patient should be achievable.[19]

Some unpleasant side effects of drugs result from their therapeutic effect, but these can be decreased. For example, diuret-

TABLE 33-9 CAUSES OF RESISTANT HYPERTENSION

Improper BP measurement

Volume overload
- Excess salt intake
- Volume retention from kidney disease
- Inadequate diuretic therapy

Drug-induced or other causes
- Nonadherence
- Illegal drugs (e.g., cocaine, amphetamines)
- Inadequate drug dosages
- Inappropriate combinations of drug therapy
- Nonsteroidal antiinflammatory drugs
- Sympathomimetics (e.g., decongestants, diet pills)
- Oral contraceptives
- Corticosteroids
- Cyclosporine and tacrolimus (Prograf)
- Erythropoietin
- Licorice (including some chewing tobacco)
- Selected over-the-counter dietary or herbal supplements and medicines (e.g., ma huang, bitter orange)

Associated conditions
- Increasing obesity
- Excess alcohol consumption

Identifiable causes of secondary hypertension

Source: National Heart, Lung, and Blood Institute: Seventh report of the Joint National Committee on Detection, Evaluation, and Treatment of High Blood Pressure (JNC-7), NIH Publication No. 04-5230, Bethesda, Md, 2004, The Institute. Retrieved from *www.nhlbi.nih.gov/guidelines/hypertension/jnc7full.pdf.*

ics cause dry mouth and frequent voiding. Sugarless gum or hard candy may help ease the dry mouth. Taking diuretics earlier in the day may limit frequent voiding during the night and preserve sleep. Side effects of vasodilators and adrenergic inhibitors decrease if the drugs are taken in the evening. Remember that BP is lowest during the night and highest shortly after awakening. Therefore drugs with a 24-hour duration of action should be taken as early in the morning as possible (e.g., 4 or 5 AM if the patient awakens to void).

Resistant Hypertension. *Resistant hypertension* is the failure to reach goal BP in patients who are taking full doses of an appropriate three-drug therapy regimen that includes a diuretic. Carefully explore reasons why the patient is not at goal BP (Table 33-9). Studies have shown that the use of *renal denervation* (destruction of overactive renal nerves) reduces BP and muscle sympathetic nerve activity in patients with resistant hypertension. The exact mechanisms underlying sympathetic neural inhibition are not clear.[20]

NURSING MANAGEMENT PRIMARY HYPERTENSION

NURSING ASSESSMENT

Table 33-10 presents subjective and objective data to obtain from a patient with hypertension.

NURSING DIAGNOSES

Nursing diagnoses and collaborative problems for the patient with hypertension include, but are not limited to, the following.

- Ineffective self-health management *related to* lack of knowledge of pathology, complications, and management of hypertension
- Anxiety *related to* complexity of management regimen

TABLE 33-10 NURSING ASSESSMENT

Hypertension

Subjective Data

Important Health Information

Past health history: Known duration and past workup of high BP; cardiovascular, cerebrovascular, renal, or thyroid disease; diabetes mellitus; pituitary disorders; obesity; dyslipidemia; menopause or hormone replacement status

Medications: Use of any prescription or over-the-counter, illicit, or herbal medications or products; previous use of antihypertensive drug therapy

Functional Health Patterns

Health perception–health management: Family history of hypertension or cardiovascular disease; tobacco use, alcohol use; sedentary lifestyle

Nutritional-metabolic: Usual salt and fat intake; weight gain or loss

Elimination: Nocturia

Activity-exercise: Fatigue; dyspnea on exertion, palpitations, exertional chest pain; intermittent claudication, muscle cramps; usual pattern and type of exercise

Cognitive-perceptual: Dizziness; blurred vision; paresthesias

Sexual-reproductive: Erectile dysfunction, decreased libido

Coping–stress tolerance: Stressful life events

Objective Data

Cardiovascular

SBP consistently >140 mm Hg or DBP >90 mm Hg, orthostatic changes in BP and pulse; bilateral BPs significantly different; abnormal heart sounds; laterally displaced, apical pulse; diminished or absent peripheral pulses; carotid, renal, or femoral bruits; peripheral edema

Gastrointestinal

Obesity (BMI ≥30 kg/m^2); abnormal waist-hip ratio

Neurologic

Mental status changes

Possible Diagnostic Findings

Abnormal serum electrolytes (especially potassium); ↑ BUN, creatinine, glucose, cholesterol, and triglyceride levels; proteinuria, microalbuminuria, microscopic hematuria; evidence of ischemic heart disease and left ventricular hypertrophy on ECG; evidence of structural heart disease and left ventricular hypertrophy on echocardiogram; evidence of arteriovenous nicking, retinal hemorrhages, and papilledema on funduscopic examination

BMI, Body mass index; *DBP,* diastolic blood pressure; *SBP,* systolic blood pressure.

- Sexual dysfunction *related to* side effects of antihypertensive medication
- Risk for decreased cardiac tissue perfusion
- Risk for ineffective cerebral tissue perfusion
- Risk for ineffective renal perfusion
- Potential complication: stroke
- Potential complication: MI

PLANNING

The overall goals for the patient with hypertension are that the patient will (1) achieve and maintain the goal BP; (2) understand and follow the therapeutic plan; (3) experience minimal or no unpleasant side effects of therapy; and (4) be confident of the ability to manage and cope with this condition.

NURSING IMPLEMENTATION

HEALTH PROMOTION. Primary prevention of hypertension is a cost-effective approach. Current recommendations for primary prevention include lifestyle modifications that prevent or delay the rise in BP in at-risk people. Following the DASH diet and reducing sodium can lower BP (see eTable 33-1). This diet is recommended for primary prevention in the general population. Dietary changes by the food industry (e.g., reducing the amount of salt in processed foods) may also be effective.

To raise awareness about the dangers of high BP, the National Heart, Lung, and Blood Institute provides web-based educational materials for health care providers, patients, and the public. (See Your Guide to Lowering High Blood Pressure at *www.nhlbi.nih.gov/hbp.*)

Individual Patient Evaluation. Hypertension is usually identified through routine screening for insurance, preemployment, and military physical examinations. You are in an ideal position to assess for the presence of hypertension, identify the risk factors for hypertension and CAD, and teach the patient about these conditions. In addition to BP measurement, a complete health assessment should include such factors as age, gender, and race; diet history (including sodium and alcohol intake); weight patterns; tobacco use; and family history of heart disease, stroke, renal disease, and diabetes mellitus. Note all medications taken, both prescribed and over-the-counter drugs. Finally, ask the patient about a previous history of high BP and the results of treatment (if any) (see Table 33-10).

Blood Pressure Measurement. BP can be measured using the oscillatory or auscultatory method.[21] Initially, take the BP in both arms to note any differences. Atherosclerosis in the subclavian artery can cause a falsely low reading on the side where the narrowing occurs. Use the arm with the highest BP and take at least two readings, a minimum of 1 minute apart (see Table 33-11). Waiting for at least 1 minute between readings allows the blood to drain from the arm and prevents inaccurate readings. Record the average pressure as the value for that visit.

Proper size and correct placement of the BP cuff are critical for accurate measurement. Place the cuff snugly around the patient's bare upper arm with the midline of the bladder of the cuff (usually marked on the cuff by the manufacturer) placed above the brachial artery. Place the patient's arm at the level of the heart during BP measurement. For BP measurements taken in the sitting position, raise and support the arm at the level of the heart. For measurements taken in a supine position, raise and support (e.g., with a small pillow) the arm at heart level. If the arm is resting on the bed, it will be below heart level.

If neither upper arm can be used to measure the BP (e.g., presence of IV lines, fistula), or if a maximum size BP cuff does not fit the upper arm, use the forearm. In this case, position the proper size cuff midway between the elbow and the wrist. Auscultate Korotkoff sounds over the radial artery or use a Doppler device to note SBP. Use of an oscillometric device on the forearm is acceptable. Forearm and upper arm BPs are not interchangeable.[21]

SAFETY ALERT

- If using the forearm for BP measurement, always document the site.
- BP cuffs that are too small or too large will result in readings that are falsely high or low, respectively.
- If bilateral BP measurements are not equal, document this finding and use the arm with the highest BP for all future measurements.

Assess for orthostatic (or postural) changes in BP and pulse in older adults, in people taking antihypertensive drugs, and in patients who report symptoms consistent with reduced BP on standing (e.g., light-headedness, dizziness, syncope). Measure serial BP and pulse with the patient in the supine, sitting, and standing positions. Initially, measure BP and pulse with the patient in the supine position after at least 2 to 3 minutes of rest. Reposition the patient in the sitting position with legs dangling and measure BP and pulse again within 1 to 2 minutes. Finally reposition the patient to the standing position and measure the BP and pulse within 1 to 2 minutes. Usually the SBP decreases slightly (less than 10 mm Hg) on standing, whereas the DBP and pulse increase slightly. A decrease of 20 mm Hg or more in SBP, a decrease of 10 mm Hg or more in DBP, and/or an increase in the HR of 20 beats/minute or more from supine to standing indicates **orthostatic hypotension.** Common causes of orthostatic hypotension include intravascular volume loss and inadequate vasoconstrictor mechanisms related to disease or medications.

TABLE 33-11 BLOOD PRESSURE MEASUREMENT

The patient should not have smoked, exercised, or ingested caffeine within 30 min before measurement.

1. Seat patient with legs uncrossed, feet on the floor, and back supported. Bare patient's arm and support it at heart level.
2. Begin measurement after patient has rested quietly for 5 min. Ask patient to relax as much as possible and not to talk during the measurement.
3. Measure and record BP in both arms initially.
4. Select the appropriate cuff size, following instructions for fit and placement according to manufacturer's recommendations.
5. Take the BP with a recently calibrated aneroid or mercury sphygmomanometer, or electronic oscillometric device. Accuracy of oscillometric devices may be limited if patients are hypertensive, are hypotensive, or have heart dysrhythmias (e.g., atrial fibrillation).
6. For auscultatory measurement, estimate SBP by palpating the radial pulse and inflating the cuff until the pulse disappears. Inflate the cuff 20-30 mm Hg above this level.
7. Deflate the cuff at a rate of 2-3 mm Hg/sec.
8. Record the SBP and the DBP. Note the SBP when the first of two or more Korotkoff sounds is heard and the DBP when sound disappears.
9. Average two or more readings (taken at intervals of at least 1 min). Obtain additional readings if the first two readings differ by more than 5 mm Hg.
10. Provide the patient (verbally and in writing) with the BP reading, BP goal, and recommendations for follow-up.

Sources: National Heart, Lung, and Blood Institute: Seventh report of the Joint National Committee on Detection, Evaluation, and Treatment of High Blood Pressure (JNC-7), NIH Publication No. 04-5230, Bethesda, Md, 2004, The Institute. Retrieved from *www.nhlbi.nih.gov/guidelines/hypertension/jnc7full.pdf*; and Seckel MA, Bradley E, Bucher L, et al: AACN practice alert: noninvasive blood pressure monitoring, 2006. Retrieved from *http://classic.aacn.org/AACN/practiceAlert.nsf/Files/NIBP/$file/Noninvasive%20BP%20Monitoring%206-2006.pdf.*
DBP, diastolic blood pressure; *SBP*, systolic blood pressure.

DRUG ALERT: Doxazosin (Cardura)

- Use caution with administration of initial dose.
- Syncope (sudden loss of consciousness) occasionally occurs 30 to 90 min after the initial dose, a too-rapid increase in dose, or addition of another antihypertensive agent to therapy.

In the acute care setting, BP measurement is usually performed to evaluate vital signs, volume status, and effects of medications, rather than to diagnose hypertension. Drugs, acute illness, bed rest, and alterations in usual diet all have an impact on BP values. Inform the health care provider of any patient with a persistent increase in BP. These patients

DELEGATION DECISIONS

Caring for the Patient With Hypertension

Many members of the health care team obtain blood pressure (BP) readings. In patients with stable hypertension, LPN/LVNs and UAP provide most of the routine BP monitoring. For patients in hypertensive crisis, the RN is responsible for titration of medications and ongoing assessment and evaluation of BP.

Role of Registered Nurse (RN)

- Develop and conduct hypertension screening programs.
- Assess patients for hypertension risk factors, and develop risk modification plans.
- Teach patients about lifestyle management and medication use.
- Evaluate the effectiveness of lifestyle management and medications in decreasing BP to acceptable levels.
- Teach about home BP monitoring, including the correct use of automatic BP monitors.
- Make appropriate referrals to other health care professionals, such as dietitians or stress management programs.
- Monitor for complications of hypertension such as coronary artery disease, heart failure, cerebrovascular disease, peripheral vascular disease, and renal disease.
- Assess the patient with hypertensive urgency or crisis for target organ disease (encephalopathy, renal insufficiency, cardiac decompensation).
- Manage the patient with hypertensive crisis, including administration of medications and evaluation for resolution of the emergency.

Role of Licensed Practical Nurse (LPN)

- Administer antihypertensive medications to stable patients.
- Monitor for adverse effects of antihypertensive medications.
- Reinforce teaching about medications and lifestyle management.

Role of Unlicensed Assistive Personnel (UAP)

- Obtain accurate BP readings in outpatient and inpatient settings.
- Report high or low BP readings immediately to RN.
- Check for postural changes in BP as directed.

should be evaluated for hypertension before discharge, if appropriate, or after discharge.[9]

Screening Programs. Screening programs in the community are widely used to check individuals for high BP. At the time of the BP measurement, give each person a written, numeric value of the reading. If necessary, explain why further evaluation is needed. Effort and resources should focus on the following: (1) controlling BP in persons already identified as having hypertension; (2) identifying and controlling BP in at-risk groups such as African Americans, obese people, and blood relatives of people with hypertension; and (3) screening those with limited access to the health care system.

Cardiovascular Risk Factor Modification. Teaching regarding CVD risk factors is appropriate for all individuals and during targeted screening programs. Modifiable cardiovascular risk factors include hypertension, obesity, diabetes mellitus, tobacco use, and physical inactivity. Discuss lifestyle modifications based on identified risk factors. (Table 34-2 discusses health-promoting behaviors for risk factor reduction.)

AMBULATORY AND HOME CARE

Your primary responsibilities for long-term management of hypertension are to assist the patient in reducing BP and adhering to the treatment plan. Your nursing actions include evaluating therapeutic effectiveness, detecting and reporting any adverse treatment effects, assessing and enhancing adherence, and patient and caregiver teaching (Table 33-12).

TABLE 33-12 PATIENT & CAREGIVER TEACHING GUIDE

Hypertension

When teaching the patient and/or caregiver about hypertension, include the following information.

General Instructions

1. Provide the patient's BP reading and explain what it means (e.g., high, low, normal, borderline). Encourage patient to monitor BP at home and instruct the patient to call health care provider if BP exceeds high or low limits set by health care provider.
2. Hypertension is usually asymptomatic and symptoms (e.g., nosebleeds) do not reliably indicate BP levels.
3. Hypertension means high BP and does not relate to a "hyper" personality.
4. Long-term therapy and follow-up care are necessary to treat hypertension. Therapy involves lifestyle changes (e.g., weight management, sodium reduction, smoking cessation, regular physical activity) and, in most cases, medications.
5. Therapy will not cure, but should control hypertension.
6. Controlled hypertension usually results in an excellent prognosis and a normal lifestyle.
7. Explain the potential dangers of uncontrolled hypertension (e.g., target organ disease).

Instructions Related to Medications

1. Be specific about the names, actions, dosages, and side effects of prescribed medications.
2. Help the patient plan regular and convenient times for taking medications and measuring BP.
3. Do not stop drugs abruptly because withdrawal may cause a severe hypertensive reaction.
4. Do not double up on doses when a dose is missed.
5. If BP increases, the patient should not increase the medication dosage before consulting with the health care provider.
6. Do not take a medication belonging to someone else.
7. Supplement diet with foods high in potassium (e.g., citrus fruits, green leafy vegetables) if taking potassium-wasting diuretics.
8. Avoid hot baths, excessive amounts of alcohol, and strenuous exercise within 3 hr of taking medications that promote vasodilation.
9. Many medications cause orthostatic hypotension. The effects of orthostatic hypotension can be reduced by rising slowly from bed, sitting on the side of the bed for a few minutes, standing slowly, and beginning to move if no symptoms develop (e.g., dizziness, light-headedness). Do not stand still for prolonged periods, do leg exercises to increase venous return, or sleep with the head of the bed raised. Do lie or sit down when dizziness occurs.
10. Many medications cause sexual problems (e.g., erectile dysfunction, decreased libido). Consult with the health care provider about changing drugs or dosages if sexual problems develop.
11. The side effects of medication(s) may decrease with time.
12. Be careful about taking potentially high-risk over-the-counter medications, such as high-sodium antacids, appetite suppressants, and cold and sinus medications. Read warning labels and consult with a pharmacist.

Home BP Monitoring. Most patients with known or suspected hypertension should monitor their BP at home. Home BP monitoring reduces the white coat effect of measurement by a health care provider. The readings are often lower than those taken in the office setting and are a better predictor of CVD risk.[22]

Patient teaching is critical to ensure accuracy. Tell patients to buy an oscillometric BP monitor that uses a cuff for the upper arm. The patient should bring the BP monitor to the office to verify proper cuff size, accuracy of the device, and the patient's technique.

INFORMATICS IN PRACTICE

Monitoring Blood Pressure

- For patients with hypertension who have a smart phone or computer access, encourage them to use applications aimed at helping them manage their care, including BP self-monitoring and appointment tracking.
- Patients enter their SBP and DBP, heart rate, and other information, including the arm measured. They also indicate whether they were standing, sitting, or lying down and time the BP was taken.
- At appointment time, you can review the reports generated from the application to assist you in determining how well the patient's BP has been controlled.

DBP, Diastolic BP; *SBP*, systolic BP.

Teach the patient to obtain a BP according to the steps in Table 33-11. Tell the patient to measure BP in the nondominant arm, or arm with the higher BP if there is a known difference between arms. Advise the patient to measure BP first thing in the morning (if possible, before taking medications) and at night before going to bed. Tell the patient to keep a log of all BP measurements and to bring the log to office visits.

For clinical decision making (e.g., adjustments in dosage, start of new drug), instruct patients to take BP readings as described for 1 week. Stable, normotensive patients should measure morning and evening BP for at least 1 week every 3 months.[22] Devices that have memory or printouts of the readings are recommended to ensure accurate reporting.[9]

Home BP readings may help achieve patient adherence by reinforcing the need to remain on therapy. However, some patients become overly concerned with the BP readings. Discourage too frequent checking of their BP. Generally, home BP monitoring should reassure the patient that the treatment is effective.

Patient Adherence. A major problem in the long-term management of the patient with hypertension is poor adherence with the prescribed treatment plan. The reasons are many and include inadequate patient teaching, unpleasant side effects of drugs, return of BP to normal range while on medication, lack of motivation, high cost of drugs, lack of insurance, and lack of a trusting relationship between the patient and the health care provider. Also assess the patient's diet, activity level, and lifestyle as additional indicators of adherence.

Individually assess patients to determine the reasons why the patient is not adhering to the treatment and develop a plan with the patient to improve adherence. The plan should be compatible with the patient's personality, habits, and lifestyle. Active patient participation increases the likelihood of adherence to the treatment plan. Measures such as including the patient in the development of a medication schedule, selecting medications that are affordable, and involving caregivers help increase patient adherence.

Substituting combination drugs for multiple drugs once the BP is stable may also facilitate adherence. Combination drugs reduce the number of pills the patient has to take each day and may reduce costs.

It is important to help the patient and caregiver understand that hypertension is a chronic illness that cannot be cured. Emphasize that it can be controlled with drug therapy, diet changes, physical activity, periodic follow-up, and other relevant lifestyle modifications.

EVALUATION

The overall expected outcomes are that the patient with hypertension will

- Achieve and maintain goal BP as defined for the individual
- Understand, accept, and implement the therapeutic plan
- Experience minimal or no unpleasant side effects of therapy

GERONTOLOGIC CONSIDERATIONS

HYPERTENSION

The prevalence of hypertension increases with age. The lifetime risk of developing hypertension is approximately 90% for middle-aged (ages 55 to 65) and older (over 65) normotensive men and women.[17] Isolated systolic hypertension (ISH) is the most common form of hypertension in people over 50 years of age. Additionally, older adults are more likely to have white coat hypertension.[9]

The pathophysiology of hypertension in the older adult involves the following age-related physical changes: (1) loss of elasticity in large arteries from atherosclerosis, (2) increased collagen content and stiffness of the myocardium, (3) increased peripheral vascular resistance, (4) decreased adrenergic receptor sensitivity, (5) blunting of baroreceptor reflexes, (6) decreased renal function, and (7) decreased renin response to sodium and water depletion.

In the older adult who is taking antihypertensive medication, absorption of some drugs may be altered as a result of decreased blood flow to the gut. Metabolism and excretion of drugs may also be prolonged.

Careful technique is important in assessing BP in older adults. Some older people have a wide gap between the first Korotkoff sound and subsequent beats. This is called the *auscultatory gap.* Failure to inflate the cuff high enough may result in underestimating SBP (see Table 33-11).

The recommended BP goals are less than 140/90 mm Hg for people 65 to 79 years of age and an SBP of 140 to 145 mm Hg for those 80 years and older. Lower goals are recommended for older adults with diabetes mellitus, kidney disease, or CAD. Preferred antihypertensive drugs are low-dose thiazides, calcium channel blockers, and RAAS blockers. A diuretic should always be the first or second drug ordered for this age-group.[17]

Because of varying degrees of impaired baroreceptor reflexes, orthostatic hypotension often occurs in older adults, especially in those with ISH. Orthostatic hypotension in this age-group is often associated with volume depletion or chronic disease states, such as decreased renal and hepatic function or electrolyte imbalance. To reduce the likelihood of orthostatic hypotension, antihypertensive drugs should be started at low doses and increased slowly. Measure BP and HR in the supine, sitting, and standing positions at every visit.

Older adults experience postprandial drops in BP. The greatest decrease occurs approximately 1 hour after eating. BP returns to preprandial levels 3 to 4 hours after eating. Avoid giving vasoactive medications with meals.[7]

After CVD, arthritis is the second most prevalent disease in older adults. The most frequently taken drugs by older adults are nonsteroidal antiinflammatory drugs (NSAIDs), both prescription and over-the-counter. Nonselective NSAIDs (e.g., ibuprofen [Advil]) and selective NSAIDs (e.g., celecoxib [Celebrex]) have caused loss of BP control and heart failure. Additionally, there is the potential for adverse renal effects and/or hyperka-

TABLE 33-13 CAUSES OF HYPERTENSIVE CRISIS

- Exacerbation of chronic hypertension
- Renovascular hypertension
- Preeclampsia, eclampsia
- Pheochromocytoma
- Drugs (cocaine, amphetamines)
- Monoamine oxidase inhibitors taken with tyramine-containing foods
- Rebound hypertension (from abrupt withdrawal of some hypertensive drugs such as clonidine [Catapres] or β-adrenergic blockers)
- Head injury
- Acute aortic dissection

lemia when NSAIDs are used with ACE inhibitors, ARBs, or aldosterone antagonists.[7]

HYPERTENSIVE CRISIS

Hypertensive crisis is a term used to indicate either a hypertensive urgency or emergency. This is determined by the degree of target organ disease and how quickly the BP must be lowered.

A *hypertensive emergency* develops over hours to days. It is a situation in which a patient's BP is severely elevated (often above 220/140 mm Hg) with clinical evidence of target organ disease. Hypertensive emergencies can cause encephalopathy, intracranial or subarachnoid hemorrhage, acute left ventricular failure, MI, renal failure, dissecting aortic aneurysm, and retinopathy.

Hypertensive urgency develops over days to weeks. This is a situation in which a patient's BP is severely elevated (usually above 180/110 mm Hg), but there is no clinical evidence of target organ disease.[23]

The rate of rise of BP is more important than the absolute value in determining the need for emergency treatment. Patients with chronic hypertension can tolerate much higher BPs than normotensive people. Prompt recognition and management of hypertensive crisis are essential to decrease the threat to organ function and life.

Hypertensive crisis occurs more often in patients with a history of hypertension who have not adhered to their medication regimens or who have been undermedicated. In such cases, rising BP is thought to trigger endothelial damage and the release of vasoconstrictor substances. A vicious cycle of BP elevation follows, leading to life-threatening damage to target organs.

Hypertensive crisis related to cocaine or crack use is a frequent problem. Other drugs such as amphetamines, phencyclidine (PCP), and lysergic acid diethylamide (LSD) can also cause hypertensive crisis that may be complicated by drug-induced seizures, stroke, MI, or encephalopathy. Table 33-13 lists causes of hypertensive crisis.

Clinical Manifestations

A hypertensive emergency is often manifested as *hypertensive encephalopathy*, a syndrome in which a sudden rise in BP is associated with severe headache, nausea, vomiting, seizures, confusion, and coma. The manifestations of encephalopathy are the result of increased cerebral capillary permeability. This leads to cerebral edema and a disruption in cerebral function. On

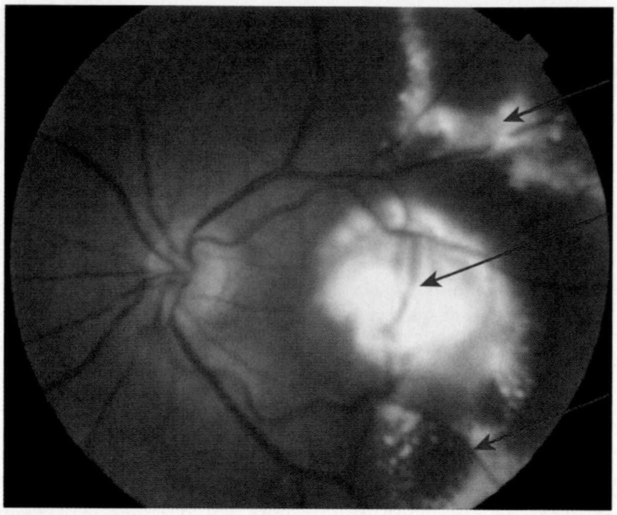

FIG. 33-4 Massive retinal exudates (indicated by *arrows*) from hypertensive retinopathy. To see what a normal retina looks like on ophthalmoscopic examination, see Fig. 21-5 on p. 377.

retinal examination, exudates, hemorrhages, and/or papilledema is found[23] (Fig. 33-4).

Renal insufficiency ranging from minor injury to complete renal failure can occur. Rapid cardiac decompensation ranging from unstable angina to MI and pulmonary edema is also possible. Patients can have chest pain and dyspnea. Aortic dissection can develop and will cause sudden, excruciating chest and back pain and possibly reduced or absent pulses in the extremities.

Patient assessment is extremely important. Monitor for signs of neurologic deficits, retinal damage, heart failure, pulmonary edema, and renal failure. The neurologic changes are often similar to those related to a stroke. However, a hypertensive crisis does not show focal or lateralizing signs often seen with a stroke.

NURSING AND COLLABORATIVE MANAGEMENT HYPERTENSIVE CRISIS

BP level alone is a poor indicator of the seriousness of the patient's condition. It is not the major factor in deciding the treatment for a hypertensive crisis. The link between elevated BP and signs of new or progressive target organ disease determines the seriousness of the situation.

Hypertensive emergencies require hospitalization, IV administration of antihypertensive drugs, and intensive care monitoring. In treatment of hypertensive emergencies, the mean arterial pressure (MAP) is often used instead of BP readings to guide and evaluate drug therapy. MAP is calculated as follows:

$$MAP = (SBP + 2\,DBP) \div 3$$

The initial goal is to decrease MAP by no more than 20% to 25%, or to decrease MAP to 110 to 115 mm Hg. If the patient is clinically stable, drugs can be titrated to gradually lower BP over the next 24 hours. Lowering the BP too quickly or too much may decrease cerebral, coronary, or renal perfusion. This could precipitate a stroke, MI, or renal failure.

Special circumstances include patients with aortic dissection. These patients should have their SBP lowered to less than 100 to 120 mm Hg as soon as possible, and if tolerated.[23] Another exception is patients with acute ischemic stroke, in whom BP is lowered to allow the use of thrombolytic agents. Finally, an elevated BP in the immediate poststroke period may be a compensatory response to improve cerebral perfusion to ischemic brain tissue. There is no clear evidence supporting the use of antihypertensive medications in these patients[1] (see Chapter 58).

IV drugs used for hypertensive emergencies include vasodilators (e.g., sodium nitroprusside [Nitropress], fenoldopam [Corlopam], nicardipine [Cardene]), adrenergic inhibitors (e.g., phentolamine [Regitine], labetalol [Normodyne], esmolol [Brevibloc]), the ACE inhibitor enalapril (Vasotec IV), and the calcium channel blocker clevidipine (Cleviprex)[23,24] (see Table 33-7). Sodium nitroprusside is the most effective IV drug to treat hypertensive emergencies. Oral agents may be given along with IV drugs to help make an earlier transition to long-term therapy.

DRUG ALERT: Labetalol (Normodyne)
- Instruct patient not to discontinue drug abruptly, since this may precipitate angina or heart failure.

Antihypertensive drugs administered IV have a rapid (within seconds to minutes) onset of action. Assess the patient's BP and pulse every 2 to 3 minutes during the initial administration of these drugs. Use an intraarterial line (see Chapter 66) or an automated, noninvasive BP machine to monitor the BP. Titrate the drug according to MAP or BP as ordered. Monitor the ECG for heart dysrhythmias and signs of ischemia or MI. Use extreme caution in treating the patient with CAD or cerebrovascular disease. Measure urine output hourly to assess renal perfusion. Patients receiving IV antihypertensive drugs may be restricted to bed. Getting up (e.g., to use the commode) may cause severe cerebral ischemia and fainting.

Ongoing assessment is essential to evaluate the effectiveness of these drugs and the patient's response to therapy. Frequent neurologic checks, including level of consciousness, pupillary size and reaction, and movement of extremities, help detect any changes in the patient's condition. Monitor cardiac, pulmonary, and renal systems for decompensation caused by the severe elevation in BP (e.g., angina, pulmonary edema, renal failure).

Hypertensive urgencies usually do not require IV medications but can be managed with oral agents. The patient with hypertensive urgency may not need hospitalization, but will require follow-up. The oral drugs most frequently used for hypertensive urgencies are captopril (Capoten), labetalol, clonidine (Catapres), and amlodipine (Norvasc)[23] (see Table 33-7). The disadvantage of oral medications is the inability to regulate the dosage moment to moment, as can be done with IV medications. If a patient with hypertensive urgency is not hospitalized, outpatient follow-up care should be arranged within 24 hours.

Once the hypertensive crisis is resolved, it is important to determine the cause. The patient will need appropriate management and teaching to avoid future crises.

DRUG ALERT: Clonidine (Catapres)
Instruct patient to do the following:
- Change positions slowly to limit orthostatic hypotension.
- Avoid hazardous activities, since the drug may cause drowsiness.
- Do not discontinue the medication abruptly to prevent rebound hypertension.

Not every patient with an elevated BP and no target organ disease will require emergent drug therapy or hospitalization. Allowing the patient to sit for 20 or 30 minutes in a quiet environment may significantly reduce BP. Oral drugs may be started or adjusted. Additional nursing interventions include encouraging the patient to verbalize any concerns or fears, answering questions regarding hypertension, and eliminating any adverse stimuli (e.g., excess noise) in the patient's environment.

CASE STUDY

Primary Hypertension

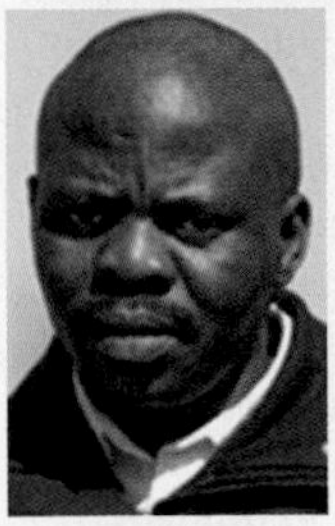

iStockphoto/Thinkstock

Patient Profile

R.L. is a 45-year-old African American man with no previous history of hypertension. At a screening clinic 2 months ago, his BP was found to be 150/95 mm Hg. His primary care provider has followed him for the past month. During this time he has been taking hydrochlorothiazide 12.5 mg/day. He is here today for a follow-up visit.

Subjective Data
- Father died of stroke at age 60
- Mother is alive but has hypertension and a history of MI
- States that he feels fine and is not a "hyper" person
- Smokes one pack of cigarettes daily for the past 28 yr
- Drinks 1-2 six-packs of beer on most Friday and Saturday nights
- Has heard that BP drugs "make you impotent"

Objective Data
Physical Examination
- Mild retinopathy (retinal arteriolar narrowing on ophthalmoscopic examination)
- BP: 166/108 mm Hg (average of two readings, 1 min apart)
- Sustained apical impulse palpable in the fourth intercostal space just lateral to the midclavicular line

Diagnostic Studies
- ECG: mild left ventricular hypertrophy
- Urinalysis: protein 30 mg/dL (0.3 g/L)
- Serum creatinine level: 1.6 mg/dL (141 mmol/L)

Collaborative Care
- Low-sodium, DASH diet
- Hydrochlorothiazide 25 mg/day PO (dosage increase)
- Nicardipine (Cardene) sustained release 30 mg PO bid (second drug added)

Discussion Questions
1. What risk factors for hypertension does R.L. have?
2. What evidence of target organ disease is present?
3. What misconceptions about hypertension should be corrected?
4. ***Priority Decision:*** Based on the assessment data, what are the priority nursing diagnoses and interventions? What are the collaborative problems?
5. ***Evidence-Based Practice:*** R.L. wants to know the most effective nonpharmacologic strategies to lower his BP. What would you tell him?

evolve Answers available at *http://evolve.elsevier.com/Lewis/medsurg.*

BRIDGE TO NCLEX EXAMINATION

The number of the question corresponds to the same-numbered outcome at the beginning of the chapter.

1. Which BP-regulating mechanism(s) can result in the development of hypertension if defective *(select all that apply)?*
   a. Release of norepinephrine
   b. Secretion of prostaglandins
   c. Stimulation of the sympathetic nervous system
   d. Stimulation of the parasympathetic nervous system
   e. Activation of the renin-angiotensin-aldosterone system
2. While obtaining subjective assessment data from a patient with hypertension, the nurse recognizes that a modifiable risk factor for the development of hypertension is
   a. a low-calcium diet.
   b. excessive alcohol consumption.
   c. a family history of hypertension.
   d. consumption of a high-protein diet.
3. In teaching a patient with hypertension about controlling the condition, the nurse recognizes that
   a. all patients with elevated BP require medication.
   b. obese persons must achieve a normal weight to lower BP.
   c. it is not necessary to limit salt in the diet if taking a diuretic.
   d. lifestyle modifications are indicated for all persons with elevated BP.
4. A major consideration in the management of the older adult with hypertension is to
   a. prevent primary hypertension from converting to secondary hypertension.
   b. recognize that the older adult is less likely to adhere to the drug therapy regimen than a younger adult.
   c. ensure that the patient receives larger initial doses of antihypertensive drugs because of impaired absorption.
   d. use careful technique in assessing the BP of the patient because of the possible presence of an auscultatory gap.
5. A patient with newly discovered high BP has an average reading of 158/98 mm Hg after 3 months of exercise and diet modifications. Which management strategy will be a priority for this patient?
   a. Medication will be required because the BP is still not at goal.
   b. BP monitoring should continue for another 3 months to confirm a diagnosis of hypertension.
   c. Lifestyle changes are less important, since they were not effective, and medications will be started.
   d. More vigorous changes in the patient's lifestyle are needed for a longer time before starting medications.
6. A patient is admitted to the hospital in hypertensive emergency (BP 244/142 mm Hg). Sodium nitroprusside is started to treat the elevated BP. Which management strategy(ies) would be appropriate for this patient *(select all that apply)?*
   a. Measuring hourly urine output
   b. Decreasing the MAP by 50% within the first hour
   c. Continuous BP monitoring with an intraarterial line
   d. Maintaining bed rest and providing tranquilizers to lower the BP
   e. Assessing the patient for signs and symptoms of heart failure and changes in mental status

1. a, c, e, 2. b, 3. d, 4. d, 5. a, 6. a, c, e

evolve

For rationales to these answers and even more NCLEX review questions, visit *http://evolve.elsevier.com/Lewis/medsurg.*

REFERENCES

*1. National Heart, Lung, and Blood Institute: *Seventh report of the Joint National Committee on Detection, Evaluation, and Treatment of High Blood Pressure (JNC-7)*, NIH Publication No. 04-5230, Bethesda, Md, 2004, The Institute. Retrieved from *www.nhlbi.nih.gov/guidelines/hypertension/jnc7full.pdf.*

2. Go AS, Mozaffarian D, Roger VL, et al: Heart disease and stroke statistics—2013 update: a report from the American Heart Association, *Circulation* 127:e6, 2013.

3. Fryar CD, Hirsch R, Eberhardt MS, et al: *Hypertension, high serum cholesterol, and diabetes: racial and ethnic prevalence differences in U.S. adults, 1999-2006*, NCHS data brief, no 36, Hyattsville, Md, 2010, National Center for Health Statistics.

4. US Department of Health and Human Services: Healthy people 2020. Retrieved from *www.healthypeople.gov.*

5. Drozda J, Messer JV, Spertus J, et al: ACCF/AHA/AMA-PCPI 2011 performance measures for adults with coronary artery disease and hypertension, *J Am Coll Cardiol* 58:316, 2011.

*6. Mosca L, Benjamin EJ, Berra K, et al: Effectiveness-based guidelines for the prevention of cardiovascular disease in women—2011 update, *Circulation* 123:1243, 2011.

7. Libby P, Bonow R, Zipes D, et al: *Braunwald's heart disease: a textbook of cardiovascular medicine*, ed 8, Philadelphia, 2008, Saunders.

8. Humes KR, Jones NA, Ramirez RR: United States Census Bureau: overview of race and Hispanic origin: 2010 census briefs. Retrieved from *www.census.gov/prod/cen2010/briefs/c2010br-02.pdf.*

*9. Pickering TG, Hall JE, Appel LJ, et al: Recommendations for blood pressure measurement in humans and experimental animals, part 1: blood pressure measurement in humans, *Hypertension* 45:142, 2005. (Classic)

10. Appel LJ: ASH position paper: dietary approaches to lower blood pressure, *J Clin Hypertension* 11:358, 2009.

11. American Heart Association: What are the symptoms of high blood pressure? Retrieved from *www.heart.org/HEARTORG/Conditions/HighBloodPressure/SymptomsDiagnosisMonitoringofHighBloodPressure/What-are-the-Symptoms-of-High-Blood-Pressure_UCM_301871_Article.jsp.*

12. National Heart, Lung, and Blood Institute: *In brief: your guide to lowering your blood pressure with DASH*, NIH Pub No 06-5834, Bethesda, Md, 2006, The Institute. Retrieved from *www.nhlbi.nih.gov/health/public/heart/hbp/dash/dash_brief.pdf.*

*13. Haskell WL, Lee I-M, Pate RR, et al: Physical activity and public health: updated recommendations for adults from the

*Evidence-based information for clinical practice.

American College of Sports Medicine and the American Heart Association, *Circulation* 116:1081, 2007.

*14. Nelson ME, Rejeski WJ, Blair SN, et al: Physical activity and public health in older adults: recommendation from the American College of Sports Medicine and the American Heart Association, *Circulation* 116:1094, 2007.

*15. Graham I, Atar D, Borch-Johnsen K, et al: European guidelines on cardiovascular disease prevention in clinical practice: executive summary; Fourth Joint Task Force of the European Society of Cardiology and other societies on cardiovascular disease prevention in clinical practice, *Eur Heart J* 28:2375, 2007.

16. Rozanski A, Blumenthal JA, Davidson KW, et al: The epidemiology, pathophysiology, and management of psychosocial risk factors in cardiac practice, *J Am Coll Cardiol* 45:637, 2005. (Classic)

*17. Aronow WS, Fleg JL, Pepine CJ, et al: ACCF/AHA 2011 expert consensus document on hypertension in the elderly, *J Am Coll Cardiol* 57:2037, 2011.

18. Olson J: *Clinical pharmacology made ridiculously simple*, ed 4, Miami, 2011, MedMaster.

19. Lehne RA: *Pharmacology for nursing care*, ed 7, St Louis, 2010, Saunders.

20. Hering D, Lambert EA, Marusic P, et al: Substantial reduction in single sympathetic nerve firing after renal denervation in patients with resistant hypertension, *Hypertension* 61:457, 2013.

*21. Seckel MA, Bradley E, Bucher L, et al: AACN practice alert: noninvasive blood pressure monitoring. Retrieved from *http://classic.aacn.org/AACN/practiceAlert.nsf/Files/NIBP/$file/Noninvasive%20BP%20Monitoring%206-2006.pdf.*

*22. Pickering TG, Miller NH, Ogedegbe G, et al: Call to action on use and reimbursement for home blood pressure monitoring: a joint scientific statement from the American Heart Association, American Society of Hypertension, and Preventive Cardiovascular Nurses Association, *Hypertension* 52:10, 2008.

23. Vidt DG: Hypertensive crises, Cleveland Clinic Center for Continuing Education. Retrieved from *www.clevelandclinicmeded.com/medicalpubs/diseasemanagement/nephrology/hypertensive-crises.*

24. Smithburger PL, Kane-Gill SL, Nestor BL, et al: Recent advances in the treatment of hypertensive emergencies, *Crit Care Nurse* 30:24, 2010.

RESOURCES

American Heart Association
www.americanheart.org

American Society of Hypertension
www.ash-us.org

National Heart, Lung, and Blood Institute
www.nhlbi.nih.gov/health/indexpro.htm

WebMD Hypertension and High Blood Pressure Community
www.exchanges.webmd.com/hypertension-and-high-blood-pressure-exchange

CHAPTER

34

I have witnessed the softening of the hardest of hearts by a simple smile.
Goldie Hawn

Nursing Management
Coronary Artery Disease and Acute Coronary Syndrome

Linda Bucher and Sharmila Johnson

evolve WEBSITE

http://evolve.elsevier.com/Lewis/medsurg

- NCLEX Review Questions
- Key Points
- Pre-Test
- Answer Guidelines for Case Study on p. 763
- Rationales for Bridge to NCLEX Examination Questions
- Case Study
  - Patient With Coronary Artery Disease and Acute Coronary Syndrome
- Nursing Care Plan (Customizable)
  - NCP 34-1: Patient With Acute Coronary Syndrome
- Concept Map Creator
- Concept Map for Case Study on p. 763
- Glossary
- Content Updates

eFigures
- eFig. 34-1: Leading causes of death for men and women
- eFig. 34-2: Cardiovascular disease mortality trends for men and women
- eFig. 34-3: Trends in deaths due to cardiovascular disease
- eFig. 34-4: Xanthomas in patients with familial hypercholesterolemia
- eFig. 34-5: What you need to know—antiplatelet therapy

eTable
- eTable 34-1: Genes Known to Contribute to Coronary Artery Disease Risk

LEARNING OUTCOMES

1. Relate the etiology and pathophysiology of coronary artery disease (CAD), angina, and acute coronary syndrome (ACS) to the clinical manifestations of each disorder.
2. Describe the nursing role in the promotion of therapeutic lifestyle changes in patients at risk for CAD.
3. Differentiate the precipitating factors, clinical manifestations, collaborative care, and nursing management of the patient with CAD and chronic stable angina.
4. Explain the clinical manifestations, complications, diagnostic study results, and collaborative care of the patient with ACS.
5. Evaluate commonly used drug therapy in treating patients with CAD and ACS.
6. Prioritize key components to include in the rehabilitation of patients recovering from ACS and coronary revascularization procedures.
7. Differentiate the precipitating factors, clinical presentation, and collaborative care of patients who are at risk for or have experienced sudden cardiac death.

KEY TERMS

acute coronary syndrome (ACS), p. 746
angina, p. 740
atherosclerosis, p. 731
chronic stable angina, p. 741
collateral circulation, p. 732
coronary artery disease (CAD), p. 731
coronary revascularization, p. 745
metabolic equivalent (MET), p. 760
myocardial infarction (MI), p. 747
percutaneous coronary intervention (PCI), p. 745
Prinzmetal's angina, p. 742
silent ischemia, p. 742
stent, p. 746
sudden cardiac death (SCD), p. 762
unstable angina (UA), p. 747

Reviewed by Marci Ebberts, RN, BSN, CCRN, STEMI Program Coordinator, St. Luke's Hospital of Kansas City, Kansas City, Missouri; Kathleen M. Hill, RN, MSN, CCNS, Clinical Nurse Specialist, Surgical Intensive Care Unit, Cleveland Clinic, Cleveland, Ohio; Christina D. Keller, RN, MSN, Instructor, Radford University School of Nursing: Clinical Simulation Center, Radford, Virginia; and Devorah Overbay, RN, MSN, CNS, NCLEX Education Specialist ATI Testing, George Fox University, Department of Nursing, Newberg, Oregon.

Cardiovascular disease is the major cause of death in the United States. (The leading causes of death are shown in eFig. 34-1, available on the website for this chapter.) Coronary artery disease (CAD) is the most common type of cardiovascular disease and accounts for the majority of these deaths.[1] Patients with CAD can be asymptomatic or develop chronic stable angina (or chest pain). Unstable angina (UA) and myocardial infarction (MI) are more serious manifestations of CAD and are termed *acute coronary syndrome* (ACS).

The American Heart Association (AHA) estimates that 1.1 million Americans have an MI each year. About one fourth of these persons die in an emergency department (ED) or before reaching a hospital. Although the mortality rate from MI has decreased because of advances in treatment, it remains the leading cause of death from all cardiovascular diseases and other conditions in general.[1]

CORONARY ARTERY DISEASE

Coronary artery disease (CAD) is a type of blood vessel disorder that is included in the general category of atherosclerosis. The term **atherosclerosis** comes from two Greek words: *athere,* meaning "fatty mush," and *skleros,* meaning "hard." This combination implies that atherosclerosis begins as soft deposits of fat that harden with age. Consequently, atherosclerosis is commonly referred to as "hardening of the arteries." Although this condition can occur in any artery in the body, the *atheromas* (fatty deposits) prefer the coronary arteries. The terms *arteriosclerotic heart disease, cardiovascular heart disease, ischemic heart disease, coronary heart disease,* and *CAD* all describe this disease process.

Etiology and Pathophysiology

Atherosclerosis is the major cause of CAD. It is characterized by deposits of lipids within the intima of the artery. Endothelial injury and inflammation play a central role in the development of atherosclerosis.

The endothelium (the inner lining of the vessel wall) is normally nonreactive to platelets and leukocytes, as well as coagulation, fibrinolytic, and complement factors. However, the endothelial lining can be injured as a result of tobacco use, hyperlipidemia, hypertension, toxins, diabetes, hyperhomocysteinemia, and infection causing a local inflammatory response[2] (Fig. 34-1, *A*).

C-reactive protein (CRP), a protein produced by the liver, is a nonspecific marker of inflammation. It is increased in many patients with CAD[3] (see Table 32-6). The level of CRP rises when there is systemic inflammation. Chronic elevations of CRP are associated with unstable plaques and the oxidation of low-density lipoprotein (LDL) cholesterol.

Developmental Stages. CAD is a progressive disease that develops over many years. When it becomes symptomatic, the disease process is usually well advanced. The stages of development in atherosclerosis are (1) fatty streak, (2) fibrous plaque, and (3) complicated lesion.

Fatty Streak. *Fatty streaks,* the earliest lesions of atherosclerosis, are characterized by lipid-filled smooth muscle cells. As streaks of fat develop within the smooth muscle cells, a yellow tinge appears.[2] Fatty streaks can be seen in the coronary arteries by age 15 and involve an increasing amount of surface area as one ages. Treatment that lowers LDL cholesterol may reverse this process (Fig. 34-1, *B*).

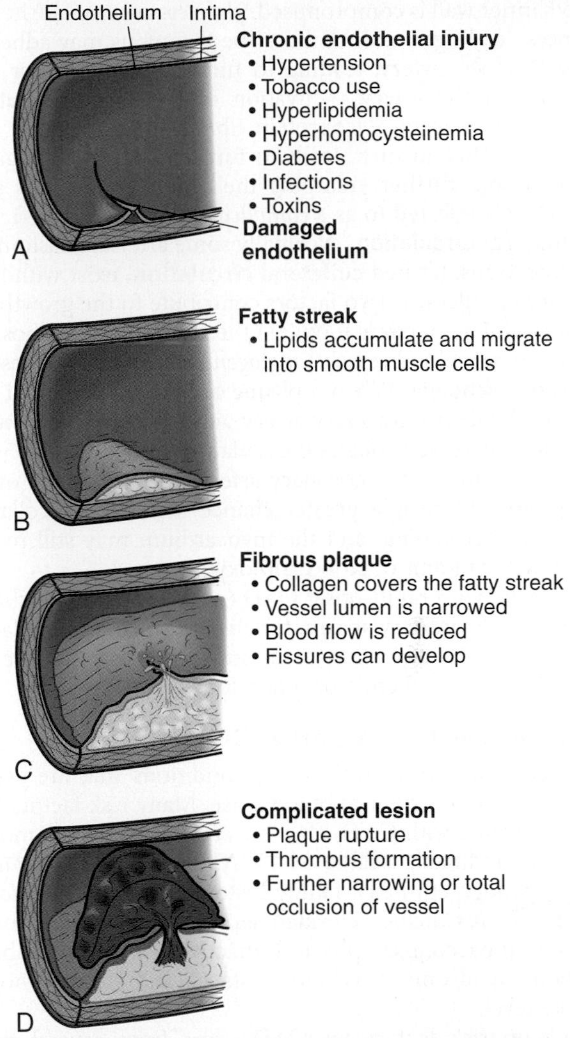

FIG. 34-1 Pathogenesis of atherosclerosis. **A,** Damaged endothelium. **B,** Fatty streak and lipid core formation. **C,** Fibrous plaque. Raised plaques are visible: some are yellow; others are white. **D,** Complicated lesion: thrombus is red; collagen is blue. Plaque is complicated by red thrombus deposition.

Fibrous Plaque. The *fibrous plaque* stage is the beginning of progressive changes in the endothelium of the arterial wall. These changes can appear in the coronary arteries by age 30 and increase with age.

Normally the endothelium repairs itself immediately. This does not happen in the individual with CAD. LDLs and growth factors from platelets stimulate smooth muscle proliferation and thickening of the arterial wall. Once endothelial injury has taken place, lipoproteins (carrier proteins within the bloodstream) transport cholesterol and other lipids into the arterial intima. Collagen covers the fatty streak and forms a fibrous plaque with a grayish or whitish appearance. These plaques can form on one portion of the artery or in a circular fashion involving the entire lumen. The borders can be smooth or irregular with rough, jagged edges. The result is a narrowing of the vessel lumen and a reduction in blood flow to the distal tissues (Fig. 34-1, *C*).

Complicated Lesion. The final stage in the development of the atherosclerotic lesion is the most dangerous. As the fibrous plaque grows, continued inflammation can result in plaque instability, ulceration, and rupture. Once the integrity of the artery's inner wall is compromised, platelets accumulate in large numbers, leading to a thrombus. The thrombus may adhere to the wall of the artery, leading to further narrowing or total occlusion of the artery. Activation of the exposed platelets causes expression of glycoprotein IIb/IIIa receptors that bind fibrinogen. This, in turn, leads to further platelet aggregation and adhesion, further enlarging the thrombus. At this stage the plaque is referred to as a *complicated lesion* (Fig. 34-1, *D*).

Collateral Circulation. Normally some arterial anastomoses or connections, termed **collateral circulation,** exist within the coronary circulation. Two factors contribute to the growth and extent of collateral circulation: (1) the inherited predisposition to develop new blood vessels *(angiogenesis)* and (2) the presence of chronic ischemia. When a plaque occludes the normal flow of blood through a coronary artery and the resulting *ischemia* is chronic, increased collateral circulation develops (Fig. 34-2). When occlusion of the coronary arteries occurs slowly over a long period, there is a greater chance of adequate collateral circulation developing, and the myocardium may still receive an adequate amount of blood and oxygen.

However, with rapid-onset CAD (e.g., familial hypercholesterolemia) or coronary spasm, time is inadequate for collateral development. Consequently, a diminished blood flow results in a more severe ischemia or infarction.

Risk Factors for Coronary Artery Disease

Risk factors are characteristics or conditions that are associated with a high incidence of a disease. Many risk factors have been associated with CAD. They are categorized as nonmodifiable and modifiable (Table 34-1). *Nonmodifiable risk factors* are age, gender, ethnicity, family history, and genetics. *Modifiable risk factors* include elevated serum lipids, elevated blood pressure, tobacco use, physical inactivity, obesity, diabetes, metabolic syndrome, psychologic states, and elevated homocysteine level.

Data on risk factors for CAD come from several major studies. In the Framingham study (one of the most widely known), men and women were observed for 20 years. Over time, it was noted that elevated serum cholesterol (greater than 240 mg/dL), elevated systolic blood pressure (BP) (greater than 160 mm Hg), and tobacco use (one or more packs a day) were positively correlated with an increased incidence of CAD.[1]

Nonmodifiable Risk Factors

Age, Gender, and Ethnicity. The incidence of CAD and MI is highest among white, middle-aged men. After age 65, the incidence in men and women equalizes, although cardiovascular

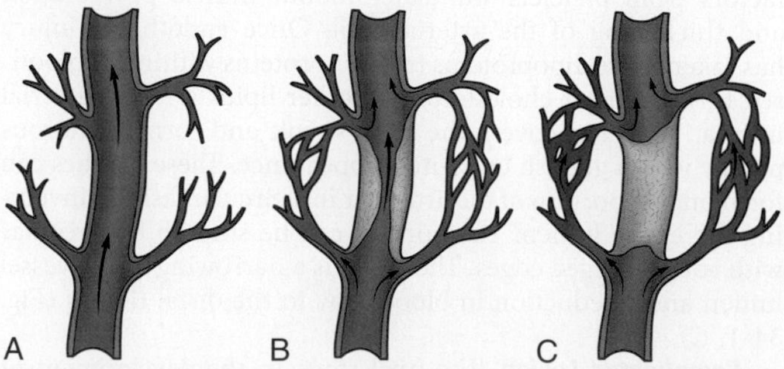

FIG. 34-2 Vessel occlusion with collateral circulation. **A,** Open, functioning coronary artery. **B,** Partial coronary artery closure with collateral circulation being established. **C,** Total coronary artery occlusion with collateral circulation bypassing the occlusion to supply blood to the myocardium.

CULTURAL & ETHNIC HEALTH DISPARITIES

Coronary Artery Disease

Whites
- White, middle-aged men have the highest incidence of coronary artery disease (CAD).

African Americans
- African Americans have an early age of onset of CAD.
- Mortality rates for African Americans ages 35 to 64 are more than twice those of whites of the same age.
- African American women have a higher incidence and death rate related to CAD than white women.

Native Americans
- Native Americans less than 35 yr of age have heart disease mortality rates twice as high as those of other Americans.
- Major modifiable cardiovascular risk factors for Native Americans are tobacco use, hypertension, obesity, and diabetes mellitus.

Hispanics
- Hispanics have lower rates of CAD than either non-Hispanic whites or African Americans.
- Hispanics have lower death rates from CAD than non-Hispanic whites.

disease causes more deaths in women than men. Additionally, CAD is present in African American women at rates higher than those of their white counterparts.[1] (See Cultural & Ethnic Health Disparities box for additional differences in CAD among ethnic groups.)

Heart disease kills almost 10 times more women than breast cancer and is the leading cause of death in women. Yet most women do not consider CAD their greatest health risk.[4] (Cardiovascular disease mortality trends for both men and women are shown in eFig. 34-2, available on the website for this chapter.) On average, women with CAD are older than men who have

TABLE 34-1 RISK FACTORS FOR CORONARY ARTERY DISEASE

Nonmodifiable Risk Factors	Modifiable Risk Factors
Increasing age	**Major**
Gender (more common in men than in women until 65 yr of age)	Serum lipids: • Total cholesterol >200 mg/dL • Triglycerides ≥150 mg/dL* • LDL cholesterol >160 mg/dL • HDL cholesterol <40 mg/dL in men or <50 mg/dL in women*
Ethnicity (more common in whites than in African Americans)	Blood pressure ≥140/90 mm Hg*
Genetic predisposition and family history of heart disease	Diabetes mellitus
	Tobacco use
	Physical inactivity
	Obesity: Waist circumference ≥102 cm (≥40 in) in men and ≥88 cm (≥35 in) in women*
	Contributing
	Fasting blood glucose ≥100 mg/dL*
	Psychosocial risk factors (e.g., depression, hostility, anger, stress)
	Elevated homocysteine levels

*Three or more of these risk factors meet the criteria for metabolic syndrome (as defined by the National Cholesterol Education Program Adult Treatment Panel III). Metabolic syndrome is discussed in Chapter 49.

GENDER DIFFERENCES

Coronary Artery Disease and Acute Coronary Syndrome

Men	Women
Coronary Artery Disease • Initial cardiac event for men is more often MI than angina. • Men report more typical signs and symptoms of angina and MI. • Men receive more evidence-based therapies (e.g., aspirin, statins, diagnostic catheterization, PCI) when acutely ill from CAD (e.g., MI) than women. • Mortality rates from CAD have fallen more rapidly for men than women.	• Women experience the onset of heart disease approximately 10 yr later than men. • CAD is the leading cause of death for women, regardless of race or ethnicity. • Initial cardiac event for women is more often angina than MI. • More women than men with MI die of sudden cardiac death before reaching the hospital. • Before menopause, women have higher HDL cholesterol levels and lower LDL cholesterol levels than men. After menopause LDL levels increase.
Acute Coronary Syndrome • Incidence of MI is highest among white, middle-aged men. • After age 65, the incidence of MI in men and women equalizes. • Men present more frequently than women with an acute MI as the first manifestation of CAD. • Men develop greater collateral circulation than women. • Men have larger-diameter coronary arteries than women. Vessel diameter is inversely related to risk of restenosis after interventions. • Standard screening for risk of sudden cardiac death (e.g., EP studies) is more predictive in men.	• Women are older than men when seen with first MI and often have more co-morbidities. • Women delay longer in seeking care and are often more ill on presentation than men. • Once a woman reaches menopause, her risk for an MI quadruples. • Fewer women than men manifest the "classic" signs and symptoms of UA or MI. • Fatigue is often the first symptom of ACS in women. • Women experience more "silent" MIs compared with men. • Among those who have an MI, women are more likely to suffer a fatal cardiac event within 1 yr than men. • Women report more disability after a cardiac event than men. • Women who have coronary artery bypass graft surgery have a higher mortality rate and more complications after surgery than men.

ACS, Acute coronary syndrome; *CAD*, coronary artery disease; *EP*, electrophysiology; *HDL*, high-density lipoprotein; *LDL*, low-density lipoprotein; *PCI*, percutaneous coronary intervention, *UA*, unstable angina.

CAD, and women are more likely to have co-morbidities (e.g., hypertension, diabetes). Most women have atypical symptoms of angina rather than MI when they experience their first cardiac event[4] (see Gender Differences box).

Genetic Link

Genetic predisposition is an important factor in the occurrence of CAD. Family history is a risk factor for CAD and MI. Most times, patients with angina or MI can name a parent or sibling who died of CAD.

The genetic basis of CAD/MI is complex and, to date, poorly understood. It is estimated that the genetic contribution to CAD/MI is as high as 40% to 60%. This proportion relates mainly to genes that control known risk factors (e.g., lipid metabolism).[5] (Genes known to contribute to CAD risk are listed in eTable 34-1, available on the website for this chapter.) See the Genetics in Clinical Practice box at right.

Major Modifiable Risk Factors

Elevated Serum Lipids. An elevated serum lipid level is one of the four most firmly established risk factors for CAD.[6] The risk of CAD is associated with a serum cholesterol level greater than 200 mg/dL (5.2 mmol/L) or a fasting triglyceride level greater than 150 mg/dL (3.7 mmol/L). (See Table 32-6 for normal serum lipid values.)

For lipids to be used and transported by the body, they must become soluble in blood by combining with proteins. Lipids combine with proteins to form lipoproteins. Lipoproteins are vehicles for fat mobilization and transport, and vary in composition. They are classified as high-density lipoproteins (HDLs), LDLs, and very-low-density lipoproteins (VLDLs).

HDLs contain more protein by weight and fewer lipids than any other lipoprotein. HDLs carry lipids away from arteries

GENETICS IN CLINICAL PRACTICE

Familial Hypercholesterolemia

Genetic Basis
- Autosomal dominant disorder.
- Mutation in low-density lipoprotein receptor *(LDLR)* gene.
- Gene codes for low-density lipoprotein (LDL) receptor that binds to LDLs.
- LDLs are the primary carriers of cholesterol in the blood. By removing LDLs from the bloodstream, the LDL receptors play a critical role in regulating cholesterol levels.
- Exists in both heterozygous (most common) and homozygous forms.

Incidence
- Heterozygotes: 1 in 500
- Homozygotes: rare

Genetic Testing
- Disorder is characterized by elevated serum LDLs.
- Serum lipid profile can be used to measure total cholesterol, triglycerides, LDLs, and high-density lipoproteins (HDLs).
- DNA testing is available.

Clinical Implications
- Common genetic disease.
- High cholesterol levels are a result of defective function of the LDL receptors.
- Plasma levels of LDLs elevated throughout life.
- Develop severe atherosclerosis in early to middle years.
- Xanthomas (fatty deposits under the surface of the skin) can occur (see eFig. 34-4, available on the website for this chapter).
- Treatment strategies include low-fat diet, exercise, and lipid-lowering medications.
- Homozygous familial hypercholesterolemia is much more severe than the heterozygous form. Cholesterol levels may exceed 600 mg/dL in these patients.

and to the liver for metabolism. This process of HDL transport prevents lipid accumulation within the arterial walls. Therefore high serum HDL levels are desirable and lower the risk of CAD.

There are two types of HDLs: HDL_2 and HDL_3. They differ by their density and apolipoprotein composition. Apolipoproteins are found on lipoproteins and activate enzyme or receptor sites that promote the removal of fat from plasma. Several types of apolipoproteins exist (e.g., apo A-I, apo B-100, apo C-I). Women produce more apo A-I than men, and premenopausal women have HDL_2 levels approximately three times greater than men. This is thought to be related to the protective effects of natural estrogen. After menopause, women's HDL_2 levels decrease and quickly near those of men.

In general, HDL levels are higher in women, decrease with age, and are low in persons with CAD. Physical activity, moderate alcohol consumption, and estrogen administration increase HDL levels.

LDLs contain more cholesterol than any of the lipoproteins and have an attraction for arterial walls. VLDLs contain both cholesterol and triglycerides, and may deposit cholesterol directly on the walls of arteries. Elevated LDL levels correlate closely with an increased incidence of atherosclerosis and CAD. Therefore low serum LDL levels are desirable.[6,7]

Certain diseases (e.g., type 2 diabetes, chronic kidney disease), drugs (e.g., corticosteroids, hormone therapy), and genetic disorders have been associated with elevated triglyceride levels. Lifestyle factors that can contribute to elevated triglycerides include high alcohol consumption, high intake of refined carbohydrates and simple sugars, and physical inactivity. When a high triglyceride level is combined with a high LDL level, a smaller, denser LDL particle is formed, which favors deposition on arterial walls. People with insulin resistance often have this pattern.

Guidelines for treating elevated LDL cholesterol are based on a person's 10-year risk for having a nonfatal MI or dying from a coronary event and his or her LDL levels. The following information generates a risk score: (1) age, (2) gender, (3) use of tobacco, (4) systolic BP, (5) use of BP medications, (6) total cholesterol, and (7) HDL cholesterol level.[7] A 10-year risk calculator is available at *http://hin.nhlbi.nih.gov/atpiii/calculator.asp?usertype=prof*.

In general, individuals with no or only one risk factor are considered at low risk for the development of CAD, and the LDL goal is less than 160 mg/dL (4.14 mmol/L). Those at very high risk have CAD and multiple risk factors. The LDL goal for this group is less than 70 mg/dL (1.8 mmol/L).[7]

Hypertension. The second major risk factor in CAD is hypertension, which is defined as a BP greater than 140/90 mm Hg or greater than 130/80 mm Hg if the patient has diabetes or chronic kidney disease.[8] Hypertension increases the risk of death from CAD 10-fold in all people. In postmenopausal women, hypertension is associated with a higher incidence of CAD than in men and premenopausal women.

Blood pressure is classified as (1) normal (BP less than 120/80 mm Hg), (2) *prehypertension* (BP of 120 to 139/80 to 89 mm Hg), (3) stage 1 hypertension (140 to 159/90 to 99 mm Hg), and (4) stage 2 hypertension (BP greater than 160/100 mm Hg).[8] The cause of hypertension in 90% of those affected is unknown, but it is usually controllable with diet and/or drugs. Therapeutic lifestyle changes should begin in people with prehypertension. Those with stage 1 or 2 hypertension often require more than one drug to reach therapeutic goals[8] (see Table 33-7). Teach all people with elevated systolic or diastolic BP the importance of achieving and maintaining target BP goals.

The stress of an elevated BP increases the rate of atherosclerotic development. This relates to the shearing stress that causes endothelial injury. Atherosclerosis, in turn, causes narrowed, thickened arterial walls and decreases the distensibility and elasticity of vessels. More force is required to pump blood through diseased arteries, and this increased force is reflected in a higher BP. This increased workload results in left ventricular hypertrophy and decreased stroke volume with each contraction. Salt intake positively correlates with elevated BP, adding volume and increasing systemic vascular resistance (SVR) to the cardiac workload. (See Chapter 33 for a complete discussion of hypertension.)

Tobacco Use. A third major risk factor in CAD is tobacco use. The risk of developing CAD is two to six times higher in those who smoke tobacco or use smokeless tobacco than in those who do not. Further, tobacco smoking decreases estrogen levels, placing premenopausal women at greater risk for CAD. Risk is proportional to the number of cigarettes smoked. Changing to lower nicotine or filtered cigarettes does not affect risk.

Nicotine in tobacco smoke causes catecholamine (i.e., epinephrine, norepinephrine) release. These neurohormones cause an increased heart rate (HR), peripheral vasoconstriction, and increased BP. These changes increase the cardiac workload. Tobacco smoke is also related to an increase in LDL level, a decrease in HDL level, and release of toxic oxygen radicals. All of these add to vessel inflammation and thrombosis.[2]

Carbon monoxide, a byproduct of combustion found in tobacco smoke, affects the oxygen-carrying capacity of hemoglobin by reducing the sites available for oxygen transport. Thus the effects of an increased cardiac workload, combined with the oxygen-depleting effect of carbon monoxide, significantly decrease the oxygen available to the myocardium. There is also some indication that carbon monoxide is a chemical irritant and causes injury to the endothelium.

The benefits of smoking cessation are dramatic and almost immediate. CAD mortality rates drop to those of nonsmokers within 12 months. However, nicotine is highly addictive, and often intensive intervention is required to assist people to quit. Individual and group counseling sessions, nicotine replacement therapy, smoking cessation medications (e.g., bupropion [Zyban], varenicline [Chantix]), and hypnosis are examples of smoking cessation strategies. (See Chapter 11, Tables 11-4 through 11-6 for information on smoking cessation.)

Chronic exposure to environmental tobacco (secondhand) smoke also increases the risk of CAD.[6] People who live in the same household as the patient should be encouraged to stop smoking. This reinforces the individual's effort and decreases the risk of ongoing exposure to environmental smoke. Pipe and cigar smokers, who often do not inhale, have an increased risk of CAD similar to those exposed to environmental tobacco smoke.

Physical Inactivity. Physical inactivity is the fourth major modifiable risk factor. Physical inactivity implies a lack of adequate physical exercise on a regular basis. An example of health-promoting regular physical activity is brisk walking (3 to 4 miles per hour) for at least 30 minutes five or more times a week.[9]

The mechanism by which physical inactivity predisposes a person to CAD is mostly still unknown. Physically active people have increased HDL levels. Exercise improves thrombolytic activity, thus reducing the risk of clot formation. Exercise may also encourage the development of collateral circulation in the heart.

Exercise training for those who are physically inactive decreases the risk of CAD through more efficient lipid metabolism, increased HDL production, and more efficient oxygen extraction by the working muscles, thereby decreasing the cardiac workload. For those individuals with CAD, regular physical activity reduces symptoms, improves functional capacity, and improves other risk factors such as insulin resistance and glucose intolerance.

Obesity. The mortality rate from CAD is statistically higher in obese persons. Obesity is defined as a body mass index (BMI) of greater than 30 kg/m^2 and a waist circumference more than 40 inches for men and more than 35 inches for women. BMI is a measure of body fat based on height and weight. It can be calculated online *(http://nhlbisupport.com/bmi/bmicalc.htm)*.

The increased risk for CAD is proportional to the degree of obesity. Obese persons may produce increased levels of LDLs and triglycerides, which are strongly related to atherosclerosis. Obesity is often associated with hypertension. There is also evidence that people who tend to store fat in the abdomen (an "apple" figure) rather than in the hips and buttocks (a "pear" figure) have a higher incidence of CAD (see Table 41-2). As obesity increases, the heart grows and uses more oxygen. In addition, there is an increase in insulin resistance in obese individuals.[2]

Contributing Modifiable Risk Factors

Diabetes Mellitus. The incidence of CAD is two to four times greater among persons who have diabetes, even those with well-controlled blood glucose levels, than the general population. The patient with diabetes manifests CAD not only more frequently but also at an earlier age.[2] There is no age difference between male or female patients with diabetes in the onset of symptoms of CAD. Diabetes virtually eliminates the lower incidence of CAD in premenopausal women.

Undiagnosed diabetes is frequently discovered at the time a person has an MI. The person with diabetes has an increased tendency toward endothelial dysfunction. This may account for the development of fatty streaks in these patients. Diabetic patients also have alterations in lipid metabolism and tend to have high cholesterol and triglyceride levels. Management of diabetes should include lifestyle changes and drug therapy to achieve a glycosylated hemoglobin (A1C or Hb A1C) level of less than 7%.[6]

Metabolic Syndrome. *Metabolic syndrome* refers to a cluster of risk factors for CAD whose underlying pathophysiology may be related to insulin resistance. These risk factors include obesity as defined by increased waist circumference, hypertension, abnormal serum lipids, and an elevated fasting blood glucose[2] (see Table 41-10). These interrelated risk factors of metabolic origin appear to promote the development of CAD. (Chapter 41 discusses metabolic syndrome.)

Psychologic States. The Framingham study provided early evidence that certain behaviors and lifestyles contribute to the development of CAD. Several behavior patterns correlated with CAD. However, the study of these behaviors remains controversial and complex. One type of behavior, referred to as type A, includes perfectionism and a hardworking, driven personality. The type A person often suppresses anger and hostility, has a sense of time urgency, is impatient, and creates stress and tension. This person may be more prone to MIs than a type B person, who is more easygoing, takes upsets in stride, knows personal limitations, takes time to relax, and is not an overachiever. However, findings from studies regarding these relationships are inconsistent.

Studies now are focusing on specific psychologic risk factors thought to increase risk of CAD. These include depression, acute and chronic stress (e.g., poverty, serving as a caregiver), anxiety, hostility and anger, and lack of social support.[10,11] In particular, depression is a risk factor for both the development and worsening of CAD. Depressed patients have elevated levels of circulating catecholamines that may contribute to endothelial injury and inflammation and platelet activation. Higher levels of depression are also associated with an increased number of adverse cardiac events.[10] More research on the treatment of depression and other negative psychologic states (e.g., anger) in patients with or at risk for CAD is needed to improve these patients' emotional and physical health.

Stressful states correlate with the development of CAD.[12] Sympathetic nervous system (SNS) stimulation and its effect on the heart are the physiologic mechanism by which stress predisposes one to the development of CAD. SNS stimulation causes an increased release of catecholamines (i.e., epinephrine, norepinephrine). This stimulation increases HR and intensifies the force of myocardial contraction, resulting in increased myocardial oxygen demand. Also, stress-induced mechanisms can cause elevated lipid and glucose levels and changes in blood coagulation, which can lead to increased atherogenesis.

Homocysteine. High blood levels of homocysteine have been linked to an increased risk for CAD and other cardiovascular diseases.[13] Homocysteine is produced by the breakdown of the essential amino acid methionine, which is found in dietary protein. High homocysteine levels possibly contribute to atherosclerosis by (1) damaging the inner lining of blood vessels, (2) promoting plaque buildup, and (3) altering the clotting mechanism to make clots more likely to occur (see Table 32-6).

Research is ongoing to determine whether a decline in homocysteine can reduce the risk of heart disease. B-complex vitamins (B_6, B_{12}, folic acid) have been shown to lower blood levels of homocysteine. Generally, a screening test for homocysteine is limited to those suspected of having elevated levels, such as older patients with pernicious anemia or people who develop CAD at an early age.

Substance Abuse. The use of illicit drugs, such as cocaine and methamphetamine, can produce coronary spasm resulting in myocardial ischemia and chest pain. Most people who are seen in the ED with drug-induced chest pain are initially indistinguishable from those with CAD. Although MI can occur, these patients more often have sinus tachycardia, high BP, angina, and anxiety.[14]

The U.S. Food and Drug Administration (FDA) prohibits the sale of dietary supplements containing ephedrine alkaloids. These compounds should be avoided because they can cause high BP, MI, and stroke.

NURSING AND COLLABORATIVE MANAGEMENT CORONARY ARTERY DISEASE

HEALTH PROMOTION

The appropriate management of risk factors in CAD may prevent, modify, or slow the progression of the disease. In the

United States during the past 30 years, there has been a gradual and persistent decline in cardiovascular-related deaths. (See eFig. 34-3, available on the website for this chapter.) The decline relates to people's efforts to become generally healthier, as well as advances in drugs and technology to treat CAD. Prevention and early treatment of heart disease must involve a multifaceted approach and needs to be ongoing throughout the life span.

IDENTIFICATION OF HIGH-RISK PEOPLE. Clinical manifestations of CAD are not apparent in the early stages of the disease. Therefore regardless of the health care setting, it is extremely important to identify people at risk for CAD. Risk screening involves obtaining a thorough health history. Question the patient about a family history of heart disease in parents and siblings. Note the presence of any cardiovascular symptoms. Assess environmental factors, such as eating habits, type of diet, and level of exercise, to elicit lifestyle patterns. Include a psychosocial history to determine tobacco use, alcohol ingestion, recent stressful events (e.g., loss of a spouse), and any negative psychologic states (e.g., anxiety, depression, anger). The place and type of employment provide important information on the kind of activity performed, exposure to pollutants or noxious chemicals, and the degree of stress associated with work.

Identify the patient's attitudes and beliefs about health and illness. This information can give some indication of how disease and lifestyle changes may affect the patient and can reveal possible misconceptions about heart disease. Knowledge of the patient's educational background can help to decide the level needed for teaching. If the patient is taking medications, it is important to know the names and dosages and if the patient is compliant with the drug regimen.

MANAGEMENT OF HIGH-RISK PEOPLE. Recommend preventive measures for all persons at risk for CAD. Risk factors such as age, gender, ethnicity, and genetics cannot be modified. However, the person with any of these risk factors can still reduce the risk of CAD by controlling the additive effects of modifiable risk factors. For example, a young man with a family history of heart disease can decrease the risk of CAD by maintaining an ideal body weight, getting adequate physical exercise, reducing intake of saturated fats, and avoiding tobacco use.

Encourage people who have modifiable risk factors to make lifestyle changes to reduce their risk of CAD. You can play a major role in teaching health-promoting behaviors (Table 34-2). For highly motivated persons, knowing how to reduce this risk may be the information they need to get started.

For persons who are less motivated to take charge of their health, the idea of reducing risk factors may be so remote that they are unable to perceive a threat of CAD. Few people desire to make lifestyle changes, especially in the absence of symptoms. First assist these patients in clarifying personal values. Then, by explaining the risk factors and having them identify their vulnerability to various risks, you may help them recognize their susceptibility to CAD. This may help patients set realistic goals and allow them to choose which risk factor(s) to change first. Some persons are reluctant to change until they begin to manifest overt symptoms or actually suffer an MI. Others, having suffered an MI, may find the idea of changing

TABLE 34-2 PATIENT & CAREGIVER TEACHING GUIDE

Reducing Risk Factors for Coronary Artery Disease

Include the following instructions when teaching risk reduction for coronary artery disease.

Risk Factor	Health-Promoting Behaviors
Hypertension	• Monitor home blood pressure (BP) and attend regular checkups. • Take prescribed medications for BP control. • Reduce salt intake (see eFig. 33-1, Your Guide to Lowering Your Blood Pressure with DASH, available on the website for this chapter). • Stop tobacco use. Avoid exposure to environmental tobacco (secondhand) smoke. • Control or reduce weight. • Perform physical activity daily.
Elevated serum lipids	• Reduce total fat intake. • Reduce animal (saturated) fat intake. • Take prescribed medications for lipid reduction. • Adjust total caloric intake to achieve and maintain ideal body weight. • Engage in daily physical activity. • Increase amount of complex carbohydrates, fiber, and vegetable proteins in diet.
Tobacco use*	• Begin a smoking cessation program. • Change daily routines associated with smoking to reduce desire to smoke. • Substitute other activities for smoking. • Ask caregivers to support efforts to stop smoking. • Avoid exposure to environmental tobacco smoke.
Physical inactivity	• Develop and maintain at least 30 min of moderate physical activity daily (minimum 5 days a week). • Increase activities to a fitness level.
Psychologic state	• Increase awareness of behaviors that are harmful to health. • Alter patterns that are conducive to stress (e.g., get up 30 min earlier so breakfast is not eaten on way to work). • Set realistic goals for self. • Reassess priorities in light of health needs. • Learn effective stress management strategies (see Chapter 7). • Seek professional help if feeling depressed, angry, anxious, etc. • Plan time for adequate rest and sleep (see Chapter 8).
Obesity†	• Change eating patterns and habits. • Reduce caloric intake to achieve body mass index of 18.5-24.9 kg/m^2. • Increase physical activity to increase caloric expenditure. • Avoid fad and crash diets, which are not effective over time. • Avoid large, heavy meals. Consider smaller, more frequent meals.
Diabetes‡	• Follow the recommended diet. • Control or reduce weight. • Take prescribed antidiabetic medications. • Monitor blood glucose levels regularly.

*Smoking cessation is discussed in Chapter 11 and Tables 11-4 through 11-6.
†See Chapter 41 for additional health-promoting behaviors.
‡See Chapter 49 for additional health-promoting behaviors.

lifelong habits still unacceptable. Help them identify such choices and respect their final decision.

PHYSICAL ACTIVITY

A physical activity program should be designed to improve physical fitness by following the FITT formula: **F**requency (how often), **I**ntensity (how hard), **T**ype (isotonic), and **T**ime (how long). Everyone should aim for at least 30 minutes of moderate physical activity on most days of the week.[9] In addition, adding weight training to an exercise program two days a week can help treat metabolic syndrome and improve muscle strength. Examples of moderate physical activity include brisk walking, hiking, biking, and swimming. Regular physical activity contributes to weight reduction, reduction in systolic BP, and, in some men more than women, increase in HDL cholesterol. The AHA has developed a program to encourage people, especially women, to increase their daily physical activity (My Heart, My Life at *www.startwalkingnow.org*).

NUTRITIONAL THERAPY

The National Heart, Lung, and Blood Institute recommends therapeutic lifestyle changes for all people to reduce the risk of CAD by lowering LDL cholesterol. These recommendations emphasize a decrease in saturated fat and cholesterol and an increase in complex carbohydrates (e.g., whole grains, fruit, vegetables) and fiber[7] (Tables 34-3 and 34-4). Fat intake should be about 30% of calories, with most coming from mono- and polyunsaturated fats (Fig. 34-3). Red meat, egg yolks, and whole milk products are major sources of saturated fat and cholesterol and should be reduced or eliminated from diets. If the serum triglyceride level is elevated, the guidelines recommend reducing or eliminating alcohol intake and simple sugars.

Omega-3 fatty acids reduce the risks associated with CAD when eaten regularly. For individuals without CAD, the AHA recommends eating fatty fish twice a week because fatty fish such as salmon and tuna contains two types of omega-3 fatty acids: eicosapentaenoic acid (EPA) and docosahexaenoic acid (DHA). Patients with CAD are encouraged to take EPA and DHA supplements with their diet. The AHA also recommends eating tofu and other forms of soybean, canola, walnut, and flaxseed because these products contain alpha-linolenic acid, which becomes omega-3 fatty acid in the body. For more information on the AHA's nutritional recommendations, see their website listed in the Resources section at the end of this chapter.

Lifestyle changes, including a low-saturated-fat, high-fiber diet; avoidance of tobacco; and increase in physical activity, can promote the reversal of CAD and reduce coronary events.

LIPID-LOWERING DRUG THERAPY

An estimated 31.9 million American adults have cholesterol levels greater than or equal to 240 mg/dL (6.2 mmol/L).[1] A complete lipid profile is recommended every 5 years beginning at age 20. The person with a serum cholesterol level greater than 200 mg/dL is at risk for CAD and should be treated. Treatment usually begins with dietary caloric restriction (if overweight), decreased dietary fat and cholesterol intake, and increased

TABLE 34-3 NUTRITIONAL THERAPY

Therapeutic Lifestyle Changes Diet

Nutrient	Recommended Daily Intake
Total fat (includes saturated fat calories)	25%-35% of total daily calories
Saturated fat	<7% of total daily calories
Cholesterol	<200 mg
Plant stanols or sterols (e.g., margarines, nuts, seeds, legumes, vegetable oils)*	2 g
Dietary fiber*	10-25 g of soluble fiber
Total calories	Only enough calories to reach or maintain a healthy weight
Physical activity	At least 30 min of a moderate-intensity physical activity (e.g., brisk walking) on most, and preferably all, days of the week

Source: Your Guide to Lowering Your Cholesterol with TLC. Retrieved from *www.nhlbi.nih.gov/health/public/heart/chol/chol_tlc.pdf.*
*Diet options for additional lowering of low-density lipoprotein (LDL).

TABLE 34-4 NUTRITIONAL THERAPY

Tips to Implement Diet and Lifestyle Recommendations

General Tips

1. Know your caloric needs to achieve and maintain a healthy weight.
2. Know the calorie content of the foods and beverages you consume.
3. Track your weight, physical activity, and calorie intake.
4. Prepare and eat smaller, more frequent meals.
5. Track your activities and, whenever possible, decrease sedentary activities (e.g., watching television, computer time).
6. Incorporate physical movement into daily activities (e.g., take extra steps when possible).
7. Do not smoke or use tobacco products.
8. If you consume alcohol, do so in moderation (i.e., no more than one drink for women or two drinks for men a day).

Tips Related to Food Choices and Preparation

1. Use the Nutrition Facts panel on food labels and ingredients list when choosing foods to buy.
2. Select frozen and canned vegetables and fruits without high-calorie sauces or added salt and sugars.
3. Replace high-calorie foods with fresh fruits and vegetables.
4. Increase fiber intake by eating beans (legumes), whole-grain products, fruits, and vegetables.
5. Use liquid vegetable oils in place of solid fats.
6. Limit beverages and foods high in added sugars (e.g., sucrose, glucose, fructose, maltose, dextrose, corn syrups, concentrated fruit juice, honey).
7. Choose foods made with whole grains (e.g., whole wheat, oats/oatmeal, rye, barley, corn, popcorn, brown rice, wild rice, buckwheat, cracked wheat, sorghum).
8. Eliminate pastries and high-calorie bakery products (e.g., muffins, doughnuts).
9. Select milk and dairy products that are either fat free or low fat.
10. Reduce salt intake by
    - Comparing the sodium content of similar products (e.g., different brands of tomato sauce) and choosing products with less sodium
    - Choosing versions of processed foods that are reduced in salt, including cereals and baked goods
    - Limiting condiments (e.g., soy sauce, ketchup)
11. Use lean cuts of meat and remove skin from poultry before cooking or eating.
12. Avoid processed meats that are high in saturated fat and sodium (e.g., deli meats).
13. Grill, bake, or broil fish, meat, and poultry.
14. Incorporate vegetable-based meat substitutes into favorite recipes (e.g., soy).
15. Consume whole vegetables and fruits in place of juices.

Adapted from Gidding SS, Lichtenstein AH, Faith MS, et al: Implementing American Heart Association pediatric and adult nutrition guidelines, *Circulation* 119:1161, 2009.

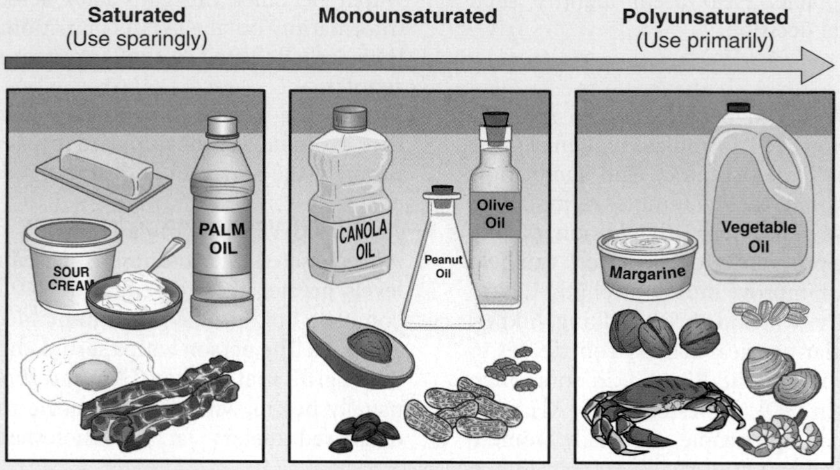

Saturated
- Animal fat (bacon, lard, egg yolk, dairy fat)
- Oils (coconut, palm oil)
- Butter
- Cream cheese
- Sour cream

Monounsaturated
- Fish oil
- Oils (canola, peanut, olive)
- Avocado
- Nuts (almonds, peanuts, pecans)
- Olives (green, black)

Polyunsaturated
- Vegetable oils (safflower, corn, soybean, flaxseed, cottonseed)
- Some fish oil, shellfish
- Nuts (walnuts)
- Seeds (pumpkin, sunflower)
- Margarine

FIG. 34-3 Types of dietary fat.

EVIDENCE-BASED PRACTICE

Translating Research into Practice

Does Dietary Fat Modification Improve Cardiovascular Disease Outcomes?

Clinical Question

For adults (P), what is the effect of dietary fat modification or reduction (I) versus placebo, usual, or control diet (C) on overall mortality and cardiovascular morbidity and mortality (O)?

Best Available Evidence

Systematic review of randomized controlled trials (RCTs)

Critical Appraisal and Synthesis of Evidence

- 48 RCTs with 60 comparisons ($n = 81,327$) of adults with or without existing cardiovascular disease. Intervention was reduced or modified dietary fat intake compared with placebo, usual, or control diet.
- Low-fat diet reduced energy intake to <30% from fat, and partially replaced fats with carbohydrates (simple or complex), protein, or fruit and vegetables.
- Modified fat diet had 30% or more energy intake from total fats with more monounsaturated or polyunsaturated fats than usual diet.

Conclusion

- Reducing saturated fat by reducing and/or modifying dietary fat reduced the risk of cardiovascular events.
- Risk for cardiovascular disease decreased in men (not women) by dietary fat modification.

Implications for Nursing Practice

- Counsel patients on modifying dietary fat intake by substituting monounsaturated or polyunsaturated fats for saturated fats.
- Assist the patient in collaboration with the dietitian to maintain long-term dietary fat changes.

Reference for Evidence

Hooper L, Summerbell C, Thompson R, et al: Reduced or modified dietary fat for preventing cardiovascular disease, *Cochrane Database Syst Rev* 7:CD002137, 2011.

P, Patient population of interest; *I*, intervention or area of interest; *C*, comparison of interest or comparison group; *O*, outcomes of interest; *T*, timing (see p. 12).

COMPLEMENTARY & ALTERNATIVE THERAPIES

*Lipid-Lowering Agents**

Agent	Evidence for Use
Garlic	Inconsistent scientific evidence for reductions in total cholesterol and low-density lipoproteins (LDLs) over short periods.
Niacin	Strong scientific evidence for increased high-density lipoproteins. Less dramatic reduction of LDLs.
Omega-3 fatty acids	Strong scientific evidence for reduction of triglyceride levels.
Psyllium	Strong scientific evidence for modest reduction in total cholesterol and LDLs.
Plant sterols	Strong scientific evidence for reduction of total cholesterol.
Red yeast rice	Strong scientific evidence for reduction of total cholesterol, LDLs, and triglycerides.
Soy	Strong scientific evidence for moderate reduction in total cholesterol and LDLs.

Based on a systematic review of scientific literature. Available at *www.naturalstandard.com*.

*Cardiovascular disease is a serious health problem. Herbal or other natural therapy should not be initiated without consultation with a health care provider. This is especially important when conventional drug therapy for cardiovascular disease is also being used.

physical activity. The guidelines for treatment of high cholesterol focus on LDL levels. Serum lipid levels are reassessed after 6 weeks of diet therapy. If they remain elevated, additional dietary options (see the Complementary & Alternative Therapies box above) and drug therapy (Table 34-5) may be considered.

DRUGS THAT RESTRICT LIPOPROTEIN PRODUCTION. The statin drugs are the most widely used lipid-lowering drugs. These drugs inhibit the synthesis of cholesterol in the liver. An unexplained result of the inhibition of cholesterol synthesis is an increase in hepatic LDL receptors. Consequently, the liver is able to remove more LDLs from the blood. In addition, statins

TABLE 34-5 DRUG THERAPY

Hyperlipidemia

Drug	Mechanism of Action	Side Effects	Nursing Considerations
Restrict Lipoprotein Production			
HMG-CoA Reductase Inhibitors (Statins)			
atorvastatin (Lipitor) fluvastatin (Lescol) lovastatin (Mevacor) pitavastatin (Livalo) pravastatin (Pravachol) simvastatin (Zocor) rosuvastatin (Crestor)	Block synthesis of cholesterol and increase LDL receptors in liver ↓ LDL ↓ Triglycerides ↑ HDL	Rash, GI disturbances, elevated liver enzymes, myopathy, rhabdomyolysis	Well tolerated with few side effects. Monitor liver enzymes and creatine kinase (if muscle weakness or pain occurs).
Niacin			
niacin (Nicobid, Niaspan) nicotinic acid (Slo-Niacin, Novo-Niacin)	Inhibits synthesis and secretion of VLDL and LDL ↓ LDL ↓ Triglycerides ↑ HDL	Flushing and pruritus in upper torso and face, GI disturbances (e.g., nausea and vomiting, dyspepsia, diarrhea), orthostatic hypotension, elevated homocysteine levels	Most side effects subside with time. Decreased liver function may occur with high doses. Taking aspirin or NSAID 30 min before drug may prevent flushing. Take drug with food. Treat elevated homocysteine levels with folic acid.
Fibric Acid Derivatives			
fenofibrate (TriCor) gemfibrozil (Lopid)	Decrease hepatic synthesis and secretion of VLDL. Reduce triglycerides by ↓ VLDL ↓ LDL ↓ Triglycerides ↑ HDL	Rashes, mild GI disturbances (e.g., nausea, diarrhea), elevated liver enzymes	May ↑ effects of warfarin (Coumadin) and some antihyperglycemic drugs. When used in combination with statins, may increase adverse effects of statins, especially myopathy.
Omega-3 Fatty Acid			
icosapent ethyl (Vascepa)	Inhibits synthesis and/or secretion of triglycerides	Arthralgia	Used for patients with severe hypertriglyceridemia (levels ≥500 mg/dL).
Increase Lipoprotein Removal			
Bile-Acid Sequestrants			
cholestyramine (Questran) colesevelam (WelChol) colestipol (Colestid)	Bind with bile acids in intestine, forming insoluble complex and excreted in feces Binding results in removal of LDL and cholesterol ↓ LDL	Unpleasant quality to taste, GI disturbances (e.g., indigestion, constipation, bloating)	Effective and safe for long-term use. Side effects diminish with time. Interfere with absorption of many drugs (e.g., digoxin, thiazide diuretics, warfarin, some antibiotics [e.g., penicillins]).
Decrease Cholesterol Absorption			
Cholesterol Absorption Inhibitor			
ezetimibe (Zetia)	Inhibits the intestinal absorption of cholesterol ↓ LDL ↑ HDL	Infrequent, but may include headache and mild GI distress	When used with a statin, LDL is further reduced. Should not be used by patients with liver impairment.

produce a small increase in HDLs and lower CRP levels.[15] Serious adverse effects of these drugs are rare and include liver damage and myopathy that can progress to rhabdomyolysis (breakdown of skeletal muscle). Liver enzymes (e.g., aspartate aminotransferase, alanine aminotransferase) are initially monitored and rechecked with any increase in dosage. Creatine kinase isoenzymes (e.g., CK-MM) are assessed if symptoms of myopathy (e.g., muscle aches, weakness) occur.[15]

DRUG ALERT

Simvastatin (Zocor)

- Increased risk for rhabdomyolysis when also used with gemfibrozil (Lopid) or niacin (Niaspan)
- Signs of rhabdomyolysis: ↑ creatine kinase levels, muscle tenderness

Niacin, a water-soluble B vitamin, is highly effective in lowering LDL and triglyceride levels by interfering with their synthesis. Niacin also increases HDL levels better than many other lipid-lowering drugs. Unfortunately, side effects of this drug are common and may include severe flushing, pruritus, gastrointestinal (GI) symptoms, and orthostatic hypotension.

DRUG ALERT

Niacin (Niaspan)

- Instruct patient that flushing (especially of face and neck) may occur within 20 minutes after taking drug and may last for 30 to 60 minutes.
- Patient can premedicate with aspirin or nonsteroidal antiinflammatory drug (NSAID) 30 minutes before administration to reduce flushing.
- Use of extended-release niacin may decrease side effects.

The *fibric acid derivatives* (see Table 34-5) work by aiding the removal of VLDLs and increasing the production of apolipoproteins A-I and A-II. They are the most effective drugs for lowering triglycerides and increasing HDL levels. They have no effect on LDLs. Although most patients tolerate the drugs well, complaints may include GI irritability. These drugs should be used with caution when combined with statin medications.

DRUG ALERT

Gemfibrozil (Lopid)

- May increase the risk of bleeding in patients taking warfarin (Coumadin)
- May increase the effects of antihyperglycemic drugs (e.g., repaglinide [Prandin])

DRUGS THAT INCREASE LIPOPROTEIN REMOVAL. The major route of elimination of cholesterol is by conversion to bile acids in the liver. Bile-acid sequestrants increase conversion of cholesterol to bile acids and decrease hepatic cholesterol. The primary effect is a decrease in total cholesterol and LDLs.

Administration of these drugs can be associated with complaints related to taste and a variety of upper and lower GI symptoms. These include belching, heartburn, nausea, abdominal pain, and constipation. The bile-acid sequestrants interfere with absorption of many other drugs (e.g., warfarin, thiazides, thyroid hormones, β-adrenergic blockers). Separating the time of administration of these drugs from that of other drugs decreases this adverse effect.[15]

DRUGS THAT DECREASE CHOLESTEROL ABSORPTION. Ezetimibe (Zetia) selectively inhibits the absorption of dietary and biliary cholesterol across the intestinal wall. It serves as an adjunct to dietary changes, especially in patients with primary hypercholesterolemia. When it is combined with a statin (e.g., ezetimibe and simvastatin [Vytorin]), even greater reductions in LDLs are found.

Drug therapy for hyperlipidemia often continues for a lifetime. New combination drug therapy (e.g., atorvastatin/ezetimibe [Liptruzet]) is available and may be considered. Concurrent diet modification is essential to minimize the need for drug therapy. The patient must fully understand the rationale and goals of treatment, as well as the safety and side effects of lipid-lowering drug therapy.

ANTIPLATELET THERAPY

Unless contraindicated (e.g., history of GI bleeding), low-dose aspirin (81 mg) is recommended for most people at risk for CAD (see eFig. 34-5, What you need to know—antiplatelet therapy, available on the website for this chapter). Current recommendations include low-dose aspirin for men over 45 years and high-risk women (i.e., those with a calculated 10-year CAD risk of more than 20%) unless contraindicated. For high-risk women who are intolerant of aspirin, clopidogrel (Plavix) can be substituted. In healthy women 65 years or older, aspirin therapy should be considered if BP is controlled and the benefit for MI prevention outweighs the risk of GI bleed or hemorrhagic stroke.[16]

GERONTOLOGIC CONSIDERATIONS

CORONARY ARTERY DISEASE

The incidence of cardiac disease is greatly increased in older adults and is the leading cause of death in older persons.[1] In the older adult, CAD is often a result of the complex interaction of nonmodifiable risk factors (e.g., age) and lifelong modifiable risk behaviors (e.g., inactivity, tobacco use). Strategies to reduce CAD risk and to treat CAD are effective in this age-group.[16]

Aggressive treatment of hypertension and hyperlipidemia stabilizes plaques in the coronary arteries of older adults, and cessation of tobacco use helps decrease the risk for CAD at any age.[16] Similarly, encourage the older patient to consider a planned program of physical activity. Activity performance, endurance, and ability to tolerate stress are improved in the older adult with physical training. Positive psychologic benefits from physical activity can include increased self-esteem and emotional well-being and improved body image. For the older adult who is obese, making modest dietary changes and slowly increasing physical activity (e.g., walking) results in more positive benefits than aiming for a significant weight loss.

When planning a physical activity program for the older adult, recommend the following: (1) longer warm-up periods, (2) longer periods of low-level activity, or (3) longer rest periods between sessions. Heat intolerance in the older adult results from a decreased ability to sweat efficiently. Teach the patient to avoid physical activity in extremes of temperature and to maintain a moderate pace. The older adult should exercise a minimum of 30 minutes on most days of the week as able.[9]

Encouraging the older patient to adopt a healthy lifestyle may increase the quality of life and reduce the risk of CAD and fatal cardiac events. Older adults face many of the same challenges as younger persons when it comes to making lifestyle changes. Older adults are more likely to consider change at two points in time: (1) when hospitalized and (2) when symptoms (e.g., chest pain) are the result of CAD and not normal aging (see Table 32-1). First, assess the older adult for readiness to change, and then help the patient select the lifestyle changes most likely to produce the greatest reduction in risk for CAD.

CHRONIC STABLE ANGINA

CAD is a progressive disease, and patients may be asymptomatic for many years or may develop chronic stable chest pain. When the demand for myocardial oxygen exceeds the ability of the coronary arteries to supply the heart with oxygen, *myocardial ischemia* occurs. **Angina,** or chest pain, is the clinical manifestation of reversible myocardial ischemia. Either an increased demand for oxygen or a decreased supply of oxygen can lead to myocardial ischemia (Table 34-6). The primary reason for insufficient blood flow is narrowing of coronary arteries by atherosclerosis. For ischemia secondary to atherosclerosis to occur, the artery is usually blocked (stenosed) 75% or more.

On the cellular level, the myocardium becomes hypoxic within the first 10 seconds of coronary occlusion. Myocardial cells are deprived of oxygen and glucose needed for aerobic

TABLE 34-6 FACTORS INFLUENCING MYOCARDIAL OXYGEN NEEDS*

Decreased Oxygen Supply	Increased Oxygen Demand or Consumption
Cardiac	
• Coronary artery spasm	• Aortic stenosis
• Coronary artery thrombosis	• Cardiomyopathy
• Dysrhythmias	• Dysrhythmias
• Heart failure	• Tachycardia
• Valve disorders	
Noncardiac	
• Anemia	• Anxiety
• Asthma	• Hypertension
• Chronic obstructive pulmonary disease	• Hyperthermia
	• Hyperthyroidism
• Hypovolemia	• Physical exertion
• Hypoxemia	• Substance abuse (e.g., cocaine, ephedrine)
• Pneumonia	

*Lists are not all-inclusive.

metabolism and contractility. Anaerobic metabolism begins, and lactic acid accumulates. Lactic acid irritates myocardial nerve fibers and transmits a pain message to the cardiac nerves and upper thoracic posterior nerve roots. This accounts for referred cardiac pain to the shoulders, neck, lower jaw, and arms. In ischemic conditions, cardiac cells are viable for approximately 20 minutes. With restoration of blood flow, aerobic metabolism resumes, contractility is restored, and cellular repair begins.

Chronic stable angina refers to chest pain that occurs intermittently over a long period with the same pattern of onset, duration, and intensity of symptoms. When questioned, some patients may deny feeling pain but describe a pressure or ache in the chest (Table 34-7). It is an unpleasant feeling, often described as a squeezing, heavy, choking, or suffocating sensation. Angina is rarely sharp or stabbing, and it usually does not change with position or breathing. Many people with angina complain of indigestion or a burning sensation in the epigastric region. Although most angina pain appears substernally, the sensation may occur in the neck or radiate to various locations, including the lower jaw, the shoulders, and the arms (Fig. 34-4). Often people complain of pain between the shoulder blades and dismiss it as not being heart related.

The pain usually lasts for only a few minutes (5 to 15 minutes) and commonly subsides when the precipitating factor is resolved (Table 34-8). Pain at rest is unusual. A 12-lead electrocardiogram (ECG) often shows ST segment depression and/or T wave inversion indicating ischemia (see Chapter 36). The ECG returns to baseline when the pain is relieved.

Chronic stable angina is controlled with medications on an outpatient basis. Because chronic stable angina is often predictable, medications are timed to provide peak effects during the

TABLE 34-7 PQRST ASSESSMENT OF ANGINA

Use the following memory aid to obtain information from the patient who has chest pain.

	Factor	Questions to Ask Patient
P	Precipitating events	What events or activities precipitated the pain (e.g., argument, exercise, resting)?
Q	Quality of pain	What does the pain feel like (e.g., pressure, dull, aching, tight, squeezing, heaviness)?
R	Radiation of pain	Where is the pain located? Does the pain radiate to other areas (e.g., back, neck, arms, jaw, shoulder, elbow)?
S	Severity of pain	On a scale of 0 to 10 with 0 indicating no pain and 10 being the most severe pain you could imagine, what number would you give the pain?
T	Timing	When did the pain begin? Has the pain changed since this time? Have you had pain like this before?

TABLE 34-8 PRECIPITATING FACTORS OF ANGINA

Physical Exertion
- Increases HR, reducing the time the heart spends in diastole (the time of greatest coronary blood flow), resulting in an increase in myocardial oxygen demand.
- Isometric exercise of the arms (e.g., raking, lifting heavy objects, snow shoveling) can cause exertional angina.

Temperature Extremes
- Increase the workload of the heart.
- Blood vessels constrict in response to a cold stimulus.
- Blood vessels dilate and blood pools in the skin in response to a hot stimulus.

Strong Emotions
- Stimulate the sympathetic nervous system, activating the stress response.
- Increase the workload of the heart.

Consumption of Heavy Meal
- Can increase the workload of the heart.
- During the digestive process, blood is diverted to the GI system, reducing blood flow in the coronary arteries.

Tobacco Use, Environmental Tobacco Smoke
- Nicotine stimulates catecholamine release, causing vasoconstriction and an increased HR.
- Diminishes available oxygen by increasing the level of carbon monoxide.

Sexual Activity
- Increases the cardiac workload and sympathetic stimulation.
- In a person with CAD, the extra cardiac workload may precipitate angina.

Stimulants (e.g., cocaine, amphetamines)
- Increase HR and subsequent myocardial oxygen demand.

Circadian Rhythm Patterns
- Related to the occurrence of chronic stable angina, Prinzmetal's angina, MI, and sudden cardiac death.
- Manifestations of CAD tend to occur in the early morning after awakening.

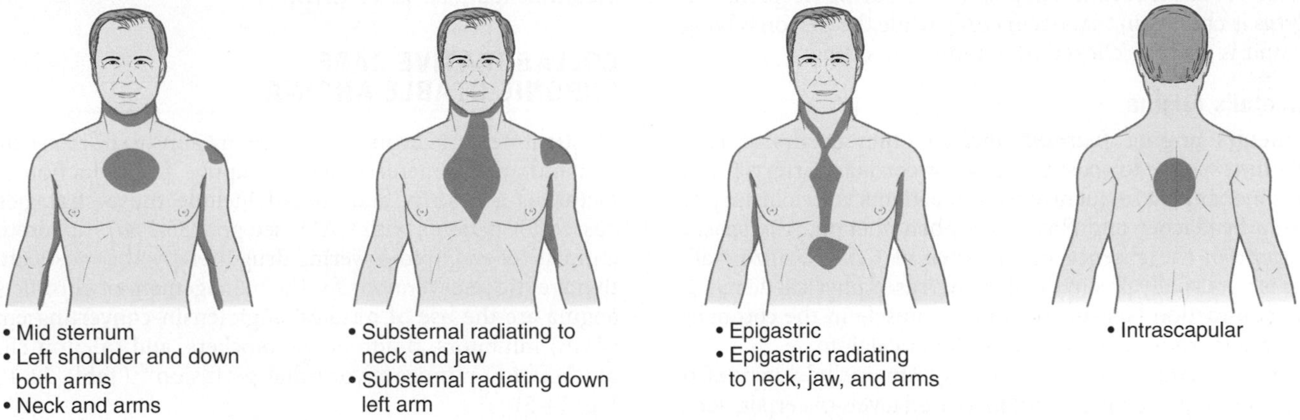

FIG. 34-4 Common locations and patterns of pain during angina or myocardial infarction.

TABLE 34-9 COMPARISON OF MAJOR TYPES OF ANGINA

Type	Etiology	Characteristics
Chronic stable angina	Myocardial ischemia, usually secondary to CAD	• Episodic pain lasting 5-15 min • Provoked by exertion • Relieved by rest or nitroglycerin
Prinzmetal's angina	Coronary vasospasm	• Occurs primarily at rest • Triggered by smoking and increased levels of some substances (e.g., histamine, epinephrine) • May occur in presence or absence of CAD
Microvascular angina	Myocardial ischemia secondary to microvascular disease affecting the small, distal branches of the coronary arteries	• More common in women • Triggered by activities of daily living (e.g., shopping, work) vs. physical exercise (exertion) • Treatment may include nitroglycerin
Unstable angina	Rupture of thickened plaque, exposing thrombogenic surface	• New-onset angina • Chronic stable angina that increases in frequency, duration, or severity • Occurs at rest or with minimal exertion • Pain refractory to nitroglycerin

time of day when angina is likely to occur. For example, if angina occurs when rising, the patient can take medication as soon as awakening and wait 30 minutes to 1 hour before engaging in activity. (See Table 34-9 for a comparison of the major types of angina.)

Silent Ischemia

Silent ischemia refers to ischemia that occurs in the absence of any subjective symptoms. Patients with diabetes have an increased prevalence of silent ischemia. This is most likely due to diabetic neuropathy affecting the nerves that innervate the cardiovascular system. When patients are monitored (e.g., Holter monitor) and silent ischemia occurs, ECG changes are revealed. Ischemia with pain or without pain has the same prognosis.

Nocturnal Angina and Angina Decubitus

Nocturnal angina occurs only at night but not necessarily when the person is in the recumbent position or during sleep. *Angina decubitus* is chest pain that occurs only while the person is lying down and is usually relieved by standing or sitting.

Prinzmetal's Angina

Prinzmetal's angina *(variant angina)* often occurs at rest, usually in response to spasm of a major coronary artery. It is a rare form of angina frequently seen in patients with a history of migraine headaches and Raynaud's phenomenon. The spasm may occur in the absence or presence of CAD. Prinzmetal's angina is not usually precipitated by increased physical demand. Strong contraction (spasm) of smooth muscle in the coronary artery results from increased intracellular calcium.

Factors causing coronary artery spasm include increased myocardial oxygen demand and increased levels of certain substances (e.g., tobacco smoke, alcohol, amphetamines). When spasm occurs, the patient experiences angina and transient ST segment elevation (see Chapter 36). The pain may occur during rapid-eye-movement (REM) sleep when myocardial oxygen consumption increases. The pain may be relieved by moderate exercise, or it may disappear spontaneously. Cyclic, short bursts of pain at a usual time each day may also occur with this type of angina. Calcium channel blockers and/or nitrates are used to control the angina.

TABLE 34-10 TREATMENT OF CHRONIC STABLE ANGINA

*Strategies for the patient with chronic stable angina should address all the treatment elements and related patient teaching in the following mnemonic:**

Element	Treatment
A	Antiplatelet/anticoagulant therapy Antianginal therapy ACE inhibitor/angiotensin receptor blocker
B	β-adrenergic blocker Blood pressure control
C	Cigarette smoking cessation Cholesterol (lipid) management Calcium channel blockers Cardiac rehabilitation
D	Diet (weight management) Diabetes management Depression screening
E	Education Exercise
F	Flu vaccination

*Modified from Smith SC, Benjamin EJ, Bonow RO, et al: AHA/ACCF secondary prevention and risk reduction therapy for patients with coronary and other atherosclerotic vascular disease: 2011 update, *J Am Coll Cardiol* 58:2432, 2011.

Microvascular Angina

In *microvascular angina,* chest pain occurs in the absence of significant coronary atherosclerosis or coronary spasm, especially in women.[2] In these patients, chest pain is related to myocardial ischemia associated with abnormalities of the coronary microcirculation. This is known as coronary microvascular disease (MVD).

Coronary MVD affects the small branches of the distal coronary arteries, whereas CAD affects larger coronary arteries. In coronary MVD, plaque can be diffuse, be evenly distributed, or develop as blockages in the tiny coronary arteries. Prevention and treatment of coronary MVD follow the same recommendations as for CAD.[2]

COLLABORATIVE CARE CHRONIC STABLE ANGINA

The treatment of chronic stable angina aims to decrease oxygen demand and/or increase oxygen supply. The reduction of risk factors is a priority and should include those strategies discussed for patients with CAD (see pp. 735-740). In addition to antiplatelet and lipid-lowering drug therapy, the most common therapeutic interventions for the management of chronic stable angina are the use of nitrates, angiotensin-converting enzyme (ACE) inhibitors, β-adrenergic blockers, and calcium channel blockers to optimize myocardial perfusion[17] (Table 34-10 and Fig. 34-5).

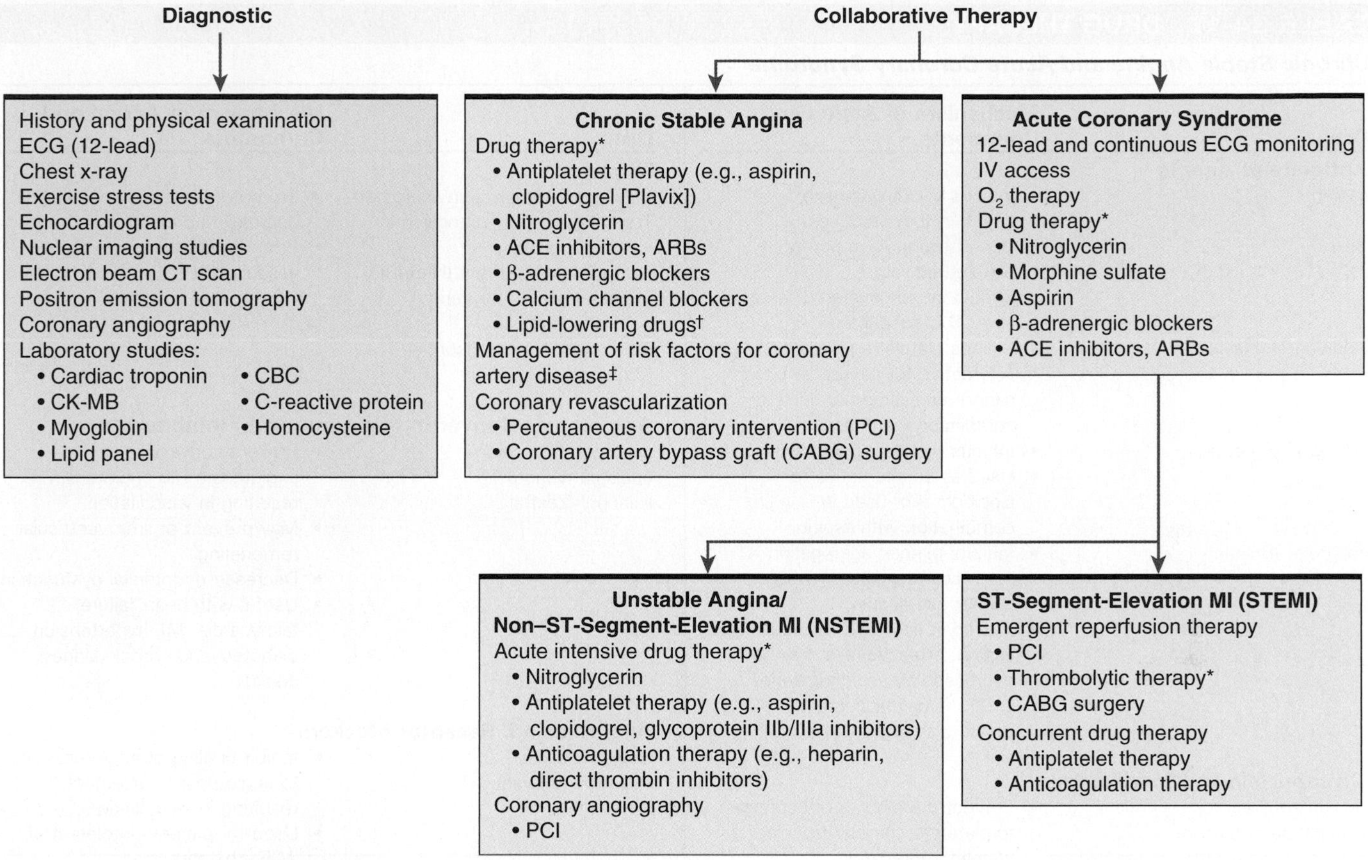

FIG. 34-5 Collaborative care: chronic stable angina and acute coronary syndrome. *ACE,* Angiotensin-converting enzyme; *ARBs,* angiotensin II receptor blockers; *CK,* creatine kinase.
*, see Table 34-11.
†, see Table 34-5.
‡, see Tables 34-2, 34-3, and 34-4.

Drug Therapy

Drug therapy for chronic stable angina aims to prevent MI and death, and reduce symptoms. Aspirin (previously discussed) is given in the absence of contraindications (Table 34-11).

Short-Acting Nitrates. Short-acting nitrates are first-line therapy for the treatment of angina. Nitrates produce their principal effects by the following mechanisms:

Dilating peripheral blood vessels: This results in decreased SVR, venous pooling, and decreased venous blood return to the heart (preload). Therefore myocardial oxygen demand is decreased because of the reduced cardiac workload.

Dilating coronary arteries and collateral vessels: This may increase blood flow to the ischemic areas of the heart. However, when the coronary arteries are severely atherosclerotic, coronary dilation is difficult to achieve.

Sublingual Nitroglycerin. Nitroglycerin (NTG) given sublingually (Nitrostat) or by translingual spray (Nitrolingual) usually relieves pain in about 3 minutes and has a duration of approximately 30 to 40 minutes. The recommended dose for the patient who has been prescribed NTG is one tablet taken sublingually (SL) or one metered spray for symptoms of angina. If symptoms are unchanged or worse after 5 minutes, tell the patient or caregiver to repeat NTG every 5 minutes for a maximum of three doses and contact EMS if symptoms have not resolved completely.[17]

Instruct the patient in the proper use of NTG. It should be easily accessible to the patient at all times. The patient should store the tablets away from light and heat sources, including body heat, to protect them from degradation. Tablets are packaged in light-resistant bottles with metal caps. Once opened, the tablets lose potency and should be replaced every 6 months.

Tell the patient to place a NTG tablet under the tongue and allow it to dissolve. If using the spray, the patient should direct it on the tongue, not inhale it. NTG should cause a tingling sensation when administered; otherwise it may be outdated. Warn the patient that a headache, dizziness, or flushing may occur. Caution the patient to change positions slowly after NTG use because orthostatic hypotension may occur.

Patients can use NTG prophylactically before starting an activity that is known to cause an anginal attack. In these cases the patient can take a tablet or spray 5 to 10 minutes before beginning the activity. Instruct the patient to report any changes in the usual pattern of pain, especially increasing frequency or nocturnal angina, to the health care provider.

Long-Acting Nitrates. Nitrates, such as isosorbide dinitrate (Isordil) and isosorbide mononitrate (Imdur), are longer acting than SL or translingual NTG. They are used to reduce the incidence of anginal attacks. The main side effect of all nitrates is headache from the dilation of cerebral blood vessels. Advise patients to take acetaminophen (Tylenol) with their nitrate to relieve the headache. Over time, the headaches may decrease, but the antianginal effect is still present.

TABLE 34-11 **DRUG THERAPY**

Chronic Stable Angina and Acute Coronary Syndrome

Drug	Mechanism of Action and Comments
Antiplatelet Agents	
aspirin	• Inhibits cyclooxygenase, which in turn produces thromboxane A_2, a potent platelet activator • Should be administered as soon as ACS is suspected
clopidogrel (Plavix)	• Inhibits platelet aggregation • Alternative for patient who cannot use aspirin or used in combination with aspirin
prasugrel (Effient)	• Inhibits platelet aggregation • Used as an alternative to clopidogrel or used in combination with aspirin
ticagrelor (Brilinta)	• Inhibits platelet aggregation • Alternative for patient who cannot use aspirin • If used in combination with aspirin, effectiveness may be decreased by aspirin dosages >100 mg/day (according to a boxed warning)
Glycoprotein IIb/IIIa Inhibitors	
abciximab (ReoPro) eptifibatide (Integrilin) tirofiban (Aggrastat)	• Prevent the binding of fibrinogen to platelets, thereby blocking platelet aggregation • Standard antiplatelet therapy in combination with aspirin for patients at high risk for unstable angina
Anticoagulant Agents	
Unfractionated Heparin*	
heparin (Hep-Lock)	• Prevents conversion of fibrinogen to fibrin and prothrombin to thrombin
Low-Molecular-Weight Heparin*	
dalteparin (Fragmin) enoxaparin (Lovenox)	• Bind to antithrombin III, enhancing its effect • Heparin–antithrombin III complex inactivates activated factor X and thrombin • Prevent conversion of fibrinogen to fibrin
Vitamin K Antagonist*	
warfarin (Coumadin)	• Interferes with hepatic synthesis of vitamin K–dependent clotting factors • Alternative for patient who cannot use aspirin or clopidogrel
Direct Thrombin Inhibitors	
bivalirudin (Angiomax) argatroban (Acova)	• Direct inhibition of the clotting factor thrombin
Nitrates	
Sublingual nitroglycerin (Nitrostat) Translingual spray nitroglycerin (Nitrolingual) nitroglycerin ointment (Nitro-Bid) Transdermal nitroglycerin (Transderm-Nitro) isosorbide dinitrate (Isordil) IV nitroglycerin (Tridil)	• Promote peripheral vasodilation, decreasing preload and afterload • Promote coronary artery vasodilation
Angiotensin-Converting Enzyme (ACE) Inhibitors†	
captopril (Capoten) enalapril (Vasotec) lisinopril (Zestril)	• Prevent conversion of angiotensin I to angiotensin II, resulting in vasodilation • May prevent or limit ventricular remodeling • Decrease endothelial dysfunction • Useful with heart failure, tachycardia, MI, hypertension, diabetes, and chronic kidney disease
Angiotensin II Receptor Blockers†	
losartan (Cozaar) valsartan (Diovan)	• Inhibit binding of angiotensin II to angiotensin I receptors, resulting in vasodilation • Used for patients intolerant of ACE inhibitors
β-Adrenergic Blockers†	
atenolol (Tenormin) carvedilol (Coreg) metoprolol (Lopressor) nadolol (Corgard)	• Inhibit sympathetic nervous stimulation of the heart • Reduce heart rate, contractility, and blood pressure • Decrease afterload
Calcium Channel Blockers†	
amlodipine (Norvasc) diltiazem (Cardizem) felodipine (Plendil) nicardipine (Cardene) verapamil (Calan)	• Prevent calcium entry into vascular smooth muscle cells and myocytes (cardiac cells) • May prevent or control coronary vasospasm • Promote coronary and peripheral vasodilation • Reduce heart rate, contractility, and blood pressure
Opioid Analgesics	
morphine (morphine sulfate)	• Functions as an analgesic and sedative • Acts as a vasodilator to reduce preload and myocardial O_2 consumption
Thrombolytic Agents	
reteplase (Retavase) alteplase (Activase) tenecteplase (TNKase)	• Breaks up fibrin meshwork in clots • Used only in ST-segment-elevation MI

*See Table 38-10.
†See Table 33-7.

Orthostatic hypotension is a complication of all nitrates. Monitor BP after the initial dose, since the venous dilation that occurs may cause a drop in BP, especially in volume-depleted patients. To limit this, patients are often scheduled an 8-hour nitrate-free period every day, usually during the night, unless the patient experiences nocturnal angina.[15] Finally, tolerance to NTG-induced vasodilation can develop.

Nitroglycerin Ointment. Nitropaste is a 2% NTG topical ointment dosed by the inch. It is placed on the upper body or arm, over a flat muscular area that is free of hair and scars. Once absorbed, it produces anginal prophylaxis for 3 to 6 hours. It is especially useful for nocturnal and unstable angina.

Transdermal Controlled-Release Nitrates. Currently two systems are available for transdermal NTG drug administration: reservoir and matrix. The reservoir system delivers the drug using a rate-controlled permeable membrane. The matrix system provides for a slow delivery of the drug through a polymer matrix. Both reservoir and matrix delivery systems offer the advantages of steady plasma levels within the therapeutic range during 24 hours, thus making only one application a day necessary. The reservoir system has the disadvantage of dose dumping if the reservoir seal is punctured or broken. An advantage of the matrix system is that there can be no dose dumping. Both systems achieve steady plasma levels by 2 hours.

DRUG ALERT

Nitroglycerin

- SL tablet must be administered under the tongue. Translingual NTG should be sprayed on the tongue.
- Instruct patient not to combine with drugs used for erectile dysfunction (e.g., sildenafil [Viagra]).
- Monitor for orthostatic hypotension because it may occur after administration.
- Use gloves to apply and remove NTG ointment or transdermal patch to avoid contact with medication.
- Never discharge cardioverter-defibrillator over NTG ointment or transdermal patch.

Angiotensin-Converting Enzyme Inhibitors. Patients with chronic stable angina who are considered high risk for a cardiac event (e.g., ejection fraction [EF] 40% or less, history of diabetes) should take an ACE inhibitor (e.g., captopril [Capoten]) indefinitely.[17] ACE inhibitors are also used for lower risk patients (e.g., patients with mildly reduced EF).

These drugs result in vasodilation and reduced blood volume. Most important, they can prevent or reverse ventricular remodeling (see p. 748). For patients who are intolerant of ACE inhibitors, angiotensin II receptor blockers (e.g., losartan [Cozaar]) are used. (ACE inhibitors and angiotensin II receptor blockers are discussed later in the chapter and in Chapter 33 and Table 33-7.)

β-Adrenergic Blockers. Patients who have left ventricular dysfunction, have elevated BP, or have had an MI should start and continue β-adrenergic blockers indefinitely.[17] These drugs decrease myocardial contractility, HR, SVR, and BP, all of which reduce the myocardial oxygen demand.

β-Adrenergic blockers have many side effects and can be poorly tolerated. Side effects may include bradycardia, hypotension, wheezing, and GI complaints. Many patients also complain of weight gain, depression, and sexual dysfunction. Patients with asthma should avoid β-adrenergic blockers. They are used cautiously in patients with diabetes, since they mask signs of hypoglycemia. β-Adrenergic blockers should not be discontinued abruptly without medical supervision. This may precipitate an increase in the frequency and intensity of angina attacks.

Calcium Channel Blockers. If β-adrenergic blockers are contraindicated, are poorly tolerated, or do not control anginal symptoms, calcium channel blockers are used.[17] These drugs are also used to manage Prinzmetal's angina. The three primary effects of calcium channel blockers are (1) systemic vasodilation with decreased SVR, (2) decreased myocardial contractility, and (3) coronary vasodilation. Most of these agents have sustained-release versions for longer action with the hope of increased patient adherence and stable blood levels of the drug.

Cardiac muscle and vascular smooth muscle cells are more dependent on extracellular calcium than skeletal muscles. Therefore these cells are more sensitive to calcium channel blocking agents. Calcium channel blockers cause smooth muscle relaxation and relative vasodilation of coronary and systemic arteries, thus increasing blood flow.

Calcium channel blockers potentiate the action of digoxin by increasing serum digoxin levels. Therefore serum digoxin levels should be closely monitored after starting calcium channel blockers. Teach the patient the signs and symptoms of digoxin toxicity (see Chapter 35).

Sodium Current Inhibitor. Ranolazine (Ranexa), a sodium current inhibitor, is used to treat chronic angina in those patients who have not achieved adequate response with other antianginals.[17] Because ranolazine prolongs the QT interval, patients with a long QT interval or who are taking QT-prolonging drugs (e.g., fluoxetine [Prozac]) should not use it. Common side effects of ranolazine include dizziness, nausea, constipation, and generalized weakness.[15]

Diagnostic Studies

When a patient has a history of CAD or CAD is suspected, a variety of studies are completed (see Fig. 34-5). After a detailed health history and physical examination, a chest x-ray is done to look for cardiac enlargement, aortic calcifications, and pulmonary congestion. A 12-lead ECG is obtained and compared with a previous tracing when possible. Certain laboratory tests (e.g., lipid profile) and diagnostic studies (e.g., echocardiogram) are done to confirm CAD and identify specific risk factors for CAD.

Measurement of coronary calcification can be useful for predicting adverse cardiac events. The degree of coronary artery calcification correlates with the severity of CAD. The calcium-score screening heart scan locates calcium deposits in atherosclerotic plaque in the coronary arteries (see Fig. 32-11). However, additional testing (e.g., stress testing) is needed to know the impact of the lesion on coronary blood flow.

For patients with known CAD and chronic stable angina, common diagnostic studies include 12-lead ECG, echocardiogram, exercise stress testing, and pharmacologic nuclear imaging. (See Chapter 32 and Table 32-6 for a discussion of these studies, including nursing considerations.)

Cardiac Catheterization. For patients with increasing symptoms or with a significant amount of myocardium that is ischemic under stress, a cardiac catheterization is ordered. Cardiac catheterization and coronary angiography provide images of the coronary circulation and identify the location and severity of any blockage.

If a coronary blockage is amenable to an intervention, **coronary revascularization** with an elective **percutaneous coronary intervention (PCI)** is done.[17] During this procedure,

EVIDENCE-BASED PRACTICE

Translating Research into Practice

Does Timing of Ambulation Affect Patient Safety After Percutaneous Coronary Intervention?

Clinical Question

Among patients following percutaneous coronary interventions (P), what is the effect of ambulation (I) early versus late (T) on bleeding and hematoma (O)?

Best Available Evidence

Meta-analysis of randomized controlled trials (RCTs)

Critical Appraisal and Synthesis of Evidence

- Five RCTs (n = 1854) of patients comparing safety of early versus late ambulation after percutaneous coronary interventions (PCIs) using a femoral artery approach.
- Early ambulation was 2-4 hr after bed rest, with late ambulation 6-20 hr after bed rest.
- Outcomes assessed were hematoma or bleeding.
- Early ambulation was not more harmful than late ambulation.

Conclusion

- Reducing bed rest time from 6-10 hr down to 2-4 hr after PCI is safe.

Implications for Nursing Practice

- Inform nursing personnel that it is safe to ambulate patients 2-4 hr after PCI is done via a femoral artery approach.
- After PCI monitor patients for signs of bleeding at the puncture site.

Reference for Evidence

Tongsai S, Thamlikitkul V: The safety of early versus late ambulation in the management of patients after percutaneous coronary interventions: a meta-analysis, *Int J Nurs Stud* 49(9):1084, 2012.

P, Patient population of interest; *I*, intervention or area of interest; *C*, comparison of interest or comparison group; *O*, outcomes of interest; *T*, timing (see p. 12).

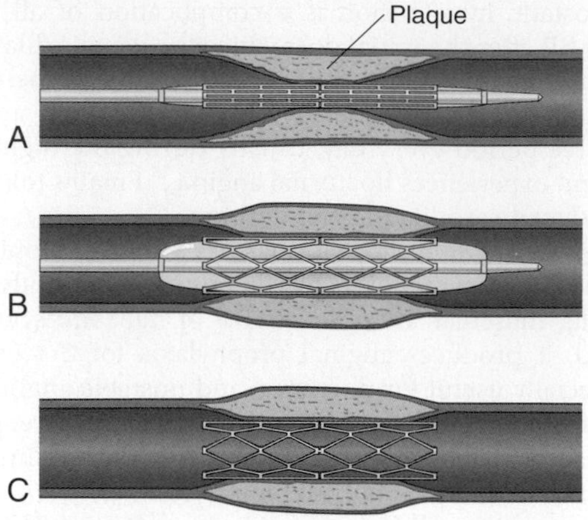

FIG. 34-6 Placement of a coronary artery stent. **A,** The stent is positioned at the site of the lesion. **B,** The balloon is inflated, expanding the stent. The balloon is then deflated and removed. **C,** The implanted stent is left in place.

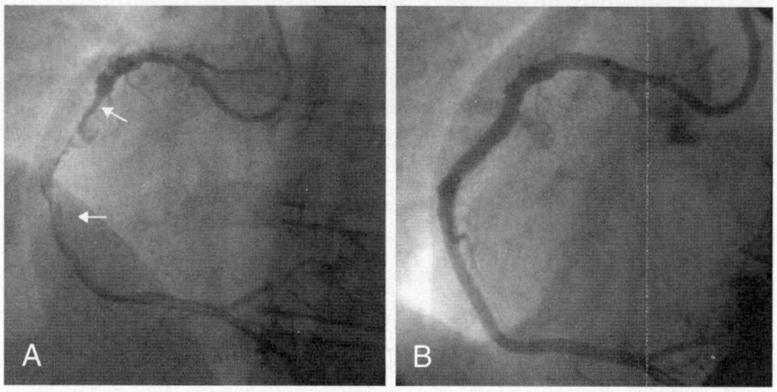

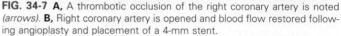

FIG. 34-7 A, A thrombotic occlusion of the right coronary artery is noted *(arrows)*. **B,** Right coronary artery is opened and blood flow restored following angioplasty and placement of a 4-mm stent.

a catheter with an inflatable balloon tip is inserted into the appropriate coronary artery. When the blockage is located, the catheter is passed through it, the balloon is inflated, and the atherosclerotic plaque is compressed, resulting in vessel dilation. This procedure is called *balloon angioplasty.*

Intracoronary stents are often inserted in conjunction with balloon angioplasty. Stents are used to treat abrupt or threatened abrupt closure and restenosis following balloon angioplasty. A **stent** is an expandable meshlike structure designed to keep the vessel open by compressing the arterial wall (Figs. 34-6 and 34-7). Because stents are thrombogenic, unfractionated heparin (UH) or low-molecular-weight heparin (LMWH) is started to maintain the open vessel. In addition, a direct thrombin inhibitor (e.g., bivalirudin [Angiomax]) and/or a glycoprotein IIb/IIIa inhibitor (e.g., tirofiban [Aggrastat]) is also used during PCI to help prevent the abrupt closure of the stents (see Table 34-11). After PCI, the patient is treated with dual antiplatelet agents (e.g., aspirin [indefinitely] and ticagrelor [Brilinta] for 12 months) until the intimal lining can grow over the stent and provide a smooth vascular surface.

Many stents are drug-eluting stents. This type of stent is coated with a drug (e.g., paclitaxel, sirolimus) that prevents the overgrowth of new intima, the primary cause of stent restenosis. Following drug-eluting stent placement, the patient continues dual antiplatelet therapy to prevent thrombus formation on the stent. Drug therapy may continue for 12 months or longer.[18]

The most serious complications from stent placement are abrupt closure and vascular injury. Other less common complications include acute MI, stent embolization, coronary spasm, and emergent coronary artery bypass graft (CABG) surgery. The possibility of dysrhythmias during and after the procedure is always present.

PCI may not be a feasible option for all patients (e.g., patients with three-vessel CAD [three different coronary arteries] and/or significant left main coronary artery disease). Coronary revascularization with CABG surgery may be recommended and is discussed later in the chapter.

ACUTE CORONARY SYNDROME

When ischemia is prolonged and not immediately reversible, **acute coronary syndrome (ACS)** develops and encompasses the spectrum of unstable angina (UA), *non–ST-segment-elevation myocardial infarction* (NSTEMI), and *ST-segment-elevation myocardial infarction* (STEMI) (Fig. 34-8). Although each remains a distinct diagnosis, this nomenclature (ACS) reflects the relationships among the pathophysiology, presentation, diagnosis, prognosis, and interventions for these disorders.

ACS is associated with deterioration of a once stable atherosclerotic plaque. The once stable plaque ruptures, exposing the intima to blood and stimulating platelet aggregation and local vasoconstriction with thrombus formation. This unstable lesion may be partially occluded by a thrombus (manifesting as UA or NSTEMI) or totally occluded by a thrombus (manifesting as

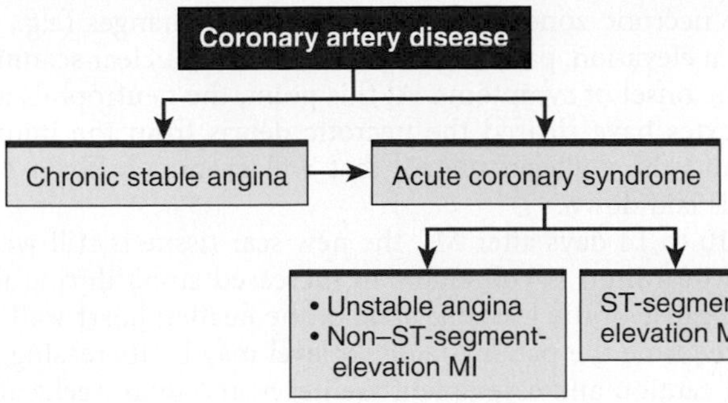

FIG. 34-8 Relationships among coronary artery disease, chronic stable angina, and acute coronary syndrome.

STEMI).[16] What causes a coronary plaque to suddenly become unstable is not well understood, but systemic inflammation (described earlier) is thought to play a role. Patients with suspected ACS require immediate hospitalization.

UNSTABLE ANGINA

Unstable angina (UA) is chest pain that is new in onset, occurs at rest, or has a worsening pattern. The patient with chronic stable angina may develop UA, or UA may be the first clinical sign of CAD. Unlike chronic stable angina, UA is unpredictable and is an emergency. The patient with previously diagnosed chronic stable angina describes a significant change in the pattern of angina. It occurs with increasing frequency and is easily provoked by minimal or no exertion, during sleep, or even at rest. The patient without previously diagnosed angina describes anginal pain that has progressed rapidly in the past few hours, days, or weeks, often ending in pain at rest.

Women seek medical attention for symptoms of UA more often than men. Despite national efforts to increase awareness, women's symptoms continue to go unrecognized as heart related. These symptoms include fatigue, shortness of breath, indigestion, and anxiety. Fatigue is the most prominent symptom. However, all these symptoms can relate to many different diseases and syndromes. Thus women often present with UA before CAD is diagnosed. (See Gender Differences box on p. 733 earlier in this chapter.)

MYOCARDIAL INFARCTION

A **myocardial infarction (MI)** occurs because of sustained ischemia, causing irreversible myocardial cell death (necrosis) (Figs. 34-9 and 34-10). Thrombus formation causes 80% to 90% of all acute MIs.[19] When a thrombus develops, there is no blood flow to the myocardium distal to the blockage, resulting in necrosis. Contractile function of the heart stops in the necrotic area(s). The degree of altered function depends on the area of the heart involved and the size of the infarction.

The acute MI process takes time. Cardiac cells can withstand ischemic conditions for approximately 20 minutes before cell death begins. The earliest tissue to become ischemic is the subendocardium (the innermost layer of tissue in the cardiac muscle). If ischemia persists, it takes approximately 4 to 6 hours for the entire thickness of the heart muscle to become necrosed. If the thrombus is not completely blocking the artery, the time to complete necrosis may be as long as 12 hours.

MIs are usually described based on the location of damage (e.g., anterior, inferior, lateral, septal, or posterior wall infarction). Most involve some portion of the left ventricle. The location of the infarction correlates with the involved coronary circulation. For example, the right coronary artery provides blood supply to the inferior wall. Blockage of the right coronary artery results in an inferior wall MI. Anterior wall infarctions result from blockages in the left anterior descending artery. Blockages in the left circumflex artery usually cause lateral and/or posterior wall MIs. Damage can occur in more than one location, especially if more than one coronary artery is involved (e.g., anterolateral MI, anteroseptal MI).

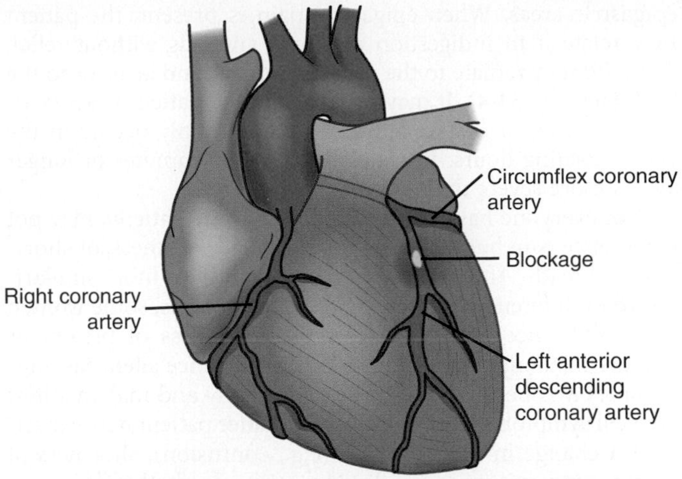

FIG. 34-9 Occlusion of the left anterior descending coronary artery, resulting in a myocardial infarction.

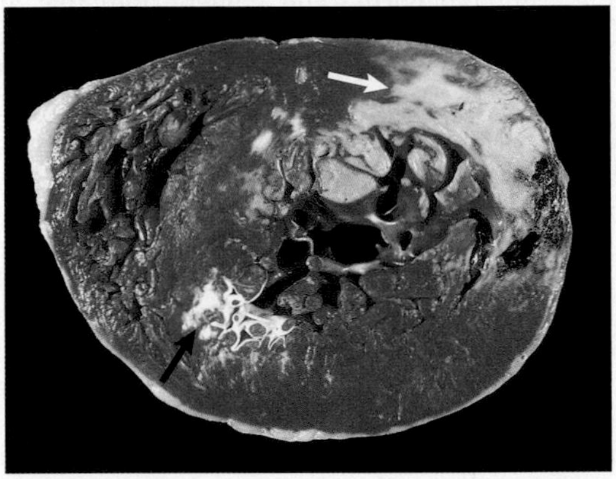

FIG. 34-10 Acute myocardial infarction in the posterolateral wall of the left ventricle. This is demonstrated by the absence of staining in the areas of necrosis *(white arrow)*. Note the scarring from a previous anterior wall myocardial infarction *(black arrow)*.

The degree of preexisting collateral circulation also influences the severity of infarction (see Fig. 34-2). An individual with a long history of CAD develops collateral circulation to provide the area surrounding the infarction site with a blood supply. This is one reason why a younger person may have a more serious first MI than an older person with the same degree of blockage.

Clinical Manifestations of Myocardial Infarction

Pain. Severe, immobilizing chest pain not relieved by rest, position change, or nitrate administration is the hallmark of an MI. Persistent and unlike any other pain, it is usually described as a heaviness, pressure, tightness, burning, constriction, or crushing. Common locations are substernal, retrosternal, or epigastric areas. When epigastric pain is present, the patient may relate it to indigestion and take antacids without relief. The pain may radiate to the neck, lower jaw, and arms or to the back (see Fig. 34-4). It may occur while the patient is active or at rest, asleep or awake. However, it commonly occurs in the early morning hours. It usually lasts for 20 minutes or longer and is more severe than usual anginal pain.

Not everyone has classic symptoms. Some patients may not experience pain but may have "discomfort," weakness, or shortness of breath. Although women and men have more similarities than differences in their acute MI symptoms, some women may experience atypical discomfort, shortness of breath, or fatigue.[20] Patients with diabetes may experience silent (asymptomatic) MIs because of cardiac neuropathy and may manifest atypical symptoms (e.g., dyspnea). An older patient may experience a change in mental status (e.g., confusion), shortness of breath, pulmonary edema, dizziness, or a dysrhythmia.

Sympathetic Nervous System Stimulation. During the initial phase of MI, the ischemic myocardial cells release catecholamines (norepinephrine and epinephrine) that are normally found in these cells. This results in release of glycogen, diaphoresis, and vasoconstriction of peripheral blood vessels. On physical examination, the patient's skin may be ashen, clammy, and cool to touch.

Cardiovascular Manifestations. In response to the release of catecholamines, BP and HR may be elevated initially. Later, the BP may drop because of decreased cardiac output (CO). If severe enough, this may result in decreased renal perfusion and urine output. Crackles, if present, may persist for several hours to several days, suggesting left ventricular dysfunction. Jugular venous distention, hepatic engorgement, and peripheral edema may indicate right ventricular dysfunction.

Cardiac examination may reveal abnormal heart sounds that may seem distant. Other abnormal sounds suggesting ventricular dysfunction are S_3 and S_4. In addition, a loud holosystolic murmur may develop and may indicate a septal defect, papillary muscle rupture, or valve dysfunction.

Nausea and Vomiting. The patient may experience nausea and vomiting. These symptoms can result from reflex stimulation of the vomiting center by the severe pain. They can also result from vasovagal reflexes initiated from the area of the infarcted myocardium.

Fever. The temperature may increase within the first 24 hours up to 100.4° F (38° C). The temperature elevation may last for as long as 1 week. This increase in temperature is due to a systemic inflammatory process caused by myocardial cell death.

Healing Process

The body's response to cell death is the inflammatory process (see Chapter 12). Within 24 hours, leukocytes infiltrate the area. The dead cardiac cells release enzymes that are important diagnostic indicators of MI. (See Serum Cardiac Markers later in this chapter.) The proteolytic enzymes of the neutrophils and macrophages begin to remove necrotic tissue by the fourth day. During this time the necrotic muscle wall is thin. The development of collateral circulation improves areas of poor perfusion and may limit the zones of injury and infarction. Once infarction takes place, catecholamine-mediated lipolysis and glycogenolysis occur. These processes allow the increased plasma glucose and free fatty acids to be used by the oxygen-depleted myocardium for anaerobic metabolism. For this reason, serum glucose levels are frequently elevated after MI.[19]

The necrotic zone is identifiable by ECG changes (e.g., ST segment elevation, pathologic Q wave) and by nuclear scanning after the onset of symptoms. At this point, the neutrophils and monocytes have cleared the necrotic debris from the injured area, and the collagen matrix that will eventually form scar tissue is laid down.

At 10 to 14 days after MI, the new scar tissue is still weak. The myocardium is vulnerable to increased stress during this time because of the unstable state of the healing heart wall. At the same time the patient's activity level may be increasing, so special caution and assessment are necessary. By 6 weeks after MI, scar tissue has replaced necrotic tissue and the injured area is considered healed. The scarred area is often less compliant than the surrounding area. This condition may be manifested by uncoordinated wall motion, ventricular dysfunction, altered conduction patterns, or heart failure (HF).

These changes in the infarcted muscle also cause changes in the unaffected myocardium. In an attempt to compensate for the damaged muscle, the normal myocardium hypertrophies and dilates. This process is called *ventricular remodeling.* Remodeling of normal myocardium can lead to the development of late HF, especially in the individual with atherosclerosis of other coronary arteries and/or an anterior MI.

Complications of Myocardial Infarction

Dysrhythmias. The most common complication after an MI is dysrhythmias, which are present in 80% to 90% of patients. Dysrhythmias are the most common cause of death in patients in the prehospital period. Any condition that affects the myocardial cell's sensitivity to nerve impulses (e.g., ischemia, electrolyte imbalances, SNS stimulation) can cause dysrhythmias. The intrinsic rhythm of the heart is disrupted. This can cause tachycardia, bradycardia, or an irregular HR, all of which adversely affect the ischemic myocardium.

Life-threatening dysrhythmias occur most often with anterior wall infarction, HF, or shock. Complete heart block develops when key portions of the conduction system are destroyed. Ventricular fibrillation, a common cause of sudden cardiac death (SCD), is a lethal dysrhythmia. It most often occurs within the first 4 hours after the onset of pain. Premature ventricular contractions may precede ventricular tachycardia and fibrillation. Life-threatening ventricular dysrhythmias must be treated immediately. (See Chapter 36 for a detailed description of dysrhythmias and their management.)

Heart Failure. *Heart failure* (HF) is a complication that occurs when the heart's pumping action is reduced. Depending on the severity and extent of the injury, HF occurs initially with subtle signs such as mild dyspnea, restlessness, agitation, or slight tachycardia. Other signs indicating the onset of HF include pulmonary congestion on chest x-ray, S_3 or S_4 heart sounds on auscultation, crackles on auscultation of breath sounds, and jugular venous distention. (The treatment of acute decompensated HF is discussed in Chapter 35.)

Cardiogenic Shock. *Cardiogenic shock* occurs when oxygen and nutrients supplied to the tissues are inadequate because of severe left ventricular failure. This occurs less often with the early and rapid treatment of MI with PCI or thrombolytic therapy. When cardiogenic shock does occur, it has a high mortality rate. Cardiogenic shock requires aggressive management. This includes control of dysrhythmias, intraaortic balloon pump (IABP) therapy, and support of contractility with vasoactive drugs. Goals of therapy are to maximize oxygen delivery, reduce oxygen demand, and prevent complications (e.g., acute kidney injury). (Cardiogenic shock is discussed in Chapter 67.)

Papillary Muscle Dysfunction. *Papillary muscle dysfunction* may occur if the infarcted area includes or is near the papillary muscle that attaches to the mitral valve (see Fig. 32-2). You should suspect papillary muscle dysfunction if you auscultate a new murmur at the cardiac apex. An echocardiogram confirms the diagnosis.

Papillary muscle rupture is a rare and life-threatening complication. It causes massive mitral valve regurgitation. Dyspnea, pulmonary edema, and decreased CO result from the back up of blood in the left atrium. This condition aggravates an already damaged left ventricle by reducing CO even further. The patient undergoes rapid clinical deterioration. Treatment includes rapid afterload reduction with nitroprusside (Nipride) and/or IABP therapy, and immediate cardiac surgery with mitral valve repair or replacement.[19] (See Chapter 37 for discussion of valve disorders.)

Ventricular Aneurysm. *Ventricular aneurysm* results when the infarcted myocardial wall is thin and bulges out during contraction. This can develop within a few days, weeks, or months. The patient with a ventricular aneurysm may experience HF, dysrhythmias, and angina. Besides ventricular rupture, which is fatal, ventricular aneurysms harbor thrombi that can lead to an embolic stroke.

Pericarditis. *Acute pericarditis,* an inflammation of the visceral and/or parietal pericardium, may result in cardiac tamponade, decreased ventricular filling and emptying, and HF. It occurs 2 or 3 days after an acute MI as a common complication of the infarction. Pericarditis is characterized by chest pain, which may vary from mild to severe and is aggravated by inspiration, coughing, and movement of the upper body. Sitting in a forward position often relieves the pain. The pain is usually different from pain associated with an MI.

Assess the patient with suspected pericarditis for the presence of a friction rub over the pericardium. The sound may be best heard with the diaphragm of the stethoscope at the mid to lower left sternal border. It may be persistent or intermittent. Fever may also be present. The patient may have hypotension and/or a narrow pulse pressure.

Diagnosis of pericarditis can be made with serial 12-lead ECGs. Typical ECG changes include diffuse ST-segment elevations. This reflects the inflammation of the pericardium. Treatment includes pain relief with NSAIDs, aspirin, or corticosteroids. (Chapter 37 discusses pericarditis.)

Dressler Syndrome. *Dressler syndrome* is pericarditis with effusion and fever that develops 4 to 6 weeks after MI. It may also occur after cardiac surgery. It is thought to be caused by an antigen-antibody reaction to the necrotic myocardium. The patient experiences pericardial pain, fever, a friction rub, pericardial effusion, and arthralgia. Laboratory findings include an elevated white blood cell count and sedimentation rate. Short-term corticosteroids are used to treat this condition.

DIAGNOSTIC STUDIES ACUTE CORONARY SYNDROME

In addition to the patient's history of pain, risk factors, and health history, the primary diagnostic studies used to determine whether a person has UA or an MI include an ECG and serum cardiac markers (see Fig. 34-5).

Electrocardiogram Findings

The ECG is one of the primary tools to diagnose UA or an MI. Changes in the QRS complex, ST segment, and T wave caused by ischemia and infarction can develop quickly with UA and MI. For diagnostic and treatment purposes, it is important to distinguish between STEMI and UA or NSTEMI. Patients with STEMI tend to have a more extensive MI that is associated with prolonged and complete coronary occlusion; a pathologic Q wave is seen on the ECG. Patients with UA or NSTEMI usually have transient thrombosis or incomplete coronary occlusion and usually do not develop pathologic Q waves. Because MI is a dynamic process that evolves with time, the ECG often reveals the time sequence of ischemia, injury, infarction, and resolution of the infarction.

The ECG must be read carefully, since changes can be subtle at first. It may also be normal or nondiagnostic when the patient comes to the ED with a complaint of chest pain. Within a few hours, the ECG may change to reflect the infarction process. For this reason, when the initial 12-lead ECG is nondiagnostic, serial 12-lead ECGs are done. (See Chapter 36 for discussion of ECG changes associated with ischemia and MI.)

Serum Cardiac Markers

Serum cardiac markers are proteins released into the blood from necrotic heart muscle after an MI (see Table 32-6). These markers are important in the diagnosis of MI. The onset, peak, and duration of levels of these markers are shown in Fig. 34-11.

Cardiac-specific troponin has two subtypes: cardiac-specific troponin T (cTnT) and cardiac-specific troponin I (cTnI). These markers are highly specific indicators of MI and have greater sensitivity and specificity for myocardial injury than creatine kinase (CK) MB (CK-MB). Serum levels of cTnI and cTnT increase 4 to 6 hours after the onset of MI, peak at 10 to 24 hours, and return to baseline over 10 to 14 days.

CK levels begin to rise about 6 hours after an MI, peak at about 18 hours, and return to normal within 24 to 36 hours. The CK enzymes are fractionated into bands. The CK-MB band is specific to myocardial cells and also helps quantify myocardial damage.

Myoglobin is released into the circulation within 2 hours after an MI and peaks in 3 to 15 hours. Although it is one of

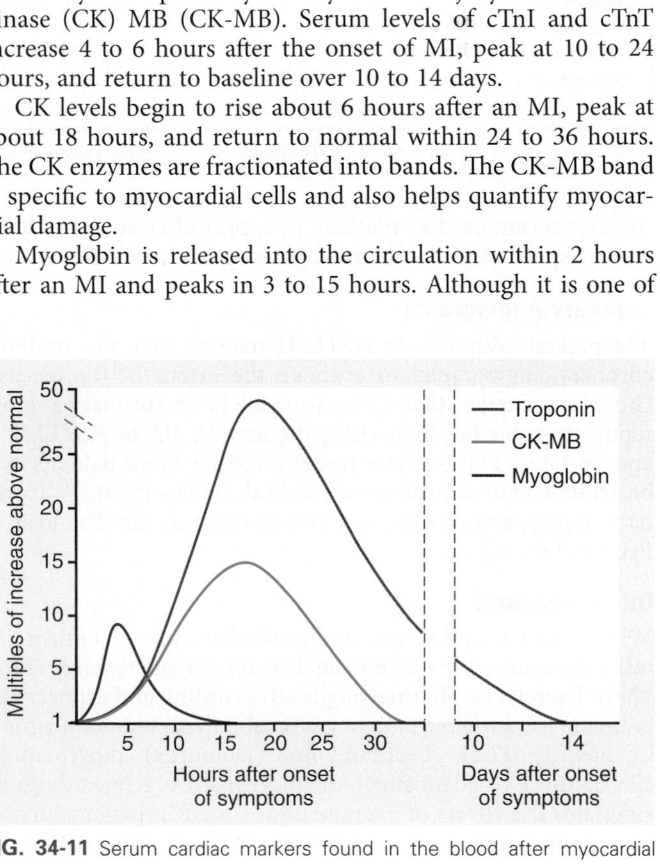

FIG. 34-11 Serum cardiac markers found in the blood after myocardial infarction.

TABLE 34-12 EMERGENCY MANAGEMENT

Chest Pain

Etiology	Assessment Findings	Interventions
Cardiovascular • Myocardial ischemia • Myocardial infarction • Dysrhythmia • Pericarditis • Aortic aneurysm • Aortic valve disease **Respiratory** • Costochondritis • Pleurisy • Pneumonia • Pneumothorax, hemothorax • Pulmonary edema • Pulmonary embolus **Chest Trauma** • Rib/sternal fracture • Flail chest • Cardiac tamponade • Hemothorax • Pulmonary contusion • Great vessel injury **Gastrointestinal** • Esophagitis • GERD • Hiatal hernia • Peptic ulcer • Cholecystitis **Others** • Stress • Strenuous exercise • Drugs (e.g., cocaine) • Acute anxiety	• Pain in chest, neck, jaw, arm, or shoulder • Cold, clammy skin • Diaphoresis • Nausea and vomiting • Epigastric pain • Indigestion, heartburn • Dyspnea, tachypnea • Weakness • Anxiety • Feeling of impending doom • Tachycardia, bradycardia • Irregular HR, murmurs • Palpitations • Dysrhythmias • Decreased or increased BP • Narrowed pulse pressure • Unequal BP readings in upper extremities • Syncope, loss of consciousness • Decreased O_2 saturation • Decreased or absent breath sounds • Pericardial friction rub	**Initial** • Assess ABCs. • Position patient upright unless contraindicated and administer O_2 by nasal cannula or non-rebreather mask. • Obtain baseline vital signs, including O_2 saturation. • Auscultate heart and breath sounds. • Obtain 12-lead ECG. • Insert two IV catheters. • Assess pain using PQRST mnemonic (see Table 34-7). • Medicate for pain as ordered (e.g., nitroglycerin, morphine). • Initiate continuous ECG monitoring and identify underlying rhythm. • Obtain baseline blood work (e.g., cardiac markers, serum electrolytes). • Obtain portable chest x-ray. • Assess for contraindications for antiplatelet, anticoagulant, or thrombolytic therapy, or PCI as appropriate. • Administer aspirin for cardiac-related chest pain unless contraindicated. • Administer antidysrhythmic drugs as indicated. **Ongoing Monitoring** • Monitor ABCs, vital signs, level of consciousness, heart and breath sounds, cardiac rhythm, and O_2 saturation. • Assess and record response to medications (e.g., decrease in chest pain) and remedicate or titrate medications (e.g., nitroglycerin) as needed. • Provide reassurance and emotional support to patient and caregiver. • Explain all interventions and procedures to patient and caregiver in simple terms. • Anticipate need for intubation if respiratory distress is evident. • Prepare for CPR and defibrillation if cardiac arrest is evident. • Anticipate need for transcutaneous pacing for symptomatic bradycardia or heart block.

ABCs, Airway, breathing, circulations; *GERD,* gastroesophageal reflux disease; *PCI,* percutaneous coronary intervention.

the first serum cardiac markers to appear after an MI, it lacks cardiac specificity. Its role in diagnosing MI is limited.

Coronary Angiography

The patient with UA or NSTEMI may or may not undergo coronary angiography to evaluate the extent of the disease. Guidelines suggest that it is reasonable to do coronary angiography on stable but high-risk patients with UA or NSTEMI. If appropriate, a PCI is performed at this time. Some patients may be treated with conservative medical management.[21,22] Coronary angiography is the only way to confirm the diagnosis of Prinzmetal's angina.

Other Measures

When the ECG and serum cardiac markers do not confirm MI, other measures for diagnosing UA are considered (see Table 32-6). Exercise or pharmacologic stress testing and echocardiogram are used when a patient has an abnormal but nondiagnostic baseline ECG. A dobutamine (Dobutrex), dipyridamole (Persantine), or adenosine (Adenocard) stress echocardiogram simulates the effects of exercise and is used in patients unable to exercise. (See Chapter 32 for additional information on cardiac assessment.)

COLLABORATIVE CARE ACUTE CORONARY SYNDROME

It is extremely important to rapidly diagnose and treat a patient with ACS to preserve cardiac muscle. Initial management of the patient with chest pain most often occurs in the ED. Table 34-12 presents the emergency care of the patient with chest pain. Obtain a 12-lead ECG and start continuous ECG monitoring. Position the patient in an upright position unless contraindicated, and initiate oxygen by nasal cannula to keep oxygen saturation above 93%. Establish an IV route to provide an access for emergency drug therapy. Give SL NTG and aspirin (chewable) if not given before arrival at the ED. Morphine sulfate is given for pain unrelieved by NTG. The patient usually receives ongoing care in a critical care unit or telemetry unit, where continuous ECG monitoring is available. Dysrhythmias are treated according to established protocols. Fig. 34-5 on p. 743 presents the collaborative care of ACS.

Monitor vital signs, including pulse oximetry, frequently during the first few hours after admission and closely thereafter. Maintain bed rest and limit activity for 12 to 24 hours, with a gradual increase in activity unless contraindicated.

For patients with ongoing angina and negative cardiac markers, dual antiplatelet therapy (e.g., aspirin and ticagrelor) and heparin (UH or LMWH) is recommended. Coronary angiography with possible PCI is considered once the patient is stabilized and angina is controlled, or if angina returns or increases in severity.[21]

For patients with STEMI or NSTEMI with positive cardiac markers, reperfusion therapy is initiated (see Figs. 34-6 and 34-7). *Reperfusion therapy* can include emergent PCI for STEMI and NSTEMI or thrombolytic (fibrinolytic) therapy for STEMI. Coronary surgical revascularization is considered for select patients (e.g., patients with diabetes and three-vessel disease [involvement of three different coronary arteries]). The goal in the treatment of MI is to salvage as much myocardial muscle as possible.

Emergent PCI

Emergent PCI is the first line of treatment for patients with confirmed MI (i.e., definitive ECG changes and/or positive cardiac markers).[23] The goal is to open the blocked artery within 90 minutes of arrival to a facility that has an interventional cardiac catheterization laboratory. In this situation the patient undergoes a cardiac catheterization to locate the blockage(s), assess the severity of the blockage(s), determine the presence of collateral circulation, and evaluate left ventricular function. During the procedure, treatment modalities (e.g., placement of drug-eluting stents) are selected. Patients with severe left ventricular dysfunction may require the addition of intraaortic balloon pump (IABP) therapy, and a small percentage of patients may require emergent CABG surgery.

The advantages of PCI include the following: (1) it provides an alternative to surgical intervention; (2) it is performed with local anesthesia; (3) the patient is ambulatory shortly after the procedure; (4) the length of hospital stay is approximately 1 to 3 days compared with the 4- to 6-day stay with CABG surgery, thus reducing hospital costs; and (5) the patient can return to work several weeks sooner after PCI, compared with a 6- to 8-week convalescence after CABG.

Advances in PCI techniques have significantly reduced the need for emergent CABG. Currently, more PCIs are performed than CABGs.[1] The most serious complication of PCI is dissection of the newly dilated coronary artery.[22] If the damage is extensive, the coronary artery could rupture, causing cardiac tamponade, ischemia and infarction, decreased CO, and possible death. There is also a danger that the infarction could be extended should a portion of the plaque dislodge and block the vessel distal to the catheter. Coronary spasm from the mechanical irritation of the catheter or balloon can occur, as well as chemical irritation from the contrast medium used to see the artery. Abrupt closure is a complication that can occur in the first 24 hours after PCI. Restenosis can also occur. Risk is greatest in the first 30 days after PCI. Nursing care of the patient following PCI is similar to that after cardiac catheterization (see Table 32-6).

Thrombolytic Therapy

Thrombolytic therapy offers the advantages of availability and rapid administration in facilities that do not have an interventional cardiac catheterization laboratory or when one is too far away to transfer the patient safely.[23] Treatment of MI with thrombolytic therapy aims to stop the infarction process by dissolving the thrombus in the coronary artery and reperfusing the myocardium. Thrombolytic therapy is given as soon as possible, ideally within the first hour and preferably within the first 6 hours after the onset of symptoms. Mortality is reduced by 25% if reperfusion occurs within 6 hours.[18,19]

Indications and Contraindications. All thrombolytics are given IV (see Table 34-11). The cost, efficacy, and ease of administration guide the choice of a thrombolytic agent. Although these drugs have different pharmacokinetics, they all open the blocked artery by lysis of the thrombus. The goal is to administer a thrombolytic within 30 minutes of the patient's arrival to a facility without an interventional cardiac catheterization laboratory. (PCI is first-line therapy in a facility with an interventional cardiac catheterization laboratory, as discussed above.)

Because all thrombolytics lyse the pathologic clot, they may also lyse other clots (e.g., a postoperative site). Therefore patient selection is important because minor or major bleeding can be a complication of therapy.[18] Inclusion criteria for thrombolytic therapy include (1) chest pain typical of acute MI 6 hours or less in duration, (2) 12-lead ECG findings consistent with acute MI, and (3) no absolute contraindications (Table 34-13). Although patients with chest pain lasting more than 6 hours and ECG changes supporting MI may be considered for thrombolytic therapy, benefits of this therapy are inconsistent.

Procedure. Each hospital has a protocol for giving thrombolytic therapy, but several factors are common. Draw blood to obtain baseline laboratory values and start two or three lines for IV therapy. All other invasive procedures are done before the thrombolytic agent is given to reduce the possibility of bleeding.

Depending on the drug selected, therapy is administered in one IV bolus or over time (30 to 90 minutes). Note the time at which therapy begins, and monitor the patient during and after administration of the thrombolytic. Evaluate heart rhythm, vital signs, and pulse oximetry and assess the heart and lungs frequently to evaluate the patient's response to therapy. Regularly assess for changes in neurologic status, since this may indicate a cerebral bleed.

TABLE 34-13 CONTRAINDICATIONS FOR THROMBOLYTIC THERAPY

Absolute Contraindications

- Active internal bleeding or bleeding diathesis (excluding menstruation)
- Known history of cerebral aneurysm or arteriovenous malformation
- Known intracranial neoplasm (primary or metastatic)
- Previous cerebral hemorrhage
- Recent (within past 3 mo) ischemic stroke
- Significant closed-head or facial trauma within past 3 mo
- Suspected aortic dissection

Relative Contraindications and Cautions

- Active peptic ulcer disease
- Current use of anticoagulants
- Pregnancy
- Prior ischemic stroke (>3 mo ago), dementia, or known intracranial pathologic condition not covered in absolute contraindications
- Recent (within 3 wk) surgery (including eye laser surgery) or puncture of noncompressible vessel
- Recent (within 2-4 wk) internal bleeding
- Serious systemic disease (e.g., advanced or terminal cancer, severe liver or kidney disease)
- Severe uncontrolled hypertension (BP >180/110 mm Hg) on presentation or chronic severe poorly controlled hypertension
- Traumatic or prolonged (>10 min) cardiopulmonary resuscitation

When reperfusion occurs (i.e., the coronary artery that was blocked is opened and blood flow is restored to the myocardium), several clinical markers may be seen. The most reliable marker is the return of the ST segment to baseline on the ECG. Other markers include a resolution of chest pain and an early, rapid rise of the serum cardiac markers within 3 hours of therapy, peaking within 12 hours. These levels increase as the necrotic myocardial cells release proteins into the circulation after perfusion is restored to the area. The presence of *reperfusion dysrhythmias* (e.g., accelerated idioventricular rhythm) is a less reliable marker of reperfusion. These dysrhythmias are generally self-limiting and do not require aggressive treatment. (See Chapter 36 for management of dysrhythmias.)

A major concern with thrombolytic therapy is reocclusion of the artery. The site of the thrombus is unstable, and formation of another clot or spasm of the artery may occur. Because of this possibility, IV heparin therapy is initiated. If another clot develops, the patient will have similar complaints of chest pain, and ECG changes will return. Patients receiving thrombolytic therapy should be transferred to a facility with PCI capabilities as soon as possible. This way, PCI can be performed if thrombolytic therapy fails.[18]

The major complication with thrombolytic therapy is bleeding. Ongoing nursing assessment is essential. Minor bleeding (e.g., surface bleeding from IV sites or gingival bleeding) is expected and controlled by applying a pressure dressing or ice packs.

SAFETY ALERT

- When thrombolytic therapy is used, bleeding may occur.
- If signs and symptoms of major bleeding occur (e.g., drop in BP, an increase in HR, a sudden change in the patient's level of consciousness, blood in the urine or stool), stop the therapy and notify the physician.

Coronary Surgical Revascularization

Coronary revascularization with CABG surgery is recommended for patients who (1) fail medical management, (2) have left main coronary artery or three-vessel disease, (3) are not candidates for PCI (e.g., lesions are long or difficult to access), (4) have failed PCI and continue to have chest pain, (5) have diabetes mellitus, or (6) are expected to have longer term benefits with CABG than with PCI.[24]

Coronary Artery Bypass Graft Surgery. CABG surgery consists of the placement of conduits to transport blood between the aorta, or other major arteries, and the myocardium distal to the blocked coronary artery (or arteries). The procedure may involve one or more grafts using the internal mammary artery, saphenous vein, radial artery, gastroepiploic artery, and/or inferior epigastric artery (Fig. 34-12).

CABG surgery requires a sternotomy (opening of the chest cavity) and *cardiopulmonary bypass* (CPB). During CPB, blood is diverted from the patient's heart to a machine where it is oxygenated and returned (via a pump) to the patient. This allows the surgeon to operate on a quiet, nonbeating, bloodless heart while perfusion to vital organs is maintained.

The internal mammary artery (IMA) is the most common artery used for bypass graft. It is left attached to its origin (the subclavian artery) but then dissected from the chest wall. Next, it is *anastomosed* (connected with sutures) to the coronary artery distal to the blockage. The long-term patency rate for IMA grafts is greater than 90% after 10 years.[24]

Saphenous veins are also used for bypass grafts. The surgeon removes the saphenous vein from one or both legs endoscopically. Sections are attached to the ascending aorta and then to a coronary artery distal to the blockage. Saphenous vein grafts do develop diffuse intimal hyperplasia. This contributes to future stenosis and graft occlusions. The use of antiplatelet therapy and statins after surgery improves vein graft patency. Patency rates of these grafts are 50% to 60% at 10 years.[24]

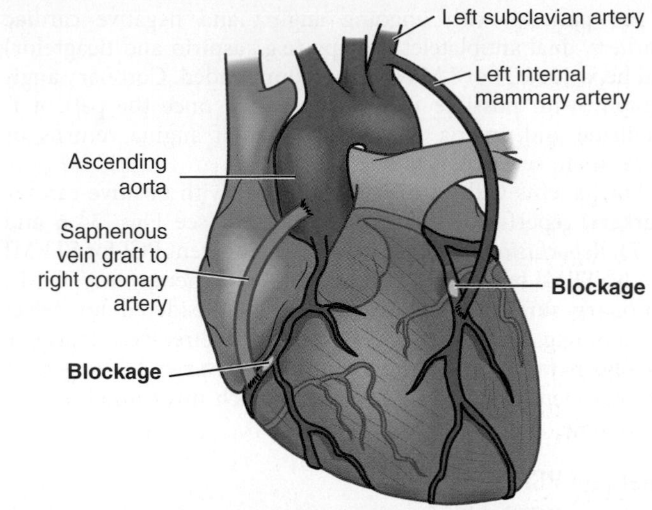

FIG. 34-12 Distal end of the left internal mammary artery is grafted below the area of blockage in the left anterior descending artery. Proximal end of the saphenous vein is grafted to the aorta, and the distal end is grafted below the area of blockage in the right coronary artery.

The radial artery is another conduit that can be used. It is a thick muscular artery that is prone to spasm. Perioperative calcium channel blockers and long-acting nitrates can control the spasms. Patency rates at 5 years are as high as 84%. There have been no reports of extremity complications (e.g., hand ischemia, wound infection) after removal of this artery.[24]

Other potential conduits include the gastroepiploic or inferior epigastric artery. However, they are rarely used, since the dissection of these arteries is extensive. This increases the length of surgery and the risk for wound complications at the harvest site, especially in an obese or diabetic patient.[24] Like the radial artery, these are also prone to spasms. One-year patency rate for the epigastric artery is 90%, and 10-year patency rate for the gastroepiploic artery is 62%.[24]

CABG surgery remains a palliative treatment for CAD and not a cure. Studies have shown improved patient outcomes, quality of life, and survival after CABG surgery. However, postoperative complications and mortality increase with age.

Women have higher operative mortality rates than men. This has been attributed to the late treatment of CAD in women because women first present with the disease at an older age and are more ill (e.g., decreased left ventricular function) at the time of surgery. Other possible factors include smaller-diameter coronary vessels and the less frequent use of the IMA.

Minimally Invasive Direct Coronary Artery Bypass. *Minimally invasive direct coronary artery bypass* (MIDCAB) offers patients with limited disease an approach to surgical treatment that does not involve a sternotomy and CPB. In many cases these patients are too high risk for traditional bypass surgery.[25] The technique requires several small incisions between the ribs. A thoracoscope is used to dissect the IMA. The heart is slowed using a β-adrenergic blocker (e.g., esmolol [Brevibloc]) or stopped temporarily with adenosine. A mechanical stabilizer immobilizes the operative site. The IMA is then sutured to the left anterior descending or right coronary artery. A radial artery or saphenous vein graft can be used if the IMA is not available.

Off-Pump Coronary Artery Bypass. The *off-pump coronary artery bypass* (OPCAB) procedure uses full or partial sternotomy to access all coronary vessels. OPCAB is performed on a beating heart using mechanical stabilizers and without CPB. It is usually reserved for patients who have limited disease but are at high risk for traditional surgery secondary to multiple co-morbidities. Patients who are typically candidates for OPCAB have a very low EF, severe lung disease, acute or chronic kidney disease, a high risk for stroke, or a calcified aorta.[25]

Robot-Assisted Cardiothoracic Surgery. This technique incorporates the use of a robot in performing CABG or mitral valve replacement. The benefits of robotic surgery include increased precision, smaller incisions, decreased blood loss, less pain, and shorter recovery time.

Transmyocardial Laser Revascularization. *Transmyocardial laser revascularization* (TMR) is an indirect revascularization procedure. It is used for patients with advanced CAD who are not candidates for traditional CABG surgery and who have persistent angina after maximum medical therapy. The procedure involves the use of a high-energy laser to create channels in the heart to allow blood flow to ischemic areas. The procedure is performed during cardiac catheterization as a percutaneous TMR or during surgery using a left anterior thoracotomy incision as an adjunct to CABG.

Drug Therapy

IV NTG, dual antiplatelet therapy (e.g., aspirin and clopidogrel), and systemic anticoagulation with either LMWH given subcutaneously or IV UH are the initial drug treatments of choice for ACS.[18,19] IV direct thrombin inhibitors may also be used if PCI is anticipated. Oral β-adrenergic blockers are given within the first 24 hours of a STEMI if there are no contraindications (e.g., HF, heart block, hypotension). ACE inhibitors are added for select patients following MI (discussed below). Calcium channel blockers or long-acting nitrates are added if the patient is already taking adequate doses of β-adrenergic blockers, cannot tolerate β-adrenergic blockers, or has Prinzmetal's angina.[18,19]

Table 34-11 and Fig. 34-5 present drug therapy for patients with ACS. These drugs are discussed on pp. 743 and 745. ACS-specific discussion of select drugs is presented in this section.

IV Nitroglycerin. IV NTG (Tridil) is used in the initial treatment of the patient with ACS. The goal of therapy is to reduce anginal pain and improve coronary blood flow. IV NTG decreases preload and afterload while increasing the myocardial oxygen supply. The onset of action is immediate. Titrate NTG to control and stop chest pain. Because hypotension is a common side effect, closely monitor BP during this time. Patients who do become hypotensive are often volume depleted and can benefit from an IV fluid bolus. Tolerance is another side effect of IV nitrate therapy. An effective strategy for this phenomenon is to titrate the dose down at night during sleep and titrate the dose up during the day.

Morphine Sulfate. Morphine sulfate is the drug of choice for chest pain that is unrelieved by NTG. As a vasodilator, it decreases cardiac workload by lowering myocardial oxygen consumption, reducing contractility, and decreasing BP and HR. In addition, morphine can help reduce anxiety and fear. In rare situations, morphine can depress respirations. Monitor patients for signs of bradypnea or hypotension, conditions to avoid in myocardial ischemia and infarction.

β-Adrenergic Blockers. β-Adrenergic blockers decrease myocardial oxygen demand by reducing HR, BP, and contractility. The use of these drugs in patients who are not at risk for complications of MI (e.g., cardiogenic shock) reduces the risk of reinfarction and the occurrence of HF. The continuation of β-adrenergic blockers indefinitely is recommended.[23] (See Table 34-11, Chapter 33, and Table 33-7 for a discussion of β-adrenergic blockers.)

Angiotensin-Converting Enzyme Inhibitors. ACE inhibitors should be started within the first 24 hours and continued indefinitely in patients recovering from STEMI of the anterior wall, with heart failure, or an EF of 40% or less.[18] The use of ACE inhibitors can help prevent ventricular remodeling and prevent or slow the progression of HF. For patients who cannot tolerate ACE inhibitors, angiotensin II receptor blockers should be considered (see Table 34-12 and Table 33-7).

Antidysrhythmic Drugs. Dysrhythmias are the most common complications after an MI. In general, they are self-limiting and are not treated aggressively unless they are life threatening (e.g., sustained ventricular tachycardia). (Chapter 36 discusses the drugs used in the treatment of dysrhythmias.)

Lipid-Lowering Drugs. A fasting lipid panel is obtained on all patients admitted with ACS. All patients with elevated triglycerides and LDL cholesterol should receive lipid-lowering drugs (see Table 34-5).

Stool Softeners. After an MI, the patient may be predisposed to constipation because of bed rest and opioid administration. Stool softeners (e.g., docusate sodium [Colace]) are given to facilitate bowel movements. This prevents straining and the resultant vagal stimulation from the Valsalva maneuver. Vagal stimulation produces bradycardia and can provoke dysrhythmias.

Nutritional Therapy

Initially, patients may be NPO (nothing by mouth) except for sips of water until stable (e.g., pain free, nausea resolved). Advance the diet as tolerated to a low-salt, low-saturated-fat, and low-cholesterol diet (see Tables 34-3 and 34-4).

NURSING MANAGEMENT
CHRONIC STABLE ANGINA AND ACUTE CORONARY SYNDROME

NURSING ASSESSMENT

Table 34-14 presents the subjective and objective data to obtain from a patient with ACS.

NURSING DIAGNOSES

Nursing diagnoses for the patient with ACS may include, but are not limited to, those presented in Nursing Care Plan 34-1.

PLANNING

The overall goals for a patient with ACS include (1) relief of pain, (2) preservation of myocardium, (3) immediate and appropriate treatment, (4) effective coping with illness-associated anxiety, (5) participation in a rehabilitation plan, and (6) reduction of risk factors. In addition, the Joint Commission has identified core measures in the management of patients with an acute MI to reflect standards of evidence-based care (available at *www.jointcommission.org/assets/1/6/Acute%20Myocardial%20Infarction.pdf*).

NURSING IMPLEMENTATION: CHRONIC STABLE ANGINA

HEALTH PROMOTION. Behaviors to reduce the risk for CAD are presented in Table 34-2 and discussed on pp. 735-740.

TABLE 34-14 NURSING ASSESSMENT
Acute Coronary Syndrome

Subjective Data
Important Health Information
Past health history: Previous history of CAD, chest pain/angina, MI, valve disease (e.g., aortic stenosis), heart failure, or cardiomyopathy; hypertension, diabetes, anemia, lung disease; hyperlipidemia
Medications: Use of antiplatelets or anticoagulants, nitrates, angiotensin-converting enzyme inhibitors, β-blockers, calcium channel blockers; antihypertensive drugs; lipid-lowering drugs; over-the-counter drugs (e.g., vitamin and herbal supplements)
History of present illness: Description of events related to current illness, including any self-treatments and response (see Table 34-8)

Functional Health Patterns
Health perception–health management: Family history of heart disease; sedentary lifestyle; tobacco use; exposure to environmental smoke
Nutritional-metabolic: Indigestion, heartburn, nausea, belching, vomiting
Elimination: Urinary urgency or frequency, straining at stool
Activity-exercise: Palpitations, dyspnea, dizziness, weakness
Cognitive-perceptual: Substernal chest pain or pressure (squeezing, constricting, aching, sharp, tingling), possible radiation to jaw, neck, shoulders, back, or arms (see Table 34-7)
Coping–stress tolerance: Stressful lifestyle, depression; anger, anxiety; feeling of impending doom

Objective Data
General
Anxious, fearful, restless, distressed

Integumentary
Cool, clammy, pale skin

Cardiovascular
Tachycardia or bradycardia, pulsus alternans (alternating weak and strong heartbeats), pulse deficit, dysrhythmias (especially ventricular), S_3, S_4, ↑ or ↓ BP, murmur

Possible Diagnostic Findings
Positive serum cardiac markers, ↑ serum lipids; ↑ WBC count; positive exercise or pharmacologic stress test and thallium scans; pathologic Q wave, ST-segment elevation, and/or T wave abnormalities on ECG; cardiac enlargement, calcifications, or pulmonary congestion on chest x-ray; abnormal wall motion with stress echocardiogram; positive coronary angiography

ACUTE INTERVENTION. If your patient experiences angina, institute the following measures: (1) position patient upright unless contraindicated and administer supplemental oxygen, (2) assess vital signs, (3) obtain a 12-lead ECG, (4) provide prompt pain relief first with a nitrate followed by an opioid analgesic if needed, and (5) auscultate heart and breath sounds. The patient will most likely be distressed and may have pale, cool, clammy skin. The BP and HR may be elevated. Auscultation of the heart may reveal an atrial (S_4) or a ventricular (S_3) gallop. A new murmur heard during an anginal attack may indicate ischemia of a papillary muscle of the mitral valve. The murmur is likely to be transient and disappear when symptoms stop.

Ask the patient to describe the pain and to rate it on a scale of 0 to 10 before and after treatment to evaluate the effectiveness of the interventions (see Table 34-7). It is important to use the same words that patients use to describe their pain. Some patients may not report pain. Assess for other manifestations of pain, such as restlessness; ECG changes; elevated HR, respiratory rate, or BP; clutching of the bed linens; or other nonverbal cues. Supportive and realistic assurance and a calm approach help reduce the patient's anxiety during an anginal attack.

AMBULATORY AND HOME CARE. Reassure the patient with a history of angina that a long, active life is possible. Prevention of angina is preferable to its treatment, and this is why teaching is important. Provide the patient with information regarding CAD, angina, precipitating factors for angina, risk factor reduction, and medications.

Patient teaching can be done in a variety of ways. One-on-one contact between you and the patient is often the most effective approach. Time spent providing daily care (e.g., administering medications) offers many teachable moments. Teaching tools such as DVDs or CDs, heart models, and printed information are important components of patient and caregiver teaching (see Chapter 4).

Assist the patient to identify factors that precipitate angina (see Table 34-8). Instruct the patient on how to avoid or control precipitating factors. For example, teach the patient to avoid exposure to extremes of weather and the consumption of large, heavy meals. If a heavy meal is eaten, instruct the patient to rest for 1 to 2 hours after the meal because blood is shunted to the GI tract to aid digestion and absorption.

Assist the patient to identify personal risk factors for CAD. Then discuss the various methods of decreasing any modifiable risk factors (see Table 34-2). Teach the patient and caregiver about diets that are low in salt and saturated fats (see Tables 34-3 and 34-4). Maintaining ideal body weight is important in controlling angina because excess weight increases myocardial workload.

Adhering to a regular, individualized program of physical activity that conditions rather than overstresses the heart is important. For example, advise patients to walk briskly on a flat surface at least 30 minutes a day, most days of the week (minimum 5) if not contraindicated.[6]

It is important to teach the patient and caregiver the proper use of NTG (see pp. 743 and 745). NTG may be used prophylactically before an emotionally stressful situation, sexual intercourse, or physical exertion (e.g., climbing a long flight of stairs).

If needed, arrange for counseling to assess the psychologic adjustment of the patient and caregiver to the diagnosis of CAD and the resulting angina. Many patients feel a threat to their identity and self-esteem and may be unable to fill their usual roles in society. These emotions are normal and real.

NURSING IMPLEMENTATION ACUTE CORONARY SYNDROME

ACUTE INTERVENTION. Priorities for nursing interventions in the initial phase of ACS include (1) pain assessment and relief, (2) physiologic monitoring, (3) promotion of rest and comfort, (4) alleviation of stress and anxiety, and (5) understanding of the patient's emotional and behavioral reactions. Patients with increased anxiety levels have a greater risk for adverse outcomes such as recurrent ischemic events and dysrhythmias.[2,12] Proper management of these priorities decreases the oxygen needs of a compromised myocardium and reduces the risk of complications. In addition, institute measures to avoid the hazards of immobility while encouraging rest.

Pain. Provide NTG, morphine, and supplemental oxygen as needed to eliminate or reduce chest pain. Ongoing evaluation and documentation of the effectiveness of the interventions are

NURSING CARE PLAN 34-1

Patient With Acute Coronary Syndrome

NURSING DIAGNOSIS* **Decreased cardiac output** *related to* altered contractility and altered heart rate and rhythm *as evidenced by* decrease in BP, elevation in HR, dyspnea, dysrhythmias, diminished pulses, peripheral edema, and/or pulmonary edema

PATIENT GOAL Maintains stable signs of effective cardiac output

Outcomes (NOC)	Interventions (NIC) and *Rationales*
Tissue Perfusion: Cardiac • Angina _____ • Dysrhythmia _____ • Tachycardia _____ • Bradycardia _____ • Profuse diaphoresis _____ • Nausea _____ • Vomiting _____ **Measurement Scale** 1 = Severe 2 = Substantial 3 = Moderate 4 = Mild 5 = None	***Cardiac Care: Acute*** • Monitor cardiac rhythm and rate and trends in blood pressure and hemodynamic parameters *to monitor for changes in cardiac output, blood pressure, and heart rhythm, which may lead to coronary hypoperfusion.* • Auscultate lungs for crackles or other adventitious sounds *that can indicate pulmonary edema.* • Monitor effectiveness of oxygen therapy (e.g., pulse oximetry) *to determine oxygenation of myocardial tissue and prevent further ischemia.* • Monitor serum cardiac markers (troponin, CK-MB levels) *to determine myocardial injury and recovery.* • Monitor neurologic, renal, and liver function *to evaluate blood perfusion to vital organs.*

NURSING DIAGNOSIS **Acute pain** *related to* an imbalance between myocardial oxygen supply and demand *as evidenced by* patient's report of severe chest pain and tightness with radiation of pain to the neck and arms, elevated cardiac markers, ECG changes supporting ST elevation MI

PATIENT GOAL Reports relief of pain

Outcomes (NOC)	Interventions (NIC) and *Rationales*
Pain Control • Uses preventive measures _____ • Uses analgesics appropriately _____ • Reports uncontrolled symptoms to health care professional _____ • Reports pain controlled _____ **Measurement Scale** 1 = Never demonstrated 2 = Rarely demonstrated 3 = Sometimes demonstrated 4 = Often demonstrated 5 = Consistently demonstrated	***Cardiac Care*** • Evaluate chest pain (e.g., PQRST [see Table 34-7]) *to accurately evaluate, treat, and prevent further ischemia.* • Monitor vital signs frequently *to determine baseline and ongoing changes.* • Obtain 12-lead ECG during pain episode *to help differentiate angina from extension of MI or pericarditis.* ***Pain Management*** • Provide the person optimal pain relief with prescribed analgesics *because pain exacerbates tachycardia and increases blood pressure.* • Consider the type and source of pain when selecting pain relief strategy *because angina responds to opioids and measures that increase myocardial perfusion.*

NURSING DIAGNOSIS **Anxiety** *related to* perceived or actual threat of death, pain, and/or possible lifestyle changes *as evidenced by* restlessness, agitation, and verbalization of concern over lifestyle changes and prognosis such as patient's statement, "What if I die? Everyone relies on me."

PATIENT GOAL Reports decreased anxiety and increased sense of self-control

Outcomes (NOC)	Interventions (NIC) and *Rationales*
Anxiety Level • Restlessness _____ • Verbalized apprehension _____ • Difficulty concentrating _____ • Distress _____ **Measurement Scale** 1 = Severe 2 = Substantial 3 = Moderate 4 = Mild 5 = None	***Anxiety Reduction*** • Observe for verbal and nonverbal signs of anxiety *to identify signs of stress and intervene appropriately.* • Identify when level of anxiety changes, *since anxiety increases the need for oxygen.* • Use a calm, reassuring approach *to avoid increasing patient's anxiety.* • Instruct patient in use of relaxation techniques (e.g., relaxation breathing, imagery) *to enhance self-control.* • Encourage caregiver to stay with patient *to provide comfort and support.* • Encourage verbalization of feelings, perceptions, and fears *to decrease anxiety and stress.* • Provide factual information concerning diagnosis, treatment, and prognosis *to decrease fear of the unknown.*
Acceptance: Health Status • Recognizes reality of health situation _____ • Adjusts to change in health status _____ • Makes decisions about health _____ **Measurement Scale** 1 = Never demonstrated 2 = Rarely demonstrated 3 = Sometimes demonstrated 4 = Often demonstrated 5 = Consistently demonstrated	***Coping Enhancement*** • Provide the patient with realistic choices about certain aspects of care *to support decision making.* • Assist the patient in identifying positive strategies *to deal with limitations and manage needed lifestyle or role changes.* • Help the patient to grieve and work through the losses of chronic illness.

*Nursing diagnoses listed in order of priority.

Continued

NURSING CARE PLAN 34-1—cont'd

Patient With Acute Coronary Syndrome

NURSING DIAGNOSIS **Activity intolerance** *related to* general weakness secondary to decreased cardiac output and poor lung and tissue perfusion *as evidenced by* patient's report of fatigue with minimal activity, inability to care for self without dyspnea, and increased heart rate

PATIENT GOAL Achieves a realistic program of activity that balances physical activity with energy-conserving activities

Outcomes (NOC)	Interventions (NIC) and *Rationales*
Activity Tolerance • Oxygen saturation with activity ____ • Pulse rate with activity ____ • Ease of breathing with activity ____ • Walking pace ____ • Ease of performing ADLs ____ **Measurement Scale** 1 = Severely compromised 2 = Substantially compromised 3 = Moderately compromised 4 = Mildly compromised 5 = Not compromised	***Cardiac Care*** • Monitor patient's response to cardiac medications, *since these medications often affect BP and pulse.* • Arrange exercise and rest periods *to avoid fatigue and to increase activity tolerance without rapidly increasing cardiac workload.* ***Energy Management*** • Help patient understand energy conservation principles (e.g., the requirement for restricted activity) *to conserve energy and promote healing.* • Teach patient and caregiver techniques of self-care that will minimize oxygen consumption (e.g., self-monitoring and pacing techniques for performance of ADLs) *to promote independence and minimize O_2 consumption.*

NURSING DIAGNOSIS **Ineffective self-health management** *related to* lack of knowledge of disease process, risk factor reduction, rehabilitation, home activities, and medications *as evidenced by* frequent questioning about illness, management, and care after discharge

PATIENT GOAL Describes the disease process, measures to reduce risk factors, and rehabilitation activities necessary to manage the therapeutic regimen

Outcomes (NOC)	Interventions (NIC) and *Rationales*
Knowledge: Cardiac Disease Management • Usual course of disease process ____ • Signs and symptoms of worsening disease ____ • Strategies to reduce risk factors ____ • Importance of completing cardiac rehabilitation program ____ • Rationale for following a low-fat, low-cholesterol diet ____ • Importance of regular exercise ____ **Measurement Scale** 1 = No knowledge 2 = Limited knowledge 3 = Moderate knowledge 4 = Substantial knowledge 5 = Extensive knowledge	***Cardiac Care: Rehabilitative*** • Encourage realistic expectations for the patient and caregiver *to promote realistic decision making.* • Instruct the patient and caregiver on appropriate prescribed and over-the-counter medications *to promote compliance with medication regimens.* • Instruct the patient and caregiver on cardiac risk factor modification (e.g., smoking cessation, diet, exercise) *to increase patient's control of the illness.* • Instruct the patient on self-care of chest pain (e.g., take nitroglycerin; if chest pain unrelieved, seek emergency medical care). • Instruct the patient and caregiver on the exercise regimen, including warm-up, endurance, and cool-down, *to reduce cardiac risk factors.* • Instruct the patient and caregiver on wound care and precautions (e.g., sternal incision or catheterization site) *to prevent infection and promote healing after invasive therapies.* • Instruct the patient and caregiver on access to emergency services available in their community *to enable them to obtain immediate care if needed.*

important. Once pain is relieved, you may have to deal with denial in a patient who interprets the absence of pain as an absence of cardiac disease.

Monitoring. Maintain continuous ECG monitoring while the patient is in the ED and intensive care unit and after transfer to a step-down or general unit. Dysrhythmias need to be identified quickly and treated. During the initial period after MI, ventricular fibrillation is the most common lethal dysrhythmia. In many patients, premature ventricular contractions or ventricular tachycardia precedes this dysrhythmia. Monitor the patient for reinfarction or ischemia by monitoring the ST segment for shifts above or below the baseline of the ECG. Silent ischemia can occur without clinical symptoms such as chest pain. Its presence places a patient at higher risk for adverse outcomes and even death. If you note ST segment changes, notify the physician. (See Chapter 36 for a complete discussion of ECG monitoring.)

Perform a physical assessment to detect deviations from the patient's baseline findings. Assess heart and breath sounds and any evidence of early HF (e.g., dyspnea, tachycardia, pulmonary congestion, distended neck veins). In addition to routine vital signs, monitor intake and output at least once a shift.

Assessment of the patient's oxygenation status is important, especially if the patient is receiving oxygen. If a nasal cannula is used to deliver oxygen, check the nares for irritation or dryness, which can cause considerable discomfort.

Rest and Comfort. It is important to promote rest and comfort with any degree of myocardial injury. Bed rest may be ordered for the first few days after an MI that involves a large portion of the ventricle. A patient with an uncomplicated MI (e.g., angina resolved, no signs of complications) may rest in a chair within 8 to 12 hours after the event. The use of a commode or bedpan is based on patient preference.

When sleeping or resting, the body requires less work from the heart than it does when active. It is important to plan nursing and therapeutic interventions to ensure adequate rest periods free from interruption. Comfort measures that can promote rest include a quiet environment, use of relaxation techniques (e.g., relaxation breathing, guided imagery), and assurance that staff are nearby and responsive to the patient's needs.

It is important that the patient understand the reasons why activity is limited but not completely restricted. Gradually increase the patient's cardiac workload through more demand-

TABLE 34-15 PHASES OF REHABILITATION AFTER ACUTE CORONARY SYNDROME

Phase I: Hospital
- Occurs while the patient is still hospitalized.
- Activity level depends on severity of angina or MI.
- Patient may initially sit up in bed or chair, perform range-of-motion exercises and self-care (e.g., washing, shaving), and progress to ambulation in hallway and limited stair climbing.
- Attention focuses on management of chest pain, anxiety, dysrhythmias, and complications.

Phase II: Early Recovery
- Begins after the patient is discharged.
- Usually lasts from 2-12 wk and is conducted in an outpatient facility.
- Activity level is gradually increased under the supervision of the cardiac rehabilitation team and with ECG monitoring.
- Team may suggest that physical activity (e.g., walking) be initiated at home.
- Information regarding risk factor reduction is provided at this time.

Phase III: Late Recovery
- Long-term maintenance program.
- Individual physical activity programs are designed and implemented at home, a local gym, or the rehabilitation center.
- Patient and caregiver possibly restructure lifestyles and roles.
- Therapeutic lifestyle changes should become lifelong habits.
- Medical supervision is still recommended.

ing physical tasks so that the patient can achieve a discharge activity level adequate for home care. Table 34-15 outlines the phases of cardiac rehabilitation.

Anxiety. Anxiety is present in all patients with ACS to some degree. Your role is to identify the source of anxiety and assist the patient in reducing it. If the patient is afraid of being alone, allow a caregiver to sit by quietly or check in with the patient frequently. If a source of anxiety is fear of the unknown, explore these concerns with the patient. For anxiety caused by lack of information, provide teaching based on the patient's stated need and level of understanding. Answer the patient's questions with clear, simple explanations.

It is important to start teaching at the patient's level rather than to present a prepackaged program. For example, patients generally are not ready to learn about the pathology of CAD. The earliest questions usually relate to how the disease affects perceived control and independence. Examples include the following.

- When will I leave the intensive care unit?
- When can I be out of bed?
- When will I be discharged?
- When can I return to work?
- How many changes will I have to make in my life?
- Will this happen again?

Tell the patient that a more complete teaching program will begin once the patient is feeling stronger. Frequently the patient may not be able to ask the most serious concern of ACS patients: Am I going to die? Even if a patient denies this concern, it is helpful for you to start a conversation by remarking that fear of dying is a common concern among most patients who have experienced ACS. This gives the patient "permission" to talk about an uncomfortable and fearful topic.

Emotional and Behavioral Reactions. Patients' emotional and behavioral reactions vary but frequently follow a predictable response pattern (Table 34-16). Your role is to understand what the patient is currently experiencing and to support the use of constructive coping styles. Denial may be a positive coping style in the early phase of recovery from ACS.

TABLE 34-16 PSYCHOSOCIAL RESPONSES TO ACUTE CORONARY SYNDROME

Denial
- May have history of ignoring signs and symptoms related to heart disease
- Minimizes severity of medical condition
- Ignores activity restrictions
- Avoids discussing illness or its significance

Anger and Hostility
- Is commonly expressed as, "Why did this happen to me?"
- May be directed at family, staff, or medical regimen

Anxiety and Fear
- Fears long-term disability and death
- Overtly manifests apprehension, restlessness, insomnia, tachycardia
- Less overtly manifests increased verbalization, projection of feelings to others, hypochondriasis
- Fears activity
- Fears recurrent chest pain, heart attacks, and sudden death

Dependency
- Is totally reliant on staff
- Is unwilling to perform tasks or activities unless approved by health care provider
- Wants to be monitored by ECG at all times
- Is hesitant to leave the intensive care or telemetry unit or hospital

Depression
- Mourns loss of health, altered body function, and changes in lifestyle
- Realizes seriousness of situation
- Begins to worry about future implications of health problem
- Shows manifestations of withdrawal, crying, apathy
- May be more evident after discharge

Realistic Acceptance
- Focuses on optimum rehabilitation
- Plans changes compatible with altered cardiac function
- Actively engages in lifestyle changes to address modifiable risk factors

Assess the support structure of the patient and caregiver. Help to determine how you can help maximize the support system. Often the patient is separated from the most significant support system at the time of hospitalization. Your role can include talking with the caregiver(s), informing them of the patient's progress, allowing the patient and the caregivers to interact as necessary, and supporting the caregivers who will provide the necessary support to the patient. Open visitation is helpful in decreasing anxiety and increasing support for the patient with ACS.[26] Social isolation has been associated with negative outcomes following MI in both men and women. It is important for you to help the patient identify additional support systems (e.g., spiritual care, Mended Hearts) that can assist after discharge.

CORONARY REVASCULARIZATION. Patients with ACS may undergo coronary revascularization with PCI or CABG surgery. The major nursing responsibilities for patient care after PCI involve monitoring for signs of recurrent angina; frequent

DELEGATION DECISIONS

Cardiac Catheterization and Percutaneous Coronary Intervention (PCI)

Role of Registered Nurse (RN)

Preprocedure

- Assess for allergies, especially to contrast medium. Perform baseline assessment, including vital signs, pulse oximetry, heart and breath sounds, neurovascular assessment of extremities (e.g., distal pulses, skin temperature, skin color, sensation).
- Teach patient and caregiver about procedure and postprocedure care.

Postprocedure

- Perform assessment and compare to baseline: vital signs, pulse oximetry, heart and breath sounds, neurovascular assessment of extremity used for procedure, assessment of catheter insertion site for hematoma or bleeding.
- Monitor ECG for dysrhythmias or other changes (e.g., ST segment elevation).
- Monitor patient for chest pain and other sources of pain or discomfort.
- Monitor IV infusions of anticoagulants, antiplatelets.
- Teach patient and caregiver about discharge medications (e.g., aspirin, prasugrel [Effient], antianginal medications).

Role of Licensed Practical/Vocational Nurse (LPN/LVN)

- Administer medications before and after the procedure (consider state nurse practice act and agency policy).
- Assess neurovascular status of involved extremity every 15 min for the first hour, then according to agency policy (consider state nurse practice act and agency policy).
- Check for bleeding at catheter insertion site every 15 min for the first hour, then according to agency policy.
- Report changes in neurovascular status of involved extremity or any bleeding to the RN.

Role of Unlicensed Assistive Personnel (UAP)

- Take vital signs and report increases or decreases in heart rate or blood pressure to RN.
- Report decreases in pulse oximetry to the RN.
- Report patient complaints of chest pain, shortness of breath, and/or any other discomfort or distress to RN.
- Assist with oral hygiene, hydration, meals, and toileting.

assessment of vital signs, including HR and rhythm; evaluation of the catheter insertion site for signs of bleeding; neurovascular assessment of the involved extremity; and maintenance of bed rest per institution policy.

For patients having CABG surgery, care is provided in the intensive care unit for the first 24 to 36 hours. Ongoing and intensive monitoring of the patient's hemodynamic status is critical. The patient will have numerous invasive lines for monitoring cardiac status and other vital organs (see Chapter 66). These include (1) a pulmonary artery catheter for measuring CO and other hemodynamic parameters, (2) an intraarterial line for continuous BP monitoring, (3) pleural and mediastinal chest tubes for chest drainage, (4) continuous ECG monitoring to detect dysrhythmias, (5) an endotracheal tube connected to mechanical ventilation, (6) epicardial pacing wires for emergency pacing of the heart, (7) a urinary catheter to monitor urine output, and (8) a nasogastric tube for gastric decompression. Most patients are extubated within 6 hours and transferred to a step-down unit within 24 hours for continued monitoring of cardiac status.

Many of the postoperative complications that develop after CABG surgery relate to the use of CPB. Major consequences of CPB are systemic inflammation, which includes complications of bleeding and anemia from damage to red blood cells and platelets, fluid and electrolyte imbalances, hypothermia as blood is cooled as it passes through the CPB machine, and infections. Focus your nursing care on assessing the patient for bleeding (e.g., chest tube drainage, incision sites), hemodynamic monitoring, checking fluid status, replacing electrolytes as needed, and restoring temperature (e.g., warming blankets).

Postoperative dysrhythmias, specifically atrial dysrhythmias, are common in the first 3 days after CABG surgery. Postoperative atrial fibrillation (AF) occurs in 20% to 50% of patients.[24] β-Adrenergic blockers should be restarted as soon as possible after surgery (unless contraindicated) to reduce the incidence of AF. Discharge is often delayed in these patients in order to begin anticoagulation therapy. (See Chapter 36 for information on treatment of AF.)

Nursing care for the patient with a CABG also involves caring for the surgical sites (e.g., chest, arm, leg). Care of the radial artery harvest site includes monitoring sensory and motor function of the distal hand. The patient with radial artery harvest should take a calcium channel blocker for approximately 3 months to decrease the incidence of arterial spasm at the arm or anastomosis site.

Care of the leg incision is minimal since endoscopy is used to harvest the vein. Management of the chest wound, which involves a sternotomy, is similar to that of other chest surgeries (see Chapter 28). Chest incisions are usually closed with Dermabond and do not require dressings. Other interventions include strategies to manage pain and prevent venous thromboembolism (e.g., early ambulation, sequential compression device) and respiratory complications (e.g., use of incentive spirometer, splinting during coughing and deep-breathing exercises). (See Chapter 20 for care of the postoperative patient.)

Postoperatively, patients may experience some cognitive dysfunction. This includes impairment of memory, concentration, language comprehension, and social integration. Patients may cry or become teary. Postoperative cognitive dysfunction (POCD) can manifest days to weeks after surgery and may remain a permanent disorder. It is seen in 40% of patients several months after cardiac surgery.[27] (POCD is discussed in Chapter 20.)

In the older patient, elective CABG is generally well tolerated. However, the incidence of postoperative complications, including dysrhythmias, stroke, and infection, is high. Although the benefits of treatment may outweigh risks in this population, complications are higher than in younger individuals.

Postoperative nursing care of the patient with a MIDCAB or OPCAB procedure is similar to that for CABG surgery patients. Pain management is important regardless of the procedure. Patients report higher levels of pain with thoracotomy incisions than a sternotomy incision. The recovery time is somewhat shorter with these procedures, and patients often resume routine activities sooner than patients who have CABG surgery.

AMBULATORY AND HOME CARE. *Cardiac rehabilitation* is the restoration of a person to an optimal state of function in six areas: physiologic, psychologic, mental, spiritual, economic, and vocational. Many patients recover from ACS physically, but do not attain psychologic well-being. All patients (e.g., those with ACS, chronic stable angina, cardiac surgery) need to be referred to a cardiac rehabilitation program. In considering rehabilitation, the patient must recognize that CAD is a chronic disease. It is not curable, nor will it disappear by itself. Therefore

EVIDENCE-BASED PRACTICE

Translating Research into Practice

Do Exercise-Based Cardiac Rehabilitation Programs Improve Outcomes?

Clinical Question

In patients with coronary heart disease (P), do exercise-based cardiac rehabilitation programs (I) versus usual care (C) reduce mortality and morbidity and improve quality of life (O)?

Best Available Evidence

Systematic review of randomized controlled trials (RCTs)

Critical Appraisal and Synthesis of Evidence

- 47 RCTs (n = 10,794) of patients with myocardial infarction (MI), angina pectoris, coronary artery bypass graft (CABG), or percutaneous transluminal coronary angioplasty (PTCA). Exercise-based cardiac rehabilitation was exercise alone or with psychosocial or educational interventions. Usual care included standard medical care and drug therapy with no structured exercise training.
- Exercise-based rehabilitation reduced overall and cardiovascular mortality, decreased hospital admissions, and improved quality of life.
- Cardiac rehabilitation did not reduce risk of recurrent MI or revascularization (CABG or PTCA).

Conclusion

- Exercise-based cardiac rehabilitation reduces risk of dying from heart disease.

Implications for Nursing Practice

- Provide assistance in accessing cardiac rehabilitation programs.
- Reinforce benefits of adhering to recommended physical activity.
- Reduce program dropout rates by motivating patients to stay engaged.

Reference for Evidence

Heran B, Chen J, Ebrahim S, et al: Exercise-based cardiac rehabilitation for coronary heart disease, *Cochrane Database Syst Rev* 7:CD001800, 2011.

P, Patient population of interest; *I*, intervention or area of interest; *C*, comparison of interest or comparison group; *O*, outcomes of interest; *T*, timing (see p. 12).

EVIDENCE-BASED PRACTICE

Applying the Evidence

J.B. is 56-year-old white man who is being discharged from the hospital after having a myocardial infarction (MI) 4 days ago. You know that he is struggling with the lifestyle changes he must make, including how to kick his cigarette habit. While you are discussing the importance of smoking cessation with him, you share information from both the best available evidence and your clinical expertise. In addition, you describe a variety of smoking cessation interventions available for his consideration.

Best Available Evidence*	Clinician Expertise	Patient Preferences and Values
Combination strategies (e.g., medication plus behavioral support) work best to help patients to stop smoking.	You have heard from several patients who have successfully stopped smoking that they tried more than one intervention at a time to stop smoking (e.g., medication plus support group, hypnotherapy plus support group).	After reviewing all the information, J.B. informs you that he is willing to start with the nicotine patch but does not want to do anything else at this time.

Your Decision and Action

As his nurse, you respect and support his decision. You document your teaching and J.B.'s response. You notify his physician of his choice and request a prescription for the nicotine patch.

References for Evidence

Carpenter MJ, Hughes JR, Gray KM, et al: Nicotine therapy sampling to induce quit attempts among smokers unmotivated to quit: a randomized clinical trial, *Arch Intern Med* 171:1901, 2011.
Joseph AM, Fu SS, Lindgren B, et al: Chronic disease management for tobacco dependence: a randomized, controlled trial, *Arch Intern Med* 171:1894, 2011.

basic changes in lifestyle must be made to promote recovery and future health. These changes often are needed when a person is middle aged or older. The patient must realize that recovery takes time. Resumption of physical activity after ACS or CABG surgery is slow and gradual. However, with appropriate and adequate supportive care, recovery is more likely to occur.

Patient Teaching. Patient teaching needs to occur at every stage of the patient's hospitalization and recovery (e.g., ED, telemetry unit, home care). The purpose of teaching is to give the patient and caregiver the tools they need to make informed decisions about their health. For teaching to be meaningful, the patient must be aware of the need to learn. Careful assessment of the patient's learning needs helps you set goals that are realistic (see Chapter 4).

The timing of the teaching is important. When patients and caregivers are in crisis (either physiologic or psychologic), they may not be interested in learning new information. Answer the patient's questions in simple, brief terms. The answers often require repetition. When the shock and disbelief accompanying a crisis subside, the patient and caregiver are better able to focus on new and more detailed information.

Limit your use of medical terminology. For example, explain that the heart, a four-chambered pump, is a muscle that needs oxygen, like all other muscles, to work properly. When blood vessels supplying the heart muscle with oxygen are blocked by plaque, less oxygen is available to the muscle. As a result, the heart cannot pump normally. It helps to have a model of the heart or to sketch a picture of what you are explaining. Literature written for a nonmedical audience is available through the AHA.

Anticipatory guidance involves preparing the patient and caregiver for what to expect in the course of recovery and rehabilitation. By learning what to expect during treatment and recovery, the patient gains a sense of control over his or her life.

The idea of perceived control is operationalized as the process by which the patient exercises choice and makes decisions by cutting back. Cutting back is one way of minimizing the psychologic and physiologic losses after MI (or any other life-changing event). For example, a middle-aged man who smokes two packs of cigarettes a day, is 20 pounds overweight, and gets no physical exercise has a seemingly overwhelming task. He may decide that he can live with a weight reduction plan and will get more exercise (although perhaps not daily) but that it is not possible for him to quit smoking. He reasons that because he is modifying two of the three risk factors, he will be healthier. Ideally, the tobacco risk factor should be a priority for this patient. If the information regarding risks and effects of tobacco use is not accepted, you must respect the patient's lifestyle choices.

TABLE 34-17 PATIENT & CAREGIVER TEACHING GUIDE

Acute Coronary Syndrome

Include the following information in the teaching plan for the patient with acute coronary syndrome and the caregiver.

- Signs and symptoms of angina and MI and what to do should they occur (e.g., take nitroglycerin)*
- When and how to seek help (e.g., contact EMS)
- Anatomy and physiology of the heart and coronary arteries
- Cause and effect of CAD
- Definition of terms (e.g., CAD, angina, MI, sudden cardiac death, heart failure)
- Identification of and plan to decrease risk factors* (see Tables 34-2, 34-3, and 34-4)
- Rationale for tests and treatments (e.g., ECG monitoring, blood tests, angiography), activity limitations and rest, diet, and medications*
- Appropriate expectations about recovery and rehabilitation (anticipatory guidance)
- Resumption of work, physical activity, sexual activity
- Measures to promote recovery and health
- Importance of the gradual, progressive resumption of activity*

*Identified by patients as most important to learn before discharge.

In addition to teaching the patient and caregiver what they wish to know, several types of information are essential in achieving optimal health. Table 34-17 presents a teaching guide for the patient with ACS.

Physical Activity. Physical activity, an integral part of rehabilitation, is necessary for optimal physiologic functioning and psychologic well-being. It has a direct, positive effect on maximal oxygen uptake, increasing CO, decreasing blood lipids, decreasing BP, increasing blood flow through the coronary arteries, increasing muscle mass and flexibility, improving the psychologic state, and assisting in weight loss and control. A regular schedule of physical activity, even after many years of sedentary living, is beneficial.[9]

One method of identifying levels of physical activity is through **metabolic equivalent (MET)** units: 1 MET is the amount of oxygen needed by the body at rest—3.5 mL of oxygen per kilogram per minute, or 1.4 cal/kg of body weight per minute. The MET determines the energy costs of various exercises (Table 34-18). Another method to determine levels of physical activity is the *Borg Rating of Perceived Exertion Scale.* This scale focuses on the patient's rating of the effort an activity requires (Table 34-19).

In the hospital the activity level is gradually increased so that by the time of discharge the patient can tolerate moderate-energy activities of 3 to 6 METs or rates activities 12 to 14 on the Borg scale. Many patients with UA that has resolved or an uncomplicated MI are in the hospital for approximately 3 or 4 days. By day 2, the patient can ambulate in the hallway and begin limited stair climbing (e.g., three or four steps). Many physicians order low-level exercise stress tests before discharge to assess readiness for discharge, optimal HR for an exercise program, and potential for ischemia or reinfarction. If tests are positive (i.e., ischemia at a low level of energy expenditure), the patient is evaluated for cardiac catheterization before discharge. If the test is negative, a catheterization may still be done before discharge or several weeks after discharge. Because of the short hospital stay, it is critical to give the patient specific guidelines for physical activity so that overexertion will not occur. It is

TABLE 34-18 ENERGY EXPENDITURE IN METABOLIC EQUIVALENTS

Low-Energy Activities (<3 METs or <3 cal/min)

Activities in Hospital
- Resting supine
- Eating
- Washing hands, face

Activities Outside Hospital
- Sweeping floor
- Painting, seated
- Driving a car
- Sewing by machine

Moderate-Energy Activities (3-6 METs or 3-5 cal/min)

Activities in Hospital
- Sitting on bedside commode
- Showering
- Using bedpan
- Walking at 3-4 mph

Activities Outside Hospital
- Ironing, standing
- Cycling at 5.5 mph on level ground
- Golfing
- General gardening
- Painting
- Ascending a flight of stairs

High-Energy Activities (6-8 METs or 6-8 cal/min)
- Walking 5 mph
- Performing carpentry
- Mowing lawn using walking mower

Very-High-Energy Activities (>9 METs or >9 cal/min)
- Cross-country skiing
- Running at >6 mph
- Cycling at >13 mph
- Shoveling heavy snow

TABLE 34-19 BORG RATING OF PERCEIVED EXERTION SCALE®*

Level of Exertion	RPE
No exertion at all	6
Extremely light	7
	8
Very light	9
	10
Light	11
	12
Somewhat hard	13
	14
Hard (heavy)	15
	16
Very hard	17
	18
Extremely hard	19
Maximal exertion	20

9 corresponds to very light exercise. For a healthy person, it is like walking slowly at his or her own pace for some minutes.

13 on the scale is somewhat hard exercise, but it still feels OK to continue.

17 (very hard) is strenuous exercise. A healthy person can still go on, but he or she really has to push himself or herself. It feels very hard, and the person is very tired.

19 on the scale is an extremely strenuous exercise level. For most people this is the most strenuous exercise they have ever experienced.

Source: Borg G: Borg's perceived exertion and pain scales, *Human Kinetics,* 1998, Champaign, Ill. © Gunnar Borg, 1970, 1985, 1994, 1998. For information about scale construction, administration, etc., see Borg's book (Borg G., 1998). Scales and instructions can be obtained for a minor fee from Dr. G. Borg. E-mail: borgperception@telia.com.

*The complete instructions on how to use this scale are available on the website for this chapter.

TABLE 34-20 PATIENT & CAREGIVER TEACHING GUIDE

FITT *Activity Guidelines After Acute Coronary Syndrome*

Include the following information in the teaching plan for the patient after an acute coronary syndrome:

Warm-up/Cool-down
Instruct the patient to perform mild stretching for 3-5 min before the physical activity and 5 min after the activity. Activity should not be started or stopped abruptly.

Frequency
Encourage the patient to perform physical activity on most days of the week.

Intensity
Activity intensity is determined by the patient's HR. If an exercise stress test has not been performed, the HR of the patient recovering from an MI should not exceed 20 beats/min over the resting HR.

Type of Physical Activity
Physical activity should be regular, rhythmic, and repetitive, using large muscles to build up endurance (e.g., walking, cycling, swimming, rowing).

Time
Physical activity sessions should be at least 30 min long. Instruct the patient to begin slowly at personal tolerance (perhaps only 5-10 min) and build up to 30 min.

important to tell the patient to "listen to what your body is saying"—the most important aspect of recovery.

Teach patients to check their pulse rate. The patient should know the limits within which to exercise. Tell the patient the maximum HR that should be present at any point. If the HR exceeds this level or does not return to the rate of the resting pulse within a few minutes, instruct the patient to stop and rest. Also instruct the patient to stop exercising and rest if chest pain or shortness of breath occurs.

In a normal, healthy person the minimum threshold for improving cardiopulmonary fitness is 60% of the age-predicted maximum HR (calculate by subtracting the person's age from 220). The ideal training target HR is 80% of maximum HR. The patient who has been physically inactive and is just beginning an exercise program should do so under supervision whenever possible.

The more important factor is the patient's response to physical activity in terms of symptoms rather than absolute HR, especially since many patients are taking β-adrenergic blockers and may not be able to reach a target HR. This point cannot be overstressed. Basic physical activity guidelines for patients after ACS follow the FITT formula (Table 34-20).

The basic categories of physical activity are isometric (static) and isotonic (dynamic). Most daily activities are a mixture of the two. *Isometric activities* involve the development of tension during muscular contraction but produce little or no change in muscle length or joint movement. Lifting, carrying, and pushing heavy objects are isometric activities. Because the HR and BP increase rapidly during isometric work, exercise programs involving isometric exercises should be limited.

Isotonic activities involve changes in muscle length and joint movement with rhythmic contractions at relatively low muscular tension. Walking, jogging, swimming, bicycling, and jumping rope are examples of activities that are predominantly isotonic. Isotonic exercise can put a safe, steady load on the heart and lungs and improve the circulation in many organs.

Discuss participation in an outpatient cardiac rehabilitation program with all patients (see Table 34-15). These programs are beneficial, but not all patients choose or are able to participate in them (e.g., location and travel limitations). Home-based cardiac rehabilitation programs can provide an alternative. Physical activity guidelines are developed for the patient, and staff maintains ongoing contact with the patient (e.g., telephone, exercise logs, Internet). Maintaining contact with the patient is one key to the success of these programs.

Older women (65 years or older) who experience MI may frequently have poor adherence to a regular physical activity program. Often these women describe continued fatigue post-MI that is poorly understood. Another factor that has been linked to poor adherence to a physical activity program after MI is depression. Depression is common among patients with CAD, especially in women.[28] Routinely screen for depression in all patients with CAD and recommend treatment as appropriate.

Resumption of Sexual Activity. It is important to include sexual counseling for cardiac patients and their partners. This often-neglected area of discussion may be difficult for both the patient and the health care provider to approach. However, the patient's concern about resumption of sexual activity after hospitalization for ACS often produces more stress than the physiologic act itself. Most of these patients change their sexual behavior not because of physical problems, but because they are concerned about sexual inadequacy, death during intercourse, and impotence. A concerned and knowledgeable health care provider could clarify any misconceptions with specific counseling.

Before providing guidelines on resumption of sexual activity, it is important to know the patient's physiologic status, the physiologic effects of sexual activity, and the psychologic effects of having a heart attack. Sexual activity for most middle-aged men and women with their usual partners is considered a moderate-energy activity equivalent to climbing two flights of stairs.[29]

You may be uncertain of how and when to begin counseling about resumption of sex. It is helpful to consider sex as a physical activity and to discuss or explore feelings in this area when other physical activities are discussed. One helpful approach is, "Many people who have had a heart attack wonder when they will be able to resume sexual activity. Has this been of concern to you?" You might also state, "Sexual activity is like other forms of activity and should be gradually resumed after MI. If your ability to perform sexually is concerning you, the energy you use is no more than walking briskly." Facilitate discussion by providing the patient with reading material on resumption of sexual activity. Say something like, "If resuming sexual activity has been of concern to you, this information should be helpful." This type of nonthreatening statement brings up the topic, allows the patient to explore personal feelings, and gives the patient an opportunity to raise questions with you or another health care provider.[28] Common guidelines are presented in Table 34-21.

The patient needs to know that the inability to perform sexually after MI is common and that sexual dysfunction usually disappears after several attempts. Reinforce the idea that

TABLE 34-21 PATIENT TEACHING GUIDE

Sexual Activity After Acute Coronary Syndrome

Include the following information in the teaching plan for the patient and his/her partner after an acute coronary syndrome:

- Sexual activity should be resumed at a level that corresponds to sexual activity before experiencing acute coronary syndrome.
- Physical training may improve the physiologic response to intercourse. Therefore daily physical activity during recovery should be encouraged.
- Consumption of food and alcohol should be reduced before intercourse is anticipated (e.g., waiting 3-4 hr after ingesting a large meal before engaging in sexual activity).
- Familiar surroundings and a familiar partner reduce anxiety.
- Masturbation may be a useful sexual outlet and may reassure the patient that sexual activity is still possible.
- Hot or cold showers should be avoided just before and after intercourse.
- Foreplay is desirable because it allows a gradual increase in heart rate before orgasm.
- Positions during intercourse are a matter of individual choice.
- Orogenital sex places no undue strain on the heart.
- A relaxed atmosphere free of fatigue and stress is optimal.
- Prophylactic use of nitrates to decrease chest pain during sexual activity may be recommended.
- Use of erectile agents (e.g., sildenafil [Viagra]) is contraindicated if taking nitrates in any form.
- Anal intercourse should be avoided because of the possibility of inducing a vasovagal response.

patience and understanding usually solve the problem. However, with the availability of drugs to correct erectile dysfunction, many male patients may be interested in using them. Caution the patient that these drugs are not to be used with nitrates because severe hypotension and even death have been reported.[15] Encourage patients to discuss the use of these drugs with their health care provider.

It is common for a patient who experiences chest pain on physical exertion to have some angina during sexual stimulation or intercourse. The patient may be instructed to take NTG prophylactically.[15] It is also helpful to have the patient avoid sex soon after a heavy meal or after excessive ingestion of alcohol, when extremely tired or stressed, or with unfamiliar partners. Patients should also avoid anal intercourse because of the likelihood of eliciting a vasovagal response.

Tell the patient that resumption of sex depends on the patient and his or her partner's emotional readiness and on the physician's assessment of the extent of recovery. It is generally safe to resume sexual activity 7 to 10 days after an uncomplicated MI.[29] However, some physicians believe that the patient should decide when he or she is ready to resume sex. Others believe that a patient must be asymptomatic when performing moderate-energy activities before resuming sexual activity.[29]

EVALUATION

Nursing Care Plan 34-1 presents the expected outcomes for the patient with an ACS.

SUDDEN CARDIAC DEATH

Sudden cardiac death (SCD) is unexpected death resulting from a variety of cardiac causes. An estimated 382,800 people experience SCD yearly.[1]

Etiology and Pathophysiology

In SCD a sudden disruption in cardiac function produces an abrupt loss of CO and cerebral blood flow. The affected person may or may not have a known history of heart disease. SCD is often the first sign of illness for 25% of those who die of heart disease.[30]

Acute ventricular dysrhythmias (e.g., ventricular tachycardia, ventricular fibrillation) cause the majority of cases of SCD. Structural heart disease accounts for 10% of the cases of SCD. Patients in this group include those with left ventricular hypertrophy, myocarditis, and hypertrophic cardiomyopathy. Hypertrophic cardiomyopathy is a risk factor for SCD, especially in young, athletic people.

Approximately 10% to 12% of cases of SCD among people less than age 45 occur in the absence of structural heart disease. These involve disturbances in the conduction system (e.g., prolonged QT syndrome, Wolff-Parkinson-White syndrome).

It is difficult to know who is at high risk for SCD. However, left ventricular dysfunction (EF less than 30%) and ventricular dysrhythmias following MI have been found to be the strongest predictors.[30] Other risk factors include history of syncope, left ventricular outflow tract obstruction (e.g., aortic stenosis), male gender (especially African American men), and family history of ventricular dysrhythmias.

Clinical Manifestations and Complications

Persons who experience SCD because of CAD fall into two groups: (1) those who did not have an acute MI and (2) those who did have an acute MI. The first group accounts for the majority of cases of SCD.[30] These victims usually have no warning signs or symptoms. Patients who survive are at risk for another SCD event because of the continued electrical instability of the heart that caused the initial event to occur.

The second, smaller group of patients includes those who have had an MI and have suffered SCD. Such patients usually have prodromal symptoms, such as chest pain, palpitations, and dyspnea. Death usually occurs within 1 hour of the onset of acute symptoms.

NURSING AND COLLABORATIVE MANAGEMENT SUDDEN CARDIAC DEATH

People who survive an episode of SCD require a diagnostic workup to determine whether they have had an MI. Thus serial analysis of cardiac markers and ECGs are done, and the patient is treated accordingly. (See section on collaborative care of ACS.) In addition, because most persons with SCD have CAD, cardiac catheterization is indicated to determine the possible location and extent of coronary artery occlusion. PCI or CABG surgery may be indicated.

Most SCD patients have a lethal ventricular dysrhythmia that is associated with a high incidence of recurrence. Thus it is useful to know when those persons are most likely to have a recurrence and what drug therapy is the most effective treatment. Assessment of dysrhythmias in these patients includes 24-hour Holter monitoring or other type of event recorder, exercise stress testing, signal-averaged ECG, and electrophysiology study (EPS).[30]

EPS is performed under fluoroscopy. Pacing electrodes are placed in selected intracardiac areas, and stimuli are selectively used to attempt to produce dysrhythmias. The patient's response to various antidysrhythmic medications is determined and monitored in a controlled environment. (Chapters 32 and 36 discuss EPS.)

The most common approach to preventing a recurrence is the use of an implantable cardioverter-defibrillator (ICD). It has been shown that an ICD improves survival compared with drug therapy alone.[30,31] (Chapter 36 discusses ICDs.) Drug therapy with amiodarone (Cordarone) may be used in conjunction with an ICD to decrease episodes of ventricular dysrhythmias.

Teaching people about the symptoms of impending cardiac arrest and the actions to take can save lives. Rapid cardiopulmonary resuscitation (CPR) (see Appendix A) and defibrillation with an automatic external defibrillator (AED), combined with early advanced cardiac life support, have greatly improved long-term survival rates for a witnessed arrest.

When caring for these patients, be alert to the patient's psychosocial adaptation to this sudden "brush with death." Many of these patients develop a "time bomb" mentality. They fear the recurrence of cardiac arrest and may become anxious, angry, and depressed. Their caregivers are likely to experience the same feelings. Patients and caregivers also may need to deal with additional issues such as possible driving restrictions, role reversal, and change in occupation. The grief response varies among patients and caregivers. Be attuned to the specific needs of the patient and caregiver and teach them accordingly while providing appropriate emotional support.

CASE STUDY

Myocardial Infarction

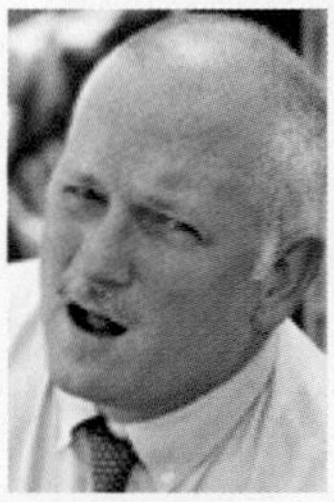

iStockphoto/Thinkstock

Patient Profile

D.M., a 51-year-old, white, successful executive, is rushed to the hospital by ambulance after experiencing crushing substernal chest pain that radiates down his left arm. He also complains of dizziness and nausea.

Subjective Data

- Has a history of chronic stable angina and hypertension
- States he is "borderline diabetic"
- Overweight but recently lost 10 pounds
- Rarely exercises
- Has three teenage children who are causing "problems"
- Recently experienced loss of best friend and business partner, who died from cancer

Objective Data

Physical Examination

- Diaphoretic, short of breath, nauseous
- BP 165/100 mm Hg, pulse rate 120/min, respiratory rate 26/min

Diagnostic Studies

- 12-lead ECG shows sinus tachycardia with ST elevation in leads II, III, aVF, V_5, V_6 with occasional premature ventricular contractions
- Cardiac-specific troponin I level elevated
- Cholesterol 350 mg/dL (9.1 mmol/L)
- Hb A1C 9.0%
- Inferolateral wall MI

Collaborative Care

Emergency Department

- Oxygen 2 L/min via nasal cannula, titrate to keep O_2 saturation above 93%
- Continuous ECG monitoring
- Aspirin 325 mg (chewable)
- Eptifibatide (Integrilin) IV
- Weight-based heparin IV
- Nitroglycerin IV, titrate to relieve chest pain; hold for systolic BP below 100 mm Hg
- Morphine 2 to 4 mg IV q5min PRN for chest pain unrelieved by nitroglycerin
- Vital signs, pulse oximetry every 10 minutes
- Preparation of patient for transfer to cardiac catheterization laboratory for possible PCI

Discussion Questions

1. Which coronary artery(ies) is (are) most likely occluded in D.M.'s coronary circulation?
2. Explain the pathogenesis of CAD. What risk factors contribute to its development? What risk factors were present in D.M.'s life?
3. What is angina? How does chronic stable angina differ from angina associated with acute coronary syndrome?
4. Explain the pathophysiologic basis for the clinical manifestations that D.M. exhibited.
5. Explain the significance of the results of the laboratory tests and the 12-lead ECG findings.
6. Provide a rationale for each treatment measure ordered for D.M.
7. ***Priority Decision:*** Based on the assessment data presented, what are the priority nursing diagnoses? Identify any collaborative problems.
8. ***Priority Decision:*** What are the priority nursing interventions for D.M. immediately after his MI? Immediately after his PCI?
9. ***Delegation Decision:*** Identify activities that can be delegated to unlicensed assistive personnel (UAP).
10. ***Evidence-Based Practice:*** Two days after an uncomplicated PCI and the placement of two stents, D.M. wants to know what the most effective strategies are to prevent another MI. Based on his clinical situation, what would you tell him?

evolve Answers and a corresponding concept map available at *http://evolve.elsevier.com/Lewis/medsurg.*

BRIDGE TO NCLEX EXAMINATION

The number of the question corresponds to the same-numbered outcome at the beginning of the chapter.

1. In teaching a patient about coronary artery disease, the nurse explains that the changes that occur in this disorder include *(select all that apply)*
   a. diffuse involvement of plaque formation in coronary veins.
   b. abnormal levels of cholesterol, especially low-density lipoproteins.
   c. accumulation of lipid and fibrous tissue within the coronary arteries.
   d. development of angina due to a decreased blood supply to the heart muscle.
   e. chronic vasoconstriction of coronary arteries leading to permanent vasospasm.
2. After teaching about ways to decrease risk factors for CAD, the nurse recognizes that additional instruction is needed when the patient says
   a. "I would like to add weight lifting to my exercise program."
   b. "I can only keep my blood pressure normal with medication."
   c. "I can change my diet to decrease my intake of saturated fats."
   d. "I will change my lifestyle to reduce activities that increase my stress."
3. A hospitalized patient with a history of chronic stable angina tells the nurse that she is having chest pain. The nurse bases his actions on the knowledge that ischemia
   a. will always progress to myocardial infarction.
   b. will be relieved by rest, nitroglycerin, or both.
   c. indicates that irreversible myocardial damage is occurring.
   d. is frequently associated with vomiting and extreme fatigue.
4. The nurse is caring for a patient who is 2 days post-MI. The patient reports that she is experiencing chest pain. She states, "It hurts when I take a deep breath." Which action would be a priority?
   a. Notify the physician STAT and obtain a 12-lead ECG.
   b. Obtain vital signs and auscultate for a pericardial friction rub.
   c. Apply high-flow oxygen by face mask and auscultate breath sounds.
   d. Medicate the patient with PRN analgesic and reevaluate in 30 minutes.
5. A patient is admitted to the ICU with a diagnosis of unstable angina. Which medication(s) would the nurse expect the patient to receive *(select all that apply)*?
   a. ACE inhibitor
   b. Antiplatelet therapy
   c. Thrombolytic therapy
   d. Prophylactic antibiotics
   e. Intravenous nitroglycerin
6. A patient is recovering from an uncomplicated MI. Which rehabilitation guideline is a priority to include in the teaching plan?
   a. Refrain from sexual activity for a minimum of 3 weeks.
   b. Plan a diet program that aims for a 1- to 2-pound weight loss per week.
   c. Begin an exercise program that aims for at least five 30-minute sessions per week.
   d. Consider the use of erectile agents and prophylactic NTG before engaging in sexual activity.
7. The most common finding in individuals at risk for sudden cardiac death is
   a. aortic valve disease.
   b. mitral valve disease.
   c. left ventricular dysfunction.
   d. atherosclerotic heart disease.

1. b, c, d, 2. a, 3. b, 4. b, 5. a, b, e, 6. c, 7. c

evolve

For rationales to these answers and even more NCLEX review questions, visit *http://evolve.elsevier.com/Lewis/medsurg*.

REFERENCES

1. Go AS, Mozaffarian D, Roger VL, et al: Heart disease and stroke statistics—2013 update: a report from the American Heart Association, *Circulation* 127:e6, 2013.
2. Huether SE, McCance KL: *Understanding pathophysiology*, ed 5, St Louis, 2012, Mosby.

*3. The Emerging Risk Factors Collaboration: C-reactive protein concentration and risk of coronary heart disease, stroke, and mortality: an individual participant meta-analysis, *Lancet* 375:132, 2010.

4. American Heart Association: Statistical fact sheet 2012 update: women and cardiovascular disease. Retrieved from *www.heart.org/idc/groups/heart-public/@wcm/@sop/@smd/documents/downloadable/ucm_319576.pdf.*
5. Musunuru K, Kathiresan S: Genetics of coronary artery disease, *Annu Rev Genomics Hum Genet* 11:91, 2010.

*6. Smith SC, Benjamin EJ, Bonow RO, et al: AHA/ACCF secondary prevention and risk reduction therapy for patients with coronary and other atherosclerotic vascular disease: 2011 update, *J Am Coll Cardiol* 58:2432, 2011.

*7. Grundy SM, Cleeman JI, Merz MB, et al: Implications of recent clinical trials for the National Cholesterol Education Program Adult Treatment Panel III Guidelines, *Circulation* 110:227, 2004.

*8. National Institutes of Health: *Seventh report of the Joint National Committee on Prevention, Detection, Evaluation, and Treatment of High Blood Pressure (JNC 7)*, pub no 03-5233, Bethesda, Md, 2003, US Department of Health and Human Services.

9. US Department of Health and Human Services (USDHHS): *2008 physical activity guidelines for Americans*, pub no U0036, Bethesda, Md, 2008, The US Department of Health and Human Services.

*10. Thombs BD, de Jonge P, Coyne JC, et al: Depression screening and patient outcomes in cardiovascular care: a systematic review, *JAMA* 300(18):2161, 2008.

*Evidence-based information for clinical practice.

*11. Brydon L, Strike PC, Bhattacharyya MR, et al: Hostility and physiological responses to laboratory stress in acute coronary syndrome patients, *J Psychosom Res* 68:109, 2010.

12. Proietti R, Mapelli D, Volpe B, et al: Mental stress and ischemic heart disease: evolving awareness of a complex association, *Future Cardiol* 7(3):425, 2011.

*13. Humphrey LL, Fu R, Rogers K, et al: Homocysteine level and coronary heart disease incidence: a systematic review and meta-analysis, *Mayo Clin Proc* 83:1203, 2008.

14. National Institute on Drug Abuse: InfoFacts: cocaine. Retrieved from *www.drugabuse.gov/publications/infofacts/cocaine.*

15. Lehne RA: *Pharmacology for nursing care*, ed 7, St Louis, 2010, Saunders.

*16. Mosca L, Benjamin EJ, Berra K, et al: Effectiveness-based guidelines for the prevention of cardiovascular disease in women 2011 update: a guideline from the American Heart Association, *J Am Coll Cardiol* 57:1401, 2011.

*17. Fihn SD, Gardin JM, Abrams J, et al: 2012 ACCF/AHA/ACP/AATS/PCNA/SCAI/STS guideline for the diagnosis and management of patients with stable ischemic heart disease: a report of the American College of Cardiology Foundation/American Heart Association Task Force on Practice Guidelines and the American College of Physicians, American Association for Thoracic Surgery, Preventive Cardiovascular Nurses Association, Society for Cardiovascular Angiography and Interventions, and Society of Thoracic Surgeons, *Circulation* 126:e354, 2012.

*18. O'Gara PT, Kushner FG, Ascheim DD, et al: 2013 ACCF/AHA guideline for the management of ST-elevation myocardial infarction: executive summary, *J Am Coll Cardiol* 61:485, 2013.

19. Bonow RO, Mann DL, Zipes DP, et al: *Braunwald's heart disease: a textbook of cardiovascular medicine*, ed 9, St Louis, 2012, Saunders.

20. Evangelista O, McLaughlin MA: Review of cardiovascular risk factors in women, *Gend Med* 6(Suppl 1):17, 2009.

*21. Jneid H, Anderson JL, Wright RS, Adams CD, et al: 2012 ACCF/AHA focused update of the guidelines for the management of patients with unstable angina/non-ST-elevation myocardial infarction (updating the 2007 guideline and replacing the 2011 focused update), *J Am Coll Cardiol* 126:875, 2012.

*22. Levine GN, Bates ER, Blankenship JC, et al: 2011 ACCF/AHA/SCAI guideline for percutaneous coronary intervention, *J Am Coll Cardiol* 58:1, 2011.

23. Krumholz HM, Anderson JL, Bachelder BL, et al: ACC/AHA 2008 performance measures for adults with ST-elevation and non ST-elevation myocardial infarction, *Circulation* 118:2596, 2008.

*24. Hillis LD, Smith PK, Anderson JL, et al: 2011 ACCF/AHA guideline for coronary artery bypass graft surgery, *J Am Coll Cardiol* 58:1, 2011.

25. Bojar RM: *Manual of perioperative care in adult cardiac surgery*, ed 5, Hoboken, NJ, 2011, Wiley-Blackwell.

26. American Association of Critical-Care Nurses: Family presence: visitation in the adult ICU (2011). Retrieved from *www.aacn.org/WD/practice/content/practicealerts/family-visitation-icu-practice-alert.content.*

27. Caza N, Taha R, Qi Y, et al: The effects of surgery and anesthesia on memory and cognition, *Prog Brain Res* 169:409, 2008.

28. Lichtman JH, Bigger T, Blumenthal JA, et al: Depression and coronary heart disease: recommendations for screening, referral, and treatment, *Circulation* 118:1768, 2008.

*29. Levine GN, Steinke EE, Bakaeen FG, et al: Sexual activity and cardiovascular disease: a scientific statement from the American Heart Association, *Circulation* 125:1058, 2012.

30. Mudawi TO, Albouaini K, Kaye GC: Sudden cardiac death: history, aetiology and management, *Br J Hosp Med* 70:89, 2009.

31. Exner DV: Implantable cardioverter defibrillator therapy for patients with less severe left ventricular dysfunction, *Curr Opin Cardiol* 24:61, 2009.

RESOURCES

American College of Cardiology
www.acc.org

American Heart Association
www.heart.org/HEARTORG/GettingHealthy/GettingHealthy_UCM_001078_SubHomePage.jsp

International Society for Minimally Invasive Cardiothoracic Surgery
www.ismics.org

Mended Hearts
www.mendedhearts.org

National Heart, Lung, and Blood Institute of the National Institutes of Health—Health Topics
www.nhlbi.nih.gov/health/health-topics/by-alpha/#

Preventive Cardiovascular Nurses Association
www.pcna.net

CHAPTER 35

A joyful heart is good medicine, but a crushed spirit dries up the bones.
Proverbs 17:22

Nursing Management
Heart Failure

Carolyn Moffa

evolve WEBSITE

http://evolve.elsevier.com/Lewis/medsurg

- NCLEX Review Questions
- Key Points
- Pre-Test
- Answer Guidelines for Case Study on p. 785
- Rationales for Bridge to NCLEX Examination Questions
- Case Study
  - Patient With Heart Failure
- Nursing Care Plan (Customizable)
  - NCP 35-1: Patient With Heart Failure
- Concept Map Creator
- Concept Map for Case Study on p. 785
- Glossary
- Content Updates

eTable

- eTable 35-1: Who Is the Patient With Heart Failure? Think FACES

LEARNING OUTCOMES

1. Compare the pathophysiology of systolic and diastolic ventricular failure.
2. Relate the compensatory mechanisms involved in heart failure (HF) to the development of acute decompensated heart failure (ADHF) and chronic HF.
3. Select appropriate nursing and collaborative interventions to manage the patient with ADHF.
4. Select appropriate nursing and collaborative interventions to manage the patient with chronic HF.
5. Describe the indications for cardiac transplantation and the nursing management of cardiac transplant recipients.

KEY TERMS

cardiac transplantation, p. 783
diastolic failure, p. 767
heart failure (HF), p. 766
paroxysmal nocturnal dyspnea (PND), p. 771
pulmonary edema, p. 770
systolic failure, p. 767

HEART FAILURE

Heart failure (HF) is an abnormal clinical syndrome that involves inadequate pumping and/or filling of the heart. It is a major health problem in the United States. This chapter discusses the management and nursing care of patients experiencing this syndrome.

HF causes the heart to be unable to provide sufficient blood to meet the oxygen needs of the tissues. In clinical practice, the terms *acute* and *chronic HF* have replaced the term *congestive HF* (CHF) because not all HF involves pulmonary congestion. However, the term *CHF* is still commonly used.[1,2]

HF is associated with numerous cardiovascular diseases, particularly long-standing hypertension, coronary artery disease (CAD), and myocardial infarction (MI). Unlike other cardiovascular diseases, HF is increasing in incidence and prevalence. This is due to improved survival after cardiac events and the growing aging population. Currently, about 5.1 million people in the United States have HF. The American Heart Association (AHA) estimates that over 600,000 new cases are diagnosed each year. HF is primarily a disease of older adults; approximately 10 in every 1000 persons over the age of 65 have HF. The incidence of HF is similar in men and women.[3]

HF is the most common reason for hospital admission in older adults. This places a significant economic burden on the health care system.[1] The complex, progressive nature of HF often results in poor outcomes, the most costly being hospital readmissions.[3]

Reviewed by Evelyn Dean, RN, MSN, ACNS-BC, CCRN, Clinical Nurse Specialist, Heart Failure Department, Mid America Heart Institute, Saint Luke's Hospital of Kansas City, Kansas City, Missouri; Carla V. Hannon, MS, APRN, CCRN, Clinical Nurse Specialist, Intensive Care Unit, Hospital of Saint Raphael, New Haven, Connecticut; Kathleen M. Hill, RN, MSN, CCNS, Clinical Nurse Specialist, Surgical Intensive Care Unit, Cleveland Clinic, Cleveland, Ohio; and Christina D. Keller, RN, MSN, Instructor, Radford University School of Nursing: Clinical Simulation Center, Radford, Virginia.

CULTURAL & ETHNIC HEALTH DISPARITIES

Heart Failure

- African Americans have a higher incidence of HF, develop HF at an earlier age, and experience higher mortality rates related to HF than whites.
- African Americans may experience more ACE inhibitor–related angioedema than whites.
- Isosorbide dinitrate/hydralazine (BiDil) is used for the treatment of HF in African Americans. This co-packaged drug is approved for use only in this ethnic group.
- Asians have an extremely high risk (15%-50%) for ACE inhibitor–related cough.

ACE, Angiotensin-converting enzyme; *HF,* heart failure.

Etiology and Pathophysiology

Hypertension and CAD are the primary risk factors for HF. Most patients with HF have a history of hypertension. The risk of HF increases with the severity of hypertension. Other factors, such as diabetes, advanced age, tobacco use, obesity, and high serum cholesterol, also contribute to the development of HF.

HF may be caused by any interference with the normal mechanisms regulating cardiac output (CO). CO depends on (1) preload, (2) afterload, (3) myocardial contractility, and (4) heart rate (HR). (Preload and afterload are discussed in Chapter 32.) Any changes in these factors can lead to decreased ventricular function and HF.

The major causes of HF may be divided into two subgroups: (1) primary causes (Table 35-1) and (2) precipitating causes (Table 35-2). Precipitating causes often increase the workload of the ventricles, resulting in an acute condition and decreased heart function.

Genetic Link

Specific genes and gene mutations have been linked to the development of hypertension, CAD, and cardiomyopathy (weakening of the heart muscle) (see Chapters 33, 34, and 37). These cardiovascular diseases are known risk factors for HF. Knowledge of why some people with these diseases are at high risk for developing HF is incomplete. Future research into the effects of these gene mutations will most likely be related to the common causes of HF.[4]

Pathophysiology of Ventricular Failure. HF is classified as systolic or diastolic failure (or dysfunction). Patients can have isolated systolic or diastolic failure or a combination of both.

Systolic Failure. Systolic failure results from an inability of the heart to pump blood effectively. It is caused by impaired contractile function (e.g., MI), increased afterload (e.g., hypertension), cardiomyopathy, and mechanical abnormalities (e.g., valvular heart disease).

The left ventricle (LV) in systolic failure loses its ability to generate enough pressure to eject blood forward through the aorta. Over time, the LV becomes dilated and hypertrophied. The hallmark of systolic failure is a decrease in the left ventricular ejection fraction (EF). The EF is defined as the amount of blood ejected from the LV with each contraction. Normal EF is 55% to 60%. Patients with systolic HF generally have an EF less than 45%. It can be as low as 10%.

Diastolic Failure. Diastolic failure is the inability of the ventricles to relax and fill during diastole. Diastolic failure is often referred to as HF with normal EF. Decreased filling of the ventricles results in decreased stroke volume and CO. Diastolic failure is characterized by high filling pressures because of stiff ventricles. This results in venous engorgement in both the pulmonary and systemic vascular systems. Diastolic failure is usually the result of left ventricular hypertrophy from hypertension (most common), myocardial ischemia, valve disease (e.g., aortic, mitral), or cardiomyopathy. However, many patients do not have an identifiable heart disease. The diagnosis of diastolic failure is made based on the presence of HF symptoms with a normal EF.[5] Diastolic failure occurs more frequently in older adults, women, and people who are obese (see Gender Differences box).

Mixed Systolic and Diastolic Failure. Mixed systolic and diastolic failure is seen in disease states such as dilated cardiomyopathy (DCM). DCM is a condition in which poor systolic function is further compromised by dilated left ventricular walls that are unable to relax (see Chapter 37). These patients often have extremely low EFs (less than 35%), high pulmonary pressures, and *biventricular failure* (both ventricles are dilated and have poor filling and emptying capacity).

The patient with ventricular failure of any type may have low blood pressure (BP), low CO, and poor renal perfusion. Poor

TABLE 35-1 PRIMARY CAUSES OF HEART FAILURE

- Coronary artery disease, including myocardial infarction
- Hypertension, including hypertensive crisis
- Rheumatic heart disease
- Congenital heart defects (e.g., ventricular septal defect)
- Pulmonary hypertension
- Cardiomyopathy (e.g., viral, postpartum, substance abuse)
- Hyperthyroidism
- Valvular disorders (e.g., mitral stenosis)
- Myocarditis

TABLE 35-2 PRECIPITATING CAUSES OF HEART FAILURE*

Cause	Mechanism
Anemia	↓ O_2-carrying capacity of the blood stimulating ↑ in CO to meet tissue demands, leading to increase in cardiac workload and increase in size of LV
Infection	↑ O_2 demand of tissues, stimulating ↑ CO
Thyrotoxicosis	Changes the tissue metabolic rate, ↑ HR and workload of the heart
Hypothyroidism	Indirectly predisposes to ↑ atherosclerosis; severe hypothyroidism decreases myocardial contractility
Dysrhythmias	May ↓ CO and ↑ workload and O_2 requirements of myocardial tissue
Bacterial endocarditis	*Infection:* ↑ metabolic demands and O_2 requirements *Valvular dysfunction:* causes stenosis and regurgitation
Pulmonary embolism	↑ Pulmonary pressure resulting from obstruction leads to pulmonary hypertension, ↓ CO
Paget's disease	↑ Workload of the heart by ↑ vascular bed in the skeletal muscle
Nutritional deficiencies	May ↓ cardiac function by ↑ myocardial muscle mass and myocardial contractility
Hypervolemia	↑ Preload causing volume overload on the RV

*List is not all inclusive.
CO, Cardiac output; *LV,* left ventricle; *RV,* right ventricle.

GENDER DIFFERENCES

Heart Failure

Men	Women
• Men experience systolic failure more frequently than women. • Men with asymptomatic systolic failure experience greater mortality benefit from ACE inhibitor therapy than women.	• Women experience diastolic failure more frequently than men. • Women have a higher risk of ACE inhibitor–related cough than men. • Women experience more digitalis-related death than men. • Women with diabetes are more predisposed to heart failure than men.

ACE, Angiotensin-converting enzyme.

exercise tolerance and heart dysrhythmias are also common. Whether a patient arrives at this point acutely from an MI or chronically from worsening cardiomyopathy or hypertension, the body's response to this low CO is to mobilize its compensatory mechanisms to maintain CO and BP.

Compensatory Mechanisms. HF can have an abrupt onset as with acute MI, or it can be a subtle process resulting from slow, progressive changes. The overloaded heart uses compensatory mechanisms to try to maintain adequate CO. The main compensatory mechanisms include (1) sympathetic nervous system (SNS) activation, (2) neurohormonal responses, (3) ventricular dilation, and (4) ventricular hypertrophy.

Sympathetic Nervous System Activation. SNS activation is often the first mechanism triggered in low-CO states. However, it is the least effective compensatory mechanism. In response to an inadequate stroke volume and CO, SNS activation increases, resulting in the increased release of catecholamines (epinephrine and norepinephrine). This results in increased HR, increased myocardial contractility, and peripheral vasoconstriction. Initially, this increase in HR and contractility improves CO. However, over time these factors are harmful, since they increase the already failing heart's workload and need for oxygen. The vasoconstriction causes an immediate increase in preload, which may initially increase CO. However, an increase in venous return to the heart, which is already volume overloaded, actually worsens ventricular performance.

Neurohormonal Response. As the CO falls, blood flow to the kidneys decreases. This is sensed by the juxtaglomerular apparatus in the kidneys as decreased volume. In response, the kidneys release renin, which converts angiotensinogen to angiotensin I (see Chapter 45 and Fig. 45-4). Angiotensin I is subsequently converted to angiotensin II by a converting enzyme made in the lungs. Angiotensin II causes (1) the adrenal cortex to release aldosterone, which results in sodium and water retention; and (2) increased peripheral vasoconstriction, which increases BP. This response is known as the renin-angiotensin-aldosterone system (RAAS).

Low CO causes a decrease in cerebral perfusion pressure. In response, the posterior pituitary gland secretes antidiuretic hormone (ADH), also called vasopressin. ADH increases water reabsorption in the kidneys, causing water retention. As a result, blood volume is increased in a person who is already volume overloaded.

Other factors also contribute to the development of HF. The production of *endothelin*, a potent vasoconstrictor produced by the vascular endothelial cells, is stimulated by ADH, catecholamines, and angiotensin II. Endothelin results in further arterial vasoconstriction and an increase in cardiac contractility and hypertrophy.

Locally, proinflammatory cytokines are released by heart cells in response to various forms of cardiac injury (e.g., MI). Two cytokines, tumor necrosis factor (TNF) and interleukin-1 (IL-1), further depress heart function by causing hypertrophy, contractile dysfunction, and cell death. Over time, a systemic inflammatory response also occurs. This accounts for the cardiac and skeletal muscle myopathy and fatigue that accompany advanced HF.

Activation of the SNS and the neurohormonal response lead to elevated levels of norepinephrine, angiotensin II, aldosterone, ADH, endothelin, and proinflammatory cytokines. Together, these factors result in an increase in cardiac workload, myocardial dysfunction, and *ventricular remodeling.* Remodeling involves hypertrophy of the ventricular myocytes, resulting in large, abnormally shaped contractile cells. This altered geometric shape of the ventricles eventually leads to increased ventricular mass, increased wall tension, increased oxygen consumption, and impaired contractility. Although the ventricles become larger, they become less effective pumps. Ventricular remodeling is a risk factor for life-threatening dysrhythmias and sudden cardiac death (SCD).

Dilation. *Dilation* is an enlargement of the chambers of the heart (Fig. 35-1, *A*). It occurs when pressure in the heart chambers (usually the LV) is elevated over time. The heart muscle fibers stretch in response to the volume of blood in the heart at the end of diastole. The degree of stretch is directly related to the force of the contraction (systole) (this is the *Frank-Starling law*). This increased contraction initially leads to increased CO and maintenance of BP and perfusion. Dilation starts as an adaptive mechanism to cope with increasing blood volume. Eventually this mechanism becomes inadequate because the elastic elements of the muscle fibers are overstretched and can no longer contract effectively, thereby decreasing the CO.

Hypertrophy. *Hypertrophy* is an increase in the muscle mass and cardiac wall thickness in response to overwork and strain (Fig. 35-1, *B*). It occurs slowly because it takes time for this increased muscle tissue to develop. Initially, the increased contractile power of the muscle fibers leads to an increase in CO and maintenance of tissue perfusion. Over time, hypertrophic heart muscle has poor contractility, requires more oxygen to perform work, has poor coronary artery circulation (tissue becomes ischemic more easily), and is prone to dysrhythmias.

Counterregulatory Mechanisms. The body's attempts to maintain balance are demonstrated by several counterregulatory processes. Natriuretic peptides (atrial natriuretic peptide [ANP] and brain, or b-type, natriuretic peptide [BNP]) are hormones produced by the heart muscle. ANP is released from the atria and BNP is released from the ventricles in response to increased blood volume in the heart.[6]

The natriuretic peptides have renal, cardiovascular, and hormonal effects. Renal effects include (1) increased glomerular filtration rate and diuresis and (2) excretion of sodium (natriuresis). Cardiovascular effects include vasodilation and decreased BP. Hormonal effects include (1) inhibition of aldosterone and renin secretion and (2) interference with ADH release. The combined effects of ANP and BNP help to counter the adverse effects of the SNS and RAAS in patients with HF.[5]

Nitric oxide (NO) is another counterregulatory substance released from the vascular endothelium in response to the compensatory mechanisms activated in HF. Like the natriuretic

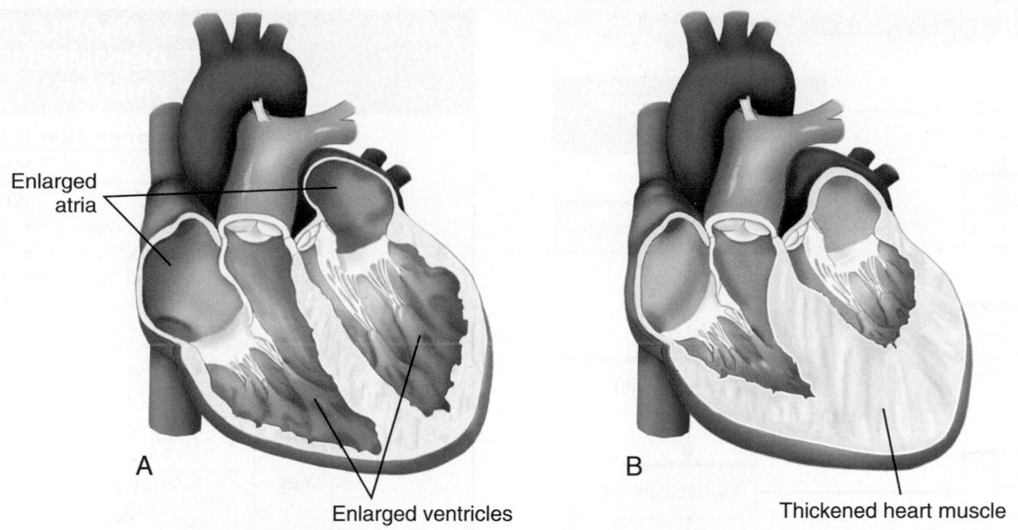

FIG. 35-1 A, Dilated heart chambers. **B,** Hypertrophied heart chambers.

peptides, NO works to relax the arterial smooth muscle, resulting in vasodilation and decreased afterload.

Cardiac compensation occurs when compensatory mechanisms succeed in maintaining an adequate CO that is needed for tissue perfusion. *Cardiac decompensation* occurs when these mechanisms can no longer maintain adequate CO and inadequate tissue perfusion results.

Types of Heart Failure

HF is usually manifested by biventricular failure, although one ventricle may precede the other in dysfunction. Normally the pumping actions of the left and right sides of the heart are synchronized, producing a continuous flow of blood. However, as a result of pathologic conditions, one side may fail while the other side continues to function normally for a time. Because of the prolonged strain, both sides of the heart eventually fail, resulting in biventricular failure (Fig. 35-2).

Left-Sided Heart Failure. The most common form of HF is left-sided HF. Left-sided HF results from left ventricular dysfunction. This prevents normal, forward blood flow and causes blood to back up into the left atrium and pulmonary veins. The increased pulmonary pressure causes fluid leakage from the pulmonary capillary bed into the interstitium and then the alveoli. This manifests as pulmonary congestion and edema.

Right-Sided Heart Failure. Right-sided HF occurs when the right ventricle (RV) fails to contract effectively. Right-sided HF causes a backup of blood into the right atrium and venous circulation. Venous congestion in the systemic circulation results in jugular venous distention, hepatomegaly, splenomegaly, vascular congestion of the gastrointestinal tract, and peripheral edema.

Right-sided HF may result from an acute condition such as right ventricular infarction or pulmonary embolism. *Cor pulmonale* (right ventricular dilation and hypertrophy caused by pulmonary disease) can also cause right-sided HF (see Chapters 28 and 29).

The primary cause of right-sided HF is left-sided HF. In this situation, left-sided HF results in pulmonary congestion and increased pressure in the blood vessels of the lung (pulmonary hypertension). Eventually, chronic pulmonary hypertension (increased right ventricular afterload) results in right-sided hypertrophy and HF.

Clinical Manifestations

Acute Decompensated Heart Failure

In acute decompensated HF (ADHF), an increase in the pulmonary venous pressure is caused by failure of the LV. This results in engorgement of the pulmonary vascular system (Fig. 35-3, *A* and *B*). As a result, the lungs become less compliant, and there is increased resistance in the small airways. In addition, the lymphatic system increases its flow to help maintain a constant volume of the pulmonary extravascular fluid. This early stage is clinically associated with a mild increase in the respiratory rate and a decrease in partial pressure of oxygen in arterial blood (PaO_2).

If pulmonary venous pressure continues to increase, the increase in intravascular pressure causes more fluid to move into the interstitial space than the lymphatics can remove. *Interstitial edema* occurs at this point (Fig. 35-3, *C*). Tachypnea develops, and the patient becomes symptomatic (e.g., short of breath). If the pulmonary venous pressure increases further, the alveoli lining cells are disrupted and a fluid containing red blood cells (RBCs) moves into the alveoli *(alveolar edema)*. As the disruption becomes worse from further increases in the pulmonary venous pressure, the alveoli and airways are flooded with fluid. This is accompanied by a worsening of the arterial blood gas values (i.e., lower PaO_2 and possible increased partial pressure of carbon dioxide in arterial blood [$PaCO_2$] and progressive respiratory acidemia).

ADHF can manifest as **pulmonary edema.** This is an acute, life-threatening situation in which the lung alveoli become filled with serosanguineous fluid (Fig. 35-3, *D*). The most common cause of pulmonary edema is left-sided HF secondary to CAD. (Other etiologic factors for pulmonary edema are listed in Table 28-25.)

Clinical manifestations of pulmonary edema are distinct. The patient is usually anxious, pale, and possibly cyanotic. The skin is clammy and cold from vasoconstriction caused by stimulation of the SNS. The patient has *dyspnea* (shortness of breath) and *orthopnea* (shortness of breath while lying down). Respiratory rate is often greater than 30 breaths/minute, and use of accessory muscles to breathe may be seen. There may be wheezing and coughing with the production of frothy, blood-tinged sputum. Auscultation of the lungs may reveal crackles, wheezes, and rhonchi throughout the lungs. The patient's HR is rapid,

PATHOPHYSIOLOGY MAP

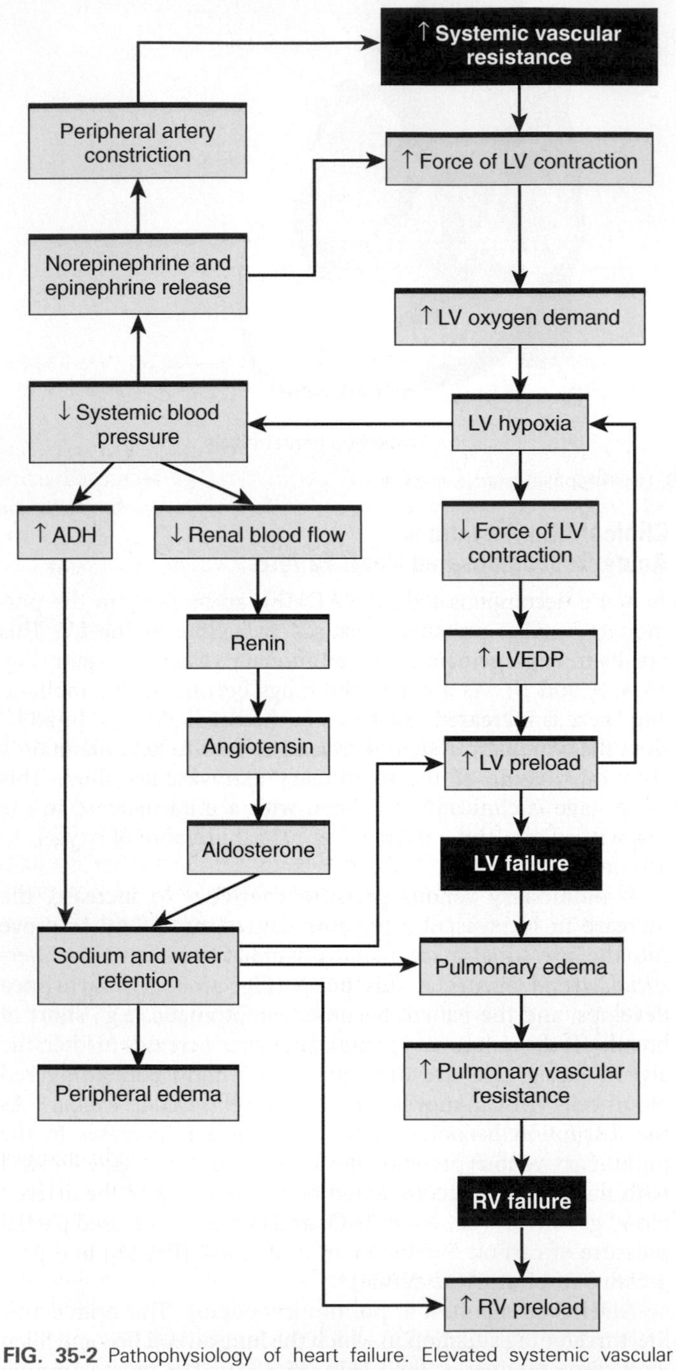

FIG. 35-2 Pathophysiology of heart failure. Elevated systemic vascular resistance results in left-sided heart failure that leads to right-sided heart failure. Systemic vascular resistance and preload are exacerbated by the renin-angiotensin-aldosterone system. *ADH,* Antidiuretic hormone; *LA,* left atrium; *LV,* left ventricle; *LVEDP,* left ventricular end-diastolic pressure; *RV,* right ventricle.

and BP may be elevated or decreased depending on the severity of the HF.

Patients with ADHF can be categorized into one of four groups based on hemodynamic and clinical status: dry-warm, dry-cold, wet-warm, and wet-cold[1] (Table 35-3). The most common presentation is the warm and wet patient. This patient has adequate perfusion (warm) but has volume overload (e.g., congestion, dyspnea, edema).

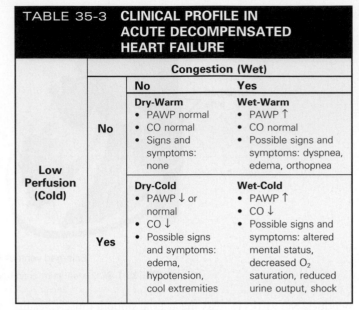

TABLE 35-3 CLINICAL PROFILE IN ACUTE DECOMPENSATED HEART FAILURE

		Congestion (Wet)	
		No	**Yes**
Low Perfusion (Cold)	**No**	**Dry-Warm** • PAWP normal • CO normal • Signs and symptoms: none	**Wet-Warm** • PAWP ↑ • CO normal • Possible signs and symptoms: dyspnea, edema, orthopnea
	Yes	**Dry-Cold** • PAWP ↓ or normal • CO ↓ • Possible signs and symptoms: edema, hypotension, cool extremities	**Wet-Cold** • PAWP ↑ • CO ↓ • Possible signs and symptoms: altered mental status, decreased O_2 saturation, reduced urine output, shock

CO, Cardiac output; *PAWP,* pulmonary artery wedge pressure.

Clinical Manifestations

Chronic Heart Failure

Chronic HF is characterized as a progressive worsening of ventricular function and chronic neurohormonal activation that results in ventricular remodeling. This process involves changes in the size, shape, and mechanical performance of the ventricle. The clinical manifestations of chronic HF depend on the patient's age, the underlying type and extent of heart disease, and which ventricle is failing to pump effectively. Table 35-4 lists the manifestations of right-sided and left-sided chronic HF. The patient with chronic HF usually has manifestations of biventricular failure. The Heart Failure Society of America (HFSA) developed the acronym FACES (*F*atigue, limitation of *A*ctivities, chest *C*ongestion/cough, *E*dema, and *S*hortness of breath) to help teach patients to identify HF symptoms[7] (see eTable 35-1 on the website for this chapter).

Fatigue. Fatigue is one of the earliest symptoms of chronic HF. The patient notes fatigue after usual activities and eventually limits these activities. The fatigue is caused by decreased CO, impaired perfusion to vital organs, decreased oxygenation of the tissues, and anemia. Anemia can result from poor nutrition, renal disease, or drug therapy (e.g., angiotensin-converting enzyme [ACE] inhibitors).

Dyspnea. Dyspnea is a common manifestation of chronic HF. It is caused by increased pulmonary pressures secondary to interstitial and alveolar edema. Dyspnea can occur with mild exertion or at rest. Orthopnea often accompanies dyspnea. Careful questioning of patients often reveals adaptive behaviors such as sleeping with two or more pillows or in a chair to aid breathing.

Paroxysmal nocturnal dyspnea (PND) occurs when the patient is asleep. It is caused by the reabsorption of fluid from dependent body areas when the patient is flat. The patient awakes in a panic, has feelings of suffocation, and has a strong desire to sit or stand up.

A cough is often associated with HF and may be the first clinical symptom. It begins as a dry, nonproductive cough and may be misdiagnosed as asthma or other lung disease. The

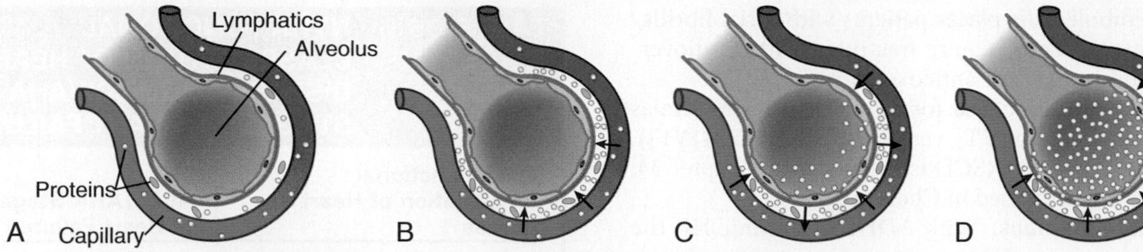

FIG. 35-3 As pulmonary edema progresses, it inhibits oxygen and carbon dioxide exchange at the alveolar-capillary interface. **A,** Normal relationship. **B,** Increased pulmonary capillary hydrostatic pressure causes fluid to move from the vascular space into the pulmonary interstitial space. **C,** Lymphatic flow increases in an attempt to pull fluid back into the vascular or lymphatic space. **D,** Failure of lymphatic flow and worsening of left-sided heart failure result in further movement of fluid into the interstitial space and into the alveoli.

TABLE 35-4 MANIFESTATIONS OF HEART FAILURE

Right-Sided Heart Failure	Left-Sided Heart Failure
Signs	
• RV heaves	• LV heaves
• Murmurs	• Pulsus alternans (alternating pulses: strong, weak)
• Jugular venous distention	• ↑ HR
• Edema (e.g., pedal, scrotum, sacrum)	• PMI displaced inferiorly and posteriorly (LV hypertrophy)
• Weight gain	• ↓ PaO_2, slight ↑ $PaCO_2$ (poor O_2 exchange)
• ↑ HR	• Crackles (pulmonary edema)
• Ascites	• S_3 and S_4 heart sounds
• Anasarca (massive generalized body edema)	• Pleural effusion
• Hepatomegaly (liver enlargement)	• Changes in mental status
	• Restlessness, confusion
Symptoms	
• Fatigue	• Weakness, fatigue
• Anxiety, depression	• Anxiety, depression
• Dependent, bilateral edema	• Dyspnea
• Right upper quadrant pain	• Shallow respirations up to 32-40/min
• Anorexia and GI bloating	• Paroxysmal nocturnal dyspnea
• Nausea	• Orthopnea (shortness of breath in recumbent position)
	• Dry, hacking cough
	• Nocturia
	• Frothy, pink-tinged sputum (advanced pulmonary edema)

LV, Left ventricle; *$PaCO_2$,* partial pressure of CO_2 in arterial blood; *PaO_2,* partial pressure of O_2 in arterial blood; *PMI,* point of maximal impulse; *RV,* right ventricle.

cough is not relieved by position change or over-the-counter cough medicine.

Tachycardia. Tachycardia is an early clinical sign of HF. One of the body's first mechanisms to compensate for a failing ventricle is to increase the HR. Because of reduced CO, the SNS is activated, which increases HR. However, this response may be blocked or reduced in patients taking β-blocker medications.

Edema. Edema is a common sign of HF. It may occur in dependent body areas (peripheral edema), liver (hepatomegaly), abdominal cavity (ascites), and lungs (pulmonary edema and pleural effusion). If the patient is in bed, sacral and scrotal edema may develop. Pressing the edematous skin with the finger may leave a transient depression *(pitting edema).* The development of dependent edema or a sudden weight gain of more than 3 lb (1.4 kg) in 2 days is often a sign of ADHF. It is important to note that not all lower extremity edema is a result of HF. Hypoproteinemia, immobility, venous insufficiency, and certain medications can cause peripheral edema.

Nocturia. A person with chronic HF who has decreased CO will also have impaired renal perfusion and decreased urine output during the day. However, when the person lies down at night, fluid moves from the interstitial spaces back into the circulatory system. In addition, cardiac workload is decreased at night while resting. These combined effects result in increased renal blood flow and diuresis. The patient may complain of having to void frequently throughout the night.

Skin Changes. Because tissue capillary oxygen extraction is increased in a person with chronic HF, the skin may appear dusky. Often the lower extremities are shiny and swollen, with diminished or absent hair growth. Chronic swelling may result in pigment changes. This causes the skin to appear brown or brawny in areas covering the ankles and lower legs.

Behavioral Changes. Cerebral circulation may be reduced with chronic HF secondary to decreased CO. The patient or caregiver may report unusual behavior, including restlessness, confusion, and decreased attention span or memory. This may also be secondary to poor gas exchange and worsening HF. It is often seen in the late stages of HF.

Chest Pain. HF can precipitate chest pain (angina) because of decreased coronary artery perfusion from decreased CO and increased myocardial work. Chest pain may accompany either ADHF or chronic HF.

Weight Changes. Many factors contribute to weight changes. First, a progressive weight gain may occur because of fluid retention. Renal failure may also contribute to fluid retention. Abdominal fullness from ascites and hepatomegaly frequently causes anorexia and nausea. As HF advances, the patient may have cardiac *cachexia* with muscle wasting and fat loss. This can be masked by the patient's edematous condition and may not be seen until after the edema subsides.

Complications of Heart Failure

Pleural Effusion. *Pleural effusion* results from increasing pressure in the pleural capillaries. A transudation of fluid occurs from these capillaries into the pleural space. (Pleural effusion is discussed in Chapter 28.)

Dysrhythmias. Chronic HF causes enlargement of the chambers of the heart. This enlargement (stretching of the atrial and ventricular walls) can cause changes in the normal electrical pathways. When numerous sites in the atria fire spontaneously and rapidly (atrial fibrillation), the organized atrial depolarization (contraction) no longer occurs. Atrial fibrillation also promotes thrombus formation within the atria. Thrombi may break loose and form emboli. This places patients with atrial fibrillation at risk for stroke. They require treatment with cardioversion, antidysrhythmics, and/or anticoagulants.

Patients with HF are also at risk for ventricular dysrhythmias (e.g., ventricular tachycardia [VT], ventricular fibrillation [VF]). VT and VF can lead to SCD. (SCD is discussed in Chapter 34, and dysrhythmias are discussed in Chapter 36.)

Left Ventricular Thrombus. With ADHF or chronic HF, the enlarged LV and decreased CO combine to increase the chance of thrombus formation in the LV. Once a thrombus has formed, it may also decrease left ventricular contractility, decrease CO, and worsen the patient's perfusion. The development of emboli from the thrombus also places the patient at risk for stroke.

Hepatomegaly. HF can lead to severe hepatomegaly, especially with RV failure. The liver becomes congested with venous blood. The hepatic congestion leads to impaired liver function. Eventually liver cells die, fibrosis occurs, and cirrhosis can develop (see Chapter 44).

Renal Failure. The decreased CO that accompanies chronic HF results in decreased perfusion to the kidneys and can lead to renal insufficiency or failure (see Chapter 47).

Classification of Heart Failure

In 1964 the New York Heart Association (NYHA) developed functional guidelines for classifying people with heart disease based on tolerance to physical activity. Because this system only reflected exercise capacity, the American College of Cardiology Foundation/AHA (ACCF/AHA) developed a staging system that identified disease progression and treatment strategies.[1] This system allows for identification of people at risk for developing HF but who do not currently have heart disease. The ACCF/AHA system encourages clinicians to actively address the patient's risk factors and treat any existing conditions to prevent further disease progression. This may help reduce the growing number of HF patients. The two systems are compared in Table 35-5.

Diagnostic Studies

Diagnosing HF is often difficult, since neither patient signs nor symptoms are highly specific, and both may mimic those associated with many other medical conditions (e.g., anemia, lung disease). Diagnostic tests for ADHF and chronic HF are presented in Table 35-6. A primary goal in diagnosis is to find the underlying cause of HF.

An endomyocardial biopsy (EMB) may be done in patients who develop unexplained, new-onset HF that is unresponsive to usual care.[8] EF is used to differentiate systolic and diastolic HF. This distinction is important to make in the early treatment of HF. EF is measured using echocardiography and/or nuclear imaging studies (see Table 32-6). Other useful diagnostic tests include electrocardiogram (ECG), chest x-ray, and heart catheterization.

Laboratory studies also aid in the diagnosis of HF. In general, BNP levels correlate positively with the degree of left ventricular failure. Many laboratories routinely measure the N-terminal prohormone of BNP (NT-proBNP). This is a more precise assay to aid in the diagnosis of HF (see Table 32-6). Levels are temporarily higher in patients receiving nesiritide (Natrecor) and may be high in patients with chronic, stable HF. Increases in BNP or NT-proBNP levels can be caused by conditions other than HF. These conditions include pulmonary embolism, renal failure, and acute coronary syndrome.

TABLE 35-5 NYHA FUNCTIONAL CLASSIFICATION OF HEART DISEASE AND ACCF/AHA STAGES OF HEART FAILURE

NYHA Functional Classification of Heart Disease	ACCF/AHA Stages of Heart Failure
Class I No limitation of physical activity. Ordinary physical activity does not cause fatigue, dyspnea, palpitations, or anginal pain.	**Stage A** Patients at high risk for HF (e.g., patients with hypertension, diabetes, metabolic syndrome) but without structural heart disease or symptoms of HF.
Class II Slight limitation of physical activity. No symptoms at rest. Ordinary physical activity results in fatigue, dyspnea, palpitations, or anginal pain.	**Stage B** Patients with structural heart disease (e.g., patients with history of MI, valve disease) but who have never shown signs or symptoms of HF.
Class III Marked limitation of physical activity but usually comfortable at rest. Less than ordinary physical activity causes fatigue, dyspnea, palpitations, or anginal pain.	**Stage C** Patients with prior or current symptoms of HF associated with known, underlying structural heart disease.
Class IV Inability to carry on any physical activity without discomfort. Symptoms of cardiac insufficiency or of angina may be present even at rest. If any physical activity is undertaken, discomfort is increased.	**Stage D** Patients with refractory HF (e.g., patients with severe symptoms at rest despite maximal medical therapy) who require specialized interventions.

Sources: The Criteria Committee of the New York Heart Association: *Nomenclature and criteria for diagnosis of diseases of the heart and great vessels,* ed 9, Boston, 1994, Little, Brown & Co. and Yancy CW, Jessup M, Bozkurt B, et al: 2013 ACCF/AHA guideline for the management of heart failure: executive summary, *Circulation* 128:e1, 2013.
ACCF/AHA, American College of Cardiology Foundation/American Heart Association; *HF,* heart failure; *MI,* myocardial infarction; *NYHA,* New York Heart Association.

Collaborative Care
Acute Decompensated Heart Failure

With the addition of new drugs and device therapies, the management of HF has dramatically changed in the past few years. Because of the large number of patients and the high cost of care related to hospital readmissions, strategies to improve outcomes have been developed. One example is the use of guideline-directed medical therapy as defined by the AACF/AHA.[1] Another example is specialized HF inpatient units with transitional programs to the outpatient setting to help manage these patients. These units are staffed with multidisciplinary HF teams, including nurses who are educated in the care of these patients. Table 35-6 lists the collaborative therapy for the patient with ADHF.

Patients with ADHF need continuous monitoring and assessment. This may be done in an intensive care unit (ICU) if the patient is unstable. In the ICU, you will monitor ECG and oxygen saturation continuously. Assess vital signs and urine output at least every hour. The patient may have hemodynamic monitoring, including intraarterial BP and pulmonary artery pressures (PAPs). If a pulmonary artery catheter is placed, eval-

TABLE 35-6 **COLLABORATIVE CARE**

Heart Failure

Both ADHF and Chronic HF	ADHF	Chronic HF
Diagnostic		
• History and physical examination • Determination of underlying cause • Serum chemistries, cardiac markers, BNP or NT-proBNP level (see Table 32-6), liver function tests, thyroid function tests, CBC, lipid profile, kidney function tests, urinalysis • Chest x-ray • 12-lead ECG • Hemodynamic monitoring • 2-dimensional echocardiogram • Nuclear imaging studies (see Table 32-6) • Cardiac catheterization	• Measurement of LV function • Endomyocardial biopsy	• Exercise stress testing
Collaborative Therapy		
• Treatment of underlying cause • Circulatory assist devices (e.g., ventricular assist device) • Daily weights • Sodium- and, possibly, fluid-restricted diet	• High Fowler's position • O_2 by mask or nasal cannula • BiPAP • Circulatory assist device: intraaortic balloon pump • Endotracheal intubation and mechanical ventilation • Vital signs, urine output at least q1hr • Continuous ECG and pulse oximetry monitoring • Hemodynamic monitoring (e.g., intraarterial BP, PAWP, CO) • Drug therapy (see Table 35-7) • Possible cardioversion (e.g., atrial fibrillation) • Ultrafiltration	• O_2 therapy at 2-6 L/min by nasal cannula if indicated • Rest-activity periods • Cardiac rehabilitation • Home health nursing care (e.g., telehealth monitoring) • Drug therapy (see Table 35-7) • Cardiac resynchronization therapy with biventricular pacing and internal cardioverter-defibrillator • LVAD • Cardiac transplantation • Palliative and end-of-life care

ADHF, Acute decompensated heart failure; *BiPAP,* bilevel positive airway pressure; *BNP,* b-type natriuretic peptide; *CO,* cardiac output; *HF,* heart failure; *LVAD,* left ventricular assist device; *NT-proBNP,* N-terminal prohormone of BNP; *PAWP,* pulmonary artery wedge pressure.

uate CO and pulmonary artery wedge pressure (PAWP). Therapy is titrated to maximize CO and reduce PAWP. A normal PAWP is generally between 8 and 12 mm Hg. Patients with ADHF may have a PAWP as high as 30 mm Hg. (Hemodynamic monitoring is discussed in Chapter 66.)

Supplemental oxygen helps increase the percentage of oxygen in inspired air. (Oxygen therapy is discussed in Chapter 29.) In severe pulmonary edema the patient may need noninvasive ventilatory support (e.g., bilevel positive airway pressure [BiPAP]) or intubation and mechanical ventilation. BiPAP is also effective in decreasing preload. (Ventilatory support is discussed in Chapter 66.)

Some patients with ADHF require hospitalization but are more stable. They are often admitted to a telemetry or stepdown unit for treatment. Assess these patients every 4 hours (e.g., vital signs, pulse oximetry) for adequate oxygenation. Record intake and output and daily weights to evaluate fluid status.

If the patient is dyspneic, place in a high Fowler's position with the feet horizontal in the bed or dangling at the bedside. This position helps decrease venous return because of the pooling of blood in the extremities. This position also increases the thoracic capacity, allowing for improved breathing.

Ultrafiltration (UF), or *aquapheresis,* is an option for the patient with volume overload.[9] It is a process to remove excess salt and water from the patient's blood. UF can rapidly remove intravascular fluid volume while maintaining hemodynamic stability. The ideal patients for UF are those with major pulmonary or systemic volume overload who have shown resistance to diuretics and are hemodynamically stable. UF also may be an appropriate adjunctive therapy for patients with HF and coexisting renal failure. (UF is discussed in Chapter 47.) Once the patient is more stable, determination of the cause of ADHF and pulmonary edema is important. Diagnosis of systolic or diastolic HF will then direct further management protocols.

Circulatory assist devices are used to manage patients with worsening HF. The intraaortic balloon pump (IABP) is a device that increases coronary blood flow to the heart muscle and decreases the heart's workload through a process called counterpulsation. It is useful in hemodynamically unstable patients because it decreases SVR, PAWP, and PAP, leading to improved CO. Ventricular assist devices (VADs) can be used to maintain the pumping action of a heart that cannot effectively contract by itself. A VAD is a battery-operated, mechanical pump that is surgically implanted. (IABPs and VADs are discussed in Chapter 66.)

Coexisting psychologic disorders, especially depression and anxiety, contribute to an increased risk of mortality and higher readmission rates and health care costs in patients with HF.[10] In addition, patients with psychologic disorders have poorer adherence to treatment and self-care.[11] Assess patients with HF for depression and anxiety and, if appropriate, initiate treatment plans.

Drug Therapy. Drug therapy is essential in treating ADHF (Table 35-7).

Diuretics. Diuretics are the mainstay of treatment in patients with volume overload. Diuretics act to decrease sodium reabsorption at various sites within the nephrons, thereby enhancing sodium and water loss. Decreasing intravascular volume with the use of diuretics reduces venous return (preload) and subsequently the volume returning to the LV. This allows the

TABLE 35-7 DRUG THERAPY

Heart Failure

Drug	Mechanism of Action
Diuretics (see Table 33-7) ***Loop Diuretics*** • furosemide (Lasix) • bumetanide (Bumex) ***Thiazide Diuretics**** • hydrochlorothiazide (HCTZ) • metolazone (Zaroxolyn) ***Potassium-Sparing Diuretics*** • spironolactone (Aldactone) • eplerenone (Inspra)	• Decrease fluid volume • Decrease preload • Decrease pulmonary venous pressure • Relieve symptoms of heart failure (e.g., edema)
Renin-Angiotensin-Aldosterone System Inhibitors (see Table 33-7) ***ACE Inhibitors*** • captopril (Capoten) • benazepril (Lotensin) • enalapril (Vasotec) ***Angiotensin II Receptor Blockers*** • losartan (Cozaar) • valsartan (Diovan)	• Dilate venules and arterioles • Improve renal blood flow • Decrease fluid volume • Relieve symptoms of heart failure • Promote reverse remodeling • Decrease morbidity and mortality
Vasodilators • hydralazine (Apresoline)* • isosorbide dinitrate/hydralazine (BiDil)* • nitrates (e.g., nitroglycerin [Nitro-Bid], isosorbide dinitrate [Isordil]) • nesiritide (Natrecor)† • nitroprusside (Nipride)†	• Reduce cardiac afterload, leading to increased CO • Dilate the arterioles of the kidneys, leading to increased renal perfusion and fluid loss • Decrease BP • Decrease preload • Relieve symptoms of heart failure (e.g., dyspnea)
β-Adrenergic Blockers* (see Table 33-7) • metoprolol (Toprol XL) • bisoprolol (Zebeta) • carvedilol (Coreg)	• Promote reverse remodeling • Decrease afterload • Inhibit SNS • Decrease morbidity and mortality
Positive Inotropes ***β-Adrenergic Agonists†*** • dopamine (Intropin) • dobutamine (Dobutrex) ***Phosphodiesterase Inhibitor†*** • milrinone (Primacor) ***Digitalis Glycoside**** • digoxin (Lanoxin)	• Increase contractility (positive inotropic effect) • Increase CO • Increase heart rate (positive chronotropic effect) • Produce mild vasodilation • Increase stroke volume and CO • Promote vasodilation
Morphine†	• Decreases anxiety • Decreases preload and afterload
Antidysrhythmic Drugs (see Table 36-9)	• Prevent or treat dysrhythmias
Anticoagulants	• Prevent thromboembolism • Recommended for patients with an ejection fraction <20% and/or atrial fibrillation

*Used for chronic HF only.
†Used for ADHF only.
ACE, Angiotensin-converting enzyme; *ADHF*, acute decompensated heart failure; *CO*, cardiac output; *SNS*, sympathetic nervous system.

LV to contract more efficiently. CO is increased, pulmonary vascular pressures are decreased, and gas exchange is improved. Loop diuretics (e.g., furosemide [Lasix], bumetanide [Bumex]) can be administered by IV push and act rapidly in the kidneys.

Vasodilators. IV nitroglycerin is a vasodilator that reduces circulating blood volume. It also improves coronary artery circulation by dilating the coronary arteries. Therefore nitroglycerin reduces preload, slightly reduces afterload (in high doses), and increases myocardial oxygen supply. When titrating IV nitroglycerin, monitor BP frequently (every 5 to 10 minutes) to avoid symptomatic hypotension.

Sodium nitroprusside (Nipride) is a potent IV vasodilator that reduces both preload and afterload, thus improving myocardial contraction, increasing CO, and reducing pulmonary congestion.[12] Complications of IV sodium nitroprusside include (1) hypotension; and (2) thiocyanate toxicity, which can develop after 48 hours of use. Sodium nitroprusside is administered in an ICU, since symptomatic hypotension is the main adverse effect.

DRUG ALERT: Sodium Nitroprusside (Nipride)
- Assess BP before administration and continuously (every 5-10 min) during administration.
- Too rapid rate of IV administration can reduce BP too quickly.
- Headache, nausea, dizziness, dyspnea, blurred vision, sweating, and restlessness can occur.

Nesiritide, administered IV, is a recombinant form of BNP and causes both arterial and venous dilation. The main hemodynamic effects of nesiritide include (1) a reduction in PAWP and (2) a decrease in systemic BP. Although classified as a vasodilator, nesiritide is also a neurohormonal blocking agent. It can be used for short-term treatment of ADHF.[1,13] Nesiritide does not require titration after the initial IV bolus. It can be given in the emergency department (ED) and non-ICU setting. Because the main adverse effect of nesiritide is symptomatic hypotension, monitor BP closely.

Morphine. Morphine sulfate reduces preload and afterload. It is frequently used in the treatment of acute coronary syndrome and HF. It dilates both the pulmonary and systemic blood vessels. Results include a decrease in pulmonary pressures and myocardial oxygen needs, and an improvement in gas exchange. When morphine is used, the patient often experiences relief from dyspnea and, consequently, the anxiety that often is associated with dyspnea.

Use morphine cautiously in patients with ADHF. Morphine is related to more adverse events, including a greater need for mechanical ventilation, more ICU admissions, prolonged hospitalization, and higher mortality rates.[14]

Positive Inotropes. Inotropic therapy increases myocardial contractility. Drugs include β-adrenergic agonists (e.g., dopamine [Intropin], dobutamine [Dobutrex], epinephrine, norepinephrine [Levophed]), the phosphodiesterase inhibitor milrinone (Primacor), and digitalis. The β-adrenergic agonists are only used as a short-term treatment of ADHF. In addition to increasing myocardial contractility and SVR, dopamine dilates the renal blood vessels and enhances urine output. Unlike dopamine, dobutamine is a selective β-adrenergic agonist and works primarily on the β_1-receptors in the heart. Dobutamine does not increase SVR and is preferred for short-term treatment of ADHF.[15]

DRUG ALERT: Dopamine (Intropin)
- Monitor IV site for signs of extravasation.
- Tissue necrosis with sloughing can occur with drug extravasation.
- High dosages may produce ventricular dysrhythmias.

Milrinone is a phosphodiesterase inhibitor that has been called an inodilator. It increases myocardial contractility (inotropic effect) and promotes peripheral vasodilation. Inhibition of phosphodiesterase increases cyclic adenosine monophosphate (cAMP). This enhances calcium entry into the cell and improves myocardial contractility. Milrinone increases CO and reduces BP (decrease afterload). Like dopamine and dobutamine, this drug is available only for IV use. Adverse effects include dysrhythmias, thrombocytopenia, and hepatotoxicity.

Digitalis is a positive inotrope that improves left ventricular function. Digitalis increases contractility but also increases myocardial oxygen consumption. Because digitalis requires a loading dose and time to work, it is not recommended for the initial treatment of ADHF.[15]

Currently, inotropic therapy is only recommended for use in the short-term management of patients with ADHF who have not responded to conventional pharmacotherapy (e.g., diuretics, vasodilators, morphine).[1]

Collaborative Care
Chronic Heart Failure

The main goals in the treatment of chronic HF are to treat the underlying cause and contributing factors, maximize CO, reduce symptoms, improve ventricular function, improve quality of life, preserve target organ function, and improve mortality and morbidity risks (see Table 35-6). The management of hypertension is discussed in Chapter 33, CAD in Chapter 34, dysrhythmias in Chapter 36, and valvular disorders in Chapter 37.

In a person with HF, oxygen saturation of the blood can be reduced because the blood is not adequately oxygenated in the lungs. Administration of oxygen improves saturation and assists in meeting tissue oxygen needs. This helps to relieve dyspnea and fatigue. Optimally pulse oximetry is used to monitor the need for and effectiveness of oxygen therapy.

Physical and emotional rest allows the patient to conserve energy and decreases the need for additional oxygen. The degree of rest recommended depends on the severity of HF. A patient with severe HF may be on bed rest with limited activity. A patient with mild to moderate HF can be ambulatory with restriction of strenuous activity. Instruct the patient to participate in prescribed activities with adequate recovery periods. A structured exercise program, such as cardiac rehabilitation, should be offered to all patients with chronic HF.

Nonpharmacologic therapies are an integral part of the care of HF patients. One therapy is *biventricular pacing* or *cardiac resynchronization therapy* (CRT). Traditional pacemakers pace one or two chambers (e.g., right atrium and/or right ventricle). In HF, neurohormonal effects and cardiac remodeling can result in dyssynchrony of the ventricular contractions. This contributes to poor CO. In CRT an extra pacing lead is placed through the coronary sinus to a coronary vein of the LV. This lead coordinates right and left ventricular contractions through biventricular pacing (Fig. 35-4). The ability to have normal electrical conduction (synchrony) between the RV and the LV increases left ventricular function and CO.

Life-threatening ventricular dysrhythmias (e.g., VT) can cause SCD. The addition of an implantable cardioverter-defibrillator (ICD) with CRT is often warranted. (Pacemakers and defibrillators are discussed in Chapter 36.)

Several mechanical options are available to sustain HF patients with deteriorating conditions, especially those awaiting cardiac transplantation. These include the IABP and VADs. However, the limitations of bed rest and the risk of infection and vascular complications preclude long-term use of IABP. VADs provide highly effective long-term support and have become standard care in many heart transplant centers. VADs are used as a bridge to transplantation. They effectively increase heart function until a donor heart becomes available. The use of a permanent, implantable VAD, known as *destination therapy*,

EVIDENCE-BASED PRACTICE
Translating Research Into Practice

Can Exercise Help Depression in Heart Failure Patients?

Clinical Question

For patients with heart failure (P), what is the effect of aerobic exercise (I) versus usual care (C) on depressive symptoms (O) at 3 and 12 mo (T)?

Best Available Evidence

Randomized controlled trial (RCT)

Critical Appraisal and Synthesis of Evidence

RCT of 82 medical centers (n = 2322) of patients with stable chronic heart failure.

- Intervention was aerobic exercise with a goal of 90 min/wk for months 1-3 followed by home exercise for ≥120 min/wk for months 4-12. Usual care was education and guideline-based heart failure care.
- Outcome measure was depressive symptoms.
- Patients engaged in aerobic exercise had fewer depressive symptoms at 3 and 12 months compared with patients receiving usual care.

Conclusion

- Exercise resulted in a significant decrease in depressive symptoms.

Implications for Nursing Practice

- Encourage patients with heart failure to discuss with their health care provider reasonable exercise goals.
- Emphasize the mental and physical benefits to patients of engaging in supervised regular aerobic exercise.

Reference for Evidence

Blumenthal J, Babyak M, O'Connor C, et al: Effects of exercise training on depressive symptoms in patients with chronic heart failure: the HF-ACTION randomized trial, *JAMA* 308:465, 2012.

P, Patient population of interest; *I*, intervention or area of interest; *C*, comparison of interest or comparison group; *O*, outcomes of interest; *T*, timing (see p. 12).

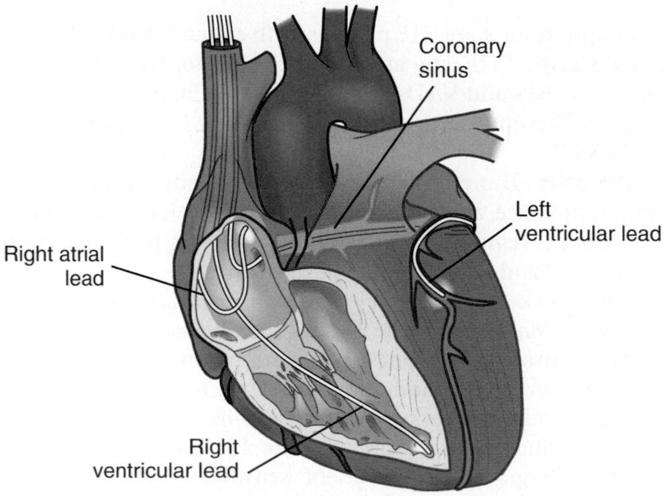

FIG. 35-4 Placement of pacing leads in cardiac resynchronization therapy.

EVIDENCE-BASED PRACTICE

Applying the Evidence

T.F. is a 62-year-old female patient recovering from an episode of acute decompensated heart failure (ADHF). Her HF is Class III in the New York Heart Association Functional Classification of Heart Disease (see Table 35-5). Her physician has recommended biventricular pacing (cardiac resynchronization therapy) for treatment of her HF symptoms. She tells you that she does not want any artificial implants, and that she has researched the use of hawthorn for treatment of her heart disease.

Best Available Evidence	Clinician Expertise	Patient Preferences and Values
Strong evidence supports the use of biventricular pacing (cardiac resynchronization therapy) to improve symptoms, exercise capacity, quality of life, ejection fraction, and survival and to decrease hospitalizations in patients like T.F.	You know the benefits of and possible complications related to biventricular pacing in patients with T.F.'s situation. You also know that there is strong evidence supporting the use of hawthorn in patients with mild to moderate HF (see Complementary & Alternative Therapies box on p. 777).	Patient does not want any artificial implants. She wants to consider alternative (herbal) therapy.

Your Decision and Action

You review the risks and benefits of biventricular pacing and herbal (hawthorn) therapy for the treatment of HF with T.F. She remains committed to the use of hawthorn—at least for a trial period. You support her decision and inform the physician of her wishes.

Reference for Evidence

Yancy CW, Jessup M, Bozkurt B, et al: 2013 ACCF/AHA guideline for the management of heart failure: executive summary, *Circulation* 128:e1, 2013.

is an option for some HF patients with advanced NYHA Functional Class IV HF who are not candidates for heart transplantation. (IABPs and VADs are discussed in Chapter 66.)

Drug Therapy. Drug therapy for chronic HF is presented in Table 35-7.

Diuretics. Diuretics are used to reduce edema, pulmonary venous pressure, and preload (see Table 33-7). If excess extracellular fluid is removed, blood volume returning to the heart can be reduced and cardiac function improved.

Diuretics act on the kidney by promoting excretion of sodium and water. Many varieties of diuretics are available. Loop diuretics (e.g., furosemide, bumetanide) are potent diuretics. These drugs act on the ascending loop of Henle to promote sodium, chloride, and water excretion. Problems in using loop diuretics include reduction in serum potassium levels, ototoxicity, and possible allergic reaction in patients sensitive to sulfa-type drugs.

Thiazide diuretics inhibit sodium reabsorption in the distal tubule, thus promoting excretion of sodium and water. They can be added to loop diuretics to obtain results if patients become resistant to loop diuretics. Thiazide diuretics also can cause severe reductions in potassium levels.

Diuretics are effective in relieving the congestive symptoms of HF. However, their use does activate the SNS and RAAS, which can exacerbate the HF syndrome. In chronic HF the lowest effective dose of diuretic should be used.

Renin-Angiotensin-Aldosterone System Inhibitors

Angiotensin-Converting Enzyme Inhibitors. ACE inhibitors are the primary drug of choice for blocking the RAAS system in HF patients with systolic failure.[1,16,17] Examples of ACE inhibitors are listed in Table 35-7. Other examples of ACE inhibitors are discussed in Chapter 33 and listed in Table 33-7.

The conversion of angiotensin I to the potent vasoconstrictor angiotensin II requires ACE (see Chapter 45, Fig. 45-4). ACE inhibitors act by blocking this enzyme, resulting in reduced levels of angiotensin II. As a result, plasma aldosterone levels are also reduced. Thus ACE inhibitors serve as neurohormonal blocking agents. Consequently, ACE inhibitors also decrease the development of ventricular remodeling by inhibiting ventricular hypertrophy.

Because CO is dependent on afterload in chronic HF, the reduction in SVR seen with the use of ACE inhibitors causes a significant increase in CO. Although the use of ACE inhibitors may decrease BP, tissue perfusion is maintained or increased as a result of improved CO. In addition, diuresis is enhanced by the suppression of aldosterone.

DRUG ALERT: Captopril (Capoten)
- Excessive hypotension and hyperkalemia may occur.
- Monitor patient for first-dose hypotension (first-dose syncope).
- Skipping doses or discontinuing the drug can result in rebound hypertension.
- Angioedema, a rare adverse effect, can develop suddenly and can be life threatening.

Major side effects of ACE inhibitors include symptomatic hypotension, intractable cough, hyperkalemia, *angioedema* (allergic reaction involving edema of the face and airways), and renal insufficiency (when ACE inhibitors are used in high doses). Aging and baseline renal insufficiency slow the metabolism of ACE inhibitors and may lead to increased serum drug levels. Carefully monitor patients taking ACE inhibitors for potential adverse effects. For example, a cough may be attributed to ACE inhibitors when, in fact, it is also a common symptom of an exacerbation of HF. It is critical that the exact cause of cough and other side effects be confirmed before stopping ACE inhibitor therapy.

Angiotensin II Receptor Blockers. For patients who are unable to tolerate ACE inhibitors, angiotensin II receptor blockers (ARBs) (see Table 33-7) are recommended.[18,19] These agents prevent the vasoconstrictor and aldosterone-secreting effects of angiotensin II by binding to the angiotensin II receptor sites.

Aldosterone Antagonists. Spironolactone (Aldactone) and eplerenone (Inspra) are aldosterone antagonists. They block the harmful neurohormonal effects of aldosterone on the heart blood vessels. They are also potassium-sparing diuretics that promote sodium and water excretion while retaining potassium. These effects occur because these agents bind to receptors at the aldosterone-dependent sodium-potassium exchange site in the distal renal tube.

DRUG ALERT: Spironolactone (Aldactone)
- Monitor potassium levels during treatment.
- Use with caution in patients taking digoxin, since hyperkalemia may reduce the effects of digoxin.
- Instruct patient to avoid foods high in potassium (e.g., bananas, oranges, dried apricots).
- Assess male patients for gynecomastia, a common side effect of long-term use of spironolactone.

β-Adrenergic Blockers. β-Adrenergic blockers directly block the negative effects of the SNS (e.g., increased HR) on the failing

COMPLEMENTARY & ALTERNATIVE THERAPIES

Hawthorn

Scientific Evidence*
- Strong evidence for its use in mild to moderate heart failure
- May inhibit angiotensin-converting enzyme
- May have a diuretic effect
- May reduce incidence of sudden cardiac death in patients with ejection fraction >25%

Nursing Implications
- May add to the effects of cardiac glycosides, antihypertensives, and cholesterol-lowering drugs
- Potentially beneficial treatment for patients who cannot or will not take prescription drugs and may offer additive benefits to established therapies

*Based on a systematic review of scientific literature. Retrieved from *www.naturalstandard.com*.

heart. They can also help in reducing the effect of renin.[19] Because β-blockers can reduce myocardial contractility, care must be taken to start slowly. Dosage is increased every 2 weeks as tolerated by the patient. Major adverse effects include edema, worsening of HF, hypotension, fatigue, and bradycardia. Three β-blockers are approved for use in HF patients: carvedilol (Coreg), bisoprolol (Zebeta), and metoprolol CR/XL (Toprol XL).[1,18]

DRUG ALERT: Carvedilol (Coreg)
- Overdosage can produce profound bradycardia, hypotension, bronchospasm, and cardiogenic shock.
- Obtain standing BP 1 hr after dosing to assess tolerance.
- Abrupt withdrawal may result in sweating, palpitations, and headaches.

Vasodilators

Nitrates. Nitrates cause vasodilation by acting directly on the smooth muscle of the vessel wall. Nitrates can be used in combination with hydralazine (Apresoline) for chronic HF management in patients who cannot tolerate ACE inhibitors or ARBs. Nitrates are of particular benefit in the management of myocardial ischemia related to HF because they promote vasodilation of the coronary arteries.

One specific problem with the use of nitrates in HF is nitrate tolerance. In addition, men with HF may experience erectile dysfunction and as a result take an erectile agent (e.g., sildenafil [Viagra]). Erectile agents are contraindicated in patients taking nitrates, since together they produce symptomatic hypotension.

BiDil. A combination drug containing isosorbide dinitrate and hydralazine (BiDil) is used for the treatment of HF in African Americans who are already being treated with standard therapy. The drug is only approved for use with this ethnic group.[20] How these two drugs work together is not fully known. As an antihypertensive agent, hydralazine relaxes the arteries and decreases the work of the heart. The antianginal agent isosorbide dinitrate relaxes the veins as well as the arteries. Isosorbide seems to work by releasing nitric oxide at the blood vessel wall, but its effect usually wears off after half a day. Hydralazine may prevent this loss of effect. Common side effects of isosorbide/hydralazine are headache and dizziness.

Positive Inotropes. Digitalis preparations (e.g., digoxin [Lanoxin]) increase the force of cardiac contraction *(inotropic action)*. They also decrease the HR *(chronotropic action)*. These actions allow for more complete emptying of the ventricles, reducing the volume remaining in the ventricles during diastole. CO increases due to the increased stroke volume from improved contractility.[19]

Patients taking a digitalis preparation are at risk for digitalis toxicity. Hypokalemia, secondary to the use of potassium-depleting diuretics (e.g., thiazides, loop diuretics), is one of the most common causes of digitalis toxicity. Low serum potassium enhances the action of digitalis, causing a therapeutic dose to reach toxic levels. Similarly, hyperkalemia inhibits the action of digitalis, resulting in a subtherapeutic dose. Both hypokalemia and hyperkalemia also cause dysrhythmias. Monitor serum potassium levels of all patients taking digitalis preparations and potassium-depleting and potassium-sparing diuretics. Other electrolyte imbalances, such as hypercalcemia and hypomagnesemia, can also precipitate digitalis toxicity. (Manifestations of electrolyte imbalances are discussed in Chapter 17.)

DRUG ALERT: Digoxin (Lanoxin)
- Monitor for signs of hypokalemia and hyperkalemia, since these can increase or decrease the effects of digoxin, respectively.
- Monitor for early signs of toxicity: anorexia, nausea and vomiting, fatigue, headache, depression, visual changes.
- Monitor for late signs of toxicity: dysrhythmias (e.g., bradycardia, atrioventricular block).

Diseases of the kidney and liver increase the risk of digitalis toxicity because most preparations are metabolized and eliminated by these organs. An older adult is especially prone to digitalis toxicity. This is because digitalis accumulation occurs sooner with decreased liver and kidney function and slowed body metabolism.

The usual treatment of toxicity consists of withholding the drug until the symptoms subside. In the case of life-threatening toxicity, IV digoxin immune Fab (ovine) (Digibind) is an antidote. The treatment of life-threatening dysrhythmias is instituted as needed (see Chapter 36).

Nutritional Therapy

Poor adherence to a low-sodium diet and failure to take prescribed medications as directed are the two most common reasons for readmissions of HF patients to the hospital.[21] Therefore it is critical that you accurately assess a patient's diet.

Diet teaching and weight management are essential to the patient's control of chronic HF. You or a dietitian should obtain a detailed diet history. Determine not only what foods the patient eats but also when, where, and how often the patient dines out. In addition, assess the sociocultural value of food. Use this information to assist the patient in making appropriate dietary choices when developing a diet plan. The National Heart, Lung, and Blood Institute provides helpful dietary guidelines for heart-healthy food preparation for people of various cultures (e.g., Hispanics, Native Americans, Asian Americans, African Americans). These are available online at *www.nhlbi.nih.gov/health/index.htm#recipes*. Diet and weight management recommendations must be individualized and culturally sensitive if the necessary changes are to be made.

The edema associated with chronic HF is often treated by dietary restriction of sodium. Teach the patient what foods are low and high in sodium and ways to enhance food flavors without the use of salt (e.g., substituting lemon juice, various spices). The degree of sodium restriction depends on the severity of the HF and the effectiveness of diuretic therapy. The Dietary Approaches to Stop Hypertension (DASH) diet is effective as a first-line therapy for many individuals with hyperten-

TABLE 35-8 **NUTRITIONAL THERAPY**

Low-Sodium Diets

General Principles

Do not add salt or seasonings containing sodium when preparing foods.*
Do not use salt at the table.*
Avoid high-sodium foods (e.g., canned soups, processed meats, cheese, frozen meals).
Limit milk products to 2 cups daily.

Sample Menu Plans for 2400-mg Sodium Diet

Breakfast	**Sodium (mg)**
⅔ cup bran cereal	161
(⅔ cup Shredded Wheat cereal)†	3
1 slice whole-wheat bread	149
1 medium banana	1
6 oz fruit yogurt, fat free	85
1 cup fat-free milk	126
2 tbs jelly	5
Coffee, 8 oz	5
Lunch	
Chicken breast sandwich	
2 slices (3 oz) chicken breast, skinless	65
2 slices whole wheat bread	299
1 slice (¾ oz) American cheese	328
(1 slice [¾ oz] Swiss cheese, natural)†	54
Large-leaf romaine lettuce	1
2 slices tomato	90
1 Tbsp mayonnaise, low fat	90
1 medium peach	7
Dinner	
¾ cup vegetarian spaghetti sauce	459
(6 oz no-salt-added tomato paste)†	260
1 cup spaghetti	1
3 tbs parmesan cheese	349
Spinach salad	
1 cup fresh spinach leaves	24
¼ cup fresh carrots (grated)	10
¼ cup fresh mushrooms (sliced)	1
2 Tbsp vinaigrette dressing	0
½ cup canned pears, juice pack	4
½ cup corn, cooked from frozen	4
Snack	
⅓ cup almonds	4
¼ cup dried apricots	3
6 oz fruit yogurt, fat free	85

*1 tsp of salt equals 2.3 g of sodium.
†Substitutes to reduce to 1500-mg sodium diet.

sion (see eTable 33-1: Your Guide to Lowering Your Blood Pressure With DASH). This diet is now also widely used for the patient with HF, with or without hypertension.

The average American adult's daily intake of sodium ranges from 7 to 15 g. A commonly prescribed diet for a patient with HF is a 2-g sodium diet (Table 35-8). All foods high in sodium (over 400 mg/serving) should be avoided. On this diet, processed meats, cheese, bread, cereals, canned soups, and canned vegetables must be limited. Teach the patient and caregiver how to read labels to look for sodium content (Fig. 35-5). The patient and caregiver should also be aware of the high sodium content of most restaurant foods.

Fluid restrictions are not commonly prescribed for the patient with mild to moderate HF. However, in moderate to severe HF and renal insufficiency, fluids are limited to less than 2 L/day.[18] Helping patients deal with thirst as a side effect of the medications is important. Suggest ice chips, gum, hard candy, or ice pops.

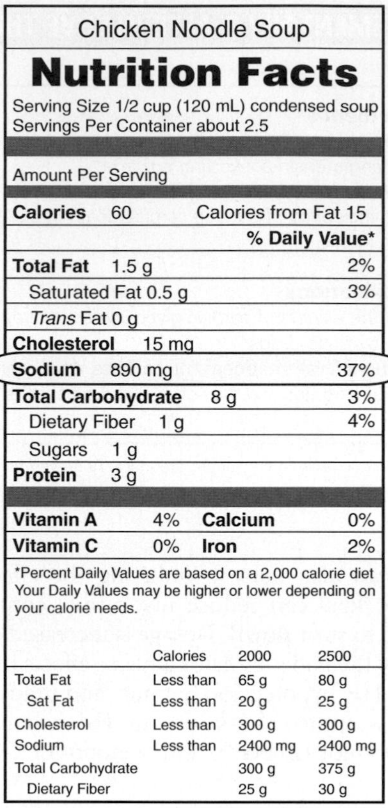
Chicken Noodle Soup
Nutrition Facts
Serving Size 1/2 cup (120 mL) condensed soup
Servings Per Container about 2.5
Amount Per Serving
Calories 60 Calories from Fat 15
% Daily Value*
Total Fat 1.5 g 2%
Saturated Fat 0.5 g 3%
Trans Fat 0 g
Cholesterol 15 mg
Sodium 890 mg 37%
Total Carbohydrate 8 g 3%
Dietary Fiber 1 g 4%
Sugars 1 g
Protein 3 g
Vitamin A 4% Calcium 0%
Vitamin C 0% Iron 2%
*Percent Daily Values are based on a 2,000 calorie diet Your Daily Values may be higher or lower depending on your calorie needs.
Calories 2000 2500
Total Fat Less than 65 g 80 g
Sat Fat Less than 20 g 25 g
Cholesterol Less than 300 g 300 g
Sodium Less than 2400 mg 2400 mg
Total Carbohydrate 300 g 375 g
Dietary Fiber 25 g 30 g

FIG. 35-5 Typical nutrition label. Note that a single serving (½ cup) provides more than one third of the daily recommended intake of sodium.

To monitor fluid status, instruct patients to weigh themselves at the same time each day, preferably before breakfast and using the same scale, while wearing the same type of clothing. This helps ensure valid comparisons from day to day and helps identify early signs of fluid retention. For patients with visual limitations, suggest scales with larger numbers or an audible response. Instruct patients to call the primary care provider if they see a weight gain of 3 lb (1.4 kg) over 2 days or a 3- to 5-lb (2.3-kg) gain over a week.[18,19]

NURSING MANAGEMENT HEART FAILURE

NURSING ASSESSMENT

Subjective and objective data that you should obtain from a patient with HF are presented in Table 35-9. Carefully review the patient's current prescription and over-the-counter medications. Assess for use of any nonsteroidal antiinflammatory drugs (NSAIDs), since they can contribute to sodium retention. In addition, review the patient's dietary habits to identify issues related to an exacerbation of HF. The patient's chronic health problems may act as exacerbating factors, affecting the plan of care and the timing and selection of therapies. For example, a patient with sleep apnea may not regularly use his or her continuous positive airway pressure device at night. This can worsen pulmonary or systemic hypertension and lead to an exacerbation of HF.

TABLE 35-9 NURSING ASSESSMENT

Heart Failure

Subjective Data

Important Health Information

Past health history: CAD (including recent MI), hypertension, cardiomyopathy, valvular or congenital heart disease, diabetes mellitus, hyperlipidemia, renal disease, thyroid or lung disease, rapid or irregular heart rate

Medications: Use of and adherence with any heart medications; use of diuretics, estrogens, corticosteroids, nonsteroidal antiinflammatory drugs, over-the-counter drugs, herbal supplements

Functional Health Patterns

Health perception–health management: Fatigue, depression, anxiety

Nutritional-metabolic: Usual sodium intake; nausea, vomiting, anorexia, stomach bloating; weight gain, ankle swelling

Elimination: Nocturia, decreased daytime urine output, constipation

Activity-exercise: Dyspnea, orthopnea, cough (e.g., dry, productive); palpitations; dizziness, fainting

Sleep-rest: Number of pillows used for sleeping; paroxysmal nocturnal dyspnea, insomnia

Cognitive-perceptual: Chest pain or heaviness; RUQ pain, abdominal discomfort; behavioral changes; visual changes

Objective Data

Integumentary

Cool, diaphoretic skin; cyanosis or pallor; peripheral edema (right-sided heart failure)

Respiratory

Tachypnea, crackles, rhonchi, wheezes; frothy, blood-tinged sputum

Cardiovascular

Tachycardia, S_3, S_4, murmurs; pulsus alternans, PMI displaced inferiorly and posteriorly, lifts and heaves, jugular venous distention

Gastrointestinal

Abdominal distention, hepatosplenomegaly, ascites

Neurologic

Restlessness, confusion, decreased attention or memory

Possible Diagnostic Findings

Altered serum electrolytes (especially Na^+ and K^+), ↑ BUN, creatinine, or liver function tests; ↑ NT-proBNP or BNP; chest x-ray demonstrating cardiomegaly, pulmonary congestion, and interstitial pulmonary edema; echocardiogram showing increased chamber size, decreased wall motion, decreased EF or normal EF with evidence of diastolic failure; atrial and ventricular enlargement on ECG; ↓ O_2 saturation

BNP, b-Type natriuretic peptide; *BUN,* blood urea nitrogen; *EF,* ejection fraction; *NT-proBNP,* N-terminal prohormone of BNP; *PMI,* point of maximal impulse; *RUQ,* right upper quadrant.

NURSING DIAGNOSES

Nursing diagnoses for the patient with HF include, but are not limited to, those presented in Nursing Care Plan 35-1.

PLANNING

The overall goals for the patient with HF include (1) a decrease in symptoms (e.g., shortness of breath, fatigue), (2) a decrease in peripheral edema, (3) an increase in exercise tolerance, (4) adherence with the medical regimen, and (5) no complications related to HF.

NURSING IMPLEMENTATION

HEALTH PROMOTION. Communication and joint decision making among the patient, caregiver, and health care team are integral to selection and delivery of high-quality, patient-centered care. Currently, there is a campaign to aggressively identify and treat risk factors for HF to prevent or slow the progression of the disease.[22] For example, teach a patient with hypertension or hyperlipidemia measures to manage BP or cholesterol with medication, diet, and exercise. Patients with valvular disease should have valve replacement planned before lung congestion develops. Coronary revascularization procedures should be considered in patients with CAD. The use of antidysrhythmic drugs or pacing therapy is indicated for patients with serious dysrhythmias or conduction disturbances. In addition, encourage patients with HF to obtain vaccinations against the flu and pneumonia.

ACUTE INTERVENTION. Many persons with HF experience one or more episodes of ADHF. When they do, they are usually admitted through the ED, initially stabilized, and then managed in an ICU, an intermediate care unit, or a specialized HF unit with continuous ECG monitoring capability.

Successful HF management depends on several important principles: (1) HF is a progressive disease, and treatment plans are established along with quality-of-life goals; (2) symptom management is controlled by the patient with self-management tools (e.g., daily weights, drug regimens, diet and exercise plans); (3) salt and, at times, water must be restricted; (4) energy must be conserved; and (5) support systems are essential to the success of the entire treatment plan.[23] Nursing Care Plan 35-1 applies to the patient with stabilized ADHF or chronic HF.

Reduction of anxiety is an important nursing function, since anxiety may increase the SNS response and further increase myocardial workload. Reducing anxiety may be facilitated by a variety of nursing interventions and the use of sedatives (e.g., benzodiazepines).

The Joint Commission has selected core measures in the management of patients with HF to reflect standards of evidence-based care[24] (available at *www.jointcommission.org/assets/1/6/Heart%20Failure.pdf*). The AHA has developed a program, Get With the Guidelines—Heart Failure, to improve adherence to standards of evidence-based care of patients hospitalized with HF.[25] Together, these approaches work to ensure high-quality care for patients with HF.

AMBULATORY AND HOME CARE. HF is a chronic illness for most persons. When a patient is diagnosed with HF, care should focus on slowing the progression of the disease. Your important nursing responsibilities include (1) teaching the patient about the physiologic changes that have occurred, (2) helping the patient adapt to both physiologic and psychologic changes, and (3) integrating the patient and the caregiver in the overall care plan. Review the signs and symptoms of HF exacerbations with the patient and caregiver and provide them with a clear action plan should symptoms occur.[18] Early detection of worsening HF may help prevent an acute episode requiring hospitalization. A patient and caregiver guide for the patient with HF is presented in Table 35-10 on p. 782.

Patients with HF are at risk for anxiety and depression.[10] Emphasize to the patient that it is possible to live a productive life with this chronic health problem. Patients with HF are usually required to take medication for the rest of their lives. This often becomes difficult because a patient may be asymp-

NURSING CARE PLAN 35-1

Patient With Heart Failure

NURSING DIAGNOSIS* **Impaired gas exchange** *related to* increased preload and alveolar-capillary membrane changes *as evidenced by* abnormal oxygen saturation, hypoxemia, dyspnea, tachypnea, tachycardia, restlessness, and patient's statement, "I am so short of breath"

PATIENT GOAL Maintains adequate O_2/CO_2 exchange at the alveolar-capillary membrane to meet O_2 needs of the body

Outcomes (NOC)

Respiratory Status: Gas Exchange

- Cognitive status ___________
- Ease of breathing ___________
- O_2 saturation ___________
- PaO_2 ___________

Measurement Scale
1 = Severely compromised
2 = Substantially compromised
3 = Moderately compromised
4 = Mildly compromised
5 = Not compromised

- Dyspnea with exertion ___________
- Dyspnea at rest ___________
- Restlessness ___________

Measurement Scale
1 = Severe
2 = Substantial
3 = Moderate
4 = Mild
5 = None

Interventions (NIC) and *Rationales*

Respiratory Monitoring

- Monitor pulse oximetry, respiratory rate, rhythm, depth, and effort of respirations *to evaluate changes in respiratory status.*
- Auscultate breath sounds, noting areas of decreased or absent ventilation and presence of adventitious sounds *to detect presence of pulmonary edema.*
- Monitor for increased restlessness, anxiety, and work of breathing *to detect increasing hypoxemia.*

Oxygen Therapy

- Administer supplemental O_2 or other noninvasive ventilator support (e.g., bilevel positive airway pressure [BiPAP]) as needed *to maintain adequate O_2 levels.*
- Monitor the O_2 liter flow rate and placement of O_2 delivery device *to ensure O_2 is adequately delivered.*
- Change O_2 delivery device from mask to nasal prongs during meals as tolerated *to sustain O_2 levels while eating.*
- Monitor the effectiveness of O_2 therapy *to identify hypoxemia and establish range of O_2 saturation.*

Positioning

- Position patient to alleviate dyspnea (e.g., semi-Fowler's position), as appropriate, *to improve ventilation by decreasing venous return to the heart and increasing thoracic capacity.*

NURSING DIAGNOSIS **Decreased cardiac output** *related to* altered contractility, altered preload, and/or altered stroke volume *as evidenced by* decreased ejection fraction, increased CVP, decreased peripheral pulses, jugular venous distention, orthopnea, chest pain, S_3 and S_4 sounds, and oliguria

PATIENT GOAL Maintains adequate blood pumped by the heart to meet metabolic demands of the body

Outcomes (NOC)

Cardiac Pump Effectiveness

- Ejection fraction ___________
- Systolic BP ___________
- Diastolic BP ___________
- Apical heart rate ___________
- 24-hr I/O balance ___________
- CVP ___________
- Peripheral pulses ___________

Measurement Scale
1 = Severely compromised
2 = Substantially compromised
3 = Moderately compromised
4 = Mildly compromised
5 = Not compromised

- Neck vein distention ___________
- Abnormal heart sounds ___________
- Dysrhythmia ___________
- Dyspnea ___________
- Peripheral edema ___________
- Pulmonary edema ___________

Measurement Scale
1 = Severe
2 = Substantial
3 = Moderate
4 = Mild
5 = None

Interventions (NIC) and *Rationales*

Cardiac Care

- Perform a comprehensive assessment of peripheral circulation (e.g., check peripheral pulses, edema, capillary refill, color, and temperature of extremity) *to determine circulatory status.*
- Note signs and symptoms of decreased cardiac output (e.g., chest pain, S_3, S_4, jugular venous distention) *to detect changes in status.*
- Monitor fluid balance (e.g., I/O and daily weight) *to evaluate renal perfusion.*
- Continuously monitor cardiac rhythm *to detect dysrhythmias.*
- Monitor for dyspnea, fatigue, tachypnea, and orthopnea *to identify involvement of respiratory system.*
- Instruct patient and caregivers on activity restriction and progression *to allay fears and anxiety.*
- Establish a supportive relationship with the patient and caregiver(s) *to promote adherence to the treatment plan.*
- Inform the patient of the purpose for and benefits of the prescribed activity and exercise.

*Nursing diagnoses are listed in order of priority.

NURSING CARE PLAN 35-1—cont'd

Patient With Heart Failure

NURSING DIAGNOSIS **Excess fluid volume** *related to* increased venous pressure and decreased renal perfusion secondary to heart failure *as evidenced by* rapid weight gain, edema, adventitious breath sounds, oliguria, and patient's statement, "My ankles are so swollen"

PATIENT GOAL Experiences reduction or absence of edema and stable baseline weight

Outcomes (NOC)	Interventions (NIC) and *Rationales*
Fluid Balance • Stable body weight ____ • Peripheral pulses ____ • Serum electrolytes ____ • BP ____ • CVP ____ • 24-hr I/O balance ____ **Measurement Scale** 1 = Severely compromised 2 = Substantially compromised 3 = Moderately compromised 4 = Mildly compromised 5 = Not compromised • Ascites ____ • Neck vein distention ____ • Peripheral edema ____ • Adventitious breath sounds ____ **Measurement Scale** 1 = Severe 2 = Substantial 3 = Moderate 4 = Mild 5 = None	***Hypervolemia Management*** • Administer prescribed diuretics, as appropriate, *to treat hypervolemia.* • Monitor for therapeutic effect of diuretic (e.g., increased urine output, decreased CVP, decreased adventitious breath sounds) *to assess response to treatment.* • Monitor potassium levels after diuresis *to detect excessive electrolyte loss.* • Weigh patient daily and monitor trends *to evaluate effect of treatment.* • Monitor intake and output *to assess fluid status.* • Monitor respiratory pattern for symptoms of respiratory difficulty *to detect pulmonary edema.* • Monitor hemodynamic status, including CVP, MAP, PAWP, if available, *to evaluate effectiveness of therapy.* • Monitor changes in peripheral edema *to assess response to treatment.*

NURSING DIAGNOSIS **Activity intolerance** *related to* imbalance between O_2 supply and demand secondary to cardiac insufficiency and pulmonary congestion *as evidenced by* dyspnea, shortness of breath, weakness, increase in heart rate on exertion, and patient's statement, "I am too tired to get out of bed; I have no energy"

PATIENT GOAL Achieves a realistic program of activity that balances physical activity with energy-conserving activities

Outcomes (NOC)	Interventions (NIC) and *Rationales*
Activity Tolerance • Pulse rate with activity ____ • O_2 saturation with activity ____ • Respiratory rate with activity ____ • Systolic BP with activity ____ • Diastolic BP with activity ____ • Ease of breathing with activity ____ • Ease of performing ADLs ____ • Skin color ____ **Measurement Scale** 1 = Severely compromised 2 = Substantially compromised 3 = Moderately compromised 4 = Mildly compromised 5 = Not compromised	***Energy Management*** • Encourage alternate rest and activity periods *to reduce cardiac workload and conserve energy.* • Provide calming diversionary activities to promote relaxation *to reduce O_2 consumption and to relieve dyspnea and fatigue.* • Monitor patient's O_2 response (e.g., pulse rate, cardiac rhythm, and respiratory rate) to self-care or nursing activities *to determine level of activity that can be performed.* • Teach patient and caregiver techniques of self-care *that will minimize O_2 consumption (e.g., self-monitoring and pacing techniques for performance of ADLs).* ***Activity Therapy*** • Collaborate with occupational and/or physical therapists *to plan and monitor activity or exercise program.* • Determine patient's commitment to increasing frequency and/or range of activities or exercise *to provide patient with obtainable goals.*

ADLs, Activities of daily living; *CVP,* central venous pressure; *I/O,* intake and output; *HF,* heart failure; *MAP,* mean arterial pressure; *PaO_2,* partial pressure of O_2 in arterial blood; *PAWP,* pulmonary artery wedge pressure.

tomatic when HF is under control. You must stress that the disease is chronic, and that medication must be continued to keep the HF under control.

Teach the patient the expected actions of the prescribed drugs and the signs of drug toxicity. Also teach the patient and caregiver how to take a pulse rate. The pulse rate should always be taken for 1 full minute. A pulse rate less than 50 beats/minute may be a contraindication to taking β-adrenergic blocker or a digitalis preparation unless directed by the health care provider. However, in the absence of symptoms (e.g., heart block, ventricular ectopy, syncope), a pulse rate less than 50 beats/minute may be acceptable. Include clear information about when a drug, especially β-blockers and digitalis, should be held and a health care provider called.

Teach the patient the symptoms of hypokalemia and hyperkalemia if diuretics that deplete or spare potassium are ordered. Frequently the patient who takes thiazide or loop diuretics is given supplemental potassium. It may also be appropriate to instruct patients in home BP monitoring, especially for those HF patients with hypertension.

TABLE 35-10 PATIENT & CAREGIVER TEACHING GUIDE

Heart Failure

Include the following instructions when teaching the patient and caregiver about the management of heart failure.

Dietary Therapy
- Consult the written diet plan and list of permitted and restricted foods.
- Examine labels to determine sodium content. Also examine the labels of over-the-counter drugs such as laxatives, cough medicines, and antacids for sodium content.
- Avoid using salt when preparing foods or adding salt to foods.
- Weigh yourself at the same time each day, preferably in the morning, using the same scale and wearing the same or similar clothes.
- Eat smaller, more frequent meals.

Activity Program
- Increase walking and other activities gradually, provided they do not cause fatigue or dyspnea. Consider a cardiac rehabilitation program.
- Avoid extremes of heat and cold.

Ongoing Monitoring
- Know the signs and symptoms of worsening heart failure (see eTable 35-1: Who Is the Patient With Heart Failure? Think FACES **[*F*atigue, limitation of *A*ctivities, chest *C*ongestion/cough, *E*dema, and *S*hortness of breath]**).
- Recall the symptoms experienced when illness began. Reappearance of previous symptoms may indicate a recurrence.
- Report immediately to health care provider any of the following:
  - Weight gain of 3 lb (1.4 kg) in 2 days, or 3-5 lb (2.3 kg) in a wk
  - Difficulty breathing, especially with exertion or when lying flat
  - Waking up breathless at night
  - Frequent dry, hacking cough, especially when lying down
  - Fatigue, weakness
  - Swelling of ankles, feet, or abdomen; swelling of face or difficulty breathing (if taking ACE inhibitors)
  - Nausea with abdominal swelling, pain, and tenderness
  - Dizziness or fainting
- Follow up with health care provider on regular basis.
- Consider joining a local support group with your family members and/or caregiver(s).

Health Promotion
- Obtain annual flu vaccination.
- Obtain pneumococcal vaccine (e.g., Pneumovax) and revaccination after 5 yr (for people at high risk of infection or serious disease).
- Develop plan to reduce risk factors (e.g., BP control, smoking cessation, weight reduction).

Rest
- Plan a regular daily rest and activity program.
- After exertion, such as exercise and ADLs, plan a rest period.
- Shorten working hours or schedule rest period during working hours.
- Avoid emotional upsets. Verbalize any concerns, fears, feelings of depression, etc., to health care provider.

Drug Therapy
- Take each drug as prescribed.
- Develop a system (e.g., daily chart, weekly pillbox) to ensure medications have been taken.
- Take pulse rate each day before taking medications (if appropriate). Know the parameters that your health care provider wants for your heart rate.
- Take BP at determined intervals (if appropriate). Know your target BP limits.
- Know signs and symptoms of orthostatic hypotension and how to prevent them (see Table 33-12).
- Know signs and symptoms of internal bleeding (bleeding gums, increased bruises, blood in stool or urine) and what to do if taking anticoagulants.
- Know own INR if taking warfarin (Coumadin) and how often to have blood monitored.

ACE, Angiotensin-converting enzyme; *INR*, international normalized ratio.

The physical therapist, occupational therapist, or you can instruct the patient in energy-conserving and energy-efficient behaviors after an evaluation of daily activities has been done. For example, once you understand the patient's daily routine, make suggestions to simplify work or modify an activity.

Exercise training (e.g., cardiac rehabilitation) improves symptoms of chronic HF but is often underprescribed. Exercise for patients with HF has been found to be safe and to improve the overall sense of well-being. It has also been correlated with mortality reduction.[25,26]

Frequently the patient needs a prescription for rest after an activity. Many hard-driving persons need the "permission" to not feel "lazy." Sometimes the patient may need to stop an activity that he or she enjoys. In such situations, help the patient explore alternative activities that cause less physical stress. Changes may be needed if situations produce an increased cardiac workload (e.g., frequent climbing of stairs). Help a patient identify areas where changes can be made and outside assistance obtained if needed.

Managing HF patients out of the hospital is a priority. Effective home health care can prevent or limit future hospitalizations by providing ongoing assessments (e.g., monitoring vital signs and weight, evaluating response to therapies).[23,27] Many agencies offer specialized programs dedicated to managing HF patients at home. For example, these programs may include the use of telehealth monitoring technology (e.g., electronic scale, BP cuff, pulse oximeter) to collect physiologic data (Fig. 35-6). The technology may also audibly ask the patient questions such as, "Are you short of breath today?" Results are transmitted telephonically or by computer to the agency. After the data are

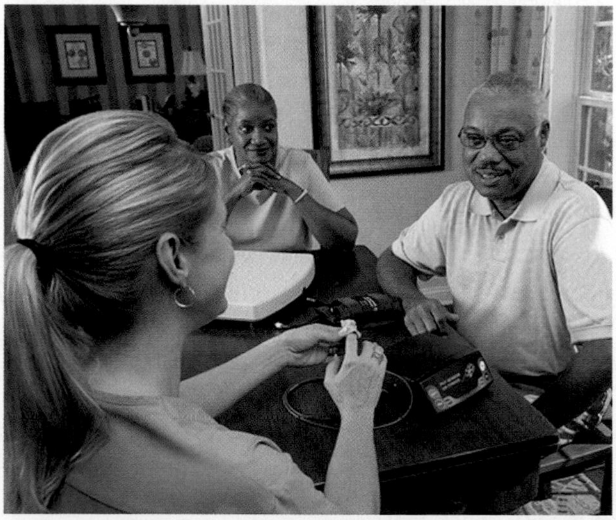

FIG. 35-6 Home-based telehealth monitoring unit.

received and reviewed, the patient may be called to further assess the situation or schedule a visit.

Home health nurses frequently work with protocols set up with the patient's health care team. The protocols enable you and the patient to identify problems, such as an increase in weight or dyspnea, as evidence of worsening HF. To prevent hospitalization, interventions can be started such as changing medications and restricting fluids. Home health nursing care of HF patients is vital in reducing the number of hospitalizations, increasing functional capacity, and improving the quality of life.

PALLIATIVE AND END-OF-LIFE CARE. Health care providers are often reluctant to refer patients with advanced HF for palliative and end-of-life care. One reason is the difficulty in assessing the prognosis of the disease and the unpredictable trajectory of HF during the last few months of life.[28] In addition, patients and caregivers may have a poor understanding of the disease and may fail to recognize HF as a terminal illness.[29]

The ACCF/AHA provides guidelines for patients with end-stage HF (stage D).[1] Health care providers in collaboration with the patient and caregiver can select either extraordinary treatment interventions (e.g., experimental surgery or drugs) or palliative and hospice care. The guidelines recommend (1) ongoing patient and caregiver education regarding prognosis and survival, (2) patient and caregiver education about options for formulating advance directives (e.g., deactivation of ICD), and (3) continuity of medical care (e.g., continuous infusion of inotropes for symptom control).[1]

Patients are eligible for hospice when a physician certifies that they are likely to have a life expectancy of 6 months or less. Unfortunately, many eligible patients are not referred to hospice. There are a number of reasons for this, including a lack of understanding of the role of hospice, lack of an identifiable terminal phase for HF, and concerns about meeting hospice referral criteria.[30] African American and Hispanic patients with HF use hospice less than whites.[31]

The seriousness of the prognosis and the actual knowledge of the expected short life span are misunderstood by many HF patients and caregivers. Many health care providers and HF patients overestimate the life expectancy.[30] When caring for these patients, attempt to identify those who may be eligible for hospice and initiate a discussion among the patient, caregiver, and health care provider.

Because patients with end-stage HF may have multiple symptoms, your care should involve ongoing assessment and evaluation of interventions for effectiveness. Strategies involve patient and caregiver support, drug therapies, and nondrug therapies. Medications are continued unless they are not tolerated. The goals of providing comfort and relieving suffering remain priorities in the care of patients with end-stage HF. (Palliative and end-of-life care are discussed in Chapter 10.)

EVALUATION

The expected outcomes for the patient with HF are presented in Nursing Care Plan 35-1.

CARDIAC TRANSPLANTATION

Cardiac transplantation is the transfer of a healthy donor heart to a patient with a diseased heart. This surgery is used to treat a variety of terminal or end-stage heart conditions (Table 35-11). Retransplantation (i.e., a second or third heart transplant) is also done. In the United States, more than 2000 cardiac transplants are done each year. However, thousands more adults would benefit from a heart transplant if more donated hearts were available. The 1-year transplant survival rate is 88% for males and 86% for females. The 5-year survival rate is 73% for males and 69% for females.[32]

TABLE 35-11 INDICATIONS AND CONTRAINDICATIONS FOR CARDIAC TRANSPLANTATION*

Indications

- End-stage heart failure refractory to medical care
- Severe, decompensated, inoperable, valvular heart disease
- Recurrent life-threatening dysrhythmias not responsive to maximal interventions, including defibrillators
- Any other cardiac abnormalities that severely limit normal function and/or have a mortality risk of more than 50% at 2 yr

Absolute Contraindications

- Chronologic age over 70 yr or physiologic age over 65 yr
- Life-threatening illness (e.g., malignancy) that will limit survival to less than 5 yr despite therapy
- Advanced cerebral or peripheral vascular disease not amenable to correction
- Active infection, including HIV infection
- Severe pulmonary disease that will likely result in the patient being ventilator dependent after transplant

Relative Contraindications

- Uncontrolled diabetes mellitus with vascular and neurologic complications
- Irreversible liver or kidney dysfunction not explained by heart failure
- Morbid obesity
- Active substance abuse (e.g., alcohol, drugs, tobacco)
- Evidence of noncompliance with accepted medical practices
- Psychologic impairment
- Lack of social support network that can make long-term commitment for patient's welfare
- Unrealistic expectations by the patient or caregiver regarding transplant, its risks, and its benefits

*These are representative examples from various heart transplant centers.

Criteria for Selection

A careful selection process ensures that hearts are distributed fairly and to those who will benefit most from the donor heart. The United Network for Organ Sharing (UNOS) is in charge of a system that gives organs fairly to people. (UNOS is discussed in Chapter 14.)

Indications and contraindications for cardiac transplantation are identified in Table 35-11. Once an individual meets the criteria for cardiac transplantation, a complete physical examination and diagnostic workup are done. In addition, the patient and caregiver undergo a comprehensive psychologic evaluation. This includes assessing coping skills, support systems, and commitment to follow the rigorous regimen that is essential to a successful transplantation. The complexity of the transplant process may be overwhelming to a patient with inadequate support systems and a poor understanding of the lifestyle changes needed after transplant.

Donor and recipient matching is based on body and heart size and an immunologic evaluation. The immunologic assessment includes ABO blood type, antibody screen, panel-reactive antibody (PRA) level, and human leukocyte antigen typing (explained in Chapter 14).

ETHICAL/LEGAL DILEMMAS

Competence

Situation

M.T., a 60-year-old man, has been awaiting heart transplantation for 6 mo. He has been a patient in intensive care for 1 mo, since he has required a ventricular assist device for his failing heart. He recently suffered a stroke, which is a complication of the device. It left him paralyzed on his right side. He is only able to answer yes/no questions by shaking his head. He has required mechanical ventilation since his stroke. For the past 2 wk, hemodialysis has been required because of renal failure. Recently, when you suction him, he has tried to prevent the ventilator tubing from being reconnected by turning his head and biting down on the endotracheal tube. Although he does not have an advance directive, his wife and daughter tell you that, on numerous occasions before these events, he expressed that he would not want to live if he lost his independence. His wife and daughter request to have the mechanical ventilator withdrawn.

Ethical/Legal Points for Consideration

- Decisional capacity for informed consent related to treatment decisions involves four elements: (1) information provided about possible treatment options must be understandable to the patient; (2) possible outcomes of the various treatment options must be explained; (3) the patient must have the capacity to deliberate about the treatment choices and their consequences; and (4) the patient's treatment decision must be freely chosen and made without coercion.
- Legal competence, as determined by the courts, has a fairly low threshold. The ability to respond to questions by signaling a yes or no may be enough to demonstrate understanding of the questions, ability to discriminate between choices, and ability to communicate choices, providing that the answers make sense and are appropriate.
- Next of kin are the legal decision makers in the absence of advance directives if he is unable to make decisions for himself. However, decisional capacity should be tested without assuming it is absent.
- Some courts have accepted past assertions of preferences, past behavior, and assertions of their parties as evidence to support end-of-life preferences in the absence of advance directives.
- You need to be knowledgeable of your hospital or agency's documentation about the local jurisdiction's laws and regulations regarding informed consent and end-of-life decision making.

Discussion Questions

1. What would you do next given M.T.'s behavior and the information you obtained from his wife?
2. What are your feelings and concerns about participating in the care of a patient for whom withdrawal of treatment will result in death?

Once a person is accepted as a transplant candidate (this may happen quickly during an acute illness or after a longer period), he or she is placed on a transplant list. Patients may wait at home and receive ongoing medical care if their condition is stable. If not, they may require hospitalization for more intensive therapy. Unfortunately, the overall waiting period for a new heart is long. Many patients die while waiting for a transplant (see Ethical/Legal Dilemmas box above).

Bridge to Transplantation

Several devices are available as a bridge to transplantation, but only two have received U.S. Food and Drug Administration (FDA) approval for heart recovery after a life-threatening cardiac event. The AB5000 Circulatory Support System and the BVS 5000 Biventricular Support System provide temporary support for one or both sides of the heart in situations where the heart has failed but has the potential to recover (e.g., reversible HF, myocarditis, acute MI). The Thoratec VAD system can also support one or both ventricles, and it is approved as a bridging device for transplantation and for recovery of the heart after cardiac surgery.

Surgical Procedure

The surgical procedure actually involves multiple surgeries. First, the donor heart is retrieved. The donor is usually someone who has suffered irreversible brain injury *(brain death)*. Most donor hearts are obtained at sites distant from the institution performing the transplant. A team of physicians, nurses, and technicians goes to the hospital of the donor to remove donated organs once brain death has been determined. The retrieved organs are transported on ice until they can be implanted. For the heart, this is optimally less than 4 hours. Often the donor heart is flown to the recipient's hospital.

Next, the donated heart is implanted into the recipient. Two different approaches are used in this surgery. In the biatrial approach the recipient's damaged heart is removed at the midatrial level and the donor heart connected at the left atrium, pulmonary artery, aorta, and right atrium. In the bicaval approach the right atrium of the recipient's heart (with the sinoatrial node and maintenance of atrial conduction) is preserved, and then the donor heart is connected. Cardiopulmonary bypass is needed during the surgical procedure to maintain oxygenation and perfusion to vital organs.

Posttransplantation

After the transplant a variety of complications can occur, including a risk for SCD. Acute rejection is an immediate posttransplant complication, and immunosuppressive therapy is the key in posttransplant management. In the first year after transplantation the major causes of death are acute rejection and infection. Later on, malignancy (especially lymphoma) and cardiac vasculopathy (accelerated CAD) are major causes of death.[32]

Most immunosuppressive regimens include corticosteroids, calcineurin inhibitors (cyclosporine [Sandimmune, Neoral], tacrolimus (Prograf), and antiproliferative drugs (mycophenolate mofetil [CellCept]). (The mechanisms of action and side effects of these and other immunosuppressants are discussed in Chapter 14 and Table 14-16.) Because of the use of immunosuppressive therapy, infection is a primary complication after transplant surgery. On a long-term basis, immunosuppressive therapy increases the risk for cancer.[32]

To detect rejection, an EMB is obtained on a weekly basis for the first month, monthly for the following 6 months, and yearly thereafter. In this procedure, a catheter is inserted into the jugular vein and moved into the RV. The catheter uses a bioptome, a device with two small cups that can be closed, to remove small samples of heart muscle.[2,32]

Nursing management throughout the posttransplant period focuses on promoting patient adaptation to the transplant process, monitoring cardiac function, managing lifestyle changes, and providing ongoing teaching of the patient and the caregiver.

CASE STUDY

Heart Failure

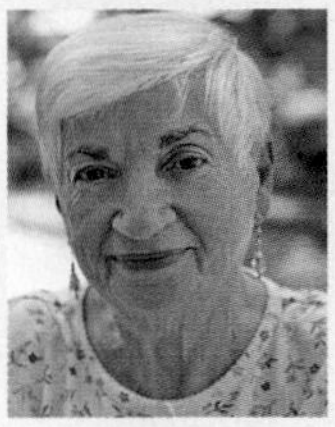

iStockphoto/
Thinkstock

Patient Profile

J.E. is a 70-year-old Hispanic woman who was admitted to the intermediate care unit with complaints of increasing shortness of breath, fatigue, and weight gain.

Subjective Data

- History of hypertension for 20 yr
- History of MI at 58 yr of age
- Has experienced increasing shortness of breath, fatigue, and an unexplained 11-lb weight gain during the past 2 wk
- Had a respiratory tract infection 2 wk ago; has persistent cough and edema in legs
- Cannot climb a flight of stairs without getting short of breath
- Sleeps with head elevated on three pillows
- Lives alone, does not always remember to take medication

Objective Data

Physical Examination

- In respiratory distress, use of accessory muscles, respiratory rate 36 breaths/min
- Systolic heart murmur
- Bilateral crackles in all lung fields
- Cyanotic lips and extremities
- Skin cool and diaphoretic

Diagnostic Studies

- Chest x-ray results: cardiomegaly with right and left ventricular hypertrophy; fluid in lower lung fields
- Echocardiogram results: EF 20%

Collaborative Care

- Furosemide (Lasix) 40 mg IV bid
- Potassium 40 mEq PO bid
- Enalapril (Vasotec) 5 mg/day PO
- Nesiritide (Natrecor) 2 mcg/kg IV bolus followed by a continuous infusion of 0.01 mcg/kg/min
- Continuous ECG monitoring
- 2-g sodium diet
- Titrate O_2 to keep O_2 saturation >93%
- Monitor intake and output, and daily weights
- Serum electrolytes; cardiac enzymes q8hr × 3

Discussion Questions

1. Explain the pathophysiology of J.E.'s heart disease and symptomatology.
2. What clinical manifestations of ADHF did J.E. exhibit?
3. What is the significance of the findings of the diagnostic studies?
4. How would a serum NT-proBNP be beneficial in the diagnosis of ADHF?
5. Provide the rationale for each of the medical orders prescribed for J.E.
6. ***Priority Decision:*** Based on the assessment data presented, what are the priority nursing diagnoses? Identify any collaborative problems.
7. ***Priority Decision:*** What are your priority nursing interventions for J.E.?
8. ***Delegation Decision:*** Which of the interventions could be delegated to unlicensed assistive personnel (UAP)?
9. ***Priority Decision:*** What priority patient teaching measures should be instituted to prevent recurrence of ADHF and prepare J.E. for discharge?
10. ***Evidence-Based Practice:*** J.E. asks you why it is so important to "watch her salt." She tells you that food tastes better with salt. How would you respond to her?

evolve Answers and a corresponding concept map available at *http://evolve.elsevier.com/Lewis/medsurg.*

BRIDGE TO NCLEX EXAMINATION

The number of the question corresponds to the same-numbered outcome at the beginning of the chapter.

1. The nurse recognizes that primary manifestations of systolic failure include
   a. ↓ EF and ↑ PAWP.
   b. ↓ PAWP and ↑ EF.
   c. ↓ pulmonary hypertension associated with normal EF.
   d. ↓ afterload and ↓ left ventricular end-diastolic pressure.
2. A compensatory mechanism involved in HF that leads to inappropriate fluid retention and additional workload of the heart is
   a. ventricular dilation.
   b. ventricular hypertrophy.
   c. neurohormonal response.
   d. sympathetic nervous system activation.
3. You are caring for a patient with ADHF who is receiving IV dobutamine (Dobutrex). You know that this drug is ordered because it *(select all that apply)*
   a. increases SVR.
   b. produces diuresis.
   c. improves contractility.
   d. dilates renal blood vessels.
   e. works on the β_1-receptors in the heart.
4. A patient with chronic HF and atrial fibrillation is treated with a digitalis glycoside and a loop diuretic. To prevent possible complications of this combination of drugs, what does the nurse need to do *(select all that apply)?*
   a. Monitor serum potassium levels.
   b. Teach the patient how to take a pulse rate.
   c. Keep an accurate measure of intake and output.
   d. Teach the patient about dietary restriction of potassium.
   e. Withhold digitalis and notify health care provider if heart rate is irregular.
5. Patients with a heart transplantation are at risk for which complications in the first year after transplantation *(select all that apply)?*
   a. Cancer
   b. Infection
   c. Rejection
   d. Vasculopathy
   e. Sudden cardiac death

1. a, 2. c, 3. c, e, 4. a, b, 5. b, c, e

evolve

For rationales to these answers and even more NCLEX review questions, visit *http://evolve.elsevier.com/Lewis/medsurg.*

REFERENCES

*1. Yancy CW, Jessup M, Bozkurt B, et al: 2013 ACCF/AHA guideline for the management of heart failure: executive summary, *Circulation* 128:e1, 2013.
2. Urden LD, Stacy KM, Lough ME: *Critical care nursing: diagnosis and management*, ed 6, St Louis, 2010, Mosby.
3. Go AS, Mozaffarian D, Roger VL, et al: Heart disease and stroke statistics—2013 update: a report from the American Heart Association, *Circulation* 127:e6, 2013.
4. Jorde LB, Carey JC, Bamshad M: *Medical genetics*, ed 4, Philadelphia, 2010, Mosby.
5. Huether S, McCance K: *Understanding pathophysiology*, ed 5, St Louis, 2012, Mosby.
*6. Silver MA, Maisel A, Yancy CW, et al: BNP Consensus Panel 2004: a clinical approach for the diagnostic, prognostic, screening, treatment monitoring, and therapeutic roles of natriuretic peptides in cardiovascular diseases, *Congest Heart Fail* 10(5 Suppl 3):1, 2004. (Classic)
7. Heart Failure Society of America: Who is the patient with heart failure? Think FACES, 2002. Retrieved from *www.hfsa.org/pdf/faces_card.pdf.* (Classic)
*8. Cooper LT, Baughman KL, Feldman AM, et al: The role of endomyocardial biopsy in the management of cardiovascular disease: a scientific statement from the American Heart Association, the American College of Cardiology, and the European Society of Cardiology, *Circulation* 116(19):2216, 2007.
9. Costanzo MR, Guglin ME, Saltzberg MT, et al: Ultrafiltration versus intravenous diuretics for patients hospitalized for acutely decompensated HF, *J Am Coll Cardiol* 49:675, 2007.
10. Diefenbeck CA: Psychosocial risk and protective factors for cardiovascular health and illness, *DNA Reporter* 34:11, 2009.
11. O'Connor C: Depression, not SSRIs linked to increased mortality in heart failure patients, *Arch Intern Med* 168:2232, 2008.
12. Mullens W, Abahams Z, Francis G, et al: Sodium nitroprusside for advanced low-output heart failure, *J Am Coll Cardiol* 52:200, 2008.
13. Dakin CL: New approaches to heart failure in the ED, *Am J Nurs* 108:68, 2008.
14. Peacock WF, Hollander JE, Diercks DB, et al: Morphine and outcomes in acute decompensated heart failure: an ADHERE analysis, *Emerg Med J* 25:205, 2009.
15. Kee JL, Hayes ER, McCuistion LE: *Pharmacology*, ed 7, St Louis, 2012, Mosby.
16. Garg R, Yusuf S: Collaborative Group on ACE Inhibitor Trials: overview of randomized trials of angiotensin-converting enzyme inhibitors on mortality and morbidity in patients with heart failure, *JAMA* 273:1450, 1995. (Classic)
17. Held ML, Sturtz M: Managing acute decompensated heart failure, *Am Nurse Today* 4:18, 2009.
*18. Lindenfeld J, Albert NM, Boehmer JP, et al: Executive summary: HFSA 2010 comprehensive heart failure practice guidelines, *J Card Fail* 16:475, 2010.
19. Ramani GV, Uber PA, Mehra MR: Chronic heart failure, *Mayo Clin Proc* 85:180, 2010.
*20. Mitchell JE, Tam SW, Trivedi K, et al: Atrial fibrillation and mortality in African American patients with heart failure: results from the African American Heart Failure Trial (A-HeFT), *Am Heart J* 162:154, 2011.
*21. Chung M, Lennie T, DeJong M, et al: Patients differ in their ability to self-monitor adherence to a low-sodium diet versus medication, *J Card Fail* 14:114, 2008.
*22. Schocken DD, Benjamin EJ, Fonarow G, et al: Prevention of heart failure: a scientific statement from the American Heart Association councils on epidemiology and prevention, clinical cardiology, cardiovascular nursing, and high blood pressure research, *Circulation* 117:2544, 2008.
*23. Hebert PL, Sisk JE, Wang JJ, et al: Cost-effectiveness of nurse-led disease management for heart failure in an ethnically diverse urban community, *Ann Intern Med* 149:540, 2008.
24. The Joint Commission: Heart failure core measure set. Retrieved from *http://www.jointcommission.org/assets/1/6/Heart%20Failure.pdf.*
25. American Heart Association: Get with the guidelines—heart failure: fact sheet. Retrieved from *www.heart.org/idc/groups/heart-public/@wcm/@hcm/@gwtg/documents/downloadable/ucm_309013.pdf.*
*26. O'Connor CM, Whellan DJ, Lee KL, et al: Efficacy and safety of exercise training in patients with chronic heart failure: HF-ACTION randomized controlled trial, *JAMA* 301:1439, 2009.
*27. Padula CA, Yeaw E, Mistry S: A home-based nurse-coached inspiratory muscle training intervention in heart failure, *Appl Nurs Res* 22:18, 2009.
28. Huynh B, Rovner A, Rich M: Identification of older patients with heart failure who may be candidates for hospice care: development of a simple four-item risk score, *J Am Geriatr Soc* 56:1111, 2008.
*29. Hemani S, Letizia M: Providing palliative care in end-stage heart failure, *J Hosp Palliat Nurs* 10:100, 2008.
30. Adler ED, Goldfinger JZ, Kalman J, et al: Palliative care in the treatment of advanced heart failure, *Circulation* 120:2597, 2009.
31. Givens JL, Tjia J, Zhou C, et al: Racial and ethnic differences in hospice use among patients with heart failure, *Arch Intern Med* 170:427, 2010.
32. Taylor D, Meiser B, Webber S, et al: The International Society of Heart and Lung Transplantation Guidelines for the Care of Heart Transplant Recipients: task force 2: immunosuppression and rejection, 2010. Retrieved from *www.ishlt.org/ContentDocuments/ISHLT_GL_TaskForce2_110810.pdf.*

*Evidence-based information for clinical practice.

RESOURCES

American Association of Cardiovascular and Pulmonary Rehabilitation
www.aacvpr.org

American Association of Heart Failure Nurses
www.aahfn.org

American College of Cardiology
www.acc.org

American Heart Association
www.heart.org

Council on Cardiovascular Nursing
www.my.americanheart.org/professional/Councils/CVN/Council-on-Cardiovascular-Nursing_UCM_320474_SubHomePage.jsp

Heart Failure Society of America
www.hfsa.org

International Society for Heart and Lung Transplantation
www.ishlt.org

Mended Hearts
www.mendedhearts.org

National Heart, Lung, and Blood Institute
www.nhlbi.nih.gov

CHAPTER

36

It is only with the heart that one can see rightly; what is essential is invisible to the eye.
Saint-Exupery

Nursing Management
Dysrhythmias

Linda Bucher

evolve WEBSITE

http://evolve.elsevier.com/Lewis/medsurg

- NCLEX Review Questions
- Key Points
- Pre-Test
- Answer Guidelines for Case Study on p. 808
- Rationales for Bridge to NCLEX Examination Questions
- Case Study
  - Patient With Atrial Fibrillation
- Concept Map Creator
- Glossary
- Content Updates

eFigure
- eFig. 36-1: Lead placement for MCL_1

eTable
- eTable 36-1: Five-Letter Pacemaker Code

LEARNING OUTCOMES

1. Examine the nursing management of patients requiring continuous electrocardiographic (ECG) monitoring.
2. Differentiate the clinical characteristics and ECG patterns of normal sinus rhythm, common dysrhythmias, and acute coronary syndrome (ACS).
3. Compare the nursing and collaborative management of patients with common dysrhythmias and ECG changes associated with ACS.
4. Differentiate between defibrillation and cardioversion, including indications for use and physiologic effects.
5. Describe the management of patients with pacemakers and implantable cardioverter-defibrillators.
6. Select appropriate interventions for patients undergoing electrophysiologic testing and radiofrequency catheter ablation therapy.

KEY TERMS

asystole, p. 795
atrial fibrillation, p. 796
atrial flutter, p. 795
automatic external defibrillator (AED), p. 802
cardiac pacemaker, p. 803
complete heart block, p. 798
dysrhythmias, p. 787
premature atrial contraction (PAC), p. 794
premature ventricular contraction (PVC), p. 799
telemetry monitoring, p. 790
ventricular fibrillation (VF), p. 800
ventricular tachycardia (VT), p. 799

This chapter describes basic principles of electrocardiographic monitoring and recognition and treatment of common dysrhythmias. In addition, it presents ECG changes that are associated with acute coronary syndrome (ACS).

RHYTHM IDENTIFICATION AND TREATMENT

Your ability to recognize normal and abnormal cardiac rhythms, called **dysrhythmias**, is an essential nursing skill.[1] Prompt assessment of dysrhythmias and the patient's response to the rhythm is critical.

Conduction System

Four properties of cardiac cells enable the conduction system to start an electrical impulse, send it through the cardiac tissue, and stimulate muscle contraction (Table 36-1). The heart's conduction system consists of specialized neuromuscular tissue located throughout the heart (Fig. 32-4, *A*). A normal cardiac impulse begins in the sinoatrial (SA) node in the upper right atrium. It spreads over the atrial myocardium via interatrial and internodal pathways, causing atrial contraction. The impulse then travels to the atrioventricular (AV) node, through the bundle of His, and down the left and right bundle branches. It ends in the Purkinje fibers, which transmit the impulse to the ventricles.

Nervous Control of the Heart

The autonomic nervous system plays an important role in the rate of impulse formation, the speed of conduction, and the strength of cardiac contraction. The components of the auto-

Reviewed by Katrina Allen, RN, MSN, CCRN, Nursing Instructor, Faulkner State Community College: Division of Nursing, Fairhope and Bay Minette, Alabama; Barbara Pope, RN, MSN, PPCN, CCRN, Critical Care Educator, Independent Consultant, Albert Einstein Healthcare Network (retired), Philadelphia, Pennsylvania; and Regina Kukulski, RN, MSN, ACNS, BC, Nurse Educator Consultant, Thomas Edison State College, Capital Health Medical Center, Trenton, New Jersey.

nomic nervous system that affect the heart are the vagus nerve fibers of the parasympathetic nervous system and nerve fibers of the sympathetic nervous system.

Stimulation of the vagus nerve causes a decreased rate of firing of the SA node and slowed impulse conduction of the AV node. Stimulation of the sympathetic nerves increases SA node firing, AV node impulse conduction, and cardiac contractility.[2]

TABLE 36-1 PROPERTIES OF CARDIAC CELLS

Property	Definition
Automaticity	Ability to initiate an impulse spontaneously and continuously
Excitability	Ability to be electrically stimulated
Conductivity	Ability to transmit an impulse along a membrane in an orderly manner
Contractility	Ability to respond mechanically to an impulse

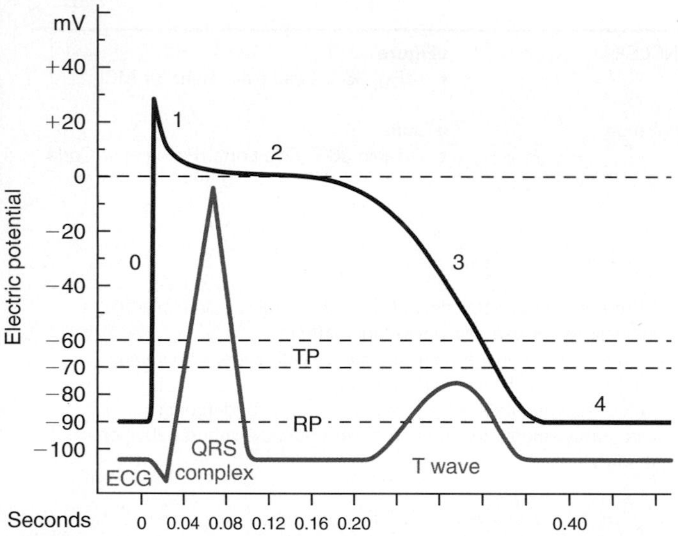

FIG. 36-1 Phases of the cardiac action potential. The electrical potential, measured in millivolts (mV), is indicated along the vertical axis of the graph. Time, measured in seconds (sec), is indicated along the horizontal axis. The action potential has five phases, labeled *0* through *4*. Each phase represents a particular electrical event or combination of electrical events. Phase 0 is the upstroke of rapid depolarization and corresponds with ventricular contraction. Phases 1, 2, and 3 represent repolarization. Phase 4 is known as complete repolarization (or the polarized state) and corresponds to diastole. *RP,* Resting membrane potential; *TP,* threshold membrane potential.

Electrocardiographic Monitoring

The *electrocardiogram* (ECG) is a graphic tracing of the electrical impulses produced in the heart. The waveforms on the ECG represent electrical activity produced by the movement of ions across the membranes of myocardial cells, representing depolarization and repolarization.

The membrane of a cardiac cell is semipermeable. This allows it to maintain a high concentration of potassium and a low concentration of sodium inside the cell. Outside the cell a high concentration of sodium and a low concentration of potassium exist. The inside of the cell, when at rest, or in the polarized state, is negative compared with the outside. When a cell or groups of cells are stimulated, the cell membrane changes its permeability. This allows sodium to move rapidly into the cell, making the inside of the cell positive compared with the outside *(depolarization).* A slower movement of ions across the membrane restores the cell to the polarized state, called *repolarization.* Fig. 36-1 describes the phases of the cardiac action potential.

The ECG has 12 recording leads. Six of the leads measure electrical forces in the frontal plane. These are bipolar (positive or negative) leads I, II, and III; and unipolar (positive) leads aVR, aVL, and aVF (Fig. 36-2, *A* and *B*). The remaining six unipolar leads (V_1 through V_6) measure the electrical forces in the horizontal plane (precordial leads) (Fig. 36-2, *C*). The 12-lead ECG may show changes suggesting structural changes, conduction disturbances, damage (e.g., ischemia, infarction), electrolyte imbalance, or drug toxicity. Obtaining 12 ECG views of the heart is also helpful in the assessment of dysrhythmias. Fig. 36-3 is an example of a normal 12-lead ECG.

One or more ECG leads can be used to continuously monitor a patient. The most common leads selected are leads II and V_1 (Fig. 36-4). A modified chest lead (MCL_1) is used when only three leads are available for monitoring (eFig. 36-1, showing MCL_1 lead placement, is available on the website for this chapter). MCL_1 is similar to V_1. Accurate interpretation of an ECG depends on the correct placement of the leads on the patient. The monitoring leads used are determined by the patient's clinical status.[3,4]

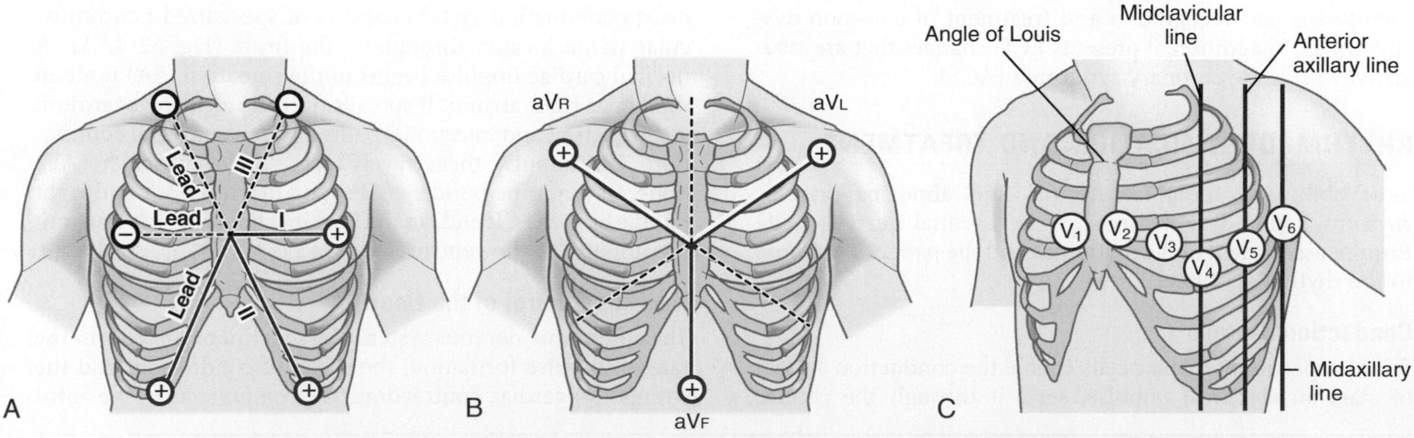

FIG. 36-2 A, Limb leads I, II, and III. These bipolar leads are located on the extremities. Illustrated are the angles from which these leads view the heart. **B,** Limb leads aVR, aVL, and aVF. These unipolar leads use the center of the heart as their negative electrode. **C,** Placement for the unipolar chest leads: *V_1,* fourth intercostal space at the right sternal border; *V_2,* fourth intercostal space at the left sternal border; *V_3,* halfway between V_2 and V_4; *V_4,* fifth intercostal space at the left midclavicular line; *V_5,* fifth intercostal space at the left anterior axillary line; *V_6,* fifth intercostal space at the left midaxillary line.

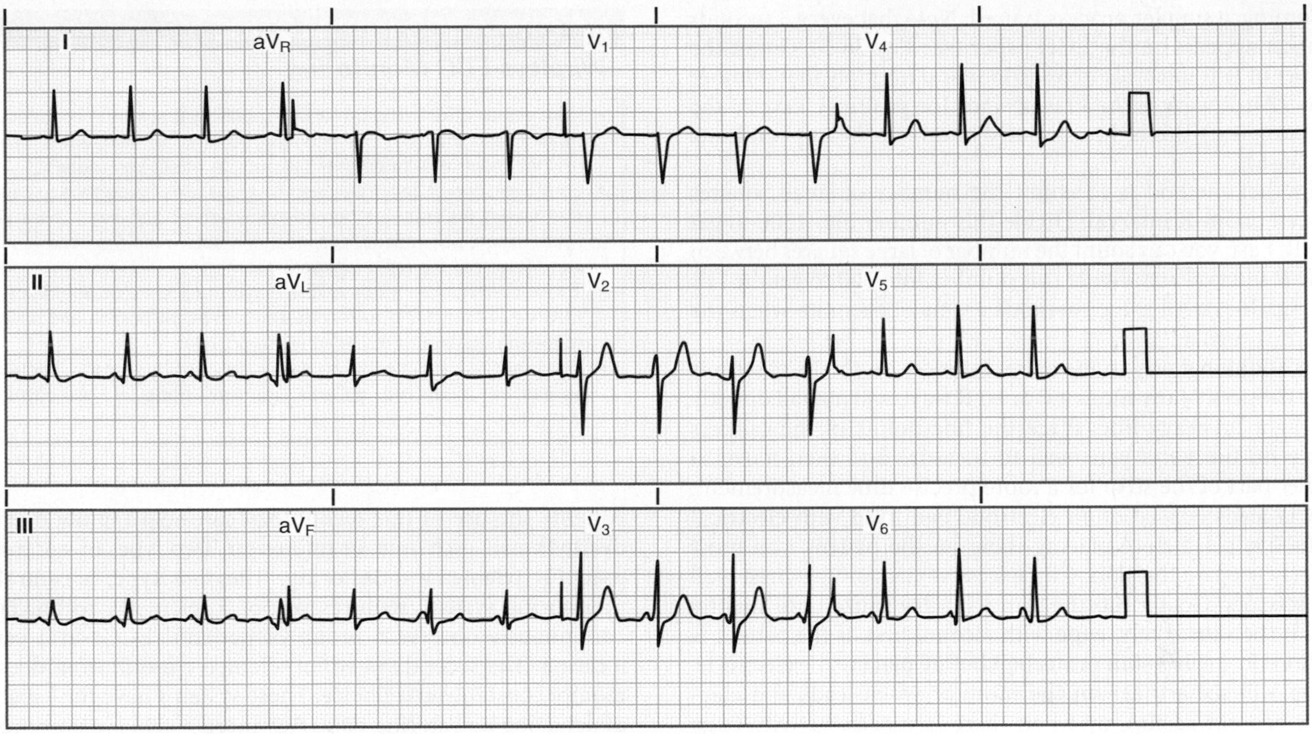

FIG. 36-3 Twelve-lead electrocardiogram showing a normal sinus rhythm.

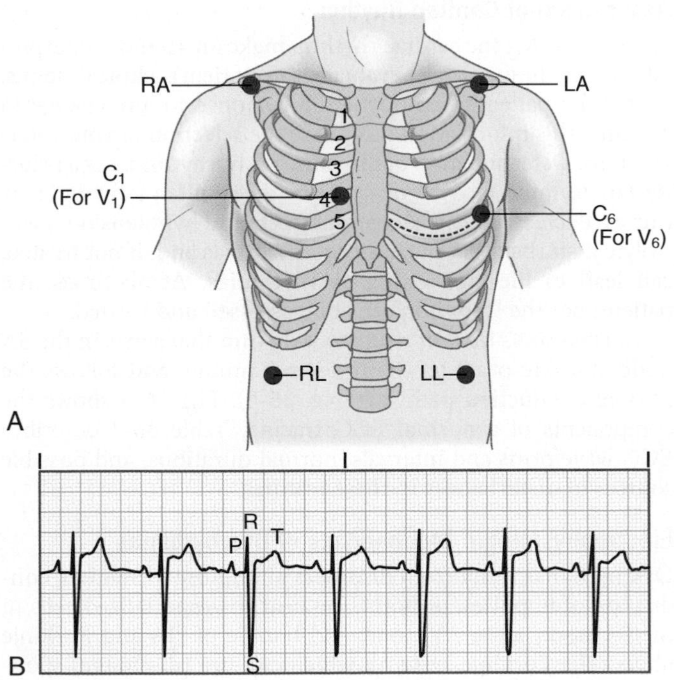

FIG. 36-4 A, Lead placement for V_1 or V_6 using a five-lead system. **B,** Typical ECG tracing in lead V_1. *C,* Chest; *LA,* left arm; *LL,* left leg; *RA,* right arm; *RL,* right leg.

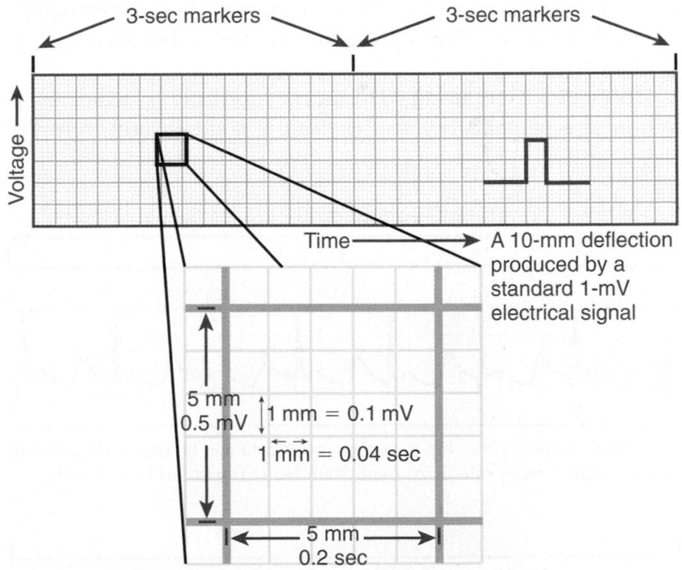

FIG. 36-5 Time and voltage on the electrocardiogram; 6-sec strip.

The monitor continuously displays the heart rhythm. ECG paper attached to the monitor records the ECG (i.e., rhythm strip). This provides a record of the patient's rhythm. It also allows for measurement of complexes and intervals and for assessment of dysrhythmias.

To correctly interpret an ECG, you measure time and voltage on the ECG paper. ECG paper consists of large (heavy lines) and small (light lines) squares (Fig. 36-5). Each large square consists of 25 smaller squares (five horizontal and five vertical). Horizontally, each small square (1 mm) represents 0.04 second. This means that one large square equals 0.20 second and that 300 large squares equal 1 minute. Vertically, each small square (1 mm) represents 0.1 millivolt (mV). This means that one large square equals 0.5 mV. Use these squares to calculate the heart rate (HR) and measure time intervals for the different ECG complexes.

You can use a variety of methods to calculate the HR from an ECG. The most accurate way is to count the number of QRS complexes in 1 minute. However, because this method is time consuming, a simpler process is used. Note that every 3 seconds a marker appears on the ECG paper (see Fig. 36-5). Count the number of R-R intervals in 6 seconds and multiply that number by 10. (An R wave is the first upward [or positive] wave of the QRS complex.) This is the estimated number of beats per minute (Fig. 36-6).

Another method is to count the number of small squares between one R-R interval. Divide this number into 1500 to get the HR. Last, you can count the number of large squares between one R-R interval and divide this number into 300 to get the HR (see Fig. 36-6). All these methods are most accurate when the rhythm is regular.[1]

An additional way to measure distances on the ECG strip is to use calipers. Many times a P or an R wave will not fall directly on a light or heavy line. Place the fine points of the calipers exactly on the parts you need to measure and then move to another part of the strip for a more precise time measurement.

ECG leads consist of an electrode pad fixed with electrical conductive gel. Before placing these on the patient, you must properly prepare the skin. Clip excessive hair on the chest wall with scissors. Gently rub the skin with dry gauze until slightly pink. If the skin is oily, wipe with alcohol first. If the patient is diaphoretic, apply a skin protectant before placing the electrode.

You will see artifact on the monitor when leads and electrodes are not secure, or when there is muscle activity (e.g., shivering) or electrical interference. *Artifact* is a distortion of the baseline and waveforms seen on the ECG (Fig. 36-7). Accurate interpretation of heart rhythm is difficult when artifact is present. If artifact occurs, check the connections in the equipment. You may need to replace the electrodes if the conductive gel has dried out.

Telemetry Monitoring. Telemetry monitoring is the observation of a patient's HR and rhythm at a site distant from the patient. The use of this technology can help rapidly diagnose dysrhythmias, ischemia, or infarction. Two types of systems are used for telemetry monitoring. The first type, a centralized monitoring system, requires you or a telemetry technician to continuously observe a group of patients' ECGs at a central location. The second system of telemetry monitoring does not require constant surveillance. These systems have the capability of detecting and storing data. Advanced alarm systems provide different levels of detection of dysrhythmias, ischemia, or infarction.

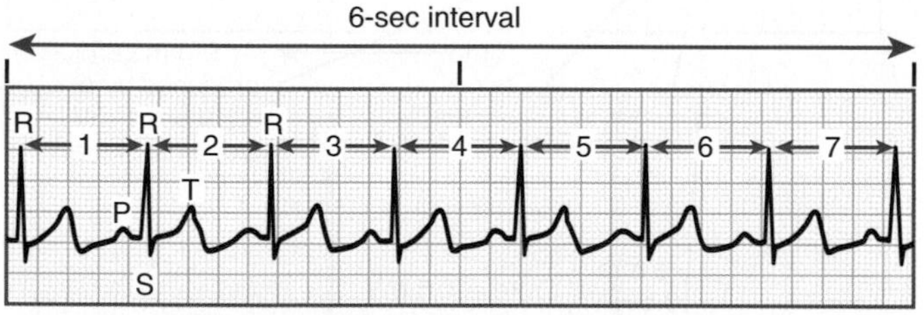

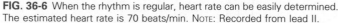

FIG. 36-6 When the rhythm is regular, heart rate can be easily determined. The estimated heart rate is 70 beats/min. NOTE: Recorded from lead II.

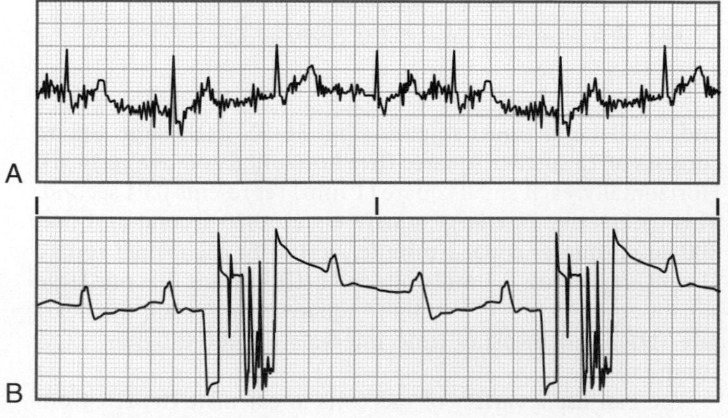

FIG. 36-7 Artifact. **A,** Muscle tremor. **B,** Loose electrodes.

INFORMATICS IN PRACTICE

Wireless ECG Monitoring

- Wireless electrocardiogram (ECG) monitoring systems continuously monitor and interpret the findings, sending an alert when patient rhythm and/or measurements fall outside of set parameters.
- Early detection of abnormal heart rhythms allows you time to assess the patient for signs of hemodynamic instability (e.g., chest pain, hypotension, palpitations, dyspnea) and determine the need to intervene (e.g., call the rapid response team).
- These systems can automatically save the pre-event portion of the ECG while continuing to record the post-event portion and send all of the information to the health care provider.
- Computerized monitoring systems are not fail-proof. Frequently assess all monitored patients for any signs of hemodynamic instability.

Assessment of Cardiac Rhythm

When assessing the cardiac rhythm, make an accurate interpretation and immediately evaluate the patient's clinical status. Assess the patient's hemodynamic response to any change in rhythm. This information will guide the selection of your interventions. Determination of the cause of dysrhythmias is a priority. For example, tachycardias may be the result of fever and may cause a decrease in cardiac output (CO) and hypotension. Electrolyte disturbances can cause dysrhythmias and, if not treated, can lead to life-threatening dysrhythmias. At all times, the patient, not the "monitor," must be assessed and treated.

Normal sinus rhythm refers to a rhythm that starts in the SA node at a rate of 60 to 100 times per minute and follows the normal conduction pathway (Fig. 36-8). Fig. 36-9 shows the components of a normal ECG tracing. Table 36-2 describes ECG waveforms and intervals, normal durations, and possible sources of disturbances in these features.

Electrophysiologic Mechanisms of Dysrhythmias

Dysrhythmias result from disorders of impulse formation, conduction of impulses, or both. The heart has specialized cells in the SA node, atria, AV node, and bundle of His and Purkinje fibers (His-Purkinje system), which can fire (discharge) spontaneously. This is termed *automaticity*. Normally, the SA node

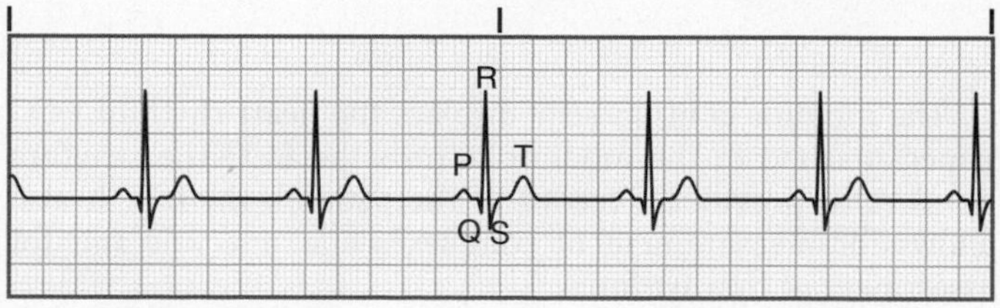

FIG. 36-8 Normal sinus rhythm. NOTE: Recorded from lead II.

is the pacemaker of the heart. It spontaneously fires 60 to 100 times per minute (Table 36-3). A secondary pacemaker from another site may fire in two ways. If the SA node fires more slowly than a secondary pacemaker, the electrical signals from the secondary pacemaker may "escape." The secondary pacemaker will then fire automatically at its intrinsic rate. These secondary pacemakers may start from the AV node at a rate of 40 to 60 times per minute or the His-Purkinje system at a rate of 20 to 40 times per minute.

Another way that secondary pacemakers can start is when they fire more rapidly than the normal pacemaker of the SA node. *Triggered beats* (early or late) may come from an *ectopic focus* or *accessory pathway* (area outside the normal conduction pathway) in the atria, AV node, or ventricles. This results in a dysrhythmia, which replaces the normal sinus rhythm.

The impulse started by the SA node or an ectopic focus must be conducted to the entire heart. The property of myocardial tissue that allows it to be depolarized by a stimulus is called *excitability*. This is an important part of the transmission of the

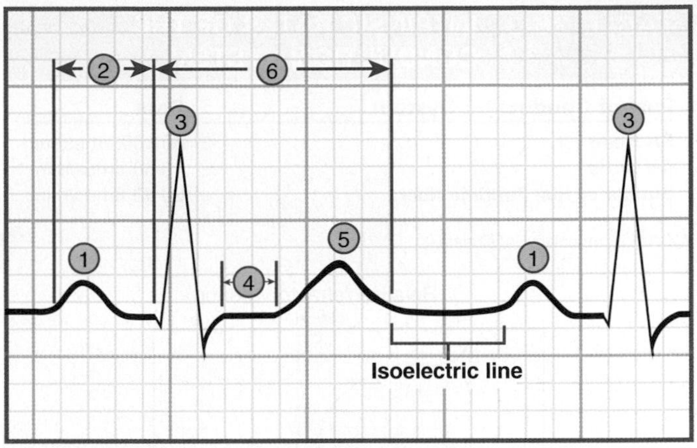

FIG. 36-9 The ECG tracing as seen in normal sinus rhythm. *1,* P wave; *2,* PR interval; *3,* QRS complex: Q wave, R wave, S wave; *4,* ST segment; *5,* T wave; *6,* QT interval. Isoelectric (flat) line or baseline represents the absence of electrical activity in the cardiac cells. (See Table 36-2 for timing of intervals.)

TABLE 36-2 ECG WAVEFORMS AND INTERVALS*

Description	Normal Duration (sec)	Source of Possible Variation
P Wave Represents time for the passage of the electrical impulse through the atrium causing atrial depolarization (contraction). Should be upright.	0.06-0.12	Disturbance in conduction within atria
PR Interval Measured from beginning of P wave to beginning of QRS complex. Represents time taken for impulse to spread through the atria, AV node and bundle of His, bundle branches, and Purkinje fibers, to a point immediately preceding ventricular contraction.	0.12-0.20	Disturbance in conduction usually in AV node, bundle of His, or bundle branches but can be in atria as well
QRS Complex		
Q wave: First negative (downward) deflection after the P wave, short and narrow, not present in several leads.	<0.03	MI may result in development of a pathologic Q wave that is wide (≥0.03 sec) and deep (≥25% of the height of the R wave)
R wave: First positive (upward) deflection in the QRS complex.	Not usually measured	
S wave: First negative (downward) deflection after the R wave.	Not usually measured	
QRS Interval Measured from beginning to end of QRS complex. Represents time taken for depolarization (contraction) of both ventricles (systole).	<0.12	Disturbance in conduction in bundle branches or in ventricles
ST Segment Measured from the S wave of the QRS complex to the beginning of the T wave. Represents the time between ventricular depolarization and repolarization (diastole). Should be isoelectric (flat).	0.12	Disturbances (e.g., elevation, depression) usually caused by ischemia, injury, or infarction
T Wave Represents time for ventricular repolarization. Should be upright.	0.16	Disturbances (e.g., tall, peaked; inverted) usually caused by electrolyte imbalances, ischemia, or infarction
QT Interval Measured from beginning of QRS complex to end of T wave. Represents time taken for entire electrical depolarization and repolarization of the ventricles.	0.34-0.43	Disturbances usually affecting repolarization more than depolarization and caused by drugs, electrolyte imbalances, and changes in heart rate

*Heart rate influences the duration of these intervals, especially those of the PR and QT intervals (e.g., QT interval shortens in duration as heart rate increases).
AV, Atrioventricular.

TABLE 36-3 INTRINSIC RATES OF THE CONDUCTION SYSTEM

Part of Conduction System	Rate
SA node	60-100 times/min
AV node	40-60 times/min
Bundle of His, Purkinje fibers	20-40 times/min

AV, Atrioventricular; *SA,* sinoatrial.

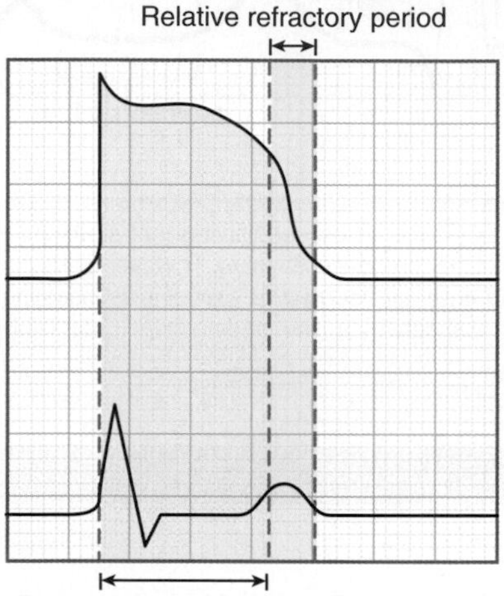

FIG. 36-10 Absolute and relative refractory periods correlated with the cardiac muscle's action potential and with an ECG tracing.

impulse from one cell to another. The level of excitability is determined by the length of time after depolarization that the tissues can be restimulated. The recovery period after stimulation is the *refractory phase* or period. The *absolute refractory phase* or period occurs when excitability is zero and the heart cannot be stimulated. The *relative refractory period* occurs slightly later in the cycle, and excitability is more likely. In states of *full excitability,* the heart is completely recovered. Fig. 36-10 shows the relationship between the refractory period and the ECG.

If conduction is depressed and some areas of the heart are blocked (e.g., by infarction), the unblocked areas are activated earlier than the blocked areas. When the block is unidirectional, this uneven conduction may allow the initial impulse to reenter areas that were previously not excitable but have recovered. The reentering impulse may be able to depolarize the atria and ventricles, causing a premature beat. If the reentrant excitation continues, tachycardia occurs.

Evaluation of Dysrhythmias

Dysrhythmias occur as the result of various abnormalities and disease states. The cause of a dysrhythmia influences the patient's treatment. Table 36-4 presents common causes of dysrhythmias. Table 36-5 presents a systematic approach to assessing a heart rhythm.

Dysrhythmias occurring in nonmonitored settings present management challenges. If the patient becomes symptomatic (e.g., chest pain), determination of the rhythm by cardiac monitoring is a high priority. Activate the emergency medical services (EMS) system. Table 36-6 outlines emergency care of the patient with a dysrhythmia.

In addition to continuous ECG monitoring during hospitalization, several other tests can assess dysrhythmias and the effectiveness of antidysrhythmia drug therapy. An electrophysiologic study, Holter monitoring, event monitoring (or loop recorder), exercise treadmill testing, and signal-averaged ECG can be performed on an inpatient or outpatient basis (see Table 32-6 for nursing care related to these tests).

An *electrophysiologic study* (EPS) can identify the causes of heart blocks, tachydysrhythmias (dysrhythmias with rates greater than 100 beats/minute), bradydysrhythmias (dysrhythmias with rates less than 60 beats/minute), and syncope. An EPS study can also locate accessory pathways and determine the effectiveness of antidysrhythmia drugs.

The Holter monitor continuously records the ECG while the patient is ambulatory and performing daily activities. The patient keeps a diary and records activities and any symptoms.

TABLE 36-4 COMMON CAUSES OF DYSRHYTHMIAS*

Cardiac Conditions
- Accessory pathways
- Cardiomyopathy
- Conduction defects
- Heart failure
- Myocardial ischemia, infarction
- Valve disease

Other Conditions
- Acid-base imbalances
- Alcohol
- Caffeine, tobacco
- Connective tissue disorders
- Drug effects (e.g., antidysrhythmia drugs, stimulants, β-adrenergic blockers) or toxicity
- Electric shock
- Electrolyte imbalances (e.g., hyperkalemia, hypocalcemia)
- Emotional crisis
- Herbal supplements (e.g., areca nut, wahoo root bark, yerba maté)
- Hypoxia
- Metabolic conditions (e.g., thyroid dysfunction)
- Near-drowning
- Sepsis, shock
- Toxins

*List is not all-inclusive.

TABLE 36-5 APPROACH TO ASSESSING HEART RHYTHM

When assessing a heart rhythm, use a consistent and systematic approach. One such approach includes the following:

1. Look for the P wave. Is it upright or inverted? Is there one for every QRS complex or more than one? Are atrial fibrillatory or flutter waves present?
2. Evaluate the atrial rhythm. Is it regular or irregular?
3. Calculate the atrial rate.
4. Measure the duration of the PR interval. Is it normal duration or prolonged?
5. Evaluate the ventricular rhythm. Is it regular or irregular?
6. Calculate the ventricular rate.
7. Measure the duration of the QRS complex. Is it normal duration or prolonged?
8. Assess the ST segment. Is it isoelectric (flat), elevated, or depressed?
9. Measure the duration of the QT interval. Is it normal duration or prolonged?
10. Note the T wave. Is it upright or inverted?

Additional questions to consider include the following:

1. What is the dominant or underlying rhythm and/or dysrhythmia?
2. What is the clinical significance of your findings?
3. What is the treatment for the particular rhythm?

TABLE 36-6 EMERGENCY MANAGEMENT

Dysrhythmias

Etiology	Assessment Findings	Interventions
See Table 36-4	• Irregular rate and rhythm; tachycardia, bradycardia • Decreased or increased blood pressure • Decreased O_2 saturation • Chest, neck, shoulder, back, jaw, or arm pain • Dizziness, syncope • Dyspnea • Extreme restlessness, anxiety • Decreased level of consciousness, confusion • Feeling of impending doom • Numbness, tingling of arms • Weakness and fatigue • Cold, clammy skin • Diminished peripheral pulses • Diaphoresis • Pallor • Palpitations • Nausea and vomiting	**Initial** • Ensure ABCs. • Administer O_2 via nasal cannula or non-rebreather mask. • Obtain baseline vital signs, including O_2 saturation. • Obtain 12-lead ECG. • Initiate continuous ECG monitoring. • Identify underlying rate and rhythm. • Identify dysrhythmia. • Establish IV access. • Obtain baseline laboratory studies (e.g., CBC, electrolytes). **Ongoing Monitoring** • Monitor vital signs, level of consciousness, O_2 saturation, and cardiac rhythm. • Anticipate need for administration of antidysrhythmia drugs and analgesics. • Anticipate need for intubation if respiratory distress is evident. • Prepare to initiate advanced cardiac life support (e.g., CPR, defibrillation, transcutaneous pacing).

ABCs, Airway, breathing, circulation.

Events in the diary are correlated with any dysrhythmias seen on the ECG. Use of event monitors has improved the evaluation of dysrhythmias in outpatients. Event monitors are recorders that the patient activates only when he or she experiences symptoms. New technology using smart phones can obtain and save ECG recordings and even detect atrial fibrillation.

Exercise treadmill testing evaluates the patient's heart rhythm during exercise. If exercise-induced dysrhythmias or ECG changes occur, they are analyzed and drug therapy evaluated.

The signal-averaged ECG identifies *late potentials* strongly suggesting that the patient may be at risk for developing serious ventricular dysrhythmias. Chapter 32 discusses the diagnostic procedures for assessment of the cardiovascular system and related nursing care.

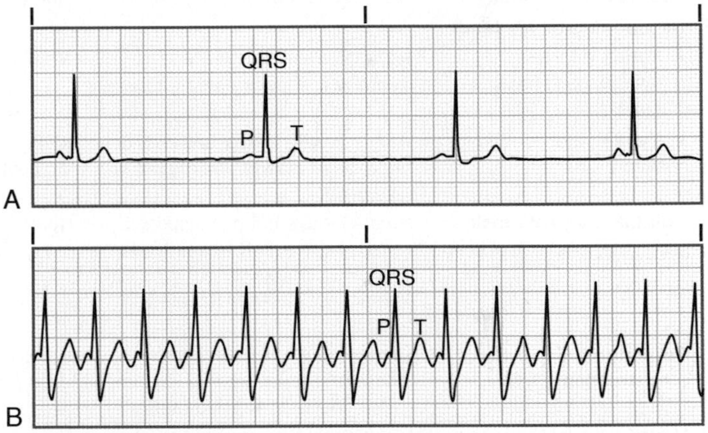

FIG. 36-11 A, Sinus bradycardia. **B,** Sinus tachycardia.

Types of Dysrhythmias

Figs. 36-11 to 36-19 provide examples of the ECG tracings of common dysrhythmias. Table 36-7 presents the descriptive characteristics.

Sinus Bradycardia. In *sinus bradycardia* the conduction pathway is the same as that in sinus rhythm but the SA node fires at a rate less than 60 beats/minute (Fig. 36-11, *A*). *Symptomatic bradycardia* refers to an HR that is less than 60 beats/minute and is inadequate for the patient's condition, causing the patient to experience symptoms (e.g., chest pain, syncope).

Clinical Associations. Sinus bradycardia may be a normal sinus rhythm in aerobically trained athletes and in some people during sleep. It also occurs in response to carotid sinus massage, Valsalva maneuver, hypothermia, increased intraocular pressure, vagal stimulation, and administration of certain drugs (e.g., β-adrenergic blockers, calcium channel blockers). Common disease states associated with sinus bradycardia are hypothyroidism, increased intracranial pressure, hypoglycemia, and inferior myocardial infarction (MI).

ECG Characteristics. In sinus bradycardia, HR is less than 60 beats/minute and the rhythm is regular. The P wave precedes each QRS complex and has a normal shape and duration. The PR interval is normal, and the QRS complex has a normal shape and duration.

Clinical Significance. The clinical significance of sinus bradycardia depends on how the patient tolerates it. Signs of symptomatic bradycardia include pale, cool skin; hypotension; weakness; angina; dizziness or syncope; confusion or disorientation; and shortness of breath.

Treatment. For the patient with symptoms, treatment consists of administration of atropine (an anticholinergic drug). If atropine (AtroPen) is ineffective, transcutaneous pacing, or a dopamine (Intropin) or epinephrine (Adrenalin) infusion is considered. Permanent pacemaker therapy may be needed. If bradycardia is due to drugs, these may need to be held, discontinued, or given in reduced dosages.

Sinus Tachycardia. The conduction pathway is the same in *sinus tachycardia* as that in normal sinus rhythm. The discharge rate from the sinus node increases because of vagal inhibition or sympathetic stimulation. The sinus rate is 101 to 200 beats/minute (Fig. 36-11, *B*).

Clinical Associations. Sinus tachycardia is associated with physiologic and psychologic stressors such as exercise, fever, pain, hypotension, hypovolemia, anemia, hypoxia, hypoglycemia, myocardial ischemia, heart failure (HF), hyperthyroidism, anxiety, and fear. It can also be an effect of drugs such as epinephrine, norepinephrine (Levophed), atropine, caffeine, theophylline (Theo-Dur), or hydralazine (Apresoline). In addition, many over-the-counter cold remedies have active ingredients (e.g., pseudoephedrine [Sudafed]) that can cause tachycardia.

TABLE 36-7 **CHARACTERISTICS OF COMMON DYSRHYTHMIAS**

Pattern	Rate and Rhythm	P Wave	PR Interval	QRS Complex
Normal sinus rhythm	60-100 beats/min and regular	Normal	Normal	Normal
Sinus bradycardia	<60 beats/min and regular	Normal	Normal	Normal
Sinus tachycardia	101-200 beats/min and regular	Normal	Normal	Normal
Premature atrial contraction	Usually 60-100 beats/min and irregular	Abnormal shape	Normal	Normal (usually)
Paroxysmal supraventricular tachycardia	150-220 beats/min and regular	Abnormal shape, may be hidden in the preceding T wave	Normal or shortened	Normal (usually)
Atrial flutter	*Atrial:* 200-350 beats/min and regular *Ventricular:* > or <100 beats/min and may be regular or irregular	Flutter (F) waves (sawtoothed pattern); more flutter waves than QRS complexes; may occur in a 2:1, 3:1, 4:1, etc., pattern	Not measurable	Normal (usually)
Atrial fibrillation	*Atrial:* 350-600 beats/min and irregular *Ventricular:* > or <100 beats/min and irregular	Fibrillatory (f) waves	Not measurable	Normal (usually)
Junctional dysrhythmias	40-180 beats/min and regular	Inverted, may be hidden in QRS complex	Variable	Normal (usually)
First-degree AV block	Normal and regular	Normal	>0.20 sec	Normal
Second-degree AV block				
• **Type I** (Mobitz I, Wenckebach heart block)	*Atrial:* Normal and regular *Ventricular:* Slower and irregular	Normal	Progressive lengthening	Normal QRS width, with pattern of one nonconducted (blocked) QRS complex
• **Type II** (Mobitz II heart block)	*Atrial:* Usually normal and regular *Ventricular:* Slower and regular or irregular	More P waves than QRS complexes (e.g., 2:1, 3:1)	Normal or prolonged	Widened QRS, preceded by ≥2 P waves, with nonconducted (blocked) QRS complex
Third-degree AV block (complete heart block)	*Atrial:* Regular but may appear irregular due to P waves hidden in QRS complexes *Ventricular:* 20-60 beats/min and regular	Normal, but no connection with QRS complex	Variable	Normal or widened, no relationship with P waves
Premature ventricular contraction (PVC)	Underlying rhythm can be any rate, regular or irregular rhythm, PVCs occur at variable rates	Not usually visible, hidden in the PVC	Not measurable	Wide and distorted
Ventricular tachycardia	150-250 beats/min and regular or irregular	Not usually visible	Not measurable	Wide and distorted
Accelerated idioventricular rhythm	40-100 beats/min and regular	Not usually visible	Not measurable	Wide and distorted
Ventricular fibrillation	Not measurable and irregular	Absent	Not measurable	Not measurable

AV, Atrioventricular.

ECG Characteristics. In sinus tachycardia, HR is 101 to 200 beats/minute and the rhythm is regular. The P wave is normal, precedes each QRS complex, and has a normal shape and duration. The PR interval is normal, and the QRS complex has a normal shape and duration.

Clinical Significance. The clinical significance of sinus tachycardia depends on the patient's tolerance of the increased HR. The patient may have dizziness, dyspnea, and hypotension because of decreased CO. Increased myocardial oxygen consumption is associated with an increased HR. Angina or an increase in infarction size may accompany sinus tachycardia in patients with coronary artery disease (CAD) or an acute MI.

Treatment. The underlying cause of tachycardia guides the treatment. For example, if the patient is experiencing tachycardia from pain, effective pain management is important to treat the tachycardia. In clinically stable patients, vagal maneuvers can be attempted. In addition, IV β-adrenergic blockers (e.g., metoprolol [Lopressor]), adenosine (Adenocard), or calcium channel blockers (e.g., diltiazem [Cardizem]) can be given to reduce HR and decrease myocardial oxygen consumption. In clinically unstable patients, synchronized cardioversion is used. (Cardioversion is discussed on p. 802.)

Premature Atrial Contraction. A **premature atrial contraction (PAC)** is a contraction starting from an ectopic focus in the atrium (i.e., a location other than the SA node) and coming sooner than the next expected sinus beat. The ectopic signal starts in the left or right atrium and travels across the atria by an abnormal pathway. This creates a distorted P wave (Fig. 36-12). At the AV node, it may be stopped (nonconducted PAC), delayed (lengthened PR interval), or conducted normally. If the signal moves through the AV node, in most cases it is conducted normally through the ventricles.

Clinical Associations. In a normal heart a PAC can result from emotional stress or physical fatigue or from the use

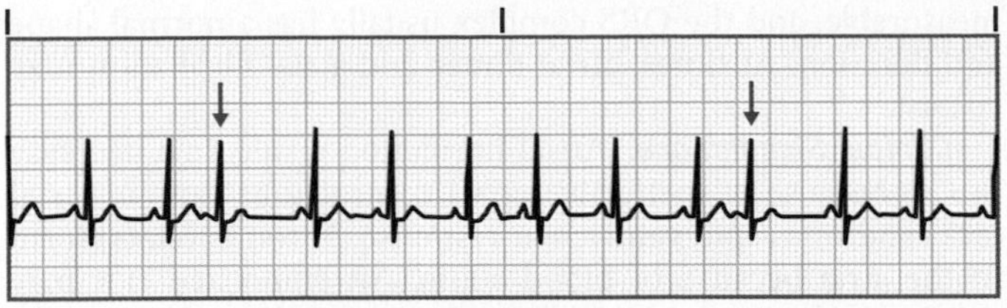

FIG. 36-12 Premature atrial contractions *(arrows)*.

of caffeine, tobacco, or alcohol. A PAC can also result from hypoxia; electrolyte imbalances; and disease states such as hyperthyroidism, chronic obstructive pulmonary disease (COPD), and heart disease, including CAD and valvular disease.

ECG Characteristics. HR varies with the underlying rate and frequency of the PAC, and the rhythm is irregular. The P wave has a different shape from that of a P wave originating in the SA node, or it may be hidden in the preceding T wave. The PR interval may be shorter or longer than the PR interval coming from the SA node, but it is within normal limits. The QRS complex is usually normal. If the QRS interval is 0.12 second or more, abnormal conduction through the ventricles occurs.

Clinical Significance. In persons with healthy hearts, isolated PACs are not significant. Patients may report palpitations or a sense that their hearts "skipped a beat." In persons with heart disease, frequent PACs may indicate enhanced automaticity of the atria or a reentry mechanism. Such PACs may warn of or start more serious dysrhythmias (e.g., supraventricular tachycardia).

Treatment. Treatment depends on the patient's symptoms. Withdrawal of sources of stimulation such as caffeine or sympathomimetic drugs may be needed. β-Adrenergic blockers may be used to decrease PACs.

Paroxysmal Supraventricular Tachycardia. *Paroxysmal supraventricular tachycardia* (PSVT) is a dysrhythmia starting in an ectopic focus anywhere above the bifurcation of the bundle of His (Fig. 36-13). Identification of the ectopic focus is often difficult even with a 12-lead ECG, since it requires recording the dysrhythmia as it starts.

PSVT occurs because of a reentrant phenomenon (reexcitation of the atria when there is a one-way block). Usually a PAC triggers a run of repeated premature beats. *Paroxysmal* refers to an abrupt onset and ending. Termination is sometimes followed by a brief period of asystole (absence of all cardiac electrical activity). Some degree of AV block may be present. PSVT can occur in the presence of Wolff-Parkinson-White (WPW) syndrome, or "preexcitation." In this syndrome, there is extra conduction or accessory pathways.

Clinical Associations. In the normal heart, PSVT is associated with overexertion, emotional stress, deep inspiration, and stimulants such as caffeine and tobacco. PSVT is also associated with rheumatic heart disease, digitalis toxicity, CAD, and cor pulmonale.

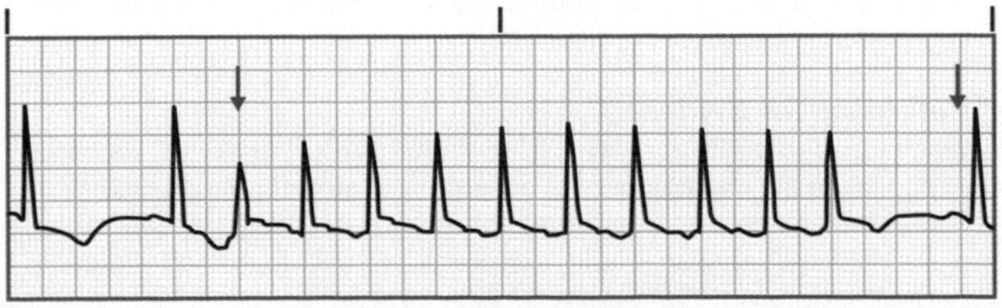

FIG. 36-13 Paroxysmal supraventricular tachycardia (PSVT). *Arrows* indicate beginning and ending of PSVT.

ECG Characteristics. In PSVT the HR is 150 to 220 beats/minute, and the rhythm is regular or slightly irregular. The P wave is often hidden in the preceding T wave. If seen, it may have an abnormal shape. The PR interval may be shortened or normal, and the QRS complex is usually normal.

Clinical Significance. The clinical significance of PSVT depends on the associated symptoms. A prolonged episode and HR greater than 180 beats/minute will cause decreased CO because of reduced stroke volume. Symptoms often include hypotension, palpitations, dyspnea, and angina.

Treatment. Treatment for PSVT includes vagal stimulation and drug therapy. Common vagal maneuvers include Valsalva, carotid massage, and coughing. IV adenosine is the drug of choice to convert PSVT to a normal sinus rhythm. This drug has a short half-life (10 seconds) and is well tolerated.[5] IV β-adrenergic blockers, calcium channel blockers, and amiodarone (Cordarone) can also be used. If vagal stimulation and drug therapy are ineffective and the patient becomes hemodynamically unstable, synchronized cardioversion is used.[6] (Cardioversion is discussed on p. 802.)

DRUG ALERT: Adenosine (Adenocard)

- Injection site should be as close to the heart as possible (e.g., antecubital area).
- Give IV dose rapidly (over 1-2 sec) and follow with a rapid 20 mL normal saline flush.
- Monitor patient's ECG continuously. Brief period of asystole is common.
- Observe patient for flushing, dizziness, chest pain, or palpitations.

If PSVT recurs in patients with WPW syndrome, radiofrequency catheter ablation of the accessory pathway is the treatment of choice.[7] (Catheter ablation therapy is discussed on p. 805.)

Atrial Flutter. Atrial flutter is an atrial tachydysrhythmia identified by recurring, regular, sawtooth-shaped flutter waves that originate from a single ectopic focus in the right atrium or, less commonly, the left atrium (Fig. 36-14, *A*).

Clinical Associations. Atrial flutter rarely occurs in a healthy heart. It is associated with CAD, hypertension, mitral valve disorders, pulmonary embolus, chronic lung disease, cor

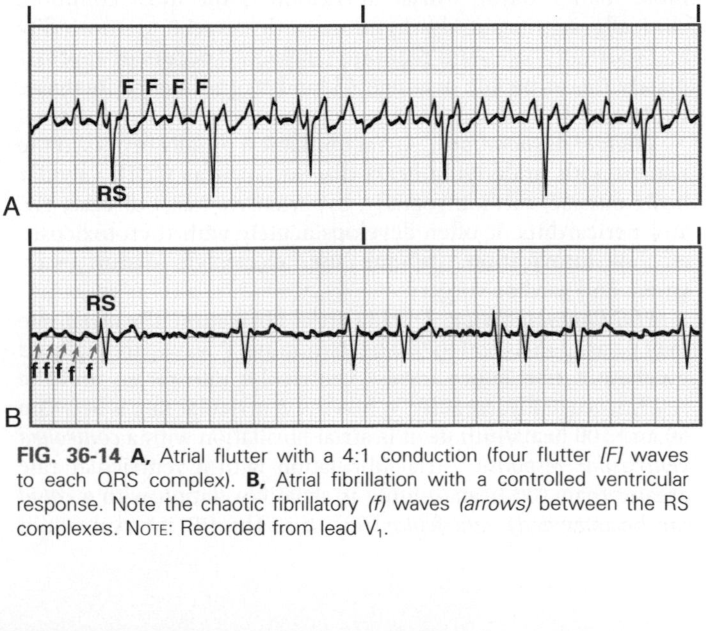

FIG. 36-14 **A,** Atrial flutter with a 4:1 conduction (four flutter *[F]* waves to each QRS complex). **B,** Atrial fibrillation with a controlled ventricular response. Note the chaotic fibrillatory *(f)* waves *(arrows)* between the RS complexes. Note: Recorded from lead V_1.

pulmonale, cardiomyopathy, hyperthyroidism, and the use of drugs such as digoxin, quinidine, and epinephrine.

ECG Characteristics. Atrial rate is 200 to 350 beats/minute. The ventricular rate varies based on the conduction ratio. In 2:1 conduction, the ventricular rate is typically found to be approximately 150 beats/minute. Atrial rhythm is regular, and ventricular rhythm is usually regular. The atrial flutter waves represent atrial depolarization followed by repolarization. The PR interval is variable and not measurable. The QRS complex is usually normal. Because the AV node can delay signals from the atria, there is usually some AV block in a fixed ratio of flutter waves to QRS complexes.

Clinical Significance. The high ventricular rates (greater than 100 beats/minute) and loss of the atrial "kick" (atrial contraction reflected by a sinus P wave) that are associated with atrial flutter decrease CO. This can cause serious consequences such as HF, especially in the patient with underlying heart disease. Patients with atrial flutter have an increased risk of stroke because of the risk of thrombus formation in the atria from the stasis of blood. Warfarin (Coumadin) is given to prevent stroke in patients who have atrial flutter.[6,7]

Treatment. The primary goal in treatment of atrial flutter is to slow the ventricular response by increasing AV block. Drugs used to control ventricular rate include calcium channel blockers and β-adrenergic blockers. Electrical cardioversion may be performed to convert the atrial flutter to sinus rhythm in an emergency (i.e., when the patient is clinically unstable) and electively. Antidysrhythmia drugs are used to convert atrial flutter to sinus rhythm (e.g., ibutilide [Corvert]) or to maintain sinus rhythm (e.g., amiodarone, flecainide [Tambocor], dronedarone [Multaq]).[5]

Radiofrequency catheter ablation is the treatment of choice for atrial flutter.[8] The procedure is done in the EPS laboratory and involves placing a catheter in the right atrium. With use of a low-voltage, high-frequency form of electrical energy, the tissue is ablated (or destroyed), the dysrhythmia is ended, and normal sinus rhythm is restored. (Catheter ablation is discussed on p. 802.)

Atrial Fibrillation. Atrial fibrillation is characterized by a total disorganization of atrial electrical activity because of multiple ectopic foci, resulting in loss of effective atrial contraction (Fig. 36-14, *B*). The dysrhythmia may be paroxysmal (i.e., beginning and ending spontaneously) or persistent (lasting more than 7 days).[9] Atrial fibrillation is the most common, clinically significant dysrhythmia with respect to morbidity and mortality rates and economic impact. It occurs in approximately 6% of people over age 65, and its prevalence increases with age.[10]

Clinical Associations. Atrial fibrillation usually occurs in the patient with underlying heart disease, such as CAD, valvular heart disease, cardiomyopathy, hypertensive heart disease, HF, and pericarditis. It often develops acutely with thyrotoxicosis, alcohol intoxication, caffeine use, electrolyte disturbances, stress, and cardiac surgery.

ECG Characteristics. During atrial fibrillation, the atrial rate may be as high as 350 to 600 beats/minute. P waves are replaced by chaotic, fibrillatory waves. Ventricular rate varies, and the rhythm is usually irregular. When the ventricular rate is between 60 and 100 beats/minute, it is atrial fibrillation with a *controlled ventricular response.* Atrial fibrillation with a ventricular rate greater than 100 beats/minute is atrial fibrillation with a *rapid (or uncontrolled) ventricular response.* The PR interval is not measurable, and the QRS complex usually has a normal shape and duration. At times, atrial flutter and atrial fibrillation may coexist.[1]

Clinical Significance. Atrial fibrillation results in a decrease in CO because of ineffective atrial contractions (loss of atrial kick) and/or a rapid ventricular response. Thrombi (clots) form in the atria because of blood stasis. An embolized clot may develop and move to the brain, causing a stroke. Atrial fibrillation accounts for as many as 17% of all strokes.[10]

Treatment. The goals of treatment include a decrease in ventricular response (to less than 100 beats/minute), prevention of stroke, and conversion to sinus rhythm, if possible. Ventricular rate control is a priority for patients with atrial fibrillation. Drugs used for rate control include calcium channel blockers (e.g., diltiazem), β-adrenergic blockers (e.g., metoprolol), dronedarone, and digoxin (Lanoxin).

For some patients, pharmacologic or electrical conversion of atrial fibrillation to a normal sinus rhythm may be considered

EVIDENCE-BASED PRACTICE

Applying the Evidence

G.D. is an 82-year-old woman with a new onset of atrial fibrillation and a history of mitral stenosis (high-risk factor). Her physician has ordered warfarin (Coumadin) to be started. You begin to teach her about the purpose and side effects of warfarin. She stops you and states that she will not take the medicine—she has heard too many stories about people bleeding from this medication. Furthermore, she tells you that she does not want to deal with the blood tests that are needed nor worry about what she eats. She states that she will continue to take her aspirin once a day as usual.

Best Available Evidence	Clinician Expertise	Patient Preferences and Values
Warfarin (Coumadin) is the drug of choice to treat patients with atrial fibrillation who have one or more high-risk factors in order to prevent stroke.	Bleeding is a potential and serious side effect of warfarin and of dual antiplatelet therapy (ASA and clopidogrel).	G.D. does not want to take warfarin or clopidogrel because she is afraid of bleeding.
For patients for whom oral anticoagulation with warfarin is considered unsuitable (e.g., patient preference), the addition of clopidogrel (Plavix) to ASA reduces the risk of major vascular events (especially stroke) but increases the risk of major hemorrhage.	When taking warfarin, INR blood levels need to be checked on a regular basis. Patients should avoid drastic changes in diet, especially foods high in vitamin K (interfere with the action of warfarin).	In addition, she does not want to change her lifestyle to accommodate the changes that would be needed to use warfarin.

Your Decision and Action

You explain the risks of not taking the prescribed medicine (warfarin) or adequate medication (adding clopidogrel to her ASA therapy). She tells you that she understands completely. You support her choice and inform the physician of her decision.

Reference for Evidence

Wann LS, Curtis AB, January CT, et al: 2011 ACCF/AHA/HRS focused update on the management of patients with atrial fibrillation (updating the 2006 guideline): a report of the American College of Cardiology Foundation/American Heart Association Task Force on Practice Guidelines, *J Am Coll Cardiol* 57:223, 2011.

ASA, Acetylsalicylic acid; *INR,* international normalized ratio.

TABLE 36-8 **DRUG THERAPY**

Anticoagulant Therapy for Atrial Fibrillation

Risk Category	Recommended Therapy
No risk factors	Aspirin, 81-325 mg/day
One moderate-risk factor	Aspirin, 81-325 mg/day, or warfarin*† (target INR 2.0-3.0)
Any high-risk factor or >1 moderate-risk factor	Warfarin* (target INR 2.0-3.0‡)
Level of Risk	**Risk Factors**
Moderate-risk factors	Age ≥75 yr Heart failure Hypertension LV ejection fraction ≤35% Diabetes mellitus
High-risk factors	Previous stroke, TIA, or embolism Mitral stenosis Prosthetic heart valve‡

Source: Wann LS, Curtis AB, January CT, et al: 2011 ACCF/AHA/HRS focused update on the management of patients with atrial fibrillation (updating the 2006 guideline): a report of the American College of Cardiology Foundation/American Heart Association Task Force on Practice Guidelines, *J Am Coll Cardiol* 57:223, 2011.

*Dabigatran (Pradaxa), a direct thrombin inhibitor, and apixaban (Eliquis) and rivaroxaban (Xarelto), factor Xa inhibitors, are oral anticoagulants approved for use in the treatment of nonvalvular atrial fibrillation only. To date, these drugs have not been incorporated into the guidelines.

†Clopidogrel (Plavix) may be added to aspirin therapy to reduce the risk of major vascular events in patients with atrial fibrillation if warfarin is considered unsuitable (e.g., patient preference, physician determines that patient cannot maintain adequate anticoagulation).

‡If prosthetic heart valve, target INR 2.5-3.5.

INR, International normalized ratio; *LV,* left ventricular; *TIA,* transient ischemic attack.

(e.g., reduced exercise tolerance with rate control drugs, contraindications to warfarin). The most common antidysrhythmia drugs used for conversion to and maintenance of sinus rhythm include amiodarone and ibutilide.[9]

Electrical cardioversion may convert atrial fibrillation to a normal sinus rhythm. If a patient is in atrial fibrillation for longer than 48 hours, anticoagulation therapy with warfarin is needed for 3 to 4 weeks before the cardioversion and for several weeks after successful cardioversion.[5] Anticoagulation therapy is necessary because the procedure can cause the clots to dislodge, placing the patient at risk for stroke. A transesophageal echocardiogram may be performed to rule out clots in the atria. If no clots are present, anticoagulation therapy may not be required before the cardioversion procedure.

If drugs or cardioversion does not convert atrial fibrillation to normal sinus rhythm, long-term anticoagulation therapy is required (Table 36-8). Warfarin is the drug of choice, and patients are monitored for therapeutic levels (e.g., international normalized ratio [INR]). Recently, alternatives to warfarin have been approved for anticoagulation therapy in patients with nonvalvular atrial fibrillation. These drugs do not require routine laboratory testing and include dabigatran (Pradaxa), apixaban (Eliquis), and rivaroxaban (Xarelto). (See Chapter 38 for discussion of anticoagulation therapy.)

For patients with drug-refractory atrial fibrillation or those who do not respond to electrical conversion, radiofrequency catheter ablation (similar to procedure for atrial flutter) and the Maze procedure are further options.[9] The Maze procedure is a surgical intervention that stops atrial fibrillation by interrupting the ectopic electrical signals that are responsible for the dysrhythmia. Incisions are made in both atria, and *cryoablation*

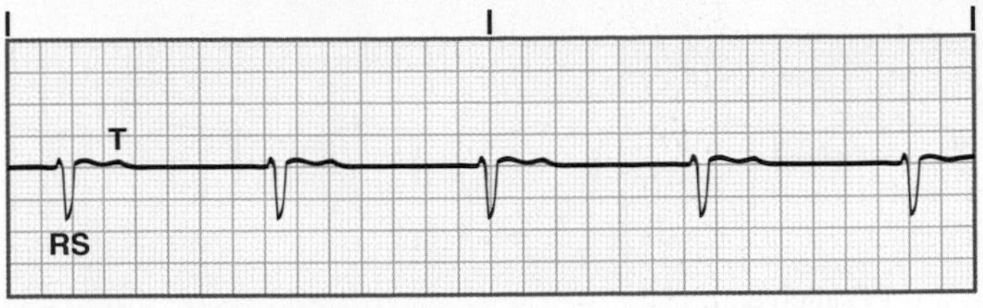

FIG. 36-15 Junctional escape rhythm. P wave is hidden in the RS complex. NOTE: Recorded from lead V_1.

(cold therapy) is used to stop the formation and conduction of these signals and restore normal sinus rhythm.[7]

Junctional Dysrhythmias. *Junctional dysrhythmias* refer to dysrhythmias that start in the area of the AV node. They result because the SA node fails to fire or the signal is blocked. When this occurs, the AV node becomes the pacemaker of the heart. The impulse from the AV node usually moves in a retrograde (backward) fashion. This produces an abnormal P wave that occurs just before or after the QRS complex or that is hidden in the QRS complex. The impulse usually moves normally through the ventricles. Junctional premature beats may occur, and they are treated in a manner similar to that for PACs. Other junctional dysrhythmias include junctional escape rhythm (Fig. 36-15), accelerated junctional rhythm, and junctional tachycardia. These dysrhythmias are treated according to the patient's tolerance of the rhythm and the patient's clinical condition.

Clinical Associations. Junctional dysrhythmias are often associated with CAD, HF, cardiomyopathy, electrolyte imbalances, inferior MI, and rheumatic heart disease. Certain drugs (e.g., digoxin, nicotine, amphetamines, caffeine) can also cause junctional dysrhythmias.

ECG Characteristics. In junctional escape rhythm the HR is 40 to 60 beats/minute. It is 61 to 100 beats/minute in accelerated junctional rhythm and 101 to 180 beats/minute in junctional tachycardia. Rhythm is regular. The P wave is abnormal in shape and inverted, or it may be hidden in the QRS complex (see Fig. 36-15). The PR interval is less than 0.12 second when the P wave precedes the QRS complex. The QRS complex is usually normal.

Clinical Significance. Junctional escape rhythms serve as a safety mechanism when the SA node has not been effective. Escape rhythms such as this should not be suppressed. Accelerated junctional rhythm is due to sympathetic stimulation to improve CO. Junctional tachycardia indicates a more serious problem. This rhythm may reduce CO, causing the patient to become hemodynamically unstable (e.g., hypotensive).

Treatment. Treatment varies according to the type of junctional dysrhythmia. If a patient has symptoms with a junctional escape rhythm, atropine can be used. In accelerated junctional rhythm and junctional tachycardia caused by drug toxicity, the drug is stopped. In the absence of digitalis toxicity, β-adrenergic blockers, calcium channel blockers, and amiodarone are used for rate control. Cardioversion should not be used.

First-Degree AV Block. *First-degree AV block* is a type of AV block in which every impulse is conducted to the ventricles but the time of AV conduction is prolonged (Fig. 36-16, *A*). After the impulse moves through the AV node, the ventricles usually respond normally.

Clinical Associations. First-degree AV block is associated with MI, CAD, rheumatic fever, hyperthyroidism, electrolyte imbalances (e.g., hypokalemia), vagal stimulation, and drugs such as digoxin, β-adrenergic blockers, calcium channel blockers, and flecainide.

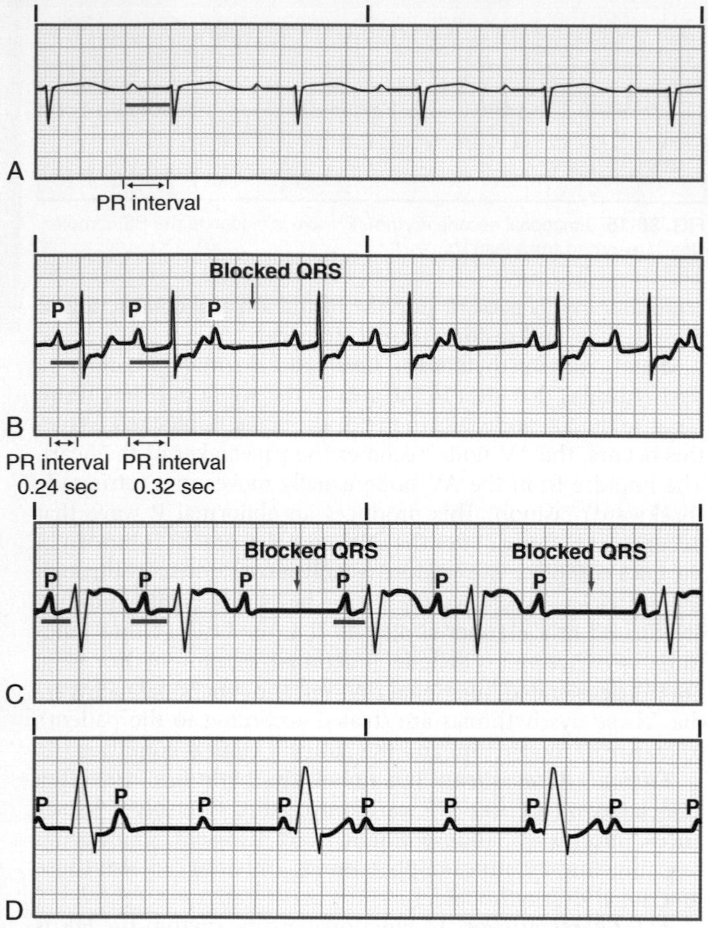

FIG. 36-16 Heart block. **A,** First-degree atrioventricular (AV) block with a PR interval of 0.40 sec. **B,** Second-degree AV block, type I, with progressive lengthening of the PR interval until a QRS complex is blocked. **C,** Second-degree AV block, type II, with constant PR intervals and variable blocked QRS complexes. **D,** Third-degree AV block. Note that there is no relationship between P waves and QRS complexes.

ECG Characteristics. In first-degree AV block, HR is normal and rhythm is regular. The P wave is normal, the PR interval is prolonged (greater than 0.20 second), and the QRS complex usually has a normal shape and duration.

Clinical Significance. First-degree AV block is usually not serious but can be a sign of higher degrees of AV block. Patients with first-degree AV block are asymptomatic.

Treatment. There is no treatment for first-degree AV block. Changes to potentially causative situations may be considered. Monitor patients for any new changes in heart rhythm (e.g., more serious AV block).

Second-Degree AV Block, Type I. *Type I second-degree AV block (Mobitz I* or *Wenckebach heart block)* includes a gradual lengthening of the PR interval. It occurs because of a prolonged AV conduction time until an atrial impulse is nonconducted and a QRS complex is blocked (missing) (Fig. 36-16, *B*). Type I AV block most commonly occurs in the AV node, but it can also occur in the His-Purkinje system.

Clinical Associations. Type I AV block may result from drugs such as digoxin or β-adrenergic blockers. It may also be associated with CAD and other diseases that can slow AV conduction.

ECG Characteristics. Atrial rate is normal, but ventricular rate may be slower because of nonconducted or blocked QRS complexes resulting in bradycardia. Once a ventricular beat is blocked, the cycle repeats itself with progressive lengthening of the PR intervals until another QRS complex is blocked. The rhythm appears on the ECG in a pattern of grouped beats. Ventricular rhythm is irregular. The P wave has a normal shape. The QRS complex has a normal shape and duration.

Clinical Significance. Type I AV block is usually a result of myocardial ischemia or inferior MI. It is generally transient and well tolerated. However, in some patients (e.g., acute MI) it may be a warning sign of a more serious AV conduction disturbance (e.g., complete heart block).

Treatment. If the patient is symptomatic, atropine is used to increase HR, or a temporary pacemaker may be needed, especially if the patient has had an MI. If the patient is asymptomatic, the rhythm is closely observed with a transcutaneous pacemaker on standby. Bradycardia is more likely to become symptomatic when hypotension, HF, or shock is present.

Second-Degree AV Block, Type II. In *type II second-degree AV block (Mobitz II heart block),* a P wave is nonconducted without progressive PR lengthening. This usually occurs when a block in one of the bundle branches is present (Fig. 36-16, *C*). On conducted beats, the PR interval is constant. Type II second-degree AV block is a more serious type of block in which a certain number of impulses from the SA node are not conducted to the ventricles. This occurs in ratios of 2:1, 3:1, and so on (i.e., two P waves to one QRS complex, three P waves to one QRS complex). It may occur with varying ratios.

Clinical Associations. Type II AV block is associated with rheumatic heart disease, CAD, anterior MI, and drug toxicity.

ECG Characteristics. Atrial rate is usually normal. Ventricular rate depends on the intrinsic rate and the degree of AV block. Atrial rhythm is regular, but ventricular rhythm may be irregular. The P wave has a normal shape. The PR interval may be normal or prolonged in duration and remains constant on conducted beats. The QRS complex is usually greater than 0.12 second because of bundle branch block.

Clinical Significance. Type II AV block often progresses to third-degree AV block and is associated with a poor prognosis. The reduced HR frequently results in decreased CO with subsequent hypotension and myocardial ischemia. Type II AV block is an indication for therapy with a permanent pacemaker.

Treatment. Insertion of a temporary pacemaker may be necessary before the insertion of a permanent pacemaker if the patient becomes symptomatic (e.g., hypotension, angina).[6,8] (Temporary pacemakers are discussed on pp. 804-805.)

Third-Degree AV Block. Third-degree AV block, or **complete heart block,** constitutes one form of AV dissociation in which no impulses from the atria are conducted to the ventricles (Fig. 36-16, *D*). The atria are stimulated and contract independently of the ventricles. The ventricular rhythm is an escape rhythm, and the ectopic pacemaker may be above or below the bifurcation of the bundle of His.

Clinical Associations. Third-degree AV block is associated with severe heart disease, including CAD, MI, myocarditis, cardiomyopathy, and some systemic diseases such as amyloidosis and progressive systemic sclerosis (scleroderma). Some drugs can also cause third-degree AV block, such as digoxin, β-adrenergic blockers, and calcium channel blockers.

ECG Characteristics. The atrial rate is usually a sinus rate of 60 to 100 beats/minute. The ventricular rate depends on the site of the block. If it is in the AV node, the rate is 40 to 60 beats/

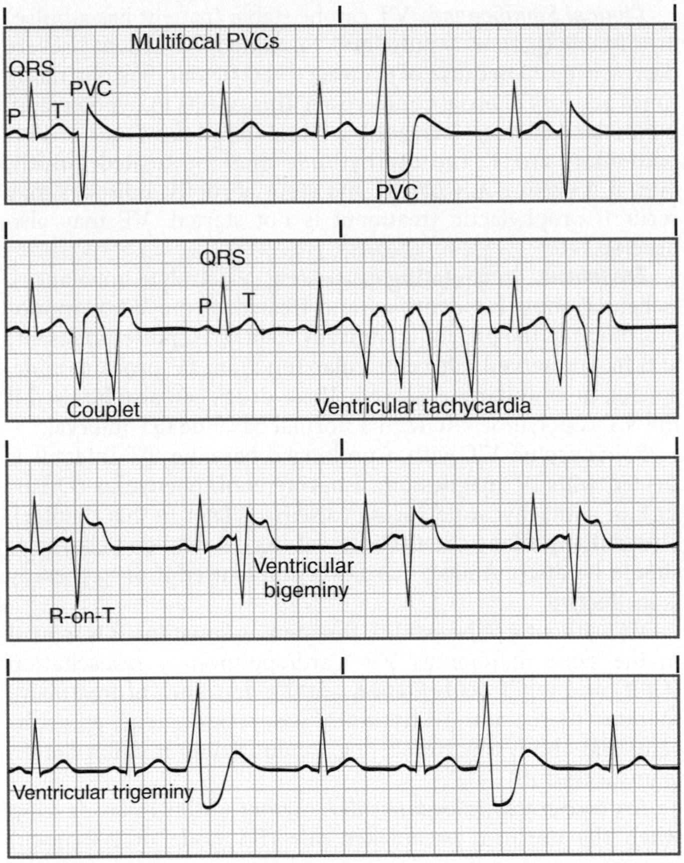

FIG. 36-17 Various forms of premature ventricular contractions (PVCs).

minute, and if it is in the His-Purkinje system, it is 20 to 40 beats/minute. Atrial and ventricular rhythms are regular but unrelated to each other. The P wave has a normal shape. The PR interval is variable, and there is no relationship between the P wave and the QRS complex. The QRS complex is normal if an escape rhythm is initiated at the bundle of His or above. It is widened if an escape rhythm is initiated below the bundle of His.

Clinical Significance. Third-degree AV block usually results in reduced CO with subsequent ischemia, HF, and shock. Syncope from third-degree AV block may result from severe bradycardia or even periods of asystole.

Treatment. For symptomatic patients, a transcutaneous pacemaker is used until a temporary transvenous pacemaker can be inserted.[8] (Types of temporary pacemakers are discussed on pp. 804-805.) The use of drugs such as atropine, dopamine, and epinephrine is a temporary measure to increase HR and support blood pressure (BP) until temporary pacing is started. Patients need a permanent pacemaker as soon as possible.

Premature Ventricular Contractions. A **premature ventricular contraction (PVC)** is a contraction coming from an ectopic focus in the ventricles. It is the premature (early) occurrence of a QRS complex. A PVC is wide and distorted in shape compared with a QRS complex coming down the normal conduction pathway (Fig. 36-17). PVCs that arise from different foci appear different in shape from each other and are called *multifocal* PVCs. PVCs that have the same shape are called *unifocal* PVCs. When every other beat is a PVC, the rhythm is called *ventricular bigeminy.* When every third beat is a PVC, it is called *ventricular trigeminy.* Two consecutive PVCs are called a *couplet.*

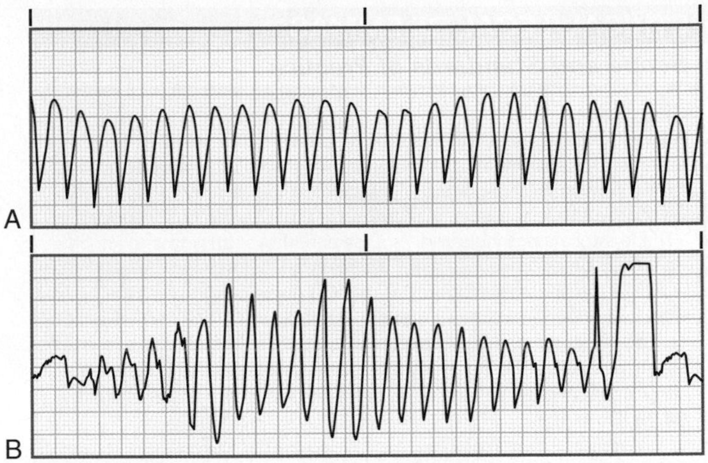

FIG. 36-18 Ventricular tachycardia. **A,** Monomorphic. **B,** Torsades de pointes (polymorphic).

Ventricular tachycardia (VT) occurs when there are three or more consecutive PVCs. *R-on-T phenomenon* occurs when a PVC falls on the T wave of a preceding beat. This is especially dangerous because the PVC is firing during the relative refractory phase of ventricular repolarization. Excitability of the cardiac cells increases during this time, and the risk for the PVC to start VT or ventricular fibrillation (VF) is great.

Clinical Associations. PVCs are associated with stimulants such as caffeine, alcohol, nicotine, aminophylline, epinephrine, isoproterenol, and digoxin. They are also associated with electrolyte imbalances, hypoxia, fever, exercise, and emotional stress. Disease states associated with PVCs include MI, mitral valve prolapse, HF, and CAD.

ECG Characteristics. HR varies according to intrinsic rate and number of PVCs. Rhythm is irregular because of premature beats. The P wave is rarely visible and is usually lost in the QRS complex of the PVC. Retrograde conduction may occur, and the P wave may be seen after the ectopic beat. The PR interval is not measurable. The QRS complex is wide and distorted in shape, lasting more than 0.12 second. The T wave is generally large and opposite in direction to the major direction of the QRS complex.

Clinical Significance. PVCs are usually not harmful in the patient with a normal heart. In heart disease, PVCs may reduce the CO and lead to angina and HF depending on frequency. Because PVCs in CAD or acute MI indicate ventricular irritability, assess the patient's physiologic response to PVCs. Obtain the patient's apical-radial pulse rate, since PVCs often do not generate a sufficient ventricular contraction to result in a peripheral pulse. This can lead to a pulse deficit.

Treatment. Treatment relates to the cause of the PVCs (e.g., oxygen therapy for hypoxia, electrolyte replacement). Assessment of the patient's hemodynamic status is important to determine if treatment with drug therapy is needed. Drug therapy includes β-adrenergic blockers, procainamide (Pronestyl), or amiodarone.

Ventricular Tachycardia. A run of three or more PVCs defines **ventricular tachycardia (VT).** It occurs when an ectopic focus or foci fire repeatedly and the ventricle takes control as the pacemaker. Different forms of VT exist, depending on QRS configuration. *Monomorphic* VT (Fig. 36-18, *A*) has QRS complexes that are the same in shape, size, and direction. *Polymorphic* VT occurs when the QRS complexes gradually change back

ETHICAL/LEGAL DILEMMAS

Scope and Standards of Practice

Situation

A young woman is admitted to the intensive care unit (ICU) from the emergency department after experiencing several episodes of nonsustained ventricular tachycardia (VT) attributed to a history of viral cardiomyopathy. While she is being stabilized in the ICU, she codes (pulseless VT) and intubation is indicated. A nurse anesthetist attempts to intubate her three times unsuccessfully. There is an unforeseen delay in the arrival of the anesthesiologist. P.F., an ICU nurse and former paramedic who is certified in advanced trauma life support (ATLS) and advanced cardiac life support (ACLS), attempts to intubate the patient and does so successfully. The next day the nursing supervisor questions P.F. about intubating the patient, since this is not within the scope of practice for an ICU nurse.

Ethical/Legal Points for Consideration

- The RN *Scope of Practice,* including rules and regulations that guide practice, are defined by individual state Boards of Nursing and can vary from state to state.
- Individual agencies also have policies and procedures that describe the scope of practice for nurses. These can be more restrictive than those of the state.
- *Scope and Standards of Practice* are also defined by professional nursing organizations (e.g., American Nurses Association, American Association of Critical-Care Nurses). These are authoritative statements that serve to define expected competent practice in various registered nurse (RN) roles (e.g., Scope and Standards for Nursing Administration).
- P.F. has had training, education, and certification beyond the usual nursing role.
- A life-threatening situation provides for extenuating circumstances.
- Negligence might have been a factor if P.F., who is a nurse with training and experience, had not acted.

Discussion Questions

1. What would you have done in this situation?
2. How would you respond to the nursing supervisor?
3. What are the legal ramifications for P.F. in this situation?
4. What are the ethical issues in this situation?

and forth from one shape, size, and direction to another over a series of beats. *Torsades de pointes* (French for "twisting of the points") is polymorphic VT associated with a prolonged QT interval of the underlying rhythm (Fig. 36-18, *B*).

VT may be sustained (longer than 30 seconds) or nonsustained (less than 30 seconds). The development of VT is an ominous sign. It is a life-threatening dysrhythmia because of decreased CO and the possibility of development of VF, which is lethal.

Clinical Associations. VT is associated with MI, CAD, significant electrolyte imbalances, cardiomyopathy, mitral valve prolapse, long QT syndrome, drug toxicity, and central nervous system disorders. This dysrhythmia can be seen in patients who have no evidence of cardiac disease.

ECG Characteristics. Ventricular rate is 150 to 250 beats/minute. Rhythm may be regular or irregular. AV dissociation may be present, with P waves occurring independently of the QRS complex. The atria may be depolarized by the ventricles in a retrograde fashion. The P wave is usually buried in the QRS complex, and the PR interval is not measurable. The QRS complex is distorted in appearance and wide (greater than 0.12 second in duration). The T wave is in the opposite direction of the QRS complex (see Fig. 36-18).

Clinical Significance. VT can be stable (patient has a pulse) or unstable (patient is pulseless). Sustained VT causes a severe decrease in CO because of decreased ventricular diastolic filling times and loss of atrial contraction. This results in hypotension, pulmonary edema, decreased cerebral blood flow, and cardiopulmonary arrest. The dysrhythmia must be treated quickly, even if it occurs only briefly and stops abruptly. Episodes may recur if prophylactic treatment is not started. VF may also develop.

Treatment. Precipitating causes (e.g., electrolyte imbalances, ischemia) must be identified and treated. If the VT is monomorphic and the patient is clinically stable (i.e., pulse is present) and has preserved left ventricular function, IV procainamide, sotalol, or amiodarone is used. These drugs can also be used if the VT is polymorphic with a normal baseline QT interval.

Polymorphic VT with a prolonged baseline QT interval is treated with IV magnesium, isoproterenol, phenytoin (Dilantin), or antitachycardia pacing (discussed later in this chapter). Drugs that prolong the QT interval (e.g., dofetilide [Tikosyn]) should be discontinued. Cardioversion is used if drug therapy is ineffective.

VT without a pulse is a life-threatening situation. It is treated in the same manner as VF. Cardiopulmonary resuscitation (CPR) and rapid defibrillation are the first lines of treatment, followed by the administration of vasopressors (e.g., epinephrine) and antidysrhythmics (e.g., amiodarone) if defibrillation is unsuccessful.[6]

An *accelerated idioventricular rhythm* (AIVR) can develop when the intrinsic pacemaker rate (SA node or AV node) becomes less than that of a ventricular ectopic pacemaker. The rate is between 40 and 100 beats/minute. It is most commonly associated with acute MI and reperfusion of the myocardium after thrombolytic therapy or angioplasty of coronary arteries. It can be seen with digitalis toxicity. In the setting of acute MI, AIVR is usually self-limiting and well tolerated, and it requires no treatment. If the patient becomes symptomatic (e.g., hypotensive, chest pain), atropine can be considered. Temporary pacing may be required. Drugs that suppress ventricular rhythms (e.g., amiodarone) should not be used, since these can terminate the ventricular rhythm and further reduce the HR.

Ventricular Fibrillation. Ventricular fibrillation (VF) is a severe derangement of the heart rhythm characterized on ECG by irregular waveforms of varying shapes and amplitude (Fig. 36-19). This represents the firing of multiple ectopic foci in the ventricle. Mechanically the ventricle is simply "quivering," with no effective contraction, and consequently no CO occurs. VF is a lethal dysrhythmia.

Clinical Associations. VF occurs in acute MI and myocardial ischemia and in chronic diseases such as HF and cardiomyopathy. It may occur during cardiac pacing or cardiac catheterization procedures because of catheter stimulation of the ventricle. It may also occur with coronary reperfusion

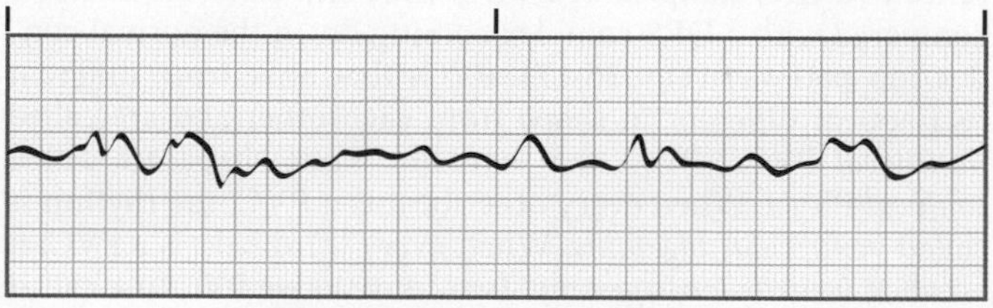

FIG. 36-19 Ventricular fibrillation.

after thrombolytic therapy. Other clinical associations are electric shock, hyperkalemia, hypoxemia, acidosis, and drug toxicity.

ECG Characteristics. HR is not measurable. Rhythm is irregular and chaotic. The P wave is not visible, and the PR interval and the QRS interval are not measurable.

Clinical Significance. VF results in an unresponsive, pulseless, and apneic state. If it is not rapidly treated, the patient will not recover.

Treatment. Treatment consists of immediate initiation of CPR and advanced cardiac life support (ACLS) with the use of defibrillation and definitive drug therapy (e.g., epinephrine, vasopressin [Pitressin]). There should be no delay in using a defibrillator once available.

Asystole. Asystole represents the total absence of ventricular electrical activity. Occasionally, P waves are seen. No ventricular contraction occurs because depolarization does not occur. Patients are unresponsive, pulseless, and apneic. Asystole is a lethal dysrhythmia that requires immediate treatment. VF may masquerade as asystole. Always assess the rhythm in more than one lead. The prognosis of a patient with asystole is extremely poor.

Clinical Associations. Asystole is usually a result of advanced cardiac disease, a severe cardiac conduction system disturbance, or end-stage HF.

Clinical Significance. Generally the patient with asystole has end-stage heart disease or has a prolonged arrest and cannot be resuscitated.

Treatment. Treatment consists of CPR with initiation of ACLS measures. These include definitive drug therapy with epinephrine and/or vasopressin, and intubation.

Pulseless Electrical Activity. *Pulseless electrical activity* (PEA) is a situation in which organized electrical activity is seen on the ECG, but there is no mechanical activity of the ventricles and the patient has no pulse. It is the most common dysrhythmia seen after defibrillation. Prognosis is poor unless the underlying cause is quickly identified and treated. The most common causes of PEA include hypovolemia, hypoxia, metabolic acidosis, hyperkalemia, hypokalemia, hypoglycemia, hypothermia, toxins (e.g., drug overdose), cardiac tamponade, thrombosis (e.g., MI, pulmonary embolus), tension pneumothorax, and trauma. Treatment begins with CPR followed by drug therapy (e.g., epinephrine) and intubation. Correcting the underlying cause is critical to prognosis.

Sudden Cardiac Death. The term *sudden cardiac death* (SCD) refers to death from a cardiac cause. Most SCDs result from ventricular dysrhythmias, specifically VT or VF. (SCD is discussed in Chapter 34.)

Prodysrhythmia. Antidysrhythmia drugs can cause life-threatening dysrhythmias similar to those for which they are given. This concept is termed *prodysrhythmia.* The patient who has severe left ventricular dysfunction is the most susceptible to prodysrhythmias. Digoxin and class IA, IC, and III antidysrhythmia drugs can cause a prodysrhythmic response.[5] The first several days of drug therapy are the vulnerable period for developing prodysrhythmias. For this reason, many oral antidysrhythmia drug regimens are started in a monitored hospital setting.

Antidysrhythmia Drugs

Table 36-9 categorizes antidysrhythmia drugs by their primary effects on the cardiac cells and the ECG.

TABLE 36-9 DRUG THERAPY

Antidysrhythmia Drugs

Drug	Actions*	Effects on ECG
Class I: Sodium Channel Blockers	Decrease impulse conduction in the atria, ventricles, and His-Purkinje system	—
Class IA disopyramide (Norpace) procainamide (Pronestyl) quinidine (Quinora)	Delay repolarization	Widened QRS and prolonged QT interval
Class IB mexiletine (Mexitil) phenytoin (Dilantin)	Accelerate repolarization	Little or no effect on ECG
Class IC flecainide (Tambocor) propafenone (Rythmol)	Decrease impulse conduction	Pronounced prodysrhythmic actions, widened QRS, prolonged QT interval
Class II: β-Adrenergic Blockers esmolol (Brevibloc) metoprolol (Lopressor) propranolol (Inderal)	Decrease automaticity of the SA node, slow impulse conduction in AV node, reduce atrial and ventricular contractility	Bradycardia, prolonged PR interval, AV block
Class III: Potassium Channel Blockers amiodarone (Cordarone) bretylium (Bretylol) dofetilide (Tikosyn) ibutilide (Corvert) sotalol† (Betapace)	Delay repolarization, resulting in prolonged duration of action potential and refractory period	Prolonged PR and QT intervals, widened QRS, bradycardia
Class IV: Calcium Channel Blockers diltiazem (Cardizem) verapamil (Calan)	Decrease automaticity of SA node, delay AV node conduction; reduce myocardial contractility	Bradycardia, prolonged PR interval, AV block
Other Antidysrhythmia Drugs adenosine (Adenocard) digoxin (Lanoxin)	Decrease conduction through AV node, reduce automaticity of SA node	Prolonged PR interval, AV block
dronedarone (Multaq)‡	Suppresses atrial dysrhythmias though mechanism is unknown	Prolonged QT interval
Magnesium	Decreases impulse conduction through AV node	AV block

*Antidysrhythmia drugs have a direct effect on the various phases of the action potential (see Fig. 36-1).
†Sotalol has both class II and class III properties.
‡Dronedarone has class I-IV properties.
AV, Atrioventricular; *SA,* sinoatrial.

Defibrillation

Defibrillation is the treatment of choice to end VF and pulseless VT. It is most effective when the myocardial cells are not anoxic or acidotic. Rapid defibrillation (within 2 minutes) is critical to a successful patient outcome. Defibrillation involves the passage of an electric shock through the heart to depolarize the cells of the myocardium. The goal is that the following repolarization

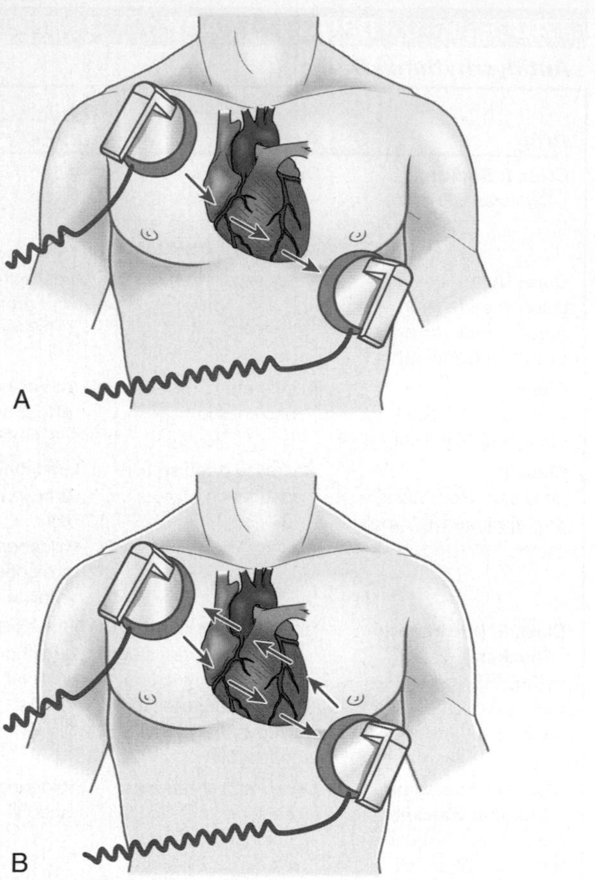

FIG. 36-20 Paddle placement and current flow in monophasic defibrillation **(A)** and biphasic defibrillation **(B)**.

of myocardial cells will allow the SA node to resume the role of pacemaker.

Defibrillators deliver energy using a monophasic or biphasic waveform. Monophasic defibrillators deliver energy in one direction, and biphasic defibrillators deliver energy in two directions (Fig. 36-20). Biphasic defibrillators deliver successful shocks at lower energies and with fewer postshock ECG abnormalities than monophasic defibrillators.

The output of a defibrillator is measured in *joules*, or watts per second. The recommended energy for initial shocks in defibrillation depends on the type of defibrillator. Biphasic defibrillators deliver the first and any successive shocks using 120 to 200 joules. Recommendations for monophasic defibrillators include an initial shock at 360 joules. After the first shock, start CPR immediately beginning with chest compressions. (CPR is discussed in Appendix A of this book.)

Rapid defibrillation can be performed using a manual or automatic device (Fig. 36-21). Manual defibrillators require you to interpret heart rhythms, determine the need for a shock, and deliver a shock. An **automatic external defibrillator (AED)** can detect heart rhythms and advise the user to deliver a shock using hands-free defibrillator pads. Proficiency in use of the AED is part of the basic life support course for health care providers. You should be familiar with the operation of the type of defibrillator used in your clinical setting.

The following general steps are taken for defibrillation: (1) CPR should be in progress until the defibrillator is available; (2) turn the defibrillator on, and select the proper energy level;

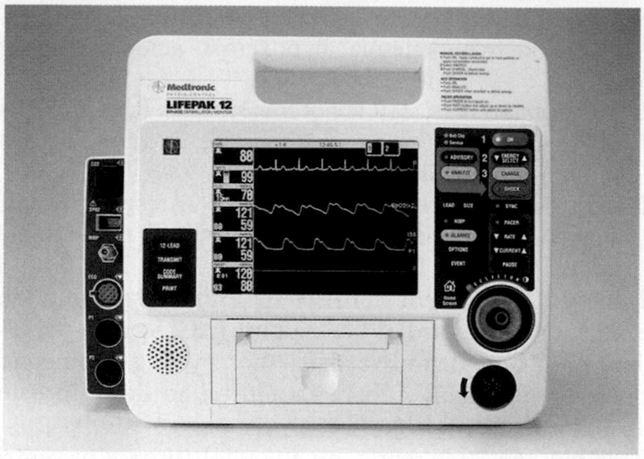

FIG. 36-21 LifePak contains a monitor, defibrillator, and transcutaneous pacemaker.

(3) check to see that the synchronizer switch is turned off (discussed below); (4) apply conductive materials (e.g., defibrillator gel pads) to the chest, one to the right of the sternum just below the clavicle, and the other to the left of the apex; (5) charge the defibrillator using the button on the defibrillator or the paddles; (6) position the paddles firmly on the chest wall over the conductive material (see Fig. 36-20); (7) call and look to see that everyone is "all clear" to ensure that personnel are not touching the patient or the bed at the time of discharge; and (8) deliver the charge by depressing buttons on both paddles simultaneously.

Hands-free, multifunction defibrillator pads are available and are placed on the chest as described above. Connect the cables from the pads to the defibrillator. Charge and discharge the defibrillator using buttons on the defibrillator. It is still essential to ensure that all personnel are clear before discharging the defibrillator.

Synchronized Cardioversion. *Synchronized cardioversion* is the therapy of choice for the patient with ventricular tachydysrhythmias (e.g., VT with a pulse) or supraventricular tachydysrhythmias (e.g., atrial fibrillation with a rapid ventricular response). A synchronized circuit in the defibrillator delivers a shock that is programmed to occur on the R wave of the QRS complex of the ECG. The synchronizer switch must be turned on when cardioversion is planned.

The procedure for synchronized cardioversion is the same as for defibrillation with the following exceptions. If synchronized cardioversion is done on a nonemergency basis (i.e., the patient is awake and hemodynamically stable), the patient is sedated (e.g., IV midazolam [Versed]) before the procedure. Strict attention to maintaining the patient's airway is critical. If a patient with supraventricular tachycardia or VT with a pulse becomes hemodynamically unstable, synchronized cardioversion should be performed as quickly as possible. Start the initial energy for synchronized cardioversion at 50 to 100 joules (biphasic defibrillator) and 100 joules (monophasic defibrillator), and increase if needed. If the patient becomes pulseless or the rhythm changes to VF, turn the synchronizer switch off and perform defibrillation.

SAFETY ALERT: Defibrillation and Cardioversion

- Check that the synchronizer switch is OFF when defibrillation is planned.
- Turn the synchronizer switch ON when cardioversion is planned.
- Be certain that personnel are "all clear" before discharging the device.

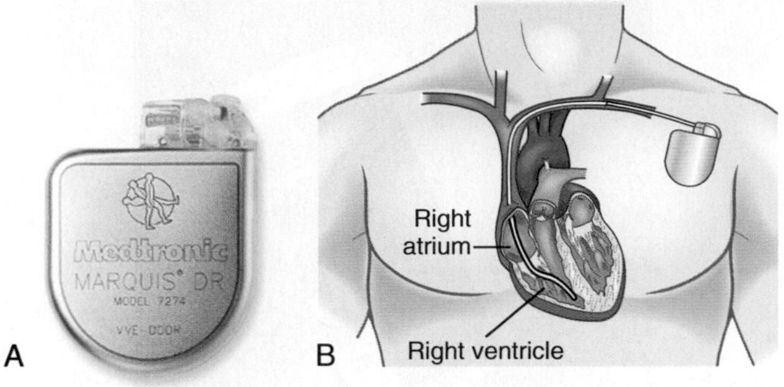

FIG. 36-22 **A,** The implantable cardioverter-defibrillator (ICD) pulse generator from Medtronic, Inc. **B,** The ICD is placed in a subcutaneous pocket over the pectoral muscle. A single-lead system is placed transvenously from the pulse generator to the endocardium. The single lead detects dysrhythmias and delivers an electric shock to the heart muscle.

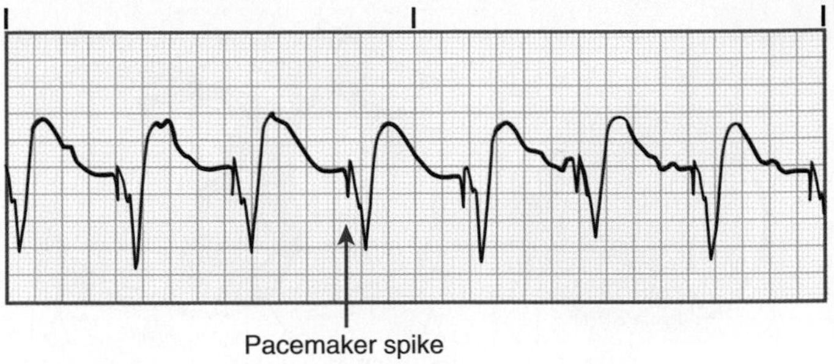

FIG. 36-23 Ventricular capture (depolarization) secondary to signal *(pacemaker spike)* from pacemaker lead in the right ventricle.

Implantable Cardioverter-Defibrillator. The *implantable cardioverter-defibrillator* (ICD) is an important technology for patients who (1) have survived SCD, (2) have spontaneous sustained VT, (3) have syncope with inducible VT or VF during EPS, or (4) are at high risk for future life-threatening dysrhythmias (e.g., have cardiomyopathy). The use of ICDs has significantly decreased cardiac mortality rates in these patients.[11]

The ICD consists of a lead system placed via a subclavian vein to the endocardium. A battery-powered pulse generator is implanted subcutaneously, usually over the pectoral muscle on the patient's nondominant side. The pulse generator is similar in size to a pacemaker. Most systems are single-lead systems (Fig. 36-22). The ICD sensing system monitors the HR and rhythm and identifies VT or VF. After the sensing system detects a lethal dysrhythmia, the device delivers a 25-joule or less shock to the patient's heart. If the first shock is unsuccessful, the device recycles and can continue to deliver shocks.

In addition to defibrillation capabilities, ICDs are equipped with antitachycardia and antibradycardia pacemakers. These devices use algorithms that detect dysrhythmias and determine the appropriate response. They can initiate *overdrive pacing* of supraventricular tachycardia and VT, sparing the patient painful defibrillator shocks. They also provide backup pacing for bradydysrhythmias that may occur after defibrillation. Preprocedure and postprocedure nursing care of the patient undergoing ICD placement is similar to the care of a patient undergoing permanent pacemaker implantation (see p. 805).

Teaching the patient who is receiving an ICD and the caregiver is extremely important. Patients experience a variety of emotions, including fear of body image change, fear of recurrent dysrhythmias, expectation of pain with ICD discharge (described as a feeling of a blow to the chest), and anxiety about going home. Encourage patients and caregivers to participate in local or online ICD support groups[12] *(www.implantable.com)*. Table 36-10 presents teaching guidelines for the patient with an ICD and the caregiver.

TABLE 36-10 PATIENT & CAREGIVER TEACHING GUIDE

Implantable Cardioverter-Defibrillator (ICD)

Include the following information in the teaching plan for a patient receiving an ICD and the patient's caregiver.

1. Follow up with cardiologist for routine checks of the function of the ICD.
2. Report any signs of infection at incision site (e.g., redness, swelling, drainage) or fever immediately.
3. Keep incision dry for 4 days after insertion or as instructed.
4. Avoid lifting arm on ICD side above shoulder until approved.
5. Discuss resuming sexual activity with your cardiologist. It is usually safe to resume sexual activity once your incision is healed.
6. Avoid driving until cleared by your cardiologist. This decision is usually based on the ongoing presence of dysrhythmias, the frequency of ICD firings, your overall health, and state laws regarding drivers with ICDs.
7. Avoid direct blows to ICD site.
8. Avoid large magnets and strong electromagnetic fields because these may interfere with the device.
9. You should not have a magnetic resonance imaging (MRI) scan unless the ICD is approved as MRI safe or there is a protocol in place for patient safety during the procedure.
10. Air travel is not restricted. Inform airport security of presence of ICD because it may set off the metal detector. If hand-held screening wand is used, it should not be placed directly over the ICD. Manufacturer information may vary regarding the effect of metal detectors on the function of the ICD.
11. Avoid standing near antitheft devices in doorways of stores and public buildings. You should walk through them at a normal pace.
12. If your ICD fires, call your cardiologist immediately.
13. If your ICD fires and you feel sick, contact the emergency medical services (EMS).
14. If your ICD fires more than once, contact EMS.
15. You should obtain and wear a Medic Alert ID or bracelet at all times.
16. Always carry the ICD identification card and a current list of your medications.
17. Consider joining an ICD support group (e.g., *www.icdsupportgroup.org*).
18. Caregivers should learn cardiopulmonary resuscitation (CPR).

Pacemakers

The artificial **cardiac pacemaker** is an electronic device used to pace the heart when the normal conduction pathway is damaged. The basic pacing circuit consists of a power source (battery-powered pulse generator) with programmable circuitry, one or more pacing leads, and the myocardium. The electrical signal (stimulus) travels from the pulse generator, through the leads, to the wall of the myocardium. The myocardium is "captured" and stimulated to contract (Fig. 36-23).

Current pacemakers are small, sophisticated, and physiologically precise. They pace the atrium and/or one or both of the ventricles. Most pacemakers are *demand pacemakers.* This means that they sense the heart's electrical activity and fire only when the HR drops below a preset rate. Demand pacemakers

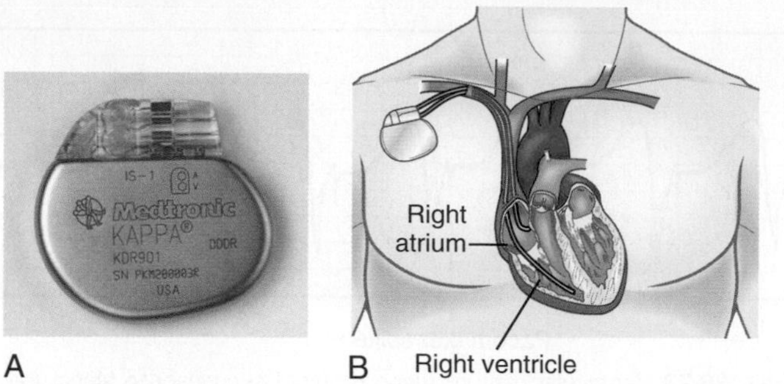

FIG. 36-24 **A,** A dual-chamber rate-responsive pacemaker from Medtronic, Inc., is designed to treat patients with chronic heart problems in which the heart beats too slowly to adequately support the body's circulation needs. **B,** Pacing leads in both the atrium and the ventricle enable a dual-chamber pacemaker to sense and pace in both heart chambers.

have two distinct features: (1) a sensing device that inhibits the pacemaker when the HR is adequate and (2) a pacing device that triggers the pacemaker when no QRS complexes occur within a preset time.[1,13]

In addition to antibradycardia pacing, devices now include antitachycardia and overdrive pacing. *Antitachycardia pacing* involves the delivery of a stimulus to the ventricle to end tachydysrhythmias (e.g., VT). Overdrive pacing involves pacing the atrium at rates of 200 to 500 impulses per minute in an attempt to terminate atrial tachycardias (e.g., atrial flutter with a rapid ventricular response). You can refer to texts on pacemaker therapy for more detailed information[13] and to eTable 36-1 for the Five Letter Pacemaker Code on the website for this chapter.

Permanent Pacemaker. A *permanent pacemaker* is implanted totally within the body (Fig. 36-24). The power source is placed subcutaneously, usually over the pectoral muscle on the patient's nondominant side. The pacing leads are placed transvenously to the right atrium and/or one or both ventricles and attached to the power source. Common reasons for insertion of a permanent pacemaker are found in Table 36-11.

Cardiac Resynchronization Therapy. *Cardiac resynchronization therapy* (CRT) is a pacing technique that resynchronizes the cardiac cycle by pacing both ventricles *(biventricular pacing)*. This promotes improvement in ventricular function (see Fig. 35-4). Most HF patients have intraventricular conduction delays causing abnormal ventricular contraction. This causes dyssynchrony between the right and left ventricles and results in reduced systolic function, pump inefficiency, and worsened HF. For patients with severe left ventricular dysfunction, CRT is combined with an ICD for maximum therapy.[14] (HF is discussed in Chapter 35.)

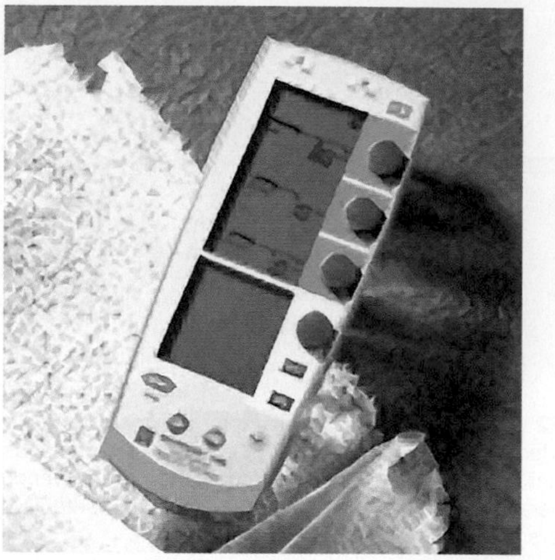

FIG. 36-25 Temporary external, dual-chamber demand pacemaker.

Temporary Pacemaker. A *temporary pacemaker* is one that has the power source outside the body (Fig. 36-25). There are three types of temporary pacemakers: transvenous, epicardial, and transcutaneous. Table 36-12 lists common reasons for temporary pacing.

A *transvenous pacemaker* consists of a lead or leads that are threaded transvenously to the right atrium and/or right ventricle and attached to the external power source (Fig. 36-26). Most temporary transvenous pacemakers are inserted in emergency departments and critical care units in emergent situations. They provide a bridge to insertion of a permanent pacemaker or until the underlying cause of the dysrhythmia is resolved.

Epicardial pacing involves attaching an atrial and ventricular pacing lead to the epicardium during heart surgery. The leads are passed through the chest wall and attached to the external power source. Epicardial pacing leads are placed prophylactically should any bradydysrhythmias or tachydysrhythmias occur in the early postoperative period.[8]

A *transcutaneous pacemaker* (TCP) is used to provide adequate HR and rhythm to the patient in an emergency situation. Placement of the TCP is a noninvasive, temporary procedure used until a transvenous pacemaker is inserted or until more definitive therapy is available.[8]

TABLE 36-11 INDICATIONS FOR PERMANENT PACEMAKERS

- Acquired AV block
- Second-degree AV block
- Third-degree AV block
- Atrial fibrillation with a slow ventricular response
- Bundle branch block
- Cardiomyopathy
  - Dilated
  - Hypertrophic
- Heart failure
- SA node dysfunction
- Tachydysrhythmias (e.g., ventricular tachycardia)

AV, Atrioventricular; *SA,* sinoatrial.

TABLE 36-12 INDICATIONS FOR TEMPORARY PACEMAKERS*

- Maintenance of adequate HR and rhythm during special circumstances such as surgery and postoperative recovery, during cardiac catheterization or coronary angioplasty, during drug therapy that may cause bradycardia, and before implantation of a permanent pacemaker
- As prophylaxis after open heart surgery
- Acute anterior MI with second- or third-degree AV block or bundle branch block
- Acute inferior MI with symptomatic bradycardia and AV block
- Electrophysiologic studies to evaluate patient with bradydysrhythmias and tachydysrhythmias

*List is not all-inclusive.
AV, Atrioventricular; *HR,* heart rate; *MI,* myocardial infarction.

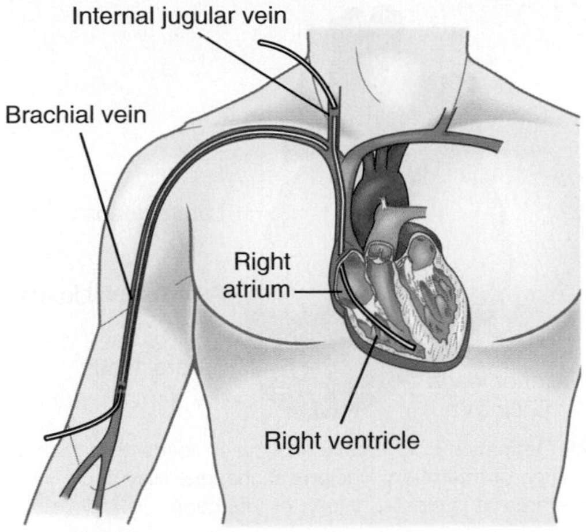

FIG. 36-26 Temporary transvenous pacemaker catheter insertion. A single lead is positioned in the right ventricle through the brachial, subclavian, jugular, or femoral vein.

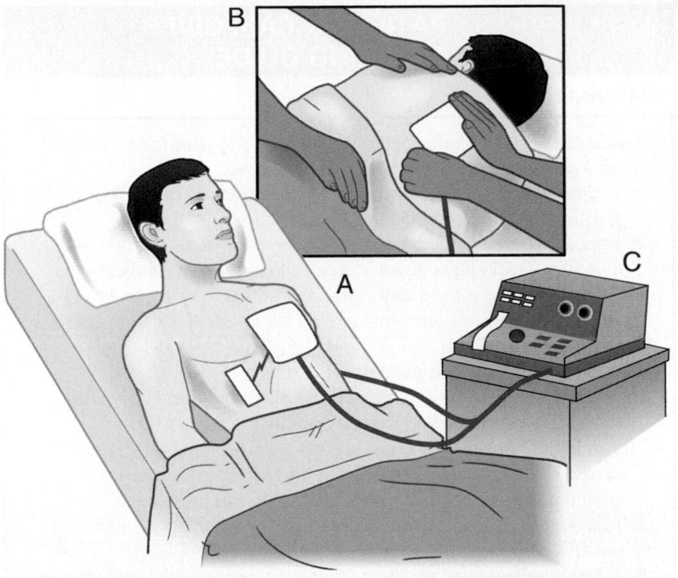

FIG. 36-27 Transcutaneous pacemaker. Pacing electrodes are placed on the patient's anterior *(A)* and posterior *(B)* chest walls and attached to an external pacing unit *(C)*.

The TCP consists of a power source and a rate- and voltage-control device that attaches to two large, multifunction electrode pads. Position one pad on the anterior part of the chest, usually on the V_4 lead position, and the other pad on the back between the spine and the left scapula at the level of the heart (Fig. 36-27). Always use the lowest current that results in a ventricular contraction (capture) to minimize patient discomfort.

Before initiating TCP therapy, it is important to tell the patient what to expect. Explain that the muscle contractions created by the pacemaker when the current passes through the chest wall are uncomfortable. Reassure the patient that the TCP is temporary and that it will be replaced by a transvenous pacemaker as soon as possible. Whenever possible, provide analgesia and/or sedation while the TCP is in use.

Monitoring of Patients With Pacemakers. Patients with temporary or permanent pacemakers are ECG monitored to evaluate the status of the pacemaker. Pacemaker malfunction primarily involves a failure to sense or a failure to capture. *Failure to sense* occurs when the pacemaker fails to recognize spontaneous atrial or ventricular activity, and it fires inappropriately. This can result in the pacemaker firing during the excitable period of the cardiac cycle, resulting in VT. Failure to sense is caused by pacer lead damage, battery failure, sensing set too high, or dislodgment of the electrode. *Failure to capture* occurs when the electrical charge to the myocardium is insufficient to produce atrial or ventricular contraction. This can result in serious bradycardia or asystole. Failure to capture is caused by pacer lead damage, battery failure, dislodgment of the electrode, electrical charge set too low, or fibrosis at the electrode tip.

Complications of invasive temporary (i.e., transvenous) or permanent pacemaker insertion include infection and hematoma formation at the insertion site, pneumothorax, failure to sense or capture, perforation of the atrial or ventricular septum by the pacing lead, and appearance of "end-of-life" battery power on testing the pacemaker. Several measures can prevent or assess for complications. These include prophylactic IV antibiotic therapy before and after insertion, postinsertion chest x-ray to check lead placement and to rule out a pneumothorax, careful observation of insertion site, and continuous ECG monitoring of the patient's rhythm.

After the pacemaker has been inserted, the patient can be out of bed once stable. Have the patient limit arm and shoulder activity on the operative side to prevent dislodging the newly implanted pacing leads. Observe the insertion site for signs of bleeding, and check that the incision is intact. Note any temperature elevation or pain at the insertion site and treat as ordered. Most patients are discharged the next day if stable.

Provide teaching in addition to observing for complications after pacemaker insertion. The patient with a newly implanted pacemaker and the caregiver may have questions about activity restrictions and fears concerning body image after the procedure. The goals of pacemaker therapy include enhancing physiologic functioning and quality of life. Emphasize this to the patient and the caregiver, and provide specific advice on activity restrictions. Table 36-13 outlines patient and caregiver teaching for the patient with a pacemaker.

After discharge, patients need to check pacemaker function on a regular basis. This can include outpatient visits to a pacemaker clinic or home monitoring using telephone transmitter devices. Another method to evaluate pacemaker performance is noninvasive program stimulation. This procedure is done on an outpatient basis in the EPS laboratory.

Radiofrequency Catheter Ablation Therapy

Radiofrequency catheter ablation therapy uses electrical energy to "burn" or ablate areas of the conduction system as definitive treatment of tachydysrhythmias. Ablation therapy is done after EPS has identified the source of the dysrhythmia. An electrode-tipped ablation catheter ablates accessory pathways or ectopic sites in the atria, the AV node, and the ventricles. Catheter ablation is considered the nonpharmacologic treatment of choice for atrial dysrhythmias resulting in rapid ventricular rates and AV nodal reentrant tachycardia refractory to drug therapy.[7,9]

The ablation procedure is successful with a low complication rate. Care of the patient after ablation therapy is similar to that of a patient undergoing cardiac catheterization (see Chapter 32 and Table 32-6).

TABLE 36-13 PATIENT & CAREGIVER TEACHING GUIDE

Pacemaker

Include the following information in the teaching plan for a patient with a pacemaker and the patient's caregiver.

1. Maintain follow-up care with your cardiologist to begin regular pacemaker function checks.
2. Report any signs of infection at incision site (e.g., redness, swelling, drainage) or fever to your cardiologist immediately.
3. Keep incision dry for 4 days after implantation, or as ordered.
4. Avoid lifting arm on pacemaker side above shoulder until approved by your cardiologist.
5. Avoid direct blows to pacemaker site.
6. Avoid close proximity to high-output electric generators, since these can interfere with the function of the pacemaker.
7. You should not have a magnetic resonance imaging (MRI) scan unless the pacemaker is approved as MRI safe or there is a protocol in place for patient safety during the procedure.
8. Microwave ovens are safe to use and do not interfere with pacemaker function.
9. Avoid standing near antitheft devices in doorways of department stores and public libraries. You should walk through them at a normal pace.
10. Air travel is not restricted. Inform airport security of presence of pacemaker because it may set off the metal detector. If hand-held screening wand is used, it should not be placed directly over the pacemaker. Manufacturer information may vary regarding the effect of metal detectors on the function of the pacemaker.
11. Monitor pulse and inform cardiologist if it drops below predetermined rate.
12. Carry pacemaker information card and a current list of your medications at all times.
13. Obtain and wear a Medic Alert ID or bracelet at all times.

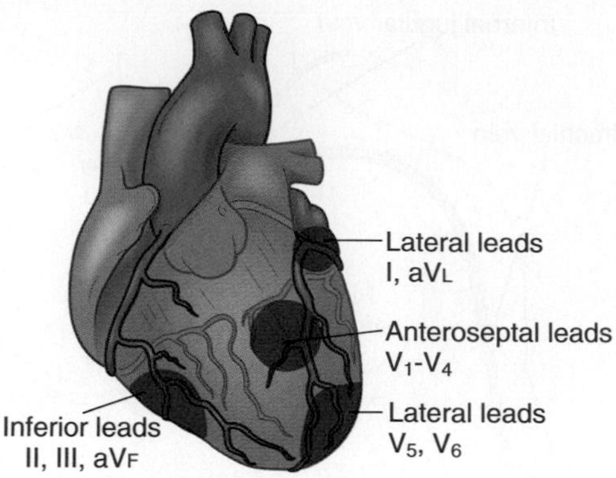

FIG. 36-28 Definitive ECG changes occur in leads that face the area of ischemia, injury, or infarction. Reciprocal changes may occur in leads facing opposite the area of ischemia, injury, or infarction.

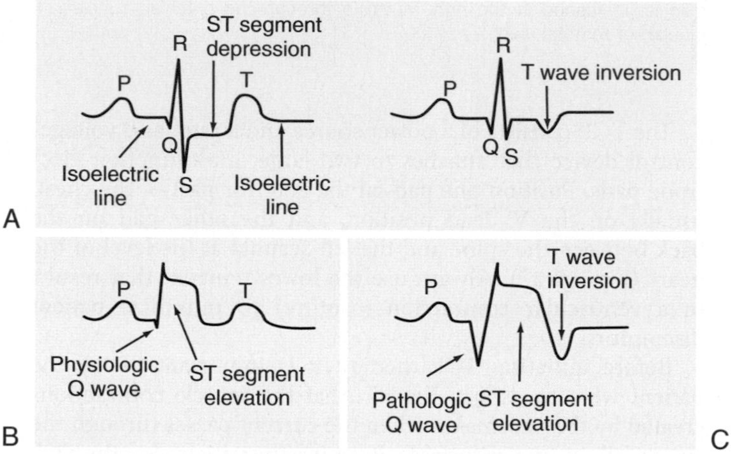

FIG. 36-29 ST segment, T wave, and Q wave changes associated with myocardial ischemia **(A)**, injury **(B)**, and infarction **(C)**.

ECG CHANGES ASSOCIATED WITH ACUTE CORONARY SYNDROME

The 12-lead ECG is a major diagnostic tool used to evaluate patients with ACS. ECG changes that occur with ACS direct many treatment decisions. The ECG changes are in response to ischemia, injury, or infarction (necrosis) of heart cells. The leads facing the area of involvement demonstrate the definitive ECG changes (Fig. 36-28). The leads facing opposite the area involved in ACS often demonstrate reciprocal (opposite) ECG changes. In addition, the pattern of ECG changes among the 12 leads provides information on the coronary artery involved in ACS (Table 36-14).

Ischemia

Typical ECG changes that are seen in myocardial ischemia include ST segment depression and/or T wave inversion (Fig. 36-29, *A*). ST segment depression is significant if it is at least 1 mm (one small box) below the isoelectric line in at least two contiguous (neighboring) leads (see Fig. 36-5). The isoelectric line is flat and represents those normal times in the cardiac cycle when the ECG is not recording any electrical activity in the heart. These times are as follows: (1) from the end of the P wave to the start of the QRS complex, (2) during the entire ST segment, and (3) from the end of the T wave to the start of the next P wave (see Fig. 36-9). Depression in the ST segment and/or T wave inversion occurs in response to an inadequate supply of blood and oxygen, which causes an electrical disturbance in the myocardial cells.[6,7] Once the patient is treated (adequate blood flow is restored), the ECG changes resolve, and the ECG returns to the patient's baseline. (See Chapter 34 for a complete discussion of ACS.)

TABLE 36-14 ECG EVIDENCE IN ACUTE CORONARY SYNDROME

	ECG Evidence		
Left Ventricle Involvement	**Leads Facing Area**	**Leads Opposite Area (Reciprocal Changes)**	**Associated Coronary Artery**
Septal wall	V_1, V_2	II, III, aVF	Left anterior descending
Anterior wall	V_2-V_4	II, III, aVF	Left anterior descending
Lateral wall, low	V_5, V_6	II, III, aVF	Left anterior descending or circumflex
Lateral wall, high	I, aVL	II, III, aVF	Circumflex
Inferior wall	II, III, aVF	I, aVL, V_5, V_6	Right coronary artery, posterior descending coronary artery

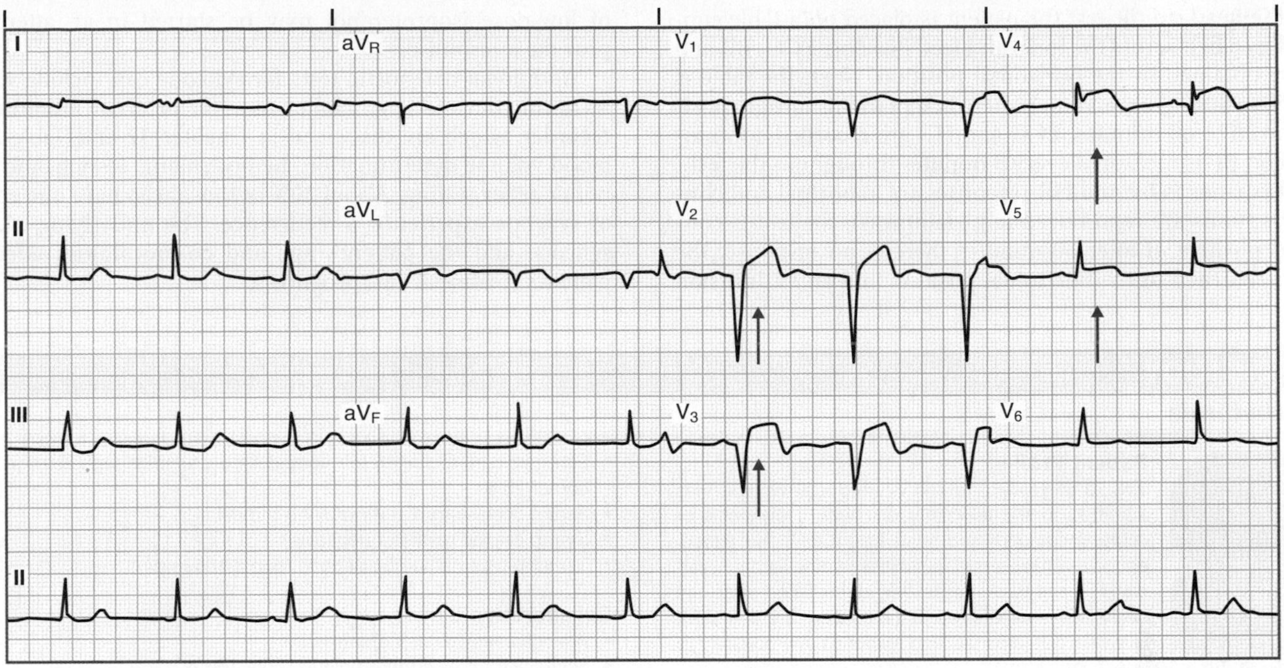

FIG. 36-30 ECG findings with anteroseptal lateral wall myocardial infarction. Normally, leads I, aVL, and V_1 to V_3 have a positive R wave. Note the pathologic Q waves in these leads and the ST segment elevation in leads V_2 to V_5 *(arrows)*.

Injury and Infarction

Myocardial injury represents a worsening stage of ischemia that is potentially reversible but may evolve to MI. The typical ECG change seen during injury is ST segment elevation. ST segment elevation is significant if it is 1 mm or more above the isoelectric line in at least two contiguous leads (Fig. 36-29, *B*). If treatment is prompt and effective, it is possible to restore oxygen to the myocardium and avoid or limit infarction. The absence of serum cardiac markers confirms this.

In addition to ST segment elevation, a pathologic Q wave may be seen on the ECG in patients with infarction (Fig. 36-29, *C*). A physiologic Q wave is the first negative deflection (wave) following the P wave. It is normally very short and narrow (see Fig. 36-9 and Table 36-2). A pathologic Q wave that develops during MI is wide (greater than 0.03 second in duration) and deep (greater than or equal to 25% of the height of the R wave).[1,7] This is referred to as a *Q wave MI*. The pathologic Q wave may be present on the ECG indefinitely.

T wave inversion related to MI occurs within hours following the event and may persist for months. The ECG changes seen in injury and MI reflect electrical disturbances in the myocardial cells caused by a prolonged lack of blood and oxygen leading to necrosis (Fig. 36-30).

Patient Monitoring

Monitoring guidelines for patients who are suspected of having ACS include continuous, multilead ECG and ST segment monitoring.[3] The leads selected for monitoring should minimally include the leads that reflect the area of ischemia, injury, or infarction.

SYNCOPE

Syncope, a brief lapse in consciousness accompanied by a loss in postural tone (fainting), is a common diagnosis of patients coming to the emergency department. The causes of syncope can be cardiovascular or noncardiovascular. The most common cause of syncope is cardioneurogenic syncope, or "vasovagal" syncope (e.g., carotid sinus sensitivity). Other cardiovascular causes relate to dysrhythmias (e.g., tachycardias, bradycardias), prosthetic valve malfunction, pulmonary emboli, and HF. Noncardiovascular causes vary and include stress, hypoglycemia, dehydration, stroke, and seizure.[14]

A diagnostic workup for a patient with syncope from a suspected cardiac cause begins with ruling out structural and ischemic heart disease. This is done with echocardiography and stress testing. In the older patient, who is more likely to have structural and ischemic heart disease, EPS is used to diagnose atrial and ventricular tachydysrhythmias and conduction disturbances causing bradydysrhythmias, all of which can cause syncope. These problems can be treated with antidysrhythmia drug therapy, pacemakers, ICDs, and/or catheter ablation therapy.

In patients without structural heart disease or in whom EPS testing is not diagnostic, the *head-up tilt-test* may be performed. Normally, an upright position results in gravity displacing 300 to 800 mL of blood to the lower extremities. Specialized nerve fibers called mechanoreceptors are located throughout the vascular system. These respond to the increased blood volume by starting a reflex increase in sympathetic stimulation and decrease in parasympathetic output. The end results are a slight increase in HR and diastolic BP, and a slight decrease in systolic BP.[15]

In cardioneurogenic syncope, the increase in venous pooling that occurs in the upright position reduces venous return to the heart. This results in a sudden, compensatory increase in ventricular contraction. This is mistaken by the brain as a hypertensive state, and consequently sympathetic stimulation is withdrawn. This produces a paradoxic vasodilation and bradycardia (vasovagal response). The end results are bradycardia, hypotension, cerebral hypoperfusion, and syncope.

In the head-up tilt-test the patient is placed on a table supported by a belt across the torso and feet. Baseline ECG, BP, and HR are obtained in the horizontal position. Next, the table is tilted 60 to 80 degrees and the patient is kept in this upright position for 20 to 60 minutes. ECG and HR are recorded continuously and BP is measured every 3 minutes throughout the test.

If the patient's BP and HR responses are abnormal and clinical symptoms are reproduced (e.g., faintness), the test is considered positive. If after 30 minutes there is no response, the table is returned to the horizontal position and an IV infusion of low-dose isoproterenol may be started in an attempt to provoke a response.

Additional diagnostic tests for syncope can include various recording devices (e.g., Holter monitor or event monitor/loop recorder, which are discussed in Chapter 32 and Table 32-6), blood volume determination, hemodynamic testing, and autonomic reflex testing. About 30% of those who have one episode of syncope experience a recurrence. The underlying cause of syncope and the patient's age and co-morbidities affect the patient's treatment and prognosis.[15]

CASE STUDY

Dysrhythmia

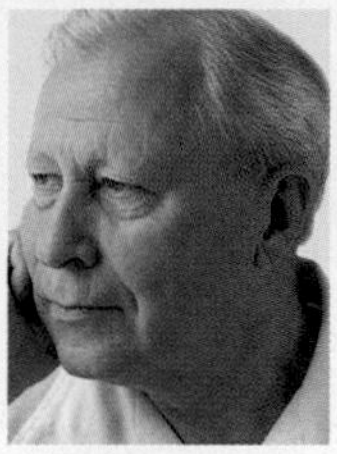

iStockphoto/Thinkstock

Patient Profile

J.M., a 68-year-old retired white postal worker, was admitted to the telemetry unit with a diagnosis of acute decompensated heart failure (HF). He experienced a cardiac arrest (pulseless ventricular tachycardia [VT]) and was successfully defibrillated after one shock. He is transferred to the cardiac care unit. J.M. is awake but lethargic, and responds appropriately to questions.

Subjective Data

- History of hypertension, coronary artery disease, two MIs, and chronic HF
- Reports shortness of breath at rest and even in an upright position

Objective Data

Physical Examination

- Appears weak, anxious
- BP 102/60 mm Hg, pulse 70/min, respirations 26/min
- Lungs: bilateral coarse crackles in the bases
- Heart: S_3 gallop at apex

Diagnostic Studies

- Continuous ECG monitoring

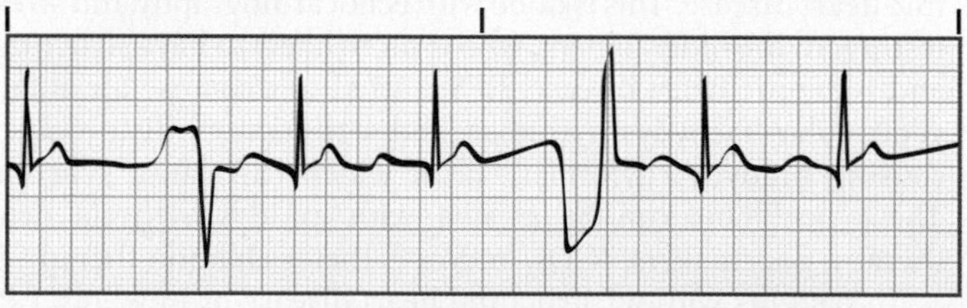

- Echocardiogram: severe left ventricular dysfunction with ejection fraction of 25%
- Serum potassium: 2.9 mEq/L (2.9 mmol/L)
- Serum cardiac markers: negative
- Serum b-type natriuretic peptide (BNP): 1852 pg/mL

Collaborative Care

- Amiodarone (Cordarone) infusion
- Scheduled for electrophysiologic study (EPS)

Discussion Questions

1. Why is J.M. at risk for sudden cardiac death?
2. Explain the rationale for using amiodarone after cardiac arrest.
3. What methods are used to assess the effectiveness of the antidysrhythmia therapy?
4. Interpret the rhythm strip and explain the significance of the other diagnostic studies.
5. Why would J.M. be a candidate for CRT and an ICD?
6. ***Priority Decision:*** Based on the assessment data provided, what are the priority nursing diagnoses?
7. ***Priority Decision:*** Based on these nursing diagnoses, what are the priority nursing interventions for J.M.?
8. ***Delegation Decision:*** Which tasks could be delegated to unlicensed assistive personnel (UAP)?
9. ***Evidence-Based Practice***: Once J.M. is stable, he is scheduled for the insertion of a CRT/ICD. On your rounds, he asks you why he needs two devices.

evolve Answers available at *http://evolve.elsevier.com/Lewis/medsurg*.

BRIDGE TO NCLEX EXAMINATION

The number of the question corresponds to the same-numbered outcome at the beginning of the chapter.

1. A patient admitted with ACS has continuous ECG monitoring. An examination of the rhythm strip reveals the following characteristics: atrial rate 74 beats/min and regular; ventricular rate 62 beats/min and irregular; P wave normal shape; PR interval lengthens progressively until a P wave is not conducted; QRS normal shape. The priority nursing intervention would be to
   a. perform synchronized cardioversion.
   b. administer epinephrine 1 mg IV push.
   c. observe for symptoms of hypotension or angina.
   d. apply transcutaneous pacemaker pads on the patient.
2. The nurse is monitoring the ECG of a patient admitted with ACS. Which ECG characteristics would be most suggestive of myocardial ischemia?
   a. Sinus rhythm with a pathologic Q wave
   b. Sinus rhythm with an elevated ST segment
   c. Sinus rhythm with a depressed ST segment
   d. Sinus rhythm with premature atrial contractions

3. The ECG monitor of a patient in the cardiac care unit after an MI indicates ventricular bigeminy with a rate of 50 beats/min. The nurse would anticipate
   a. performing defibrillation.
   b. treating with IV amiodarone.
   c. inserting a temporary transvenous pacemaker.
   d. assessing the patient's response to the dysrhythmia.
4. The nurse prepares a patient for synchronized cardioversion knowing that cardioversion differs from defibrillation in that
   a. defibrillation requires a lower dose of electrical energy.
   b. cardioversion is indicated to treat atrial bradydysrhythmias.
   c. defibrillation is synchronized to deliver a shock during the QRS complex.
   d. patients should be sedated if cardioversion is done on a non-emergency basis.
5. Which patient teaching points should the nurse include when providing discharge instructions to a patient with a new permanent pacemaker and the caregiver *(select all that apply)?*
   a. Avoid or limit air travel.
   b. Take and record a daily pulse rate.
   c. Obtain and wear a Medic Alert ID or bracelet at all times.
   d. Avoid lifting arm on the side of the pacemaker above shoulder.
   e. Avoid microwave ovens because they interfere with pacemaker function.
6. Important teaching for the patient scheduled for a radiofrequency catheter ablation procedure includes explaining that
   a. ventricular bradycardia may be induced and treated during the procedure.
   b. a catheter will be placed in both femoral arteries to allow double-catheter use.
   c. the procedure will destroy areas of the conduction system that are causing rapid heart rhythms.
   d. a general anesthetic will be given to prevent the awareness of any "sudden cardiac death" experiences.

1. c, 2. c, 3. d, 4. d, 5. b, c, d, 6. c

evolve

For rationales to these answers and even more NCLEX review questions, visit *http://evolve.elsevier.com/Lewis/medsurg.*

REFERENCES

1. Wesley K: *Huszar's basic dysrhythmias and acute coronary syndrome*, ed 4, St Louis, 2011, Mosby Jems.
2. Patton KT, Thibodeau GA, Douglas MM: *Essentials of anatomy and physiology*, St Louis, 2012, Mosby.
*3. American Association of Critical-Care Nurses: AACN practice alert: ST segment monitoring. Retrieved from *www.aacn.org/wd/practice/content/st-segment-practice-alert.pcms?menu=practice.*
*4. American Association of Critical-Care Nurses: AACN practice alert: dysrhythmia monitoring. Retrieved from *www.aacn.org/wd/practice/content/dysrhythmia-monitoring-practice-alert.pcms?menu=practice.*
5. Lehne RA: *Pharmacology for nursing care*, ed 7, St Louis, 2010, Mosby.
6. Sinz E, Navarro K, Soderberg ES, editors: *Advanced cardiovascular life support: provider manual*, Dallas, 2011, American Heart Association.
7. Carlson KK: *Advanced critical care nursing*, St Louis, 2009, Saunders.
8. American Association of Critical-Care Nurses: *Core curriculum for progressive care nurses*, St Louis, 2010, Saunders.
*9. Wann LS, Curtis AB, January CT, et al: 2011 ACCF/AHA/HRS focused update on the management of patients with atrial fibrillation (updating the 2006 guideline): a report of the American College of Cardiology Foundation/American Heart Association task force on practice guidelines, *J Am Coll Cardiol* 57:223, 2011.
10. Go AS, Mozaffarian D, Roger VL, et al: Heart disease and stroke statistics—2013 update: a report from the American Heart Association, *Circulation* 127:e6, 2013.
*11. Tracy CM, Epstein AE, Darbar D, et al: 2012 ACCF/AHA/HRS focused update of the 2008 guidelines for device-based therapy of cardiac rhythm abnormalities: a report of the American College of Cardiology Foundation/American Heart Association Task Force on Practice Guidelines, *Circulation* 126:1784, 2012.
12. Dunbar SB, Dougherty CM, Sears SF, et al: Educational and psychological interventions to improve outcomes for recipients of implantable cardioverter defibrillators and their families: a scientific statement from the American Heart Association, *Circulation* 126:2146, 2012.
13. Barold SS, Stroobandt RX, Sinnaeve AF: *Cardiac pacemakers and resynchronization step-by-step*, ed 2, Hoboken, NJ, 2010, Wiley-Blackwell.
*14. McAlister FA, Ezekowitz J, Dryden DM, et al: Cardiac resynchronization therapy and implantable cardiac defibrillators in left ventricular systolic dysfunction, AHRQ Pub No 07-E009. Retrieved from *www.ahrq.gov/downloads/pub/evidence/pdf/defib/defib.pdf.* (Classic)
15. Cleveland Clinic: Syncope care and treatment. Retrieved from *http://my.clevelandclinic.org/heart/disorders/electric/syncope.aspx.*

RESOURCES

Additional resources for this chapter are listed after Chapter 34 on p. 765 and Chapter 35 on p. 786.

*Evidence-based information for clinical practice.

CHAPTER

37

One of the hardest things is having words in your heart that you can't utter.
James Earl Jones

Nursing Management

Inflammatory and Structural Heart Disorders

Nancy Kupper and De Ann F. Mitchell

evolve WEBSITE

http://evolve.elsevier.com/Lewis/medsurg

- NCLEX Review Questions
- Key Points
- Pre-Test
- Answer Guidelines for Case Study on p. 830
- Rationales for Bridge to NCLEX Examination Questions
- Case Study
  - Patient With Rheumatic Fever and Heart Disease
- Nursing Care Plans (Customizable)
  - eNCP 37-1: Patient With Infective Endocarditis
  - eNCP 37-2: Patient With Valvular Heart Disease
- Concept Map Creator
- Glossary
- Content Updates
- Audio
  - Pericardial Friction Rub

eFigures

- eFig. 37-1: Mitral stenosis and vegetation
- eFig. 37-2: Mitral stenosis with classic "fish mouth" orifice
- eFig. 37-3: Types of cardiomyopathy

LEARNING OUTCOMES

1. Differentiate the etiology, pathophysiology, and clinical manifestations of infective endocarditis and pericarditis.
2. Describe the collaborative care and nursing management of the patient with infective endocarditis and pericarditis.
3. Describe the etiology, pathophysiology, and clinical manifestations of myocarditis.
4. Describe the collaborative care and nursing management of the patient with myocarditis.
5. Differentiate the etiology, pathophysiology, and clinical manifestations of rheumatic fever and rheumatic heart disease.
6. Describe the collaborative care and nursing management of the patient with rheumatic fever and rheumatic heart disease.
7. Relate the pathophysiology to the clinical manifestations and diagnostic studies for the various types of valvular heart disease.
8. Describe the collaborative care and nursing management of the patient with valvular heart disease.
9. Relate the pathophysiology to the clinical manifestations and diagnostic studies for the different types of cardiomyopathy.
10. Compare the nursing and collaborative management of patients with different types of cardiomyopathy.

KEY TERMS

Reviewed by Katrina Allen, RN, MSN, CCRN, Nursing Instructor, Faulkner State Community College: Division of Nursing, Fairhope and Bay Minette, Alabama; Tracy H. Knoll, RN, MSN, Nursing Instructor, Chamberlain College of Nursing, St. Louis, Missouri; and Tammy Ann Ramon, RN, MSN, Nursing Instructor, Delta College, University Center, Michigan.

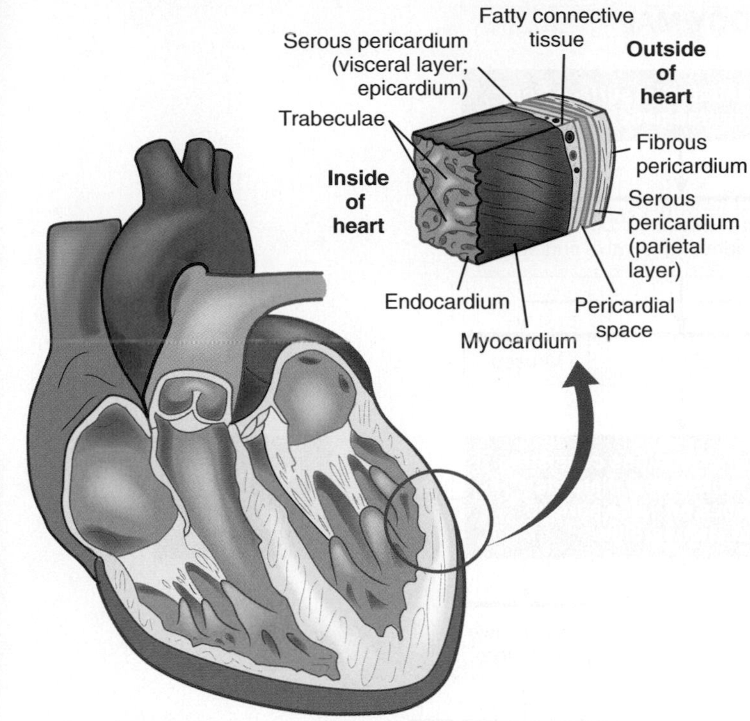

FIG. 37-1 Layers of the heart muscle and pericardium. The section of the heart wall shows the fibrous pericardium, the parietal and visceral layers of the serous pericardium (with the pericardial sac between them), the myocardium, and the endocardium.

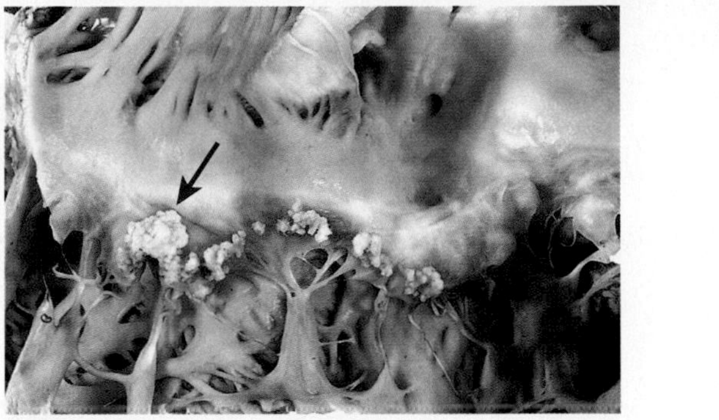

FIG. 37-2 Bacterial endocarditis of the mitral valve. The valve is covered with large, irregular vegetations *(arrow)*.

This chapter describes the pathophysiology and management of patients experiencing select inflammatory and structural heart disorders. In addition, the nursing care required to manage the needs of these patients is presented.

INFLAMMATORY DISORDERS OF HEART

INFECTIVE ENDOCARDITIS

Infective endocarditis (IE) is an infection of the endocardial layer of the heart. The *endocardium* is the innermost layer of the heart (Fig. 37-1) and heart valves. Therefore IE affects the valves. Treatment of IE with antibiotic therapy has improved the prognosis of this disease. Though relatively uncommon, an estimated 10,000 to 15,000 new cases of IE are diagnosed in the United States each year.[1]

Classification

IE can be classified as subacute or acute. The *subacute form* typically affects those with preexisting valve disease and has a clinical course that may extend over months. In contrast, the *acute form* typically affects those with healthy valves and manifests as a rapidly progressive illness. IE can also be classified based on the cause (e.g., IV drug abuse IE [IVDA IE], fungal endocarditis) or site of involvement (e.g., prosthetic valve endocarditis [PVE]).

Etiology and Pathophysiology

The most common causative organisms of IE, *Staphylococcus aureus* and *Streptococcus viridans,* are bacterial. Other possible pathogens include fungi and viruses.[2] IE occurs when blood turbulence within the heart allows the causative organism to infect previously damaged valves or other endothelial surfaces. This can occur in individuals with a variety of underlying cardiac and noncardiac conditions (Table 37-1).

TABLE 37-1 RISK FACTORS FOR ENDOCARDITIS*

Cardiac Conditions
- Prior endocarditis
- Prosthetic heart valves
- Acquired valve disease (e.g., mitral valve prolapse with regurgitation, calcified aortic stenosis)
- Cardiac lesions (e.g., ventricular septal defect, asymmetric septal hypertrophy)
- Rheumatic heart disease (e.g., mitral valve regurgitation)
- Congenital heart disease
- Pacemakers
- Marfan's syndrome
- Cardiomyopathy

Noncardiac Conditions
- Hospital-acquired bacteremia
- IV drug abuse

Procedure-Associated Risks
- Intravascular devices (e.g., pulmonary artery catheters)
- Procedures listed in Table 37-2

*List is not all-inclusive.

Vegetations, the primary lesions of IE, consist of fibrin, leukocytes, platelets, and microbes that stick to the valve surface or endocardium (Fig. 37-2). The loss of parts of these fragile vegetations into the circulation results in *emboli.* As many as 50% of patients with IE experience systemic embolization. This occurs from left-sided heart vegetation moving to various organs (e.g., brain, kidneys, spleen) and to the extremities, causing limb infarction. Right-sided heart lesions move to the lungs, resulting in pulmonary emboli.

The infection may spread locally and damage the valves or their supporting structures. This causes dysrhythmias, valve dysfunction, and eventual invasion of the myocardium, leading to heart failure (HF), sepsis, and heart block (Fig. 37-3).

At one time rheumatic heart disease was the most common cause of IE. However, now it accounts for less than 20% of cases. The main contributing factors to IE include (1) aging (more than 50% of older people have aortic stenosis [AS]), (2) IVDA, (3) use of prosthetic valves, (4) use of intravascular devices resulting in health care–associated infections (e.g., methicillin-resistant *S. aureus* [MRSA]), and (5) renal dialysis.[3]

PATHOPHYSIOLOGY MAP

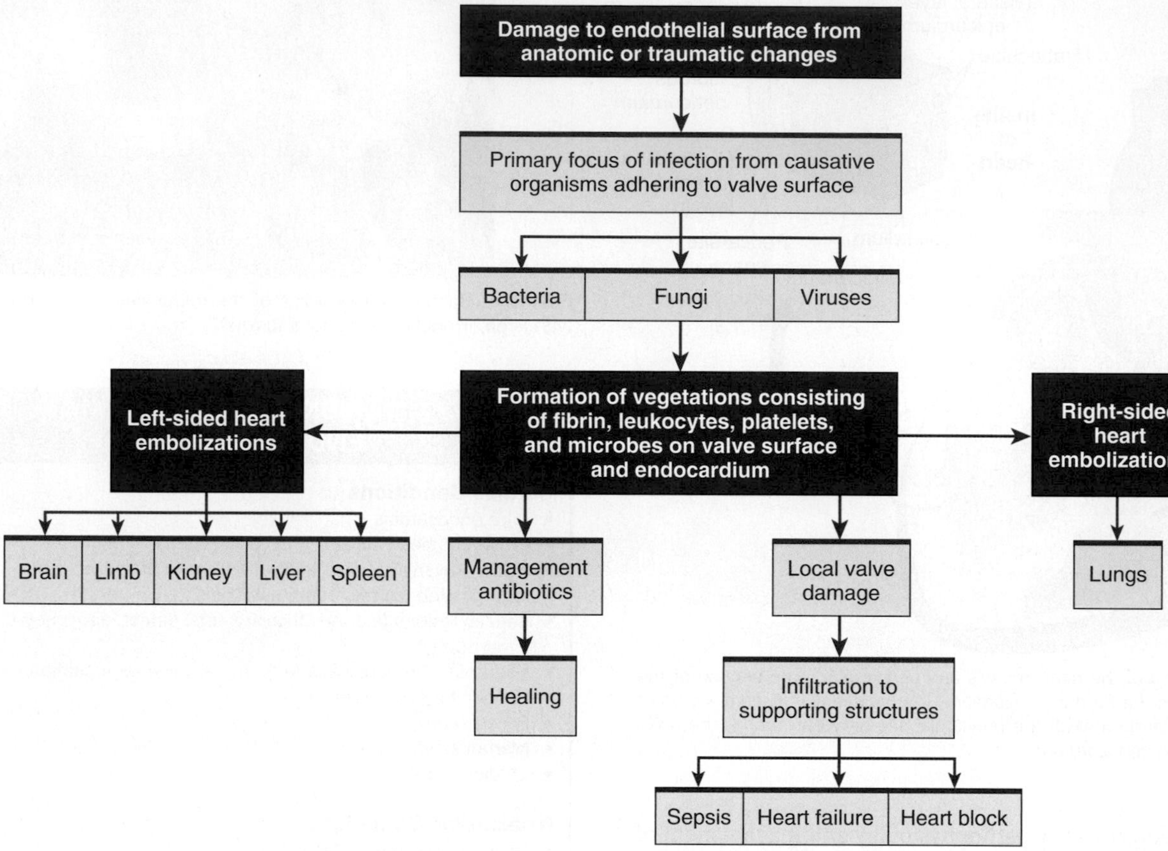

FIG. 37-3 Pathogenesis of infective endocarditis.

Clinical Manifestations

The clinical manifestations of IE are nonspecific and can involve multiple organ systems. Low-grade fever occurs in more than 90% of patients. Other nonspecific manifestations include chills, weakness, malaise, fatigue, and anorexia. Arthralgias, myalgias, back pain, abdominal discomfort, weight loss, headache, and clubbing of fingers may occur in subacute forms of endocarditis.

Vascular manifestations of IE include *splinter hemorrhages* (black longitudinal streaks) that may occur in the nail beds. Petechiae may result from fragmentation and microembolization of vegetative lesions. They can occur in the conjunctivae, lips, buccal mucosa, and palate and over the ankles, feet, and antecubital and popliteal areas. *Osler's nodes* (painful, tender, red or purple, pea-size lesions) may be found on the fingertips or toes. *Janeway's lesions* (flat, painless, small, red spots) may be seen on the palms and soles. Funduscopic examination may reveal hemorrhagic retinal lesions called *Roth's spots*.

The onset of a new or changing murmur is noted in most patients with IE. The aortic and mitral valves are most often affected. Murmurs are usually absent in tricuspid endocarditis because right-sided heart sounds are too low to be heard. HF occurs in up to 80% of patients with aortic valve endocarditis and in approximately 50% of patients with mitral valve endocarditis.[4]

Clinical manifestations secondary to embolization may be present in various body organs. Embolization to the spleen may cause sharp, left upper quadrant pain and splenomegaly, local tenderness, and abdominal rigidity. Embolization to the kidneys may cause flank pain, hematuria, and renal failure. Emboli may lodge in small peripheral blood vessels of the arms and legs and may cause ischemia and gangrene. Embolization to the brain may cause neurologic damage resulting in hemiplegia, ataxia, aphasia, visual changes, and change in the level of consciousness. Pulmonary emboli may occur in right-sided endocarditis and cause dyspnea, chest pain, hemoptysis, and respiratory arrest.

Diagnostic Studies

The patient's recent health history is important in assessing IE. Ask patients if they have had any recent (within the past 3 to 6 months) dental, urologic, surgical, or gynecologic procedures, including normal or abnormal obstetric delivery. Document any previous history of IVDA, heart disease, recent cardiac catheterization, cardiac surgery, intravascular device placement, renal dialysis, or infections (e.g., skin, respiratory, urinary tract).

Two blood cultures drawn 30 minutes apart from two different sites will be positive in more than 90% of patients. Culture-negative endocarditis is often associated with antibiotic usage within the previous 2 weeks, or results from a pathogen not easily detected by standard culture procedures. Negative cultures should be kept for 3 weeks if the clinical diagnosis remains endocarditis because of the possibility of slow-growing organisms. A mild leukocytosis occurs in acute IE (uncommon in subacute). The erythrocyte sedimentation rate (ESR) and C-reactive protein (CRP) levels may also be elevated.

Major criteria to diagnose IE include at least two of the following: positive blood cultures, new or changed heart murmur, or intracardiac mass or vegetation noted on echocardiography.[5] Echocardiography is valuable in the diagnostic workup for a patient with IE when the blood cultures are negative, or for the patient who is a surgical candidate and has an active infection. Transesophageal echocardiogram and two- or three-dimensional (2-D or 3-D) transthoracic echocardiograms can detect vegetations on the heart valves.[6]

A chest x-ray is done to detect *cardiomegaly* (an enlarged heart). An electrocardiogram (ECG) may show first- or second-degree atrioventricular (AV) block. Heart block occurs because the cardiac valves lie close to conductive tissue, especially the AV node. Cardiac catheterization may be used to evaluate valve functioning and to assess the coronary arteries when surgical intervention is being considered.[7]

Collaborative Care

Prophylactic Treatment. The situations and conditions requiring antibiotic prophylaxis are presented in Table 37-2.

Drug Therapy. Accurate identification of the infecting organism is the key to successful treatment of IE. Long-term treatment is necessary to kill dormant bacteria within the valvular vegetations. Complete elimination of the organism generally takes weeks, and relapses are common.

Initially, patients are hospitalized and IV antibiotic therapy, based on blood cultures, is started. The effectiveness of therapy is assessed with subsequent blood cultures. Cultures that remain positive indicate inadequate or inappropriate selection of antibiotic, aortic root or myocardial abscess, or the wrong diagnosis (e.g., an infection elsewhere).

Fungal endocarditis and PVE respond poorly to antibiotic therapy alone. Early valve replacement followed by prolonged (6 weeks or more) antibiotics is recommended in these situations. Valve replacement (discussed later in this chapter) has become an important adjunct procedure in the management of IE.

Fever may persist for several days after treatment has been started and can be treated with aspirin, acetaminophen (Tylenol), ibuprofen (Motrin), fluids, and rest. Complete bed rest is usually not indicated unless the temperature remains elevated or there are signs of HF. Endocarditis coupled with HF responds poorly to drug therapy and valve replacement and is often life threatening.

TABLE 37-2 ANTIBIOTIC PROPHYLAXIS TO PREVENT ENDOCARDITIS

Target Groups for Prophylactic Antibiotics

People with the following heart conditions should receive prophylactic antibiotics when they have the conditions or procedures listed below.

- Prosthetic heart valve or prosthetic material used to repair heart valve
- Previous history of infectious endocarditis
- Congenital heart disease (CHD)*
  - Unrepaired cyanotic CHD (including palliative shunts and conduits)
  - Repaired congenital heart defect with prosthetic material or device for 6 mo after the procedure
  - Repaired CHD with residual defects at the site or adjacent to the site of prosthetic patch or prosthetic device
- Cardiac transplantation recipients who develop heart valve disease

Conditions or Procedures Requiring Antibiotic Prophylaxis

When the target groups have the following conditions or procedures, they need prophylactic antibiotics.

- Oral
  - Dental manipulation involving the gums or roots of the teeth
  - Dental manipulation involving puncture of the oral mucosa
  - Dental extractions or implants
  - Prophylactic teeth cleaning with expected bleeding
- Respiratory
  - Respiratory tract incisions (e.g., biopsy)
  - Tonsillectomy and adenoidectomy
- Gastrointestinal and genitourinary
  - Wound infection
  - Urinary tract infection

*Except for the conditions listed above, prophylaxis is no longer recommended for any form of CHD.

Source: Habib G, Hoen B, Tornos P, et al: Guidelines on the prevention, diagnosis and treatment of infective endocarditis (new version 2009): the Task Force on the Prevention, Diagnosis, and Treatment of Infective Endocarditis of the European Society of Cardiology (ESC), *Eur Heart J* 30:2369, 2009.

NURSING MANAGEMENT INFECTIVE ENDOCARDITIS

NURSING ASSESSMENT

Subjective and objective data that you should obtain from a patient with IE are presented in Table 37-3. Assess vital signs together with heart sounds to detect a murmur, a change in a preexisting murmur, and extra sounds (e.g., S_3).

Arthralgia, which is common in IE, may involve multiple joints and be accompanied by myalgias. Assess the patient for joint tenderness, decreased range of motion (ROM), and muscle tenderness. Examine the patient for petechiae, splinter hemorrhages, and Osler's nodes. Complete a general systems assessment to determine any hemodynamic or embolic complications.

NURSING DIAGNOSES

Nursing diagnoses for the patient with IE may include, but are not limited to, the following:

- Decreased cardiac output *related to* altered heart rhythm, valvular insufficiency, and fluid overload
- Activity intolerance *related to* generalized weakness, arthralgia, and alteration in oxygen transport secondary to valvular dysfunction

Additional information on nursing diagnoses is presented in eNursing Care Plan 37-1 available on the website for this chapter.

PLANNING

The overall goals for the patient with IE include (1) normal or baseline heart function, (2) performance of activities of daily living (ADLs) without fatigue, and (3) knowledge of the therapeutic regimen to prevent recurrence of endocarditis.

NURSING IMPLEMENTATION

HEALTH PROMOTION. The incidence of IE can be decreased by identifying individuals who are at risk for the disease (see Tables 37-1 and 37-2). Assessment of the patient's history and an understanding of the disease process are crucial for planning and implementing appropriate health promotion strategies.

Teaching the patient at high risk for IE helps reduce the incidence and recurrence of the disease. Teaching is crucial for the patient's understanding of and adherence to the treatment

TABLE 37-3 NURSING ASSESSMENT
Infective Endocarditis

Subjective Data
Important Health Information
Past health history: Valvular, congenital, or syphilitic cardiac disease, including valve repair or replacement; previous endocarditis, childbirth, staphylococcal or streptococcal infections, hospital-acquired bacteremia
Medications: Immunosuppressive therapy
Surgery or other treatments: Recent obstetric or gynecologic procedures; invasive techniques, including catheterization, cystoscopy, intravascular procedures; recent dental or surgical procedures; GI procedures (e.g., endoscopy)

Functional Health Patterns
Health perception–health management: IV drug abuse, alcohol abuse; malaise
Nutritional-metabolic: Weight gain or loss; anorexia; chills, diaphoresis
Elimination: Bloody urine
Activity-exercise: Exercise intolerance, generalized weakness, fatigue; cough, dyspnea on exertion, orthopnea; palpitations
Sleep-rest: Night sweats
Cognitive-perceptual: Chest, back, or abdominal pain; headache; joint tenderness, muscle tenderness

Objective Data
General
Fever

Integumentary
Osler's nodes on extremities; splinter hemorrhages under nail beds; Janeway's lesions on palms and soles; petechiae of skin, mucous membranes, or conjunctivae; purpura; peripheral edema, finger clubbing

Respiratory
Tachypnea, crackles

Cardiovascular
Dysrhythmia, tachycardia, new murmurs, S_3, S_4; retinal hemorrhages

Possible Diagnostic Findings
Leukocytosis, anemia, ↑ ESR, ↑ CRP and cardiac enzymes; positive blood cultures; hematuria; echocardiogram showing chamber enlargement, valvular dysfunction, and vegetations; chest x-ray showing cardiomegaly and pulmonary infiltrates; ECG demonstrating ischemia and conduction defects; signs of systemic embolization or pulmonary embolism

CRP, C-reactive protein; *ESR*, erythrocyte sedimentation rate.

regimen. Tell the patient to avoid people with infection, especially upper respiratory tract infection, and to report cold, flu, and cough symptoms. Stress the importance of avoiding excessive fatigue and the need to plan rest periods before and after activity. Good oral hygiene, including daily care and regular dental visits, is also important. Instruct the patient to inform health care providers performing certain invasive procedures of the history of IE. Be certain the patient understands the importance of prophylactic antibiotic therapy before certain invasive procedures. Refer the patient with a history of IVDA for drug rehabilitation.

AMBULATORY AND HOME CARE. A patient with IE has many problems that require nursing management (see eNursing Care Plan 37-1 on the website for this chapter). IE generally requires treatment with antibiotics for 4 to 6 weeks. After initial treatment in the hospital, the patient may continue treatment at home if hemodynamically stable and adherent. Assess the home setting for adequate support. Patients who receive outpatient IV antibiotics require vigilant home nursing care.

Assessment findings are often nonspecific (see Table 37-3) but can help with the treatment plan. Fever, chronic or intermittent, is a common early sign. Instruct the patient or caregiver about the importance of monitoring body temperature. Persistent temperature elevations may mean that the drug therapy is ineffective. Patients with IE are at risk for life-threatening complications, such as stroke, pulmonary edema, and HF. Teach patients and caregivers to recognize signs and symptoms of these complications (e.g., change in mental status, dyspnea, chest pain, unexplained weight gain).

The patient with IE needs adequate periods of physical and emotional rest. Bed rest may be necessary when the patient has fever or complications (e.g., heart damage). Otherwise the patient may ambulate and perform moderate activity. To prevent problems related to reduced mobility, tell the patient to wear elastic compression stockings, perform ROM exercises, and deep breathe and cough every 2 hours.

The patient may experience anxiety and fear associated with the illness. You must recognize this and implement strategies to help the patient cope with the illness.

Monitor laboratory data to determine the effectiveness of the antibiotic therapy. Ongoing monitoring of the patient's blood cultures is necessary to ensure destruction of the infecting organism. Assess IV lines for patency and signs of complications (e.g., phlebitis). Administer antibiotics as scheduled, and monitor the patient for any adverse drug reactions.

Management also focuses on teaching the patient and caregiver the nature of the disease and on reducing the risk of reinfection. Explain to the patient the relationship of follow-up care, good nutrition, and early treatment of common infections (e.g., colds) to maintain health. Instruct the patient about symptoms that may indicate recurrent infection (e.g., fever, fatigue, chills). Tell the patient to notify the health care provider if any of these symptoms occur. Finally, inform the patient about the importance of prophylactic antibiotic therapy before certain invasive procedures (see Table 37-2).

EVALUATION

The expected outcomes are that the patient with IE will
- Maintain adequate tissue and organ perfusion
- Maintain normal body temperature
- Report an increase in physical and emotional comfort

Additional information on expected outcomes for the patient with IE are presented in eNursing Care Plan 37-1 on the website for this chapter.

ACUTE PERICARDITIS

Pericarditis is a condition caused by inflammation of the pericardial sac (the pericardium).The pericardium is composed of the inner serous membrane (visceral pericardium) and the outer fibrous (parietal) layer (see Fig. 37-1). The pericardial space is the cavity between these two layers. Normally it contains 10 to 15 mL of serous fluid. The pericardium serves an anchoring function, provides lubrication to decrease friction during systolic and diastolic heart movements, and assists in preventing excessive dilation of the heart during diastole. It may be congenitally absent or surgically removed.

TABLE 37-4 COMMON CAUSES OF PERICARDITIS

Infectious
- Viral: Coxsackie A and B virus, echovirus, adenovirus, mumps, hepatitis, Epstein-Barr, varicella zoster, human immunodeficiency virus
- Bacterial: Pneumococci, staphylococci, streptococci, *Neisseria gonorrhoeae, Legionella pneumophila, Mycobacterium tuberculosis,* septicemia from gram-negative organisms
- Fungal: *Histoplasma, Candida* species
- Others: Toxoplasmosis, Lyme disease

Noninfectious
- Uremia
- Acute myocardial infarction
- Neoplasms: Lung cancer, breast cancer, leukemia, Hodgkin's lymphoma, non-Hodgkin's lymphoma
- Trauma: Thoracic surgery, pacemaker insertion, cardiac diagnostic procedures
- Radiation
- Dissecting aortic aneurysm
- Myxedema

Hypersensitive or Autoimmune
- Dressler syndrome
- Postpericardiotomy syndrome
- Rheumatic fever
- Drug reactions (e.g., procainamide [Pronestyl], hydralazine [Apresoline])
- Rheumatologic diseases: Rheumatoid arthritis, systemic lupus erythematosus, systemic sclerosis (scleroderma), ankylosing spondylitis

Etiology and Pathophysiology

Common causes of acute pericarditis are listed in Table 37-4. Most often the cause of acute pericarditis is *idiopathic* (unknown), with a variety of suspected viral causes. The coxsackie B virus is the most commonly identified virus.[8]

Pericarditis in the patient with an MI may be described as two distinct syndromes. The first is *acute pericarditis,* which may occur within the initial 48 to 72 hours after an MI. The second is *Dressler syndrome* (late pericarditis), which appears 4 to 6 weeks after an MI (see Chapter 34). An inflammatory response is the characteristic pathologic finding in acute pericarditis. There is an influx of neutrophils, increased pericardial vascularity, and eventually fibrin deposition on the epicardium (Fig. 37-4).

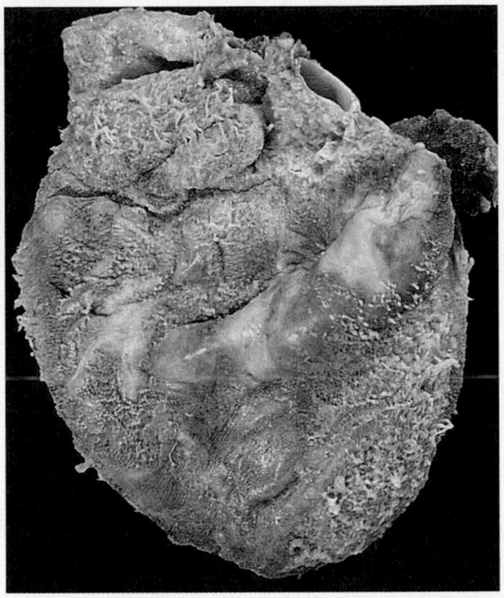

FIG. 37-4 Acute pericarditis. Note shaggy coat of fibers covering surface of heart.

Clinical Manifestations

In acute pericarditis, clinical manifestations include progressive, frequently severe, sharp chest pain. The pain is generally worse with deep inspiration and when lying supine. It is relieved by sitting up and leaning forward. The pain may radiate to the neck, arms, or left shoulder, making it difficult to differentiate from angina. One distinction is that the pain from pericarditis can be referred to the trapezius muscle (shoulder, upper back), since the phrenic nerve innervates this region. The dyspnea that accompanies acute pericarditis is related to the patient's need to breathe in rapid, shallow breaths to avoid chest pain and may be aggravated by fever and anxiety.

The hallmark finding in acute pericarditis is the *pericardial friction rub.* The rub is a scratching, grating, high-pitched sound believed to result from friction between the roughened pericardial and epicardial surfaces. It is best heard with the stethoscope placed at the lower left sternal border of the chest with the patient leaning forward. Since it is difficult to distinguish a pericardial friction rub from a pleural friction rub, ask the patient to hold his or her breath. If you still hear the rub, then it is cardiac. It may require frequent attempts to identify because pericardial friction rubs are often intermittent and short lived.

Complications

Two major complications that may result from acute pericarditis are pericardial effusion and cardiac tamponade. *Pericardial effusion* is a build-up of fluid in the pericardium. It can occur rapidly (e.g., chest trauma) or slowly (e.g., tuberculosis pericarditis). Large effusions may compress nearby structures. Pulmonary tissue compression can cause cough, dyspnea, and tachypnea. Phrenic nerve compression can induce hiccups, and compression of the laryngeal nerve may result in hoarseness. Heart sounds are generally distant and muffled, although blood pressure (BP) usually is maintained.

Cardiac tamponade develops as the pericardial effusion increases in volume. This results in compression of the heart. The speed of fluid accumulation affects the severity of clinical manifestations. Cardiac tamponade can occur acutely (e.g., rupture of heart, trauma) or subacutely (e.g., secondary to renal failure, malignancy).

The patient with cardiac tamponade may report chest pain and is often confused, anxious, and restless. As the compression of the heart increases, there is decreased cardiac output (CO), muffled heart sounds, and narrowed pulse pressure. The patient develops tachypnea and tachycardia. Neck veins usually are markedly distended because of increased jugular venous pressure, and pulsus paradoxus is present. *Pulsus paradoxus* is a decrease in systolic BP during inspiration that is exaggerated in cardiac tamponade. (See Table 37-5 for the measurement technique.) In a patient with a slow onset of a cardiac tamponade, dyspnea may be the only clinical manifestation.

Diagnostic Studies

The ECG is useful in the diagnosis of acute pericarditis, with changes noted in approximately 90% of the cases. The most

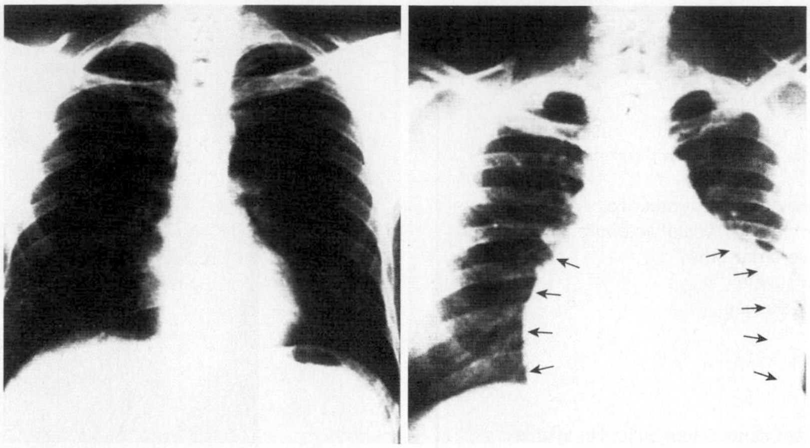

FIG. 37-5 A, X-ray of a normal chest. **B,** Pericardial effusion is present, and the cardiac silhouette is enlarged with a globular shape *(arrows).*

TABLE 37-5 MEASUREMENT OF PULSUS PARADOXUS

1. Position the patient in a semirecumbent position.
2. Instruct patient to breathe normally.*
2. Using a manually operated blood pressure (BP) cuff, determine systolic BP.
3. Inflate BP cuff at least 20 mm Hg above systolic BP.
4. Deflate cuff slowly until you hear the first Korotkoff sound during expiration, and note the pressure.
5. Continue to slowly deflate cuff until you hear sounds throughout the respiratory cycle (inspiration and expiration), and note the pressure.
6. Determine the difference between the measurements taken in steps 4 and 5. This will equal the amount of paradox:

Sounds heard on expiration at	110 mm Hg
Sounds heard throughout cycle at	– 82 mm Hg
Amount of paradox	28 mm Hg

The difference is normally <10 mm Hg. If the difference is >10 mm Hg, cardiac tamponade may be present.

*Ask the patient to breathe slowly and deeply to reveal this finding when pulsus paradoxus is not severe.

TABLE 37-6 COLLABORATIVE CARE

Acute Pericarditis

Diagnostic	Collaborative Therapy
• History and physical examination: pericardial friction rub, pulsus paradoxus • Laboratory: CRP, ESR, white blood cell count • Electrocardiogram • Chest x-ray • Echocardiogram • Computed tomography • Magnetic resonance imaging • Pericardiocentesis, pericardial window • Pericardial biopsy	• Treatment of underlying disease • Bed rest • Nonsteroidal antiinflammatory drugs • Corticosteroids • Pericardiocentesis (for tamponade) • Pericardial window (for tamponade or ongoing pericardial effusion)

CRP, C-reactive protein; *ESR,* erythrocyte sedimentation rate.

sensitive ECG changes include diffuse (widespread) ST segment elevations. This reflects the abnormal repolarization that develops secondary to the pericardial inflammation. You need to differentiate these changes from the ST changes seen with MI. (See Chapter 36 for more information on ECG monitoring.)

Echocardiographic findings are most useful in determining the presence of a pericardial effusion or cardiac tamponade. Methods such as Doppler imaging and color M-mode assess diastolic function and diagnose constrictive pericarditis (discussed later in the chapter). Computed tomography (CT) and magnetic resonance imaging (MRI) provide for visualization of the pericardium and pericardial space. Chest x-ray findings are generally normal, but cardiomegaly may be seen in a patient who has a large pericardial effusion (Fig. 37-5).

Common laboratory findings include leukocytosis and elevation of CRP and ESR. Troponin levels may be elevated in patients with ST segment elevation and acute pericarditis, which could indicate concurrent myocardial damage. The fluid obtained during pericardiocentesis or the tissue from a pericardial biopsy may be studied to determine the cause of the pericarditis.

Collaborative Care

Management of acute pericarditis is aimed at identifying and treating the underlying problem and symptoms (Table 37-6). Antibiotics treat bacterial pericarditis, and nonsteroidal antiinflammatory drugs (NSAIDs) (e.g., salicylates [aspirin], ibuprofen) control the pain and inflammation. Corticosteroids are generally reserved for patients with pericarditis secondary to systemic lupus erythematosus, patients already taking corticosteroids for rheumatologic or other autoimmune conditions, or patients who do not respond to NSAIDs. They are used cautiously because of their numerous side effects (see Chapter 50). Colchicine (Colsalide), an antiinflammatory drug used for gout, can be used for patients who have recurrent pericarditis.[9]

Pericardiocentesis is usually performed for pericardial effusion with acute cardiac tamponade, purulent pericarditis, and suspected neoplasm. Hemodynamic support for the patient being prepared for the pericardiocentesis may include administration of volume expanders and inotropic agents (e.g., dopamine [Intropin]) and the discontinuation of any anticoagulants. The procedure is performed rapidly and safely using a percutaneous approach that is guided by echocardiography (Fig. 37-6). A needle is inserted into the pericardial space to remove fluid for analysis and to relieve cardiac pressure. Complications from pericardiocentesis include dysrhythmias, further cardiac tam-

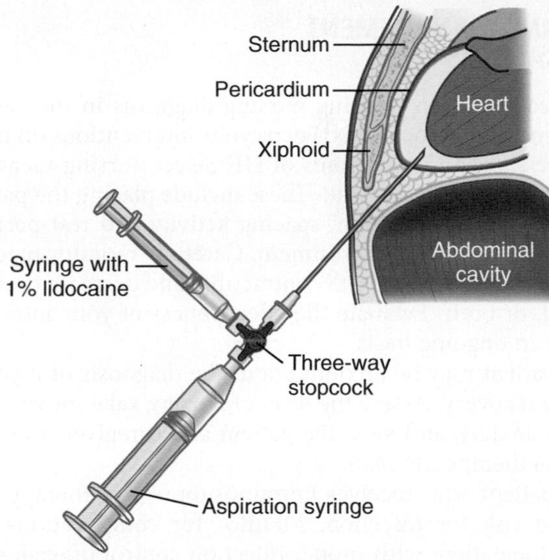

FIG. 37-6 Pericardiocentesis performed under sterile conditions in conjunction with electrocardiogram (ECG) and hemodynamic measurements.

ponade, pneumomediastinum, pneumothorax, myocardial laceration, and coronary artery laceration.

A *pericardial window* can be used for diagnosis or for drainage of excess fluid. It involves cutting a "window" or portion of the pericardium. This allows the fluid to drain continuously into the peritoneum or chest.

NURSING MANAGEMENT ACUTE PERICARDITIS

The management of the patient's pain and anxiety during acute pericarditis is your primary nursing consideration. Assess the pain to distinguish the pain of myocardial ischemia (angina) from the pain of pericarditis (see Table 34-7). Pericarditic pain is usually located in the precordium or left trapezius region and has a sharp, pleuritic quality that increases with inspiration. Pain is often relieved when the patient sits up or leans forward, and is worse when lying supine. The ECG can aid in distinguishing these types of pain. In acute pericarditis there are diffuse ST segment elevations. In myocardial ischemia there are usually localized ST segment changes. In addition, in acute pericarditis serial ECGs do not show evolving changes like those with MI.

Pain relief measures include keeping the patient on bed rest with the head of the bed elevated to 45 degrees and providing an overbed table for support. Antiinflammatory medications can help control the pain. However, because of the risk of gastrointestinal (GI) bleeding, administer these drugs with food or milk and instruct the patient to avoid alcohol. Other medications, such as a proton pump inhibitor (e.g., pantoprazole [Protonix]), may be ordered to decrease stomach acid.

Anxiety-reducing measures for the patient with acute pericarditis include providing simple, complete explanations of all procedures and possible causes of the pain. These explanations are particularly important for the patient whose diagnosis of acute pericarditis is being established and for the patient who has previously experienced angina or an acute MI.

The patient with acute pericarditis is at risk for cardiac tamponade and decreased CO. Monitor for the signs and symptoms of tamponade and prepare for possible pericardiocentesis.

CHRONIC CONSTRICTIVE PERICARDITIS

Etiology and Pathophysiology

Chronic constrictive pericarditis results from scarring with consequent loss of elasticity of the pericardial sac. It usually begins with an initial episode of acute pericarditis and is characterized by fibrin deposition with a clinically undetected pericardial effusion. Reabsorption of the effusion slowly follows, with progression toward the chronic stage. This involves fibrous scarring, thickening of the pericardium from calcium deposition, and eventual destruction of the pericardial space. The fibrotic, thickened, and adherent pericardium encases the heart, thereby impairing the ability of the atria and ventricles to stretch adequately.

Clinical Manifestations and Diagnostic Studies

Manifestations of chronic constrictive pericarditis occur over time and mimic those of HF and cor pulmonale. Decreased CO accounts for many of the clinical manifestations, including dyspnea on exertion, peripheral edema, ascites, fatigue, anorexia, and weight loss. The most prominent finding on physical examination is jugular venous distention (JVD). Unlike with cardiac tamponade, the presence of pulsus paradoxus (greater than 10 mm Hg) is not common.

ECG changes are often nonspecific in chronic constrictive pericarditis. The heart on the chest x-ray may be normal or enlarged depending on the degree of pericardial thickening and the presence of a pericardial effusion. 2-D echocardiography findings may reveal a thickened pericardium, but without a large pericardial effusion. CT and MRI provide measurement of pericardial thickness and assessment of diastolic filling patterns.

NURSING AND COLLABORATIVE MANAGEMENT CHRONIC CONSTRICTIVE PERICARDITIS

Unless the patient is free of symptoms or the condition is inoperable, the treatment of choice for chronic constrictive pericarditis is a *pericardiectomy*. This involves complete resection of the pericardium through a median sternotomy with the use of cardiopulmonary bypass (see Chapter 34). Some patients show immediate improvement after surgery, but others may take weeks. The prognosis improves when surgery is performed before the patient becomes clinically unstable.

MYOCARDITIS

Etiology and Pathophysiology

Myocarditis is a focal or diffuse inflammation of the myocardium. Possible causes include viruses, bacteria, fungi, radiation therapy, and pharmacologic and chemical factors. Coxsackie A and B viruses are the most common etiologic agents. Autoimmune disorders (e.g., polymyositis) also have been associated with the development of myocarditis. It may also be idiopathic. Myocarditis is frequently associated with acute pericarditis, particularly when it is caused by coxsackie B virus.[10]

When the myocardium becomes infected, the causative agent invades the myocytes and causes cellular damage and necrosis. The immune response is activated, and cytokines and oxygen free radicals are released. As the infection progresses, an autoimmune response is activated. This causes further destruction of myocytes. Myocarditis results in cardiac dysfunction and has been linked to the development of dilated cardiomyopathy (discussed later in this chapter).

Clinical Manifestations

The clinical features of myocarditis are variable, ranging from a benign course without any overt manifestations to severe heart involvement or sudden cardiac death (SCD). Fever, fatigue, malaise, myalgias, pharyngitis, dyspnea, lymphadenopathy, and nausea and vomiting are early systemic manifestations of the viral illness.

Early cardiac signs appear 7 to 10 days after viral infection. These include pleuritic chest pain with a pericardial friction rub and effusion because pericarditis often accompanies myocarditis. Late cardiac signs relate to the development of HF and may include an S_3 heart sound, crackles, JVD, syncope, peripheral edema, and angina.

Diagnostic Studies and Collaborative Care

The ECG changes for a patient with myocarditis are often nonspecific but may reflect associated pericardial involvement (e.g., diffuse ST segment changes). Dysrhythmias and conduction disturbances may be present. Laboratory findings are often inconclusive. They may include mild to moderate leukocytosis and atypical lymphocytes, increased ESR and CRP levels, elevated levels of myocardial markers such as troponin, and elevated viral titers. The virus is generally present in tissue and pericardial fluid samples only during the initial 8 to 10 days of illness.

Histologic confirmation of myocarditis is through an *endomyocardial biopsy.* A biopsy done during the first 6 weeks of acute illness is most diagnostic. This is the period in which lymphocytic infiltration and myocyte damage are present. Nuclear scans, echocardiography, and MRI are used to assess cardiac function.

The treatment for myocarditis consists of managing associated heart symptoms. Angiotensin-converting enzyme (ACE) inhibitors and β-adrenergic blockers are used if the heart is enlarged or to treat HF (see Chapter 35). Diuretics reduce fluid volume and decrease preload. If hypotension is not present, IV medications such as nitroprusside (Nitropress) and milrinone (Primacor) reduce afterload and improve CO by decreasing systemic vascular resistance. Digoxin (Lanoxin) improves myocardial contractility and reduces the heart rate. However, it is used cautiously in patients with myocarditis because of the heart's increased sensitivity to the adverse effects of this drug (e.g., dysrhythmias) and the potential toxicity. Anticoagulation therapy reduces the risk of thrombus formation from blood stasis in patients with a low ejection fraction (EF).

DRUG ALERT: Digoxin (Lanoxin)

- Use cautiously in patients with myocarditis, since the condition predisposes patients to drug-related dysrhythmias and toxicity.

Because myocarditis may have an autoimmune basis, immunosuppressive agents have been used to reduce myocardial inflammation and prevent irreversible myocardial damage. However, the use of these agents for the treatment of myocarditis remains controversial.[11]

General supportive measures for management of myocarditis include oxygen therapy, bed rest, and restricted activity. In cases of severe HF, intraaortic balloon pump therapy and ventricular assist devices may be required (see Chapters 35 and 66).

NURSING MANAGEMENT MYOCARDITIS

Decreased CO is an ongoing nursing diagnosis in the care of the patient with myocarditis. Focus your interventions on managing the signs and symptoms of HF. Select nursing measures to decrease cardiac workload. These include placing the patient in a semi-Fowler's position, spacing activity and rest periods, and providing a quiet environment. Carefully monitor medications that increase the heart's contractility and decrease preload, afterload, or both. Evaluate the effectiveness of your interventions on an ongoing basis.

The patient may be anxious about the diagnosis of myocarditis and recovery. Assess the level of anxiety, take measures to decrease anxiety, and keep the patient and caregiver informed about the therapeutic plan.

The patient who receives immunosuppressive therapy is at increased risk for infection. Monitor for complications and provide the patient with proper infection control procedures.

Most patients with myocarditis recover spontaneously, although some may develop dilated cardiomyopathy (discussed later in this chapter). If severe HF occurs, the patient may require heart transplantation.

RHEUMATIC FEVER AND RHEUMATIC HEART DISEASE

Rheumatic fever (RF) is an acute inflammatory disease of the heart potentially involving all layers (endocardium, myocardium, and pericardium). **Rheumatic heart disease** is a chronic condition resulting from RF that is characterized by scarring and deformity of the heart valves.

Etiology and Pathophysiology

RF is a complication that occurs as a delayed result (usually after 2 to 3 weeks) of a group A streptococcal pharyngitis. Symptoms of RF appear to be related to an abnormal immunologic response to group A streptococcal cell membrane antigens.[12] RF affects the heart, skin, joints, and central nervous system (CNS).

RF has declined in developed countries because of the effective use of antibiotics to treat streptococcal infections. However, it remains an important public health problem in developing countries.[12] Rheumatic heart disease, caused by RF, primarily affects young adults.

Cardiac Lesions and Valve Deformities. About 40% of RF episodes are marked by carditis, meaning that all layers of the heart (endocardium, myocardium, and pericardium) are involved (see Fig. 37-1). This gives rise to the term *rheumatic pancarditis.*

Rheumatic endocarditis is found mainly in the valves, with swelling and erosion of the valve leaflets. Vegetation forms from deposits of fibrin and blood cells in areas of erosion (see eFig. 37-1 on the website for this chapter). The lesions initially create thickening of the valve leaflets, fusion of commissures and chordae tendineae, and fibrosis of the papillary muscle. Valve leaflets may become calcified, resulting in stenosis. The less mobile valve leaflets may not close properly, resulting in regurgitation. The mitral and aortic valves are most commonly affected.

Nodules, called *Aschoff's bodies,* are formed by a reaction to inflammation with swelling and destruction of collagen fibers. As the Aschoff's bodies age, they become more fibrous, and scar

TABLE 37-7 MODIFIED JONES CRITERIA FOR DIAGNOSING RHEUMATIC FEVER

Major Criteria
- Carditis
- Monoarthritis or polyarthritis
- Sydenham's chorea
- Erythema marginatum
- Subcutaneous nodules

Minor Criteria
- Clinical findings: Fever, polyarthralgia
- Laboratory findings: ↑ ESR, ↑ WBC count, ↑ CRP
- ECG findings: Prolonged PR interval

Evidence of Group A Streptococcal Infection
- Laboratory findings: ↑ Antistreptolysin-O titer, positive throat culture, positive rapid antigen test for group A streptococci

Source: American Heart Association: Scientific statement: proceedings of the Jones criteria workshop, *Circulation* 106:2521, 2002.
CRP, C-reactive protein; *ESR,* erythrocyte sedimentation rate.

tissue forms in the myocardium. Rheumatic pericarditis develops and affects both layers of the pericardium. The layers become thickened and covered with a fibrinous exudate. A serosanguineous pericardial effusion may develop. When healing occurs, fibrosis and adhesions develop that partially or completely destroy the pericardial sac. These pathophysiologic changes in the heart can begin during an initial attack of RF. Recurrent infections cause further structural damage.

Extracardiac Lesions. The lesions of RF are systemic and involve the skin, joints, and CNS. Painless subcutaneous nodules, arthralgias or arthritis, and chorea may develop.

Clinical Manifestations

A cluster of signs and symptoms, including laboratory findings, leads to the diagnosis of RF. Established criteria provide a basis for diagnosis.[13] The presence of two major criteria or one major and two minor criteria plus evidence of a preceding group A streptococcal infection indicate a high probability of RF (Table 37-7).

Major Criteria. *Carditis* is the most important manifestation of RF and results in three signs: (1) a heart murmur or murmurs of mitral or aortic regurgitation, or mitral stenosis; (2) cardiac enlargement and HF secondary to myocarditis; and (3) pericarditis resulting in muffled heart sounds, chest pain, pericardial friction rub, or signs of effusion.

Monoarthritis or *polyarthritis* is the most common finding in RF. The inflammatory process affects the synovial membranes of the joints, causing swelling, heat, redness, tenderness, and limitation of motion. The larger joints, particularly the knees, ankles, elbows, and wrists, are most frequently affected.

Sydenham's chorea is the major CNS manifestation of RF. It is often a delayed sign occurring several months after the initial infection. It is characterized by involuntary movements, especially of the face and limbs; muscle weakness; and disturbances of speech and gait.

Erythema marginatum lesions are a less common feature of RF. The bright pink, nonpruritic, maplike macular lesions occur mainly on the trunk and proximal extremities, and may be exacerbated by heat (e.g., warm bath).

Subcutaneous nodules, usually associated with severe carditis, are firm, small, hard, painless swellings located over extensor surfaces of joints, particularly the knees, wrists, and elbows.

TABLE 37-8 COLLABORATIVE CARE
Rheumatic Fever

Diagnostic
- History and physical examination
- Laboratory findings (see Table 37-7)
- Chest x-ray
- Echocardiogram
- Electrocardiogram

Collaborative Therapy
- Bed rest
- Antibiotics
- Nonsteroidal antiinflammatory drugs
- Salicylates
- Corticosteroids

Minor Criteria. Minor clinical manifestations (see Table 37-7) are frequently present and are helpful in diagnosing the disease. The minor criteria are used as supplemental data to confirm the presence of RF when only one major criterion is present.

Evidence of Infection. In addition to the major and minor criteria, there must also be evidence of a preceding group A streptococcal infection. Table 37-7 lists the various laboratory tests used to confirm evidence of infection.

Complications

A complication that can result from RF is *chronic rheumatic carditis.* It results from changes in valvular structure that may occur months to years after an episode of RF. Rheumatic endocarditis can result in fibrous tissue growth in valve leaflets and chordae tendineae with scarring and contractures. The mitral valve is most frequently involved. The aortic and tricuspid valves may also be affected.

Diagnostic Studies and Collaborative Care

No single diagnostic test exists for RF. An echocardiogram may show valvular insufficiency and pericardial fluid or thickening.[14] A chest x-ray may show an enlarged heart if HF is present. The most consistent ECG change is delayed AV conduction as evidenced by a prolonged PR interval.

Treatment consists of drug therapy and supportive measures (Table 37-8). Antibiotic therapy does not change the course of the acute disease or the development of carditis. It does eliminate residual group A streptococci remaining in the tonsils and pharynx and prevents the spread of organisms to close contacts. Salicylates, NSAIDs, and corticosteroids are the antiinflammatory agents most widely used in the management of RF. All are effective in controlling the fever and joint manifestations. Salicylates or NSAIDs are used when arthritis is the main manifestation, and corticosteroids are used if severe carditis is present.

NURSING MANAGEMENT
RHEUMATIC FEVER AND RHEUMATIC HEART DISEASE

NURSING ASSESSMENT

Table 37-9 presents the subjective and objective data that you should obtain from a patient with RF and rheumatic heart disease.

Inspect the patient's skin for subcutaneous nodules and erythema marginatum. This involves palpating for subcutaneous nodules over all bony surfaces and along extensor tendons of

TABLE 37-9 NURSING ASSESSMENT

Rheumatic Fever and Rheumatic Heart Disease

Subjective Data

Important Health Information

Past health history: Recent streptococcal infection, previous history of rheumatic fever or rheumatic heart disease

Functional Health Patterns

Health perception–health management: Family history of rheumatic fever; malaise

Nutritional-metabolic: Anorexia, weight loss

Activity-exercise: Palpitations; generalized weakness, fatigue; ataxia

Cognitive-perceptual: Chest pain; widespread joint pain and tenderness (especially large joints)

Objective Data

General

Fever

Integumentary

Subcutaneous nodules and erythema marginatum

Cardiovascular

Tachycardia, pericardial friction rub, muffled heart sounds; murmurs; peripheral edema

Neurologic

Chorea (involuntary, purposeless, rapid motions; facial grimaces)

Musculoskeletal

Signs of monoarthritis or polyarthritis, including swelling, heat, redness, limitation of motion (especially of knees, ankles, elbows, shoulders, wrists)

Possible Diagnostic Findings

Cardiomegaly on chest x-ray; prolonged PR interval on ECG; valve abnormalities, chamber dilation, and pericardial effusion on echocardiogram; ↑ antistreptolysin-O titer, positive throat culture, positive rapid antigen test for group A streptococci; ↑ ESR, ↑ CRP, leukocytosis

CRP, C-reactive protein; *ESR,* erythrocyte sedimentation rate.

the hands and feet. The nodules range in size from 1 to 4 cm and are hard, painless, and freely movable. Erythema marginatum can occur on the trunk and inner aspects of the upper arm and thigh. The erythematous maculae do not itch and are flat. Assess for these bright pink maculae in good light because the rash is difficult to observe, especially in dark-skinned patients.

NURSING DIAGNOSES

Nursing diagnoses for the patient with RF and rheumatic heart disease may include, but are not limited to, the following:

- Decreased CO *related to* valve dysfunction or HF
- Activity intolerance *related to* arthralgia or arthritis secondary to joint pain, pain from pericarditis, and HF
- Ineffective self–health management *related to* lack of knowledge concerning possible disease sequelae and the need for long-term prophylactic antibiotic therapy

PLANNING

The goals for a patient with RF and rheumatic heart disease include (1) normal or baseline heart function, (2) resumption of daily activities without joint pain, and (3) verbalization of the ability to manage the disease sequelae.

NURSING IMPLEMENTATION

HEALTH PROMOTION. RF is a preventable cardiovascular disease. It involves early detection and immediate treatment of group A streptococcal pharyngitis. Adequate treatment of streptococcal pharyngitis prevents initial attacks of RF. Treatment with oral penicillin V (Penicillin VK) or amoxicillin (Moxatag) for 10 days is recommended. If the patient is allergic to penicillin, a narrow-spectrum cephalosporin (e.g., cephalexin [Keflex]), clindamycin (Cleocin), or azithromycin (Zithromax) is used.[15] Therapy requires strict adherence to the full course of treatment. Your role is to teach the community to seek medical attention for symptoms of streptococcal pharyngitis and to emphasize the need for prompt and adequate treatment.

ACUTE INTERVENTION. The primary goals of managing a patient with RF are to (1) control and remove the infecting organism; (2) prevent cardiac complications; and (3) relieve joint pain, fever, and other symptoms. Administer antibiotics as ordered to treat the streptococcal infection. Teach the patient that completing the full course of antibiotics is vital to successful treatment. Administer salicylates, NSAIDs, and corticosteroids as prescribed, and monitor fluid intake as appropriate.

Promoting optimal rest is essential to reduce cardiac workload and the body's metabolic needs. A priority nursing goal is relief of joint pain. Position painful joints for comfort and in proper alignment. Heat may be applied and salicylates or NSAIDs administered for joint pain.

After the acute symptoms have subsided, the patient without carditis can ambulate. If the patient has carditis with HF, strict bed rest restrictions apply (see Chapter 35 for care of a patient with HF). Encourage nonstrenuous activities once recovery has begun.

AMBULATORY AND HOME CARE. Secondary prevention aims at stopping the recurrence of RF. Teach the patient with a history of RF about the disease process, possible sequelae, and the need for continuous antibiotic prophylaxis.

Prior history of RF makes the patient more susceptible to a second attack after a streptococcal infection. The best prevention is treatment with prophylactic antibiotics. Patients with RF without carditis require prophylaxis until age 20 and for a minimum of 5 years. Patients with rheumatic carditis and residual heart disease (e.g., persistent valve disease) need longer-term and even life-long prophylaxis.[13]

Teach the patient about good nutrition, hygienic practices, and adequate rest. Caution the patient about the possible development of heart valve disease. Teach the patient to seek medical attention if symptoms such as excessive fatigue, dizziness, palpitations, unexplained weight gain, or exertional dyspnea develop.[16]

EVALUATION

The expected outcomes for the patient with RF and rheumatic heart disease include

- Ability to perform ADLs with minimal fatigue and pain
- Adherence to treatment regimen
- Expression of confidence in managing disease
- Prevention of complications

VALVULAR HEART DISEASE

The heart contains two AV valves (mitral and tricuspid) and two semilunar valves (aortic and pulmonic), which control unidirectional blood flow (see Fig. 32-1). Valvular heart disease is

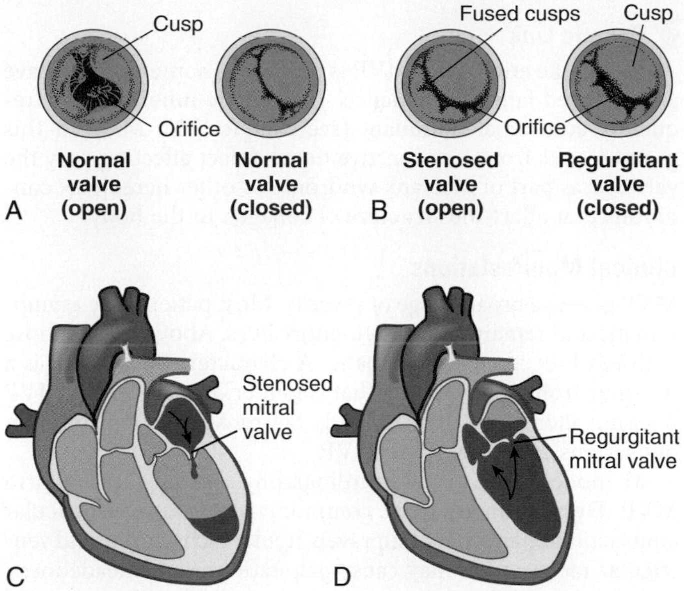

FIG. 37-7 Valvular stenosis and regurgitation. **A,** Normal position of the valve leaflets, or cusps, when the valve is open and closed. **B,** Open position of a stenosed valve *(left)* and closed position of regurgitant valve *(right)*. **C,** Hemodynamic effect of mitral stenosis. The stenosed valve is unable to open sufficiently during left atrial systole, inhibiting left ventricular filling. **D,** Hemodynamic effect of mitral regurgitation. The mitral valve does not close completely during left ventricular systole, permitting blood to reenter the left atrium. At the same time, blood is moving forward through the aortic valve.

defined according to the valve or valves affected and the type of functional alteration: stenosis or regurgitation (Fig. 37-7).

The pressure on either side of an open valve is normally equal. However, in a stenotic valve, the valve opening is smaller. The forward flow of blood is impaired. This creates a difference in pressure on the two sides of the open valve. The amount of **stenosis** (constriction or narrowing) is seen in the pressure differences (i.e., the higher the difference, the greater the stenosis). In **regurgitation** (also called *incompetence* or *insufficiency*), incomplete closure of the valve results in the backward flow of blood.

Valve disorders occur in children and adolescents mainly from congenital conditions. Valvular heart disease remains prevalent because of an increased number of older adults who have some form of cardiovascular disease. AS and mitral regurgitation (MR) are common valve disorders in older adults. Other causes of valve disease in adults include disorders related to acquired immunodeficiency syndrome and the use of some antiparkinsonian drugs.[17]

MITRAL VALVE STENOSIS

Etiology and Pathophysiology

Most cases of adult mitral valve stenosis result from rheumatic heart disease. Rheumatic mitral stenosis is widespread in developing countries. Less common causes are congenital mitral stenosis, rheumatoid arthritis, and systemic lupus erythematosus. Rheumatic endocarditis causes scarring of the valve leaflets and the chordae tendineae. Contractures and adhesions develop between the commissures (the junctional areas). The stenotic mitral valve takes on a "fish mouth" shape because of the thickening and shortening of the mitral valve structures (see eFig. 37-2 on the website for this chapter). These deformities block

TABLE 37-10 MANIFESTATIONS OF VALVULAR HEART DISEASE

Type	Manifestations
Mitral valve stenosis	Dyspnea on exertion, hemoptysis; fatigue; atrial fibrillation on ECG, palpitations, stroke; loud, accentuated S_1; low-pitched, diastolic murmur
Mitral valve regurgitation	*Acute:* Generally poorly tolerated; new systolic murmur with pulmonary edema and cardiogenic shock developing rapidly *Chronic:* Weakness, fatigue, exertional dyspnea, palpitations; an S_3 gallop, holosystolic murmur
Mitral valve prolapse	Palpitations, dyspnea, chest pain, activity intolerance, syncope; or holosystolic murmur
Aortic valve stenosis	Angina, syncope, dyspnea on exertion, heart failure; normal or soft S_1, diminished or absent S_2, systolic murmur, prominent S_4
Aortic valve regurgitation	*Acute:* Abrupt onset of profound dyspnea, chest pain, left ventricular failure and cardiogenic shock *Chronic:* Fatigue, exertional dyspnea, orthopnea, PND; water-hammer pulse; heaving precordial impulse; diminished or absent S_1, S_3, or S_4; soft high-pitched diastolic murmur, Austin Flint murmur
Tricuspid and pulmonic stenosis	*Tricuspid:* Peripheral edema, ascites, hepatomegaly; diastolic low-pitched murmur with increased intensity during inspiration *Pulmonic:* Fatigue, loud midsystolic murmur

PND, Paroxysmal nocturnal dyspnea.

the blood flow and create a pressure difference between the left atrium and the left ventricle during diastole. Left atrial pressure and volume increase. This causes higher pulmonary vasculature pressure. The overloaded left atrium places the patient at risk for atrial fibrillation. In chronic mitral stenosis, pressure overload occurs in the left atrium, the pulmonary bed, and the right ventricle.

Clinical Manifestations

The primary symptom of mitral stenosis is exertional dyspnea caused by reduced lung compliance (Table 37-10). Heart sounds include a loud first heart sound and a low-pitched, diastolic murmur (best heard at the apex with the stethoscope). Less frequently, patients may have hoarseness (from atrial enlargement pressing on the laryngeal nerve), hemoptysis (from pulmonary hypertension), chest pain (from decreased CO and coronary perfusion), and seizures or a stroke (from emboli). Fatigue and palpitations from atrial fibrillation may also occur. Emboli can arise from blood stasis in the left atrium secondary to atrial fibrillation.[18]

MITRAL VALVE REGURGITATION

Etiology and Pathophysiology

Mitral valve function depends on intact mitral leaflets, mitral annulus, chordae tendineae, papillary muscles, left atrium, and left ventricle. A defect in any of these structures can result in regurgitation. Most cases of mitral regurgitation (MR) are caused by MI, chronic rheumatic heart disease, mitral valve prolapse, ischemic papillary muscle dysfunction, and IE. MI with left ventricular failure increases the risk for rupture of the chordae tendineae and acute MR.

MR allows blood to flow backward from the left ventricle to the left atrium because of incomplete valve closure during systole. Both the left ventricle and left atrium must work harder to preserve an adequate CO. In acute MR the sudden increase in pressure and volume transmits to the pulmonary bed. This results in pulmonary edema and, if untreated, cardiogenic shock. In chronic MR the additional volume results in left atrial enlargement, left ventricular dilation and hypertrophy, and, finally, a decrease in CO.

Clinical Manifestations

The clinical course of MR is determined by the nature of its onset (see Table 37-10). Patients with acute MR have thready, peripheral pulses and cool, clammy extremities. A low CO may mask a new systolic murmur. Rapid assessment (e.g., cardiac catheterization) and intervention (e.g., valve repair or replacement) are critical.

Patients with chronic MR may remain asymptomatic for many years. Initial symptoms of left ventricular failure may include weakness, fatigue, palpitations, and dyspnea that gradually progress to orthopnea, paroxysmal nocturnal dyspnea, and peripheral edema. Increased left ventricular volume leads to an audible third heart sound (S_3), even with normal left ventricular function. The murmur is a loud holosystolic murmur at the apex radiating to the left axilla. Patients with asymptomatic MR must be monitored carefully. Surgery (valve repair or replacement) should be considered before significant left ventricular failure or pulmonary hypertension develops.[19]

MITRAL VALVE PROLAPSE

Etiology and Pathophysiology

Mitral valve prolapse (MVP) is an abnormality of the mitral valve leaflets and the papillary muscles or chordae that allows the leaflets to prolapse, or buckle, back into the left atrium during systole (Fig. 37-8). It is the most common form of valvular heart disease in the United States. It affects both genders equally.[20]

The use of the term *prolapse* can be misleading because it is used even when the valve is working normally. MVP is usually benign, but serious complications can occur, including MR, IE, SCD, HF, and cerebral ischemia.

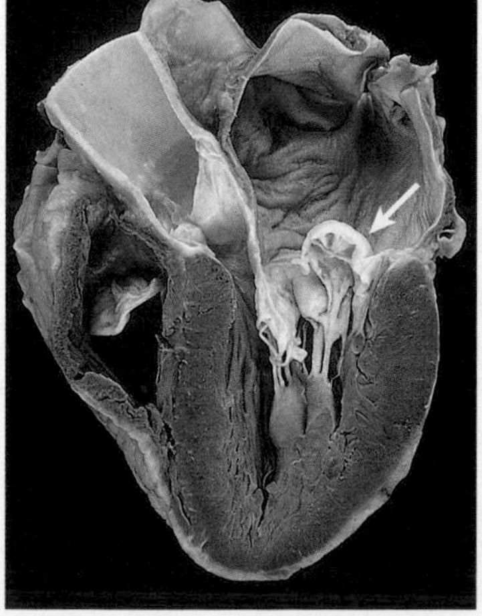

FIG. 37-8 Mitral valve prolapse. In this valvular abnormality, the mitral leaflets have prolapsed back into the left atrium. They also demonstrate hooding *(arrow)*. The left ventricle is on the right.

Genetic Link

Although the etiology of MVP is unknown, some patients have an increased familial incidence. The genetic inheritance is frequently autosomal dominant (see Chapter 13). MVP in this group results from a connective tissue defect affecting only the valve, or as part of Marfan's syndrome or other hereditary conditions that affect the structure of collagen in the body.

Clinical Manifestations

MVP covers a broad range of severity. Most patients are asymptomatic and remain so for their entire lives. About 10% of those with MVP become symptomatic. A characteristic of MVP is a murmur from regurgitation that is louder during systole. MVP does not alter S_1 or S_2 heart sounds. Severe MR is an uncommon but serious complication of MVP.

M-mode and 2-D echocardiography are used to confirm MVP. Dysrhythmias, most commonly premature ventricular contractions, paroxysmal supraventricular tachycardia, and ventricular tachycardia, may cause palpitations, light-headedness, and dizziness. IE may occur in patients with MR associated with MVP.

Patients may or may not have chest pain. The cause of the chest pain is not known. It may be the result of abnormal tension on the papillary muscles. If chest pain occurs, episodes tend to occur in clusters, especially during periods of emotional stress. Dyspnea, palpitations, and syncope may occasionally accompany the chest pain and do not respond to antianginal treatment (e.g., nitrates). β-Adrenergic blockers may be prescribed to control palpitations and chest pain. Encourage the patient to stay hydrated, exercise regularly, and avoid caffeine.

Patients with MVP generally have a benign, manageable course unless problems related to MR develop. No accepted medical therapy appears to delay the need for valve surgery in this group.[20] A teaching plan for patients with MVP is presented in Table 37-11.

AORTIC VALVE STENOSIS

Etiology and Pathophysiology

Congenital **aortic stenosis (AS)** is generally found in childhood, adolescence, or young adulthood. In older adults, AS is a result of RF or degeneration that may have an etiology similar to that of coronary artery disease. It affects 3% of people over

TABLE 37-11 PATIENT & CAREGIVER TEACHING GUIDE

Mitral Valve Prolapse

Include the following information in the teaching plan for a patient with mitral valve prolapse (MVP) and the patient's caregiver.

- Take medications as prescribed (e.g., β-adrenergic blockers to control palpitations, chest pain).
- Adopt healthy eating habits and avoid caffeine because it is a stimulant and may exacerbate symptoms.
- If you use diet pills or other over-the-counter drugs, check for common ingredients that are stimulants (e.g., caffeine, ephedrine), since these can exacerbate symptoms.
- Begin (or maintain) an exercise program to achieve optimal health.
- Contact the health care provider or emergency medical services (EMS) if symptoms develop or worsen (e.g., palpitations, fatigue, shortness of breath, anxiety).

65 years of age.[21] In rheumatic valve disease, fusion of the commissures and secondary calcification cause the valve leaflets to stiffen and retract, resulting in stenosis. If AS occurs due to rheumatic heart disease, mitral valve disease accompanies it. Isolated AS is usually nonrheumatic in origin. The incidence of rheumatic aortic valve disease has been decreasing, but degenerative stenosis is increasing as the population ages.

AS causes obstruction of flow from the left ventricle to the aorta during systole. The effect is left ventricular hypertrophy and increased myocardial oxygen consumption because of the increased myocardial mass. As the disease progresses and compensatory mechanisms fail, reduced CO leads to decreased tissue perfusion, pulmonary hypertension, and HF.

Clinical Manifestations

Symptoms of AS (see Table 37-10) develop when the valve orifice becomes about one third its normal size. Symptoms include the classic triad of angina, syncope, and exertional dyspnea, reflecting left ventricular failure.[21] The prognosis is poor for patients with symptoms and those whose valve obstruction is not fixed. Nitroglycerin is used cautiously to treat angina, since the drug can significantly reduce BP and worsen chest pain. Auscultation of AS typically reveals a normal or soft S_1, a diminished or absent S_2, a systolic murmur, and a prominent S_4.

DRUG ALERT: Nitroglycerin (Nitro-Bid)
- Use cautiously in patients with AS, since significant hypotension may occur.
- Chest pain can worsen due to a decrease in preload and drop in BP.

AORTIC VALVE REGURGITATION

Etiology and Pathophysiology

Aortic regurgitation (AR) may be the result of primary disease of the aortic valve leaflets, the aortic root, or both. Trauma, IE, or aortic dissection can cause acute AR, which constitutes a life-threatening emergency. Chronic AR is generally the result of rheumatic heart disease, a congenital bicuspid aortic valve, syphilis, or chronic rheumatic conditions such as ankylosing spondylitis or reactive arthritis.

AR causes retrograde (backward) blood flow from the ascending aorta into the left ventricle during diastole. This results in volume overload. The left ventricle initially compensates for chronic AR by dilation and hypertrophy. Myocardial contractility eventually declines, and blood volume in the left atrium and pulmonary bed increases. This leads to pulmonary hypertension and right ventricular failure.

Clinical Manifestations

Patients with acute AR have sudden manifestations of cardiovascular collapse (see Table 37-10). The left ventricle is exposed to aortic pressure during diastole. The patient develops severe dyspnea, chest pain, and hypotension indicating left ventricular failure and cardiogenic shock, a life-threatening emergency.

Patients with chronic, severe AR develop a *water-hammer pulse* (a strong, quick beat that collapses immediately). Heart sounds may include a soft or absent S_1, S_3, or S_4; and a soft, high-pitched diastolic murmur.

The patient with chronic AR generally remains asymptomatic for years. Exertional dyspnea, orthopnea, and paroxysmal nocturnal dyspnea develop only after considerable heart dysfunction has occurred (see Table 37-10). Angina occurs less frequently than in AS.

TRICUSPID AND PULMONIC VALVE DISEASE

Etiology and Pathophysiology

Diseases of the tricuspid and pulmonic valves are uncommon, with stenosis occurring more frequently than regurgitation. *Tricuspid stenosis* occurs almost exclusively in patients who have RF or who abuse IV drugs. Tricuspid stenosis results in right atrial enlargement and elevated systemic venous pressures. *Pulmonic stenosis* is almost always congenital and results in right ventricular hypertension and hypertrophy (see Table 37-10).

DIAGNOSTIC STUDIES FOR VALVULAR HEART DISEASE

Diagnosis of valvular heart disease includes data from the patient's history and physical examination and a variety of tests (Table 37-12). A CT scan of the chest with contrast is the gold standard for evaluating aortic disorders.[22] An echocardiogram reveals valve structure, function, and heart chamber size. Transesophageal echocardiography and Doppler color-flow imaging help diagnose and monitor valvular heart disease progression. Real-time 3-D echocardiography can help assess mitral valve and congenital heart disease. Chest x-ray reveals the heart size, altered pulmonary circulation, and valve calcification. An ECG identifies heart rate, rhythm, and any ischemia or ventricular hypertrophy. Cardiac catheterization detects pressure changes in the cardiac chambers, records pressure differences across the valves, and measures the size of valve openings.

TABLE 37-12 COLLABORATIVE CARE

Valvular Heart Disease

Diagnostic
- History and physical examination
- Chest x-ray
- CBC
- Electrocardiogram
- Echocardiography (Doppler and transesophageal)
- Cardiac catheterization

Collaborative Therapy

Nonsurgical
- Prophylactic antibiotic therapy (see Table 37-2)
  - Rheumatic fever
  - Infective endocarditis (see Table 37-2)
- Sodium restriction
- Medications to treat or control HF
  - Vasodilators* (e.g., nitrates, ACE inhibitors)
  - Positive inotropes (e.g., digoxin)
  - Diuretics
  - β-Adrenergic blockers
- Anticoagulation therapy (see Table 38-10)
- Antidysrhythmia drugs
- Percutaneous transluminal balloon valvuloplasty
- Percutaneous valve replacement

Surgical
- Valve repair
  - Commissurotomy (valvulotomy)
  - Valvuloplasty
  - Annuloplasty
- Valve replacement

*Use cautiously in patients with aortic stenosis.
ACE, Angiotensin-converting enzyme; *HF*, heart failure.

COLLABORATIVE CARE OF VALVULAR HEART DISEASE

Conservative Therapy

An important aspect of conservative management of valvular heart disease is prevention of recurrent RF and IE (see Table 37-12). Treatment depends on the valve involved and disease severity. It focuses on preventing exacerbations of HF, acute pulmonary edema, thromboembolism, and recurrent endocarditis. HF is treated with vasodilators, positive inotropes, β-adrenergic blockers, diuretics, and a low-sodium diet (see Chapter 35).

Anticoagulant therapy prevents and treats systemic or pulmonary emboli. It is used prophylactically in patients with atrial fibrillation. Atrial dysrhythmias are common and treated with calcium channel blockers, β-adrenergic blockers, antidysrhythmia drugs, or electrical cardioversion (see Chapter 36).

Percutaneous Transluminal Balloon Valvuloplasty. An alternative treatment for some patients with valvular heart disease is the *percutaneous transluminal balloon valvuloplasty* (PTBV) procedure. During PTBV, the fused commissures are split open. Balloon valvuloplasty is used for mitral, tricuspid, and pulmonic stenosis, and less often for AS. The procedure is done in the cardiac catheterization laboratory. It involves threading a balloon-tipped catheter from the femoral artery or vein to the stenotic valve. The balloon is inflated in an attempt to separate the valve leaflets. A single- or double-balloon technique may be used for the PTBV procedure. Currently, the use of a single Inoue balloon with hourglass shape allows sequential inflation (Fig. 37-9). This technique is the most popular because it is easy and has good results with few complications (e.g., left ventricular perforation). The PTBV procedure is generally indicated for older adults and for those who are poor surgery candidates. The long-term results of PTBV are similar to those of surgical commissurotomy.

Similar to PTBV, the Sapien Transcatheter Heart Valve (THV) is approved for select patients with AS. The THV is inserted through the femoral artery and moved to the heart. It is released and expanded with a balloon in the location of the aortic valve. This procedure is limited to patients who are eligible for surgery, but who are at high risk for surgical complications (e.g., patients with multiple comorbidities).[23]

Surgical Therapy. The decision for surgical intervention depends on the patient's clinical state using the New York Heart Association classification system for functional disability (see Table 35-5). The type of surgery can be valve repair or valve replacement. The procedure that is used depends on the valves involved, the pathology and severity of the disease, and the patient's clinical condition. All types of valve surgery are palliative, not curative, and patients require lifelong health care.

Valve Repair. Valve repair is usually the surgical procedure of choice. It has a lower operative mortality rate than valve replacement and is often used in mitral or tricuspid valvular heart disease.[24,25] Although valve repair avoids the risks of replacement, it may not restore total valve function.

Mitral *commissurotomy (valvulotomy)* is the procedure of choice for patients with pure mitral stenosis. The less precise closed method of commissurotomy has generally been replaced by the open method. In the *closed procedure* the surgeon inserts a transventricular dilator through the apex of the left ventricle into the opening of the mitral valve. The direct vision procedure, or *open procedure,* requires the use of cardiopulmonary bypass. The surgeon removes thrombi from the atrium and makes a commissure incision. Next, the fused chordae are separated by splitting the papillary muscle and debriding the calcified valve.

Open surgical *valvuloplasty* involves repair of the valve by suturing the torn leaflets, chordae tendineae, or papillary muscles. It is primarily used to treat mitral or tricuspid regurgitation.

Minimally invasive valvuloplasty surgery involves a ministernotomy or parasternal approach. It may include robotic and thoracoscopic surgical systems. Results compare with those of

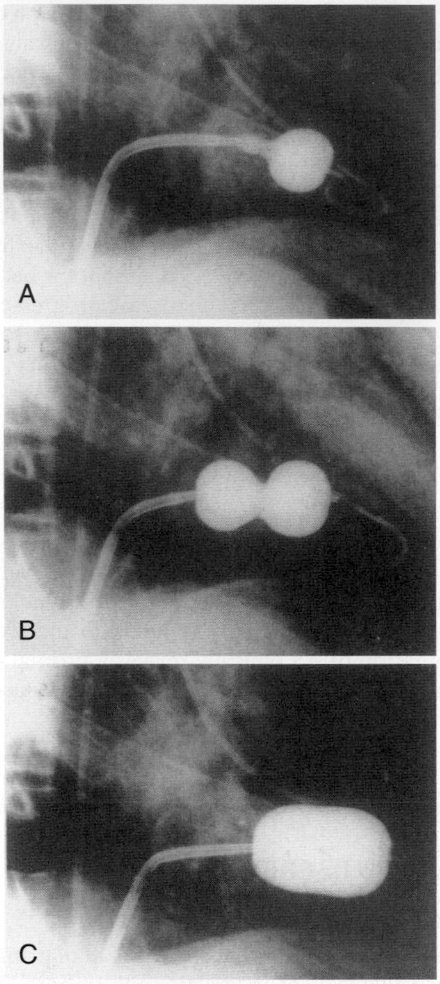

FIG. 37-9 Mitral valvuloplasty performed by the Inoue technique. The catheter is placed in the mitral valve and the distal part of the Inoue balloon inflated **(A).** The balloon is then pulled back in the mitral valve and inflated for 10 to 15 sec under fluoroscopic control **(B)** until the waist of the balloon is no longer visible **(C)** and the balloon falls back into the left atrium.

INFORMATICS IN PRACTICE

Heart Surgery DVD or CD

- Many patients prefer to watch DVDs or listen to CDs instead of reading pamphlets. For a patient facing heart surgery, using a video can be an effective tool to use when teaching the patient and caregiver what to expect before and after the procedure.
- Remember that the DVD or CD is not the teacher.
- Beforehand discuss what the DVD or CD will cover and encourage the patient and caregiver to write down questions or note what they do not understand.
- After the patient and caregiver view or listen to the material, be available to answer any questions they have. Reinforce important information from the DVD or CD.

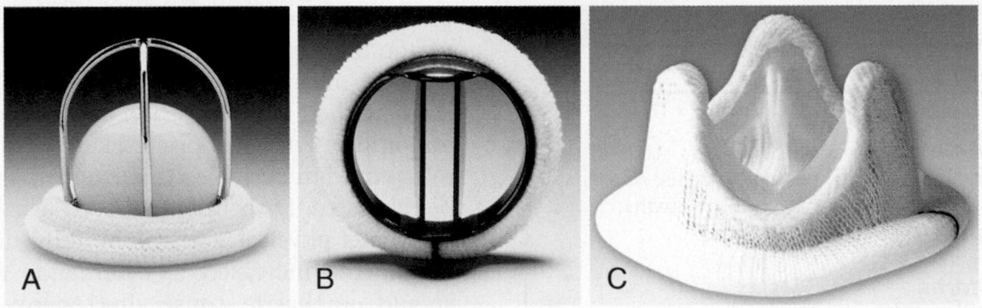

FIG. 37-10 Types of prosthetic heart valves. **A,** Starr-Edwards caged ball valve. **B,** St. Jude bi-leaflet valve. **C,** Carpentier-Edwards porcine valve.

ETHICAL/LEGAL DILEMMAS

Do Not Resuscitate

Situation

J.L., a 68-year-old man, is admitted for a second mitral valve surgery and coronary artery bypass graft surgery. He did not adhere to the treatment plan after his original surgery 7 years ago. You are worried about his future adherence with medications, diet, and exercise. His kidneys are failing and he is on dialysis, making him a high-risk surgical patient. The patient and caregivers want all possible treatment and refuse to discuss Do Not Resuscitate (DNR) orders.

Ethical/Legal Points for Consideration

- Based on their expertise, health care providers have the right to refuse to provide treatment that offers no benefit to the patient.
- Advance directives do not include a DNR order. If the patient is unable to speak for himself or herself, a DNR order can be initiated only by the attending physician or agent and usually depends on evidence of the patient's preferences.
- If there is an advance directive refusing resuscitation, the health care provider is required to act accordingly but is not compelled to enact a DNR without clear direction from the patient or proxy.
- Patient adherence with past treatment plans is not a factor that must be considered in DNR decisions. Many circumstances related to nonadherence are outside the patient's control such as financing, transportation, availability of assistance, and declining physical and medical capabilities.
- If there is disagreement about the patient's treatment plan, a referral can be made to an ethics committee, or the patient can seek treatment from another provider.

Discussion Questions

1. How can a lack of understanding or limited financial resources contribute to nonadherence with the plan of care?
2. What type of information should be provided to a patient and caregiver in discussions about DNR orders? Who should provide this information?
3. Who can initiate a referral to an ethics committee?

the open procedure. In addition, shorter lengths of stay, fewer blood transfusions, less pain, and lower risk of sternal infection and postoperative atrial fibrillation have been reported.[26]

For patients with mitral or tricuspid regurgitation, further valve repair or reconstruction using annuloplasty is an option. *Annuloplasty* involves reconstruction of the annulus, with or without the aid of prosthetic rings (e.g., a Carpentier ring).

Valve Replacement. Valve replacement may be required for mitral, aortic, tricuspid, and occasionally pulmonic valve disease. A wide variety of prosthetic valves are currently available. Desirable valves are nonthrombogenic and durable, and create minimal stenosis. Prosthetic valves are categorized as mechanical or biologic (tissue) valves (Fig. 37-10).

Mechanical valves are manufactured from artificial materials and consist of combinations of metal alloys, pyrolytic carbon, and Dacron. *Biologic valves* are constructed from bovine, porcine, and human (cadaver) heart tissue and usually contain some man-made materials. A "decellularizing" process removes the cadaver cells from the valve. This lowers the risk of immune response and tissue rejection. Biologic valves are asymmetric in shape and produce a more natural pattern of blood flow compared with mechanical valves. Asymmetric mechanical valve prototypes are being tested.[27]

Mechanical prosthetic valves are more durable and last longer than biologic valves. However, they have an increased risk of thromboembolism and require long-term anticoagulation therapy. The main complication of mechanical valves is bleeding from the use of anticoagulants. Biologic valves do not require anticoagulation therapy because of their low thrombogenicity. However, they are less durable and tend to cause early calcification, tissue degeneration, and stiffening of the leaflets. Either type of prosthetic valve can leak and cause endocarditis. Minimally invasive aortic valve replacement uses a transcatheter or transapical approach and is the surgical choice for patients at high risk for traditional surgery.[28,29]

Long-term anticoagulation is needed for those patients with biologic valves who have atrial fibrillation. Some patients with biologic valves or annuloplasty with prosthetic rings may need anticoagulation the first few months after surgery until the suture lines are covered by endothelial cells (endothelialized).

The choice of valves depends on many factors. For example, if a patient cannot take an anticoagulant (e.g., women of childbearing age), a biologic valve is considered. A mechanical valve may be best for a younger patient because it is more durable. For patients over age 65, durability is less important than the risks of bleeding from anticoagulants, so most receive a biologic valve.

NURSING MANAGEMENT VALVULAR DISORDERS

NURSING ASSESSMENT

Table 37-13 presents the subjective and objective data to obtain from an individual with valve disease.

NURSING DIAGNOSES

Nursing diagnoses for the patient with valvular heart disease may include, but are not limited to, the following:

- Decreased CO *related to* valvular incompetence
- Excess fluid volume *related to* fluid retention secondary to valvular-induced HF
- Activity intolerance *related to* insufficient oxygenation secondary to decreased CO and pulmonary congestion

TABLE 37-13 NURSING ASSESSMENT

Valvular Heart Disease

Subjective Data

Important Health Information

Past health history: Rheumatic fever, infective endocarditis; congenital defects, myocardial infarction, chest trauma, cardiomyopathy; syphilis, Marfan's syndrome, streptococcal infections

Functional Health Patterns

Health perception–health management: IV drug abuse; fatigue

Activity-exercise: Palpitations; generalized weakness, activity intolerance; dizziness, fainting; dyspnea on exertion, cough, hemoptysis, orthopnea

Sleep-rest: Paroxysmal nocturnal dyspnea

Cognitive-perceptual: Angina or atypical chest pain

Objective Data

General

Fever

Integumentary

Diaphoresis, flushing, cyanosis, clubbing; peripheral edema

Respiratory

Crackles, wheezes, hoarseness

Cardiovascular

Abnormal heart sounds, including murmurs, S_3, and S_4; dysrhythmias, including atrial fibrillation, premature ventricular contractions; tachycardia; ↑ or ↓ in pulse pressure; hypotension, water-hammer or thready peripheral pulses

Gastrointestinal

Ascites, hepatomegaly, unexplained weight gain

Possible Diagnostic Findings

Cardiomegaly on chest x-ray; ECG abnormalities specific to involved valve; echocardiogram (valve abnormalities and chamber dilation); cardiac catheterization (abnormalities in valves, chamber pressures, cardiac output, and blood flow depending on involved valve)

Additional information on nursing diagnoses is presented in eNursing Care Plan 37-2 available on the website for this chapter.

PLANNING

The overall goals for the patient with valve disease include (1) normal heart function, (2) improved activity tolerance, and (3) an understanding of the disease process and health maintenance measures.

NURSING IMPLEMENTATION

HEALTH PROMOTION. Diagnosing and treating streptococcal infections and providing prophylactic antibiotics for patients with a history of RF are critical to prevent acquired rheumatic valve disease. The patient at risk for endocarditis and any patient with certain cardiac conditions must also receive prophylactic antibiotics (see Table 37-2).

The patient must adhere to prescribed therapies. The individual with a history of RF, endocarditis, and congenital heart disease should know the symptoms of valvular heart disease so early medical treatment may begin.

ACUTE INTERVENTION AND AMBULATORY AND HOME CARE. A patient with progressive valvular heart disease may require outpatient care or hospitalization for management of HF, endocarditis, embolic disease, or dysrhythmias. HF is the most common reason for ongoing medical care.

Your role is to implement therapeutic interventions and evaluate their effects. Design activities considering the patient's limitations. An appropriate exercise plan can increase cardiac tolerance, but activities that cause fatigue and dyspnea should be restricted. Discourage tobacco use. Tell the patient to avoid strenuous physical exercise because damaged valves may not handle the increased CO demand. Your patient's care plan should emphasize conserving energy, setting priorities, and taking planned rest periods. Referral to a vocational counselor may be needed if the patient has a physically or emotionally demanding job.

Perform ongoing cardiac assessments to monitor the effectiveness of medications. Teaching the actions and side effects of drugs is important to increase adherence. The patient must understand the importance of prophylactic antibiotic therapy to prevent IE (see Table 37-2). If the valve disease was caused by RF, ongoing prophylaxis to prevent recurrence is necessary.

When valvular heart disease can no longer be managed medically, surgical intervention is necessary (see Chapter 34 for the care of a patient having heart surgery). The patient who is on anticoagulation therapy (e.g., warfarin [Coumadin]) after surgery for valve replacement must have the international normalized ratio (INR) checked regularly to determine proper dosage and adequacy of therapy. INR values of 2.5 to 3.5 are therapeutic for patients with mechanical valves.

Teaching instructions related to anticoagulation therapy are found in Table 38-14. The patient must know that valve surgery is not a cure, and that regular follow-up with a health care provider is required. Also, teach the patient when to seek medical care. Any manifestations of infection, HF, signs of bleeding, and planned invasive or dental procedures require the patient to notify the health care provider. Finally, encourage patients to obtain and wear a Medic Alert bracelet.

EVALUATION

The expected outcomes for a patient with valvular heart disease are presented in eNursing Care Plan 37-2 available on the website for this chapter.

CARDIOMYOPATHY

Cardiomyopathy (CMP) is a group of diseases that directly affect myocardial structure or function. A diagnosis of CMP is based on the patient's clinical manifestations and noninvasive and invasive diagnostic procedures.

CMP can be classified as primary or secondary. *Primary CMP* refers to those conditions in which the etiology of the disease is idiopathic. The heart muscle in this case is the only part of the heart involved, and other cardiac structures are unaffected. In *secondary CMP* the cause of the myocardial disease is known and is secondary to another disease process. Common causes of secondary CMP are listed in Table 37-14.

Three major types of CMP are dilated, hypertrophic, and restrictive. Each type has its own pathogenesis, clinical presentation, and treatment protocols (Tables 37-15 and 37-16). CMP can lead to cardiomegaly and HF. It is the primary reason that heart transplants are performed.

Takotsubo cardiomyopathy (TCM) is a transient cardiac syndrome that mimics acute coronary syndrome. Patients often are

TABLE 37-14 CAUSES OF CARDIOMYOPATHY

Dilated
- Cardiotoxic agents: alcohol, cocaine, doxorubicin (Adriamycin)
- Coronary artery disease
- Genetic (autosomal dominant)
- Hypertension
- Metabolic disorders
- Muscular dystrophy
- Myocarditis
- Pregnancy
- Valve disease

Hypertrophic
- Aortic stenosis
- Genetic (autosomal dominant)
- Hypertension

Restrictive
- Amyloidosis
- Endomyocardial fibrosis
- Neoplastic tumor
- Post-radiation therapy
- Sarcoidosis
- Ventricular thrombus

TABLE 37-15 COMPARISON OF TYPES OF CARDIOMYOPATHY

Dilated	Hypertrophic	Restrictive
Major Manifestations		
Fatigue, weakness, palpitations, dyspnea	Exertional dyspnea, fatigue, angina, syncope, palpitations	Dyspnea, fatigue
Cardiomegaly		
Moderate to severe	Mild to moderate	Mild
Contractility		
Decreased	Increased or decreased	Normal or decreased
Valvular Incompetence		
Atrioventricular (AV) valves, especially mitral	Mitral valve	AV valves
Dysrhythmias		
Sinus tachycardia, atrial and ventricular dysrhythmias	Atrial and ventricular dysrhythmias	Atrial and ventricular dysrhythmias
Cardiac Output		
Decreased	Normal or decreased	Normal or decreased
Outflow Tract Obstruction		
None	Increased	None

seen with chest pain, have ST segment elevation on ECG, and have elevated cardiac enzyme levels consistent with an MI. However, when the patient undergoes cardiac angiography, there is no significant coronary artery disease. TCM is an acute, stress-related syndrome that is more common in postmenopausal women. Normal cardiac function returns in days or weeks after supportive therapy.[30]

DILATED CARDIOMYOPATHY

Etiology and Pathophysiology

Dilated cardiomyopathy is the most common type of CMP, with a prevalence of 5 to 8 cases per 100,000 people in the United States. It causes HF in 25% to 40% of cases, occurs more frequently in middle-aged African Americans and men, and has a genetic link in 30% of cases. Dilated CMP often follows an infectious myocarditis. Some evidence links dilated CMP

TABLE 37-16 COLLABORATIVE CARE

Cardiomyopathy

Diagnostic
- History and physical examination
- Electrocardiogram
- b-Type natriuretic peptide (BNP)
- Chest x-ray
- Echocardiogram
- Nuclear imaging studies
- Cardiac catheterization
- Endomyocardial biopsy

Collaborative Therapy
- Drug therapy
  - Nitrates (except in hypertrophic CMP)
  - β-Adrenergic blockers
  - Antidysrhythmics
  - ACE inhibitors
  - Diuretics
  - Digitalis (except in hypertrophic CMP unless used to treat atrial fibrillation)
  - Anticoagulants (if indicated)
- Ventricular assist device
- Cardiac resynchronization therapy
- Implantable cardioverter-defibrillator
- Surgical correction
- Heart transplantation

ACE, Angiotensin-converting enzyme; *CMP*, cardiomyopathy.

with an autoimmune process.[31] Alcoholic dilated CMP is underrecognized and has unique presentation, treatment, and outcomes.[32] Other common causes of dilated CMP are listed in Table 37-14.

Dilated CMP is characterized by a diffuse inflammation and rapid degeneration of myocardial fibers. This results in ventricular dilation, impaired systolic function, atrial enlargement, and stasis of blood in the left ventricle. SCD from ventricular dysrhythmias is a leading cause of death in idiopathic dilated CMP.[33] *Cardiomegaly* results from ventricular dilation (Fig. 37-11). This causes contractile dysfunction in spite of an enlarged chamber size. In contrast to HF, the walls of the ventricles do not hypertrophy (see eFig. 37-3 on the website for this chapter).

Clinical Manifestations

The signs and symptoms of dilated CMP may develop acutely after a systemic infection or slowly over time. Most people eventually develop HF. Symptoms can include decreased exercise capacity, fatigue, dyspnea at rest, paroxysmal nocturnal dyspnea, and orthopnea. As the disease progresses, the patient may experience dry cough, palpitations, abdominal bloating, nausea, vomiting, and anorexia. Signs can include an abnormal S_3 and/or S_4, dysrhythmias, heart murmurs, pulmonary crackles, edema, weak peripheral pulses, pallor, hepatomegaly, and JVD. Decreased blood flow through an enlarged heart promotes stasis and blood clot formation, and may lead to systemic embolization.

Diagnostic Studies

The diagnosis of dilated CMP is based on the patient's history and exclusion of other causes of HF. Doppler echocardiography is the basis for the diagnosis of dilated CMP in the majority of patients. The chest x-ray may show cardiomegaly with signs of

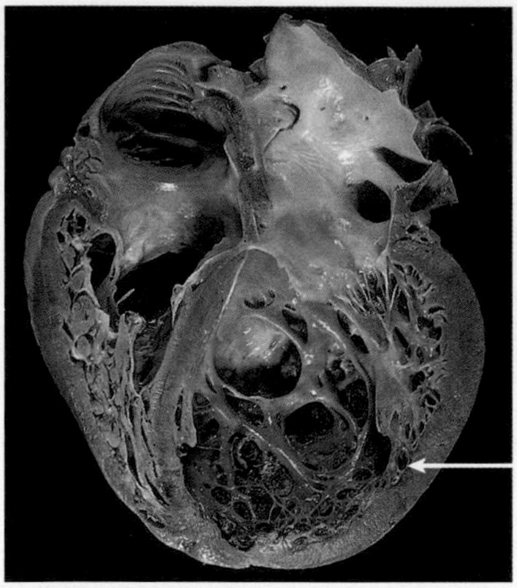

FIG. 37-11 Dilated cardiomyopathy. The dilated left ventricular wall has thinned *(arrow)*, and the chamber size and volume are increased.

pulmonary venous hypertension and pleural effusion. The ECG may reveal tachycardia, bradycardia, and dysrhythmias with conduction disturbances. Laboratory studies may show elevated serum levels of b-type natriuretic peptide (BNP) in the presence of HF.

Cardiac catheterization confirms or rules out coronary artery disease, and multiple gated acquisition (MUGA) nuclear scan determines EF. EF less than 20% is associated with a 50% mortality rate within 1 year. Endomyocardial biopsy is done at the time of the right-sided heart catheterization to identify any infectious organisms in heart tissue.

NURSING AND COLLABORATIVE MANAGEMENT DILATED CARDIOMYOPATHY

Interventions focus on controlling HF by enhancing myocardial contractility and decreasing preload and afterload. This is similar to the management of chronic HF. Treatment guidelines are based on the specific stage of disease progression (see Table 35-5). Treatment of patients with Class IV (stage D) HF is more palliative than curative.

Several different types of drugs are available to manage HF (see Table 35-7). Nitrates (e.g., nitroglycerin [Nitrol]) and diuretics (e.g., furosemide [Lasix]) decrease preload, and ACE inhibitors (e.g., captopril [Capoten]) reduce afterload. β-Adrenergic blockers (e.g., metoprolol [Lopressor]) and aldosterone antagonists (e.g., spironolactone [Aldactone]) control the neurohormonal stimulation that occurs in HF. Dysrhythmias are treated with antidysrhythmics (e.g., amiodarone) as indicated (see Chapter 36). Anticoagulation therapy reduces the risk of systemic embolization from clots. These may form in the heart chambers secondary to atrial fibrillation.

Drug and nutritional therapy and cardiac rehabilitation may help (1) alleviate symptoms of HF and (2) improve CO and quality of life. A patient with secondary dilated CMP must be treated for the underlying disease process. For example, the patient with alcohol-related dilated CMP must abstain from all alcohol. (See Chapter 11 for a discussion on addictive behaviors and Chapter 35 for a discussion on HF.)

Unfortunately, dilated CMP does not respond well to therapy, and patients experience multiple episodes of HF. Patients are often hospitalized for infusions of dobutamine (Dobutrex) or milrinone followed by aggressive diuresis. Sometimes these treatments are done on an outpatient basis or in the home under nursing supervision. After treatment, many patients experience an improvement in symptoms that lasts several weeks. The use of statins (e.g., atorvastatin [Lipitor]) in ischemic and idiopathic dilated CMP does increase survival, improve cardiac function, and reduce inflammatory markers[34,35] (see Table 34-5). Additionally, trimetazidine (Vastarel), a metabolic modulator, improves cardiac function and glucose control in diabetic patients with dilated CMP.[36]

Patients also may benefit from nondrug therapies. A ventricular assist device (VAD) allows the heart to rest and recover from acute HF. It may also serve as a bridge to heart transplantation. Additionally, cardiac resynchronization therapy and an implantable cardioverter-defibrillator are used in appropriate patients (see Chapter 35).

The patient with terminal or end-stage CMP may consider heart transplantation. The use of a permanent, implantable VAD, known as destination therapy, is an option for patients with advanced disease who are not candidates for heart transplantation (see Chapter 35). Currently, approximately 50% of heart transplantations are performed for treatment of CMP. Cardiac transplant recipients have a good prognosis. However, donor hearts are difficult to obtain, and many patients with dilated CMP die while awaiting heart transplantation.

Patients with dilated CMP are very ill people with a grave prognosis who need expert nursing care. Observe for signs and symptoms of worsening HF, dysrhythmias, embolic formation, and drug responsiveness. The goals of therapy are to keep the patient at an optimal level of functioning and out of the hospital. Always include caregivers when planning a patient's care. Encourage caregivers to learn cardiopulmonary resuscitation (CPR). Instruct them on when and how to access emergency care.

Home health and hospice nursing can provide the patient and caregiver with palliative care. This includes interventions to maximize and maintain functional status or end-of-life care to prepare for a peaceful death.

HYPERTROPHIC CARDIOMYOPATHY

Etiology and Pathophysiology

Hypertrophic cardiomyopathy is asymmetric left ventricular hypertrophy without ventricular dilation. In one form of the disease the septum between the two ventricles becomes enlarged and obstructs the blood flow from the left ventricle. It is termed *hypertrophic obstructive cardiomyopathy* (HOCMP) or *asymmetric septal hypertrophy* (ASH).

Although hypertrophic CMP can be idiopathic, about half of all cases have a genetic basis characterized by inappropriate myocardial hypertrophy.[37] Early identification is important (see Table 37-14). Hypertrophic CMP occurs less commonly than dilated CMP and is more common in men than in women. It is usually diagnosed in young adults and, most often, in active, athletic individuals. Hypertrophic CMP is the most common cause of SCD in otherwise healthy young people. It accounts for 3% of deaths in young competitive athletes.[38,39]

The four main characteristics of hypertrophic CMP are (1) massive ventricular hypertrophy; (2) rapid, forceful contraction of the left ventricle; (3) impaired relaxation (diastole); and (4) obstruction to aortic outflow (not present in all patients). Ventricular hypertrophy is associated with a thickened intra-

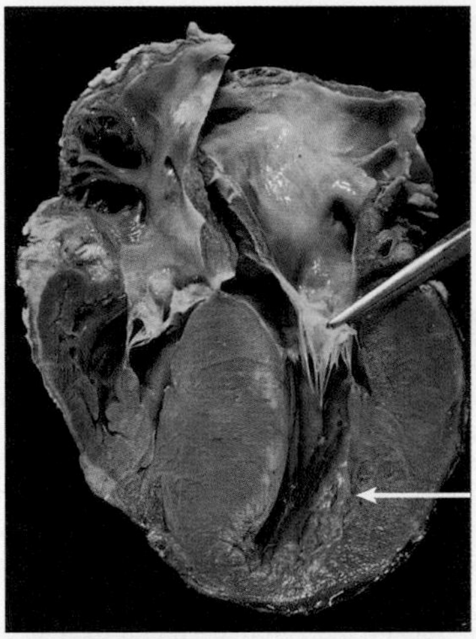

FIG. 37-12 Hypertrophic cardiomyopathy. There is marked left ventricular hypertrophy *(arrow)*, and the chamber size and volume are decreased.

ventricular septum and ventricular wall (Fig. 37-12; also see eFig. 37-3 on the website for this chapter). The end result is impaired ventricular filling as the ventricle becomes noncompliant and unable to relax. The primary defect of hypertrophic CMP is diastolic dysfunction from left ventricular stiffness. Decreased ventricular filling and obstruction to outflow can result in decreased CO, especially during exertion.

Clinical Manifestations

Patients with hypertrophic CMP may be asymptomatic or may have exertional dyspnea, fatigue, angina, and syncope. The most common symptom is dyspnea, which is caused by an elevated left ventricular diastolic pressure. Fatigue occurs because of the resultant decrease in CO and in exercise-induced flow obstruction. Angina can occur and is most often caused by the increased left ventricular muscle mass or compression of the small coronary arteries by the hypertrophic ventricular myocardium. The patient may also have syncope, especially during exertion. Syncope is most often caused by an increase in obstruction to aortic outflow during increased activity. This results in decreased CO and cerebrovascular circulation. Syncope can also be caused by dysrhythmias. Common dysrhythmias include supraventricular tachycardia, atrial fibrillation, ventricular tachycardia, and ventricular fibrillation. Any of these dysrhythmias may lead to syncope or SCD (see Chapters 34 and 36).

Diagnostic Studies

Clinical findings on examination may be unremarkable. However, on palpation of the chest the apical impulse can be exaggerated and displaced to the left. Auscultation may reveal an S_4 and a systolic murmur between the apex and the sternal border at the fourth intercostal space. ECG findings usually indicate ventricular hypertrophy, ST-T wave abnormalities, prominent Q waves in the inferior or precordial leads, left axis deviation, and ventricular and atrial dysrhythmias (see Chapter 36).

The echocardiogram is the primary diagnostic tool to confirm hypertrophic CMP. The echocardiogram may also demonstrate wall motion abnormalities and diastolic dysfunction. Cardiac catheterization and nuclear stress testing may also be helpful in diagnosing and guiding the treatment of hypertrophic CMP.

NURSING AND COLLABORATIVE MANAGEMENT HYPERTROPHIC CARDIOMYOPATHY

Goals of care are to improve ventricular filling by reducing ventricular contractility and relieving left ventricular outflow obstruction. These can be done with the use of β-adrenergic blockers (e.g., metoprolol) or calcium channel blockers (e.g., verapamil [Calan]). Digitalis is considered if needed to treat atrial fibrillation. Amiodarone or sotalol (Betapace) are effective antidysrhythmia medications. However, their use does not prevent SCD. For patients at risk for SCD, a cardioverter-defibrillator is needed (see Chapter 36).

AV pacing is helpful for patients with hypertrophic CMP and outflow obstruction. When the ventricles are paced from the apex of the right ventricle, septal depolarization occurs first. This allows the septum to move away from the left ventricular wall and reduces the degree of obstruction of the outflow tract.

Some patients may be candidates for surgical treatment of their hypertrophied septum. The indications for surgery include severe symptoms unresponsive to therapy with marked obstruction to aortic outflow. The surgery is termed a *ventriculomyotomy and myectomy.* It involves cutting into the thickened septal muscle and removing some of the ventricular muscle. Most patients have an improvement in symptoms and exercise tolerance after surgery.

An alternative nonsurgical procedure to reduce symptoms and the left ventricular outflow obstruction is alcohol-induced, percutaneous transluminal septal myocardial ablation (PTSMA). This procedure consists of injecting alcohol into the first septal artery branching off the left anterior descending artery. This causes ischemia and septal wall infarction. Ablation of the septal wall decreases the obstruction to flow, and the patient's symptoms decrease. The procedure improves HF symptoms and exercise capacity 3 months after ablation.[40] Potential complications of PTSMA include conduction disturbances (e.g., heart block) and MI.

Nursing interventions for hypertrophic CMP focus on relieving symptoms, observing for and preventing complications, and providing emotional support. Focus your teaching on helping patients avoid strenuous activity and dehydration. Any activity that causes an increase in systemic vascular resistance (thus increasing the obstruction to forward flow) is dangerous and should be avoided. Rest and elevation of the feet to improve venous return to the heart can manage chest pain in these patients. Vasodilators such as nitroglycerin may worsen the chest pain by decreasing venous return and further increasing obstruction of blood flow from the heart.

RESTRICTIVE CARDIOMYOPATHY

Etiology and Pathophysiology

Restrictive cardiomyopathy is the least common type of CMP. It is a disease of the myocardium that impairs diastolic filling and stretch (see eFig. 37-3 on the website for this chapter). Systolic function remains unchanged. Although the specific etiology of restrictive CMP is unknown, a number of pathologic processes may be involved in its development. Myocardial fibrosis, hypertrophy, and infiltration produce stiffness of the ventricular wall with loss of ventricular compliance. Secondary causes of restrictive CMP include amyloidosis, endocardial fibrosis, sarcoidosis, fibrosis of different etiology, and radiation to the thorax. With restrictive CMP, the ventricles are resistant to filling and therefore demand high diastolic filling pressures to maintain CO.

Clinical Manifestations and Diagnostic Studies

Classic manifestations of restrictive CMP are fatigue, exercise intolerance, and dyspnea. These occur because the heart cannot increase CO by increasing the heart rate without further compromising ventricular filling. Additional symptoms may include angina, orthopnea, syncope, and palpitations. The patient may have signs of HF, including dyspnea, peripheral edema, weight gain, ascites, hepatomegaly, and JVD.

The chest x-ray may be normal, or it may show cardiomegaly from right and left atrial enlargement. Pleural effusions and pulmonary congestion may be seen in the patient with progression to HF. The ECG may reveal a mild tachycardia at rest. The most common dysrhythmias are supraventricular (atrial fibrillation) or AV block. Echocardiography may reveal a left ventricle that is normal size with a thickened wall, slightly dilated right ventricle, and dilated atria. Endomyocardial biopsy, CT scan, and nuclear imaging may help in the diagnosis.

NURSING AND COLLABORATIVE MANAGEMENT RESTRICTIVE CARDIOMYOPATHY

Currently, there is no specific treatment for restrictive CMP. Interventions are aimed at improving diastolic filling and the underlying disease process. Treatment includes conventional therapy for HF and dysrhythmias. Heart transplant may also be a consideration. Nursing care is similar to the care of a patient with HF. As in the treatment of patients with hypertrophic CMP, teach the patient to avoid situations that impair ventricular filling and increase systemic vascular resistance, such as strenuous activity and dehydration.

Nursing care of a patient with CMP includes individualized teaching based on the patient's clinical manifestations. All patients with CMP are at risk for IE from any procedure that may cause bacteremia. Instruct the patient on the need for prophylactic antibiotics (see Table 37-2). A general patient and caregiver teaching guide is presented in Table 37-17.

TABLE 37-17 PATIENT & CAREGIVER TEACHING GUIDE

Cardiomyopathy

Include the following information in the teaching plan for a patient with cardiomyopathy and the patient's caregiver.

1. Take all medications as prescribed and regularly follow up with health care provider.
2. Follow a low-sodium diet (if ordered) and read all product labels (food and over-the-counter drugs) for sodium content.
3. Drink six to eight glasses of water a day unless fluids are restricted.
4. Achieve and maintain a reasonable weight and avoid large meals.
5. Avoid alcohol, caffeine, diet pills, and over-the-counter cold medicines that may contain stimulants.
6. Balance activity and rest periods.
7. Avoid heavy lifting or vigorous isometric exercises, and check with health care provider for exercise guidelines.
8. Use stress management techniques: relaxation breathing, guided imagery (see Chapter 7).
9. Report any signs of heart failure to health care provider, including weight gain, edema, shortness of breath, and increased fatigue.
10. Encourage caregivers to learn CPR because of the potential for cardiac arrest (see Appendix A).
11. Access emergency medical services according to the health care provider's instructions.

CPR, Cardiopulmonary resuscitation.

CASE STUDY

Valvular Heart Disease

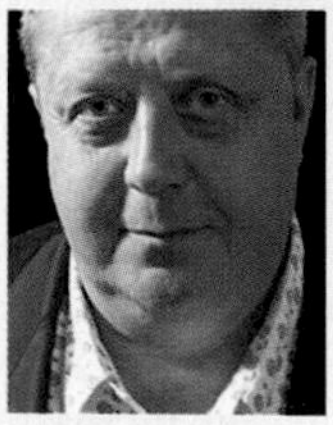

Jupiterimages/ Photos.com/Thinkstock

Patient Profile

R.B., a 50-year-old white man, is admitted to the hospital for valvular heart disease.

Subjective Data

- Reports past history of IV drug abuse
- Reports current regular alcohol intake approximately 1 pint of whiskey per day
- Complains of chest pain with minimal exertion
- Recently unemployed
- States he is short of breath and cannot sleep lying flat
- States he is tired and irritable all the time
- States he cannot afford medications
- Smokes a pack of cigarettes a day

Objective Data

Physical Examination

- Third heart sound (S_3)
- Loud holosystolic murmur of mitral regurgitation
- Edentulous (secondary to periodontal disease)
- Vital signs: temperature 99.0°F (37.2°C); pulse 110, irregular; respirations 24; BP 104/58

Diagnostic Studies

- ECG shows atrial fibrillation with a rapid ventricular response.
- Chest x-ray reveals pulmonary congestion and cardiomegaly.
- Transesophageal echocardiography shows left atrial and ventricular hypertrophy and mitral and aortic regurgitation.

Discussion Questions

1. Identify the cause and course of R.B.'s disease based on his history and current examination.
2. Differentiate between mitral and aortic regurgitation.
3. What medical treatments or surgical procedures will R.B. probably require as his condition worsens?
4. ***Priority Decision:*** On the basis of the assessment data provided, what are the priority nursing diagnoses?
5. ***Priority Decision:*** Identify the priority nursing interventions for R.B.
6. ***Delegation Decision:*** Identify those tasks that you could delegate to unlicensed assistive personnel (UAP).
7. ***Evidence-Based Practice***: R.B. asks you why he needs to be on "blood thinners" after his valves are replaced.

evolve Answers available at *http://evolve.elsevier.com/Lewis/medsurg.*

BRIDGE TO NCLEX EXAMINATION

The number of the question corresponds to the same-numbered outcome at the beginning of the chapter.

1. Assessment of an IV cocaine user with infective endocarditis should focus on which signs and symptoms *(select all that apply)*?
   a. Retinal hemorrhages
   b. Splinter hemorrhages
   c. Presence of Osler's nodes
   d. Painless nodules over bony prominences
   e. Painless erythematous macules on the palms and soles
2. The nurse is caring for a patient with chronic constrictive pericarditis. Which assessment finding reflects a more serious complication of this condition?
   a. Fatigue
   b. Peripheral edema
   c. Jugular venous distention
   d. Thickened pericardium on echocardiography
3. A patient is admitted with myocarditis. While performing the initial assessment, the nurse may find which clinical signs and symptoms *(select all that apply)*?
   a. Angina
   b. Pleuritic chest pain
   c. Splinter hemorrhages
   d. Pericardial friction rub
   e. Presence of Osler's nodes
4. Priority nursing management for a patient with myocarditis includes interventions related to
   a. meticulous skin care.
   b. antibiotic prophylaxis.
   c. tight glycemic control.
   d. oxygenation and ventilation.
5. When teaching a patient about the long-term consequences of rheumatic fever, the nurse should discuss the possibility of
   a. valvular heart disease.
   b. pulmonary hypertension.
   c. superior vena cava syndrome.
   d. hypertrophy of the right ventricle.
6. Which is a priority nursing intervention for a patient during the acute phase of rheumatic fever?
   a. Administration of antibiotics as ordered
   b. Management of pain with opioid analgesics
   c. Encouragement of fluid intake for hydration
   d. Performance of frequent active range-of-motion exercises
7. Which clinical finding would most likely indicate decreased cardiac output in a patient with aortic valve regurgitation?
   a. Reduction in peripheral edema and weight
   b. Carotid venous distention and new-onset atrial fibrillation
   c. Significant pulsus paradoxus and diminished peripheral pulses
   d. Shortness of breath on minimal exertion and a diastolic murmur
8. A patient is diagnosed with mitral stenosis and new-onset atrial fibrillation. Which interventions could the nurse delegate to unlicensed assistive personnel (UAP) *(select all that apply)*?
   a. Obtain and record daily weight.
   b. Determine apical-radial pulse rate.
   c. Observe for overt signs of bleeding.
   d. Obtain and record vital signs, including pulse oximetry.
   e. Teach the patient how to purchase a Medic Alert bracelet.
9. Which diagnostic study best differentiates the various types of cardiomyopathy?
   a. Echocardiography
   b. Arterial blood gases
   c. Cardiac catheterization
   d. Endomyocardial biopsy
10. The nurse is caring for a patient newly admitted with heart failure secondary to dilated cardiomyopathy. Which intervention would be a priority?
   a. Encourage caregivers to learn CPR.
   b. Consider a consultation with hospice for palliative care.
   c. Monitor the patient's response to prescribed medications.
   d. Arrange for the patient to enter a cardiac rehabilitation program.

1. a, b, c, e; 2. c; 3. a, b, d; 4. d; 5. a; 6. a; 7. d; 8. a, c, d; 9. a; 10. c

evolve

For rationales to these answers and even more NCLEX review questions, visit *http://evolve.elsevier.com/Lewis/medsurg.*

REFERENCES

1. Wu K-S, Lee S, Tsai H-C, et al: Non-nosocomial healthcare-associated infective endocarditis in Taiwan: an underrecognized disease with poor outcomes, *BMC Infect Dis* 11(221):1, 2011.
2. Lomas J, Martinez-Marcos F, Plata A, et al: Healthcare-associated infective endocarditis: an undesirable effect of healthcare universalization, *Clin Microbiol Infect* 16(11):1683, 2010.
3. Birchenough E, Moore C, Stevens K, et al: Buttonhole cannulation in adult patients on hemodialysis: an increased risk of infection? *Nephrology Nurs J* 37(5):491, 2010.
4. Cunha B, D'Elia A, Pawar N, et al: Viridans streptococcal *(Streptococcus intermedius)* mitral valve subacute bacterial endocarditis (SBE) in a patient with mitral valve prolapse after a dental procedure: the importance of antibiotic prophylaxis, *Heart Lung* 39(1):65, 2010.
5. Buppert C: NP sued for failure to diagnosis (sic) endocarditis—$1 million settlement, *J Nurs Pract* 7(10):872, 2011.
6. McDermott B, Cunha B, Choi D, et al: Transthoracic echocardiography (TEE): sufficiently sensitive screening test for native valve infective endocarditis (IE), *Heart Lung* 40:358, 2010.
7. Cleveland Clinic: Cardiac catheterization, 2012. Retrieved from *http://my.clevelandclinic.org/heart/services/tests/invasive/ccath.aspx.*
8. Petrov D: Sudden onset of chest pain associated with PR-segment depression in ECG, *Heart Lung* 38(5):440, 2009.
9. Kuo I, Pearson GJ, Koshman SL: Colchicine for the primary and secondary prevention of pericarditis: an update, *Ann Pharmacother* 43(12):2075, 2009.

10. Metzger T, Anderson M: Myocarditis: a defect in central immune tolerance? *J Clin Invest* 121(4):125, 2011.
11. Myocarditis—new treatments, 2011. Retrieved from *www.ccspublishing.com/journals3a/myocarditis.htm*.
12. Parks T: Erratum: underdiagnosis of acute rheumatic fever in primary care settings in a developing country, *Trop Med Int Health* 15(3):384, 2010.
13. Mayo Clinic Staff: Rheumatic fever, 2011. Retrieved from *www.mayoclinic.com/health/rheumatic-fever/DS00250/METHOD+print*.
*14. Simsek Z, Karakelleoglu S, Gündogdu F, et al: Evaluation of left ventricular function with strain/strain rate imaging in patients with rheumatic mitral stenosis, *Anatolian J Cardiol* 10(4):328, 2010.
15. Shulman ST, Bisno AL, Clegg HW, et al: Clinical practice guideline for the diagnosis and management of group A streptococcal pharyngitis: 2012 update by the Infectious Diseases Society of America, *Clin Infect Dis* 55:e86, 2012.
16. Mosby's Nursing Consult, Patient Information: Rheumatic fever, 2012. Retrieved from *www.nursingconsult.com/nursing/patient-education/full-text?handout_id=45551&docId=10087&tab=cond&otherid=48822&english=true&filter_id=47523&filter_by=Rheumatology&sort_by=title&sort_order=asc&page=1&title=&requestUri=filter&story_title=Rheumatic+Fever&parentpage=&secondpage=&searchId=&searchTerm=*.
17. Surapaneni P, Vinales K, Najib M, et al: Valvular heart disease with the use of fenfluramine-phentermine, *Tex Heart Inst J* 38(5):581, 2011.
18. Maganti K, Rigolin V, Sarano M, et al: Valvular heart disease: diagnosis and management, *Mayo Clin Proc* 85(5):483, 2009.
19. Madden S: An alternative treatment approach to mitral regurgitation, *Nurs Stand* 26(13):40, 2011.
20. Gemignani A, Ferri F, Wu W: Mitral valve prolapse. In Ferri F, editor: *Ferri's clinical advisor: 5 books in 1*, Philadelphia, 2012, Mosby.
21. Michelena H, Abel M, Suri R, et al: Intraoperative echocardiography in valvular heart disease: an evidence-based appraisal, *Mayo Clin Proc* 85(7):646, 2010.
22. Bachore T, Hranitzky P, Patel M: Heart disease. In McPhee SJ, Papadakis MA, editors: *Lange 2011 current medical diagnosis and treatment*, ed 50, New York, 2011, McGraw-Hill Medical.
23. U.S. Food and Drug Administration: FDA expands approved use of Sapien artificial heart valve. Retrieved from *www.fda.gov/NewsEvents/Newsroom/PressAnnouncements/ucm323478.htm?source=govdelivery*.
24. Mitral Valve Repair Center at the Mount Sinai Hospital: Mitral valve repair, 2011. Retrieved from *www.mitralvalverepair.org/content/view/64*.
25. Mitral Valve Repair Center at the Mount Sinai Hospital: Mitral valve repair vs. replacement rates, 2011. Retrieved from *www.mitralvalverepair.org/content/view/72*.
26. Mitral Valve Repair Center at the Mount Sinai Hospital: Minimally invasive heart surgery center, 2011. Retrieved from *www.mitralvalverepair.org/content/view/16*.
27. Science Daily: New design for mechanical heart valves, 2011. Retrieved from *www.sciencedaily.com/releases/2011/11/111122113212.htm*.
28. Held ML: Transcatheter aortic valve replacement: new hope for patients with aortic stenosis, *Am Nurse Today* 7(5):11, 2012.
29. Cleveland Clinic: Diseases and conditions—heart valve disease—percutaneous interventions, 2012. Retrieved from *http://my.clevelandclinic.org/heart/percutaneous/percutaneousValve.aspx*.
30. Bradbury B, Cohen F: Early postoperative Takotsubo cardiomyopathy: a case report, *AANA J* 79(3):181, 2011.
31. Xiao H, Wang M, Du Y, et al: Arrhythmogenic autoantibodies against calcium channel lead to sudden death in idiopathic dilated cardiomyopathy, *Eur J Heart Fail* 13:264, 2011.
32. Lamari A, Dattilo G, Morabito G, et al: A dilated alcoholic cardiomyopathy, *Int J Cardiol* 149(3):95, 2009.
33. Samanta S, Vijayverghia R, Vaiphei K: Isolated idiopathic right ventricular dilated cardiomyopathy, *Indian J Pathol Microbiol* 54(1):164, 2011.
*34. Nagueh S, Lombardi R, Tan Y, et al: Atorvastatin and cardiac hypertrophy and function in hypertrophic cardiomyopathy: a pilot study, *Eur J Clin Invest* 40:976, 2010.
35. Kostner K: Statin therapy for hypertrophic cardiomyopathy: too good to be true? *Eur J Clin Invest* 40:965, 2010.
36. Wafa S: Clinical benefits of trimetazidine in diabetic patients with coronary artery disease, *Heart Metab* 48:23, 2010.
37. Wang L, Seidman J, Seidman C: Narrative review: harnessing molecular genetics for the diagnosis and management of hypertrophic cardiomyopathy, *Ann Intern Med* 152(8):513, 2010.
*38. Hypertrophic Cardiomyopathy Association: 2011 ACCF/AHA guidelines for the diagnosis and treatment of hypertrophic cardiomyopathy: a report of the American College of Cardiology Foundation /American Heart Association Task Force on Practice Guidelines. Retrieved from *www.4hcm.org/2011_accf_aha_guidelines.html*.
39. Wilson M, Chandra N, Papadakis M, et al: Hypertrophic cardiomyopathy and ultra-endurance running—two incompatible entities? *J Cardiovasc Magnetic Res* 13(77):1, 2011.
40. Otto A, Aytemir K, Okutucu S, et al: Cyanoacrylate for septal ablation in hypertrophic cardiomyopathy, *J Interv Cardiol* 24(1):77, 2011.

RESOURCES

American Association of Cardiovascular and Pulmonary Rehabilitation
www.aacvpr.org

American College of Cardiology
www.acc.org

American Heart Association
www.heart.org/HEARTORG

Hypertrophic Cardiomyopathy Association
www.4hcm.org

Mayo Clinic
www.mayoclinic.com/health/cardiomyopathy/DS00519

Mended Hearts
www.mendedhearts.org

National Heart, Lung, and Blood Institute
www.nhlbi.nih.gov

Percutaneous Transvenous Mitral Valvuloplasty
www.ptmv.org

YourHeartValve.com
www.yourheartvalve.com

*Evidence-based information for clinical practice.

CHAPTER

38

The best and most beautiful things in the world cannot be seen or even touched. They must be felt within the heart.
Helen Keller

Nursing Management
Vascular Disorders

Deirdre D. Wipke-Tevis and Kathleen A. Rich

evolve WEBSITE

http://evolve.elsevier.com/Lewis/medsurg

- NCLEX Review Questions
- Key Points
- Pre-Test
- Answer Guidelines for Case Study on p. 859
- Rationales for Bridge to NCLEX Examination Questions
- Concept Map Creator
- Glossary
- Content Updates
- Case Studies
  - Patient With Abdominal Aortic Aneurysm
  - Patient With Chronic Peripheral Artery Disease
- Nursing Care Plans (Customizable)
  - eNCP 38-1: Patient With Peripheral Artery Disease of the Lower Extremities
  - eNCP 38-2: Patient After Surgical Repair of the Aorta

eTables

- eTable 38-1: Drugs, Vitamins, Minerals, and Supplements That Interact With Oral Anticoagulants
- eTable 38-2: Sample Venous Thromboembolism Protocol/Order Set

LEARNING OUTCOMES

1. Relate the major risk factors to the etiology and pathophysiology of peripheral artery disease (PAD).
2. Describe the clinical manifestations, collaborative care, and surgical and nursing management of PAD of the lower extremities.
3. Plan appropriate nursing care for the patient with acute arterial ischemic disorders of the lower extremities.
4. Differentiate the pathophysiology, clinical manifestations, collaborative care, and nursing management of thromboangiitis obliterans (Buerger's disease) and Raynaud's phenomenon.
5. Differentiate the pathophysiology, clinical manifestations, and collaborative care of different types of aortic aneurysms.
6. Select appropriate nursing interventions for a patient undergoing an aortic aneurysm repair.
7. Describe the pathophysiology, clinical manifestations, collaborative care, and nursing management of aortic dissection.
8. Evaluate the risk factors predisposing patients to the development of superficial vein thrombosis and venous thromboembolism (VTE).
9. Differentiate between the clinical characteristics of superficial vein thrombosis and VTE.
10. Compare and contrast the collaborative care and nursing management of patients with superficial vein thrombosis and VTE.
11. Prioritize the key aspects of nursing management of the patient receiving anticoagulant therapy.
12. Relate the pathophysiology and clinical manifestations to the collaborative care of patients with varicose veins, chronic venous insufficiency, and venous leg ulcers.

KEY TERMS

acute arterial ischemia, p. 839
aneurysm, p. 841
aortic dissection, p. 845
chronic venous insufficiency (CVI), p. 857
critical limb ischemia, p. 837
deep vein thrombosis (DVT), p. 847
intermittent claudication, p. 834
peripheral artery disease (PAD), p. 833
post-thrombotic syndrome (PTS), p. 849
Raynaud's phenomenon, p. 840
superficial vein thrombosis (SVT), p. 847
thromboangiitis obliterans (Buerger's disease), p. 840
varicose veins, p. 856
venous thromboembolism (VTE), p. 847
venous thrombosis, p. 847
Virchow's triad, p. 847

Problems of the vascular system include disorders of the arteries, veins, and lymphatic vessels. Arterial disorders are classified as atherosclerotic, aneurysmal, and nonatherosclerotic vascular diseases. Atherosclerotic vascular disease is divided into coronary, cerebral, peripheral, mesenteric, and renal artery disease.[1] This chapter discusses peripheral artery disease; aortic aneurysm and dissection; and venous diseases, specifically venous thromboembolism and chronic venous insufficiency.

PERIPHERAL ARTERY DISEASE

Peripheral artery disease (PAD) involves thickening of artery walls, which results in a progressive narrowing of the arteries

Reviewed by Patricia Hong, RN, MA, Senior Lecturer, University of Washington, School of Nursing, Seattle, Washington; Teri Lynn Kiss, RN, MS, MSSW, CCRN, Director, Medical Unit–2 South and Patient Quality Resources, Fairbanks Memorial Hospital, Fairbanks, Alaska; and Tara McMillan-Queen, RN, MSN, ANP, GNP, Faculty II, Mercy School of Nursing, Charlotte, North Carolina.

GENDER DIFFERENCES

Vascular Disorders

Men

- Thromboangiitis obliterans (Buerger's disease) occurs predominantly in men <40 yr of age.
- Abdominal aortic aneurysms (AAAs) are more common in men than women.
- Men with AAAs are more likely to undergo endovascular aneurysm repair or open aneurysm repair than women.
- Aortic dissection affects men more often than women.

Women

- Women with low lifetime recreational activity are at greater risk for peripheral artery disease (PAD) than similar men.
- Older women experience the classic signs of intermittent claudication less often than men.
- Women with PAD experience faster functional decline and greater mobility loss than men with PAD.
- Raynaud's phenomenon occurs primarily in women between 15 and 40 yr of age.
- Women with AAAs are at higher risk for rupture and have a higher in-hospital mortality rate than men.
- Women undergoing open aneurysm repair and endovascular aneurysm repair have higher 30-day mortality and readmission rates than men of similar age.
- Risk for venous thromboembolism (VTE) is greater in women over age 35 who use tobacco and oral contraceptives or oral hormone therapy (HT), are pregnant or postpartum, or have a family history of VTE.
- Risk for varicose veins is greater in women who use oral contraceptives or HT or are pregnant.

of the upper and lower extremities. The risk for PAD increases with age; it usually become symptomatic in the sixth to eighth decades of life. In persons with diabetes mellitus, PAD occurs much earlier. About 6% of adults ages 40 years and older and 13% of adults ages 60 years and older have PAD.[2] PAD prevalence is higher in women, and non-Hispanic African Americans.[3,4]

PAD is strongly related to other types of cardiovascular disease (CVD) and their risk factors. Patients with PAD have a significantly higher risk of mortality (in general), CVD mortality, and major coronary events.[5] Thus PAD is a marker of advanced systemic atherosclerosis. Patients with PAD are more likely to have coronary artery disease and/or cerebral artery disease. Unfortunately, most Americans are not familiar with PAD, nor are they aware of PAD risk factors and complications.[6] In general, PAD remains underdiagnosed and undertreated.

Etiology and Pathophysiology

The leading cause of PAD is *atherosclerosis,* a gradual thickening of the *intima* (the innermost layer of the arterial wall) and *media* (middle layer of the arterial wall). This results from the deposit of cholesterol and lipids within the vessel walls and leads to progressive narrowing of the artery. Although the exact cause(s) of atherosclerosis are unknown, inflammation and endothelial injury play a major role (see Chapter 34).

Significant risk factors for PAD include tobacco use, diabetes, hyperlipidemia, elevated C-reactive protein, and uncontrolled hypertension, with the most important being tobacco use. Nicotine is a vasoconstrictor, and tobacco smoke impairs transport and cellular use of oxygen, and increases blood viscosity and homocysteine levels. Other risk factors include family history, hypertriglyceridemia, increasing age, hyperhomocysteinemia, hyperuricemia, obesity, sedentary lifestyle, and stress.[4,7] Women with low lifetime recreational activity are at greater risk for PAD than similar men.[8]

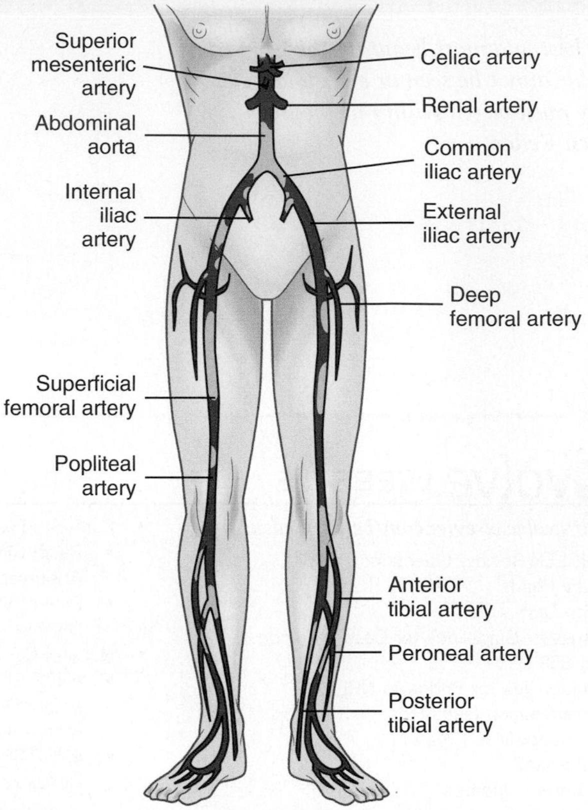

FIG. 38-1 Common anatomic locations of atherosclerotic lesions (shown in *yellow*) of the abdominal aorta and lower extremities.

Atherosclerosis more commonly affects certain segments of the arterial tree. These include the coronary (see Chapter 34), carotid (see Chapter 58), and lower extremity arteries. Clinical symptoms occur when vessels are 60% to 75% blocked.

PERIPHERAL ARTERY DISEASE OF THE LOWER EXTREMITIES

Lower extremity PAD may affect the iliac, femoral, popliteal, tibial, or peroneal arteries, or any combination of these arteries (Fig. 38-1). The femoral popliteal area is the most common site in nondiabetic patients. Patients with diabetes tend to develop PAD in the arteries below the knee. In advanced PAD, multiple levels of occlusions are found.

Clinical Manifestations

Generally, the severity of the clinical manifestations depends on the site and extent of the blockage and the amount of collateral circulation. The classic symptom of lower extremity PAD is **intermittent claudication,** which is ischemic muscle pain that is caused by exercise, resolves within 10 minutes or less with rest, and is reproducible.[9] The ischemic pain is a result of the buildup of lactic acid from anaerobic metabolism. Once the patient stops exercising, the lactic acid is cleared and the pain subsides. PAD of the iliac arteries produces claudication in the buttocks and thighs. Calf claudication indicates femoral or popliteal artery involvement. Only about 10% of patients with PAD display the classic symptom of intermittent claudication. Older

TABLE 38-1 COMPARISON OF PERIPHERAL ARTERY AND VENOUS DISEASE

Characteristic	Peripheral Artery Disease	Venous Disease
Peripheral pulses	Decreased or absent	Present, may be difficult to palpate with edema
Capillary refill	>3 sec	<3 sec
Ankle-brachial index	≤0.90	>0.90
Edema	Absent unless leg constantly in dependent position	Lower leg edema
Hair	Loss of hair on legs, feet, toes	Hair may be present or absent
Ulcer		
• Location	Tips of toes, foot, or lateral malleolus	Near medial malleolus
• Margin	Rounded, smooth, looks "punched out"	Irregularly shaped
• Drainage	Minimal	Moderate to large amount
• Tissue	Black eschar or pale pink granulation	Yellow slough or dark red, "ruddy" granulation
Pain	Intermittent claudication or rest pain in foot Ulcer may or may not be painful	Dull ache or heaviness in calf or thigh Ulcer often painful
Nails	Thickened; brittle	Normal or thickened
Skin color	Dependent rubor, elevation pallor	Bronze-brown pigmentation Varicose veins may be visible
Skin texture	Thin, shiny, taut	Skin thick, hardened, and indurated
Skin temperature	Cool, temperature gradient down the leg	Warm, no temperature gradient
Dermatitis	Rarely occurs	Frequently occurs
Pruritus	Rarely occurs	Frequently occurs

women experience it less often than men.[10] If PAD involves the internal iliac arteries, erectile dysfunction may result.

Paresthesia, or numbness or tingling, in the toes or feet may result from nerve tissue ischemia. True peripheral neuropathy occurs more often in patients with diabetes (see Chapter 49) and in those with long-standing ischemia. Neuropathy produces severe shooting or burning pain in the extremity. It does not follow particular nerve roots and may be present near ulcerated areas. Gradual, reduced blood flow to neurons produces loss of both pressure and deep pain sensations. Thus patients may not notice lower extremity injuries.

The limb's physical appearance provides important information about blood flow. The skin becomes thin, shiny, and taut, and hair loss occurs on the lower legs. Pedal, popliteal, or femoral pulses are diminished or absent. Pallor (blanching of the foot) develops in response to leg elevation *(elevation pallor).* Conversely, *reactive hyperemia* (redness of the foot) develops when the limb is in a dependent position *(dependent rubor)* (see Table 38-1).

As PAD progresses and involves multiple arterial segments, continuous pain develops at rest. *Rest pain* most often occurs in the foot or toes and is aggravated by limb elevation. Rest pain occurs when blood flow is insufficient to meet basic metabolic requirements of the distal tissues. Rest pain occurs more often at night because cardiac output tends to drop during sleep and the limbs are at the level of the heart. Patients often try to achieve pain relief by dangling the leg over the side of the bed or sleeping in a chair. This allows gravity to maximize blood flow.

The patient with chronic rest pain, ulceration, or gangrene has *critical limb ischemia.* Critical limb ischemia may lead to amputation if untreated. Every attempt is made to save the limb with surgical or endovascular revascularization. If a patient is not a candidate for revascularization and/or if revascularization is not technically possible, medical treatment is required.[11]

Complications

Lower extremity PAD progresses slowly. Prolonged ischemia leads to atrophy of the skin and underlying muscles. Even minor trauma to the feet (e.g., stubbing one's toe, blister from shoes) can result in delayed healing, wound infection, and tissue necrosis, especially in the diabetic patient. Arterial (ischemic) ulcers most often occur over bony prominences on the toes, feet, and lower legs (Table 38-1). Nonhealing arterial ulcers and gangrene are the most serious complications. Amputation may be needed if adequate blood flow is not restored or if severe infection occurs. If PAD is present for an extended period, collateral circulation may prevent gangrene of the extremity. Uncontrolled pain and severe, spreading infection are indicators that an amputation is needed in individuals who are not candidates for revascularization.

Diagnostic Studies

Various tests can assess blood flow and outline the vascular system (Table 38-2). Doppler ultrasound with duplex imaging maps blood flow throughout the entire region of an artery. When palpation of a peripheral pulse is difficult because of severe PAD, the Doppler ultrasound can determine the degree of blood flow. A palpable pulse and a Doppler pulse are not equivalent, and the terms are not interchangeable. *Segmental blood pressures* (BPs) are obtained (using Doppler ultrasound and a sphygmomanometer) at the thigh, below the knee, and at ankle level while the patient is supine. A drop in segmental BP of greater than 30 mm Hg suggests PAD. Angiography and magnetic resonance angiography delineate the location and extent of PAD (see Table 32-6).

The *ankle-brachial index* (ABI) is a PAD screening tool. It is performed using a hand-held Doppler. The ABI is calculated by dividing the ankle systolic BPs by the higher of the left and right brachial systolic BPs. PAD guidelines recommend uniform reporting of ABI results[12] (Table 38-3). In very elderly patients and those with diabetes, the arteries often are calcified and noncompressible. This results in a falsely elevated ABI. ABI measurement is not recommended immediately after revascularization surgery or on distal bypass grafts because of the risk of graft thrombosis.[13]

Collaborative Care

Table 38-2 summarizes the collaborative care for a patient with PAD.

Risk Factor Modification. The first treatment goal in treating PAD is to reduce CVD risk factors in all patients with PAD regardless of the severity of symptoms.[14] Risk factors need to be

TABLE 38-2 COLLABORATIVE CARE

Peripheral Artery Disease

Diagnostic
- Health history and physical examination, including palpation of peripheral pulses
- Doppler ultrasound studies
- Segmental blood pressures
- Ankle-brachial index (see Table 38-3)
- Duplex imaging
- Angiography
- Magnetic resonance angiography

Collaborative Therapy
- Cardiovascular disease risk factor modification
  - Tobacco cessation
  - Regular physical exercise
  - Achieve or maintain ideal body weight
  - Follow Dietary Approaches to Stop Hypertension (DASH) diet (see eTable 33-1)
  - Tight glucose control in diabetics
  - Tight blood pressure control
  - Treatment of hyperlipidemia and hypertriglyceridemia (see Table 34-5)
  - Antiplatelet agent (aspirin or clopidogrel [Plavix])
  - Angiotensin-converting enzyme inhibitors (see Table 33-7)
- Treatment of claudication symptoms
  - Structured walking or exercise program
  - Cilostazol (Pletal)
- Nutrition therapy
- Proper foot care (see Table 49-21)
- Percutaneous transluminal balloon angioplasty with or without stent
- Percutaneous transluminal atherectomy
- Percutaneous transluminal cryoplasty
- Peripheral artery bypass surgery
- Patch graft angioplasty, often in conjunction with bypass surgery
- Endarterectomy (for localized stenosis but rarely done)
- Thrombolytic therapy or mechanical clot extraction therapy (for acute ischemia only)
- Sympathectomy (for pain management only)
- Amputation

TABLE 38-3 INTERPRETATION OF ANKLE-BRACHIAL INDEX RESULTS

Ankle-Brachial Index (ABI)	Clinical Significance
≥1.40	Noncompressible arteries
1.00-1.40	Normal ABI
0.91-0.99	Borderline ABI
≤0.90	Abnormal ABI
Classification of PAD Severity	
0.90-0.71	Mild PAD
0.71-0.41	Moderate PAD
≤40	Severe PAD

PAD, Peripheral artery disease.

modified with both drug therapy and lifestyle changes (see Tables 34-3 to 34-5).

Tobacco cessation is essential to reduce the risk of CVD events, PAD progression, and death. This is a complex and difficult process with a high incidence of smoking relapse. Comprehensive tobacco cessation strategies are recommended (see Tables 11-4 to 11-6).

Diabetes is a major risk factor for PAD and increases the risk of amputation in these patients. It is recommended that diabetic patients maintain a glycosylated hemoglobin (Hb A1C) below 7.0% and, optimally, as near as possible to 6.0%.[15] (Chapter 49 discusses diabetes mellitus.)

Aggressive lipid management is essential for all patients with PAD.[14] Both dietary interventions and drug therapy are needed. Statins (e.g., simvastatin [Zocor]) lower low-density lipoprotein (LDL) and triglyceride levels and reduce CVD morbidity and mortality risks.[16] Unfortunately, as many as 70% of people with PAD do not take a statin and have elevated LDL levels.[2]

Hypertension is a well-known risk factor for PAD progression, as well as other CVD events (e.g., stroke, myocardial infarction [MI], heart failure). Guidelines for the management of hypertension in persons with PAD include BP less than 140/90 mm Hg.[2,14] In PAD patients with diabetes or renal insufficiency, BP less than 130/80 mm Hg is recommended.[15]

Initial antihypertensive therapy includes thiazides and angiotensin-converting enzyme (ACE) inhibitors (e.g., ramipril [Altace]). Lifestyle changes are encouraged and include reducing dietary sodium and following the Dietary Approaches to Stop Hypertension (DASH) diet. (Chapter 33 discusses hypertension.)

Drug Therapy. Antiplatelet agents are considered critical for reducing the risks of CVD events and death in PAD patients. Oral antiplatelet therapy should include 75 to 100 mg/day of aspirin for patients with asymptomatic PAD and 75 to 325 mg/day of aspirin for patients with symptomatic PAD.[11,12] Aspirin-intolerant patients may take clopidogrel (Plavix) daily.

Combination antiplatelet therapy with aspirin and clopidogrel is not typically recommended, but may be used in symptomatic PAD patients at high risk for CVD events.[12] Anticoagulants (e.g., warfarin [Coumadin]) are not recommended for the prevention of CVD events in PAD patients.

DRUG ALERT: Clopidogrel (Plavix) and Omeprazole (Prilosec)
- Antiplatelet effect of clopidogrel is reduced by about half when given with omeprazole.
- This increases the risk of MI and stroke.

Two drugs are available to treat intermittent claudication: cilostazol (Pletal) and pentoxifylline (Trental). Cilostazol, a phosphodiesterase inhibitor, inhibits platelet aggregation and increases vasodilation. It is recommended as first-line drug therapy for patients with intermittent claudication who do not respond to exercise therapy or stop using tobacco.[11] Cilostazol does not reduce CVD morbidity and mortality risks, so antiplatelet therapy is also needed.

DRUG ALERT: Cilostazol (Pletal)
- Contraindicated in patients with heart failure of any severity.

Exercise Therapy. The primary nondrug treatment for intermittent claudication is tobacco cessation in combination with a formal, supervised exercise training program. Exercise improves walking ability. Lack of exercise and impaired walking ability in PAD patients is related to low quality of life.[17] Encouragement of participation in exercise is particularly important for women with PAD, since women experience faster functional decline and greater mobility loss than men with PAD.[17] In addition, women with PAD are more likely to have a history of limited recreational activities.[8]

Walking is the most effective exercise for PAD patients. A supervised PAD rehabilitation program is an effective means of improving exercise performance. Such programs typically include exercise for 30 to 60 minutes/day, 3 to 5 times/week, for 3 to 6 months. Supervised treadmill exercise training improves walking performance and quality of life in PAD patients, whether or not they have claudication.[17]

A home exercise program is an effective alternative to supervised rehabilitation. Encourage slow, progressive physical activity after a warm-up period. Instruct the patient to walk to the point of discomfort, stop and rest, and then resume walking until the discomfort recurs. Walking should be done for 30 to 40 minutes/day, 3 to 5 times/week. An exercise therapy program should also be implemented in PAD patients after surgical interventions (discussed later in this chapter).

Nutritional Therapy. Teach PAD patients to adjust their dietary intake so that their body mass index (BMI) is less than 25 kg/m^2 and their waist circumference is less than 40 inches for men and less than 35 inches for women.[18] Recommend a diet high in fruits, vegetables, and whole grains and low in cholesterol, saturated fat, and salt (see Chapters 34 and 35).

Complementary and Alternative Therapies. Patients taking antiplatelet agents, nonsteroidal antiinflammatory drugs (NSAIDs) (e.g., ibuprofen [Motrin]), and anticoagulants (e.g., warfarin) should consult with their health care provider before taking any dietary or herbal supplements because of potential interactions and bleeding risks[19] (see the Complementary & Alternative Therapies box on p. 851).

Care of the Leg With Critical Limb Ischemia. **Critical limb ischemia** is a condition characterized by chronic ischemic rest pain lasting more than 2 weeks, arterial leg ulcers, or gangrene of the leg as a result of PAD.[12] Optimal therapy is revascularization via bypass surgery. If this is not feasible, percutaneous transluminal angioplasty (PTA) is recommended in patients with a life expectancy of 2 years or less.[12] Patients with critical limb ischemia who are not candidates for surgery or PTA may be treated with prostanoids (e.g., iloprost [Ventavis]). These drugs may decrease rest pain and improve ulcer healing. Patients with critical limb ischemia should continue CVD risk factor reduction and antiplatelet therapy to reduce the risk of a CVD event.

Conservative management of critical limb ischemia includes protecting the extremity from trauma, decreasing ischemic pain, preventing and controlling infection, and improving perfusion. Carefully inspect, cleanse, and lubricate both feet to prevent cracking of the skin and infection. Avoid soaking the patient's feet to prevent skin *maceration* (or breakdown). If ulceration is present, keep the affected foot clean and dry. Cover any ulcers with a dry, sterile dressing to maintain cleanliness. Deep ulcers can be treated with a variety of wound care products, but healing is unlikely without increased blood flow.

Encourage the patient to select soft, roomy, and protective footwear and avoid extremes of heat and cold. Keep the patient's heels free of pressure. You can do this by placing a pillow under the calves so that the heels are off the mattress. Commercially available devices can also provide heel protection. Administering opioid analgesics and placing the bed in the reverse Trendelenburg position may control pain and increase perfusion to the lower extremities.

Spinal cord stimulation may be helpful in managing pain and preventing amputation in patients with critical limb ischemia. Other promising strategies include gene therapy and endothelial progenitor cell therapy to stimulate blood vessel growth *(angiogenesis)*.[20]

Interventional Radiology Catheter-Based Procedures. Interventional radiology catheter-based procedures are alternatives to open surgical approaches for treatment of lower extremity PAD. These procedures take place in a catheterization laboratory rather than in an operating room. Determining which intervention to use depends on blockage location and lesion type and severity.

All these procedures are similar to angiography in that they involve the insertion of a specialized catheter into the femoral artery. The *percutaneous transluminal angioplasty* (PTA) procedure uses a catheter that contains a cylindric balloon at the tip. The end of the catheter is moved to the narrowed (stenotic) area of the artery. The balloon is then inflated, compressing the atherosclerotic intimal lining.[21]

Stents, expandable metallic devices, are positioned within the artery immediately after the balloon angioplasty is done. The stent acts as a scaffold to keep the artery open. The stents may be covered with Dacron or a drug-eluting agent (e.g., paclitaxel) to reduce restenosis by limiting the amount of new tissue growth in the stent.

Atherectomy is the removal of the obstructing plaque. A directional atherectomy device uses a high-speed cutting disk that cuts long strips of the atheroma. Laser atherectomy uses ultraviolet energy to break up the atheroma. Orbital or rotational atherectomy catheters have a diamond-coated tip that rotates at a high speed (similar to a dentist drill). These crush the calcium within the atheroma into particles smaller than a blood cell.

Cryoplasty combines two procedures: PTA and cold therapy. A specialized balloon is filled with liquid nitrous oxide, which changes from liquid to gas as it enters the balloon. Expansion of the gas results in cooling to 14° F (−10° C). The cold limits restenosis by reducing smooth muscle cell activity.[22] Preprocedure and postprocedure nursing care is the same as for a diagnostic angiography. Antiplatelet agents are needed after the procedure to reduce the risk of restenosis. Long-term, low-dose aspirin therapy (75 to 100 mg/day) or clopidogrel (75 mg/day) is recommended. Restenosis rates depend on the procedure performed, lesion type and length, and target vessel characteristics. Immediate postprocedure success rates are high (greater than 95%) for iliac and femoral interventions.[23]

Surgical Therapy. Various surgical approaches can be used to improve blood flow beyond a blocked artery. The most common is peripheral artery bypass surgery with an autogenous (native) vein or synthetic graft to bypass, or carry blood around, the lesion (Fig. 38-2). Synthetic grafts typically are used for long bypasses such as an axillary-femoral bypass. When a person's own vein is not available, human umbilical vein or a composite sequential bypass graft (native vein plus synthetic graft) is an alternative.[14] PTA with stenting may also be used in combination with bypass surgery. Other surgical options include *endarterectomy* (opening the artery and removing the obstructing plaque) and *patch graft angioplasty* (opening the artery, removing plaque, and sewing a patch to the opening to widen the lumen).

Amputation may be required if tissue necrosis is extensive, gangrene or osteomyelitis develops, or all major arteries in the limb are blocked, precluding the possibility of successful surgery.[20] Every effort is made to preserve as much of the limb as possible to improve the potential for rehabilitation. (Amputation is discussed in Chapter 63.)

NURSING MANAGEMENT
LOWER EXTREMITY PERIPHERAL ARTERY DISEASE

NURSING ASSESSMENT

Table 38-4 presents subjective and objective data that you should obtain from a patient with PAD.

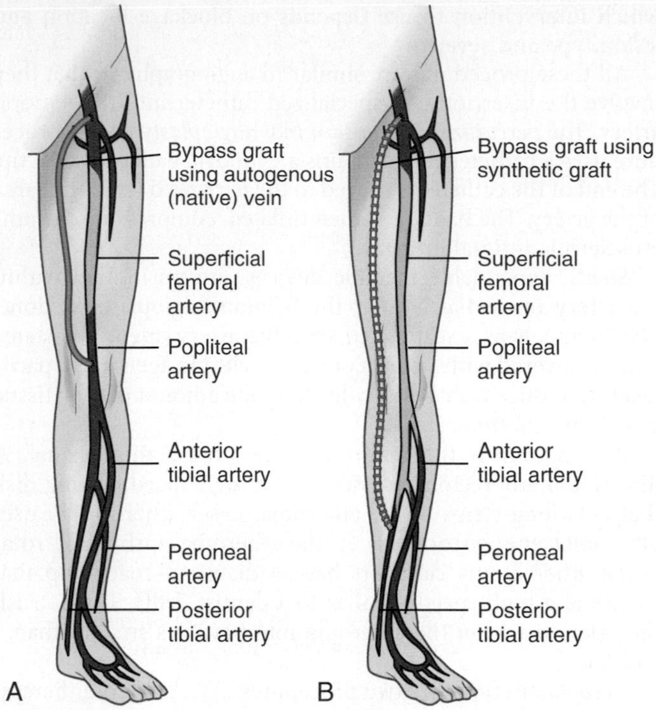

FIG. 38-2 A, Femoral-popliteal bypass graft around an occluded superficial femoral artery. **B,** Femoral–posterior tibial bypass graft around occluded superficial femoral, popliteal, and proximal tibial arteries.

NURSING DIAGNOSES

Nursing diagnoses for the patient with PAD may include, but are not limited to, the following:

- Ineffective peripheral tissue perfusion *related to* deficient knowledge of contributing factors
- Activity intolerance *related to* imbalance between oxygen supply and demand
- Ineffective self-health management *related to* lack of knowledge of disease and self-care measures

Additional information on nursing diagnoses for the patient with PAD of the lower extremities is presented in eNursing Care Plan 38-1 on the website for this chapter.

PLANNING

The overall goals for the patient who has lower extremity PAD include (1) adequate tissue perfusion; (2) relief of pain; (3) increased exercise tolerance; and (4) intact, healthy skin on the extremities.

NURSING IMPLEMENTATION

HEALTH PROMOTION. Assess the patient for CVD risk factors and provide instructions on how to control them (see Tables 34-2 to 34-4). Also teach diet modification to reduce the intake of cholesterol, saturated fat, and refined sugars; proper care of the feet; and avoidance of injury to the extremities. Encourage patients with positive family histories of cardiac, diabetic, or vascular disease to obtain regular follow-up care.

ACUTE INTERVENTION. After surgical or radiologic intervention, the patient is moved to a recovery area for observation. Check the operative extremity every 15 minutes initially and then hourly for color, temperature, capillary refill, presence of peripheral pulses, and sensation and movement. Loss of palpable pulses or a change in the Doppler sound over a pulse requires immediate notification of the physician or radiologist and prompt intervention. Postoperative ABI measurements are not recommended as they place the patient at risk for graft thrombosis.[13] Compare all assessment findings with the patient's baseline and with findings in the opposite limb.

TABLE 38-4 NURSING ASSESSMENT

Peripheral Artery Disease

Subjective Data

Important Health Information

Past health history: Tobacco use, diabetes mellitus, hypertension, hyperlipidemia, hypertriglyceridemia, hyperuricemia, impaired renal function, obesity; ↑ high-sensitivity C-reactive protein, homocysteine, or lipoprotein (a) [Lp(a)] levels; positive family history, sedentary lifestyle, stress

Functional Health Patterns

Health perception–health management: Family history of cardiovascular disease; tobacco use, including exposure to environmental smoke

Nutritional-metabolic: High sodium, saturated fat, and cholesterol intake; elevated Hb A1C

Activity-exercise: Exercise intolerance

Cognitive-perceptual: Buttock, thigh, or calf pain that is precipitated by exercise and that subsides with rest (intermittent claudication) or progresses to pain at rest; burning pain in forefeet and toes at rest; numbness, tingling, sensation of cold in legs or feet; progressive loss of sensation and deep pain in extremities

Sexuality-reproductive: Erectile dysfunction

Objective Data

Integumentary

Loss of hair on legs and feet; thick toenails; pallor with elevation; dependent rubor; thin, cool, shiny skin with muscle atrophy; skin breakdown and arterial ulcers, especially over bony areas; gangrene

Cardiovascular

Decreased or absent peripheral pulses; feet cool to touch; capillary refill >3 sec; bruits may be present at pulse sites

Neurologic

Mobility or sensation impairment

Possible Diagnostic Findings

Arterial stenosis evident with duplex imaging, ↓ Doppler pressures, ↓ ankle-brachial index, angiography indicative of peripheral atherosclerosis

Many PAD patients have a history of chronic ischemic rest pain and may have developed a tolerance to opioids. Thus aggressive pain management may be needed postoperatively.

After the patient leaves the recovery area, continue to monitor perfusion to the extremities. Assess for potential complications such as bleeding, hematoma, thrombosis, embolization, and compartment syndrome. A dramatic increase in pain, loss of previously palpable pulses, extremity pallor or cyanosis, decreasing ABIs, numbness or tingling, or a cold extremity suggests blockage of the graft or stent. Report these findings to the physician immediately. Women, particularly African American women, experience more graft failure and amputation after lower extremity bypass surgery than men.[6]

Avoid placing the patient in a knee-flexed position except for exercise. Turn the patient and position frequently with pillows to support the incision. On postoperative day 1, assist the patient out of bed several times daily. Discourage prolonged sitting with leg dependency, since it may cause pain and edema, increase the risk of venous thrombosis, and place stress on the suture lines. If edema develops, position the patient supine and elevate the leg above heart level. Occasionally, elastic compression stockings are used to help control leg edema. Walking even short distances is desirable. The use of a walker may be helpful, especially in frail, older patients.

Surgical site infection (SSI) after lower extremity revascularization occurs in about 11% of cases. Women develop SSIs more often than men. Careful postoperative assessment and wound care are important. SSIs are associated with early graft loss, reoperation, and sepsis.[24] If no complications occur, discharge can be anticipated 3 to 5 days after surgery.

AMBULATORY AND HOME CARE. Assess for CVD risk factors and be alert for opportunities to teach health promotion strategies to patients and their caregivers (see Chapters 4 and 34). Continued tobacco use dramatically decreases the long-term patency rates of grafts and stents and increases the risk of an MI or stroke. Long-term therapy with aspirin or clopidogrel is recommended for patients after surgery. Patients having distal peripheral bypass surgery (i.e., below the knee) using synthetic graft materials are given dual antiplatelet therapy (clopidogrel plus aspirin) for 1 year, followed by lifelong single antiplatelet therapy.

Encourage supervised exercise training after a successful revascularization. Explain that exercise improves a number of CVD risk factors, including hypertension, hyperlipidemia, obesity, and glucose levels. Teach foot care to all patients with PAD. Meticulous foot care is especially important in the diabetic patient with PAD (see Table 49-21). Diabetic neuropathy increases the patient's risk for injury and results in delay in seeking treatment. Instruct patients to inspect their legs and feet daily for mottling, changes in skin color or texture, and reduction in hair growth. Show patients how to check skin temperature and capillary refill and to palpate pulses. Emphasize that they must report any changes in these findings or the development of ulceration or inflammation to their health care provider. Thick or overgrown toenails and calluses are potentially serious and require regular attention by a health care provider (e.g., podiatrist). Patients who have poor eyesight, back problems, obesity, or arthritis may need help with foot care. Encourage patients to wear clean, all-cotton or all-wool socks and comfortable shoes with rounded (not pointed) toes and soft insoles. Tell patients to lace shoes loosely and to break in new shoes gradually (Table 38-5).

EVALUATION

The expected outcomes for the patient with PAD of the lower extremities include

- Adequate peripheral tissue perfusion
- Increased activity tolerance
- Knowledge of disease and treatment plan

Additional information on the expected outcomes for the patient with PAD of the lower extremities are presented in eNursing Care Plan 38-1 (available on the website for this chapter).

TABLE 38-5 PATIENT & CAREGIVER TEACHING GUIDE

Peripheral Artery Bypass Surgery

Include the following information in the teaching plan for a patient undergoing peripheral artery bypass surgery and the patient's caregiver.

1. Reduce risk factors by stopping the use of all tobacco products, controlling blood glucose levels (if diabetic) and blood pressure, lowering cholesterol and triglyceride levels, achieving or maintaining ideal body weight, and exercising regularly.
2. Provide rationales, basic action, and anticipated duration of medications such as antiplatelets, antihypertensives, lipid-lowering therapy, and pain medication.
3. Eat healthy—it is essential to recovery. Drink plenty of fluids, eat a well-balanced diet (e.g., foods high in protein, vitamins C and A, and zinc; high-fiber foods; fresh fruits and vegetables), eat fewer high-fat foods, and reduce salt intake.
4. Participate in a supervised exercise program or take a daily walk. In the beginning, take several short walks a day and rest between activities. Gradually increase your walking to 30 to 40 min/day, 3 to 5 days/wk.
5. Care for feet and legs. Inspect feet and wash them daily. Wear clean cotton or wool socks and well-fitting shoes. File toenails straight across. Avoid sitting with legs crossed, extreme hot and cold temperatures, and prolonged standing.
6. Follow routine postoperative wound care that includes keeping incision clean and dry; do not disturb Steri-Strips (if present).
7. Monitor for signs and symptoms of impaired healing or infection of the leg incision, and notify health care provider if any of the following occurs:
   - Prolonged drainage or pus from the incision
   - Increased redness, warmth, pain, or hardness along incision
   - Separation of wound edges
   - Temperature >100° F (37.8° C)
8. Keep all follow-up appointments with health care provider.
9. Notify health care provider immediately of increased leg or foot pain or a change in the color or temperature of leg or foot.

ACUTE ARTERIAL ISCHEMIC DISORDERS

Etiology and Pathophysiology

Acute arterial ischemia is a sudden interruption in the arterial blood supply to a tissue, an organ, or an extremity that, if left untreated, can result in tissue death. It is caused by embolism, thrombosis of a preexisting atherosclerotic artery, or trauma. *Embolization* of a thrombus from the heart is the most frequent cause of acute arterial occlusion. Heart conditions in which thrombi can develop include infective endocarditis, mitral valve disease, atrial fibrillation, cardiomyopathies, and prosthetic heart valves. Noncardiac sources of emboli include aneurysms, ulcerated atherosclerotic plaque, recent endovascular procedures, and venous thrombi.

The thrombi become dislodged and may travel anywhere in the systemic circulation if they originate in the left side of the heart. Most emboli block an artery of the lower extremity in areas where vessels branch (e.g., iliofemoral, popliteal, tibial) or there is atherosclerotic narrowing. Sudden local thrombosis may occur at the site of an atherosclerotic plaque. Hypovolemia (e.g., shock), hyperviscosity (e.g., polycythemia), and hypercoagulability (e.g., chemotherapy) predispose an individual to thrombotic arterial occlusion.[25]

Traumatic injury to the extremity itself may cause partial or total blockage. Acute arterial occlusion may also develop as a result of arterial dissection in the carotid artery or aorta or as a result of a procedure-related arterial injury (e.g., after angiography).

Clinical Manifestations

Clinical manifestations of acute arterial ischemia include the *"six Ps": pain, pallor, pulselessness, paresthesia, paralysis,* and *poikilothermia* (adaptation of the limb to the environmental temperature, most often cool). Without immediate intervention, ischemia may progress to tissue necrosis and gangrene within a few hours. If you detect these signs, immediately notify the physician. Paralysis is a late sign of acute arterial ischemia and signals the death of nerves supplying the extremity. Foot drop occurs as a result of nerve damage. Because nerve tissue is extremely sensitive to hypoxia, limb paralysis or ischemic neuropathy may persist even after revascularization.

Collaborative Care

Early treatment is essential to keep the affected limb viable during acute arterial ischemia. Anticoagulant therapy with IV unfractionated heparin (UH) is started to prevent thrombus growth and inhibit further embolization.[11] In patients undergoing embolectomy, UH should be followed by long-term anticoagulation with warfarin (see discussion of other anticoagulant options later in this chapter).

To restore blood flow, the thrombus is removed as soon as possible. Options consist of surgical thrombectomy (recommended procedure), percutaneous catheter-directed thrombolytic therapy, percutaneous mechanical thrombectomy with or without thrombolytic therapy, or surgical bypass.

If surgical thrombectomy is not possible, percutaneous catheter-directed thrombolytic therapy using tissue plasminogen activator (tPA [alteplase]) or urokinase (Kinlytic) is recommended. A catheter is inserted into the femoral artery and moved to the site of the clot, and the thrombolytic drug is infused. Thrombolytic agents work by directly dissolving the clot over a period of 24 to 48 hours. (Chapter 34 discusses thrombolytic therapy.) Another type of catheter may act as a mechanical thrombectomy device, meaning it is also designed to remove or fragment the thrombus.[26] Surgical revascularization may be used in a patient with trauma (e.g., laceration of the artery) or with significant arterial blockage. Amputation is reserved for patients with ischemic rest pain and tissue loss in whom limb salvage is not possible. If the patient remains at risk for further embolization from a persistent source (e.g., chronic atrial fibrillation), long-term oral anticoagulation is recommended to prevent further acute arterial ischemic episodes[27] (see Table 38-10 later in this chapter).

THROMBOANGIITIS OBLITERANS

Thromboangiitis obliterans (Buerger's disease) is a nonatherosclerotic, segmental, recurrent inflammatory disorder of the small- and medium-sized arteries and veins of the upper and lower extremities. Rarely, systemic manifestations of the disease may involve cerebral, coronary, mesenteric, pulmonary, and/or renal arteries. The disease occurs mostly in young men (less than 45 years of age) with a long history of tobacco and/or marijuana use and chronic periodontal infection, but without other CVD risk factors (e.g., hypertension, hyperlipidemia, diabetes).[28]

In the acute phase of Buerger's disease, an inflammatory thrombus forms and blocks the vessel. Over time, the thrombus becomes more organized and the inflammation subsides.[28] During the chronic phase, thrombosis and fibrosis occur in the vessel, causing tissue ischemia. The symptoms of Buerger's disease often are confused with PAD and other autoimmune diseases (e.g., scleroderma). Patients may have intermittent claudication of the feet, hands, or arms. As the disease progresses, rest pain and ischemic ulcerations develop. Other signs and symptoms may include color and temperature changes of the limbs, paresthesia, superficial vein thrombosis, and cold sensitivity.

There are no laboratory or diagnostic tests specific to Buerger's disease. Diagnosis is made based on age of onset; history; clinical symptoms; involvement of distal vessels; presence of ischemic ulcerations; and exclusion of autoimmune disease, diabetes, thrombophilia (inherited tendency to clot), and other source of emboli.[28]

The mainstay of treatment for Buerger's disease is the complete cessation of tobacco and marijuana use in any form. Use of nicotine replacement products is contraindicated. Patients must choose between their tobacco or marijuana and their affected limb, but not both. Conservative management includes avoiding limb exposure to cold temperatures, a supervised walking program, antibiotics to treat any infected ulcers, and analgesics to manage the ischemic pain. Teach patients to avoid trauma to the extremities.

A variety of drugs have been tried to treat Buerger's disease (e.g., calcium channel blockers, cilostazol, sildenafil [Viagra]), but evidence supporting their use is lacking. One promising drug has been IV iloprost. This has been shown to improve rest pain, promote healing of ischemic ulcers, and decrease the need for amputation.[28]

Surgical options include *sympathectomy* (transection of a nerve, ganglion, and/or plexus of the sympathetic nervous system), implantation of a spinal cord stimulator, and bypass surgery. Sympathectomy and implantation of a spinal cord stimulator can improve distal blood flow and reduce pain, but neither alters the inflammatory process. Bypass surgery typically is not an option because of the involvement of smaller, distal vessels but may be used in selected patients with severe ischemia. Painful ulcerations may require finger or toe amputations. Amputation below the knee may occur in severe cases. The rate of amputation in patients who continue tobacco or marijuana use after diagnosis is much higher than in those who stop.[28,29]

RAYNAUD'S PHENOMENON

Raynaud's phenomenon is an episodic vasospastic disorder of small cutaneous arteries, most often involving the fingers and toes. It occurs primarily in young women (typically between 15 and 40 years of age), and it is more common in women than men. The pathogenesis of Raynaud's phenomenon is due to abnormalities in the vascular, intravascular, and neuronal mechanisms that cause an imbalance between vasodilation and vasoconstriction.[30]

Raynaud's phenomenon may occur in isolation or in association with an underlying disease (e.g., rheumatoid arthritis, scleroderma, systemic lupus erythematosus). Other contributing factors include occupation-related conditions, such as use of vibrating machinery or work in cold environments, exposure to heavy metals (e.g., lead), and hyperhomocysteinemia.[30] Diagnosis is based on persistent symptoms for at least 2 years. Patients with Raynaud's phenomenon should have routine follow-up to monitor for development of connective tissue or autoimmune diseases.[31]

Raynaud's phenomenon is characterized by vasospasm-induced color changes of fingers, toes, ears, and nose (white, blue, and red). Decreased perfusion results in pallor (white). The digits then appear cyanotic (bluish purple) (Fig. 38-3). These changes are followed by rubor (red), caused by the hyperemic response that occurs when blood flow is restored. The patient usually describes coldness and numbness in the vasoconstrictive phase. This is followed by throbbing, aching pain,

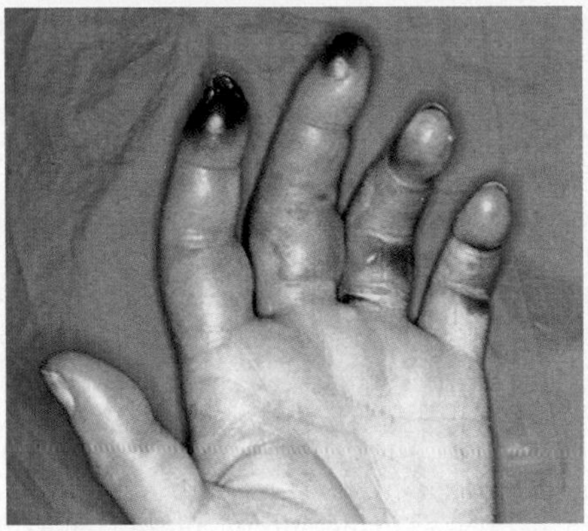

FIG. 38-3 Raynaud's phenomenon.

tingling, and swelling in the hyperemic phase. An episode usually lasts only minutes but in severe cases may persist for several hours. Exposure to cold, emotional upsets, tobacco use, and caffeine often bring on symptoms.

After frequent, prolonged attacks the skin may become thickened and the nails brittle. Occasionally, complications include *punctate* (small hole) lesions of the fingertips and superficial gangrenous ulcers in advanced stages.

The primary focus of nursing management of Raynaud's phenomenon is patient teaching. Focus your instructions on preventing recurrent episodes. Tell patients to wear loose, warm clothing as protection from the cold, including gloves when handling cold objects. At all times, patients should avoid temperature extremes. Immersing hands in warm water often decreases the vasospasm. The patient should stop using all tobacco products and avoid caffeine and other drugs that have vasoconstrictive effects (e.g., cocaine, amphetamines, ergotamine, pseudoephedrine). Finally, provide patients with stress management strategies as appropriate.

When conservative management is ineffective, drug therapy is considered. Sustained-release calcium channel blockers (e.g., nifedipine [Procardia]) are the first-line drug therapy.[31] Calcium channel blockers relax smooth muscles of the arterioles by blocking the influx of calcium into the cells. This reduces the frequency and severity of vasospastic attacks.

Prompt intervention is needed for patients with digital ulceration and/or critical ischemia. Treatment options include IV prostanoid therapy (e.g., iloprost), antibiotics, analgesics, and possibly an endothelin receptor antagonist (e.g., bosentan [Tracleer]) and surgical debridement of necrotic tissue.[31] Sympathectomy is considered only in advanced cases.

AORTIC ANEURYSMS

The aorta is the largest artery and supplies oxygen, nutrients, and blood to all vital organs. One of the most common problems affecting the aorta is an **aneurysm,** which is a permanent, localized outpouching or dilation of the vessel wall. Aneurysms occur in men more often than in women, and the incidence increases with age. Aneurysms may occur in more than one location. Peripheral artery aneurysms can also develop but are not common.

Etiology and Pathophysiology

Aortic aneurysms may involve the aortic arch and thoracic and/or abdominal aorta. Three fourths of aortic aneurysms occur in the abdominal aorta (Fig. 38-4) and one fourth in the thoracic aorta. About 1.1 million adults between 55 and 84 years of age have an abdominal aortic aneurysm (AAA).[32] Most AAAs occur below the renal arteries. An abdominal aorta larger than 3 cm in diameter is considered aneurysmal. Growth rates are unpredictable, but the larger the aneurysm, the greater the risk of rupture.

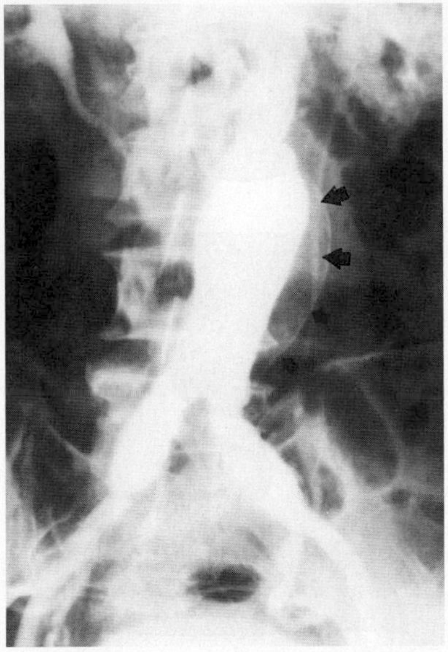

FIG. 38-4 Angiography demonstrating fusiform abdominal aortic aneurysm. Note calcification of the aortic wall *(arrows)* and extension of the aneurysm into the common iliac arteries.

A variety of disorders are associated with aortic aneurysms. The primary causes are classified as degenerative, congenital, mechanical (e.g., penetrating or blunt trauma), inflammatory (e.g., aortitis [Takayasu's arteritis]), or infectious (e.g., aortitis [*Chlamydia pneumoniae,* human immunodeficiency virus]).

Risk factors for aortic aneurysms include age, male gender, hypertension, coronary artery disease, family history, high cholesterol, lower extremity PAD, carotid artery disease, previous stroke, tobacco use, and excess weight or obesity. Male gender, older age, and tobacco use are the most important risk factors. Whites and Native Americans have a higher risk of AAA development than African Americans, Hispanics, and Asian Americans.[32]

Genetic Link

The development of aortic aneurysm and dissection has a strong genetic component. The familial tendency is related to a number of congenital anomalies. Examples include bicuspid aortic valve, coarctation of the aorta, Turner syndrome, autosomal dominant polycystic kidney disease, specific collagen defects (e.g., Ehlers-Danlos syndrome), and premature breakdown of vascular elastic tissue (e.g., Loeys-Dietz syndrome, Marfan's syndrome).[33]

Classification

Aneurysms are classified as true or false aneurysms (Fig. 38-5, *A* to *C*). A *true aneurysm* is one in which the wall of the artery forms the aneurysm, with at least one vessel layer still intact. True aneurysms are further subdivided into fusiform and saccular types. A *fusiform aneurysm* is circumferential and relatively uniform in shape. A *saccular aneurysm* is pouchlike with

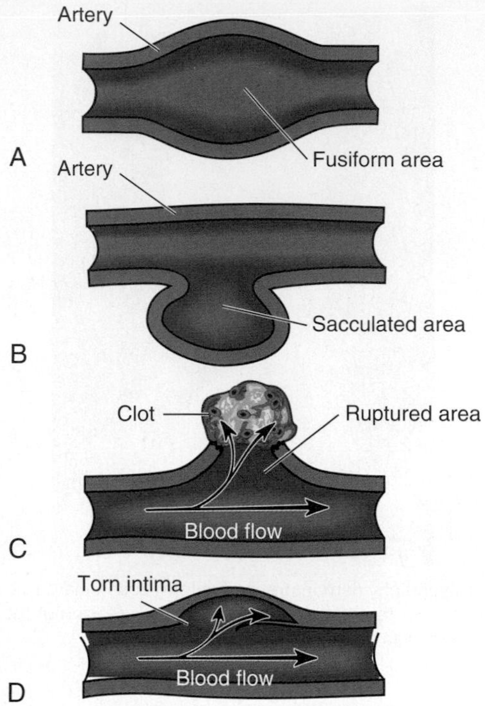

FIG. 38-5 A, True fusiform abdominal aortic aneurysm. **B,** True saccular aortic aneurysm. **C,** False aneurysm, or pseudoaneurysm. **D,** Aortic dissection.

a narrow neck connecting the bulge to one side of the arterial wall.

A *false aneurysm,* or *pseudoaneurysm,* is not an aneurysm but a disruption of all arterial wall layers with bleeding that is contained by surrounding anatomic structures. False aneurysms may result from trauma, infection, peripheral artery bypass graft surgery (at the site of the graft-to-artery anastomosis), or arterial leakage after removal of cannulae (e.g., femoral artery catheters, intraaortic balloon pump devices).[33]

Clinical Manifestations

Thoracic aortic aneurysms (TAAs) are often asymptomatic. When present, symptoms include deep, diffuse chest pain that may extend to the interscapular area. Ascending aorta and aortic arch aneurysms can produce angina from decreased blood flow to the coronary arteries and hoarseness from pressure on the laryngeal nerve. Pressure on the esophagus can cause dysphagia. If the aneurysm presses on the superior vena cava, decreased venous return can result in jugular venous distention (distended neck veins) and edema of the face and the arms.

AAAs also are often asymptomatic and frequently found during routine physical examinations or evaluations for an unrelated problem (e.g., abdominal x-ray, computed tomography [CT] scan). A pulsatile mass in the periumbilical area slightly to the left of the midline may be present. Bruits may be auscultated over the aneurysm. Physical findings may be more difficult to detect in obese individuals.

AAA symptoms may mimic pain associated with abdominal or back disorders. Compression of nearby anatomic structures and nerves may cause symptoms such as back pain, epigastric discomfort, and altered bowel elimination. Occasionally, aneurysms spontaneously embolize plaque, causing *"blue toe syndrome"* (patchy mottling of the feet and toes in the presence of palpable pedal pulses).

Complications

Rupture of an aneurysm is the most serious complication. If rupture occurs into the retroperitoneal space, bleeding may be controlled by surrounding anatomic structures, preventing exsanguination and death. In this case the patient often has severe back pain and may or may not have back or flank ecchymosis *(Grey Turner's sign).* If rupture occurs into the thoracic or abdominal cavity, more than 90% of patients will die from massive hemorrhage.[4] The patient who reaches the hospital will be in hypovolemic shock with tachycardia, hypotension, pale clammy skin, decreased urine output, altered level of consciousness, and abdominal tenderness. (Shock is discussed in Chapter 67.) In this situation, simultaneous resuscitation and immediate surgical repair are necessary.

Diagnostic Studies

Chest x-rays are done to reveal abnormal widening of the thoracic aorta. An abdominal x-ray may show calcification within the aortic wall. An electrocardiogram (ECG) may rule out MI, since thoracic aneurysm or dissection symptoms can mimic angina. Echocardiography assesses the function of the aortic valve. Ultrasound is useful for aneurysm screening and to monitor aneurysm size. A CT scan is the most accurate test to determine the length and cross-sectional diameter and the presence of thrombus in the aneurysm. Magnetic resonance imaging (MRI) also may be used to diagnose and assess the location and severity of aneurysms. *Angiography* provides helpful information by using contrast imaging to map the entire aortic system. (Chapter 32 and Table 32-6 discuss angiography.)

Collaborative Care

The goal of both medical and surgical management is to prevent aneurysm rupture. Early detection and prompt treatment are essential. Conservative therapy of small, asymptomatic AAAs (4.0 to 5.5 cm) is the best practice.[34] This consists of risk factor modification (ceasing tobacco use, decreasing BP, optimizing lipid profile) and annual monitoring of aneurysm size using ultrasound, CT, or MRI. Growth rates may be lowered with β-adrenergic blocking agents (e.g. propranolol [Inderal]), statins (e.g., simvastatin), and antibiotics (e.g., doxycycline).[33]

Surgical repair is recommended in patients with asymptomatic aneurysms 5.5 cm in diameter or larger. Surgical intervention may occur sooner if the patient has a genetic disorder (e.g., Marfan's, Ehlers-Danlos syndrome), the aneurysm expands rapidly, it becomes symptomatic, or the risk of rupture is high.[12] A careful review of body systems is necessary to identify any co-morbidities, especially of the lungs, heart, or kidney, because they can influence the patient's surgical risk. Correction of existing carotid or coronary artery blockages may be needed before the aneurysm is repaired.

Surgical Therapy. For elective surgery, the patient is well hydrated, and any electrolyte, coagulation, and hematocrit abnormalities are corrected preoperatively. If the aneurysm has ruptured, emergent surgical intervention is required.

The open aneurysm repair (OAR) involves a large abdominal incision through which the surgeon (1) cuts into the diseased aortic segment, (2) removes any thrombus or plaque, (3) sutures a synthetic graft to the aorta proximal and distal to the aneurysm, and (4) sutures the native aortic wall around the graft to

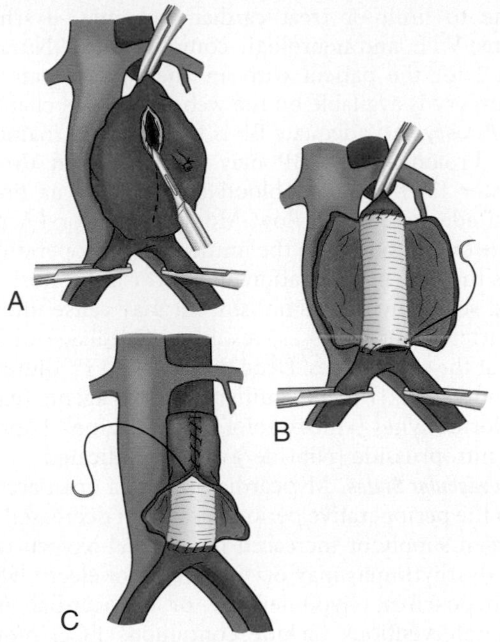

FIG. 38-6 Surgical repair of an abdominal aortic aneurysm. **A,** Incising the aneurysmal sac. **B,** Insertion of synthetic graft. **C,** Suturing native aortic wall over synthetic graft.

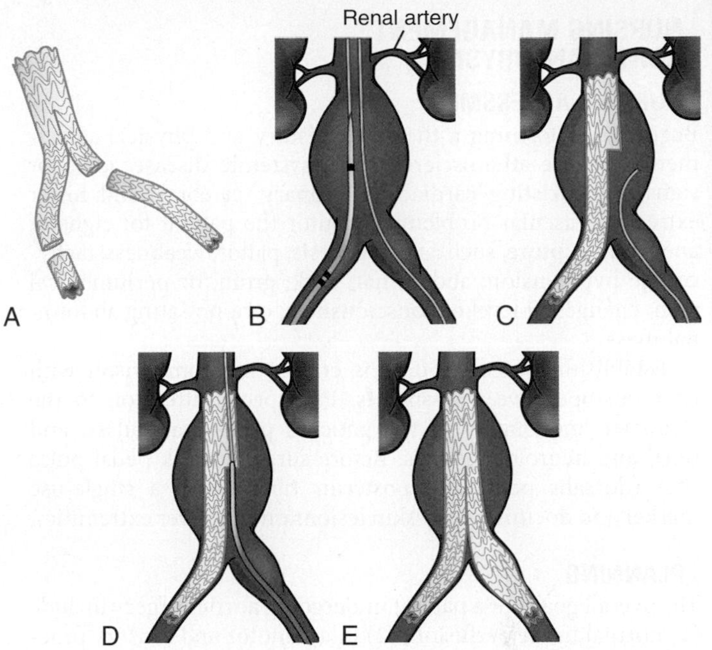

FIG. 38-7 Bifurcated (two-branched) endovascular stent grafting of an aneurysm. **A,** Insertion of a woven polyester tube (graft) covered by a tubular metal web (stent). **B,** The stent graft is inserted through a large blood vessel (e.g., femoral artery) using a delivery catheter. The catheter is positioned below the renal arteries in the area of the aneurysm. **C,** The stent graft is slowly released (deployed) into the blood vessel. When the stent comes in contact with the blood vessel, it expands to a preset size. **D,** A second stent graft can be inserted in the contralateral (opposite) vessel if necessary. **E,** Fully deployed bifurcated stent graft.

act as a protective cover (Fig. 38-6). If the iliac arteries are also aneurysmal, a bifurcated graft replaces the entire diseased segment. With saccular aneurysms, it may be possible to excise only the bulbous lesion, repairing the artery by primary closure (suturing the artery together) or by application of an autogenous or synthetic patch graft.

All OARs require aortic cross-clamping proximal and distal to the aneurysm. Most resections are done in 30 to 45 minutes, after which the clamps are removed and blood flow is restored. If the cross clamp must be applied above the renal arteries, adequate renal blood flow after clamp removal should be determined before closure of the abdominal incision. The risk of postoperative renal complications such as acute kidney injury increases in patients who have OAR of AAAs above the level of the renal arteries.

Endovascular Graft Procedure. Minimally invasive endovascular aneurysm repair (EVAR) is an alternative to conventional OAR. Patients must meet certain eligibility criteria to be candidates for EVAR. These include iliofemoral vessels that will allow for safe graft insertion and vessels of sufficient length and width to support the graft.[33]

EVAR involves the placement of a sutureless aortic graft into the abdominal aorta inside the aneurysm via the femoral artery. The graft, a Dacron cylinder consisting of several sections, is supported with multiple rings of flexible wire (Fig. 38-7). The main section of the graft is bifurcated and delivered through a femoral artery catheter. The second part of the graft is inserted through the opposite femoral artery. When all graft components are in place, they are released (deployed) against the vessel wall by balloon inflation. The blood then flows through the endovascular graft, thus preventing further expansion of the aneurysm. The aneurysmal wall will shrink over time because the blood is now being diverted through the endograft.

Complications. EVAR is less invasive than OAR. However, over time both techniques have similar rates of morbidity and mortality.[12,35]

The most common complication of AAA repair is *endoleak,* the seepage of blood back into the old aneurysm. This may be the result of an inadequate seal at either graft end, a tear through the graft fabric, or leakage between overlapping graft segments. Repair may require coil embolization (insertion of beads) for hemostasis.

Other potential complications include aneurysm growth above or below the graft, aneurysm rupture, aortic dissection, bleeding, renal artery occlusion caused by stent migration, graft thrombosis, incisional site hematoma, and incisional infection. Patients undergoing EVAR must have regular follow-up visits and routine CT or MRI scans for the rest of their lives to monitor for complications. Graft dysfunction may require conversion to an open surgical repair.

A potentially lethal complication in an emergency repair of a ruptured AAA is the development of *intraabdominal hypertension* (IAH) with associated *abdominal compartment syndrome* (ACS).[36] Persistent IAH reduces blood flow to the viscera. ACS refers to the impaired end-organ perfusion caused by IAH and resulting multisystem organ failure.

ACS occurs in about one fourth of cases of ruptured OARs and EVARs. It has a mortality rate up to 70%.[37] IAH is confirmed by measuring the patient's intraabdominal pressure indirectly through a catheter and transducer system, typically by using an indwelling urinary catheter. Treatment goals include control of situations that lead to IAH such as head of bed elevation, hemodynamic instability, and uncontrolled pain and anxiety. A percutaneous catheter decompression may be required in the patient with severe ACS to reduce intraabdominal pressure.[38]

NURSING MANAGEMENT AORTIC ANEURYSMS

NURSING ASSESSMENT

Begin by performing a thorough history and physical assessment. Because atherosclerosis is a systemic disease, look for signs of coexisting cardiac, pulmonary, cerebral, and lower extremity vascular problems. Monitor the patient for signs of aneurysm rupture, such as diaphoresis; pallor; weakness; tachycardia; hypotension; abdominal, back, groin, or periumbilical pain; changes in level of consciousness; or a pulsating abdominal mass.

Establishing baseline data is critical for comparison with later postoperative assessments. Pay special attention to the character and quality of the patient's peripheral pulses, and renal and neurologic status. Before surgery, mark pedal pulse sites (dorsalis pedis and posterior tibial) with a single-use marker and document any skin lesions on the lower extremities.

PLANNING

The overall goals for a patient undergoing aortic surgery include (1) normal tissue perfusion; (2) intact motor and sensory function; and (3) no complications related to surgical repair, such as thrombosis, infection, or rupture.

NURSING IMPLEMENTATION

HEALTH PROMOTION. To promote overall health, encourage the patient to reduce CVD risk factors (see Table 34-2), including controlling BP, ceasing tobacco use (see Chapter 11), increasing physical activity, and maintaining normal body weight and serum lipid levels. These measures also help ensure continued graft patency after surgical repair.

ACUTE INTERVENTION. During the preoperative period, provide emotional support and teaching to the patient and the caregiver. Preoperative teaching includes a brief explanation of the disease process, the planned surgical procedure(s), preoperative routines, what to expect immediately after surgery (e.g., recovery room, tubes and drains), and usual postoperative timelines. Specific preoperative routines vary by agency and surgeon. In general, aortic surgery patients have a bowel preparation (e.g., laxatives, enemas) and skin cleansing with an antimicrobial agent the day before surgery, have nothing by mouth (NPO) after midnight the day of surgery, and receive IV antibiotics immediately before the incision is made. If appropriate, a preoperative visit to the intensive care unit (ICU) may be helpful to the patient and caregiver. Patients with a history of CVD should receive a β-adrenergic blocker (e.g., metoprolol [Lopressor]) preoperatively to reduce morbidity and mortality.

Postoperatively, aortic surgery patients typically go to an ICU for 24 to 48 hours for close monitoring. When the patient arrives in the ICU, various devices are in place. These include an endotracheal tube for mechanical ventilation, an arterial line, a central venous pressure (CVP) or pulmonary artery (PA) catheter, peripheral IV lines, an indwelling urinary catheter, and a nasogastric (NG) tube. The patient needs continuous ECG and pulse oximetry monitoring. If the thorax is opened during surgery, chest tubes will be in place. Pain medication is given via epidural catheter or patient-controlled analgesia (PCA).

In addition to the usual goals of care for a postoperative patient (e.g., maintaining adequate respiratory function, fluid and electrolyte balance, and pain control [see Chapter 20]), check for graft patency and renal perfusion. Also watch for and intervene to limit or treat cardiac ischemia, dysrhythmias, infections, VTE, and neurologic complications. eNursing Care Plan 38-2 for the patient with an aneurysm repair or other aortic surgery is available on the website for this chapter.

Graft Patency. An adequate BP is important to maintain graft patency. Prolonged low BP may result in graft thrombosis. Administer IV fluids and blood components as ordered to maintain adequate blood flow. Monitor CVP or PA pressures and urine output hourly in the immediate postoperative period to assess the patient's hydration and perfusion status.

Avoid severe hypertension, since it may cause undue stress on the arterial anastomoses, resulting in leakage of blood or rupture at the suture lines. Drug therapy with IV diuretics (e.g., furosemide [Lasix]) or IV antihypertensive agents (e.g., labetalol [Normodyne], metoprolol, hydralazine [Apresoline], sodium nitroprusside [Nipride]) may be indicated.

Cardiovascular Status. Myocardial ischemia or infarction may occur in the perioperative period because of decreased myocardial oxygen supply or increased myocardial oxygen demands. Cardiac dysrhythmias may occur because of electrolyte imbalances, hypoxemia, hypothermia, or myocardial ischemia. Nursing interventions include continuous ECG monitoring; frequent electrolyte and arterial blood gas determinations; administration of oxygen, IV antidysrhythmic and antihypertensive medications, and electrolytes as needed; adequate pain control; and resumption of heart medications.

Infection. A prosthetic vascular graft infection is a relatively rare but potentially life-threatening complication. Nursing interventions to prevent infection include administering a broad-spectrum antibiotic as prescribed. Assess temperature regularly, and promptly report elevations. Monitor laboratory data for an elevated white blood cell (WBC) count, which may be the first indication of an infection. Ensure adequate nutrition, and assess the surgical incision for signs of infection (e.g., redness, swelling, drainage). Keep surgical incisions clean and dry and perform wound care as ordered.

Use strict aseptic technique in the care of all IV, arterial, and CVP or PA catheter insertion sites, since these are ports of entry for bacteria. Meticulous perineal care for the patient with an indwelling urinary catheter and early catheter removal are essential to minimize the risk of urinary tract infection.

Gastrointestinal Status. After OAR, postoperative ileus may develop as a result of anesthesia and the handling of the bowel during surgery. The intestines may become swollen and bruised, and peristalsis ceases for variable intervals. A retroperitoneal surgical approach can be used to decrease the risk of bowel complications.

An NG tube may be placed during surgery and connected to low, intermittent suction to decompress the stomach, prevent aspiration of stomach contents, and decrease pressure on suture lines. Record the amount and character of the NG output. While the patient is NPO, provide oral care frequently. Ice chips or lozenges can help soothe a dry or irritated throat. Assess for bowel sounds every 4 hours. The passing of flatus signals returning bowel function and should be noted. Encourage early ambulation, since this can help the return of bowel function. A postoperative ileus rarely lasts beyond the fourth postoperative day.

If the blood supply to the bowel is disrupted during surgery, temporary ischemia or infarction (death) of intestinal tissue may result. Clinical manifestations of this rare but serious complication include absent bowel sounds, fever, abdominal distention and pain, diarrhea, and bloody stools. If bowel infarction occurs, immediate reoperation is necessary to restore blood flow, with likely resection of the infarcted bowel.

Neurologic Status. Neurologic complications can occur after aortic surgery. When the ascending aorta and aortic arch are involved, assess the patient's level of consciousness, pupil size and response to light, facial symmetry, tongue position, speech, upper extremity movement, and quality of hand grasps (see Chapter 57). When the descending aorta is involved, perform a neurovascular assessment of the lower extremities. Record all assessments and report changes from baseline to the physician immediately.

Peripheral Perfusion Status. The location of the aneurysm determines what type of peripheral perfusion assessment is done. Check and record all peripheral pulses hourly for several hours and then routinely, based on agency policy. When the ascending aorta and aortic arch are involved, assess the carotid, radial, and temporal artery pulses. For surgery of the descending aorta, assess the femoral, popliteal, posterior tibial, and dorsalis pedis pulses (see Fig. 32-6). You may need a Doppler to assess peripheral pulses. Check skin temperature and color, capillary refill time, and sensation and movement of the extremities (see Chapter 32).

Occasionally, lower extremity pulses may be absent for a short time after surgery because of vasospasm and hypothermia. A decreased or absent pulse together with a cool, pale, mottled, or painful extremity may indicate embolization or graft occlusion. Report these findings to the physician immediately. Graft occlusion requires reoperation if identified early. Thrombolytic therapy may also be considered. In some patients, pulses may have been absent before surgery because of coexistent PAD. It is essential to compare your findings with the preoperative status to determine the cause of a decreased or absent pulse and the proper treatment.

Renal Perfusion Status. The patient will have an indwelling urinary catheter after surgery. In the immediate postoperative period, record hourly urine output. Further evaluate renal function by monitoring daily blood urea nitrogen (BUN) and serum creatinine levels. CVP and PA pressures also provide important information about hydration status. Maintain accurate fluid intake and output and record daily weights until the patient resumes a regular diet.

Decreased renal perfusion can occur from embolization of the aortic thrombus or plaque to one or both of the renal arteries. This causes ischemia of one or both kidneys. Hypotension, dehydration, prolonged aortic clamping during surgery, or blood loss also can lead to decreased renal perfusion. Irreversible renal failure may occur after surgery, particularly in high-risk people (e.g., patients with diabetes). (Acute kidney injury is discussed in Chapter 47.)

AMBULATORY AND HOME CARE Instruct the patient and caregiver to gradually increase activities once home. Fatigue, poor appetite, and irregular bowel habits are common. Teach the patient to avoid heavy lifting for 6 weeks after surgery. Any redness, swelling, increased pain, drainage from incisions, or fever greater than 100° F (37.8° C) should be reported to a health care provider.

Teach the patient and caregiver to look for changes in color or warmth of the extremities. Patients and caregivers can learn to palpate peripheral pulses to assess changes in their quality.

Sexual dysfunction in male patients is common after aortic surgery. Preoperatively, document baseline sexual function and recommend counseling as appropriate. A referral to a urologist may be useful if erectile dysfunction occurs.

EVALUATION

Expected outcomes for the patient who undergoes aortic surgery include the following:

- Patent arterial graft with adequate distal perfusion
- Adequate urine output
- No signs of infection

AORTIC DISSECTION

Aortic dissection, often misnamed *"dissecting aneurysm,"* is not a type of aneurysm. Rather, dissection results from the creation of a false lumen between the intima (inner lining) and the media (middle layer) of arterial wall (Figs. 38-5, *D,* and 38-8). Classification of the aortic dissection is based on anatomic location (ascending versus descending aorta) and duration of onset (acute versus chronic). Approximately two thirds of dissections involve the ascending aorta and are acute in onset.[39] Chronic dissections almost always involve the descending aorta.

Etiology and Pathophysiology

Most experts link nontraumatic aortic dissection to degenerated elastic fibers in the arterial wall. Chronic hypertension hastens this process. In aortic dissection a tear develops in the inner layer of the aorta. Blood surges through this tear into the middle layer of the aorta, causing the inner and middle layers to separate (dissect). If the blood-filled channel ruptures through the outside aortic wall, aortic dissection is often fatal.

As the heart contracts, each pulsation increases the pressure on the damaged area, which further increases the dissection. Extension of the dissection may cut off blood supply to critical areas such as the brain, kidneys, spinal cord, and extremities. The false lumen may remain patent, become thrombosed (clotted), rejoin the true lumen by way of a distal tear, or rupture.

Aortic dissection affects men 2 to 5 times more often than women and occurs most frequently in the sixth and seventh decades of life.[39] Predisposing factors include age, aortitis (e.g., syphilis), blunt or iatrogenic trauma, congenital heart disease (e.g., bicuspid aortic valve), connective tissue disorders (e.g., Marfan's syndrome), cocaine or methamphetamine use, history of heart surgery, atherosclerosis, male gender, pregnancy, and hypertension.[33] Younger patients are more likely to have a bicus-

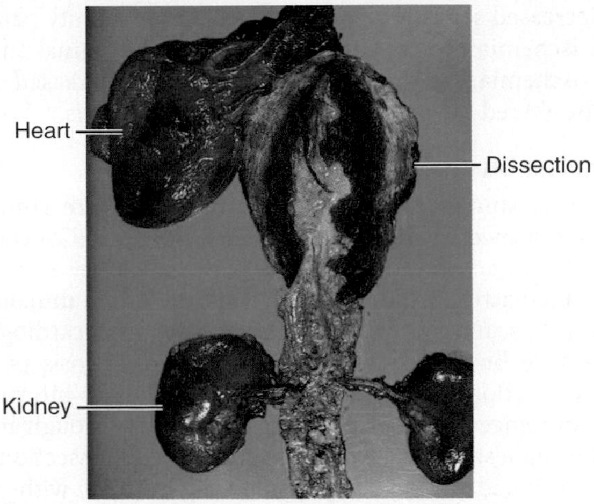

FIG. 38-8 Aortic dissection of the thoracic aorta.

pid aortic valve, Marfan's syndrome, prior aortic valve surgery, or recent trauma. Nearly half of all dissections in women younger than 40 years occur during pregnancy.

Clinical Manifestations

Most patients with an acute ascending aortic dissection report abrupt onset of excruciating chest and/or back pain radiating to the neck or shoulders. Patients with acute descending aortic dissection are more likely to report pain located in their back, abdomen, or legs. The pain is frequently described as "sharp" and "worst ever," or as "tearing," "ripping," or "stabbing."

Dissection pain can be differentiated from MI pain, which is more gradual in onset and has increasing intensity. As the dissection progresses, pain may migrate. Older patients are less likely to have abrupt onset of chest or back pain and more likely to have hypotension and vague symptoms. Some patients have a painless aortic dissection, emphasizing the importance of the physical examination.

If the aortic arch is involved, the patient may exhibit neurologic deficits. These include altered level of consciousness, weakened or absent carotid and temporal pulses, and dizziness or syncope. An ascending aortic dissection usually produces some degree of disruption in blood flow in the coronary arteries and aortic valve insufficiency. The patient may develop angina; MI; and a new high-pitched, heart murmur. In severe cases, these complications can result in left heart failure with the development of dyspnea, orthopnea, and pulmonary edema. When either subclavian artery is involved, radial, ulnar, and brachial pulse quality and BP readings may be different between the left and right arms. As the dissection progresses down the aorta, the abdominal organs and the lower extremities demonstrate evidence of decreased tissue perfusion.

Complications

A severe and life-threatening complication of an acute ascending aortic dissection is *cardiac tamponade*. This occurs when blood from the dissection leaks into the pericardial sac. Clinical manifestations of tamponade include hypotension, narrowed pulse pressure, jugular venous distention, muffled heart sounds, and pulsus paradoxus (see Chapter 37).

The aorta may rupture because it is weakened by the dissection. Hemorrhage may occur into the mediastinal, pleural, or abdominal cavities. Aortic rupture typically results in exsanguination and death. Dissection can lead to occlusion of the blood supply to vital organs. Spinal cord ischemia leads to weakness and decreased sensation to complete lower extremity paralysis. Renal ischemia can lead to renal failure. Abdominal (mesenteric) ischemia can cause abdominal pain, decreased bowel sounds, altered bowel function, and bowel necrosis.

Diagnostic Studies

Diagnostic studies to detect aortic dissection are similar to those for suspected aneurysms (Table 38-6). An ECG can help rule out cardiac ischemia. A chest x-ray may show a widening of the mediastinum and pleural effusion. Three-dimensional (3-D) CT scanning and transesophageal echocardiography (TEE) have become the standard for the diagnosis of acute aortic dissection. A CT scan can provide valuable information on the presence and severity of the dissection. Although an MRI has the highest accuracy for detecting aortic dissection, it is contraindicated in some patients (e.g., those with metal implants, hemodynamically unstable patients).[39]

TABLE 38-6 COLLABORATIVE CARE

Aortic Dissection

Diagnostic	Collaborative Therapy

• Health history and physical examination
• ECG
• Chest x-ray
• CT scan with 3-D reconstruction
• Transesophageal echocardiogram
• Magnetic resonance imaging
	• Bed rest
	• Pain relief with opioids
	• Blood transfusion (if necessary)
	• Drug therapy (see Table 33-7)
	  • IV β-adrenergic blockers (e.g., esmolol [Brevibloc], propranolol [Inderal])
	  • IV calcium channel blockers
	  • Angiotensin-converting enzyme inhibitors
	  • Sodium nitroprusside (Nipride)
	• Surgical aortic resection and repair
	• Endovascular aortic dissection repair

Collaborative Care

Patients with acute aortic dissection are managed in the ICU. The initial goals of therapy for acute aortic dissection without complications are heart rate (HR) and BP control and pain management. HR and BP control reduces aortic wall stress by decreasing systolic BP and myocardial contractility (see Table 38-6). An IV β-adrenergic blocker (e.g., esmolol [Brevibloc]) is titrated to a target HR of 60 beats/minute or less. A calcium channel blocker (e.g., diltiazem [Cardizem], verapamil [Calan]) can be used to lower HR if a β-adrenergic blocker is contraindicated. An IV ACE inhibitor (e.g., enalapril [Vasotec]) may also be used. Reducing the HR, BP, and myocardial contractility limits extension of the dissection. Morphine is the preferred analgesic because it decreases sympathetic nervous system stimulation and relieves pain. Supportive treatment for an acute aortic dissection serves as a bridge to surgery.

Conservative Therapy. The patient with an acute or chronic descending aortic dissection without complications can be treated conservatively. Conservative treatment includes pain relief, HR and BP control, and CVD risk factor modification.

Endovascular Dissection Repair. Endovascular repair of acute descending aortic dissections with complications (e.g., hemodynamic instability) and chronic descending aortic dissection with complications (e.g., peripheral ischemia) is a treatment option. Endovascular dissection repair is similar to EVAR. However, a temporary lumbar drain may be inserted for cerebrospinal fluid removal to reduce spinal cord edema and help prevent paralysis.[40]

Surgical Therapy. An acute ascending aortic dissection is considered a surgical emergency. Otherwise, surgery is indicated when conservative therapy is ineffective or when complications (e.g., heart failure) occur. Open surgical repair is recommended for patients with a chronic dissection who have a connective tissue disorder and a descending thoracic aortic diameter greater than 5.5 cm.[33] The aorta is fragile after dissection. Thus surgery is delayed for as long as possible to allow time for edema to decrease and to permit clotting of the blood in the false lumen. Surgery involves resection of the aortic segment containing the intimal tear and replacement with a synthetic graft. Even with prompt surgical intervention, the in-hospital mortality rate of acute aortic dissection is high.[39] Causes of death include aortic rupture, mesenteric ischemia, MI, sepsis, and multiorgan failure.

NURSING MANAGEMENT AORTIC DISSECTION

Preoperatively, nursing management includes keeping the patient in bed in a semi-Fowler's position and maintaining a quiet environment. These measures help to keep the HR and the systolic BP at the lowest possible level that maintains vital organ perfusion (typically HR less than 60 beats/minute; systolic BP less than 120 mm Hg). Administer opioids and sedatives as ordered. To prevent extension of the dissection, manage pain and anxiety because they can cause elevations in the HR and systolic BP.

Administration and titration of IV antihypertensive agents require careful supervision, including continuous ECG and intraarterial BP monitoring (see Chapters 36 and 66). Monitor vital signs frequently, sometimes as often as every 2 to 3 minutes, until target HR and BP are reached. Observe for changes in peripheral pulses and signs of increasing pain, restlessness, and anxiety. If the arteries branching off the aortic arch are involved, decreased cerebral blood flow may alter the patient's level of consciousness. Postoperative care is similar to that after OAR (see earlier section on nursing management of aortic aneurysms).

In preparation for discharge, focus on patient and caregiver teaching. All patients with a history of aortic dissection, regardless of location or treatment approach, require long-term medical care to control HR and BP. Patients must understand that they need to take antihypertensive drugs daily for the rest of their lives. β-Adrenergic blockers (e.g., metoprolol) are used to control HR and BP and decrease myocardial contractility. It is important that patients understand the drug regimen and potential side effects (e.g., dizziness, depression, fatigue, erectile dysfunction). Tell the patient to discuss any side effects with the health care provider before discontinuing the drug. Follow-up with regularly scheduled MRIs or CTs is essential. The most common cause of death in long-term survivors is aortic rupture from redissection or aneurysm formation. Instruct patients that if the pain or other symptoms return, they should activate emergency medical services (EMS) for immediate care.

VENOUS DISORDERS

PHLEBITIS

Generally, every hospitalized patient has an IV catheter inserted for giving fluids and/or drugs. *Phlebitis* is inflammation of the walls of small cannulated veins of the hand or arm. Clinical signs and symptoms include pain, tenderness, warmth, erythema, swelling, and a palpable cord.[41] Phlebitis risk factors are mechanical irritation from the catheter, infusion of irritating medications, and catheter location. Phlebitis is rarely infectious and usually resolves quickly after catheter removal. If edema is present, elevate the extremity to promote reabsorption of fluid into the vasculature. Apply warm, moist heat and administer oral NSAIDs (e.g., diclofenac [Voltaren]) or topical NSAIDs (e.g., diclofenac gel [Solaraze]) to relieve pain and inflammation.

VENOUS THROMBOSIS

Venous thrombosis involves the formation of a thrombus in association with inflammation of the vein. It is the most common disorder of the veins and is classified as either superficial vein thrombosis or deep vein thrombosis. **Superficial vein thrombosis (SVT)** is the formation of a thrombus in a superficial vein, usually the greater or lesser saphenous vein. **Deep vein thrombosis (DVT)** is a disorder involving a thrombus in a deep vein, most commonly the iliac and femoral veins. **Venous thromboembolism (VTE)** is the preferred terminology and represents the spectrum of pathology from DVT to pulmonary embolism (PE) (Table 38-7). (Chapter 28 discusses PE.)

TABLE 38-7 COMPARISON OF SUPERFICIAL VEIN THROMBOSIS AND VENOUS THROMBOEMBOLISM

	Superficial Vein Thrombosis	Venous Thromboembolism (VTE)
Usual location	Typically, superficial leg veins (e.g., varicosities). Occasionally superficial arm veins.	Deep veins of arms (e.g., axillary, subclavian), legs (e.g., femoral), pelvis (e.g., iliac, inferior or superior vena cava), and pulmonary system.
Clinical findings	Tenderness, itchiness, redness, warmth, pain, inflammation and induration along the course of the superficial vein. Vein appears as a palpable cord. Edema rarely occurs.	Tenderness to pressure over involved vein, induration of overlying muscle, venous distention. Edema. May have mild to moderate pain, deep reddish color to area caused by venous congestion. NOTE: Some patients may have no obvious physical changes in the affected extremity.
Sequelae	If untreated, clot may extend to deeper veins and VTE may occur.	Embolization to lungs (pulmonary embolism) may occur and may result in death.* Pulmonary hypertension and post-thrombotic syndrome with or without venous leg ulceration may develop.

*See Chapter 28 for clinical findings related to pulmonary embolism.

SVT has been considered a benign disorder. However, recent data indicate that SVT may be more serious. Nearly 25% of patients with SVT may also have VTE at the time of diagnosis. Further, between 5% and 10% of SVT patients are at risk for developing thromboembolic complications in the future.[42]

Etiology

Three important factors (called **Virchow's triad**) in the etiology of venous thrombosis are (1) venous stasis, (2) damage of the endothelium (inner lining of the vein), and (3) hypercoagulability of the blood (Fig. 38-9). The patient at risk for the development of VTE usually has predisposing conditions to these three disorders (Table 38-8).

Venous Stasis. Normal venous blood flow depends on the action of muscles in the extremities and the functional adequacy of venous valves, which allow flow in one direction. *Venous stasis* occurs when the valves are dysfunctional or the muscles of the extremities are inactive. Venous stasis occurs more frequently in people who are obese or pregnant, have chronic heart failure or atrial fibrillation, have been traveling on long trips without regular exercise, have a prolonged surgical procedure, or are immobile for long periods (e.g., spinal cord injury, fractured hip, limb paralysis).[43]

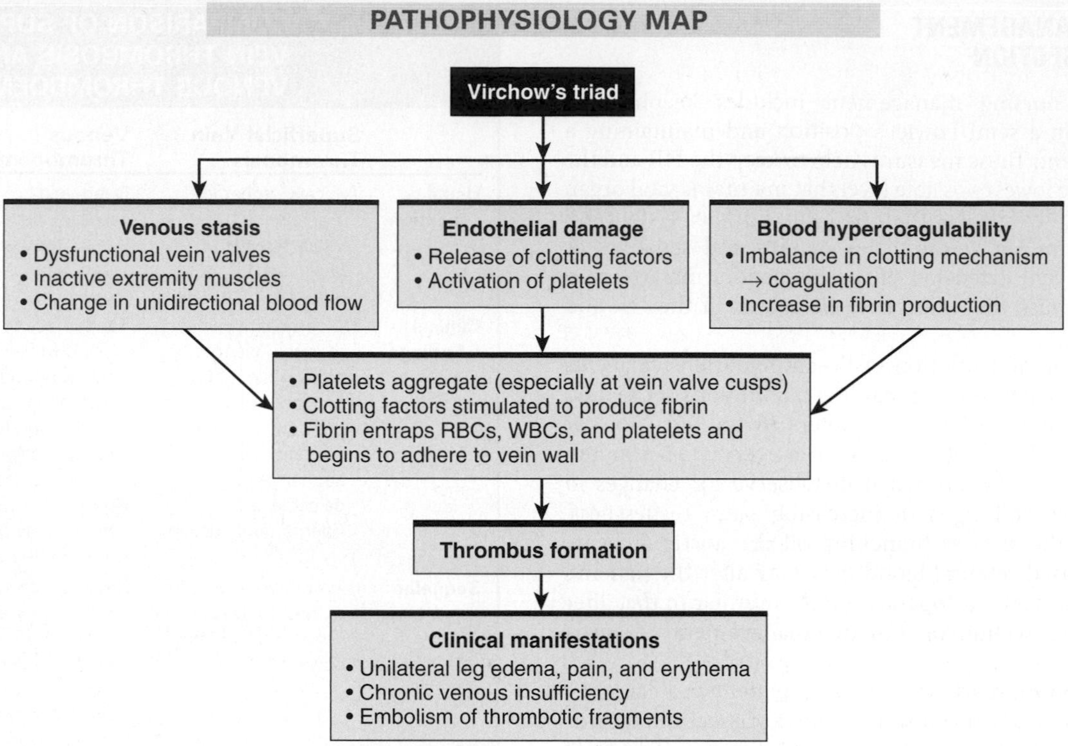

FIG. 38-9 Pathophysiology of venous thromboembolism.

TABLE 38-8 RISK FACTORS FOR VENOUS THROMBOEMBOLISM

Venous Stasis
- Advanced age
- Atrial fibrillation
- Chronic heart failure
- Obesity
- Orthopedic surgery (especially hip or lower extremity)
- Pregnancy and postpartum period
- Prolonged immobility
  - Bed rest
  - Fractured leg or hip
  - Long trips without adequate exercise
  - Spinal cord injury or limb paralysis
- Stroke
- Varicose veins

Endothelial Damage
- Abdominal and pelvic surgery (e.g., gynecologic or urologic surgery)
- Caustic or hypertonic IV medications
- Fractures of the pelvis, hip, or leg
- History of previous venous thromboembolism
- Indwelling, peripherally inserted, central vein catheter
- IV drug abuse
- Trauma

Hypercoagulability of Blood
- Antiphospholipid antibody syndrome
- Antithrombin III deficiency
- Dehydration or malnutrition
- Elevated (clotting) factor VIII or lipoprotein (a)
- Erythropoiesis-stimulating drugs (e.g., epoetin alfa [Procrit])
- Factor V Leiden or prothrombin gene mutation
- High altitudes
- Hormone therapy
- Hyperhomocysteinemia
- Malignancies (especially breast, brain, hepatic, pancreatic, and gastrointestinal)
- Nephrotic syndrome
- Oral contraceptives, especially in women >35 yr who use tobacco
- Polycythemia vera
- Pregnancy and postpartum period
- Protein C deficiency
- Protein S deficiency
- Sepsis
- Severe anemias
- Tobacco use

Endothelial Damage. Damage to the endothelium of the vein may be caused by direct (e.g., surgery, intravascular catheterization, trauma, burns) or indirect (chemotherapy, diabetes, sepsis) injury to the vessel.[43] Damaged endothelium stimulates platelet activation and starts the coagulation cascade. This predisposes the patient to thrombus development.

Hypercoagulability of Blood. Hypercoagulability of blood occurs in many disorders, including severe anemias, polycythemia, malignancies (e.g., cancers of the breast, brain, pancreas, and gastrointestinal tract), nephrotic syndrome, hyperhomocysteinemia, and protein C and S deficiency.[43] A patient with sepsis is predisposed to hypercoagulability because of endotoxins that are released. Some medications (e.g., corticosteroids, estrogens) predispose a patient to thrombus formation.

Women of childbearing age who take estrogen-based oral contraceptives or postmenopausal women on oral hormone therapy (HT) are at increased risk for VTE.[43] Women who use oral contraceptives and tobacco double their risk. Smoking causes hypercoagulability by increasing plasma fibrinogen and homocysteine levels and activating the intrinsic coagulation pathway. Women who use tobacco and oral contraceptives, are over 35 years old, and have a family history of VTE are at an extremely high risk for VTE. In women with a known thrombophilia, the benefits of HT, tamoxifen (Nolvadex), or raloxifene (Evista) must be weighed against the risk for VTE.

Pathophysiology

Localized platelet aggregation and fibrin entrap red blood cells (RBCs), WBCs, and more platelets to form a thrombus. A frequent site of thrombus formation is the valve cusps of veins, where venous stasis occurs. As the thrombus enlarges, increased numbers of blood cells and fibrin collect behind it. This produces a larger clot with a "tail" that eventually blocks the lumen of the vein.

If a thrombus only partially blocks the vein, endothelial cells cover the thrombus and stop the thrombotic process. If the thrombus does not become detached, it undergoes lysis or becomes firmly organized and adherent within 5 to 7 days. The organized thrombus may detach and result in an embolus. Turbulence of blood flow is a major contributing factor to embolization. The thrombus can become an embolus that flows through the venous circulation to the heart and lodges in the pulmonary circulation, becoming a PE (see Fig. 28-11).

Superficial Vein Thrombosis

Clinical Manifestations. The patient with SVT may have a palpable, firm, subcutaneous cordlike vein (see Table 38-7). The area surrounding the vein may be itchy, tender or painful to the touch, reddened, and warm. A mild temperature elevation and leukocytosis may be present. Extremity edema may or may not occur. Lower extremity SVT often involves one or more varicose veins.

Risk factors for SVT include increased age; pregnancy; obesity; malignancy; thrombophilia; estrogen therapy; recent sclerotherapy (e.g., treatment for varicose veins); long-distance travel; and a history of CVI, SVT, or VTE.[42] SVT also can occur in persons with endothelial alterations (e.g., Buerger's disease). SVT also may be unprovoked.

Collaborative Care. Duplex ultrasound is used to confirm the diagnosis (clot 5 cm or larger) and to rule out clot extension to a deep vein.[44,45] For patients with a lower leg SVT, treatment consists of low-molecular-weight heparin (LMWH) for 45 days or a prophylactic dose of fondaparinux (Arixtra).[44] If the SVT affects a very short vein segment (less than 5 cm) and is not near the saphenofemoral junction, anticoagulants may not be necessary and oral NSAIDs can ease symptoms. Additional interventions to relieve SVT symptoms include telling the patient to wear elastic compression stockings, apply topical NSAIDS, and perform mild exercise such as walking.[46]

Venous Thromboembolism

Clinical Manifestations. The patient with lower extremity VTE may or may not have unilateral leg edema, pain, tenderness with palpation, dilated superficial veins, a sense of fullness in the thigh or the calf, paresthesias, warm skin, erythema, or a systemic temperature greater than 100.4° F (38° C) (see Table 38-7). If the inferior vena cava is involved, both legs may be edematous and cyanotic. About 5% to 10% of VTEs involve the upper extremity veins and may extend into the internal jugular vein or superior vena cava.[44] If the superior vena cava is involved, similar symptoms may occur in the arms, neck, back, and face. Diagnosis of an initial VTE is based on clinical assessment combined with D-dimer testing and duplex ultrasound.[47]

Complications. The most serious complications of VTE are PE, post-thrombotic syndrome, and phlegmasia cerulea dolens. (See Chapter 28 for discussion of PE.)

Post-thrombotic syndrome (PTS) occurs in 20% to 50% of patients despite adequate anticoagulant therapy. It results from chronic venous hypertension caused by valvular destruction (from inflammation and scarring), stiff noncompliant vein walls, and persistent venous obstruction. Symptoms include pain, aching, heaviness, swelling, cramps, itching, and tingling.[48,49] Clinical signs include persistent edema, increased pigmentation, eczema, secondary varicosities, and *lipodermatosclerosis* (Fig. 38-10). Venous ulceration can occur with severe PTS. Manifestations of PTS typically begin within 2 years of a VTE.[48,49] Risk factors include persistent leg symptoms 1 month after VTE, VTE located near the iliofemoral junction, extensive VTE, recurrent VTE, obesity, older age, and female gender. Sequential compression devices (SCDs) may be used for patients with severe PTS.[50]

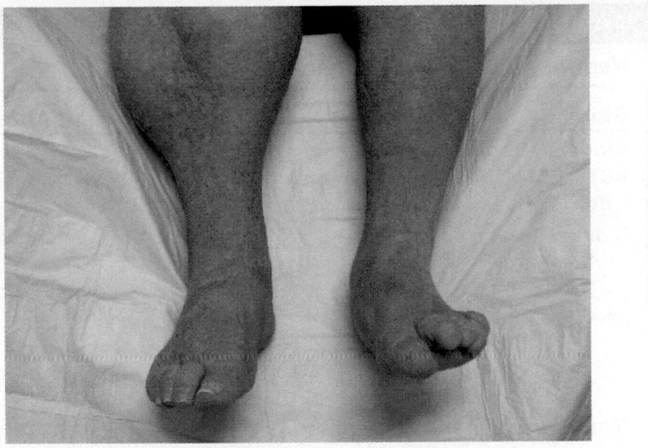

FIG. 38-10 Lipodermatosclerosis. Skin on lower leg becomes scarred, and the leg becomes tapered like an "inverted bottle." Hallmark signs of lipodermatosclerosis are leathery skin, brown discoloration, hyperpigmentation and hypopigmentation, and circumferential or near circumferential scarring and shrinking of the extremity.

Phlegmasia cerulea dolens (swollen, blue, painful leg), a rare complication, may develop in a patient in the advanced stages of cancer. It results from severe lower extremity VTE(s) that involve the major leg veins, causing near-total occlusion of venous outflow. Patients typically experience sudden, massive swelling; deep pain; and intense cyanosis of the extremity. If untreated, the venous obstruction causes arterial occlusion and gangrene and requires amputation.

Diagnostic Studies. Table 38-9 presents the various diagnostic studies used to determine the site or location and extent of a VTE.

Collaborative Care

Prevention and Prophylaxis. VTE prophylaxis is a core measure of high-quality health care in hospitalized surgical patients. The Joint Commission's core measures for the care of patients with VTE can be found at *www.jointcommission.org/core_measure_sets.aspx*. In addition, it is recommended that hospitals have a thromboprophylaxis policy that addresses VTE prevention on admission of all adult patients. As many as 60% of patients at risk for VTE do not receive appropriate thromboprophylaxis.[51]

In patients at risk for VTE, a variety of interventions are used. These are based on such factors as bleeding and thrombosis risk, past medical history, current medications, medical diagnoses, scheduled procedures, and patient preferences.[52] Early and aggressive mobilization based on the patient's condition is the easiest and most cost-effective method to decrease VTE risk. Patients on bed rest need to change position every 2 hours. Unless contraindicated, teach patients to flex and extend their feet, knees, and hips every 2 to 4 hours while awake. Patients who are able to get out of bed need to be in a chair for meals and ambulate at least four to six times per day as tolerated. Tell the patient and caregiver about the importance of these measures. Early and frequent ambulation is sufficient prophylaxis for very low VTE–risk patients undergoing minor surgical procedures.[53] Anticoagulation and mechanical prophylaxis

TABLE 38-9 DIAGNOSTIC STUDIES

Venous Thromboembolism*

Study	Description and Abnormal Findings
Blood Laboratory Studies	
ACT, aPTT, INR, bleeding time, Hgb, Hct, platelet count	Alterations if patient has underlying blood dyscrasia (e.g., increased Hgb and Hct in patient with polycythemia).
D-dimer	Fragment of fibrin formed as result of fibrin degradation and clot lysis. Elevated results suggest venous thromboembolism (VTE). *Normal results:* <250 ng/mL (<250 mcg/L)
Fibrin monomer complex	Forms when concentration of thrombin exceeds that of antithrombin. Presence is evidence of thrombus formation and suggests VTE. *Normal results:* <6.1 mg/L
Noninvasive Venous Studies	
Venous compression ultrasound	Evaluation of deep femoral, popliteal, and posterior tibial veins. *Normal finding:* Veins collapse with application of external pressure. *Abnormal finding:* Veins fail to collapse with application of external pressure. Failure to collapse suggests a thrombus.
Duplex ultrasound	Combination of compression ultrasound with spectral and color flow Doppler. Veins examined for respiratory variation, compressibility, and intraluminal filling defects to help determine location and extent of thrombus (most widely used test to diagnose VTE).
Invasive Venous Studies	
Computed tomography venography (CTV)	Uses spiral CT to evaluate veins in the pelvis, thighs, and calves after injection of venous phase contrast material. Uses less contrast material than traditional venography. May be performed simultaneously with CT angiography of pulmonary vessels for patients being evaluated for VTE.
Magnetic resonance venography	Uses magnetic resonance imaging with specialized software to evaluate blood flow through veins. Can be done with or without contrast. Highly accurate for pelvic and proximal veins. Less accurate for calf veins. Can distinguish acute and chronic thrombus.
Contrast venography (phlebogram)	X-ray determination of location and extent of clot using contrast media to outline filling defects. Identifies the presence of collateral circulation. Once the gold standard but currently rarely performed.

*See Table 28-26 for diagnostic studies for pulmonary embolism.
ACT, Activated clotting time; *aPTT,* activated partial thromboplastin time; *INR,* international normalized ratio.

are not recommended for acutely ill medical patients at low risk for VTE.

Elastic compression (antiembolism) stockings (e.g., thromboembolic deterrent [TED] hose) are a part of VTE prevention in hospitalized patients. When fitted correctly (both size and length) and worn properly and consistently from admission until discharge or full mobility, these stockings decrease VTE risk.[54] Proper use means the toe hole is under the toes, the heel patch is over the heel, the thigh gusset is on the inner thigh (thigh length only), and there are no wrinkles. The stockings are not to be rolled down, cut, or otherwise altered. Thigh-length stockings prevent proximal VTE better than knee-length stockings.[55] If the stockings are not fitted and worn correctly, venous return is impeded. This may promote the development of VTE and skin breakdown. VTE prevention is enhanced if elastic compression stockings are used along with anticoagulation.

Sequential compression devices (SCDs) are inflatable garments wrapped around the legs. They apply external pressure to the lower extremities by means of an electric pump. SCDs may or may not be used with elastic compression stockings. Like elastic compression stockings, ensure correct fit by accurately measuring the extremities. SCDs will not be effective if they are not applied correctly; if the fit is incorrect; or if the patient does not wear the device continuously except during bathing, skin assessment, and ambulation. SCDs are not worn when a patient has an active VTE because of the risk of PE. VTE prevention is enhanced if SCDs are used along with anticoagulation.[56]

Drug Therapy. Anticoagulants are used routinely for VTE prevention and treatment. The regimen depends on the patient's VTE risk. The goal of anticoagulant therapy for VTE prophylaxis is to prevent clot formation. The goals for treatment of a confirmed VTE are to prevent new clot development, spread of the clot, and embolization.[57]

Three major classes of anticoagulants are available: (1) vitamin K antagonists (VKA), (2) thrombin inhibitors (both indirect and direct), and (3) factor Xa inhibitors[58] (Table 38-10). Anticoagulant therapy does not dissolve the clot. Clot lysis begins naturally through the body's intrinsic fibrinolytic system (see Chapter 30).

Vitamin K Antagonists. The oral anticoagulant for long-term or extended anticoagulation is warfarin, a VKA. Warfarin inhibits activation of the vitamin K–dependent coagulation factors II, VII, IX, and X, as well as the anticoagulant proteins C and S. (Fig. 30-4 displays the clotting pathways, and clotting factors are listed in Table 30-2.) Warfarin begins to take effect in 48 to 72 hours. It then takes several more days to achieve a maximum effect. Thus an overlap of a parenteral anticoagulant (e.g., UH or LMWH) and warfarin typically is required for 5 days. The level of anticoagulation is monitored daily using the international normalized ratio (INR). The INR is a standardized system of reporting prothrombin time (PT) (Table 38-11, p. 852). The antidote for warfarin-related bleeding is vitamin K or Kcentra (Prothrombin Complex Concentrate [Human]).

Take a careful history before starting warfarin. Do not give antiplatelets or NSAIDs with warfarin, since these drugs

TABLE 38-10 DRUG THERAPY

Anticoagulant Therapy

Drug	Route of Administration	Comments
Vitamin K Antagonists (VKA)		
warfarin (Coumadin)	PO	INR is used for monitoring therapeutic levels. Administer at the same time each day. Variations of certain genes (e.g., *CYP2CP, VKORC1*) may influence response to the drug. *Antidote*: Vitamin K. For major VKA-related bleeding, treatment with four-factor prothrombin complex concentrate and IV vitamin K is recommended over fresh frozen plasma.
Thrombin Inhibitors: Indirect		
Unfractionated heparin (UH) heparin sodium (Hep-Lock, Liquaemin, Calciparine)	Continuous IV Intermittent IV Subcutaneous	Therapeutic effects measured at regular intervals by the aPTT or ACT. Monitor complete blood counts at regular intervals and titrate according to parameters. If administering subcutaneously, inject deep into subcutaneous tissue (preferably into the abdominal fatty tissue or above the iliac crest), inserting the entire length of the needle. Hold skinfold during injection but release before removing needle. Do not aspirate. Do not inject intramuscularly. Do not rub site after injection. Rotate sites. *Antidote*: Protamine
Low-molecular-weight heparin (LMWH) enoxaparin (Lovenox) tinzaparin (Innohep) dalteparin (Fragmin) nadroparin (Fraxiparine)	Subcutaneous	Routine coagulation tests typically not required. Monitor complete blood count at regular intervals. Do not expel air bubble before administering subcutaneously. Follow remaining administration guidelines as described above for UH. Reduced dosage needed in patients with renal impairment. Use extreme caution in patients with a history of HIT. *Antidote:* Protamine neutralizes the effects of LMWH.
Thrombin Inhibitors: Direct		
Hirudin derivatives lepirudin (Refludan) bivalirudin (Angiomax) desirudin (Iprivask)	 IV or subcutaneous IV IV or subcutaneous	Therapeutic effect measured by ACT or aPTT. Used in patients with HIT when anticoagulation is still required. *Antidote*: None
Synthetic thrombin inhibitors argatroban (Acova) dabigatran (Pradaxa)	 IV Subcutaneous	Therapeutic effect measured by aPTT. Used in patients at risk for or with HIT. Used for VTE prevention in joint replacement surgery. VTE treatment option and for stroke prevention in nonvalvular atrial fibrillation. *Antidote:* None
Factor Xa inhibitors fondaparinux (Arixtra) rivaroxaban (Xarelto)	 Subcutaneous PO	Routine coagulation tests not required. Monitor complete blood count and creatinine at regular intervals. Do not expel air bubble before administering. Follow remaining administration guidelines as described for UH. Both drugs approved for VTE prophylaxis and treatment. For surgical patients, initial dose should be given no earlier than 6 hr postoperatively. Use with caution in older patients and patients with impaired renal function. May cause thrombocytopenia. If uncontrollable bleeding occurs, treatment with recombinant factor VIIa may be effective. *Antidote:* None

ACT, Activated clotting time; *aPTT,* activated partial thromboplastin time; *HIT,* heparin-induced thrombocytopenia; *INR,* international normalized ratio; *VTE,* venous thromboembolism.

increase bleeding risk.[58] Many other drugs, vitamins, minerals, and dietary and herbal supplements also interact with warfarin (see eTable 38-1, available on the website for this chapter, and the Complementary & Alternative Therapies box on the right). A diet that frequently varies in vitamin K intake (e.g., green leafy vegetables) can make it hard to achieve and maintain a target INR level.

Genetic variants in the genes *VKORC1* and cytochrome P450 2C9 *(CYP2C9)* may influence how some people respond to warfarin (see Table 13-5). Although genetic testing is available, pharmacogenetic-based dosing is not recommended in clinical practice at this time.[59]

Thrombin Inhibitors: Indirect. *Indirect thrombin inhibitors* are divided into two major classes: UH and LMWHs. UH (e.g., heparin [Hep-Lock]) affects both the intrinsic and common pathways of blood coagulation by way of the plasma antithrombin. Antithrombin inhibits thrombin-mediated conversion of fibrinogen to fibrin by affecting factors II (prothrombin), IX, X, XI, and XII (see Fig. 30-4).

COMPLEMENTARY & ALTERNATIVE THERAPIES

Herbal and Dietary Supplements That May Affect Clotting

Scientific Evidence

There is evidence that the following herbs and dietary supplements may affect blood clotting: bilberry, black cohosh, chamomile, chondroitin sulfate, DHEA, feverfew, garlic, ginger, ginkgo biloba, ginseng, goldenseal, green tea, melatonin, niacin, omega-3 fatty acids, psyllium, red yeast rice extract, saw palmetto, soy, turmeric.

Nursing Implications

- Inform patients that taking these herbs, or dietary supplements may increase their risk of bleeding.
- Caution patients with bleeding disorders about the use of these herbs and dietary supplements. Advise them that they should consult with their health care provider before using these substances.

DHEA, Dehydroepiandrosterone.

TABLE 38-11 TESTS OF BLOOD COAGULATION

Drugs Monitored	Normal Value	Therapeutic Value
International normalized ratio (INR)	0.75-1.25	2-3
Vitamin K antagonists (e.g., warfarin [Coumadin])		
Activated partial thromboplastin time (aPTT)	25-35 sec	46-70 sec
• Unfractionated heparin (e.g., heparin [Hep-Lock])		
• Hirudin derivatives (e.g., bivalirudin [Angiomax])		
• Synthetic thrombin inhibitors (e.g., argatroban [Acova], dabigatran [Pradaxa])		
Activated clotting time (ACT)	70-120 sec*	>300 sec
• Unfractionated heparin		
• Hirudin derivatives		
• Synthetic thrombin inhibitors		
Anti–factor Xa		
• Low-molecular-weight heparin (e.g., enoxaparin [Lovenox])	0 U/mL	0.6-1.0 U/mL
• Factor Xa inhibitors (e.g., fondaparinux [Arixtra], rivaroxaban [Xarelto])	0 U/mL	0.2-1.5 U/mL

*Varies based on type of system and test reagent or activator used.

Heparin can be given subcutaneously for VTE prophylaxis or by continuous IV infusion for VTE treatment. When given IV, heparin requires frequent monitoring of clotting status as measured by activated partial thromboplastin time (aPTT) (see Table 38-11). Protamine sulfate reverses the effect of heparin.

One serious side effect of heparin is *heparin-induced thrombocytopenia* (HIT). HIT is an immune reaction to heparin. It causes a severe, sudden reduction in the platelet count along with a paradoxic increase in venous or arterial thrombosis. HIT is diagnosed by measuring the presence of heparin antibodies in the blood. Treatment requires immediately stopping heparin therapy and, if further anticoagulation is required, using a nonheparin anticoagulant (e.g., fondaparinux).[60] Another side effect of long-term heparin therapy is osteoporosis.

LMWHs (e.g., nadroparin [Fraxiparine]) are derived from UH. They have more bioavailability, more predictable dose response, longer half-life, and fewer bleeding complications than UH. LMWHs are less likely to cause HIT and osteoporosis. LMWHs typically do not require ongoing anticoagulant monitoring and dose adjustment. Protamine neutralizes the effect of LMWH.

Thrombin Inhibitors: Direct. *Direct thrombin inhibitors* are classified as hirudin derivatives or synthetic thrombin inhibitors. Hirudin is manufactured through recombinant deoxyribonucleic acid (DNA) technology. It binds specifically with thrombin and directly inhibits its function without causing plasma protein and platelet interactions. Hirudin derivatives (e.g., lepirudin [Refludan], bivalirudin [Angiomax]) are administered by continuous IV infusion. Lepirudin is approved for prophylaxis or treatment of patients with HIT. Bivalirudin is approved for HIT patients undergoing percutaneous coronary angioplasty. Anticoagulant activity is monitored using aPTT or activated clotting time (ACT) (see Table 38-11). There is no antidote for hirudin derivatives if bleeding occurs.

Argatroban (Acova), a synthetic direct thrombin inhibitor, inhibits thrombin. It is used as an alternative to heparin for the prevention and treatment of HIT and for known HIT patients who require percutaneous coronary interventions. Dabigatran (Pradaxa), an oral direct thrombin inhibitor, is used for VTE prevention after elective joint replacement, for stroke prevention in nonvalvular atrial fibrillation, and as a treatment option in VTE. The effects of argatroban and dabigatran are not reversible. Anticoagulant effect is monitored for both medications using aPTT or ACT.

Factor Xa Inhibitors. *Factor Xa inhibitors* inhibit factor Xa directly or indirectly, producing rapid anticoagulation. Fondaparinux is used for both VTE treatment and prophylaxis. It is given subcutaneously. Coagulation monitoring or dose adjustment is not needed, although the drug's anticoagulant activity can be measured using anti-Xa assays (see Table 38-11). If uncontrollable bleeding occurs, recombinant factor VIIa may be useful. Fondaparinux is contraindicated in patients with renal insufficiency. Rivaroxaban (Xarelto) is an oral factor Xa inhibitor used for VTE prevention.

Anticoagulant Therapy for VTE Prophylaxis. For VTE prophylaxis in the hospitalized medical patient at risk for thrombosis who is not bleeding, low-dose UH, LMWH, or fondaparinux is used. If the patient is at low VTE risk, drug prophylaxis is not needed. Patients with moderate VTE risk (e.g., general, gynecologic, urologic surgery) should receive either UH or LMWH. Patients with high VTE risk (e.g., trauma) should receive UH or LMWH until discharge. Patients having abdominal or pelvic surgery for cancer or major orthopedic surgery (e.g., total knee or hip replacement) should be prescribed VTE prophylaxis for up to 35 days after discharge.[59,61] (See eTable 38-2 for a sample VTE protocol/order set on the website for this chapter.)

Anticoagulant Therapy for VTE Treatment. Patients with confirmed VTE should receive initial treatment with either LMWH, UH, fondaparinux, or rivaroxaban. Oral VKA therapy is also started and continued for 3 months. A therapeutic INR is maintained between 2.0 and 3.0. Daily administration of only LMWH for 3 months is another option. Patients with multiple co-morbidities, complex medical issues, or a very large VTE usually are hospitalized for treatment. Parenteral administration of UH is the typical initial treatment. Depending on the

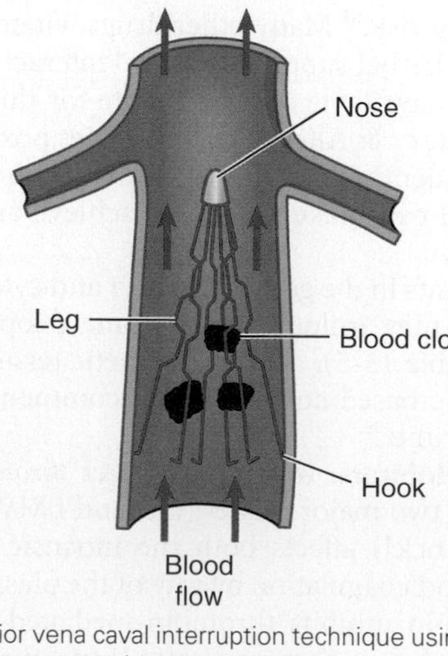

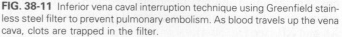

FIG. 38-11 Inferior vena caval interruption technique using Greenfield stainless steel filter to prevent pulmonary embolism. As blood travels up the vena cava, clots are trapped in the filter.

EVIDENCE-BASED PRACTICE

Applying the Evidence

You are caring for H.B., a 78-year-old Native American woman who is being discharged on enoxaparin (Lovenox) following a knee replacement. Her granddaughter will be her primary caregiver. You are preparing to teach her granddaughter how to inject the medication, since H.B. has limited dexterity in her hands because of arthritis. Her granddaughter tells you that H.B. is a modest woman and will not permit her to expose H.B.'s abdomen. She asks if the injection can be given in her arm.

Best Available Evidence	Clinician Expertise	Patient Preferences and Values
Enoxaparin (per the package literature) should be administered by deep subcutaneous injection in the abdomen. Injection sites should be rotated.	Some patients have told you that they used alternate sites for injection of enoxaparin, specifically the thighs and upper arms. You do not have any evidence about the efficacy of the drug when alternate sites are used.	H.B. states she does not want to expose herself to her granddaughter. The granddaughter expresses a desire to support her grandmother's need for modesty.

Your Decision and Action

You discuss the importance of following the drug manufacturer's recommendations regarding site selection with H.B. and her granddaughter. You further explain that there is no evidence on whether alternate sites are equally effective. H.B.'s granddaughter states she is the only one available to do this and she needs to respect her grandmother's wishes. You teach the granddaughter how to inject enoxaparin in H.B.'s upper arms and to alternate the sites and arms. You inform the physician of H.B.'s decision and document your teaching and related conversation.

Reference for Evidence

Lovenox. Retrieved from *www.lovenox.com/consumer/default.aspx.*

clinical presentation and home situation, patients may be safely and effectively managed as outpatients.

Thrombolytic Therapy for VTE Treatment. Another treatment option for patients with a thrombus is catheter-directed administration of a thrombolytic drug (e.g., urokinase, tPA). Catheter-directed thrombolysis dissolves the clot(s), reduces the acute symptoms, and decreases the incidence of PTS. Other catheter-based interventions such as angioplasty, stents, or mechanical thrombectomy can be used along with thrombolytic drug therapy. (Chapter 34 discusses thrombolytic therapy.)

Surgical Therapy. Although most patients are managed medically, a small number of patients undergo surgery. Surgical options include open venous thrombectomy and inferior vena cava interruption. *Venous thrombectomy* involves the removal of a thrombus through an incision in the vein. Anticoagulant therapy is recommended after venous thrombectomy.

Vena cava interruption devices (e.g., Greenfield, Vena Tech, TrapEase filters) can be inserted percutaneously through the right femoral or right internal jugular veins. The filter device is opened, and the spokes penetrate the vessel walls (Fig. 38-11). The filters act as a "sieve-type" device, permitting filtration of clots without interruption of blood flow. Complications after the insertion of the device are rare but include air embolism, improper placement, migration of the filter, and perforation of the vena cava with retroperitoneal bleeding. Over time, venous congestion can occur from a buildup of trapped clots. These can clog the filter and completely block the vena cava, requiring filter removal and replacement. A filter device is recommended with proximal VTE of the leg if anticoagulant therapy is contraindicated due to an increased risk of bleeding. Patients with a filter device are at increased risk of developing a VTE. If the bleeding risk resolves, a course of anticoagulant therapy is suggested.[62]

TABLE 38-12 NURSING ASSESSMENT

Venous Thromboembolism

Subjective Data

Important Health Information (see Table 38-8)

Past health history: Trauma to vein, intravascular catheter (e.g., peripherally inserted central catheter), varicose veins, pregnancy or recent childbirth, bacteremia, obesity, prolonged bed rest, irregular heartbeat (e.g., atrial fibrillation), COPD, HF, cancer, coagulation disorders and hypercoagulable states, systemic lupus erythematosus, MI, spinal cord injury, stroke, prolonged travel, recent bone fracture, dehydration

Medications: Use of estrogens (including oral contraceptives, hormone therapy), tamoxifen (Nolvadex), raloxifene (Evista), corticosteroids, excessive amounts of vitamin E, erythropoiesis-stimulating drugs

Surgery or other treatments: Any recent surgery, especially orthopedic, gynecologic, gastric, or urologic; previous surgery involving veins; central venous catheter

Functional Health Patterns

Health perception–health management: IV drug abuse, tobacco use, obesity

Activity-exercise: Inactivity

Cognitive-perceptual: Pain in area on palpation or ambulation

Objective Data

General

Fever, anxiety, pain

Integumentary

Increased size of extremity when compared with other side; taut, shiny, warm skin, erythematous, tender to palpation; no physical changes in the affected extremity in some patients

Cardiovascular

Distention and warmth of superficial veins in affected area; edema and cyanosis of extremities, neck, back, and face (if superior vena cava involvement)

Possible Diagnostic Findings

Leukocytosis, abnormal coagulation, anemia or ↑ hematocrit and RBC count, ↑ D-dimer level, positive venous compression on duplex ultrasound study; positive CTV, magnetic resonance venogram, or contrast venogram study

COPD, Chronic obstructive pulmonary disease; *CTV,* computed tomography venogram; *HF,* heart failure; *MI,* myocardial infarction; *RBC,* red blood cell.

NURSING MANAGEMENT VENOUS THROMBOEMBOLISM

NURSING ASSESSMENT

Table 38-12 presents the subjective and objective data to obtain from a patient with VTE.

NURSING DIAGNOSES

Nursing diagnoses and collaborative problems for the patient with VTE include, but are not limited to, the following:

- Acute pain *related to* venous congestion, impaired venous return, and inflammation

- Ineffective health maintenance *related to* lack of knowledge about disorder and its treatment
- Risk for impaired skin integrity *related to* altered peripheral tissue perfusion
- Potential complication: bleeding *related to* anticoagulant therapy
- Potential complication: PE *related to* embolization of thrombus, dehydration, and immobility

PLANNING

The overall goals for the patient with VTE include (1) pain relief, (2) decreased edema, (3) no skin ulceration, (4) no bleeding complications, and (5) no evidence of PE.

NURSING IMPLEMENTATION

ACUTE INTERVENTION. Focus your nursing care for the patient with VTE on prevention of emboli formation and reduction of inflammation. Review with the patient any medications, vitamins, minerals, and dietary and herbal supplements being taken that may interfere with anticoagulant therapy (see eTable 38-1 on the website for this chapter and the Complementary & Alternative Therapies box on p. 851). Depending on the anticoagulant ordered, monitor INR, aPTT, ACT, anti–factor Xa levels, complete blood count (CBC), creatinine, factor X levels, hemoglobin, hematocrit, platelet levels, and/or liver enzymes.[63] Monitor platelet counts for patients getting UH or LMWH to assess for HIT. Titrate doses of UH, warfarin, and direct thrombin inhibitors based on results of blood studies and physician-ordered parameters. Direct thrombin inhibitors may need adjustment for patients with renal or liver dysfunction. Always check the results of appropriate tests before starting, giving, or changing anticoagulant therapy.

DRUG ALERT: Anticoagulant Therapy

- Tell patient to avoid taking aspirin, NSAIDs, fish oil supplements, garlic supplements, ginkgo biloba, and certain antibiotics (e.g., sulfamethoxazole and trimethoprim [Bactrim]).
- Instruct patient to report any signs of bleeding (e.g., black or bloody stools, bloody urine, coffee-ground or bloody vomit, nosebleeds).
- Assess for signs of bleeding (e.g., hypotension, tachycardia, hematuria, melena, hematemesis, petechiae, ecchymosis).

Monitor for and reduce the risk of bleeding that may occur with anticoagulant therapy (Table 38-13). Be aware that the risk of bleeding is greater in persons receiving LMWH or UH with an active gastroduodenal ulcer, prior bleeding history, low platelet count, hepatic or renal failure, rheumatic disease, cancer, or age greater than 85 years.[64] Patients receiving warfarin with an INR of 5.0 or more are also at increased risk for bleeding. In the event of anticoagulation above target goals, give reversal agents (e.g., protamine, vitamin K) or make dosage adjustments as ordered. In the event of major VKA-related bleeding, rapid treatment with four-factor prothrombin complex concentrate and IV vitamin K is recommended over fresh frozen plasma.

SAFETY ALERT

- Observe closely for any signs of bleeding:
  - Epistaxis and bleeding gingivae
  - Blood (visible or occult) in emesis, urine, stool, sputum
  - Oozing or visible bleeding from trauma site or surgical incision
  - Excessive menstrual bleeding
- Monitor vital signs for changes: decreased BP, increased HR
- Avoid intramuscular (IM) injections.
- Assess for mental status changes, especially in the older patient, since this may indicate cerebral bleeding.

TABLE 38-13 NURSING INTERVENTIONS FOR PATIENTS TAKING ANTICOAGULANTS

Assessment

- Monitor vital signs as indicated.
- Examine urine and stool for overt and occult signs of blood.
- Inspect skin frequently, especially under any splinting devices.
- Evaluate platelet count for signs of heparin-induced thrombocytopenia.
- Evaluate appropriate laboratory coagulation tests for target therapeutic levels.
- Evaluate lower extremity for ecchymosis or hematoma development if sequential compression device used.
- Perform assessments frequently to observe for signs and symptoms of bleeding (e.g., hypotension, tachycardia) or clotting.
- Notify the health care provider of any abnormalities in assessments, vital signs, or laboratory values.

Injections

- Avoid intramuscular injections.
- Minimize venipunctures.
- Use small-gauge needles for venipunctures unless ordered therapy requires a larger gauge.
- Apply manual pressure for at least 10 min (or longer if needed) on venipuncture sites.

Patient Care

- Avoid restrictive clothing.
- Apply moisturizing lotion to skin.
- Use electric razors, not straight razors.
- Perform physical care in a gentle manner.
- Instruct patient not to forcefully blow nose.
- Avoid removing or disrupting established clots.
- Humidify O_2 source if supplemental O_2 is ordered.
- Use soft toothbrushes or foam swabs for oral care.
- Reposition the patient carefully at regular intervals.
- Limit tape application. Use paper tape as appropriate.
- Administer stool softeners to avoid hard stools and straining.
- Lubricate tubes (e.g., suction catheter) adequately before insertion.
- Avoid restraints if possible. Use only soft, padded restraints if needed.
- Use support pads, mattresses, bed cradles, and therapeutic beds as indicated.
- Apply elastic compression stockings or sequential compression devices as ordered and with attention to proper size, application, and use.
- Perform risk for fall and skin breakdown assessments per agency policy and implement safety measures as needed.

Early ambulation when compared with bed rest does not increase the short-term risk of a PE in patients with VTE. In addition, early ambulation after acute VTE results in a more rapid decrease in edema and limb pain, fewer PTS symptoms, and better quality of life. Teach the patient and caregiver the importance of physical activity and assist the patient to ambulate several times a day. For patients with acute VTE with severe edema and limb pain, bed rest with limb elevation may initially be prescribed.

AMBULATORY AND HOME CARE. Focus discharge teaching on modification of VTE risk factors, use of elastic compression stockings, importance of monitoring laboratory values, medication instructions, and guidelines for follow-up. Once the edema is resolved, measure the patient for custom-fit elastic compression stockings. Stocking use (or sleeves in the case of an upper

DELEGATION DECISIONS

Caring for the Patient With Venous Thromboembolism (VTE)

All members of the health care team have important roles in preventing and managing VTE.

Role of Registered Nurse (RN)
- Assess patients for VTE risk and monitor for VTE in at-risk patients.
- Develop a plan of care to prevent VTE.
- Teach hospitalized patients who are at risk for VTE about preventive measures such as increasing mobility, using elastic compression stockings and sequential compression devices, and taking anticoagulant medications.
- Assess for the use of dietary supplements or herbs that may affect the coagulation status before the initiation of anticoagulant therapy.
- Monitor for adverse effects of anticoagulant use.
- Evaluate the effect of anticoagulant medications by monitoring appropriate laboratory results.
- Assess for complications of VTE, including pulmonary embolism (PE) and chronic venous insufficiency.
- Provide discharge teaching about use of elastic compression stockings and anticoagulant medication instructions (including diet, necessary laboratory testing, and administration of subcutaneous anticoagulants if needed).
- Teach the patient and caregiver the clinical manifestations of PE and the need to contact the EMS if these occur.
- Teach safety precautions to prevent falls or other injuries that might result in bleeding.
- Provide instructions about the use of pressure to stop bleeding and that the EMS should be contacted for persistent bleeding.
- Teach the patient about lifestyle measures to prevent VTE, including leg exercises, ambulation, and avoidance of nicotine and oral contraceptives.

Role of Licensed Practical/Vocational Nurse (LPN/LVN)
- Administer prescribed oral, subcutaneous, and IV anticoagulants (consider state nurse practice act and agency policies regarding administration of high-alert medications and IV medications).
- Measure patients for elastic compression stockings and/or sequential compression devices.

Role of Unlicensed Assistive Personnel (UAP)
- Reposition patients who are on bed rest at least every 2 hr.
- Remind patients about the need to flex and extend the legs and feet every 2 hr while in bed.
- Assist ambulatory patients to ambulate at least 4 to 6 times daily.
- Assist patients with putting on elastic compression stockings.
- Apply sequential compression devices.

extremity VTE) is recommended for at least 2 years after a VTE to support the vein walls and valves and decrease swelling and pain.[44,49] Regular use of elastic compression stockings reduces the incidence of mild PTS. Unfortunately, getting the patient to adhere to wearing stockings is a challenge. Address individual risk factors for VTE (e.g., obesity) and barriers to stocking use (e.g., lack of knowledge, depression) to improve patient adherence.[65]

If appropriate, tell the patient to stop smoking and avoid all nicotine products. Instruct the patient to avoid constrictive clothing. If appropriate, tell women with a history of VTE to stop oral contraceptives or HT. Teach patients to limit standing or sitting in a motionless, leg-dependent position. During long train or plane rides, encourage patients to frequently exercise the calf muscles and take short walks around the cabin. For those at high risk for VTE who are planning a long trip, recommend properly fitted, knee-high elastic compression stockings during travel to decrease edema and VTE risk. Aspirin or anticoagulant use is not suggested for long-distance travelers. Teach the patient and caregiver about signs and symptoms of PE such as sudden onset of dyspnea, tachypnea, and pleuritic chest pain. (Chapter 28 discusses PE.) They should contact EMS if these symptoms occur.

TABLE 38-14 PATIENT & CAREGIVER TEACHING GUIDE

Anticoagulant Therapy

Include the following information in the teaching plan for a patient receiving anticoagulant therapy and the patient's caregiver.

1. Give reasons for and action of anticoagulant therapy and how long therapy will last.
2. Take medication at the same time each day (preferably in afternoon or evening).
3. Depending on medication prescribed, obtain blood tests to assess therapeutic effect of the drug and whether change in drug dosage is needed.
4. Contact emergency medical services immediately for any of the following adverse side effects of drug therapy:
   - Blood in urine or stool; or black, tarry stools
   - Vomiting blood, coffee-ground emesis
   - Unusual bleeding from gums, skin, or nose, or heavy menstrual bleeding
   - Severe headaches or stomach pains
   - Chest pain, shortness of breath, palpitations (heart racing)
   - Weakness, dizziness, mental status changes
   - Cold, blue, or painful feet
5. Avoid any trauma or injury that might cause bleeding (e.g., vigorous brushing of teeth, contact sports, rollerblading, use of straight razor).
6. Avoid all aspirin-containing drugs and nonsteroidal antiinflammatory drugs.
7. Limit alcohol intake to small to moderate amounts (12 oz beer, 4 oz wine, 1 oz hard liquor/day).
8. Wear a Medic Alert device indicating what anticoagulant is being taken.
9. Avoid frequent changes in eating habits, such as dramatically increasing foods high in vitamin K (e.g., broccoli, spinach, kale, greens). Do not take supplemental vitamin K.
10. Consult with health care provider before beginning or discontinuing any medication, vitamin, mineral, or dietary or herbal supplement (see Complementary & Alternative Therapies box).
11. Inform all health care providers, including dentist, of anticoagulant therapy.
12. Correct dosing is essential. Provide supervision if patient experiences confusion or cognitive impairment.

Instruct the patient and the caregiver about drug dosage, actions, and side effects; the need for routine blood tests; and what symptoms need immediate medical attention (Table 38-14). Devices are available for home monitoring of INR. Teach patients taking LMWH or fondaparinux and their caregivers how to give the drug subcutaneously. Active or young patients need to avoid contact sports and high-risk (for trauma) activities (e.g., skiing). Teach older patients about safety precautions to prevent falls (e.g., avoid use of throw rugs). Instruct the patient and caregiver to apply pressure for 10 to 15 minutes if bleeding occurs (e.g., nosebleed).

A well-balanced diet is important. Teach patients taking warfarin to follow a consistent diet of foods containing vitamin K and to avoid any supplements containing vitamin K (e.g., vitamins, green tea). Instruct the patient to avoid excessive amounts of vitamin E and alcohol. Encourage proper hydration to prevent additional hypercoagulability of the blood, which may occur with dehydration.

The overweight patient needs to not only limit caloric intake but also increase physical activity to achieve and maintain desired weight. A balanced program of rest and exercise also improves venous return. Help the patient develop an exercise program with an emphasis on walking and swimming. Water exercise is particularly beneficial because of the gentle, even pressure of the water. A 6-month exercise program improves quality of life and reduces PTS.[66]

EVALUATION

The expected outcomes for the patient with VTE include

- Minimal to no pain
- Intact skin
- No signs of hemorrhage or occult bleeding
- No signs of respiratory distress

VARICOSE VEINS

Varicose veins, or *varicosities,* are dilated (3 mm or larger in diameter), tortuous subcutaneous veins commonly found in the saphenous vein system.[67] Varicosities may be small and harmless or large and bulging. *Primary varicose veins* (idiopathic) are due to a congenital weakness of the veins and are more common in women. *Secondary varicose veins* typically result from a previous VTE. Secondary varicose veins also may occur in the esophagus (esophageal varices), vulva, spermatic cords (varicoceles), and anorectal area (hemorrhoids), and as abnormal arteriovenous (AV) connections. *Reticular veins* are smaller varicose veins that appear flat, less tortuous, and blue-green in color. *Telangiectasias* (often referred to as spider veins) are small visible vessels (generally less than 1 mm in diameter) that appear bluish black, purple, or red.

Etiology and Pathophysiology

The etiology of varicose veins is multifactorial. Superficial veins in the lower extremities become dilated and tortuous in response to increased venous pressure. Risk factors include family history of venous disease, weakness of the vein structure, female gender, use of oral contraceptives or HT, tobacco use, increasing age, obesity, pregnancy, history of VTE, venous obstruction resulting from extrinsic pressure by tumors, thrombophilia, or occupations that require prolonged standing or sitting.[67] Although the exact etiology remains unknown, it is thought that the vein valve leaflets are stretched and become incompetent (do not fit together properly). Incompetent vein valves allow backward blood flow, particularly when the patient is standing. This results in increased venous pressure and further venous distention.

Clinical Manifestations and Complications

Discomfort from varicose veins varies among people and tends to be worse after episodes of SVT. Many patients are concerned about cosmetic disfigurement. The most common varicose vein symptoms include a heavy, achy feeling or pain after prolonged standing or sitting, which is relieved by walking or limb elevation. Some patients feel pressure or complain of an itchy, burning, tingling, throbbing, or cramplike leg sensation. Swelling, restless or tired legs, fatigue, and nocturnal leg cramps also may occur.

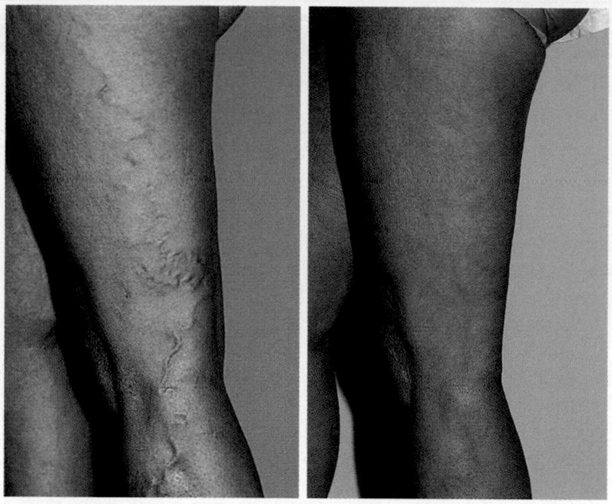

A B

FIG. 38-12 A, Lateral aspect of varicose veins before treatment. **B,** Lateral aspect of varicose veins 2 years after initial treatment with sclerotherapy.

SVT is the most frequent complication of varicose veins. It may occur spontaneously or after trauma, surgical procedures, or pregnancy. Rare complications include rupture of the varicose veins resulting in external bleeding and skin ulcerations.

Diagnostic Studies and Collaborative Care

Superficial varicose veins can be diagnosed by appearance. A duplex ultrasound can detect obstruction and reflux in the venous system. Treatment usually is not indicated if varicose veins are only a cosmetic problem. If CVI develops, care involves rest with limb elevation; elastic compression stockings; and exercise, such as walking. Two herbal therapies used for varicose vein treatment are horse chestnut seed extract (HCSE) *(Aesculus hippocastanum)* and butcher's broom *(Ruscus aculeatus).*[68] Venoactive drugs (e.g., diosmin, hesperidin, rutosides [Venoruton]) with compression therapy are recommended for patients with varicose veins experiencing pain and swelling.

Sclerotherapy involves the injection of a substance (e.g., hypertonic saline, polidocanol, glycerine) that destroys venous telangiectasias, reticular veins, and superficial varicose veins 5 mm in diameter or smaller (Fig. 38-12). Direct IV injection of a sclerosing agent causes inflammation and results in thrombosis of the vein. This procedure is performed in an office setting and causes minimal discomfort. Potential complications include itching, pain, blistering, edema, inflammation, hyperpigmentation, tissue necrosis, recurrence of varicosities, SVT, and VTE.[69] After injection, a thigh-high elastic compression stocking is worn or an elastic bandage is applied to the leg for several days to maintain pressure over the vein. Long-term compression therapy is advised to help prevent further varicosities.

Other noninvasive options for the treatment of venous telangiectasias include laser therapy and high-intensity pulsed-light therapy. Laser or light therapy is used for isolated small telangiectasias or for patients in whom sclerotherapy is contraindicated or has been ineffective. Laser treatment typically requires more than one session, scheduled at 6- to 12-week intervals. Vascular lasers work by heating the hemoglobin in the vessels, resulting in vessel sclerosis. Potential complications of these therapies include pain, blistering, hyperpigmentation, and superficial erosions.

Surgical intervention is indicated for recurrent SVT or when CVI cannot be controlled with conservative therapy. The traditional surgical intervention involves ligation of the entire vein (usually the greater saphenous vein) and removal of its incompetent branches. An alternative but time-consuming technique is ambulatory phlebectomy. This involves pulling the varicosity through a "stab" incision followed by excision of the vein. Transilluminated powered phlebectomy involves the use of a tissue resector to destroy the varices and removes the pieces via aspiration. Potential complications include bleeding, bruising, and infection. In up to 30% of patients, a new vein forms to replace the one removed.

A less invasive procedure is endovenous ablation of the saphenous vein. Ablation involves the insertion of a catheter that emits energy. This causes collapse and sclerosis of the vein.[70] Potential complications include bruising, tightness along the vein, recanalization (reopening of the vein), and paresthesia. Endovenous ablation also may be done in combination with ligation or phlebectomy.

NURSING MANAGEMENT VARICOSE VEINS

Prevention is a key factor related to varicose veins. Instruct the patient to avoid sitting or standing for long periods, maintain ideal body weight, take precautions against injury to the extremities, avoid wearing constrictive clothing, and walk daily.

After vein ligation surgery, encourage the patient to deep breathe, which promotes venous return. Check the extremities regularly for color, movement, sensation, temperature, edema, and quality of pedal pulses. Some bruising and discoloration are normal. Postoperatively, elevate the legs 15 degrees to limit edema. Apply elastic compression stockings. Remove them every 8 hours for short periods and then reapply.

Long-term management of varicose veins is directed toward improving circulation and appearance, relieving discomfort, and avoiding complications and ulceration. Varicose veins can recur in other veins after surgery. Teach the patient the proper use and care of custom-fitted elastic compression stockings. The patient should apply stockings in bed before rising in the morning. Emphasize the importance of periodic positioning of the legs above the heart. The overweight patient may need assistance with weight loss. The patient with a job that requires long periods of standing or sitting needs to frequently flex and extend her or his hips, legs, and ankles and change positions.

CHRONIC VENOUS INSUFFICIENCY AND VENOUS LEG ULCERS

Chronic venous insufficiency (CVI), a common problem in women and older adults, is a condition that develops when leg veins and valves fail to keep blood moving forward. This results in *ambulatory venous hypertension*. CVI can lead to *venous leg ulcers* (formerly called *venous stasis ulcers* or *varicose ulcers*). Although CVI and venous leg ulcers are not life-threatening diseases, they are painful, debilitating, and costly conditions that adversely affect the quality of patients' lives.

Etiology and Pathophysiology

Both long-standing primary varicose veins and PTS can progress to CVI. As a result of ambulatory venous hypertension, serous fluid and RBCs leak from the capillaries and venules into the tissue. This produces edema and chronic inflammatory changes. Enzymes in the tissue eventually break down RBCs, causing the release of *hemosiderin*, which causes a brownish skin discoloration. Over time, the skin and subcutaneous tissue around the ankle are replaced by fibrous tissue, resulting in thick, hardened, contracted skin. Although the causes of CVI are known, the exact pathophysiology of venous leg ulcers is unknown.

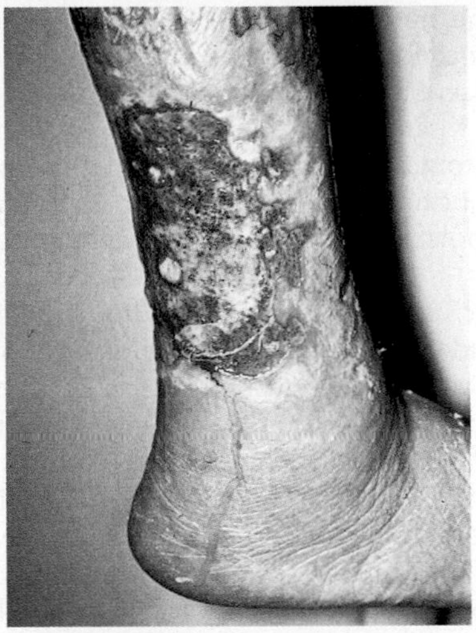

FIG. 38-13 Venous leg ulcer.

Clinical Manifestations and Complications

In individuals with CVI the skin of the lower leg is leathery, with a characteristic brownish or "brawny" appearance from the hemosiderin deposition. Edema usually has been persistent for a prolonged period. Eczema, or "stasis dermatitis," is often present, and itching is a common complaint (see Table 38-1).

Venous ulcers classically are located above the medial malleolus (Fig. 38-13). The ulcer is often quite painful, particularly when edema or infection is present. Pain may be worse when the leg is in a dependent position. If the venous ulcer is untreated, the wound becomes wider and deeper, increasing the likelihood of infection. Severe complications can include osteomyelitis and malignant changes.[71] On rare occasions, severe CVI with long-standing nonhealing venous ulcers may result in the need for amputation.

Collaborative Care

Compression is essential for CVI treatment, venous ulcer healing, and prevention of ulcer recurrence. A variety of options are available for compression therapy. These include custom-fitted elastic compression stockings, elastic tubular support bandages, a Velcro wrap (CircAid), SCDs, a paste bandage (Unna boot) with an elastic wrap, and multilayer (three or four) bandage systems (e.g., Profore).[71] There are benefits to each type of compression therapy. Evaluate patients individually when choosing a compression method. Before starting compression therapy, assess the arterial status to make sure that PAD is not also present. An ABI of less than 0.9 suggests PAD, and the patient should not have high levels of compression therapy.

Moist environment dressings are the basis of wound care. A variety of these dressings are available, including transparent film dressings, hydrocolloids, hydrogels, foams, alginates, gauze, and combination dressings.[72] Dressing decisions should be based on wound characteristics, cost, and clinician judgment. (Chapter 12 and Table 12-10 discuss dressings.)

Evaluate the nutritional status of a patient with a venous ulcer. A balanced diet with adequate protein, calories, and nutrients is essential. Foods high in protein (e.g., meat, beans, cheese, tofu), vitamin A (green leafy vegetables), vitamin C (citrus fruits, tomatoes, cantaloupe), and zinc (meat, seafood) are most important for healing. For patients with diabetes, maintaining normal blood glucose levels assists the healing process.

Routine use of antibiotics is not indicated. Clinical signs of infection include change in quantity, color, or odor of the drainage; pus; erythema of the wound edges; change in sensation around the wound; warmth around the wound; increased local pain, edema, or both; dark-colored granulation tissue; induration around the wound; delayed healing; and cellulitis. If signs of infection occur, obtain a wound culture before starting antibiotic therapy. The usual treatment for infection is debridement, wound excision, and systemic antibiotics. A number of antimicrobial dressings (e.g., cadexomer iodine, silver) are available.

If the ulcer does not heal with conservative therapy, pentoxifylline or micronized purified flavonoid fraction (Daflon) is recommended with compression therapy to improve healing.[67] Other treatments may include coverage with a skin replacement or substitute such as split-thickness skin grafts, cultured keratinocyte grafts, or artificial bioengineered skin. When used with compression therapy, a bilayer artificial skin (e.g., Apligraf or Orcel) can increase ulcer healing more than a simple dressing and compression.[73] (Chapter 25 discusses skin grafting.) Although grafts may aid with healing, they do not replace the need for lifelong compression therapy.

An herbal therapy used for CVI treatment is horse chestnut seed extract (HCSE). Escins (the active ingredient) reduce leg pain, itching, and swelling.[68] Minor side effects associated with HCSE include dizziness, gastrointestinal complaints, headache, and pruritus. The value of HCSE in venous ulcer healing and recurrence is not known.

NURSING MANAGEMENT
CHRONIC VENOUS INSUFFICIENCY AND VENOUS LEG ULCERS

Long-term management of venous leg ulcers should focus on teaching the patient self-care measures. Demonstrate the correct application of elastic compression stockings, and have the patient "show back" the skill. Prescription elastic compression stockings should be worn daily to reduce the occurrence of CVI. Stress the importance of regular replacement every 4 to 6 months. Instruct the patient and caregiver to avoid trauma to the limbs, and teach them proper foot and leg care to avoid additional skin trauma. Patients with CVI have dry, flaky, itchy skin because of stasis dermatitis. Daily moisturizing decreases itching and prevents cracking of the skin. Venous dermatitis may result from contact with sensitizing products such as antibacterial agents (e.g., gentamicin); additives in bandages or dressings (e.g., adhesives); ointments containing lanolin, alcohols, or benzocaine; and over-the-counter creams or lotions with fragrance or preservatives.[71] Assess the wound for signs of infection with each dressing change.

Be certain to discuss activity guidelines and proper limb positioning. Instruct patients with CVI with or without a venous ulcer to avoid standing or sitting for long periods. Standing or sitting with the legs in a dependent position decreases blood flow to the lower extremities. Also instruct patients to frequently elevate their legs above the level of the heart to reduce edema. Encourage patients to begin a daily walking program once an ulcer heals.

DELEGATION DECISIONS
Caring for the Patient With Chronic Venous Insufficiency

Many patients with chronic venous insufficiency and venous ulcers are cared for in an outpatient setting. In this case the registered nurse (RN) does an initial assessment of the wound, develops the plan of care, and periodically evaluates the patient and venous ulcer. Much of the routine wound care is done by unlicensed assistive personnel (UAP) and licensed practical/vocational nurses (LPN/LVNs).

Role of Registered Nurse (RN)
- Assess patients with venous insufficiency for increases in edema, stasis dermatitis, and venous stasis ulcers.
- Assess patient's diet and nutritional status and make referrals as necessary to a dietitian.
- Choose appropriate options for compression therapy and wound care.
- Evaluate for the effectiveness of therapies and need for alternative approaches.
- Teach patient and family about the pathophysiology, clinical manifestations, complications, and treatment of venous insufficiency.

Role of Licensed Practical/Vocational Nurse (LPN/LVN)
- Administer prescribed analgesics, antibiotics, or other medications.
- Apply compression devices.
- Provide wound care for chronic venous ulcers (consider state nurse practice act and agency policy).

Role of Unlicensed Assistive Personnel (UAP)
- Assist patients in elevating extremities to reduce edema and pain.
- Apply elastic wraps or compression stockings, as directed by the RN.
- Provide wound care for chronic venous ulcers (consider state nurse practice act and agency policy).

CASE STUDY

Peripheral Artery Disease

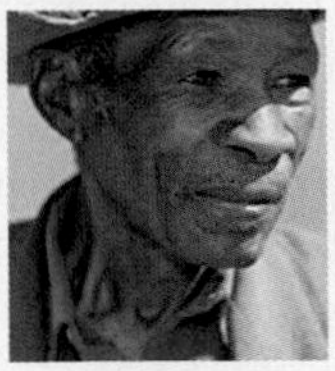

iStockphoto/Thinkstock

Patient Profile

S.J., a 76-yr-old African American man, is admitted to the hospital with rest pain in both legs and a nonhealing ulcer of the big toe on the right foot.

Subjective Data

- History of a myocardial infarction, stroke, hypertension, heart failure, and type 1 diabetes mellitus
- Underwent a left femoral-popliteal bypass 5 yr ago
- Has a 45 pack-yr history of tobacco use
- Has been using insulin for 30 yr
- Complains of sudden, intense increase in right foot pain for past 2 hr
- Has slept in recliner with right leg in dependent position for several months

Current Medications

- furosemide 40 mg/day PO
- isosorbide dinitrate/hydralazine hydrochloride (BiDil) 1 tablet q8hr
- aspart (NovoLog) insulin with meals
- glargine insulin 50 U/day subcutaneously
- diltiazem sustained release 240 mg/day PO
- aspirin 325 mg/day PO
- Fish oil daily (self-prescribed)

Objective Data

Physical Examination

- BP 148/92 mm Hg; irregular apical HR 90/min, respiratory rate 22/min, temperature 97.9° F (36.6° C)
- Alert and oriented but anxious, no apparent physical or mental deficits from previous stroke
- Has a diminished right femoral pulse, popliteal pulse by Doppler only, posterior tibial pulse by Doppler only, and dorsalis pedis pulse absent (not palpable or present by Doppler); left leg pulses are weakly palpable
- Right leg ABI: 0.20; left leg ABI: 0.68
- Has a 2-cm necrotic ulcer on tip of right big toe
- Has thickened toenails; shiny, thin skin on legs; and hair absent on both lower legs
- Right foot is very cool, pale, and mottled in color with decreased sensation
- No peripheral edema present
- Bedside glucose measurement 298 mg/dL (last meal 4 hr before admission)

Discussion Questions

1. Assess S.J.'s risk factors for peripheral artery disease (PAD).
2. Differentiate S.J.'s signs and symptoms of chronic PAD and acute arterial ischemia.
3. Identify the possible cause(s) for the sudden, intense increase in right foot pain.
4. How would you interpret S.J.'s ABI findings?
5. What additional diagnostic tests can be performed to assess the extent of his PAD?
6. Given the physical examination data, what initial medication(s) would you expect the physician to prescribe?
7. What treatment modalities are possible for S.J.?
8. ***Priority Decision:*** What are the priority nursing responsibilities in caring for S.J.?
9. ***Delegation Decision:*** Identify activities that can be delegated to unlicensed assistive personnel.
10. ***Priority Decision:*** Based on the assessment data presented, what are the priority nursing diagnoses? Are there any collaborative problems?
11. ***Evidence-Based Practice:*** When teaching S.J., what evidence-based advice would you give him regarding the use of dietary supplements such as fish oil?

evolve Answers available at *http://evolve.elsevier.com/Lewis/medsurg.*

BRIDGE TO NCLEX EXAMINATION

The number of the question corresponds to the same-numbered outcome at the beginning of the chapter.

1. A 50-year-old woman weighs 95 kg and has a history of tobacco use, high blood pressure, high sodium intake, and sedentary lifestyle. When developing an individualized care plan for her, the nurse determines that the most important risk factors for peripheral artery disease (PAD) that need to be modified are
   a. weight and diet.
   b. activity level and diet.
   c. tobacco use and high blood pressure.
   d. sedentary lifestyle and high blood pressure.
2. Rest pain is a manifestation of PAD that occurs due to a chronic
   a. vasospasm of small cutaneous arteries in the feet.
   b. increase in retrograde venous blood flow in the legs.
   c. decrease in arterial blood flow to the nerves of the feet.
   d. decrease in arterial blood flow to the leg muscles during exercise.
3. A patient with infective endocarditis develops sudden left leg pain with pallor, paresthesia, and a loss of peripheral pulses. The nurse's initial action should be to
   a. elevate the leg to promote venous return.
   b. start anticoagulant therapy with IV heparin.
   c. notify the physician of the change in peripheral perfusion.
   d. place the bed in reverse Trendelenburg to promote perfusion.
4. Which clinical manifestations are seen in patients with either Buerger's disease or Raynaud's phenomenon *(select all that apply)?*
   a. Intermittent fevers
   b. Sensitivity to cold temperatures
   c. Gangrenous ulcers on fingertips
   d. Color changes of fingers and toes
   e. Episodes of superficial vein thrombosis
5. A patient is admitted to the hospital with a diagnosis of abdominal aortic aneurysm. Which signs and symptoms would suggest that his aneurysm has ruptured?
   a. Sudden shortness of breath and hemoptysis
   b. Sudden, severe low back pain and bruising along his flank
   c. Gradually increasing substernal chest pain and diaphoresis
   d. Sudden, patchy blue mottling on feet and toes and rest pain
6. Priority nursing measures after an abdominal aortic aneurysm repair include
   a. assessment of cranial nerves and mental status.
   b. administration of IV heparin and monitoring of aPTT.
   c. administration of IV fluids and monitoring of kidney function.
   d. elevation of the legs and application of elastic compression stockings.

7. The first priority of collaborative care of a patient with a suspected acute aortic dissection is to
   a. reduce anxiety.
   b. control blood pressure.
   c. monitor for chest pain.
   d. increase myocardial contractility.
8. The patient at highest risk for venous thromboembolism (VTE) is
   a. a 62-year-old man with spider veins who is having arthroscopic knee surgery.
   b. a 32-year-old woman who smokes, takes oral contraceptives, and is planning a trip to Europe.
   c. a 26-year-old woman who is 3 days postpartum and received maintenance IV fluids for 12 hours during her labor.
   d. an active 72-year-old man at home recovering from transurethral resection of the prostate for benign prostatic hyperplasia.
9. Which are probable clinical findings in a person with an acute lower extremity VTE *(select all that apply)?*
   a. Pallor and coolness of foot and calf
   b. Mild to moderate calf pain and tenderness
   c. Grossly diminished or absent pedal pulses
   d. Unilateral edema and induration of the thigh
   e. Palpable cord along a superficial varicose vein
10. The recommended treatment for an initial VTE in an otherwise healthy person with no significant co-morbidities would include
   a. IV argatroban (Acova) as an inpatient.
   b. IV unfractionated heparin as an inpatient.
   c. subcutaneous unfractionated heparin as an outpatient.
   d. subcutaneous low-molecular-weight heparin as an outpatient.
11. A key aspect of teaching for the patient on anticoagulant therapy includes which instructions?
   a. Monitor for and report any signs of bleeding.
   b. Do not take acetaminophen (Tylenol) for a headache.
   c. Decrease your dietary intake of foods containing vitamin K.
   d. Arrange to have blood drawn routinely to check drug levels.
12. In planning care and patient teaching for the patient with venous leg ulcers, the nurse recognizes that the most important intervention in healing and control of this condition is
   a. sclerotherapy.
   b. using moist environment dressings.
   c. taking horse chestnut seed extract daily.
   d. applying elastic compression stockings.

1. c, 2. c, 3. c, 4. b, c, d, 5. b, 6. c, 7. b, 8. b, 9. b, d, 10. d, 11. a, 12. d

evolve

For rationales to these answers and even more NCLEX review questions, visit *http://evolve.elsevier.com/Lewis/medsurg.*

REFERENCES

1. Creager MA, Belkin B, Bluth EI, et al: 2012 ACCF/AHA/ACR/SCAI/SIR/STS/SVM/SVN/SVS key data elements and definitions for peripheral atherosclerotic vascular disease: a report of the American College of Cardiology Foundation/American Heart Association Task Force on Clinical Data Standards, *Circulation* 125:395, 2012.
*2. Pande RL, Perlstein TS, Beckman JA, et al: Secondary prevention and mortality in peripheral artery disease National Health and Nutrition Examination Study, 1999 to 2004, *Circulation* 124:17, 2011.
3. Widner JM: Peripheral arterial disease and disability from NHANES 2001-2004 data, *J Vasc Nurs* 29:104, 2011.
4. Go AS, Mozaffarian D, Roger VL, et al: Heart disease and stroke statistics—2013 update: a report from the American Heart Association, *Circulation* 127:e6, 2013.
*5. Arain FA, Ye Z, Bailey KR, et al: Survival in patients with poorly compressible leg arteries, *J Am Coll Cardiol* 59:400, 2012.
*6. Hirsch AT, Allison MA, Gomes AS, et al: A call to action: women and peripheral artery disease: a scientific statement from the American Heart Association, *Circulation* 125:1449, 2012.
*7. Ix JH, Biggs ML, Kizer JR, et al: Association of body mass index with peripheral arterial disease in older adults: the Cardiovascular Health Study, *Am J Epidemiol* 174:1036, 2011.
*8. Wilson AM, Sadrzadeh-Rafie AH, Myers J, et al: Low lifetime recreational activity is a risk factor for peripheral arterial disease, *J Vasc Surg* 54:427, 2011.
9. Huether SE, McCance KL: *Understanding pathophysiology*, ed 5, St Louis, 2012, Mosby.
*10. Egorova NN, Vouyouka AG, Quin J, et al: Analysis of gender-related differences in lower extremity peripheral arterial disease, *J Vasc Surg* 51:372, 2010.
*11. Alonso-Coello P, Bellmunt S, McGorrian C, et al: Antithrombotic therapy in peripheral artery disease: antithrombotic therapy and prevention of thrombosis, ed 9: American College of Chest Physicians evidence-based clinical practice guidelines, *Chest* 141:e669S, 2012. doi: 10.1378/chest.11-2307.
*12. Rooke TW, Hirsch AT, Misra S, et al: 2011 ACCF/AHA focused update of the guideline for the management of patients with peripheral artery disease (updating the 2005 guideline): a report of the American College of Cardiology Foundation/American Heart Association Task Force on Practice Guidelines, *J Am Coll Cardiol* 8:2020, 2012.
13. Aboyans V, Criqui MH, Abraham P, et al: Measurement and interpretation of the ankle-brachial index: a scientific statement from the American Heart Association, *Circulation* 126:2890, 2012.
*14. Hirsch AT, Haskal ZJ, Hertzer NR, et al: ACC/AHA 2005 practice guidelines for the management of patients with peripheral arterial disease (lower extremity, renal, mesenteric, and abdominal aortic): a collaborative report from the American Association for Vascular Surgery/Society for Vascular Surgery, Society for Cardiovascular Angiography and Interventions, Society for Vascular Medicine and Biology,

*Evidence-based information for clinical practice.

Society of Interventional Radiology, and the ACC/AHA Task Force on Practice Guidelines, *Circulation* 113:e463, 2006. (Classic)
15. American Diabetes Association: Standards of medical care in diabetes—2012, *Diabetes Care* 35(Suppl):S11, 2012.
16. Saratzis A, Kitas GD, Saratzis N, et al: Can statins suppress the development of abdominal aortic aneurysms? A review of the current evidence, *Angiology* 61:137, 2010.
17. Hamburg NM, Balady GJ: Exercise rehabilitation in peripheral artery disease: functional impact and mechanisms of benefit, *Circulation* 123:87, 2011.
*18. National Heart, Lung, and Blood Institute: *Clinical guidelines on the identification, evaluation, and treatment of overweight and obesity in adults: the evidence report,* NIH Pub No 98-4083, Bethesda, MD, 1998, National Institutes of Health. (Classic)
19. Tachjian A, Maria V, Jahangir A: Use of herbal products and potential interactions in patients with cardiovascular diseases, *J Am Coll Cardiol* 55:515, 2010.
20. Varu VN, Hogg ME, Kibbe MR: Critical limb ischemia, *J Vasc Surg* 51:230, 2010.
21. Nanjundappa A, Jain A, Cohoon K, et al: Percutaneous management of chronic critical limb ischemia, *Cardiol Clin* 29:395, 2011.
22. Gandhi S, Sakhuja R, Slovut DP: Recent advances in percutaneous management of iliofemoral and superficial femoral artery disease, *Cardiol Clin* 29:381, 2011.
*23. Ahimastos AA, Pappas EP, Bultner PG, et al: A meta-analysis of the outcome of endovascular and noninvasive therapies in the treatment of intermittent claudication, *J Vasc Surg* 64:1511, 2011.
*24. Greenblatt DY, Rajamanickam V, Mell MW: Predictors of surgical site infection after open lower extremity revascularization, *J Vasc Surg* 54:433, 2011.
25. Ouriel K, Kasyap V: Acute limb ischemia. In Jaff M, White C, editors: *Vascular disease: diagnostic and therapeutic approaches,* Minneapolis, 2011, Cardiotext.
26. Lyden SP: Endovascular treatment of acute limb ischemia: review of current plasminogen activators and mechanical thrombectomy devices, *Perspect Vasc Surg* 22:219, 2010.
*27. You JJ, Singer DE, Howard PA, et al: Antithrombotic therapy for atrial fibrillation: antithrombotic therapy and prevention of thrombosis, 9th ed: American College of Chest Physicians evidence-based clinical practice guidelines, *Chest* 141:e531S, 2012.
28. Piazza G, Creager MA: Thromboangiitis obliterans, *Circulation* 121:1858, 2010.
*29. Japanese Circulation Society Joint Working Group: Guideline for management of vasculitis syndrome—JCS 2008, *Circulation* 75:474, 2011.
30. Lazzerini PE, Capecchi PL, Bisogno S, et al: Homocysteine and Raynaud's phenomenon: a review, *Autoimmun Rev* 9:181, 2010.
31. Herrick AL: Contemporary management of Raynaud's phenomenon and digital ischaemic complications, *Curr Opin Rheumatol* 23:555, 2011.
*32. Kent KC, Zwolak RM, Egorova NN, et al: Analysis of risk factors for abdominal aortic aneurysm in a cohort of more than 3 million individuals, *J Vasc Surg* 52:539, 2010.
*33. Hiratzka LF, Bakris GL, Beckman JA, et al: 2010 ACCF/AHA/AATS/ACR/ASA/SCA/SCAI/SIR/STS/SVM guidelines for the diagnosis and management of patients with thoracic aortic disease: a report of the American College of Cardiology Foundation/American Heart Association Task Force on Practice Guidelines, American Association for Thoracic Surgery, American College of Radiology, American Stroke Association, Society of Cardiovascular Anesthesiologists, Society for Cardiovascular Angiography and Interventions, Society of Interventional Radiology, Society of Thoracic Surgeons, and Society for Vascular Medicine, *J Am Coll Cardiol* 55:e27, 2010.
*34. Filardo G, Powell JT, Martinez MAM, et al: Surgery for small asymptomatic abdominal aortic aneurysms, *Cochrane Database Syst Rev* 3:CD001835, 2012.
*35. Egorova NN, Vouyouka AG, McKinsey JF, et al: Effect of gender on long-term survival after abdominal aortic aneurysm repair based on results from the Medicare national database, *J Vasc Surg* 54:1, 2011.
36. Ganeshanantham G, Walsh SR, Varty K: Abdominal compartment syndrome in vascular surgery—a review, *Int J Surg* 8:181, 2010.
37. Gidlund KD, Wanhainen A, Björck M: Intra-abdominal hypertension and abdominal compartment syndrome after endovascular repair of ruptured abdominal aortic aneurysm, *Eur J Vasc Endovasc Surg* 41:742e, 2011.
38. Cheatham ML, Safcsak K: Percutaneous catheter decompression in the treatment of elevated intraabdominal pressure, *Chest* 140(6):1428, 2011.
39. Nordon IM, Hinchliffe RJ, Loftus IM, et al: Management of acute aortic syndrome and chronic aortic dissection, *Cardiovasc Intervent Radiol* 34:890, 2011.
*40. Thrumurthy SG, Karthikesalingam A, Patterson BO, et al: A systematic review of mid-term outcomes of thoracic endovascular repair (TEVAR) of chronic type B aortic dissection, *Eur J Vasc Endovasc Surg* 42:632, 2011.
41. Ho KH, Cheung DS: Guidelines on timing in replacing peripheral intravenous catheters, *J Clin Nurs* 21:1499, 2012.
*42. van Langevelde K, Lijfering WM, Rosendaal FR, et al: Increased risk of venous thrombosis in persons with clinically diagnosed superficial vein thrombosis: results from the MEGA study, *Blood* 118:4239, 2011.
43. Reitsma PH, Versteeg HH, Middeldorp S: Mechanistic view of risk factors for venous thromboembolism, *Arterioscler Thromb Vasc Biol* 32:563, 2012.
*44. Kearon C, Akl EA, Comerota AJ, et al: Antithrombotic therapy for VTE disease: antithrombotic therapy and prevention of thrombosis, ed 9: American College of Chest Physicians evidence-based clinical practice guidelines, *Chest* 141:e419S, 2012.
45. Decousus H, Bertoletti L, Frappé P, et al: Recent findings in the epidemiology, diagnosis and treatment of superficial-vein thrombosis, *Thrombosis Res* 127:S81, 2011.
*46. Di Nisio M, Wichers IM, Middeldorp S: Treatment for superficial thrombophlebitis of the leg, *Cochrane Database Syst Rev* 3:CD004982, 2012.
*47. Bates SM, Jaeschke R, Stevens SM, et al: Diagnosis of DVT: antithrombotic therapy and prevention of thrombosis, 9th ed: American College of Chest Physicians evidence-based clinical practice guidelines, *Chest* 141:e351S, 2012.
48. Henke PK, Comerota AJ: An update: etiology, prevention, and therapy of postthrombotic syndrome, *J Vasc Surg* 53:500, 2011.
49. Crumley C: Post-thrombotic syndrome patient education based on the health belief model: self-reported intention to comply with recommendations, *J WOCN* 38:648, 2011.

*50. Cohen J, Akl E, Kahn S: Pharmacologic and compression therapies for postthrombotic syndrome: a systematic review of randomized controlled trials, *Chest* 141(2):308, 2012.
51. Bergmann J-F, Cohen AT, Tapson VF, et al: Venous thromboembolism risk and prophylaxis in hospitalized medically ill patients, *Thromb Haemost* 103:736, 2010.
*52. Kahn SR, Lim W, Dunn AS, et al: Prevention of VTE in nonsurgical patients: antithrombotic therapy and prevention of thrombosis, 9th ed: American College of Chest Physicians evidence-based clinical practice guidelines, *Chest* 141:e195S, 2012.
*53. Gould MK, Garcia DA, Wren SM, et al: Prevention of VTE in nonorthopedic surgical patients: antithrombotic therapy and prevention of thrombosis, 9th ed: American College of Chest Physicians evidence-based clinical practice guidelines, *Chest* 141:e227S, 2012.
*54. Sachdeva A, Dalton M, Amaragiri SV, et al: Elastic compression stockings for prevention of deep vein thrombosis, *Cochrane Database Syst Rev* 7:CD001484, 2010.
*55. CLOTS Trial Collaboration: Thigh-length versus below-knee stockings for deep venous thrombosis prophylaxis after stroke, *Ann Intern Med* 153:553, 2010.
*56. Kakkos SK, Caprini JA, Geroulakos G, et al: Combined intermittent pneumatic leg compression and pharmacological prophylaxis for prevention of venous thromboembolism in high-risk patients, *Cochrane Database Syst Rev* 3:CD005258, 2011.
*57. Garcia DA, Baglin TP, Weitz JI, et al: Parenteral anticoagulants: antithrombotic therapy and prevention of thrombosis, ed 9: American College of Chest Physicians evidence-based clinical practice guidelines, *Chest* 141:e24S, 2012.
*58. Ageno W, Gallus AS, Wittkowsky A, et al: Oral anticoagulant therapy: antithrombotic therapy and prevention of thrombosis, 9th ed: American College of Chest Physicians evidence-based clinical practice guidelines, *Chest* 141:e44S, 2012.
*59. Guyatt GH, Akl EA, Crowther M, et al: Executive summary: antithrombotic therapy and prevention of thrombosis, 9th ed: American College of Chest Physicians evidence-based clinical practice guidelines, *Chest* 141:7S, 2012.
*60. Linkins LA, Dans AL, Moores LK, et al: Treatment and prevention of heparin-induced thrombocytopenia: antithrombotic therapy and prevention of thrombosis, 9th ed: American College of Chest Physicians evidence-based clinical practice guidelines, *Chest* 141:e495S, 2012.
*61. Falck-Ytter Y, Francis CW, Johanson NA, et al: Prevention of VTE in orthopedic surgery patients: antithrombotic therapy and prevention of thrombosis, 9th ed: American College of Chest Physicians evidence-based clinical practice guidelines, *Chest* 141:e278S, 2012.
*62. Young T, Tang H, Hughes R: Vena caval filters for the prevention of pulmonary embolism, *Cochrane Database Syst Rev* 2:CD006212, 2010.
*63. Holbrook A, Schulman S, Witt DM, et al: Evidence-based management of anticoagulant therapy: antithrombotic therapy and prevention of thrombosis, ed 9: American College of Chest Physicians evidence-based clinical practice guidelines, *Chest* 141:e152S, 2012.
*64. Decousus H, Tapson VF, Bergmann JF, et al: Factors at admission associated with bleeding risk in medical patients: findings from the IMPROVE investigators, *Chest* 139:69, 2011.
*65. Finlayson K, Edwards H, Courtney M: The impact of psychosocial factors on adherence to compression therapy to prevent recurrence of venous leg ulcers, *J Clin Nurs* 19:1289, 2010.
*66. Kahn SR, Shrier I, Shapiro S, et al: Six-month exercise training program to treat post-thrombotic syndrome: a randomized controlled two-centre trial, *Can Med Assoc J* 183:37, 2011.
*67. Gloviczki P, Comerota AJ, Dalsing MC, et al: The care of patients with varicose veins and associated chronic venous diseases: clinical practice guidelines of the Society for Vascular Surgery and the American Venous Forum, *J Vasc Surg* 53:2S, 2011.
*68. Pittler MH, Ernst E: Horse chestnut seed extract for chronic venous insufficiency, *Cochrane Database Syst Rev* 9:CD003230, 2010.
*69. Tisi PV, Beverley C, Rees A: Injection sclerotherapy for varicose veins, *Cochrane Database Syst Rev* 5:CD001732, 2011.
*70. Nesbitt C, Eifell RKG, Coyne P, et al: Endovenous ablation (radiofrequency and laser) and foam sclerotherapy versus conventional surgery for great saphenous vein varices, *Cochrane Database Syst Rev* 10:CD005624, 2011.
71. Collins L, Seraj S: Diagnosis and treatment of venous ulcers, *Am Fam Physician* 81:989, 2010.
*72. Palfreyman SSJ, Nelson EA, Lochiel R, et al: Dressings for healing venous leg ulcers, *Cochrane Database Syst Rev* 1:CD001103, 2010.
*73. Jones JE, Nelson EA: Skin grafting for venous leg ulcers, *Cochrane Database Syst Rev* 1:CD001737, 2010.

RESOURCES

American Heart Association
www.heart.org/HEARTORG
American Venous Forum
www.veinforum.org
Cochrane Peripheral Vascular Diseases Group
www.pvd.cochrane.org
Mayo Clinic Heart and Blood Vessels Center: Peripheral Artery Disease
www.mayoclinic.com/health/peripheral-arterial-disease/DS00537/
Society for Clinical Vascular Surgery
http://scvs.org
Society for Vascular Nursing
www.svnnet.org
Society for Vascular Surgery
www.vascularweb.org
Vascular Disease Foundation
www.vdf.org
Venous Disease Coalition
http://venousdiseasecoalition.org

CASE STUDY

Managing Multiple Patients

Introduction

You are working on the cardiovascular stepdown unit and have been assigned to care for the following six patients. You have one LPN and a UAP who are assigned to help you.

Patients

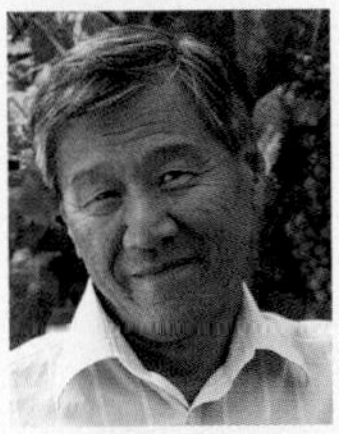

Jupiterimages/Banana-Stock/Thinkstock

L.P. is a 63-year-old Asian American man who was brought to the ED with complaints of chest pain, shortness of breath (SOB), palpitations, and dizziness. L.P.'s CK-MB and troponin levels are within normal limits. His ECG showed atrial fibrillation with a rapid ventricular response. He has been on IV diltiazem (Cardizem) and IV heparin for 24 hours. Although his heart rate has decreased to 102 bpm, the atrial fibrillation persists.

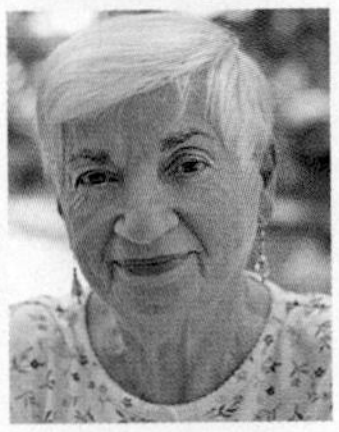

iStockphoto/Thinkstock

J.E. is a 70-year-old Hispanic woman admitted with complaints of increasing shortness of breath, fatigue, and weight gain. She has a systolic murmur and bilateral crackles. Her ejection fraction is 20%. She is currently receiving IV Lasix, oral potassium and enalapril (Vasotec), and a continuous infusion of nesiritide (Natrecor). She is receiving O_2 at 6 L per nasal cannula for an O_2 saturation greater than 93%. Her initial set of cardiac enzymes were normal.

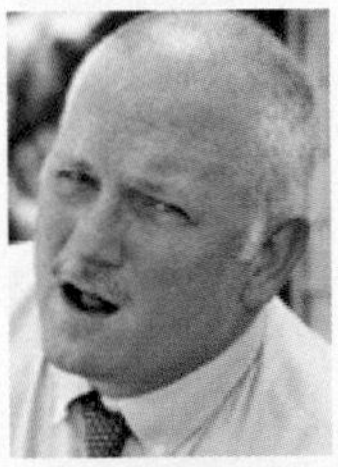

iStockphoto/Thinkstock

D.M. is a 51-year-old white man who was rushed to the hospital by ambulance after experiencing crushing substernal chest pain that radiated down his left arm. His ECG demonstrated marked ST segment elevation in the inferior leads. Cardiac catheterization within 60 minutes of admission showed a 90% blockage of his LAD. Coronary angioplasty was performed and a stent inserted. He is now 2 days post-PTCA and has no recurrence of his chest pain.

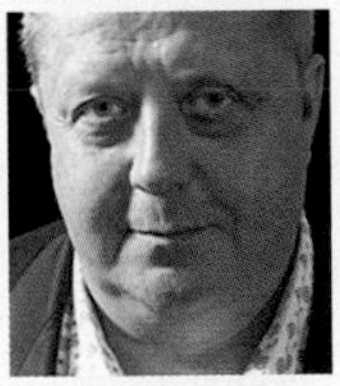

Jupiterimages/Photos.com/Thinkstock

R.B. is a 50-year-old white man admitted for valvular heart disease with a history of IV drug use and alcohol abuse. He complains of chest pain with minimal exertion. He has atrial fibrillation with a rapid ventricular response. His rhythm converted to normal sinus rhythm after receiving IV amiodarone. Transesophageal echocardiography shows left atrial and ventricular hypertrophy and mitral and aortic regurgitation.

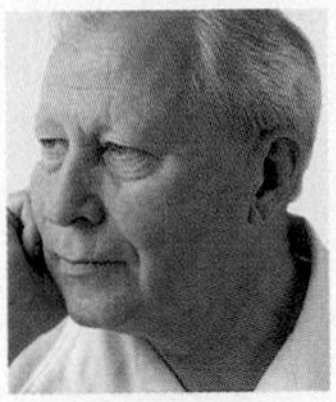

iStockphoto/Thinkstock

J.M. is a 68-year-old white man originally admitted 3 days ago with a diagnosis of acute decompensated HF. He had a cardiac arrest (pulseless VT) and was successfully defibrillated after one shock. He underwent electrophysiology studies, culminating in the implantation of an implantable cardiodefibrillator (ICD). He now is being treated for his heart failure.

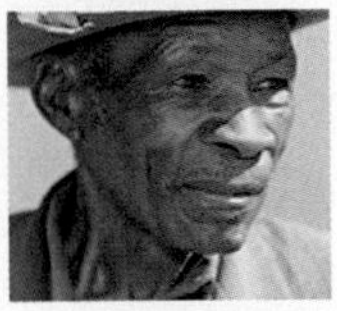

iStockphoto/Thinkstock

S.J. is a 76-year-old African American man admitted with rest pain in both legs and a nonhealing ulcer of the big toe on the right foot. He has a history of an MI, stroke, hypertension, heart failure, and type 1 diabetes mellitus. He underwent a left femoral-popliteal bypass 5 years ago. His right foot is very cool, pale, and mottled in color with decreased sensation. He has a diminished right femoral pulse, a right popliteal and posterior tibial pulse by Doppler only, and his right dorsalis pedis pulse is absent (not palpable or present by Doppler). His left leg pulses are weakly palpable. His right leg ABI: 0.20; left leg ABI: 0.68.

Management Discussion Questions

1. ***Priority Decision:*** After receiving report, which patient should you see first? Second? Provide a rationale for your decision.
2. ***Delegation Decision:*** Which tasks could you delegate to the UAP *(select all that apply)*?
   a. Monitor L.P.'s heparin infusion.
   b. Teach D.M. about activity restriction post-PTCA.
   c. Administer prescribed medications to R.B. and J.M.
   d. Report changes in pain or sensation of S.J.'s legs.
   e. Hook up J.M. to 12-lead ECG and monitor for any dysrhythmias.
3. ***Priority and Delegation Decision:*** As you are assessing L.P., the LPN informs you that S.J. is diaphoretic and complaining of chest pain. Which initial action would be most appropriate?
   a. Ask the LPN to notify S.J.'s health care provider.
   b. Have the LPN administer prescribed nitroglycerin to S.J.
   c. Leave L.P.'s room to perform a focused assessment on S.J.
   d. Finish assessing L.P. while the UAP obtains a 12-lead ECG on S.J.

Case Study Progression

S.J. rates his chest pain as a 9/10. His blood pressure is 110/70, heart rate 110, respiratory rate 26, and O_2 93% on room air. You obtain a 12-lead ECG and administer 0.4 mg SL nitroglycerin with minimal pain relief after 5 minutes. The 12-lead ECG demonstrates new ST elevation in leads II, III, and aVF.

4. Which interventions would you expect the health care provider to order for S.J. *(select all that apply)?*
   a. IV nitroglycerin
   b. IV morphine sulfate
   c. Emergent cardiac catheterization
   d. Furosemide 40 mg IV push STAT
   e. Increase O_2 flow rate to 12 L/minute
5. Which statement would you include in patient teaching regarding ICDs with J.M. and his family?
   a. Avoid air travel.
   b. Avoid driving for 6 weeks.
   c. Avoid any sexual activity in case the ICD discharges.
   d. Avoid standing near antitheft devices in doorways of stores and public buildings.
6. Knowing the mechanism of action for nesiritide, you prioritize monitoring of J.E.'s
   a. blood pressure.
   b. respiratory rate.
   c. b-Natriuretic peptide (BNP) level.
   d. troponin and CK-MB laboratory values.
7. ***Management Decision:*** You ask the UAP to take D.M.'s vital signs before and after having him walk 300 feet. When reviewing the patient's chart, you note documentation of the patient's walk but not his vital signs. What is your best initial action?
   a. Report the incident to the charge nurse for follow-up.
   b. Talk to the UAP to discuss why the vital signs were not documented.
   c. Walk D.M. yourself again and take his vital signs pre- and post-activity.
   d. Ask the LPN to ambulate D.M. and obtain his vital signs before and after.

evolve Answers and rationales available at *http://evolve.elsevier.com/Lewis/medsurg.*

ILLUSTRATION CREDITS

CHAPTER 1

Fig. 1-4, Courtesy Elizabeth Burkhart, RN, MPH, PhD, Chicago, Ill. **Fig. 1-6,** Courtesy Kathryn Bowles. From Moser DK, Riegel B: *Cardiac nursing: a companion to Braunwald's heart disease,* St Louis, 2008, Saunders. **Fig. 1-7,** Adapted from Courtlandt CD, Noonan L, Leonard GF: Model for improvement—part 1: A framework for health care quality, *Pediatric Clinics of North America* 56:757, 2009.

CHAPTER 2

Fig. 2-1, From McGinnis JM, Williams-Russo P, Knickman JR: The case for more active policy attention to health promotion, *Health Affairs* 21:78, 2002. **Fig. 2-2,** From *www.cdc.gov/vitalsigns.* **Fig. 2-9,** From Giger JN: *Transcultural nursing,* ed 6, St Louis, 2013, Mosby.

CHAPTER 3

Figs. 3-1, 3-4, Courtesy Linda Bucher, RN, PhD, CEN, CNE, Staff Nurse, Virtua Memorial Hospital, Mt. Holly, N.J. **Fig. 3-3,** From Seidel HM, Ball JW, Dains JE, Flynn JA: *Mosby's guide to physical examination,* ed 7, St Louis, 2011, Saunders.

CHAPTER 4

Figs. 4-2, 4-3, 4-4, Courtesy Linda Bucher, RN, PhD, CEN, CNE, Staff Nurse, Virtua Memorial Hospital, Mt. Holly, N.J.

CHAPTER 5

Fig. 5-1, From Woog P: *The chronic illness trajectory framework: the Corbin and Strauss nursing model,* New York, 1992, Springer. **Fig. 5-7,** Adapted from Fulmer T: The geriatric nurse specialist role: a new model, *Nursing Management* 22:91, 1991. © Copyright Lippincott Williams & Wilkins, *http://lww.com.* **Fig. 5-10,** Redrawn from Benzon J: Approaching drug regimens with a therapeutic dose of suspicion, *Geriatric Nursing* 12(4):1813, 1991.

CHAPTER 8

Fig. 8-4, Modified from LaFleur Brooks M: *Exploring medical language: a student-directed approach,* ed 8, St Louis, 2012, Mosby. **Fig. 8-5,** From Goldman L, Schafer AI: *Goldman's Cecil medicine,* ed 24, Philadelphia, 2012, Saunders.

CHAPTER 9

Fig. 9-1, Developed by McCaffery M, Pasero C, Paice JA. Modified from M McCaffery, C Pasero: *Pain: clinical manual,* ed 2, St Louis, 1999, Mosby. **Fig. 9-7,** From DeLee JC, Drez D, Miller MD: *DeLee and Drez's orthopaedic sports medicine: principles and practices,* ed 3, Philadelphia, 2009, Saunders.

CHAPTER 10

Fig. 10-1, Courtesy Kathleen A. Pollard, RN, MSN, CHPN, Phoenix, Ariz. **Fig. 10-4,** From Rick Brady, Riva, Md.

CHAPTER 12

Fig. 12-5, From Bale S, Jones V: *Wound care nursing: a patient-centered approach,* ed 2, St Louis, 2006, Mosby. **Fig. 12-6,** From Hayden RJ, Jebson PJL: Wrist arthrodesis, *Hand Clinics,* 21(4): 631-640, 2005. **Figs. 12-7, 12-8,** Reproduced with kind permission from Dr. C. Lawrence, Wound Healing Research Unit, Cardiff. In S Bale, V Jones, editors: *Wound care nursing: a patient-centered approach,* ed 2, St Louis, 2006, Mosby. **Fig. 12-9,** Courtesy Robert B. Babiak, RN, BSN, CWOCN, San Antonio, Tex. **Fig. 12-10,** From Perry AG, Potter PA, Elkin MK: *Nursing interventions and clinical skills,* ed 5, St Louis, 2012, Mosby. **Fig. 12-11,** From Abai B, Zickler RW, Pappas PJ, et al: Lymphorrhea responds to negative pressure wound therapy, *Journal of Vascular Surgery* 45(3):610-613, 2007.

CHAPTER 13

Figs. 13-1, 13-2, Adapted from *The New Genetics.* National Institute of General Medical Science. National Institutes of Health. US Department of Health and Human Services.

CHAPTER 14

Figs. 14-8, 14-9, From Morison MJ: *Nursing management of chronic wounds,* Edinburgh, 2001, Mosby. **Fig. 14-13,** From McKenry L, Tessier E, Hogan M: *Mosby's pharmacology in nursing,* St Louis, 2006, Mosby.

CHAPTER 15

Fig. 15-5, From Emond R, Welsby P, Rowland H: *Colour atlas of infectious diseases,* ed 4, Edinburgh, 2003, Mosby. **Fig. 15-6,** From Friedman-Kien AE: *Color atlas of AIDS,* Philadelphia, 1989, Saunders. **Fig. 15-7,** Set of slides published in 1992 by Jon Fuller, MD and Howard Libman, MD at Boston University School of Medicine, Boston, Mass. **Fig. 15-8,** From the Centers for Disease Control and Prevention. Courtesy Jonathan W.M. Gold, MD, New York. **Fig. 15-9,** From James WD, Berger T, Elston D: *Andrews' diseases of the skin: clinical dermatology,* ed 11, St Louis, 2011, Saunders.

CHAPTER 16

Fig. 16-1, Adapted from Kumar V, Abbas AK, Fausto N, et al: *Robbins and Cotran pathologic basis of disease,* ed 8, Philadelphia, 2010, Saunders. **Fig. 16-3,** Adapted from Stevens A, Lowe J: *Pathology: an illustrated review in colour,* ed 2, London, 2000, Mosby. **Fig. 16-4,** Adapted from Fidler IT: The pathogenesis of cancer metastasis: the "seed and soil" hypothesis revisited, *Nature Reviews. Cancer* 3:453-458, 2003. **Fig. 16-7,** From Shimizu N, Masuda H, Yamanaka H, et al: Fluorodeoxyglucose positron emission tomography scan of prostate cancer bone metastases with flare reaction after endocrine therapy, *Journal of Urology* 161(2): 609, 1999. **Fig. 16-11,** From Weinzweig N, Weinzweig J: *The mutilated hand,* Philadelphia, 2005, Mosby. **Figs. 16-12, 16-13,** Courtesy Jormain Cady, Virginia Mason Medical Center, Seattle, Wash. **Fig. 16-18,** From Forbes CD, Jackson WF: *Colour atlas and text of clinical medicine,* ed 3, London, 2003, Mosby.

CHAPTER 17

Fig. 17-1, Modified from Copstead-Kirkhorn LC, Banasik JL: *Pathophysiology,* ed 4, St Louis, 2010, Mosby. **Figs. 17-4, 17-6, 17-7,** From Patton KT, Thibodeau GA: *Anatomy and physiology,* ed 8, St Louis, 2013, Mosby. **Fig. 17-14,** From McCance KL, Huether SE: *Pathophysiology: the biologic basis for disease in adults and children,* ed 6, St Louis, 2010, Mosby.

CHAPTER 18

Fig. 18-1, Courtesy Susan R. Volk, RN, MSN, CCRN, CPAN, Staff Development Specialist, Christiana Care Health System, Newark, Del.

CHAPTER 19

Fig. 19-1, Courtesy Greg McVicar. **Fig. 19-2,** Courtesy Swedish Edmonds Hospital, Edmonds, Wash. Photograph by Amy Wesley. **Fig. 19-4,** Courtesy The Methodist Hospital, Houston, Tex. Photograph by Donna Dahms, RN, CNOR. **Fig. 19-5,** Courtesy Covidien, Mansfield, Mass.

CHAPTER 20

Fig. 20-5, Courtesy Christine R. Hoch, RN, MSN, Nursing Instructor, Delaware Technical Community College, Newark, Del.

CHAPTER 21

Figs. 21-1, 21-3, 21-6, Modified from Patton KT, Thibodeau GA: *Anatomy and physiology,* ed 8, St Louis, 2013, Mosby. **Fig. 21-4,** From Kanski JJ: *Clinical ophthalmology: a synopsis,* ed 2, New York, 2009, Butterworth-Heinemann. **Fig. 21-5,** From Newell FW: *Ophthalmology: principles and concepts,* ed 7, St Louis, 1992, Mosby. **Fig. 21-7, *B, C,*** from Swartz MH: *Textbook of physical diagnosis: history and examination,* ed 6, Philadelphia, 2010, Saunders.

CHAPTER 22

Figs. 22-1, 22-2, 22-3, 22-4, 22-5, 22-8, Courtesy Cory J. Bosanko, OD, FAAO, Eye Centers of Tennessee, Crossville, Tenn. **Fig. 22-9,** From Flint P, Haughey B, Lund V, Niparko JK, editors: *Cummings otolaryngology: head and neck surgery,* ed 5, St Louis, 2010, Mosby.

CHAPTER 23

Fig. 23-2, From Patton KT, Thibodeau GA, Douglas M: *Essentials of anatomy and physiology,* St. Louis, 2012, Mosby. **Figs. 23-3, 23-6,** From Habif TP: *Clinical dermatology: a color guide to diagnosis and therapy,* ed 5, St Louis, 2009, Mosby. **Figs. 23-4, 23-8,** From Gawkrodger D, Ardern-Jones MR: *Dermatology,* ed 5, Edinburgh, 2012, Churchill Livingstone. **Figs. 23-5, 23-7, 23-10,** From Graham-Brown R, Bourke J, Cunliffe T: *Dermatology: fundamentals of practice,* Edinburgh, 2008, Mosby Ltd. **Fig. 23-9,** From Hurwitz S: *Clinical pediatric dermatology: a textbook of skin disorders of childhood and adolescence,* ed 2, Philadelphia, 1993, Saunders.

CHAPTER 24

Figs. 24-1, 24-11, From Habif TP: *Clinical dermatology: a color guide to diagnosis and therapy,* ed 5, St Louis, 2010, Mosby. **Fig. 24-2,** From The Skin Cancer Foundation, New York, N.Y. **Figs. 24-3, 24-12,** From Graham-Brown R, Bourke J, Cunliffe T: *Dermatology: fundamentals of practice,* Edinburgh, 2008, Mosby Ltd. **Figs. 24-4, 24-8,** From Swartz MH: *Textbook of physical diagnosis: history and examination,* ed 6, Philadelphia, 2010, Saunders. **Figs. 24-5, 24-9,** From Gawkrodger D, Ardern-Jones MR: *Dermatology,* ed 5, Edinburgh, 2012, Churchill Livingstone. **Fig. 24-6,** From Habif TP: *Clinical dermatology: a color guide to diagnosis and therapy,* ed 4, St Louis, 2004, Mosby. **Figs. 24-7, 24-10,** From James WD, Berger T, Elston DMD: *Andrews' diseases of the skin,* ed 11, Philadelphia, 2011, Saunders. **Fig. 24-13,** Courtesy Peter Bonner, Placitas, N. Mex. **Fig. 24-14,** From Pastorek N, Bustillo A: Deep plane facelift, *Facial Plastic Surgery Clinics of North America* 13:433-449, 2005.

CHAPTER 25

Figs. 25-1, 25-2, 25-8, 25-9, 25-11, 25-12, Courtesy Judy A. Knighton, Toronto, Canada. **Fig. 25-6,** From American Association of Critical-Care Nurses: *AACN advanced critical care nursing,* St Louis, 2009, Mosby. **Fig. 25-14,** Courtesy Linda Bucher, RN, PhD, CEN, CNE, Staff Nurse, Virtua Memorial Hospital, Mt. Holly, N.J.

CHAPTER 26

Fig. 26-1, Redrawn from Price SA, Wilson LM: *Pathophysiology: clinical concepts of disease processes,* ed 6, St Louis, 2003, Mosby. **Figs. 26-2, 26-3, 26-8, 26-9,** Redrawn from Thompson JM, McFarland GK, Hirsch JE, Tucker SM: *Mosby's clinical nursing,* ed 5, St Louis, 2002, Mosby. **Fig. 26-4, *A,*** From Dantzker DR, Bone RC, George RB, editors: *Pulmonary and critical care medicine,* vol 1, St Louis, 1993, Mosby. **Fig. 26-4, *B,*** From Albertine KH, Williams MC, Hyde DM: Anatomy of the lungs. In RJ Mason, VC Broaddus, JF Murray, et al, editors: *Murray and Nadel's textbook of respiratory medicine,* ed 4, Philadelphia, 2005, Saunders. **Fig. 26-10,** Redrawn from Beare PG, Myers JL: *Adult health nursing,* ed 3, St Louis, 1998, Mosby. **Fig. 26-11, *A,*** Courtesy Olympus America Inc, Melville, N.Y. **Fig. 26-12,** Redrawn from Du Bois RM, Clarke SW: *Fiberoptic bronchoscopy in diagnosis and management,* Orlando, 1987, Grune & Stratton.

CHAPTER 27

Fig. 27-1, *A,* Courtesy Boston Medical, Westborough, Mass. **Fig. 27-1, *B,*** From Roberts JR, Hedges JR: *Clinical procedures in emergency medicine,* ed 5, Philadelphia, 2009, Saunders. **Fig. 27-4,** From Potter PA, Perry AG: *Basic nursing: essentials for practice,* ed 7, St Louis, 2011, Mosby. **Fig. 27-5, *D,*** Courtesy Dale Medical Products, Inc, Plainville, Mass. **Fig. 27-8,** Courtesy Passy-Muir, Inc, Irvine, Calif. **Fig. 27-11,** From Eggers G, Flechtenmacher C, Kurzen J, Hassfeld S: Infiltrating basal cell carcinoma of the neck 34 years after irradiation of an haemangioma in early childhood. A case-report, *Journal of Cranio-maxillofacial Surgery* 33:199, 2005. **Fig. 27-12, *A,*** Courtesy Wade Hampton.

CHAPTER 28

Fig. 28-2, From Damjanov I, Linder J: *Anderson's pathology,* ed 10, St Louis, 1996, Mosby. **Fig. 28-3,** From Kumar V, Abbas AK, Aster JC, Fausto N: *Robbins and Cotran pathologic basis of disease,* ed 8, Philadelphia, 2010, Saunders. **Fig. 28-8,** From Atrium Medical Corporation, Hudson, N.H. **Fig. 28-9, *A,*** Courtesy and © Copyright Becton, Dickinson and Company. **Fig. 28-11,** From the teaching collection of the Department of Pathology, University of Texas Southwestern Medical School, Dallas, Tex. In V Kumar, AK Abbas, JC Aster, N Fausto, editors: *Robbins and Cotran pathologic basis of disease,* ed 8, Philadelphia, 2010, Saunders.

CHAPTER 29

Fig. 29-1, Adapted from McCance KL, Huether SE, editors: *Pathophysiology: the biologic basis for disease in adults and children,* ed 6, St Louis, 2010, Mosby. **Fig. 29-3,** Redrawn from Price SA, Wilson LM: *Pathophysiology: clinical concepts of disease processes,* ed 6, St Louis, 2003, Mosby. **Fig. 29-4,** Modified from National Heart, Lung, and Blood Institute: *Expert Panel Report 3: Guidelines for the diagnosis and management of asthma.* National Asthma Education and Prevention Program, The Institute, 2007. **Figs. 29-5, 29-7,** From Potter PA, Perry AG, Stockert P, Hall A: *Basic nursing: essentials for practice,* ed 7, St. Louis, 2011, Mosby. **Figs. 29-12, 29-13,** Courtesy Nellcor Puritan Bennett, Inc, Pleasanton, Calif. **Fig. 29-15,** Courtesy Smiths Medical North America. **Fig. 29-17, *C,*** From Kumar V, Abbas AK, Aster JC, Fausto N: *Robbins and Cotran pathologic basis of disease,* ed 8, Philadelphia, 2010, Saunders.

CHAPTER 30

Figs. 30-1, 30-2, Modified from Patton KT, Thibodeau GA: *Anatomy and physiology,* ed 8, St Louis, 2013, Mosby. **Fig. 30-7,** Modified from Herlihy B, Maebius N: *The human body in health and illness,* ed 4, Philadelphia, 2011, Saunders.

CHAPTER 31

Fig. 31-4, Modified from McCance KL, Huether SE: *Pathophysiology: the biologic basis for disease in adults and children,* ed 6, St Louis, 2010, Mosby. **Figs. 31-6, 31-8, 31-10,** From Forbes CD, Jackson WF: *Colour atlas and text of clinical medicine,* ed 3, London, 2003, Mosby. **Fig. 31-12,** Modified from McKinney ES, James SR, Murray SS, Nelson K: *Maternal-child nursing,* Philadelphia, 2000, Saunders. **Fig. 31-13,** From Hoffman AV, Pettit JE: *Color atlas of clinical hematology,* ed 4, Philadelphia, 2009, Mosby. **Fig. 31-15,** From Cotran RS, Kumar V, Abbas AK: *Robbins pathologic basis of disease,* ed 6, Philadelphia, 1999, Saunders.

CHAPTER 32

Figs. 32-9, 32-12, From Drake RL, Vogl AW, Mitchell AWM: *Gray's anatomy for students,* ed 2, Philadelphia, 2010, Churchill Livingstone. **Fig. 32-10,** From Otto C: *Textbook of clinical echocardiography,* ed 3, St Louis, 2004, Saunders. **Fig. 32-11,** From Libby P et al: *Braunwald's heart disease: a textbook of cardiovascular medicine,* ed 8, St Louis, 2008, Saunders.

CHAPTER 33

Fig. 33-2, From Kumar V, Cotran RS, Robbins SL: *Robbins basic pathology,* ed 8, Philadelphia, 2007, Saunders. **Fig. 33-3,** From US Department of Health and Human Services: *Seventh report of the Joint National Committee on Prevention, Detection, Evaluation, and Treatment of High Blood Pressure (JNC 7),* Washington, DC, 2003, National Institutes of Health. **Fig. 33-4,** From Kliegman RM, Behrman RE, Jenson HB, Stanton B: *Nelson textbook of pediatrics,* ed 18, Philadelphia, 2011, Saunders.

CHAPTER 34

Fig. 34-7, From Zipes DB, Libby P, Bonow RO, Braunwald E: *Braunwald's heart disease: a textbook of cardiovascular medicine,* ed 7, St Louis, 2005, Saunders. **Fig. 34-10,** From Kumar V, Abbas AK, Aster JC, Fausto N: *Robbins and Cotran pathologic basis of disease,* ed 8, Philadelphia, 2010, Saunders.

CHAPTER 35

Fig. 35-2, Modified from Huether SE, McCance KL: *Understanding pathophysiology,* ed 3, St Louis, 2004, Mosby. **Fig. 35-3,** Modified from Urden LD, Stacy KM, Lough ME: *Critical care nursing: diagnosis and management,* ed 6, St Louis, 2010, Mosby. **Fig. 35-6,** Used with permission from Honeywell HomMed.

CHAPTER 36

Fig. 36-5, Modified from Wesley K: *Basic dysrhythmias and acute coronary syndromes,* ed 4, St Louis, 2011, Mosby JEMS. **Fig. 36-10,** Modified from Urden LD, Stacy KM, Lough ME: *Critical care nursing: diagnosis and management,* ed 6, St Louis, 2010, Mosby. **Fig. 36-21,** Courtesy Medtronic Physio-Control, Redmond, Wash. **Figs. 36-22, *A*, 36-24, *A*, 36-25,** Courtesy Medtronic, Inc., Minneapolis, Minn. **Fig. 36-29,** From Bucher L, Melander S: *Critical care nursing,* Philadelphia, 1999, Saunders.

CHAPTER 37

Fig. 37-1, Modified from Patton KT, Thibodeau GA: *The human body in health and disease,* ed 5, St Louis, 2010, Mosby. **Figs. 37-2, 37-4,** From Damjanov I, Linder J: *Pathology: a color atlas,* St Louis, 2000, Mosby. **Fig. 37-5,** From Guzzetta CE, Dossey BM: *Cardiovascular nursing: holistic practice,* St Louis, 1992, Mosby. **Fig. 37-7,** From McCance KL, Huether SE: *Pathophysiology: the biologic basis for disease in adults and children,* ed 6, St Louis, 2010, Mosby. **Figs. 37-8, 37-11, 37-12,** From Kumar V, Abbas AK, Aster JC, Fausto N: *Robbins and Cotran pathologic basis of disease,* ed 8, Philadelphia, 2010, Saunders. **Fig. 37-9,** From Crawford MH, DiMarco JP, Paulus WJ: *Cardiology,* ed 3, Edinburgh, 2010, Mosby Ltd. **Fig. 37-10,** From Bonow RO, Mann DL, Zipes DP, Libby P: *Braunwald's heart disease: a textbook of cardiovascular medicine,* ed 9, Philadelphia, 2012, Saunders.

CHAPTER 38

Figs. 38-3, 38-13, From Kamal A, Brockelhurst JC: *Colour atlas of geriatric medicine,* ed 2, 1991, Mosby-Year Book-Europe. **Fig. 38-4,** Courtesy Jo Menzoian, Boston, Mass. **Fig. 38-8,** From Damjanov I, Linder J, editors: *Anderson's pathology,* ed 10, St Louis, 1996, Mosby. **Fig. 38-10,** From Etufugh CN, Phillips TJ: Venous ulcers, *Clinics in Dermatology,* 25(1):125, 2007. **Fig. 38-12,** From Goldman MP, Guex JJ, Weiss RA: *Sclerotherapy: treatment of varicose and telangiectatic leg veins,* ed 5, Philadelphia, 2011, Mosby.

CHAPTER 39

Fig. 39-2, From Patton KT, Thibodeau GA: *Anatomy and physiology,* ed 8, St Louis, 2013, Mosby. **Figs. 39-9, 39-10,** From Drake RL, Vogl W, Mitchell AWM: *Gray's anatomy for students,* ed 2, Edinburgh, 2010, Churchill Livingstone. **Fig. 39-11,** From Given Imaging, Inc, Norcross, Ga.

CHAPTER 40

Fig. 40-1, US Department of Agriculture, Center for Nutrition Policy and Promotion: Guidance on Use of USDA's MyPlate and Statements about Amounts of Food Groups Contributed by Foods on Food Product Labels, Washington, DC. **Fig. 40-2,** US Department of Health and Human Services, Nutrition Facts Label, Silver Spring, Md. **Fig. 40-3,** From Morgan SL, Weinsier RL: *Fundamentals of clinical nutrition,* ed 2, St Louis, 1998, Mosby. **Fig. 40-4,** From Kamal A, Brockelhurst JC: *Color atlas of geriatric medicine,* ed 2, St Louis, 1991, Mosby. **Fig. 40-5,** Adapted from Ukleja A, Freeman KL, Gilbert K, and the ASPEN Board of Directors: Standards for nutrition support: adult hospitalized patients, *Nutrition in Clinical Practice* 25:403, 2010. **Fig. 40-7,** Redrawn from Mahan LK, Arlin M: *Krause's food, nutrition, and diet therapy,* ed 8, Philadelphia, 1992, Saunders.

CHAPTER 41

Fig. 41-6, From Shermak MA: Contouring the epigastrium, *Aesthetic Surgery Journal* 25:506, 2005.

CHAPTER 42

Fig. 42-1, Modified from McKenry L, Tessier E, Hogan M: *Mosby's pharmacology in nursing,* ed 22, St Louis, 2006, Mosby. **Fig. 42-4,** Modified from Doughty DB, Jackson DB: *Mosby's clinical nursing series: gastrointestinal disorders,* St Louis, 1993, Mosby. **Figs. 42-6, 42-8, 42-9,** Modified from Price SA, Wilson LM: *Pathophysiology: clinical concepts of disease processes,* ed 6, St Louis, 2003, Mosby. **Figs. 42-10, 42-15,** From Kumar V, Abbas AK, Aster JC, Fausto N: *Robbins and Cotran pathologic basis of disease,* ed 8, Philadelphia, 2010, Saunders.

CHAPTER 43

Fig. 43-6, Courtesy David Bjorkman, MD, University of Utah School of Medicine, Department of Gastroenterology. In McCance KL, Huether SE: *Pathophysiology: the biologic basis for disease in adults and children,* ed 6, St Louis, 2010, Mosby. **Fig. 43-8,** Modified from McCance KL, Huether SE: *Pathophysiology: the biologic basis for disease in adults and children,* ed 6, St Louis, 2010, Mosby. **Fig. 43-14, *A* and *B*,** From Zitelli BJ, McIntire SC, Nowalk AJ: *Zitelli and Davis' atlas of pediatric physical diagnosis,* ed 6, Philadelphia, 2012, Saunders. **Fig. 43-14, *C*,** From Swartz MH: *Textbook of physical diagnosis: history and examination,* ed 6, Philadelphia, 2010, Saunders. **Fig. 43-16,** From Townsend CM, Beauchamp RD, Evers BM, et al: *Sabiston textbook of surgery: the biological basis of modern surgical practice,* ed 19, Philadelphia, 2012, Saunders.

CHAPTER 44

Figs. 44-1, 44-8, 44-13, From Butcher GP: *Gastroenterology: an illustrated colour text,* London, 2004, Churchill Livingstone. **Figs. 44-2, 44-3,** From McCance KL, Huether SE: *Pathophysiology: the biologic basis for disease in adults and children,* ed 6, St Louis, 2010, Mosby. **Figs. 44-4, 44-10, *B*, 44-14,** From Kumar V, Abbas AK, Aster JC, Fausto N: *Robbins and Cotran pathologic basis of disease,* ed 8, Philadelphia, 2010, Saunders. **Figs. 44-5, 44-7,** Adapted from Huether SE, McCance KL: *Understanding pathophysiology,* ed 5, St Louis, 2012, Mosby. **Fig. 44-10, *A*,** From Kumar V, Abbas AK, Fausto N: *Robbins and Cotran pathologic basis of disease,* ed 7, Philadelphia, 2005, Saunders. **Fig. 44-12,** From Stevens A, Lowe J: *Pathology: illustrated review in colour,* ed 2, London, 2000, Mosby.

CHAPTER 45

Fig. 45-3, Modified from Thibodeau GA, Patton KT: *The human body in health and disease,* ed 4, St Louis, 2005, Mosby. **Fig. 45-4,** Modified from Herlihy B, Maebius N: *The human body in health and disease,* ed 4, Philadelphia, 2011, Saunders. **Fig. 45-5,** Modified from Thibodeau GA, Patton KT: *Anatomy and physiology,* ed 6, St Louis, 2007, Mosby. **Figs. 45-6, 45-8,** From Brundage DJ: *Renal disorders,* St Louis, 1992, Mosby. **Fig. 45-10, *A,*** Courtesy Circon Corporation, Santa Barbara, Calif.

CHAPTER 46

Figs. 46-2, 46-4, From Kumar V, Abbas AK, Aster JC, Fausto N, et al: *Robbins and Cotran pathologic basis of disease,* ed 8, Philadelphia, 2010, Saunders. **Fig. 46-5, *A,*** From Stevens A, Lowe JS, Scott I: *Core pathology: illustrated review in color,* ed 3, London, 2009, Mosby Ltd. **Figs. 46-5, *B,* and 46-6,** From Bullock N, Doble A, Turner W, Cuckow P: *Urology: an illustrated colour text.* London, 2008, Churchill Livingstone. **Fig. 46-7, *A,*** From Brundage DJ: *Renal disorders,* St Louis, 1992, Mosby. **Figs. 46-7, *B,* and 46-8, 46-9, *B,*** From Kumar V, Abbas AK, Fausto N: *Robbins and Cotran pathologic basis of disease,* ed 7, Philadelphia, 2005, Saunders. **Fig. 46-9, *A,*** From Stevens A, Lowe J: *Pathology: illustrated review in colour,* ed 2, London, 2000, Mosby. **Figs. 46-12, 46-14, 46-15,** Courtesy Lynda Brubacher, Virginia Mason Hospital, Seattle, Wash.

CHAPTER 47

Fig. 47-1, From Stevens A, Lowe J: *Pathology: illustrated review in colour,* ed 2, London, 2000, Mosby. **Fig. 47-6,** Courtesy Mary Jo Holechek, Baltimore, Md. **Fig. 47-7,** Courtesy Baxter Healthcare Corporation, McGaw Park, Ill. **Figs. 47-9, 47-11, *B, C,*** Courtesy Dr. Stephen Van Voorst, MD. **Fig. 47-10, *A,*** Courtesy Quinton Instrument Co., Seattle, Wash. **Fig. 47-13,** From NxStage Medical, Inc, Lawrence, Mass.

CHAPTER 48

Figs. 48-1, 48-6, Modified from Patton KT, Thibodeau GA: *Anatomy and physiology,* ed 8, St Louis, 2013, Mosby. **Fig. 48-3,** Modified from McCance KL, Huether SE: *Pathophysiology: the biologic basis for disease in adults and children,* ed 6, St Louis, 2010, Mosby. **Fig. 48-8,** From Thibodeau GA, Patton KT: *The human body in health and disease,* ed 4, St Louis, 2005, Mosby.

CHAPTER 49

Figs. 49-11, 49-13, From Kumar V, Abbas AK, Aster JC, Fausto N: *Robbins and Cotran pathologic basis of disease,* ed 8, Philadelphia, 2010, Saunders. **Fig. 49-12,** Modified from Urden LD, Stacy KM, Lough ME: *Critical care nursing: diagnosis and management,* ed 6, St Louis, 2010, Mosby. **Figs. 49-15, 49-16,** From Chew SL, Leslie D: *Clinical endocrinology and diabetes: an illustrated colour text,* Edinburgh, 2006, Churchill Livingstone.

CHAPTER 50

Fig. 50-1, Courtesy Linda Haas, Seattle, Wash. **Fig. 50-3,** Modified from Urden LD, Stacy KM, Lough ME: *Critical care nursing: diagnosis and management,* ed 6, St Louis, 2010, Mosby. **Fig. 50-6,** From Forbes CD, Jackson WF: *Colour atlas and text of clinical medicine,* ed 3, London, 2003, Mosby. **Figs. 50-7, 50-12, 50-13,** From Chew SL, Leslie D: *Clinical endocrinology and diabetes: an illustrated colour text,* Edinburgh, 2006, Churchill Livingstone. **Fig. 50-9,** Courtesy Paul W. Ladenson, MD, The Johns Hopkins University and Hospital, Baltimore, Md. From HM Seidel, JW Ball, JE Dains, GW Benedict, editors: *Mosby's guide to physical examination,* ed 6, St Louis, 2006, Mosby. **Fig. 50-10,** From Seidel HM, Ball JW, Dains JE, Benedict GW: *Mosby's guide to physical examination,* ed 6, St Louis, 2006, Mosby.

CHAPTER 51

Figs. 51-1, 51-2, 51-4, 51-5, 51-7, Modified from Patton KT, Thibodeau GA: *Anatomy and physiology,* ed 8, St Louis, 2013, Mosby. **Fig. 51-3,** Modified from McKenry L, Tessier E, Hogan M: *Mosby's pharmacology in nursing,* St Louis, 2006, Mosby. **Fig. 51-8, *A,*** From Abrahams P, Marks S, Hutching R: *McMinn's color atlas of human anatomy,* ed 5, Philadelphia, 2003, Saunders. **Fig. 51-8, *B,*** From Symonds EM, MacPherson MB: *Color atlas of obstetrics and gynecology,* London, 1994, Mosby Wolfe.

CHAPTER 52

Fig. 52-1, Data from American Cancer Society: How to perform a breast self-exam, revised October 2011. *www.cancer.org/Cancer/BreastCancer/MoreInformation/BreastCancerEarlyDetection/breast-cancer-early-detection-acsrecsbse.* **Fig. 52-2,** From Adam A, Dixon AK, Grainger RG, et al: *Grainger and Allison's diagnostic radiology,* ed 5, St Louis, 2008, Churchill Livingstone. **Fig. 52-5,** From Donegan WL, Spratt JS: *Cancer of the breast,* ed 3, Philadelphia, 1988, Saunders. **Fig. 52-7,** From Swartz MH: *Textbook of physical diagnosis: history and examination,* ed 6, Philadelphia, 2010, Saunders. **Fig. 52-10,** Courtesy Brian Davies, MD. From Fortunato N, McCullough S: *Plastic and reconstructive surgery,* St Louis, 1998, Mosby. **Fig. 52-11, *A,*** Modified from Cameron J: *Current surgical therapy,* ed 5, St Louis, 1995, Mosby. **Fig. 52-11, *B,*** Courtesy Brian Davies, MD. From Fortunato N, McCullough S: *Plastic and reconstructive surgery,* St Louis, 1998, Mosby.

CHAPTER 53

Fig. 53-1, From Marx J, Walls R, Hockberger R: *Rosen's emergency medicine: concepts and clinical practice,* ed 7, St Louis, 2010, Mosby. **Figs. 53-2, 53-7, 53-8, *B,*** From Morse S, Moreland A, Holmes K, editors: *Atlas of sexually transmitted diseases and AIDS,* London, 1996, Mosby-Wolfe. **Figs. 53-3, *A,* and 53-6,** From Cohen J, Powderly WG: *Infectious diseases,* ed 2, St Louis, 2004, Mosby. **Figs. 53-3, *B,* and 53-5,** From Mandell GL, Bennett JE, Dolin R: *Mandell, Douglas, and Bennett's principles and practice of infectious diseases,* ed 7, Philadelphia, 2010, Churchill Livingstone. **Fig. 53-4,** From Forbes CD, Jackson WF. *Color atlas and text of clinical medicine,* ed 3, London, 2003, Mosby. **Figs. 53-8, *A, C,* and 53-10, *C,*** From Centers for Disease Control and Prevention. Courtesy Susan Lindsley. **Fig. 53-9,** From Centers for Disease Control and Prevention. Courtesy Dr. Hermann. **Fig. 53-10, *A,*** From Centers for Disease Control and Prevention. Courtesy Joe Millar. **Fig. 53-10, *B,*** From Centers for Disease Control and Prevention. Courtesy Dr. Wiesner.

CHAPTER 54

Fig. 54-3, From Katz V: *Comprehensive gynecology,* ed 5, St Louis, 2007, Mosby. **Fig. 54-4,** From Kumar V, Abbas AK, Aster JC, Fausto N: *Robbins and Cotran pathologic basis of disease,* ed 8, Philadelphia, 2010, Saunders. **Fig. 54-5,** Modified from Stenchever MA, Droegemueller W, Herbst AL, Mishell D Jr: *Comprehensive gynecology,* ed 4, St Louis, 2001, Mosby. **Fig. 54-6,** From McCance KL, Huether SE: *Pathophysiology: the biologic basis for disease in adults and children,* ed 6, St Louis, 2010, Mosby. **Fig. 54-7,** From Symonds EM, McPherson MBA: *Colour atlas of obstetrics and gynecology,* London, 1994, Mosby. **Fig. 54-8,** From Kumar V, Abbas A, Fausto N: *Robbins and Cotran pathologic basis of disease,* ed 7, Philadelphia, 2005, Saunders. **Fig. 54-9,** From Drake RL, Vogl W, Mitchell AWM: *Gray's anatomy for students,* ed 2, Edinburgh, 2010, Churchill Livingstone. **Fig. 54-10,** Modified from Phipps WJ, Sands JK, Marek JF: *Medical-surgical nursing: concepts and clinical practice,* ed 6, St Louis, 1999, Mosby. **Fig. 54-12,** Modified from Seidel HM, Ball JW, Dains JE, Flynn JA: *Mosby's guide to physical examination,* ed 7, St Louis, 2011, Mosby. **Fig. 54-13, *B,*** From Huffman JW: *Gynecology and obstetrics,* Philadelphia, 1962, Saunders. **Fig. 54-14, *B,*** From Townsend CM: *Sabiston textbook of surgery,* ed 18, St Louis, 2009, Mosby.

CHAPTER 55

Fig. 55-3, From Townsend CM, Beauchamp RD, Evers BM, Mattox KL: *Sabiston textbook of surgery,* ed 19, Philadelphia, 2012, Saunders. **Fig. 55-5,** From Mettler F: *Essentials of radiology,* ed 2, Philadelphia, 2004, Saunders. **Fig. 55-7, *B*,** From Abeloff MD, Armitage JO, Niederhuber JE, Kastan MB, editors: *Abeloff's clinical oncology,* ed 4, 2008, Churchill Livingstone. **Fig. 55-10,** From Swartz MH: *Textbook of physical diagnosis,* ed 6, Philadelphia, 2010, Saunders. **Fig. 55-11,** From Seidel HM, Ball JW, Dains JE, Flynn JA: *Mosby's guide to physical examination,* ed 7, St Louis, 2011, Mosby.

CHAPTER 56

Figs. 56-1, 56-8, 56-9, 56-10, Modified from Thibodeau GA, Patton KT: *Anatomy and physiology,* ed 8, St Louis, 2013, Mosby. **Fig. 56-2,** Modified from Thibodeau GA, Patton KT: *Anatomy and physiology,* ed 6, St Louis, 2007, Mosby. **Fig. 56-6,** From Herlihy B: *The human body in health and illness,* ed 4, St Louis, 2011, Saunders. **Fig. 56-7,** Redrawn from McCance KL, Huether SE: *Pathophysiology: the biologic basis for disease in adults and children,* ed 6, St Louis, 2010, Mosby. **Figs. 56-11, 56-12,** Courtesy DaiWai Olson, RN PhD, CCRN, Dallas, Tex. **Fig. 56-14,** From Chipps E, Clanin N, Campbell V: *Neurologic disorders,* St Louis, 1992, Mosby. **Fig. 56-15,** From Fuller G, Manford M: *Neurology: an illustrated colour text,* ed 3, New York, 2010, Churchill Livingstone.

CHAPTER 57

Fig. 57-4, Modified from McCance KL, Huether SE: *Pathophysiology: the biologic basis for disease in adults and children,* ed 6, St Louis, 2010, Mosby. **Fig. 57-7,** Modified from Copstead-Kirkhorn LC, Banasik JL: *Pathophysiology,* ed 5, St Louis, 2013, Mosby. **Fig. 57-9,** Courtesy Meg Zomorodi, RN, PhD, CNL, Raleigh, N.C. **Fig. 57-13, *C*,** From Bingham BJG, Hawke M, Kwok P: *Clinical atlas of otolaryngology,* St Louis, 1992, Mosby. **Fig. 57-15,** From Copstead-Kirkhorn LC, Banasik JL: *Pathophysiology,* ed 4, St Louis, 2010, Mosby. **Fig. 57-16,** From Kumar V, Abbas AK, Aster JC, Fausto N: *Robbins and Cotran pathologic basis of disease,* ed 8, Philadelphia, 2010, Saunders. **Fig. 57-17,** From Stevens A, Lowe J: *Pathology: illustrated review in colour,* ed 2, London, 2000, Mosby.

CHAPTER 58

Fig. 58-3, From Kumar V, Abbas AK, Aster JC, Fausto N: *Robbins and Cotran pathologic basis of disease,* ed 8, Philadelphia, 2010, Saunders. **Fig. 58-11,** Modified from Hoeman SP: *Rehabilitation nursing,* ed 2, St Louis, 1995, Mosby. **Fig. 58-12,** From Forbes CD, Jackson WF: *Colour atlas and text of clinical medicine,* ed 3, London, 2003, Mosby.

CHAPTER 59

Fig. 59-4, From Stevens A, Lowe J: *Pathology: illustrated review in colour,* ed 2, London, 2000, Mosby. **Fig. 59-7,** From Lehne RA: *Pharmacology for nursing care,* ed 8, St Louis, 2013, Saunders. **Fig. 59-8,** From Aminoff MJ, Daroff RB: *Encyclopedia of the neurological sciences,* Waltham, Mass., 2003, Academic Press. **Fig. 59-11,** From Sanders DB, Massey JM: Clinical features of myasthenia gravis. In AG Engel, editor: *Neuromuscular junction disorders: handbook of clinical neurology,* New York, 2008, Elsevier.

CHAPTER 60

Fig. 60-5, From Roberts GS: *Neuropsychiatric disorders,* London, 1993, Mosby-Wolfe. **Fig. 60-6,** Modified from Stern TA: *Massachusetts General Hospital comprehensive clinical psychiatry,* Philadelphia, 2008, Mosby.

CHAPTER 61

Fig. 61-1, Modified from Patton KT, Thibodeau GA: *Anatomy and physiology,* ed 8, St Louis, 2013, Mosby. **Fig. 61-2,** Courtesy Joe Rothrock, Media, Pa. **Fig. 61-3,** From Forbes CD, Jackson WF: *Color atlas and text of clinical medicine,* ed 3, London, 2003, Mosby. **Fig. 61-4,** Modified from Marciano FF, Greene KA, Apostolides PJ, et al: Pharmacologic management of spinal cord injury: review of the literature, *BNI Quarterly* 11(2):11, 1995. In KL McCance, SE Huether, editors: *Pathophysiology: the biologic basis for disease in adults and children,* ed 5, St Louis, 2006, Mosby. **Fig. 61-5, *A, B, C*,** From Copstead-Kirkhorn LC, Banasik JL: *Pathophysiology,* ed 5, St Louis, 2014, Mosby. **Fig. 61-7,** From American Spinal Injury Association/International Medical Society of Paraplegic (ASIA/IMOSP): *International standards for neurological functional classification of spinal cord injury patients* (revised), Chicago, 2002, The Association. **Figs. 61-8, 61-12,** Courtesy Michael S. Clement, MD, Mesa, Ariz. **Fig. 61-11,** Modified from Urden LD, Stacy KM, Lough ME: *Priorities in critical care nursing,* ed 6, St Louis, 2012, Mosby.

CHAPTER 62

Fig. 62-1, *A*, From Herlihy B, Maebius N: *The human body in health and illness,* ed 4, Philadelphia, 2011, Saunders. **Figs. 62-1, *B*, 62-6,** From Patton KT, Thibodeau GA: *Anatomy and physiology,* ed 8, St Louis, 2013, Mosby. **Fig. 62-5,** From Patton KT, Thibodeau GA, Douglas M: *Essentials of anatomy and physiology,* St Louis, 2012, Mosby. **Fig. 62-7, *A*,** From Wilson SF, Giddens JF: *Health assessment for nursing practice,* ed 5, St Louis, 2013, Mosby. **Fig. 62-7, *B*,** From Barkauskas V, Baumann L, Stoltenberg-Allen K, et al: *Health and physical assessment,* ed 2, St Louis, 1998, Mosby. **Fig. 62-8,** From Zitelli BJ, McIntire SC, Nowalk AJ: *Zitelli and Davis' atlas of pediatric physical diagnosis,* ed 6, St Louis, 2012, Mosby. **Fig. 62-9,** From Miller MD, Howard RF, Plancher KD: *Surgical atlas of sports medicine,* Philadelphia, 2003, Saunders.

CHAPTER 63

Fig. 63-2, From Buttaravoli P: *Minor emergencies,* ed 3, Philadelphia, Saunders, 2012. **Fig. 63-4, *A*,** From David Lintner, MD, Houston, Tex., *www.drlintner.com.* **Fig. 63-4, *B, C*,** Courtesy Peter Bonner, Placitas, N. Mex. **Figs. 63-9, 63-20,** Courtesy Mary Wollan, RN, BAN, ONC, Spring Park, Minn. **Fig. 63-12,** From Maher AB, Salmond SW, Pellino T, editors: *Orthopaedic nursing,* ed 3, Philadelphia, 2002, Saunders. **Fig. 63-13, *A*,** Courtesy Howmedica, Inc, Allendale, Pa. **Fig. 63-13, *B*,** From Canale ST, Beaty JH: *Campbell's operative orthopaedics,* ed 12, Philadelphia, 2013, Mosby. **Fig. 63-14,** From Jeremy Lewis, MD. Dallas, Tex. **Fig. 63-15,** From Browner BD, Jupiter JB, Levine AM, Trafton P: *Skeletal trauma: fractures, dislocations, ligamentous injuries,* ed 4, Philadelphia, 2009, Saunders. **Fig. 63-16,** Mettler FA: *Essentials of radiology,* ed 2, Philadelphia, 2005, Saunders. **Fig. 63-21,** Courtesy R.A. Weinstein, Denver, Colo.

CHAPTER 64

Fig. 64-2, From Thibodeau GA, Patton KT: *The human body in health and disease,* ed 5, St Louis, 2010, Mosby. **Fig. 64-3,** From Damjanov I, Linder J: *Anderson's pathology,* ed 10, St Louis, 1996, Mosby. **Figs. 64-6, 64-7,** From Canale ST, Beaty JH: *Campbell's operative orthopaedics,* ed 12, Philadelphia, 2013, Mosby. **Fig. 64-9, *A*,** From Phillips N: *Berry & Kohn's operating room technique,* ed 12, St Louis, 2013, Mosby. **Fig. 64-9, *B*,** Courtesy MA Mir. In Kanski JJ: *Clinical diagnosis in ophthalmology,* St Louis, 2006, Mosby.

CHAPTER 65

Fig. 65-1, *D*, From Forbes CD, Jackson WF: *Color atlas and text of clinical medicine,* ed 3, London, 2003, Mosby. **Fig. 65-3, *D*,** From Canale ST, Beaty JH: *Campbell's operative orthopaedics,* ed 12, Philadelphia, 2013, Mosby. **Fig. 65-6,** Courtesy John Cook, MD. From Goldstein, BG, Goldstein AE: *Practical dermatology,* ed 2, St Louis, 1997, Mosby. **Fig. 65-7,** From Marx J, Hockberger R, Walls R: *Rosen's emergency medicine,* ed 7, Philadelphia, 2009, Mosby. **Fig. 65-8,** From Kim DH, Henn J, Vaccaro AR, Dickman C: *Surgical anatomy and techniques to the spine,* Philadelphia, 2006, Saunders. **Figs. 65-10, 65-13,** From Firestein GS, Budd RC, Gabriel SE, McInnes IB: *Kelley's textbook of rheumatology,* ed 9, Philadelphia, 2012, Saunders. **Fig. 65-12,** From Zitelli BJ, Davis HW: *Atlas of pediatric physical diagnosis,* ed 4, St Louis, 2002, Mosby.

CHAPTER 66

Fig. 66-1, From Avera Health, Sioux Falls, S. Dak. **Fig. 66-2,** Courtesy Spacelabs Medical, Redmond, Wash. **Fig. 66-5,** From Darovic GO, Vanriper S, Vanriper J: Fluid-filled monitoring systems. In GO Darovic: *Hemodynamic monitoring,* ed 2, Philadelphia, 1995, Saunders. **Figs. 66-6, 66-9, 66-10,** Modified from Urden LD, Stacy KM, Lough ME: *Critical care nursing: diagnosis and management,* ed 6, St Louis, 2010, Mosby. **Fig. 66-14,** ***A,*** From Beare PG, Myers JL: *Adult health nursing,* ed 3, St Louis, 1998, Mosby.

CHAPTER 67

Figs. 67-2, 67-3, 67-4, 67-5, Modified from Urden LD, Stacy KM, Lough ME: *Critical care nursing: diagnosis and management,* ed 6, St Louis, 2010, Mosby.

CHAPTER 68

Fig. 68-6, From Wilson SF, Giddens JF: *Health assessment for nursing practice,* ed 4, St Louis, 2009, Mosby. **Fig. 68-7,** From American Association of Critical Care Nurses: *AACN advanced critical care nursing,* St Louis, 2009, Mosby. **Fig. 68-8,** Courtesy Richard Arbour, RN, MSN, CCRN, CNRN, CCNS, FAAN and Anna Kirk, RN, MSN. **Fig. 68-11,** From Cohen J, Powderly WG: *Infectious diseases,* ed 2, St Louis, 2004, Mosby.

CHAPTER 69

Figs. 69-2, 69-3, Courtesy Cameron Bangs, MD. From Auerbach PS, Donner HJ, Weiss EA: *Field guide to wilderness medicine,* ed 2, St Louis, 2003, Mosby. **Fig. 69-6,** From Roberts JR, Hedges JR: *Clinical procedures in emergency medicine,* ed 5, Philadelphia, 2009, Saunders. **Fig. 69-7,** Photo used with the permission of the American Red Cross.

A

NOTE: Disorder names and key terms are in **boldface**. Page numbers in **boldface** indicate main discussions. Page numbers followed by f, t, or b indicate figures, tables, and boxes, respectively.

B

C

D

E

H

J

K

L

N

O

P

Q

R

ABBREVIATIONS

ABG	arterial blood gas
ACE	angiotensin-converting enzyme
ACLS	advanced cardiac life support
ACS	acute coronary syndrome
ACTH	adrenocorticotropic hormone
ADH	antidiuretic hormone
AED	automatic external defibrillator
AIDS	acquired immunodeficiency syndrome
AKA	above-knee amputation
AKI	acute kidney injury
ALI	acute lung injury
ALL	acute lymphocytic leukemia
ALS	amyotrophic lateral sclerosis
AMI	acute myocardial infarction
ANA	antinuclear antibody
ANS	autonomic nervous system
AORN	Association of periOperative Room Nurses
APD	automated peritoneal dialysis
aPTT	activated partial thromboplastin time
ARDS	acute respiratory distress syndrome
ATN	acute tubular necrosis
BCLS	basic cardiac life support
BKA	below-knee amputation
BMI	body mass index
BMR	basal metabolic rate
BMT	bone marrow transplantation
BPH	benign prostatic hyperplasia
BSE	breast self-examination
BUN	blood urea nitrogen
CABG	coronary artery bypass graft
CAD	coronary artery disease; circulatory assist device
CAPD	continuous ambulatory peritoneal dialysis
CAVH	continuous arteriovenous hemofiltration
CBC	complete blood count
CCU	coronary care unit; critical care unit
CDC	Centers for Disease Control and Prevention
CIS	carcinoma in situ
CKD	chronic kidney disease
CLL	chronic lymphocytic leukemia
CML	chronic myelocytic leukemia
CMP	cardiomyopathy
CN	cranial nerve
CNS	central nervous system
CO	cardiac output
COPD	chronic obstructive pulmonary disease
CPAP	continuous positive airway pressure
CPR	cardiopulmonary resuscitation
CRRT	continuous renal replacement therapy
CRNA	certified registered nurse anesthetist
CSF	cerebrospinal fluid
CT	computed tomography
CVA	cerebrovascular accident; costovertebral angle
CVAD	central venous access device
CVI	chronic venous insufficiency
CVP	central venous pressure
D&C	dilation and curettage
DDD	degenerative disk disease
DI	diabetes insipidus
DIC	disseminated intravascular coagulation
DJD	degenerative joint disease
DKA	diabetic ketoacidosis
DM	diabetes mellitus; diastolic murmur
DRE	digital rectal examination
DVT	deep vein thrombosis
ECF	extracellular fluid
ECG	electrocardiogram
ED	emergency department; erectile dysfunction
EEG	electroencephalogram
EMG	electromyogram
EMS	emergency medical services
ENT	ear, nose, and throat
ERCP	endoscopic retrograde cholangiopancreatography
ERT	estrogen replacement therapy
ESKD	end-stage kidney disease
ESR	erythrocyte sedimentation rate
ET	endotracheal
FEV	forced expiratory volume
FRC	functional residual capacity
FUO	fever of unknown origin
GCS	Glasgow Coma Scale
GERD	gastroesophageal reflux disease
GFR	glomerular filtration rate
GH	growth hormone
GI	glycemic index
GTT	glucose tolerance test
GU	genitourinary
GYN, Gyn	gynecologic
HAI	health care–associated infection
HAV	hepatitis A virus
Hb, Hgb	hemoglobin
HBV	hepatitis B virus
Hct	hematocrit
HCV	hepatitis C virus
HD	hemodialysis, Huntington's disease
HDL	high-density lipoprotein
HF	heart failure
HIV	human immunodeficiency virus
H&P	history and physical examination
HPV	human papillomavirus
HSCT	hematopoietic stem cell transplantation
IABP	intraaortic balloon pump
IBS	irritable bowel syndrome
ICP	intracranial pressure
I&D	incision and drainage
IE	infective endocarditis
IFG	impaired fasting glucose
IGT	impaired glucose tolerance
INR	international normalized ratio
IOP	intraocular pressure
IPPB	intermittent positive-pressure breathing
ITP	idiopathic thrombocytopenic purpura
IUD	intrauterine device
IV	intravenous
IVP	intravenous push; intravenous pyelogram
JVD	jugular venous distention
KS	Kaposi sarcoma
KUB	kidney, ureters, and bladder (x-ray)
KVO	keep vein open
LAD	left anterior descending
LDL	low-density lipoprotein